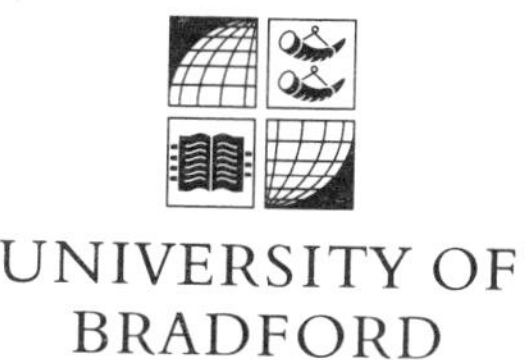

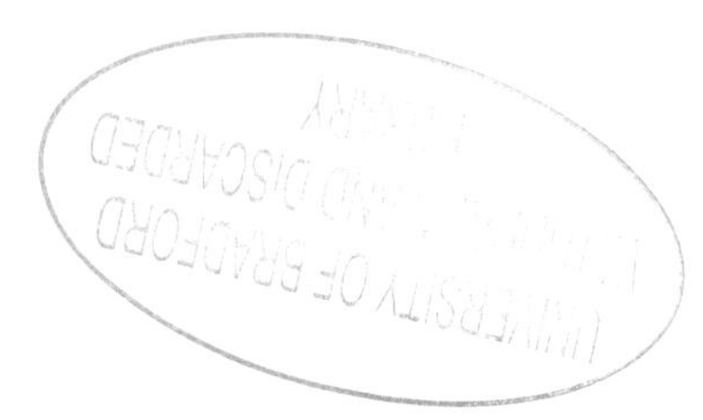

TOXICOLOGY

TOXICOLOGY

Edited by

Hans Marquardt
Department of Toxicology
Hamburg University Medical School and
Department of Toxicology and Environmental
Medicine of the Fraunhofer Society
Hamburg, Germany

Siegfried G. Schäfer
Solvay Pharmaceuticals
Hannover, Germany and
Department of Toxicology
Hamburg University Medical School
Hamburg, Germany

Roger McClellan
Chemical Industry Institute of Toxicology
Research Triangle Park
North Carolina

Frank Welsch
Chemical Industry Institute of Toxicology
Research Triangle Park
North Carolina

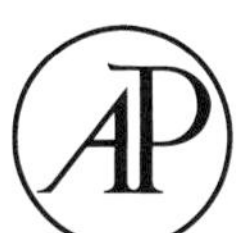

Academic Press
San Diego London Boston New York Sydney Tokyo Toronto

Front cover photograph: The monument of Paracelsus, father of toxicology, who lived worked in Salzburg, Austria and who also is buried there. Photograph taken by Dr. Herbert V. Levinsky. Background copyright Digital Stock Incorporated 1999.

This book is printed on acid-free paper. ∞

Academic Press
A Division of Harcourt, Inc.
525 B Street, Suite 1900, San Diego, California 92101-4495, USA
http://www.apnet.com

Academic Press
24-28 Oval Road, London NW1 7DX, UK
http://www.hbuk.co.uk/ap/

Library of Congress Catalog Card Number: 98-89314

International Standard Book Number: 0-12-473270-4

PRINTED IN THE UNITED STATES OF AMERICA
99 00 01 02 03 04 MM 9 8 7 6 5 4 3 2 1

Contents

CHAPTER

4

Xenobiotic Metabolism

FRANZ OESCH AND MICHAEL ARAND

CHAPTER

5

Free Radicals and Reactive Oxygen Species

MAGED YOUNES

CHAPTER

6

Genetic Toxicology

DAVID J. BRUSICK

CHAPTER

7

Chemical Carcinogenesis

HANS MARQUARDT

CHAPTER

8

Tumor Promotion

ROLF SCHULTE-HERMANN, BRIGITTE MARIAN, AND WILFRED BURSCH

CHAPTER

9

Transgenic Rodent Models

KENNETH R. TINDALL AND RAYMOND W. TENNANT

CHAPTER

10

Receptor Toxicology

MARTIN GÖTTLICHER

CHAPTER

11

Mechanisms of Toxicology: Programmed Cell Death (Apoptosis)

DOROTHEE CHARLOTTE DARTSCH

CHAPTER

12

Mixtures

JOHN P. GROTEN, FLEMMING R. CASSEE, PETER J. VAN BLADEREN, CHRIS T. DE ROSA, AND VICTOR J. FERON

PART

II

ORGAN TOXICITY

CHAPTER

13

The Liver

REGINE KAHL

CHAPTER

14

The Kidney

CONSTANTIN COJOCEL AND EDWARD A. LOCK

CHAPTER

15

Respiratory Tract

HARTWIG MUHLE AND ROGER O. MCCLELLAN

CHAPTER

16

Blood and Blood-Forming Organs

PETER EYER AND REINHARD KLIMMEK

CHAPTER

17

Immune System

REINHARD NEUBERT AND DIETHER NEUBERT

CHAPTER

18

Skin

NANCY A. MONTEIRO-RIVIERE AND JIM E. RIVIERE

CHAPTER

19

The Eye

DORIS A. SCHWINDT AND HANS F. MERK

CHAPTER

20

Nervous System

KLAUS ANDREAS AND DAVID E. RAY

CHAPTER

21

Reproduction and Development

DIETHER NEUBERT, BIRGIT JÖDICKE, AND FRANK WELSCH

CHAPTER

22

Endocrine System—Adrenal Cortex, Thyroid, and Pancreas

MICHAEL J. THOMAS AND JOHN A. THOMAS

CHAPTER

23

Gastrointestinal Tract

KLAUS SCHÜMANN, BERND ELSENHANS, AND ELMAR RICHTER

CHAPTER

24

Cardiovascular System

PAUL J. BOOR

PART

III

TOXICOLOGY OF COMPOUNDS

CHAPTER

25

Hydrocarbons

GÜNTER KOSS AND IRENE TESSERAUX

CHAPTER

26

Halogenated Hydrocarbons

HERMANN M. BOLT AND JÜRGEN T. BORLAK

CHAPTER

27

Fluorocarbons

STEPHEN MAGDA

CHAPTER

28

Pesticides

RANDY L. ROSE, ERNEST HODGSON, AND R. MICHAEL ROE

CHAPTER

29

Dioxin and Dioxin-like Polychlorinated Hydrocarbons and Biphenyls

GÜNTER KOSS AND DETLEF WÖLFLE

CHAPTER

30

Aromatic Amines, Nitroarenes, and Heterocyclic Aromatic Amines

GABRIELE SABBIONI AND ELMAR RICHTER

CHAPTER

31

N-Nitroso Compounds

WERNER KOEHL AND GERHARD EISENBRAND

CHAPTER

32

Metals

SIEGFRIED G. SCHÄFER, RONALD L. F. DAWES, BERND ELSENHANS, WOLFGANG FORTH, AND KLAUS SCHÜMANN

CHAPTER

33

Gases

PETER EYER

CHAPTER

34

Fibers

DAVID B. WARHEIT, GEORGIA A. HART, AND THOMAS W. HESTERBERG

CHAPTER

35

Chemical and Biological Agents

LADISLAUS SZINICZ AND STEVEN I. BASKIN

CHAPTER

36

Active and Passive Smoking

DIETRICH HOFFMANN AND ERNST L. WYNDER

CHAPTER

37

Cosmetic Toxicology

JOHN F. CORBETT, RAJ K. SHARMA, AND WILLIAM E. DRESSLER

CHAPTER

38

Polymers

ECKHARD LÖSER AND GISELA STROPP

CHAPTER

39

Radiation

R. J. MICHAEL FRY, ULRICH F. W. HAGEN, JOHANN KUMMERMEHR, AND R. JULIAN PRESTON

CHAPTER

40

Natural Compounds

JOHANNES WESTENDORF

CHAPTER

41

Bacterial Toxins

HANS BIGALKE AND HANS-HERBERT WELLHÖNER

PART

IV

APPLICATIONS OF TOXICOLOGY

CHAPTER

42

Biomonitoring in Occupational Medicine

HUGO W. RÜDIGER

CHAPTER

43

Water

RICHARD J. BULL

CHAPTER

44

Risk Assessment in Environmental Remediation

THOMAS E. RODRIGUEZ AND DENNIS JAMES PAUSTENBACH

CHAPTER

45

Ecotoxicology

HEIDI FOTH

CHAPTER

46

Food Toxicology: Legal Aspects

DAVID G. HATTAN AND ALAN M. RULIS

CHAPTER

47

Food: Compound Related Aspects

WERNER GRUNOW

CHAPTER

48

Toxicological Evaluation Methods for the Registration of Chemicals

HEINZ-PETER GELBKE, BERNHARD HILDEBRAND, AND EDWARD J. KERFOOT

CHAPTER

49

In Vitro Methods

HORST SPIELMANN AND ALAN M. GOLDBERG

CHAPTER

50

Regulatory Toxicology

ARPAD SOMOGYI, GIO B. GORI, AND KLAUS E. APPEL

PART

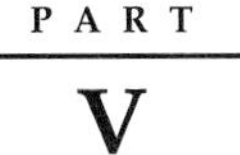

V RISK ASSESSMENT

CHAPTER

51

Risk Assessment and Preventive Hazard Minimization

DIETHER NEUBERT

CHAPTER

52

Toxicity Equivalents and Their Use in Hazard and Risk Assessment

STEPHEN SAFE

PART

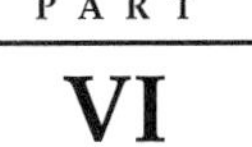

VI APPENDIX

Appendix: Threshold Values and Recommendations

INGA OLLROGE

Contributors

Numbers in parentheses indicate the pages on which the authors' contributions begin.

Bruce N. Ames (1) Division of Biochemistry and Molecular Biology, University of California at Berkeley, Berkeley, California 94720

Klaus Andreas (463) Institute of Pharmacology and Toxicology, Technical University Dresden, University Hospital, 01109 Dresden, Germany

Klaus E. Appel (1139) Federal Institute for Health Protection of Consumers and Veterinary Medicine, 14191 Berlin, Germany

Michael Arand (83) Institute of Toxicology, University of Mainz, 55131 Mainz, Germany

Steven I. Baskin (851) Division of Pharmacology, U.S. Army Medical Research Institute of Chemical Defense, Aberdeen Proving Ground, Maryland 21010

Hans Bigalke (1109) Medizinische Hochschule Hannover, Institut für Toxicologie, Zentrum Pharmakologie und Toxikologie, 30625 Hannover, Germany

Hermann M. Bolt (645) Institute of Occupational Physiology, University of Dortmund, 44139 Dortmund, Germany

Paul J. Boor (587) Department of Pathology, University of Texas Medical Branch, Galveston, Texas 77555

Jürgen T. Borlak (645) Fraunhofer Institute of Toxicology and Aerosol Research, 30625 Hannover, Germany

David J. Brusick (127) Covance Laboratories, Inc., Vienna, Virginia 22182

Richard J. Bull (1041) Pacific Northwest National Laboratory, Richland, Washington 99352

Wilfred Bursch (179) Institute of Cancer Research, University of Vienna, 1090 Vienna, Austria

Flemming R. Cassee (257) National Institute of Public Health and the Environment, Laboratory of Health Effects Research, 3720 BA Bilthoven, The Netherlands

Constantin Cojocel (297) Hoechst Marion Roussel, 65812 Bad Soden am Taunus, Germany

John F. Corbett (899) Bristol-Myers Squibb Worldwide Beauty Care, Scientific and Technical Affairs, Stamford, Connecticut 06922

Dorothee Charlotte Dartsch (245) Department of Toxicology and Environmental Medicine of the Fraunhofer Society, 20146 Hamburg, Germany

R. L. F. Dawes (755) Solvay Pharmaceuticals, 1381 CP Weesp, The Netherlands

Chris T. De Rosa (257) Division of Toxicology, Agency for Toxic Substances and Disease Registry, U.S. Department of Health and Human Services, Atlanta, Georgia 30333

William E. Dressler (899) Bristol-Myers Squibb Worldwide Beauty Care, Stamford, Connecticut 06922

Gerhard Eisenbrand (743) Department of Food Chemistry and Environmental Toxicology, University of Kaiserslautern, 67663 Kaiserslautern, Germany

Bernd Elsenhans (573, 755) Walther Straub Institute of Pharmacology and Toxicology, Ludwig Maximilians University, 80336 Munich, Germany

Peter Eyer (349, 805) Walther Straub Institute of Pharmacology and Toxicology, Ludwig Maximilians University, 80336 Munich, Germany

Victor J. Feron (257) TNO Nutrition and Food Research Institute, 3700 AJ Zeist, The Netherlands

Burckhard Fichtl (43) Walther Straub Institute of Pharmacology and Toxicology, Ludwig Maximilians University, 80336 Munich, Germany

Wolfgang Forth (755) Walther Straub Institute of Pharmacology and Toxicology, Ludwig Maximilians University, 80336 Munich, Germany

Heidi Foth (1067) Institute of Environmental Toxicology, Martin Luther University of Halle-Wittenberg, 06097 Halle, Germany

R. J. Michael Fry (937) Life Sciences Division, Oak Ridge National Laboratory, Oak Ridge, Tennessee 37830

Heinz-Peter Gelbke (1116) Department of Toxicology, BASF, 67056 Ludwigshafen, Germany

Lois Swirsky Gold (1) Division of Biochemistry and Molecular Biology, University of California at Berkeley, Berkeley, California 94720

Alan M. Goldberg (1139) Center for Alternatives to Animal Testing, Johns Hopkins University, Baltimore, Maryland 21202

Gio B. Gori (1139) The Health Policy Center, Bethesda, Maryland 20816

Martin Göttlicher (231) Karlsruhe Research Center, Institute for Genetics, Karlsruhe, Germany

John P. Groten (257) TNO Nutrition and Food Research Institute, Toxicology Division, 3700 AJ Zeist, The Netherlands

Werner Grunow (1103) Bundesinstitut für gesundheitlichen Verbraucherschutz und Veterinärmedizin, 14195 Berlin, Germany

Ulrich F. W. Hagen (937) Karwinskistrasse 64, 81247 Munich, Germany

Gerald Hajian (25) Schering-Plough Research Institute, Kenilworth, New Jersey 07033

Georgia A. Hart (833) Health Safety and Environmental Department, Schuller International, Inc., Littleton, Colorado 80162

David G. Hattan (1087) Division of Health Effects Evaluation, Office of Premarket Approval, U.S. Food and Drug Administration Center for Food Safety and Applied Nutrition, Washington, DC 20204

Thomas W. Hesterberg (833) Health Safety and Environmental Department, Schuller International, Inc., Littleton, Colorado 80162

Bernhard Hildebrand (1116) Department of Toxicology, BASF, 67056 Ludwigshafen, Germany

Ernest Hodgson (663) Department of Toxicology, North Carolina State University, Raleigh, North Carolina 27695

Dietrich Hoffmann (898) Naylor Dana Institute for Disease Prevention, American Health Foundation, Valhalla, New York 10595

Ludwig A. Hothorn (25) University of Hannover, 30149 Hannover, Germany

Birgit Jödicke (491) 35581 Wetzlar-Münchholzhausen, Germany

Regine Kahl (273) Institute of Toxicology, University of Düsseldorf, 40225 Düsseldorf, Germany

Edward J. Kerfoot (1116) Product Regulations and Toxicology, BASF, Southgate, Michigan 48195

Reinhard Klimmek (349) Walther Straub Institute of Pharmacology and Toxicology, Ludwig Maximilians University, 80336 Munich, Germany

Werner Koehl (743) Department of Toxicology, Henkel, 40191 Düsseldorf, Germany

Günter Koss (603, 699) Department of Labor, Health and Social Affairs, 20148 Hamburg, Germany; and Department of Toxicology, Hamburg University Medical School, 20146 Hamburg, Germany

Johann Kummermehr (937) Institute for Radiobiology, National Center for Environment and Health, 85758 Neuherberg, Germany

Edward A. Lock (297) Central Toxicology Laboratory, Zeneca Ltd., Alderley Park, Macclesfield, Cheshire SK10 4TJ, United Kingdom

Eckhard Löser (919) Institute of Industrial Toxicology, Bayer, 42096 Wuppertal, Germany

Stephen Magda (657) Solvay Pharmaceuticals, 30002 Hannover, Germany

Brigitte Marian (179) Institute of Cancer Research, University of Vienna, 1090 Vienna, Austria

Hans Marquardt (151) Department of Toxicology, Hamburg University Medical School, 20146 Hamburg, Germany; and Department of Toxicology and Environmental Medicine of the Fraunhofer Society, 20146 Hamburg, Germany

Roger O. McClellan (331) Chemical Industry Institute of Toxicology, Research Triangle Park, North Carolina

Hans F. Merk (459) Department of Dermatology and Allergology, University Hospital, RWTH Aachen, 52074, Germany

Dietrich Milles (11) Center for Social Policy Research, University of Bremen, 28334 Bremen, Germany

Nancy A. Monteiro-Riviere (439) Center for Cutaneous Toxicology and Residue Pharmacology, North Carolina State University, Raleigh, North Carolina 27606

Hartwig Muhle (331) Fraunhofer Institute of Toxicology and Aerosol Research, 30625 Hannover, Germany

Diether Neubert (371, 491, 1153) Department of Toxicology, Institute of Clinical Pharmacology and Toxicology, Benjamin Franklin Medical Center, Free University of Berlin, 14195 Berlin, Germany

Reinhard Neubert (371) Groupement de Rechereche Scientifique et Médicale AHCRAA, Département Neurochirurgie, 74000 Annecy, France

Franz Oesch (83) Institute of Toxicology, University of Mainz, 55131 Mainz, Germany

Inga Ollroge (1201) Department of Labor, Health, and Social Affairs, 20148 Hamburg, Germany

Dennis James Paustenbach (1057) Exponent, Menlo Park, California

R. Julian Preston (937) Chemical Industry Institute of Toxicology, Research Triangle Park, North Carolina 27709

David E. Ray (463) Neurotox Section, MRC Toxicology Laboratory, University Leicester, Leicester LE13YD, England

Elmar Richter (573, 729) Walther Straub Institute of Pharmacology and Toxicology, Ludwig Maximilians University, 80336 Munich, Germany

Jim E. Riviere (439) Center for Cutaneous Toxicology and Residue Pharmacology, North Carolina State University, Raleigh, North Carolina 27606

Thomas E. Rodriguez (1051) McLaren–Hart, Philadelphia, Pennsylvania 19133

R. Michael Roe (663) Department of Entomology and Toxicology, North Carolina State University, Raleigh, North Carolina 27695

Randy L. Rose (663) Department of Toxicology, North Carolina State University, Raleigh, North Carolina 27695

Hugo W. Rüdiger (1027) Department of Occupational Medicine, University of Vienna, 1090 Vienna, Austria

Alan M. Rulis (1087) Office of Premarket Approval, U.S. Food and Drug Administration Center for Food Safety and Applied Nutrition, Washington, DC 20204

Gabriele Sabbioni (729) Walther Straub Institute of Pharmacology and Toxicology, Ludwig Maximilians University, 80336 Munich, Germany

Stephen H. Safe (1191) Department of Veterinary Physiology and Pharmacology, Texas A & M University, College Station, Texas 77843

Siegfried G. Schäfer (755) Solvay Pharmaceuticals, 30002 Hannover, Germany; and Department of Toxicology, Hamburg University Medical School, 20146 Hamburg, Germany

Rolf Schulte-Hermann (179) Institute of Cancer Research, University of Vienna, 1090 Vienna, Austria

Klaus Schümann (573, 755) Walther Straub Institute of Pharmacology and Toxicology, Ludwig Maximilians University, 80336 Munich, Germany

Doris A. Schwindt (459) Department of Dermatology and Allergology, University Hospital, RWTH 52074 Aachen, Germany

Raj K. Sharma (899) Bristol-Myers Squibb Worldwide Beauty Care, Scientific and Technical Affairs, Stamford, Connecticut 06922

Arpad Somogyi (1139) Federal Institute for Health Protection of Consumers and Veterinary Medicine, 14191 Berlin, Germany

Horst Spielmann (1139) National Center for Documentation and Evaluation of Alternatives to Animal Experiments, 12277 Berlin, Germany

Gisela Stropp (919) Institute of Industrial Toxicology, Bayer, 42096 Wuppertal, Germany

Ladislaus Szinicz (851) Institut für Pharmakologie und Toxikologie, Akademie des Sanitäts und Gesundheitswesens der Bundeswehr, 85748 Garching–Hochbrück, Germany

Raymond W. Tennant (217) Laboratory of Environmental Carcinogens, NIEHS, Research Triangle Park, North Carolina 27709

Irene Tesseraux (603) Department of Labor, Health, and Social Affairs, 20148 Hamburg, Germany

John A. Thomas (559) Department of Pharmacology, The University of Texas Health Science Center, San Antonio, Texas 78284

Michael J. Thomas (559) Department of Internal Medicine, Division of Endocrinology, University of North Carolina School of Medicine, Chapel Hill, North Carolina 27599

Kenneth R. Tindall (217) Laboratory for Environmental Carcinogens, NIEHS, Research Triangle Park, North Carolina 27709

Peter J. van Bladeren (251) TNO Nutrition and Food Research Institute, 3700 AJ Zeist, The Netherlands

David B. Warheit (833) Haskell Laboratory, E. I. du Pont de Nemours & Company, Newark, Delaware 19714

Hans-Herbert Wellhöner (1009) Medizinische Hochschule, Zentrum Pharmakologie und Toxikologie, 30625 Hannover, Germany

Frank Welsch (491) Chemical Industry Institute of Toxicology, Research Triangle Park, North Carolina 27709

Johannes Westendorf (959) Department of Toxicology, University Medical School, 20146 Hamburg, Germany

Detlef Wölfle (699) Federal Institute for Health Protection of Consumers and Veterinary Medicine, 14191 Berlin, Germany; and Department of Toxicology, Hamburg University Medical School, 20146 Hamburg, Germany

Ernst L. Wynder (898) Naylor Dana Institute for Disease Prevention, American Health Foundation, Valhalla, New York 10595

Maged Younes (111) International Programme on Chemical Safety, World Health Organization, 1211 Geneva 27, Switzerland

Preface

Toxicology, the science of poisons and poisonous activities, is an applied science. It describes chemical and biological interactions that have acute and chronic health-threatening effects, particularly on humans. It aims at quantifying these effects in order to detect, treat, and possibly prevent any damage. Thus, this discipline is challenged to make a significant scientific contribution to preventive medicine. ("The ultimate goal in medicine is to achieve to die young as late as possible," E. Wynder.) This was not always the case. The Greek words for bow and medicinal drug are "toxon" and "pharmakon"; hence, arrow poison is "toxon pharmakon." The historian Herodotus used the word "toxikon" for poison arrow. Combining this with "logos" for science gives the term "toxicology."

The study of poisons was an aspect of many ancient cultures (e.g., Egyptians—cardiac glycosides; Chinese—opium alkaloids; Incas—coca and strychnos alkaloids; Greeks—hemlock), and toxicology thus was descriptive and empirical. In contrast, modern toxicology, with an emphasis on mechanisms of action and toxicokinetics, is a fundamentally new science that is influencing medicine and greatly improving society. The 1990s particularly have seen a rapid expansion of knowledge regarding the biological basis of toxic reactions in response to exposure to xenobiotics. Molecular and cell biology have revealed a wealth of information on cellular mechanisms, such as signal pathways, as well as an increasing understanding of the consequences of loss of these controls. Emerging techniques, such as the use of transgenic animals, promise to stimulate continued progress. However, while toxicology has developed beyond describing reactions to compounds and is increasingly successful in unraveling the cellular and molecular bases of such reactions, the methods and practices of health risk assessment are mostly underdeveloped and have made little specific use of the mechanistic approaches to toxicology. Nevertheless, the ultimate goal of toxicological research is to provide a rational basis for judgments with regard to the potential health hazards of chemical exposure for humans and the environment. Because risk assessment is a process that has an impact on society at large, it must be based on a foundation as sound as possible, and the lack of incorporation of mechanistic insights, which in addition are often rather weak, must be of utmost concern to all toxicologists.

Toxicology is one of the few scientific disciplines that increase our knowledge in ways that might find major and often immediate public responses. The fears of chemical hazards to human health and the environment are important public issues—at least in our highly industrialized societies. The fear of chemicals is not new. As Pliny the Elder commented in the first century BC: "We use so many poisons to adjust the wine to our taste—and then we wonder why this does not do us any good." However, the massive "intrusion of chemistry into the human habitat" can no longer be denied. It forces us to confront the issue.

In future history books, the second half of the 20th century will be recorded as the era of synthetic chemistry. Beginning in the 1940s, we witnessed an explosive development of new industrial technologies and an integration of synthetic chemicals into our personal lives. In the United States alone, almost 600,000 chemical products are in use. About 70,000 of these products surround us daily, and the numbers are rising continuously. These substances have qualitatively and quantitatively different effects that may threaten our health. Initially, this type of chemistry was viewed positively as a benefit to our lives. Society has become more suspicious, however, due to wake-up calls such as Rachel Carson's book *The Silent Spring* (1962). Although people in the industrialized parts of the world enjoy much longer and qualitatively richer lives, the public no longer sees science and technology only as valuable allies; rather, they view them, at least in part, as enemies of nature.

Public pressure has led to strict legislation with respect to chemical exposure, both in the environment and in the work place. Naturally, we all should welcome this development and demand that human welfare and the environment be protected. However, it is also uncontested that industry must be encouraged to invest in research to develop new materials and products that will be beneficial to all of us. The toxicological risk assessment—the evaluation of risks to human health and the environment from exposure to chemicals—is more and more a matter of sitting on the fence between these two postulates; it also stands on shaky scientific ground. On the one hand, chemical analytical techniques are capable of determining unimaginably small trace amounts of most chemicals, both synthetic and natural. The analytical results are often linked to symptoms induced by large doses of the respective compounds—without considering that analytical data and disease-related doses possibly differ by several orders of magnitude. Without such quantitative considerations of effect and risk assessment, however, the analytical findings are meaningless. On the other hand, toxicology does not always keep pace with advances in analytical technology. Despite huge gains in knowledge during the 1990s, it is unquestionable that, despite impressive progress, both our understanding of the mechanisms of toxicity and particularly our ability to assess risks quantitatively are very limited.

One can certainly quarrel over whether the increase in the use of chemicals—cosmetics, laundry detergents, food preservatives—is necessary, but this debate is irrelevant. These products are part of our lives and will stay with us into the forseeable future. The responsibility of toxicology is to ensure that humans are not subjected to unnecessary risks through exposure to these chemicals.

The foundation of toxicology is and will be for the forseeable future animal experiments that can point out potential hazards for the purpose of preventive health protection. For years, alternative methods have been advocated to replace intact animals by applying test systems other than intact organisms. However, these methods are valuable tools for special studies, but nothing more. The development of defined breeds of laboratory animals, as well as methods for their maintenance, has made it possible to carry out reproducible experiments. This must be viewed as the real beginning of experimental toxicology.

The most important principle of toxicology is the realization by Paracelsus that there are no toxic substances, only toxic dosages (applications) of compounds. In his third Carinthian Defence, Paracelsus made it quite clear that poison cannot be defined as a substance per se; rather, the same substance might be both poisonous and nonpoisonous: "Only the dose determines when a thing is not a poison." According to Paracelsus, we should define poison as a mechanism of action that is associated with both the chemical compound and the dose. Toxicologists are therefore confronted with the fact that—with exception of genotoxic compounds—any chemical is toxic above a certain threshold concentration (even 100 g of sodium chloride may be deadly), but not toxic at all below a threshold. This problem can only be solved by carefully analyzing the underlying mechanisms of action and the conditions that lead to toxicity. Threshold concentrations such as the no adverse effect level (NOAEL) are derived from toxicological investigations and, under the consideration of factors of (un)certainty, lead to human exposures that are tolerable from a toxicological point of view—that is, threshold values or guidelines such as the accepted daily intake (ADI).

The priority of modern toxicology is the detection of possible health hazards caused by the contamination of water, soil, air, and food. This poses especially difficult problems, as we are dealing here with biological activities of substances present in minute quantities. Initially, toxicology treated cases of acute poisoning after relatively high levels of exposure (Orfila, 1814). The clinical picture is characterized by more or less typical symptoms, a characteristic course of disease, and an obvious chronological relationship between intake of a compound and beginning of the disease; the effects are to a large extent reversible and the threshold values described above are applicable. Since the 1950s, toxicology has been mainly concerned with assessment and treatment of chronic intoxication and long-term effects of exogenous substances taken up in trace amounts. This development is due mainly to the identification of a new type of toxic effect, namely, the interaction of chemicals with genetic material.

The damage caused by these genotoxic effects—mutagenicity and carcinogenicity—is to a large extent irreversible and possibly occurs even with exposure to minute concentrations. The (often only theoretical) possibility that long-term exposure to minute doses might induce cancer has caused public fear and uncertainty. However, we all know very well that chemicals are acutely poisonous in high doses.

1. Five of 100,000 children die every year from accidental poisoning, especially from household chemicals. This risk is commonly accepted.
2. Most of our fellow citizens, however, are afraid of

a 1:1,000,000 risk (probability), if it exists at all, of developing cancer from exposure to asbestos in schools and demand a "cleanup," although it is exactly this measure that may cause the real asbestos threat.

Assessing the potential dangers of carcinogens is especially difficult. Presumably, there are multiple reasons that a normal cell may be transformed into a cancer cell. The underlying mechanisms of action are mostly unknown, and the test assays are inadequate in many ways. Nevertheless, there are certain basics of risk assessment. According to Paracelsus, exposure to concentrations below a threshold value is harmless. At present, such threshold values cannot be defined for carcinogens that interact with genetic material. Here, the experimentally unproven principle of stochastic effects is valid. It says that the probability of damage by a foreign compound declines with decreasing concentrations but will never be zero as long as a single molecule is still present. However, for a large number of nongenotoxic carcinogens in our environment—such as saccharin or some chlorinated hydrocarbons—there is no reason that we should not follow the rule of Paracelsus. We can no longer watch passively as it is declared reasonable that test results obtained with exorbitantly high dosages are extrapolated to the ppb or ppt range (1 part per billion or trillion) of normal environmental concentrations (comparable to a cube of sugar dissolved in Lake Geneva, Switzerland). If the one molecule hypothesis of carcinogenesis were correct, we all would be dead from cancer at an early age: Natural carcinogens occur normally in food at levels 10,000 times higher than those of residues of synthetic chemicals, and carcinogens are produced in food by ordinary cooking procedures. Furthermore, each cell normally contains elements that are carcinogenic, such as arsenic, cadmium, and uranium. Obviously, the toxicological assessment of both the chemicals and the specific situations in which humans are exposed to chemicals requires expert knowledge and great experience. The simple extrapolation of data from animal experiments to humans without considering the differences between species and mechanisms of action and without considering dose–response relationships inevitably leads to great uncertainties. "Extrapolation is more than using carbon paper" (A. F. Rahde). The assessment of the health risks from the exposure to chemicals must be based on established scientific knowledge. We can no longer tolerate irrationality when dealing with chemicals. Chemophobia, which is so much in the limelight, is often far from scientific reality: "Alarm is sounded long before it is clear what exactly we must be warned about—and those who paint the gloomiest pictures are trusted the most" (H. Rüdiger).

Humans are exposed to xenobiotics when using compounds with both beneficial and toxic effects (drugs) or to chemicals that have only toxic potentials. Xenobiotics generally show dose-dependent toxicity. The huge diversity in the use of and exposure to these potentially toxic xenobiotics has resulted in the cooperation of scientists from many disciplines with inevitably differing approaches. Thus, the study of toxicology can be divided into various fields, such as food, occupational medicine, environmental studies, and drug development.

Experimental toxicology collects data that are partly descriptive, but which also contribute to an understanding of the mechanism of the toxic effects observed. Thus, toxicological studies are performed not only in laboratories of the chemical and pharmaceutical industries, but also in research institutes concerned with biochemistry, physiology, pharmacology, cell biology, and pharmaceutical research.

Regulatory toxicology assesses the results of toxicological investigations with regard to the potential risk to humans and the environment. The existence of regulatory toxicology has resulted in the establishment of a large number of standardized or core study protocols. The quality of the data generated is maintained and guaranteed by the implementation of GLP (good laboratory practice) rules and the certification of the relevant laboratories by the responsible authorities. Standardization and the transparent documentation of the methods, animal strains, cell lines, and bacterial strains used are necessary to guarantee comparability of the data. Regulatory toxicology estimates the potential risk of exposure to xenobiotics of humans or the environment. Often only animal data are available for extrapolation to define an acceptable safety margin for public health. Risk represents the probability that a given xenobiotic will induce adverse effects or even severe damage; it is the reciprocal of safety. In other words, safety corresponds to the expectation of an acceptable risk under specified exposure conditions. The acceptable risk, however, must be defined on a case by case basis.

Thus, for example, an extremely toxic xenobiotic handled in a well-controlled manner will be less dangerous than a moderately toxic material released without appropriate control or assimilated in an uncontrolled manner. The assimilation of the material is a function of the exposure route and the physicochemical properties of the compound, which will have a major effect on the amount of compound absorbed and the exposure time. Toxicokinetic studies provide information about bioavailability, distribution to target organs, metabolism, and elimination. Investigation of the metabolism of a compound can give valuable insights into the mechanism of toxicity, such as in the case of the hepatotoxicity of acetaminophen or the porphyrinogenic effect of lead.

When toxicology is considered in depth, it becomes clear that the old concept of "toxicology is the pharmacology of high doses" is incomplete. In contrast, numerous actions and methods employed in toxicology have no relevance in pharmacology, examples being mutagenicity and carcinogenicity. These actions are, however, of the utmost importance in evaluating new chemical entities before their human exposure can be considered.

As a rule, the effects of xenobiotics are a function of dose, duration, and frequency of exposure. Toxicology discriminates among four categories of exposure, independent of the route of administration: (i) acute, (ii) subacute, (iii) subchronic, and (iv) chronic. *Acute* uptake indicates a single exposure lasting less than 24 hours, whereas the other categories describe repeated administrations. A *subacute* exposure describes repeated administrations of up to 28 days. *Subchronic* exposure reflects repeated administrations between 1 and 3 months. Exposure for more than 3 months is designated *chronic.*

Symptoms observed after repeated exposures may differ substantially from those observed after a single dose. For example, acute benzene exposure results in effects on the central nervous system, whereas leukemia is the prominent adverse event after prolonged exposure. Another well-known example is ethanol (ethyl alcohol, or alcohol), which after a single overdose mainly shows central nervous effects, for instance, disturbance of movements, euphoria, and unconsciousness, in addition to nausea, vomiting, and even death. Chronic abuse of alcohol results in liver cirrhosis, polyneurophathia, liver cancer, and addiction. Furthermore, symptoms resulting from acute toxic effects may be delayed, being observed only after several days, such as in the case of acetaminophen intoxication. This time lag can result in an acute intoxication being underestimated or even not being recognized by a practitioner.

Test strategies and requirements vary considerably according to the intended use of the compounds under consideration, whether for human use (e.g., drugs, food additives, and cosmetics) or bulk industrial production. Regulatory authorities have well-defined toxicological requirements for both classes of compounds.

Repeated or continuous exposure to xenobiotics may result in *tolerance,* that is, reduced effects due to prior exposure to the same or a chemically related compound. There are two possible causes of tolerance: the target organ is presented with a less toxic metabolite of the parent compound following modulation of metabolism, or the susceptibility of the target organ is reduced. The detailed mechanisms for these phenomena often need to be elucidated. Tolerance is observed for both drugs and other xenobiotics such as carbon tetrachloride. In the latter case, the trichloromethyl radical, the reactive metabolite responsible for hepatotoxicity, is formed to a lesser extent after repeated exposure. The heavy metal cadmium provides another example. Repeated uptake results in the induction of a cadmium-binding protein called metallothionein. As long as the concentration of free cadmium ions is practically zero, the symptoms of cadmium poisoning generally remain absent.

A further aspect of the toxicity of a compound is its *reversibility,* as shown by two classes of insecticides, carbamates and alkylated phosphates. For example, carbamate intoxication leads to reversible inhibition of acetylcholinesterase activity; however, the enzyme is reactivated after a few hours. In contrast, alkylated phosphates bind irreversibly to the same enzymes. The symptoms are identical in both intoxications. However, in the latter case, the acetylcholinesterase cannot be reactivated, and *de novo* erythropoesis is necessary. Consequently, the symptoms will persist much longer in the case of alkylated phosphate intoxication and therapeutic measures must be substantially different.

The *interaction* between two or more compounds can play an important role. Interaction can result in either an increase or a decrease in the toxic effects of a compound. A toxic effect is *additive* if, after simultaneous administration of two or more xenobiotics, it is the sum of the individual effects; this occurs, for example, after exposure to two different organophosphates. A *synergistic* effect will produce more severe symptoms than would be expected from the toxicities of the individual compounds; this is observed in the hepatotoxicity of carbon tetrachloride when it is given in the presence of ethanol. *Potentiation* occurs when a compound showing little or no toxicity markedly increases the toxicity of a second compound. As an example, isopropanol alone shows no hepatotoxicity; however, co-administration of isopropanol and carbon tetrachloride provokes hepatotoxic effects much more severe than would be expected from carbon tetrachloride alone.

Two compounds can interact to antagonize one another's effects. This phenomenon is the basis of *antidote* therapy. If two compounds counteract one another with regard to physiological effects, but not necessarily by the same mechanism of action, a *func-*

tional antagonism is involved. For example, several classes of compounds induce convulsions, which are antagonized by diazepam, but diazepam does not necessarily compete for the same binding site or receptor as the convulsant. *Chemical antagonism* occurs if a well-defined chemical reaction inactivates the toxic xenobiotic. Dimercaprol (British Anti-Lewisite, BAL) chelates arsenic, lead, and mercury ions, producing a nontoxic metal complex. By this simple chemical reaction, the chelating agent withdraws the toxic metal ions from the target organ and facilitates excretion. Competition for bonding to the same receptor is called *receptor antagonism;* an overdose of morphine can be antagonized by naloxone, and an overdose of benzodiazepam by flumenazil, as in each case both compounds are competing for the same receptor. In practice, however, the antagonist must be shown to have no deleterious pharmacodynamic effect. An antidote acting through a receptor antagonism does not necessarily compete with the xenobiotic directly. Atropine can be used to treat organophosphate poisoning, which causes accumulation of the neurotransmitter acetylcholine, by blocking the acetylcholine receptor.

As a result of developing strategies in drug research, such as combinatorial chemistry and high throughput screening (HTS), toxicology has developed an additional focus, involving mainly mechanistically oriented *in vitro* screening. These new pharmacological screening strategies allow the testing of several hundred thousand new chemical entities each year per laboratory. Consequently, an increasing demand for new test systems for use in early qualitative decision making in the development of new chemical entities can be expected. These screening systems will probably be focused mainly on mechanistically oriented toxicology with clearly defined target organs. *Predictive in vitro toxicology* should fulfill at least five criteria:

1. Target-related toxicity should correlate with the structure of the compounds and potential effects, for example, organ toxicity or metabolic effects.
2. Prediction of targets for epigenetic risk factors for carcinogenicity should be achieved.
3. A good correlation between results from *in vitro* and *in vivo* test systems should be demonstrated.
4. Test systems should have a low incidence of false negatives results.
5. An automatization of toxicological *in vitro* screening should be possible.

Much effort will be required to meet these goals. However, substantial progress is expected.

The responsibility that toxicology as a science has to humanity and the technological achievements of the chemical industry should encourage us to develop this discipline further, using great care and critical expertise. It is essential that any risk assessment be based on the best science available. The dramatic developments in toxicology and the substantial progress in cell and molecular biology must be integrated into toxicological risk assessment. Above all, the critical information must be communicated to the general public. More than ever before, physicians, chemists, and other scientists must become familiar with toxicological knowledge and the principles of toxicological safety assessment. This book is dedicated to this goal.

H. Marquardt, S. G. Schäfer, R. McClellan, F. Welsch

Introduction

BRUCE N. AMES, LOIS SWIRSKY GOLD

Division of Biochemistry and Molecular Biology and National Institutes of Environmental Health Sciences Center, University of California at Berkeley, Berkeley, California

In this introductory essay we raise four issues in the fuzzy interface between toxicology, nutrition, public health, and government regulations.

PARACELSUS TO PARASCIENCE: THE DOSE/TRACE MAKES THE POISON

About 50% of all chemicals—whether natural or synthetic—that have been tested in standard, high-dose animal cancer tests are rodent carcinogens (Table 1). What are the explanations for this high percentage? In standard cancer tests, rodents are given a chronic, near-toxic dose: the maximum tolerated dose (MTD). Evidence is accumulating that cell division caused by the high dose itself, rather than the chemical per se, can contribute to cancer in these tests. High doses can cause chronic wounding of tissues, cell death, and the consequent chronic cell division of neighboring cells, which is a risk factor for cancer. Each time a cell divides, the probability increases that a mutation will occur, thereby increasing the risk for cancer. At the low levels to which humans are usually exposed, such increased cell division does not occur. In addition, tissues injured by high doses of chemicals have an inflammatory immune response involving the activation of white cells in response to cell death. Activated white cells release mutagenic oxidants (including peroxynitrite, hypochlorite, and hydrogen peroxide). Therefore, the very low levels of chemicals to which humans are exposed through water pollution or synthetic pesticide residues may pose no or minimal cancer risks.

Is the high positivity rate due to selecting more suspicious chemicals to test, which is a likely bias because cancer testing is both expensive and time-consuming, and it is prudent to test suspicious compounds? One argument against selection bias is the high positivity rate for drugs (Table 1) because drug development tends to select chemicals that are not mutagens or expected carcinogens. A second argument against selection bias is that the knowledge needed to predict carcinogenicity in rodent tests is highly imperfect, even now after decades of testing results have become available on which to base predictions. For example, a prospective prediction exercise was conducted by several experts in 1990 in advance of the 2-year NTP bioassays. There was a wide disagreement among them on which chemicals would be carcinogenic when tested and the level of accuracy varied by expert, thus indicating that predictive knowledge is highly uncertain.

It seems likely that a high proportion of all chemicals, whether synthetic or natural, might be "carcinogens" if administered in the standard rodent bioassay at the maximum tolerated dose, primarily due to the effects of high doses on cell division and DNA damage. Without additional data on how a chemical causes cancer, the interpretation of a positive result in a rodent bioassay is highly uncertain. The induction of cancer could be the result of the high doses tested.

In regulatory policy, the virtually safe dose (VSD), corresponding to a maximum hypothetical risk of one cancer in a million, is estimated from bioassay results using a linear model that assumes cancer causation is directly proportional to dose and that there are no unique effects of high doses. To the extent that carci-

TABLE 1 Proportion of Chemicals Evaluated as Carcinogenic

	Proportion	Percent
Chemicals tested in both rats and mice[a]	330/559	(59%)
Naturally occurring chemicals	73/127	(57%)
Synthetic chemicals	257/432	(59%)
Chemicals tested in rats and/or mice[a]		
Chemicals in Carcinogenic Potency Database	668/1275	(52%)
Natural pesticides	35/64	(55%)
Mold toxins	14/23	(61%)
Chemicals in roasted coffee	19/28	(68%)
Innes negative chemicals retested[a,b]	16/34	(47%)
Physician's Desk Reference (PDR)		
Drugs with reported cancer tests[c]	117/241	(49%)
FDA database of drug submissions[d]	125/282	(44%)

[a]From Gold, L. S. *et al.* (1997).
[b]The 1969 study by Innes *et al.* is frequently cited as evidence that the proportion of carcinogens is low, as only 9% of 119 chemicals tested (primarily pesticides) were positive. However, these tests, which were only in mice with few animals per group, lacked the power of modern tests. Of the 34 Innes negative chemicals that have been retested using modern protocols, 16 were positive.
[c]Davies and Monro (1995).
[d]Contrera *et al.* (1997). 140 drugs are in both the FDA and PDR databases.

nogenicity in rodent bioassays is due to the effects of high doses for the nonmutagens and a synergistic effect of cell division at high doses with DNA damage for the mutagens, then this model is inappropriate.

EVEN RACHEL CARSON WAS MADE OF CHEMICALS: NATURAL VERSUS SYNTHETIC CHEMICALS

About 99.9% of the chemicals humans ingest are natural. The amounts of synthetic pesticide residues in plant foods are insignificant compared to the amount of natural pesticides produced by plants themselves. Of all dietary pesticides that humans eat, 99.99% are natural: they are chemicals produced by plants to defend themselves against fungi, insects, and other animal predators. Each plant produces a different array of such chemicals.

On average, Americans ingest roughly 5000 to 10,000 different natural pesticides and their breakdown products. Americans eat about 1500 mg of natural pesticides per person per day, which is about 10,000 times more than they consume of synthetic pesticide residues.

Even though only a small proportion of natural pesticides have been tested for carcinogenicity, 35 of the 63 tested are rodent carcinogens. Naturally occurring pesticides that are rodent carcinogens are ubiquitous in fruits, vegetables, herbs, and spices (Table 2).

Cooking foods produces about 2000 mg per person per day of burnt material that contains many rodent carcinogens and many mutagens. By contrast, the residues of 200 synthetic chemicals measured by FDA, including the synthetic pesticides thought to be of greatest importance, average only about 0.09 mg per person per day. In a single cup of coffee, the natural chemicals that are known rodent carcinogens are about equal in weight to a year's worth of synthetic pesticide residues that are rodent carcinogens, even though only 3% of the natural chemicals in roasted coffee have been adequately tested for carcinogenicity (Table 3). This does not mean that coffee or natural pesticides are dangerous but rather that assumptions about high-dose animal cancer tests for assessing human risk at low doses need reexamination. No diet can be free of natural chemicals that are rodent carcinogens.

Gaining a broad perspective about the vast number of chemicals to which humans are exposed can be helpful when setting research and regulatory priorities. Rodent cancer tests provide little information about how a chemical causes cancer or about its effects at a low dose. The assumption that synthetic chemicals are hazardous has led to a bias in testing, such that synthetic chemicals account for 77% (432 of 559) of the chemicals tested chronically in both rats and mice (Table 1). The natural world of chemicals has never been tested systematically. One reasonable strategy is to use a rough index to compare and rank possible carcinogenic hazards from a wide variety of

TABLE 2 Carcinogenicity in Rodents of Natural Plant Pesticides Tested[a]

Carcinogens ($N = 35$)
Acetaldehyde methylformylhydrazone, Allyl isothiocyanate, Arecoline.HCl, Benzaldehyde, Benzyl acetate, Caffeic acid, Catechol, Clivorine, Coumarin, Crotonaldehyde, Cycasin and methylazoxymethanol acetate, 3,4-dihydrocoumarin, Estragole, Ethyl acrylate, N^2-γ-Glutamyl-*p*-hydrazinobenzoic acid, Hexanal methylformylhydrazine, *p*-Hydrazinobenzoic acid.HCl, Hydroquinone, 1-Hydroxyanthraquinone, Lasiocarpine, D-Limonene, 8-Methoxypsoralen, *N*-Methyl-*N*-formylhydrazine, α-Methylbenzyl alcohol, 3-Methylbutanal methylformylhydrazone, Methylhydrazine, Monocrotaline, Pentanal methylformylhydrazone, Petasitenine, Quercetin, Reserpine, Safrole, Senkirkine, Sesamol, Symphytine

Noncarcinogens ($N = 28$)
Atropine, Benzyl alcohol, Biphenyl, D-Carvone, Deserpidine, Disodium glycyrrhizinate, Emetine.2HCl, Ephedrine sulphate, Eucalyptol, Eugenol, Gallic acid, Geranyl acetate, β-*N*-[γ-l(+)-Glutamyl]-4-hydroxy-methylphenylhydrazine, Glycyrrhetinic acid, *p*-Hydrazinobenzoic acid, Isosafrole, Kaempferol, DL-Menthol, Nicotine, Norharman, Pilocarpine, Piperidine, Protocatechuic acid, Rotenone, Rutin sulfate, Sodium benzoate, Turmeric oleoresin, Vinblastine

Rodent carcinogen sources
Absinthe, Allspice, Anise, Apple, Apricot, Banana, Basil, Beet, Broccoli, Brussels sprouts, Cabbage, Cantaloupe, Caraway, Cardamom, Carrot, Cauliflower, Celery, Cherries, Chili pepper, Cinnamon, Cloves, Cocoa, Coffee, Collard greens, Comfrey herb tea, Coriander, Corn, Currants, Dill, Eggplant, Endive, Fennel, Garlic, Grapefruit, Grapes, Guava, Honey, Honeydew melon, Horseradish, Kale, Lemon, Lentils, Lettuce, Licorice, Lime, Mace, Mango, Marjoram, Mint, Mushrooms, Mustard, Nutmeg, Onion, Orange, Paprika, Parsley, Parsnip, Peach, Pear, Peas, Black pepper, Pineapple, Plum, Potato, Radish, Raspberries, Rhubarb, Rosemary, Rutabaga, Sage, Savory, Sesame seeds, Soybean, Star anise, Tarragon, Tea, Thyme, Tomato, Turmeric, Turnip

[a]Fungal toxins are not included. Reprinted from Gold *et al.*, In *Food Chemical Risk Analysis* (D. Tennant, ed.), pp. 267–295, © 1997 Aspen Publishers, Inc.

chemical exposures at levels that humans typically receive, and then to focus on those that rank highest. Ranking is a critical first step that can help to set priorities for selecting chemicals for long-term cancer tests, studies on mechanism, epidemiological research, and regulatory policy. Although one cannot say whether the ranked chemical exposures are likely to be of major or minor importance in human cancer, it is not prudent to focus attention on the possible hazards at the bottom of a ranking if, using the same methodology to identify hazard, there are numerous common human exposures with much greater possible hazards. Our analyses are based on the HERP index (Human Exposure/Rodent Potency), which indicates what percentage of the rodent carcinogenic potency a human receives from a given daily lifetime exposure. A ranking based on standard regulatory risk assessment would be similar.

TABLE 3 Carcinogenicity in Rodents of Natural Chemicals in Roasted Coffee[a]

Positive ($N = 19$)
Acetaldehyde, Benzaldehyde, Benzene, Benzofuran, Benzo[*a*]pyrene, Caffeic acid, Catechol, 1,2,5,6-Dibenzanthracene, Ethanol, Ethylbenzene, Formaldehyde, Furan, Furfural, Hydrogen peroxide, Hydroquinone, Limonene, Styrene, Toluene, Xylene

Not positive ($N = 8$)
Acrolein, Biphenyl, Choline, Eugenol, Nicotinamide, Nicotinic acid, Phenol, Piperidine

Uncertain: Caffeine

Yet to test: ~1000 chemicals

[a]Gold *et al.* (1997).

Overall, the analyses have shown that HERP values for some historically high exposures in the work place (e.g., butadiene and tetrachloroethylene) and some pharmaceuticals (e.g., clofibrate) rank high, and that there is an enormous background of naturally occurring rodent carcinogens in the average consumption of common foods that casts doubt on the relative importance of low-dose exposures to residues of synthetic chemicals such as pesticides. A committee of the National Research Council of the National Academy of Sciences, recently reached similar conclusions about natural vs synthetic chemicals in the diet and called for further research on natural chemicals.

The possible carcinogenic hazards from synthetic pesticides are minimal compared to the background of nature's pesticides, though neither may be a hazard at the doses consumed. Analysis also indicates that many ordinary foods would not pass the regulatory criteria used for synthetic chemicals. Caution is necessary in drawing conclusions from the occurrence in the diet of natural chemicals that are rodent carcinogens. It is not argued here that these dietary exposures are necessarily of much relevance to human cancer. The data call for a reevaluation of the utility of animal cancer tests in protecting the public against minor hypothetical risks.

It is often assumed that because natural chemicals are part of human evolutionary history, whereas synthetic chemicals are recent, the mechanisms that have evolved in animals to cope with the toxicity of natural chemicals will fail to protect against synthetic chemicals. This assumption is flawed for several reasons:

1. Humans have many natural defenses that buffer against normal exposures to toxins and these are usually general, rather than tailored for each specific chemical. Thus they work against both natural and synthetic chemicals. Examples of general defenses include the continuous shedding of cells (the surface layers of the mouth, esophagus, stomach, intestine, colon, skin, and lungs are discarded every few days); DNA-repair enzymes, which repair DNA that was damaged from many different sources; and detoxification enzymes of the liver and other organs, which generally target classes of chemicals rather than individual chemicals. That human defenses are usually general, rather than specific for each chemical, makes good evolutionary sense. The reason that predators of plants evolved general defenses is presumably to be prepared to counter a diverse and ever-changing array of chemicals in plants in an evolving world; if a herbivore had defenses against only a set of specific plant pesticides, it would be at a great disadvantage in obtaining new food when favored foods became scarce or evolved new chemical defenses.

2. Various natural toxins, which have been present throughout vertebrate evolutionary history, nevertheless cause cancer in vertebrates. Mold toxins, such as aflatoxin, have been shown to cause cancer in rodents and other species, including humans (Table 1). Many of the common elements are carcinogenic to humans at high doses (e.g., salts of cadmium, beryllium, nickel, chromium, and arsenic) despite their presence throughout evolution. Furthermore, epidemiological studies from various parts of the world show that certain natural chemicals in food may be carcinogenic risks to humans; for example, the chewing of betel nuts with tobacco caused oral cancer.

3. Humans have not had time to evolve a "toxic harmony" with all of their dietary plants. The human diet has changed markedly in the last few thousand years. Indeed, very few of the plants that humans eat today (e.g., coffee, cocoa, tea, potatoes, tomatoes, corn, avocados, mangoes, olives, and kiwi fruit) would have been present in a hunter–gatherer's diet. Natural selection works far too slowly for humans to have evolved specific resistance to the chemicals in these newly introduced plants.

4. DDT is often viewed as the typically dangerous synthetic pesticide because it concentrates in tissues and persists for years, being slowly released into the bloodstream. DDT, the first synthetic pesticide, eradicated malaria from many parts of the world, including the United States. It was effective against many vectors of disease such as mosquitoes, tsetse flies, lice, ticks, and fleas. DDT was also lethal to many crop pests and significantly increased the supply and lowered the cost of food, making fresh nutritious foods more accessible to poor people. DDT was also of low toxicity to humans. A 1970 National Academy of Sciences report concluded: "In little more than two decades DDT has prevented 500 million deaths due to malaria, that would otherwise have been inevitable." There is no convincing epidemiological evidence, nor is there much toxicological plausibility, that the levels of DDT normally found in the environment are likely to be a significant contributor to human cancer. DDT was unusual with respect to bioconcentration and, because of its chlorine substituents, it takes longer to degrade in nature than most chemicals; however, these are properties of relatively few synthetic chemicals. In addition, many thousands of chlorinated chemicals are produced in nature and natural pesticides also can bioconcentrate if they are fat soluble. Potatoes, for example, naturally contain the fat-soluble neurotoxins solanine and chaconine, which can be detected in the bloodstream of all potato eaters. High levels of these potato neurotoxins have been shown to cause birth defects in rodents.

5. Since no plot of land is immune to attack by insects, plants need chemical defenses—either natural or synthetic—to survive pest attack. Thus, there is a trade-off between naturally occurring pesticides and synthetic pesticides. One consequence of the disproportionate concern about synthetic pesticide residues is that some plant breeders develop plants to be more insect-resistant by making them higher in natural toxins. A recent case illustrates the potential hazards of this approach to pest control. When a major grower introduced a new variety of highly insect-resistant celery into commerce, people who handled the celery developed rashes when they were subsequently exposed to sunlight. Some detective work found that the pest-resistant celery contained 6200 parts per billion (ppb) of carcinogenic (and mutagenic) psoralens instead of the 800 ppb present in common celery.

ERRORS OF OMISSION: TOXICITY OF INSUFFICIENT MICRONUTRIENTS

Hormonal factors, dietary imbalances, infection and inflammation, and genetic factors, none of which involve a carcinogenic chemical, are major contributors to cancer.

TABLE 4 Review of Epidemiological Studies on Cancer Showing Protection by Consumption of Fruits and Vegetables[a]

Cancer site	Fraction of studies showing significant cancer protection	Median relative risk of low-quarter vs. high-quarter consumption
Epithelial		
Lung	24/25	2.2
Oral	9/9	2.0
Larynx	4/4	2.3
Esophagus	15/16	2.0
Stomach	17/19	2.5
Pancreas	9/11	2.8
Cervix	7/8	2.0
Bladder	3/5	2.1
Colorectal	20/35	1.9
Miscellaneous	6/8	—
Hormone-dependent		
Breast	8/14	1.3
Ovary, endometrim	3/4	1.8
Prostate	4/14	1.3
Total	129/172	

[a]Block *et al.* (1992).

The high consumption of fruits and vegetables is associated with a lower risk of degenerative diseases including cancer, cardiovascular disease, cataracts, and brain dysfunction. Over 200 epidemiological studies have been reviewed that show, with great consistency, an association between the low consumption of fruits and vegetables and cancer incidence (Table 4).

The quarter of the population with the lowest dietary intake of fruits and vegetables has roughly twice the cancer rate of the quarter with the highest intake for most types of cancer (lung, larynx, oral cavity, esophagus, stomach, colorectal, bladder, pancreas, cervix, and ovary). In the United States, 80% of children and adolescents and 68% of adults did not meet the intake recommended by the National Cancer Institute and the National Research Council of five servings of fruits and vegetables per day.

Publicity about hundreds of minor hypothetical risks, such as pesticide residues, can result in a loss of perspective about what is important: half the public does not know that fruit and vegetable consumption is a major protection against cancer. Fruits and vegetables are of major importance for reducing cancer; if they become more expensive because of reduced use of synthetic pesticides, then consumption will decline and cancer is likely to increase. People with low incomes eat fewer fruits and vegetables and spend a higher percentage of their income on food.

Folic acid deficiency, one of the most common vitamin deficiencies among people consuming few dietary fruits and vegetables, causes extensive chromosome breaks in human genes. Approximately 10% of the U.S. population has a folate level lower than that at which chromosome breaks occur. In two small studies of low-income (mainly African-American) elderly and adolescents done nearly 20 years ago, nearly half had folate levels this low although the issue should be reexamined. The rate of chromosome breaks in humans is reduced by folate administration. Chromosome breaks could contribute to the increased risk of cancer and cognitive defects associated with folate deficiency in humans. Folate deficiency also damages human sperm, causes neural tube defects in the fetus, and causes about 10% of U.S. heart disease. Diets deficient in fruits and vegetables are commonly low in folate, antioxidants (e.g., vitamin C), and many other micronutrients, and result in DNA damage and higher cancer rates.

Antioxidants, such as vitamin C (whose dietary source is fruits and vegetables), vitamin E, and selenium, protect against oxidative damage from normal metabolism, smoking, and inflammation. Because radiation causes oxidative damage, insufficiency of dietary antioxidants is a radiation mimic.

Deficiency of any one of nine dietary micronutrients—folic acid, niacin, iron, zinc, selenium, and vitamins B6, B12, C, and E—appear to act as radiation mimics in breaking DNA and chromosomes or causing oxidative damage to DNA or both. Some of these micronutrients come from fruits and vegetables and could account for a good part of their protective effect against cancer.

Many other micronutrients whose main dietary sources are other than fruits and vegetables, also are likely to play a significant role in the prevention and repair of DNA damage, and thus are important to the maintenance of long-term health. Deficiency of vitamin B12 (found in about 10% of U.S. elderly) causes a functional folate deficiency, the accumulation of homocysteine, a risk factor for heart disease, and probably chromosome breaks. Strict vegetarians are at increased risk of developing a vitamin B12 deficiency. Niacin contributes to the repair of DNA breaks. As a result, dietary insufficiencies of niacin (15% of some populations are deficient), folate, and antioxidants may act together to increase DNA damage. There is also evidence that low intake (<50% recommended daily allowance) of zinc, iron, selenium, or vitamin B6 (7–20% of the U.S. population is low in each) can lead to DNA damage. Half of the U.S. population may be low in at least one of these nine micronutrients. Optimizing micronutrient intake (through better diets, fortification of foods, or multivitamin–mineral pills) can have a major impact on health at a low cost. Increasing research in this area and efforts to increase micronutrient intake and more balanced diets should be high priorities for public policy.

DAMAGE BY DISTRACTION: REGULATING LOW HYPOTHETICAL RISKS

Synthetic hormone mimics have become an environmental issue. Hormonal factors are important in cancer, as mentioned above. The book *Our Stolen Future* (Colburn *et al.*, 1996) claims that traces of synthetic chemicals, such as pesticides with weak hormonal activity, may contribute to cancer and reduce sperm counts. The book ignores the fact that our normal diet contains natural chemicals that have estrogenic activity millions of times higher than that due to the traces of synthetic estrogenic chemicals and that lifestyle factors can markedly change the levels of endogenous hormones. The low levels of human exposure to residues of industrial chemicals are toxicologically implausible as a significant cause of cancer or of reproductive abnormalities, especially when compared to the natural background. In addition, it has not been shown convincingly that sperm counts are declining, and even if they were there are many more likely causes, such as smoking and diet.

Because there is no risk-free world and resources are limited, society must set priorities based on benefits and cost-effectiveness in order to save the most lives. The EPA projected in 1991 that the cost to society of U.S. environmental regulations in 1997 would be about $140 billion per year (about 2.6% of the gross national product). Most of this cost is to the private sector. Several economic analyses by others have concluded that current expenditures are not cost-effective; that is, resources are not being used so as to save the most lives per dollar. One estimate is that the United States could prevent 60,000 deaths per year by redirecting the same dollar resources to more cost-effective programs. For example, the median toxin-control program costs 146 times more per year of life saved than the median medical-intervention program. This difference is likely to be greater because cancer-risk estimates for toxin-control programs are worst-case hypothetical estimates, and the true risks at low dose are often likely to be zero. Rules regulating air and water pollution are necessary (e.g., it was a public health advance to phase lead out of gasoline) and clearly cancer prevention is not the only reason for regulations. However, worst-case assumptions in risk assessment represent a policy decision, not a scientific one, and they confuse attempts to allocate money effectively for public health.

Regulatory efforts to reduce low-level human exposures to synthetic chemicals because they are rodent carcinogens are expensive; they aim to eliminate minuscule concentrations that now can be measured with improved techniques. These efforts are distractions from the major task of improving public health through increasing scientific understanding of how to prevent cancer (e.g., what aspects of diet are important), increasing public understanding of how lifestyle influences health, and improving our ability to help individuals alter their lifestyles.

Why has the government focused on minor hypothetical risks at huge cost? A recent article in *The Economist* (December 20, 1997) had fairly harsh judgment:

> Predictions of ecological doom, including recent ones, have such a terrible track record that people should take them with pinches of salt instead of lapping them up with relish. For reasons of their own, pressure groups, journalists and fameseekers will no doubt continue to peddle ecological catastrophes at an undiminishing speed . . . . Environmentalists are quick to accuse their opponents in business of having vested interests. But their own incomes, their fame and their very existence can depend on supporting the most alarming versions of every environmental scare. 'The whole aim of practical politics,' said H.L. Mencken, 'is to keep the popu-

lace alarmed—and hence clamorous to be led to safety—by menacing it with a series of hobgoblins, all of them imaginary.' Mencken's forecast, at least, appears to have been correct.

Aaron Wildavsky discusses worst-case risk assessment in his book *But Is It True: A Citizen's Guide to Environmental Health and Safety Issues.*

> We should be guided by the probability and extent of harm, not by its mere possibility. The search for possibilities is endless and it trivializes the subject. There is bound to be great diversion of resources without reducing substantial sources of harm. Consternation is created but health is not enhanced . . . . Weak causes are likely to have weak effects. Our search should be for strong causes with palpable effects, like cigarette smoking. They are easier to find and their effects are much more important to control . . . . The past necessity of proving harm has been replaced by a reversal of causality: now the individuals and businesses must prove that they will do no harm. My objection to this . . . is profound: our liberties are curbed and our health is harmed.

Acknowledgments

This essay has been adapted in part from Ames and Gold, *FASEB J.* **11,** 1041–1052 (1997) and Ames, *Toxicol. Lett.* **102/103,** 5–18 (1998) with permission from Elsevier Science. For detailed literature, the reader is referred to both publications.

Bibliography

Block, G. *et al.* (1992). *Nutr. and Cancer* **18,** 1–29.

Contrera, J., *et al.* (1997). *Regul Toxicol. Pharmacol.* **25,** 130–145.

Davies, T., and Monro, A. (1995). *J. Am. Coll. Toxicol.* **14,** 90–107.

Gold, L. S., *et al.* (1997). In *Handbook of Carcinogenic Potency and Genotoxicity Databases* (L. S. Gold and E. Zeiger, eds.) pp. 661–685. CRC Press, Boca Raton, Florida.

Gold, L. S., *et al.* (1997a). In *Food Chemical Risk Analysis* (D. Tennant, ed.), pp. 267–295. Aspen Publishers, Gaithersburg, Maryland.

Innes, J., *et al.* (1969). *J. Natl. Cancer Inst.* **42,** 1101–1114.

PART I

FUNDAMENTALS

CHAPTER

1

History of Toxicology

DIETRICH MILLES
Center for Social Policy Research, University of Bremen, Bremen, Germany

It has been known for centuries that substances affect the human body. From earliest times, people have wanted to know which substances support which bodily functions, whether they calm or paralyze them, lead to healing or death, and how they do so. It was established that the effects of a substance depended on its state: liquid or powder, in work or building materials or in foodstuffs, or through radiation. A long-lasting argument flared up as to whether substances are inherently effective or only in specific quantities. There was research into why different substances work differently on different people, in different environments, in different combinations. History supplies us not only with much evidence about the most important problems of toxicology, which vary with time, but also about the continuing efforts to approach its tasks in a responsible way, both scientifically and practically. The following introduction can deal with only some of the more important endeavors.

TOXICOLOGY—THE SCIENCE OF POISON

The word "toxicology" comes from the Greek word for poison (*toxicon*) and scientific study (*logos*) and was coined in the 17th century. To begin with, toxicology developed as an empirical science linked to medicine. The great turning point for the science came through Paracelsus, who worked on chemical processes in life functions and who emphasized the importance of the quantity of a substance: "Was ist das Allein die Dosis macht, daß ein ding gifft ist" ("Is there anything that is not poison? Everything is poison, and nothing is without poison. The dose alone makes a thing poisonous").

Toxicology was originally an empirical science, and did not evolve into a volumetric science until the emergence of chemistry and analytical science. The disciplines of pharmacy, chemistry, and toxicology branched off from medicine with the development of methods. At the University of Leiden in the Netherlands, Hermann Boerhaave, in a pathbreaking move, combined the chairs of medicine, botany, and chemistry from 1718 to 1729, while H. M. Bracken at the University of Minnesota subsumed under the subject of medical remedies ("materia medica"), phramacognosy, pharmacology, toxicology, and pharmacy in 1859. Towards the end of the 19th century, the disciplines of pharmacology and toxicology, linked until then, were separated due to the growth of the chemical industry and chemical products.

The distinct object of scientific inquiry in the ancient and the medieval world was "pharmakon," and there was no differentiation between cure and poison. In more modern times, we find in Zedler's universal encyclopedia (1735), under the heading "poison," "that which is very damaging, if not necessarily fatal, to the human body, when body parts come into contact with it, internally or externally." Louis Lewin, a distinguished chronicler in this field, differentiated in 1907 among four main types of poison: (1) inflammatory or caustic poisons, (2) poisons causing metabolic disturbance, (3) poisons of the nervous system, and (4) poisons of the blood. Through this differentiation of the types of poison, he attempted to define the subject matter of toxicology as regards causes and effects.

Leading figures who from the end of the 19th century onwards defined the outlines in the field of toxicology typified the close relationships that extended beyond the boundaries of the subject. Lewin belonged to this generation (as did K. B. Lehmann, J. Abel, R. Kobert, T. H. Legge, L. Teleky, and others), who, at an intersection between medicine, pharmacology, pharmacy, chemistry, ergonomics, and technology, combined exact research into effect through analysis of cause and preventative reasoning. Thus, the Zurich toxicologist and forensic medical expert Heinrich Zangger, with the chlorine-gas attacks of the First World War still fresh in his mind, demanded in 1920 that guaranteed levels of safety be achieved through scientific identification of risk and through statistical examination: "Risk and its scientific control must remain in step." Medicine could then encourage and keep pace with technological advancement without undue risk, in particular without "scientifically establishable, chronic, permanent, unseen, degenerative damage to mankind." Meeting this challenge, toxicology has taken up its place in the ranks of the acknowledged sciences.

EARLY FUNDAMENTAL DEVELOPMENTS

The use of poisons and active substances dates from the earliest days of human evolution. Primitive man certainly instinctively avoided poisonous substances just as animals do and particularly feared the bite of poisonous animals. From such an animal instinct we can also infer the use of remedies taken internally; naturally occurring substances could be taken to help maintain physical and spiritual balance.

Primitive peoples used laxatives, emetics, enemas, fumigants, medicinal baths, and sudorifics. Narcotics are among the first plant-based active substances for which there is evidence. The first collections of information about the effects of compounds from various plants (among them aconite, arsenic, and opium) were made in Persia and China. The Ebers Papyrus lists over 800 substances used in Egypt 2000 years ago. In the 16th century B.C. opium, hyoscyamus (henbane), scilla, aloe, mint, calamus, juniper, cassia, sandalwood, myrrh, styrax, wine, honey, antimony, verdigris, iron, and animal organs, and secretions were used as medical remedies. Reports from the Trojan War (12th century B.C.) mention the use of wine laced with opium for the wounded.

The conditions for recovery or harm attributed to remedies and poisons lay beyond people's lives. The particular effects of substances could be easily understood as mystical concepts. "Harmful magic" was used to explain symbolic poisons and remedies, and "foreign bodies" their effects. This kind of understanding is illustrated by their attitudes toward plants surrounded in mystery, like mandrake (containing the alkaloids scopolamine, atropine, and hyoscyamine), which was as famous as it was poisonous; the same applies to opium poppies and hemlock.

Within the framework of primitive magic ideas of taboo, the concepts of poison and sin fused together. Both of these led to contagion and poisoning. Through efforts to purge sin, through cleansing such as blood-letting, the attempt to combat disease finally became a rational and logical act. In ancient Greece there was no strict dividing line between poisons and cures. Instead, an additional classification, such as "harmful" or "fatal," was necessary. Not until the writings of Hippocrates is there a stricter differentiation between *pharmakon* (collections of herbal or plant-based remedies, e.g., anaesthetizing sponges) and foodstuffs.

Significant experiments with medical remedies were made by Heraclides of Tarentum (1st century B.C.). At this time various minor tyrants were extremely interested in research into poisons and their antidotes, which could put the life of a dictator at risk or save it. The most famous of these was King Mithridates VI of Pontus (132–63 B.C.), who not only stood up to the Romans, but who tested out poisons on condemned criminals and tried to achieve immunity for himself by repeated small doses. An antidote named after him (Mithridatium, an electuary) was still being used in the Middle Ages. Important discoveries were made by Pedanios Dioscorides (64 A.D.) who knew lead chloride (Chlorblei), zinc oxide, sodium carbonate, sulphide of arsenic, and indigo, and who described the process by which mercury is obtained from cinnabar and the manufacture of lead acetate, limewater, and copper sulphate.

But there was another specialized use for toxic properties: In Athens, drinking the juice of hemlock was chosen as the death penalty for political criminals. In the 16th century we find aconite being used for an execution in the presence of Pope Clement VII. The most horrific effects of poison (Zyklon B) were seen in the gas chambers of the German concentration camps. Even today in some states of the U.S. (in Utah and Delaware, for example), the death penalty is carried out with lethal injections, in others with gas.

Greek doctors, whom the Romans at first denounced as quacks, disseminated medical knowledge throughout the Roman Empire with the support of Julius Caesar. The earliest preserved compilation on the subject of medical remedies from the first century A.D. handed down to us over 1000 remedies. Particularly worthy of mention is Galenos of Pergamon (129–199 A.D.), who in his comprehensive review of medical knowledge in the ancient world also described pharmaceutical preparations in the form of tinctures, extracts, ointments, and so on, which were kept in stock. His doctrines were based on the theory of the pathology of the humors, according to which illnesses are caused by evil fluids, the humors, and can be treated according to the principle of opposites as well as by cleansing of the body, mainly through enemas and blood-letting. His theories were fundamental, too, to monastic medicine and remained unchanged until the advent of Paracelsus.

FROM ALCHEMY TO THE DEVELOPMENT OF A PURE SCIENCE

The early history of toxicology can be written as the history of pharmaceutics, but also as the history of forensic medicine. Priests and rulers, villains and assassins—all used poisons and were interested in the effects of poison from the point of view of perpetrator and victim. Sure knowledge and the correct diagnosis were, however, dependent on detection of the poison. But the examination of corpses was bound up in ancient times with religious and mystic taboos; the *corpus iuris civilis* (439 A.D.) did not permit obduction. It was not until the 15th century that the Catholic church allowed postmortem examinations for scientific purposes; in practice the taboos mentioned are still in effect today. As the numbers of murders by poisoning and the pursuit of the, mainly female, poisoners increased, and citizens increasingly felt the need to feel secure, there finally grew too the public desire for cases of poisoning to be cleared up.

To begin with, substances were used in many combinations based on Greek and Arab traditions—this continued into the Middle Ages. Along with henbane, mandrake, opium, and hemlock, alcohol gained in importance. Early mixtures consisted of powdered plants and heavy metals, in particular mercury and arsenic. The recipes for these mixtures were handed down to more recent times and took on new significance in the battle against syphilis, which spread through Europe like an epidemic after the return of Christopher Columbus. A further contributor to its spread was the army of the French king, Charles VIII. The treatment of the condition was as disastrous as it was ineffective. Arsenic compounds played a leading pharmaceutical role for a long time. Even Hippocrates recommended a paste containing arsenic sulfide in the treatment of excrescences. The infamous Aqua Tofana (white arsenic boiled with lead and antimony), was in its time a favorite with murderers.

Alchemy, which held sway in the Middle Ages and which came originally from Arabia, was strongly linked to metallurgy. It was thought that mercury could be changed into gold using the "philosopher's stone," and "elixirs of life" were concocted from heavy metals. In the course of such experimentation tin chloride was discovered in 1604 by Andreas Libavius. In 1662 tartar emetic was discovered by Adrian v. Mynsicht, and at the beginning of the same century Johann R. Glauber (1604–1670) discovered Glauber's salt. He named the sodium sulfate, which he was the first to create, "sal mirabile"—the wonder salt.

The transition to the chemical synthesis of effective medical remedies took place in the Renaissance and was linked to Theophrastus Bombastus von Hohenheim (1493–1541), known as Paracelsus. His work was not based on juices and their balance, but on effective natural elements and analogous chemical principles: salt (solid, permanent), sulfur (inflammable), quicksilver (pertaining to Mercury—changeable, active). Paracelsus recommended treating the sick body with compensatory metal salts such as sublimate, lead acetate, silver nitrate, arsenic sulfide, and also salts of antimony, bismuth, zinc, and gold. Antimony in particular was vehemently argued over in the 16th and 17th centuries. In disputes of this kind, people eventually became convinced that it was feasible to use artificially manufactured substances for medical purposes. Paracelsus viewed the human organism as a kind of laboratory that took in food and other substances, processed them, and excreted them. Extracts and tinctures were therefore investigated to see how they would work in this "laboratory." In this way he developed the concept of effective quantities, still valid today—"dosis sola facit venenum" ("the dose alone makes a thing poisonous").

Up until this time, folk medicine had been of great daily and practical significance. Persons who were in contact with nature and who observed animals were considered to be knowledgeable about the efficacy of different herbs, and this knowledge was recorded and passed on. Luther spoke strongly in his "Tischreden" (Colloquia Doct.): "I am astonished that God has set such high and noble medicine in dung; for we know from experience that pig manure stops the flow of blood. Horse manure can be used for pleurisy. Human dung heals wounds and hemorrhagic smallpox. Donkey manure is needed, among other things, for bloody dysentery, and cow dung with preserved

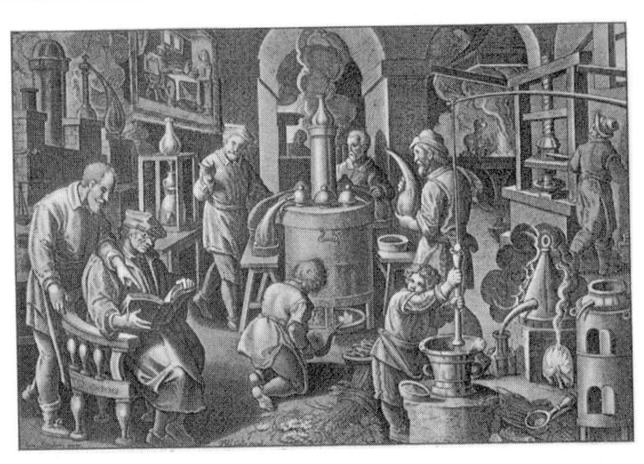

FIGURE 1 An apothecary's laboratory, 1560. Copper engraving from Ph.Galle after Stradamus around 1560, Sociopolitical Archive of Centre for Social Policy Research, University Bremen.

roses can be used for epilepsy in children." Luther was referring to a dubious increase in the wealth of available remedies that owed their existence to the so-called "Drecksapotheke" (filthy pharmacy) of Kristian Frantz Paullini (1696).

At that time universities were extended in the direction of natural sciences. While the earlier medical colleges (the first of which was set up in Salerno, by Naples) worked essentially from collections of books and translations, that is to say with the received wisdom of classical and Arab medicine, analytical endeavors now began. In 1533 the first chair of botany or materia medica was established in the medical faculty at the University of Padua. In 1609, Moritz, Landgrave of Hesse, appointed his personal physician, Johannes Hartmann (1568–1631), to the new professorship of "Chymiatrie" and thus established chemistry as an academic discipline, initially within the medical faculty. Such initiatives met with initial apprehension that chemical experiments and products could lead to health problems for local residents and neighbors, and corresponded to the unpleasant experiences that the common man (as opposed to the members of the noble ruling classes or the well-off middle classes) had undergone during medical treatment at the hands of contemporary physicians.

The results of scientific research and the development of more accurate methods led gradually, however, to an acceptance of scientific procedure, from which medicine also eventually profited. In 1628 William Harvey discovered the circulation of blood. In 1661 Robert Boyle (1627–1691) published his treatise "The Sceptical Chymist," in which he took a critical view of the accuracy and conclusiveness of many experiments. Georg Ernst Stahl (1659–1734), after making his own investigations, accused the alchemists of sloppy science and laid down precise methods of chemical research. The new developments took on visible form with the founding of the University of Halle in 1694, in which philosophy and natural sciences were brought together on the principle of freedom of thought and freedom of instruction.

A further thrust in the development of the sciences came through the discovery of America. While it is not clear whether the syphilis which raged through Europe in 1495, and which increased the importance of mercury, was brought by Columbus, some efficacious medical remedies were the result of his discovery—ipecac and cinchona, for example, were brought to Europe and promoted the demand and trade in pharmaceutical substances. In this period, which was ushered in by Paracelsus and which was characterized by the success of scientific modes of thought, toxicology was consolidated as a distinct field.

ACADEMIC QUALIFICATION AND THE PRACTICAL APPLICATION OF TOXICOLOGICAL KNOWLEDGE AT THE BEGINNING OF THE INDUSTRIAL AGE

The success of scientific modes of thought brought with it a demand for scientific–academic qualification. The trend in the Age of Enlightenment was that academic qualification should mean above all, training people to be socially and vocationally useful. In connection with this new direction in society towards, among other things, the advancement of trade and industry, there followed the founding of university chairs. Under the influence of Justus von Liebig (1803–1873), the investigation of the causes of natural phenomena came to the foreground; chemistry in particular promoted the study of cause and effect.

In the 18th century, toxicology developed in the context of chemistry as a pure science and in the context of pharmacy as an applied science. It was taught, for example, by Georg Augustin Bertele (1767–1818), professor of pharmacy, toxicology, pharmacology, and the study of chemical formulae at the medical faculty in Landshut (which was later moved to Munich) and by his successor, Johannes Buchner (1783–1852). In the British colonies in North America, toxicology continued to be subsumed under the rubric of materia medica until 1765, when the first medical school was established at the College of Philadelphia.

At the level of practice and business, mechanical–economical chemistry developed. Under cameralism, the theory and practice of a well-ordered community at the end of the 18th century, manufacturing and factories took on great social significance. The profitable application of chemical principles to arts and crafts was at the center of this development. In the association between medicines produced for business profit and the health risks of particular trades, toxicology found a new emphasis. Henceforth it could be seen as an applied science, moving in step with the rapid industrial boom.

In occupational toxicology significant connections became apparent, which went along with very obvious risks and health impairment. This was so in mines, particularly in the case of carbon monoxide poisoning, but also in metal-processing industries (especially for lead and mercury). The Italian physician Bernardo Ramazzini (1633–1714) described in 1700 the diseases of craftsmen and artists so thoroughly and systematically that his work was translated into five languages and remained a textbook of occupational hygiene for a century.

Laurent Lavoisier (1743–1794) continued to concentrate on working empirically with substances and developed chemical research mainly on the basis of speculative experimental research (in the manner of Isaac Newton) and following the axiom of the conservation of matter. His "Traité Elémentaire de Chimie" appeared in 1789 and was to remain into the 19th century a shining example of what a chemistry textbook should be.

The industrial manufacture of Glauber's salt from rock salt and sulfuric acid used materials and their actions to a specific end. In the process, the technique

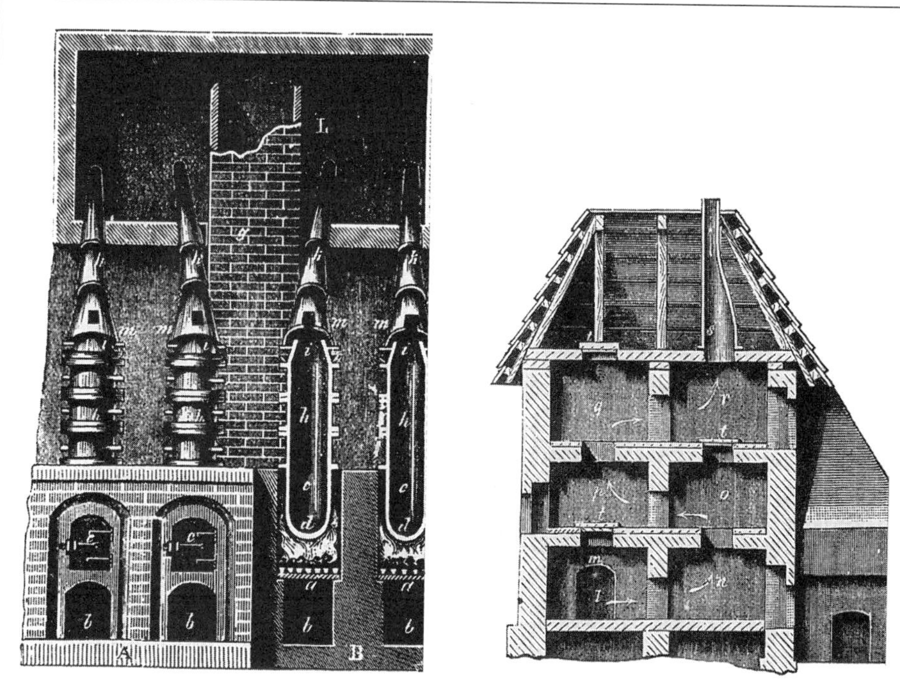

FIGURE 2 Poison processing towers and collection chambers for arsenious acid. From Hermann Scelenz (1911). Zur Geschichte der parmazeutish-chemischen Destilliergeräte. Hildescheim: Georg Olms, 1964, pp. 114, 115.

of making soda from sodium sulfate and coal was discovered. Along with sulfuric acid, soda was an all purpose material whose principal source was the soda lakes in Egypt. Now in 1790, with Nicolas Leblanc (1724–1806) and the process he developed, there began a chapter that is often described as the conquest of chemical discovery. The physician Leblanc, however, was a successful practical chemist for a short time only—only until his patrons were condemned to death and his soda factory was confiscated by a revolutionary tribunal. Leblanc committed suicide in the poorhouse.

In 1813 Mathieu J. B. Orfila summarized the results of specific toxic effects, added what was known to be possible in the way of precise detection of poison and in his "Traité de toxicologie générale" made a systematic compilation of the level of knowledge at the time.

CHEMISTRY AND THE CHEMICAL INDUSTRY IN THE NINETEENTH CENTURY

With technical production and the control of chemical activity, pharmacology became a new pure science. It kept pace with the most important advances that were being made in experimental physiology, especially under the influence of Johannes Müller (1801–1858) and his assistants. Unlike medicine, the methods of pharmacology were not dependent on investigations made at the sickbed. In 1802 the association between medical theory and pharmacology took an important step forward when the French apothecary Jean-Francois Derosne isolated the first crystalline "opium salt" (as a mixture of at least two alkaloids). The apothecary Friedrich Wilhelm Sertürner from Paderborn (1783–1841) created morphium from opium in 1804 and recognized in 1817 that the alkaline product is the physiologically active constituent of opium. At the beginning of the 19th century Parisian pharmacists (among them Pierre-Joseph Pelletier and Joseph-Bienaimé Caventou) discovered the substances chlorine, bromine, and iodine, and isolated quinine, caffeine, codeine, strychnine, and others. The state of learning was summarized by the physiologist François Magendie (1783–1855) who at the same time influenced research into the specific effects of substances in clinical medicine via his pupil Claude Bernard (1813–1878).

An important turning point, although it cannot be precisely dated, was the systematic pharmacological screening of synthetically produced molecules. In this way, pharmacologically effective substances could be made available in the form of preparations for therapeutic purposes, such as, for example, Serullass iodoform (1829) chloroform, obtained by both Soubeiran and Liebig at the same time in 1831.

As the importance of medicine and pharmacology grew, so did that of toxicology as an applied science. One of the influences on this development, along with pharmacy, continued to be the analytic impulse coming from forensic medicine.

Throughout history there has been an abundance of spectacular cases of murder through poison, from the female poisoner Locusta, who worked for Nero, to Teofania di Adamo, who was executed in Palermo in 1633 for murders using her Aqua Tofania (white arsenic boiled with lead and antimony), to Gesche Gottfried, who killed at least fifteen people and in 1831 was the last female criminal to be publicly beheaded in Bremen. During the 19th century most of the world-famous cases of systematic poisoning on a grand or a small scale involved the use of arsenic compounds, above all arsenious acid. As late as 1926 a nurse who had poisoned twelve people with arsenic was executed in Paris. J. Marsh took a significant step forward in 1832 when he invented an apparatus to show the level of arsenic present and was thus able to prove the use of the poison before an English court. The court, however, refused to recognise his evidence. It was not until 1840 that the Marsh apparatus given long-lasting recognition when it was used by the Parisian forensic medical expert Orfila in a sensational murder-by-poison trial in France.

Forensic medicine was initially taught, for example by Johann Peter Frank (1745–1821) in Pavia and Vienna, along with surgery. Around 1770 the Vienna School developed pharmacological and clinical experiments (Anton de Haen worked with opium, bearberry (*arctostaphylus uva ursi*), and cinchona). In 1804 it set up a separate professorship in a historical combination of state medicine and pharmacology, and in 1818 it established its own institute within the general hospital. The most important impetus came from Franz Cölestin Schneider (1812–1897) who succeeded, for example, in separating out arsenic in 1851 and who, like Pettenkoffer, worked towards combining chemistry and medicine. Out of this too grew the toxicological orientation of forensic medicine, for which Graz (Adolf Schauenstein 1827–1891) and Vienna (Ernst Ludwig 1842–1915, full professor of medical chemistry, 1874) were the main centers. In Zurich, in contrast, the disciplines were in competition, and as a consequence physiological chemistry was not offered until 1887 and Max Cloetta was not made associate professor of pharmacology until 1901. Cloetta represented a group of subjects, among them toxicology.

With Sertürner's isolation of pure morphine there began a new phase in cases of poisoning in which arsenic was supplanted by alkaloids, whose presence in a corpse could not at first be proved. The number of possible poisons rose rapidly, while their detection during a postmortem examination grew ever more difficult. Carl Remigius Fresenius (1818–1897), on the other hand, was already demanding in 1844 that contradictory scientific presentations of evidence should be standardized and improved on. A spectacular trial took place in Belgium in 1851 (Count Bocarmé had poisoned his brother-in-law with nicotine) during which Jean Servais Stas succeeded in separating the alkaloids from body tissue by the removal of protein by alcohol and by ether extraction. Subsequently detection methods for countless alkaloids were developed. This "isolation of the poisonous substance" remained one of the cornerstones of forensic medicine and toxicology.

At the end of the 17th and beginning of the 18th century, a stricter scientific training for pharmacists was considered increasingly important. As early as 1779, the apothecary Johann Christian Wiegleb founded an institute for the teaching of pharmaceutics in Langensalza; more were established in the following years. The private institute of Johann Bartholomäus Trommsdorf in Erfurt (founded 1795) was famous; it served as a model for other institutes. In 1826 Liebig founded a private pharmaceutical–technological school in Gießen. Out of the larger pharmacies the first factories grew; Trommsdorf set up the first chemical–pharmaceutical factory in Erfurt in 1813, and his pupil Merck did the same in Darmstadt in 1827.

There was a close and fruitful connection between the academic science of the universities and commercial practice, illustrated, for example, by the relationship between Justus Liebig and Heinrich Emanuel Merck in the 1830s. In 1827 Merck began the factory production of morphine using the dried latex of opium poppy capsules. In the same year the Prussian government issued an edict that allowed doctors and pharmacists to obtain from factories medicines that were difficult to make. In England in 1844, William Brockedon compressed tablets out of a dry powder; shortly afterwards the pharmaceutical trade began to deal in gelatin capsules and coated tablets, followed by ampoules. There was a significant boom in the industrial production of medicines after 1870.

The development of pharmacology was one of the main reasons for an expansion in toxicology at university level in the second half of the 19th century. In 1847 Rudolf Buchheim founded his pharmacological laboratory in Dorpat, initially on a private basis, and introduced experimentation on animals. In the footsteps of Buchheim, who in 1860 set up the state institute for pharmacology, followed Rudolf Boehm, Hans Horst Meyer, and Rudolf Kobert. The center of emphasis shifted later with Oswald Schmiedeberg (1838–1921) to the newly established model university of Strasbourg. Out of private institutions, which were called "laboratories" until the 1870s, developed professorates and institutes in all the larger universities, in which toxicological approaches and concerns were also taken into account. S. Weir Mitchell, under the influence of Claude Bernard, carried out in 1858 a series of experimental studies on the toxicology of snake venoms and arrow poisons.

In the mid-1880s the systematic linking up of university scientific research with industrial laboratory work began. The intensity of research and specialization towards the end of the 19th century posed new problems for the integration of toxicology, particularly as a result of the growing independence of chemistry and pharmacology. As far as practical application was concerned, the scientific fields of pharmacy, toxicology, and food chemistry were integrated in certain pharmaceutical institutes, like the one in Marburg, which was developed by Robert Wilhelm Bunsen (1811–1899). In the USA, similar research institutes were founded based on the German example, beginning with Johns Hopkins University's 1876 Chair in Experimental Pharmacology.

In the latter third of the 19th century, a marked advance took place in mathematical and natural science teaching and research. The Chemistry Congress in Karlsruhe in 1860 stimulated an economic, scientific, and technical thrust forward that was scientifically strengthened by the benzol theory of 1865. The foundations of the theory, laid by August Kekulé (1829–1896), opened up the way for empirical, methodological searches for new dyestuffs. Certain scientific advances were influenced by the laboratories of the chemical industry. Hoechst, for example, appointed in 1883 the university professor A. Laubenheimer, who carried out bacteriological and serological research in close association with Emil A. Behring (1854–1917) and Paul Ehrlich (1854–1914). In 1876 the American Chemical Society was founded. In the wake of conflicts during the 1890s between more academically and more industrially oriented chemists, this body developed into four specialized organizations: the Division of Industrial and Engineering Chemistry (1907), the American Society for Pharmacology and Experimental Therapeutics (1908), the American Society for Agricultural and Food Chemistry (1908), and the American Oil Chemists Society (1909). In addition, an American Institute of Chemical Engineers was founded.

The toxicological implications of the revolutionary scientific and industrial developmental tendencies were already apparent at the end of the 19th century, but a blind eye was turned in the hope of manufacturing effective substances synthetically and systemati-

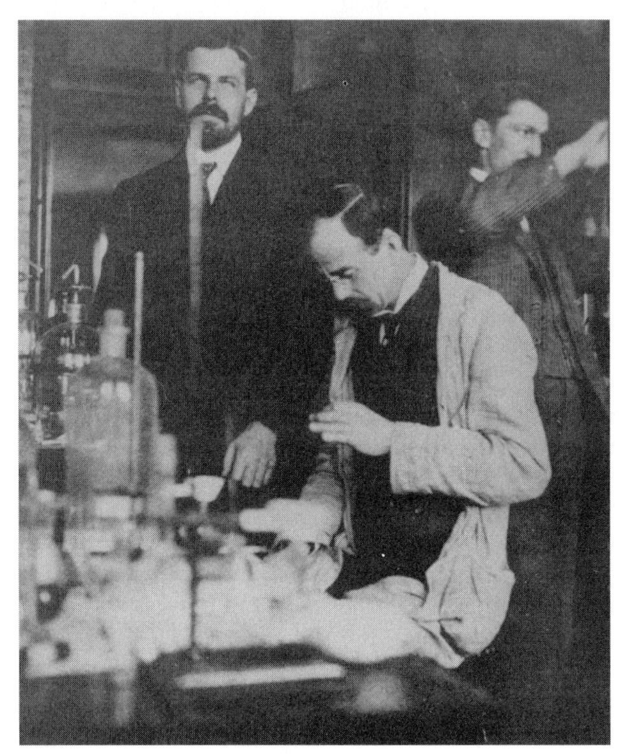

FIGURE 3 John Abel (seated) and colleagues at Johns Hopkins Laboratory, 1901.

cally. John J. Abel (1857–1938) studied in Germany under Carl Ludwig in Leipzig and Oswald Schmiedeberg in Strasbourg and became a founding father of pharmacology in the USA. Rudolf Kobert summarized the developments that had taken place in pharmacological knowledge at the end of the 19th century in two important textbooks, in which he emphasized the metabolic changes in the human organism through resorption, neutralization, oxidation, reduction, fission, conjugation, synthesis, secretion, and excretion. In his opinion, pharmacology was the fundamental science that was the impetus behind the applied branches of toxicology and pharmacotherapy.

SUBSTANCE EFFECTS—USES AND LIMITS

In the field of applied medical science, Charles Turner Thackrah (1795–1833) was the first to fashion an overview of studies in industrial hygiene, "The Effects of Arts, Trades and Professions on Health and Longevity" (1831), a pathbreaking study of worker health risks in England. A more useful and practical development arose from the association between chemistry, pharmacology, toxicology, and hygiene, as practiced by Max Pettenkofer (1818–1901). In 1852 the pharmacist and physician became a full professor of medical chemistry in Munich and in 1865 was appointed to the first professorship in experimental hygiene, also in Munich. Working in collaboration with Carl Voit, he began research on the exchange of gases between the organism and its environment.

Commercial developments augmented toxicological knowledge, which went beyond the knowledge of pharmacological agents and included all procedures. Hermann Eulenberg published the first summaries of results of experimental research on harmful and poisonous gases in 1865 and 1876, but had to admit that in practice one had to rely more on one's sense of smell than on chemistry. Ludwig Hirt (1844–1907) published in the 1870s the first modern standard work on occupational medicine, which took as its starting point substances harmful to health.

The varying intensity and duration of cases of poisoning directed speculative attention to the difference between the substance itself and the affected individuals. In this regard Pettenkofer and his followers were particularly interested in the connection between the quantity of the substance and the body's processing of it. "Limits of toxicity," and "limits of tolerance," and the first limits for dangerous concentrations were calculated, among them the carbon dioxide concentration established in 1883 by Max Gruber. Karl Bernhard Lehmann (1858–1940) began in 1884 his research into the most important industrial gases. His institute in Würzburg (founded in 1887) became the foremost center of toxicological research. Up to the beginning of the Second World War he established the limits of concentration of over one hundred substances. Lehmann recognized, among other things, that in some gases relative habituation can occur, while others can cause increasingly severe reactions. In the USA, lists of harmful concentrations of gases had been established in 1912 and 1921. In 1927 the American Chemical Society published limits for 25 noxious gases concerning acute toxic affects and the "maximum concentration allowable for prolonged exposure." In 1946, the American Conference of Governmental Industrial Hygienists established 144 threshold-limit values for specific vapors, dusts, fumes, and mists.

At the turn of the century, pharmaceutical products became increasingly important in the development of the chemical industry. The manufacture of drugs shifted from the pharmacies to the factories and required precise analysis. As late as the beginning of the 19th century, the preferred method was experimentation on a small range of animals, the effects of which were as accurately described as possible, followed by a conclusion based on analogy with humans. Changes in behavior and secretions were noted. The tendency of the development was away from application according to symptoms and empirical discovery and toward systematically creating compounds and testing them.

The close association between commerce and medicine was henceforth influential in encouraging a connection, based on practical application, between toxicology and pharmaco-therapy. There was, for example, a collaboration between the firm of Hoechst and Paul Ehrlich, who was engaged in research into nontoxic arsenic compounds at the turn of the century. Chemotherapy, too, is linked with Ehrlich's name. His motto was: "Corpora non agunt, nisi fixata." In the 1880s Ehrlich was the first to establish the classification of leucocytes using a dye technique that is still in use today, and he was the founder of modern hematology. Ehrlich developed together with John N. Lanlay the drug-receptor theory, which in the 1930s was further developed by A. J. Clark.

In addition to the rapid developments in the field of pharmaceutics, important discoveries were made in the 19th century regarding the manufacture of indigo, sulfuric acid, ammonia, and chlorine, which influenced toxicology from the standpoint of occupational hygiene. From the 1890s onwards, chlorine was one of the keystones of organic synthesis. It made possible the use of chlorinated substances in the form of solvents, synthetic materials, wood preservatives, insecticides, herbicides, and so on. The decisive step for the future importance of pesticide toxicology was taken. Also decisive was the fact that the largescale availability of hydrogen chloride paved the way for the production of thermoplastic synthetic substances—polyvinyl chloride and polyvinyl acetate. The toxicity of these substances did not become significant until much later.

Many of the substances that were needed for industrial production were known to be dangerous, those used in the production of fuchsin, for example. At the Hoechst works in 1867, no less than 2.15 tons of 70% arsenious acid were processed. One could, however, according to Carl Duisberg, not only take measures to combat the dangers, but even remove them entirely, if the appropriate apparatus were used. Nevertheless, in 1903, more than 50 cases of aniline cancer were diagnosed among the workers at Badische Anilin- und Soda-Fabrik (BASF).

Thus the chemical industry at an early stage integrated medical knowledge and medical experts into the production to protect and select the workforce. Carl Knaps became the first factory physician at BASF in 1866; Wilhelm Grandhomme was appointed to the Hoechst works in 1874. These doctors assessed the toxicity of the raw materials, the factory buildings and installations, and the intermediate and the end products. The doctors of the large-scale chemical industries were of profound importance for the state of knowledge and the setting up of the areas of responsibility of the occupational hygiene authorities. In 1908, for example, the chemical industry set up the medical wing of BASF, out of which grew the "institute for occupational hygiene and toxicology." In collaboration with the employers' liability insurance association of the chemical industry, an occupational toxicology institute for research into and treatment of occupational disease was set up within the Ludwigshafen city hospital. In the context of the laws governing social insurance, in particular the laws regarding accident insurance (e.g., the U.S. Occupational Hazards Act of 1889 and the British Workman's Compensation Act of 1906), toxicological questions had to be settled by expert opinion. The experiences of the First World War reinforced efforts of this kind, which found their expression in the inclusion of coverage for occupational disease—at first mainly occupational poisoning—in accident insurance. In England and the U.S., this authority lay predominately with government agencies (e.g., in the U.K., the Chief Inspector of Factories, created in 1896 and headed by Thomas Legge; and in the USA the Office of Industrial Hygiene and Sanitation, set up in 1919). The strengths of these agencies lay in field research and statistics rather than in laboratory research. In the Public Health Service, studies on industrial toxicology were carried out from 1919. In particular, Alice Hamilton conducted exemplary studies, for example, of the lead industry and of mercury poisoning in the felt hat industry. In 1919, she became the first female faculty member at Harvard University.

In Germany, toxicology experts, for example Louis Lewin, were caught in the sociopolitical struggle between labor and capital. Louis Lewin (1850–1929), assistant to Voit and Pettenkofer in Munich, qualified as a lecturer in pharmacology, toxicology, and hygiene in Berlin in 1881. His Jewish background was a particular hindrance to his career. He delivered his lectures in an apartment, which he had converted into an institute of pharmacology and toxicology. In addition to pharmacology and the effects and side effects of the newest drugs, he was engaged in toxicological work, which included occupational poisoning and how to prove a case of poisoning before a court. Lewin was one of the first teachers at an institute of higher learning to regularly take his students on visits to factories, in particular to chemical plants.

The International Association for the Statutory Protection of Workers, predecessor to the International Labor Office, acting on the advice of the occupational hygiene expert Theodor Sommerfeld, in particular, drew up a "List of Poisons" with the following aims: the obligation of doctors and hospitals to inform the authorities in the event of occupational poisoning, the preservation of the independence of company doctors, the obligatory registration of the production and use of commercial poisons, the institution of special morbidity identification papers for persons working with poisons, the promotion of toxicological research and teaching in medical science, the institution of special training for toxicologists, the expert supervision of work where poisons are used, and the institution of rules regarding hours of work for those employed in this field.

In these practical functions of occupational toxicology, findings were often made that were of far-reaching importance but that were only properly appreciated in other contexts. Thus the blister-like swellings in workers using fuchsin in an aniline factory had been described, but L. Rehn in 1895 traced these to the workers' exposure to aniline and fuchsin. For the first time the specific organotropic carcinogenic effects of chemical substances had appeared at a distance from the point at which they were caused. The first investigation of asbestos cases was conducted in 1906 by Montague and Murray, but did not bear policy consequences. The gap between initial scientific analyses and definite assessment in terms of occupational hygiene remained a practical difficulty for toxicology. K. B. Lehmann, for example, could give as early as 1898 a clinical picture of the disease chlorine-related acne among chemical workers involved in electrolysis. Later, after accidents in the 1950s, this was recognized as a symptom of massive exposure to dioxin.

Noise, vibration, air pollution (through smoke, soot, dust, foul smells, and toxic gases), ground pollution (through residue and wastewater) continued to be analyzed and assessed following Pettenkofer's tradition. The law "aerum corrumpere non licet," laid down by the *corpus iuris civilis* in the 17th century, was always relevant and topical in the period of industrialization, with its smoke from foundry chimneys, smog, and, above all, the toxic gases and vapors from factories.

In the field of food hygiene, too, we find important developments in the 19th century. A continual problem was, of course, alcohol. Earlier considered in many respects a remedy (to aid digestion), alcohol came to be seen from the 17th century onwards as a symbol of immoral behavior. Both public houses and pharmacies were now forbidden to sell brandy and beer on Sundays between and after the church services. Coffee, too, was originally considered a medical remedy, but its inclusion in the books of the apothecaries was short-lived. Soon it was being denounced as a new vice, was subject to taxes, and at the end of the 18th century was forbidden entirely. Looking at the matter from the point of view of economics, Frederick the Great considered it better to let the population re-accustom itself to beer. Food hygiene became increasingly important in Germany in the 1860s and 1870s, especially in the context of increasing amounts of "fake" foodstuffs, which became easier to detect with more effective methods in the 1830s. In 1879 the German Reich issued a decree concerning commerce in foodstuffs, alcohol, tobacco, stimulants, and utensils involved in food preparation. Initial attempts at standardization in the U.S. occurred, for example, from 1901 at the Bureau of Standards, which made progress with the use of accurate methods of analysis. Under the auspices of the Pure Food and Drug Act, the Department of Agriculture began in 1906 to research toxicological questions. During the 1930s, above all in association with the mass production of canned goods, the Department of Agriculture's Food and Drug Administration carried out studies of the toxicity of substances used as food additives or that occurred as impurities in foods (e.g., insecticide residues). This was the beginning of broad-based campaigns, including among others the 1936 long-term project on the chronic toxicity of lead and arsenic and the Food, Drug, and Cosmetic Act of 1938.

Towards the end of the 19th century, research that was done into the problems of alcoholism and also into toxicomania took into account the aspect of addiction as well as that of depravation and underlined the connection between hygiene and efforts to improve public health.

Toxicology contributed to the recognition and minimization of several causes of danger to health present in foodstuffs. Food toxicology gained international recognition through scandals, when, for example, the hygienic conditions (or lack of them) in the meat-processing plants in Chicago became known. Another example is that of meat preservation. Until the beginning of the 20th century, meat was cured with a mixture of salt and saltpeter. J. Haldane established in 1901 that the desired red coloring of meat could be achieved by reducing the added nitrate to nitrite. The meat curers now began to use salt mixtures with pure nitrite. After curing salt with sodium nitrite came on the market in 1916, there were cases of poisoning, including a case of mass poisoning of 34 people, including a child who died, in Leipzig. Thereafter, the use of nitrite in curing was banned in Germany. The 1927 law relating to foodstuffs was drawn up on the basis of a list of prohibited additives, the criminally negligent use of which was punishable by law. The list was amended in 1958 to contain a "positive list" of all the specifically admissible substances.

There were difficulties with the analysis of those threats to health that have a long period of latency and complex causes. The carcinogenic effect of arsenic on humans was known because of its frequent use and was described as early as 1822. After the First World War, winegrowers combated the larvae of the grape moth with sprays containing arsenic. The risk of exposure was, however, limited to a period of a few days, and the toxicity of the related copper–arsenic compounds was known both to industry and to the authorities. In 1924 there were numerous reports from the Kaiserstuhl area of cases of arsenic poisoning and also of cancer. Franz Koelsch (1876–1940) pondered the question why workers in metallurgical plants and chemical factories, with greater exposure to these substances, almost never suffered from carcinomas or diseases of the liver. Severe chronic arsenic poisoning was also found among coopers, publicans, and winetasters. Only years later was the significance of the latency period recognized, when H. von Pein established in 1943 that 15 years or more can elapse between hyperkeratosis and the emergence of cancer, and that chronic arsenic poisoning can increase the organism's tendency to develop cancer. The assessment of arsenic poisoning in winegrowing remained a problem for toxicologists, however, because of the possibility of the misuse of alcohol.

Another famous example was the synthesis of dichlorodiphenyl-trichloroethane (DDT), which was carried out by the German chemist O. Zeidler as early as 1874, although the practical uses of the substance were not recognized until the Second World War when it was used as an insecticide. For this, the Swiss scientist Paul-Hermann Müller won the Nobel Prize for Physiology and Medicine in 1948. In 1972 special legislation was introduced to ban the use of the substance as an insecticide because of its unusual biological half-life. It had been realized that DDT (DDE) accumulates in the food chain. The scientific assessment of its practical application and use, missing in this case, became the central task of toxicology.

The seedtime of American industrial laboratories was the 1920s. The chemical industry, regarded as either a sort of glorified drugstore or as the producer of cheap and nasty substitutes, suddenly became the creator of new values. New close contacts between the chemical industry and the universities helped improve the heretofore somewhat suspect reputation of the drug industry. The chemical industry—and within it applied toxicology—developed in two spurts in the mid 20th century. First, the experience of the significance of Germany's poison gases and patented chemical technologies during the First World War, as well as the lessons learned from the analysis of and often dangerous application of petroleum in the booming interwar oil industry, boosted the importance of hygiene engineers and toxicologists in the U.S. Second, after the Second World War, in connection with the economic expansion, a boom in industrial hygiene and research into public health occurred, for instance, the Controlling Chemical Hazard reports conducted from 1945 to 1947 by the Bureau of Labor Studies. This development, in which German exiles also participated, culminated in the Occupational Safety and Health Act of 1970.

From the middle of the 20th century onwards, experimental research on isolated organs and cell cultures was growing. This required specialized knowledge and made the practical generalization of the results difficult. Especially in regard to the statistical evaluation of the experiments, the quality of experimental planning and the collection and biometric processing of data have become an increasingly significant methodological problem. This is reflected today in the guidelines on "Good Laboratory Practice" (GLP).

A qualitatively new problem for toxicology arose with the discovery of radioactivity by H. Becquerel. Soon after this "sensational discovery," loss of hair and a decrease in the size of tumors were noticed among its biological effects. Once radium had been isolated by Marie and Pierre Curie, research into radiation and radioactive damage went hand in hand. The great attraction of X-rays and radioactivity initially masked the harmful effects of ionized radiation, to which Marie Curie herself fell victim. Safety precautions were called for as early as 1906, and in 1929 the International Commission on Radiological Protection was formed. The dosimeter for ionized radiation was originally developed for therapeutic purposes and later extended to cover all radiation effects. It was recognized early on that special limitations were necessary in the case of radiation damage to skin (Holthausen, 1936), to prevent genetic mutation in living creatures (Regaud and Dubreuil, 1908; Muller, 1927) and to avoid inducing cancer (Marie, 1910; Hesse 1911). In 1956 in the USA a threshold was set for genetic risk in the population (10 R in the first 30 years of life). The risks of radiation have become particularly significant in recent years, for sociopolitical reasons.

It must be borne in mind that there have been spectacular incidents in industrial production that have put great social pressure on toxicology, such as the mining disaster at Courrièrs in 1906, the chemical explosions in Ludwigshafen-Oppau in 1921 and in Buna in 1925, the smog disaster in the Maastaal in 1930, the mass poisoning due to a drug containing diethylene glycol in 1937, the fish poisoning in the Japan Kiushu due to industrial mercury residues dumped in the sea in 1953, the fetal poisoning caused by thalidomide from 1958–1961, the Santa Barbara oil spill in 1969, the trichlorphenol (dioxin) accident in Seveso in 1969, Love Canal in 1978, Three Mile Island in 1979, the poisonous gas explosion in the pesticides plant in Bhopal in 1984, the Institute of West Virginia in 1985, the admixture of diethylene glycol into Austrian wines in 1985, the introduction of 400 liters of herbicide into the canals and the Rhine river in Basel in 1986, and Tschernobyl in 1986. This pressure is not always conducive to good science.

Pharmacologists have always been interested in poisons, but in recent decades toxicology has become a separate discipline entirely, mainly on the basis of physiological and biochemical foundations. Still today, the subject of toxicology is found above all in the realm of biochemistry.

In forensic medicine, toxicological examinations are done in institutes of legal medicine and also in various bureaus of criminal investigation run by the German Bundesländer. There was reciprocal action among the demands of judicial presentation of evidence, analytic methods, and the quality of the institutes in which forensic toxicological work was being carried out.

In Zurich the medicolegal laboratory set up by Heinrich Zanggers became an official part of the university when he was appointed to an associate professorship there in 1906. In addition, there was the biochemical institute founded by Johann Bonifaz Flaschenträger (1894–1957).

Independent departments of toxicology were not established in universities until the 1960s. Environmental problems, above all, brought about the realization that the harmful effects of impurities on a healthy organism must be independently recognized, assessed, and prevented.

THE SCOPE OF TOXICOLOGY IN HISTORIC TERMS

"The question *why* is the mother of all science," said the philosopher Arthur Schopenhauer in 1813, and thus was formulated the guiding principle for the methodology of toxicology. The history of toxicology is the account of the endeavors made to answer that question qualitatively and quantitatively in a causal analytic way. It must be said, however, that the overlapping interpretations and evaluations of toxic effects are not part of the actual field of toxicology but represent indications and questions that toxicology must pass on to the fields of medicine, hygiene, or politics.

Oswald Schmiedeberg differentiated strictly between the "effects" and the "consequences" of substances. This differentiation characterizes the systematic orientation of toxicology. In its fundamental research into effects, toxicology was oriented towards medicine (physiology), chemistry and pharmacology. In the practical applied research into consequences, toxicology was oriented towards pharmacy, forensic medicine, the chemical industry, and hygiene.

In a good historical survey written in 1925, Louis Lewin described toxicology in the widest sense as the study of life under the conditions that are known to cause illness. He believed that there were numerous variations in the conditions that cause illness and their corresponding physical malfunctions. The specific knowledge and experience that toxicology has developed can be used in the appraisal of the impact of these illnesses from a chemical, physical, and medical standpoint. Distinguished exponents classified the field of toxicological work as the common responsibility of civilized beings. As Lewin put it in 1922, "Anyone who is in the possession of an object which could be harmful to others is obliged to reduce or remove the possibility of that harm."

Bibliography

Ackerknecht. E. (1979). "Geschichte der Medizin." 4th ed. Enke, Stuttgart.

Amberger-Lahrmann, M., and Schmähl, D. (eds.) (1987). "Gifte: Geschichte der Toxikologie." Springer, Berlin.

Artelt, W. (1937). "Studien zur Geschichte der Begriffe 'Heilmittel' und 'Gift'." J. A. Barth, Leipzig.

Beyerlein, B. (1991). "Die Entwicklung der Pharmazie zur Hochschuldiziplin: Ein Beitrag zur Universitäts- und Sozialgeschichte." Wissenschaft, Verlagsgesellschaft, Stuttgart.

Chen, K. K. (ed.) (1969). "The American Society for Pharmacology and Experimental Therapeutics, Incorporated: The First Sixty Years, 1908–1969." ASPET, Bethesda, MD.

Cowen, D. L., and Helfand, W. H. (1990) "Pharmacy—An Illustrated History." Abrams, New York.

Doull, J. (1984). The past, present, and future of toxicology. *Pharmacol. Review* **36,** 15–18.

Doull, J., Klassen, C. D., and Amder, M. O. (1980). *The Basic Science of Poison* (J. Doull *et al.*, eds.) MacMillan, New York.

Earles, M. P. (1961). "Studies in the Development of Experimental Pharmacology in the Eighteenth and Early Nineteenth Centuries." London, University College.

Fischer-Homberger, E. (1983). "Medizin vor Gericht: Gerichtsmedizin von der Renaissance bis zur Aufklärung." Luchterhand, Bern.

Fye, W. B. (1987). "The Development of American Physiology. Scientific Medicine in the Nineteenth Century." Johns Hopkins University Press, Baltimore, MD.

Hamilton, A. (1925). "Industrial Poisons in the United States." MacMillan, New York.

Issekutz, B. (1971). "Die Geschichte der Arzneimittelforschung." Akadémiai Kiadó, Budapest.

Koelbing, H. M. (1985). "Die ärztliche Therapic: Grundzüge ihrer Geschichte." Darmstadt.

Lewin, L. (1922). "Die Gifte in der Weltgeschichte. Toxikologische, allgemeinverständliche Untersuchungen der historischen Quellen." J. Springer, Berlin.

de Malcissye, J. (1991). "Histoire du poison." F. Bourin, Paris.

Müller, R. K. (1986). "Dokumente zur Entwicklung der Toxikologie im 19. Jahrhundert." Akademie Verlagsgeselleschaft, Leipzig.

Parnham, M. J., and Bruinvels, J. (1983). *Discoveries in Pharmacology vol. 2.* Elsevier, Amsterdam, New York, Oxford.

Parascandola, J. (1990). "The Development of American Pharmacology." Johns Hopkins University Press, Baltimore, MD.

Perrine, D. M. (1996). "The Chemistry of Mind-Altering Drugs: History, Pharmacology and Cultural Context." American Chemical Society, Washington, D.C.

Sprung, W.-D. (1990). "Zur Geschichte von Pharmakologie und Toxikologie; Rudolf Kobert und seine Zeit; wissenschaftshistorische Beiträge zum Rudolf-Kobert-Symposium am 26, und 27, Oktober 1990 in Rostock." -University Abt. Wissenschaftspublizistik, Rostock.

Teleky, L. (1948) "History of Factory and Mine Hygiene." Columbia University Press, New York.

Tansey, T. (1948). The history of toxicology. The long and short of it. *Human & Experimental Toxicology,* **6,** 459–460.

Thackray, A. *et al.* (1985). "Chemistry in America 1876–1976." Reidel, Dordrecht.

Weindling, P. (ed.) (1985). "The Social History of Occupational Health." Helm, London.

Wetzel, W. (1991). "Naturwissenschaften und chemische Industrie in Deutschland: Voraussetzungen und Mechanismen ihres Aufstiegs im 19, Jahrhundert." F. Steiner, Stuttgart.

CHAPTER

2

Biostatistics in Toxicology

LUDWIG A. HOTHORN,* GERALD HAJIAN†

*University of Hannover, Hannover, Germany

†Schering–Plough Research Institute, Kenilworth, New Jersey

PRINCIPLES

This chapter covers the use of biostatistical methods in toxicology. Toxicology as a science is multifaceted; therefore, the methods presented are limited to regulatory toxicology studies. These studies are usually conducted according to national or international guidelines for the proof of safety for new drugs or chemicals. The problems are discussed from a biostatistical point of view. Selected simple statistical methods are described and demonstrated in small teaching examples, without need of computer programs.

At the end of a toxicological study, a decision about whether the new drug or chemical is harmless, harmful, or harmless up to a specified dose is made. Decision making requires a confirmatory type of statistical method given by the following criteria:

- A priori definition of an experimental design (frequently chosen according to guidelines).
- A priori definition of the necessary number of animals or sample sizes (frequently determined according to recommendations).
- A priori definition of the statistical test to be used and the upper limits of false positive (type I error α) and false negative (type II error β) decision rates.

The statistical methods can be classified into estimation (e.g., the estimation of LD_{50}) and testing (e.g., high dose versus negative control). The latter represents the emphasis of this chapter.

According to standard statistical techniques, the traditional null hypothesis of no difference in the effect between the treated and negative control group is tested.

Null hypothesis
H_0: effect of control group $\geq$ effect of dose group

Alternative hypothesis
H_A: effect of control group $<$ effect of dose group

Failing to reject the null hypothesis (i.e., when the p value is greater than 0.05), often leads to the conclusion that the evidence is in favor of safety (harmless). However, the most frequent testing theory is based on the falsification principle. Therefore, how the decision rule is set up in terms of the null and alternative hypotheses makes a big difference. Two approaches have to be distinguished: proof of hazard (null hypothesis of no difference) and proof of safety (alternative hypothesis of no relevant difference). In the first approach, the probability of erroneously concluding hazard (the producer's risk) will be controlled and in the second the probability of erroneously concluding safety (the consumer's risk) is limited. For drug-safety assessment, the consumer's risk (i.e., erroneously overlooking a toxic effect) should be controlled primarily. However, some difficulties still exist, for example, the a priori definition of the minimal relevant safety difference in a multiple endpoint case, and the approach represents a break from tradition. Therefore, the classical proof of hazard will be described here. However, a toxicological study must have a reasonable chance of detecting a relevant treatment effect. Consequently, the sample size should be based on the type I and type II errors, and underlying variability, and the specific size of effects considered appropriate by the toxicologist. Moreover, in the case that the test failed to reject the null hypothesis, the type II error (or the power = 1 type II error) has to be reported.

Experimental design before the start of a study is important. Two aspects will be discussed here: sample size estimation, and choice of the many-to-one layout. However, in regulatory toxicology a minimum demand for sample size and number of dose groups is recommended by the guidelines. Another major objective of experimental design is dose selection. This is a very difficult task in real toxicological studies, and is not only dependent on statistical arguments. Therefore, this will not discussed here.

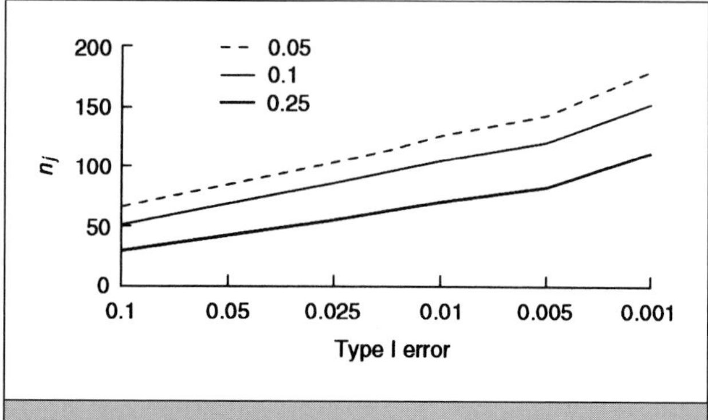

FIGURE 1 Relationship $n_j = f(\alpha, \beta, \sigma/\delta = 2$, one-sided) for the t-test.

Sample Size Estimation

For a defined design and test the relationship between type I error α and type II error β is

$$\beta = f(n_j, \delta, \sigma, \alpha),$$

where δ denotes the minimal relevant difference, n_j the sample size per group, and σ^2 the variance. Type II error increases with smaller sample sizes n_j and/or increasing variance σ and/or smaller relevant difference δ and/or smaller α levels. As a simple example, sample-size estimation is demonstrated for the t test with assumed Gaussian distribution and equal sample sizes and variances:

$$n_j = (2\sigma^2/\delta^2)(z_{1-\alpha} + z_{1-\beta})^2$$

with $z_{1-\alpha} \ldots (1 - \alpha)$ quantile of normal distribution.

Sample-Size Estimation for a Subchronic Toxicity Study

For the serum variable, alkaline phosphatase (AP) in Wistar rat is known from historical controls to have a coefficient of variation (CV) equal to 36.5% (variance $\sigma^2 = 71$). Assuming a relevant safety difference $\delta = 4.2$ (i.e., 50% of the standard deviation) one-sided testing for an increase, sample sizes n_j are necessary for several levels of type II (0.05, 0.10, 0.25) and type I error (see Fig. 1).

In practice, such a blind sample-size estimation is often impossible because an unrealistically large sample size number would be calculated. A more pragmatic approach is the estimation of the type II error or the minimal detectable difference based on the sample sizes recommended by guidelines. Moreover, for each animal, multiple endpoints with different variances are measured. Based on the idea that a comparable type II error rate is important, the estimation of an endpoint-specific type I error rate is also possible. For the different endpoint (e.g., serum protein), an α level of 1.1% instead of 5% would have to be used to ensure the same β level.

Sometimes, the direction of the effect is known a priori; that is, only an increase of tumor rates represents the experimental question in a carcinogenicity study. Two minimize type II error, one-sided testing should be performed. If a two-sided test is used, a marked increase in sample size is necessary. In the above example, $n_{\text{one-sided}} = 32$, but $n_{\text{two-sided}} = 44$ is necessary.

In the many-to-one design, an increase in the sample size of the control will be used according to the statistical optimality rule $n_K = \sqrt{k}\, n_D$, where k denotes the number of dose groups. However, this rule holds true only in the case of variance homogeneity (which is questionable in toxicological studies, a priori) and the exact $\sqrt{k}$ rule is not necessary. For the typical three- or four-dose experiment, simply doubling the sample size is sufficient. Thus, the control sample size can be divided into two independent randomized controls, possibly stratified on pretest conditions (e.g., body weights). In the case of dichotomous data, such as mortality or tumor rates, the sample size n_i also depends on the spontaneous rate of the controls p_C (see Fig. 2).

Therefore, detection sensitivity increases with lower spontaneous rates. The minimum sensitivity occurs when is $p_C = 0.5$. In a carcinogenicity study based on a balanced false-positive–false-negative ratio, animal strains with the spontaneous rate of the target tumor greater than zero and smaller than about 10% should be selected. Unfortunately, the target tumor seldom can be defined a priori, because numerous tumors with rather different spontaneous rates must be taken into account. Therefore, an animal

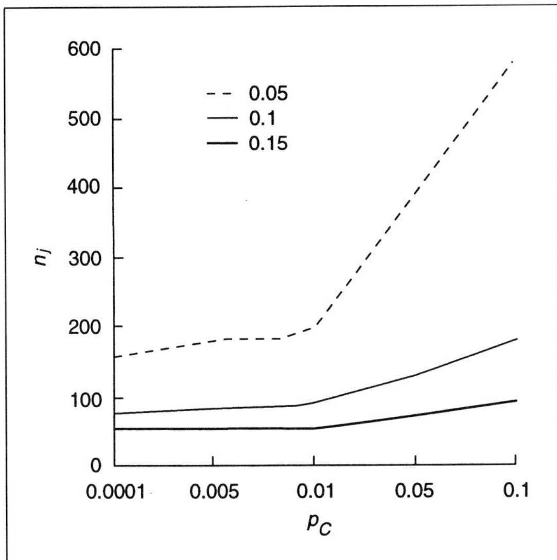

FIGURE 2 Sample-size estimation for the asymptotic test for comparing two proportions (one-sided, $\alpha = 0.05$, $\beta = 0.20$) as a function of spontaneous rate p_C and $\Delta p(0.05; 0.01; 0.15)$.

strain with an average small spontaneous rate across all tumor types should be selected.

Experimental Design

The many-to-one design *treatments versus negative control* (i.e., $k + 1$ experimental groups) is applied to all toxicological studies, with the exception of acute toxicity studies. Usually, this one-way layout is included in a factorial design with the factors of litter, sex, and time. Assuming an interaction between these factors in advance, an independent analysis is done for a dose effect by each factor separately. Therefore, only methods for the one-way design are described here and the following types can be distinguished:

- Unrestricted design: $C^-, T_1, \ldots, T_k$, with T_j denoting different treatments (e.g., different substances, application forms, or combinations of substances).
- Dose–response design: $C^-, D_1, \ldots, D_k$, with D_j denoting different doses; $C^- = 0 < D_1 < \cdots < D_k$ (k not too large, i.e., $\in \{2, 3, 4\}$).
- Extended design including a positive control: C^-, $D_1, \ldots, D_k, C^+$.
- Complex design: $C^-, C^0, S_A\ (D_1, \ldots, D_k)$, $S_B\ (D_1, \ldots, D_k), C^+$, where C^0 denotes an empty control (without any administration), and $S_{A,B}$ denote several substances.

For the first type, comparisons of treatments versus negative control (many-to-one procedures) are used. For the second type, the following can be distinguished:

- Dose–response analysis based on selected complex models (e.g., single hit model) and testing selected model parameters. Unfortunately, there is no possibility for the separation of model and lack-of-fit. According to the slogan "all models are wrong, some are helpful," independent model selection for the typical three- or four-dose design is difficult and the routine use of this approach cannot be recommended.
- Dose–response analysis with comparison procedures for ordered alternatives. A priori assumption that the rejection of the null hypothesis will be according to an increasing trend only:

$$H_0: \quad \mu_C = \mu_{D_1} = \mu_{D_2} = \cdots = \mu_{D_k}$$

$$H_A: \quad \mu_C \leq \mu_{D_1} \leq \mu_{D_2} \leq \cdots \leq \mu_{D_k} \quad \text{with at least } \mu_C < \mu_{D_k}$$

Weaker assumptions are used (monotonic increasing, without knowledge of the kind of shape); therefore, this method is more robust.

Comparison Procedures "Control versus k Treatments or Doses"

In several publications, numerous statistical approaches for many-to-one designs in toxicology were described. Two concepts should be distinguished:

- Pairwise tests (t tests, u tests) "control versus group j," each independent at level α. Here, the principle of an experimental type I error rate is violated and no order information is used. Independent of the number of groups, a minimum type II error rate is guaranteed.
- Multiple comparison procedures guarantee an experimental type I error rate, but depending on the number of groups, the type II error rate will increase. If a priori monotonicity of the dose–response can be assumed, either procedures for order restriction or trend tests within the closure test principle should be used to decrease the type II error.

However, the following approaches should be avoided:

- Pairwise tests "each against each other" using t or u tests, because the experimental α level will be strongly violated.

TABLE 1 Recommendations for Pairwise Tests

Endpoint	Example	Two-sample test
Parametric, homogeneous variances	Hemoglobin	t test
Parametric, heterogeneous variances	Erythrocytes	Welch t test
Nonparametric, continuous	ASAT	u test, asymptotic version
Nonparametric, discrete with ties	Number of micronuclei	u test, permutative version
Dichotomous	Mortality rate	Fisher's or Barnard's test

- All-pair comparisons procedures (e.g., the well-known Tukey procedure) because the many-to-one structure is ignored and type II errors increase dramatically.
- "Omnibus" global tests (e.g., Kruskal and Wallis (1952) test or F test) because the rejection of the null hypothesis only shows heterogeneity among the groups in an unknown structure.
- Test hierarchies consisting of test on distribution, omnibus test, and procedures because, from the viewpoint of type II error, they are not free of contradiction.

The choice depends on the type of endpoint, which is shown for pairwise tests in Table 1 and many-to-one procedures in Table 2 (the tests and procedures used are explained in the examples).

Stepwise modifications of most procedures are now available. They guarantee smaller type II errors. However, no simultaneous confidence intervals are generally available. Until now, only "mean value statistics" (e.g., t test or Dunnett's procedure) have been considered in this paper. Frequently in toxicological studies, a responder–nonresponder behavior can be observed. Tests on means are based on the principle of 100% responders. For cases where responders are less than 100%, tests for Lehmann alternatives can be used. In this case, we assume that the treatment consists of a proportion of p nonresponders (i.e., the same behavior as control group animals) and a proportion $(1 - p)$ of pathologically reacting animals. Such a mixing distribution can be detected by larger variances, which is exactly what is frequently observed in toxicology studies: increasing variances with increasing effects (see Conover and Salsburg, 1988).

Robustness

The tests and procedures should be robust against violation of their assumptions, that is, no increase of type I or type II error rates due to real data problems. Real data are characterized by violations of the Gaussian distribution and/or the variance homogeneity assumption. Unfortunately, in small-sample-size studies, a reliable test for a distribution is impossible. Either such a test can be performed on historical controls or a nonnormal distribution is assumed a priori, leading to nonparametric methods. However, numerous investigations have revealed that under different distribution types usually observed in toxicology, the parametric tests and procedures are relatively robust. In contrast, both parametric and nonparametric methods are very sensitive to heterogenous variances, especially when combined with unbalancedness (high variances and unequal small sample sizes). Variance

TABLE 2 Recommendations for Many-to-One Procedures

Endpoint	Without restriction of the alternative hypothesis	Ordered alternative hypothesis
Parametric	Dunnett (1955) procedure	A priori ordered procedure based on t tests or contrasts
Nonparametric	Steel (1959) procedure	A priori ordered procedure based on u tests or Jonckheere (1954) trend tests
Dichotomous	Passing (1984) procedure	A priori ordered procedure based on Fisher tests or Armitage (1955) trend tests

heterogeneity can be simply tested on the concurrent study (e.g., using the F test or the Levene 1960 test). The Levene test has the added benefit of being robust under skewed distributions and hence is recommended. If the variance homogeneity is markedly violated, procedures based on common mean-square error should not be used. Simply α-adjusted Welch t tests can be used instead.

Reporting of "Significances"

The results of significance tests or procedures can be reported as:

- Significant or not significant as a dichotomous decision.
- Symbols (e.g., * $p \leq 0.05$, ** $p \leq 0.01$, *** $p \leq 0.001$).
- p values (the smallest possible empirical type I error rate).
- Confidence intervals for the differences control versus treatment j.

While p values are the shortest representation and are now up-to-date, parametric confidence intervals $[x_{\text{lower}}; x_{\text{upper}}]$ contain the most information. The distance from zero is a measure of the magnitude of violation of the null hypothesis; the width is a measure of variance, sample size, dimension k, and type I error α. Confidence intervals are scale variant (endpoint-specific interpretation is easy) and can be used in the safety approach (a posteriori defined minimal relevant difference δ). For Dunnett's procedure (see the section on Chronic Toxicity) the two-sided $(1-\alpha)$-confidence interval is

$$[\bar{x}_j - \bar{x}_C - d_{k,\nu,\rho_{Cj},1-\alpha}\sqrt{s^2(1/n_j + 1/n_C)};$$

$$\bar{x}_j - \bar{x}_C + d_{k,\nu,\rho_{Cj},1-\alpha}\sqrt{s^2(1/n_j + 1/n_C)}],$$

where $d_{k,\nu,\rho_{Cj},1-\alpha}$ denotes the $(1-\alpha)$-quantile of the multivariate t distribution with correlation ρ_{Cj}. Selected quantiles are given in Table 3 (calculated using the PROBMC function in SAS).

Descriptive Statistics

Not only should the results of significance tests or procedures (p values or confidence intervals) be reported, but also group-specific location, scale measures, and sample sizes. Either parametric statistics (mean and standard deviation) or nonparametric (median and percentiles) should be chosen.

ACUTE TOXICITY

The objective of an acute toxicity study is the estimation of the toxicity of a compound after the single administration of increasing doses to estimate, among others, the lethal dose for 50% of the animal population: LD_{50}. A randomized one-way design (independent for each sex) with the factor dose at the levels $D_1 < D_2 < \cdots < D_k$ will be used. The endpoint is the number of dead animals r_j in group j after a predefined observation time (e.g., 48 h) in relation to the number of animals at risk (e.g., group sample size n_j). This mortality rate $p_j = r_j/n_j$ represents a dichotomous variable and the statistical problem consists in the estimation of the dose–response relationship with the following steps:

- Transformation of p_j into an approximate normally distributed variable y_j.
- Logarithmic transformation of the dose D_j into $x_j = \log D_j$.
- Parameter estimation in the linear model $y_j = a + b\,x_j$.
- Estimation of the LD_{50} by inverse transformation:

TABLE 3 Selected 95%-Quantiles of the Multivariate t Distribution and Normal Distribution (equal correlation coefficients $1/\sqrt{2}$; n_j = const.)

	One-sided		Two-sided	
Degree of freedom ν	$k = 2$	$k = 3$	$k = 2$	$k = 3$
10	2.15	2.34	2.57	2.76
15	2.07	2.24	2.44	2.61
20	2.03	2.19	2.38	2.54
30	1.99	2.32	2.15	2.47
60	1.95	2.10	2.27	2.41
120	1.93	2.08	2.24	2.38
∞ (multivariate normal distribution)	1.92	2.09	2.21	2.35

$p_j \longrightarrow 0.5\ (= 50\%) \longrightarrow y_j = 0 \longrightarrow x_j \longrightarrow \mathrm{LD}_{50}.$

- Estimation of the two-sided $(1 - \alpha)$ confidence interval for LD_{50}.

In the statistical literature, the problem of different transformations of dichotomous variables is discussed. However, for the estimation of a central parameter like LD_{50}, the choice is not critical because well-known transformation methods, such as

Probit: $\mathrm{probit}(r_j/n_j) = \Phi^{-1}(r_j/n_j)$ with Φ^{-1} inverse of normal distribution,

Logit: $\mathrm{logit}(r_j/n_j) = \ln[(r_j/n_j)/1 - (r_j/n_j)]$, and

Angular: $\mathrm{angular}(r_j/n_j) = \arcsin\sqrt{r_j/n_j}$,

differ markedly only for $p_j < 0.1$ and $p_j > 0.9$. Because of the simple numerical property of the logit transformation, we will describe its use. Parameters can be estimated by the iterative maximum likelihood method, the method of moments, and the weighted least-square method. The last is simple and will be demonstrated here. A correction of the transformation

$$y_j = \ln\left(\frac{r_j + n_j/40}{n_j - r_j + n_j/40}\right)$$

is necessary because $p_j = 0$ and $p_j = 1$ are possible. Because $\mathrm{var}(y_j) \approx p_j(1 - p_j)/n_j$, the variance homogeneity assumption is violated and hence the weighted least-squares estimation with the weights $w_j = n_j(p_j + n_j)(1 - p_j^2)$ should be used with the asymptotic estimators

$$a = \bar{y} - b\bar{x}$$

$$\text{with } \bar{y} = \left(\sum_{j=1}^{k} w_j y_j\right) \Big/ \left(\sum_{j=1}^{k} w_j\right)$$

$$\text{and } \bar{x} = \left(\sum_{j=1}^{k} w_j y_j\right) \Big/ \left(\sum_{j=1}^{k} w_j\right)$$

where

$$b = \left(\sum_{j=1}^{k} w_j(y_j - \bar{y})(x_j - \bar{x})\right) \Big/ \left(\sum_{j=1}^{k} w_j(x_j - \bar{x})^2\right).$$

The estimation for the LD_{50} is simply $\mathrm{LD}_{50} = \exp(-a/b)$. The two-sided $(1 - \alpha)$ confidence interval of the LD_{50} is the *quotient of two variables* a/b and is given by Fieller's theorem:

$$\mathrm{CI}(\mathrm{LD}_{50}) = \exp(-\frac{a}{b} \pm z_{1-\alpha/2}\sqrt{\mathrm{Var}(\mathrm{LD}_{50})})$$

with

$$\mathrm{Var}(\mathrm{LD}_{50}) = \left[\frac{1}{\sum_{j=1}^{k} w_j} + \mathrm{LD}_{50} - \frac{\bar{x}^2}{\sum_{j=1}^{k} w_j(x_j - \bar{x})^2}\right] / b^2$$

Numerous computer programs are available to produce these computations. Other relevant practical methods are nonparametric and sequential approaches for the estimation of approximate toxicity limits that reduce the number of experimental animals needed.

CHRONIC TOXICITY

Introduction

The objective of a repeated toxicity study is to estimate the toxicity and side effects of a new substance after repeated administration of increasing doses. Multiple comparisons of all the endpoints in treated groups versus the negative control group C^- determines the toxicological effects. The duration of administration varies from 10 days to 2 years, depending on the objective in relation to clinical trials and international regulatory recommendations.

The usual design is the completely randomized three-factorial layout:

SUBSTANCE × SEX × TIME
(where × denotes cross classification)

As levels for the factor substance, either treatments T_j (e.g., different substances, different application routes) or dose groups D_j are used in a many-to-one design:

$$C^-, T_1, \ldots, T_k \quad \text{or} \quad C^-, D_1, \ldots, D_k$$

As levels of the factor time, the measurement time points $t_1, t_2, \ldots, t_T$ are used; these are frequently nonequidistant. A typical characteristic of chronic toxicity studies is the simultaneous estimation of different measurements and findings for each individual animal (e.g., body weight, hematology, clinical chemistry parameters, urine analysis, organ weights, and clinical and histopathological findings). Although a multivariate analysis is possible, the state of the art is the univariate analysis done separately for each endpoint.

The primary problem for statistical analysis is the proof of substance effect by comparing the effect of the dose or treatment group with that of the negative control group. Although the three-way layout can be analyzed by standard analysis of variance methods, including the interactions dose × time and dose ×

TABLE 4 Repeated Toxicity Study with Number of Animals Dead after 6-Month Duration					
	0	**10 mg/kg**	**50 mg/kg**	**100 mg/kg**	**Σ**
Number of animals dead, r_j	0	1	6	8	$r. = 19$
Number of animals at risk, n_j	40	20	20	20	$n. = 100$
Mortality rate, p_j	0.10	0.05	0.30	0.40	

sex, many-to-one comparisons frequently will be performed separately for each time point and sex.

Analysis of Mortality

Two types of mortality data can be distinguished: one with time dependence and the other without time dependence. The first case typically occurs in long-term studies (i.e., comparison of survival functions), while the second one occurs in short-term studies. In the last case, both the number of dead animals at the end of the study r_j and the number of animals at risk n_j are recorded (Table 4). The comparison of the proportion of the negative control $p_C = r_C/n_C$ with the proportion in the treatment groups p_j can be performed with the many-to-one procedure. Assuming a monotone dose–response relationship, the trend test can be used within a closure test principle according to Marcus *et al.* (1976).

Many-to-One Comparison Procedure for Dichotomous Variables (Passing, 1984)

$$dp_j = (p_j - p_C)/\sqrt{r.(1 - r./n.)(1/n_j + 1/n_C)(n./(n. - 1))} \quad \text{for each } j \in \{1, \ldots, k\}$$

with

$$p_j = r_j/n_j \quad r. = \textstyle\sum_{j=C}^{k} r_j \text{ and } n. = \sum_{j=C}^{k} n_j$$

TABLE 5 Selected 95%-Quantiles of the t Distribution and Normal Distribution		
ν	**One-sided**	**Two-sided**
12	1.782	2.179
14	1.761	2.145
16	1.746	2.120
18	1.734	2.101
20	1.725	2.086
40	1.684	2.021
60	1.671	2.000
∞ (normal distribution)	1.6449	1.9600

and

$$dp_{10\,\mathrm{mg/kg}} = (0.05 - 0.10)/\sqrt{(19(1 - 19/100)(1/20 + 1/40)(100/100 - 1)} = -0.46$$

$$dp_{50\,\mathrm{mg/kg}} = 1.85$$

and

$$dp_{100\,\mathrm{mg/kg}} = 2.78$$

The null hypothesis of equality of the mortality rates of the treatment groups in comparison to the negative control will be rejected if the test statistic is larger than the quantile of the multivariate t distribution $t_{k,\mathrm{one/two\text{-}sided},1-\alpha}$ (see Table 3). Only $dp_{100\,\mathrm{mg/kg}} = 2.78$ is larger than the quantile $t_{k=3,\mathrm{one\text{-}sided},1-\alpha=0.95} = 2.09$, and hence we can conclude that there is an increase of mortality in the 100 mg/kg group.

Trend Test For Dichotomous Variables (Armitage, 1955)

$$ta = \frac{\sum_{j=C}^{k} D_j(r_j - (n_j r./n.)}{\sqrt{\begin{array}{l} r.(n. - r.)/(n.(n. - 1)) \\ \times \sum_{j=C}^{k} n_j\left(D_j - \left(\sum_{j=C}^{k} n_j D_j/n.\right)\right)^2 \end{array}}}$$

$$ta = \frac{\begin{array}{l} 0 + 10(1 - 20 \times 19/100) \\ + 50(6 - 20 \times 19/100) \\ + 100(8 - 20 \times 19/100) \end{array}}{\sqrt{\begin{array}{l} (19(100 - 19)/100 \times 99)(40(0 - 32)^2 \\ + 20(10 + 32)^2 + 20(50 - 32)^2 \\ + 20(100 - 32)^2 \end{array}}}$$

$$= 3.29.$$

The null hypothesis of equality of the mortality rates will be rejected if the test statistic is larger than the quantile of the normal distribution $z_{1-\alpha}$ (see Table 5).

TABLE 6 Analysis of Body-Weight Data by the t Test and AUC Approach

t	Body weight/g	
	Control	Dose
0	203, 206, 201, 196, 201	177, 183, 209, 189, 185
1	239, 243, 244, 239, 251	205, 209, 221, 191, 207
4	302, 291, 287, 291, 315	233, 251, 268, 227, 251
8	388, 371, 383, 371, 413	277, 322, 357, 270, 329
13	411, 391, 401, 399, 390	355, 299, 391, 311, 351

Because $ta = 3.29$ is larger than the quantile $z_{0.95} = 1.6449$, the null hypothesis can be rejected and a dose trend in mortality can be assumed. The closure principle can be used here to detect the minimum effective dose simply by conditional step-down testing of k, $k-1, k-2, \ldots, 1$ dimensional trend tests, each at level α (if the null hypothesis in the jth dimension can be rejected, the $(j-1)$ dimensional trend test can be tested; otherwise, the procedure stops and the minimum effective dose is j). In the example for the four-dimensional trend test (global test) the null hypothesis can be rejected. The test statistic for the three-dimensional trend test is 2.27 and again larger than 1.6449. Therefore, the two-dimensional trend test can be conducted and because this test value is 0.65, the minimum effective dose is 50 mg/kg.

Analysis of Body Weight

Two types of body weight data can be distinguished: (1) only a few measurements (e.g., weekly in a 4-week study) and (2) growth curves based on numerous measurements (from a 2-y carcinogenicity study). In the first case, individual differences from the baseline are calculated and separate tests at each time point are appropriate. This approach could also be used in the second case; however, the large number of tests will increase the global false-positive rate. Body weight-versus-time relationships are important in long-term studies because this noninvasive simple method has a large predictive value for potential toxic effects. The problem is the comparison of the growth curve of the negative control versus those of the treatment or dose groups under the conditions of nonequidistant measurements and, dose- and time-dependent drop out due to mortality. Three simple approaches will be recommended here:

- Fitting a nonlinear growth curve model with the smallest possible number of parameters and testing between selected parameters for treatment effects.
- Assuming the repeated measures are multivariate vectors and using multiple endpoint test in its stabilized version.
- Transformation into an univariate individual variable in the sense of an integral measure of the growth curve using the area-under-the-curve (AUC) technique for the global time interval $(0,T)$ or selected time intervals (t_1, t_2). AUC can be computed simply by trapezoidal rule.

In Table 6, the t test and the AUC approach are demonstrated for a small number of real data. Only a part of the raw data from a 90-day study on female rats is presented. The test is one-sided for a decrease.

t Test for Differences to Baseline

Differences in week 4;

Control: 99, 85, 86, 95, 114

Dose: 56, 68, 59, 39, 66

The p value of the t test is 0.0004 and the null hypothesis can be rejected.

AUC Approach

Individual AUC estimation using trapezoidal rule between t_0 and t_{end} (0th and 13th weeks):

$$\mathrm{AUC} \approx (m_0(t_1 - t_0) + m_1(t_2 - t_0) + m_2(t_3 - t_1) + \cdots + m_{end}(t_{end} - t_{end-1})/2.$$

For the first animal in the control, the AUC is

$$(203{*}1 + 239{*}4 + 302{*}7 + 388{*}9 + 411{*}5)/2$$

For all other animals, the AUCs are:

Control: 4410, 4254.5, 4319, 4261.5, 4538.5

Dose: 3448, 3584.5, 4068.5, 3263.5, 3743

TABLE 7 Subchronic Toxicity Study on Wistar Rat, Endpoint Alkaline Phosphatase

Group	n_j	Alkaline phosphatase	Mean	SD
Control	12	17.3, 23.0, 22.5, 10.0, 21.6, 19.7, 17.7, 20.0, 17.9, 20.9, 24.3, 19.9	20.317	2.216
D_{low}	12	23.9, 19.2, 24.1, 19.1, 17.4, 21.9, 24.1, 24.0, 20.7, 21.9, 23.1, 16.9	21.358	2.660
D_{high}	10	24.2, 31.3, 30.7, 17.4, 27.9, 25.7, 18.1, 21.9, 25.9, 19.8	24.290	4.939

Now the mean values and standard deviations from these transformed values are calculated. Because the variance is heterogeneous, the Welch t test was used.

$$t = \frac{\bar{x}_D - \bar{x}_C}{\sqrt{s_D^2/n_D + s_C^2/n_C}}$$

with

$$\nu = \frac{(s_D^2/n_D + s_C^2/n_C)^2}{(s_D^2/n_D)^2/(n_D - 1) + (s_C^2/n_C)^2/(n_C - 1)}$$

With the modified degrees of freedom $\nu = 5$, a p value of 0.0021 results; that is, the integral of the body weight–time relationship from the beginning to the end is significantly reduced.

Analysis of Continuous Variables

The choice of the procedure depends on the type of design, type of endpoint, and the possibility of order restriction. In Table 7, the endpoint alkaline phosphatase was measured in a many-to-one design.

Parametric Many-to-One Procedure (Dunnett, 1955)

$$d_j = \frac{\bar{x}_j - \bar{x}_C}{\sqrt{\text{MSE}(1/n_j + 1/n_C)}} \quad \text{for both } j \text{ (i.e., } D_{\text{low}}, D_{\text{high}})$$

$$\text{with MSE} = \frac{\sum_{j=C}^{k} \sum_{i=1}^{n_j} x_{ij}^2 - \dfrac{\sum_{j=C}^{k} x_{j.}^2}{n_j}}{\sum_{j=C}^{k} (n_j - 1)}$$

$$\text{and } \nu = \sum_{j=K}^{k} (n_j - 1)$$

$$\text{and } \rho_{Cj} = 1/\sqrt{n_j/(n_C + n_j)}$$

TABLE 8 Selected Values f for Nonparametric, Two-Sided $1 - \alpha = 95\%$ Tolerance Intervals for $p = 90$ or 95% of the Population[a]

Sample size of historical controls	Value f	
	$p = 90\%$	$p = 95\%$
30	1	1
50	2	1
100	5	2
200	13	5
300	22	9
400	30	13
500	39	17

[a]According to Hahn and Meeker, "Statistical Intervals," Copyright © 1991. Adapted by permission of John Wiley & Sons, Inc.

The null hypothesis for group j is rejected if $d_j > d_{k,\nu,\text{one/two-sided},\rho_{Cj},1-\alpha}$, where $d_{k,\nu,\text{one/two-sided},\rho_{Cj},1-\alpha}$, denotes the quantile of the multivariate t distribution with degree of freedom ν and correlation coefficients ρ_{Cj} (see Table 3). The values of the statistics are

$$d_{D_{\text{high}}} = \frac{(24.29 - 20.317)}{\sqrt{11.33(1/12 + 1/10)}} = 2.74$$

and

$$d_{D_{\text{low}}} = \frac{(21.358 - 20.317)}{\sqrt{11.33(1/12 + 1/12)}} = 0.756 \quad \text{(with MSE} = 11.33)$$

Because $d_{k=2,\nu=31,\text{one-sided},\rho=.707;0.74,1-\alpha=0.95} = 1.983$ (estimated by the PROBMC function in SAS; the approximate table value is 1.99; see Table 3), the high dose is increased with respect to control. The stepwise procedure is as follows: (1) first order the test statistics d_j, (2) then compare the largest test statistics with the quantile $d_{k,\nu,\text{one/two-sided},\rho_{Cj},1-\alpha}$, (3) if and only if this null hypothesis is rejected, compare the next largest test statistics with the quantile $d_{k-1,\nu,\text{one/two-sided},\rho_{Cj},1-\alpha}$ (i.e., compare with the k, $(k-1)$, $(k-2)$, . . . , one-dimensional quantile instead of only the k-dimensional quantities). This approach decreases the type II error.

Nonparametric Many-to-One Procedure (Steel, 1959) Pairwise Ranking {C,D$_j$}, Asymptotic Version:

$$ds_j = \frac{\sum_{i=1}^{n_j} R_{ij} - n_j(n_j + n_C + 1)/2}{\sqrt{n_C n_j (n_j + n_C + 1)/12}}$$

with R_{ij} . . . pairwise ranking of C and D_j

The null hypothesis is rejected for group j if $ds_j > d_{k,\nu=\infty,\text{one/two-sided},\rho_{Cj},1-\alpha}$ (see Table 3). The pairwise ranking works for the low dose with respect to the control group as follows: (1) rank the pooled sample from 1 to $(n_C + n_j)$ (mid-ranks for equal values):

C: 3.0, 18.0, 17.0, 1.0, 14.0, 9.0, 5.0, 11.0, 6.0, 13.0, 24.0, 10.0

D_{low}: 20.0; 8.0, 22.5, 7.0, 4.0, 15.5, 22.5, 21.0, 12.0, 15.5, 19.0,

(2) For the low dose, the rank sum is 169, (3) the test statistic is:

$$ds_{D_{\text{low}}} = \frac{169 - 12 \cdot 25/2}{\sqrt{12 \cdot 12 \cdot 25/12}} = 0.87$$

and

$$ds_{D_{\text{low}}} = \frac{146 - 10 \cdot 23/2}{\sqrt{12 \cdot 10 \cdot 23/12}} = 2.04,$$

(4) with the quantile $d_{2,\infty,0.95} = 1.92$, the null hypothesis can be rejected for the comparison with the high dose only.

Assuming a priori monotonic ordering, a simple procedure on ordered t tests (each at level α) should be demonstrated (so-called pairwise contrasts):

$$t_j = \frac{\bar{x}_j - \bar{x}_C}{\sqrt{\text{MSE}(1/n_j + 1/n_C)}}$$

$$t_{D_{\text{low}}} = 0.756; \quad t_{D_{\text{high}}} = 2.744$$

The procedure starts with $t_{D_{\text{high}}}$. If $t_{D_{\text{high}}} > t_{\nu,1-\alpha}$, proceed with the next lower dose; otherwise the procedure stops. Because $t_{D_{\text{high}}} = 2.744 > 1.696$, the global null hypothesis can be rejected and we proceed with D_{low}. Because $t_{D_{\text{low}}} = 0.756 < 1.696$, the procedure stops. This procedure guarantees experimental type I error and can be extended to any kind of pairwise contrast, that is, to nonparametric or dichotomous ones.

Moreover, we describe a simple score test for Lehmann alternatives for the groups C and D_{high} briefly. First the raw data are ranked into R_{ji} and transformed into

$$y_{ji} = (R_{ji}/(N + 1))^4,$$

where $N = n_1 + n_2$ denotes the global sample size. For example, the first value of D_{high} group is

$$R_{1,D_{\text{high}}} = 16 \longrightarrow y_{1,D_{\text{high}}} = (16/23)^4 = 0.234.$$

Using this transformed value, simple t tests are performed. In the example $\bar{y}_{D_{\text{high}}} = 0.330$, $s_{D_{\text{high}}} = 0.307$, and $\bar{y}_C = 0.068$, $s_c = 0.093$, and a p value of 0.0082 results. In this example, no mixing distribution of "responder and nonresponder" seems to exist because the p value of the t test on the raw data results in the same magnitude ($p = 0.0063$).

Analysis of Organ Weights

The specific problem in the analysis of organ weights is that changes in organ weights can be effected by changes in body weight (e.g., a decrease in liver organ weight can be caused by the test substance or by a decrease in body weight). The pragmatic solution for this problem is the analysis of both absolute and relative (organ weight/body weight) organ weights. From a statistical point of view, the analysis of this quotient assumes a linear relationship between the organ-versus-body weight and variance proportionality. Frequently, however, this is not the case (e.g., for the allometric function of organ weight = $a \cdot$ body weight^b, different values were observed for brain $b = 0.16$ and for prostate $b = 2.13$). Several alternative approaches have been published, including the analysis of covariance (with the covariate body weight). However, the simple concept of relative organ weights mentioned is routinely used.

Analysis of the Recovery Period

In some chronic studies, the test of reversibility becomes an important objective. Therefore, a subpopulation of at least one high-dose group and the control group are observed for some period of time (e.g., the recovery period) after the end of substance administration. For noninvasive measures (e.g., body weight and hematology parameters) paired tests should be used for the comparison between dosing and recovery periods in the same animals.

Analysis of Histopathological Findings

A biostatistical analysis of macroscopic and microscopic findings is frequently not done. However, selected histopathological findings may represent the primary endpoints. Moreover, a basic contradiction can be observed; the predictive value of easy and precise measurable variables is low, but it is high for the findings with the lowest possible information content: yes or no. Most of the findings are irreversible, but some clinical findings are reversible. For the latter, either the time of the first observation or the time period of the occurrence can be analyzed. The majority of the other findings can be analyzed as simple proportions. Here, the methodology of mortality rates (see the preceding section) or crude tumor rates (see the subsection Carcinogenicity Studies) can be used. Sometimes, histopathological findings are graded. Here, special tests for ordered categorical data should be used, preferably permutative versions.

Use of Reference Values

An inherent problem in the application of statistical significance tests in toxicology is the sometimes occurring contradiction between statistical significance and biological relevance. Several controversial approaches are discussed in the literature to overcome this problem. A simple approach is the additional use of reference or normal values. The rule is simple: first characterize what is "normal" and then classify the individual values into normal and nonnormal categories. A large proportion of nonnormal values will support the statistical significance.

TABLE 9 Number of Resorptions and Implantations in Control and D_{high}

		Litter									
		1	2	3	4	5	6	7	8	9	10
C	r_{Ci}	2	2	1	0	0	1	1	0	1	0
	n_{Ci}	12	14	11	12	13	9	10	12	13	14
D	r_{Di}	5	3	3	2	7	3	1	4		
	n_{Di}	6	13	12	13	11	10	15	11		
Transformation to $y_{ji} = r_{ji}/n_{ji}$											
		1	2	3	4	5	6	7	8	9	10
C	y_{Ci}	0.167	0.143	0.091	0	0	0.111	0.100	0	0.07	0
D	y_{Di}	0.833	0.231	0.250	0.154	0.636	0.300	0.067	0.364	7	

In regulatory toxicology, relatively good conditions exist for the estimation of normal values, since a large number of negative control animal data are available under standardized conditions (e.g., animals' housing, and analysis devices). From a statistical point of view, reference values can be categorized into those for a single future value, for a group (e.g., by the median) and for s values out of n_j of a group.

Here, only nonparametric reference values will be considered since the well-known parametric ones $[\bar{x} - 3s; \bar{x} + 3s]$ are very sensitive to a violation of the normal distribution assumption. A two-sided nonparametric reference region, including with $(1 - \alpha)$ probability $p100\%$ of the single values X_{ji} of an actual experiment, is

$$[X_{(f)}, X_{(n-f+1)}].$$

The parameter f can be found in Table 8 and the $X_{(\,)}$ represents the ordered single values of the historical controls from the smallest to the largest. The reference region is simply the f-smallest and the $(n - f + 1)$-largest value of this sample. The decision nonnormal is simply if $X_{ji} < X_{(f)}$ or $X_{ji} > X_{(n-f+1)}$ occurs.

REPRODUCTIVE TOXICOLOGY

For simplicity, the scheme of the most widely used teratogenicity study for estimation of blasto- and embryotoxic and teratogenic effects is presented in Fig. 3. From this scheme, some particularities found in comparison to the other toxicological studies follow.

- A hierarchical design: female $\supset$ litter $\supset$ fetus finding.
- The experimental unit "female" is not completely randomized according to the procedure of mating.
- The application of the substance occurs to the randomized sample unit "female," but most of the findings are on the fetuses.
- Numerous interactions occur (e.g., between the fetuses within a litter or concurrence between fetal mortality and the malformation rate, that is, the malformation rate could be biased by a large mortality rate).
- The primary endpoints are only discrete (e.g., the number of malformed fetuses per global number of fetuses).

Three statistical approaches can be distinguished according to these particularities:

- *Per fetus analysis:* Assume the fetus is the experimental unit. The independence assumption is violated and the false-positive rate is increased dramatically because of the pseudo increase in sample size. This approach should not be recommended.
- *Per litter analysis:* Assume the litter as the experimental unit, taking into account the interactions between the fetuses. This approach fits the biological background; however, the statistical methods (e.g., beta-binomial model) are complicated and frequently not robust.
- *Quasi per litter analysis:* This simple compromise is based on the transformation of the findings per litter $y_{ji} = r_{ji}/n_{ji}$, followed by a nonparametric test. Table 9 demonstrates this approach for the number of resorptions r_{ji} in relation to the number of implantations per litter (for control and high dose only). According to the transformed values y_{ij}, the permutative u test was used and a one-sided p value = 0.001 was found; that is, the rate of resorptions in the high dose is significantly increased with respect to the control.

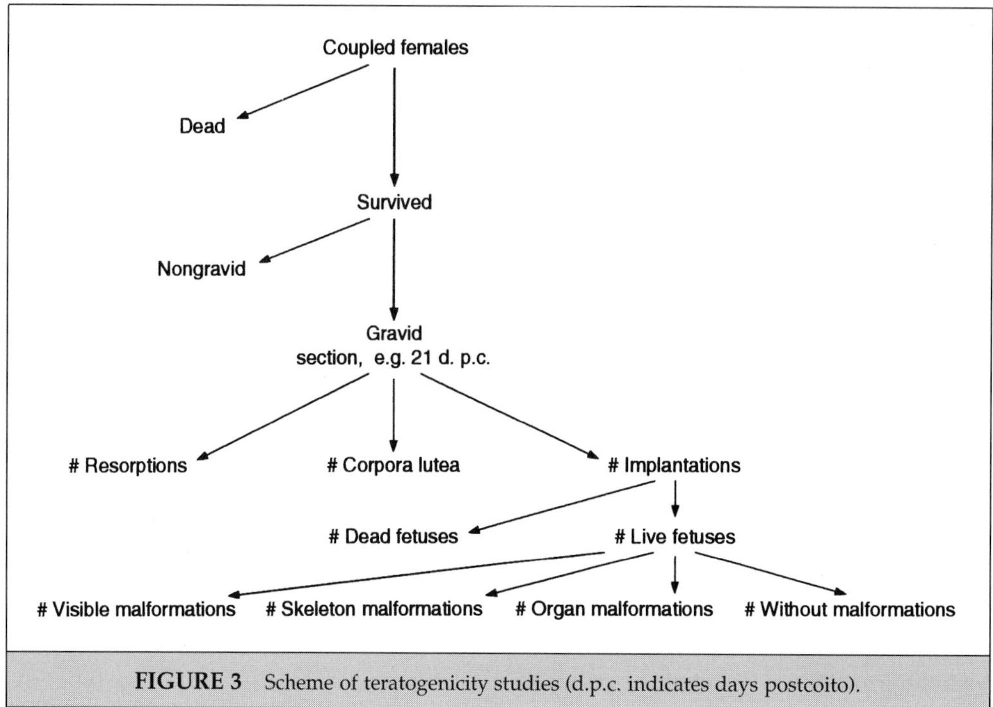

FIGURE 3 Scheme of teratogenicity studies (d.p.c. indicates days postcoito).

MUTAGENICITY STUDIES

To determine a potential mutagenic effect of a test substance, a testing battery consisting of several assays (e.g., salmonella–microsome (Ames), micronucleus, chromosome aberration, or HGPRT) is used. The most commonly used standardized assay is the salmonella–microsome (Ames) assay; hence its statistical analysis will be discussed as an example.

The objective of this assay is the determination of a potential gene-mutagenic effect of a substance after the single administration of several doses on histidine-free agar plates with specially modified *Salmonella typhimurium* bacteria strains. The numbers of grown visible colonies (revertants) of the dose groups are compared with those of the negative and positive controls. Several strains are used with different sensitivities for the different DNA mutagenic mechanisms, for example, base change mutation (TA 100 strain) or frameshift mutation (TA 98 strain).

TABLE 10 Biostatistical Analysis of Salmonella–Microsome (Ames) Assay Data on TA 100

j	Dose	Revertants	$\bar{x}_j$
0	0	80, 83, 79	80.7
1	0.01	92, 88, 78	86.0
2	0.02	96, 102, 98	98.7
3	0.04	104, 103, 95	100.7
4	0.08	94, 97, 99	96.7
5	0.16	93, 87, 91	90.3

The design is a completely randomized one-way layout $[C-, D_1, \ldots, D_k, C+]$, where the number of doses is between 3 and 6. Because the false-negative rate increases dramatically with too-low doses, the doses must be selected so that a nonmonotonic dose–response relationship occurs due to the interaction of mutagenic and cell-toxic effects. Therefore, the shape of the dose–response must be assumed to be an "umbrella."

Three statistical approaches can be distinguished:

- A formal twofold rule. That is, the effect is relevant if the mean values of two consecutive doses or the highest nontoxic dose are greater than 2 × the mean of the negative control (see, e.g., Cariello and Piegorsch 1996).
- A dose–response model. An example is the "single hit model,"

$$p(D_j) = (1 - \exp(-(a_1 + a_2 D_j)))\exp(-a_3 D_j),$$

  where the parameters a_1, a_2, and a_3 are to be estimated from the data.
- A suitable trend test that is robust against nonmonotonicity at high doses as well as the distribution of the revertants.

TABLE 11 Selected 95% Quantiles of the Jonckheere Trend Test[a]

Number of groups (incl. C)	n = const = 3	n = const = 4	n = const = 5
3	22	36	54
4	40	67	100
5	62	104	160
6	90	154	234

[a]Lehmann (1975).

In several publications, the distribution of the number of revertants is used in parametric models. However, even for the historical controls, this is difficult. Therefore, we use nonparametric tests for the discrete (including tied) endpoints with small sample sizes, called permutative versions. Simpson and Margolin (1986) published a Jonckheere trend test with a predetermined change point, while a simple partial order procedure using u tests can be found in Neuhäuser and Hothorn (1995).

Both the twofold and Simpson and Margolin (1986) approaches with Salmonella–microsome (Ames) assay data are demonstrated in Table 10. For the twofold rule there is no effect because there is no mean $\bar{x}_j > 161.4$ $(= 2 \cdot 80.7)$. For the Simpson and Margolin (1986) approach, the change point q is calculated as:

TABLE 12 Mortality Data from a Carcinogenicity Study on Rats with a Duration of Two Years[a]

Control, $n_0 = 50$			D_{high}, $n_0 = 50$		
Week	Died	$W_C(t)$	Week	Died	$W_{D_{\text{high}}}(t)$
0	—	1.0	0	—	1.0
52	1	0.98	44	3	0.94
53	1	0.96	53	4	0.86
63	2	0.92	56	1	0.84
75	1	0.90	62	1	0.82
94	2	0.86	63	2	0.78
99	3	0.80	75	3	0.72
101	1	0.78	76	1	0.70
102	4	0.70	83	2	0.66
103	2	0.66	91	2	0.62
			94	4	0.54
			95	1	0.52
			99	3	0.48
			101	1	0.46
			102	1	0.44
			103	4	0.36

[a]Control and high dose only.

$$q = \max_{h \le j \le k} k \ge 1: \sum_{h=C}^{j} U_{hj} > c_j \quad \text{with } c_j = 0.5 n_j N_{j-1}$$

where U_{hj} denotes the Mann–Whitney counts for group h vs group j and $N_j = n_j$.

j	U	$\sum U_{hj}$	c_j	*Result*
1	U_{C1}	3	4.5	—
2	$U_{C2} + U_{12}$	18	9	
3	$U_{C3} + U_{13} + U_{23}$	24	13.5	
4	$U_{C4} + U_{14} + U_{24} + U_{34}$	23	18	max j
5	$U_{C5} + U_{15} + U_{25} + U_{35} + U_{45}$	15	22.5	

Here, the change point is $q = 4$. The Jonckheere trend test until q is

$$\text{JT}^q = \sum_{i=C}^{q-1} \sum_{j=i+1}^{q} U_{ij}$$

$$\begin{aligned} \text{JT}^q &= U_{C1} + U_{C2} + U_{C3} + U_{C4} + U_{12} + U_{13} + U_{14} \\ &\quad + U_{23} + U_{34} \\ &= 3 + 9 + 9 + 9 + 9 + 9 + 9 + 6 \\ &\quad + 3 + 2 = 68. \end{aligned}$$

This test value must be compared with the quantile $r_{k=5,n=3,1-\alpha=0.95} = 61$. Selected values for the quantiles of the Jonckheere trend test are given in Table 11. Because $\text{JT}^q = 68 > 62$, the null hypothesis is rejected (p value of the permutative test $p = 0.004$). If the Jonckheere trend test had been used for all doses, ignoring the nonmonotonicity,

$$\text{JT} = \sum_{i=C}^{k-1} \sum_{j=i+1}^{k} \text{U}_{ij}$$

$$\begin{aligned} \text{JT} &= U_{C1} + U_{C2} + U_{C3} + U_{C4} + U_{C5} + U_{12} \\ &\quad + U_{13} + U_{14} + U_{15} + U_{23} + U_{24} + U_{25} \\ &\quad + U_{34} + U_{35} + U_{45} \\ &= 3 + 9 + 9 + 9 + 9 + 9 + 9 + 9 + 6 \\ &\quad + 6 + 3 + 0 + 2 + 0 + 0 = 83 \end{aligned}$$

the null hypothesis would not be rejected (quantile $r_{k=6,n=3,1-\alpha=0.95} = 90$; see Table 11).

TABLE 13 Analysis of Tumors without Mortality Adjustment: Males with Benign Leydig-Cell Tumors

	C	1 mg/kg	3 mg/kg	10 mg/kg
$n_{\text{Leydig cell tumor}}$	1	4	3	5
n_0	100	50	50	50
$n_{\text{autolysis}}$	1	0	0	0
$n_{\text{died before 6 months}}$	2	1	0	2
$n_{\text{under tumor risk}}$	97	49	50	48

CARCINOGENICITY STUDIES

The objective of a carcinogenicity study is the estimation of a carcinogenic effect over a lifetime administration of a substance. The long life is accomplished by the use of specific pathogen-free animals, germ-free environment, standard diet, constant temperature, and constant moisture in animals' housing. In this discussion, only terminal killing will be assumed. Whereas serial sacrifies allow for more precise conclusions, the statistical methodology is complicated and beyond the scope of this discussion.

The carcinogenic effect can be determined by:

- Comparing the tumor incidences (or tumor–time relationships) between dose and control groups (primary objective).
- Comparing the survival functions between dose and control groups (secondary objective).
- Comparing additional measures, like body weight, food consumption, hematology, clinical chemistry, and nonneoplastic histopathological findings (tertiary objective).

We will only discuss the primary and secondary objectives. The analysis of the additional measures can be done in analogy to the chronic studies.

Analysis of Mortality

On the one hand, dose-dependent mortality is a criterion for substance effect; on the other hand, mortality and tumor growth are correlated; that is, mortality is the inherent effect of extensive tumor growth, but non-tumor-caused mortality is a competitor to tumor formation.

First for all animals, the cause of death must be evaluated (sometimes by histopathological examination):

1. Died according to the study protocol
2. Killed in extremes (moribund)
3. Killed according to the study protocol
4. Died not according to the study protocol (e.g., artifacts or erroneous manipulation during narcosis or gavaging)

Animals of category 4 will be removed before the analysis; animals of categories 2 and 3 are censored (i.e., nominal date of death ≠ unknown spontaneous date of death). The statistical problem consists in the comparison of the survival functions between dose groups and the control. Frequently, a dose trend can be assumed. Model-based (e.g., proportional-hazard model) or model-free (e.g., nonparametric tests for censored data using generalized Wilcoxon statistics) assumptions can be used.

Graphical representation of the product–limit estimator of the survival functions (and if possible the confidence curves) is helpful (Table 12). Statistical differences between these survival-time functions can be estimated by confidence intervals or special tests for censored data.

Kaplan and Meier (1958) Estimator

$$W_j(t) = \prod_k (1 - x_{jk}/n_{jk})$$

where t denotes the different times t_k (e.g., 52, 53, or 63 weeks), x_{jk} is the number of death in group j at time t_k, and n_{jk} is the number of animals in group j at risk of dying at t_k. For example, for the high-dose-group results until week 44, $W_{D_{\text{high}}}(1) = (1 - 3/50) = 0.94$; until week 53, $W_{D_{\text{high}}}(2) = 0.94{*}(1 - 4/47) = 0.86$.

Analysis of Tumors

The principles of tumor development can be illustrated by

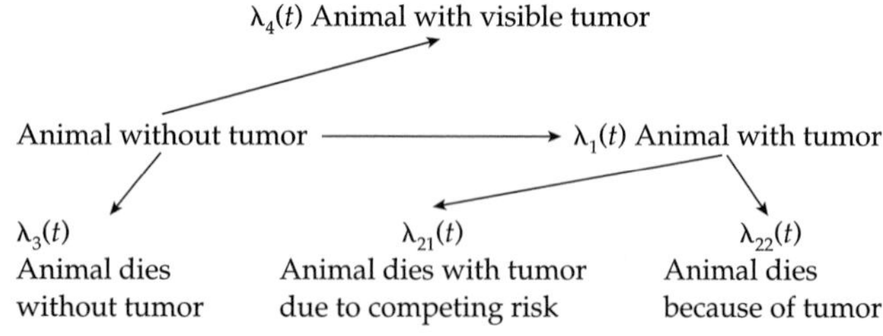

where $\lambda_i(t)$ denotes the probabilities from one level to another. The definition of "carcinogenic risk" is a multisource problem.

- Increased incidence of a dose group with respect to the negative control (increased tumor risk $\lambda_1(t)$).

- Increased prevalence of a dose group with respect to the negative control, where prevalence is the probability (tumor exists | animal is living).
- Reduction of latency time of a tumor of a dose group with respect to the negative control where latency time is $t \mid \lambda_1(t) = 0$.
- Increased incidence of visible tumors (i.e., increased risk of $\lambda_4(t)$).
- Observation of untypical tumor sites for the used strain.
- Increased degree of metastazation or multiple tumors within one site.

Tumors should be classified as:

- Mortality-independent tumors (e.g., tumors that are visible or found palpation). The latency time can be predicted with more or less precision.
- Internal tumors found during macroscopic or microscopic examination.

1. fatal tumors (i.e., cause of the animal's death)
2. incidental tumors (i.e., not the cause of the animal's death)

Competing risks could be other tumors, non-neoplastic reasons, or preprotocol sacrifice. Other classification criteria are

- Benign tumors.
- Malignant tumors.
- Tumors of an organ system (e.g., tumors in the sexual system).
- Tumors of an organ (e.g., liver tumors).
- Tissue-specific organs (e.g., bronchial adenoma).

These tumor findings can be analyzed using mortality-unadjusted (crude proportions) or mortality-adjusted methods. Independent of the magnitude of the global mortality differences, a mortality-adjusted analysis is necessary. Crude proportions (percentages) can be used; however, the statistical results might be biased.

TABLE 14 Analysis of an Incidental Tumor

Time interval	Definition	C	D_{low}	D_{high}
81–104 weeks	Number of tumors	0	0	2
	Number of animals at tumor risk	15	14	19
Terminal sacrifice	Number of tumors	0	1	0
	Number of animals at tumor risk	37	31	26

Analysis of Tumor Incidences without Mortality Adjustment

Here, the data of a $2 \times (k + 1)$ contingency table are analyzed.

	Control	*Dose*$_1$	$\cdots$	*Dose*$_k$	*Total*
Number of animals with tumor	r_C	r_{D1}	$\cdots$	r_{Dk}	$r.$
Number of animals without a tumor	o_C	o_{D1}	$\cdots$	o_{Dk}	$o.$
$\sum$ = animals under tumor risk	n_C	n_{D1}	$\cdots$	n_{Dk}	$n.$

Usually, separate pairwise comparisons of treated animals versus the negative control are performed by a one-sided approximate χ^2 two-sample test for proportions with continuity correction. Because of the small sample sizes and tumor rates, an exact test should be done (e.g., Fisher's or Barnard's test). Even more appropriate are many-to-one procedures for proportions; see the Passing (1984) procedure.

The correct definition of the number of animals under tumor risk is important. Normally, from the initial sample sizes n_0, the number of animals that died very early (i.e., before a predefined time, such as 12 months or before the first tumor was observed will be subtracted). This will also be done for the animals that are not autopsied (because, e.g., of autolysis or cannibalism). Therefore, the organ-specific number under risk is normally different.

Because the decision for a biologically relevant tumor effect is valid if a monotonic dose–response exists, a trend test should be used. Here again, the Armitage (1955) trend test can be used. Tumor incidences are analyzed in this way (Table 13). Because of small animal and tumor numbers, the exact version of the Armitage (1955) trend test was used.

The one-sided p values is 0.016; hence a dose-dependent increase of Leydig cell tumor can be assumed.

In a carcinogenicity study, multiple tumor sites are to be analyzed simultaneously. Up to about 30 to 50 sites are examined because an a priori definition of a target tumor site is seldom possible. Therefore, a multiple-testing problem exists. Some statistical procedures exist to treat this problem, but a simple decision rule according to Haseman (1983) can also be used: A relevant effect is valid if the p value is less than 0.05

for a common tumor (spontaneous rate > 1%); the p value should be less than 0.025 for a rare tumor (spontaneous rate < 1%).

Tumor findings can also be reported as total number of tumors, number of benign tumors, number of malignant tumors, number of tumors of an organ system, and the number of tumors in an organ. Again, the increased false-positive rate should be taken into account.

Mortality-Adjusted Tumor Analysis

For fatal tumors, the null hypothesis assumes that the risk of dying is equal to the risk of developing a tumor and that this risk is the same for all groups. Therefore, all surviving animals and animals that died because of a competing risk are censored. Data should be simply arranged in a stratified $2 \times (k + 1)$ contingency table, where the strata represent the order of mortality time (e.g., as experimental weeks). The responder r_{ji} is the number of animals with a selected fatal tumor (i.e., tumor-site specific or pooled) and n_{ji} is the number of animals at tumor risk in this time interval.

The risks of mortality for animals without a tumor and those with an incidental tumor are assumed to be equal. The null hypothesis is: All animals within a selected time interval have the same probability of an incidental tumor regardless of the treatment. Therefore, an analogous stratified table similar to the fatal-tumor table exists. However, the number of animals at tumor risk in a particular time period is the number of animals that died or were sacrified in that time period. Suitable time intervals should be chosen so that the number of animals at tumor risk is not zero for any treatment group. This can be accomplished by methods that are data-driven (ad hoc runs according to Peto *et al.* 1980) or with an a priori definition (e.g., for rats, time intervals should be defined according to the National Toxicology Program (NTP) into 0–12, 12–18, 18–20, 20–22, and 22–24 months and terminal sacrifice intervals). The latter is much simpler and more reproducible, and is recommended. Combined analysis of both fatal and incidental tumors is also possible. In Table 14, a real data example is analyzed in this way. The animals at tumor risk in the time interval are those animals that died or were killed. Because of the small number of animals at risk and the small number of tumors, a permutative test is recommended. Here a stratified Armitage (1955) trend test was used and a p value of 0.07 (asymptotic version) was calculated by the program STATXACT (Metha *et al.*, 1995). Combined analysis of both fatal and incidental tumors is also possible.

BIOSTATISTICS IN REGULATORY TOXICOLOGY

The good laboratory practice (GLP) regulations have had a deep influence on the conduct of regulatory toxicology studies. The major principles, standard operating procedures (SOPs) and validation, are also applicable to the statistics. Hence, for biostatistical analysis, SOPs should be worked out and only validated software should be used.

Bibliography

Armitage, P. (1955). Tests for linear trends in proportions and frequencies. *Biometrics* **11,** 375–386.

Cariello, N. F., and Piegorsch, W. W. (1996). The Ames assay: The two-fold rule revisited. *Mutation Res.* **369,** 23–31.

Conover, W. J., and Salsburg, D. S. (1988). Locally most powerful tests for detecting treatment effects when only a subset of patients can be expected to respond to treatment. *Biometrics* **44,** 188–196.

Dunnett C. W. (1955). A multiple comparison procedure for comparing several treatments with a control. *J. Am. Statist. Ass.* **50,** 1096–1121.

Hahn G. J., and Meeker, W. Q. (1991). "Statistical Intervals." John Wiley and Sons, New York. pp. 75–99.

Haseman, J. (1983). A re-examination of false-positive rates for carcinogenicity studies. *Fund. Appl. Toxicol.* **3,** 334–339.

Hsu, J. C. (1996). "Multiple Comparisons." Chapman & Hall, New York.

Jonckheere, A. R. (1954). A distribution-free k-sample test against ordered alternatives. *Biometrika* **41,** 133–145.

Kaplan, E. L., and Meier, P. (1958). Nonparametric estimation from incomplete observations. *J. Am. Statist. Ass.* **53,** 457–481.

Lin, K. K., and Ali, M. W. (1994). Statistical review and evaluation of animal tumorigenicity studies. *In* "Statistics in the Pharmaceutical Industry" (C. R. Buncher and J. Y. Tsay, eds.), pp. 19–57. M. Dekker, New York.

Kruskal, W. H., and Wallis, W. A. (1952). Use rank on one-criterion variance analysis. *J. Am. Statist. Ass.* **47,** 583–621.

Lehmann, E. L. (1975). "Nonparametrics." Holden-Day, New York. p. 429.

Levene H. (1960). Robust tests for equality of variance. *In* "Contributions to Probability and Statistics," pp. 278–292. Stanford University Press.

Marcus, R., Peritz, E., and Gabriel, K. B. (1976). On closed testing procedures with special reference to ordered analysis of variance. *Biometrika.* **63,** 655–660.

Mehta C, and Patel N. (1995). StatXact 3 for Windows. Cytel Software Corp., Cambridge.

Neuhäuser, M., and Hothorn, L. A. (1995). Auswertung der Dosis-Wirkungs-Abhängigkeit des Ames Mutagenitätsassay bei direkter Kontrolle des Konsumentenrisikos. *In* "Medizin. Informatik, Biometrie und Epidemiologie, Vol. 80, Medizinische Forschung und ärztliches Handeln" MVM Medizin Verlag, München (H. J. Trampisch and S. Lange, eds.), pp. 113–116.

Neuhäuser, M, and Hothorn, L. A. (1997). Trend tests for dichotomous endpoints. *Drug Information J.* **30,** 463–469.

Passing, H. (1984). Exact simultaneous comparisons with control in a rxc contingency table. *Biometr. J.* **26,** 643–654.

Peto, R. *et al.* (1980). Guidelines for simple, sensitive significance tests for carcinogenic effects in long-term animal experiments. *In* "Long-Term and Short-Term Screening Assays for Carcinogens: A Critical Appraisal," IARC monographs supplement 2, pp. 311–426. IARC Lyon.

Simpson, D. G., and Margolin, B. H. (1986). Recursive nonparametric testing for dose-response relationship subject to downturns at high doses. *Biometrika* **73,** 589–596.

Steel, R. G. D. (1959). A multiple comparison sign test: Treatments vs. control. *J. Am. Statist. Ass.* **54,** 767–775.

CHAPTER

3

Principles of Toxicokinetics

BURCKHARD FICHTL

Walther Straub Institute of Pharmacology and Toxicology, Ludwig Maximilians University, Munich, Germany

INTRODUCTORY REMARKS

The effects of any foreign compound (xenobiotic) acting on the body of man or animals depend on the pharmacodynamic and pharmacokinetic properties of the substance. Pharmacodynamics (Greek φαρμακον = drug, poison; δυναμισ = strength, power) deals with the effects that a substance exerts and the mechanisms of action, and thus describes "what a substance does to the body." Both the magnitude and the time course of effects also depend on the fate of a substance in the body. Pharmacokinetics (Greek κινειν = to move) deals with the time course of the concentrations of a substance in the body, which is the net result of the interplay between absorption, distribution, and elimination. Pharmacokinetics thus describes "what the body does to the substance."

What Is Toxicokinetics?

According to Case (1993), the term "toxicokinetics" was apparently first used in a paper published by a Russian author in 1937. Since then, the term toxicokinetics has gained in popularity, but its use has not been very consequent (see the examples given in Table 1). In recent years, there appears to be a tendency to restrict its use to preclinical toxicology studies. It may be questioned, however, whether the peculiarities of these studies, such as the use of different animal species and rather high doses, merit toxicokinetics being regarded as a special discipline. For instance, kinetic aspects may be of importance also in toxicological studies concerned with the effect of low doses of environmental chemicals in humans. One should not lose sight of the fact that toxicokinetics—in any form—is essentially based on pharmacokinetic principles that apply to any xenobiotic, be it a drug used for therapeutical purposes or a toxicant. In order to avoid possible embarrassment, in the present chapter we will largely rely on the neutral term "kinetics."

Pharmco(toxico)kinetic Parameters

The fate of a drug (or any xenobiotic) in the body may be characterized by the LADME scheme (Fig. 1.) If a drug is administered in a drug product, it must be liberated first. If not injected directly into the circulation, a drug must be absorbed from an absorption site (e.g., gastrointestinal fluid or intramuscular or subcutaneous injection site). After entering the systemic circulation, the drug is distributed via the blood stream to the tissues and will eventually reach its site(s) of action. To a certain extent, most substances become reversibly bound to plasma proteins and/or tissue constituents. A substance may be degraded by metabolism (biotransformation) and ultimately it is excreted from the body. During the processes of absorption, distribution, metabolism, and excretion, a drug has to permeate biological membranes. Drugs cross membranes mainly by passive diffusion. According to Fick's law, the diffusion rate is directly proportional to the concentration gradient across a membrane. Furthermore, it depends on the lipid solubility of the substance in question. For an ionizable drug, lipid solubility depends on its pK_a value and the pH of body fluids. Obviously, the fate of a sub-

TABLE 1 Is There a Discipline Toxicokinetics and If So What Is It?	
Definition	**Source**
"Toxicokinetics is . . . the application of pharmacokinetic principles to the investigation of toxicity and other adverse effects of drugs."	Yacobi *et al.* (1989)
"The primary purpose of toxicokinetics is to provide information on the rate, extent, and duration of exposure of the test animal species to the test compound during the course of a toxicity study."	Chasseaud (1993)
Toxicokinetics may be defined as "the generation of pharmacokinetic data either as an integral component in the conduct of nonclinical toxicity studies or in specially designed supportive studies, in order to assess system exposure."	ICH2 (1993)
"Toxicokinetics is a unique expansion of the science of pharmacokinetics. The major difference between the two disciplines, of course, is that toxicokinetic studies are generally carried out at much higher doses than those used in pharmacokinetic studies."	Welling (1995)
"Toxicokinetics is a subdiscipline of pharmacokinetics dealing with the absorption, distribution, metabolism, and elimination of xenobiotics at doses higher than those expected to produce therapeutic effects."	Dahlem *et al.* (1995)

stance is a highly complex issue and for a detailed discussion of the numerous factors involved the reader should refer to standard pharmacology textbooks.

Given the aforementioned complexities, it may appear rather forward when kineticists dare to characterize the different stages of the LADME scheme by use of a few kinetic parameters. The principal kinetic parameters used to describe absorption, distribution, metabolism, and excretion are bioavailability, volume of distribution, and clearance. The principal kinetic parameters used to describe the time course of drug concentrations are half-life, the area under the concentration time curve (AUC), and the maximal and minimal concentrations in plasma. The latter four parameters may be viewed as "secondary" parameters because they depend on the "primary" parameters of bioavailability, volume of distribution, and clearance.

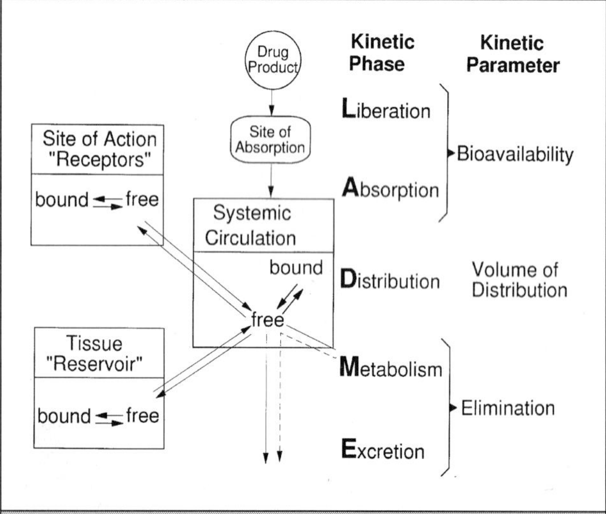

FIGURE 1 Schematic representation of the fate of a drug in the body (LADME scheme).

PRINCIPAL KINETIC PARAMETERS

The following discussion concerns the principal kinetic parameters that allow us to describe the time course of a drug in the body. Measurement of drugs is to a large extent limited—at least in humans—to the determination of concentrations in blood or plasma and in the excreta, such as urine or feces. Plasma, besides being a convenient sampling site, appears to be a rational "reference fluid" for kinetic calculations. Both when a drug is injected directly into the blood or is absorbed from a site of administration, it first enters the plasma space. From plasma, it can enter the blood cells and be eventually distributed via the blood stream to the different body tissues. It is a tenet basic to pharmacokinetics that it is the concentration in plasma water ("free" or "unbound" concentration) that equilibrates with the concentration at the site(s) of action. Ideally, therefore, kinetic calculations should be based on this concentration. However, the determination of the free concentration requires tedious and time-consuming procedures, such as equilibrium dialysis, ultrafiltration, and gel filtration. Thus, in practice kinetic calculations are largely based on the total concentrations in plasma.

Volume of Distribution

The volume of distribution (V) is a parameter that relates the total amount (A) of a drug in the body to its concentration in plasma (C), i.e.,

$$A = V \cdot C \tag{1}$$

or

$$V = \frac{A}{C} \tag{2}$$

As a parameter relating an amount (e.g., mg) to a concentration (e.g., mg/liter), it has the dimension of volume, usually given in liters, or when referenced to body weight, in liters per kilogram. Average values of the apparent volume of distribution for selected drugs are compiled in Table 2. The numerical values cover a wide range, extending over several orders of magnitude. It is important to realize that the volume of distribution as defined in Eq. (1) does not necessarily correspond to the real volume into which the drug distributes.

Depending on the ability of a drug to permeate capillary walls and cell membranes, three major distribution spaces are available in the body: the plasma, the extracellular volume (i.e., plasma plus interstitial fluid), and total body water (plasma plus interstitial fluid plus intracellular fluid). The plasma volume of a "standard" 70-kg man is about 3 liters on the average, corresponding to about 0.04 liters/kg body weight. The volume of extracellular fluid is 15 liters (about 0.2 liters/kg) and total body water amounts to about 42 liters (0.6 liters/kg). As can be seen from the data given in Table 2, calculated distribution volumes of drugs may be far in excess of total body water. For example, chlorpromazine has a distribution volume of 20 liters/kg (Table 2), or 1400 liters in a 70-kg man. Most drugs do not evenly distribute in the body. If a large amount is sequestered in tissues or fat, a given dose will result in a much lower plasma concentration than would be anticipated if the drug distributed in body water only. Therefore, calculation of the distribution volume according to Eq. (2) may result in *apparent* distribution volume that exceeds the physiological distribution space (Fig. 2).

In interpreting numerical values of the volume of distribution, one also must consider that most drugs are to a certain extent bound to plasma proteins. The calculated apparent volume of distribution depends not only on the magnitude of the real distribution spaces, but also on the relative extent of binding in plasma and tissues (Fig. 3) This explains why, for most drugs, the apparent distribution volume does not correspond to one of the major physiological dis-

TABLE 2 Examples for the Apparent Volume of Distribution (*V*) of Selected Compounds[a]

Compound	V
Heparin	0.06
Insulin	0.08
Tolbutamide	0.1
Warfarin	0.2
Ampicillin	0.3
Theophylline	0.4
Isoniazid	0.6
Phenytoin	0.6
Ethanol	0.65
Paracetamol	1.0
Pentobarbital	1.8
Procainamide	2.0
Morphine	2.0
Quinidine	2.3
Propranolol	3.0
Lidocaine	3.0
Meperidine	3.5
Digoxin	7.0
Imipramine	15.0
Chlorpromazine	20.0

[a]The values are referenced to body weight (liters/kg).

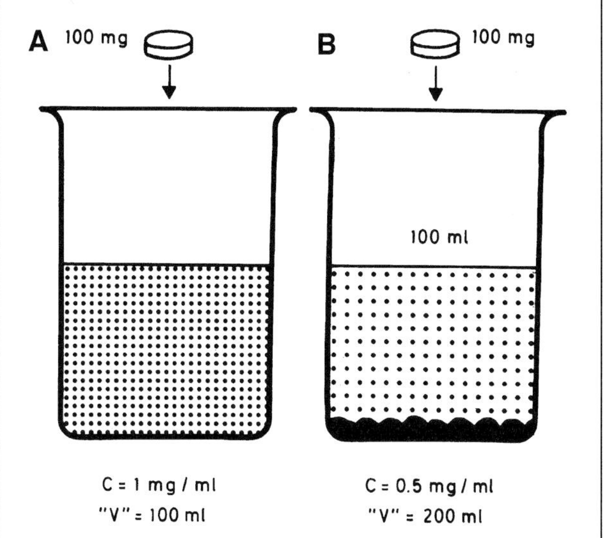

FIGURE 2 The concept of the apparent volume of distribution. In this simplified model the body is represented as a beaker filled with water. (A) An amount (*A*) of 100 mg of a drug is dissoluted in 100 ml yielding a concentration (*C*) of 1 mg/ml. According to the equation $V = A/C$, the volume of distribution is calculated as 100 mg/(1 mg/ml) = 100 ml, which equals the real distribution space. (B) Again 100 mg is administered. Part of this drug is accumulated in tissues (represented in the model by precipitation at the bottom of the beaker). Therefore, the resulting concentration is lower than in the previous experiment. Calculation in this case results in 100 mg/(0.5 mg/ml) = 200 ml, yielding an apparent distribution volume that greatly exceeds the real distribution space.

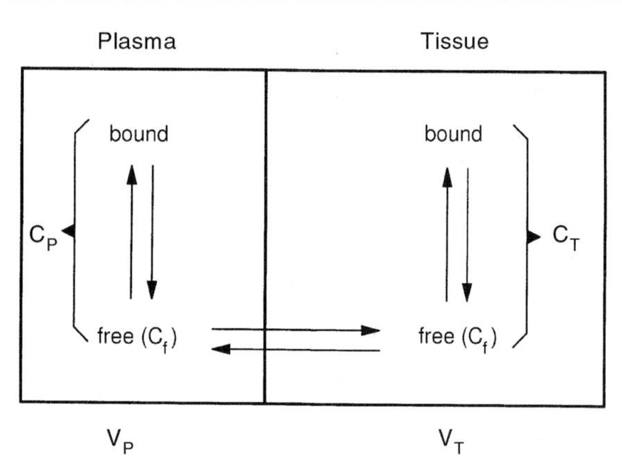

FIGURE 3 Dependence of the apparent volume of distribution on plasma and tissue binding. The body is represented by a simple model consisting of a plasma and a tissue compartment, having the volumes V_P and V_T, respectively. The total concentrations in plasma and tissue are C_P and C_T. Both in plasma and in tissue, part of the drug is reversibly bound (e.g., to albumin or tissue proteins); the respective free (unbound) fractions are f_P and f_T. Only the free molecules can cross the barrier between plasma and tissue. After equilibrium is obtained the free concentration (C_f) in plasma and tissues is equal. The total amount in the body is given by $A = V_P \cdot C_P + V_T \cdot C_T$ and according to the definition (Eq. (1)) the volume of distribution is $V = A/C_P = V_P + V_T \cdot (C_T/C_P)$. With $C_P \cdot f_P = C_f$ and $C_T \cdot f_T = C_f$, it follows that $C_T/C_P = f_P/f_T$, thus yielding $V = V_P + V_T \cdot (f_P/f_T)$. It should be noted that V is the calculated *apparent* volume of distribution, whereas V_P and V_T are *real* volumes. According to the relationship derived, several typical cases may be discerned:

1. No binding in plasma or tissue: $f_P = f_T = 1 -> V = V_P + V_T$ (i.e., the apparent volume of distribution equals the real distribution space (example ethanol; cf. Table 2).
2. Extent of binding in plasma is higher than in tissue: $f_P < f_T -> V < V_P + V_T$ (i.e., the apparent volume of distribution is lower than the real distribution space (example: heparin).
3. Extent of binding in plasma is lower than in tissue: $f_P > f_T -> V > V_P + V_T$ (i.e., the apparent volume of distribution exceeds the real distribution space (example: chlorpromazine).
4. Equal extent of binding in plasma and tissue: $f_P = f_T -> V = V_P + V_T$ (i.e., the apparent volume of distribution equals the real distribution space (example: phenytoin).

tribution spaces and why its numerical value can assume virtually any value in between or even in excess of total body water (see Table 2). Despite these limitations, the concept of the apparent volume of distribution is extremely useful for practical purposes. If its numerical value is known, one can calculate, using Eq. (1), the dose that will result in a certain (therapeutic or toxic) concentration in plasma.

Volume Terms in Pharmacokinetics

In the foregoing discussion, it was tacitly assumed that a steady state between the concentrations in plasma and tissues had been obtained. This does not necessarily imply that the concentrations are the same throughout the body, but rather that the concentrations in plasma and tissues equilibrate so rapidly that they vary with time in parallel. The body behaves as a single "compartment." For some drugs, this assumption of one-compartment kinetics is a reasonable approximation. In this case, the definition of the volume of distribution given by Eq. (1) is unequivocal. The calculated volume term is equivalent to the "volume of distribution at steady state" (V_{ss}). For many drugs, however, the time course of distribution must be taken into account. Under these circumstances the volume of distribution as calculated by Eq. (1) is no longer constant, but depends on the time.

Suppose a drug is injected intravenously. Immediately after injection the whole amount of the drug resides in plasma. The quotient between the amount in plasma and the initially high plasma concentration (the "initial volume of distribution") is low (Fig. 4). Later on, the drug distributes from plasma to tissues and only after distribution is complete does the steady state volume of distribution, which exceeds the initial distribution volume apply. If the redistribution from tissues to plasma is slow, then the tissue concentrations lag behind the plasma concentrations and a pseudo-equilibrium is obtained, during which the ratio between the amount in the body and the plasma concentration is higher than in true equilibrium; that is, the calculated volume of distribution exceeds the volume of distribution at steady state. For reasons discussed in the following, this volume term calculated during the elimination phase is called V_{area}, V_β, or V_z.

Clearance

The clearance is a measure of the body's ability to eliminate a substance. The term "elimination" subsumes both the actual removal of a substance from the body by excretion and the conversion of a substance by metabolism (Fig. 5). The major pathways for excretion of unchanged substances are excretion by the kidneys into the urine, secretion into the bile with subsequent passage through the gut and excretion into the feces, and exhalation from the lungs. Occasionally a compound may be secreted from the blood directly into the gut lumen, as has been observed with thallium ions. Small amounts can be removed from

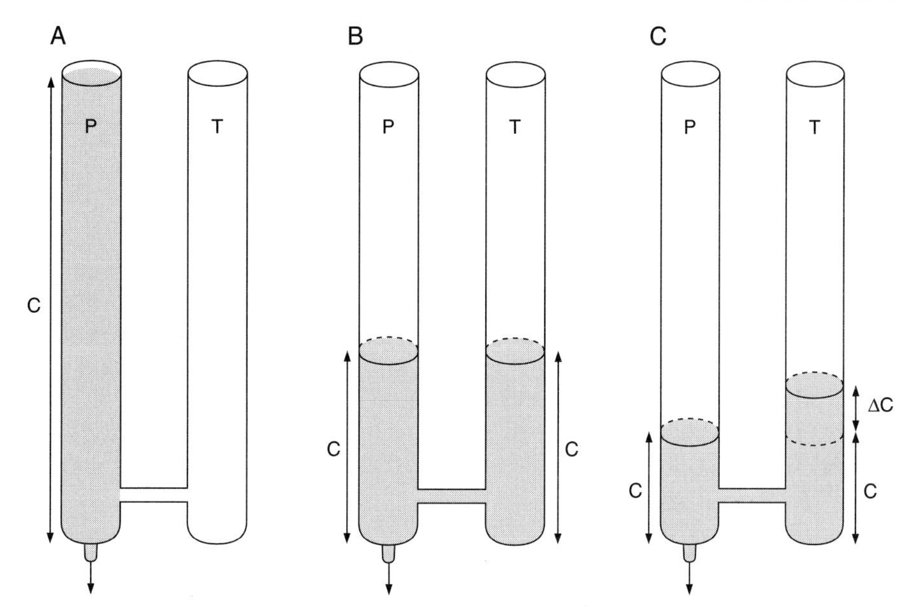

FIGURE 4 The different types of distribution volumes. The meaning of the different volume terms used in pharmacokinetics can be visualized by a model using water containers. The height of the water column represents the concentration (C) of a drug in plasma (P) or tissue (T). The amount of water in the containers is given by the product $C \cdot B$, where B denotes the base area of the respective container (B_P and B_T, respectively). The volume of distribution is calculated according to Eq. (2) as the quotient between the total amount in the system and the plasma concentration. (A) First a certain amount of water is poured into the "plasma" (corresponding to an intravenous bolus dose). Immediately after the "injection" the drug (water) is contained only in the "plasma." The initial volume of distribution at this moment in time is calculated as $V_{\text{initial}} = (C \cdot B_P/C) = B_P$. (B) The water distributes from "plasma" to "tissue." When equilibrium between the two compartments is attained (i.e., no net transfer occurs) the volume of distribution at steady state is given by

$$V_{ss} = \frac{C \cdot B_P + C \cdot B_T}{C} = B_P + B_T.$$

(C) Since the water drains from the "plasma," the "concentration" (height of water column) will diminish in both compartments. If the redistribution from "tissue" to "water" is slow compared to the elimination from the "plasma," the water level in "tissue" will lag behind. Thus the volume of distribution during the elimination phase (usually denoted as V_z) is

$$V_z = \frac{C \cdot B_P + (C + \Delta C) \cdot B_T}{C} = B_P + B_T \cdot \left(1 + \frac{\Delta C}{C}\right).$$

Hence $V_{\text{initial}} < V_{ss} < V_z$. Adapted from Fichtl *et al.* (1996).

the body by excreta such as saliva, milk, tears, or desquamated epithelial cells. From the kinetic point of view, a substance is also eliminated when it has been changed into something else (i.e., a metabolite), although the metabolites may still be present in the body. The metabolities are ultimately removed from the body by excretion. Metabolism occurs primarily in the liver, but other organs are also capable of metabolizing foreign compounds (Fig. 5).

The concept of clearance to characterize the ability of the kidneys to eliminate a substance has been used by physiologists for a long time. However, all other ("nonrenal") processes involved in the elimination of foreign compounds can also be characterized by a clearance. The total clearance (CL) of a compound is the sum of the renal (CL_R) and nonrenal (CL_{NR}) clearance. By definition the clearance is a proportionality constant relating the elimination rate (amount per

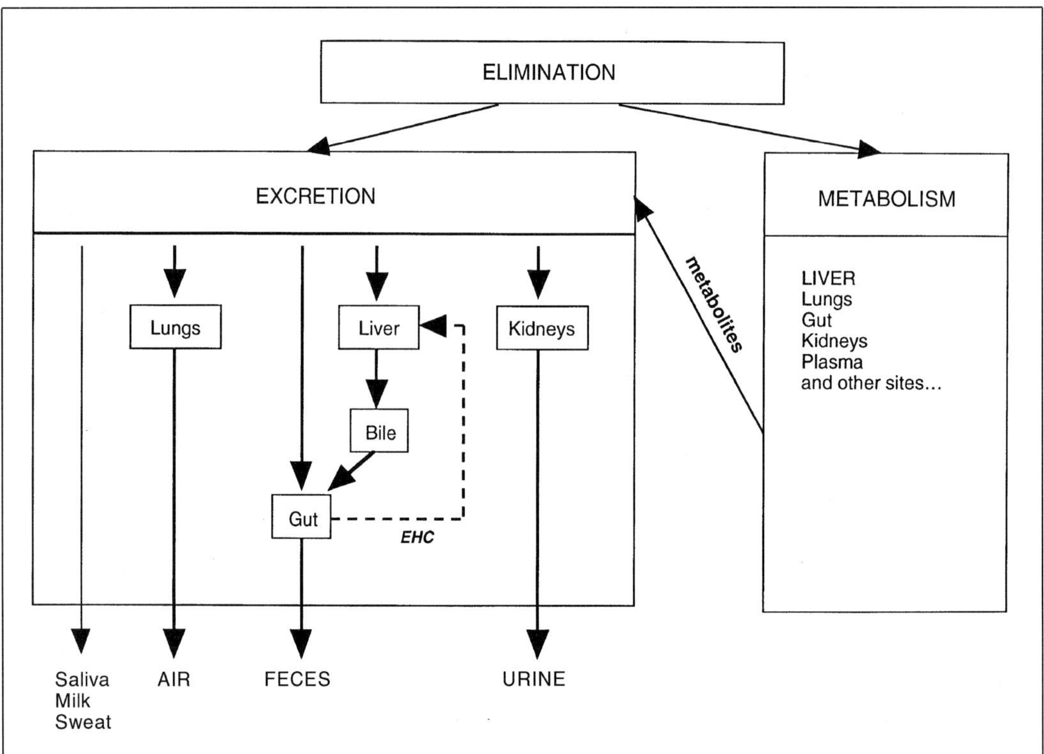

FIGURE 5 Pathways of elimination. Foreign compounds are eliminated from the body by excretion. From the kinetic point of view a substance is also eliminated when it has changed into something else by metabolism (biotransformation). The metabolites are ultimately removed from the body by excretion. Occasionally a substance excreted via bile into the small intestine may be reabsorbed during the passage of the gut (EHC, enterohepatic cycling).

unit of time, A/t) of a compound to its concentration in plasma (C),

$$\frac{A}{t} = \mathrm{CL} \cdot C \tag{3}$$

or as a differential equation,

$$-\frac{dA}{dt} = \mathrm{CL} \cdot C. \tag{4}$$

Clearance values can also be calculated based on the concentration in another reference fluid, such as the free (unbound) concentration in plasma water or the concentration in whole blood. From the defining equation, it is apparent that the clearance has the dimension of volume per time, usually given as ml/min ($\mathrm{ml} \cdot \mathrm{min}^{-1}$) or liters/h ($\mathrm{liters} \cdot \mathrm{h}^{-1}$). When referenced to (i.e., divided by) body weight, the units are $\mathrm{ml} \cdot \mathrm{min}^{-1} \cdot \mathrm{kg}^{-1}$ or $\mathrm{liters} \cdot \mathrm{h}^{-1} \cdot \mathrm{kg}^{-1}$.

To visualize the concept of clearance, it is often stated that the clearance can be viewed as the volume of plasma (or another reference fluid) that is cleared of a substance per time unit. However, the essential meaning of clearance becomes more apparent if it is conceived simply as a parameter that allows for the calculation of the elimination rate of a substance at a given plasma concentration.

Renal Clearance

Three mechanisms are involved in renal elimination: glomerular filtration, tubular secretion, and tubular reabsorption (Fig. 6). The renal plasma flow (RPF) is 600 ml/min on average. One-fifth of this volume is filtered during the passage of plasma through the capillaries of the glomeruli, thus yielding a glomerular filtration rate (GFR) of about 120 ml/min. The estimated effective pore radius of the glomeruli is 3 nm. Molecules having a high molecular mass (MM $>$ 60,000), such as albumin or hemoglobin, can virtually not pass the renal filter membranes. On the other hand, any solute not bound to plasma proteins and having a MM $<$ 15,000 is freely filtered in the same proportion as the water.

After filtration, most of the water is reabsorbed during the passage of the tubular system. If, for in-

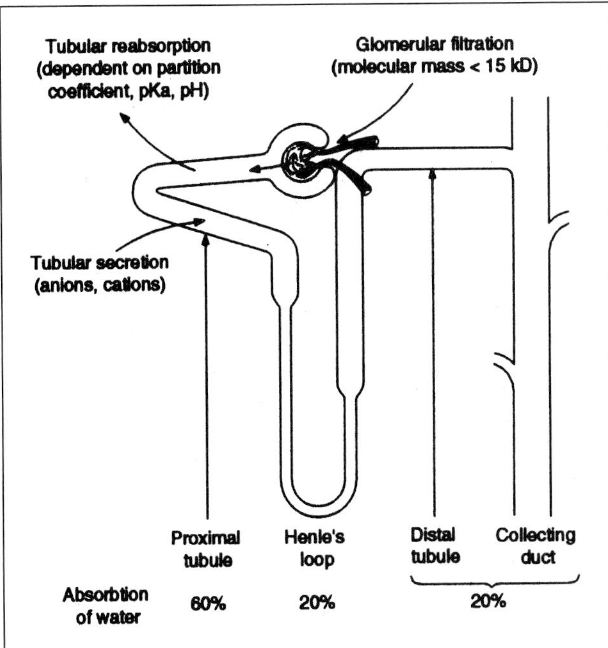

FIGURE 6 Scheme of a nephron, the functional unit of the kidneys. Adapted from Fichtl *et al.* (1996).

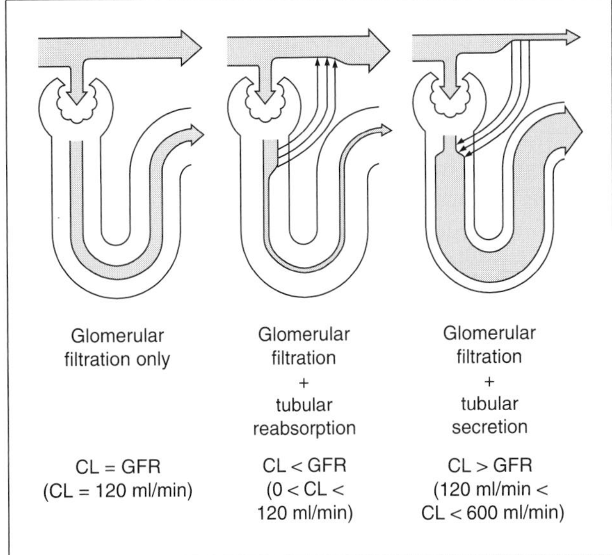

FIGURE 7 Renal clearance as a resultant of glomerular filtration rate (GFR) and tubular handling. The scheme applies to any substance that can be freely filtered (molecular mass <15 kDa, no binding to plasma proteins). Adapted from Fichtl *et al.* (1996).

stance, the urine output is 1.5 liters per day, more than 99% of the glomerular filtrate (120 ml/min, corresponding to about 170 liters/day) has been reabsorbed. Accordingly, polar solutes that cannot cross the epithelial cells of the renal tubulus will be concentrated during the tubular passage, their concentration in the urine exceeding that in plasma by a factor of 100 or more.

The elimination rate of such a compound is given by the product of GFR and the plasma concentration C. Substituting into Eq. (3) yields

$$\frac{A}{t} = \mathrm{GFR} \cdot C = \mathrm{CL}_R \cdot C$$

or

$$\mathrm{CL}_R = \frac{\mathrm{GFR} \cdot \mathrm{C}}{\mathrm{C}} = \mathrm{GFR}. \qquad (5)$$

In other words, the renal clearance of a polar compound that is excreted solely by glomerular filtration and not bound to plasma proteins equals the glomerular filtration rate (cf. Fig. 7). It is possible, therefore, to determine the glomerular filtration rate by measuring the renal clearance of substances meeting these requirements (e.g., inulin or creatinine).

Lipophilic compounds can be reabsorbed during the passage of the renal tubules. Accordingly, the amount eventually excreted in the urine is lower than the amount filtered and their renal clearance is below the glomerular filtration rate (Fig. 7). Tubular reabsorption occurs mainly by passive diffusion, depending on the concentration gradient between the tubulus lumen and the plasma water. Essentially, only the lipophilic uncharged form of weak bases or acids can be reabsorbed. Thus their renal clearance is dependent on the respective pK value and urine pH. While glomerular filtration rate is normally held fairly constant by autoregulation mechanisms of the perfusion pressure in the glomeruli, the extent of water reabsorption, and consequently urinary flow, may vary appreciably. As previously discussed, for polar drugs not reabsorbed in the tubule, the total amount filtered is ultimately excreted. For such compounds, variations in the urine flow rate due to variations in the amount of water reabsorbed will affect only the *concentration* in the urine. The *amount* excreted, the excretion rate, and consequently the renal clearance are not influenced by urine flow.

On the other hand, tubular reabsorption of lipophilic compounds may be influenced by the urine flow rate since it is facilitated by low flow rates. For a substance that is rapidly reabsorbed (i.e., that can "follow" the water), renal clearance is low and approaches the urinary flow rate. Diuretics or fluid therapy can alter the renal clearance of substances subject to tubular reabsorption.

Many endogenous substances and foreign compounds not only are filtered in the glomeruli, but also can be secreted from the blood into the tubular lumen by active transport processes. The tubular cells possess transport systems for organic acids and bases. Examples of compounds that are considerably secreted by glucuronide and sulfate conjugates are uric acid, furosemide, and penicillins. For drugs that are handled in this manner, renal clearance exceeds the glomerular filtration rate (Fig. 7). If the secretion is fast enough, virtually all of the substance in the plasma is cleared during the passage through the kidneys. If the substance is not reabsorbed in the tubule its excretion rate is

$$\frac{A}{t} = \mathrm{RPF} \cdot C = \mathrm{CL}_R \cdot C \tag{6}$$

or

$$\mathrm{CL}_R = \mathrm{RPF}. \tag{7}$$

That is, the renal clearance equals the renal plasma flow (RPF). *p*-Aminohippuric acid (PAH) is handled in this manner and can be used to measure RPF.

Metabolic Clearance

Drug metabolism or biotransformation is another important route of elimination. The reactions are usually divided into two phases. Phase I reactions involve oxidation, reduction, and hydrolysis. Phase I reactions may both decrease and increase the biological activity of compounds. Inactive compounds (pro-drugs) can be transformed into active ones (e.g., parathion to paraoxon). In phase II reactions, also denoted as synthetic reactions, an endogenous substance is attached to the parent drug or to a phase I metabolite. Examples are the conjugation of a compound with glucuronic acid, sulfate, acetate, methyl groups, and glycine. Most conjugates are inactive, a notable exemption being morphine-6-glucuronide which is more effective than its parent compound. As discussed above, lipophilic drugs cannot be cleared by the kidneys effectively. Many biotransformation reactions decrease the lipophilicity of the respective compounds. The polar metabolites can be excreted by the kidneys and other excretory pathways.

In principle the activity of drug-metabolizing enzymes can be described by the Michaelis–Menten equation (cf. Fig. 8),

$$v = \frac{v_{max} \cdot C}{K_m + C}. \tag{8}$$

The rate of metabolism (amount metabolized or

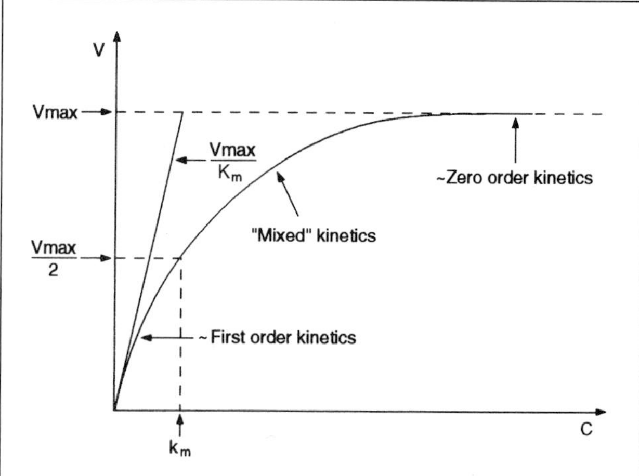

FIGURE 8 Elimination according to Michaelis–Menten kinetics. The relationship between the reaction velocity v (the amount of a substance that is metabolized per time unit) and the concentration C is hyperbolic. At concentrations below the Michaelis constant K_m is approximately linearly related to C.

"eliminated" per time unit) is given by the parameter v, the velocity of the reaction. Using the notation introduced above, Eq. (8) is equivalent to

$$v = -\frac{dA}{dt} = \frac{v_{max} \cdot C}{K_m + C}. \tag{9}$$

For most drugs encountered in clinical practice, the concentrations achieved at the sites of metabolism are well below the Michaelis constant, that is, $C \ll K_m$. In this case, Eqs (8) and (9) reduce to

$$v = \frac{v_{\max}}{K_m} \cdot C \tag{10}$$

and

$$-\frac{dA}{dt} = \frac{v_{\max}}{K_m} \cdot C \tag{11}$$

respectively. Obviously, Eq. (11) is analogous to Eq. (4); under these circumstances ($C \ll K_m$), the elimination rate due to metabolism is proportional to the concentration. The proportionality constant is the clearance that is determined by the ratio $v_{\max}/K_m$. Thus the elimination of drugs by metabolic conversion can also be described by the clearance concept defined by Eq. (4).

Occasionally drugs are administered in a dosage range that yields concentrations near to or above the Michaelis constant (e.g., phenytoin). Even higher concentrations may be encountered in drug overdose or intoxication by other foreign compounds. Under these circumstances, the enzymes become saturated and the concept of a constant clearance no longer applies. When the enzymes are saturated, the elimination rate is constant ($=v_{max}$) and independent of the plasma concentration. This in turn means that the clearance calculated as the (amount eliminated per time unit)/ C is dependent on the concentration and hence the time. The consequences of saturable or "nonlinear" elimination will be dealt with later.

Clearance and "Area under the Curve" (AUC)

In principle, the clearance can be measured according to the defining equation (Eq. (3)) by sampling the amount eliminated over a certain time period (A/t) and dividing by the plasma concentration (C). This is a frequently used approach to determine the renal clearance of a substance, since it is relatively easy to measure the amount excreted into urine. On the other hand, it may be difficult or even impossible to measure the amount eliminated via other pathways. Fortunately, the total clearance of a substance can be determined solely from the time course of plasma concentrations without having to resort to sampling at all possible sites of elimination. When the plasma concentrations are plotted against time, the area under the concentration time curve (AUC) may be calculated. Obviously, the magnitude of the total AUC (from zero to infinity) depends on the amount of a substance that has entered the body; higher doses will result in higher concentrations. It is important to realize that the AUC is also dependent on clearance. If a drug is slowly cleared from the body, higher concentrations are measured than if it is eliminated more rapidly.

Provided that linear kinetics apply, the following relationship between AUC, drug dose (D), and clearance (CL) holds (Fig. 9),

$$\text{AUC} = \frac{F \cdot D}{\text{CL}}, \tag{12}$$

where F is the fraction of the dose that has been absorbed. Strictly speaking, F is the fraction of the dose that has entered the systemic circulation, as discussed in more detail under bioavailability.

Equation (12) provides a convenient means of determining the total clearance of a substance. For instance if a substance is introduced directly into plasma by intravenous injection ($F = 1$) and the resulting plasma concentrations are measured, the total clearance can be calculated by dividing the intravenous dose (D_{iv}) by AUC,

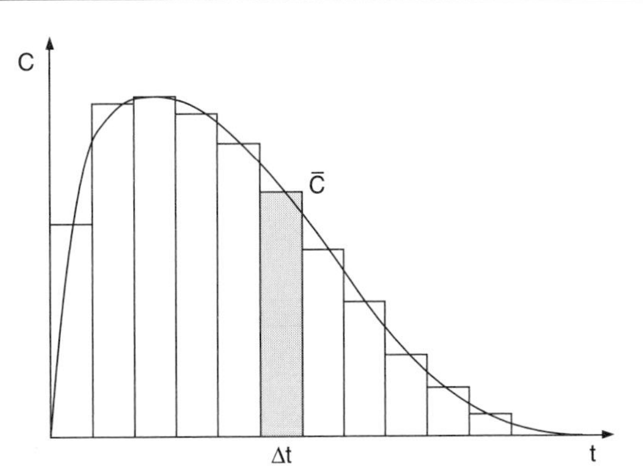

FIGURE 9 The relation between clearance and AUC. The curve represents the time course of plasma concentrations (C) after administering a certain dose (D) of a drug. The elimination follows first-order kinetics (i.e., the amount eliminated per time unit is directly proportional to C); the proportionality constant is the clearance CL (cf. Eq. (4)). The amount (ΔA) that is eliminated in a small time interval (Δt) is then given by $\Delta A = \text{CL} \cdot \bar{C} \cdot \Delta t$, $\bar{C}$ is the average plasma concentration during the time interval Δt. The product $\bar{C} \cdot \Delta t$ is represented by the area of the shaded rectangle. The total amount eventually eliminated (A_e) can be assessed by summing up all rectangles, $A_e = \text{CL} \cdot \Sigma\bar{C} \cdot \Delta t$. With decreasing interval width, this sum approaches the AUC. Mathematically this is equivalent to the integration $A_e = \text{CL} \cdot \int_0^\infty C \cdot dt = \text{CL} \cdot \text{AUC}$. If the drug is not irreversibly retained in the body, the total amount eventually eliminated (A_e) equals the fraction of the dose ($F \cdot D$) that has been absorbed. Hence, AUC = $(F \cdot D)/\text{CL}$. Adapted from Fichtl *et al.* (1996).

$$\text{CL}_{\text{tot}} = \frac{D_{\text{iv}}}{\text{AUC}_{\text{iv}}}. \tag{13}$$

Should a drug be eliminated by different pathways, the total clearance is the sum of the clearance terms for the individual elimination processes.

The renal clearance can be calculated from the fraction of the absorbed dose that is eliminated unchanged in urine. If the urine is collected completely over a sufficient time, the total amount eventually eliminated in urine (U_e) can be measured and renal clearance can be calculated in analogy to Eq. (13) as

$$\text{CL}_{\text{ren}} = \frac{U_e}{\text{AUC}}. \tag{14}$$

The nonrenal or extrarenal clearance is then given by the difference between total and renal clearance.

Half-Life and First-Order Elimination

If a drug is eliminated with a constant clearance, its elimination rate can be described by the differential equation given previously in Eq. (4),

$$-\frac{dA}{dt} = \mathrm{CL} \cdot C$$

Taking into account the relationship between the amount of a drug in the body and its volume of distribution in Eq. (1) we can write

$$-V \cdot \frac{dC}{dt} = \mathrm{CL} \cdot C \tag{15}$$

or

$$-\frac{dC}{dt} = \frac{\mathrm{CL}}{V} \cdot C \tag{16}$$

and with the substitution

$$k = \frac{\mathrm{CL}}{V} \tag{17}$$

we obtain

$$-\frac{dC}{dt} = k \cdot C. \tag{18}$$

When the rate of elimination and, consequently, the decrease of plasma concentration are proportional to the current concentration in plasma, the elimination is said to follow first-order kinetics. This designation arises from the exponent of C in the differential equation describing the kinetics. The equation can be written as $-(dC/dt) = k \cdot C = k \cdot C^1$. Similarly, the kinetics is said to be zero-order if the elimination rate is constant, that is, $-dC/dt) = k = k \cdot C^0$.

Integrating Eq. (18) yields

$$C = C_0 \cdot e^{-k \cdot t}. \tag{19}$$

Thus the decrease of the plasma concentration can be described by an exponential function with the first-order rate constant k. The exponential decay of the plasma concentration resulting from first-order kinetics is shown in Fig. 10A. At first the elimination rate is high; the concentration decreases rapidly. With decreasing plasma concentrations, the elimination rate slows down (cf. Eq. (4)), resulting in the typical curvature of the concentration–time plot. A process following first-order kinetics can be described by a half-life, which is the time taken by the plasma concentration to fall to half its value (Fig. 10). Equation (19) may be linearized to facilitate the determination of half-life. Taking the logarithm of both sides, Eq. (19) becomes

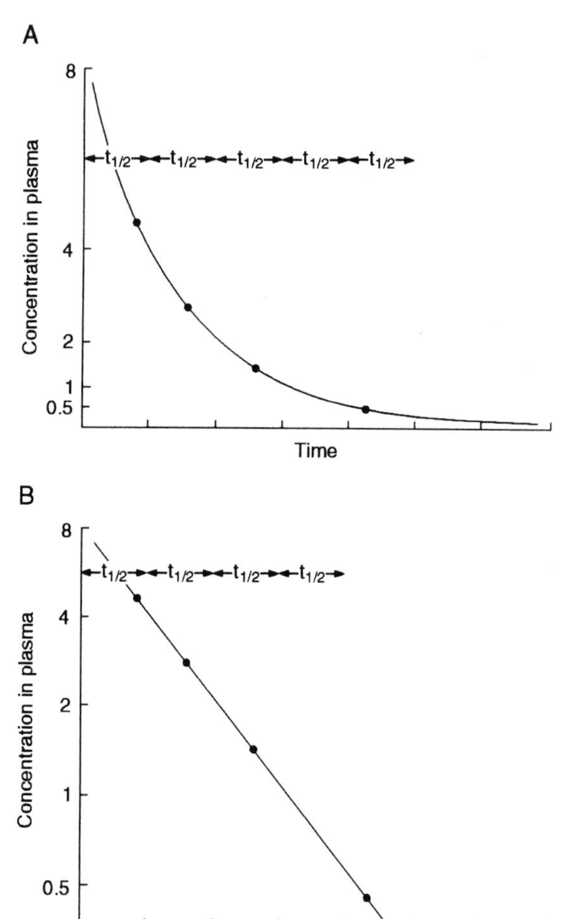

FIGURE 10 Plasma concentration–time profile of a drug eliminated by first-order kinetics. (A) Linear plot: The elimination rate decreases proportional to the plasma concentration, thus resulting in a curvature of the plot. The half-life ($t_{1/2}$) is the time needed for the plasma concentration to fall to half its value. If first order kinetics apply $t_{1/2}$ is a constant. In real life only discrete points of the curve are available, which makes the precise estimation of $t_{1/2}$ difficult. (B) Semilogarithmic plot: If the concentrations are plotted on a logarithmic scale the curve is linearized and the data points are centered about a straight line. Adapted from Fichtl *et al.* (1996).

$$\ln C = \ln C_0 \cdot e^{-k \cdot t}. \tag{20}$$

Hence,

$$\ln C = -k \cdot t + \ln C_0. \tag{21}$$

Thus when plotting the (natural) logarithm of the concentrations against time, a straight line is obtained (Fig. 10B) with the slope $-k$ and the intercept ln C_0.

Half-Life as a "Hybrid" Kinetic Parameter

Half-life is probably the most "popular" kinetic parameter. Nevertheless, misconceptions are common when interpreting its meaning. It is important to realize that half-life depends not only on the efficiency of the elimination processes (i.e., the clearance), but also on the distribution volume of a substance. Looking at the simple kinetic model depicted in Fig. 4, we have a situation analogous to first-order elimination. The water is driven out by the hydrostatic pressure, which is proportional to the height of the water column. Thus the rate at which the water level decreases is proportional to the current water level and can be described by a half-life. The amount of water eliminated per time unit depends on the height of the water column and the width of the outlet. The greater the diameter of the outlet (i.e., the clearance), the more rapidly the water runs out, that is, the shorter the half-life. However, the half-life depends not only on the width of the outlet but also on the dimensions of the system. Suppose we repeat the experiment in a system where the water reservoirs have twice the base area as before. The amount eliminated per time unit at a given water level is the same as before, depending only on the height of the water column and the width of the outlet. However, the system contains twice the amount of water; that is, the "volume of distribution" has doubled. Therefore the water level will decrease at a slower pace than before; it will take double the previous time to empty the reservoirs.

The quantitative relationship between half-life, clearance and distribution volume can be easily derived. After one half-life, the initial concentration has decreased to half its value. Substituting into Eq. (19) we obtain

$$\frac{C_0}{2} = C_0 \cdot e^{-k \cdot t_{1/2}} \tag{22}$$

or

$$\frac{1}{2} = e^{-k \cdot t_{1/2}} \tag{23}$$

and taking the logarithm of both sides,

$$-\ln 2 = -k \cdot t_{1/2}. \tag{24}$$

Hence,

$$t_{1/2} = \frac{\ln 2}{k} \tag{25}$$

and together with Eq. (17) we obtain, finally,

$$t_{1/2} = \ln 2 \cdot \frac{V}{CL} \tag{26}$$

Considering that the natural logarithm of 2 can be approximated as ln 2 = 0.693 . . . or ln 2 ≈ 0.7, Eq. (26) for practical purposes may be rewritten as

$$t_{1/2} = 0.7 \cdot \frac{V}{CL}. \tag{27}$$

The longer the half-life, the greater the volume of distribution; and the shorter the half-life, the greater the clearance. Table 3 summarizes the kinetic parameters of diazepam and warfarin. Although the ability of the body to eliminate these drugs as assessed by the clearance is eight times higher for diazepam, the half-lives of both drugs are approximately equal. According to Eq. (26), this is explained by the about eightfold-greater distribution volume of diazepam.

The half-life is the resultant of two parameters that may vary independently, and as such it may be viewed as a compound or "hybrid" parameter. Obviously the same reasoning applies to the rate constant for elimination (cf. Eq. (17)).

TABLE 3 Kinetic Parameters of Diazepam and Warfarin[a]

	Diazepam	Warfarin	Ratio
Volume of distribution (liter·kg^{-1})	1.1	0.14	7.9
Clearance (liters·h^{-1}·kg^{-1})	0.023	0.0027	8.5
Half-life time (h)	43	37	1.2

[a]Data from Benet *et al.* (1995).

[b]Despite marked differences in volume of distribution and clearance, the half-life is approximately the same for both drugs.

The fact that the parameters used to characterize the time course of a drug in plasma are compound parameters must be considered, for instance, when interpreting a half-life that is longer than normal. A prolonged half-live may result from a decrease in clearance (e.g., in renal insufficiency or liver disease) or from an increase of distribution volume (for a lipophilic drug, e.g., due to an increase of body fat). Furthermore, half-life may be "normal" even if the parameters determining its value are grossly altered. A notable example is the interaction between digoxin and quinidine. It has been reported that quinidine markedly enhances the plasma concentrations of digoxin in patients treated with this drug. Quinidine decreases both the clearance and the distribution volume of digoxin. In some patients both parameters decrease in the same proportion, resulting in an unchanged half-life. Thus a normal half-life does not preclude anomalous kinetic behavior.

Consulting the relevant literature, one may come across statements such as: "According to the relationship CL $= k \cdot V$, the clearance depends on the distribution volume and the elimination rate constant or its reciprocal, the half-life." Obviously this is a gross misunderstanding. It stands to reason that the clearance can be *calculated* according to

$$\mathrm{CL} = k \cdot V \tag{28}$$

if k and V are known. However, the clearance does not *depend* on them. Equation (28), despite being a mathematically correct transformation of Eq. (17), does not describe the factual relationship between the parameters.

Terminal Half-Life and Dominant Half-Life

When a drug is injected intravenously, it is in general not confined to the plasma space. Lipophilic compounds readily pass through the capillary walls and may accumulate in tissues. Even polar substances can leave the plasma through "pores" in the capillary wall and distribute at least in the extracellular fluid. If tissue distribution is not extensive, the initial mixing up between plasma and extracellular fluid may occur so fast that this distribution phase is not seen by the measured plasma concentrations. In this case, the time course of plasma concentrations can be described by a single exponential term like Eq. (19). The drug is said to obey single-compartment kinetics. Frequently however, two or more phases become apparent when the plasma concentrations are plotted on a logarithmic scale (Fig. 11). In the first phase, often denoted as α-phase, the drug is removed from plasma not only by elimination but also due to extensive distribution into the tissues, and the concentration time curve is steep (cf. Fig. 4; this phase corresponds to the transition from scenario A to B). When the distribution phase is completed, the concentrations decrease together in all parts of the body and the decrease of the plasma concentrations is due to elimination only. This postdistributive phase, often denoted as elimination phase or β-phase, corresponds to the situation depicted in Fig. 4C. Mathematically, the concentration–time curve shown in Fig. 11 can be described by a sum of two exponentials,

$$C = A \cdot e^{-\alpha \cdot t} + B \cdot e^{-\beta \cdot t} \tag{29}$$

and the drug is said to follow two-compartment kinetics.

Provided the processes involved in absorption, distribution, and elimination are all first-order reactions, these processes, too, can be characterized by rate constants or half-lives, respectively, and the time course of plasma concentrations can be described by a sum of exponentials even in cases where multicompartment kinetics apply or after extravasal administration. If more than two exponentials are needed to describe the concentration–time curve, a different notation is often used for the constants,

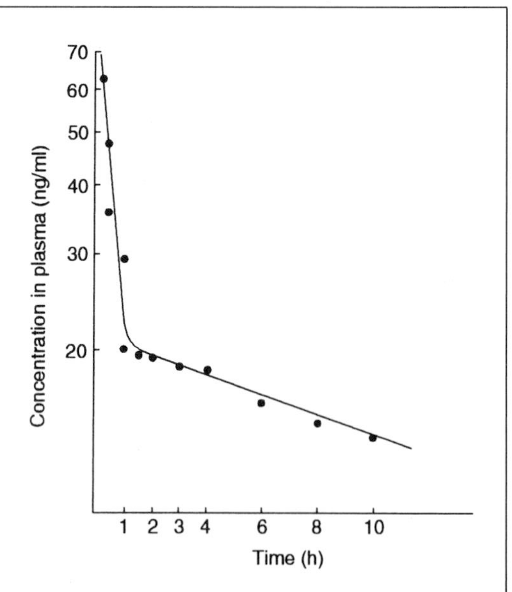

FIGURE 11 Plasma concentrations of verapamil following an intravenous bolus dose of 10 mg. When the concentrations are plotted on a logarithmic scale, two distinct phases are apparent; a rapid initial "distribution" or α-phase is followed by the slower "elimination" or β-phase. Data from Hamann *et al.* (1984).

$$C = P_1 \cdot e^{-\lambda_1 \cdot t} + P_2 \cdot e^{-\lambda_2 \cdot t} + \cdots + P_z \cdot e^{-\lambda_z \cdot t} \quad (30)$$

Depending on the notation used, the terminal (slowest) phase of the concentration–time curve is called the β-phased or z-phase. Consequently, the volume term applying during this phase (cf. Fig. 4C) is called V_β or V_z.

Since each phase of the concentration–time curve is characterized by a rate constant, the corresponding half-life can be calculated according to Eq. (25) as

$$t_{1/2}(1) = \ln 2/\lambda_1$$
$$t_{1/2}(2) = \ln 2/\lambda_2$$
$$\vdots$$
$$t_{1/2}(z) = \ln 2/\lambda_z$$

The half-life of the terminal phase, $t_{1/2}(\beta)$ or $t_{1/2}(z)$ is called the *terminal half-life.*

When the concentration–time curve can be fitted by a sum of exponentials, the total AUC may be calculated from the constants as

$$\text{AUC} = \frac{P_1}{\lambda_1} + \frac{P_2}{\lambda_2} + \cdots + \frac{P_z}{\lambda_z}. \quad (31)$$

The half-life of the phase that according to Eq. (31), contributes most to the AUC is also called the dominant half-life. Frequently, the terminal half-life is also the dominant half-life. Notable exceptions are the aminoglycoside antibiotics. Following the injection of gentamicin, the plasma concentrations decrease from a half-life of about 2–3 h to rather low values, compatible with single-compartment kinetics. After repeated administration, slowly accessible sites in tissues are "filled up." At this stage, the fast α-phase is followed by a β-phase (Fig. 12) with an appreciably longer half-life (>50 h). During the β-phase the slow redistribution of gentamicin from the "deep" compartment is rate limiting for the elimination.

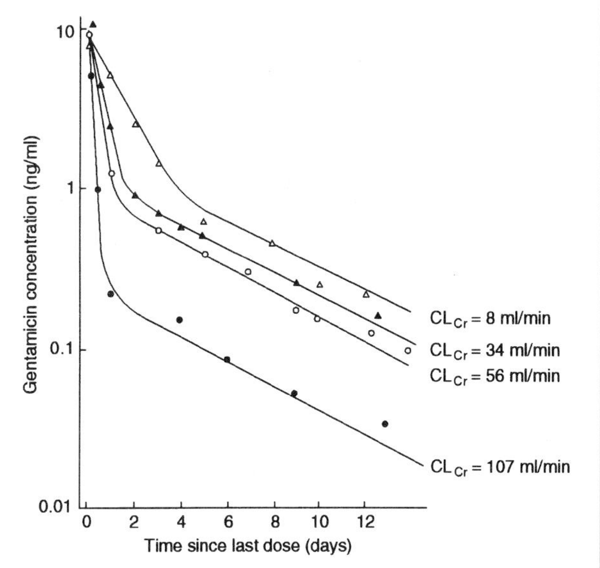

FIGURE 12 Concentration time profile of gentamicin in serum of patients with different renal function. The patients were treated for several days with gentamicin. The measured plasma concentrations after the last dose (symbols) could be fitted using a biexponential equation (solid lines). Obviously the half-life during the initial phase depends on renal function: The lower the creatinine clearance (CL_{Cr}), the longer the half-life. On the other hand, the terminal half-life does not vary appreciably among the patients. During this phase the slow redistribution of gentamicin from tissues is rate limiting for the elimination. Data from Schentag *et al.* (1977).

Bioavailability

If a drug is administered directly into the blood stream (e.g., by intravenous injection or infusion), the entire dose reaches the circulation. The venous blood passes through the right part of the heart and the lungs and returns to the left part of the heart. Via the arteries, the blood is distributed to the different organs and tissues (Fig. 13). In general, the entire dose administered intravenously is available for distribution in the body. Exceptions are drugs that are extensively metabolized in plasma or the lungs. For instance, up to 95% of an intravenous dose of certain prostaglandines may be metabolized during the first passage through the lungs.

Following other routes of application, a drug or toxicant has to be absorbed in order to reach the general circulation. The rate and extent of absorption are influenced by the rate and extent to which a substance is liberated from a drug product and becomes dissolved. During the process of absorption, the agent has to pass biological membranes such as the epithelia of the skin and mucous membranes, and the capillary endothelium (Fig. 13). Thus the rate and extent of absorption depend also on the ability of an agent to pass biological membranes. Even if the entire dose of a drug has been absorbed, it is not necessarily "available." Frequently drugs are administered by the oral route. The blood draining from the stomach, intestines, and the upper part of the rectum has to pass through liver, where appreciable amounts can be metabolized or excreted in the bile during the passage of the blood (Fig. 14). The extraction of a drug from the blood may be so extensive that most of the drug is removed from the blood during the first passage through the liver ("first-pass effect"). For instance, glycerol trinitrate is completely absorbed after oral administration; however, virtually none of the

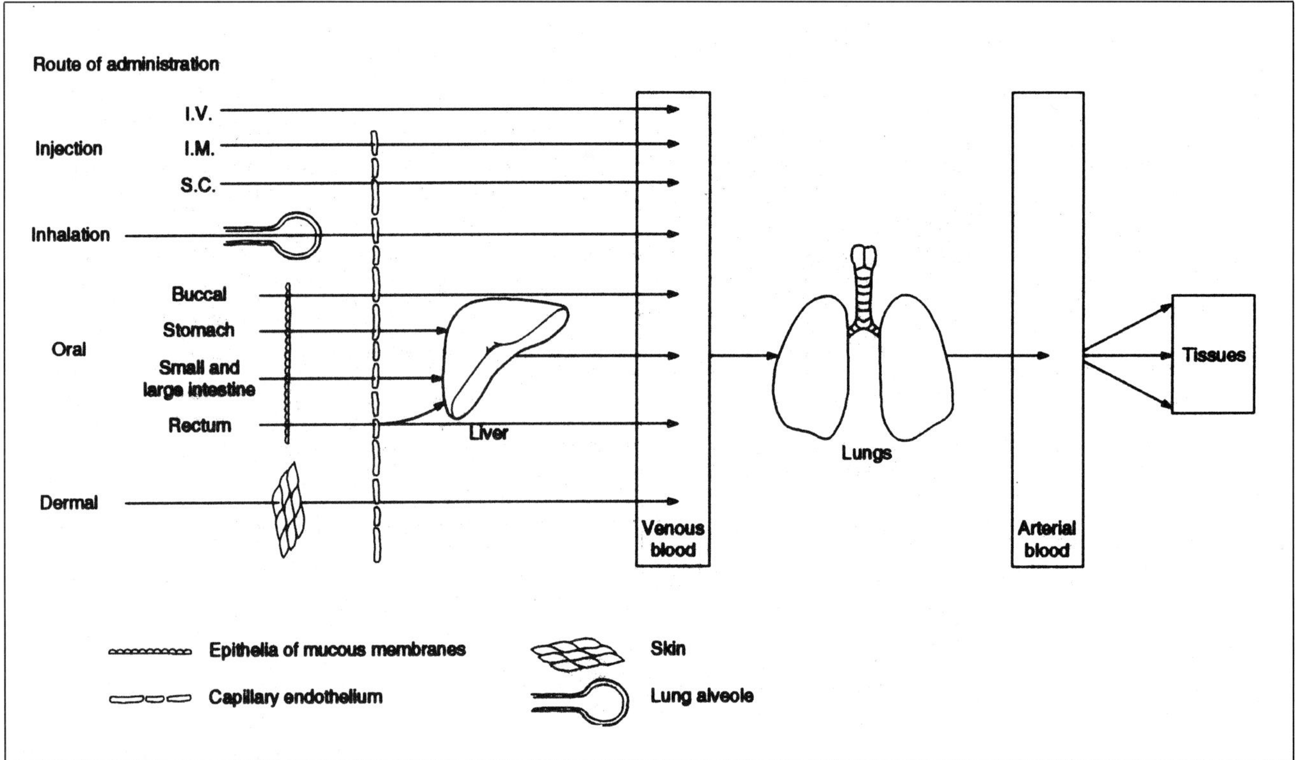

FIGURE 13 Scheme of absorption pathways. Unless a substance is directly injected into the blood stream, it will have to pass (several) biological membranes before it enters the central venous blood pool. It should be noted that after oral administration, a substance absorbed from the stomach, intestines, or the upper part of the rectum has to pass through the liver.

amount absorbed arrives in the general circulation due to complete first-pass metabolism. It is necessary, therefore, to administer glycerol trinitrate sublingually. From the oral cavity, the agent is absorbed into the veins, bypassing the liver. A "presystemic" metabolism of substances may also occur in the mucosa of the gastrointestinal tract (Table 4).

Bioavailability is a term used to describe the rate and extent to which a substance ultimately becomes available after liberation, absorption, and first-pass elimination and as such embraces more than the term absorption. According to the classic definition (Food and Drug Administration, 1977), "bioavailability means the rate and the extent to which the active drug ingredient or therapeutic moiety is absorbed from a drug product and becomes available at the site of drug action." For several reasons, however, this definition is not suitable for practical purposes. Two parameters, rate and extent, are intermingled in one notion. For many substances, the site of action is not known; drugs may exert their effects at several different sites; and even if the site of action is known, it is rarely accessible in the living organism, especially in humans. The measurement of bioavailability is, therefore, based on a more pragmatic definition in which bioavailability refers to the fraction of the administered dose that enters the general circulation.

Assessment of Bioavailability

In most cases, the extent to which a substance enters the circulation is more important than the rate. The extent of bioavailability is defined as the fraction (F) of an administered dose that enters the systemic circulation. If a drug is administered intravenously, its bioavailability is said to be 100% or $F = 1$. It should be noted that this again is a pragmatic definition. As discussed above, in rare cases the "true" availability of an intravenous dose may be lower due to first-pass elimination during the passage through the lungs.

The measurement of the extent of bioavailability after extravasal administration is based on Eq. (12), which states that the AUC is proportional to the amount that has entered the plasma. It should be noted that in deriving the equation (cf. Fig. 9) no

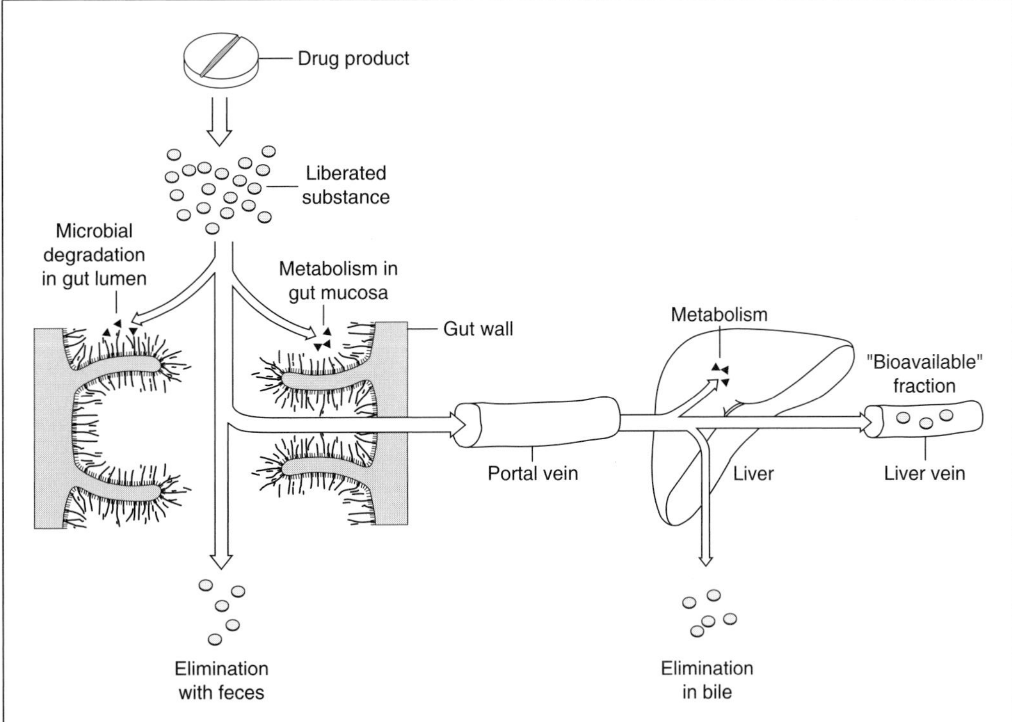

FIGURE 14 Bioavailability and presystemic metabolism. Only that part of an orally administered dose that arrives unchanged in the central venous blood pool is "bioavailable." Bioavailability depends on absorption and presystemic metabolism in the gut and liver. Usually a drug has to be liberated from a drug product. Thus the properties of the respective galenic preparation may also affect the bioavailability. Adapted from Fichtl *et al.* (1996).

TABLE 4 Examples of Drugs That Are Subject to Presystemic Metabolism

Compound	Presystemic metabolism: Hepatic	Presystemic metabolism: Gastrointestinal
Acetylic salicylic acid	+	+
Dihydroergotamine	+	
L-Dopa	+	
Estradiol	+	+
Glyceryl trinitrate	+	
Hydralazine	+	
Imipramine	+	
Isoprenaline	+	+
Lidocaine	+	
Metoprolol	+	
Pentazocine	+	
Pethidine	+	
Propranolol	+	
Salicylamide	+	+
Verapamil	+	

assumption was made as to the route of administration; Eq. (12) holds for any route of administration. For instance, if a drug is administered intravenously the concentration–time profile is quite different from that obtained after administering the drug per os. The AUC, however, is the same provided that the same amount has entered the circulation (Fig. 15). If only a part of the extravascular dose enters the circulation, the AUC is correspondingly lower. Hence the extent of bioavailability after extravascular application may be calculated by comparing the AUC with the AUC obtained after intravenous injection of the same dose (Fig. 16).

When a drug is administered extravascularly, absorption occurs simultaneously with distribution and elimination. The observed time course of the plasma concentrations is the resultant of all three events. Usually a peak in the concentration–time profile is seen. Both the time (t_{max}) at which the maximum concentration (C_{max}) is observed and the magnitude of C_{max} depend on the rate of absorption. In practice the rate of bioavailability is often characterized simply by specifying t_{max} and C_{max} (Fig. 16).

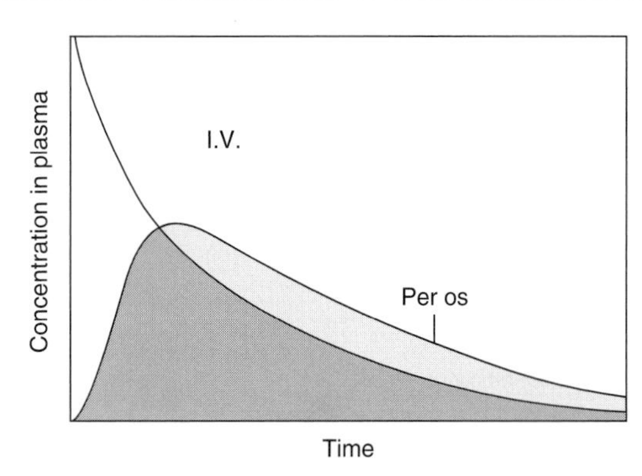

FIGURE 15 The principle of "corresponding areas." The concentration time profile in plasma depends on the route of administration. Provided the same amount of a substance has entered the plasma the area under the concentration time curve (AUC) is the same. This principle, Dost's law, is named after the German pediatricist and pharmacokinetic pioneer of the 1950s. Adapted from Fichtl *et al.* (1996).

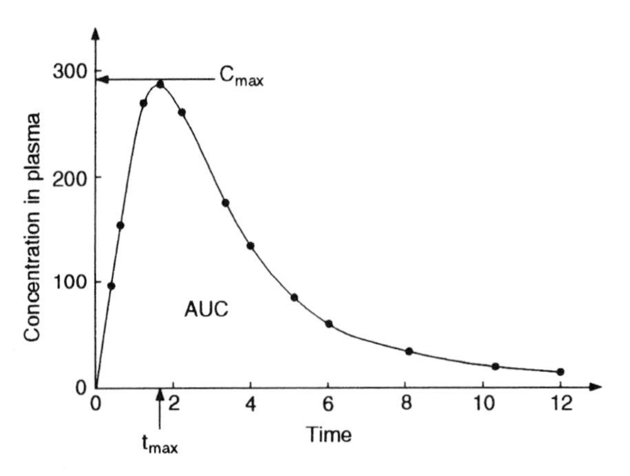

FIGURE 16 Parameters used for the assessment of bioavailability. By definition the extent of bioavailability after intravenous injection of a substance is regarded as 100% (F = 1). Since the amount of a drug that has entered the systemic plasma is proportional to the area under the plasma-concentration time curve (AUC) and to clearance (cf. Fig. 9), the bioavailability after extravasal (ev) administration can readily be estimated by comparing the AUC after extravascular dosing to that after intravenous (iv) administration of the same dose, $F = AUC_{ev} \cdot CL_{ev}/AUC_{iv} \cdot CL_{iv}$. If the extravascular and the intravenous dose are both administered in the same individual, the clearance terms cancel out and the equation can be simplified to read as follows $F = AUC_{ev}/AUC_{iv}$. The bioavailability calculated with reference to an intravenous dose is usually termed *absolute bioavailability*. When comparing the bioavailability of a substance from two different galenic preparations A and B the *relative bioavailability* is given by comparing the respective AUCs obtained after the administration of A and of B, $F = AUC_A/AUC_B$ The rate of bioavailability may be characterized by stating the maximal concentration C_{max} and the corresponding time t_{max}. Two preparations of a drug are said to be bioequivalent if they do not differ with respect to AUC, C_{max}, and t_{max}. A difference of not more than 20–25% is usually regarded as acceptable when stating bioequivalence. Adapted from Fichtl *et al.* (1996).

KINETIC MODELS

Compartmental Analysis

The origins of pharmacokinetics go back to the 1920s and 1930s. Since then, compartment models have been used extensively in pharmacokinetic analysis. In these models the body is treated as consisting of several interconnecting compartments (Fig. 17). A compartment may be viewed as an ideal volume in which the rate of mixing is rapid compared to the rate of entry or leaving, resulting in a uniform concentration within it. If the kinetics of distribution and elimination are linear, that is, the rates are directly proportional to the respective concentrations, the processes can be characterized by appropriate rate constants. The mathematical solution of the pertinent differential equations results in concentration–time profiles corresponding to a series of exponentials (cf. Eq. (30)). The simplest model is the one-compartment model, which is suited to describing the kinetics of drugs that distribute rapidly throughout the body. This does not necessarily imply that the concentrations are the same in all regions of the body, but if distribution is swift enough, the concentrations in all parts of the body run parallel to the plasma concentration and the body behaves as a kinetically homogenous unit. Frequently the assumption of at least two or more compartments is necessary to describe the observed plasma concentration (Fig. 11).

One of the reasons for the popularity of compartment models is the fact that the underlying mathematics is rather simple. The parameters P_i and λ_i in Eq. (30) can readily be obtained by curve fitting, using graphical methods (e.g., "curve-stripping," "peeling," and "feathering"; see Fig. 18) or appropriate computer programs. It must be kept in mind, however, that the compartments are abstract entities that do not correspond to a real anatomical space in the body. Even if the concentration–time profile in plasma perfectly fits to a sum of exponentials, it is difficult or impossible to predict the concentrations in any other tissue of the body.

Noncompartmental Analysis

Essentially we have used a noncompartmental approach in the discussion of the principal kinetic

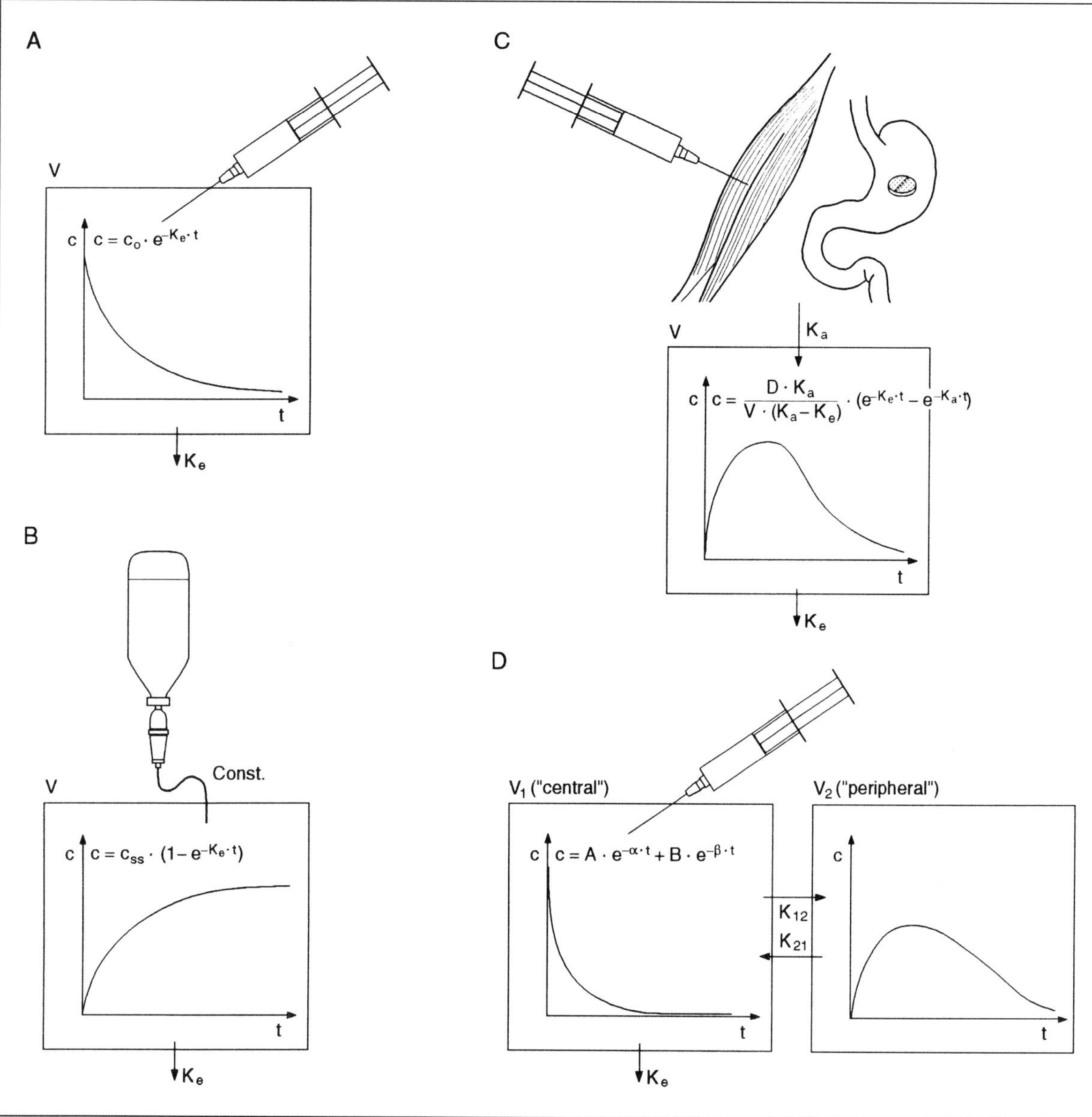

FIGURE 17 Examples of compartment models used in pharmacokinetics. (A) *One-compartment model, intravenous injection.* In the one-compartment model the body is conceived as consisting of one single kinetically homogenous compartment. Elimination occurs by first-order kinetics. After an intravenous bolus dose (*D*), the substance is assumed to instantaneously distribute in the volume *V*. The concentration time profile is then given by a simple exponential function, which is characterized by the initial concentration $C_0 = D/V$ and the elimination rate k_e (or the corresponding half-life, respectively). (B) *One-compartment model, intravenous infusion.* The graph illustrates the concentration time course when a substance is administered by a constant-rate infusion. Eventually a steady state concentration is achieved; the time to achieve steady state depends on the rate constant for elimination. This is discussed in more detail in the section dealing with drug dosing. (C) *One-compartment model, extravascular administration.* After extravascular administration (p.o., i.m. s.c.), the concentration time profile is influenced by the rate and extent of absorption. If absorption obeys first-order kinetics (rate constant k_a) the plasma concentrations are described by a simple biexponential equation (Bateman equation). In most cases absorption is more rapid than elimination, and the rate constant associated with the terminal phase of the plasma concentrations is k_e. If absorption is slow (i.e., $k_a \ll k_e$), absorption becomes rate limiting for the decrease of the plasma concentrations and the terminal phase reflects k_a (flip-flop phenomenon). (D) *Multicompartment models.* Frequently the assumption of two or more compartments has to be made to adequately describe the concentration time profile in plasma. The distribution between the compartments is assumed to follow first-order kinetics. As shown here for the two-compartment model, the concentration time profile may be fitted by a sum of exponentials. From the constants *A, B, α, β*, the rate constants for the transfer between the fictitious compartments ("micro constants") and the time course of the amount in the "peripheral" compartments can be calculated. Adapted from Fichtl *et al.* (1996).

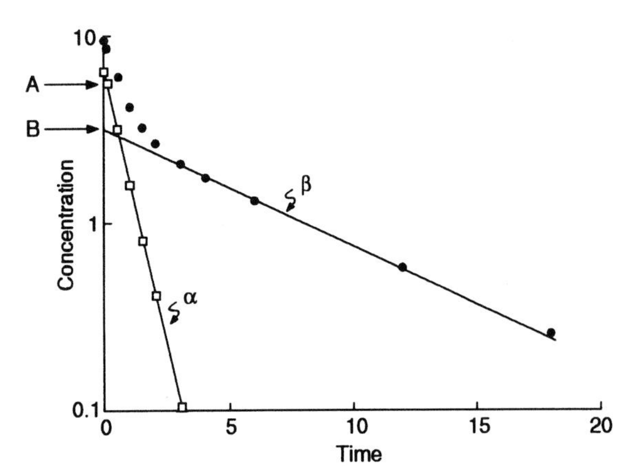

FIGURE 18 "Feathering" of a multiexponential curve. If the plasma concentrations can be described by a sum of exponentials, the parameters determining the equation may be obtained by the method known as "feathering" (also termed "stripping," "peeling" or the method of residuals) as is exemplified here for a function of the type $C = A \cdot e^{-\alpha \cdot t} + B \cdot e^{-\beta \cdot t}$, with $\alpha > \beta$. The concentrations are plotted on a logarithmic scale. At later time points ($t > 5\ t_{1/2}(\alpha)$) the first term of the equation approaches zero. Thus β and the parameter B can be obtained from the slope and the intercept of a regression line through the late data points. At earlier time points the difference (residual) between this line and the measured concentration is $A \cdot e^{-\alpha \cdot t}$. Plotting the residuals (□) results in a straight line from which α and A are obtained. It stands to reason that curve fitting is nowadays preferably done by nonlinear regression using appropriate computer programs. Nevertheless, graphical curve fitting is useful for quickly obtaining estimates of the parameters, which may be used as starting values for computer programs or to assess the plausibility of published data.

parameters describing the absorption, distribution, and elimination. It was possible to define and determine bioavailability, volume of distribution, and clearance without having to resort to a specific compartment model. Only a single assumption is necessary, namely, that the processes involved follow first-order kinetics. The determination of the parameters does not require sophisticated mathematics or curve fitting and is largely based on the measurement of the area under the plasma concentration–time curve. A convenient and practical means to assess the AUC is the numerical approximation by the trapezoidal rule (Fig. 19).

Statistical Moments and Mean Residence Time

In recent years the "model-independent" analysis based on AUC measurements has been complemented by applying the statistical moment theory to pharmacokinetics. This approach was introduced into pharmacokinetics in the late 1970s and, in contrast to the "classic" compartmental kinetics, is often denoted as "modern" pharmacokinetics. It should be pointed out, however, that it is only its application to pharmacokinetics that is new. It has been used for years in chemical engineering and the concept of the mean residence time was described as early as 1931 by the American physiologist Hamilton. A detailed discussion of statistical moment theory is beyond the scope of this chapter and the reader is referred to the pertinent literature.

In principle, statistical moment theory interprets the time course of drug concentrations in plasma as a statistical distribution curve resulting from a stochastic process. If a drug is introduced into the body it is not possible to predict the time span a single molecule will spend in the organism. Using statistical methods it is, however, possible to make predictions concerning the average fate of the population. It can be shown for instance that the mean residence time (MRT) of the molecules in body is given by

$$\mathrm{MRT} = \frac{\int_0^\infty C \cdot t \cdot dt}{\int_0^\infty C \cdot dt} = \frac{\mathrm{AUMC}}{\mathrm{AUC}}. \tag{32}$$

The integral in the numerator of Eq. (32) is the entire area under a plot of $C \cdot t$ versus time (t). The product $C \cdot t$ is called the first moment of the concentration–time curve and accordingly the corresponding area is denoted as the area under the first-moment curve (AUMC). Undoubted statistical moment theory bears great potential for model independent kinetic analysis. Thus it is possible to further characterize the time course of a drug in the body by calculating appropriate mean absorption and transit times. Another useful relation that allows the model independent determination of the volume of distribution at steady state (V_{ss}) following a single intravenous bolus dose is given in Fig. 19. Despite the appealing simplicity of the model-independent methods, their use is somewhat limited by the fact that they require "good" data and frequent sampling to prevent large estimation errors. Nevertheless, the authors of a standard textbook on pharmacokinetics dare to predict that "these trends in pharmacokinetics . . . may make compartmental analysis a matter of historical interest" (Gibaldi and Perrier, 1982).

Physiological Pharmacokinetic Models

Another approach taken in pharmacokinetic analysis is the use of physiological models. Those models

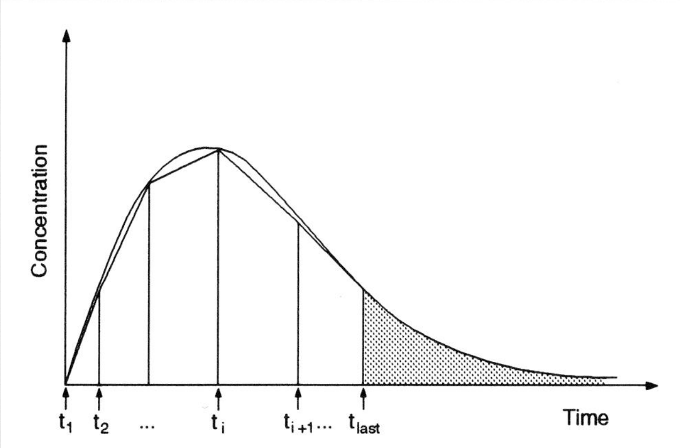

FIGURE 19 Model-independent assessment of AUC and other basic kinetic parameters. The area under the plasma concentration time curve (AUC) can be approximated with reasonable precision by using the trapezoidal rule. The data points are connected by straight lines. The area of the trapezoid between two consecutive data points is $[(C_{i+1} + C_i)/2] \cdot (t_{i+1} - t_i)$ and summing yields $AUC = 1/2\ \Sigma(C_{i+1} + C_i) \cdot (t_{i+1} - t_i)$. The residual area after the last measured concentration (C_{last}) is given by C_{last}/λ_z. The area under the first moment curve (AUMC) can be evaluated in an analogous manner by plotting the products $C_i \cdot t_i$ versus time. The residual area is

$$\frac{C_{last}}{\lambda_z}\left(t_{last} + \frac{1}{\lambda_z}\right).$$

If the plasma concentrations can be fitted by a sum of exponentials AUC and AUMC may be calculated as $AUC = \Sigma(P_i/\lambda_i)$ and $AUMC = \Sigma(P_i/\lambda^2_i)$, respectively. The rate constant λ_z and the corresponding half-life $t_{1/2}$ can be obtained directly from a log-linear plot of the plasma concentrations (cf. Fig. 18). Further we can calculate: mean resident time, MRT = AUMC/AUC; clearance, $CL = D_{iv}/AUC$; volume of distribution, $V_\beta = V_z = V_{area} = D_{iv}/(AUC \cdot \lambda_z)$; steady state volume of distribution, V_{ss} = CL/MRT; and after extravascular administration bioavailability, $F = AUC_{ev}/AUC_{iv}$.

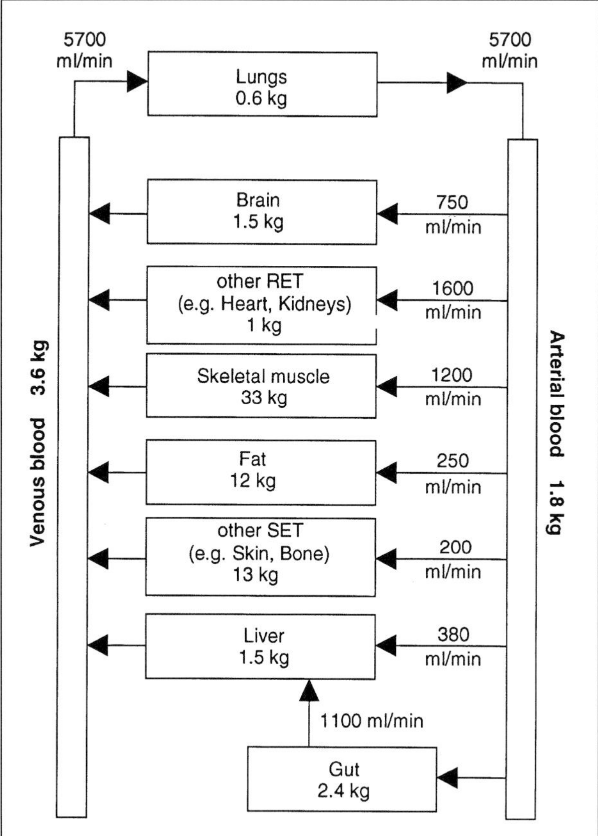

FIGURE 20 Example of a typical physiologically based pharmacokinetic model. Besides organ weight and blood flow, additional data such as the respective extraction ratio and tissue–plasma partition coefficient may be needed for a thorough description of the fate of a drug. RET, rapidly equilibrating tissues; SET, slowly equilibrating tissues.

are based on a more realistic representation of the body and comprise at least the major organs (Fig. 20). They also incorporate numerous parameters, such as the actual values of tissue size, blood flow through the organs, permeability of membranes, binding of drug to plasma proteins and tissue constituents, drug partitioning into lipids, and organ clearances.

Writing the appropriate rate equations and integrating them provides a framework for the more or less complete description of drug kinetics. Physiological modeling has been successfully applied to several drugs and toxicants (Table 5). By use of physiological models important questions may be addressed that cannot be tackled with compartmental models. Notable examples are the influence of circulatory changes such as hemorrhagic shock on drug kinetics, the influence of fat content of the growing organism on the kinetics of lipophilic organochlorine compounds, or the accessibility of crucial organs to anticancer drugs.

KINETIC PRINCIPLES OF DRUG DOSING

Most therapeutic and toxic effects exerted by drugs or toxicants depend on the concentration of the respective agent at its site of action. In many cases the site of action is not known or not accessible for measurement. For many substances, however, the ranges of plasma concentration that are necessary for a therapeutic effect or are associated with toxicity are known. The use of pharmacokinetic principles may help in answering the question, "What is the appro-

TABLE 5 Examples of Drugs and Toxic Compounds for Which Physiologically Based Kinetic Models Have Been Described

Compound	Species	References
Actinomycin D	Dog	Lutz *et al.* (1977a)
Cytarabine	Mouse, monkey, human	Dedrick *et al.* (1973)
Digoxin	Rat	Harrison and Gibaldi (1977)
Mercaptopurine	Rat, human	Terlikkis *et al.* (1977)
Methotrexate	Mouse, rat, human	Bischoff *et al.* (1970, 1971)
Morphine	Rat	Gabrielsson and Paalzow (1983)
Salicylate	Dog	Chen *et al.* (1978)
Chlorinated biphenyls	Rat	Lutz *et al.* (1977b)
Dichloromethane, carbon monoxide	Rat, human	Andersen *et al.* (1991)
Polychlorinated dibenzo-*p*-dioxins and dibenzofurans	Rat, hamster, monkey	Carrier *et al.* (1995)
Styrene, styrene-7,8-oxide	Mouse, rat, human	Csanády *et al.* (1994)
Tetrachloroethylene	Mouse, rat, human	Reitz *et al.* (1996)
Toluene	Human	Pierce *et al.* (1996)
Trichloroethylene and metabolites	Mouse	Abbas and Fisher (1997)

priate dose to achieve a desired plasma concentration?" Before we can answer the question, we have to clarify which type of dose is needed, a loading dose or a maintenance dose. If a specified concentration has to be achieved by a single dose an appropriate loading dose (D_L) has to be administered. As is immediately apparent from Eq. (1), the loading or initial dose necessary to achieve the plasma concentration C depends on the distribution volume that has to be "loaded." In case of extravascular administration, the bioavailability (F) must also be taken in account, thus yielding

$$F \cdot D_L = C \cdot V$$

or

$$D_L = \frac{C \cdot V}{F}. \tag{33}$$

The maintenance dose is the dose needed to maintain the plasma concentration within a given range. It is important to realize that the maintenance dose is linked to time. When asking for the appropriate maintenance dose, we have to calculate essentially a maintenance dosing rate such that it equals the amount that is eliminated per time unit from the body. The dosing rate needed to maintain a given plasma concentration can be achieved by a continuous infusion or in a series of repetitive doses.

Constant Rate Infusion

Figure 21 shows the time course of plasma concentrations during a constant-rate infusion. At the beginning there is a rapid increase of the plasma concentration. As the concentration increases, the rate of elimination increases according to the principle of first-order elimination and the rise of the concentration slows down. Eventually a steady state concentration (C_{ss}) is attained. In steady state, the infusion rate (R) equals the elimination rate, which is given by Eq. (3). Thus

$$R = C_{ss} \cdot \mathrm{CL}. \tag{34}$$

Equation (34) provides another convenient means to determine the clearance from a single measurement of C_{ss}. An important conclusion can be drawn from Eq. (34). The dose rate needed to maintain a certain plasma concentration is determined by the clearance. It is independent of the volume of distribution.

Time to Reach Steady State

Suppose the infusion is stopped. After one half-life ($t_{1/2}$), the concentration has decreased to half its value, after 2 $t_{1/2}$ to 1/4, after 3 $t_{1/2}$ to 1/8, after 4 $t_{1/2}$ to 1/16, after 5 $t_{1/2}$ to 1/32 (i.e., to less than 3% of the initial value). Obviously after 4 to 5 half-lives, elimination is almost complete. This rule of thumb applies to all processes that can be characterized by a half-life. Interestingly, the time needed to attain the steady state also depends on the elimination half-life as is explained in Fig. 21. Thus when a drug is administered at a constant rate, it takes 4 to 5 half-lives to attain the intended plasma concentration. If the steady state concentration is too high or lower than intended, the dose rate has to be changed. Again it will take 4 to 5 half-lives to establish the new steady state. For drugs with a long half-life, such as digitoxin ($t_{1/2}$ = 7 days), the time necessary to achieve steady state may be too long. In that case a loading dose may be administered that produces the intended target concentration, which is then maintained by the infusion (Fig. 21).

It should be noted that the time to steady state is solely a function of half-life and does not depend on the infusion rate. As discussed above (cf. Eq. (26)), the half-life is dependent on volume of distribution and clearance. If a given infusion rate is applied in an individual having a higher volume of distribution, it takes longer to reach at the steady state since half-life is longer. The steady state concentration ultimately attained, however, will be the same as in a subject with lower distribution volume. If the same infusion rate is applied in an individual having a higher clearance, the half-life and hence the time to steady state will be shorter than in a subject with lower clearance, and a lower steady state concentration is established.

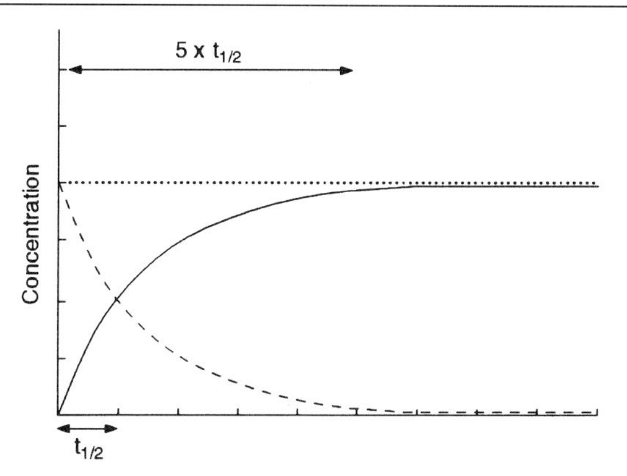

FIGURE 21 Concentration time profile in plasma during a constant-rate infusion. When a drug is administered continually, the plasma concentrations increase. According to the principle of first-order kinetics, the elimination rate increases with increasing plasma concentrations and eventually a steady state is achieved (solid line). If the infusion is stopped, the plasma concentrations decrease, the time course of the decrease is determined by the half-life. After five half-lives, elimination is almost complete. It is important to realize that the (elimination) half-life time determines also the time needed to attain the steady state. Suppose the steady state concentration is established by an appropriate loading dose and then maintained by the infusion (dotted line). The elimination of the loading dose (dashed line) is obviously matched by the infusion rate, and thus both are governed by the same half-life. Adapted from Fichtl *et al.* (1996).

Summing up, it may be stated that the time to steady state depends on half-life and thus on the distribution volume and the clearance but is independent of the infusion rate. The steady state concentration eventually attained depends only on the infusion rate and the clearance. It is independent of the volume of distribution.

First-Order Elimination and Drug Dosing

The fact that most drugs—at least in the therapeutic concentration range—are eliminated according to first-order kinetics is of utmost importance for drug treatment. As we have seen, if a drug is continuously administered a steady state is achieved, since the elimination rate increases with increasing plasma concentrations until it matches the dose rate. According to Eq. (34) the steady state concentration is directly proportional to the dose rate. Suppose a drug that is eliminated by zero-order kinetics; that is, the elimination rate is constant. A given plasma concentration could only be maintained if the infusion rate exactly matches the elimination rate. If the infusion rate were only slightly higher than the elimination rate, the plasma concentration would steadily rise, eventually reaching toxic levels. If the infusion rate were only slightly lower than the elimination rate, the concentrations would steadily decrease, eventually approaching zero. A maintenance therapy with this drug would not be practical. Phenytoin is a notorious example. The metabolism of this drug may become saturated, approaching zero-order kinetics. In this case a small increase in the dosing rate may result in a disproportional increase of the steady state concentration (Fig. 22).

Multiple-Dose Administration

In clinical practice repetitive doses are usually administered to maintain the plasma concentration within the therapeutic range. Essentially the same principles as above apply in this case. The dosing rate is given by the maintenance dose D_M and the dosing interval τ.

The relationship between the dosing rate D_M/τ and the average plasma concentration ($\bar{C}_{ss}$) during the dosing interval is analogous to Eq. (34),

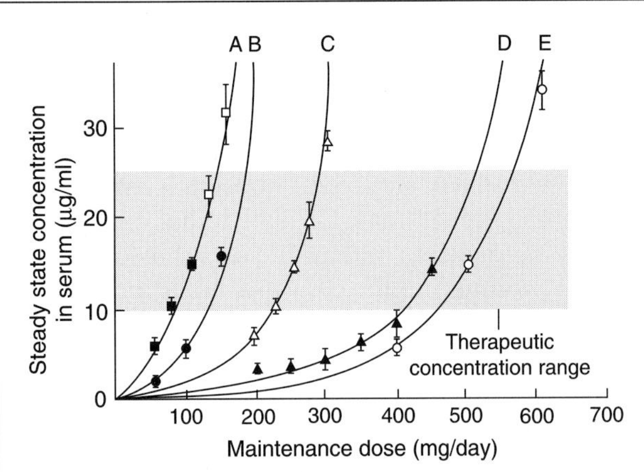

FIGURE 22 Nonlinear relationship between maintenance dose of phenytoin and steady state concentration in plasma. In the five patients, the steady state concentrations resulting from increasing maintenance doses increased more than proportional. In patient C, for instance, an increase in the daily dose from 200 to 300 mg (+50%) produced an about fourfold increase in the steady state concentration (+300%). Adapted from Fichtl *et al.* (1996).

$$\frac{F \cdot D_{M}}{\tau} = \overline{C}_{ss} \cdot CL$$

or

$$\frac{D_{M}}{\tau} = \frac{\overline{C}_{ss} \cdot CL}{F}. \tag{35}$$

Figure 23 shows the concentration–time profiles in plasma when a drug is administered either by a constant-rate infusion or by repetitive doses. When multiple doses are applied, the plasma concentrations during a dose interval oscillate between a peak (C_{max}) and a trough (C_{min}) level. Provided the dosing rate is the same, that is, $D_M/\tau = R$, the concentrations oscillate around the line obtained after infusion. The average concentration is the same as that obtained during the infusion and it depends solely on the dosing rate and the clearance but is independent of the distribution volume. Nevertheless, the distribution volume has also to be taken into account when designing a multiple-dose regimen, at least for drugs with a narrow therapeutic index. Suppose the same maintenance dose is applied to two individuals having the same clearance but different distribution volumes. The average concentration is the same in both individuals since it is determined by the clearance. However, in the subject with the lower distribution volume, higher peak concentrations will result. Furthermore, the lower distribution volume implies a shorter half-life; that is, the concentrations decrease to lower trough levels. Thus the extent of the swing between C_{max} and C_{min} depends on the distribution volume. It is higher the lower the volume of distribution. Undue oscillations of the plasma concentrations may be avoided by proper adjustment of the dose regimen. If for instance both the maintenance dose and the dose interval are reduced by half, the dosage rate D_M/τ and hence the average plasma concentration remain the same, but the fluctuation between C_{max} and C_{min} is halved (Fig. 23).

Multiple Dosing and Drug Accumulation

When a drug is administered repeatedly, each dose adds to the remainder of the previous dose and the drug is said to accumulate. The accumulation may be described in terms of dose rate and clearance, as shown before. Another useful concept is the accumulation rate (AR) or accumulation index. The accumulation ratio may be defined as the ratio of the average concentration at steady state to the average concentration during the first dose interval,

$$AR = \frac{\overline{C}_{ss}}{\overline{C}_{1}} = \frac{1}{1 - 2^{\tau/t_{1/2}}}. \tag{36}$$

The relation usually given for the accumulation rate (Eq. (36)) is exact only for drugs exhibiting single-compartment kinetics and if absorption is rapid. A simpler relationship to assess the extent of accumulation can be derived when comparing the amount of drug that is in the body during the steady state (A_{ss})

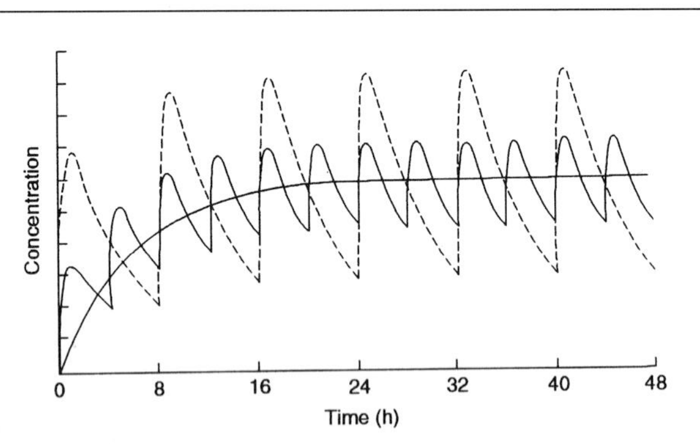

FIGURE 23 Dependence of the fluctuations of the plasma concentration on dose regimen. The thick solid line represents the plasma concentrations obtained during a constant rate infusion (e.g., R = 25 mg/h). When a maintenance dose (D_M) of 200 mg is administered at a dose interval (τ) of 8 h (dashed line) the fluctuations between maximal and minimal concentration are greater than after administering 100 mg every 4 h (thin solid line). The average dose rate (D_M/τ or R) is the same (25 mg/h or 600 mg/day) for all three dosage regimens and, therefore, the average concentrations at steady state are the same. Adapted from Fichtl *et al.* (1996).

to the amount that was absorbed from the first dose (A_1). Using Eqs. (1), (35), and (26) we obtain

$$A_{ss} = \overline{C}_{ss} \cdot V = \frac{F \cdot D_M}{\tau \cdot \mathrm{CL}} \cdot V = \frac{F \cdot D_M \cdot \tau_{1/2}}{\tau \cdot 0.7}. \quad (37)$$

The amount absorbed from the first dose is

$$A_1 = F \cdot D_M. \quad (38)$$

Thus the accumulation rate becomes

$$\mathrm{AR} = \frac{A_{ss}}{A_1} = \frac{t_{1/2}}{\tau \cdot 0.693}$$

or approximately

$$\mathrm{AR} \approx 1.5 \cdot \frac{t_{1/2}}{\tau}. \quad (39)$$

Both Eq. (36) and Eq. (39) indicate that the accumulation ratio depends on the ratio between the dose interval and half-life, but the inherent information is easier to grasp from Eq. (39). If a given maintenance dose is administered at shorter dose intervals, a greater fraction of the dose remains at the end of the dose interval and adds to the next dose. Stated in another way, when the dose interval is fixed, a drug will accumulate more the longer its half-life. For instance the accumulation rate of digitoxin ($t_{1/2} \approx 7$ days) when administered once daily ($\tau = 1$ day) is 10.5; that is, the amount present in steady state is about 10 times higher than the amount administered with the first dose.

NONLINEAR KINETICS

If the processes involved in the absorption, distribution, and elimination of a compound are first-order reactions, then the kinetics is said to be linear. In this case the amount entering the body, the AUC, C_{max}, and C_{min}, are directly proportional to the dose. A plot versus dose will result in a straight line (i.e., they are linearly related to the dose administered). Therefore, concentration–time profiles obtained after the administration of different doses (by the same route) are superimposable when normalized to dose (Fig. 24). Linear kinetics implies also that kinetic parameters such as bioavailability, volume of distribution, clear-

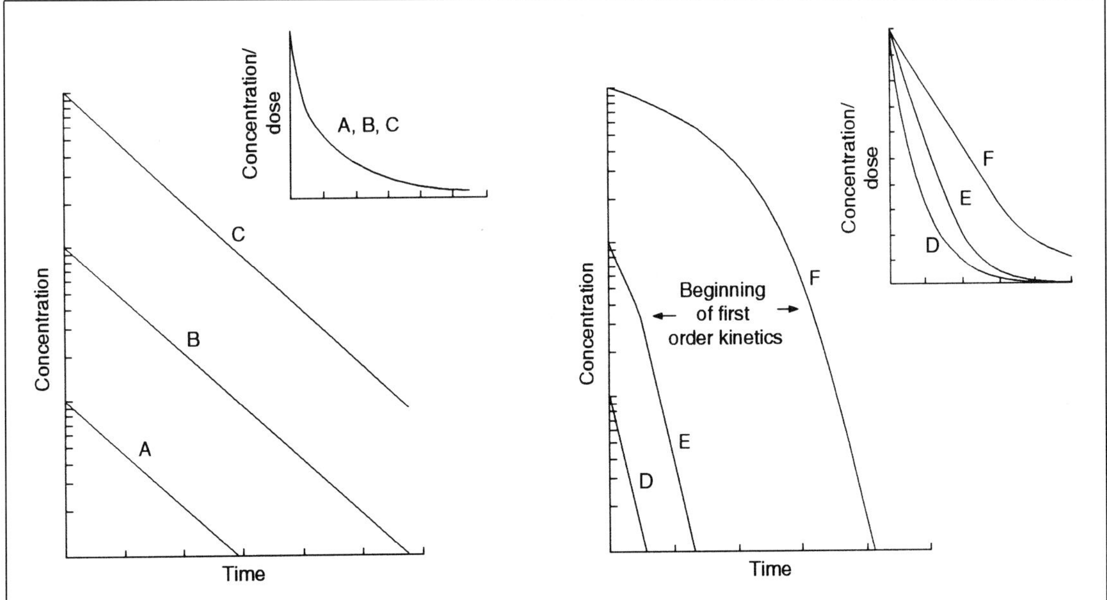

FIGURE 24 Linear versus nonlinear kinetics. The plots simulate for two hypothetical drugs the plasma concentrations resulting from different doses. If kinetics is linear, the plasma concentrations are proportional (i.e., linearily related) to increasing doses (A–C). When the plasma concentrations are normalized to (i.e., divided by) dose, the plots are superimposable and independent of the dose (small insert). Furthermore, plotting the concentrations on a linear scale (small insert) results in curvature of the plot. For a drug exhibiting nonlinear kinetics the concentration–time profiles are dose dependent and no longer superimposable (D–F). At high concentrations, half-life is not time invariant. Half-life does not become constant before the concentrations have dropped to a level where first-order kinetics apply (E, F). On a linear scale, the plot of concentrations obtained after high doses (insert, line F) first results in a straight line; curvature becomes apparent only at low concentrations. Concentration–time profiles of this kind are typically observed when elimination pathways become saturated at high concentrations.

ance, and half-life are constants and do not depend on dose or concentration. If nonlinear kinetics prevails, the principle of superposition no longer holds and kinetic parameters may change as a function of dose (or concentration) and time (Fig. 24). The main reason for nonlinear kinetics is the saturation of specific processes such as metabolism, carrier mediated transport, or protein binding. Thus nonlinearities are usually a problem of high doses. Nonlinear kinetics is rare with drugs administered at usual therapeutic doses. In drug overdose and in safety evaluation studies where multiples of the usual therapeutic doses are applied, nonlinear kinetics are probably more the rule than the exception. A thorough treatment of the complex mathematics and the numerous causes of nonlinear kinetics is beyond the scope of this chapter; the reader is referred to the pertinent literature. To continue, we will exemplify some of the more common reasons for nonlinear kinetics.

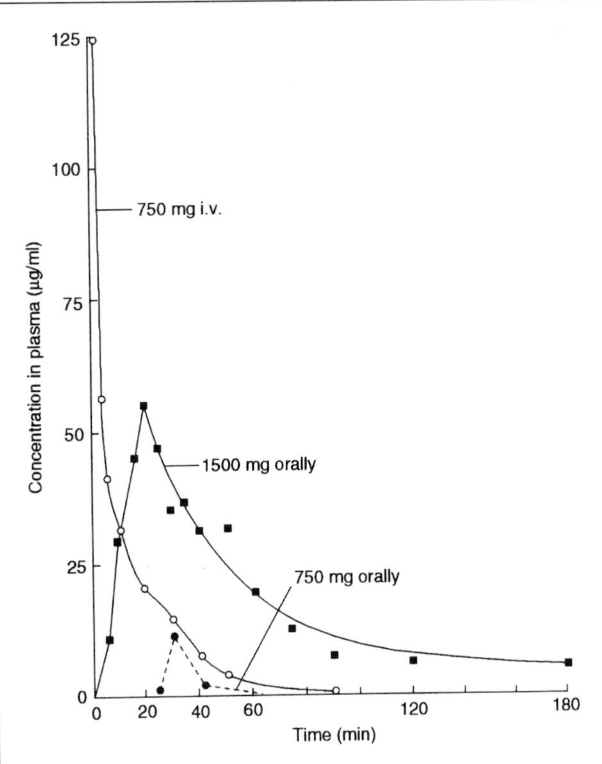

FIGURE 25 Dose-dependent bioavailability of fluorouracil. In a patient the plasma concentrations of fluorouracil were measured after intravenous and oral administration. Since fluorouracil is subject to a pronounced first-pass effect, the AUC after 750 mg given orally is much lower than after intravenous injection of the same dose. If the oral dose is doubled the AUC increases about 13-fold, which reflects saturation of first-pass metabolism at the higher dose. Data from Christophidis *et al.* (1978). Adapted from Fichtl *et al.* (1996).

Nonlinear Bioavailability

Poor solubility in gastrointestinal fluid may result in a less than proportional increase in the amount that enters the systemic circulation as the dose is increased. Known examples are phenytoin and griseofulvin. On the other hand, saturation of presystemic metabolism may result in a greater than proportional increase in plasma concentrations, as has been observed for drugs such as fluorouracil, hydralazine, propranolol, and verapamil (Fig. 25). It stands to reason that the possibility of nonlinear bioavailability has to be considered in safety evaluation studies. It may be necessary to ascertain the relationship between bioavailability and dose.

Nonlinear Distribution

Many drugs are bound to plasma proteins and tissue constituents. At low concentrations binding is linear; that is, the ratio between the bound and free concentration is constant and independent of the concentration. If the binding sites become saturated, the ratio between bound and free concentration decreases with increasing concentration and kinetic parameters calculated from total concentration become concentration dependent. In this case parameters based on free concentrations are often less affected. For instance, if a dose of 100 mg results in a plasma concentration of 1 mg/liter the apparent volume of distribution is 100 liters. If binding is linear, a dose of 400 mg will result in a plasma concentration of 4 mg/liter again yielding an apparent distribution volume of 100 liters. The amount of drug contained in the plasma is 12 mg (assuming a plasma volume of 3 liters). Suppose binding sites become satured at the high dose. In this case a lower plasma concentration will result, let us say 2 mg/liter, and the calculated apparent volume is 200 liters. Now only 6 mg is being held in plasma while the remaining 6 mg distributes to the tissues. Because this amount is only a small fraction of the dose, the free concentration will only marginally be affected and the volume of distribution in relation to the free concentration is almost the same as in the case of linear binding.

A similar setup applies to the clearance. Suppose a drug is excreted by glomerular filtration. Because only unbound molecules can be filtered, the elimination rate is given by the product of the glomerular filtration rate and the free concentration in plasma ($GFR \cdot C_f$). The clearance is calculated by using Eq. (3) as

$$\mathrm{CL} = \frac{\mathrm{GFR} \cdot C_f}{C}$$

or

$$\mathrm{CL} = \mathrm{GFR} \cdot f_P. \tag{40}$$

Thus the clearance based on the total concentration C depends on the free fraction f_P. If 90% of the drug in plasma is bound, (i.e., $f_P = 0.1$), the clearance is 12 ml/min. If binding becomes saturated and decreases to let us say 50% ($f_p = 0.5$), the clearance increases to 60 ml/min. On the other hand, the clearance in relation to the free concentration equals the GFR (120 ml/min) and does not depend on the extent of binding.

Nonlinear Elimination

Saturation of metabolism is probably the most common cause of nonlinear elimination. According to the Michaelis–Menten equation (cf. Eq. (8)), metabolism becomes saturated when the concentrations approach and exceed K_m. If $C \gg K_m$ the elimination rate is constant ($=v_{max}$); that is, zero-order kinetics prevail. The typical concentration–time profile of a substance that is eliminated by Micheaelis–Menten kinetics was shown in Fig. 24. If the concentrations are plotted on a logarithmic scale, curvature occurs and the half-life is not constant but is concentration and time dependent. It should be noted, however, that at low concentrations, which are below K_m, the kinetics is linear (i.e., first-order). It is to be anticipated that saturation of metabolism is a frequent scenario in drug overdose, but it may occur even in the therapeutic concentration range with drugs such as phenytoin or salicylates. When metabolism becomes saturated, small changes in the dosing rate may produce disproportionally high steady state concentrations, as was exemplified for phenytoin (Fig. 22). Ethanol is the classic example of a toxicant that is eliminated by zero-order kinetics, even after moderate doses. The plasma concentrations of ethanol that are achieved when ethanol is ingested for recreational use are well above K_m, which is about 0.1 g/liter.

STEREOSELECTIVE KINETICS

Many xenobiotics are chiral and their stereoisomers usually differ greatly with respect to effects and efficacy since targets such as receptors, carriers, or enzymes may be able to discriminate between molecules that differ in steric configuration. It has been estimated that at least 25% of the drugs on the market are racemates. Frequently, the therapeutic activity resides in only one of the enatiomers. Thus, the patient is exposed to "isomeric ballast" that, despite being devoid of therapeutic activity, may add to unwanted effects or toxicity.

Stereoisomers may appreciably differ with respect to kinetics. If a racemic mixture is administered, the concentration–time profile of the isomers is different and their proportion changes continuously. Thus the concentration of a racemic mixture in a biological fluid is often a virtually meaningless concept. As has been pointed out (Ariens, 1992), kinetic parameters based on racemate concentrations are of the same "quality" as is the age or weight of a four-person family and "astereognosis" pollutes not only the patient with isomeric ballast but also the scientific literature.

Enantiomers and Diastereomers

In any discussion of stereoselective kinetics, it is useful to recall the concepts of enantiomers and diastereomers. Atoms with four different substituents are called chiral centers (from the Greek $\chi\epsilon\iota\rho$ = hand). Two steric conformations of a molecule containing a chiral center are possible, and these are termed enantiomers. One enantiomer is the mirror image of the other. Chiral molecules rotate the plane of polarized light and the enantiomeres may be characterized by the direction of that rotation as (+) or (−) (formerly also *d* or *l*; from the Latin *dexter* = right, *leavus* = left). Other nomenclatures are based on the actual steric arrangement of the substituents at the chiral center (*D*–*L* nomenclature according to Fisher; and *R*–*S* nomenclature according to Cahn, Ingold and Prelog; from the Latin *rectus* = right, *sinister* = left). Should a molecule contain two chiral centers, then four different conformations are possible. The pairs *S*/*S* and *R*/*R* or *S*/*R* and *R*/*S* are enantiomers. On the other hand, *S*/*S* and *R*/*R* are not mirror images (enantiomers) of *S*/*R* or *R*/*S*. Stereoisomers that are not enantiomers are termed diastereomers. As opposed to enantiomers, diastereomers may differ appreciably with respect to physicochemical properties such as solubility in water or lipids. This may also influence their kinetic behavior. For enantiomers stereoselective disposition is to anticipated only if stereoselective processes are involved.

Stereoselective Absorption, Distribution, and Excretion

Absorption of xenobiotics occurs mainly by means of passive diffusion. Difference between enantiomers are to be anticipated only if specific carrier molecules are involved in the absorption process. Examples are L-dopa and L-methotrexate, whose bioavailability is greater than that of the respective D-isomers. In rare cases, binding to plasma proteins may be stereoselective, which affects the distribution of a drug (cf. the example of verapamil dealt with in the following). The excretion of drugs by filtration in the kidneys is not stereoselective. Conceivably, carrier-mediated excretory processes, such as tubular secretion, may be stereoselective. Pertinent experimental data, however, are virtually absent. One of the rare well-documented examples refers to the diastereomers quinine and quinidine. The antiarrhythmic quinidine is more effectively secreted by the renal tubules than the antimalarial quinine, resulting in an about four times greater renal clearance. Given the present state of knowledge, based on experimental evidence that is scarce at best, it would appear that major differences between enantiomers with respect to absorption, distribution, and excretion are rare.

Stereoselective Metabolism

On the other hand, stereoselective metabolism is not uncommon and may profoundly influence the kinetics of an agent. Stereoselective metabolism affects not only the clearance but also the bioavailability if a drug is subject to first-pass metabolism. The complexities resulting from stereoselective kinetics may be exemplified by verapamil. Table 6 gives the pharmacokinetic parameters of (*R*)- and (*S*)-verapamil. Verapamil is eliminated by stereoselective metabolism. The (metabolic) clearance and the volume of distribution of (*S*)-verapamil are both about twice as high as that of the (*R*)-enantiomer. The greater volume of distribution can be explained by the lower extent of plasma binding (higher f_P) of (*S*)-verapamil (cf. Fig. 3). On the other hand, the half-life is almost the same for both enantiomers, which is to be anticipated when recalling the relation given by Eq. (26). The slower metabolism of the (*R*)-enantiomer results in a less pronounced first-pass effect and a corresponding higher bioavailability. The differences in the kinetics of the verapamil enantiomers provide an explanation for an observation that at first glance might appear puzzling. During investigations with racemic verapamil, it was observed that the concentration–response curve obtained following intravenous administration was different from that after oral application. After oral administration, about three times higher plasma concentrations were needed to achieve the same effect. The (*R*)-enantiomer is much less effective than the (*S*)-enantiomer. Since the bioavailability of (*R*)-verapamil is about 2.5 times greater than that of (*S*)-verapamil, a correspondingly greater fraction of verapamil in plasma is in the less active form following oral administration. As the example shows "effective concentrations" based on the measurement of racemate concentrations are questionable.

Another point of interest is the fact that variables such as age or gender may differently affect the kinetics of enantiomers as investigation with mephobarbital will show. This drug is used in several countries for the treatment of epilepsy. The results (Table 7) merit attention in several respects. First there is an enormous difference in the kinetics of the two enantiomers. In all study groups both AUC and half-life of the (*S*)-enantiomer are 10 to 100 times greater than the corresponding values for the (*R*)-enantiomer. Furthermore, there are pronounced age- and gender-related differences in the kinetics of (*R*)-mephobarbital, AUC, and half-life, varying between groups by a factor of 3 to 10. On the other hand, the kinetic parameters of (*S*)-mephobarbital did not vary greatly between groups, except for a shorter half-life in the group of young males.

TABLE 6 Stereoselective Kinetics of Verapamil[a]

Isomer	*F* (%)	Ratio *S*/*R*	V (liters · kg^{-1})	Ratio *S*/*R*	f_P (%)	Ratio *S*/*R*	Cl (liters · kg^{-1} · h^{-1})	Ratio *S*/*R*	$t_{1/2}$ (h)	Ratio *S*/*R*
(*R*), (+)-Verapamil	50		2.7		6.4		0.6		4.1	
		0.4		2.3		1.7		1.8		1.2
(*S*), (−)-Verapamil	20		6.4		11		1.1		4.8	
Racemate	38		3.4				0.85		3.8	

[a]The data for bioavailability (*F*), volume of distribution, (*V*), free fraction in plasma (f_p), clearance (CL), and half-life ($t_{1/2}$) were determined in healthy volunteers; mean values, for $t_{1/2}$ harmonic mean. Data from Echizen and Eichelbaum (1986).

VARIABILITY OF KINETIC PARAMETERS

The kinetic behavior of a substance is characterized by a specific set of kinetic parameters. It is important to realize that the value of kinetic parameters depends not only on the substance in question but also on the individual to whom a substance is administered, and as such may be subject to appreciable interindividual variability. Kinetic parameters depend on the species and the genetic disposition of an individual and may change with age or in disease. Furthermore, substances may interact at any stage of the LADME scheme. An exhaustive treatment of the virtually innumerable possibilities cannot be given here; the discussion will be focused on selected issues of major importance, such as kinetics at the extremes of age and in diseases of the kidneys and liver. Table 8 summarizes the changes in the principal kinetic parameters that are to be anticipated under these circumstances. This synopsis should be regarded as a memory aid rather than as an exact description. Before discussing the contents of the table in more detail, some general remarks seem appropriate. In most cases, changes of the clearance are of greater importance than changes of distribution volume. There are two reasons for this. First, the clearance is the parameter that together with the dose rate determines the extent to which a substance accumulates in the body. Changes in the volume of distribution affect only the fluctuations around the average concentration and generally they are only of interest for drugs with a narrow range of therapeutic concentrations and/or a narrow margin between therapeutic and toxic concentrations (narrow therapeutic index). The second and even more important reason is the fact that the clearance may vary over a much wider range than the volume of distribution. For instance, the elimination of aminoglycoside antibiotics such as gentamicin occurs almost entirely in the kidneys. In a completely anuric patient, the clearance drops to some 3% of normal; that is, clearance has changed by a factor of 33. Variations of this degree are impossible for the distribution volume; it rarely changes more than twofold. The volume of distribution cannot decrease to zero, whereas clearance can.

Another point to be kept in mind is the hybrid character of half-life. A proper interpretation of a changed half-life depends on the underlying reason. For instance, if half-life is prolonged due to a decreased clearance, it may be necessary to adjust the dosage rate. If half-life is prolonged due to an increased distribution volume, it may be necessary to adjust a loading dose; the dosage rate needed to maintain a given average concentration will remain be unaffected.

Finally it should be stressed that experimental evidence as to the influence of the parameters mentioned on the disposition of toxic compounds is meager. Thus the following discussion heavily relies on examples from drug therapy. Nevertheless, the general principles also apply to toxic compounds.

Kinetics in Kidney and Liver Disease

Because the kidneys and liver are the major sites of drug elimination, diseases of these organs can profoundly affect the clearance. Kidney disease may impair both glomerular filtration and tubular excretion of drugs. Usually the reduction of the glomerular filtration rate approximately parallels the reduction of tubular functions. It is possible, therefore, to assess the reduction of the renal clearance of drugs by mea-

TABLE 7 Stereoselective Kinetics of Mephobarbital[a]

	Young men	Young women	Elderly men	Elderly women
(*R*)-Mephobarbital				
$t_{1/2}$ (h)	3.1	7.0	10.7	9.6
AUC ($\mu g \cdot ml^{-1} \cdot h$)	1.3	8.0	8.2	15.5
(*S*)-Mephobarbital				
$t_{1/2}$ (h)	51	85	95	96
AUC ($\mu g \cdot ml^{-1} \cdot h$)	142	178	150	172

[a]After an oral dose of 400 mg (*S*)-mephobarbital or (*R*)-mephobarbital the plasma concentrations were measured in young and elderly men and in young and elderly women. (Young, 18 to 25 years old; elderly, more than 60 years old). Obviously both isomers differ appreciably with respect to kinetics and the effect of age and gender. Data from Hooper and Qing (1990).

TABLE 8 Synopsis of the Possible Influences of Age and Diseases of the Elimination Organs on Principal Kinetic Parameters[a]

	Newborn infant	Children	Elderly	Kidney disease	Liver disease
Bioavailability	•		= ↑ (f.p.)		↑ (f.p.)
Volume of distribution	• (ΔPB)	(ΔPB)	• (ΔPB)	(ΔPB)	(ΔPB)
Renal clearance	↓	↓ (≈BSA)	↓	↓	
Hepatic clearance	↓	↑ (≈BSA)	•		= or ↓
Half-life	Changes depend on changes in distribution volume and clearance				

[a]The symbols indicate the changes with respect to values in healthy young adults and apply to distribution volumes and clearances referenced to body weight. Thus the absolute value of drug clearance is lower in children than in adults, relative to body weight, the clearance is higher in children. Symbols: =, parameter unchanged; •, parameter may be affected; ↓, parameter decreased; ↑, parameter increased; f.p., applies to drugs subject to marked first-pass effect; ΔPB, change in plasma protein binding; BSA, body surface area.

suring the creatinine clearance. In clinical practice, frequently the plasma creatinine concentration has to act as substitute for the creatinine clearance (Fig. 26). This is essentially an application of Eq. (3). Creatinine is a metabolite constantly produced by skeletal muscle. Thus the steady state concentration of creatinine in plasma is inversely proportional to creatinine clearance.

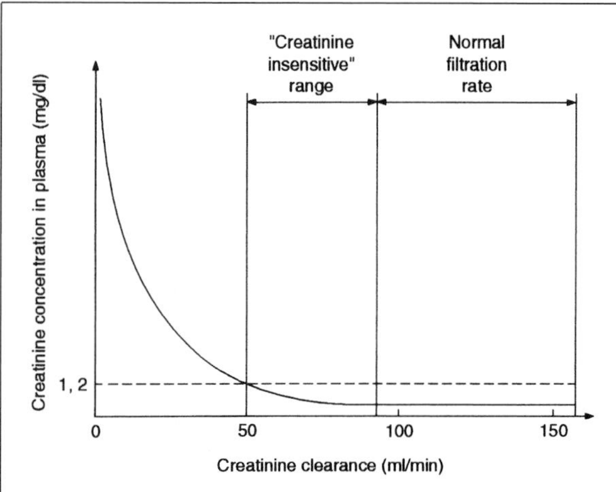

FIGURE 26 Dependence of plasma creatinine concentration on creatinine clearance. In kidney disease, the degree of renal impairment may be assessed from the glomerular filtration rate. A decrease in the glomerular filtration rate is reflected in a decreased creatinine clearance, which in turn increases plasma creatinine concentrations. The hyperbolic relationship may pose practical problems when assessing creatinine clearance from a measurement of plasma creatinine concentration. In a range between normal values (>100 ml/min) and about 50 ml/min, a change in creatinine clearance only slightly affects plasma creatinine concentration ("creatinine insensitive" range). Given the inevitable interindividual variability, a markedly compromised renal function may thus be compatible with normal creatinine concentrations (<1.2 mg/dl). Adapted from Fichtl *et al.* (1996).

The situation becomes more complicated with liver disease. Metabolic pathways may be differently affected by different types of liver disease (Table 9). Even in severe liver disease, the metabolism of drugs may occur at the normal rate, and there is no simple means of assessing the degree of impairment (if any) of metabolic clearance. The only "rule" that can be given is to watch out and be careful.

Special caution is warranted if drugs that are subject to a high hepatic first-pass effect are administered in liver disease since their bioavailability may dramatically increase. The more a drug is normally extracted by the liver, the more its bioavailability may increase when extraction decreases. Take as an example a drug for which 90% is normally extracted by the liver. At the extreme, its bioavailability may increase from 10 to 100% (i.e., 10-fold). If 95% is normally extracted, bioavailability may vary 20-fold. Furthermore, even a moderate impairment of liver function that only slightly affects the clearance may result in a large increase in bioavailability (Fig. 27). Accordingly, in liver disease, this type of drug may prove more dangerous to the patient after oral application than after parenteral administration. The problem may be aggravated in liver cirrhosis, where functional liver cells are replaced by connective tissue. Under these conditions, appreciable amounts of a drug normally extracted from blood during the liver passage may escape metabolism even if the metabolic capacity of the remaining liver cells is normal.

TABLE 9 Examples illustrating the Influence of Liver Diseases on Drug Biotransformation

Disease	Biotransformation decreased	Biotransformation unchanged
Cirrhosis	Ampicillin Diazepam Lidocain Pethidine	Tolbutamide Oxazepam
Viral hepatitis	Diazepam Hexobarbital Pethidine Warfarin	Oxazepam Phenytoin Lidocain

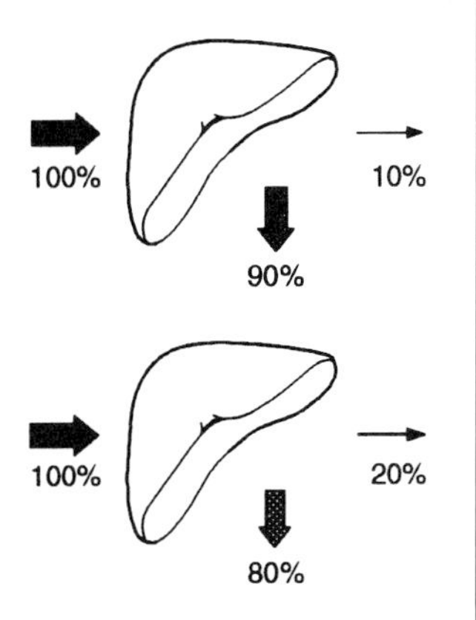

FIGURE 27 Dependence of bioavailability on the extent of first-pass elimination. If during liver passage 90% of a drug is removed from blood, the bioavailability is 10%. If the extraction by the liver decreases from 90 to 80% (−10%) the bioavailability is doubled (+100%). For substances subject to a high first-pass effect, even relatively small changes in first-pass extraction may result in large changes of bioavailability. Adapted from Fichtl *et al.* (1996).

Kinetics in the Elderly

Age may affect both the quantity and the quality of drug effects. For instance aged people are more sensitive to many drugs acting on the central nervous system and sedatives may elicit paradoxical excitement reactions in the elderly. Frequently, however, an apparent higher "sensitivity" of the elderly is the result of age-related pharmacokinetic changes. The involutional processes associated with aging result in a host of anatomical and physiological changes, which may affect the kinetics of a substance (Table 10). In recent years the possible impact of age on drug kinetics has received increased attention, as is reflected in an increasing number of pertinent publications. Aged people are prone to multimorbidity, which may add to pharmacokinetic variability and the often unavoidable multiple-drug treatment increases the possibility of drug interactions. Therefore it may be difficult to decide whether a reported change of a kinetic parameter in age is actually due to age, and conflicting or apparently contradictory findings are not uncommon. Furthermore, one has to realize that aging is a continual process and the chronological age may be a poor predictor of biological age. It is not surprising, therefore, that age-related changes of kinetic parameters are subject to pronounced interindividual variability. It should also be realized that predictions concerning the impact of age on kinetics that are theoretically "deduced" from altered anatomy and physiology, or are based on animal experiments, may prove to be erroneous.

Bioavailability

This very point is aptly illustrated by the impact of age on drug absorption. Despite the numerous alterations in anatomy and physiology of the gastrointestinal tract (cf. Table 10), drug absorption is not appreciably impaired in old age. Occasionally, the rate of absorption may be decreased. A reduced extent of bioavailability is observed for substances that are absorbed by special transport systems such as glucose or folic acid. A notable exception are drugs subject to first-pass metabolism. It is to be anticipated that even moderate decreases in liver function occurring in the elderly may result in an increased bioavailability. Experimental evidence supports this contention (Table 11).

Volume of Distribution

Age-related changes in body composition (cf. Table 10) may influence the distribution volume. Their practical importance, however, is frequently exaggerated. It should be noted that the proportion of these changes is relatively small. An appreciable change is observed only for body fat, which may result in a higher distribution volume of lipophilic compounds. It is necessary, however, to guard against sweeping generalizations. In fact, the distribution volume of substances such as diazepam, nitrazepam, pethidine, or thiopentone may increase in the elderly. On the other hand, the distribution volume of compounds

TABLE 10 Examples of Age-Related Changes Which Could Affect Kinetics[a]

Kinetic Parameter Affected	Age-Induced Change[b]
Absorption, bioavailability	Surface area of gastointestinal mucosa ↓
	Blood flow through splanchnic area ↓
	Acid production in stomach ↓
	Gastric emptying ↓
	Peristalsis ↓
Volume of distribution	Muscle mass ↓ (−20%)
	Body fat ↑ (+ 50 to 100%)
	Total body water ↓ (−20%)
	Albumin ↓ (−20%)
Hepatic clearance, bioavailability (first-pass effect)	Liver mass ↓ (−40%)
	Liver perfusion ↓ (−50%)
	Enzyme activity ↓ (?)
	Enzyme induction ↓ (?)
Renal clearance	Renal blood flow ↓ (−50%)
	Glomerular filtration rate ↓ (−50%)
	Tubular secretion ↓

[a]For some entries the change in the elderly (70–90 y) with respect to the younger (20–30 y) is given as a percentage. Given the wide variability in the respective sources, these figures should be regarded as rough approximations, illustrating the possible range of changes.

[b]Symbols: ↓ decreased or slower in the elderly; ↑ increased in the elderly.

such as phenothiazines, tricyclic antidepressants, or verapamil is not substantially affected by an increase of body fat. These drugs are lipophilic compounds that are positively charged at physiological pH values. Such "amphiphilic" compounds accumulate preferentially in tissues rich in phospholipds.

Renal Clearance

Renal function decreases with increasing age (cf. Table 10). As a rule of thumb, one may assume that the renal clearance of drugs in people over 65 years of age is approximately halved. In principle, the clearance may be assessed by the creatinine clearance. The approximation of the creatinine clearance based on the plasma creatinine concentration may be misleading. In the elderly, creatinine production decreases and the plasma creatinine concentration may as a result appear apparently normal, despite a decrease in clearance.

Metabolic Clearance

With respect to metabolic clearance, things again become more complicated. As is apparent from Table 12, the metabolism of drugs in the aged may be unchanged, decrease, or rarely even increase. Virtually no generalizations can be made as to the impact of age on metabolic clearance. It has been suggested that mainly phase I reactions of drug metabolism are affected by age, whereas the effect of aging on phase II reactions, such as glucuronidation, is less pronounced. In recent years, however, an increasing number of exceptions to this "rule" have become evident. At present the mechanisms involved in age-related decreases of drug metabolism are not well understood. It is difficult to separate the effect of aging from confounding factors such as environmental influences, concomitant disease, or drug therapy. The changes observed can only be partially explained by age-related physiological changes in liver mass or liver blood flow, and no firm conclusions can be drawn concerning the age-related changes in the activity of drug-metabolizing enzymes. Similarly it is still a matter of debate whether age is associated with an altered response to inhibition or induction of drug metabolism.

Kinetics in Children

In relation to body weight, the (maintenance) dose of drugs in children is usually higher than in adults. The dosage requirements in children to achieve the

TABLE 11 Influence of Age on Bioavailability of Drugs Subject to a First-Pass Effect

Drug	Bioavailability in young [age in years]	Bioavailability in elderly [age in years]	Ratio young/ elderly	Sources
Clomethiazol[b]	5–16% [25–28]	70–90% [68–70]		Nation *et al.* (1977)
Nalbuphine	11% (8–20) [23–32]	44% (19–99) [65–90]	4.0	Jaillon *et al.* (1989)
Lidocain	13% (4–21) [20–34]	27% (12–52) [73–87]	2.1	Cusack *et al.* (1985)
Verapamil	23% (10–42) [33–70]	38% (9–83) [85–93]	1.65	Storstein *et al.* (1984)
Propranolol	30% [29 ± 2][c]	55% [78 ± 3][c]	1.83	Castleden and George (1979)
Nifedipine	46 ± 2%[c] [22–35]	61 ± 7%[c] [73–83]	1.32	Robertson *et al.* (1988)

[a]The extent of the first-pass effect may decrease in the elderly resulting in a marked increase in bioavailability. The lower the bioavailability, the greater the possible increase, a finding that has to be anticipated (cf. Fig. 27).

[b]Approximate value (iv and po data not measured in the same patients).

[c]$\bar{x} \pm$ SD.

same concentrations as in adults correlate better with body surface than with body weight. It is often maintained that this "surface rule" can be explained by difference in drug distribution between children and adults. This line of argument, however, is conceptually wrong. According to Eq. (35), the "surface rule" can be explained only if clearance correlates to body surface area. It has been common knowledge for quite some time that renal clearance correlates with body surface (Fig. 28) and obviously this also applies to the metabolic clearance of many drugs. If the body is approximated by a sphere having radius r, then its volume and hence its weight is proportional to r^3. The surface will vary in proportion to r^2, as does clearance. If r is halved, the weight drops to 1/8, whereas a surface-related parameter such as the clearance drops only to 1/4. In other words, in a small body the clearance is higher with respect to body weight, and consequently the maintenance dose that has to be administered per kilogram of body weight is higher in children than in adults (Fig. 29). It should be stressed that the "surface rule" is to be regarded as an explanation for the relatively higher dose that is often required for children and not as a universal guide to drug dosing in children, since there are notable exceptions to this rule (e.g. codeine, morphine).

Kinetics in the Neonate

The disposition of drugs in the neonate differs from that in children or adults. The absorption of drugs may be slower. The distribution volume may be affected by the relatively higher water content of the neonate's body. The extracellular volume (about 40% of body weight) is twice as high as in adults. Frequently the extent of drug binding to plasma proteins is lower than in adults. The major problem, however, is the fact that all processes determining the clearance are immature at birth. The maintenance dose of all drugs must therefore be much lower than in children, even when calculated in relation to body weight (cf. Fig. 29). The maturation of the excretory function takes up to 6 months (Fig. 30). Quite obviously, the utmost caution should be exercised when administering drugs to neonates. In addition to careful monitoring of drug effects, the determination of plasma concentrations is advisable when drugs with a low therapeutic index are to be used.

Changes in Plasma Protein Binding

Numerous factors may influence the extent of drug binding to plasma proteins. Protein binding may vary with age and is subject to change in many disease states. A decreased binding is frequently observed in liver and kidney disease, which at least in part may be due to the accumulation of endogenous substances interfering with binding. For most drugs, albumin is the major drug-binding protein in plasma, and any disease affecting its concentration may affect the extent of binding. Several basic drugs are extensively bound to α_1-acid glycoprotein (orosomucoid). The concentration of this protein increases markedly following surgery or in inflammatory disease. Furthermore, a drug may displace another drug from binding sites.

Consequences of Altered Drug Binding

The consequences of altered drug binding are frequently exaggerated. Although abundantly evident, changes in protein binding usually appear to be of minor importance. For most drugs the rate of elimination is determined by the free concentration in plasma because only the unbound molecules can be filtered in the kidney or can pass the membranes of tubulus and liver cells (restrictive elimination). Should a drug be administered continuously, the free concentration will increase until the elimination rate matches the dosing rate. In other words, the free concentration ultimately attained is regulated by the dosing rate and the clearance of the unbound drug. The total concentration depends on the amount that can be bound at a given free concentration and is determined by the affinity of the drug to the binding proteins and their binding capacity. If a drug is administered at the same dosing rate in two subjects differing only with respect to plasma binding, the free concentration that can equilibrate with the concentration at the site of action(s) is the same in both patients and the drug effects are not dependent on the extent of plasma binding. At a given free concentration, however, the total concentration will be higher in the subject with higher plasma protein binding.

TABLE 12 Changes in Clearance of Metabolized Drugs in the Elderly[a,b]

Increased clearance	Unchanged clearance	Decreased clearance
PHENYTOIN	**Acetaminophen**	**Acetaminophen**
THEOPHYLLINE	Acetanilide	**Antipyrine**
Thiopentone	Acetylic salicyclic acid	Carbenoxolone
Tolbutamide	**Antipyrine**	Quinidine
	Diazepam	Quinine
	Diclofenac	Chlordiazepoxid
	Digitoxin	Clobazam
	Diphenhydramine	Clomethiazole
	Ethanol	Desmethyldiazepam
	Flunitrazepame	**Diazepam**
	Heparin	Indocyanine green
	Labetalol	**Lidocaine**
	Lidocaine	**Lorazepam**
	Lorazepam	Norepinephrine
	Lormetazepam	Nortriptyline
	Nitrazepam	Pethidine
	Midazolam	**PHENYTOIN**
	Oxazepam	Piroxicam
	PHENYTOIN	**Propranolol**
	Prazosin	**THEOPHYLLINE**
	Propranolol	Verapamil
	Propylthiouracil	
	Temazepam	
	THEOPHYLLINE	
	Thiopentone	
	Tolbutamide	
	Warfarin	

[a]For the drugs in boldface apparently contradictory findings have been reported.

[b]Reprinted from *Pharmacology and Therapeutics* **36,** Loi and Vestal, Drug metabolism in the elderly, pp. 131–149, Copyright 1988, with permission from Elsevier Science.

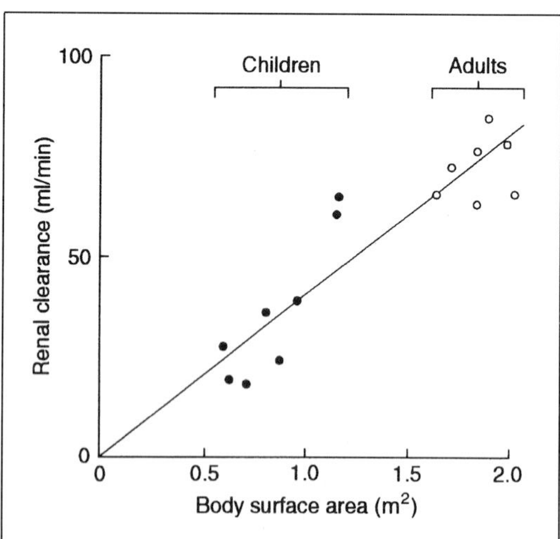

FIGURE 28 Renal clearance in children and adults. As shown here for the renal clearance of urea the renal clearance correlates with body surface area (v. Slyke *et al.*, (1928). Adapted from Fichtl *et al.* (1996).

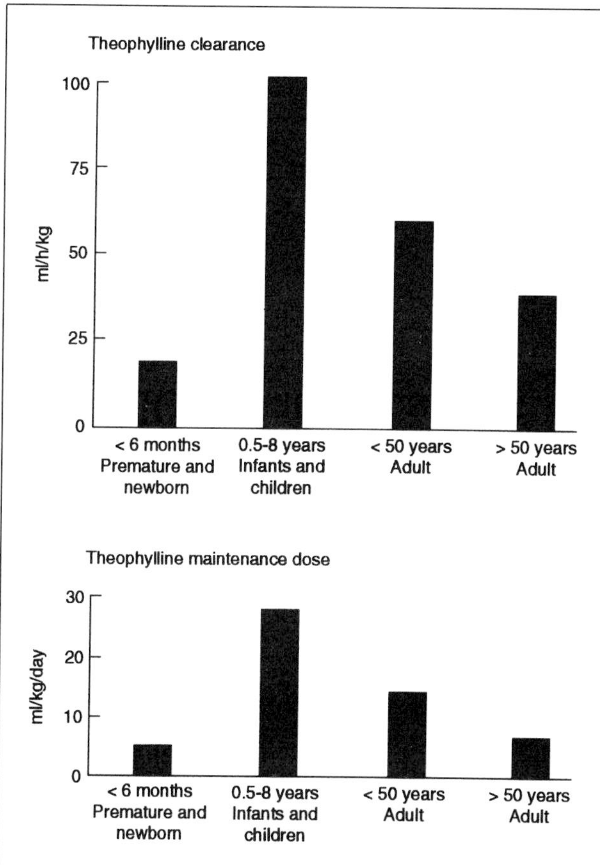

FIGURE 29 Clearance and maintenance dose of theophylline as influenced by age. As exemplified for theophylline, drug clearance referenced to body weight is usually higher in children than in adults and a correspondingly higher maintenance dose per kg is needed for children to achieve the same plasma concentration. This does not apply to the newborn, since their elimination pathways are immature (cf. Fig. 30). Adapted from Fichtl *et al.* (1996).

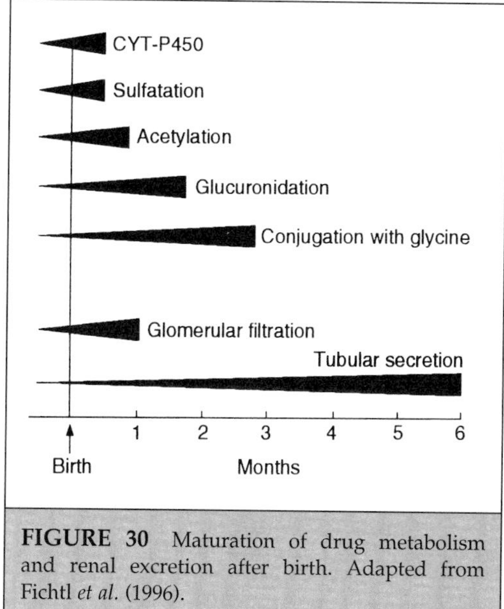

FIGURE 30 Maturation of drug metabolism and renal excretion after birth. Adapted from Fichtl *et al.* (1996).

The same applies if the extent of binding is changed, for example, due to displacement by another drug (Fig. 31). The molecules displaced from binding sites increase the free concentration. The molecules that are now unbound may leave the plasma and distribute at least in the extracellular volume, which dampens the increase of the unbound concentration. Furthermore, according to the principle of first-order elimination, an increase in the free concentration implies an increased elimination rate. Eventually the original free concentration is restored. Because fewer molecules are now bound, the ultimate outcome of the displacement interaction will be characterized by a decreased total concentration, an increased free fraction (f_p) and an unchanged free concentration. This must to be considered in therapeutic drug monitoring, where usually total concentrations are measured. If the extent of binding changes, then the total concentration will change; the free (effective) concentration remains unaltered.

Despite speculation to the contrary aired in numerous review articles and textbooks, there is essentially no convincing evidence that pure drug displacement interactions are of clinical relevance. While scrutinizing alleged examples such as the interaction between phenylbutazone and oral anticoagulants, it becomes apparent that in addition to displacement, other kinetic changes are involved, such as an inhibition of elimination.

Before putting aside displacement interactions, two points of caution seem appropriate. The aforementioned reasoning does not necessarily apply to highly toxic compounds such as bilirubin. In newborns it has been observed that after displacement of bilirubin from plasma proteins, even the transient increase of free bilirubin (cf. Fig. 31) can result in severe brain damage (kernicterus). Undoubtedly, however, additional factors are involved, such as the increased bilirubin production from fetal erythrocyte degradation and decreased blood–brain barrier. Furthermore the outcome of a drug displacement interaction may be different if a drug is nonrestrictively eliminated; that is, its elimination rate depends not on the free concentration but on the total concentration in plasma. Substances with a high-first pass effect provide typical examples. If the extraction from the blood is extensive,

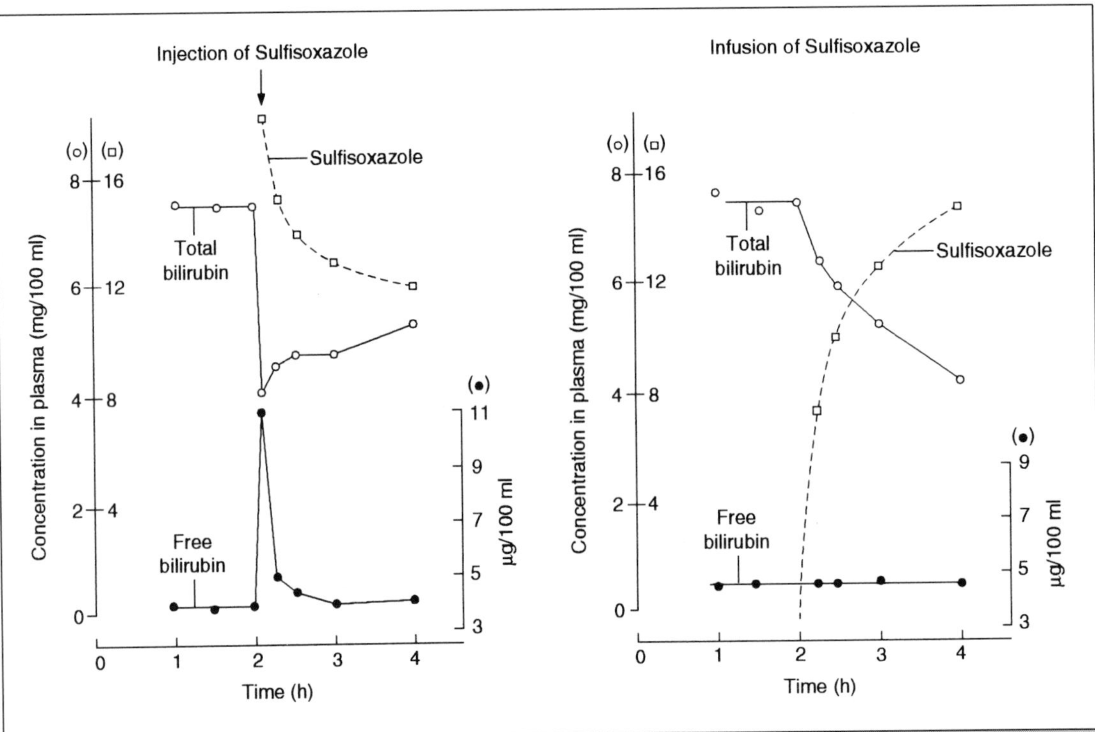

FIGURE 31 Consequences of displacement from plasma protein binding. In this experiment (Oie and Levy, 1979), bilirubin, which is extensively bound in plasma (>99.9%; i.e., $f_P < 0.001$) was infused in rats. Sulfonamides such as sulfisoxazol displace bilirubin from its binding sites. Following a bolus injection of sulfisoxazol (left panel), resulting immediately in high plasma concentrations, the free concentration of bilirubin rises transiently and the total concentration is decreased. When sulfisoxazol is administered as a constant rate infusion (right panel), its concentrations gradually increase and the displacement of bilirubin occurs more slowly. In this case, the redistribution and elimination of the bilirubin molecules set free from their binding sites is so rapid that no increase in the free concentration is observed. Adapted from Fichtl *et al.* (1996).

the free concentration may decrease rapidly during the passage of the liver and an appreciable part of the bound molecules is also set free. In this case, the elimination rate is little affected by the extent of binding. Accordingly, it is the total concentration that is regulated by dosing rate and elimination rate, and a decrease of the fraction bound would result in an increased free concentration (Fig. 32B). At present, experimental evidence for this type of displacement interaction is not available. This may be partially explained by the fact that, due to the high interindividual variability in first-pass extraction, drugs of this type must have a reasonable margin of safety. Furthermore, an increase in the free fraction will increase the first-pass effect, that is, decrease the bioavailability after oral administration (Fig. 32C). The dependence of bioavailability on the extent of binding may be appreciated when recalling Fig. 27. If a drug is highly extracted by the liver, an increase in the free fraction will only slightly increase the elimination rate. A small increase in the elimination rate, however, results in an appreciable decrease in the fraction that becomes available.

SPECIES DIFFERENCES IN KINETICS

Valerian is an aphrodisiac for tom cats but a sedative in humans. Acetylaminofluorene is highly carcinogenic in rats but not in guinea pigs. The same dose (in mg/kg) of hexobarbitone injected to dogs may result in a sleeping time 30 times longer than it does in mice. These examples demonstrate—and they can be augmented at will—that the effects of drugs or toxicants may differ among species, both qualitatively and quantitatively. True qualitative differences in pharmacodynamics (or toxicodynamics) are not very common among mammalian species. Essential ana-

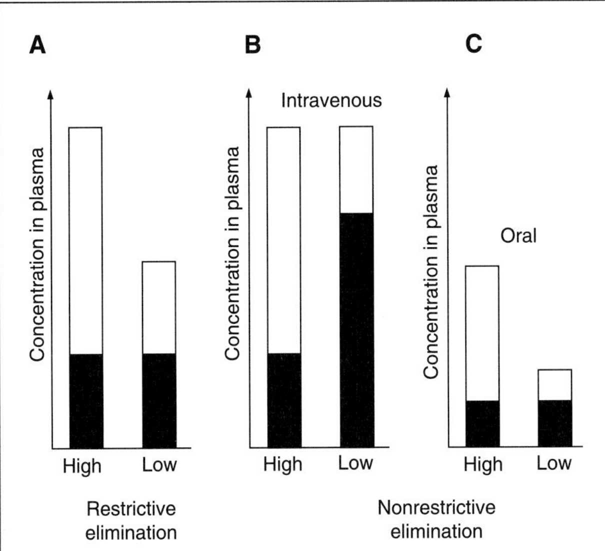

FIGURE 32 Influence of plasma protein binding on steady state concentrations in plasma. (A) For a drug with restrictive elimination (i.e., the elimination rate is determined by the free concentration in plasma), a decreased binding results in a decrease of total concentration, the free concentration remains unchanged (cf. Fig. 31). (B) If the extraction rate in the liver is high, the elimination rate depends on total concentration (i.e., elimination is not restricted to the free fraction in plasma). The total concentration is then independent of the binding, and a decrease in binding results in an increased free concentration. (C) After oral administration a drug that is highly extracted in the liver has a low bioavailability (high first-pass effect). For a drug with a high first-pass effect, a slight increase in hepatic extraction due to diminished binding results in a large decrease of bioavailability. Thus the eventual outcome of a decrease in binding after oral administration is a decreased total concentration and little change in the free concentration. Symbols: high, high plasma protein binding; low, low plasma protein binding; ■, free concentration in plasma; ⬓, total concentration in plasma. From Rowland and Tozer, "Clinical Pharmacokinetics," © 1989 Lippincott Williams & Williams, with permission.

tomical structure, basic physiology, and major biochemical pathways tend to be similar across species. An important exception is the biotransformation of foreign compounds. Frequently, an apparent species difference in the pharmacodynamic effects is due to a species difference in the biotransformation of that substance. For instance, a metabolite is responsible for the carcinogenic action of acetylaminofluorene. This metabolite is produced in rats but not in guinea pigs.

Species-related quantitative differences in the action of xenobiotics may be due to differences in target-cell sensitivity, resulting in a different concentration–effect relationship. Frequently, however, they reflect species differences in kinetics, as is illustrated by the example regarding sleeping times. When the animals awake from the hexobarbitone anesthesia, the plasma concentrations are approximately the same, both in the mice and in the dogs. However, the time it takes for the plasma concentrations to drop to that level is longer in dogs. Due to the slower metabolism, the half-life of hexobarbitone is appreciably higher in this species. Species differences are not only observed in the metabolism of drugs but may affect all stages of the LADME scheme.

Species Differences in Absorption and Bioavailability

Absorption may be affected by species differences in gastrointestinal anatomy and physiology. Furthermore, feeding habits may influence factors such as the pH value or the rate at which different parts of the gastrointestinal tract are emptied. In this respect carnivores (e.g., cats and dogs) appear to be more similar to humans than herbivores (e.g., horses and cattle). Another point that has to be considered is the different composition of the gastrointestinal bacterial flora. The rat has considerable numbers of bacteria in the forestomach and upper parts of the small intestine. In humans and in carnivora, the gastrointestinal flora resides mainly in the large intestine. In the stomachs of ruminants, a large number of bacteria capable of metabolizing drugs are present. This explains why cattle are largely insensitive to orally ingested E605 or atropine. It stands to reason that species differences in first-pass metabolism may affect bioavailability. The bioavailability of diazepam and flunitrazepame, being approximately 85 to 100% in humans, is only minute in dogs. This is due to pronounced presystemic metabolism in the gut wall and the liver. Incidentally, the bioavailability of a substance from a galenic preparation that has been optimized for humans may be different in animals.

Species Differences in Distribution Volume

It is obvious that the distribution volume of a substance may vary enormously among species of different body size. Since the organ volumes in different species correlate with body weight (Table 13), these differences largely disappear if the volume of distribution is related to body weight (i.e., is expressed as liters $\cdot$ kg^{-1}). When normalized to weight, the (average) distribution volumes measured in humans and in other species that are frequently used in toxicolog-

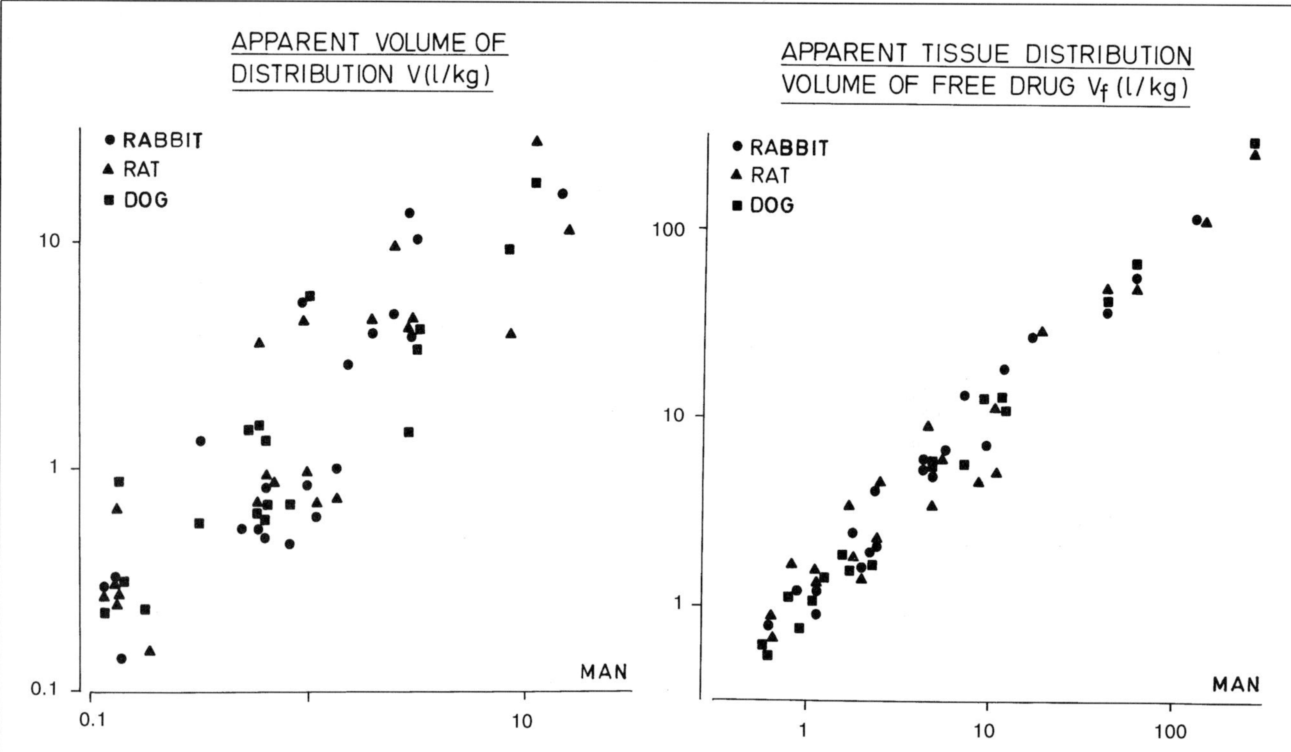

FIGURE 33 Correlation between the distribution volume of drugs in different species. The plots refer to a series of miscellaneous drugs for which data for the volume of distribution and the extent of plasma protein binding in man and three other species were available from the literature. The distribution volumes reported extend over several orders of magnitude. As is apparent from the left panel, the distribution volumes in man correlate to a certain extent to the distribution volumes in animals; there is, however, considerable scatter. With respect to humans, the distribution volumes in animals may vary by a factor of 10 or more (note the logarithmic scale). In order to eliminate the variability due to species differences in plasma binding the equation given in Figure 3 may be rearranged:

$$\frac{(V - V_P)}{f_P} = \frac{V_T}{f_T} = V_f.$$

Thus from the apparent volume of distribution V, the plasma volume V_P, and the free fraction in plasma f_P, a term V_f can be calculated that depends on tissue volume and tissue binding only. V_f may be viewed as distribution volume of free drug in tissues. When plotting V_f much closer correlations are observed (right panel). With respect to man, the values of V_f vary between species by a factor of two at the most (Fichtl *et al.*, 1991).

ical studies, such as rats, dogs, and rabbits, often vary not more than by a factor of two to three. It appears that larger variations are mainly due to species differences in plasma protein binding (Fig. 33). Species differences in plasma protein binding are fairly common and variations in free fraction up to 20-fold have been observed. As previously discussed (cf. Fig. 3), the apparent volume of distribution depends not only on the real volumes accessible to a substance, but also on the extent to which a compound becomes bound to plasma and tissues. Given the limited experimental evidence available at present, it appears that unspecific binding to tissues varies less across species than binding to plasma proteins. Since usually only a small fraction of the total amount in the body resides in plasma, the volume of distribution referenced to the free concentration is not greatly affected by differences in plasma binding. The possibility of species-dependent protein binding should be taken into account when comparing "toxic" concentrations based on total concentration in plasma. For instance, it has been found that the hematotoxicity of the anticancer drug etoposide correlates better with the free rather than with the total concentration in plasma. The unbound fraction of etoposide is 0.63 in dog and 0.52 in rats, but only 0.048 in humans. Thus at a given free concentration, the total concentration in humans will be about 10 to 12 times higher than in rats or dogs.

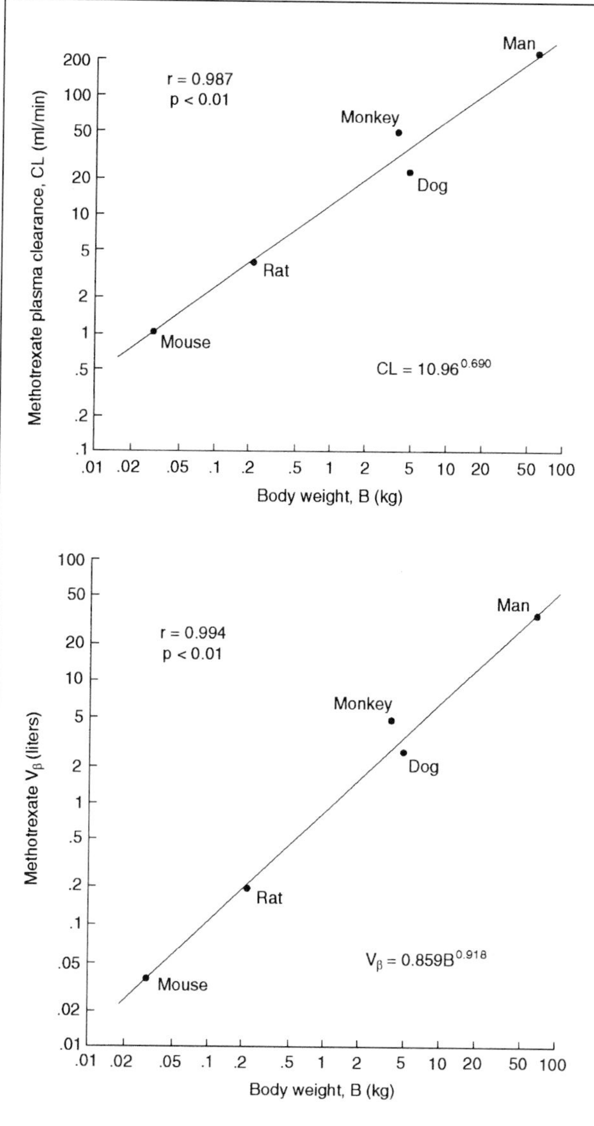

FIGURE 34 Allometric scaling of the clearance and distribution volume of methotrexate. When pharmacokinetic parameters obtained in different species are plotted against body weight, the relationship can often be described by a power function ("allometric" equation), which on a double logarithmic scale will be a straight line. After Boxenbaum (1982), with permission.

Species Differences in Clearance

Clearance is obviously dependent on body size as well. Exceptions notwithstanding, when related to body weight (i.e. expressed as liters $\cdot$ h^{-1} $\cdot$ kg^{-1}) clearance tends to be higher in smaller animals. Body surface area has been proven to be a better correlate of clearance than body weight. With respect to renal clearance, body size is the main source of interspecies variability. Differences in tubular handling of drugs may also contribute to species differences in renal clearance. The tubular reabsorption of weak organic acids or bases, for instance, is influenced by the pH value in the tubular lumen, which differs between carnivores (urinary pH 5.5–7) and herbivores (pH 7–8). Nevertheless, the renal clearance of substances that are mainly excreted by filtration can be reasonably well predicted using the allometric approach outlined below. On the other hand, metabolic clearance may vary greatly among species even when the differences in body size are taken into account. The differences may be due to unique metabolic pathways that are present or absent in a given species (e.g., poor glucuronidation in cats, poor acetylation in dogs) or may reflect differences in the activity of drug-metabolizing enzymes. Regarding drugs that are primarily eliminated by metabolism using cytochrome P_{450}, marked species differences in the metabolic clearance are commonplace.

Species Extrapolation

Species extrapolation, that is, the scaling of pharmacokinetic parameters from animal to human is of great relevance in drug development and toxicology. For instance, animal scale up may aid in selecting an appropriate first-time-in-human dose or in establishing an appropriate dose regimen for toxicity studies in experimental animals. One approach is the use of physiological models. Their practical applicability, however, is limited because of the inherent complexities and the data needed to completely characterize these models is seldom available. Another approach is the use of allometric methods. Allometric literally means "being of a different measure." Based on the seminal work of Adolph (1949) and subsequent investigations, it has become apparent that the weight of many organs and many physiological variables are closely related to body weight by the power equation

$$X = a \cdot BW^b, \qquad (41)$$

where a and b are constants and X is the parameter that depends on body weight (BW). It should be noted that the numerical values for X and BW refer to the average values (population means) in a species. When plotting both X and BW on a logarithmic scale, a

TABLE 13 Examples of Allometric Equations Relating Physiological Properties to Body Weight (BW) in Mammals

Parameter	Allometric Equation
Organ weight (g)	
Plasma	$0.043 \times BW^{0.99}$
Skeletal muscle	$0.046 \times BW^{1.01}$
Kidneys	$0.022 \times BW^{0.84}$
Liver	$0.086 \times BW^{0.89}$
Intestines	$0.087 \times BW^{0.91}$
Heart	$0.002 \times BW^{1.04}$
Lungs	$0.032 \times BW^{1.10}$
Renal clearance (ml/h)	
Creatinine	$4.2 \times BW^{0.69}$
Inulin	$1.74 \times BW^{0.77}$
PAH	$5.4 \times BW^{0.80}$
Physiological periods (h)	
Heartbeat duration	$1.19 \times 10^{-5} \times BW^{0.27}$
Breath duration	$4.7 \times 10^{-5} \times BW^{0.28}$

[a]Data from Mordenti (1986) and Adolph (1949).

straight line results with the slope b. For many organs, the allometric exponent b is close to 1 (cf. Table 13), which means that their weight varies in the same proportion as does body weight. In other words, the ratio X/BW is constant and independent of body weight. If $b < 1$, then the parameter X decreases less rapidly than does BW, which in turn means that the ratio X/BW is higher in small animals, as is the case for the body surface area ($b = 0.66$). Many rate parameters, such as blood flow rates, oxygen consumption, and glomerular filtration rate, are related to body weight with an allometric exponent in the range of 0.66 to 0.8. In an attempt to rationalize the better correlation with body surface area, it is often maintained that the smaller organism has a relatively higher surface and thus needs proportional higher "metabolic rates" to maintain homeostasis. It should be stressed, however, that allometric relations are purely empirical. Since parameters such as organ volumes, blood flow rates, and filtration rate are major determinants of drug disposition, it is not surprising that allometric equations can also be used to describe the relation between kinetic parameters and body weight. Close correlations that allow reasonably accurate extrapolations to other species can be expected for drugs such as methotrexate (Fig. 34), which are mainly eliminated by the kidneys and are not extensively bound to plasma proteins. Often the allometric exponent relating the distribution volume to body weight is close to 1 and for clearance is close (but not necessarily equal) to 0.66 (Table 14). This means that the clearance correlates better with body surface area than with body weight.

Assuming "typical" allometric exponents of 1 and 0.7 for distribution volume and clearance, respectively, and recalling Eq. (26), we can deduce that the

TABLE 14 Examples of Allometric Parameters Obtained from Interspecies Scaling of Kinetic Parameters[a,b]

Parameter	Compound	Coefficient[a]	Exponent[b]
Volume of distribution	Antipyrine	0.756	0.963
	Cyclophosphamide	0.883	0.989
	Methotrexate	0.859	0.918
	Aztreonam	0.234	0.906
	Cefoperazone	0.221	0.913
Clearance	Antipyrine	8.16	0.885
	Cyclophosphamide	16.7	0.754
	Methotrexate	10.9	0.690
	Aztreonam	4.45	0.665
	Cefoperazone	6.69	0.571
Half-life	Antipyrine	74.5	0.296
	Cyclophosphamide	36.6	0.236
	Methotrexate	54.6	0.228
	Aztreonam	32.6	0.186
	Cefoperazone	38.8	0.212

[a]The kinetic parameters X measured in different species were fitted using the equation $X = a \cdot BW^b$, where BW is body weight.
[b]Data from Ings (1990).

allometric expression for the dependence of half-life on body weight is something like

$$t_{1/2} \approx \frac{V}{CL} \approx BW^{1-0.7}$$

or

$$t_{1/2} \approx BW^{0.3}. \qquad (42)$$

It should be pointed out incidentally that an allometric exponent of approximately 0.3 applies also to biological periods such as heart beat and breath duration (Table 13).

Equation (42) indicates that a drug is eliminated more rapidly in small animals; that is, the smaller the animal, the shorter the half-life. This ought to be taken into account in toxicity studies using small animals. Ideally the dosage regimen should result in concentration–time profiles equivalent to those observed in humans. The dosage rate necessary to result in the same AUC can be calculated from the respective clearances in humans and animals. In order to mimic the time course in humans, it is also necessary to achieve the same ratio between half-life and dose interval. Suppose a drug with a half-life of 12 h is administered in humans twice daily. Assuming an allometric exponent of 0.25, the half-life in a mouse will be about 7 times shorter, that is, the order of 2h. Administering the drug every 2 h is impracticable for chronic toxicity studies in mice.

Bibliography

Abbas, R., and Fisher, J. W. (1997). A physiologically based pharmacokinetic model for trichloroethylene and its metabolites, chloral hydrate, trichloroacetate, dichloroacetate, trichloroethanol, and trichloroethanol glucuronide in B6C3F1 mice. *Toxicol. Appl. Pharmacol.* **147,** 15–30.

Adolph, E. F. (1949). Quantitative relations in the physiological constitutions of mammals. *Science* **109,** 579–585.

Andersen, M. E., Clewell, H. J., Gargas, M. L., MacNaughton, M. G., Reitz, R. H., Nolan, R. J., and McKenna, M. J. (1991). Physiologically based pharmacokinetic modelling with dichloromethane, its metabolite, carbon monoxide, and blood carboxyhemoglobin in rats and humans. *Toxicol. Appl. Pharmacol.* **108,** 14–27.

Ariens, E. J. (1992). Chirality in pharmacokinetics and therapeutic drug monitoring. *In* "Recent Developments in Therapeutic Drug Monitoring and Clinical Toxicology" (I. Sunshine, ed.), pp. 257–264. Marcel Dekker, New York.

Benet, L. Z., Oie, S., and Schwartz, J. (1995). Design and optimization of dosage regimens; Pharmacokinetic data. In "Goodman & Gilman's The Pharmacological Basis of Therapeutics," 9th ed., pp. 1707–1792. McGraw-Hill, New York.

Bischoff, K. B., Dedrick, R. L., Zaharko, D. S., and Longstreth, J. A. (1971). Methotrexate pharmacokinetics. *J. Pharm. Sci.* **60,** 1128–1133.

Boxenbaum, H. (1982). Interspecies scaling, allometry, physiological time, and the ground plan of pharmacokinetics. *J. Pharmacokin. Biopharm.* **10,** 201–227.

Carrier, G., Brunet, R. C., and Brodeur, J. (1995). Modeling and toxicokinetics of polychlorinated dibenzo-p-dioxins and dibenzofurans in mammalians, including humans. *Toxicol. Appl. Pharmacol.* **131,** 253–276.

Case, D. E. (1993). ICH-2 and development of "Note for Guidance on Toxikokinetics." *J. Toxicol. Sci.* **18,** 213–216.

Castleden, C. M., and George, C. F. (1979). The effect of ageing on the hepatic clearance of propranolol. *Br. J. Clin. Pharmacol.* **7,** 49–54.

Chasseaud, L. F. (1993). Role of toxicokinetics in toxicity testing. *In* "Drug Toxicokinetics" (P. G. Welling and F. A. da Iglesia, eds.), pp. 105–142. Marcel Dekker, New York.

Chen, C. N., Coleman, D. L., Andrade, J. D., and Temple, A. R. (1978). Pharmacokinetic model for salicylate in cerebrospinal fluid, blood, organs, and tissues. *J. Pharm. Sci.* **67,** 38–41.

Christophidis, N., Vajda, F. J. E., Lucas, I., Drummer, O., Moon, W. J., and Louis, W. J. (1978). Fluorouracil therapy in patients with carcinoma of the large bowel: A pharmacokinetic comparison of various routes of administration. *Clin. Pharmacokin.* **3,** 330–336.

Csánady, G. A., Mendrala, A. L., Nolan, R. J., and Filser, J. G. (1994). A physiologic pharmacokinetic model for styrene and styrene-7,8-oxide in mouse, rat, and man. *Arch. Toxicol.* **68,** 143–157.

Cusack, B., O'Malley, K., Lavan, J., Noel, J., and Kelly, J. G. (1985). Protein binding and disposition of lignocaine in the elderly. *Eur. J. Clin. Pharmacol.* **29,** 323–329.

Dahlem, A. M., Allerheiligen, S. R., and Vodicnik, M. J. (1995). Concomitant toxicokinetics: Techniques for and interpretation of exposure data obtained during the conduct of toxicology studies. *Toxicol. Pathol.* **23,** 170–178.

Dedrick, R. L., Forrester, D., Cannon, J. N., El Dareer, S. M., and Mellett, B. (1973). Pharmacokinetics of 1-β-D-arabinofuranosylcytosine (ARA-C) deamination in several species. *Biochem. Pharmacol.* **22,** 2405–2417.

Echizen, H., and Eichelbaum, M. (1986). Clinical pharmacokinetics of verapamil, nifedipine and diltiazem. *Clin. Pharmacokin.* **11,** 425–449.

Fichtl, B., Füllgraff, G., Neumann, H.-G., Wollenberg, P., Forth, W., Henschler, D., and Rummel, W. (1996). Allgemeine Pharmakologie und Toxikolgie. *In* "Allgemeine und spezielle Pharmakologie und Toxikolgie" (W. Forth *et al.*, eds.), 7th ed., pp. 3–102. Spektrum Akademischer Verlag, Heidelberg.

Fichtl, B., v. Nieciecki, A., Walter, K. (1991). Tissue binding versus plasma binding of drugs: General principles and pharmacokinetic consequences. *Adv. Drug. Res.* **20,** 117–166.

Food and Drug Administration (FDA) Division of Biopharmaceutics. (1977). Bioavailability protocol guideline for ANDA and NDA submission.

Gabrielsson, J. L., and Paalzow, L. K. (1983). A physiological pharmacokinetic model for morphine disposition in the pregnant rat. *J. Pharmacokin. Biopharm.* **11,** 147–163.

Gibaldi, M., and Perrier, D. (1982). "Pharmacokinetics," 2nd ed. Marcel Dekker, New York.

Hamann, S. R., Blouin, R. A., and McAllister, R. G. (1984). Clinical pharmacokinetics of verapamil. *Clin. Pharmacokin.* **9,** 26–41.

Harrison, L., and Gibaldi, M. (1977). Physiologically based pharmacokinetic model for digoxin distribution and elimination in the rat. *J. Pharm. Sci.* **66,** 1138–1142.

Hooper, W. D., and Qing, M. S. (1990). The influence of age and gender on the stereoselective metabolism and pharmacokinetics of mephobarbital, in humans. *Clin. Pharmacol. Ther.* **48,** 633–640.

ICH2 (1993). "International Conference on Harmonisation Safety Topic S3: Toxicokinetics Note for Guidance on Toxicokinetics. A

Guidance for Assessing Systemic Exposure in Toxicity Studies." EFPIA, Draft 10, Brussels.

Ings, R. M. J. (1990). Interspecies scaling and comparison in drug development and toxicokinetics. *Xenobiotica* **20,** 1201–1231.

Jaillon, P., Gardin, M. E., Lecocq, B., Richard, M. O., Meignan, S., Blondel, Y., Grippat, J. C., Bergnieres, J., and Vergnoux, O. (1989). Pharmacokinetics of nalbuphine in infants, young healthy volunteers, and elderly patients. *Clin. Pharmacol. Ther.* **46,** 226–233.

Labaune, J.-P. (1989). "Handbook of Pharmacokinetics. Toxicity Assessment of Chemicals." Ellis Horwood Ltd., Chichester.

Loi, C.-M., and Vestal, R. E. (1988). Drug metabolism in the elderly. *Pharmacol. Ther.* **36,** 131–149.

Lutz, R. J., Galbraith, W. M., Dedrick, R. L., Shrager, R., and Mellett, L. B. (1977a). A model for the kinetics of distribution of actinomycin-D in the beagle dog. *J. Pharmacol. Exp. Ther.* **200,** 469–478.

Lutz, R. J., Dedrick, R. L., Matthews, H. B., Eling, T. E., and Anderson, M. W. (1977b). A preliminary pharmacokinetic model for several chlorinated biphenyls in the rat. *Drug. Metab. Disp.* **5,** 386–396.

Mordenti, J. (1986). Man versus beast: Pharmacokinetic scaling in mammals. *J. Pharm. Sci.* **75,** 1028–1040.

Nation, R. L., Vine, J., Triggs, E. J., and Learoyd, B. (1977). Plasma level of chlormethiazole and two metabolites after oral administration to young and aged human subjects. *Eur. J. Clin. Pharmacol.* **12,** 137–145.

National Academy (1987). "Pharmacokinetics in Risk Assessment; Drinking Water and Health." National Academy Press, Washington D.C.

Pierce, C. H., Dillis, R. L., Morgan, M. S., Nothstein, G. L., Shen, D. D., and Kalman, D. A. (1996). Interindividual differences in $^2H_8$-toluene toxicokinetics assessed by a semiempirical physiologically based model. *Toxicol. Appl. Pharmacol.* **139,** 49–61.

Reitz, R. H., Gargas, M. L., Mendrala, A. L., and Schumann, A. M. (1996). In vivo and in vitro studies of perchlorethylene metabolism for physiologically based pharmacokinetic modelling in rats, mice, and humans. *Toxicol. Appl. Pharmacol.* **136,** 289–306.

Robertson, D. R. C., Waller, D. G., Renwick, A. G., and George, C. F. (1988). Age-related changes in the pharmacokinetics and pharmacodynamics of nifedipine. *Br. J. Clin. Pharmacol.* **25,** 297–305.

Rowland, M. (1986). Physiologic pharmacokinetic models and inter-animal species scaling. *In* "Pharmacokinetics: Theory and methodology" (M. Rowland and G. Tucker, eds.), pp. 69–88.

Rowland, M., and Tozer, T. N. (1989). "Clinical Pharmacokinetics. Concepts and Applications," 2nd ed. Lea & Febiger, Philadelphia, PA.

Schentag, J. J., Jusko, W. J., Plaut, M. E., Cumbo, T. J., Vance, J. W., and Abrytyn, E. (1977). Tissue persistence of gentamicin in man. *JAMA* **238,** 327–329.

Storstein, L., Larsen, A., Midtbo, K., and Soevareid, L. (1984). Pharmacokinetics of calcium blockers in patients with renal insufficiency and in geriatric patients. *Acta Med. Scand.* **(suppl.) 681,** 25–30.

Tterlikkis, L., Ortega, E., Solomon, R., and Day, J. L. (1977). Pharmacokinetics of mercaptopurine. *J. Pharm. Sci.* **66,** 1454–1457.

van Rossum, J. M. (ed.) (1977). "Handbook of Experimental Pharmacology, Vol. 47, Kinetics of Drug Action." Springer Verlag, Berlin.

Welling, P. G. (1995). Differences between pharmacokinetics and toxicokinetics. *Toxicol. Pathol.* **23,** 143–147.

Welling, P. G., and Balant, L. P. (eds.) (1994). "Handbook of Experimental Pharmacology, Vol. 110, Pharmacokinetics of Drugs." Springer Verlag, Berlin.

Yacobi, A., Skelly, J. P., and Batra, V. K. (1989). "Toxicokinetics and New Drug Development." Pergamon Press, New York.

Yacobi, A., Skelly, J. P., Shah, V. P., and Benet, L. Z. eds. (1993) "Integration of Pharmacokinetics, Pharmacodynamics and Toxicokinetics in Rational Drug Development." Plenum, New York.

C H A P T E R

4

Xenobiotic Metabolism

FRANZ OESCH, MICHAEL ARAND
Institute of Toxicology, University of Mainz, Mainz, Germany

INTRODUCTION

Why Xenobiotic Metabolism?

Each day, our bodies take up significant amounts of material that are used neither as energy substrates nor as building blocks for biological matrices. Uptake of such xenobiotica occurs mainly with the food but also by inhalation or transdermally. If these compounds accumulated in the organism, the resulting body burden would be enormous. Thus, efficient mechanisms for the excretion of such compounds that have their roots very early in the evolution of life have developed.

The two major elimination pathways in humans are excretion via bile and excretion via urine. For volatile compounds, exhalation can represent the dominant mechanism of excretion. In some cases, secretion into the mother's milk may be of toxicological significance. Both renal and biliary elimination require water-soluble substrates and become increasingly efficient with rising polarity of the compound to be excreted. While some xenobiotics are sufficiently water soluble for excretion, many lipophilic components cannot be directly excreted and would accumulate if not processed to more polar derivatives. This is presumed to be the main reason that a complex network of xenobiotic-metabolizing enzymes has evolved. In higher animals, the major location for xenobiotic metabolism within the body is the liver, but a number of other organs, such as kidney, gut, and lung, are also proficient in the metabolism of foreign compounds.

Demands

Three major demands should ideally be met by a xenobiotic-metabolizing enzyme system:

- The metabolites should have sufficient water solubility to allow efficient excretion via bile or urine.
- The metabolites should not have adverse biological activity, to avoid toxicological effects.
- The enzyme system should have a broad substrate specificity, to be able to deal with any newly encountered compound.

It is obviously not possible to fulfill all these criteria at the same time. For instance, there are many lipophilic compounds, such as polycyclic aromatic hydrocarbons, that are chemically almost inert. The first step of their transformation in the phase I or functionalization phase of xenobiotic metabolism (see the following) leads to chemically more reactive metabolites. A typical example, epoxidation of polycyclic aromatic hydrocarbons, yields electrophiles, including several of high chemical reactivity. On the one hand, these metabolites can be rapidly conjugated to the nucleophile glutathione by enzymatic or nonenzymatic conjugation to result in readily water-soluble metabolites. On the other hand, these compounds also react very quickly with cellular macromolecules, in particular with proteins and DNA, which renders these metabolites potentially cytotoxic and genotoxic. In most instances, the efficacy of the secondary metabolism of these compounds by glutathione *S*-transferases and epoxide hydrolases is sufficient to keep the toxicity of the intermediary metabolites at an acceptable level. However, there are quite a number of examples where xenobiotic metabolism actually leads to toxification.

The Plant–Animal Chemical Warfare

While the defense of the body against the accumulation of lipophilic junk is the likely primary cause for the development of a xenobiotic-metabolizing system, there is at least one additional driving force for the evolution of this complex enzyme network. This is plant–animal chemical warfare. Most animals are herbivores, profiting from plants' ability to transform sunlight into chemical energy. Plants defend themselves against being eaten by animals by a variety of mechanisms, including physical (e.g., solid bark, formation of thorns) and chemical (e.g., alkaloids, saponines, terpenes) weapons. It is the vast amount of different toxic secondary metabolites in plants that force herbivores to extend their xenobiotic-metabolizing enzyme system to digest the plants. There are metabolism pathways that appear to have evolved exclusively for this purpose since they do not increase the water solubility of the respective compounds. N-acetylation, for instance, is well suited to terminating the biological activity of compounds carrying an amino group as a determinant of their toxicity. However, this usually leads to an increase in lipophilicity of the respective metabolites, which sometimes causes harmful effects. A famous example of drugs that can be toxified by N-acetylation is the case of the bacteriostatic sulfonamides, which are more prone to precipitate in the kidney tubules after acetylation.

Toxicological Implication

Xenobiotic metabolism is an issue of major significance for the toxicology of chemical compounds. For drugs under development, one of the first things to be assessed is their metabolism in order to understand their kinetics after they enter the organism and to identify possible biologically active metabolites. It is important to realize that both the extent and the quality of the xenobiotic metabolism strongly depends on quite a number of factors. The most obvious are the species differences in metabolism, which pose the severe problem of limited transferability of the results obtained in toxicological experiments to the human situation. Next, there are the inherent characteristics of a given individual, such as sex, age, and genetic predisposition, which represent important determinants of xenobiotic metabolism. And finally, an indefinite number of environmental factors can modulate the expression and/or activity of xenobiotic-metabolizing enzymes. Chemical compounds themselves are often capable of inducing, repressing, inhibiting, or activating these enzymes. Nutritional behavior and dietary factors other than xenobiotics also have a proven effect on the metabolic competence. Disease states, such as infections, chronic liver disease, or simply fever, can alter the capacity of the foreign compound metabolism significantly.

CLASSIFICATION OF XENOBIOTIC-METABOLIZING ENZYMES

The Phase Concept of Xenobiotic Metabolism

The metabolism of a given compound often proceeds in several sequential steps. A common strategy of the organism to improve the water solubility of foreign compounds is to conjugate lipophilic substrates with hydrophilic building blocks, such as glucuronic acid, glutathione, and sulfate. This conjugation step requires the presence of a suitable functional group in the molecule that often has to be introduced or uncovered by one or more steps. In the classical model of xenobiotic metabolism, this functionalization is called phase I, while conjugation is termed phase II (Fig. 1). Depending on the nature of the introduced functional groups, these groups can be classified as being either electrophilic or nucleophilic. Typical structures with an electrophilic carbon are epoxide functions and α,β-unsaturated carbonyl groups. Important nucleophilic moieties are alcoholic or phenolic hydroxyl groups, amino and sulfhydryl functions, or carboxylic groups.

Depending on their individual chemical reactivity, electrophiles can have a significant cytotoxic and/or mutagenic potential, due to their ability to react with electron-rich partners, in particular proteins, RNA, and DNA. In contrast, nucleophilic metabolites do not usually attack endogenous macromolecules by covalent interaction and are thus, in general, less dangerous. However, they are quite often the determinants of the biological activity of a given compound. Acutely toxic effects of xenobiotics and/or their metabolites can depend upon the presence of specific nucleophilic groups in the respective molecule.

Conjugation reactions usually terminate either the potential of electrophiles to react with proteins and

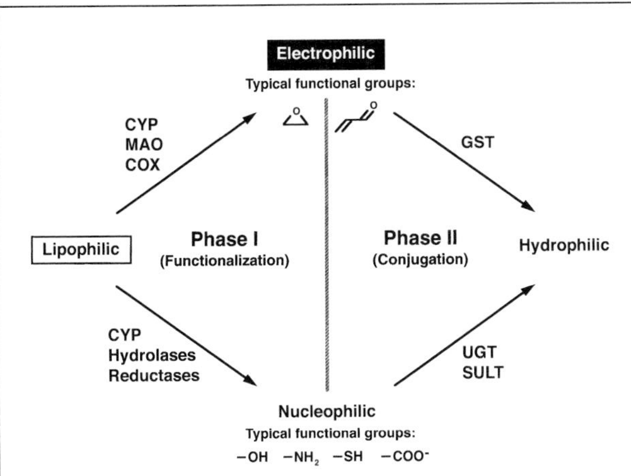

FIGURE 1 The phase model of xenobiotic metabolism. Metabolism of lipophilic foreign compounds typically proceeds in sequential steps. In phase I, the compounds are functionalized via introduction or liberation of nucleophilic or electrophilic anchor groups by oxidoreductases or hydrolases. These anchor groups then allow phase II of xenobiotic metabolism conjugation of strongly polar endogenous building blocks, such as glucuronic acid and glutathione, to the compounds. The resulting metabolites are usually readily water soluble and can be excreted via bile or urine. The conjugation reaction often terminates the biological activity of compounds, such as the genotoxic effects of many electrophiles or the pharmacological effects of many therapeutic drugs.

DNA or the ability of nucleophiles to interact with a biological receptor. At the same time, they strongly increase the water solubility of the compound in most instances. That is why conjugation reactions can be regarded as the major detoxification step in the metabolism of xenobiotics. However, there are exceptions. Glutathione conjugation can strongly increase the electrophilic reactivity of vicinal dihaloalkanes, enzymatic sulfate ester formation with hydroxymethylated aromatic compounds leads to mutagenic species, and the glucuronidation of morphine at the enolic hydroxy group (position 6) leaves the resulting metabolite pharmacologically active. Thus, the system obviously does not react perfectly in each setting.

General Characteristics of Xenobiotic-Metabolizing Enzymes

How does the organism fulfill the demand to take care of any possible compound entering the body, and what are the trade-offs? The obvious need for a broad substrate specificity is fulfilled in two ways. Usually, the different enzymes exclusively or predominantly involved in the metabolism of xenobiotics (i) have a broad substrate specificity and (ii) build large (super)families of enzymes with distinct but overlapping substrate specificities.

Xenobiotic-metabolizing enzymes are, in general, rather slow catalysts. With a reported maximum turnover of about 10^4 min^{-1}, glutathione *S*-transferases are among the fastest of these, but this is still very slow compared to, for instance, carboanhydrase, with an approximate turnover of 4×10^7 min^{-1}.

The facts that there are a large number of different xenobiotic-metabolizing enzymes in a single organism (probably hundreds) and that the individual enzymes are comparatively slow catalysts reveals the need for an economical way to provide the necessary amounts of each of these under conditions when they are required. This may be one reason that many xenobiotic-metabolizing enzymes are substrate-inducible. In fact, a broad substrate specificity and inducibility by foreign compounds can be regarded as the two main characteristics of a typical xenobiotic-metabolizing enzyme.

Enzymes Implicated in Xenobiotic Metabolism

The phase I–functionalization phase of the xenobiotic metabolism is carried out by two major groups of enzymes, namely, oxidoreductases and hydrolases. The oxidoreductases include the quantitatively most important superfamily of xenobiotic-metabolizing enzymes, the cytochrome P450-dependent monooxygenases (CYP), as well as flavin-containing monooxygenases (FMO), monoamine oxidases (MAO), and cyclooxygenases (COX), all of which introduce oxygen into or remove electrons from their substrates, with few exceptions. Dehydrogenases and reductases, among which alcohol dehydrogenases, aldehyde dehydrogenases, and carbonyl reductases play a role in xenobiotic metabolism, add or remove hydrogen to or from the target molecule. The hydrolases comprise families of enzymes specialized in the hydrolysis of either esters, amides, epoxides, or glucuronides.

The phase II–conjugation phase of the xenobiotic metabolism is carried out by transferases. Electrophilic substrates are taken over by the glutathione *S*-transferases. Nucleophilic substrates, (i.e., those with hydroxy, sulfhydryl, amino, or carboxyl groups) are metabolized by UDP-glucuronosyltransferases (UGT), sulfotransferases (SULT), acetyltransferases (AT), acyl-CoA amino acid *N*-acyltransferase, and methyl transferases (Table 1).

TABLE 1 Major Pathways in the Metabolism of Xenobiotics

Phase I metabolism: functionalization

Predominant function: conversion of apolar, lipophilic compounds into more polar, more hydrophilic compounds; introduction or liberation of functional groups that can be used for conjugation in the subsequent phase II of xenobiotic metabolism.

A. Oxidation: expoxidation; hydroxylation; O-, N-, or S-dealkylation; substitution of heteroatoms by oxygen; dehydrogenation

B. Reduction: azo reduction; nitro reduction; reduction of carbonyl compounds

C. Hydrolysis: ester hydrolysis; amide hydrolysis; epoxide hydrolysis[a]

Phase II metabolism: conjugation

Conjugation of xenobiotics or their phase I metabolites with endogenous building blocks. The resulting products are often significantly more hydrophilic than the corresponding substrates, usually readily water soluble and easily excretable.

A. Glutathione conjugation
B. Glucuronidation
C. Sulfation
D. Acetylation
E. Conjugation to amino acids
F. Methylation

[a]By some regarded as conjugation to water and thus grouped among the phase II metabolism.

CHARACTERIZATION OF INDIVIDUAL XENOBIOTIC-METABOLIZING ENZYMES

Phase I Enzymes (A): Oxidoreductases

Cytochromes P450 (CYP:EC 1.14.14.1)

Systematics and Nomenclature

The cytochromes P450 or cytochrome P450-dependent monooxygenases represent a large superfamily of enzymes, many of which play a prominent role in the metabolism of foreign compounds. In eucaryotes, the cytochromes P450 are membrane-bound enzymes, residing mainly in the endoplasmic reticulum where these heme–thiolate proteins form a complex with the cytochrome P450 reductase. They can be retrieved for experimental purposes in the microsomal fraction, the 100,000*g* sediment of the postmitochondrial supernatant of tissue homogenates.

Historically, CYP have been identified on the basis of their absorbance maximum at 450 nm, after reduction and complex formation with carbon monoxide. It soon became evident that this membrane-bound pigment plays a major role in the oxidative metabolism of a large number of exogenous and endogenous compounds. Subsequently, the multiplicity of individual CYP was uncovered by the differential inducibility of CYP-dependent enzymatic activities by foreign compounds and later by the isolation of distinct isoenzymes. Today, in the age of gene-sequence analysis, the number of individual CYP isoenzymes as well as their phylogenetic relationship can be studied in greater detail. So far, 38 different functional CYP genes have been identified in humans. On the basis of sequence similarity, these are grouped into 14 different families, each containing a variable number of subfamilies. In general, enzymes within a family share more than 40% amino acid sequence identity, while enzymes within a subfamily are more than 55% identical. However, these values hold true in general only for a comparison among mammalian species. The official recommendation by the P450 Nomenclature Committee proposes the capitalized root symbol CYP (*cy*tochrome *P*450) for all members of the superfamily, followed by an arabic number for the family and a capital letter for the subfamily, followed by a second arabic number designating the individual isoenzyme. Thus, CYP1A1 is the correct name for the first enzyme in the subfamily A of the cytochrome P450 family 1. If it is possible to assign the orthologous enzymes in different organisms with sufficient precision, that is, if there is significantly higher sequence similarity between these orthologous forms from different species than there is between any of these and a second related enzyme within the same species, the enzymes from different organisms receive the same designation, as is the case for CYP family 1 members. In contrast, if the homology between two isoenzymes within a given species is higher than it is to the most closely related enzyme in another species, then assignment of orthologous forms is impossible and all sequences within the subfamily are subsequently numbered, usually in the order of their discovery. This is the case with many enzymes from CYP families 2, 3, and 4. Because the human genome is not completely analyzed, the findings in other species may serve as estimates of the possible number of human CYP genes that can be expected.

At present, 57 functional CYP genes have been reported in the rat and 68 different CYP genes have been identified in *Caenorhabditis elegans,* a nematode of which about 60% of its genome has been analyzed. Thus, we can expect about 100 CYP genes in this comparatively simple organism. The current development in this field can be followed via the Internet, either at the Web site of the P450 Gene Superfamily Nomenclature Committee (http://drnelson.utmem.

edu/nelsonhomepage.html) or at another excellent Web site (http://www.icgeb.trieste.it/p450).

Enzymatic Mechanism

The prominent activity of CYP is, as implied by its name monooxygenase, the transfer of one oxygen atom from molecular oxygen to an organic substrate. The remaining oxygen atom is reduced to water during the reaction, the required reducing equivalents coming from the cofactor NADPH. The final result of a CYP-catalyzed oxidation is usually an epoxidation, hydroxylation, desaturation, or dealkylation or a heteroatom oxygenation or replacement by oxygen. In some cases, the enzyme may act as a reductase. Multiply halogenated alkanes, for instance, can undergo CYP-mediated reductive dehalogenation.

The CYP-catalyzed oxygenation proceeds by a number of sequential steps (Fig. 2). There is evidence that CYP forms a multimeric complex in the endoplasmic membrane with the flavoprotein NADPH–P450 reductase. The CYP itself carries a heme as the prosthetic group, with an iron as the central atom, which is in the ferric form [Fe^{3+}] and, in most CYP isoenzymes, is predominantly in the low-spin configuration in its d^5 orbitals. Binding of a substrate molecule in the catalytic pocket of the enzyme in many cases seems to trigger the conversion of the iron from the low-spin to the high-spin configuration, which in turn, favors the reduction of the ferric [Fe^{3+}] to the ferrous [Fe^{2+}] form of CYP by the NADPH–P450 reductase in a one-electron transfer reaction. In this state, the iron can bind molecular oxygen to form an $Fe^{2+}-O_2$ complex. This is reduced again in a further one-electron transfer step, either directly by the NADPH–P450 reductase or sometimes by the soluble cytochrome b_5, which itself has to be activated by the NADH-dependent cytochrome b_5 reductase. Now the complex is in a highly activated form ($Fe^{2+}-O_2^-$) that can transfer oxygen to the substrate or, alternatively, release active oxygen species, for instance, hydrogen peroxide, and thereby start cytotoxic processes such as lipid peroxidation. The oxygen transfer to the substrate is, of course, the main route, but proceeds via unstable intermediates difficult to analyze. It is generally accepted that heterolytic scission of the O–O bond and binding of two protons lead to the formation of a water molecule and a $(FeO)^{3+}$ intermediate with a high oxygen-transfer potential, which in the final step oxygenates the substrate.

A few important conclusions can be drawn from this mechanism: (i) many, but not all, CYP can bind and activate oxygen only after substrate binding has occurred, which protects the organism from the potentially destructive generation of reactive oxygen species by CYP; (ii) because of their capability to activate oxygen, CYP can per se represent a toxic challenge for the organism, especially in the presence of competitive inhibitors that may bind to the active site of the protein and thereby initiate the oxygen activation without being able to undergo oxidation; and (iii) NADPH and, in some cases, NADH are necessary cofactors for the reaction and processes that change the redox state of the cell potentially interfer with the efficiency of the CYP-dependent metabolism.

Cytochrome P450 Isozymes with Implication in Xenobiotic Metabolism

CYP families 1–3 harbor the major players in the CYP-mediated drug metabolism in mammalian species (Table 2). The CYP1 family currently comprises three known members in humans, CYP1A1, CYP1A2, and CYP1B1. CYP1A1 is the classical isoenzyme involved in the metabolism of polycyclic aromatic hydrocarbons (PAH), a large group of relevant potentially carcinogenic pollutants. While they are themselves chemically almost inert, their oxidative metabolic transformation leads to mutagenic intermediates. Figure 3 shows the different metabolic steps that lead to the formation of the ultimate carcinogenic metabolite of the model PAH benzo[*a*]pyrene, the benzo[*a*]pyrene-7,8-dihydrodiol-9,10-epoxide. Both of the CYP-mediated reactions of this cascade can be carried out by CYP1A1. Many of the usually planar lipophilic PAHs can induce their own metabolism by CYP1A1 by increasing the transcription of the gene via the aryl hydrocarbon receptor (Ah receptor). Under normal conditions, CYP1A1 is essentially absent from human liver but can be found in a number of other tissues, including lymphocytes, lung, and placenta.

CYP1A2, in contrast, is in humans found almost exclusively in the liver. Like the CYP1A1, it is inducible by planar PAHs. On average, about 10% of the total liver CYP is CYP1A2, but the level of expression differs considerably among individuals. Quite a large number of procarcinogens are metabolically activated by this isoenzyme, including aromatic amines such as the protein pyrolysis products 2-amino-3-methylimidazo[4,5-*f*]quinoline (IQ) and 2-amino-1-methyl-6-phenylimidazo[4,5-*b*]pyridine (PhIP), polycyclic aromatic hydrocarbons, and the strongly hepatocarcinogenic mycotoxin aflatoxin B_1. Of practical toxicological importance is the fact that CYP1A2 significantly contributes to the metabolic inactivation of caffeine. Therefore, CYP1A2 inhibitors, such as furafyline and fluvoxamine, can strongly reduce the caf-

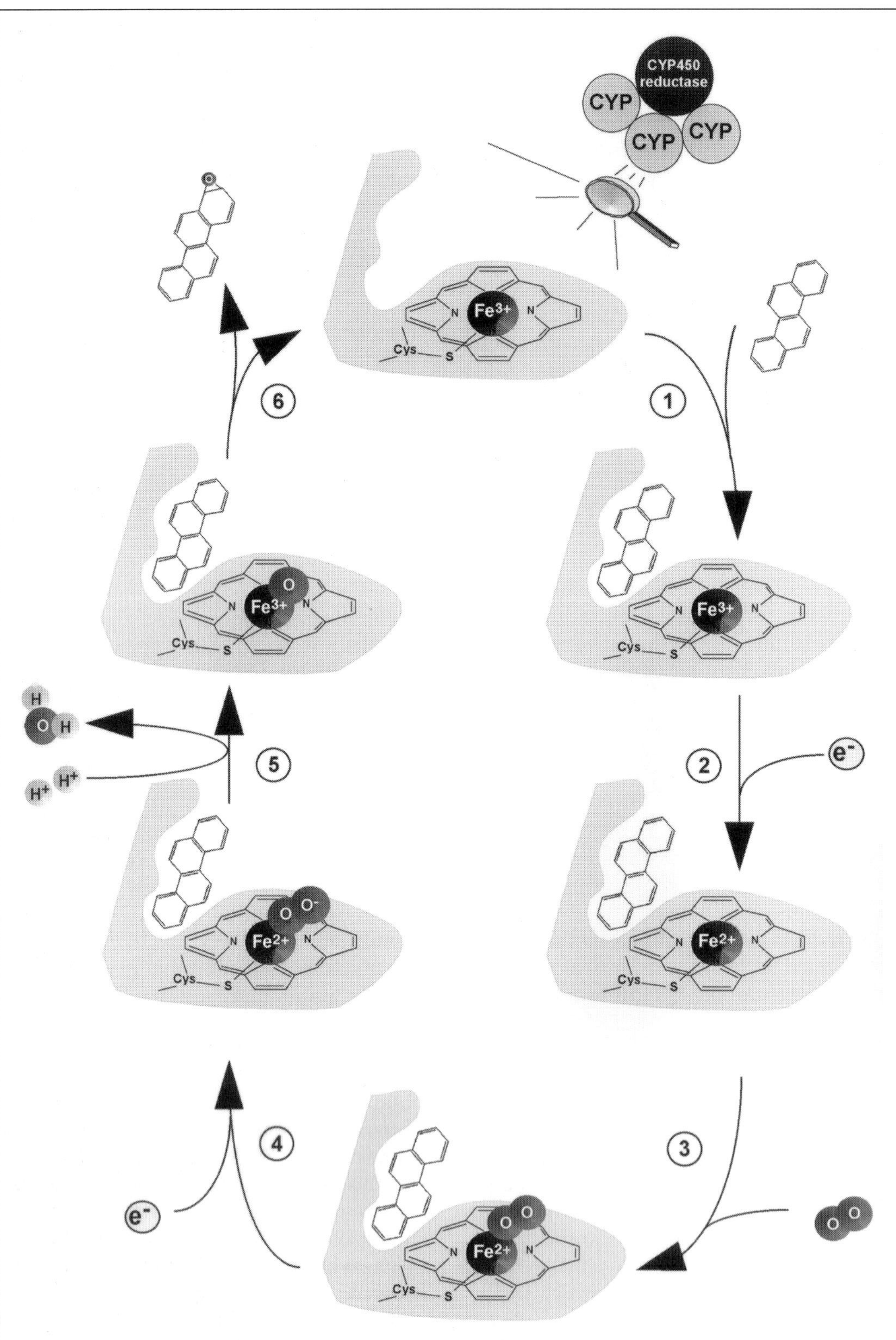

FIGURE 2 Cytochrome P450 (CYP)-mediated oxidation. (1) A substrate molecule, such as chrysene in the present case, binds in the catalytic pocket of the enzyme and supports the conversion of the heme iron from the low-spin to the hight-spin configuration; (2) the ferric [Fe^{3+}] form of CYP is reduced to the ferrous [Fe^{2+}] form by NADPH–P450 reductase in a one-electron transfer reaction; (3) the iron [Fe^{2+}] binds molecular oxygen; (4) a second one-electron reduction, either by NADPH–P450 reductase or by cytochrome b_5, leads to the highly activated [Fe^{2-} – O^-_2]; (5) heterolytic scission of the O—O bond and binding of two protons lead to the release of a water molecule; (6) the unstable $(FeO)^{3+}$ intermediate oxygenates the substrate, which is subsequently released from the enzyme.

TABLE 2 Important Human Xenobiotic-Metabolizing Cytochrome P450 Isoenzymes

Isoenzyme	Organ[a]	Relevant substrates (selection)	Relation to animal cytochromes P450
CYP1A1	Multiple	Polycyclic aromatic hydrocarbons (PAH)	Orthologous forms with similar biochemical characteristics in vertebrates
CYP1A2	Liver	Aromatic amines, PAH, phenacetin, caffeine, warfarin, aflatoxin B_1	Orthologous forms with similar biochemical characteristics in vertebrates
CYP2A6	Liver	Coumarin, 6-aminochrysene, aflatoxin B_1, nitrosamines	No clear relationship to a specific animal CYP
CYP2B6	Liver	Cyclophosphamide, nicotine	In contrast to the rat CYP2B1 that is strongly inducible (e.g., by phenobarbital) and thereby becoming a major hepatic CYP in this species, CYP2B6 has been found only in rather small amounts in human liver and does not seem to play an important role in xenobiotic metabolism
CYP2C8	Liver	Taxol, retinoids	No clear relationship to a specific animal CYP
CYP2C9	Liver, kidney	Diclofenac, ibuprofen, phenytoin, tolbutamide	No clear relationship to a specific animal CYP
CYP2C19	Liver	(*S*)-Mephenytoin, omeprazole	No clear relationship to a specific animal CYP
CYP2D6	Liver	Debrisoquin, propranolol, dextromethorphan	No clear relationship to a specific animal CYP
CYP2E1	Liver, gastro-intestinal tract	Ethanol, benzene, dimethylnitrosamine, chlorzoxazone	Orthologous enzymes in other species, the only subfamily member in human and many animals
CYP3A4	Liver, small intestine	Acetaminophen, benzphetamine, nifedipine, steroid hormones, erythromycin, aflatoxin B_1	Several very closely related isoenzymes in man (CYP3A3, CYP3A5, and CYP3A7) make it impossible to assign orthologous forms in other species; otherwise, the biochemical characteristics resemble those of animal CYP3A enzymes

[a]Primarily identified in the indicated organ, but possibly also expressed in other locations.

feine tolerance of individuals with an initially high CYP1A2 activity.

The recently identified isoenzyme CYP1B1 shares some of the characteristics of the CYP1A family in that it is PAH-inducible and metabolizes some polycyclic aromatic hydrocarbons. However, there are not many reports on this new CYP to date. A possible marker activity for its expression may be the 4-hydroxylation of β-estradiol.

The CYP2 family is the largest CYP family in mammals. The isoenzymes of major toxicological significance in human are CYP2A6, CYP2C8, CYP2C9, CYP2C19, CYP2D6, and CYP2E1. Although not expressed at a high level in human liver ($<5\%$ of total CYP), CYP2A6 may be of significance because of its ability to activate the carcinogens 6-aminochrysene and aflatoxin B_1, as well as some tobacco-specific nitrosamines. The 7-hydroxylation of coumarin can be taken as a diagnostic enzyme activity for this isozyme.

CYP2B family members were discovered very early and represent important isoenzymes in many model animals, especially in rat and rabbit. However, the single human CYP2B member discovered so far, CYP2B6, is only poorly expressed in the liver and does not seem to possess any major importance in the xenobiotic metabolism. It appears that members of the CYP2C family substitute for this. They constitute about 20% of the human liver CYP content, at least

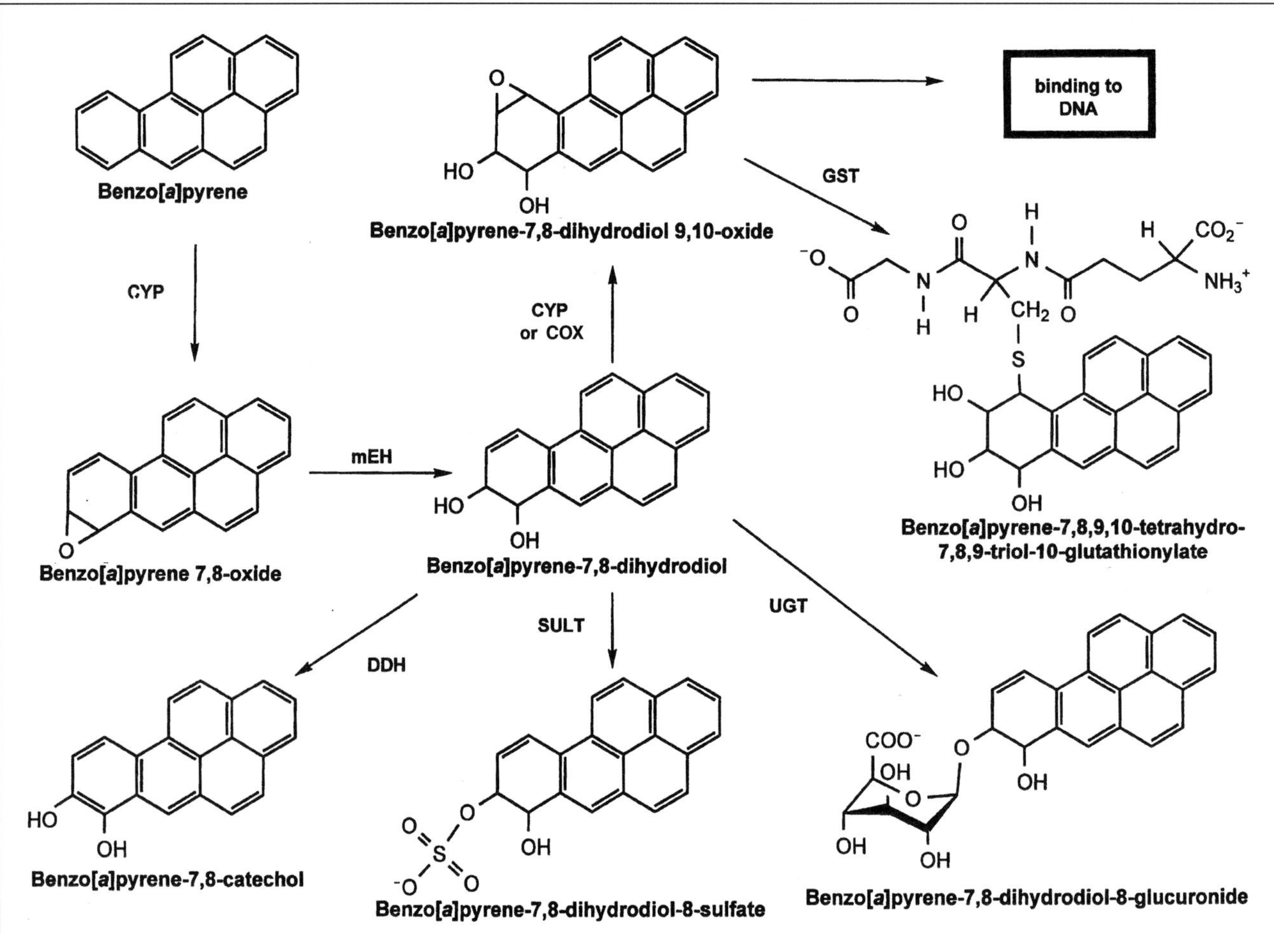

FIGURE 3 Selected metabolism pathways of benzo[*a*]pyrene. Benzo[*a*]pyrene is metabolized to many primary, secondary, and tertiary metabolites. The example shows the activation pathway to the ultimate carcinogenic metabolite, benzo[*a*]pyrene-7,8-dihydrodiol 9,10-oxide. In a first step, cytochrome P450-mediated oxidation leads to the corresponding 7,8-epoxide, which is subsequently hydrolyzed by microsomal epoxide hydrolase to the 7,8-dihydrodiol. At this stage, conjugation to glucuronic acid or sulfate, oxidation to the catechol, or spontaneous isomerization to the phenol (not shown) can sequester the metabolite from the final activation step (i.e., the oxidation to the diol epoxide by cytochromes P450 or prostaglandin synthase (COX)). The diol epoxide is a highly mutagenic compound that is not a substrate for epoxide hydrolase. Conjugation to glutathione leads to detoxification, but this metabolic step is not fast enough to abolish the genotoxic effect.

some of them are inducible by drugs such as phenobarbital and rifampicin, and they metabolize a large number of chemical compounds (Table 2).

A particularly important CYP in human is CYP2D6, known as debrisoquine hydroxylase. The expression of this isoenzyme, which usually represents about 5% of the liver CYP content, is polymorphic, due to a number of functionally inactive alleles. It is responsible for the metabolism of a plethora of drugs, and lack of CYP2D6 activity can lead to significantly prolonged half-lives of these drugs. About 7% of the Caucasian population suffers from this defect and therefore must be aware of potentially toxic effects caused by standard doses of the compounds. Furthermore, there are reports of a statistically significant correlation between CYP2D6 genotype and the incidence of certain forms of Parkinson syndrome, a disease that can result, for instance, from chemically induced degeneration of dopaminergic neurons in the central nervous system. While several other CYP isoenzymes and other xenobiotic-metabolizing enzymes are also subject to polymorphisms, the case of CYP2D6 is probably the most relevant for acute drug toxicity.

CYP2E1 is the only member of the CYP2E subfamily in most species, including human. The enzyme is capable of metabolizing a broad range of substrates that have in common a relatively small molecular size, such as ethanol, benzene, several alkylnitrosamines, and acetaminophen. In the presence of excess substrate, the half-life of the protein is considerably increased, leading to an accumulation of enzyme protein after some time. In some cases, this is potentiated by a concomitant stimulation of the transcription rate of the *CYP2E1* gene. The fact that the heme iron of CYP2E1 is, even in the absence of substrate, predominantly in the high-spin state and thus capable of generating active oxygen species has led to the concept that ethanol-induced liver injury may be—at least in part—a consequence of oxidative damage caused by ethanol-induced enhanced CYP2E1 levels.

Four different isoenzymes have been identified in the human CYP3 family, the most important of them being CYP3A4. It is usually the most abundant CYP in human liver, accounting for about 30% of the total amount. At the same time, this enzyme displays an extraordinarily broad substrate specificity, including many kinds of steroid hormones, macrolide antibiotics, alkaloids, benzodiazepines, dihydropyridines, warfarin, polycyclic aromatic hydrocarbon-derived dihydrodiols, and aflatoxin B_1. Furthermore, the enzyme is inducible, for instance, by dexamethasone, rifampicin, and phenobarbital. This once led to one of the most spectacular cases of drug–drug interactions, inducing the metabolism of contraceptive steroids to such an extent that quite a number of unwanted pregnancies were observed in tuberculosis patients who had been simultaneously treated with contraceptives and rifampicin. CYP3A4 may fairly be regarded as the most important human CYP.

Flavin-Containing Monooxygenases (FMOs; EC 1.14.13.8)

The second family of microsomal oxidative xenobiotic-metabolizing enzymes with a broad substrate specificity contains the flavin-containing monooxygenases. Despite the significant overlap in function with the CYP enzymes, the mechanisms of action of the two kinds of monooxygenases are fundamentally different. In contrast to many CYP isoenzymes, the FMOs bind and activate molecular oxygen before the substrate binds to the enzyme. In the first step of the catalytic cycle (Fig. 4), the prosthetic group of FMO, the flavin adenine dinucleotide (FAD); is reduced by NADPH to form $FADH_2$. At this stage, the $NADP^+$ remains bound to the enzyme. In the second step, molecular oxygen is incorporated into the prosthetic group, resulting in the formation of the hydroperoxide FADH-4α-OOH. Now, the enzyme is able to transfer oxygen to a suitable substrate. After oxygenation of the substrate, a water molecule is released, leaving the FAD in its oxidized form. Finally, $NADP^+$ dissociates from the enzyme, which is thus ready to undergo the next catalytic cycle.

How does the organism protect itself against the potentially destructive force of an armed FMO that forms before the oxygen acceptor binds? First, the oxygen transfer potential of FMO is much lower than that of CYP, restricting acceptor substrates to "soft" nucleophiles, usually molecules containing sulfur or nitrogen as a hetero atom. The major FMO-catalyzed reactions are therefore *N*-oxide and *S*-oxide formation. Second, important endogenous soft nucleophiles, such as glutathione, amino acids, and polyamines, are protected from metabolism by FMO because charged molecules, in general, are poor FMO substrates if the single charged group within the molecule is not itself the acceptor site for the oxygen or if the molecule carries more than one charged group.

Five single-member FMO subfamilies, termed FMO1–5, have been described to date. These isoenzymes share about 50–60% amino acid sequence identity. All FMO subfamilies are present in human. The respective genes all map to chromosome 1q and, thus, probably represent a gene cluster. Due to the instability of FMOs, there are only few reports on the substrate specificity of the human isoenzymes. Among the compounds known to be oxidized by human FMO are (*S*)-nicotine, phenothiazine derivatives, and cimetidine. Table 3 gives on overview of the substrate spectrum of pig liver FMO1, which has been studied more extensively. However, it must be pointed out that there is evidence indicating a substantially broader substrate specificity of this enzyme than of the human FMOs.

There is no indication of any inducibility of FMO by foreign compounds. The prominent isoenzyme in human liver is FMO3. FMO2 was first described in the lung of experimental animals, whereas in humans it is the prominent form in the kidney. In addition to the liver, FMO1 has also been found in kidney and intestine. The major locations of FMO4 and FMO5 have not been identified because they are detectable only in traces in a number of different human tissues.

A genetic disorder called the "fish odor" syndrome is the result of a FMO deficiency. The syndrome is caused by the inability of a respective individual to metabolize trimethylamine to its *N*-oxide, a reaction that is carried out exclusively by FMO. People suffering from this deficiency excrete and exhale the unmetabolized amine, which is highly volatile and smells like rotten fish, a circumstance that results in severe social problems. The responsible isoenzyme has not been identified yet. Because all FMO genes reside on the same chromosome, possibly in close proximity to

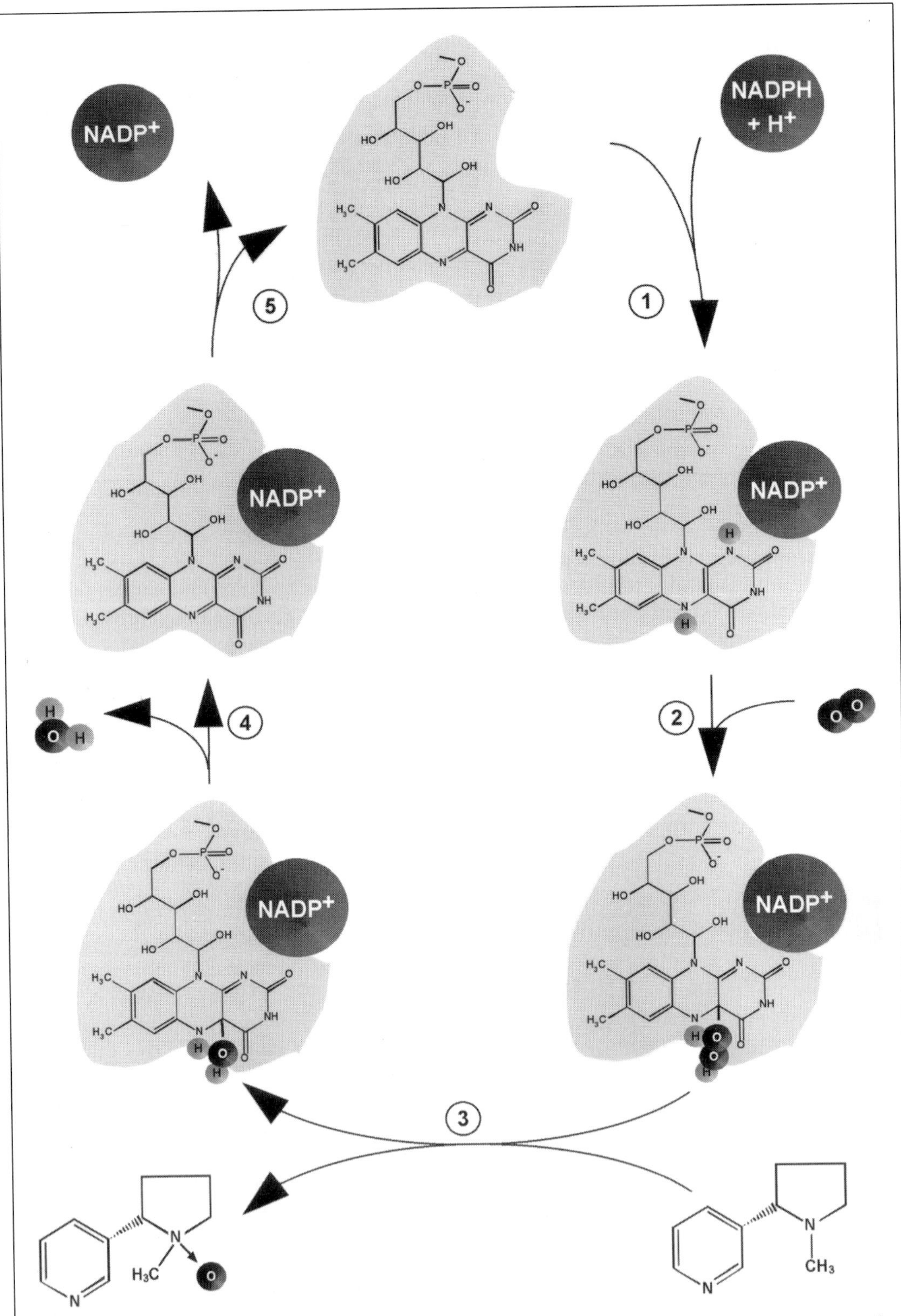

FIGURE 4 Flavin-containing monooxygenase-mediated oxidation. In contrast to many CYP isoenzymes, the FMOs bind and activate molecular oxygen before the substrate binds to the enzyme. (1) NADPH binds to the enzyme and reduces the prosthetic group flavin adenine dinucleotide (FAD; only the riboflavin part is presented in the figure) to $FADH_2$; at this stage, the $NADP^+$ remains bound to the enzyme; (2) molecular oxygen is incorporated into the prosthetic group, resulting in the formation of the hydroperoxide FADH-4α-OOH; (3) oxygen is transferred to the substrate, nicotine in the present case; (4) a water molecule is released, leaving the FAD in its oxidized form; (5) $NADP^+$ dissociates from the enzyme.

TABLE 3 Substrate Specificity of Pig Liver Flavin-Containing Monooxygenase FMO1

Organic nitrogen compounds
Secondary and tertiary acyclic and cyclic amines
N-Alkyl- and *N*, *N*,-dialkyl arylamines
Hydrazines
Organic sulfur-containing compounds
Mercaptopurines, -pyrimidines, and -imidazoles
Cyclic and acyclic sulfides and disulfides
Thioamides, thiocarbamides, dithiocarbamides, dithioacids
Other organic substrates
Phosphines
Boronic acid
Selenides
Selenocarbamides
Inorganic compounds
Sulfur, sulfides, thiocyanates
Iodine, iodides, hypoiodites

each other, it is quite likely that more than one FMO gene is affected in this phenotype.

Monoamine Oxidases (MAOs; EC 1.4.3.4)

Monoamine oxidases are flavoproteins of the outer mitochondrial membrane. They exist in two isoforms, MAO-A and MAO-B, which share about 70% sequence identity on the amino acid level. Both forms are almost ubiquitous in the mammalian organism. In humans, MAO-A appears to be absent from blood platelets, lymphocytes, and chromaffin cells, while MAO-B is only poorly expressed in placenta. Organs with particularly high enzymatic activity are the central nervous system and the liver. MAO has primarily endogenous function in inactivating monoamine neurotransmitters, such as serotonine and dopamine, by oxidative desamination. Likewise, the enzyme is capable of using a number of xenobiotic primary, secondary, or tertiary amines as substrates to generate an aldehyde, ammonia or an amine, and hydrogen peroxide:

$$R^1CH_2NR^2R^3 + O_2 + H_2O \longrightarrow R^1CHO + HNR^2R^3 + H_2O_2.$$

The amount of hydrogen peroxide produced by this reaction can reach toxicologically relevant levels. Prominent examples of foreign compounds metabolized by MAO are some β-adrenergic antagonists, such as propranolol. Serotonin is preferentially metabolized by MAO-A, while β-phenyl ethylamine is a better substrate for MAO-B. The latter enzyme also acts more efficiently than MAO-A on most tertiary amines and prefers highly lipophilic substrates.

A MAO substrate of significant toxicological relevance is 1-methyl-4-phenyl-1,2,3,6-tetrahydropyridine (MPTP). It is metabolized via the intermediate 1-methyl-4-phenyl-2,3-dihydropyridinium ($MPDP^+$) to the 1-methyl-4-phenyl pyridinium (MPP^+). MPP^+ is taken up by the nigrostriatal dopaminergic neurons through their high-affinity re-uptake system and blocks the mitochondrial metabolism, thereby killing these cells. The loss of these dopaminergic neurons leads to Parkinson disease. The selectivity of the neurotoxicity depends upon the fact that within the neurons, only MAO can metabolize MPTP, while in other tissues CYP- and FMO-catalyzed detoxification reactions compete with MAO for the substrate. While MPTP itself is an experimental chemical, there are related compounds, such as β- carboline and tetrahydroisoquinoline, that are present in minor concentrations in the food. Whether they behave similarly to MPTP and are thereby of relevance for the development of the idiopathic Parkinson syndrome remains to be clarified.

Cyclooxygenases (COX: EC 1.14.99.1)

Cyclooxygenase, also called prostaglandin synthase, is a membrane-bound protein of the endoplasmic reticulum. This enzyme metabolizes arachidonic acid in a two-step process to prostaglandin H_2 (see Fig. 5). In a first reaction, two molecules of oxygen are incorporated into the unsaturated fatty acid to create a cyclic peroxide (endoperoxide) moiety and a hydroperoxide function. The resulting intermediate is called prostaglandin G_2. In the second step, the hydroperoxide group is converted to a hydroxyl group, resulting in the formation of prostaglandin H_2. In this second reaction, many organic compounds are able to serve as an oxygen acceptor or electron donor, provided they are sufficiently lipophilic and have a low redox potential, like many phenolic compounds and aromatic amines, and therefore many drugs are potential substrates for COX. The extent to which a compound may be co-oxidized by COX can be estimated from the influence of its substituents at the aromatic ring system on the redox potential of the compound. For example, substitution of the aromatic ring with electron-withdrawing groups reduces the rate of metabolism of *N*-methyl aniline derivatives by COX. Similarly, acetylation of aromatic amines to amides reduces the reactivity of a compound as a potential substrate of COX.

During co-oxidation, some substrates acquire the state of a radical. Radicals are characterized by the presence of an unpaired electron and therefore are usually highly reactive. They can either dimerize or

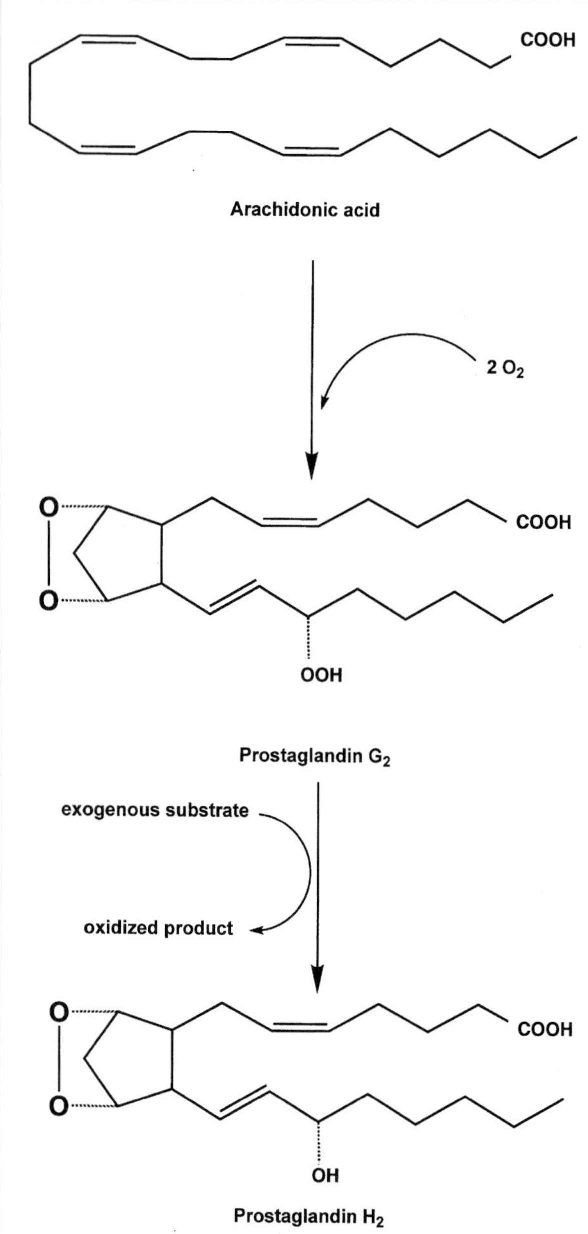

FIGURE 5 Cyclooxygenase-mediated cooxidation. In the first Step (A) of prostaglandin H_2 synthesis, two molecules of oxygen are incorporated into arachidonic acid, forming the cyclic peroxide (endoperoxide) prostaglandin G_2, which also contains a hydroperoxy group. In second step (f), this hydroperoxide group is converted to a hydroxyl group, resulting in the formation of prostaglandin H_2. During this reaction, the oxygen can be transferred to an exogenous acceptor substrate.

react with other molecules to yield new radicals. In this way, they can initiate lipid peroxidation or can bind to cellular proteins or DNA.

A second, slightly different, activation pathway can also be mediated by COX. Prostaglandin G_2 is capable—over a number of intermediate steps—of forming a peroxyl radical. This reactive compound can epoxidize a variety of substrates, including polycyclic aromatic hydrocarbons and aflatoxin B_1. An interesting aspect of this activation pathway is that the metabolites sometimes have the inverse geometry of the analogous species evolving from the CYP-metabolism. Thus, (+)-benzo[*a*]pyrene-7,8-diol is metabolized to (+)-*syn*-benzo[*a*]pyrene-7,8-diol-9,10-epoxide by CYP and to (−)-*anti*-benzo[*a*]pyrene-7,8-diol-9,10-epoxide by COX. This can be taken to analyze the contributions of these two different oxidoreductases to the metabolism in a respective sample.

Two isoenzymes, COX-1 and COX-2, have been identified. COX-1 is a constitutively expressed enzyme, whereas COX-2 is an inducible form up-regulated in inflammation. Quite a number of extrahepatic tissues that are low in CYP are rich in COX, which is believed to be of significance for the carcinogenic effect of aromatic amines in these organs, for example, kidney, gastrointestinal tract, brain, lung, and urinary bladder. Ram seminal vesicles have become the standard source for the purification and analysis of COX because of the particularly high content in COX.

Dehydrogenases and Reductases

One of the foreign compounds that most frequently enters the human body in significant amounts is ethanol. It is metabolized by an alcohol dehydrogenase (ADH; EC 1.1.1) to the toxic intermediate acetaldehyde, which is further metabolized by an aldehyde dehydrogenase (EC 1.2.1) to acetic acid. The metabolic transformation of ethanol to acetaldehyde is one of the few xenobiotic metabolism pathways that follows zero-order kinetics, due to the rapid saturation of the responsible enzyme. This is explained by the fact that a blood alcohol concentration of 0.1‰, where the zero-order kinetic becomes apparent, already corresponds to a substrate concentration in the millimolar range. The second step of the described metabolic cascade, the aldehyde dehydrogenase-mediated oxidation to acetic acid, can be efficiently inhibited by the drug disulfiram (Antabus). Therefore, it is used to support the treatment of alcohol addicts. After intake, the toxic acetaldehyde accumulates and provokes headache and nausea, which is supposed to keep the patient from further ingestion of alcohol. Many other aldehydes, such as the α,β-unsaturated aldehydes arising from lipid peroxidation, also have a considerable toxic potential. Therefore, aldehyde dehydrogenase is, in general, a detoxifying enzyme. The most prominent exception is the metabolism of methanol via formaldehyde to formic acid. Formic acid appears to be the decisive toxic principle of methanol, leading first to blindness through edema of the retina and eventually to death. The suitable antidote is ethanol, because ethanol has the much higher affinity to the alcohol dehydrogenase. Thus, keeping a constant level of ethanol in the body allows the unmetabolized excretion of methanol and prevents the metabolic formation of the formic acid.

The family of medium-chain alcohol dehydrogenases currently comprises six classes of dimeric enzymes in mammals. A class in this sense describes a group of enzymes with common physicochemical and biochemical characteristics. Class I contains the classic liver ADH and the subunits α, β, and γ. Class II is characterized by the π subunit and is also present in liver, although less abundantly. Class III is known as the glutathione-dependent formaldehyde dehydrogenase. Its subunit is designated χ. Class IV, with the subunit σ, interestingly is most abundant in the stomach. It is the enzyme with the highest activity toward ethanol and is strongly implicated in the metabolism of this compound. Two further classes of medium-chain alcohol dehydrogenases have been characterized on the bases of subunit structure, but otherwise little is known about these.

The short-chain dehydrogenases are implicated mainly in steroid metabolism in mammals. However, the 3α-hydroxysteroid dehydrogenase (3α-HSD) of rat and human has been shown to be able to oxidize vicinal dihydrodiols of polycyclic aromatic hydrocarbons via the corresponding catechols to the respective quinones and has therefore also been termed dihydrodiol dehydrogenase. This reaction is of potential significance in polycyclic aromatic hydrocarbon metabolism, because it sequesters the prebay dihydrodiols of polycyclic aromatic hydrocarbon away from their critical activation pathway (end product is the ultimate carcinogenic dihydrodiol bay-region epoxide) to form catechols and/or quinones instead (Fig. 3). Although this can be regarded as a protective metabolic function against the formation of genotoxic metabolites, the formation of quinones is itself a potentially toxic process; these compounds are frequently able to undergo redox cycling, thereby compromising the intracellular redox status. Thus, the role of dihydrodiol dehydrogenase is not exclusively beneficial. A well-documented example of the toxic consequences of a catechol formation is naphthalene-induced cataract formation, where the generation of 1,2-dihydroxynaphthalene is the critical step in the toxification of the compound. Remarkably, the dihydrodiol dehydrogenase activity is not necessarily restricted to 3α-HSD. In rabbit liver, at least eight clearly distinct enzymes display dihydrodiol dehydrogenase activity, one of them being the 3α-hydroxysteroid dehydrogenase. In contrast, in rat liver the 3α-HSD is the single enzyme known to be proficient in dihydrodiol dehydrogenase activity. Like 3α-HSD, 11β-hydroxysteroid dehydrogenase (11β-HSD) has recently been reported to be involved in the metabolism of xenobiotics, acting as a carbonyl reductase. In particular 4-(methylnitrosamino)-1-(3-pyridyl)-butan-1-one (NNK), a tobacco-specific and highly mutagenic nitrosamine, is a documented substrate of 11β-HSD. It has been suggested that the activation of NNK to the ultimate mutagenic metabolite can be circumvented by conjugation to glucuronic acid after 11β-HSD-mediated reduction of the keto function.

Another reductase of toxicological relevance is NAD(P)H quinone oxidoreductase (NQOR; EC 1.6.99.2), formerly called DT-diaphorase. NQOR is a dimeric flavoprotein. Two isoenzymes have been identified; one, NQOR-1, is inducible by TCDD. The enzymatic kinetics of NQOR follow an ordered "ping-pong" mechanism, working by a sequential formation of two different binary complexes. First, an enzyme–cofactor complex is formed, leading to the reduction of the prosthetic group of the enzyme. NADH and NADPH are equally well suited as electron donors for NQOR. After subsequent dissociation of the enzyme–cofactor complex, the substrate binds to the enzyme and is reduced, and the product is finally released. Therefore, the enzymatic reaction can be significantly inhibited by high concentrations of either the substrate or the cofactor. Relevant natural inhibitors are coumarin derivatives, such as warfarine.

It is important to point out that there are significant species differences in the relevance of NQOR for the metabolism of xenobiotics. In the rat, NQOR appears to be the most important enzyme for the reduction of many quinones. In humans, however, a less specific carbonyl reductase is of higher quantitative importance.

NQOR acts on its substrate by a two-electron transfer mechanism and thereby circumvents the formation of the highly reactive semiquinone radicals. However, NQOR is also capable of reducing aromatic nitro compounds to aromatic hydroxyl amines, precursors of highly genotoxic reactive esters.

Phase I Enzymes (B): Hydrolases

Esterases (EC 3.1.1) and Amidases (EC 3.5.1)

Carboxylic esters are, in general, enzymatically hydrolyzed more rapidly than the corresponding amides. Both reactions are catalyzed by the same enzymes, despite the assignment of different enzyme class numbers due to the two different activities. Historically, the esterases are grouped according to their interaction with the toxicologically important organophosphates into A-, B-, and C-esterases. A-esterases hydrolyze organophosphates, while B-esterases are strongly inhibited by these compounds. C-esterases do not interact with organophosphates.

Esters derived from aromatic compounds are preferred substrates of A-esterases, sometimes called aryl esterases. The toxicologically most important substrates of these esterases are the organophosphates, widely used as insecticides. The susceptibility of insects to these toxins is different from that of mammals due to the lack of A-esterases in nonvertebrates.

The B-esterases represent a large heterogeneous group of enzymes. The prominent member is acetylcholinesterase, the enzyme responsible for the termination of cholinergic neurotransmission. The general enzymatic mechanism of B-esterases has been well known for a long time. Studies on the three-dimensional structure of acetylcholinesterase from the electric fish *Torpedo californica* have improved our understanding of it. B-esterases act on their substrates by means of a catalytic triad, composed of three amino acid residues of the peptide chain that are brought into close proximity to each other by the overall fold of the protein, the α/β hydrolase fold. In the first step of the catalytic process, a serine residue acts as the catalytic nucleophile by binding covalently to the carbonyl component of the substrate ester, leading to a transesterification and release of the alcoholic component of the substrate molecule. In the second step, a water molecule in the active center of the enzyme is activated to a hydroxyl anion by proton abstraction through a charge-relay system, formed by a histidine residue supported by the side chain of an acidic amino acid, either aspartate or glutamate. This hydroxyl anion hydrolyzes the enzyme–substrate ester to liberate the free carboxylate and to regenerate the enzyme. Because organophosphates are mechanism-based inhibitors of these enzymes, their toxic effects are best described as an overshooting activity of the cholinergic system. The inhibitory effect of the organophosphates is based on the fact that the enzyme phosphoserine ester formed between B-esterases and organophosphates hydrolyzes very slowly, if at all, and thus the enzyme is not regenerated.

A specific B-esterase localized in the central nervous system is differentially susceptible to different organophosphates, being resistant to paraoxon but sensitive to mipafox inhibition. This enzyme is the target for an organophosphorus-induced delayed polyneuropathy (OPIDP) and is thus called the neuropathy target esterase (NTE). Possibly, the combined use of organophosphorus-based insecticides and pyridostigmine, an acetylcholinesterase inhibitor used as an antidote against anticholinergic chemical weapons, is implicated in neurological disorders observed in some Gulf War veterans. A B-esterase predominantly expressed in the liver, sometimes called the "unspecific carboxyl esterase," is responsible for the hydrolysis of a large variety of xenobiotic esters and amides, including a number of anaesthetic and antiarrhythmic drugs. This enzyme is polymorphic in humans. Individuals lacking the enzyme activity display a strongly extended half-life of the drug suxamethonium, which is used as a neuromuscular-blocking drug.

Little information is available on the C-esterases. They prefer acetyl esters and are therefore also called acetyl esterases. Typical substrates are 4-nitrophenyl acetate, propyl chloroacetate, and fluorescein diacetate.

Epoxide Hydrolases (EHs; EC 3.3.2.3)

Epoxide hydrolases are a group of functionally related enzymes that catalyze the hydrolytic cleavage of oxirane rings. The two mammalian EHs with implications for xenobiotic metabolism are microsomal epoxide hydrolase (mEH) and soluble epoxide hydrolase (sEH). Despite the lack of significant sequence similarity of their amino acid sequences (<15%), these two enzymes are phylogenetically related and belong to the ancient family of α/β hydrolase fold enzymes, sharing a common three-dimensional structure that harbors a catalytic triad (see the previous discussion) in its center. This observation has led to a new concept of the mechanism of enzymatic epoxide hydrolysis. It had been believed for a long time that epoxide hydrolases act on epoxides by activating water, which, in turn, attacks the epoxide ring. The membership of epoxide hydrolases in the α/β hydrolase fold enzymes, on the other hand, suggested a two-step mechanism for EHs. Meanwhile, a clear picture has evolved from experimental analyses (Fig. 6). The catalytic triad of epoxide hydrolases is composed of an aspartate as the catalytic nucleophile and a histidine–aspartate pair (sEH) or a histidine–glutamate pair (mEH) as the water-activating charge-relay system. In the first step of the reaction, the epoxide ring of the substrate is attacked by the aspartate to form an intermediate enzyme–substrate ester. In the second step, this ester is hydrolyzed by a water molecule activated by proton abstraction through the histidine–acidic amino acid pair. This releases the product of the enzymatic reaction, a vicinal (*trans-*, if applicable) diol, and renders the enzyme ready for the next substrate turnover. The second step of this reaction appears to be rate-limiting.

The toxicological importance of the epoxide hydrolases is obvious: the oxirane ring, the essential struc-

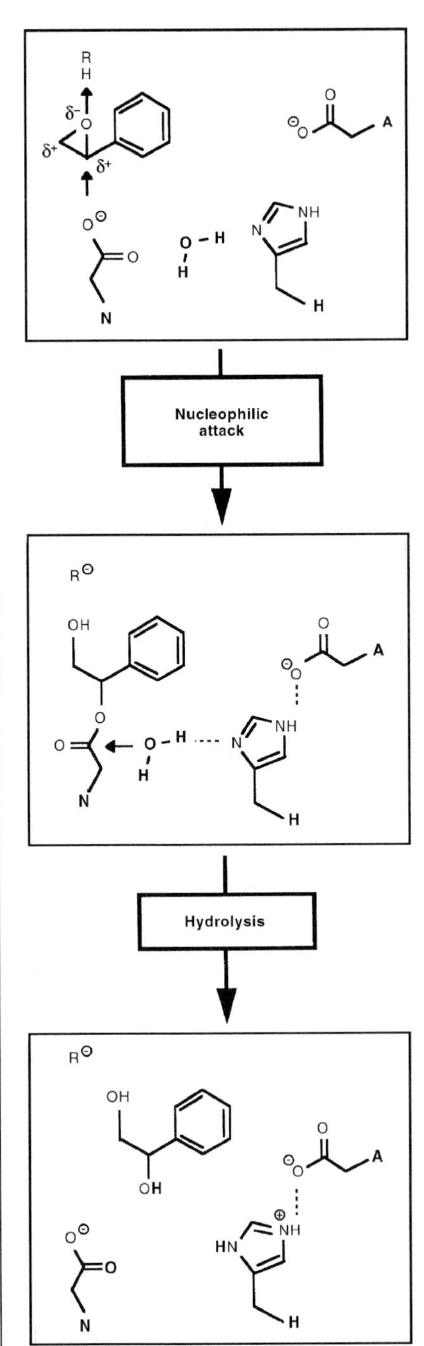

FIGURE 6 Enzymatic epoxide hydrolysis. In the first step, the catalytic nucleophile aspartate (N) attacks the oxirane ring of the substrate (here styrene oxide) to form the respective enzyme–substrate ester intermediate. Subsequently, a water molecule is activated through proton abstraction by a charge relay system composed of a histidine (H) and an acidic side chain (A), leading to hydrolysis of the intermediate and liberation of the final product.

tural element of epoxides, is a highly strained, three-member ring system. Furthermore, the C–O bonds in the ring are polarized. Depending on the substitution pattern at the two carbon atoms, epoxides are more or less reactive electrophilic compounds that can potentially form DNA-base adducts.

The mEH, an enzyme of the endoplasmic reticulum, is strongly expressed in the liver of humans and other mammals. In addition, it is widely expressed in many other tissues. Particularly high amounts have been found in the human adrenal gland. The enzyme is inducible by a number of foreign compounds, such as phenobarbital, *trans*-stilbene oxide, and Aroclor 1254. It is proficient in hydrolyzing a large number of different epoxides. Major structural requirements for an mEH substrate are sufficient lipophilicity and lack of *trans*-substitution at the oxirane ring. Among the typical substrates are metabolites from polycyclic aromatic hydrocarbons or drugs, such as phenytoin and carbamazepine. Almost paradoxical is the fact that epoxide hydrolysis can be detrimental in some instances. The mEH-catalyzed hydrolysis of the benzo[*a*]pyrene-7,8-epoxide, for instance, prevents its isomerization to the corresponding 7- or 8-phenol, products of comparatively low toxicity. Instead, benzo[*a*]pyrene-7,8-dihydrodiol is formed, a compound that can be further metabolized by a variety of enzymes to the highly mutagenic benzo[*a*]pyrene-7,8-dihydrodiol-9,10-epoxide, which itself is not a substrate for epoxide hydrolases (Fig. 3). Thus, mEH indeed increases the mutagenicity of benzo[*a*]pyrene in the presence of the appropriate monooxygenases (i.e., monooxygenases with a substantial component of oxidative attack at the 7,8-position of benzo[*a*]pyrene).

The sEH is predominantly expressed in liver, kidney, heart, and brain; yet it is found in low amounts in a variety of other organs as well. It is located in the cytosol and a significant proportion is located in the matrix of peroxisomes, small organelles, that harbor a large variety of different metabolic functions, for example, long-chain fatty acid degradation, plasmalogen synthesis, and urate oxidation. A significant number of peroxisomal enzymes produce hydrogen peroxide. The fact that sEH is present in peroxisomes and that sEH is exclusively inducible by peroxisome proliferators, a group of compounds that induce peroxisomal β-oxidation and concomitantly hydrogen peroxide production, suggests a protective role of sEH against hydrogen peroxide-induced oxidative damage. Indeed, fatty acid epoxides which can arise as secondary products from lipid peroxidation, are good substrates for the sEH. On the other hand, some of these fatty acid epoxides, such as those derived from arachidonic acid or linolenic acid, have been proposed to act by themselves or as precursors in signal transduction, which points to a possible regulatory function of sEH. A recent report on the increased cytotoxicity of the sEH metabolite 9,10-dihydroxyoctadec-12-enoic acid compared to that of the parent compound leukotoxin suggests a central role of sEH in the pathogenesis of multiple-organ failure, in particular, adult respiratory distress syndrome (ARDS), which apparently develops as a consequence of a massive leukotoxin overproduction by leukocytes.

The role of sEH in xenobiotic metabolism may be regarded as complementary to that of the mEH. In contrast to mEH, sEH is only poorly active, if at all, toward the epoxides derived from most polycyclic aromatic hydrocarbons. On the other hand, the enzyme readily hydrolyzes many *trans*-substituted epoxides, such as *trans*-stilbene oxide and *trans*-ethyl styrene oxide.

Unlike the mEH, sEH reveals large interspecies differences. Rat sEH displays a particularly low level of expression in the liver, reaching only 0.01% of the total soluble protein in this organ under normal conditions. In contrast, the enzyme is highly abundant in mouse liver, making up about 0.3% of the soluble protein. In addition, the mouse enzyme is about three times more active. In human, sEH represents about 0.1% of the soluble liver proteins and displays a specific enzymatic activity in the range of that of the rat enzyme.

Other Hydrolases

Among other hydrolases present in the human organism, glycosidases and sulfatases deserve attention with respect to xenobiotic metabolism. The endogenous sulfatases and glycosidases, in particular the β-glucuronidases, have some potential to act on the respective conjugates of xenobiotic compounds, although they are known to accept glycosaminoglycans and steroids as their physiological substrates. The gut flora, as yet still a poorly investigated population of microorganisms, obviously is quite proficient in deconjugating many compounds that are excreted via the bile in form of glucuronides or sulfates. This can lead to enterohepatic circulation of conjugated compounds because the deconjugation products are often reabsorbed from the gut. In some cases, the aglycons of natural compounds are toxic or mutagenic, and deglycosylation is required to exert their biological effects. A good example is that of the cycad plant, containing the procarcinogenic glycoside cycasin. After oral uptake, germ free rats do not suffer any long-term effects of cycasin, whereas rats with a normal gut flora develop tumors in the liver, kidney, and intestine, due to the liberation of the genotoxic aglycon methyl azoxymethanol.

Phase II Enzymes: Transferases

Glutathione S-Transferases (GSTs, EC 2.5.1.18)

Glutathione transferases conjugate the endogenous nucleophile glutathione (Fig. 7) to a large array of electrophilic compounds. Because sufficient electrophilicity appears to represent an important prerequisite of a given substrate to exert a genotoxic effect, GSTs are important safeguards of the organism against chemical carcinogenesis. The majority of GSTs are soluble dimeric enzymes that belong to a single large superfamily of proteins. In addition, there are at least two membrane-bound glutathione-dependent enzymes, one of which is designated the microsomal GST and is involved in the metabolism of xenobiotic compounds.

While glutathione can already react spontaneously with many electrophiles, GST can strongly enhance the rate of conjugation, essentially by deprotonating the sulfhydryl group of GSH and properly orienting substrate and GSH toward each other in a way that facilitates their interaction proper for conjugation. The highly specific GSH binding site of cytosolic GST is called the G-site, while the less-selective binding site for the mostly hydrophobic substrates is called the H-site. In contrast to most of the other xenobiotic-metabolizing enzymes, cytosolic GSTs have been extensively studied by X-ray crystallography, and these analyses have drawn a clear picture of the architecture and structure–function relationship of GST. GST subunits are two-domain proteins. A small N-terminal α–β domain that resembles the structure of the previously resolved glutathione peroxidase and the bacterial thioredoxin is followed by a larger domain composed of five α-helices (Fig. 8). Both domains contribute to the dimerization. Each of the two G-sites of the native enzyme is composed of several domain-I residues from one subunit and one or two domain-II residues from the other subunit. Thus, dimerization is essential for the catalytic activity of GST. The H-site, in contrast, is formed by domain-I and domain-II residues from within the same subunit. Multiple electrostatic interactions tightly fix glutathione in the G-site. A major determinant of the activation of GSH apparently is a conserved tyrosine residue near the N-terminus of GST (position 6–8), that hydrogen-bonds to the thiolate anion, thereby stabilizing this reactive state.

Glutathione conjugation leads to a strong increase in the water solubility of the resulting metabolites compared to the parent compounds, due to the three

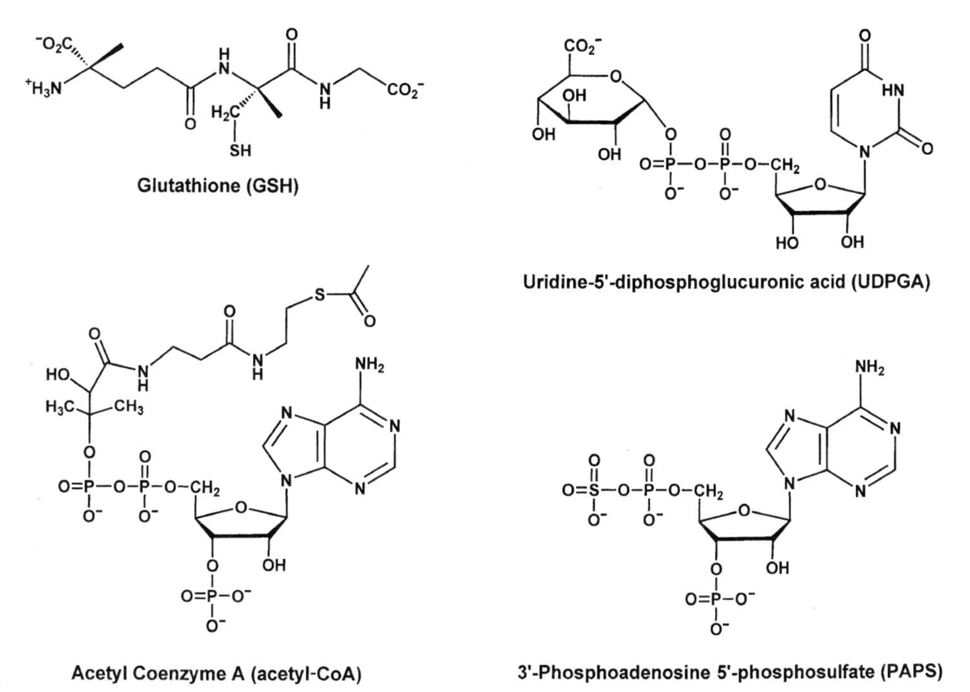

Glutathione (GSH)

Uridine-5'-diphosphoglucuronic acid (UDPGA)

Acetyl Coenzyme A (acetyl-CoA)

3'-Phosphoadenosine 5'-phosphosulfate (PAPS)

FIGURE 7 Cofactors of conjugating enzymes.

charged moieties of glutathione. These metabolites are released from the cells by an active transport system that belongs to the mdr (multidrug resistance) protein complex. This is important for the efficiency of GST-catalyzed detoxification because the GST are often strongly product-inhibited. Glutathione conjugates are usually further processed before their terminal excretion. First, the glutamate is cleaved off by γ-glutamyltranspeptidase and, subsequently, glycine is released by the action of aminopeptidase M. The resulting cysteinyl conjugate is then usually N-acetylated to form the mercapturic acid derivative, the final metabolite. In some cases, β-lyase converts the cysteinyl conjugates to the sulfhydryl metabolite, a reaction that represents a toxification rather than a detoxification step. The gene superfamily of cytosolic GST can be divided into six families (historically called classes): the α (alpha), μ (mu), π (pi), θ (theta), σ (sigma), and κ (kappa) families (Table 4). The mature dimeric proteins arise either by homodimer formation or by heterodimerization of closely related members from within the same family. The confusion about the naming of individual GST isoenzymes has often obscured for the uninitiated the identity of individual GST isoenzymes in reports from different laboratories, but a recent recommendation for a nomenclature system promises a more systematic and transparent labeling. It proposes to use the stem GST for the enzyme, preceded by a small roman letter for the species (r for rat, h for human, etc.) and followed by a capital roman letter for the family (A for α, K for κ, M for μ, P for π, S for σ, and T for θ). Individual subunits are designated with an arabic number, with two numbers connected with a hyphen giving the subunit composition of an enzyme. Thus, hGSTM2-2 is the homodimer of the human μ family subunit 2. Caution must be taken in interspecies comparison when using this nomenclature system because, in contrast to the situation with the CYP enzymes, the number of a given isoenzyme from one species does not necessarily reflect its relationship to the isoenzyme with the same name from another species. Especially in the μ family, the valid assignment of orthologous enzymes (see cytochromes P450) between, for example, human and rodent species, is not possible.

Several different types of reactions are catalyzed by GST. A prominent activity of GST is the nucleophilic substitution of electron-withdrawing substituents at carbon atoms. A good example is the broad spectrum substrate 1-chloro-2,4-dinitrobenzene (CDNB) that is readily conjugated by all GSTs, with the exception of those from the θ family, resulting in the formation of the metabolite *S*-(2,4-dinitrophenyl)glutathione and the by-product hydrochloric acid.

A second important type of reaction catalyzed by GST is the nucleophilic addition of GSH, either to

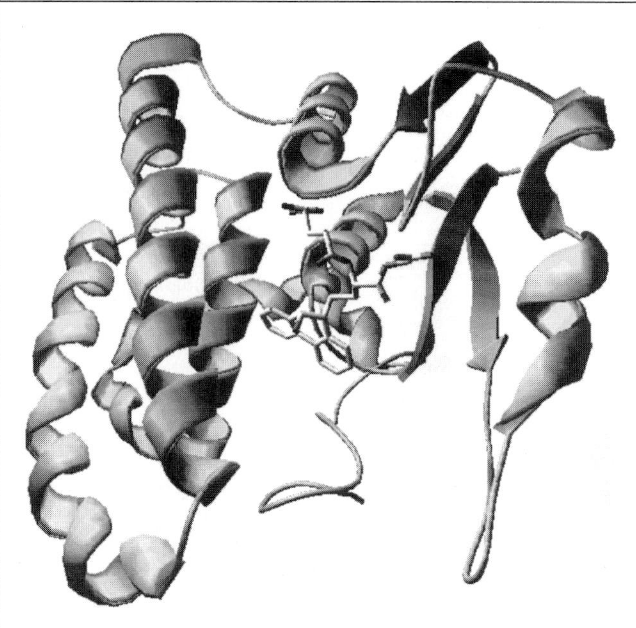

FIGURE 8 The three-dimensional structure of glutathione *S*-transferase. One subunit of the rat GSTM1 is shown, with the glutathione adduct of phenanthrene-5,6-oxide bound in the catalytic site. The view is directed toward the dimerization surface of the subunit. The right half of the protein represents the N-terminal α–β domain and the left half shows the C-terminal α helix bundle. Note that the glycyl end of the glutathionyl moiety sticks out of the plane toward the invisible second subunit that forms part of the cosubstrate binding pocket. The coordinates are taken from Ji *et al.* (1992).

epoxides by opening of the oxirane ring or to α,β-unsaturated carbonyl compounds via Michael addition. Many epoxides are good substrates for individual GST isoenzymes. For instance, GSTP1 from most species has been shown to possess high activity for the conjugation of benzo[*a*]pyrene-7,8-diol-9,10-epoxide, an ultimate carcinogen arising from benzo[*a*]pyrene metabolism (see Fig. 3). Likewise, aflatoxin-8,9-epoxide is detoxified by GSH conjugation. Of pathophysiological significance is the GST-mediated formation of leukotriene C_4, the glutathione conjugate of the endogenous epoxide leukotriene A_4. Leukotriene C_4 and its metabolite, leukotriene D_4 are pharmacologically active components of SRS-A, the slow-reacting substance of anaphylaxis, which plays an important role in the pathogenesis of anaphylaxis and asthma bronchiale. A typical α,β-unsaturated carbonyl substrate undergoing Michael addition is ethacrynic acid, a very good substrate for the mitochondrial isoenzyme GSTK1. A particularly high turnover rate has been reported for rGSTA4-4 (the former rat GST 8-8, or Y_k-Y_k) with the lipid peroxidation product 4-hydroxynon-2-enal, also a Michael substrate, which points to an important role of GST in protection against oxidative stress.

A third type of GST-catalyzed reaction is the reduction of another type of peroxidation products, namely, organic hydroperoxides. These are converted to the corresponding alcohols under intermediate formation of the sulfenic acid of GSH, which in turn reacts spontaneously with a second GSH molecule to form GSSG. In contrast to the separate enzyme glutathione peroxidase, a selenoprotein that also accepts organic hydroperoxides, GSTs are unable to reduce hydrogen peroxide.

A fourth type of reaction catalyzed by GST is the isomerization of organic compounds. For instance, GST-mediated isomerization leads to the formation of Δ^4-androstene dione from Δ^5-androstene dione. However, the significance of GST-catalyzed isomerization reactions is not well understood. Often, GSH conjugation represents a detoxification process, because the electrophilic potential of the substrate is frequently lost in the resulting product. However, there are at

TABLE 4 List of the Cytosolic Glutathione *S*-Transferase Isoenzymes from Rat, Including Typical Substrates[a]

Isoenzyme	Selective substrate
Alpha family	
GSTA1-1	Δ^5-Androstene-3, 17-dione
GSTA2-2	Δ^5-Androstene-3, 17-dione
GSTA3-3	
GSTA4-4	4-Hydroxynon-2-enal
GSTA5-5	Alflatoxin B_1 *exo*-8,9-epoxide
Mu family	
GSTM1-1	1,2-Dichloro-4-nitrobenzene
GSTM2-2	*trans*-Stilbene oxide
GSTM3-3	1,2-Dichloro-4-nitrobenzene
GSTM4-4	
GSTM4-5	
GSTM6-6	
Pi family	
GSTP1-1	(+)-*anti*-Benzo[*a*]pyrene-7,8-diol-9,10-epoxide
Theta family	
GSTT1-1	1,2-Epoxy-3-(4-nitrophenoxy)propane
GSTT2-2	Menaphthyl sulfate
Sigma family	
GSTS1-1	Prostaglandine H (isomerization)
Kappa family	
GSTK1-1	Ethacrynic acid

[a]This list includes only homodimers. In general, the properties of heterodimeric forms almost stochiometrically reflect the subunit composition, probably because the substrate binding site (H-site) is formed by a single subunit. The following heterodimers have been observed: GSTA1-2, GSTA1-3, GSTA2-3, GSTA3-5, GSTM1-2, GSTM1-3, GSTM2-3, GSTM3-5. A general substrate for all GSTs, with the exception of the theta GSTs (GSTT1-1 and GSTT2-2), is 1-chloro-2,4-dinitrobenzene (CDNB).

least two mechanisms by which GST can toxify xenobiotics. Both of these toxication pathways involve halogenated hydrocarbons. Vicinal dihaloalkanes, such as dibromoethane, can be enzymatically conjugated to GSH, preferentially by the isoenzyme GSTT1. The resulting metabolite can undergo a spontaneous intramolecular nucleophilic substitution reaction, resulting in the release of the second bromine as a bromide anion and the formation of a highly reactive thiiranium ion. The thiiranium can be regarded as the thioanalogon of an epoxide. Its chemical reactivity is strongly enhanced by the positive charge of the heteroatom, and the respective compounds are powerful genotoxins.

The second toxication pathway is particularly relevant for the organic solvent perchloroethylene. Metabolism by the β-lyase of its cysteine adduct, formed from its glutathione conjugate, gives rise to the formation of a highly cytotoxic and carcinogenic thioketene.

A variety of polymorphisms for individual GST isoenzymes have been reported. Most prominent are the cases of GSTM1 and GSTT1, for which a homozygous null allele (i.e., the absence of a functional gene) has been reported in about 50% and 15%, respectively, of the Caucasian population. Lack of a functional GSTM1 positively correlates with an increased risk for bladder cancer and, possibly, for lung cancer. A functionally active GSTT1 enzyme seems to be a protective factor against a myelodysplastic syndrome.

UDP-Glucuronosyltransferases (UGTs; EC 2.4.1.17)

Conjugation to glucuronic acid is the quantitatively most important phase II reaction. The UDP-glucuronosyltranferases are a superfamily of membrane-bound enzymes that catalyze the conjugation of α-D-UDP-glucuronic acid (UDPGA; see Fig. 7) to a large variety of compounds to form β-D-glucuronides. Hydroxyl, thiol, amino, hydroxylamino, and carboxyl groups can serve as the anchor for the glucuronic acid conjugation. Even C-glucuronides can be formed, provided the hydrogen of the involved C–H bond of the substrate is sufficiently mobile. An example is phenylbutazone, which can be glucuronidated at a carbon atom flanked by two carbonyl functions. From their chemical nature, the substrate moieties engaged in the glucuronic acid conjugation are nucleophilic. In line with this, the majority of the UGT substrates are not genotoxic, at least not directly. The anchor groups listed above are often important determinants of the biological activities of drugs and toxins, because they are frequently involved in the interaction of these compounds with biological structures, such as receptors and enzymes. In most cases, glucuronic acid conjugation substantially increases the hydrophilicity of a substrate and terminates its biological effect. Only very few glucuronides (e.g., morphine-O^6-glucuronide) retain the biological activity. Therefore, UGTs are of prominent importance for the detoxication of many acutely toxic compounds.

The currently known UGTs can be divided into two families. Family 2 is further subdivided into the subfamilies 2A and 2B. The subfamily UGT2B comprises by far the most UGT genes identified to date, the products of which are mainly implicated in steroid metabolism. In contrast, only one gene has currently been identified for the subfamily UGT2A. The protein has a particularly broad substrate specificity, including many terpene alcohols. Because it is highly expressed in the nasal mucosa, it is believed to be involved in the termination of odor reception.

Especially interesting is the situation of the family UGT1. The single gene of this family encodes at least 10 different proteins. Due to the presence of as many different transcription start sites, a number of different primary transcripts can be derived from the same gene. Splicing of these different transcripts results in mRNAs that differ from each other only in the sequence of their first exon and are identical in the sequences of the following exons 2 to 5. Because the N-terminal parts of the resulting proteins corresponding to the variable exon 1 contain the substrate binding domains of these UGTs, the corresponding individual UGTs differ substantially from each other with respect to their substrate specificities. These range from the endogenous metabolite bilirubin to pharmacologically active compounds (e.g., morphine) to carcinogen precursors (e.g., benzo[*a*]pyrene-7,8-diol). A genetic defect in this single gene can therefore have dramatic consequences. Heritable human diseases are attributed to this, such as Crigler–Najjar syndrome and Gilbert syndrome. In particular, the intrinsic hyperbilirubinemia that results from the reduced or lost capacity to conjugate bilirubin can lead to an early death (Crigler–Najjar type 1). The Gunn rat is a model for this disease because it is lacking any UGT1 family protein due to a mutation in exon 2 of the gene. Because rats are much more tolerant than humans to high plasma levels of bilirubin, these animals can survive and represent a tool with which to study the consequences of a lack of the respective UGT activities.

UGTs are resident proteins of the endoplasmic reticulum (ER). Their synthesis is directed to the ER by an N-terminal hydrophobic signal peptide that is cleaved off during the maturation of the protein. UGTs are retained in the ER membrane by a C-terminal membrane anchor sequence, followed by a stop transfer signal. The orientation of the catalytic center thus is toward the lumen of the ER. The co-substrate UDPGA is supplied by a transport system apparently involving two separate components. UDPGA is shuttled into the ER lumen by a carrier that exchanges it with UDP-*N*-acetylglucosamine (UDP-GlcNAc). UDP-GlcNAc is pumped into the ER lumen by a countertransporter, simultaneously translocating uridine monophosphate from the ER lumen to the cytosol. This transport mechanism can become the rate-limiting step during *in vitro* analysis of UGT activities in liver microsomes. Activity can be stimulated by adding UDP-GlcNAc, but the best results are usually obtained by permeabilization of the phospholipid membranes with optimized amounts of detergents to give the enzyme free access to its co-substrate. Among the many UGT-catalyzed reactions, few enhance the toxicity of the substrates, as does the glucuronidation of some nonsteroidal antiinflammatory drugs (NSAID). The resulting ester glucuronides can undergo a reaction called acyl migration, that is, the intramolecular *trans*-esterification from the C1 hydroxy group of the glucuronic acid to the C2 hydroxy group. This process can proceed further to the C3 and C4 hydroxy groups. Under these conditions, ring opening of the sugar moiety can lead to the formation of an aldehyde group at C1 that can react with primary amino groups in proteins, such as lysine side chains, to form the corresponding Schiff's bases. A subsequent Amadori rearrangement can finally lead to a stable protein adduct, which may give rise to an allergic reaction, a typical unwanted side effect of some NSAID. Finally, it should be mentioned that glucuronic acid conjugation can also result in enhanced genotoxicity of metabolites in a few cases. Glucuronidation of aromatic hydroxylamines leads to the formation of a moderately good leaving group that tends to dissociate from the molecule under mildly acidic conditions, as is usually present in the urine, to generate the free glucuronic acid and a strongly electrophilic aryl nitrenium ion with a high genotoxic potential. Therefore, glucuronidation supports the formation of bladder tumors from aryl hydroxylamines by constituting the transport form of the carcinogen. However, it must be pointed out that the alternative conjugation reactions for these compounds, namely, sulfation and acetylation, form better leaving groups that can separate from the molecule at neutral pH.

Sulfotransferases (SULTs; EC 2.8.2)

Sulfotransferases catalyze the transfer of a sulfonyl group from the co-substrate 3′-phosphoadenosine 5′-phosphosulfate (PAPS; Fig. 7) to nucleophilic acceptor substrates. In the metabolism of xenobiotics, SULTs have a substrate spectrum similar to that of the UGTs, with the exception that they do not conjugate carboxylic acids. As a general rule, SULTs are lower in K_M and V_{max} than UGT. Thus, they have high affinity to their substrates but only limited turnover capacity. This leads quite often to the situation that a compound is preferentially glucuronidated at high concentration but sulfated at low concentration. This is also reflected in the concentrations of the respective co-substrates; while the PAPS concentration in the human liver is about 50 μM, UDPGA is present in a roughly 10-fold higher concentration. In contrast to the membrane-bound UGT, xenobiotic-metabolizing SULTs are soluble enzymes localized in the cytoplasm. On the basis of their primary structure, the SULTs with implications for the metabolism of foreign compounds can be divided into three families. Family 1, the former aryl sulfotransferases, prefers phenolic substrates; family 2 enzymes, previously called hydroxysteroid sulfotransferases, act mainly on alcoholic compounds. The single member of family 3 known to date readily sulfonates alkyl amines.

An important detoxication function of SULT is the efficient conjugation of small amounts of xenobiotics, which leads to their inactivation and rapid excretion, due to the enhanced hydrophilicity of the resulting metabolite. Sulfoconjugation represents also an important activation mechanism for several different types of procarcinogens. First, the previously mentioned aromatic hydroxylamines that can arise from aromatic amine oxidation (e.g., by CYP1A2-mediated hydroxylation) serve as substrates for SULT. The resulting aromatic *N,O*-sulfate esters readily decompose to give the genotoxic nitrenium ions. In a similar fashion, sulfation of benzylic alcohols leads to the formation of highly reactive carbenium ions after spontaneous loss of the sulfate group. That this is, indeed, a relevant activation pathway *in vivo* is underlined by the observation that mice with an inherited deficiency in the PAPS synthesis are less prone to developing liver cancer after treatment with the hepatocarcinogen 1′-hydroxysafrol than are mice with a normal PAPS metabolism.

Acetyltransferases (ATs; EC 2.3.1)

The two acetyltransferases with major implication in the metabolism of drugs and foreign compounds are *N*-acetyltransferases 1 and 2 (NAT-1 and NAT-2). Both enzymes catalyze the acetyl transfer from acetyl-CoA (Fig. 7) to amines or hydroxylamines. The two closely related enzymes share about 80% sequence identity in humans but differ significantly in their substrate specificity. Typical substrates for NAT-1 are 4-aminobenzoic acid and 4-aminosalicylic acid, while NAT-2 readily acetylates a large variety of common drugs, such as caffeine, hydralazine, isoniazide, sulfamethazine, and procainamide. Both enzymes are capable of metabolizing aromatic amines, such as benzidine, 4-aminobiphenyl, 2-naphthylamine, and 2-aminofluorene. Acetyl transfer by NAT proceeds by an ordered ping-pong mechanism. First, the acetyl group of acetyl-CoA is transferred to the enzyme, which subsequently binds and acetylates the substrate molecule.

Because the metabolites of NAT reactions are usually less hydrophilic than their parent compounds, the function of these enzymes seems to be primarily the inactivation of biologically active compounds, possibly alkaloid-like substrates. Their role in the detoxication of the procarcinogenic aromatic amines is ambivalent: N-acetylation of the parent compound, the aromatic amine itself, is a detoxication reaction, because it competes with the activation of the parent compound by oxidative metabolism. However, if N-oxidation takes place first, the resulting hydroxylamine is also a substrate for NAT, and formation of the *N,O*-acetate ester finally results in the formation of a reactive nitrenium ion. Thus, the balance between good and evil is at least in part determined by the relative velocities of the oxidative to the acetylation pathway. In humans, this leads to a high interindividual variability in risk because the expression level of the major enzyme implicated in the oxidation of aryl amines, CYP1A2, differs dramatically between individuals, and NAT-2, which often is quantitatively very important in this reaction, is polymorphic in humans. Some individuals, called slow acetylators, are very low in the acetylation of aromatic amines and their metabolites. While a high CYP1A2 level generally leads to a higher genotoxicity of aromatic amines, it appears that the acetylator phenotype may be decisive for the organ selectivity of tumor formation. It has been observed that slow acetylators are more susceptible to aryl amine-induced bladder cancer, whereas rapid acetylators have a higher risk of developing aryl amine-induced colorectal cancer. The latter observation may be because heterocyclic aryl amines arising from amino acids during food preparation such as PhiP (2-amino-6-methylimidazo[4,5-*b*]pyridine), are poor substrates for both NATs, but the corresponding hydroxylamines can be activated to carcinogens by NAT-2. The NAT-2 polymorphism also has consequences for the metabolism of certain drugs. Isoniazide, for instance, has a significantly prolonged half-life in the slow acetylator phenotype, which can lead to accumulation and toxic effects of the drug. The acetylator phenotype can be assessed using caffeine as an *in vivo* probe. The amount of caffeine present in one strong cup of coffee is sufficient for this purpose. The indicative parameter is the ratio between the two metabolites 5-acetylamino-6-amino-3-methyl uracil (AAMU) and 1-methyl xanthine (1X). A ratio of AAMU/1X greater than 2 is indicative of a rapid acetylator.

Acyl-CoA Amino Acid N-Acyl Transferase (EC 2.3.1) and Methyl Transferase (EC 2.1.1)

The conjugation of xenobiotics with amino acids is mainly of historical interest; the first xenobiotic metabolite ever reported was hippuric acid, the glycine conjugate of benzoic acid discovered by Keller in his own urine after having swallowed a substantial amount of benzoic acid. Since then, other amino acid conjugates, mainly containing glycine, asparagine, or glutamine, have been identified. The first step in conjugating a xenobiotic carboxylic acid to an amino acid is to activate it by formation of the respective xenobiotic CoA thioester. From this, the carboxylic acid can be transferred to the amino group of the amino acid. The physiological relevance of this process is as yet poorly understood, and it is of no toxicological relevance so far.

Sporadically, methyl transfer can be of importance in the metabolism of xenobiotics. Thus, nicotine can be methylated to the *N*-methylnicotinium ion, β-lyase products of the glutathione conjugation pathway can be detoxified by methylation of the free SH group, or some catechol-type compounds can be O-methylated by catechol *O*-methyltransferase, thereby preventing the formation of toxic quinones. The different enzymes involved in these reactions are mainly specialized on endogenous substrates. The co-substrate for these reactions is usually *S*-adenosylmethionine.

FACTORS INFLUENCING XENOBIOTIC METABOLISM

Modulation of Expression and Activity of Xenobiotic-Metabolizing Enzymes

In general, there are four ways by which a compound can influence the contribution of a specific xenobiotic-metabolizing enzyme to the biotransformation process.

- Induction of the expression of the enzyme protein.
- Repression of the expression of the enzyme protein.
- Direct activation of the enzymatic function.
- Direct inhibition of the enzymatic function.

Especially well investigated is enzyme induction. Substrate induction is a strategy for economically meeting the demand for a pluripotent xenobiotic metabolism without wasting too many resources, by constitutively synthesizing all components of the enzymatic arsenal that are necessary to cover the required broad substrate specificity. Usually, application of an inducer does not lead to the enhanced expression of a single enzyme but rather to an increased expression level of a set of enzymes that can act synergistically to a given challenge.

In the strict sense, the term induction refers to an increased amount of gene product due to an enhanced transcription rate. Yet the term is often used to describe any process that eventually leads to an increased concentration of enzyme protein in the target tissue. Therefore, processes leading to an enhanced stability of the protein and/or mRNA are included in this more loose definition of enzyme induction. The two classic prototypes of enzyme inducers are the hypnotic drug phenobarbital (PB) and the carcinogen 3-methylcholanthrene (MC). The fact that these two compounds differentially affected the activities of CYP and UGT toward individual substrates was an early indication of the multiplicity of these enzymes, that is, the existence of isoenzymes. A number of other inducer prototypes affecting different sets of enzymes were identified, such as a group of synthetic steroids, with pregenolone-16α-carbonitrile being the model compound; the peroxisome proliferators (e.g., fibrate-type drugs and phthalate esters); or the antioxidant-type inducers (e.g., *tert.*-butylated hydroxytoluene and ethoxyquin) (Table 5). The molecular mechanism underlying the enzyme induction frequently involves the activation of a nuclear transcription factor by the respective inducer. An exception to this general mechanism is the substrate-induction of CYP2E1, which is, at least in part, due to the stabilization of the protein. There is evidence that substrate binding to the active site of the enzyme inhibits phosphorylation of the protein. Apparently, phosphorylation leads to rapid degradation of the enzyme protein; hence, substrate binding prolongs its half-life and, therefore, the enzyme protein level.

Induction of xenobiotic-metabolizing enzymes is often most pronounced in, but not exclusively restricted to, the liver. It is also observed in kidney, lung, gut, brain, skin, and placenta. The increase in drug-metabolizing capacity leads to the phenomenon of pharmacokinetic tolerance. This is an important mechanism of drug–drug interaction. An intriguing example is the simultaneous (and obsolete) treatment with the anticoagulant warfarin and the hypnotic drug phenobarbital. After 1 to 2 days, the phenobarbital treatment will lead to a strong increase in CYP2C and CYP3A enzymes, thereby increasing the warfarin metabolism and reducing its plasma concentrations. The necessary dose adjustment can result in a fatal outcome when the phenobarbital treatment is discontinued. The decrease in the activity of the previously induced enzymes, which takes place within a few days after withdrawal of the inducer, will lead to significantly enhanced warfarin plasma concentrations that may result in internal bleeding with an eventually lethal outcome.

Repression of xenobiotic-metabolizing enzyme expression has been less frequently observed than induction but can be of importance. Sometimes induction of one set of drug-metabolizing enzymes is at the

TABLE 5 Prototypes of Inducers of Xenobiotic-Metabolizing Enzymes

Prototype	Examples	Structural requirements	Affected xenobiotic-metabolizing enzymes
3-Methylcholanthrene	2,3,7,8-Tetrachlorodibenzo-*p*-dioxin; *β*-naphthoflavone benzo[*a*]pyrene; 3,3′,4,4′-tetrachlorobiphenyl	Planar, hydrophobic compounds;	CYP1A1, CYP1A2, CYP1B1 GSTA1 UGT1*06 NQOR1
Phenobarbital	Many drugs and pesticides	Bulky, hydrophobic compounds	several CYP2B, CYP2C and CYP3A isoenzymes CYP450 oxidoreductase mEH several GST isoenzymes several UGT isoenzymes
Peroxisome proliferators	Fibrate-type hypolipidemic drugs, such as clofibrate; plasticizers of the phthalate-type; tiadenol; perfluorinated fatty acids	No clear structural characteristics (carboxylic acids or precursors of these, unable to undergo regular *β*-oxidation?)	GYP4A UGT1*01 sEH mEH (weak)
Pregenonolone-16*α*-carbonitrile	synthetic glucocorticoids; tris-acetyl oleandomycine; rifampicin	?	CYP3A CYP2B (variable) mEH
Ethanol	Isoniazide; acetone	?	CYP2E1
Butylated hydroxytoluene	Butylated hydroxyanisol; ethoxyquin	No general structural characteristics (antioxidant/oxidant function required?)	mEH NQOR several GST isoenzymes several UGT isoenzymes CYP isoenzymes?

expense of the expression of another set of these enzymes. For instance, some peroxisome proliferators significantly decrease the relative expression of several GST and CYP isoenzymes, while inducing CYP4A1, UGT1*01, and sEH. Another relevant observation is that cytokines, such as interleukin 1*β*, interleukin 6, and interferon *γ*, significantly down-regulate the expression of several CYP isoenzymes. Therefore, inflammatory processes may substantially alter the capacity for the metabolism of xenobiotics and also lead to a qualitative change in the metabolite pattern.

Inhibition of enzyme activities can be accomplished either by direct interaction with the enzyme protein, which can result in isozyme-specific inhibition, or by cofactor depletion affecting a whole group of enzymes. Impressive effects of enzyme inhibition have been reported. Furafylline, a potent inhibitor of CYP1A2, strongly reduced the caffeine tolerance of healthy volunteers, leading to significant signs of intoxication from their regular coffee intake. Naringenin and related flavonoids are inhibitors of CYP3A4 at dosages that can be reached by drinking a glass of grapefruit juice. It has been suggested that this reduces the susceptibility to chemical carcinogens that are activated by this isoenzyme. However, the toxicity of nifedipine-related calcium antagonists and other CYP3A4-metabolized drugs may be significantly enhanced by this effect.

Activation of xenobiotic-metabolizing enzyme activities by direct interaction with the protein has been observed in few cases. For instance, isoquinoline and clotrimazole, among other compounds, reportedly activate the *in vitro* activity of mEH toward styrene oxide by a factor of 5. Diethyl ketone and structurally related solvents strongly enhance the activity of UGT2B3, the 17*β*-hydroxysteroid UGT, toward 2-aminophenol, thereby shifting the substrate pattern of the enzyme.

Interindividual Differences

Interindividual differences in xenobiotic-metabolizing enzyme activities complicate their analysis. Several factors other than the above-described exogenous modulators additionally contribute to this phenomenon. First, sex and developmental stage are two determinants that can easily be assessed. Sex differences in the expression of drug-metabolizing enzymes are frequent in many laboratory animal species but are not usually pronounced in humans. There are, for instance, sex-specific CYP isoenzymes in the CYP2A, CYP2C, and the CYP3A subfamilies in the rat. In the human, no sex-specific CYP isoenzymes are known, but quantitative differences in the expression of xenobiotic-metabolizing enzymes may play a role. Of forensic interest is the observation that females have a lower alcohol clearance than males. Ontogenetic development of drug-metabolizing capacities has received some attention. CYP activities already are detectable in the human fetus around the fourth month of pregnancy, while they appear in rodents only around 4 days before delivery. Acetylation and sulfation also develop very early in humans. In contrast, the glucuronidation capacity for the heme-degradation product bilirubin appears to be underdeveloped in the neonate, causing severe problems in the case of neonatal erythroblastosis and resulting in a pronounced neonatal jaundice.

A major cause of interindividual differences in drug metabolism is polymorphism of the involved enzyme. An increasing number of human xenobiotic-metabolizing enzymes are reported to be polymorphic, that is, to exist in different allelic forms with more or less pronounced different characteristics of the respective gene product in a considerable part (>1%) of the population (Table 6). Several of these polymorphisms have a proven impact on the susceptibility to chemical carcinogenesis, as discussed previously for the individual enzymes. The prevalence of these polymorphisms displays considerable ethnic variations.

TABLE 6 Polymorphic Xenobiotic-Metabolizing Enzymes

Established polymorphism	Suspected polymorphism
CYP1A1	FMO
CYP2A6	UGT2B7
CYP2C9	SULT1A3
CYP2C18	
CYP2C19	
CYP2D6	
CYP2E1	
mEH	
NAT1	
NAT2	
GSTM1	
GSTP1	
GSTT1	
UGT1	

Species Differences

Most types of drug-metabolizing enzymes were already present early in evolution. This implies a close relationship between the higher animals in terms of their ability to metabolize foreign compounds. However, every species has its specific habitat and was under an individual selection pressure in terms of xenobiotic metabolism, mainly dictated by its preferred diet. This has led to considerable species differences in foreign-compound metabolism. Cats, for instance, being exclusively carnivores, almost completely lack the ability to glucuronidate xenobiotics, probably because they do not need to deal extensively with compounds of plant origin, such as flavonoids or alkaloids. For less obvious reasons, pigs are slow in the sulfation of xenobiotics, and dogs are particularly poor acetylators. The rat displays an extremely low expression of sEH in the liver.

It is obvious from these examples that it is very important to choose the correct species for the analysis of the metabolism of a drug in order to make sensible predictions for the human situation. For instance, testing a compound carrying a primary amino group with dog as the model species bears the danger of missing relevant metabolites derived from acetylation of the drug. A good example of using an unsuitable species is the case of a study performed in cynomolgus monkeys, attempting to assess the carcinogenic potency of heterocyclic amines present in cooked meat. These primates are, in general, a good animal model because they are closely related to humans. In this case, however, they turned out to be a very poor choice because they lack CYP1A2, the enzyme needed to activate most of the relevant heterocyclic arylamines. Thus, the study gave false negative results with several of the compounds under investigation. In contrast, these mutagens turned out to be potent carcinogens in the marmoset, a primate with a significant hepatic CYP1A2 expression.

Relevant species differences can also occur at the level of the regulation of enzyme expression. A prominent example is that of the peroxisome proliferators (see previous discussion), a heterogeneous group of compounds inducing a specific subset of enzymes while at the same time leading to an increase in the number and size of peroxisomes. Peroxisomes are organelles harboring a large number of metabolism pathways, several of which produce hydrogen peroxide in stoichiometric amounts. Among these, the peroxisomal β-oxidation is co-induced together with several xenobiotic-metabolizing enzymes by peroxisome proliferators. A couple of years after the observation that peroxisome proliferation results from treatment with the respective compounds, an increased number of hepatocellular carcinomas were observed in the treated animals. For a short while this raised severe concerns because some of the compounds were already in wide use as hypolipidemic agents in human drug therapy. Soon it turned out that the peroxisome proliferation, which was thought to be the reason for the increased incidence of liver cancer, was a species-specific effect that did not occur to a significant extent in humans. Therefore, the hypolipidemic drugs known to induce liver cancer in mice and rat are still in use as human therapeutics.

Stereoselectivity

Enzymes are chiral molecules and therefore usually interact with their substrates in a highly stereo- and enantioselective manner. Unlike most compounds of biological origin, chiral drugs produced by chemical processes are still prepared as the racemic mixtures, in most cases. However, the desired pharmacological activity often resides predominantly or exclusively in one of the two enantiomers. Moreover, metabolism usually discriminates between the optical antipodes. Significant enantioselective metabolism has been reported for nitrogen mustard-derived cytostatic drugs, such as cyclophosphamide and ifosfamide; for some β-adrenergic antagonists, for instance, metoprolol; and for a variety of other drugs. Similarly, metabolism pathways leading to the activation of procarcinogens display stereoselectivity. A particularly unfortunate example is that of the bioactivation of benzo[*a*]pyrene to the corresponding 7,8-dihydrodiol-9,10-epoxide (Fig. 3). Four chiral centers are present in the molecule (carbon atoms 7, 8, 9, and 10), resulting in four possible isomers (the fact that the conformation at position 7 relative to position 8 usually is *trans* and that at position 9 relative to position 10 must be *cis* reduces the number of possible isomers from 16 to 4). Of these, the (+)-*anti*-enantiomer with the absolute configuration 7*R*,8*S*,9*S*,10*R* not only has the highest mutagenic and carcinogenic potential but also is the most abundant diolepoxide formed during the mammalian metabolism of benzo[*a*]pyrene.

In addition to its toxicological implication, the regio- and stereoselectivity in xenobiotic metabolism can be used for diagnostic purposes. An impressive example is the metabolism of testosterone by rat CYP isoenzymes. The more than 10 diagnostic metabolites resulting from metabolism of testosterone by rat liver microsomes can be separated by HPLC to generate a metabolic fingerprint that allows the simultaneous determination of several CYP isoenzymes.

Bibliography

Arand, M., Grant, D. F., Beetham, J. K., Friedberg, T., Oesch, F., and Hammock, B. D. (1994). Sequence similarity of mammalian epoxide hydrolases to the bacterial haloalkane dehalogenase and other related proteins—Implication for the potential catalytic mechanism of enzymatic epoxide hydrolysis. *FEBS Lett.* **338,** 251–256.

Arand, M., Wagner, H., and Oesch, F. (1996). Asp^{333}, Asp^{495}, and His^{523} form the catalytic triad of rat soluble epoxide hydrolase. *J. Biol. Chem.* **271,** 4223–4229.

Armstrong, R. N. (1987). Enzyme-catalyzed detoxication reactions: Mechanisms and stereochemistry. *CRC Crit. Rev. Biochem.* **22,** 39–88.

Armstrong, R. N. (1991). Glutathione S-transferases: Reaction mechanism, structure, and function. *Chem. Res. Toxicol.* **4,** 131–140.

Awasthi, Y. C., Sharma, R., and Singhal, S. S. (1994). Human glutathione *S*-transferases. *Int. J. Biochem.* **26,** 295–308.

Badawi, A. F., Stern, S. J., Lang, N. P., and Kadlubar, F. F. (1996). Cytochrome P-450 and acetyltransferase expression as biomarkers of carcinogen–DNA adduct levels and human cancer susceptibility. *Prog. Clin. Biol. Res.* **395,** 109–140.

Beetham, J. K., Grant, D., Arand, M., Garbarino, J., Kiyosue, T., Pinot, F., Oesch, F., Belknap, W. R., Shinozaki, K., and Hammock, B. D. (1995). Gene evolution of epoxide hydrolases and recommended nomenclature. *DNA Cell Biol.* **14,** 61–71.

Bock, K. W. (1991). Roles of UDP-glucuronosyltransferases in chemical carcinogenesis. *Crit. Rev. Biochem. Mol. Biol.* **26,** 129–150.

Brockmöller, J., Cascorbi, I., Kerb, R., and Roots, I. (1996). Combined analysis of inherited polymorphisms in arylamine *N*-acetyltransferase 2, glutathione *S*-transferases M1 and T1, microsomal epoxide hydrolase, and cytochrome P450 enzymes as modulators of bladder cancer risk. *Cancer Res.* **56,** 3915–3925.

Burchell, B., McGurk, K., Brierley, C. H., and Clarke, D. J. (1997). UDP-Glucuronosyltransferases. *In* "Comprehensive Toxicology" (F. P. Guengerich ed.), Vol. 3, pp. 401–435. Elsevier, Amsterdam.

Burchell, B., Nebert, D. W., Nelson, D. R., Bock, K. W., Iyanagi, T., Jansen, P. L. M., Lancet, D., Mulder, G. J., Chowdhury, J. R., Siest, G., Tephly, T. R., and Mackenzie, P. I. (1991). The UDP-glucuronosyltransferase gene superfamily—suggested nomenclature based on evolutionary divergence. *DNA Cell Biol.* **10,** 487–494.

Cameron, A. D., Sinning, I., Lhermite, G., Olin, B., Board, P. G., Mannervik, B., and Jones, T. A. (1995). Structural analysis of human alpha-class glutathione transferase A1-1 in the apo-form and in complexes with ethacrynic acid and its glutathione conjugate. *Structure* **3,** 717–727.

Cashman, J. R. (1995). Structural and catalytic properties of the mammalian flavin-containing monooxygenase. *Chem. Res. Toxicol.* **8,** 165–181.

Cashman, J. R., Perotti, B. Y. T., Berkman, C. E., and Lin, J. (1996). Pharmacokinetics and molecular detoxication. *Environ. Health Perspect.* **104,** 23–40.

Chen, H. W., Sandler, D. P., Taylor, J. A., Shore, D. L., Liu, E., Bloomfield, C. D., and Bell, D. A. (1996). Increased risk for myelodysplastic syndromes in individuals with glutathione transferase theta 1 (GSTT1) gene defect. *Lancet* **347,** 295–297.

Coles, B., and Ketterer, B. (1990). The role of glutathione and glutathione transferases in chemical carcinogenesis. *Crit. Rev. Biochem. Mol. Biol.* **25,** 47–70.

Coon, M. J., Vaz, A. D. N., and Bestervelt, L. L. (1996). Cytochrome P450. 2. Peroxidative reactions of diversozymes. *FASEB J.* **10,** 428–434.

Coughtrie, M. W. H. (1996). Sulphation catalysed by the human cytosolic sulphotransferases—Chemical defence or molecular terrorism? *Hum. Exp. Toxicol.* **15,** 547–555.

Dekant, W., and Vamvakas, S. (1996). Biotransformation and membrane transport in nephrotoxicity. *Crit. Rev. Toxicol.* **26,** 309–334.

Dirr, H., Reinemer, P., and Huber, R. (1994). X-ray crystal structures of cytosolic glutathione *S*-transferases—Implications for protein architecture, substrate recognition and catalytic function. *Eur. J. Biochem.* **220,** 645–661.

Estabrook, R. W. (1996). The remarkable P450s: A historical overview of these versatile hemeprotein catalysts. *FASEB J.* **10,** 202–204.

Fernandez-Salguero, P. M., and Gonzalez, F. J. (1996). Targeted disruption of specific cytochromes P450 and xenobiotic receptor genes. *In* "Cytochrome P450" (E. F. Johnson and M. R. Waterman eds.), Vol. 272, pp. 412–430. Academic Press, San Diego, CA.

Friedberg, T., and Wolf, C. R. (1996). Recombinant DNA technology as an investigative tool in drug metabolism research. *Adv. Drug Delivery Rev.* **22,** 187–213.

Fujii-Kuriyama, Y., Imataka, H., Sogawa, K., Yasumoto, K.-I., and Kikuchi, Y. (1992). Regulation of CYP1A1 expression. *FASEB J.* **6,** 706–710.

Goeptar, A. R., Commandeur, J. N. M., van Ommen, B., van Bladeren, P. J., and Vermeulen, N. P. E. (1995). Metabolism and kinetics of trichloroethylene in relation to toxicity and carcinogenicity. Relevance of the mercapturic acid pathway. *Chem. Res. Toxicol.* **8,** 3–21.

Goldstein, J. A., and de Morais, S. M. F. (1994). Biochemistry and molecular biology of the human CYP2C subfamily. *Pharmacogenetics* **4,** 285–299.

Gonzalez, F. J., and Gelboin, H. V. (1994). Role of human cytochromes P450 in the metabolic activation of chemical carcinogens and toxins. *Drug Metab. Rev.* **26,** 165–183.

Gonzalez, F. J., and Lee, Y. H. (1996). Cytochromes P450. 6. Constitutive expression of hepatic cytochrome P450 genes. *FASEB J.* **10,** 1112–1117.

Guengerich, F. P. (1995). Human cytochrome P450 enzymes. *In* "Cytochrome P450—Structure, Mechanism, and Biochemistry" (P. R. Ortiz de Montellano, ed.), 2nd ed., pp. 473–535. Plenum Press, New York.

Guengerich, F. P., Gillam, E. M. J., and Shimada, T. (1996). New applications of bacterial systems to problems in toxicology. *Crit. Rev. Toxicol.* **26,** 551–583.

Hankinson, O. (1995). The aryl hydrocarbon receptor complex. *Ann. Rev. Pharmacol. Toxicol.* **35,** 307–340.

Hayes, J. D., and Pulford, D. J. (1995). The glutathione *S*-transferase supergene family: Regulation of GST and the contribution of the isoenzymes to cancer chemoprotection and drug resistance. *Crit. Rev. Biochem. Mol. Biol.* **30,** 445–600.

Ji, X., Zhang, P., Armstrong, R. N., and Gilliland, G. L. (1992). The three-dimensional structure of a glutathione *S*-transferase from the mu gene class enzyme 3-3 and glutathione at 2.2 Å resolution. *Biochemistry* **31,** 10169–10184.

Jörnvall, H., and Höög, J.-O. (1995). Nomenclature of alcohol dehydrogenases. *Alcohol Alcoholism* **30,** 153–161.

Kawajiri, K., and Hayashi, S.-I. (1996). The CYP1 family. *In* "Cytochromes P450—Metabolic and Toxicological Aspects" (C. Ioannides, ed.), pp. 77–97. CRC Press, Boca Raton, FL.

Ketterer, B. (1996). Effects of genetic polymorphism and enzyme induction in the glutathione *S*-transferase family on chemical safety and risk assessment. *Environ. Toxicol. Pharmacol.* **2,** 157–160.

Lacourciere, G. M., and Armstrong, R. N. (1993). The catalytic mechanism of microsomal epoxide hydrolase involves an ester intermediate. *J. Am. Chem. Soc.* **115,** 10466–10467.

Mackenzie, P. I., Mojarrabi, B., Meech, R., and Hansen, A. (1996). Steroid UDP-glucuronosyltransferases: Characterization and regulation. *J. Endocrinol.* **150,** S79–S86.

Mannervik, B., and Danielson, H. (1988). Glutathione transferase—Structure and catalytic activity. *Crit. Rev. Biochem.* **23,** 283–337.

Mannervik, B., Awasthi, Y. C., Board, P. G., Hayes, J. D., di Ilio, C., Ketterer, B., Listowsky, I., Morgenstern, R., Muramatsu, M., Pearson, W. R., Pickett, C. B., Sato, K., Widersten, M., and Wolf, C. R. (1992). Nomenclature for human glutathione transferases. *Biochem. J.* **282,** 305–306.

Maser, E., Richter, E., and Friebertshauser, J. (1996). The identification of 11 β-hydroxysteroid dehydrogenase as carbonyl reductase of the tobacco-specific nitrosamine 4-(methylnitrosamino)-1-(3-pyridyl)-1-butanone. *Eur. J. Biochem.* **238,** 484–489.

Maurel, P. (1996). The CYP3 family. *In* "Cytochromes P450—Metabolic and Toxicological Aspects" (C. Ioannides, ed.), pp. 241–270. CRC Press, Boca Raton, FL.

Moghaddam, M. F., Grant, D. F., Cheek, J. M., Greene, J. F., Williamson, K. C., and Hammock, B. D. (1997). Bioactivation of leukotoxins to their toxic diols by epoxide hydrolase. *Nature Med.* **3,** 562–566.

Morgan, E. T., Thomas, K. B., Swanson, R., Vales, T., Hwang, J., and Wright, K. (1994). Selective suppression of cytochrome P-450 gene expression by interleukins 1 and 6 in rat liver. *Biochim. Biophys. Acta* **1219,** 475–483.

Nebert, D. W., and McKinnon, R. A. (1994). Cytochrome P450: Evolution and functional diversity. *Prog. Liver Dis.* **12,** 63–97.

Nebert, D. W., McKinnon, R. A., and Puga, A. (1996). Human drug-metabolizing enzyme polymorphisms: effects on risk of toxicity and cancer. *DNA Cell Biol.* **15,** 273–280.

Nedelcheva, V., Persson, I., and Ingelman-Sundberg, M. (1996). Genetic polymorphism of human cytochrome P450 2E1. *In* "Cytochrome P450" (E. F. Johnson and M. R. Waterman, eds.), Vol. 272, pp. 218–225. Academic Press, San Diego, CA.

Nelson, D. R., Koymans, L., Kamataki, T., Stegeman, J. J., Feyereisen, R., Waxman, D. J., Waterman, M. R., Gotoh, O., Coon, M. J., Estabrook, R. W., Gunsalus, I. C., and Nebert, D. W. (1996). P450 superfamily: Update on new sequences, gene mapping, accession numbers and nomenclature. *Pharmacogenetics* **6,** 1–42.

Oesch, F., Oesch-Bartlomowicz, B., Arens, J., Fändrich, F., Vogel, E., Friedberg, T., and Glatt, H. (1994). Mechanism-based predictions of interactions. *Environ. Health Perspect.* **102,** 5–9.

Owens, I. S., and Ritter, J. K. (1995). Gene structure at the human UGT1 locus creates diversity in isozyme structure, substrate specificity, and regulation. *In* "Progress in Nucleic Acid Research and Molecular Biology" (W. E. Cohn and K. Moldave, eds.), Vol. 51, pp. 305–338. Academic Press, San Diego, CA.

Prough, R. A., Linder, M. W., Pinaire, J. A., Xiao, G. H., and Falkner, K. C. (1996). Cytochromes P450. 8. Hormonal regulation of hepatic enzymes involved in foreign compound metabolism. *FASEB J.* **10,** 1369–1377.

Ronis, M. J. J., Lindros, K. O., and Ingelman-Sundberg, M. (1996). The CYP2E family. *In* "Cytochromes P450—Metabolic and Toxicological Aspects" (C. Ioannides, ed.), pp. 211–239. CRC Press, Boca Raton, FL.

Sakaguchi, M., and Omura, T. (1993). Topology and biogenesis of microsomal cytochrome P-450s. *In* "Medicinal Implications in Cytochrome P-450 Catalyzed Biotransformations" (K. Ruckpaul and H. Rein, eds.). Akademie Verlag, Berlin.

Schmidt, J. V., and Bradfield C. A. (1996). Ah receptor signaling pathways. *Annu. Rev. Cell Dev. Biol.* **12,** 55–89.

Smith, C. A. D., Smith, G., and Wolf, C. R. (1994). Genetic polymorphisms in xenobiotic metabolism. *Eur. J. Cancer A* **30,** 1921–1935.

Sogawa, K., Matsushita, N., Ema, M., and Fujii-Kuriyama, Y. (1994). DNA-binding regulatory factors and inducible expression of the P4501A1 gene. *In* "Cytochrome P450" (M. C. Lechner, ed.), pp. 75–80. John Libbey Eurotext, Montrouge, France.

Vistisen, K., Poulsen, H. E., and Loft, S. (1992). Foreign compound metabolism capacity in man measured from metabolites of dietary caffeine. *Carcinogenesis* **13,** 1561–1568.

Waterman, M. R. (1996). Introduction: Transcription and regulation of activities of cytochromes P450 metabolizing endogenous substrates. *FASEB J.* **10,** 1455.

Weinshilboum, R., and Aksoy, I. (1994). Sulfation pharmacogenetics in humans. *Chem. Biol. Interact.* **92,** 233–246.

Whitlock, J. P., Okino, S. T., Dong, L. Q., Ko, H. S. P., Clarke-Katzenberg, R., Qiang, M., and Li, H. (1996). Cytochromes P450. 5. Induction of cytochrome P4501A1: A model for analyzing mammalian gene transcription. *FASEB J.* **10,** 809–818.

CHAPTER

5

Free Radicals and Reactive Oxygen Species

MAGED YOUNES

International Programme on Chemical Safety, World Health Organization, Geneva, Switzerland

INTRODUCTION

Free radicals are chemical entities characterized by a high reactivity. The formation of free radicals during the metabolism of xenobiotics is therefore an important mechanism of action through which some toxic agents may cause cellular damage. Free radicals can react in several ways, including the addition to double bonds, the reaction with nucleophilic groups (thiols, amines), the abstraction of hydrogen atoms from biomolecules, and the formation of dimers. The interaction of free radicals with cellular components may lead to the formation of secondary radicals derived from proteins, lipids, or nucleic acids. These may, in turn, react with other cellular macromolecules, and initiate and thus maintain a chain reaction. Consequently, cellular damage may be exacerbated to a large extent. The consequences of free radical reactions with cellular constituents are variable in nature. Radicals may have immediate effects, such as cellular necrosis and, eventually, fibrosis. They may, however, also result in delayed long-term effects, for example, tumorigenesis. The type of manifestation of toxicity and the degree of damage depend on the nature of the free radical species involved, the biological site of radical formation, and the type of chemical interaction with cellular constituents.

WHAT ARE FREE RADICALS?

Free radicals are defined chemical entities (atoms, molecules, ions) that possess one or more unpaired electrons. An unpaired electron occupies an atomic or molecular orbital on its own. The presence of unpaired electrons provides radicals, apart from specific chemical characteristics, with particular physical properties. Thus, free radicals are paramagnetic, and this property can be used to detect them by means of electron spin resonance spectrometry (ESR).

Free radicals can be formed from neutral molecules through uptake or release of an electron. One further possibility of radical formation lies in the homolytic cleavage of a covalent bond, a reaction that normally requires a substantial amount of energy. Free radicals can thus be anionic, cationic, or neutral species, carrying a net negative charge or a net positive charge or being electrically neutral (Fig. 1). Despite the fact that the formation of free radicals in chemical systems generally requires extreme conditions, several compounds both of natural and of synthetic nature are easily converted to radical species under conditions that may be encountered in biological systems.

OXYGEN FREE RADICALS AND NONRADICAL REACTIVE OXYGEN SPECIES

Molecular oxygen, in its ground state, is a biradical. The outer "antibinding" molecular orbitals ($2p\pi^*$) are occupied by an unpaired electron each. Both electrons have a parallel spin, an arrangement that characterizes a "triplet state" (triplet oxygen, $^3O_2$). In contrast to molecular oxygen, most organic molecules have a "singlet" ground state. This means that their outer electrons possess antiparallel spin. Molecules in the singlet state can only react with their equals; any

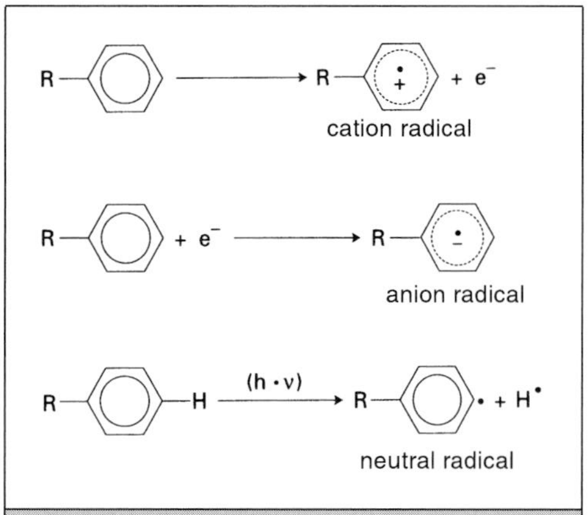

FIGURE 1 Possible radical formations.

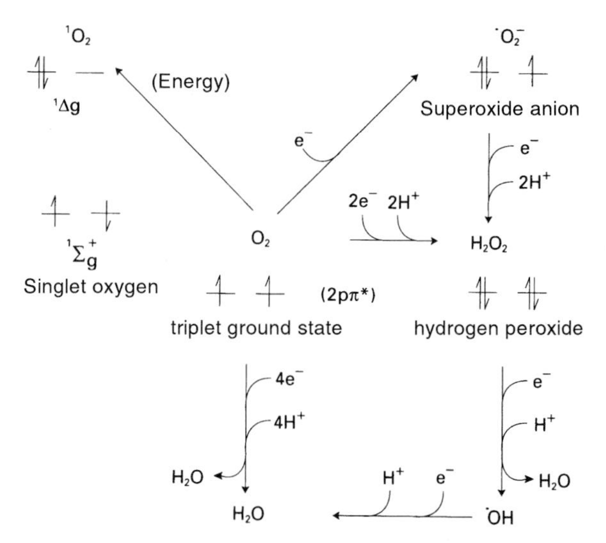

FIGURE 2 Activation of molecular oxygen and electron distribution in the outer antibinding molecular orbitals (2pπ*). Molecular oxygen has a triplet ground state. The outer antibinding molecular orbitals are occupied by one electron each, both having parallel spin. Therefore, reactions with organic molecules, which generally have a singlet ground state, are not possible. To initiate such a reaction, oxygen must be activated, be it through uptake of energy and formation of singlet molecular oxygen or by uptake of electrons.

chemical reaction would require the addition of a pair of electrons with antiparallel spin, as binding molecular orbitals can only be occupied by two electrons with antiparallel spin (spin-paired electrons). Because molecular oxygen has a triplet ground state, reactions with organic molecules cannot take place directly; they are "spin forbidden." For a reaction between a triplet molecule (oxygen) and a singlet molecule (organic substrate) to proceed, one electron must undergo a spin conversion. This, however, is a much slower process than the lifetime of a collision complex between oxygen and any oxidizable substrate. Therefore, oxygen is a weak oxidant in its ground state.

One-electron reduction of oxygen, in contrast to the type of reaction described previously, does not involve spin conversion; thus, it predominates over two-electron reduction pathways, even in biological systems. In fact, consecutive one-electron reductions of molecular oxygen take place in cellular systems leading to the formation of the superoxide anion radical, $\cdot O_2^-$, hydrogen peroxide, H_2O_2, the hydroxyl radical, $\cdot OH$, and, finally, water, H_2O (Fig. 2). $\cdot O_2^-$, H_2O_2, and $\cdot OH$ are better oxidants than triplet oxygen. They are too reactive to be tolerated in living cells and are therefore kept under control by a variety of cellular defence mechanisms. Other possibilities for oxygen activation include complex formation between molecular oxygen and transition metal ions, and spin inversion, a reaction that requires energy and that leads to the formation of singlet oxygen ($^1O_2$). Both pathways can also be undergone in biological systems.

The Superoxide Anion Radical

The uptake of one electron by molecular oxygen results in the formation of the superoxide anion radical (Fig. 2). Its reactivity stems from a number of chemical characteristics. First, superoxide is a strong base and can therefore abstract protons from a variety of compounds. Second, O_2^- is a potent reducing agent; it can reduce quinones reversibly to semiquinones and transition metal ions such as Fe^{3+} and Cu^{2+} into their reduced forms (Fe^{2+} and Cu^+). Third, the superoxide ion is a nucleophile and may thus readily interact with a number of electrophilic agents. Finally, it is an oxidant, though a weak one. Superoxide may initiate oxidation reactions, for example, of molecules such as ascorbic acid or epinephrine (adrenaline), following hydrogen abstraction due to its basicity.

Hydrogen Peroxide and the Hydroxyl Radical

During the stepwise one-electron reduction of molecular oxygen, hydrogen peroxide is the second intermediate. It may, however, also be generated directly via a two-electron reduction of molecular oxygen (Fig. 2). Hydrogen peroxide is a stable molecule that is generated as an end product of a variety of oxidative reactions in living cells. It may, in fact, act as both as an oxidizing and as a reducing agent.

Though not a radical per se, H_2O_2 is a source of hydroxyl radicals ($\cdot OH$), generated following interaction with transition metal ions ("Fenton"-type reactions),

$$H_2O_2 + Fe^{2+} \longrightarrow Fe^{3+} + \cdot OH + OH^-$$

or through reaction with a multiplicity of other agents (e.g., the air pollutants NO or NO_2),

$$NO + H_2O_2 \longrightarrow \cdot OH + HONO$$

$$NO_2 + H_2O_2 \longrightarrow \cdot OH + HONO_2.$$

The hydroxyl radical is a highly reactive oxidizing agent that can react with a wide variety of organic molecules. It can abstract a hydrogen atom from essentially any hydrogen–carbon bond and undergo addition reactions with aromatic systems at a reaction rate close to diffusion limit.

Singlet Molecular Oxygen

Singlet molecular oxygen is formed through spin conversion of one of the two unpaired electrons of the triplet ground state oxygen molecule ($^3\Sigma_g{}^-O_2$) (Fig. 2). This process requires energy. Two forms of singlet oxygen are known: $^1\Sigma_g{}^+O_2$, in which the paired electrons with antiparallel spin occupy one antibinding molecular orbital each; and $^1\Delta_g\ O_2$, where the paired outer electrons are located on one of the two antibinding $2p\pi^*$ molecular orbitals (Fig. 2). $^1\Sigma_g{}^+O_2$ requires that higher energy be formed and can be generated only in the gas phase. $^1\Delta_gO_2$, in contrast, can be formed in aqueous solutions, though its lifetime in water is as low as 2 μs. Although singlet oxygen is not a free radical, it is a reactive oxygen species with strong oxidative properties due to the lack of spin restriction. The formation of singlet oxygen in biological systems has long been disputed. There is adequate evidence today that $^1\Delta_g\ O_2$ is generated during some physiological and pathophysiological reactions (e.g., during phagocytosis or prostaglandin biosynthesis).

Interconversion Reactions of Reactive Oxygen Species

A primary oxygen radical with relatively low toxicity may undergo a number of interconversion reactions resulting in the formation of more reactive oxygen species of higher toxicity. Superoxide anions undergo a spontaneous or, more rapidly, an enzymatically catalyzed disproportionation (dismutation) reaction generating molecular oxygen and hydrogen peroxide.

$$\cdot O_2^- + O_2^- + 2H^+ \longrightarrow H_2O_2 + O_2$$

O_2^- and H_2O_2 may interact with transition metal ions (e.g., Fe^{3+}/Fe^{2+} or Cu^{2+}/Cu^+) in a series of reactions resulting, finally, in the formation of hydroxyl radicals.

$$Me^{n+} + \cdot O_2^- \longrightarrow Me^{(n-1)+} + O_2$$

$$Me^{(n-1)+} + H_2O_2 \longrightarrow Me^{n+} + \cdot OH + OH^-$$

The net result of both reactions is a transition-metal-catalyzed reaction of superoxide anions and hydrogen peroxide, which was postulated in 1934 by Haber and Weiss (therefore, the "Haber–Weiss reaction").

$$\cdot O_2^- + H_2O_2 \xrightarrow{Me^{n+}/Me^{(n-1)+}} O_2 + \cdot OH + OH^-$$

H_2O_2 may also interact with hypochlorite, which in turn is produced via the oxidation of chloride by hydrogen peroxide. This reaction results in the formation of $^1\Delta_g\ O_2$, and takes place in polymorphonuclear leukocytes where it is catalyzed by a specific enzyme, myeloperoxidase.

Biological Sources of Oxygen Radicals and Other Reactive Oxygen Species

Oxygen free radicals and nonradical reactive oxygen species, primarily superoxide and hydrogen peroxide, are produced in a number of biological processes (Table 1). The most simple biological systems are soluble cell constituents that can activate molecular oxygen during autoxidation reactions. This group comprises, among others, thiols, hydroquinones, flavins, catecholamines, tetrahydropterins, hemoproteins, and transition metal ions. Various soluble enzymes generate superoxide and hydrogen peroxide by reducing molecular oxygen in their catalytic cycles. Examples of such enzymes are xanthine oxidase, aldehyde oxidase, tryptophan dioxygenase, dihydroorotete dehydrogenase, and diamine oxidase. Membrane-bound enzymes and electron transport systems can also release oxygen radicals and related reactive oxygen species. Thus, superoxide and, consequently, hydrogen peroxide are produced by the mitochondrial electron transport system. The source of superoxide radicals is most likely the ubiquinone–cytochrome *b* complex, not the cytochrome oxidase.

Xenobiotic-metabolizing enzymes located in the endoplasmic reticulum and the nuclear membrane are also capable of activating molecular oxygen. This was shown to be the case for the cytochrome P450-dependent monooxygenases, the NADPH-dependent cytochrome reductases, and the flavin-dependent monooxygenases. Phagocyting cells are another major biological source of reactive oxygen.

Toxic agents have also been identified that cause damage by recruiting phagocytic cells, which, in turn,

TABLE 1 Some Biological Systems Capable of Activating Molecular Oxygen

Enzymes	Xanthine oxidase
	Aldehyde oxiodase
	Prostaglandin synthase
	Galactose oxidase
	Dopamine-β-hydroxylase
	Diamine oxidase
	Cytochrome P450-dependent monooxygenases
Autoxidation reactions	Catecholamines
	Thiols
	Hemoproteins
	Tetrahydropterins
	Hydroquinones
	Flavins
Complex systems	Phagocyting cells
	Microsomal electron transport chain
	Mitochondrial electron transport chain

generate reactive oxygen species. One prominent example is asbestos, which can activate alveolar macrophages and polymorphonuclear leukocytes. At the same time, however, asbestos fibers contain iron ions, which catalyze the formation and interconversion of oxygen radicals and other reactive oxygen species.

The formation of oxygen radicals and related reactive oxygen species in biological systems is controlled by a number of physiological antioxidative defence mechanisms. Generally, cellular constituents are thus well protected. Under certain conditions, however, the rate of formation of reactive oxygen species may exceed the capacity of antioxidative systems. As a consequence, reactive oxygen species may undergo oxidative damage; an "oxidative stress" is observed. Besides its apparent importance for some biological processes like aging and inflammation reactions, oxidative stress is supposed to play a role in the pathogenesis of a number of diseases, including acute pancreatitis, postischemic syndrome, tumorigenesis (particularly tumor promotion), atherosclerosis, and diabetic angiopathy.

ORGANIC FREE RADICALS

Organic free radicals are formed during metabolism of a number of xenobiotics. The prototype of a compound that is metabolized yielding a carbon-centered free radical is carbon tetrachloride, CCl_4. It undergoes a reductive dehalogenation reaction catalyzed by cytochrome P450-dependent monooxygenases (Fig. 3). The molecule is first reduced (electron uptake); then a chloride ion is abstracted. This sequence of reactions results in the formation of the reactive trichloromethyl radical (CCl_3), which can undergo additional reactions with macromolecules and abstract hydrogen atoms from other (bio)molecules. It may also interact with molecular oxygen forming the much more reactive trichloromethylperoxyl radical ($\cdot OOCCl_3$).

Similar to carbon tetrachloride, other halogenated hydrocarbons may also undergo reductive dehalogen-

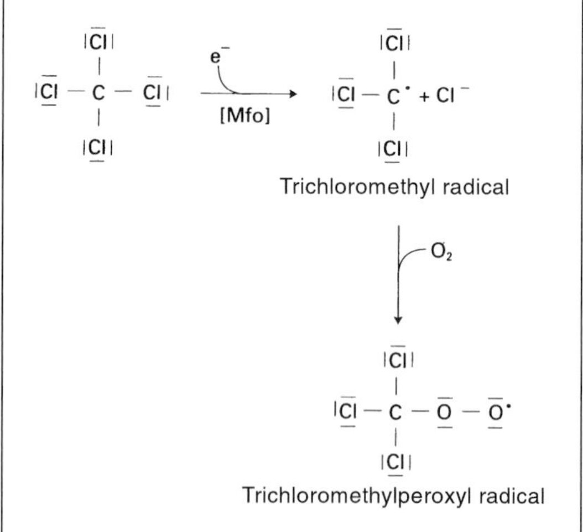

FIGURE 3 Radical formation through reductive dehalogenation of carbon tetrachloride (CCl_4). Carbon tetrachloride undergoes first a cytochrome P450-dependent monooxygenase-catalyzed one-electron reduction. Following the release of a chloride ion, the trichloromethyl radical is formed. This radical may react with molecular oxygen to form the trichloromethyl peroxyl radical.

ation reactions. Apart from other halogenated methanes (e.g., bromotrichloromethane ($BrCCl_3$)), this is the case with the gasoline additive 1,2-dibromoethane and the anaesthetic halothane.

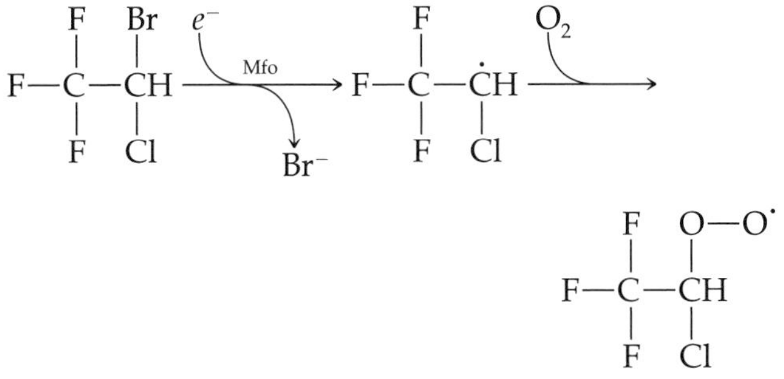

$$F_3C\text{—}CHBrCl \xrightarrow[\;Br^-]{e^-,\ \text{Mfo}} F_3C\text{—}\dot{C}HCl \xrightarrow{O_2} F_3C\text{—}CH(Cl)\text{—}O\text{—}O^{\bullet}$$

Organic free radicals are formed not only through reductive pathways, but also by oxidation reactions. This is, for example, the case with phenyl hydrazines, which are capable of exerting hemolytic effects following a hemoglobin-catalyzed metabolic conversion. This hemolytic effect is a consequence of the formation of free radicals according to the following reaction scheme (of phenylhydrazine, itself a prototype).

$$Ph\text{—}NH\text{—}NH_2 \xrightarrow{Hb} Ph\text{—}N{=}NH \quad \text{(Phenyl diazine)}$$

$$O_2 + Ph\text{—}\overline{N}{=}\overline{N}H \longrightarrow \cdot O_2^- + Ph\text{—}N{=}N\cdot + H^+ \quad \text{(Phenyl diazinyl radical)}$$

$$Ph\text{—}N{=}N\cdot \longrightarrow N_2 + Ph\cdot \quad \text{(Phenyl radical)}$$

Oxygen activation (generation of superoxide) occurs during one of the reactions of this metabolic sequence. Such a reaction is not confined to phenyl hydrazines, though. A number of exogenous and endogenous compounds were shown to activate oxygen, forming oxygen free-radical species once they undergo a one-electron transfer reaction yielding radical intermediates. These radical intermediates are well capable of transferring single electrons onto molecular oxygen, resulting in the formation of superoxide (and, subsequently, other reactive oxygen species). Prototypes of such compounds are quinones, such as adriamycin and structurally related cytostatistics; aflatoxin B_1 and metabolites of polycyclic aromatic hydrocarbons.

Quinones can undergo an univalent reduction reaction giving rise to a semiquinone radical. Semiquinoid metabolites are highly reactive and may interact with biological macromolecules through covalent binding. They can also transfer an electron onto molecular oxygen, producing superoxide radical anions. During such a reaction, the quinone is regenerated and may undergo a further enzyme-catalyzed one-electron reduction. A reaction cycle is thus initiated, during which oxygen is continuously activated—a "redox cycle" (Fig. 4). The uptake of a second electron by the semiquinone or the direct two-electron reduction of the parent quinone results in the formation of

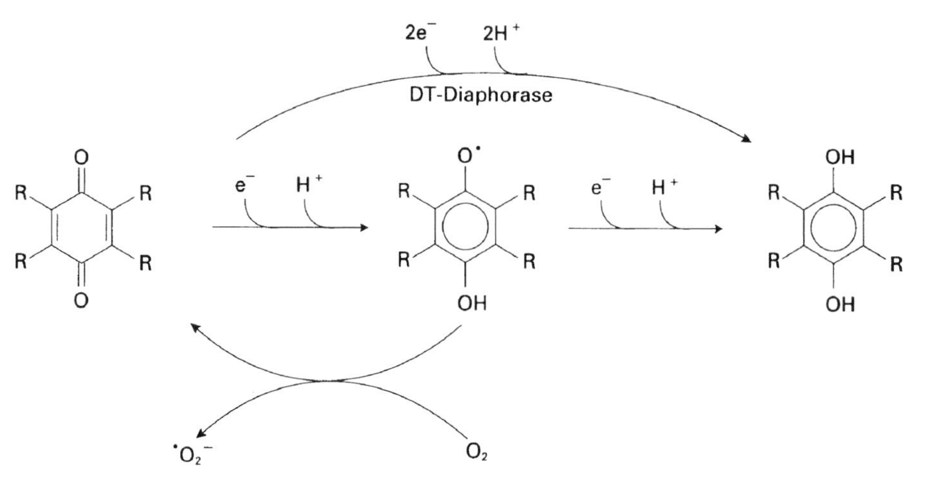

FIGURE 4 Quinone reduction and redox cycling. Quinones (and related quinoid compounds) can undergo one-electron reduction reactions yielding a semiquinone. This may transfer an electron onto molecular oxygen, forming superoxide and regenerating the quinoid structure. Such a redox cycle leads to a continuous generation of superoxide radicals. Further reduction of the semiquinone to the respective hydroquinone, as well as the direct two-electron reduction of the quinone (a reaction catalyzed by the DT-diaphorase), interrupt the redox cycle.

the respective hydroquinone. The divalent reduction of quinones occurs physiologically in a reaction catalyzed by a specific enzyme, the DT-diaphorase. This enzyme has an antioxidative cytoprotective function since its action leads to avoiding the generation of reactive semiquinones and, consequently, reactive oxygen species.

The analgetic and antipyretic drug acetaminophen (paracetamol) undergoes a bioactivation reaction similar to that of a semiquinoid intermediate, although the occurrence of a redox cycle in this case is still unproved. Paracetamol, the *N*-acetyl-*p*-aminophenol, undergoes a one-electron oxidation to yield the *N*-acetyl-*p*-benzosemiquinone imine (NAPSQI). NAPSQI can reduce molecular oxygen to superoxide, being oxidized to the *N*-acetyl-*p*-benzoquinone imine (NAPQI), or be oxidized in an enzyme-catalyzed reaction yielding the same product (Fig. 5). Both the semiquinoid and the quinoid metabolites are reactive. They have both been causally related to the hepatotoxicity of paracetamol. Under normal physiological conditions, reactive metabolites of paracetamol are inactivated through conjugation with endogenous glutathione (GSH), yielding the 3-(glutathion-*S*-yl)paracetamol. Following the release of the glycyl and the glutamyl moieties, and the N-acetylation of the cysteine conjugate, paracetamol is excreted renally as a mercapturic acid. It is only after endogenous glutathione has been depleted that cellular macromolecules can be arylated by reactive metabolites of paracetamol. It is unclear to what extent oxidative mechanisms are also responsible for paracetamol cytotoxicity.

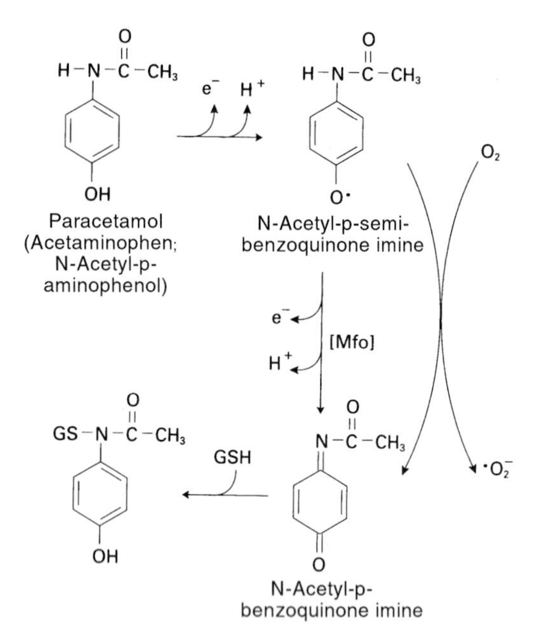

FIGURE 5 Formation of reactive intermediates during the metabolism of paracetamol (acetaminophen). Paracetamol undergoes a mixed-function oxidase (Mfo)-catalyzed oxidation. The release of one electron results in the generation of the *N*-acetyl-*p*-benzosemiquinone imine. The loss of a second electron (through enzymatic oxidation or transfer onto molecular oxygen) yields the reactive *N*-acetyl-*p*-benzoquinone imine. Both metabolites are considered responsible for the cytotoxicity of paracetamol. They are both inactivated through conjugation with glutathione (GSH). Only after depletion of endogenous GSH stores does cytotoxicity become evident.

A number of nonquinoid compounds can also undergo one-electron transfer reactions, making them subject to possible redox cycling. Among these compounds can be found several nitroaromatic compounds ($Ar{-}NO_2$) (e.g., chemotherapeutic agent nitrofurantoin and nifurtimox, an agent used to treat Chaga's disease, transmitted by *Trypanosoma cruci*). The univalent reduction of such nitroaromatic compounds results in the formation of nitro anion radicals (Fig. 6), which, in turn, react with molecular oxygen, yielding superoxide with the nitro group being regenerated.

$$Ar{-}NO_2 \xrightarrow{e^-} Ar{-}NO_2^{\dot{-}}$$

$$Ar{-}NO_2^{-}\cdot + O_2 \longrightarrow Ar{-}NO_2 + \cdot O_2^-$$

Bipyridinium herbicides of the paraquat type also belong to the group of nonquinoid compounds that are capable of initiating a redox cycle. Paraquat is transformed through a univalent reduction reaction to a pyridinium cation radical (Fig. 6), which transfers an electron onto molecular oxygen, regenerating the parent compound and generating superoxide.

$$PQ^{++} \xrightarrow{e^-} PQ^{\dot{+}}$$

$$PQ^{+}\cdot + O_2 \longrightarrow PQ^{++} + \cdot O_2^-$$

Several enzymes can catalyze such one-electron transfer reactions (mainly reduction reactions). Among those are NADPH–cytochrome *c* reductase, NADH–cytochrome b_5 reductase, xanthine oxidase, and aldehyde oxidase.

Free radical species are also found in complex pollutant mixtures. For example, free radicals can be detected in cigarette smoke and in soot. Among the radicals detected, nitrogen oxides and other nitro radicals, alkyl (R·), alkoxyl (RO·) and peroxyl (ROO·)

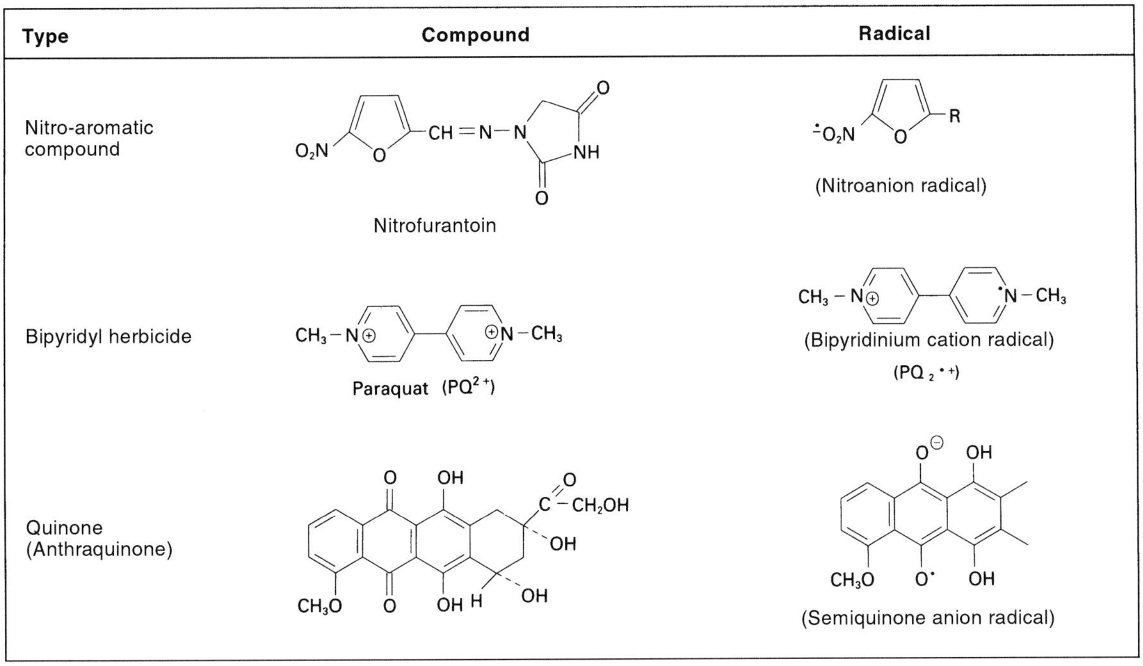

Type	Compound	Radical
Nitro-aromatic compound	Nitrofurantoin	(Nitroanion radical)
Bipyridyl herbicide	Paraquat (PQ^{2+})	(Bipyridinium cation radical) ($PQ_2^{\cdot +}$)
Quinone (Anthraquinone)		(Semiquinone anion radical)

FIGURE 6 Examples of one-electron oxidation–reduction reactions of organic compounds.

radicals, as well as sulfite ($SO_3^{\cdot -}$), sulfate ($SO_4^{\cdot -}$), and peroxysulfate radicals ($SO_5^{\cdot -}$).

BIOLOGICAL EFFECTS OF FREE RADICALS

The organ-directed toxic effects of a variety of compounds are thought to be mediated by radical intermediates. Examples are given in Table 2. The particular toxicity of free radicals is a consequence of their high reactivity. In principle, free radicals can react with virtually all vital molecules in living cells. This can lead to metabolic and structural alterations, which may, under certain conditions, lead to cell death. Free radicals have also been associated with more complex toxic processes, including reproductive toxicity and tumorigenesis. In the context of the latter, it has recently been reported that superoxide is a mediator of the *ras* oncogene, transmitting mitogenic signaling.

Due to the diversity of biologically generated free radicals and their different properties, it is difficult to generalize about their biological effects. Such effects will vary depending on the site of radical formation, the lifetime of the radical(s), and the nature of the target molecule with which the radical interacts. General observations can be made concerning the reactions of free radicals with specific cellular molecules, however. Free radicals can react with low-molecular-weight biomolecules like neurotransmitters or coenzymes and, consequently, inactivate them. One prominent example of such a reaction being of physiological relevance is the inactivation of superoxide with nitric oxide. In fact, nitric oxide (NO) itself is a free radical. It is produced physiologically from L-arginine and molecular oxygen in a reaction catalyzed by a dioxygenase, the nitric oxide synthetase. At low concentrations, NO mediates many physiological processes, for example, vasodilatation, neurotransmission, and immune response. At high concentrations, however, it exerts cytotoxic and genotoxic (DNA damage) effects. Also, the reaction product of nitric oxide and superoxide, the peroxynitrite ($ONOO^-$) is highly reactive. It damages proteins by reacting with tyrosine moieties and oxidizes thiols.

Macromolecules and cellular membranes are particularly vulnerable to free-radical damage. On reacting with these, they may lose their physiological reactivity resulting, ultimately, in cell death. The interaction of free radicals and nonradical reactive oxygen species with polysaccharides like hyaluronic acid, a major constituent of extracellular fluids, results in depolymerization of the macromolecule. Such a degradative process seems to play a role in inflam-

TABLE 2 Examples of Compounds That Exert Toxic Effects through Activation of Molecular Oxygen

Compound	Target organ	Mechanism of action
Paraquat	Lung	Selective accumulation; enzymatic reduction to bipyridinium cation; oxygen activation
Alloxan	Pancreas	Selective accumulation in β-cells; autoxidation of reduced form (dialuric acid); oxygen activation
Adriamycin	Heart	Reduction to semiquinone radical; oxygen activation
Bleomycin	Lung	Interaction with iron ions; redox-cycling of complex
6-Hydroxydopamine	Nervous system (peripheral adrenergic and central catecholaminergic neurons)	Autoxidation with quinone formation; covalent binding and oxygen activation
Paracetamol (acetaminophen)	Liver	Oxidation to *N*-acetyl-*p*-benzoquinone imine; further oxidation to quinone imine (oxygen activation?); covalent binding
Carbon tetrachloride	Liver	Reductive dehalogenation to trichloromethyl radical; covalent binding and lipid peroxidation
Ethanol	Liver	Oxygen activation (aldehyde oxidase reaction); inhibition of anaerobic energy conservation reactions

matory reactions of the joints; mucopolysaccharides of synovial fluid are degraded through the action of reactive oxygen species produced by phagocytes.

In the following sections, reactions of free radicals with proteins, nucleic acids, and lipids will be described in some detail.

Interactions of Free Radicals with Proteins

Free radicals have a high affinity to molecules with nucleophilic character. This is also the case with unsaturated and sulfur-containing amino acids like tryptophan, tyrosine, phenylalanine, histidine, methionine, and cysteine and thus with proteins. Organic free radicals and related electrophilic metabolites can bind covalently to cellular proteins. Such binding is not random but, rather, selective with respect to proteins targeted. A number of compounds that are metabolized to free radicals were shown to undergo covalent binding with proteins. Examples include carbon tetrachloride, halothane, paracetamol (acetaminophen), and adriamycin. Covalent binding was also evident for compounds, the reactive metabolites of which are electrophilic epoxides rather than free radicals (e.g., vinyl chloride, trichloroethylene, and other halogenated alkanes).

Covalent binding to proteins may lead to a loss of the macromolecule's biological function; that is, enzymes may be unable to exert their catalytic function and specific receptors may be inactivated. A covalent binding of a reactive metabolite to a protein may also initiate allergic reactions, since a protein that has been structurally modified by a "foreign" metabolite might exhibit antigenic characteristics.

Amino acids can undergo oxidative damage if they interact with oxygen free radicals and nonradical reactive oxygen species. This is true for unsaturated and sulfur-containing amino acids, as well as those that are relatively "resistant" like proline and lysine, which are subject to hydroxylation by hydroxyl radicals in a nonenzymatic reaction. Even peptide bonds can be subject to oxidative modification by reactive oxygen species. The consequence of such oxidative protein modifications, in general, is a loss of physiological function, as in the case of covalent binding of reactive organic metabolites to proteins. As free radicals are capable of initiating chain reactions, cross-linking of soluble and/or membrane-bound proteins, yielding dimers or larger aggregates, may occur. This leads to an amplification of the primary reaction. For example, interaction of reactive oxygen species with tryptophan results in the formation of *N*-formylkyneurine, which easily interacts with protein amino groups in a Schiff-base reaction between proteins. Similarly, cross-links may be formed between proteins and lipids or between lipids only. The direct consequence is a change in higher order structure of the protein (e.g., in the quarternary structure), which, in turn, results in a loss of biological function. A further effect of oxygen free radicals on proteins is the possible initiation of depolymerization reactions of structural proteins like collagen.

The vulnerability of a given protein with regard to radical-induced damage depends on its amino acid composition, the relevance of reactive (e.g., nucleophilic) amino acids for its physiological function, and/or its higher order structure, and the extent to which radical-induced damage can be repaired. An example of such a repair reaction is the reduction of radical-induced disulfide moieties or methionine sulfoxide groups, which are formed through oxidation of the cysteine thiol group or the methionine thioether group, respectively.

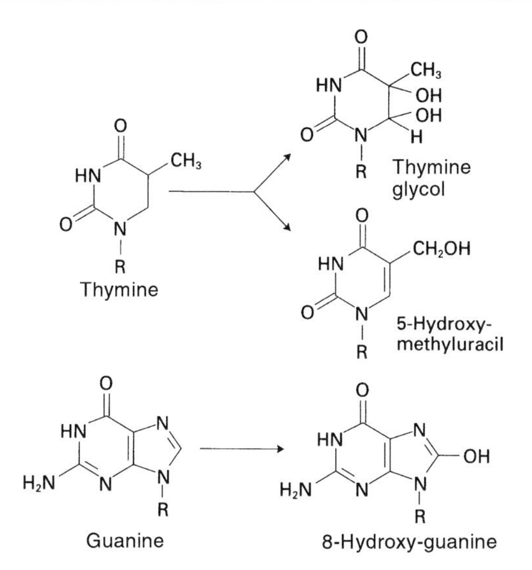

FIGURE 7 Modifications of DNA bases by reactive oxygen species. Nucleobases can undergo oxidative modifications by interacting with reactive oxygen species. In the case of thymine, reaction products are mainly thymine glycol and 5-hydroxymethyl uracil, in the case of guanine, mainly 8-hydroxy guanine.

Interaction of Free Radicals with Nucleic Acids

Besides covalent binding to proteins, radical intermediates produced during the metabolism of organic xenobiotics can react with nucleic acids, in particular with nucleobases, resulting in their damage. Such damage has been observed with a number of compounds in the case of DNA, many of which are cytostatic agents. A prominent example is adriamycin, which, like other anthracycline derivatives, is metabolized to a semiquinone that binds to DNA. Another mechanism of DNA damage by such compounds is based on their capability to activate molecular oxygen when undergoing redox cycling. Nucleic acid damage through redox cycling and generation of reactive oxygen species is not restricted to those compounds metabolized to semiquinones. Bleomycin, another cytostatic agent, for example, forms a complex with iron ions, which in turn is subjected to redox cycling.

Oxygen radicals can damage nucleic acids in two different ways. On the one hand, hydroxyl radicals can react with the sugar–phosphate backbone of nucleic acids, resulting in strand scissions and possibly chromosome breakage. On the other hand, reactive oxygen species may oxidatively modify the sugar moiety (e.g., deoxyribose in the case of DNA) or the different bases. Examples of oxidatively modified nucleobases are thymine glycol, 5-hydroxymethyl uracil, and 8-hydroxyguanine (Fig. 7).

Oxidative damage of nucleic acids can result in cell death (mainly through apoptosis), as is the case with radiation damage. Oxidative modifications of DNA can represent a process of tumor initiation, similar to the alkylation–arylation of nucleobases by organic radicals or other reactive metabolites. Besides their possible role in tumor initiation, oxygen free radicals and related reactive oxygen species have been implicated in the process of tumor promotion.

Interaction of Free Radicals with Lipids—Lipid Peroxidation

Lipids are also subject to reactions with free radicals. On the one hand, free-radical metabolites, particularly lipophilic ones, can bind covalently to lipids; on the other hand, they can initiate an oxidative chain reaction. Lipids containing several double bonds like polyunsaturated fatty acids (PUFAs) and cholesterol may, thus, be subject to oxidative damage. In the case of membrane phospholipids, such peroxidative destruction of their PUFAs generally result in an impairment of the function of cellular and/or subcellular membranes. This functional impairment may lead to cell death.

The process of lipid peroxidation is a chain reaction (Fig. 8). Polyunsaturated fatty acids (labeled LH) generally possess isolated double bonds; The C–H bond in the allylic position is "activated" and therefore par-

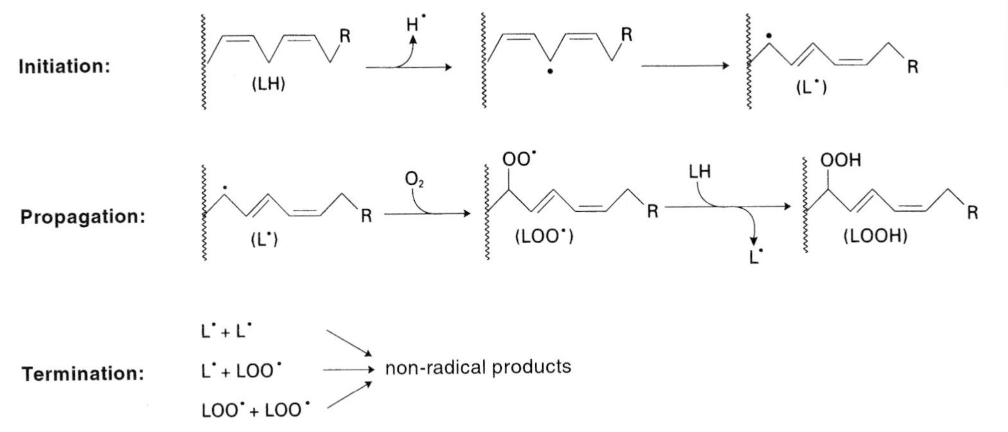

FIGURE 8 Schematic presentation of lipid peroxidation. The peroxidation of membrane phospholipids is initiated by the abstraction of a hydrogen atom from the allylic C–H bond of a polyunsaturated fatty acid, resulting in the formation of a lipid alkyl radical (L·). The lipid alkyl radical adds molecular oxygen to yield a lipid peroxyl radical (LOO·), which, in turn, abstracts a hydrogen atom from a neighboring fatty acid. A lipid hydroperoxide and a new lipid alkyl radical are formed. A chain reaction is thus maintained and is only terminated upon interaction of radical intermediates with each other.

ticularly vulnerable to oxidation reactions. Hydrogen atoms in such positions can react with free radicals (and other reactive "initiators") and are thus easily split (abstracted) from the C–H bond. This reaction, the initiation reaction, results in the formation of a lipid alkyl radical (L·).

$$LH + X\cdot \longrightarrow L\cdot + XH$$

This step is followed by an isomerization reaction leading to the transformation of an isolated double bond into a conjugated one. During the "propagation" reaction sequence that follows, the lipid alkyl radical reacts with molecular oxygen (which is a biradical by nature). A lipid peroxyl radical (LOO·) is produced, which, in turn, can abstract a hydrogen atom from a neighboring unsaturated fatty acid yielding a semistabile hydroperoxide and a new lipid alkyl radical. As a consequence, the process of lipid peroxidation may proceed in an autocatalytical manner.

$$L\cdot + O_2 \longrightarrow LOO\cdot$$

$$LOO\cdot + LH \longrightarrow LOOH + L\cdot$$

The chain reaction stops when the termination reactions take place (Fig. 8). These are reactions between two radical intermediates, resulting in the generation of nonradical products.

While molecular oxygen in its ground state is not capable of initiating the autocatalytic peroxidation of membrane phospholipids, oxygen radicals and other reactive oxygen species, including ozone, are. Superoxide anion radicals themselves cannot easily abstract hydrogen atoms from PUFAs in membrane phospholipids. They can produce ·OH or ·OH-like radicals in a metal (mainly Fe^{3+}/Fe^{2+})-catalyzed reaction, which in turn can initiate lipid peroxidation. Superoxide radicals can also form reactive complexes with transition metal ions, which can also act as initiators of lipid peroxidation. In the case of iron, the perferryl ion $[Fe^{2+} - O_2] \rightarrow [Fe^{3+} - \cdot O_2^-]$ and a $Fe^{2+}/O_2/Fe^{3+}$-complex have been proposed.

Substances that undergo redox cycling, such as adriamycin, paraquat, and nitrofurantoin, can activate oxygen and, consequently, initiate lipid peroxidation. Lipid peroxidation can also be initiated by paracetamol (acetaminophen), which is metabolized to a semiquinone imine intermediate capable of generating superoxide radicals. With these compounds, as in the case of enzymatically produced oxygen radicals, conversion of less reactive primary radicals (e.g., superoxide anion radicals) into more potent oxidants (e.g., ·OH radicals) in a transition-metal-catalyzed reaction seems to be a prerequisite for initiating lipid peroxidation reactions.

Besides oxygen radicals, several organic free radicals are well capable of abstracting a hydrogen atom from a polyunsaturated fatty acid and thus of initiating lipid peroxidation. The best studied example is that of carbon tetrachloride. Both the trichloromethyl radical (CCl_3) and the more reactive trichloromethyl peroxyl radical ($\cdot OOCCl_3$) are capable of initiating a peroxidative degradation of polyunsaturated fatty acids in membrane phospholipids. Other compounds that are capable of initiating lipid peroxidation without the intermediacy of reactive oxygen species besides other halogenated methanes, include polychlorinated biphenyls (PCBs), halothane, choroacetamide, polychlorinated dibenzo-*p*-dioxins (PCDDs), 1,2-dibromoethane, and 1,1-dichloroethylene.

As described previously, transition metal ions play an important role in initiating lipid peroxidation. Besides Fe^{3+}/Fe^{2+}, copper and mercury ions, as well as vanadate and chromate ions, can also initiate the peroxidation of membrane phospholipids. The role of metal ions is not restricted to the initiation reaction, however. They can also interact with semistabile lipid hydroperoxides, which are formed in the course of peroxidation reactions. Such reactions result in the generation of secondary radicals.

$$\mathrm{LOOH} + \mathrm{Fe}^{2+} \longrightarrow \mathrm{LO}\cdot + \mathrm{OH}^- + \mathrm{Fe}^{3+}$$

$$\mathrm{LOOH} + \mathrm{Fe}^{3+} \longrightarrow \mathrm{LOO}\cdot + \mathrm{H}^+ + \mathrm{Fe}^{2+}$$

These secondary alkoxyl and peroxyl radicals can, again, abstract hydrogen atoms from polyunsaturated fatty acids leading to a "reinitiation" of the chain reaction. Peroxidative damage of membrane phospholipids can, thus, be considerably exacerbated.

Apart from membrane phospholipids and cholesterol, other lipophilic biomolecules are vulnerable to peroxidative damage. Retinol (vitamin A) can undergo peroxidative degradation, yielding a variety of biologically inactive products. Lipoproteins can also be peroxidized. The peroxidation of low-density lipoproteins (LDL) is thought to be a key step in the pathogenesis of atherosclerosis.

Biological Consequences of Free Radical Damage

Primary reactions of free radicals with cellular molecules can cause further reactions. In biological membranes, for example, lipid peroxidation may result in an interaction of neighboring phospholipids. During chain termination reactions, alkyl, alkoxyl, or peroxyl radicals in neighboring molecules may combine, resulting in the formation of lipid–lipid cross-links. This may lead to an impairment of membrane functions. Radical intermediates formed by membrane proteins through direct interaction with free radicals or during lipid peroxidation (through the reaction of a lipid peroxyl radical with the protein) can also interact with phospholipid-derived radicals, yielding protein–lipid bridges. Finally, protein radicals may react with each other, generating protein–protein binding. The consequences of such changes of membrane structure are variable.

Several morphological alterations of cellular membrane structure have been described following free-radical damage. Thus, a dissociation of bound ribosomes has been observed in the endoplasmic reticulum. Membrane aggregation, deformation, and breakage, as well as loss of intramembranous particles, have been detected in the endoplasmic reticulum and in other organelles (e.g., mitochondria and lysosomes). Free radicals may, under extreme exposure conditions, lead to swelling and lysis of mitochondria. Lysosomes can also be subject to lysis under conditions of oxidative stress. This results in a release of hydrolytic enzymes which, in turn, may degrade functional macromolecules and cause secondary damage.

Peroxidation of membrane structures often leads to a functional impairment of membrane-bound proteins. This is the case with enzymes (glucose-6-phosphatase, UDP-glucuronyltransferase, cytochrome P450-dependent monooxygenases), electron transport proteins (e.g., the mitochondrial respiratory chain), and receptors. In this context, the inhibition of membrane-bound ATP-dependent calcium-transport proteins seems to be of particular relevance to cell damage, since it results in an intracellular accumulation of Ca^{2+}. Intracellular calcium accumulation has been postulated as a final irreversible step leading to cell damage through various toxic agents. Compounds that cause an oxidative stress (e.g., CCl_4, $BrCCl_3$, and 1,1-dichloroethylene) were shown to inhibit Ca^{2+}-ATPases of the endoplasmic reticulum both *in vivo* and *in vitro*. This inhibitory effect was accompanied by an oxidation of protein thiols.

Side products of lipid peroxidation can also exert toxic actions, even at sites more distant from the primary peroxidation event. Malondialdehyde and a large group of hydroxyalkenals, primarily 4-hydroxynonenal, are best known. Such aldehydes can interact with protein thiols, in the case of 4-hydroxynonenal, for example, according to the following scheme.

$$\mathrm{CH_3{-}(CH_2)_4{-}CH(OH){-}CH{=}CH{-}CHO} \xrightarrow{\mathrm{Prot{-}Cys{-}SH}}$$

$$\mathrm{CH_3{-}(CH_2)_4{-}CH{-}CH(S{-}Cys{-}Prot){-}CH_2{-}CHOH} \quad \text{(ring closed through O between the first CH and CHOH)}$$

Another common reaction is the formation of Schiff

bases by reacting with amino groups in proteins. In the case of malondialdehyde, intermolecular cross-links can thus be formed.

$$H_2C\begin{matrix} \diagup CHO \\ \diagdown CHO \end{matrix} + \begin{matrix} H_2N\text{—Prot} \\ H_2N\text{—Prot} \end{matrix} \longrightarrow H_2C\begin{matrix} \diagup CH{=}\overline{N}\text{—Prot} \\ \diagdown CH{=}\overline{N}\text{—Prot} \end{matrix} + 2\,H_2O$$

The consequence of such reactions is a functional impairment of the respective enzymes, receptors, or structural proteins. Aldehydes were also shown to inhibit protein biosynthesis and to increase the osmotic fragility of lysosomes and other subcellular organelles. They can also react with nucleic acids. Malondialdehyde exerted mutagenic effects both on *Salmonella typhimurium* (Ames test) and on primary cultures of rat fibroblasts.

CELLULAR DEFENCE MECHANISMS AGAINST FREE RADICALS

In living cells, several lines of defence, both enzymatic and nonenzymatic, against damage by free-radical or nonradical reactive oxygen species are found. These systems are capable of interacting directly with and inactivating initiating species, of interferring with oxidative processes, or of repairing damage that has already occurred (Table 3; Fig. 9).

Protective Enzyme Systems

Superoxide anion radicals are detoxified and kept under control through the action of superoxide dismutases, a family of metalloenzymes. These enzymes catalyze the disproportionation (dismutation) of superoxide ions.

$$\cdot O_2^- + \cdot O_2^- + 2H^+ \longrightarrow H_2O_2 + O_2$$

The second-order rate constant of this reaction is around 2×10^{-9} liter $mol^{-1}\ s^{-1}$, which is near diffusion limit.

In eukaryotic cells, two forms exist: a cytosolic copper- and zinc-containing enzyme and a mitochondrial manganese-containing enzyme. The fact that these enzymes are present in high concentrations in all tissues, together with their high catalytic efficiency, provides a high degree of cellular protection against superoxide anion radicals under normal conditions. In liver, the steady state concentration of free superoxide is thus maintained at levels as low as 10^{-11}–10^{-12} mol/liter. Different enzyme systems are capable of detoxifying hydrogen peroxide. In peroxisomes, catalase, a tetrameric hemoprotein, catalyzes the disproportionation of H_2O_2.

$$H_2O_2 + H_2O_2 \longrightarrow 2H_2O + O_2$$

The cytosolic selenium-containing glutathione peroxidase, a tetrameric protein, catalyzes the reduction of hydrogen peroxide by the tripeptide glutathione (GSH).

$$H_2O_2 + 2\ GSH \longrightarrow 2H_2O + GSSG$$

The action of these H_2O_2-scavenging enzymes results in the cellular concentration of hydrogen peroxide staying at 10^{-7}–10^{-9} mol/liter. As the concentrations of both superoxide and hydrogen peroxide are normally very low, it is highly improbable that secondary radicals like ·OH are produced under physiological conditions.

Organic free radicals and electrophilic metabolites of organic molecules can react directly with glutathione. Such reactions may be catalyzed by the glutathione *S*-transferases, a group of cytosolic enzymes with overlapping substrate specificity. These enzymes can also serve as selenium-independent glutathione peroxidases capable of reducing organic hydroperoxides already formed.

$$ROOH + 2\ GSH \longrightarrow GSSG + ROH + H_2O$$

This reaction can also be catalyzed by the selenium-

TABLE 3 Enzymatic Defense Mechanisms Against Reactive Oxygen Species

Enzyme	Oxygen species	Reaction catalyzed
Superoxide dismutases	$\cdot O_2^-$	$\cdot O_2^- + \cdot O_2^- + 2H^+ \rightarrow H_2O_2 + O_2$
Catalase	H_2O_2	$H_2O_2 + H_2O_2 \rightarrow 2H_2O + O_2$
Glutathione peroxidase	H_2O_2 ROOH	$H_2O_2 + 2\ GSH \rightarrow 2\ H_2O + GSSG$ $ROOH + 2\ GSH \rightarrow GSSG + ROH + H_2O$

Compound	Structure	Function
Ascorbic acid (Vit C)	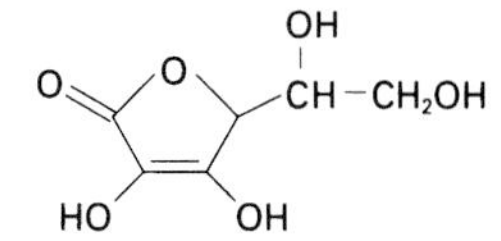	Scavenging of •O_2-, •OH, singlet oxygen and H_2O_2; Regeneration of α-tocopherol.
Glutathione	γ-Glu-Cys-Gly	Co-substrate for GSH-peroxidases; Interaction with •OH, •O_2- and organic radicals; Regeneration of protein thiols and α-tocopherol.
Carotinoids (β-carotin; Vit A)	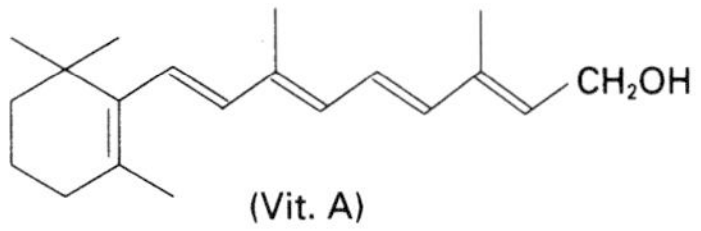 (Vit. A)	Scavenging of singlet oxygen.
α-Tocopherol (Vit E)	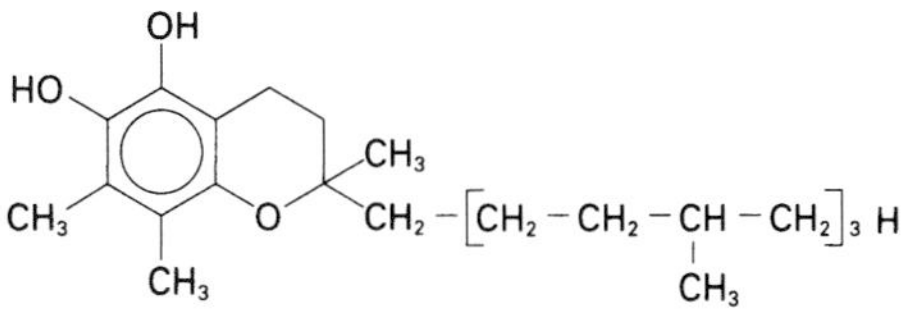	Antioxidative action through interaction with alkoxyl and peroxyl radicals; Interruption of chain propagation reactions of perioxidative processes.
Uric acid	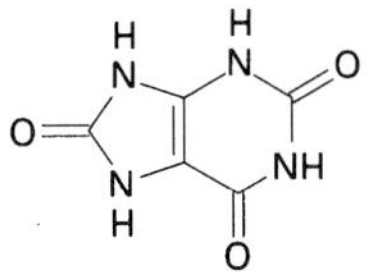	Scavenging of •OH, singlet oxygen and ROO•.

FIGURE 9 Nonenzymatic defense mechanisms against free radicals and nonradical reactive oxygen species.

dependent GSH-peroxidase, besides its capability to act on hydrogen peroxide as a substrate, unlike the selenium-independent enzyme. Another glutathione peroxidase of particular biological relevance is a selenoenzyme that specifically catalyzes the glutathione-mediated reduction of hydroperoxides in membrane phospholipids ("phospholipid hydroperoxide glutathione peroxidase").

To maintain the physiologically high ratio of reduced to oxidized glutathione (GSH/GSSG), glutathione disulfide generated in the GSH-peroxidase reaction must be reduced again. This function is fulfilled by the NADPH-dependent enzyme glutathione reductase, which catalyzes the following reaction.

$$\text{GSSG} + 2\,\text{NADPH} \longrightarrow 2\,\text{GSH} + 2\,\text{NADP}$$

The main source of NADPH is the glucose-6-phosphate dehydrogenase reaction.

An enzyme that prevents the formation of reactive oxygen species during the course of metabolism of a number of xenobiotics is the DT-diaphorase (NADPH–quinone oxidoreductase) mentioned previously. This enzyme catalyzes the two-electron reduction of various quinones and thus prevents the formation of semiquinones via one-electron transfer reactions. In the absence of semiquinoid structures, redox cycling of quinoid compounds cannot take place and oxygen radicals are not produced.

Nonenzymic Protective Systems

Among the low-molecular-weight cellular antioxidants, glutathione plays a central role. This thiol-containing tripeptide (γ-glutamyl-cysteinyl-glycine) is present in virtually all living cells in high concentrations. Apart from its function as a co-substrate of the glutathione peroxidases and transferases, glutathione can react directly with free radicals like O_2^-, ·OH, RO·, and ROO·. In such reactions, the thiol group loses a hydrogen atom, resulting in the generation of a thiyl radical.

$$R\cdot + GSH \longrightarrow RH + GS\cdot$$

Thiyl radicals can, in turn, combine to form glutathione disulfide (oxidized glutathione).

$$GS\cdot + GS\cdot \longrightarrow H_2O + AH\cdot$$

They can also react with other cellular molecules, however. This explains why glutathione can act as a pro-oxidant under certain conditions and even exert cytotoxic and mutagenic activity. Under physiological conditions, however, the antioxidant, radical scavenging capacity of glutathione prevails.

Ascorbic acid (vitamin C) is another water-soluble radical scavenger of high biological relevance. Ascorbic acid (AH_2) can react with oxygen radicals, generating the semidehydroascorbate radical ($AH\cdot$).

$$\cdot OH + AH_2 \longrightarrow H_2O + AH\cdot$$

$$\cdot O_2^- + H^+ + AH_2 \longrightarrow H_2O_2 + AH\cdot$$

The semidehydroascorbate radical disproportionates, generating ascorbate (AH_2) and dehydroascorbate (A).

$$2\,AH\cdot \longrightarrow A + AH_2$$

Apart from its ability to react with free radicals, ascorbate in the presence of transition metal ions (Fe^{3+}, Cu^{2+}) can act as a pro-oxidant. This is due to the fact that ascorbate can reduce these ions, producing ionic transition-metal species capable of interacting with hydrogen peroxide in a Fenton-type reaction to generate hydroxyl radicals. As with glutathione, the antioxidative properties of ascorbate are more prominent under physiological conditions.

Beside glutathione and ascorbate, other soluble molecules like uric acid and taurine have also been shown to exert an antioxidative activity. Their physiological relevance as free-radical scavengers is still unclear, however.

Among the lipophilic antioxidants, the tocopherols, primarily α-tocopherol (vitamin E), play a central role. Their main structural characteristics are a 6-chromanol ring and an isoprenoid, lipophilic side chain. The chromanol group is capable of reacting with peroxyl and alkoxyl radicals (mainly in peroxidized membrane phospholipids) and thus of inhibiting the propagation of peroxidative chain reactions.

$$ROO\cdot + VitE{-}OH \longrightarrow ROOH + VitE{-}O\cdot$$

Thus, tocopherols are potent inhibitors of lipid peroxidation. The active form of α-tocopherol is regenerated through reduction of the vitamin E radical. Ascorbic acid and/or glutathione seems to serve as the physiological reducing agents.

$$VitE{-}O\cdot + GSH \longrightarrow VitE{-}OH + GS\cdot$$

$$VitE{-}AH_2 \longrightarrow VitE{-}OH + AH\cdot$$

Apart from its antioxidative properties, vitamin E seems to play a role in maintaining selenium in an enzymatically active form, a vital function of high relevance for the activity of selenium-dependent enzymes, mainly glutathione peroxidase.

β-Carotin (provitamin A) is found in the membranes of certain tissues (e.g., the retina) in high concentrations. Its antioxidative capacity is, on the one hand, a consequence of its ability to inactivate singlet molecular oxygen. On the other hand, β-carotin can react directly with free radicals (e.g., with peroxyl radicals). In this manner, β-carotin is capable of interrupting peroxidative chain reactions like vitamin E.

CONCLUSION

Free radicals are generated during a number of physiological processes, as well as under certain pathophysiological conditions. They represent the toxic principle of a variety of xenobiotics, because their high reactivity makes them capable of interacting with vital cellular molecules like membrane phospholipids, DNA, and functional proteins, resulting eventually in an impairment of their function. A number of cellular defence mechanisms have the potential of inactivating free radicals (and related activated species). The degree of free-radical damage will ultimately depend on the balance between radical formation and radical inactivation.

Bibliography

Cohen, S. D., Pumford, N. R., Khairallah, E. A., Boekelheide, K., Pohl, L. R., Amouzadeh, H. R., and Hinson, J. A. (1996). Selective protein covalent binding and target organ toxicity. *Toxicol. Appl. Pharmacol.* **143,** 1–12.

Cotgreave, I. A., Moldéus, P., and Orrenius, S. (1988). Host biochemical defense mechanisms against prooxidants. *Annu. Rev. Pharmacol. Toxicol.* **28,** 189–212.

Feig, D. I., Reid, T. M., and Loeb, L. A. (1994). Reactive oxygen species in tumorigenesis. *Cancer Res. (Suppl.)* **54,** 1890s–1894s.

Grace, P. A. (1994). Ischemia-reperfusion injury. *Br. J. Surgery* **81,** 637–647.

Guyton, K. Z., and Kensler, T. W. (1993). Oxidative mechanisms in carcinogenesis. *Br. Med. Bulletin* **49,** 523–544.

Halliwell, B., and Gutteridge, J. M. C. (1989). "Free Radicals in Biology and Medicine." 2nd ed. Clarendon Press, Oxford.

Horton, A. A., and Fairhurst, S. (1987). Lipid peroxidation and mechanisms of toxicity. *CRC Crit. Rev. Toxicol.* **128,** 27–79.

Irani, K., Xia, Y., Zweier, J. L., Sollott, S. J., Der, C. J., Fearon, E. R., Sundaresan, M., Finkel, T., and Goldschmidt-Clermont, P. J. (1997). Mitogenic signalling mediated by oxidants in ras-transformed fibroblasts. *Science* **275,** 1649–1652.

Janssen, Y. M. W., Van Houten, B., Borm, P. A. J., and Mossman, B. T. (1993). Cell and tissue responses to oxidative damage. *Lab. Invest.* **69,** 261–274.

Kamp, D. W., Graceffa, P., Pryor, W. A., and Weitzman, S. A. (1992). The role of free radicals in asbestos-induced diseases. *Free Rad. Biol. Med.* **12,** 293–315.

Nathan, C. (1991). Mechanisms and modulation of macrophage activation. *Behring Inst. Mitt.* **88,** 200–207.

Reilly, P. M., Schiller, H. J., and Bulkley, G. B. (1991). Pharmacologic approaches to tissue injury mediated by free radicals and other reactive oxygen metabolites. *Am. J. Surgery* **161,** 480–503.

Riley, J. C. M., and Behrman, H. R. (1991). Oxygen radicals and reactive oxygen species in reproduction. *Proc. Soc. Exp. Biol. Med.* **198,** 781–791.

Rosen, G. M., Pou, S., Ramos, C. L., Cohen, M. S., and Britigan, B. E. (1995). Free radicals and phagocytic cells. *FASEB J.* **9,** 200–209.

Sies, H. (ed.)(1985). "Oxidative Stress." Academic Press, London.

Spiteller, G. (1993). Review: On the chemistry of oxidative stress. *J. Lipid Mediat.* **7,** 199–221.

Younes, M., and Siegers, C.-P. (1984). Interrelation between lipid peroxidation and other hepatotoxic events. *Biochem. Pharmacol.* **33,** 2001–2003.

CHAPTER

6

Genetic Toxicology

DAVID J. BRUSICK
Covance Laboratories, Vienna, Virginia

INTRODUCTION

The initial justification for genetic testing was best articulated by Alexander Hollaender in the late 1960s. It was based on concerns about the effects of environmental mutagens on the integrity of the human genome. Consequently, testing schemes used to evaluate environmental agents were predominantly *in vivo* and directed toward effects on germ cells (e.g., the rodent, dominant lethal assay and the *Drosophila* sex-linked recessive lethal assay).

In 1970, Bruce Ames, as well as other microbial geneticists, developed rapid screens for mutation in which reverse mutation could be easily detected on a single petri dish. These assays quickly replaced the more traditional animal and insect tests because they were inexpensive, provided rapid results, and demonstrated that a diverse set of environmental chemicals (i.e., food colors, pharmaceutical products, and pesticides) was capable of inducing genetic alterations. This approach to screening chemicals and mixtures was the beginning of what became known as "genetic toxicology."

Using methods and systems like the Ames test, genetic toxicologists quickly demonstrated a strong association between positive results in the bacteria and carcinogenic activity in rodents. From 1975 until 1985, much of the attention of genetic toxicology was diverted from assessing germ cell risk to screening chemicals for possible carcinogenic activity. *In vitro* test methods proliferated and test batteries were adopted to screen large numbers of chemicals and other physical agents for their ability to induce DNA adducts, DNA repair, DNA strand breaks, and mutations.

During the last decade, genetic toxicology has shifted its focus and regained some perspective on the larger issue of genomic integrity. Many investigators in this field are now focused on developing information about a chemical's reactivity with an organism's DNA and what that reactivity may mean to the ultimate viability of that organism or its progeny.

One of the goals of genetic toxicology continues to be the identification of DNA damage at doses capable of leading to adverse health effects in the exposed organisms. In the regulatory toxicology arena, the organisms of primary concern are humans.

Genotoxicity is not a rare phenomenon. In mammals, endogenous processes, as well as exposure to exogenous agents, result in the induction of thousands of DNA lesions per cell per hour. Error-free DNA repair will eliminate the vast majority of this damage, but the possibility for induction of new alterations does exist. The role of the genetic toxicologist is to understand the dynamics and significance of DNA-damage and -repair processes in the context of anticipated human exposure to genotoxicants, as well as the kinetics involved in the transformation of DNA lesions into stable heritable mutations. Once mutagenic agents are identified, genetic toxicologists, working with other biomedical and environmental scientists, can determine the level of risk from exposure and devise means to manage the risk by elimination of the agents from the environment or reduction of exposure to them.

BASIC GENETIC MECHANISMS

Gene Structure

The hereditary informational molecules of all living systems, with the exception of some viruses that use RNA, are composed of DNA, and those organisms that store their hereditary information in RNA go through a DNA-intermediate during replication. Some common characteristic features of DNA molecules are listed in Table 1.

The simplest complete functional unit in a DNA molecule is called a gene. Gene composition varies with organism; in humans, however, the size of a small gene, such as a neuropeptide gene, may contain as few as 100 nucleotides. A large human gene could be in the range of 2,000,000 nucleotides in length. Most of what is known about the structure and function of genes has been acquired from studies with bacteria or bacteriophages, although knowledge about the molecular biology of DNA replication and regulation in mammalian cells has increased dramatically during the past decade. The differences between the genes of prokaryotic (bacteria) and eukaryotic (plant and animal cells) organisms center primarily on their number, location on the respective chromosome entities, and mechanisms of gene regulation (Table 2). In prokaryotic cells there is a single chromosome entity with little or no differentiation along the DNA molecule so far as function is concerned. Eukaryotic cells, on the other hand, have DNA with nonfunctional, repeated sequences in or on some genes; these cells also have regions of noncoding DNA (called introns) between coding sequence (called exons). The function of repeated DNA sequences and intron regions is not known. The nucleotide composition and the mechanisms by which information encoded in a gene is transformed into gene products appear to be universal. This assumption of universality has been confirmed by genetic engineering studies in which genes continue to function properly after having been transplanted from human cells to bacterial cells or from bacterial cells to plant cells.

In eukaryotic cells the process of gene expression follows the pattern shown in Fig. 1. Enzymes located in the nucleus of the cell excise intron regions and splice the coding sequence back together. The resulting mRNA is transported to ribosomes in the cytoplasm for translation. Intron regions are not found in prokaryotic DNA. DNA repair processes are also influenced by transcription activity. DNA segments undergoing transcription into mRNA show higher rates of DNA repair than nontranscribed regions of the macromolecule.

Somatic and Germ-Cell Characteristics

Mammals and many other multicellular organisms are composed of two cell types, somatic cells and germ cells. Somatic cells constitute the major portion of the mammalian organism. The genomes of somatic cells are generally diploid (i.e., having two complete sets of chromosomes). While genetic damage to somatic cells may be transmitted to daughter cells following mitotic cell division, it is not transmissible to subsequent generations. Virtually all *in vitro* mammalian cell assays used in genetic toxicology employ somatic cell types as target organisms.

Germ cells, the second cell type, form a unique cell population in multicellular organisms and play a spe-

TABLE 1 Basic Biochemical Characteristics of Double-Stranded DNA
DNA consists of two purines (guanine, adenine) and two pyrimidines (thymine and cytosine).
A nucleotide pair consists of one purine and one pyrimidine [adenine–thymine (AT) or guanine–cytosine (GC)].
Nucleotide pairs are connected to a double-helix molecule by sugar–phosphate backbone linkages and hydrogen bonding.
The AT base pair is held by two hydrogen bonds, and the GC is held by three.
The distance between each base pair in a molecule is 3.4 Å, producing 10 nucleotide pairs per turn of the DNA helix.
The number of adenine molecules must equal the number of thymine molecules in a DNA molecule. The same relation exists for guanine and cytosine molecules. The ratio of AT to GC base pairs, however, may vary in DNA from species to species.
The two strands of the double helix are complementary and antiparallel with respect to the polarity of the two sugar–phosphate backbones, one strand being 3′–5′ and the other 5′–3′ with respect to the terminal OH group on the ribose sugar.
DNA replicates by a semiconservative method in which the two strands separate and each is used as a template for the synthesis of a new complementary strand.
The rate of DNA nucleotide polymerization during replication is approximately 600 nucleotides per second. The helix must unwind to form templates at a rate of 3600 rpm to accommodate this replication rate.
The DNA content of cells is variable (1.8×10^9 D for *Escherichia coli* to 1.9×10^{11} D for human cells).

TABLE 2 Characteristics of DNA in Prokaryotic and Eukaryotic Cell Types

Prokaryotic cells	Eukaryotic cells
Primarily haploid	Primarily diploid
DNA uncomplexed	DNA complexed with proteins forming chromosomes
DNA nonlocalized in the cell cytoplasm	DNA localized primarily within the nucleus of the cell
No morphologic stages in DNA replication	DNA replication described by mitotic cycle consisting of specific cytologic stages
DNA often found as a closed circle	DNA found in linear chromosomes
Replication not associated with cellular organelles	Replication and separation of chromosome associated with cellular organelles called centrioles
All genes encoded in the DNA are functional	Repetitive, nonfunctional gene sequences are common
Spacer sequences have not been identified.	Noncoding spacer sequences identified as introns occur along the DNA model

cialized role in sexual reproduction. Mature germ cells are derived from diploid stem cells in gonadal tissues, and following meiosis, carry a haploid set of chromosomes. Mutations in germ cells result in a broad array of heritable genetic diseases, congenital malformations, and other disorders in subsequent generations. The incidence of heritable genetic damage in the total number of germ cells residing in a population (species) is called the genetic load.

Mutations are classified as recessive or dominant, depending upon their expression in the diploid state. Dominant mutations are expressed when a single mutant allele is present. A large proportion of human genetic diseases, however, are associated with recessive mutant genes and are expressed only when two mutant alleles (one contributed by each parent) are present in the homozygous condition. Recessive mutations are maintained in the gene pool in the heterozygous state and are carried in that configuration by individuals who are phenotypically normal. The inability to easily identify heterozygous carriers of mutant alleles is one of the primary factors preventing the human genetic burden from being eliminated or even reduced.

DNA ALTERATIONS RESULTING IN GENOTOXIC EFFECTS IN CELLS

DNA replication and repair are not flawless processes, and in rare instances, they lead to "spontaneous" genetic damage. Spontaneous genetic damage occurs at a predictable rate per gene for most organisms. Other genetic damage is produced by endogenous and exogenous agents that interact with DNA and are therefore classified as genotoxicants. Some examples of endogenous agents are free radicals and peroxides produced during oxidative metabolism, and biologically produced aldehydes and ketones.

Classification of Genotoxic Effects

DNA damage may be classified into several broad categories based on the nature (presumed mechanism) of the DNA change. The following is one classification.

A. *DNA disruption damage* involves the breakage of and/or interchange of DNA segments between chromosomal structures. This type of damage may be visible through cytologic analysis of condensed chromosomes. Although genotoxins such as alkylating agents induce DNA disruption damage, a characteristic of its occurrence is that it may also be caused by secondary mechanisms that do not target nucleic acids specifically (e.g., processes that result in cell stress, such as high temperature.)

B. *Microlesions* are nonvisible alterations occurring at the nucleotide level. Nucleotide damage generally produces point mutations through base-pair substitution or insertion–delection or it may induce recombination between sister chromatids. Microlesions are

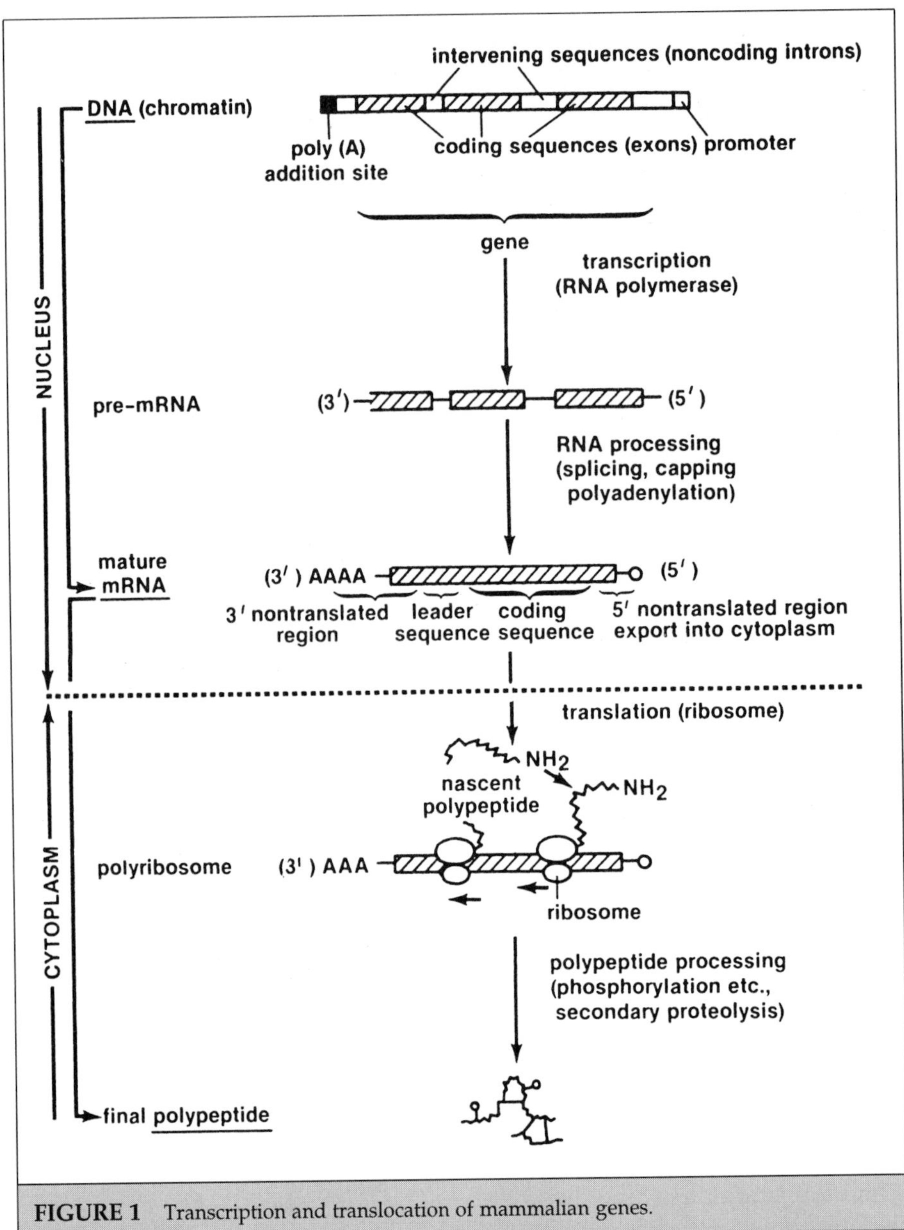

FIGURE 1 Transcription and translocation of mammalian genes.

generally induced by agents that specifically target nucleic acids (e.g., electrophilic agents).

Some biological effects may be induced by other mechanisms that do not fall readily into either of the two mechanisms here. Examples of such genotoxic damage might be aneuploidy–polyploidy and morphological cell transformation.

Normal DNA base pairings are shown in Fig. 2. Adenine and thymine form two hydrogen bonds, and guanine and cytosine form three. Hydrogen bonds are weak electrostatic forces involving oxygen and nitrogen atoms at specific sites on the purine and pyrimidine molecules. If electrophilic chemical species covalently bind to portions of the DNA bases involved in the formation of hydrogen bonds, these covalently bound species (adducts) can produce electron shifts from the H-bonding sites to areas within the molecules giving rise to opportunities for short-lived mispaired bases (e.g., A:C or G:T). If this mispairing occurs before or during a DNA replication cycle, the result may be the substitution of an incorrect base pair for the original pair (base-pair-substitution-type mutation). The period of time between exposure and the initiation of cell division (DNA replication) is the period in which DNA damage may be fixed in the ge-

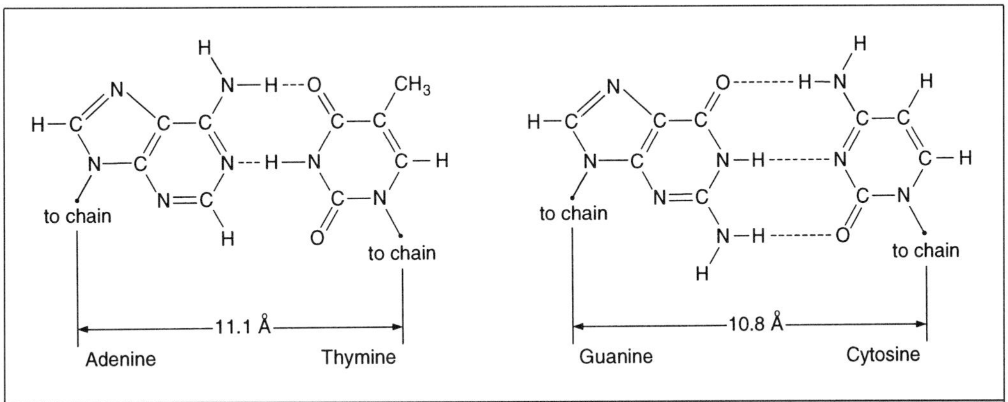

FIGURE 2 Hydrogen bonding of nucleotides normally found in DNA.

nome of the target organism. This period is called the "expression period" in most *in vitro* mutation assay designs. Unrepaired damage may be transformed into mutations, which will be expressed following the expression period. If mutant selection is introduced during the expression period, many DNA lesions will result in cell death and the yield of mutants will be relatively low.

Base-pair addition–deletion mutations, also called frameshift mutations, result from the addition or deletion of one or a few nucleotide pairs from the nucleotide sequence in an exon or gene. Because the codon sequence reads in one direction and is nonpunctuated, the loss or gain of a single base pair changes the reading frame of the gene—hence, frameshift mutation. This type of mutagenic mechanism is illustrated in Fig. 3. The production of frameshift mutations has been hypothesized to occur from misrepair of mismatched nucleotides. Both frameshift and base-pair substitution gene mutations result in alterations in translation of mRNA into the proper sequence of amino acids in the gene products and produce a mutant cell or organism, as illustrated in Fig. 4.

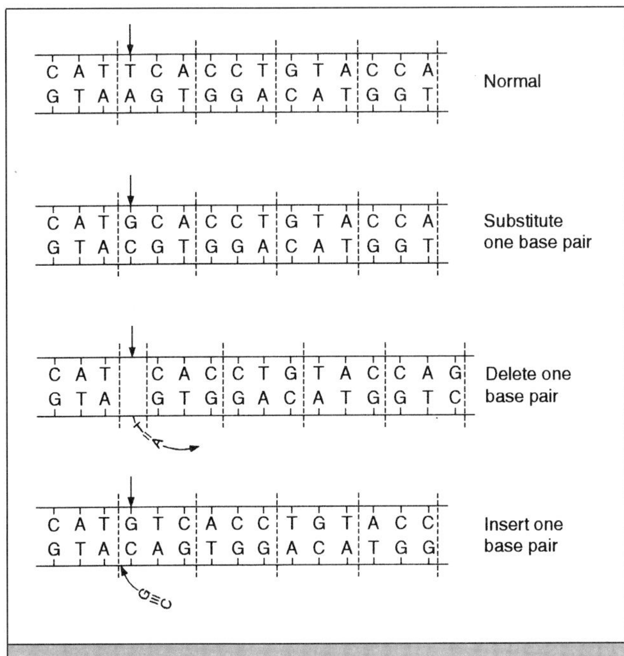

FIGURE 3 The steps involved in the generation of base-pair addition–delection (frameshift) mutations.

DNA is visible microscopically as a chromosome. Figure 5 illustrates the generalized anatomy of a chromosome. The chromosome illustrated is typical of a metaphase-stage structure and the anatomy shows distinctive bands as a result of giemsa staining. Mammalian chromosomes have a constriction known as the centromere. To either side of the centromere are the chromosome arms, which terminate in a structures called telomeres. The dark G+ bands represent highly condensed DNA and are areas of little or no gene expression (transcription). The light G− bands represent active genomic areas where gene expression (transcription) is occurring. The telomeric regions at the ends of the chromosome structures are important for chromosome stability. Telomeres consist of repeat units of a small number of nucleotides that stabilize the linear DNA molecule. At each cell division, chromosomes lose small amounts of telomeric DNA. The ability of the cell to replace the lost DNA with telomerase determines whether the cell continues to proliferate or, if the DNA loss reaches a critical level, stops dividing.

Microscopically visible DNA disruption damage is subdivided into changes in chromosome number (gain or loss of single chromosomes or sets of chromosomes) and changes in chromosome structure

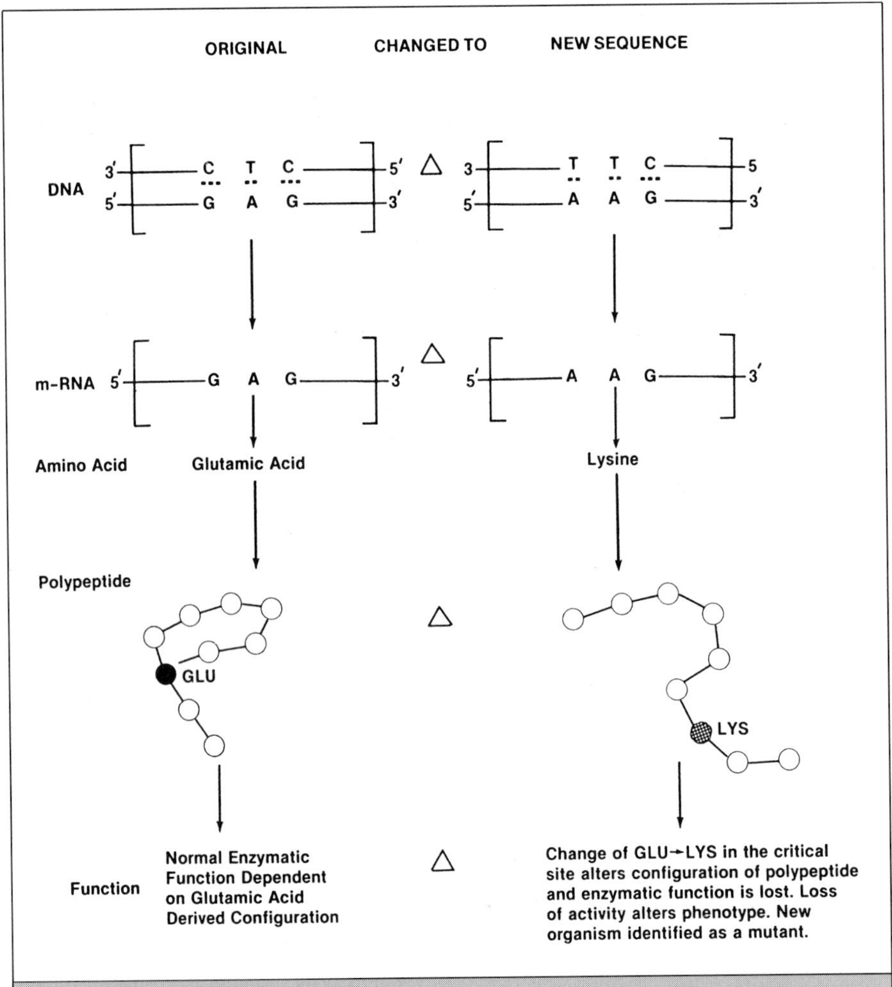

FIGURE 4 The relationship between base-pair mutations in the DNA and the production of altered proteins in mutant gene products.

(breaks, deletions, and rearrangements). Each type of chromosome change has a characteristic morphometric description so that a reasonably high degree of uniformity can be maintained when scoring for such changes. Variations in chromosome number can result from incomplete dissociation of single or entire sets of chromosomes at metaphase, resulting aneuploidy or polyploidy. A wide range of *in vitro* and *in vivo* methods are designed to assess chromosome breakage and numerical changes.

In addition to the tests that specifically measure nucleotide substitutions and chromosome alterations, a separate group of microlesion tests have been developed to measure DNA binding, DNA repair, sister chromatid exchange (SCE), and mitotic recombination. These phenomena are all associated with processes leading to stable genetic damage and have been proposed as tests indicating genetic hazard.

Repair of DNA Damage

The fidelity and integrity of genetic information in organisms are maintained by several types of enzymatic DNA repair. The characteristic of "self-repair" is unique to DNA and illustrates how important the integrity of this molecule is to the survival of an organism. Table 3 summarizes the general types of repair processes that exist in organisms. Components of DNA repair operate consititutively in organisms and other types are adaptive or inducible following some interaction with genotoxicants.

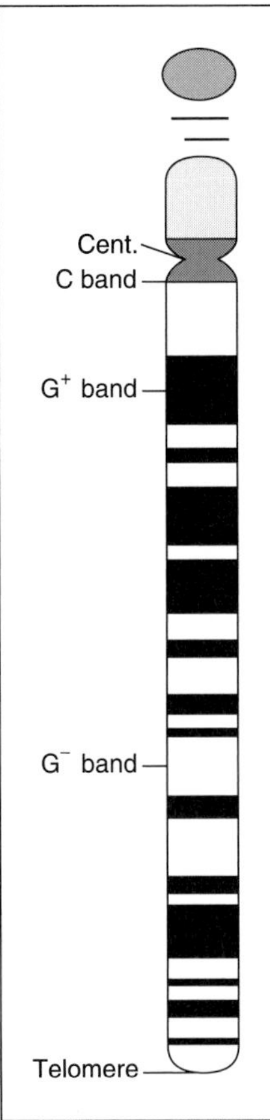

FIGURE 5 The anatomy of a mammalian chromosome. The illustration includes the centromere (cent.), regions of transcribed DNA (G^- bands), regions of nontranscribed DNA (G^+ band), and telomeric regions.

DNA damage is induced by both environmental agents and normal cellular proceses of DNA replication or oxidative stress. Some estimates of endogenous damage and repair capacities for human cells are given in Table 4. As indicated, endogenous cellular repair capacities are more than adequate to compensate for background damage; however, massive or frequent environmental exposures to genotoxic agents may saturate the endogenous capacity leading to primary DNA damage (e.g., DNA adducts, single- or double-strand breaks, or loss of DNA bases).

TABLE 3 Classification and Properties of Excision Repair Process

Class	Properties
Constitutive	The level of repair enzymes is fixed at a certain level of production; increased incidence of DNA lesions does not lead to greater repair enzyme activity
Inducible	Repair enzyme levels respond to the number of DNA lesions; for example, chronic pretreatment of cells with low levels of alkylating agents enhances the repair of lesions with a higher "challenge" level of the same agent
Error-free	The DNA repair process consists of an accurate base replacement, resulting in no net change in the DNA once the repair process is complete
Error-prone	The repair process is not accurate and aberrant DNA sequences are produced by the repair polymerase; new mutations may result as a consequence

The common feature of repair processes is the ability to remove and replace damaged segments of DNA. Therefore, if a DNA lesion can be repaired prior to mutation fixation, the net effect of the DNA damage may be nil. This is especially true following intermittent low-level exposure where repair enzymes are not fully saturated by excessive numbers of damaged DNA sites. DNA adducts are not all recognized or repaired equally by excision repair. The size of an adduct and the effect that an adduct has on the conformation of DNA determines how readily it is detected by the repair enzymes and is subsequently excised. Thus, it is not advisable to use the number of adducts per cell as a predictor of damage or genetic hazard unless definitive information is available about the elimination kinetics for the specific adducts.

Test systems measuring some parameter of the DNA repair process have been used as screens to detect primary DNA damage. Normal organisms are capable of some type of DNA repair activity following chemical insult; thus, stimulation or induction of repair activity following chemical treatment at sublethal concentrations is a good general indicator that the target organism has experienced DNA-directed toxicity.

Studies of DNA repair kinetics indicate that once premutational lesions have been induced in the DNA, both error-prone and error-free repair processes are activated. Error-prone repair processes generate nu-

TABLE 4 Estimates of Human Endogenous DNA Damage and Repair Processes

Type of damage	Estimated occurrences of damage per hour per cell[a]	Maximal repair rate, base pair per hour per cell[a]
Depurination	1000	[a]
Depyrimidination	55	[a]
Cytosine deamination	15	[a]
Single-stranded breaks	5000	2×10^5
N^7-Methylguanine	3500	[a]
O^6-Methylguanine	130	10^4
Oxidation products	120	10^5

[a]Actual values have been determined but estimates indicate capacities in excess of twice the endogenous induction rate.

cleotide mismatches (i.e., A:C or G:T) that actually produce *de novo* mutations. Error-free repair replaces the damaged DNA site with a correct nucleotide sequence.

The fidelity of repair depends on the degree to which the two different processes are involved. Factors that determine whether error-prone or error-free pathways predominate include the target species, cell type involved, chemical mutagen, and the specific DNA lesion induced. Some data suggest that the error-free repair pathways predominate at low exposure levels and that error-prone pathways come into play only following saturation of the error-free enzymes.

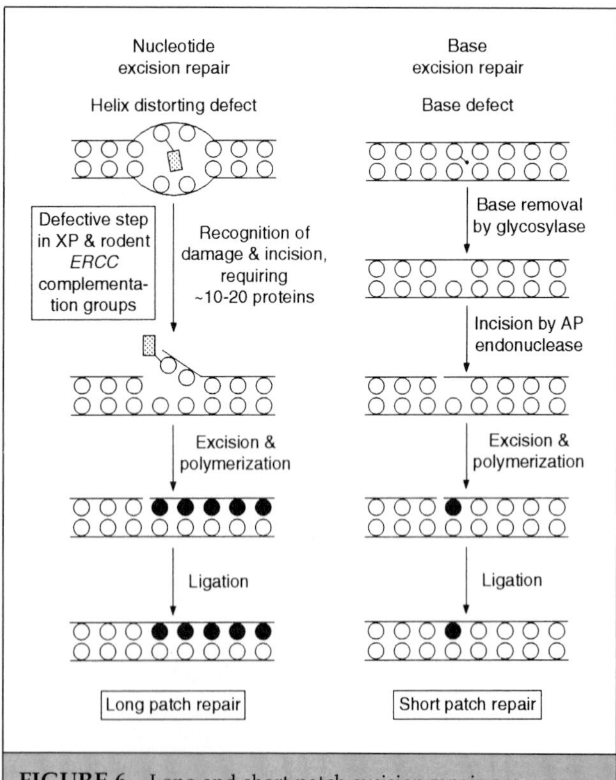

FIGURE 6 Long and short patch excision repair processes.

The basic processes of excision repair, the primary repair mechanisms for chemical damage, are shown in Fig. 6. The enzyme complex responsible for excision repair of bulky adducts consists of several proteins. Some are 3′ and 5′ endonucleases that cleave the DNA at either side of damage and an exonuclease that cuts out the damaged region (approximately 30 nucleotides in length), including nucleotides to either side. The correct bases are replaced by a DNA polymerase using editing functions to ensure the correct bases are incorporated into the repair patch. DNA ligase seals the repair patch. There are two general processes of nucleotide excision repair. One type is called global genomic repair (GGR), which removes lesions throughout the genome. A second type, called transcription coupled repair (TCR), is characterized by excision repair occurring in functionally expressed genes and only on the transcribed DNA strand. GGR and TCR differ in capacity across mammalian species.

Occasionally, even in error-free repair, incorrect bases are incorporated by the polymerase, resulting in mismatched bases that do not properly hydrogen-bond. A second system, called mismatch repair, recognizes non-hydrogen-bonding base pairs, and one segment of the DNA duplex is excised and filled by the polymerase. This is a "second chance" repair process to improve the accuracy of the process.

Repair of mutational damage has been shown to be inducible by low-level exposures to DNA-damaging agents. Inducibility of repair processes above the constitutive levels will increase the magnitude of expo-

TABLE 5 DNA Repair Generalizations

DNA repair is tissue and species specific (e.g., human capacity approximately 10-fold greater than mouse).
DNA repair is increased in genes involved in transcription (e.g., chromosome loops).
DNA adducts are repaired with different efficiencies (e.g., bulk > small).
Effects of DNA repair are tied closely to cell stringency and apoptosis.

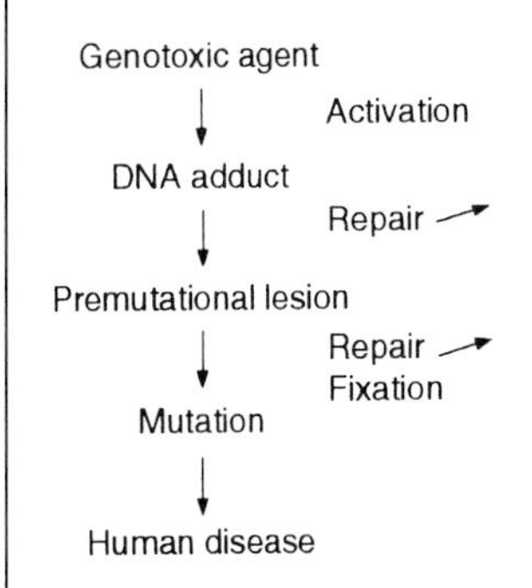

FIGURE 7 The hypothetical process from exposure to genotoxin to the induction of genetic disease in humans. Repair processes can eliminate the formation of mutations that produce disease.

sure required to exceed the intrinsic capacity, producing a "threshold" for mutation, and produce a protective effort for subsequent exposures. Theoretical assumptions and data from studies of repair support the belief that at background or low exposure levels an error-free removal of alkyl groups from DNA can be virtually 100% effective. Thus, one observes survival shoulders and nonlinear kinetics for mutation induction in repair-proficient cells and the loss of apparent "no effect" regions in repair-deficient cells.

Because of the influence that species- and cell-specific genetic backgrounds have on repair capacity, an appreciation of the variability of DNA repair in somatic and germ cells of humans, as well as in the animal models used in assessing genetic risk, is essential. Several general characteristics of mammalian DNA repair are summarized in Table 5.

RELATIONSHIP OF GENOTOXIC DAMAGE TO TOXICITY

DNA damage in somatic cells has been implicated in several different manifestations of toxicity such as:

- Oncogenesis—both inherited and carcinogen-induced forms.
- Teratogenesis—somatic mutations in differentiating cell populations.
- Sterility or semisterility—inactivation of spermatogenesis and/or chromosome translocations.
- Atherosclerosis—somatic mutation in cells lining blood vessels.
- Aging—cumulative mutation in somatic tissues.

Inherited germ-cell mutations are associated with a wide range of human diseases and disorders and are transmitted by reproduction from one generation to the next. Human disease and death records indicate that the mutational basis for this genetic disease burden in humans is the consequence of mutations and chromosomal effects affecting approximately 5% of all newborns. Environmental mutagens contribute an as yet unknown addition to this rate. Figure 7 illustrates the presumed pathway leading from exposure to induced genetic diseases, ranging from new cases of dominant and recessive syndromes to initiation of cancer or congenital anomalies.

Genotoxicants and Carcinogenesis

In the early 1970s, Bruce Ames introduced a microbial assay detecting reverse mutation combined with an *in vitro* metabolic activation system. This technique appeared to offer a rapid inexpensive solution to the identification of chemical carcinogens. The Ames test, as it became known worldwide, was the forerunner of a broad array of submammalian and mammalian cell assays developed as screens for mammalian carcinogens. The rationale for the use of these methods was based on investigations indicating that properties associated with the transformed (malignant) cell phenotype were encoded in the DNA. Studies conducted in the late 1970s demonstrated that DNA isolated from transformed mouse cells could be purified of other contaminants, cut into discrete fragments by bacterial restriction enzymes, and transfected into "normal" cells, resulting in the conversion of "normal" cells to a malignant-appearing phenotype. Investigators conducting these experiments ultimately identified a series of genes in the restriction fragments (proto-oncogenes) responsible for transforming the cells. Proto-oncogens are highly conserved genes found in most eukaryotic organisms and some, such as the *ras*, *myc*, and *neu* genes, are known to be activated to oncogenes by base-pair substitution mutations or chromosome aberrations. Additional loci have been discovered that code for tumor-suppressor molecules (e.g., p53 gene and retinoblastoma gene). The suppressor molecules, which prevent cell proliferation, become inactive following mutation in the genes coding for them. Consequently, it is logical to expect that screens for genotoxic agents would be an effective method of detecting carcinogenic agents. The initial focus of the use of genetic toxicology in carcinogen detection was to correlate the results of specific genotoxicity tests (or batteries of tests) with responses of chemicals classified as carcinogens on the basis of long-term tests using mice or rats. Animal cancer classifications are typically consensus responses derived from multiple tests employing at least two rodent species. Concordance between rodent carcinogenicity and results in the Ames test ranged from 90 to 95% in early validation studies conducted during the late 1970s. By 1984, however, the concordance had dropped to just over 60%. These data raised questions about the importance of mutation in the cancer process in rodents.

Two explanations for the reduction in concordance between genotoxcity tests and rodent cancer have been proposed:

- Insufficient or inappropriate metabolic capacities in the *in vitro* models.
- The role of induced cell proliferation as a "nongenotoxic" mechanism for tumor induction.

However, the factor that had the most influence was the selection of chemicals used in the comparisons. Studies, in the early to mid-1970s showing high concordance employed test chemicals clustered in the group of electrophilic carcinogens, which were often multispecies (mouse and rat) carcinogens. Reports of lower concordance employed groups of chemicals not selected for electrophilic properties, with a better balance of carcinogens and noncarcinogens, and with high proportion of nongenotoxic carcinogens that were less likely to be multispecies carcinogens.

A consequence of the *in vivo–in vitro* concordance analyses has been the identification of an ancillary role for genotoxicity tests. The new role involves using genotoxicity to select the most appropriate risk-assessment model for extrapolation of rodent data to humans. Rodent *in vivo* carcinogens producing positive effects in multiple genetic tests are considered genotoxic, in contrast to agents causing carcinogenesis *in vivo* with predominantly negative results in genetic test batteries. This classification scheme of genotoxic and nongenotoxic carcinogens is used to explain the mechanisms of tumor initiation and as an aid in the selection of the most appropriate data extrapolation model for cancer risk assessment. The risk to mammals from genotoxic carcinogens would be assessed using a no-threshold linear risk-analysis model. Nongenotoxic carcinogenic agents might be subjected to a threshold analysis. While conceptually this scheme appears reasonable, a better understanding of carcinogenic processes is necessary to support a broad application of the concept to risk assessment. The use of genetic tests as part of an assessment for carcinogenic potential can be justified by mechanistic considerations but not from the results of correlation studies because the methods used to define the carcinogenic and mutagenic activities of chemicals are incompatible with achieving high concordance.

Effects of Mutagen on the Human Gene Pool

Induction of genetic damage in the germ-cell lines of plant and animal species has the potential of creating serious adverse consequences for the health and survival of those organisms. In humans, genetic damage is a cause of hereditary diseases, cancer, congenital anomalies, and even reduced life expectancy.

The genes needed to produce the current human population were acquired from the generations of previous gene pools. The gene pool is the sum total of genes, at a given point in time in the reproductively active population of a species, that are available for transmission to the next generation. Deleterious genes are present in the gene pool at a set frequency, as evidenced by predictable rates of recurring genetic diseases in the human species. The origin of this genetic burden (genetic load) is not known, but it contributes significantly to human health care costs. The genetic load carried in the human gene pool consists of the alteration frequencies shown in Table 6.

The majority of the alterations comprising the human genetic load is inherited, but in each generation

TABLE 6 Types of DNA Damage Contributing to the Human Genetic Load

Type of genetic damage	Rate (per thousand newborn)
Chromosome abnormalities	6.7
Autosomal mutations	5.0
Sex-linked mutations	1.5
Polygenic syndromes (congenital abnormalities)	35.0
Total	48.2 (~5%)

a small number of new mutations arise from spontaneous mechanisms and from unavoidable environmental exposures to radiation, fossil fuel combustion products, mycotoxins, and other ubiquitous genotoxicants.

Genetic disease in humans appears to be produced by the same classes of mutations identified in animal models: (a) chromosome abnormalities resulting in stable changes in chromosome number or structure, (b) dominant gene mutations in which only a single mutant allele (of the normal gene pair) is required to produce the disease, (c) recessive gene mutations in which both alleles of the pair must be mutant for expression of the trait, or (d) polygenic damage in which the mutant phenotype is determined by the interaction of several genes. Based on data from human genetics and experimental models in mice, the existence of human mutagens can be hypothesized but no agents have been proven to increase the heritable mutational load in humans. Because of technical limitations associated the logistics of identifying appropriate exposed populations and reliable mutant genotype detection in first generation offspring, it is virtually impossible to conduct human epidemiology studies for the purpose of identifying human mutagens. As a consequence, genetic toxicology's role in safety assessment has historically been limited to chemical screening and conducting *in vivo* tests for hazard identification.

Intrinsic Differences Affecting Susceptibility to Genotoxic Effects

Unlike the animals used as experimental models in toxicology testing, the human population is heterogeneous and consists of subpopulations with a considerable range of susceptibilities to chemical-induced effects. Parameters such as metabolic variability, DNA-repair capacity, and genetic predisposition can influence the severity of a given exposure to a known genotoxic agent.

As stated earlier, DNA repair in all organisms is controlled by a complex genetic system of structural and regulatory genes, and little is known about the basis of human variability; however, human mutations resulting in diseases such as xeroderm pigmentosum (XP) provide some insight. Diseases such as XP are the result of mutations in genes that are part of the human DNA repair complex. Individuals with XP lack one of the enzyme functions of the excision repair process and often experience high levels of intrinsic DNA damage and cancer. Cancer susceptibility among XP genotypes is believed to be a consequence of the unrepaired genetic damage, which can be as much as 100 times greater than non-XP individuals. Other human syndromes associated with reduced repair capacity (e.g., ataxia telangiectasia, Blooms syndrome, and Fanconi's anemia) are inherited traits that may also exhibit increased cancer risk. Thus, the wide range of variability in such important components of genotoxicity as DNA-repair capacity leads to a conclusion that estimates of hazard to genotoxic chemicals based on animal data are likely to have large margins of error.

GENETIC TOXICOLOGY TESTING STRATEGIES AND DATA EVALUATION

Genetic toxicology assessments seldom consist of a single assay. Due to the multiplicity of mechanisms involved in mutation induction, most use a battery of several tests to determine the genotoxic properties of an agent. Test batteries may consist of screening tests, hazard assessment tests, or both. It is important at the outset of testing to carefully define the objectives desired in a testing program. Prescreening to prioritize agents for further testing will require different types of tests than would be used to quantify somatic-cell hazard to humans.

After conducting the tests, the more complex task is that of interpreting the results generated from the test battery. A compound may be defined as genotoxic using the criterion that it is "an agent that produces a positive response (e.g., mutation, unscheduled DNA synthesis (UDS), or chromosome breakage) in a bioassay measuring any genetic endpoint." Although this definition considers virtually all forms of damage to DNA to define an agent as genotoxic, "genotoxicity" should not be interpreted a priori as an indication of hazard or risk. The label "genotoxic" is only a convenient method of classifying all chemicals, into groups called genotoxic or nongenotoxic according to their DNA reactivity. Additional information beyond this initial classification is necessary to address concerns of genetic hazard to somatic or germ cells. Thus, *in vitro* tests or test batteries are used to either prescreen for potential biological activity or to identify genetic hazards, but human risk can only be developed with appropriate animal-screening tests and/or epidemiology studies.

Test results are interpreted on both an individual-test basis (i.e., positive or negative in the specific assay) and on a test-battery basis. Most decisions made for regulatory purposes are based on the response profile from a battery of tests specified by regulations or guidelines. The international scientific community has proposed a number of genetic test batteries for the evaluation of new chemicals, pesticides, food additives, and pharmaceutical products.

CONSIDERATIONS FOR ASSAY SELECTION

Regulatory Standards

Conventional study designs for routine genetic toxicology assays have been published by the EPA, Organization for Economic Co-operation and Development (OECD), Canadian Health and Welfare, and European Community. Most test batteries include at minimum the Ames test, a test for *in vitro* cytogenetic analysis, and, usually, an *in vivo* test for cytogenetic damage. Other tests may be included to expand the profile on the agent if there were positive results or if human exposure was anticipated to be very high. It is also possible to add tests that may be particularly informative for specific chemical classes.

A standard core battery of tests for pharmaceuticals has been proposed under the International Committe for Harmonization (ICH) processes. This battery usually consists of the Ames test, the mouse micronucleus test, and either the mouse lymphoma test (with colony sizing) or an *in vitro* test for chromosome aberrations. On rare occasions where an additional *in vivo* study is requested, a rat test for DNA repair (UDS) may be conducted.

Development of a standard core test battery of the type proposed by ICH has raised a number of issues regarding which genotoxic endpoints are relevant to hazard assessment and which tests also should be conducted. The two tests agreeable to all participants in the harmonization process were the Ames test for gene mutation and the *in vivo* micronucleus for chromosome breakage. The use of *in vitro* tests for chromosome analysis and gene mutation were more controversial. While the proposed core battery has not been given final approval by the ICH committee, there was agreement that the mouse lymphoma assay could serve as an *in vitro* measure of gene mutation and chromosome aberrations, since induction of mutation at the target gene (thymidine kinase) could be induced by either base-pair substitution mutation or chromosome deletions.

Description of Core Battery Test Methods

The Ames test uses several histidine-requiring mutants of the bacteria *Salmonella typhimurium* and one mutant strain of *Escherichia coli*. None of the mutant strains will form colonies on culture medium not supplemented with histidine (in the case the *Salmonella*) or tryptophan (in the case of the *E. coli*). Each mutant strain carries a mutation with a different altered nucleotide sequence that can undergo back mutation (reversion) by spontaneous or induced reversion of the altered nucleotides. Use of multiple strains ensures that a broad range of nucleotides will be available for chemical interactions. To perform the assay, approximately 10^8 cells of a particular mutant strain are added to tubes containing warm agar and a specified amount of the test agent. Contents from half of the tubes are then poured onto individual minimal agar plates that will only support the growth of revertant (mutant) cells. A suspension of rat liver microsomes plus P450 cofactors (S9 mix metabolic activation) is added to each of the remaining tubes before pouring the contents onto minimal agar plates. Following a 3-day incubation period at 37°C, the number of colonies growing on each plate in the control groups (positive and vehicle) and the treated groups are counted. If the test agent, or a metabolite, is mutagenic, there will be an increase in the number of revertant (histidine-independent) colonies on the treatment plates. The Ames test measures base-pair substitution and frameshift mutations.

The Mouse Lymphoma test is a second test measuring gene mutation. This test employs cells from a continuous culture of mouse lymphoma cells called L5178Y. The cells are heterozygous for the thymidine kinase (TK+/−) gene, which is involved in nucleotide transport. The heterozygous TK+/− cells have a functional kinase, which will transport exogenous nucleotides into the cells to synthesize DNA. If a toxic nucleotide analog (e.g., 6-thioguanine or trifluorothymidine) is added to the medium, the analog is transported into the cells, producing cell death. When the mutant allele in the heterozygous state undergoes spontaneous or induced mutation to yield a homozygous mutant cell (TK−/−) it will be resistant to toxic analogs and will grow, forming a colony of resistant cells. In the mouse lymphoma assay, TK+/− cells are incubated in culture medium with escalating concentrations of the test agent, both with and without the hepatic microsome preparation (S9 mix), for several hours, followed by an expression period of several days. After incubation in expression medium, about 10^6 cells are placed in soft agar containing trifluorothymidine and incubated at 37°C for several days. Colonies are counted in the control (positive and vehicle) plates and in the treatment plates. If the test agent is a mutagen, the number of mutant colonies will be higher in the treatment plates. Because this is a eukaryotic organism containing chromosomes, TK+/− cells can undergo mutation to TK−/− cells through base-pair substitution or frameshift mutations, as well as through chromosome damage (i.e., deletions or translocations). It has been hypothesized that small mutant colonies are the result of chromosome damage and large mutant colonies the result of base-pair changes. Therefore, colony sizing may be an important part of a mouse lymphoma protocol. Recently a microwell version of this assay has been developed and is used interchangeably with the soft-agar plate method.

Chromosome damage *in vivo* is measured in the mouse or rat. Hemopoetic cells (either bone marrow or circulating lymphocytes) can be used to look for micronuclei. Micronuclei are chromosome remnants produced during cell division in cells with broken chromosomes. If a chromosome fragment is not connected to the spindle apparatus during mitosis, it may remain behind in one daughter cell. In bone-marrow cells, which are precursors to red blood cells, the normal nucleus is lost and micronuclei are the only DNA-staining body in the cells. In lymphocytes, the micronuclei are small DNA-staining bodies in the cytoplasm. Micronuclei form spontaneously at about 1 per 1000 bone marrow cells. If an agent breaks chromosomes (i.e., clastogenic), the number of micronuclei per 1000 cells scored will increase. A typical micronucleus study in mice involves at least three dose levels of test agent and at least two harvest times. A second harvest time is included to detect micronuclei if the normal cell cycle is delayed by the test agent exposure (bone-marrow toxicity). Each dose group usually consists of five male and five female animals. Typically 1000 bone marrow cells are scored per animal. The route of administration may vary but should mimic the route of anticipated human exposure.

In vitro chromosome-damage tests are conducted if the mouse lymphoma assay is not used. These tests look for chromosome breakage and rearrangements in cells from continuous lines, such as CHO (chinese hamster ovary) or V79 cells. Cultured human lymphocytes may also be used in place of the continuous cell lines. These tests are conducted in tissue culture medium both with and without the hepatic microsome preparation (S9 mix). Cells are arrested in metaphase and placed on slides. The cells are stained for DNA, and the frequency of chromosome breaks, gaps, and rearrangements in the treated and control cells are scored.

Some of the issues raised about how tests should be conducted have not been resolved. Decisions on the proper methods for high-dose selection, automatic repetition of *in vitro* tests, use of both male and female animals for the micronucleus assay, and verification of target tissue exposure for *in vivo* tests are still under active review.

Table 7 summarizes some of the limitations of test batteries such as the ICH core battery. The specific comments made for each test would be applicable to its use in other batteries as well. In fact, there is probably no ideal battery for all applications. Validation data developed by the National Institute for Environmental Health Sciences (NIEHS) in which *in vitro* methods were assessed for carcinogen identification suggests that the Ames test, used alone, provides the most reliable prediction of rodent carcinogenicity.

Identification of Genetic Hazard

Most commercially available pharmaceutical products, consumer products, industrial chemicals, and food substances have been subjected to genetic screening. Consequently, the amount of published genetic toxicology data is enormous and is probably greater than that for any other area of safety assessment. A major portion of the existing database in genetic toxicology consists of results from submammalian and mammalian *in vitro* tests. Unfortunately, most of those data are of little value in evaluating human hazard or

TABLE 7 Problems Encountered with Conventional Testing Batteries

All lesions found in humans are not detected by assays
- Aneuploidy
- DNA methylation
- Transposons

Production of genetic damage in humans may involve divergent mechanisms not found in current assays
- Repeat sequences
- Homozygosity
- Splice site mutations (not possible in prokaryotes)

Locus specificity may affect detection of some chemicals
- Hot spots (ras, p53 codons) important in humans will be absent

Repair mechanisms may differ
- O^6 Demethylase lower in some cell lines than in primary human tissues
- Coding vs noncoding sequences are repaired differently

In vitro to *in vivo* extrapolation
- *In vitro* dose setting at concentrations that are not achievable *in vivo*
- Cell cycle stringency affects differences between *in vivo* and *in vitro* conditions unknown
- Phase I and II metabolism absent *in vitro*

risk following exposure to the agents tested. *In vivo* screening tests are required to establish hazard and to estimate risk to somatic- or germ-cell populations. *In vivo* screening tests can be applied alone or as a follow-up to analogous *in vitro* tests. Because of cost and issues of sensitivity, most *in vivo* tests are conducted to confirm positive *in vitro* prescreening test results. The general interpretation applied to *in vivo* results when following *in vitro* tests is that *in vivo* results should take precedence over *in vitro* results if the design of the *in vivo* study is adequate to detect weak responses, and evidence can be provided that the test article or its metabolites have access to the target tissue. Positive *in vivo* responses confirming *in vitro* data should be viewed as adequate evidence for genetic hazard. Quantitative data from somatic- or germ-cell studies conducted in animal models may then be used to estimate the level of risk.

DATA ANALYSIS AND INTERPRETATION

Data Analysis Issues

Reliance on test batteries places a unique burden on the genetic toxicologist when it is time to evaluate the data. Testing batteries range from a relatively small number of tests, such as the proposed ICH battery of three tests, to the Environmental Protection Agency's Federal Insecticide Fungicide Rodenticide Act (FIFRA) testing scheme, which may require five or more tests. It is unusual to obtain totally uniform negative or positive response profiles from these batteries. More common are data showing isolated positive responses. Such isolated positives may be true indicators of test-specific effects or they may be spurious responses generated as a consequence of technical errors or study-design deficiencies. Unfortunately, it is not always easy to distinguish between an isolated true positive genetic effect and a spurious positive.

Many investigations have reviewed the occurrence of nonreproducible positive effects, especially in *in vitro* test methods. The conclusions from these investigations are that most test methods have intrinsic rates of sporadic nonreproducible positive effects. The following are some of the causes for such effects.

1. **Toxicity.** Setting appropriate dose levels for genetic toxicity tests has been controversial and good rules have not yet been developed for all tests. Using the concept of setting the high dose based on a maximum-tolerated concentration, investigators run the risk of producing cytotoxic effects in the target organisms, which may indirectly lead to results that appear to be DNA reactive. The most common occurrence of this situation is with *in vitro* chromosome-aberration assays. If cell toxicity results in pleotropic effects including the destruction of chromosomal integrity, it will be visible as damage in cells that attempt to complete mitosis. These spurious effects are not the consequence of DNA-specific reactivity but are more typically reflect high-dose-only responses.

2. **Treatment condition dependent.** Cells in culture are affected by environmental conditions such as temperature, pH, osmolality, and other factors that will result in cellular stress. For example, several reports have demonstrated that low pH and high osmotic conditions (from NaCl and other ionic components of media or control vehicles) can produce chromosome aberrations, SCEs, gene mutation, and morphological cell transformation *in vitro*. Such effects are seldom encountered *in vivo* due to homeostatic control mechanisms. Consequently, regulation of environmental conditions during *in vitro* exposures is important and should be monitored, recorded, and reported with each study.

3. **Inappropriate sample size.** Study designs that fail to provide adequate sample sizes per dose group for scoring events, such as micronuclei, cell transformation, SCEs, nuclear-grain counts, could produce a single positive effect that cannot be reproduced. Proper statistical design input is critical to assay reproducibility.

4. **Assay evaluation rules.** Some tests, especially microbial plate assays such as the Ames test, rely on evaluation rules rather than on statistical analysis to declare the results positive or negative. As a consequence, marginal effects in treated groups may be classified as negative in one trial and positive in a repeat trial, due to slight shifts in the response within a treatment group or in the spontaneous background. Because this variation exists, some regulatory agencies have built automatic independent repeat trials into their guideline requirements.

Unless it is possible to identify a specific cause for isolated positive responses, the more conservative approach is to evaluate the body of positive and negative data using a weight-of-evidence approach. This approach can be performed qualitatively by conducting a sufficient number of tests to see a clear pattern of either positive or negative responses. With a relatively large body of data, isolated positive effects from *in vitro* tests may be considered spurious and the agent declared nongenotoxic. It is difficult to apply the same weight-of-evidence approach if the isolated positive response is from a well-conducted *in vivo* study. *In vivo* responses should be evaluated as indicators of hazard, and additional pharmacology and toxicokinetic data should be included in the assessment.

Interpretation Issues

There are two types of interpretation issues. The first involves the appropriateness of the test models used in a battery, and the second is the relevance of the findings in the genetic test to potential adverse effects in exposed humans.

Examples of the first issue are the knowledge that (a) some cells lines such as the CHO lines used in many *in vitro* tests have reduced repair capacity (e.g., lower endogenous levels of O^6-demethylase) compared to normal human cells and may therefore be unusually susceptible to specific genotoxins, and (b) most of the cell lines used to measure chromosome aberrations (e.g., CHO, V79, and CHL [chinese hamster lung]) exhibit high degrees of intrinsic chromosome instability and may not be reliable models for measuring induced aberrations. Substitution of primary cell cultures (e.g., lymphocytes) in place of cell lines in these tests produces more reliable data. Other concerns have been raised about mechanistic similarities between morphological cell transformation *in vitro* in C3H 10T1/2 cells or Syrian hamster embryo cells (SHE assay) and true cell transformation leading to tumor induction in mammals. These assays have been adopted primarily on the basis of concordance studies and not on mechanistic relevance.

The second issue is the one of extrapolation from short-term genetic assays to estimates of hazard or risk in human populations exposed to the test agents. Without an ability to conduct epidemiology studies to verify extrapolation, a number of assumptions are required to make estimates of hazard or risk. The following is a short list of variables that are critical to any extrapolation process but are often not considered in developing genetic toxicology data.

1. *Metabolic variability between the test organism and the organism of concern.* In order for genetic toxicology data to be used in regulatory toxicology decisions of hazard or risk, it will become necessary to integrate the test results with information about the *in vivo* fate of the chemical and its pharmacology.

2. Dose rate affects the impact of exposure to genotoxins. In general, a total individual daily dose administered in intermittent exposures at relatively low levels will have an entirely different (i.e., lower) effect on the organism than the same total daily dose administered by a single acute bolus administration. Similar problems exist for route of exposure. Bioavailability can vary significantly with exposure route.

3. DNA repair varies across tissues within a species as well as across species. Global genomic repair capacities in mice have been estimated to be a factor of 10 lower than those in humans. Such differences should be considered when making extrapolations from animal tests to humans.

Whether the endpoint of concern is mutation in proto-oncogenes or tumor suppressor genes in somatic tissues or gene mutation in spermatogonia, the variability in factors listed here must be considered in reaching conclusions of genotoxic hazard and risk.

GENETIC RISK ASSESSMENTS

Assessing human risk to mutagenic substances represents a formidable task. There is so far no conclusive proof of showing chemical-induced mutation in human germ cells; however, mutagens can alter rodent germ cells and quantitative estimates of induced mutation rates per gene locus or the dose required to double a specific mutation rate have to be calculated from results of the *in vivo*-specific-locus or heritable-translocation assays. These estimates may be of limited value in calculating human risk or in setting safe exposure levels because they are based on male gametes and, in the case of specific-locus assay, generally on premeiotic stem cells (spermatogonia). The data do not reflect the risk to later cell stages in spermatogenesis or in female germ cells. Estimates of mutation in postmeiotic sperm and from female gametes will become available; but even so, other important biological variables would interfere with reliable risk estimates and extrapolation between species.

While differences in DNA-repair capacities from species to species are potentially the most confounding parameter when determining germ-cell damage, other factors such as similarities or differences in endocrine profiles, gene structure, mutation specificity, mutation expression, and disease homology between rodents and humans will make extrapolation tenuous. In addition, post-zygotic repair of damaged sperm is a factor that can greatly affect genetic risk.

Exposure assessment is a critical component of risk assessment. Exposure may occur by different routes and duration; however, most *in vivo* mutagenicity studies used in hazard assessment are dosed in bolus by the oral or intraperitoneal routes. Information derived from the physical–chemical properties of the agent, its concentration in environmental matrices, and exposure modeling are important factors that must be included in the development of quantitative risk assessments.

EXTRAPOLATION OF SOMATIC CELL RESPONSES TO GERM CELLS

Several groups have attempted to evaluate *in vitro* and *in vivo* somatic-cell assays to determine those that would most closely predict the germ-cell effects of a mutagenic substance. The differences between these two cell types and their accessibility by chemicals has proven resistant to most approaches. Thus, it is difficult to conclude that nongerm-cell assays are either qualitatively or quantitatively able to predict responses in germ cells.

At present, the only reliable method to define germ-cell risk is to conduct *in vivo* studies that employ male and female germ cells as targets.

In the 1970s, scientists proposed an indirect approach to risk analysis that utilizes the assumption of parallelism in dosimetry and cell mutation to predict germ-cell mutation in exposed humans. The method, referred to as the "parallelogram" approach, makes direct measurements of germ-cell and somatic-cell DNA dosimetry in animals and combines this information with measured germ-cell dosimetry measures to estimate the germ-cell mutation (Fig. 8). If gonadal dosimetry data are available for humans, this approach could be used to calculate germ cell mutation estimates for humans from direct measurement of blood levels of the test agent and somatic cell mutation rates (i.e., mutation in peripheral lymphocytes). The outcome of this type of analysis would be a calculated estimate of germ-cell mutation rate for humans. Application of the "parallelogram" method for indirect genetic-risk assessment will incorporate a number of assumptions that increase the uncertainty of final assessment.

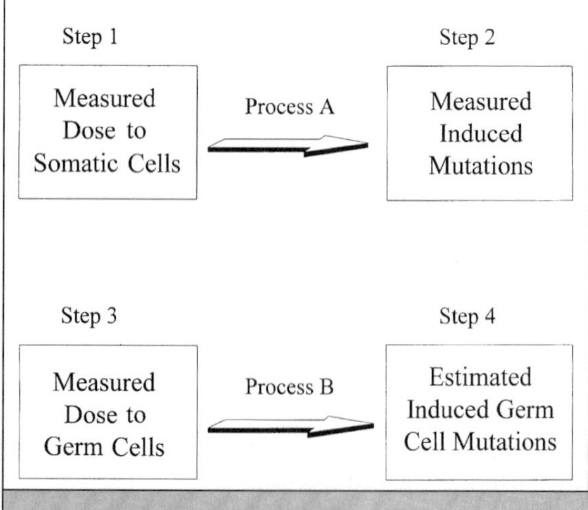

FIGURE 8 Diagrammatic representation of the parallelogram method of estimating germ cell risk using somatic results and target site dosimetry. This method has been used with rodent and human data to develop probable mutation risks.

NEW TECHNOLOGY AND ITS PLACE IN GENETIC TESTING

Current Technology and Its Limitations

By 1980 over 150 different tests for genotoxicity were available and had at least contributed some data to scientific journals. Many of the tests were redundant, but each method had a champion who attempted to define the unique value of the particular technique or target organism. The following decade saw extensive efforts to validate and evaluate the best test or set of tests for the purposes of detecting relevant genotoxins (carcinogens and/or germ-cell mutagens). In the process several valuable lessons have been learned.

1. Many test methods are very sensitive and respond positively to rodent carcinogens; however, the tests do not discriminate agents based on DNA reactivity and they also respond to agents that are not carcinogenic or mutagenic. Examples of such tests are *in vitro* SCE measures, and alkaline elution and other measures of DNA single- and double-strand breakage.
2. Several test methods worked extremely well in the laboratory of the "inventor" but did not reliably transfer to other testing laboratories. Notable among those methods are the *in vitro* morphological cell transformation assays.
3. The array of mechanisms detected by the available tests may not include mechanisms that are prevalent in mammalian systems. Examples of such deficiencies are tests that reliably measure aneuploidy, induction of random repeat errors, transpositions, or effects of DNA methylation.
4. There is a general lack of feasible methods to assess quantitative genetic hazard or risk using the combination of *in vitro* and *in vivo* exposure conditions encountered in most test batteries. Explaining why one test method supersedes another for hazard identification is a major issue in the interpretation of test battery data.

Several actions were taken in an attempt to resolve the issues listed here. The most dramatic was a reduction in test methods requested by regulatory agencies. Genetic toxicology was simplified for the purposes of regulatory toxicology safety testing. Most agencies expect to see a limited test battery consisting of tests for gene mutation and chromosome aberrations. The ICH core battery of tests is the best example of this approach, and this battery is expected to become the international standard for most testing requirements. Other tests measuring mechanisms such as *in vitro* cell transformation, DNA breakage and repair, mitotic recombination, and DNA-adduct formation are now used in basic research or as supplemental methods to support or explain findings from core battery results. Many tests that were found to have little relevance to genotoxic hazard or were difficult to replicate in different laboratories are seldom used in regulatory toxicology screening.

Weight-of-evidence methods have been developed to evaluate complex response patterns from test batteries. Some of the methods, such as the mutagenic activity profiles created by the International Commission for the Protection against Environmental Mutagen and Carcinogens (ICPEMC), have been validated with large data sets and encoded into computer software.

The technical deficiencies indicated in the list have not been resolved. Thus if one uses the International Committee for Harmonization core battery as an example of the methods employed to screen environmental agents and/or new products for their genotoxic activity in exposed humans, the potential limitations are significant. The tests included in the battery do not provide a full coverage of mechanisms known to occur in higher mammals and can potentially fail to detect agents that may be relevant to elements of the human genome. In addition, the battery has no method that detects gene mutation *in vivo*. This is a serious deficiency when attempting to confirm or extrapolate the results from the Ames test to organisms with eukaryotic DNA and chromosome structure.

Proposed New Methods for Genetic Testing

Table 8 lists several methods or techniques that have become widely available during the past 5 years and appear to be directly applicable to gaps identified in the existing methods used in genetic toxicology.

Specific tests have been developed as a consequence of the technology. These new methods are currently being evaluated and validated as either replacements or additions to the current test batteries.

Transgenic Models for Mutation Detection

Transgenic animals for mutation detection were developed in 1990 using shuttle vector technology. The two models that are commercially available are compared in Table 9. In both models, a gene from the

TABLE 8 Technologies Leading to the Development of New Genetic Testing Methods

Method	Properties	*In vivo* tests
Polymerase chain reaction (PCR)	Specific gene amplification that permits isolation, amplification, and analysis of specific endogenous mammalian genes	Gene mutation at the HGPRT gene in mice and rats
Shuttle vectors	Engineer specific DNA sequences into a rescuable vector that can integrate into the host organism's genomic DNA	Transgenic mice and rat models for gene mutation
DNA gel electrophoresis	Use of various types of gels to EPA-rate DNA on the basis of size or base composition	COMET assay for DNA strand breakage Gene mutation using single-strand conformated polymorphism
Fluorescent immunochemical straining combined with *in situ* hybridization	Use of fluorescent stains attached to specific nucleotide sequences to identify gene locations	Highly specific chromosome mapping and tests to detect small deletions and rearrangements

TABLE 9 Characteristics of Two Commercially Available Transgenic Model Systems

MutaMouse	Big Blue Mouse
80 copies of the *gt101ac* Z shuttle vector	80 copies of *lac* I reporter gene per diploid genome
40-merconcatemers (head-to-tail) chromosome 3	*lac* I target DNA is 1080 bp in length
lac Z target DNA is 3126bp in length	Nontranscribed target gene
Nontranscribed target gene	Visual selection of mutants
Positive selection system for mutant identification	Rat model also available

lactose operon of *E. coli* was combined with DNA sequences from λ phage to form a recoverable shuttle vector (Fig. 9). The shuttle vector was micro-injected into fertilized mouse ova, which were subsequently placed back into the uteri of pseudo-pregnant dams. Founder animals with integrated shuttle vectors were recovered and used to develop stable homozygous strains of mice (and rats) from which the target *lac* genes can be recovered and analyzed for mutation following *in vivo* exposure.

Studies using transgenic animals are conducted as illustrated in Fig. 10. The transgenic animals can be exposed to the test agent using any route of administration and duration. DNA containing the recoverable shuttle vector can be isolated from virtually any cell type in the treated animal. Table 10 provides examples of the range of data for different tissues. Validation studies with transgenic models have demonstrated that they are reliable and relevant. For example, studies of known rodent carcinogens have demonstrated tissue-specific mutation associated with the target organs where tumors develop. Both transgenic models show very close concordance with the Ames test for known genotoxic carcinogens (>90% and can, therefore, serve as a confirmatory test for the Ames or other *in vitro* gene mutation screens.

There are limitations associated with the transgenic models (e.g., poor detection of chromosome deletions or rearrangements); however, these limitations do not restrict the value of this technology in genetic testing, particularly in combination with other *in vivo* assays, such as the mouse micronucleus test. Other transgenic models are being developed with shuttle vectors that avoid some of the limitations identified in the *lac* gene models.

Gene Amplification Approaches to Mutation Detection

Development of the polymerase chain reaction (PCR) has resulted in the ability to select specific DNA sequences and create millions of copies of them rapidly and inexpensively. PCR technology has had its greatest impact in other areas of biotechnology but has also been used to develop some new methods of mutation analysis. Two such models appear promis-

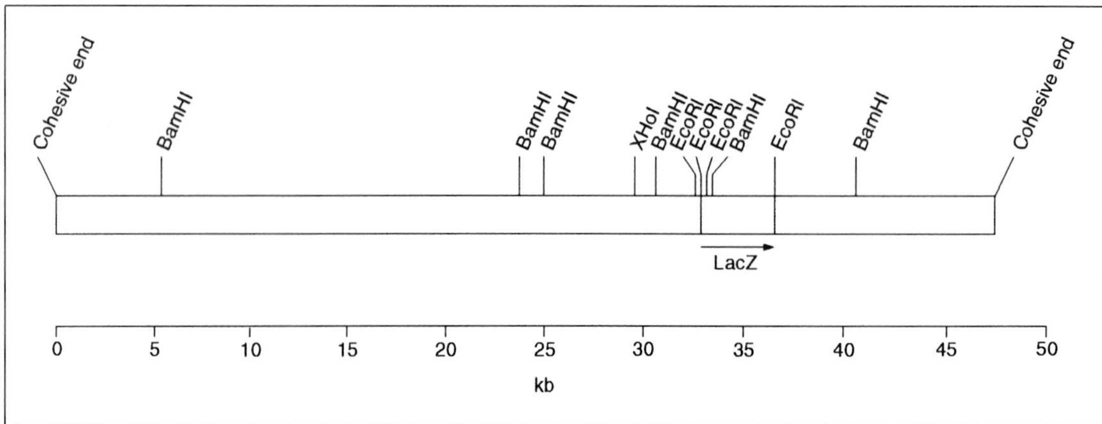

FIGURE 9 The shuttle vector used to produce the MutaMouse transgenic model for mutation detection. The vector consists of the *lac* Z gene from *E. coli* with lambda phage genes on either end. The vector is rescuable from mammalian DNA with lambda packaging extracts.

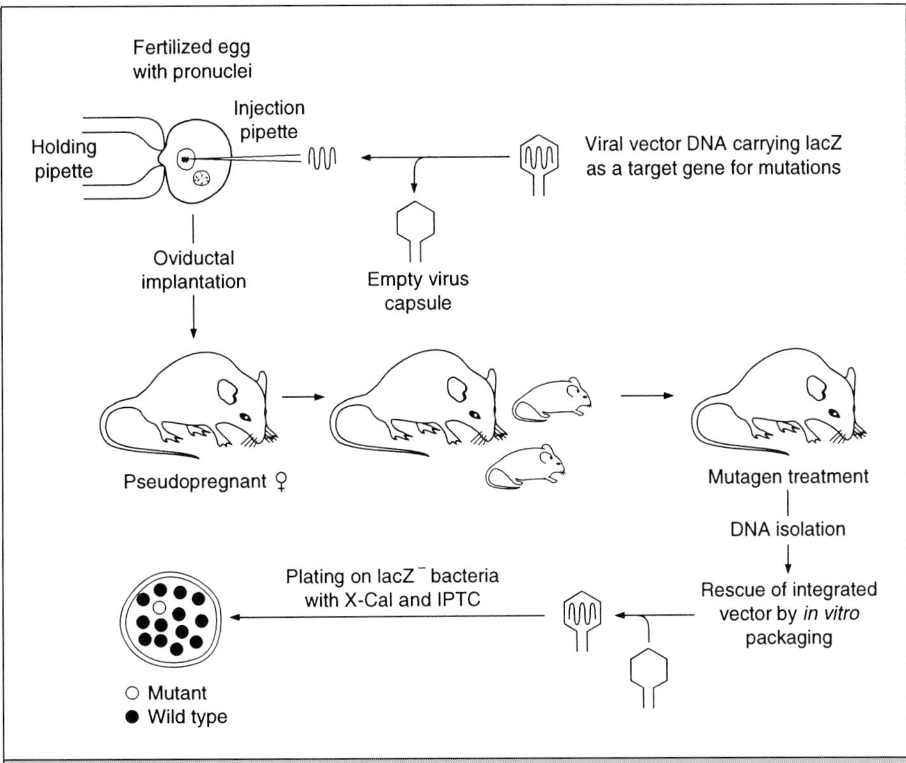

FIGURE 10 Outline of the production of a transgenic mouse through microinjection. The animal containing a rescuable shuttle vector can be used as a model for *in situ* mutation with DNA isolated from cells of any tissue and mutants observed *ex vivo*.

ing as methods to detect mutation *in vivo* and are compared to the transgenic model. The advantages of these methods over transgenic models are that the target DNA sequences are endogenous in origin rather than transplanted from other organisms, the technology can be applied to any mammalian system

TABLE 10 Examples of the Range of Chemicals Tested for Mutation Induction in Transgenic Mice

Agent	Model	Tissue	Response
2-Acetylaminofluorence	*lac* I	Liver	+
O-Anisidine	*lac* I	Bladder	+
Benzo[*a*]pyrene	*lac* I	Lung	+
1,3-Butadiene	*lac* I/*lac* Z	Lung, bone marrow	+
Dimethylnitrosamine	*lac* I/*lac* Z	Liver	+
Ethylene oxide	*lac* I	Lung, spleen	+
Ethylnitrosourea	*lac* I/*lac* Z	Liver, bone marrow	+
Phenobarbital	*lac* I	Liver	−
Urethane	*lac* I	Lung	+
Benzene	*lac* I	Spleen	+
Acetone	*lac* I/*lac* Z	Skin	−
Acrylamide	*lac* Z	Bone marrow	+
Mitomycin C	*lac* Z	Bone marrow	+
Procarbazine	*lac* Z	Bone marrow	+
Heptachlor	*lac* I	Liver	−

TABLE 11 New Methods for Mutation Identification *in Vivo*

Single-strand conformation polymorphism, PCR (SSCP/PCR)
In vivo technique, any organ possible
Nonselective mutant identification
Gradient gel electrophoresis, PCR (GGE/PCR)
In vivo, spleen T-cells
Selective (resistance to 6-thioguanine)
Detects one to several base-pair changes
Can sequence mutants to identify altered site(s)
Trangenic systems
In vivo, any organ possible
Selective system to isolate mutants
Detects one to hundreds of base-pair changes
Can sequence mutants to identify altered site(s)
Special mouse strains required

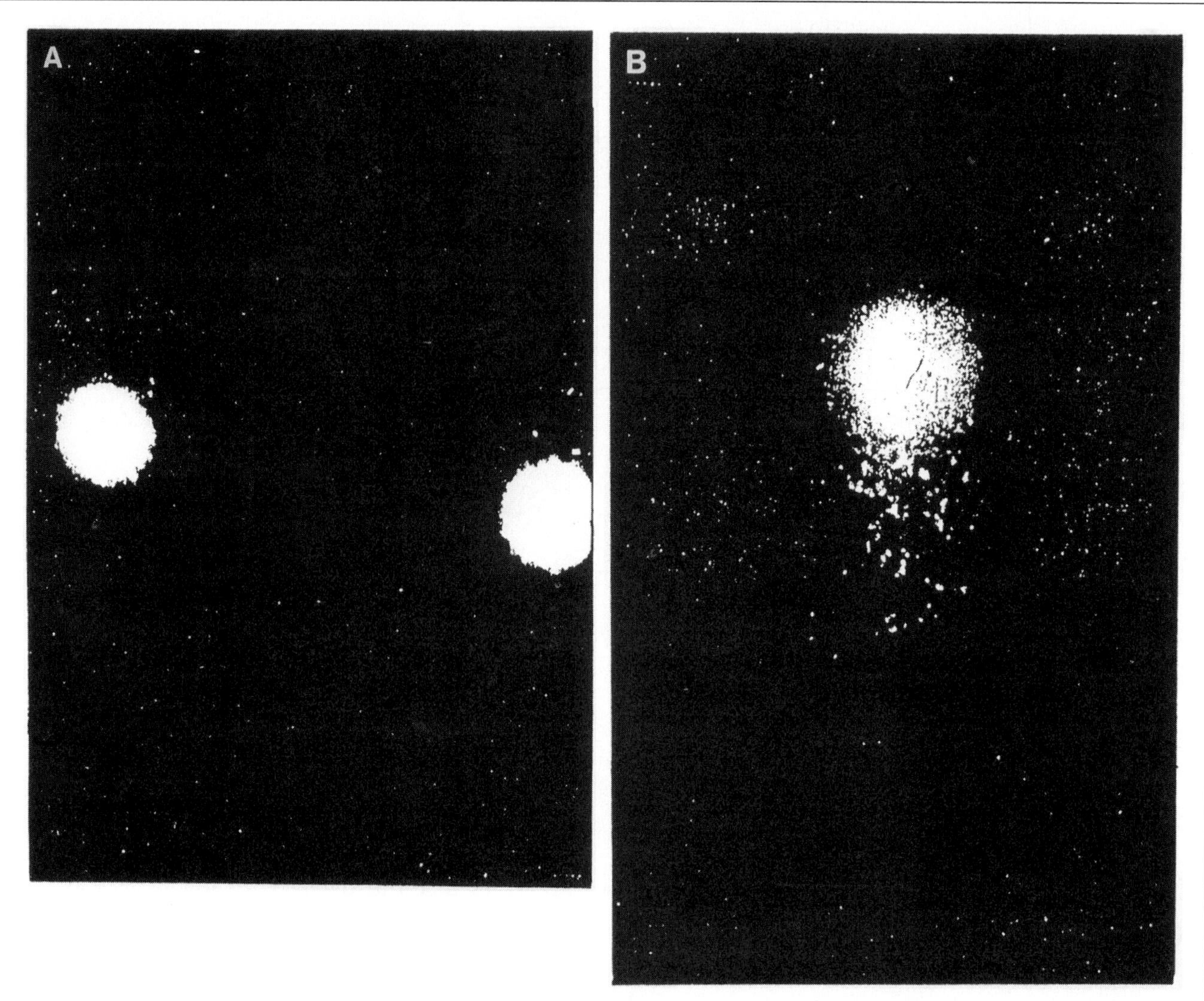

FIGURE 11 COMET assay can be seen as a tail of fragmented DNA. (A) Control cells are stained, but no tail is evident. (B) Moderate DNA damage results in a small tail.

from mouse to primate, and the types of damage detected are relatively unrestricted to specific mechanisms (although DNA deletions are not detected). Table 11 compares the two PCR methods with the transgenic models developed for *in vivo* gene mutation.

Single-Cell Gel Electrophoresis (COMET) Assay

This technique is dependent on the analysis of DNA integrity in single cells. The advantage of this method on approach is that the source of the cells is almost unrestricted. The basis of the test is that if single- or double-strand breaks are induced in DNA *in situ* when cells are isolated, treated to denature nucleic acids, and placed in an electric field, DNA will migrate from the negative to the positive charge at a rate related to the length of the DNA. Fragmented DNA pieces migrate rapidly and, when stained, form a tail on the cells similar to that of a comet (Fig. 11). The COMET assay is a very versatile technique and can be used *in vitro* or *in vivo*.

The use of this method increased dramatically from 1994 through 1996 but has slowed somewhat due to technical problems associated with the sensitivity of the method to stress-induced positive effects occurring during the isolation and fixation steps of the methods. Interpretation of the results from this test might be compromised by cytotoxic effects from normal processes, such as programmed cell death (apoptosis). Extreme care must be taken during these steps of the procedure to eliminate false-positive effects.

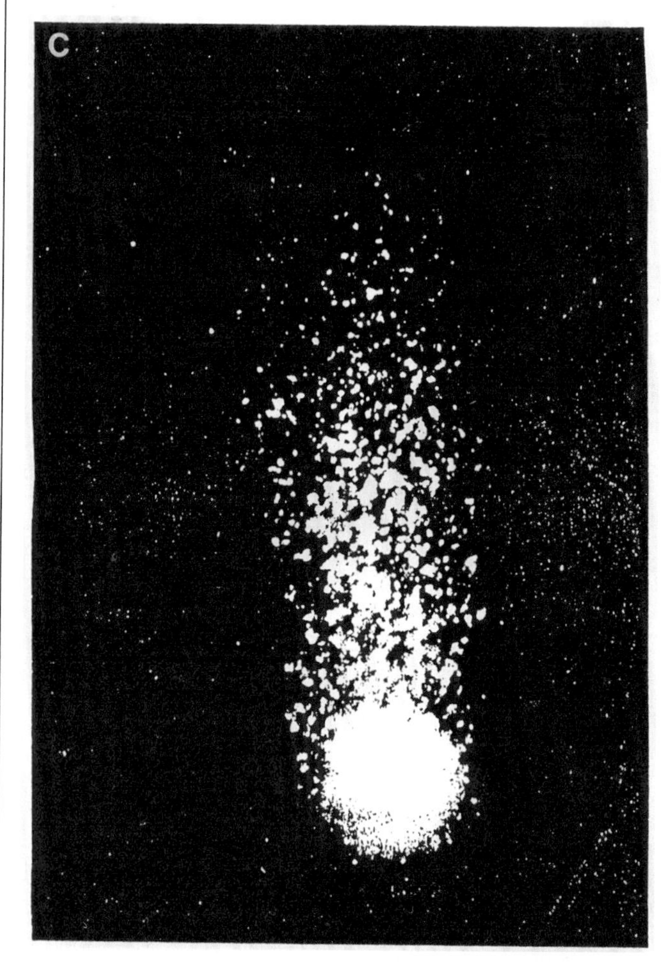

FIGURE 11 (*Continued*) (C) Substantial DNA breakage results in a long tail.

Some of the limitations and advantages of the COMET assay are listed in Table 12.

The introduction of one or more of these *in vivo* methods, or others that are in development, would significantly improve the relevance of test batteries such as the International Committee for Harmonization core battery. *In vivo* data from the mouse micronucleus and, for example, a transgenic-mutation assay conducted using the anticipated route of human exposure, coupled with toxicokinetic data from the site of cell harvest, could provide a realistic set of results upon which quantitative hazard or risk decisions might be made.

TABLE 12 Single Cell Assay Measuring Primary DNA Damage

Advantages
In vivo and *in vitro*
Rapid indication of amount of DNA breakage by length of tail
Nonspecific indicator of genotoxicity
Sensitive
Disadvantages
Complicated by toxicity and programmed cells death (apoptosis)
Possibly too sensitive—stress induced DNA breakage in animals
Conditions may be tissue specific
Not specific for heritable effects

CONCLUSION

Genetic toxicology provides important information about the biological activity of new chemicals planned for introduction into the marketplace and thus their potential appearance in the environment as general environmental agents. The methods used are versatile and can be adapted to most chemical forms (e.g., solids, liquids, and gases) and even extracts and/or mixtures of chemicals. *In vivo* models are available for confirmation of *in vitro* results and to develop information related to genetic hazard potential. New models using PCR or shuttle vectors have improved the ability of the genetic toxicologist to conduct relevant hazard assessments. Risk analysis for the induction of genetic disease is possible using models such as the parallelogram or the ICPEMC model using mouse-heritable-translocation or specific-locus test data.

Bibliography

Ames, B. N., Durston, W. E., and Lee, F. D. (1973). Carcinogens are mutagen: A simple test system combining liver homogenates for activation and bacteria for detection. *Proc. Natl. Acad. Sci. USA* **70,** 2281.

Ames, B. N., McCann, J., and Yamasaki, E. (1975). Methods for detecting carcinogens and mutagen with the Salmonella mammalian microscome mutagenicity test. *Mutat. Res.* **31,** 347–364.

Anderson, M. W., Maronpot, R. R., and Reynolds, S. H. (1988). Role of oncogenes in chemical carcinogenesis: Extrapolation from rodents to humans. *In* "Methods for Detecting DNA Damaging Agents in Humans" (H. Bartsch *et al.*, eds.), pp. 477–485. IARC Scientific Publications No. 89, Lyon.

Ashby, J., and Purchase, I. F. H. (1988). Reflections on the declining ability of the Salmonella assay to detect rodent carcinogens as positive. *Mutat. Res.* **205,** 51–58.

Balajee, A. S., Dominguez, I., Natarajan, A. T. (1995). Construction of Chinese hamster chromosome specific DNA libraries and their use in the analysis of spontaneous chromosome rearrangements indifferent cell lines. *Cytogenet. Cell Genet.* **70,** 95–101.

Barbacid, M. (1987). Mutagen, oncogenes and cancer. *In* "Oncogenes and Growth Factors" (R. A. Bradshaw and S. Prentis, eds.) pp. 90–99. Elsevier, Amsterdam.

Brusick, D. J. (1987a). "Principles of Genetic Toxicology." Plenum Press, New York.

Brusick, D. J. (1987b). Implications of treatment-condition-induced GENOTOXICITY for chemical screening and data interpretation. *Mutat. Res.* **189,** 1–6.

Brusick, D. J. (1989). Role of metabolism in short-term test development. *Environ. Mol. Mutagen.* **14 Suppl. 16,** 60–65.

Brusick, D. J. (1991). A proposed method for assembly and interpretation of short-term test data. *Environ. Health Perspect.* **96,** 101–111.

Burnet, F. M. (1974). "Intrinsic Mutagenesis: A Genetic Approach to Aging." Medical & Technical Publishing, Lancaster, England.

Butterworth, B. (1996). The integrity of the human gene pool. *Environ. and Mol. Mutagen.* **28,** 1–2.

Butterworth, B., Conolly, R., and Morgan, K. (1995). A strategy for establishing mode of action of chemical carcinogens as a guide for approaches to risk assessments. *Cancer Lett.* **93,** 129–146.

Canadian Health and Welfare. (1986). Guidelines on the use of mutagenicity tests in the toxicological evaluation of chemicals. *Environ. Mol. Mutagenesis* **11,** 261–304.

Dolle, M., Martus, H. J., Gossen, J., Boerrigter, M., and Vijg, J. (1996). Evaluation of a plasmid-based transgenic mouse model for detecting *in vivo* mutations. *Mutagenesis* **11,** 111–118.

European Economic Community. (1983). EEC Official Journal of the European Communities, Th Amendment to Directive 67/548/EEC, Annex VII, 15.10.79, and Annex V, EEC Directive 79-831, part B, Toxicological Methods of Annex VIII, Draft, July 1983.

Ehling, U. H. (1988). Quantification of the genetic risk environmental mutagen. *Risk Analysis* **8,** 45–56.

Ehling, U. H., Averbeck, D., Cerutti, P. A., Friedman, J., Greim, H., Kolbye, A. C., Jr., and Mendelsohn, M. L. (1983). Review of the evidence for the presence or absence of thresholds in the induction of genetic effects by genotoxic chemicals. *Mutat. Res.* **123,** 281–341.

EPA Office of Pesticides and Toxic Substances. (1982). Health Effects Test Guidelines. EPA Publication 560/682-001. National Technical Information Service, Springfield, Virginia.

Evans, H. J. (1990). Cytogenetics: overview. *In* "Mutation and the Environment, Part B" (M. L. Mendelsohn and R. J. Albertini, eds.) pp. 301–323. Wiley-Liss, Inc., New York.

Favor, J., Layton, D., Sega, G., Wassom, J., Burkhart, J., Douglas, G., Dearfield, K., and Brusick, D. (1995). Genetic risk extrapolation from animal data to human disease. *Mutation Res.* **330,** 23–34.

Gorelick, N. J. (1995). Overview of mutation assays in transgenic mice for routine testing. *Environ. and Mol. Mutagenesis* **25,** 218–230.

Gossen, J., Deleeuw, W., Tan, C., Zwarthoff, E., Berends, F., Lohman, P., Knock, D., and Viig, J. (1989). Efficient rescue of integrated shuttle vectors from transgenic mice: A model for studying mutations *in vivo*. *Proc. Nat. Acad. Sci. USA* **86,** 7971–7975.

Heflich, R., Mittelstaedt, A., Manjanatha, M., Lyn-Cook, L., and Aidoo, A (1996). DNA sequence analysis of hprt mutations in lymphocytes from Sprague-Dawley rats treated with 7,12-dimethylbenz[a]anthracene. *Environ. and Mol. Mutagen.* **28,** 5–12.

Holden, H. E., Majeska, J. B., and Studwell, D. (1997). A direct comparison of mouse and ratbone marrow and blood as target tissues in the micronucleus assay. *Mutat. Res.* **391,** 87–89.

ICPEMC. (1990). The possible involvement of somatic mutations in the development of atheriosclerotic plaques. *Mutat. Res.* **239,** 143–148.

Kier, L. D., Brusick, D. J., Auletta, A. E., Von Halle, E. S., Brown, M. M., Simmon, V. F., Dunkel, V., McCann, J., Mortelmans, K., Prival, M., Rao, T. K., and Ray, V. (1986). The Salmonella typhimurium/mammalian microsomal assay: A report of the U.S. EPA Gene-Tox Program. *Mutat. Res.* **168,** 69–240.

Knudsen, A. G., Jr. (1973). Mutation and human cancer. *Adv. Cancer Res.* **17,** 317–352.

McCann, J., Choi, E., Yamasaki, E., and Ames B. N. (1975). Detection of carcinogens as mutagens in the Salmonella/microsome test: Assay of 300 chemicals. *Proc. Natl. Acad. Sci. USA,* **72,** 5135–5139.

Mendelsohn, M. L., Moore, D. H., II, Lohman, P. H. M. (1992). A method for comparing and combining short-term genotoxicity test data: Results and interpretation. *Muation Res.* **266,** 43–60.

NAS. (1989). Biological significance of DNA adducts and protein adducts. *In* "Drinking Water and Health" Vol. 9, pp. 6–37. National Academy Press, Washington, D.C.

Nohmi, M. K., Suzuki, H., Matsui, M., Yamada, M., Watanabe, M., Suzuki, M., Horiya, N., Ueda, O., Shibuya, T., Ikeda, H., and Sofuni, T. (1996). A new transgenic mouse mutagenesis test system using Spi and 6 thioguanine selections. *Environ. and Mol. Mutagen.* **28,** 465–470.

Organization for Economic Co-operation and Development. (1981; revised May 1983). "Guidelines for Testing of Chemicals." OECD.

Pienta, R. J., Kuschner, L. M., and Russell, L. S. (1984). The use of short-term tests and limited bioassays in carcinogenicity testing. *Regul. Toxicol. Pharmacol* **4,** 249–260.

Rhomberg, L., Dellarco, V., Siegel-Scott, C., Dearfield, K., and Jacobson-Kram, D. (1990). Quantitative estimation of the genetic risk associated with the induction of heritable transolcations at low-dose exposure: Ethylene oxide as an example. *Environ. and Mol. Mutagen.* **16,** 104–125.

Samson, L., and Schwartz, J. L. (1980). Evidence for an adaptive DNA repair pathway in CHO and human skin fibroblast cell lines. *Nature* **287,** 861–863.

Setlow, R. B. (1978). Repair deficient human disorders and cancer. *Nature* **271,** 713–717.

Short, J. M., Kohler, S. W., Provost, G. S., Ferik, A., and Kretz, P. L. (1990). The use of lambda phage shuttle vectors in transgenic mice for development of a short-term mutagenicity assay. *In* "Mutation and the Environment Part A" (M. Mendelsohn and R. Albertini, eds.), pp. 355–367. Wiley-Liss Inc., New York.

Singh, N. P., McCoy, M. T., Tice, R. R., and Schneider, E. L. (1988). A simple technique for quantitation of low leveles of DNA damage in individual cells. *Exp. Cell Res.* **175,** 184–191.

Sobels, F. H. (1982). Extrapolation from experimental test systems for evaluation of genetic risks in man. *In* "Progress in Mutation Research" (K. C. Bora *et al.,* eds.), Vol. 3 pp. 323–327. Elsevier, Amsterdam.

Turturro, A., and Hart, R. W. (1984). DNA repair mechanisms in aging. *In* "Comparative Pathology of Major Age-Related Diseases" D. G. Scarpelli and G. Migaki, eds.), p. 1946. Mark R. Liss, New York.

UNEP. (1992). *In* "Assessing the Risk of Genetic Damage" (D. J. Brusick *et al.,* eds.). Lewis Publishers, Boca Raton.

Wolff, S., Afzal, V., and Olivieri, G. (1990). Inducible repair of cytogenetic damage to human lymphocytes: Adaption to low-level exposures to DNA-damaging agents. *In* "Mutation and the Environment, Part B" (M. L. Mendelsohn and R. J. Albertini, eds.), pp. 397–405. Wiley-Liss, Inc., New York.

Young, R., Oveisistork, F., Harrington-Brock, K., Schalkowsky, S., Moore, M., and Myhr, B. (1991). Quantitative size analysis of L5178Y $TK^{+/-}$ mutant colonies in soft agar; An interlaboratory comparison. *Environ. Mol. Mutagenen.* **17 Suppl. 19,** 79.

CHAPTER

7

Chemical Carcinogenesis

H. MARQUARDT

Department of Toxicology, Hamburg University Medical School, Hamburg, Germany, and Department of Toxicology and Environmental Medicine of the Fraunhofer Society, Hamburg, Germany

INTRODUCTION

Cancer is without doubt one of the most urgent problems of contemporary medical science. It is the nature of cancer that the carcinogenic events are irreversible. Translated into human experience, cancer is a tragical irrevocable fate (Bauer, 1963), at least in most cases. The Greek word for cancer, καρχινοσ (carcinos, *i.e.*, new growth), goes back to Hippocrates, while the Latin word, *cancer*, goes back to Celsius. "Like a crab which extends its extremities outward from all parts of its body," said Galen, "in this disease, the veins swell up and spread out, forming a similar figure" (Bauer, 1963). However, it is a also said that cancer got its name from the fact that it stubbornly attaches itself to the attacked parts like a crab to its prey (Paulus of Aegina). Cancer probably exists as long as multicellular organisms do; tumors were observed in the bones of dinosaurs and cancer in humans was known to the ancient Egyptians.

Cancer is defined as a malignant tumor (or swelling) that grows in an autonomous and excessive way and has certain pathological characteristics, such as cellular atypia, invasive growth, and, frequently, metastasizing capacity (formation of daughter growths). In contrast to the orderly, always regulated growth of cells in a normal organism—like the regeneration of liver or the contact inhibition of isolated cells grown in culture—growth controls are abolished during the malignant growth of tumor cells.

Hence, the growth of malignant tumors is invasive and infiltrating, causing the destruction of the surrounding tissues. By contrast, benign tumors grow expansively on their own. The fate of many cancer patients depends on the metastasizing capacity of the primary tumor. A metastasis is a daughter tumor that is spatially separated from the primary tumor. It is viewed as an unambiguous sign of malignancy since most types of cancer develop metastases.

In most countries of the world, cancer is the second leading cause of death next to cardiovascular diseases (Table 1). In the United States alone, estimates of the number of new cancer cases for the year 1994 indicate that 1,208,000 individuals will be diagnosed with cancer and that 538,000 cancer-associated deaths will occur.

Although ionizing irradiation, infectious biological material, and genetic determinants also play a role in causing cancer, we know today that the majority of human tumor incidences are caused by chemical substances in the environment. This statement includes the optimistic message that preventive medicine—through reduced exposure to such substances by changes in food and lifestyle—can lead to reduced cancer incidences (Tables 2–3).

The following facts indicate the causal significance of exogenous noxious substances in cancer causation. First, more than 90% of all cancers arise preferentially in epithelial tissues that are in direct contact with the environment (e.g., skin, intestinal tract, urogenital system, and bronchial tree). Second, cancer is generally and typically a disease of old age (approximately 75% of all malignancies appear after the 60th year of life). Of etiological significance are, particularly, chemicals and combinations of chemicals, such as diet, cigarette smoke, and alcohol (Table 3).

Connections between cancer and exogenous noxious influences have been known for a long time

TABLE 1 Cancer as a Substantial Cause of Death

Incident	Casualties[a]
Poliomyelitis (in 1952)	3300
Korean War (3 y)	34,000
Vietnam War (6 y)	41,000
Car accidents (1974)	46,400
Second World War (4 y)	292,000
Cancer (1975)	365,000

[a]Numbers refer exclusively to the U.S.A. or to Americans.

(based on geographical pathology, which describes different incidences of tumors in different parts of the world; shifts of incidences in immigrants; occupational cancer in workers of the chemical industry). The Japanese are particularly well studied with respect to geographical differences in cancer incidences. In the Japanese population, the incidence of stomach cancer is 40% in Japan but only 21% in Hawaii; the incidence of colon cancer is 5% in Japan but 19% in Hawaii; the incidence of breast cancer is 13% in Japan but 44% in Hawaii. With respect to etiology, the connections between lung cancer and cigarette smoking and between liver carcinoma and aflatoxin-contaminated food are the ones that have been best investigated.

It should be taken into consideration, however, that epidemiological studies are more difficult to carry out than standard toxicology studies. Due to long latency periods, the carcinogenic effects usually present themselves only many decades after the relevant exposure. Retrospective or prospective studies associated with occupational exposure are relatively easy (Table 4). Here the extent of exposure is much greater and well known, and only a defined group of people is in contact with them.

Studies of foreign substances (xenobiotics) in our environment are particularly difficult. These substances are ubiquitous and occur mostly in very low concentrations. However, these environmental contaminants may be particularly important as cancer causes; with the advent of advanced technology, new chemicals enter the environment, although at relatively low levels. (It has been estimated that the number of organic chemicals that are brought into the environment may include more than 100,000 compounds, and that in our daily life we are exposed to about 70,000 compounds.)

Observing a correlation between environmental factors and cancer development in humans or in experimental models, however, is only one aspect of studying chemical carcinogenesis. In addition to the etiology, the other aspects are important, such as, the underlying mechanisms that lead to malignant trans-

TABLE 2 Cancer Casualties vs Chemical Therapy—the Potential of Preventive Medicine[a]

	Cancer casualties (per y)	Chemotherapy-induced cures (per y)
Children, adolescents	Approx 8,000	Approx 3,000
Adults	Approx 400,000	Max 10,000
Related to smoking	Approx 100,000	

[a]Reduction of exposure to carcinogens; U.S.A. data, 1985.

TABLE 3 Estimated Cancer Mortalities in the U.S.A.

Cause	Target organ	Percent
Cigarettes	Lung, bladder, possibly others	35
Alcohol	Esophagus, oral cavity	3
Diet (fiber–fat content, pyrolysis products, etc.)	Intestine, breast, pancreas, prostate, ovary	35
Nitrosamines (nitrite)	Stomach	3
Mycotoxins (aflatoxins)	Liver	4
Sunlight	Skin (melanoma)	2
Occupation (various carcinogens)	Urinary bladder, liver	2
Lifestyle and occupation (cigarettes, work)	Lung	4
Iatrogenic (irradiation, medication)	Blood (leukemia, etc.)	2
Genetic disposition	Eye (retinoblastoma)	1
Virus (papilloma virus, HTLV-1)	Blood (lymphoma, etc.)	4

TABLE 4 Workplace Carcinogens

Agent	Location of tumor	Industry
Aromatic amines	Urinary bladder	Rubber
Arsenicals	Lung, skin	Glass, metals, pesticides
Asbestos	Lung, mesothelioma	Insulation
Benzene	Leukemia	Solvent, gasoline
Diesel exhaust	Lung	Engine operation
Nickel	Lung	Metals
Vinyl chloride	Liver	Plastics
Hair dyes	Bladder	Hairdressers
Mineral oils	Skin	Metals

formation (initiation) and especially the pathogenesis of the disease, namely the development from the initiated cell to the clinical manifestation of a metastasizing tumor (promotion, progression). Today, chemical carcinogenesis is viewed as a multistep process with a latency period of many years. Clearly, knowledge about these mechanisms is critical for the control and prevention of human cancer.

HISTORIC REVIEW

In the Ebers papyrus, long before the advent of modern times, there is a very detailed etiological and clinical description of bladder cancer in farmers living in the Nile valley (bilharziosis). As we know today, this is caused by a nematode (*Schistosomum haematobium*); but the question is still open whether chemical substances or tissue irritations (irritation-induced cancer or "Reizkrebs" Schmähl, 1981) are at the root of the problem. It can be assumed with some certainty that Paracelsus (1493–1541) was the first to view a chemical substance, namely, realgar or arsenic disulfide (As_4S_4), as the cause of lung cancer in the miners of Schneeberg and Joachimsthal, Germany. In 1700, Ramazzini (1633–1714) described the high incidence of breast cancer in nuns. In 1761, the English physician, botanist, and writer John Hill (1716–1775) described six cases of polyps and cancer of the nasal mucosa after long-term use of snuff. In 1775, Percival Pott (1714–1788) described soot as the cause of skin cancer on the scrotum and thighs of London chimney sweeps. Hence, Pott was the first to observe a chemical cause of cancer in a distinct professional group. In 1795, T. von Soemmering (1755–1830), an anatomy professor in Mainz and Munich, published a paper on lip cancer in pipe smokers.

In the 19th century, it became known that occupational exposure to chemical substances is an important cause of human cancer (Table 5). Skin tumors occur after exposure to arsenic (noted by I. A. Paris in 1822) and paraffin or tar (R. von Volkmann in 1875), while urinary bladder tumors occur in fuchsine workers (L. Rehn in 1895).

The early 20th century can be regarded as the beginning of experimental cancer research. The Japanese pathologist K. Yamagiwa (1863–1930), with his assistant Ichikawa, is regarded as its pioneer. He was able to produce, for the first time, a chemically-induced tumor in an animal experiment (tar cancer of the skin—a late experimental confirmation of Pott's observation). He himself described his reaction to this

TABLE 5 Historical Foundations of Chemical Carcinogenesis

Suspected carcinogen	Organ	Discovered by	Year
Snuff	Nose	Hill	1761
Soot	Scrotum	Pott	1775
Pipe smoking	Lip	Soemmering	1795
Coal tar	Skin	von Volkmann	1875
Dyes (aromatic amines)	Urinary bladder	Rehn	1895
X rays	Skin	van Trieben	1902
Radioactive watch colors	Bones	Martland	1929
Cigarette smoking	Lung, bladder	Lickint	1930
Asbestos	Lung	Gloyne	1932
Sunlight	Skin	Molesworth	1937
Chromates	Airways	Pfeil	1935
Butter yellow (4-dimethylaminoazobenzene)	Liver	Kinosita	1936
Cadmium	Prostate gland	Kipling, Waterhouse	1967
Diethylstilbestrol	Genital tract (via placenta)	Herbst	1970

achievement as follows: "Cancer was produced! Proudly I walked a few steps." His discovery demonstrated that, in principle, the experimental investigation of chemical carcinogenesis was possible.

More investigations followed, by the English team around Sir Ernest Kennaway and by J. Hieger (in 1930) and J. W. Cook (in 1933), respectively, at the Chester Beatty Institute in London, working on polycyclic aromatic hydrocarbons as tar components; by W. C. Hueper and co-workers (in 1938) and T. Yoshida (in 1933), working on aromatic amines; and by A. Lacassagne (in 1932), working on estrogen (a confirmation of Ramazzini's observation). The studies by T. Boveri (in 1914; somatic mutation theory of tumor formation), by P. Rous and J. G. Kidd (in 1941) and I. Berenblum and P. Shubik (in 1947) on tumor promotion, by H. Druckrey (in 1949) on the irreversibility of chemical carcinogenesis, and by J. and E. Miller (in 1969) on metabolic activation represent the foundations of today's knowledge and hypotheses on chemical carcinogenesis—the precise mechanisms of which we still do not understand, despite the explosive gain in knowledge during the past decades. The following statement by the pathologist H. Ribbert (in 1906) is still valid: "No subject in pathology is more vigorously discussed at the moment than the formation of tumors."

TABLE 6 Proven Human Carcinogens
Chemicals
Aflatoxins
4-Aminobiphenyl
Arsenic (compounds)
Benzene
Benzidine
Beryllium (compounds)
Bis(chloromethyl) ether
Cadmium
Chromium(VI) (compounds)
Coal tar, soot
Mineral oils
Mustard gas
2-Naphthylamine
Nickel (compounds)
Vinyl chloride
Substances abuse
Alcohol
Betel nuts
Cigarettes
Dusts and fibers
Asbestos
Silica
Soots
Talcum
Wood dusts
Chronic infections
Helicobacter pylori
Hepatitis B, C
Human immunodeficiency virus
Opisthorchis (liver fluke)
Papilloma virus
Schistosomes

CHEMICAL CARCINOGENS—STRUCTURE AND FUNCTION

Chemical carcinogens are defined as substances that induce cancer; that is, they are responsible for:

- The induction of tumors not observed in control animals.
- The increased incidence of tumors also occurring in control animals.
- The early development of tumors that occur only later in control animals.
- The increased multiplicity of tumors.

Tumors of epithelial origin are called carcinomas, while those of mesenchymal origin are called sarcomas.

Until 1962, more than 500 chemical substances (about 20% of all substances tested for chronic toxicity) had been shown to have carcinogenic potential in animal experiments. In 1997, the WHO International Agency for Research on Cancer, Lyon, listed 74 proven human carcinogens, 56 compounds probably carcinogenic to humans, and 225 compounds possibly carcinogenic to humans out of 836 evaluated agents. Of the 74 proven human carcinogens, 13 were related to industrial processes, 20 to the working environment, 25 to medical drugs, and 5 to cultural habits; and 7 were biological agents. Substances inducing the entire process of tumor formation—when given in sufficient doses and without additional measures—are called complete carcinogens (solitary carcinogens), whereas initiating or promoting substances trigger only certain steps of the multistep process of chemical carcinogenesis. In contrast to directly acting carcinogens, indirectly acting carcinogens require metabolic activation.

Chemical carcinogens belong to very different classes of chemical substances, such as, inorganic and organic substances, fiber and plastic materials, and hormones (Table 6). A considerable number of pharmaceutical products have also been shown, or are suspected, to induce cancer in humans (Table 7). Based on their chemical and biological activities, the chemical carcinogens can be classified into two

TABLE 7 Drugs as Human Carcinogens

Proven	Possible
Alkylating agents (cyclophosphamide, melphalan)	Anthraquinones
Diethylstilbestrol	Anthracyclines
Estrogens	Anabolics
Immunosuppressants (azathioprine, cyclosporin A)	Antimetabolites
8-Methoxypsoralen plus UV light	Chloramphenicol
Oral contraceptives	Clofibrate
Phenacetin-containing analgesic mixtures	Metromidazole
Tamoxifen	Niridazole
	Phenobarbital
	Reserpine
	Senecio alkaloids

groups (Table 8), DNA-reactive genotoxic substances and epigenetic nongenotoxic substances. (The latter description is operational. It is based on the fact that these substances do not show any activity in the conventional mutagenesis assays but display other biological activities that might be the cause of their carcinogenicity.) Though this division is significant for the assessment of carcinogens as a human health risk, it is often difficult to verify in practice.

TABLE 8 Chemical Carcinogens

Type	Example
Genotoxic carcinogens	
Direct carcinogens (without metabolic activation)	Alkylating agents
Indirect carcinogens (after metabolic activation)	Polycyclic hydrocarbons, aromatic amines, nitrosamines, natural substances (mycotoxins)
Inorganic carcinogens	Nickel, chromium, cadmium, arsenic
Epigenetic carcinogens	
Cytotoxic carcinogens	Nitrilotriacetate, butylated hydroxyanisole or hydroxytoluene (BHA, BHT)
Tumor promoters	Tetradecanoylphorbolacetate (TPA), phenobarbital, chlorinated hydrocarbons (DDT, TCDD)
Hormones	Estradiol, diethylstilbestrol
Immunosuppressants	Azathioprine, cyclosporin A
Peroxisome proliferators	Clofibrate,phthalates
Solid bodies or particles	Asbestos, plastic foils (wood dust)

Genotoxic Carcinogens— Mutagenesis

These substances interact with cellular macromolecules, particularly DNA, and are mutagenic.

Direct Carcinogens: Active without Metabolic Activation

This group includes halogenated substances, nitrosamides, and nitrourea (Fig. 1). These substances are chemically reactive (electrophilic) and interact spontaneously with cellular macromolecules and particularly with DNA (DNA adducts) (i.e., they are alkylating agents). They do not occur in nature but are used in the chemical industry or as cancer-therapeutic agents, disinfectants, and insecticides. Above all, they are active as irritants (e.g., to the skin, lung). These substances are often extremely potent carcinogens, frequently with transplacental activity. This group also includes therapeutically used platinum compounds.

Indirect Carcinogens—Active after Metabolic Activation

The majority of genotoxic carcinogens belong to this group. Since the capacity for metabolic activation of these substances is species-specific as well as individual- and organ-specific, the biological activity of these substances often shows a distinct species and organ specificity. With the exception of polycyclic hydrocarbons, which induce skin tumors after dermal application, they are mainly systemically acting carcinogens. This class includes synthetic and natural substances.

Polycyclic Aromatic Hydrocarbons

Polycyclic hydrocarbons are ubiquitous contaminants of the environment (Fig. 2). They arise as combustion products and are present, for example, in soot, tar, coal, petroleum, oils, car exhaust fumes, and tobacco smoke. Carcinogenic hydrocarbons were the first pure chemicals for which a carcinogenic activity could be demonstrated experimentally. They act locally (e.g., on the skin), as well as systemically. All species are sensitive to the carcinogenic activity of these substances, although big differences exist among species. (Rodents are particularly sensitive. Only petroleum oil, but not the pure substances, were shown to be active in monkeys.)

A distinct structure–function relationship could be demonstrated for hydrocarbons. The addition of benzene rings to the noncarcinogenic anthracene (to yield four- to six-ring systems), as well as the substitution of rings by methyl groups (7,12-dimethyl-

Nitrogen mustard

Bis(chloromethyl) ether

Dimethyl sulfate

β-Propiolactone

Diepoxybutane

Ethyleneimine

Methanesulfonic acid methylester

N-Methyl-N′-nitro-N-nitrosoguanidine

N-methyl-N-nitrourea

Diaminedichloro-platinum II, DDP

FIGURE 1 Direct genotoxic carcinogens (alkylating agents). These carcinogens act directly without metabolic activation.

benz[*a*]anthracene), lead to an increase in activity. Hydrocarbons must be converted metabolically into reactive electrophilic "ultimate" carcinogens (binding to DNA and other nucleophilic macromolecules) (Fig. 3).

The metabolic activation of hydrocarbons occurs through epoxidation. Originally, the K region (A. Pulman) of hydrocarbon molecules was thought to be essential for metabolic activation based on its high electron density and reactivity. The bay region of the molecule and the formation of dihydrodiol-epoxides (P. L. Grover and P. Sims; D. Jerina) in the bay region are thought to be essential for metabolic activation. Responsible for this metabolic activation is the microsome (endoplasmatic reticulum)-bound cytochrome P450 enzyme system (P450 1A1; substrate-inducible). The detoxification of these substances is mediated by epoxide hydrolases and conjugations. Hence, their biological activity depends on the balance between activation and detoxification in the target cell (species and organ specificity).

Nitro analogs of carcinogenic polycyclic aromatic hydrocarbons (1-nitropyrene) have gained special interest as components of diesel emission. They are very strong mutagens but also act as carcinogens. However, it is not clear whether the established carcinogenicity of diesel emission (in the lungs of rats) is caused

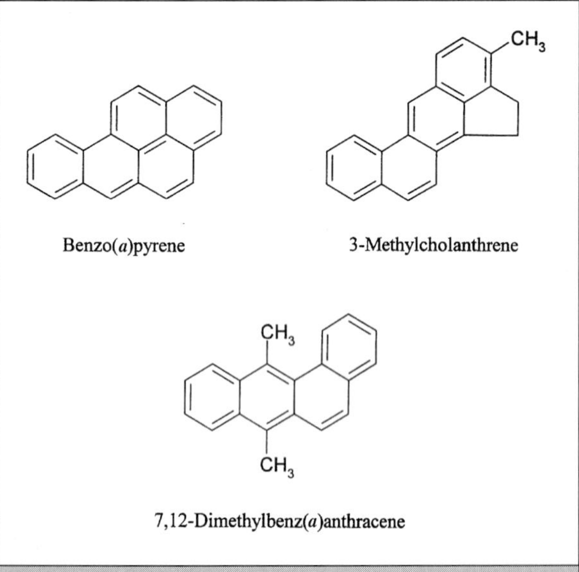

FIGURE 2 Carcinogenic polycyclic aromatic hydrocarbons. These polycyclic aromatic hydrocarbons are highly lipophilic compounds that are derived from phenanthrene.

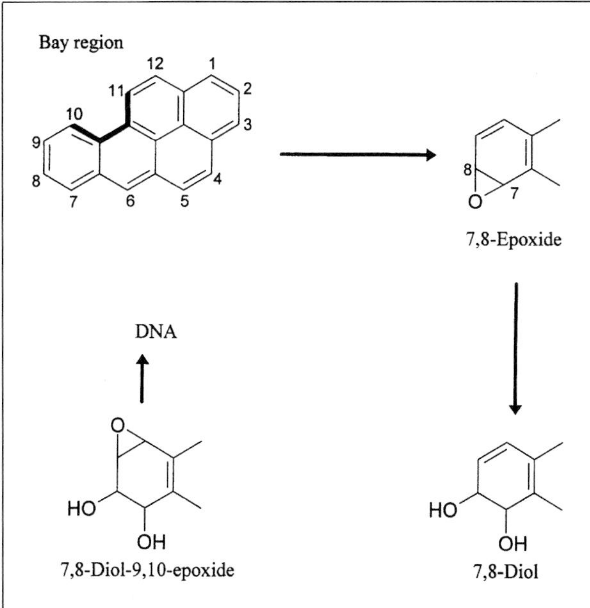

FIGURE 3 Metabolic activation for benzo[*a*]pyrene. Shown here are only the metabolic reactions leading to the "ultimate" carcincogen, the reactive diol-epoxide in the characteristic bay region.

by such components or, rather, by soot particles (irritation-induced tumors).

Aromatic Amines

Aromatic amines (arylamines), (Fig. 4) consist of aromatic hydrocarbons that contain amino groups as substituents. With the exception of some complex compounds formed by pyrolysis (Fig. 6), they do not occur in nature but are synthesized as dyes, antioxidants, and precursors of pharmaceutical products. Usually, they do not act locally; they are carcinogenic after metabolic activation, act systemically, and show significant species differences. In rodents, many of these substances induce liver cancer and urinary bladder cancer, particularly in males, and breast cancer in females.

The metabolic activation (Fig. 5) of these substances is mediated by the microsome (endoplasmatic reticulum)-bound cytochrome P450 enzyme system (P450 1A2) and depends on initial N-hydroxylation to form the corresponding hydroxyl amines. Such *N*-hydroxy substances are extremely toxic to the hematopoietic system. Further activation to form the ultimate carcinogens takes place mostly in the liver, mediated by the following enzymes:

- Sulfotransferase: Sulfate ester formation.

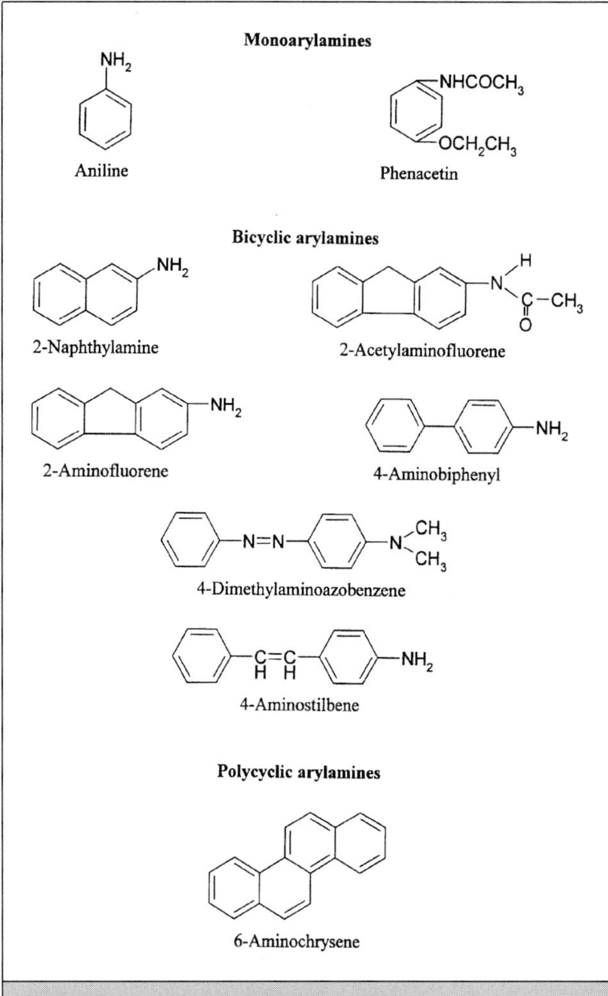

FIGURE 4 Carcinogenic aromatic amines.

- *N*-Acetyltransferase (also detoxification reaction): This enzyme is polymorphic in humans (there are rapidly and slowly activating individuals), whereas acetylation is fast in hamsters and slow in dogs and rats. These kinetic differences are important for the toxic activity of these substances.
- Prostaglandin H synthetase: Further detoxification takes place through phase II reactions (e.g., glucuronidation).

In contrast to the abundance of experimental studies on homocyclic amines, there are far fewer investigations on heterocyclic analogs.

- Quinolines induce hepatocellular carcinoma and hemangioendothelioma in rats and mice, as well as skin tumors. 4-Nitroquinoline-*N*-oxide is carcinogenic in a variety of organs.
- Particularly through the work of Sugimura, new and potent mutagenic and carcinogenic heterocyclic

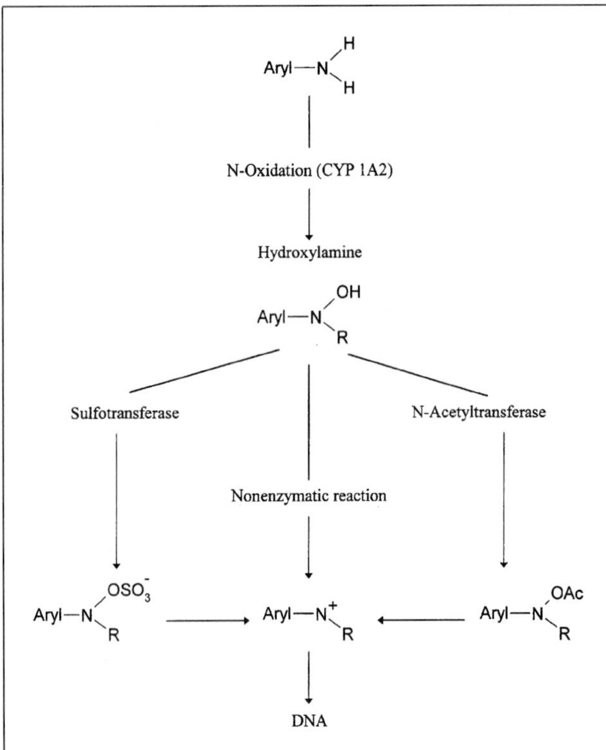

FIGURE 5 Metabolic activation of aromatic amines. Illustration of the most important metabolic reactions leading to ultimate carcinogens.

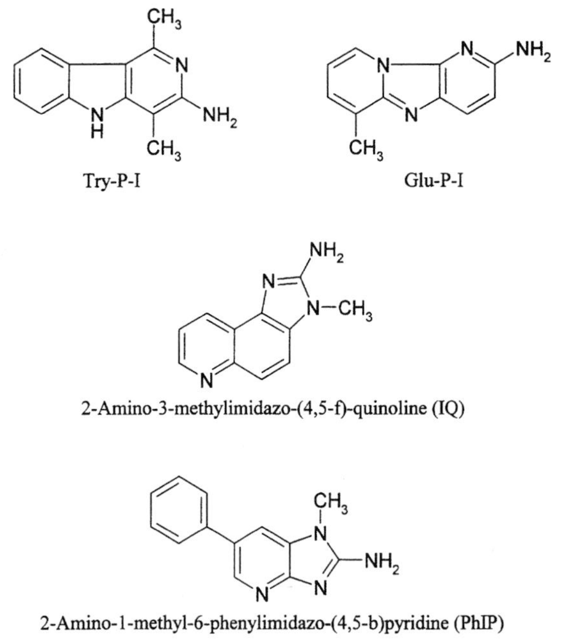

Try-P-I

Glu-P-I

2-Amino-3-methylimidazo-(4,5-f)-quinoline (IQ)

2-Amino-1-methyl-6-phenylimidazo-(4,5-b)pyridine (PhIP)

FIGURE 6 Carcinogenic heterocyclic amines. These carcinogens are formed as pyroplytic products from amino acids in protein-containing food.

amines were discovered as pyrolytic products of amino acids (after cooking protein-containing food or frying meat and fish) (Fig. 6). For example, they are formed from tryptophan (Trp-P-I) and glutamic acid (Glu-P-I). These amines also include imidazoquinolines (IQ) and pyridoindol-amines (PhIP).

Qualitatively, the latter substances are with all probability carcinogenic to humans, but their quantitative risk is controversial. They are discussed as causative for human breast cancer. Furthermore, epidemiological studies point to a connection between colon cancer and the consumption of fried meat.

Nitrofurans (some of which have antibacterial activity) usually show strong carcinogenic activity. FANFT [*N*-4-(5-nitro-2-furyl)-2-thiazolylformamide] induces bladder cancer; AF2[2-(2furyl)-3-(5-nitro-2-furyl)acrylamid], formerly used as food additive in Japan, induces stomach cancer in rats.

N-Nitroso Compounds

With respect to structure and function, *N*-nitrosamides are distinct from *N*-nitrosamines. Nitrosamides react spontaneously, nitrosamines only after enzymatic oxidation. These substances occur both naturally and as synthetic products (e.g., in solvents; in cigarette smoke and food).

Nitrosamines are divided into symmetric, asymmetric, and cyclic compounds (Fig. 7). These *N*-nitroso compounds are characterized by a distinct organotropism (due to their metabolic activation). They induce tumors in every species tested so far.

Nitrosamines are also formed endogenously, namely, in the acidic environment of the stomach from secondary amines (derived from proteins during cooking and frying) by reaction with nitrite (contained in pickle salt; in the saliva, nitrite is formed by bacteria from nitrate derived from fertilizer). The formation of nitrosamines is discussed as causative for human stomach cancer:

- Orally administered *N*-nitroso compounds induce stomach tumors. Stomach cancer is more frequent in nitrite-rich regions and in Japan (amines in fish are easily nitrosated).
- The nitrosating reaction can be inhibited by vitamin C. Nutrition poor in vitamin C and human stomach cancer are more frequent in the north than in the south (Scandinavia vs Italy, Canada vs Florida). The significant reduction in human stomach cancer during the last decades (>50%) can be associated

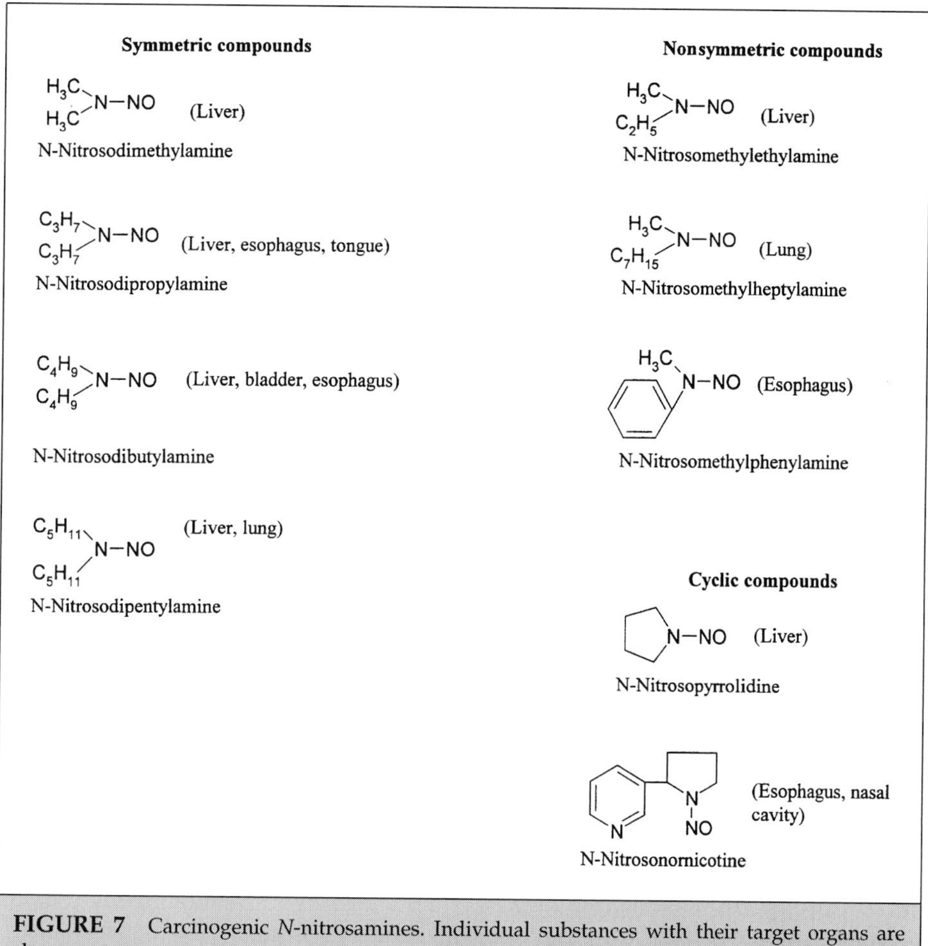

FIGURE 7 Carcinogenic *N*-nitrosamines. Individual substances with their target organs are shown.

with the increased consumption of fresh fruits and vegetables.

Also tertiary and quaternary amines, when present together with nitrite, can lead to the formation of *N*-nitroso compounds some of which are carcinogenic.

Nitrosamines are metabolically activated by oxidation at a C atom next to the amino group. Through enzymatic α-C-hydroxylation (cytochrome P450 2E1), reactive electrophilic metabolites are formed as the ultimate carcinogens (alkyldiazohydroxide, diazonium ion). Mainly N^7-alkylguanines are formed as reaction products with DNA, although it can be safely assumed that O^6-alkylguanine and O^4- and O^2-alkylthymidine (miscoding) are essential for the carcinogenic activity.

In contrast to the indirectly acting nitrosamines, the nitrosamides are reactive compounds that decompose in aqueous solution and, therefore, act directly. These substances usually induce tumors locally at the site of application. After IV injection, however, *N*-nitrosomethyl urethane also induces lung tumors transplacentally, while *N*-methyl-*N*-nitrosourea induces malignant tumors of the brain, bone marrow, and peripheral nerves.

This group of carcinogens also includes *N*-nitrosodialkylhydroxylamines and dialkylhydazines. Among these is cycasin (present in the flour of the cycad seed); its active metabolite, methylazoxymethanol, is released by the β-glycosidases of intestinal bacteria. It induces tumors of the liver, kidney, and intestine (colon). The organ specificity of hydrazines is not clear. Hydrazine induces lung tumors in mice and rats; 1,2-dimethylhydrazine induces via methylazoxymethanol the tumor spectrum of this compound, whereas 1,2-diethylhydrazine induces liver and lung tumors. To this group of substances also belong isoniazid (INH, isonicotylhydrazine, used in tuberculosis therapy), which induces lung tumors in mice, and the cancer chemotherapeutic agent, Natulan (procarbazine).

Other Indirect Genotoxic Carcinogens

Nitroalkyl compounds: The inhalation of 2-nitropropan causes liver tumors.

Aldehydes: Formaldehyde is used primarily in the production of synthetic resins and plastics. It is formed during combustion processes (indoor pollution) but also endogenously in small amounts as a normal metabolite in mammalian organisms. The substance is mutagenic and induces a high incidence of nasal-cavity tumors in rats after excessive exposure (14.3 ppm for 24 months). This carcinogenic effect, however, is assessed as "abnormal regeneration" after local ulceration and thus occurs only after high exposures (threshold value). The mostly negative results of epidemiological studies support this view. Based on the data, it must be concluded that the human cancer risk after occupational and, most of all, domestic exposure is nonexistent or so low that it remains indiscernible. Formaldehyde is the main metabolite of N-methylated compounds (such as hexamethylphosphoramide) after their microsomal oxidation. Acetaldehyde and glutaraldehyde must be viewed similarly.

Carbamates: Ethyl carbamate (urethane) is a potent carcinogen, which in mice and other species can induce lung tumors and also tumors of the liver, skin, and the hematopoietic system.

Halogenated hydrocarbons: Many of these substances are widely distributed as industrial chemicals and environmental contaminants. This group contains very different substances. Chloroform and carbon tetrachloride induce liver tumors, but they do not have genotoxic activity. Halogenated olefines (such as tri- and tetrachloroethylene, hexachlorobutadiene, and dichloroacetylene) induce kidney carcinoma in rodents. An important role in their metabolic activation is played by β-lyase (e.g., enzymatic cleavage of cysteine adducts). Polyhalogenated cyclic hydrocarbons (DDT, aldrin, dieldrin, and other pesticides; polychlorinated biphenyls; polychlorinated dibenzodioxins; and dibenzofurans) should be mentioned here. They, too, are carcinogens in animal experiments; although they do not have genotoxic activity, they are very active tumor promoters. The significance of these promoting compounds for human carcinogenesis is unresolved.

Vinyl chloride (monochloroethylene), the monomer of PVC, and acrylonitrile (vinyl nitrile) are mutagenic and carcinogenic after metabolic activation (epoxide, oxirane). In exposed humans, vinyl chloride induces especially hemangiosarcoma of the liver.

1,2-Dichloroethane is carcinogenic and toxic after metabolic activation, similar to 1,1-dichloroethane (vinylidene chloride).

Chlorohydrines (3-chloro-1,2-propandiol and 1,3-dichloro-2-propanol) are formed, for example, in seasonings through hydrochloric hydrolysis of plant proteins. These substances are genotoxic and carcinogenic in rats.

Natural Compounds

Some potent carcinogens are formed by microorganisms or in plants. The structures of these substances are very diverse, but all of them require metabolic activation (Fig. 8).

Mycotoxins: Carcinogenic mycotoxins are metabolites of molds that grow on food and fodder. Apart from patulin (formed by *Penicillium* and *Aspergillus* species), sterigmatocystine (*Aspergillus*), luteoskyrin, and cyclochlorotin (*Penicillium*), they include particularly the aflatoxins (*Aspergillus flavus*). The latter mycotoxins attracted attention as pathogens through the die-off of turkeys in England in 1960, after they were fed oil from moldy Brazilian peanuts. Aflatoxin B_1 is metabolically activated through epoxidation (cytochrome P450 3A4) and is one of the most potent liver carcinogens in the rat and various other species, but—with the exception of newborns—not in the mouse (species-specificity of chemical carcinogenesis). Less potent analogs are the aflatoxins B_2, G_1, and G_2. In some regions of Africa, liver cancer is widespread in humans. In these regions (subtropic and tropic), a high content of aflatoxins in the food has been observed, but also a wide distribution of hepatitis B (HBV). If the risk of hepatocellular carcinomas without recognizable exposure is 1, this risk is increased to 2 after aflatoxin exposure, to 5 with HBV infection, and to 60 with simultaneous HBV infection and aflatoxin exposure.

Bacterial carcinogens: Only few antibiotics have been investigated for carcinogenic activity. They are mostly used as medical drugs. Antineoplastic antibiotics of the anthracycline type (e.g., daunomycin, adriamycin) are genotoxic and carcinogenic. The same is true for the antineoplastic agent streptozotocin (*Strep-*

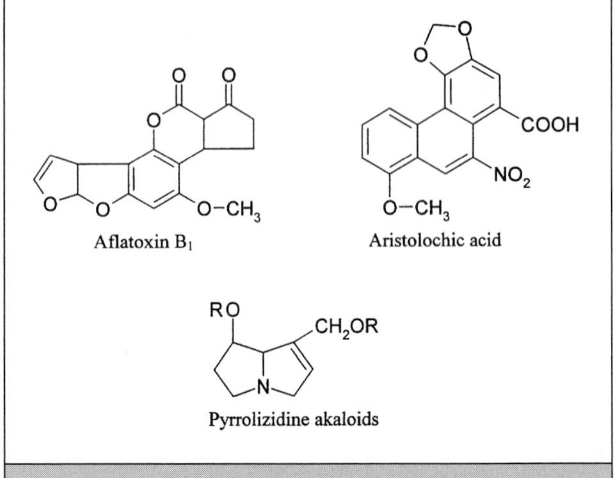

Aflatoxin B_1

Aristolochic acid

Pyrrolizidine akaloids

FIGURE 8 Carcinogenic natural compounds.

tomyces; diabetogenic through pancreatic β-cell toxicity), a methylnitrourea analog. In rats, azaserine *(Streptomyces)* induces pancreas and kidney tumors; ethionine *(E. coli)* induces liver tumors; and elaiomycin *(Streptomyces)* induces tumors of the brain, uterus, kidney, intestine, and stomach.

Plant carcinogens: Here again, the high carcinogenic potential (to lung, larynx, esophagus, oral cavity, pharynx, pancreas, bladder, and kidney) of cigarette smoking must be emphasized. Cigarette smoke contains a multitude of genotoxic substances (hydrocarbons, nitrosamines, formaldehyde, and cadmium), as well as tumor promoters (phenol and terpene). Just as alarming are the substances from chewing betel, from the fruit of the Indio-Malayan betel nut palm. Among others, plant carcinogens include safrole (liver), senecio alkaloids (pyrrolizidines; liver), constituents of the bracken fern (*Pteridium aquilinum,* "Adlerfarn"; urinary bladder), cycasin, aristolochic acid (*Aristolochia clematis,* "Osterluzei"; stomach, kidney), and plant anthraquinones.

Pharmaceutical Products

Pharmaceutical products that are carcinogenic in humans are listed in Table 7. In addition, it should be mentioned that numerous drugs are amines and, as such, can be nitrosated (for example, cimetidine).

Inorganic Substances

Uranium, polonium, plutonium, radium, and radon gas are carcinogenic due to their radioactivity. Many metal ions are genotoxic or induce mutations through errors during the semiconservative synthesis of DNA (DNA replication). Accordingly, titanium, nickel, cadmium, chromium VI, beryllium, and some of their compounds, and possibly also mercury, possess carcinogenic activity mainly at the site of exposure (subcutaneous application and inhalation). Nickel and combinations of chromates(VI), hematite, and nickel(II) (dust, powder) are carcinogenic in humans (lung; mainly occupational exposure).

Inorganic arsenic compounds, such as arsenic trioxide, are carcinogenic in mice. Based on epidemiological studies, they are strongly suspected to be also carcinogenic in humans (for winegrowers: skin, lung, liver). In this connection, the genotoxic and carcinogenic potential of wood dust (e.g., from oak, beech; nasal cancer) should be emphasized. The exact mechanism of action is not known for these substances. Apart from their direct genotoxic capacity, indirect oxidative cell damage, as well as their tumor-promoting potential (such as kidney carcinogenesis in rats after exposure to nickel), are discussed in this connection.

Manganese, magnesium, calcium, zinc, and iron, and also chelating agents (diethyldithiocarbamate (DDC) or ethylenediaminetetraacetic acid (EDTA)), can act as antagonists against metal-induced toxicity and carcinogenesis. Especially selenium and selenium compounds—on the one hand, extremely toxic and mutagenic (without any hint of carcinogenicity in humans) and, on the other hand, anticarcinogenic (antioxidative)—have stirred public interest. In physiological concentrations (through food uptake), selenium and selenium compounds inhibit chemically induced carcinogenesis (breast, colon, skin) in animal experiments. Corresponding studies in patients yielded contradictory results. Whereas higher serum levels of selenium correlated with lower cancer incidences in some epidemiological studies, the contrary was true in other studies, particularly for stomach–intestinal and prostate cancer.

Epigenetic Nongenotoxic Carcinogens

Epigenetic or nongenotoxic carcinogens are defined as carcinogenic substances for which a DNA reaction cannot be demonstrated but which show other biological effects that could be the basis for their carcinogenicity (e.g., disturbance of homeostasis; Table 8). These biological effects include cytotoxicity (increased regenerative cell proliferation), chronic inflammatory reactions, hormonal influences, immunological processes, and tumor promotion.

At one time, this concept of epigenetic chemical carcinogenesis would not have been accepted. However, increasing numbers of nongenotoxic substances have been shown to possess carcinogenic activity. (Even lactose increases the incidence of pheochromocytoma in rats.) These observations necessitate the acceptance of the concept, which poses important questions with respect to the mechanisms involved, as well as serious problems with respect to assessing the implications for our health (i.e., threshold value). Interestingly, we are confronted with such xenobiotics particularly in environmental toxicology—dioxins, phthalates, dichloromethane, saccharin, butylated hydroxyanisole, and asbestos.

Cytotoxicity and Cell Proliferation: Mitogenesis

It has been known for a long time that induced cell proliferation (as in regenerating liver) enhances the carcinogenic activity of chemical compounds (Table 9). Therefore, toxic effects leading to cell death and subsequently to regeneration are an important factor when assessing the carcinogenic potential of a substance.

TABLE 9 Increased Cell Proliferation as Risk Factor in Carcinogenesis, Some Substances and Their Target Organs

Factor	Target
Hormones	
ACTH	Adrenal gland
Estrogens, progesterone	Uterus, mammary gland
Gonadotropins	Ovary, testis, pituitary
Testosterone	Prostate gland
TSH (increased after goitrogenic substances)	Thyroid gland
Pharmaceuptical products	
Oral contraceptives, anabolic steroids	Liver
Analgesics	Renal pelvis
Diuretics	Kidney
Infectious agents	
Hepatitis B	Liver
Schistosoma haematobium	Urinary bladder
Schistosoma japonicum	Colon
C. sinensis, O. viverini	Gall bladder
Epstein–Barr virus	Lymph nodes (Burkitt's lymphoma)
M. tuberculosis	Lung
Helicobacter pylori	Stomach
Chemical substances	
Betel nut	Oral cavity
Bile acids	Small intestine
Saturated fatty acids	Colon
Salt	Stomach
Tobacco	Oral cavity, lung, bladder, etc.
Saccharin, uracil, melamine, tetraphthalic acid and other xenobiotics causing urinary stones	Urinary bladder
Dichlorobenzene, trimethylpentane (lead-free gasoline), perchloroethylene, limonene and other xenobiotics binding to the $\alpha_{2\mu}$-globulin of male rats	Kidney
Butylated hydroxyanisole, propionic acid	Stomach
Nitrilotriacetate	Kidney
Physical influences (mechanical trauma)	
Asbestos	Lung, pleura (mesothelioma)
Stone formation	Gall bladder, urinary bladder
Chronic inflammation	
Ulcers	Skin
Chronic ulcerative colitis	Colon

Naturally, these observations also have implications for the assessment of our test procedures designed to detect carcinogenic effects of chemicals (e.g., bioassays using the maximum tolerated dose, MTD).

Tumor Promoters

The phenomenon of tumor promotion was discovered and defined based on the role of chronic inflammation and wound healing during carcinogenesis (R. Virchow). Tumor promoters were defined by I. Berenblum as substances that, without being carcinogens themselves, increase the cancer incidence after exposure to carcinogenic (initiating) substances. They either increase the number of tumors per animal and/or shorten the latency period of carcinogenesis. They show this activity when applied repeatedly after an initiating carcinogen (in the mouse, even when application is started one year after initiation, which proves the irreversibility of initiation). Tumor promoters are neither electrophilic nor do they react with DNA, and they are not metabolically activated.

Tumor promotion is a biological phenomenon that is both species- and organ-specific. It was first discovered in mouse skin. It is mostly investigated in rat liver. The term tumor promotion is purely descriptive; the underlying mechanisms are mostly unknown and certainly manifold. The phenomenon probably is based on the clonal expansion of initiated cells (mitogenesis); it seems to be reversible and, possibly, dependent on a threshold dose. Certain tumor promoters (tetradecanoylphorbolacetate) interact with mitogenesis-related cellular signal transduction pathways. The focal changes in enzyme patterns observed during hepatocarcinogenesis, the benign papillomas during skin carcinogenesis, and the benign polyps during colon carcinogenesis are possibly tissue manifestations of a promoting influence. It is worth mentioning here that after the phase of initiation (irreversible transformation of a normal cell into an initiated premalignant cell) and the phase of promotion, there must follow a phase of progression (genetic or epigenetic mechanisms) before a malignant tumor becomes clinically manifest.

As the mechanisms of tumor promotion are still unknown, we only have few test methods for demonstrating the tumor-promoting potential of chemicals (*in vivo:* induction of papillomas in mouse skin, of foci in rat liver, of lung tumors in mouse strains with high spontaneous incidence of lung tumors; *in vitro:* cellular transformation, inhibition of intercellular communication via gap junctions, or possibly also an increase in hepatocyte proliferation). The concept of tumor promotion is disputed; since all tumor promoters may also induce tumors on their own (pro-

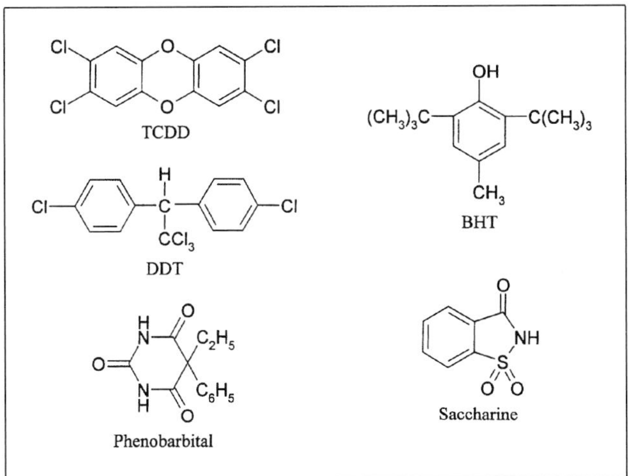

FIGURE 9 Important substances with promoting activity.

motion of spontaneously transformed cells?), synergistic effects might be involved, too.

The phenomenon of cocarcinogenesis (application immediately prior to or together with the initiator) must be viewed as distinct from tumor promotion. Silicon dioxide, for example, is cocarcinogenic with benzo(a)pyrene in the larynx, trachea, and lung. The following mechanisms of action are possibly responsible for this principle: increased uptake or metabolic activation of the carcinogen, depletion of nucleophiles, and inhibition of DNA repair.

Today, the following carcinogens are believed to act through tumor promotion (Fig. 9): tetradecanoylphorbolacetate (TPA) and other croton oil constituents (from the seeds of *Croton tiglium* and other Euphorbiaceae), phenobarbital, chlorinated hydrocarbons (DDT and other organochlorinated pesticides), polychlorinated and polybromated biphenyls, polychlorinated dibenzo-*p*-dioxins and dibenzofurans (such as TCDD), saccharin, and butylated hydroxyanisole (BHA) or butylated hydroxytoluene (BHT). (The toxic effects of TCDD are mostly mediated by binding to the cytosolic Ah receptor, which regulates the genetic expression of cytochromes, growth and differentiation factors, etc.; the affinity of TCDD for the Ah receptor is greater in rodent cells than in human cells.) Also regarded as tumor promoters are unsaturated fatty acids in the case of pancreatic carcinogenesis (initiated by azaserine in rats) and orotic acid in the case of liver carcinogenesis. These substances induce hypertrophy and hyperplasia of pancreas or liver.

Hormones

Hormones induce tumors in various target tissues (e.g., mammary tumors in dogs after long-term treatment with progesterone or progesterone–estrogen combinations; pituitary and mammary tumors in rats and mice after long-term treatment with estrogens or progesterones; and endometrial carcinoma after chronic treatment with dopamine). Generally, the hormonal effect requires extremely high doses and long treatment periods. Pharmaceutical products or chemical substances that influence the endogenous hormone production can also be effective. Generally, the carcinogenic effect is preceded by excessive hyperplasia of the target organ or the pituitary gland (synthesis of stimulating hormones) (Table 9). Similarly, disturbances in the hormonal equilibrium can lead to tumor formation (e.g., antithyroid goitrogenic substances, like thiourea, cause thyroid tumors in rodents through TSH secretion).

The mechanism of action of hormone-induced carcinogenesis is unknown. However, all cancer-inducing hormones stimulate cell proliferation in their corresponding target organ. Some hormones (e.g., thyroid hormones, estrogens) bind to cellular receptors, which, by binding to specific DNA sequences, affect the expression of genes regulating growth and differentiation. The thyroid hormone receptor has been identified as the product of the proto-oncogene c-*erbA*, and thyroid hormone seems to play a role in the formation of tumors in laboratory animals, as well as breast cancer and other tumors in humans. For some estrogens, at least for the synthetic estrogen diethylstilbestrol, which transplacentally induces vaginal tumors in humans, a genotoxic activity could be demonstrated in addition. The extent to which environmental estrogens or "endocrine disruptors" contribute to human cancer incidence remains to be determined.

Immunosuppressive Agents

Both in humans (transplantation patients) and in laboratory animals, immunosuppressants may cause leukemia or lymphoma and, less frequently, solid tumors: e.g., azathioprine, 6-mercaptopurine, and cyclosporin A (increased incidence of kidney tumors after exposure to streptozotocin). In this connection, it should be mentioned that chemically induced tumors are immunogenic. Antigens associated with methylcholanthrene-induced tumors elicit exquisite specificity; for instance, even two sarcomas induced in the same mouse did not cross-react immunogenically.

Peroxisomes and Peroxisome Proliferators

There are approximately 100 nontoxic substances that increase the number of peroxisomes in the rat liver and induce rat liver tumors. Peroxisomes are organelles that are present in the cytoplasm of almost all eukaryotic cells, but particularly in hepatocytes. Their biological significance lies in the catabolism of long-chain fatty acids (the preferred substrate of peroxisomal β-oxidation). In addition, peroxisomes play a role in the metabolism of cholesterols and, possibly, in chemical thermogenesis and in maintaining a constant body weight. The entire hepatic peroxisomal enzyme activity in humans is only a quarter of that found in rats. The oxidases present in peroxisomes are of particular toxicological significance. Their catalytic activity leads to the release of H_2O_2 and, thereby, free oxygen radicals (genotoxic "oxidative stress"). There is perhaps a causal relationship between this capacity of peroxisomal oxidases and carcinogenesis, although this hypothesis is controversial: peroxisome proliferators often also induce cell proliferation in the liver and act as tumor promoters. The peroxisome proliferators include lipid-lowering agents, such as clofibrate and fenofibrate, plasticizers (phthalates), and solvents (1,1,2-trichloroethylene)—all substances that have not been shown to be genotoxic. There is no epidemiological evidence that peroxisome proliferators induce liver tumors in humans.

Carcinogenesis Induced by Foreign Bodies and Solids

Platelets of plastic material (organic polymers) may induce sarcomas at the site of application when applied subcutaneously. This effect depends solely on the physical properties of surfaces; the material is inactive as a powder. Here, too, chronic inflammatory reactions and increased cell proliferation are presumably the underlying mechanisms. Therefore, H. Selye (in 1961) attributed this type of carcinogenesis to "local stress." But other causes are also discussed, such as the production of free radicals by macrophages.

Asbestos dust (particularly blue asbestos or crocidolite) induces mesothelioma (malignant tumor of the pleura) after exposure by inhalation and, together with cigarette smoke, lung tumors. Here again, the external properties of the fibers (fiber length $>5\ \mu m$, fiber diameter $<3 \mu m$) play a major role. These fibers have a very long biological half-life. There is absolutely no doubt that the high asbestos concentrations ($>$100,000 fibers/m^3 of air) that were once measured at some workplaces have carcinogenic potential in humans. There is no epidemiological evidence, however, that this is also true for low or below-detection-limit concentrations, like those occurring in buildings that are now cleaned up because asbestos was used during their construction (caution: this results in mobilization of previously fixed fibers). As a result of preventive measures at the workplace, asbestosis is now a rare disease. Apart from this, a genotoxic–mutagenic activity of asbestos could not be demonstrated (although, depending on the content of iron, which increases the redox potential, active oxygen species were implicated as cause for asbestos-induced toxicity). Therefore, as with other epigenetic carcinogens, a threshold value must be considered for the epigenetic carcinogenesis due to asbestos.

There is some evidence that, like asbestos, other artificial mineral fibers, such as, rock wool, glass fibers, ceramic fibers, and also crystalline silicon dioxide (quartz), have carcinogenic potential. However, the fact that these fibers do not induce fibrosis and are only short-lived, does not support this view.

It should be mentioned in this connection that, when inhaled, soot and other particles, like titanium dioxide, zeolites, talcum, also induce lung tumors and, in some studies, pheochromocytoma (carcinogenesis by "irritation"). It is still not clear whether the lung tumors observed in rats after exposure to diesel emissions result from "irritation" by soot particles (particle overload inhibiting lung clearance, threshold value) or from exposure to genotoxic substances contained in the emissions. Frequently, the induction of lung tumors by foreign bodies is preceded by chronic granulomatous inflammation of the lung (like in asbestosis and silicosis). Furthermore, animal experiments suggest that foreign bodies (including intrauterine devices, IUDs) have a tumor-promoting effect.

Carcinogens in the Human Environment

Polycyclic Aromatic Hydrocarbons

For a long time, these substances were considered to be the most important environmental carcinogens altogether, or "humanity's fateful substances" (Bauer, 1963). They are created during each combustion process (including the incomplete combustion of organic material) and occur almost exclusively as mixtures (carcinogenic as well as noncarcinogenic and tumor-promoting substances), although often in different compositions (with benzo [*a*]pyrene as Leitmotif). For example, 280 polycyclic hydrocarbons have been demonstrated in cigarette smoke, 146 in motor vehicle exhaust, 108 in flue gas from oil heating, about 150 in crude mineral oil samples, and 106 in coal tar. They are also constituents of fossil fuels. Consequently, energy production for heating and traffic, as well as industrial combustion processes must be regarded as the most important sources of hydrocarbon emission (Table 10).

Accordingly, polycyclic hydrocarbons are usually found as air pollutants attached to soot particles and, after sedimentation, in water, soil, and vegetable food.

TABLE 10 Sources of Hydrocarbon Emission[a]

Source	Amount
Traffic	47%
Household heating	16%
Energy-producing plants	18%
Industry	19%
Chemical industry	2%
Hydrocarbon emission	16.6 million metric tons

[a]West Germany, 1982.

For example, 1400 metric tons per day were registered in the air above Los Angeles; the resulting human uptake of benzo[*a*]pyrene per day was equivalent to smoking one cigarette.

Though these substances are found as pollutants in our food, they are also created *de novo* during the thermic preparation of food (e.g., by roasting, frying, baking, deep frying, and smoking) and by migration from the packaging material. In Germany, the amount of benzo[*a*]pyrene in smoked meats is restricted to 1 μg/kg. The consumption of a grilled 200-g steak leads to the uptake of about 10 μg of benzo[*a*]pyrene. In Germany, the yearly benzo[*a*]pyrene uptake by food is estimated to be 0.35 to 1.2 mg per person. Another important source of exposure to these substances is smoking (0.4–0.8 μg benzo[*a*]pyrene per 20 cigarettes).

Aromatic Amines

The importance of mutagenic and carcinogenic heterocyclic amines has already been mentioned. They are created, for example, via the Maillard reaction as pyrolytic products during food preparation. Aromatic amines in cigarette smoke must be considered to be causally related to urinary bladder cancer in humans. Smokers of black tobacco, which has a high content of aromatic amines, have approximately a three-fold greater risk of developing bladder cancer than smokers of light tobacco.

N-Nitroso Compounds–Nitrosamines, Nitrosamides

In the human environment, these potent chemical carcinogens are often found in food and are created by the exogenous reaction of nitrate/nitrite with amines. The first experimental evidence for such contaminants came in 1969, through an investigation into the cause of the widespread deaths of sheep fed with nitrite-treated fish meal. The nitrosating reaction also occurs endogenously in the organism (particularly at the acidic pH in the stomach) with nitrate (from fertilizer converted into nitrite by bacteria in the saliva) or nitrite (pickling) and nitrosable amines (in food, daily uptake approximately 1 μg of dimethylnitrosamine; also from pharmaceutical products).

Apart from this, *N*-nitroso compounds are present in tobacco smoke (approximately 0.5 μg of dimethylnitrosamine or 10–20 μg of nitrosamines per 20 cigarettes; 10–40 times this concentration is in the sidestream smoke), but also in cosmetics (in Germany, the approved maximum is 50 ppb) and at certain workplaces, (e.g., in the rubber industry, chemical industry, metal-processing plants, and in areas working with hydraulic liquids).

Tumors as a Result of Lifestyle

It should be emphasized here that, apart from identifiable chemical substances, lifestyles play a special role in the genesis of human cancer. The following should be mentioned in particular: smoking, diet (e.g., alcohol: cancer of the esophagus), and physical activity.

With respect to diet, it is often said that, apart from identifiable chemicals, its composition represents a major risk factor (Table 3: 35%, range: 10–70%). Of particular importance are residues, such as, pharmaceuticals (antibiotics) and pesticides, food additives, such as, preservatives (butylated hydroxyanisole or hydroxytoluene), and mold infestation. In 1988, the United States Academy of Sciences estimated that 20,000 cases of malignant tumors per year can be attributed to the lifelong consumption of pesticide residues in food. The consumption of food additives in the United States is approximately 1.5 kg/person/year. Diets with high fat content (approximately 40% of calories taken up as fat) are connected with tumors of the colon, breast, prostate, ovary, endometrium, and pancreas. On the other hand, a diet rich in vegetables and fruit protects against cancers of the digestive and respiratory tract. Also discussed is a connection between fiber content of the diet and colon cancer. Reliable data supporting these hypotheses are missing. The health risk caused by smoking and alcohol abuse, however, is beyond doubt.

Anticarcinogenesis– Chemoprevention

A large number of substances can inhibit or suppress carcinogenesis (Table 11). The related findings usually stem from animal experiments, while the underlying mechanisms of action are mainly hypothetical. Their relevance to human health is a future research topic.

TABLE 11 Chemical Anticarcinogens

Type of inhibition	Substances (examples)
Inhibition of the nitrosating reaction (formation of nitroso compounds)	Ascorbic acid, tocopherols, phenols (such as caffeic acid)
Inhibition of metabolic activation, activation of carcinogen detoxification, scavenger of ultimate carcinogens	Phenols (butylated hydroxyanisole or hydroxytoluene), indoles, coumarines, flavones, diterpenes, dithiocarbamates, phenothiazines, barbiturates
Hormone receptor antagonists	Tamoxifen
Blockers of hormone synthesis	Finasteride
Inhibition of carcinogenesis, inhibition of tumor promotion, induction of differentiation	Retinoids, carotenoids, selenium compounds, protease inhibitors, inhibitors of arachidonic acid metabolism, phenols (butylated hydroxyanisole), aspirin, NSAIDs

METABOLIC ACTIVATION

The covalent modification of DNA by chemical (genotoxic) carcinogens plays a major role in the initiation of carcinogenesis and, possibly, also in tumor promotion and tumor progression. By interacting with DNA replication, these modifications may lead to mutations and, potentially, to cancer. Most of the chemical carcinogens, however, are chemically relatively inert. Before they can undergo reactions with nucleophilic groups of cellular macromolecules, they must be metabolically activated to turn into electrophilic "ultimate carcinogens."

Many different reactions and enzymes participate in the metabolic activation of carcinogens. To a high degree, this metabolic activation is species-, individual-, and organ-specific, and its induction and inhibition are substrate-dependent. At least in part, this variability poses major, still unsolved problems for the quantitative extrapolation of risks from experimental model systems to humans. The experimental findings concerning a carcinogenic potential have only qualitative validity for human health.

It should be mentioned in this connection that all cell culture-based model systems (mutation and transformation assays) are insufficient with respect to their capacity to metabolize xenobiotics. This deficit must be compensated for by adding external metabolizing systems (such as liver homogenate, microsomal fraction), by co-culture with metabolically active cells (primary hepatocytes), or by transfecting indicator cells with cDNA coding for the metabolism. The carcinogen-activating enzymatic reactions are of a multiple nature.

Oxidative Reactions

- Heteroatomic oxidation, particularly at the nitrogen atom, affects especially aromatic amines (leading, in the DNA, to C^8-guanyl adducts). (Oxidation at the phosphorus atom often leads to detoxification.)
- Epoxide formation affects polycyclic aromatic hydrocarbons, olefines, vinyl chloride, styrene, trichloroethylene, and aflatoxin B_1.
- C-hydroxylation affects nitrosamines (leading in the DNA to, quantitatively, mainly N^7 -alkylguanine; qualitatively and of mutagenic significance, mainly O^6 -alkylguanine and O^4/O^2 -alkylthymidine) and dialkyltriazenes. Further activation (estragole, 7,12-dimethylbenz[*a*]anthracene) may occur by subsequent sulfation.
- N-dealkylation of *N,N*-dimethylarylamines and pyrrolizidine alkaloids.

These reactions are catalyzed by microsomal P450 proteins (monooxygenases; at least 40 proteins are known): P450 1A1,—polycyclic hydrocarbons (benzo[*a*]pyrene); P450 1A2—aromatic amines; P450 2E1—benzene, styrene, vinyl chloride, ethyl carbamate, trichloroethylene, chloroform, carbon tetrachloride, nitrosamines, dichloropropane; and P450 3A4—aflatoxin, estradiol, 1-nitropyrene, pyrrolizidines. Flavone-containing monooxidases activate thioles and amines, while peroxidases activate mainly arylamines.

Reductions

Reductions lead to the activation of carbon tetrachloride, dinitropyrene (diesel emission), and nitroimidazole. Azo dyes are detoxified this way.

Conjugations

- Reactions with glutathione are primarily detoxification reactions, but polyhalogenated hydrocarbons and 1,2-dihaloalkanes are activated by this mechanism.

- Acetylations activate many hydroxylated compounds and detoxify aromatic amines. *N*-Acetyltransferases show a marked genetic polymorphism, which was discovered during the 1950s through the observation of interindividual variability in the metabolism of isoniazid. Subjects were classified as fast and slow acetylators and family studies demonstrated the genetic basis of this metabolic polymorphism. Since N-acetylation (NAT2) is a detoxifying step in the metabolism of aromatic amines, slow acetylators are at higher risk of developing bladder cancer (a suggestion that has been confirmed by epidemiologic studies). On the other hand, fast acetylators have been found to be at increased risk of developing colorectal cancer, possibly since some carcinogenic heterocyclic aromatic amines (i.e., pyrolytic products in food) may form DNA adducts via local (colon) *N*-acetyltransferase activation (NAT1), which also shows a genetic polymorphism. Though similar genetic polymorphisms exist in several enzymes that catalyze carcinogen activation or detoxification, epidemiological data linking a particular phenotype to increased or decreased cancer risk are often lacking.
- Sulfate esterification by sulfotransferases activate 2-acetylaminofluorene and 7,12-dimethylbenz[*a*]anthracene.
- Glucuronidation by UDP-glucuronosyltransferases affects *N*-hydroxyarylamines (metabolites of 4-aminobiphenyl), 2-naphthylamine, and some heterocyclic amines (pyrolytic products).
- Microsomal and cytosolic epoxide hydroxylases (epoxide hydrolysis) usually catalyze detoxification reactions; *in vitro*, however, metabolites of polycyclic aromatic hydrocarbons are activated. The significance of this latter observation is not clear.

MECHANISMS OF ACTION

Carcinogenesis (Fig. 10) is seen today as a multistep process that consists at least of the following mechanistically different phases, operationally defined as initiation, promotion, and progression. Thus, malignant cells develop progressively through new cell populations with increasing growth potential. After a latency period of years or decades, these phases lead from the initial transformation of a normal cell to the clinically manifest tumor. R. van Potter considered cancer as the result of a carcinogen-induced irreversible block in the terminal differentiation of a stem cell, whereby initiation is the irreversible conversion of a normal cell to a premalignant state. Without a stimulus to proliferate, this cell is kept under control by the surrounding normal cells. During promotion, the initiated cell is clonally amplified; this process seems to be partly reversible. The underlying proliferative stimuli are growth factors, solid bodies, wounds, and the death of cells and tissues. Skin papillomas during skin carcinogenesis, foci during liver carcinogenesis, and polyps during colon carcinogenesis are considered to be manifestations of this process (possibly the formation of arterial plaques during atherogenesis, too). Due to further genetic and epigenetic factors (activation of proto-oncogenes, such as c-*myc*), the malignant cell emerges during the irreversible phase of pro-

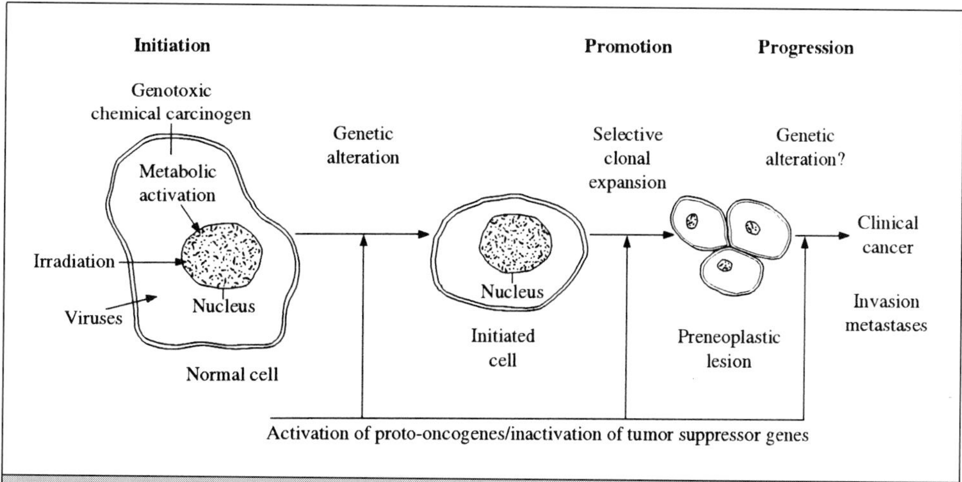

FIGURE 10 Phases of chemical carcinogenesis. Carcinogenesis is a multistep process that involves various genetic and epigenetic mechanisms, as well as (proto-)oncogenes and tumor-suppressor genes. Adapted with permission from Harris (1991).

TABLE 12 Familial Cancer Susceptibility[a]

	Risk of lung cancer	
	Normal family	Family with hereditary lung cancer
No cigarettes	1	4
Exposure to cigarettes	5.2	13.6

[a]In families with increased cancer risk, the cancer incidence is increased in both spontaneous and chemically induced carcinogenesis (relative risk factors).

gression. It is characterized by invasive growth and the formation of metastases.

Under the influence of the somatic mutation theory of T. Boveri (in 1914), carcinogenesis had almost been equated with mutagenesis, and mutation assays took center stage in developing test strategies for assessing the carcinogenic potential of chemicals. The modern view holds that carcinogenesis involves more than just mutagenesis and that cancer formation has its origin in genetic events (mutagenesis) as well as epigenetic events (mitogenesis).

After application of a chemical carcinogen, tumors are formed; their number and latency period depend on the dose of the carcinogen. In that regard, the law of Paracelsus, namely that the toxic effect depends on the dose, applies also to carcinogenesis.

It should be pointed out here that, apart from hereditary cancer syndromes (retinoblastoma, Wilms tumors) and recessive DNA-repair-defect syndromes (xeroderma pigmentosum), there also exists in certain instances a genetic or familial cancer predisposition (e.g., well-known cases of increased cancer incidence in families, such as stomach cancer in the Napoleon family). Many types of cancer seem to cluster in families due to a familial genetic susceptibility to cancer. This predisposition also exists for the susceptibility to chemical carcinogens (Table 12). Today, 5% of all breast cancer cases are considered to be hereditary. The mechanisms underlying these observations are still unknown, but at least the metabolism of carcinogens and the repair of DNA are genetically determined. The genetic epidemiology, (i.e., the study of a genetic predisposition for carcinogenesis) is one of the most important fields of cancer research. Thus, it has been demonstrated that the existence of cancer gene loci predisposes for familial polyposis (chromosome 5), medullary thyroid carcinoma (chromosome 10), melanoma (chromosome 9), pheochromocytoma (chromosome 10), and breast and ovary cancer (chromosome 17). It is interesting to note that the expression of such genes seems also to be ethnically determined. In recent years, several cancer-predisposing genes have been identified, which, when altered, can confer a very high risk of various human cancers (Table 13). Often, these tumors occur much earlier in life than environmentally induced cancers.

Furthermore, it should be mentioned that there exists also endogenous–spontaneous mutagenesis (and possibly carcinogenesis). During the normal metabolism of amino acids, sugars, and oxygen, reactive mutagenic species are formed, the mutagenic activity of which can be fixed in the genome by DNA replication. Polymerase errors (i.e., mutations) may occur during recombination but also during DNA repair or semiconservative DNA replication. As "adaptive mutagenesis," these processes possibly play an important

TABLE 13 Inherited Mutations in Genes That Predispose for a High Cancer Risk

Cancer	Gene	Type of gene
Breast, ovary	BRCA1	Tumor suppressor
Breast	BRCA2	Tumor suppressor
Breast, brain, sarcomas (Li-Fraumeni syndrome)	p53	Tumor suppressor
Colon	APC	Tumor suppressor
Colon	MSH2, MLH1	Tumor suppressor
Colon	PMS1, 2	Tumor suppressor
Melanoma	MTS1	Tumor suppressor
Retinoblastoma	RB	Tumor suppressor
Thyroid	RET	Oncogene
Wilms tumor	WT1	Tumor suppressor
Melanoma	p16	Tumor suppressor

role in evolution. Cancer as a result of mutations is possibly the price the individual organism has to pay for germ-line mutations that contribute to the survival of the species.

Genotoxicity

DNA Interaction—DNA Adducts and Mutations

A genotoxic chemical carcinogen is either electrophilic or it is converted to an electrophilic "ultimate" carcinogen by metabolic activation. These reactive species react covalently with DNA and other macromolecules and, thus, lead to structural and functional alterations in the DNA (mutation).

The following facts speak for a causal relationship between these reactions and the initiation of chemical carcinogenesis. All genotoxic carcinogens induce mutations and DNA repair processes; inherited defects in DNA repair (such as in the genetic disease xeroderma pigmentosum) predispose an individual to tumor formation; and practically all malignancies show chromosomal aberrations. In principle, two types of mutation are considered here, base-pair substitutions (methylation of a DNA base) and frameshift mutations (a shift in the reading frame, e.g., by intercalation of a molecule between the base pairs of the DNA and subsequent recombination).

Quantitatively, the formation of DNA adducts varies with different carcinogens, with different organs, and also within the genome ("hot spots"). Proliferating cells are particularly sensitive to interactions between the DNA and chemical mutagens. DNA adducts persist over long periods of time, partly until clinical cancer is manifest. By means of transgenic cell lines with defined DNA repair functions, the biological significance of DNA adduct formation could be demonstrated in a particularly impressive way. The formation of DNA adducts inhibits the synthesis of DNA and other macromolecules and leads to cell death, DNA repair processes, clastogenesis (including sister chromatid exchange), mutagenesis, teratogenesis (including transplacental carcinogenesis), and malignant transformation.

Today, the internal carcinogen load of an individual can be measured by the determination of DNA adducts, using specific antibodies or the ^{32}P-postlabeling method. The close relationship between mutagenic and carcinogenic activities of the genotoxic carcinogens has lead to the development of many genotoxicity assays (e.g., mutation assays, DNA repair assays) for the assessment of the carcinogenic potential of chemicals.

It should be mentioned that DNA adducts of genotoxic xenobiotics have also been causally implicated in chronic degenerative diseases, such as atherosklerosis and cardiomyopathies. Thus, detection of DNA adducts may provide a useful biomarker of the biologically active dose not only in carcinogenesis but also in other chronic diseases.

DNA Repair

Most alterations of the DNA are quickly corrected by a variety of DNA repair processes. Animal cells have pathways for direct reversal of damage in a single enzymic step, for recombinational repair of daughter strand gaps and for SOS repair. Different enzymatic DNA-repair processes thus guarantee the integrity of the genome, but their molecular mechanisms are not understood in detail. The essential role played by DNA-repair processes in the prevention and reduction of chemical carcinogenesis is illustrated by autosomal recessive genetic diseases in humans where defects in DNA repair are correlated with an increase in cancer incidence. Examples are xeroderma pigmentosum (skin cancer, sensitivity to UV light), Fanconi's anemia (leukemia), ataxia telangiectasia (lymphoma, sensitivity to X rays), Bloom's syndrome (various types of tumors, sensitivity to many agents), and, more common, hereditary nonpolyposis colorectal cancer.

Since genotoxic chemical carcinogens are able to induce DNA-repair processes, DNA repair assays also serve as indicators for previous DNA damage and for the carcinogenic potential of a chemical. Partial hepatectomy as well as repeated application of nitrosamines lead to the induction of DNA repair. Nevertheless, both processes increase the tumor incidence. There is no doubt, therefore, that the connection between DNA repair and carcinogenesis is complex (there is also "error-prone" DNA repair). These complexities include the fact that the induction of DNA repair is dependent on the class of chemical carcinogen, the sequence specificity of DNA alkylation, and also on the affected cells and organs (organ specificity of chemical carcinogenesis). For example, DNA alkylations seem to occur and persist especially within oncogenes. The repair of methylnitrourea-induced DNA adducts is particularly slow in the brain—the target organ of this carcinogen—compared to liver and kidney. Therefore, in addition to severe defects in DNA repair, large differences in the ability to repair DNA exist in the general population and such genetic polymorphisms influencing rate and fidelity of DNA repair may be one explanation for interindividual differences in cancer risk and species-, individual- and organ-specific differences in chemical carcinogenesis.

Oncogenes and Tumor Suppressor Genes

The somatic mutation theory of cancer (Boveri) has been confirmed by the cloning of genes that are altered (mutated) in tumors but not in normal tissue. Some of these mutated and thus activated genes confer their products with new functions (oncogenes), while the function of other gene products are lost as a consequence of genetic alterations (tumor suppressor genes). Cell culture and animal studies provided direct confirmation that such genes are involved in the process of multistage carcinogenesis, (i.e., at least in initiation and progression). These genes encode proteins that often play opposing and complementary roles. Proto-oncogenes often activate the cell cycle and thus stimulate cell division. Tumor suppressor genes code for genes leading to inhibition of cell division (i.e., they block cell proliferation).

Mutated proto-oncogenes (i.e., oncogenes) cause the stimulatory proteins to be overactive (i.e., the cells proliferate excessively). Mutation of tumor suppressor genes leads to inactivation of their gene products and may thus deprive cells of restraints of proliferation. The most common alteration found in human cancer, for instance, are mutations of the tumor suppressor gene p53; cells that have lost p53 activity can escape DNA repair and cell death (apoptosis) and proliferate. Mutations of p53 are known in aflatoxin-induced hepatocellular carcinomas (mutation, AGG → AGT in codon 249), tobacco-induced lung tumors (mutation, G → T in various codons), vinyl chloride-induced hemangiosarcomas of the liver (mutation, A:T → T:A in various codons), and aromatic amine-induced bladder cancer (mutation, G:C base pairs in various codons). There are today a great number of (until now unconfirmed) reports that the mutational patterns of tumor genes in primary tumors are of diagnostic value and of prognostic significance. Many such regulatory genes are known today (Table 14).

TABLE 14 Proto-Oncogenes and Tumor Suppressor Genes

Localization or Target	Gene	Tumor type
	Oncogenes	
Plasma membrane and growth factors or their receptors	PDGF (platelet-derived growth factor)	Brain
	erb-B (epidermal growth factor)	Brain, breast
	neu	Breast, ovary
	RET	Thyroid
Cytosol or plasma membrane/ signaling pathways	K-ras	Many
	H-ras	Many
	N-ras	Leukemia
	abl	
	raf	
	src	
Nucleus/activation of growth-stimulating genes	c-myc	Breast, stomach, lung, leukemia
	fos	
	myb	
Others	bcl-2 (blocks apoptosis)	Lymphomas
	Tumor suppressor genes	
Cytoplasm	APC	Colon, stomach
	NF1	Leukemia, nervous system
	NF2	Brain
Nucleus	RB	Retinoblastoma, bladder, lung, breast
	p53 (induces apoptosis)	Many tumor types
	WT1	Kidney
Others	BRCA1,2	Breast

Telomerase

Telomerase is an enzyme associated with cellular immortality (i.e., a hallmark of cancer). Telomerase rebuilds telomers, that is, the TTAGGG-repeated ends of chromosomes that regulate the number of divisions a cell can undergo. Germ-line cells express telomerase and are immortal; normal cells loose enzyme activity (and thus chromosomal integrity by the shortening of the telomers) when they mature. During carcinogenesis, a rare somatic cell may escape programmed senescence due to the shortening of the telomers, and the following extended cell survival (immortality) of such a cell may provide opportunities for the accumulation of additional genomic insults and progressive neoplastic evolution. Evidence exists that telomerase expression is considerably lower in normal (even renewal) tissues than in cancerous tissues (thus, telomerase might have potential as biomarker for the early detection of cancer).

Epigenetic Mechanisms—Effects on Growth Regulation

The postulated mechanisms of individual classes of epigenetic carcinogens have been discussed previously. The following deals briefly with some general mechanisms.

Cell Death and Cell Proliferation—Mitogenesis

Toxic effects of chemical substances associated with the induction of hyperplasia and regeneration (cell proliferation) are often closely related to their carcinogenic effect. Thus, differences in cell proliferation between target cells often are responsible for the species-specificity of carcinogenesis. It has been known for many years that, in the regenerating liver, the effect of chemical carcinogens is enhanced when DNA replication is increased. Infections or foreign bodies, as well as stones in gall bladder, kidney, and urinary bladder, increase cell proliferation in the affected organs or tissues and lead to nongenotoxic carcinogenesis (Table 9). In the male rat, the interaction of chemical substances, such as unleaded gasoline, 1,4-dichlorobenzene, α-limonene, isophorone, dimethylmethylphosphonate, hexachloroethane, and *tert*.-butyl alcohol, with $\alpha_{2\mu}$-globulin, which leads to a toxic accumulation of this protein in the nephron, seems to be particularly important in the case of kidney carcinogenesis. The $\alpha_{2\mu}$-nephropathy leads to tubular necrosis and, as a result, to regenerative cell proliferation. Therefore, the carcinogenic effect of these agents is directed toward the kidney of the male rat only. In humans, this protein does not exist. However, this hypothesis is in dispute. Some chemicals (the antiepileptic gabapentin, lindane, and trimethylpentane) induce this nephropathy and, nevertheless, do not induce kidney cancer; moreover, exposure to aviation fuels may increase the kidney cancer risk in humans.

Therefore apart from the induction of DNA damage, the induction of mitogenesis plays a key role in the process of chemical carcinogenesis. The induction of mitogenesis may lead by itself to mutations and to the inhibition of intercellular communication. On the other hand, nonproliferating mature neurons are not targeted by chemical carcinogenesis. Accordingly, the hyperplasia-associated toxic effect of nongenotoxic substances must be regarded as an indicator of possible carcinogenic potential. The compensating induction of cell proliferation after cell death leads primarily to increased mitogenesis and—due to errors during DNA synthesis and mitosis—possibly to secondary mutations in the dividing cells (Fig. 11), particularly because DNA repair processes are less active during DNA replication and mitosis. However, it is extremely important to note that such induced secondary processes might be associated with a threshold dose.

Cancer as a Disorder of Cellular Differentiation and Apoptosis

Obviously, there exists a close relationship between cellular proliferation on the one hand and terminal differentiation on the other. It has been assumed for quite some time that transforming substances interfere with cellular differentiation and, thereby cause uncontrolled growth. For example, they may block the differentiation of stem cells (teratocarcinoma). On the other hand, the induction of terminal differentiation may cause the transformed cells to lose their malignant phenotype (Fig. 12). The latter hypothesis has led to a new concept of cancer therapy. It should be noted that DNA methylation can affect the normal function of growth regulatory genes by mutagenic and epigenetic mechanisms.

Examples supporting this hypothesis are the induction of differentiation and simultaneous loss of malignancy in hematopoietic tumor cell lines, or the induction of myogenic determination and loss of tumorigenicity in transformed mouse fibroblasts.

Growth, differentiation, and programmed cell death (apoptosis) control the homeostasis of multicellular organisms. Disturbances of the balance between cell survival and apoptosis contribute to many diseases and pathological processes and are critical in carcinogenesis. Programmed cell death, apoptosis, is genetically controlled (for instance, induced by the

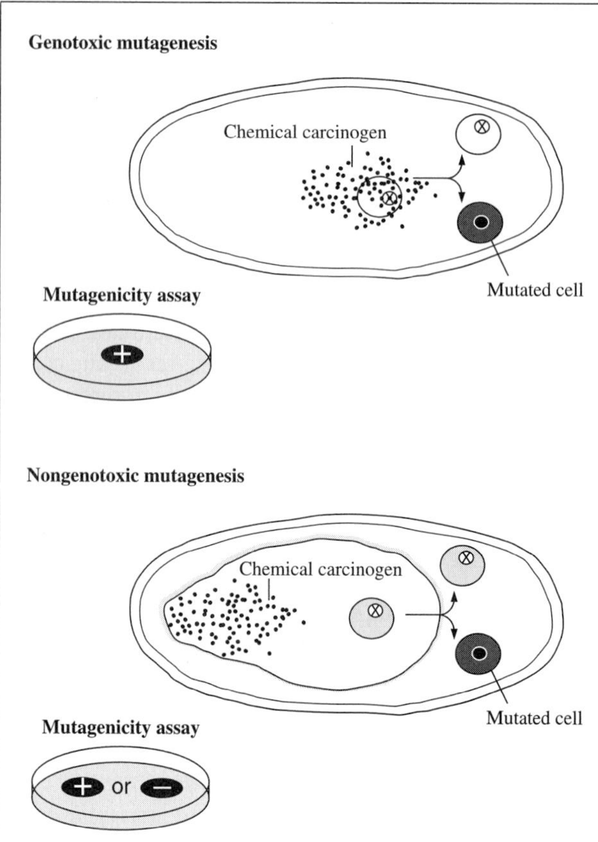

FIGURE 11 Mechanisms of genotoxic and nongenotoxic mutagenesis. In genotoxic mutagenesis, the chemical carcinogen is present within the initiated cell, where it reacts with DNA. In nongenotoxic mutagenesis, the chemical carcinogen is not necessarily present in the mutated cells; the mutation is caused secondarily by influences coming from the surrounding tissue (pear-shaped area). * indicates chemical carcinogen. (From Ashby and Leigibl (1992). Commentary: Transgenic mouse mutation assay. *Environ. Molec. Mutagen.* **20,** Copyright © Wiley-Liss, Inc. Adapted by permission of Wiley-Liss, Inc., a subsidiary of John Wiley & Sons, Inc.)

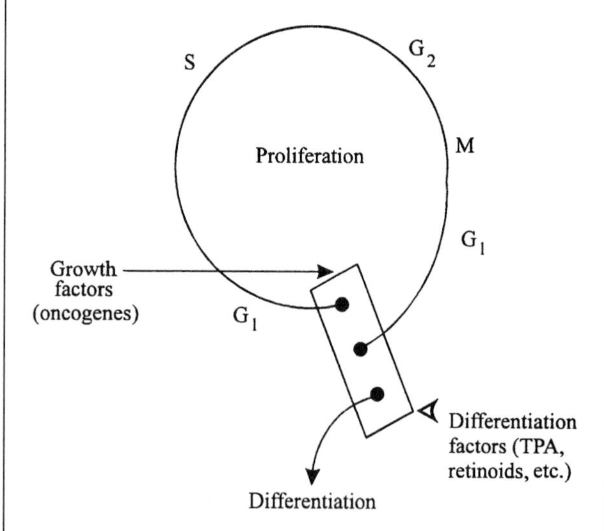

FIGURE 12 Proliferation (malignant phenotype) vs. differentiation. The cells are either in the cell cycle (driven by growth factors), or they differentiate under the influence of differentiation factors. The two processes are reversible: proliferation can be converted in differentiation, and vice versa. (From Block, 1984, with permission.)

p53 gene product and inhibited by the *bcl-2* gene product) and induced also by extrinsic factors, including certain carcinogens. It must be differentiated from cytotoxically induced necrosis. Treatments leading to an increase in apoptosis may eliminate DNA-damaged cells and initiated cells, as well as counter clonal expansion and suppress tumor growth. Alternatively, treatments inhibiting apoptotic processes may enhance the survival and expansion of precancerous cell populations. Agents such as 1,2-dichloroethylene, dimethylnitrosamine, and thioacetamide or retinoids are capable of inducing apoptosis while many nongenotoxic carcinogens (such as TPA, phenobarbital, TCDD, and other tumor promotors, peroxisome proliferators, cyproterone acetate and dichloroacetic acid) suppress apoptosis. Indeed, tumor promotors are considered cell survival factors (Fig. 13).

Cellular Signal Transduction—Cancer Genes and Receptor-Mediated Carcinogenesis

The malignant transformation of a cell leads to a tumor cell, which is generally characterized by uncontrolled growth; hence, it destroys the surrounding tissue by infiltration. Signal transduction pathways, such as the second-messenger pathway (second messengers, such as cyclic nucleoside phosphates, diacylglycerol, prostaglandins) represent a control mechanism by which the cells adapt to their environment and control their growth and differentiation.

The receptors involved are found mainly on the cell membrane, but also in the cytoplasm, on the nuclear membrane, or even on chromosomes (Table 14). Some receptors are ubiquitous and present on practically every cell; others are highly specific. Receptors for steroid hormones, thyroid hormones, retinoids, and vitamin D are soluble cytosolic DNA-binding proteins that regulate the transcription of specific genes. By contrast, receptors for peptides, like insulin or epidermal growth factor (EGF), are cell-membrane receptors that, for example, lead to the activation of mitosis via tyrosine phosphorylations. G-proteins (guanine nucle-

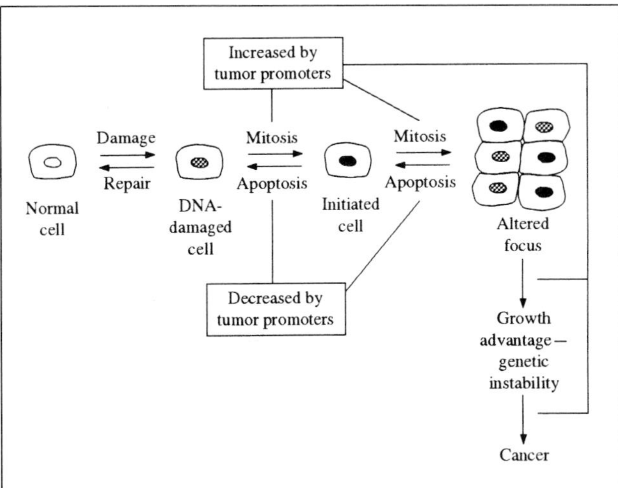

FIGURE 13 Mechanisms of tumor promoters. (From Roberts *et al.*, 1997, with permission.)

otide-binding proteins) as receptors activate various second-messenger pathways (adenylcyclase pathways, inositol phosphate pathways) and, thereby, cellular proliferation. Growth and differentiation are regulated particularly by protein kinases (multigene family—protein kinase C, PKC) and phosphatases, which are activated through the signal transduction pathways mentioned here.

Due to the high affinity of these receptors for their ligands, already tiny amounts of receptor-binding xenobiotics may influence the signal transduction pathways and, thereby, proliferation and differentiation. Some genotoxic carcinogens (polycyclic hydrocarbons, nitrosamines), as well as nongenotoxic carcinogens (dioxins such as TCDD; peroxisome proliferators; the antihistamine methapyrilene) and tumor promoters (TPA, which activates PKC; teleocidine; aplysiatoxin) interact with such receptors. These findings have led to the hypothesis that by binding to such receptors, carcinogens can irreversibly induce abnormal cell responses, such as abnormal proliferative behavior. Carcinogen–receptor interactions are influenced by ligand metabolism, receptor polymorphisms, receptor isoforms, and receptor levels and may also explain organ- and species-specific carcinogenesis, as well as the dependence of the carcinogen-susceptibility of organs and species on development and age of the animals.

Several factors regulate the behavior of cells and especially their proliferative capacity by means of signal transduction pathways and subsequently, for example, by tyrosine-specific kinases (PKC). Apart from growth factors (like EGF), such factors include tumor genes, oncogenes and tumor-suppressor genes (Table 14). Proto-oncogenes are normal cellular genes (*myc, fos, ras,* and at least 30 others) that may lead to abnormal regulation of growth and differentiation and to malignant transformation when falsely activated by point mutation, chromosomal translocation, or gene amplification. By contrast, tumor suppressor genes (like the p53 gene on chromosome 17p13 or the retinoblastoma gene) are normal cellular genes that may yield the same result when falsely inactivated. As discussed above, chemical carcinogens can activate proto-oncogenes and inactivate tumor suppressor genes. Some oncogene products have been identified as receptors for growth factors. In certain cases, it has also been shown that the cooperation of several oncogene products (such as the membrane-bound ras protein and the nuclear myc protein) is required for the induction of malignant transformation.

Changes in cellular signal transduction and the activation of proto-oncogenes or inactivation of tumor suppressor genes are regarded as possible common mechanisms of action of both genotoxic and epigenetic carcinogens. The identification of changes on this level of genetic and epigenetic cooperation will be important in throwing some light on the still unknown causal mechanisms of chemical carcinogenesis. The genetic and epigenetic mechanisms do not exclude each other; rather they act together in the multistep and multicause process of chemical carcinogenesis.

Oxidative DNA Damage

In the case of certain nongenotoxic carcinogens, DNA damage is induced by "oxidative stress." This could represent a common mechanism of action for chemical carcinogens. It is widely assumed that about 1 million of such incidents of DNA damage exist in the genome of a rat liver cell. About 100,000 new incidents of damage arise every day, and these may lead to mutations as well as cytotoxicity and, thereby, to regenerative cell proliferation. For example, activation of proto-oncogenes may result from mismatching caused by 8-hydroxydeoxyguanosine, which is a lesion commonly observed after oxidative stress. Enzymatic reduction (by catalase) of reactive species (hydrogen peroxide, superoxide radicals), as well as DNA repair, minimizes the induction of these lesions so that cells can survive such a massive damage. Oxidative stress can be induced by inflammatory processes (e.g., macrophages) and irradiation, and also by chemical substances like metals (e.g., iron and copper, neither of which is carcinogenic), peroxisome proliferators, polyphenols and quinones (butylated hydroxyanisole), and tumor promoters (e.g., TPA, which has a limited carcinogenic potential).

In this connection, it should be mentioned that endogenously or exogenously generated nitric oxide has also facilitated tumor growth by interacting with reactive oxygen species.

Methods for the Identification of Carcinogenic Potential

The methods available for assessing the carcinogenic potential of chemicals with the objective of minimizing the human exposure to carcinogens are based on our limited understanding of the mechanisms of chemical carcinogenesis. By employing diverse experimental test procedures, qualitative extrapolations to humans are feasible, but such extrapolations are almost impossible for the quantitative determination of the human health risk. Only in very rare cases do we have acceptable epidemiological data that could allow us to quantitatively assess, at least approximately, the human health risk after exposure to carcinogens. The problems encountered in epidemiological studies are partly due to our lack of knowledge about the external and, above all, internal exposure of individuals and, in part, to the latency period of chemical carcinogenesis. If toxicokinetic data are considered, important deductions toward the carcinogenic potential can often be made from the **chemical structure** of a xenobiotic substance.

In Vitro Short-Term Tests—Genotoxicity Assays

Of particular importance for the carcinogenic potential of xenobiotics is their chemical reactivity. This can be directly estimated, for example, by the determination of DNA adducts with the sensitive ^{32}P-postlabeling technique or indirectly by using genotoxicity assays.

Most of these assays use mutagenicity or other cellular responses to DNA damage (DNA repair) as endpoint. During the past decades, numerous such test methods have been developed.

With the help of genotoxicity assays, valuable information on individual substances and on their mechanisms of action could be deduced in special cases. In general, however, the efficiency of these assays in indicating a carcinogenic potential is very limited. Many carcinogens do not show mutagenic activity in conventional *in vitro* mutagenicity assays. The multistep process of carcinogenesis is more than just mutagenesis (and many chemical carcinogens are not genotoxic). Mutations per se may not be sufficient for tumorigenesis. Thus, in p53-knockout mice, tumors are formed by inhibition of apoptosis; nonpolyposis colorectal cancer patients show numerous mutations in all tissues but very few tumors only; mutagens induce DNA damage and/or mutations in many tissues but their carcinogenic effect is evident in very few only. These insights imply that the simplistic view that one agent causes cancer must be altered: multiple actions of cooperating compounds must be detected. In addition, there are mutagens that, so far, have failed to show any carcinogenicity. These facts significantly limit the validity of *in vitro* short-term tests for carcinogenic potential. It is unlikely that the activity in genotoxicity tests corresponds exactly with the carcinogenicity in laboratory animals or humans, respectively. Furthermore, these test are unsuited for the identification of carcinogens that act through nongenotoxic mechanisms.

Genotoxicity assays are well suited to identifying carcinogens with electrophilic genotoxic potential and, hence, play an important role in risk assessment. Genotoxicity has toxic effects beyond carcinogenicity and, therefore, represents a separate endpoint in the toxicological examination of chemicals.

In order to classify a chemical as potentially genotoxic, two assays are usually sufficient. These may have a high sensitivity, indeed. Of course, a substance cannot be classified as carcinogenic simply on the basis of its positive activity in such *in vitro* tests. It is up to research to clarify to what extent it may be more valid to employ *in vivo* mutagenicity tests, including those using transgenic animals.

Genotoxicity assays may contribute to the classification of carcinogens as being nongenotoxic. However, it must be emphasized that the classification of a substance as nongenotoxic carcinogen (Table 15) is far more difficult than the classification as genotoxic carcinogen. It requires the analysis of the complete toxicological profile (acute toxicity; understanding the mechanisms of action, i.e., uncovering events that might be at the root of the carcinogenic potential). This realization has implications for the assessment of risks.

Transformation assays must be viewed differently. They register as endpoints the transformation of a "normal cell" into a tumor cell and, like chemical carcinogenesis, are based on a multistep process (effects of oncogenes and tumor-suppressor genes; interaction with cellular differentiation). They are also different from genotoxicity assays with respect to their capacity to register the carcinogenic potential of

TABLE 15 Assays to Screen Nongenotoxic Carcinogens

Mechanism-based assays
- Gap-junctional intercellular communication
- Modified gene expression/differentiation
- Immortalisation of cells
- Aberrant cell proliferation, induction of ornithine decarboxylase, etc.

Transformation assays
- SHE, BALB/c-3T3, CH_3-10T1/2, CH3-M2

Newborn rodents

Transgenic rodents
- Muta Mouse (lacZ)
- Big Blue Mice: induced mitogenesis
- p53-heterozygous knockout mouse
- human c-Ha-*ras* or v-Ha-*ras* transgenic mice

chemicals. These assays are able to identify nongenotoxic carcinogens and tumor promoters (TPA, TCDD) (Table 16). However, it is still not known why human cells, unlike rodent cells, are very rarely transformed in culture.

In Vivo Carcinogenesis Assays— Bioassays

Carcinogenesis assays in rodents currently represent the important and absolutely essential bioassay for uncovering the carcinogenic potential of chemicals. Available for this purpose are limited (short-term) assays (induction of skin tumors in mice, lung tumors in A/Heston or A/J mice, breast tumors in female Sprague–Dawley rats, and foci in rat liver), as well as the classical chronic bioassay.

The classical whole-animal carcinogenesis assay in rodents (duration at least 2 y in rats, 1.5 y in mice) has recently been criticized as being nonrepresentative for carcinogenic activities in humans, especially because of the use of the maximum tolerated dose (MTD). Without doubt, this assay has its uncertainties with respect to the extrapolation of high experimental doses to the mostly low doses of normal human exposure:

- It is not known whether rodents are a representative model system.
- It has not been proven that a linear dose–activity relationship exists.
- Synergistic effects are not taken into account.
- Protective effects (metabolic detoxification and DNA repair) are possibly exhausted by high doses.
- High doses (MTD) induce toxic (lethal) effects, which may lead to regeneration by increased cell proliferation (mitogenesis favors chemical carcinogenesis).

TABLE 16 Examples of Transforming Nongenotoxic Carcinogens

Amitrol	Arsenic compounds
Asbestos	5-Azacytidine
Benzene	Diethylstilbestrol
17β-Estradiol	Ethionine
Vincristine	

There are no data, however, that directly prove the existence of such discrepancies between rodents and humans. On the contrary,

- All substances known to have carcinogenic activity in humans are also positive in rodent bioassays, often even with comparable doses and identical organ specificity.
- Although numerous chemical substances are carcinogenic in laboratory animals but not in humans, many human carcinogens have only been discovered because of their carcinogenicity in animal experiments (e.g., aflatoxin, diethylstilbestrol, 4-aminobiphenyl, and vinyl chloride).
- The carcinogenic effect of chemical substances in rodent bioassays is not observed only with substances of obvious toxicity.
- None of the 143 rodent carcinogens has been proven to be noncarcinogenic in humans.

With respect to carcinogenic activity, the chronic bioassays cannot be expected to correlate completely with the human situation, neither in a qualitative nor in a quantitative sense. Its interpretation calls for a complete analysis of the toxicological profile of a substance (weight of evidence approach; especially species-comparative toxicokinetic studies). Studies on the mechanisms of action are indispensable. Nevertheless, with respect to risk assessment and in view of our available knowledge, it seems important to distinguish between genotoxic (electrophilically reactive) and nongenotoxic (epigenetically active) substances once they have been identified in animal experiments as potential carcinogens.

It must be emphasized also that the use of general toxicity findings to evaluate the carcinogenic potential or risk of compounds is fraught with uncertainty; available data do not support a general correlation between chemically induced toxicity and carcinogenicity.

Risk Assessment

Chronic carcinogenesis bioassays with whole animals represent the foundation for assessing the human health risk of exposure. The complexity of the mechanisms underlying chemical carcinogenesis and our lack of knowledge in this regard complicate the evaluation of data obtained from animal experiments. The qualitative extrapolation of experimental data to humans depends on the analysis of the entire toxicological profile of a substance. Quantitative extrapolations are currently not possible. There is no doubt that cancer incidence and the latency period (after which the chemically induced tumors become clinically manifest) are dosage-dependent. Numerous examples in humans can be quoted in support of this; they stem from radiation biology (bone tumors following exposure to radium, thorotrast-induced liver tumors) as well as chemical carcinogenesis (bladder cancer after exposure to 2-naphthylamine, mesothelioma after exposure to asbestos). The cancer risk after exposure to very low doses, however, is controversial. The stochastic theory, though never validated, holds that the risk becomes less likely with decreasing doses, but it will never be zero.

According to this theory—which does not accept threshold values—the cancer risk after chemical exposure is calculated from animal experiments (with the MTD); that is, the calculation is done according to the nonthreshold linear relationship model. It is, therefore, possible that the real risks are widely overestimated. Against this model speaks also the fact that, despite the intrusion of chemistry into our world (we are exposed daily to approximately 70,000 chemicals), the cancer incidence in the industrial world did not significantly increase after the Second World War. A rational risk extrapolation from the high doses of experimental studies to the mostly low doses of normal human exposure will only be possible once we understand the mechanisms of chemical carcinogenesis.

The findings concerning the mechanisms of action, especially the existence of genotoxic and nongenotoxic carcinogens, have significant implications for risk assessment (Fig. 14).

- Threshold values cannot be provided for genotoxic carcinogens. Nevertheless, the carcinogenic effect of such substances shows a clear dose–effect relationship with respect to tumor incidence and latency period. It is a fact that most of the identified human carcinogens induce cancer only after exposure to high doses.
- There are good reasons for the assumption that threshold values do exist for nongenotoxic carcinogens; their control may, therefore, follow standard practices of toxicological analysis (e.g., NOAEL, no observable adverse effect level; uncertainty factor; ADI, acceptable daily intake). This approach, however, requires a careful recording and analysis of those biological and toxicological effects of substances that precede carcinogenesis. At least nongenotoxic carcinogenesis is, therefore, a dosage phenomenon like any other toxic effect and not a "yes or no" property of the chemical substance.

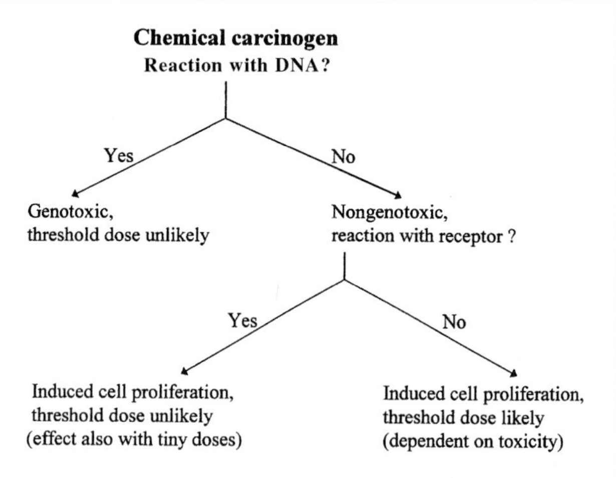

FIGURE 14 Classification of chemical carcinogens. (From Cohen and Ellwein, 1991, with permission.)

Apart from this, genotoxic carcinogens seem to be more potent, while nongenotoxic carcinogens probably represent a smaller risk to human health (Tables 17–18). Mitogenesis affects the carcinogenicity of both, genotoxic and nongenotoxic (epigenetic) carcinogens (Fig. 11). (When tested within the MTD range, genotoxic carcinogens induce cytotoxicity through DNA damage and, thereby, regenerative cell proliferation. Nongenotoxic carcinogens, too, may indirectly act as mutagens by inducing cytotoxicity and regenerative cell proliferation.) Thus, in the case of genotoxic carcinogens, there is an amplifying interaction (mutagenesis and mitogenesis) involved in the process of carcinogenesis. This explains why genotoxic carcinogens have a greater carcinogenic potential (Table 18). In contrast to nongenotoxic carcinogens, they often induce tumors in several species and in a larger number of organs (81% of carcinogens that induce tumors in rats and mice and in several organs are also mutagens). The significance of mutagenesis as a causal factor might also explain the high sensitivity of rodent assays (MTD): 50% of the several hundreds of substances tested in these assays yielded positive re-

TABLE 17 Properties of Chemical Carcinogens[a]

	Genotoxic carcinogens	Nongenotoxic carcinogens
Active after single exposure	Sometimes	No
Active after subtoxic doses	Frequently	No
Dose–effect relationship	Yes	Yes
Threshold dose	Very low or none	Relatively high
Species specificity	Several species	Only very few species
Transplacental activity	Yes	No
Human cancer hazard	Yes?	No?

[a]From Williams (1987), with permission.

TABLE 18 Susceptibility of Humans to Some Nongenotoxic Mechanisms of Carcinogenesis in Rodents[a]

Target tissue	Mechanism in rodents	Human susceptibility
Kidney	$\alpha_{2\mu}$-Globulinopathy	Nil: no $\alpha_{2\mu}$-globulin
Liver	Peroxisome proliferators	None to date: hepatocytes unresponsive *in vitro*
	Chlorinated hydrocarbons and phenobarbital-like enzyme inducers	None to date: hepatocytes unresponsive *in vitro*
Thyroid	Goitrogenic	None to date: thyroid gland is relatively insensitive to TSH
	Liver enzyme inducers (reduce T3/T4, increase TSH)	None to date: thyroid gland is relatively insensitive to TSH
Mesovarium	β-agonists (in rats)	None to date at therapeutic dose levels (exposure too low or absence of receptor?)
Mammary	Increased prolactin secretion (dopamine antagonists)	Unlikely: negligible role for prolactin
	Increased estrogen	Likely: if exposure is elevated and prolonged
Uterus	Decreased prolactin secretion (dopamine agonists)	Unlikely: different endocrine control of endometrial activity
Stomach	Prolonged gastrin secretion (H_2 antagonists, proton pump inhibitors)	Unlikely: gastrin secretion not elevated in a sustained manner under therapeutic exposure conditions
Testis	Prolonged LH secretion	Possible
Bladder, kidney, stomach, skin	Chronic irritation	Unlikely: exposure necessary to cause prolonged inflammation (factors include pH, Na^+ crystal formation, or anything causing cell proliferation) will not be tolerated
Lymphatic system and other tissues	Immunosuppression	Likely: if exposure is prolonged and causes immunosuppression

[a]From Monro (1993), with permission.

sults, but only 35 substances or groups of substances could be identified as human carcinogens. (These data are not directly comparable; cancer mortalities are not recorded in bioassays, while tumor incidences are not recorded in human populations.)

CONCLUSION

"What we know is a drop, what we do not know—an ocean" (Isaac Newton). In spite of significant gains in knowledge, we are still moving mainly in the dark when dealing with the quantitative importance of risk factors in chemical carcinogenesis (Table 3), the mechanisms of action of chemical carcinogens (Table 8), and, hence, their detection and the assessment of their risks to human health. The basic understanding, especially of the mechanisms of nongenotoxic carcinogenesis, is still missing.

We have to accept that life has its advantages as well as its risks. Security exists if we consider a risk as being acceptable—which may be an individual or a social decision. In a highly industrialized society, the activities of one individual certainly include disadvantages to other members of society. Rigid restrictions, including those applying to industrial activities, without compelling reasons lead easily to far-reaching losses to society. This is especially true for chemical carcinogens and their regulation.

The simplistic public concerns for environmental and industrial carcinogens pushes too far into the background the role that our lifestyles (not only smoking) play in human carcinogenesis and, thus, also any effective preventive measures of the individual.

Bibliography

Ashby, I., and Leigibl, U. (1992). Commentary: Transgenic mouse mutation assay. *Environ. Mole. Mutagen.* **20,** 145–147.

Barrett, J. C. (1993). Mechanisms of multistep carcinogenesis and risk assessment. *Environ. Health Persp.* **100,** 9–20.

Barrett, J. C. (1995). Mechanisms for species differences in receptor-mediated carcinogenesis. *Mutat. Res.* **333,** 189–202.

Bauer, K. H. (1963). "Das Krebsproblem." Springer Verlag, Berlin.

Bloch, A. (1984). Induced cell differentiation in cancer therapy. *Cancer Treatment Repts* **68,** 199–205.

Clayson, D. B. (1962). "Chemical Carcinogenesis." J. A. Churchill, Ltd., London.

Clayson, D. B., and Iverson, F. (1996). Cancer risk assessment at the crossroads: The need to turn to a biological approach. *Regul. Toxicol. Pharmacol.* **24,** 45–59.

Cohen, S. M., and Ellwein, L. B. (1991). Genetic error, cell proliferation and carcinogenesis. *Cancer Res.* **51,** 6493–6505.

Cooper, C. S., and Grover, P. L. (eds.) (1990). "Chemical Carcinogenesis and Mutagenesis I/II," Handbook of Experimental Pharmacology, Vol. 94 I/II. Springer Verlag, Berlin.

Elespuru, R. K. (1996). Future approaches to genetic toxicology risk assessment. *Mutat. Res.* **365,** 191–204.

Goldsworthy, T. L., Conolly, R. B., and Frausson-Stehen, R. (1996). Apoptosis and cancer risk assessment. *Mutat. Res.* **365,** 71–90.

Gonzalgo, M. L., and Jones, P. A. (1997). Mutagenic and epigenetic effects of DNA methylation. *Mutat. Res.* **368,** 107–118.

Grover, P. L. (ed.) (1979). "Chemical Carcinogens and DNA." CRC Press, Boca Raton, FL.

Harris, C. C. (1991). Chemical and physical carcinogenesis: Advances and perspectives for the 1990s. *Cancer Res.* **51,** 5023s–5044s.

Kayser, D. (ed.) (1986). "Kurzzeittests zum Nachweis von Kanzerogenen, BGA-Schriften." MMV Medizin Verlag, München.

Klassen, C. D. (ed.) (1996). "Casarett and Doull's Toxicology," 5th ed. Pergamon Press, New York.

Monro, A. (1993). The paradoxical lack of interspecies correlation between plasma concentrations and chemical carcinogenicity. *Regul. Toxicol. Pharmacol.* **18,** 115–135.

Office of Science and Technology Policy (1985). Chemical carcinogens. *Federal Register* **14.3,** 10371–10442.

Prehn, R. T. (1994). Cancers beget mutations versus mutations beget cancers. *Cancer Res.* **54,** 5296–5300.

Roberts, R. A., *et al.* (1997). Perturbation of the mitosis/apoptosis balance: A fundamental mechanism in toxicology. *Fundamen. Appl. Toxicol.* **38,** 107–115.

Rosenkranz, H. S., and Klopman, G. (1993). Structural evidence for a dichotomy in rodent carcinogenesis: Involvement of genetic and cellular toxicity. *Mutat. Res.* **303,** 83–89.

Schmähl, D. (ed.) (1981). "Maligne Tumore, Entstehung—Wachstum—Chemotherapie." Editio Cantor, Aulendorf.

Sell, S., and Pierce, G. B. (1994). Maturation arrest of stem differentiation is a common pathway for the cellular origin of teratocarcinomas and epithelial cancers. *Lab. Invest.* **70,** 6–20.

Tomatis, L. *et al.* (1997). Avoided and avoidable risks of cancer. *Carcinogenesis* **18,** 97–105.

Trosko, J. E. (1997). Challenge to the simple paradigm that "carcinogens" are "mutagens" and to the in vitro and in vivo assays used to test the paradigm. *Mutat. Res.* **373,** 245–249.

Williams, G. M. (1987). Definition of a human cancer hazard. *In* "Nongenotoxic Mechanisms in Carcinogenesis" (B. E. Butterworth and T. J. Slaga, eds.), Banbury Report no. 25, pp. 367–378. Cold Springs Habor Laboratory.

CHAPTER

8

Tumor Promotion

R. SCHULTE-HERMANN, B. MARIAN, and W. BURSCH
Institute of Tumorbiology–Cancer Research, University of Vienna, Austria

STAGES OF CARCINOGENESIS

Initiation and Promotion—Early Discoveries

In 1917 Yamagiwa and Ishikawa demonstrated that tar can induce cancer in experimental animals. This discovery paved the way for mechanistic investigations of carcinogenesis. The isolation of polycyclic aromatic hydrocarbons from tar yielded compounds with a specific carcinogenic effect. This contrasted with the earlier view that cancer is induced unspecifically by chronic injury and inflammation. In the early 1940s Rous, Beerenblum, Mottram, and others investigated carcinogenesis on mouse skin induced by polycyclic aromatic hydrocarbons and by a strong skin irritant obtained from Euphorbia plants, croton oil. At low doses, both factors alone had no effect, but when combined, the same low doses produced numerous tumors. The sequence of treatments was crucial; tumors formed only when *first* the aromatic hydrocarbon and *then* croton oil was administered. The reverse sequence had no effect (Fig. 1). It was concluded that tumorigenesis in skin depended on two inherently different processes—initiation and promotion.

Likewise, carcinogenesis in other organs was found to require the action of different factors. Soon after their discovery, estrogens were shown to produce mammary cancer in mice (Lacassagne in 1932). This carcinogenic effect was seen in mouse strains with high spontaneous rates of mammary cancer, but not in strains with low rates. Obviously, the carcinogenic effect of estrogens depended on the presence of (genetically transmitted) susceptibility to cancer formation in the mammary gland. Genetically determined susceptibility may correspond to initiation; hormones were considered as "conditional carcinogens" (Butenandt; Hecker). Furthermore, hormones were found to promote tumor development after initiation by chemical carcinogens or radiation in a variety of organs.

In the last few decades the validity of the initiation–promotion concept has been demonstrated in a number of different organs. It was expanded to the multistage concept of carcinogenesis. It integrates the earlier, appearingly antagonistic concepts of cancer causation by chronic irritation (Virchow) or by somatic mutation (Boveri, Bauer). Thus, chemical compounds have been important tools in elucidating the complex biological processes involved in carcinogenesis.

Evolution of Cancer

The multistage concept implies that normal body cells are not transformed immediately or by a single event into malignant cells. Rather malignant cells develop stepwise via a sequence of intermediary cell populations whose phenotypes deviate increasingly from the original cell (Fig. 2). Histological correlates of intermediary populations, such as foci of altered cells or benign tumors, adenoma, and papilloma, in a variety of organs of animals and humans have been described.

Each of the various intermediary cell populations is considered to originate from single cells. They constitute clones ("clonal genesis" of tumors). The inter-

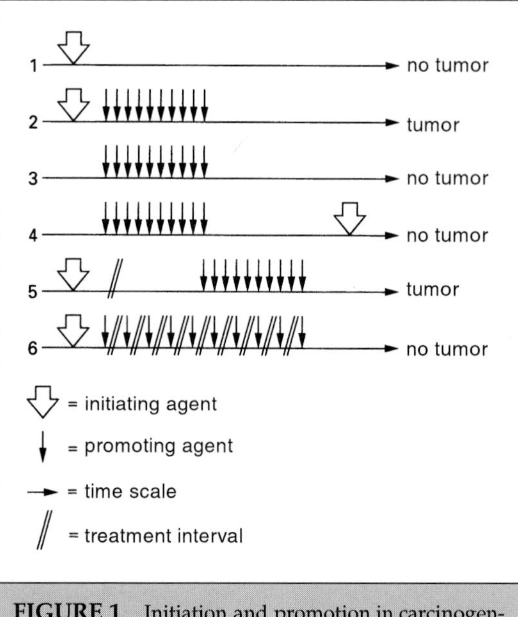

FIGURE 1 Initiation and promotion in carcinogenesis (from Boutwell, 1964, modified with permission of S. Karger AG, Basel).

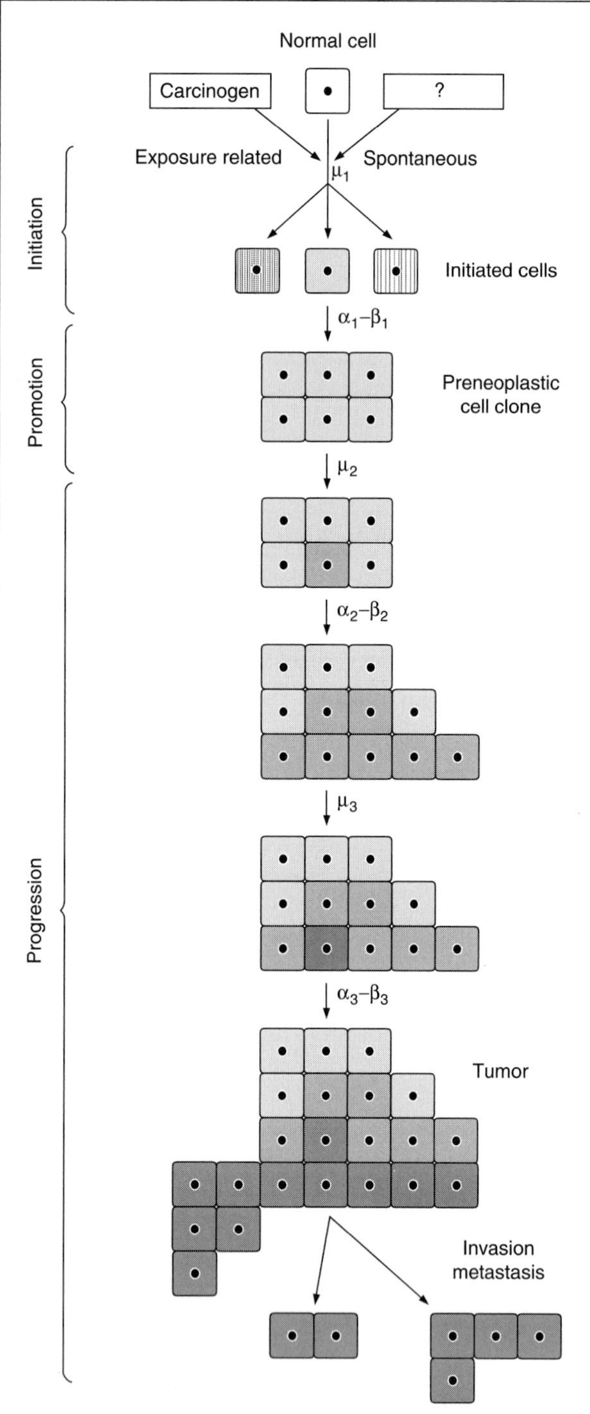

FIGURE 2 Multistage concept of carcinogenesis. Initiation results from exposure to certain noxes (e.g., genotoxic chemicals, ionizing radiation) or for unknown reasons ("spontaneously"). There may appear different types of initiated cells. In the figure one of these is promoted to form a clone of initiated (preneoplastic) cells. Subsequently, further cell clones with increasing phenotypic (and genotypic) deviation develop up to frank malignancy. Abbreviations: $\mu_{1,2,3}$: rates of initiation or further transformation; $\alpha_{1,2,3}$: rates of cell proliferation; $\beta_{1,2,3}$: rates of cell death.

mediary cell populations grow more rapidly than the tissue of origin (preferential or selective growth). This proliferative advantage is low in early populations and becomes manifest with promotion, while growth of later populations is further increased, frequently independent of promotion. However, even some cancers require the presence of promoting factors. Thus, certain cancers of the breast and prostate stop growing after estrogen or androgen deprivation, and even regress.

The sequential formation of a series of new cell clones can explain why in most cases cancer development requires a long latency phase constituting a considerable fraction of the life-span of the organism. The overall rate of cancer formation is determined by the rate of *formation* of new cell phenotypes (μ in Fig. 2). μ increases with the size of the population at risk. Hence the *growth rate* of intermediary cell populations (α-β in Fig. 2) is a second very important determinant of cancer development. A third determinant is the *number* of sequential intermediary populations (or stages) until appearance of the malignant cell. These determinants can be used for mathematical modeling of carcinogens. Chemical compounds can modify the rate of carcinogenesis by affecting mutation frequency, growth rate, or expression of phenotypic deviations.

What is the driving force behind the appearingly directed development from normal to malignant cells? The underlying principle is the same as in evolution of life; (stochastic) formation of *new cell pheno-*

types and *selection* of those able to escape from inhibitory mechanisms in the organism. Although the evolution of cancer cells usually results in death of the host, from an evolutionary point of view this is not a disadvantage because most cancers develop beyond the reproductive age.

Initiation

Initiation and promotion are operationally defined in the context of each other, mainly on the basis of experimental work with mouse skin, rat liver, and a few other tissues. Initiation is produced by complete or incomplete carcinogens (see following). The essence of initiation is a proliferation advantage over normal cells in the presence of tumor promoters. Initiation alone does not lead, or only slowly leads, to tumor formation. The lag phase between initiation and the beginning of promotion can be short or long; obviously initiation is a persistent alteration and is transmitted to daughter cells (Fig. 2).

Initiation is a rare event. In animal experiments even high doses of genotoxic carcinogens yield only relatively few initiated cells. In rat liver following treatment with a high dose of nitrosamine only one of 10^6 liver cells is initiated. Apparently, initiation requires a very specific kind of damage. Furthermore, in some tissues only a small fraction of cells can be initiated (stem cells in renewing tissues). Initiation can occur rapidly. One single dose of short-lived carcinogens such as methyl- or ethylnitrosourea may produce initiation in susceptible tissues (pulse carcinogenesis).

Initiation seems to require cell replication. Therefore developing organisms in embryonal and perinatal stages usually are much more susceptible to carcinogenic effects than adults. Incomplete carcinogens such as methylnitrosourea have little if any initiating activity in the liver of adult animals; however, if liver growth is stimulated by partial hepatectomy shortly before methylnitrosourea, liver cells become quite susceptible to initiation by this agent. The late G_1 and early S phase are the most sensitive phases of the cell cycle. This is probably due to incomplete DNA repair before DNA replication, which results in mispairing of bases in the daughter strand, mutations, and (presumably) initiation.

The efficiency of initiation depends on the state of differentiation of the target tissue. During maturation of the mamma, a window of high sensitivity for initiation by carcinogens exists (see the following section on Tumor Promotion, Mammary Gland).

Mechanistically, in many cases initiation is due to mutations of DNA or of chromosomes. Initiating noxes frequently have genotoxic or mutagenic activity. Presumably, a mutation of some proto-oncogene or tumor suppressor gene, such as described in Chapter 7, may be the crucial event in initiation. However, no genetic alterations specifically associated with initiation have been found. Some inborn gene alterations (e.g., defects in tumor suppressor genes) similar to initiation enhance the susceptibility of tissues to promoters (see the following sections on Tumor Promotion, Colon; Mammary Gland).

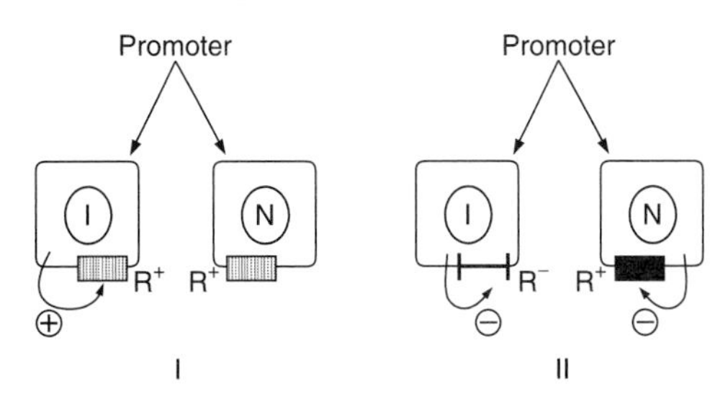

FIGURE 3 Cooperation between initiation and promoter effects, two hypothetical models. Model I: Initiation results in synthesis of a growth-stimulating signal ⊕. The promoter induces or activates a receptor (R^+) recognizing this signal. The initiated cell thereby stimulates itself in an autocrine way. Model II: Initiation leads to the disappearance or insensitivity of a receptor (R^-). This protects the initiated cell from inhibitory signals ⊖ released by the tumor promoter. Abbreviations: I, initiated cell; N, normal cell.

A nonmutational (i.e., epigenetic) origin of initiation is possible, at least in some types of cancer. Heritability of initiation to daughter cells does not exclude this possibility. Most differentiated cells transmit their phenotype to daughter cells without "fixation" by mutations. Specific changes in the methylation pattern of DNA may be one of the epigenetic mechanisms involved. The hypothesis of "Imprinting" cells, (e.g., by diethylstilbestrol), as discussed in the following section on Tumor Promotion, Other Sexual Organs, may serve to illustrate the concept of epigenetic initiation.

Genetic and functional alterations causing an initiated state of cells appear to be diverse. Cells can gain a proliferative advantage by an enhanced or sustained response to stimulatory signals during tumor promotion or by a reduced response to inhibitory effects (Fig. 3). More details are described in the following.

Promotion

Tumor promotion is operationally defined as a process accelerating and enhancing the formation of tumors after initiation. The essence of promotion is the selective multiplication of initiated cells (Fig. 2). Promotion before or without initiation has no tumorigenic effect (Fig. 1). Promotion always requires a prolonged period of action, which may last weeks, months, or years. The effect of promotion may disappear again after termination of treatment. Promoter doses below a certain threshold are not effective. Therefore tumor promotion, at least in early stages, is considered reversible. These characteristics contrast sharply with characteristics of initiation (Fig. 1; Table 1).

Tumor promotion is frequently associated with enzyme induction and growth or with tissue damage in the affected organs. Genotoxic events and mutations apparently are not necessary for promotion. A high degree of organ specificity is an important characteristic of many tumor-promoting agents, in contrast to initiation, which may occur in several organs in parallel. Therefore, tumor promotion may determine the target organ of carcinogenic action. Some agents may act as promoters in one organ, but as antipromoters in another organ (Table 2). In contrast to these rather specific actions, over-caloric nutrition has a broad promoting effect on tumor development in numerous organs (see the following sections on Tumor Promotion).

Originally, the definition of tumor promoters implied the absence of initiating activity. This understanding is abandoned because the *absence* of a biological effect cannot be proven. In fact, virtually all tumor promoters tested in long-term studies at high doses produced tumors without preceding initiating treatment (see the previous section).

TABLE 1 Characteristics of Tumor-Promoting Effects

Enhancement and acceleration of tumor development (higher yield, shorter lag phase)
Synergistic (over-additive) effects if combined with initiating carcinogens
Organ specificity (frequently)
Growth stimulation in target organ (regenerative, adaptive or hormonally induced = receptor mediated)
Preferential (selective) growth of cancer prestages
Enhanced expression of the "preneoplastic phenotype" of tumor prestages
Reversibility[a]
Threshold[a]
Long duration required

[a]Not yet generally proven.

Progression

The sequence initiation to promotion produces only *pre*neoplastic lesions and *benign* tumors. Their transformation into malignant lesions is termed progression (Fig. 2). Thus, more than one genetic lesion appears to be necessary for malignancy. In most cancers genotypic and phenotypic alterations do not reach a fixed endpoint but show increasing autonomy and potential for metastasis. This continued alteration and enhancement of the malignant phenotype is also called progression (by Foulds). Induction of mutations by genotoxic carcinogens can lead to progression. A variety of changes in growth-controlling genes have been found in progressing tumors; the sequence of changes seems variable.

An inherent instability of the genome is a characteristic of progressed lesions. Mutations of the tumor suppressor gene p53 may be involved in genome instability. The p53 gene contributes to monitoring and repair of DNA damage; it delays progress to the S-phase of the cell cycle until DNA repair is completed. The p53 gene was therefore named "guardian of the genome." In many human tumors, it is inactivated by mutation. This may result in more rapid accumulation of genetic damage and accelerate progression. Likewise, defects in mismatch repair mechanisms that correct base alterations in DNA may result in enhanced mutation rates and genome instability.

Complete and Incomplete Carcinogens

Many chemical carcinogens have both initiating and promoting activity. They are termed complete carcinogens. Examples are carcinogenic polycyclic hydrocarbons, nitrosamines, and aromatic amines. On the other hand, methyl- and ethylnitrosourea and urethane (previously used as hypnotic) in most models had only initiating activity. Such agents are called incomplete carcinogens. Certain agents can act as complete carcinogens in one organ, in others only as initiators. Thus, acetylaminostilben produces tumors in the zymbal gland of the rat (a sebaceous gland at the ear duct region), but not in mamma, liver, and kidney; induction of initiated cells in these organs was shown by treatment with target-specific promoters, which yielded numerous tumors (Table 2). Cisplatinum, an important cytostatic drug and genotoxin, produced tumors in the lung, but not in skin of mice. Application of the skin tumor promoter croton oil resulted in the appearance of numerous skin papillomas indicating the formation of initiated cells in skin by cisplatinum. It is possible that many of the geno-

TABLE 2 Tumor Promoters Determine the Target Organ of Carcinogenic Effects

Initiating carcinogen	Promoter	Target organ
Nitrosomethylurea	Phenobarbital	Liver, thyroid gland
	Saccharin	Bladder
4-Acetylaminostilbene	None	Zymbal gland[a]
	Phenobarbital, DDT	Liver
	Diethylstilbestrol	Mamma, liver
	β-cyclodextrin	Kidney
Nitrosodiethylamine	Phenobarbital	Liver, thyroid gland
	Barbital	Liver, kidney
2-Acetylaminofluorene	Phenobarbital	Liver
	Saccharin	Bladder
	Methylthiouracil	Thyroid gland
	Butylhydroxyanisol	Bladder: promotion
		Liver: *antipromotion*

[a] A sebaccous gland at the ear-duct region.

toxic carcinogens in human environment at the low doses present have purely initiating effects.

Modification of Carcinogenesis (co-, anti-, syn-carcinogenesis)

Multiple interactions at the various stages of carcinogenesis can modify the formation of cancer. Some chemicals and biological events can increase or decrease the susceptibility to initiating effects without being carcinogenic themselves (co- and anticarcinogenesis). (The original definition of co-carcinogenesis included promotion, but this use has been abandoned.) Co-carcinogenic effects may result from induction of enzymes activating procarcinogens, from inhibition of inactivating enzymes, or from increase of cell replication. Co-carcinogenesis differs from syn-carcinogenesis, where the effect of one carcinogen is enhanced by a second carcinogen; for syn-carcinogenesis, the sequence of agents is not important. Co- and syn-carcinogenesis should not be mixed up with promotion, which is effective only after initiation. If the nature of the modifying effect is unclear, the term "enhancement" may be appropriate.

RELATION BETWEEN TUMOR PROMOTERS AND NONGENOTOXIC CARCINOGENS

Nongenotoxic or epigenetic carcinogens lead to formation of tumors without exhibiting detectable mutagenic or genotoxic activity in the majority of test systems. The human carcinogens asbestos, diethylstilbestrol, estrogens, cyclosporine, and others can be categorized into this class. Animal experiments have identified numerous additional nongenotoxic carcinogens, including various trophic hormones (Table 3).

There is a close relationship between nongenotoxic carcinogens and tumor promoters.

1. Almost all members of both groups of agents share the ability to induce or accelerate growth in their target organ. This may result from regenerative or adaptive–hormonal mechanisms. The effects are frequently organ specific and reversible; they have to persist for prolonged periods of time in order to produce tumors.
2. The known tumor promoters are carcinogenic even if given alone (i.e., without initiating treatment). Conversely, compounds first identified as nongenotoxic carcinogens usually show tumor promoting activity if tested in two-stage protocols. Saccharin (rat urinary bladder tumors) and limonene (male rat kidney tumors) represent two well-studied examples.

Thus, a clear discrimination between tumor promoters and nongenotoxic carcinogens is not possible. Rather, the classification of a compound largely depends on the experimental protocol to which the compound was subjected.

Assuming that nongenotoxic carcinogens are merely tumor promoters, one has to ask for the origin of initiation. Possible answers could be that the compound may initiate by genotoxic effects undetectable

TABLE 3 Some Tumor Promoters and Nongenotoxic Carcinogens That Induce Hormonal Imbalance, Cell Proliferation, and Hyperplasia and upon Chronic Treatment May Lead to Tumors

Substance	Primary effect	Hormone or nervous function increased	Target organ for chronic hyperplasia and tumor induction
Omeprazol (ATPase inhibitor)	Reduced secretion of gastric acid	Gastrin	Stomach: enterochromaffine cells
Bromocriptin (dopamine agonist)	Hypophysis: reduced secretion of prolactin	Estrogen	Endometrium
Estrogen, haloperidol (dopamine antagonist)	Hypophysis	Prolactin	Mamma
Estrogen, inhibitors of androgen synthesis	Hypophysis	LH	Testicles: Leydig cells
Methylthiouracil, inhibition of thyroid gland	Thyroid gland: reduction of T_4 synthesis	TSH	Thyroid gland: follicular cells
Reserpin	Emptying of catecholamine stores	Nervous stimulation (splanchnicus)	Adrenal gland
Cyclosporin	Decrease of T-lymphocytes		B-cell lymphomas

in current test systems, or by epigenetic mechanisms, or indirectly via enhanced proliferative activity resulting in enhanced replication errors, mutation, and initiation (Table 4). Furthermore, initiated cells may occur spontaneously due to a genetic or environmental background. If promoted, these spontaneous initiated cells will develop into tumors. Histological studies suggest the occurrence of preneoplastic lesions in various target organs of nongenotoxic carcinogens. In rodent liver such foci increased in size and number with increasing age. Promoting nongenotoxic carcinogens had pronounced carcinogenic effects in old but not in young animals.

KINETIC AND MECHANISTIC ASPECTS

Growth and Cell Replication

Growth events can be assigned to three categories (Table 5), depending on the physiological state and on the stimulus. All three types may contribute to tumor promotion. Chemical agents with promoting activity induce either regenerative or hyperfunctional (adaptive) growth.

According to the proliferative behavior of their cells, tissues in the adult organism are designated as renewing, static (expanding), or stable. In renewing tissues (skin, mucosal epithelia, blood cells, and immune cells), differentiated cells do not proliferate and have a limited life span. Dying cells are continuously replaced by proliferation and differentiation of undifferentiated stem cells. In skin and mucosa, these are located in the basal cell layer or in intestinal crypts; blood-forming stem cells are found in the bone marrow. Cell loss, functional demand, and hormonal stimuli may enhance the rate of proliferation of stem cells. Stem cells are the target for initiation in these tissues.

Static tissues (liver, thyroid gland, and kidney tubules) exhibit low cell turnover in the healthy adult organism. Cell losses or functional load or hormonal stimulation can induce the formation of new cells, which mainly originate from differentiated cells of the tissue and not from stem cells. Differentiated cells can be initiated. After hormonal or functional stimulation, organ enlargement and hyperplasia are maintained as long as the stimulation is effective. However, the en-

TABLE 4 Dual Role of Cell Proliferation in Carcinogenesis

Formation of mutations

- Transformation of promutagenic DNA damage in mutations (e.g., DNA-adducts → mispairing of bases during replication)

Errors during DNA replication → spontaneous mutations (Fidelity of DNA replication is <100%)

Multiplication of initiated and (pre)neoplastic cells

- → Formation of clones of initiated and (pre)neoplastic cells
- → Enhanced probability for progression to malignant phenotype
- → Tumor growth

TABLE 5 Categories of Growth

Fetal and perinatal growth; Stem-cell-dependent growth
→ Steadily high rates of cell replication
Regenerative growth
Cell loss by acute or chronic toxicity
→ Replacement by enhanced cell replication
Adaptive and hormonally induced growth (hyperfunctional growth)
Cell replication enhanced, but only initially until new steady state is reached
→ Chronic hyperplasia, "growth pressure" during entire period of stimulation, regression after end of stimulation (by active cell death, apoptosis)

hanced cell replication is restricted to the first few days of treatment. Subsequently cells become resistent to the mitogenic effects but still show enhanced function (e.g., enhanced enzyme activity). This "mitosuppressed" state may result from a feedback system that monitors the DNA content or cell number of the organ and prevents cell multiplication beyond physiological needs. Possibly, initiated cells escape from this mitosuppressed state (see the following). The presence of the stimulus ensures survival of the excessive cells; after withdrawal, organ hypertrophy and hyperplasia are reversible (Fig. 4). Functional increases are also reversible.

Cells of stable tissues (e.g., neurons) do not proliferate in the adult organism and are no longer responsive to tumor induction. (Brain tumors in the adult are of mesenchymal, not neuronal origin.)

Cell replication is important at various stages of carcinogenesis (Table 4); it is a prerequisite for formation of mutations and of initiated cells. Because of some, albeit low, infidelity of genome replication, mutations may occur in the absence of genotoxic chemicals or radiation. This may lead to spontaneous initiation in an occasional cell (Fig. 2). Furthermore, cell replication is essential for the growth of initiated and (pre)neoplastic cell populations. However, high cell proliferation per se does not necessarily mean high cancer risk. During embryogenesis tumors are rarely formed despite of high rates of cell replication. In the adult organism, some tissues such as the small intestine show high proliferative activity, but rarely develop malignant tumors, in remarkable contrast to the large bowel. Likewise, not every increase of cell proliferation by chemicals is necessarily associated with an enhanced risk for tumor promotion or carcinogenesis.

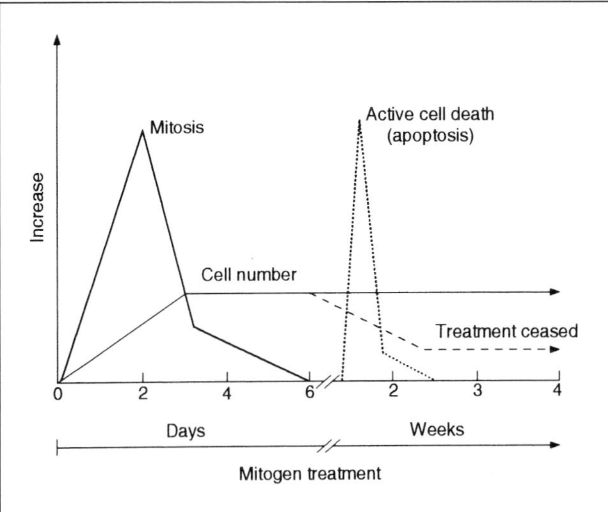

FIGURE 4 Cell proliferation and hyperplasia after functional–hormonal stimuli. Regression after end of stimulation.

Cell Death, Apoptosis

The growth rate of cell populations is principally determined by the difference between birth rates (α) and death rates (β) of cells ($\alpha - \beta$ = net growth rate). Traditionally cell death has been viewed as a passive degenerative phenomenon. An actively controlled, programmed or "suicide" cell death was first observed during regression of excessive embryonal tissues and later in the adult organism. Active cell death counteracts mitosis to maintain homeostasis of cell number in organs. It serves to eliminate excessive cells during involution of organs, such as after withdrawal of mitogens (Fig. 4). Also, damaged cells are eliminated by active mechanisms unless essential cellular functions such as ATP synthesis or maintenance of ion gradients are seriously harmed. This active type of cell death is mostly referred to as apoptosis. Originally the definition of apoptosis was based on a specific morphology (condensation followed by fragmentation and heterophagy). This does not cover other types of active cell death, such as the type characterized by autophagic–lysosomal intracellular degradation. Therefore the terms active or programmed cell death should be preferred unless specific evidence of apoptotic death is available.

Preneoplastic and tumor cell populations are characterized by a shift in the balance of birth and death of cells favoring clonal expansion $(\alpha_{Tu} - \beta_{Tu}) > (\alpha_{no} - \beta_{no})$. Active cell death frequently is not decreased in tumors and preneoplastic lesions but may occur at much higher rates than in the tissue of origin, although in growing tumors replication rates exceed death rates. Thus, in many tumors, cell turnover is more rapid than in normal tissue. Active cell death may also eliminate some of the initiated cells formed spontaneously or from carcinogen exposure (Fig. 5). Therefore, the regulation of cell survival is pivotal for development and growth of tumors.

Tumor promoters may inhibit active cell death in initiated or neoplastic cells and thereby accelerate the accumulation of these cells and enhance the incidence of cancer. This survival factor activity of tumor promoters is part of their growth-stimulatory effect (Fig. 6).

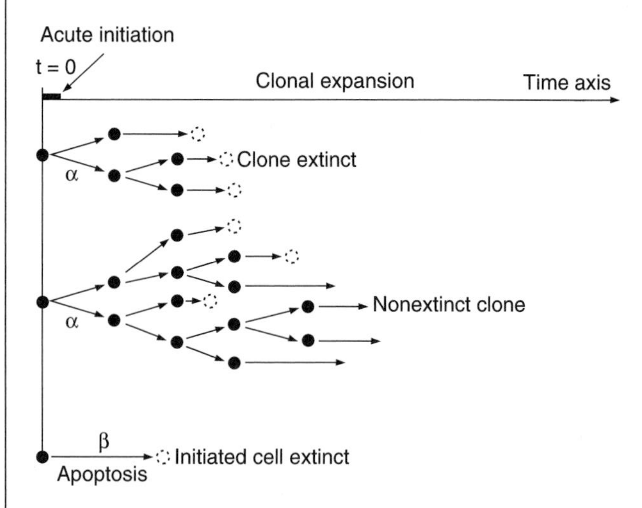

FIGURE 5 Relevance of cell birth and death for clonal expansion and extinction. Only initiated cells are shown. Cells may either divide or undergo death. If all cells in a clone die, the clone becomes extinct. The probability of this occuring is high when the clone is small. From Luebeck *et al.* (1995), modified.

Mathematical Models of Carcinogenesis

Mathematical models may help to elucidate the development of cancer. Earlier models assumed that malignant tumors arise from a single cell via a sequence of irreversible steps. The "linearized multistage model of Armitage and Doll adequately describes the incidence of many adult human carcinomas and is still used for risk assessment of carcinogenic chemicals. However, these earlier models do not take into account growth of intermediate cell populations and hence the effects of tumor promotion. More recent approaches such as the "two-mutation clonal expansion model" by Moolgavkar and co-workers include both the multistage nature of carcinogenesis and variations in growth rates of intermediate (initiated) cell populations. Rates of formation of intermediate or malignant cell types ($\mu 1$, $\mu 2$, ...) (Fig 2), of cell division (α), and of cell death (or differentiation) (β) are used in these models. An important aspect is that initiated cells may die if β is greater than 0 ($\beta > 0$). The probability of a clone being extinguished is determined by the ratio of birth and death rates $\beta{:}\alpha$. If $\beta > \alpha$, then the (asymptotic) probability of elimination is 1 (Fig. 5). The number of cells (clone size) determines the time necessary for extinction. Thus, inclusion of cell kinetics (α and β) provides a basis for mathematical modeling the effect of tumor promotion and its reversibility.

Signals Regulating Growth

Multicellular organisms have developed a network of signaling mechanisms to adapt growth and function of individual cells to the needs of the entire organism. Growth and death factors are either generated distantly from the target organ and distributed via the bloodstream (endocrine control) or generated in closer proximity (paracrine control). Autocrine signals are produced by the target cells themselves.

These signals tightly control cell replication and cell death in a dual way (i.e., by stimulation and inhibition). A number of growth factors stimulate replication and at the same time inhibit death, that is, act as survival factors. Conversely, replication-inhibiting factors may induce cell death (Fig. 6).

Extracellular signal molecules are recognized by specific receptors located either on the surface or inside of the cell. Some membrane receptors contain a protein kinase domain at the intracellular region, phosphorylating tyrosine or serine–threonine in proteins. Other membrane receptors generate intracellular signals via G proteins or second messengers such as cAMP or diglycerides. Intracellular signals eventually will modulate transcription rates of growth-regulating genes. Receptors for more lipophilic signal molecules such as steroid and thyroid hormones, which diffuse through the cell membrane, are located within the cell. They are nuclear transcription factors that are activated by binding of the signal molecule, subsequently bind to specific recognition sites called "response elements" in target genes, and regulate their transcription.

Intracellular second messengers and signal transduction cascades activated by extracellular mitogenic or death factors are closely interconnected, thereby providing precise control of the life and death decision of the cell. Some proto-oncogenes such as c-*myc* and c-*fos* seem to activate regulatory cascades for both

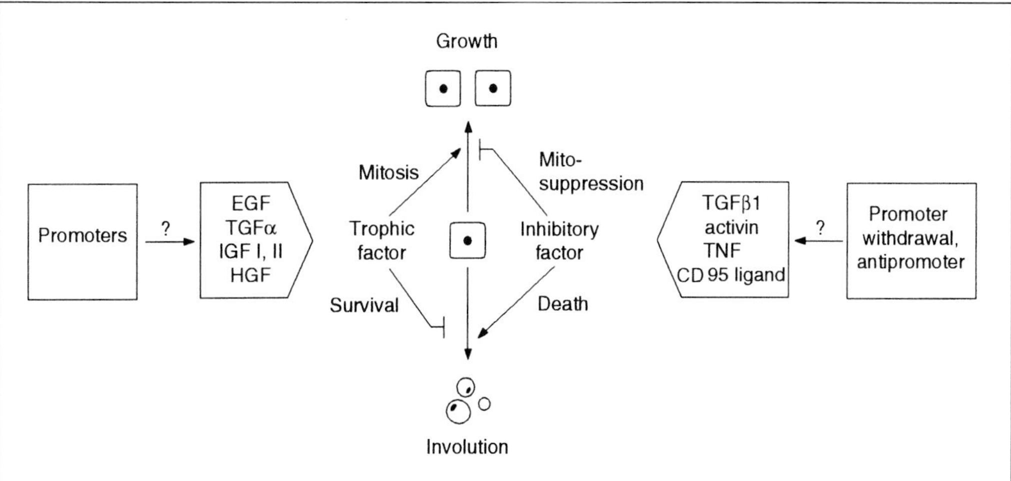

FIGURE 6 Regulation of birth and death of cells. The balance between replication and death of cells is tightly controlled according to the physiological needs of the organism. Some mitogenic growth factors also act as survival factors. Examples are transforming growth factor α (TGF α), epidermal growth factor (EGF), or insulin-like growth factors I and II (IGF I, II). Mitosis-inhibiting factors may induce cell death, for example, transfoming growth factor $\beta1$ (TGF $\beta1$), activin A, and tumor necrosis factor (TNF α, β). A further important death signal is the ligand to the CD 95 (= fas, Apo I) receptor. Tumor promoters interfere with mechanisms maintaining the balance between birth and death of cells. Schulte-Hermann *et al.* (1995), modified.

suicide and replication. To survive, the suicide program of cells must be continuously suppressed by extracellular survival factors or by intrinsic factors such as BCL2. During the G1 phase of the cell cycle, there is a checkpoint regulating further progression to the S phase but may also drive cells into death. The p53 gene product, the retinoblastoma protein, cyclin E, and other proteins seem to be involved in the control of these events.

Exogenous promoters interfere with this growth-regulatory network in multiple ways. Some mimic endogenous growth signals and bind to receptors; others modulate the phosphorylation status of proteins in signal cascades. Still other promoters affect growth of target cells only secondarily, while their primary effects may be cytotoxic and/or occur in other organs (Table 3). Specific agents are described in the following sections on Tumor Promotion.

Intercellular Communication through Gap Junctions

One way of signaling between cells is to exchange small regulatory molecules through gap junctions, channels in the plasma membrane. They provide an open connection between the cytoplasm of neighboring cells allowing an exchange of molecules up to approximately 1000 Da. The channels consist of proteins called connexins. Specific connexins occur in different cell types. The regulation of gap-junctional communication occurs either rapidly by opening and closing of channels or in a protracted way via connexin synthesis (Fig. 7).

Many tumor cells were found to communicate via gap junctions with each other, but not with normal cells. Restitution of gap junctional communication between normal and transformed fibroblasts suppressed the transformed (malignant) phenotype. It was concluded that lack of intercellular communication can lead to uncontrolled growth. A variety of different tumor promoters inhibited intercellular communication *in vitro* in test cells. These agents include phorbol ester, diglycerides, phenobarbital, and DDT.

Phenotypically altered liver foci exhibited a reduction of liver specific connexin (Cx 32); treatment with tumor promoters resulted in a further decrease which was reversible after stop of treatment (Pitot, 1990). Studies on isolated tissue specimens (*ex vivo*) suggested a reduced exchange of test compounds between individual focus cells. Inhibition of communication of initiated or preneoplastic cells with their normal neighbors could be a mechanism of escape from the growth inhibitory environment in a resting tissue.

To what extent inhibition of gap-junctional intercellular communication by tumor promoters may be im-

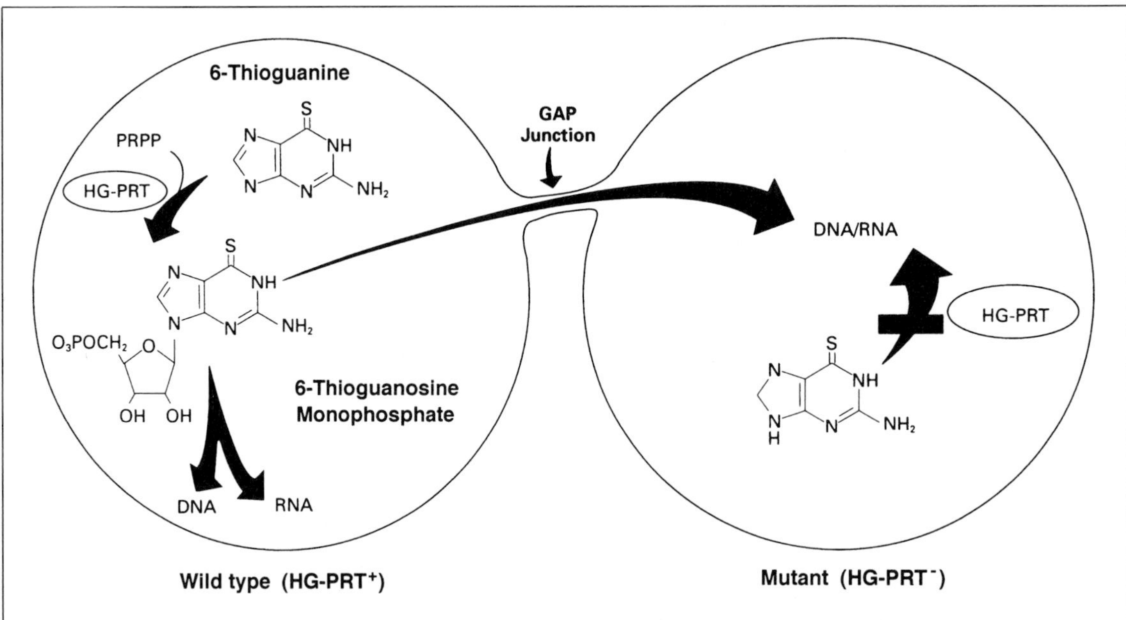

FIGURE 7 Intercellular communication by gap junctions (GJIC). Schematic illustration of metabolic cooperation. The pretoxin 6-thioguanine is activated to a toxic metabolite by hypoxanthine–guanine phosphoribosyltransferase (HG-PRT). HG-PRT$^-$ mutant cells survive in a medium containing 6-thioguanine. If cocultured with sensitive wild-type cells, the toxic metabolite will spread through gap junctions into the resistant cells, which consequently die. Reproduced from Trosko *et al.* (1982), with permission.

portant for carcinogenesis can not be evaluated, because almost all observations were made *in vitro* with a limited number of different cell types. It seems questionable whether results with one cell type can be extrapolated to others because tumor promotion in most cases appears to be highly cell type specific.

TUMOR PROMOTION IN SPECIFIC ORGANS

Skin

Experimental Models

Polycyclic aromatic hydrocarbons (PAH), such as dimethylbenzanthracene or methylcholanthrene, are mostly used as initiators, but many other carcinogens are equally effective (Table 6). They are administered locally to the skin, but are also effective if administered systemically; for example, single doses of cisplatin or urethane given parenterally produce initiated keratinocytes that respond to subsequent tumor promotion. In many skin tumors of the mouse (both papillomas and carcinomas) mutations of the Ha-*ras* gene have been demonstrated. They mostly involve codon 12 or 61 and are characteristic of the initiator used (Table 6). Normal keratinocytes obtained from skin adjacent to the tumors do not contain these mutations, indicating that they are caused by the initiator in individual basal cells to which they confer a selective growth advantage. For recovery from cellular damage the initiator might have caused, at least one week is allowed to pass before promotion treatment starts.

The tumor promoter administered locally causes irritation and hyperplasia after one single treatment. For tumor production, however, the treatment must be continued for several weeks, when premalignant papillomas are first observed. Depending on the dose

TABLE 6 Initiators in Mouse Skin

	ras Mutation	
Initiator	Codon	Mutation
Dimethylbenzanthracene	61	A = >T
Methylcholanthrene	61/13	A = >T/G = >T
Methylnitronitrosoguanidine	12	G = >A
Ethylnitrosourea	12	G = >A
Urethane	61	A = >T
Cisplatin	61	A = >T
UV light	61	C = >A/A = >T

applied, both tumor incidence (number of animals with tumors) and tumor yield (number of tumors per animal) reach a maximum after about 12–20 weeks (Fig. 8).

For efficient tumor formation it is crucial that the intervals between promoter applications do not exceed a certain time period. Apparently, each dose must be applied while the previous one is still effective (Fig. 9), indicating that the effects of a single promoter administration are reversible. In addition, subdivision of the efficient doses into smaller portions results in a loss of promoting activity; obviously the effects of small subthreshold doses are not additive and every single promoter dose has to exceed a certain threshold level (Fig. 9).

This causes a remarkable contrast between complete carcinogens and tumor promoters; if dose vs latency period is plotted on a log–log scale, the dose–effect relationship is linear for complete carcinogens but sigmoid for tumor promoters, indicating the existence of a threshold dose for tumor promoters.

Tumor-Promoting Substances, Wounding

The first skin tumor promoter identified was croton oil, a skin irritant obtained from the seeds of *Croton tiglium,* an Euphorbiacea, that had been in use as a strong laxative. Several related plant species (Euphorbiaceae and Thymelaceae) contain similar compounds. During the 1960s a series of structurally related compounds was isolated from croton oil. They are tricyclic diterpene alcohols, esterified with different fatty acids at positions 12 and 13 (phorbol esters) (Fig. 10). Their isolation in a pure chemically defined form has since allowed elucidation of their basic biological and biochemical effects.

In contrast to its esters, phorbol alcohol by itself is ineffective both as irritant and as tumor promoter, and even small changes in the ring structure of the esters abolish the tumor-promoting effectivity. All active promoters have a 4β-configuration, while 4α-phorbol esters are inactive. Methylation of the OH residue at position 4 also yields a promoter with very low activity. Modification of the fatty acid residues modulates promoting activity (Table 7). The optimal side chains are saturated fatty acids with 10–14 carbon atoms, the most active ester being 12-*O*-tetradecanoyl phorbol 13-acetate (TPA). Unsaturated side chains result in a qualitative shift of the activity (see the following section on conversion).

Several other diterpenes, as well as chemically unrelated compounds, also have promoting activity in mouse skin (Table 6; Fig. 10). Like the phorbol esters, they cause stable hyperplasia and inflammation in the skin.

A full-thickness wound involving both epithelium and connective tissue has strong tumor-promoting activity. It causes epidermal hyperplasia, growth response, and inflammation. Endogenous growth factors like TGFα, TGFβ, and FGF, which are involved in the process of wound healing, stimulate connective tissue and epidermal proliferation and may have tumor-promoting activity. Superficial wounding that does not involve the connective tissue has much weaker promoting activity.

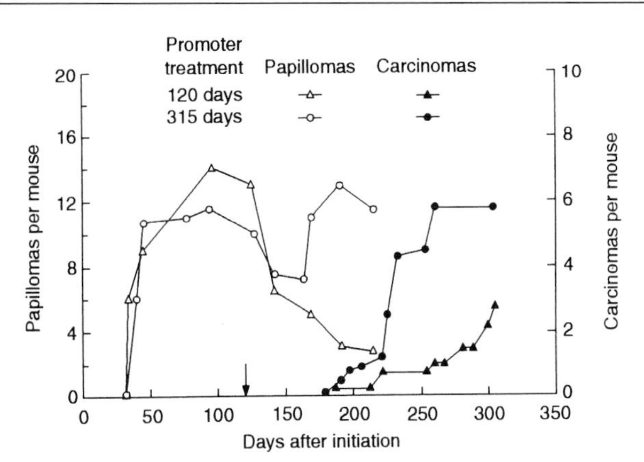

FIGURE 8 Tumor induction by phorbol esters in mouse skin. Initiation was performed using 25 μg DMBA applied locally. Two weeks later 2.5 μg TPA dissolved in 0.2 ml acetone was applied three times per week for 120 or 315 days. Tumor induction is shown as tumor yield; tumor incidence follows the same kinetics. After 120 days of treatment, most of the papillomas regress (open triangles). Carcinomas do not appear before day 175 and are less numerous than the papillomas (closed triangles). Longer treatment causes persistence of papillomas and enhances induction of carcinomas (open and closed circles). Burns *et al.* (1978).

Tumor Progression

Prolonged treatment with TPA induces persistent papillomas and subsequent formation of carcinomas, indicating that it supports tumor progression. Carcinomas are mostly basal cell carcinomas and squamous cell carcinomas and arise within papillomas or in adjacent areas. If promotion treatment is terminated after the appearance of papillomas, most of these are reversible. However, some carcinomas arise without further treatment, although with a much lower yield (Fig. 8). Progression of papillomas to carcinomas can be enhanced by local administration of

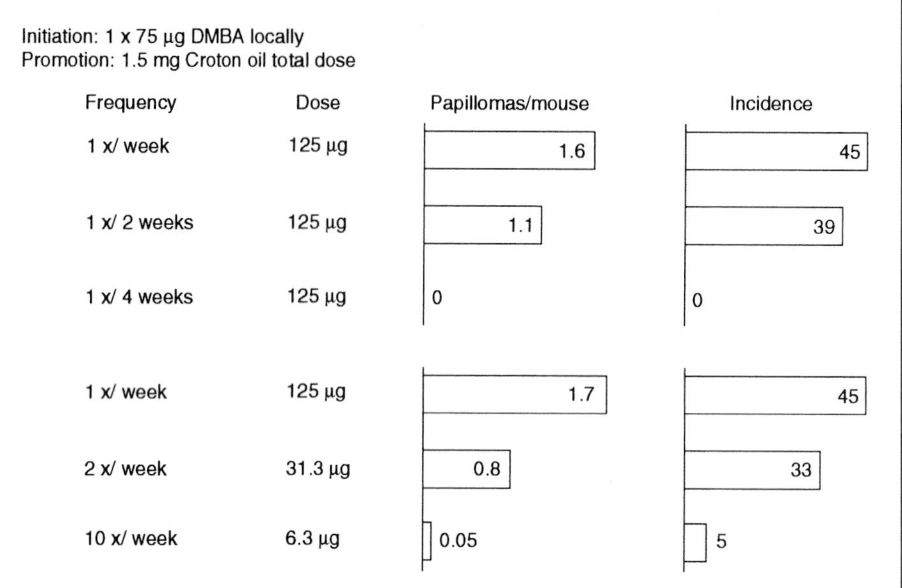

FIGURE 9 Reversibility and threshold of promoting action in mouse skin. Initiation was performed by application of 75 μg DMBA in one dose and promotion with a total dose of 1.5 mg croton oil. The effects of different treatment schedules on tumor incidence and yield were compared. Prolongation of the interval between two applications to 2 weeks reduced tumor development, applications with a 4-week interval were completely ineffective. Splitting the dose per week (63 μg) into 10 single doses of 6.3 μg each almost abolished the promoting effect (Boutwell, 1964; reproduced with permission of S. Karger AG, Basel).

carcinogens like ethylnitrosourea or methylnitrosonitroguanidine. Phorbol esters, such as TPA and several peroxides (e.g., benzoyl peroxide), are also effective as progressors.

Conversion

Diterpene tumor promoters containing polyunsaturated side chains like 12-*O*-retinoylphorbol 13-acetate (RPA) or mezerein (Fig. 10) do not promote when applied alone after initiation. However, if one or two doses of TPA are given before RPA or mezerein subsequent, treatment with these agents is as effective as continuous TPA treatment. Apparently TPA has an additional effect that is not exerted by other tumor promoters. The effect is called conversion. It can also be observed if performed before initiation and it persists for several weeks, so that the process is not classified as part of tumor promotion, which, by definition, takes place after initiation. The clastogenic activity of TPA might be responsible for its convertogenic effect, as it is shared by several other converting factors (e.g., methyl methanesulfonate, wound healing, TGFβ).

Effects and Mechanisms

Generally, the biochemical and biological effects of phorbol esters involve proliferation and differentiation control, lipid metabolism, and induction of inflammation. A single dose of TPA applied to mouse skin causes a wave of proliferation in the basal cells and the induction of proliferation-related genes (ornithine decarboxylase, c-*myc*, c-*fos*, histone, and actin). The number of dark cells, a subpopulation of basal cells that are regarded as stem cells, increases. High doses can cause abscess, cell damage, and leukocyte infiltration.

Chronic treatment causes stable hyperplasia and chronic inflammation. Characteristically, proliferation, which is normally restricted to the basal layer, extends to several skin layers (cf., "adaptive growth"). Growth regulation and keratin gene expression change to a pattern regarded as "dedifferentiated." Suitable doses of TPA can cause the formation of new hair follicles in mouse skin, a process involving "retrodifferentiation."

Comparison of a large number of phorbol esters has shown that all active promoters cause both prolif-

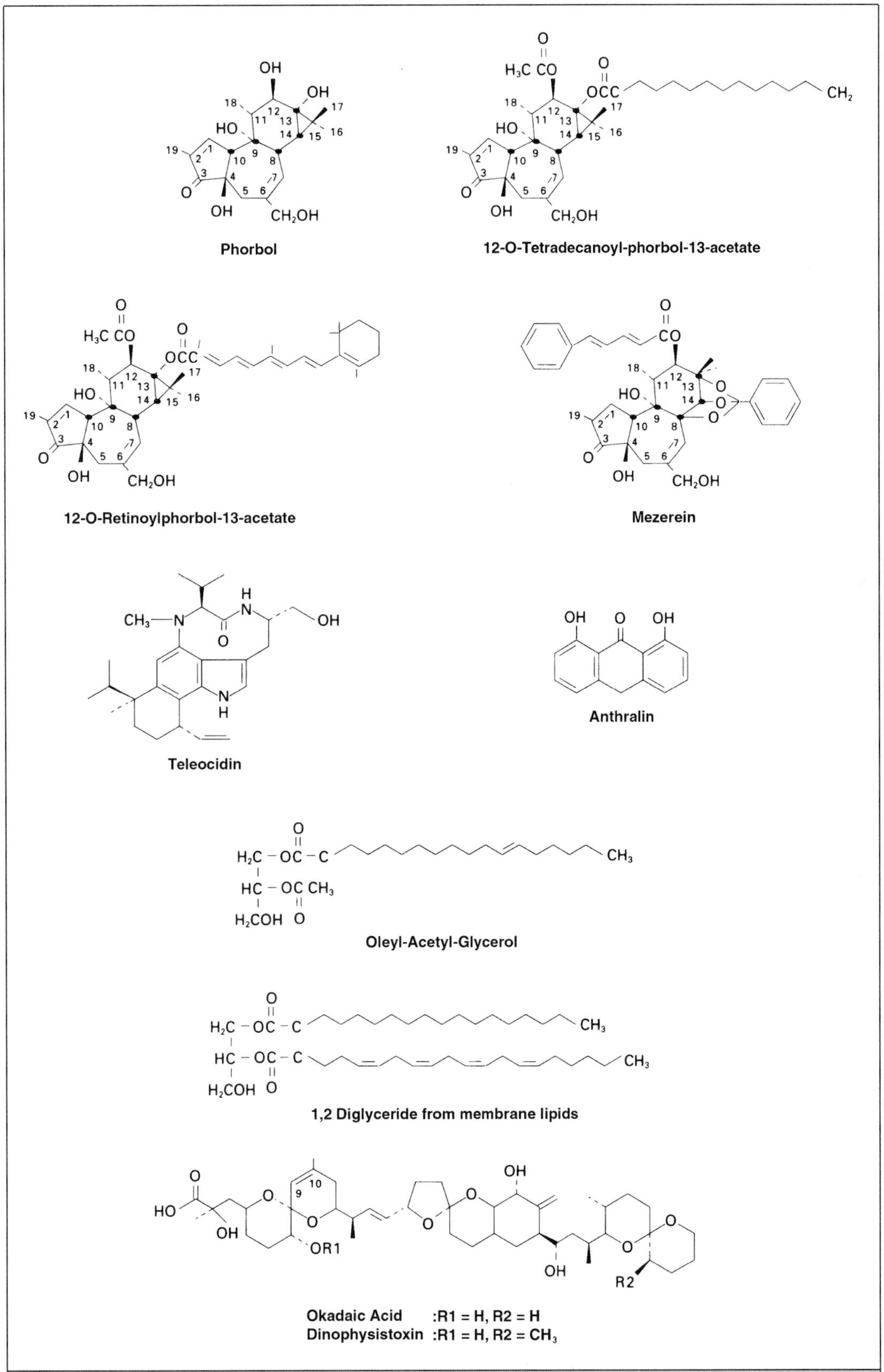

Phorbol

12-O-Tetradecanoyl-phorbol-13-acetate

12-O-Retinoylphorbol-13-acetate

Mezerein

Teleocidin

Anthralin

Oleyl-Acetyl-Glycerol

1,2 Diglyceride from membrane lipids

Okadaic Acid :R1 = H, R2 = H
Dinophysistoxin :R1 = H, R2 = CH_3

FIGURE 10 Chemical structures of selected skin tumor promoters.

TABLE 7 Skin Tumor Promoters

Promoter	Potency	Promoter	Potency
12-O-Tetradecanoyl phorbol 13-acetate	++++	Fatty acids	+
12-O-Retinoylphorbol 13-acetate	+++	Detergents	+
Phorboldidecanoate	+++	Tobacco smoke condensates	++
Mezerein	++	Benzoyl peroxide	++
Teleocidine	++++	Benzo [*a*] pyrene	++
1,2-Diglycerides	++	7-Bromomethylbenz-[*a*]anthracene	+++
Okadaic acid	++++	TCDD	++
Anthraline	++	UV light (UVA)	+ (?)
Phenole	+		

eration and inflammation, but not all mitogenic and irritant substances are tumor promoters.

Large species and strain specific differences have been observed in the sensitivity to tumor induction by an initiation–promotion regimen. Mice are particularly responsive, but different strains show dramatic differences in tumor response. The SENCAR mouse, an in-bred strain specifically developed for high susceptibility, shows the highest sensitivity followed by the strains CD-1 > BalbC > C57/bl > DBA. Rats and hamsters show little or no tumor response. Sensitivity to tumor induction closely corresponds to sensitivity to the induction of stable hyperplasia in chronically treated skin areas, underlining the importance of a sustained proliferative response for tumor formation.

TPA treatment causes rapid alterations in lipid metabolism of keratinocytes. Both degradation and synthesis of phosphatidylcholine are stimulated. Phospholipase A2 is activated and liberates arachidonic acid, the substrate of cyclooxygenases (COX) and lipoxygenases. Consequently, synthesis and secretion of their products, namely prostaglandins PGE2 and PGF2α, as well as of linear arachidonic acid derivatives (hydroxyeicosatetraenoic acid, or HETE), are increased (Fig. 11). The expression of the inducible cyclooxygenase isoenzyme COX-2 is also stimulated by TPA. Prostaglandin synthesis is restricted to specific short time periods after the treatment, and inhibition prevents both cell proliferation and tumor development, suggesting a crucial role for the prostaglandins in tumor development.

Direct interaction of phorbol esters with DNA has not been observed. They do, however, inhibit superoxide dismutase, an enzyme necessary for detoxification of free radicals arising from lipoxygenase action. This results in a clastogenic effect of phorbol esters and might indirectly cause DNA damage. Clastogenic activity is necessary for conversion and tumor progression, processes supported by phorbol esters with saturated side chains. Phorbol esters carrying unsaturated side chains are not clastogenic because their side chains interact with and trap oxygen radicals. They also lack converting activity (see previous discussion).

The process of tumor promotion can be inhibited by a large variety of substances. Retinoic acid, a substance acting on the differentiation of keratinocytes, is in this group, as well as the inhibitors of ornithine decarboxylase and inhibitors of proteases and anti-inflammatory drugs (Table 8).

In Vitro Effects of Phorbol Esters and Other Skin Tumor Promoters

In tissue culture, TPA can cause similar effects in many cell types. It stimulates cell proliferation and induces expression of growth-related genes. It confers a transformed phenotype to normal fibroblasts, supporting growth to higher densities under reduced serum conditions and in semisolid agar medium. These effects are completely reversible upon withdrawal of the phorbol ester.

Phorbol esters also inhibit cell communication through gap junctions in many cell types (see previous section). They may inhibit or stimulate differentiation, depending on the cell type. Cell type specificity has to be taken into account when using *in vitro* assays for tumor promoters. The cell culture model used should be as close as possible to the *in vivo* target cells.

The high biological activity of phorbol esters, as well as the distinct structure–activity relationship, caused an intensive search for a receptor that would

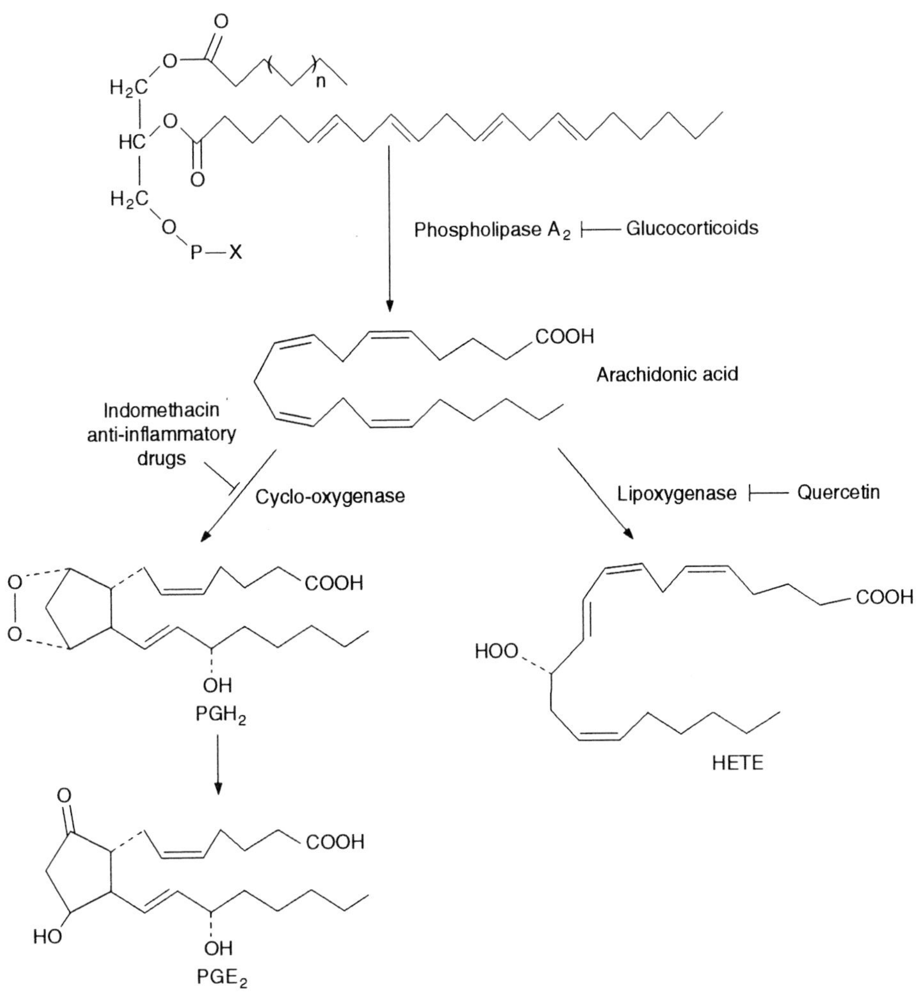

FIGURE 11 Arachidonic acid metabolism. Arachidonic acid can be metabolized by lipoxygenase and cyclcoxygenase producing linear oxidation products or prostaglandins, respectively. Many of these products are inflammation mediators. Inhibition of the enzymes inhibits skin tumor promotion.

mediate the pleiotropic effects of the promoter. This receptor was found to be protein kinase C (PKC), a serine–threonine kinase activated by lipids and Ca^{2+} and that is involved in signal transduction pathways in all cells investigated. Physiological signals cause hydrolysis of membrane lipids to produce 1,2-diglycerides (1,2-DG), the physiological activators of PKC. Subsequently activated PKC phosphorylates proteins of a cellular signal cascade, which eventually induces expression of growth regulatory genes. Due to their structural similarity to 1,2-DG, phorbol esters bind to and activate PKC (Fig. 12). Because phorbol esters have a much longer biological half-life than 1,2-DG, the activation is stronger and prolonged and ultimately causes degradation of PKC by proteolytic enzymes (down-regulation). The tumor-promoting activity of phorbol esters and other diterpene tumor promoters correlates with their affinity to PKC.

Okadaic acid, a tumor promoter as effective as TPA, does not react with PKC, but inhibits the serine–threonine phosphatases PP1 and PP2a. It also causes hyperphosphorylation of regulatory cellular proteins. The cellular mechanisms of action of most other tumor promoters are not known.

The mutated ras protein present in many skin tumors might further enhance PKC activation. Ras proteins activate phospholipases that produce 1,2-DG, not only from phosphatidylinositol (PI) but also from phosphatidylcholine (PC). As PC is more abundant in cell membranes than PI, more 1,2-DG becomes avail-

TABLE 8 Inhibitors of Skin Tumor Promotion

Response	Compound
Differentiation	Vitamin A analogs, butyrate
Inhibition of inflammation	Cortisol, indomethacine
Inhibition of thromboxane synthesis	Imidazolphenol, imidazolacetophenone
Inhibition of lipoxygenase	Quercetin
Protease inhibition	Antipain, leupeptine
Inhibition of protein kinase C	Staurosporine

able and PKC activation is increased. Thus, mutated ras and TPA enhance the function of the same stimulatory signal cascade, which may explain the synergism of initiation and promotion in the skin model (Fig. 12).

Relevance for Humans

Skin cancers are the most common of all human cancers, with about 1 million new cases per year in the United States. There are three groups, resulting from the three major cell types in the epidermis: basal cells, squamous cells, and melanocytes. Fortunately, the majority of the cases are basal-cell and squamous-cell carcinomas, which can easily be treated surgically and have a very good prognosis. Only a small fraction of the cases are highly malignant melanomas, which cause most skin cancer deaths (38,000 new cases and about 7,000 deaths/y in the United States).

Phorbol esters and related diterpenes are natural constituents of many plants and phytotherapeutic drugs. Most of these drugs, however, are no longer used and probably do not play a role in the etiology of human skin cancers. However, there may be some risk for carcinogenesis of internal organs; esophagus, stomach, and gut may be target organs. Epidemiological observations from western Europe or the United States dealing with phorbol esters in different malignant diseases are not available.

More important as causative factors in human skin carcinogenesis are UV exposure and sunburn. Particularly in children, sunburn is an important risk factor for skin cancer development later in life. It favors

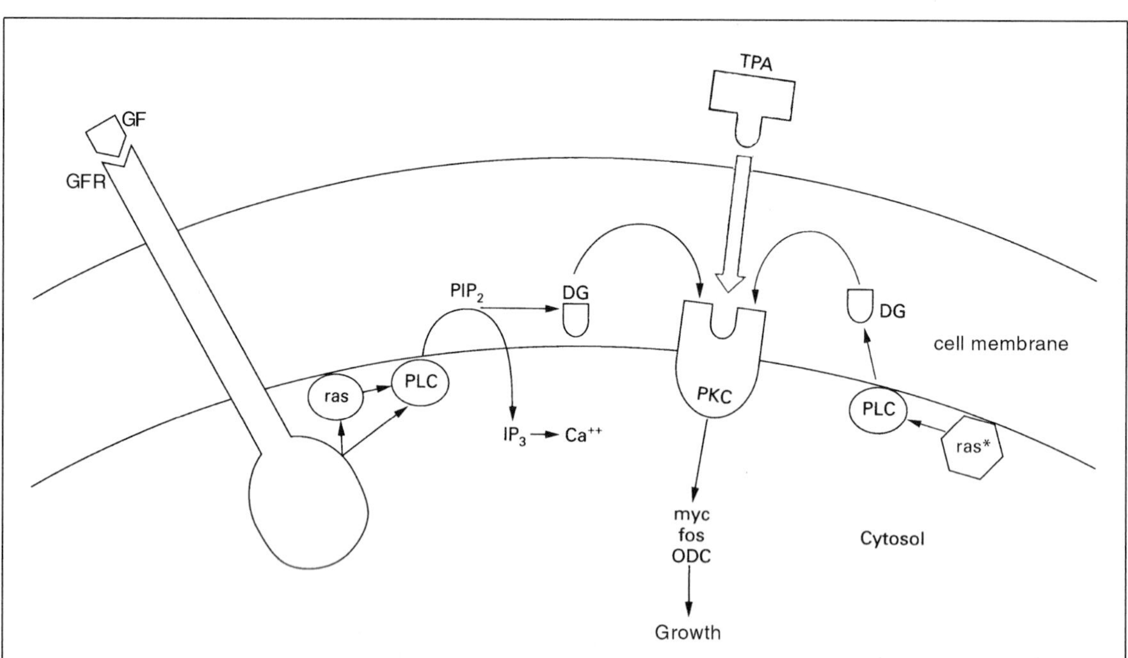

FIGURE 12 Activation of protein kinase C by physiological signals and by phorbol esters. Normal growth factor signals (GF and GFR) cause hydrolysis of inositolphospholipids (PIP_2) by phospholipase C (PLC), producing 1, 2-diglycerides (DG) and inositol phosphate (IP_3). The DG activates protein kinase C (PKC) transiently before it is reused for synthesis of membrane lipids. The activation can be mediated directly by the receptor or via activation of the ras pathway. Consequently, mutated ras proteins (ras*) as present in many skin tumors can enhance the activation. Phorbol esters like TPA activate PKC directly. Due to their chemical stability, phorbol esters cause hyperactivation of the kinases.

development of naevi, which are considered as preneoplastic lesions in human skin. UV light causes DNA damage and mutations. In many human skin cancers, mutation of the p53 gene has been identified. The gene p53 is thought responsible for cell-cycle arrest in damaged cells and for induction of apoptosis. This mutation may be crucial for initiation, especially if aquired at an early age. It inhibits apoptosis after further DNA damage, while nonmutated damaged cells are removed from the tissue. The consequence will be clonal expansion of mutated cells during the regenerative proliferation phase (promotion) and retention of DNA damage, causing accumulation of mutated genes (progression).

Skin cancer risk depends not only on the duration and intensity of irradiation, but also on the type of skin and the induction of a sunburn reaction. In addition, tumor development requires repeated UV irradiation over longer periods of time, a characteristic of tumor promotion. The promotion phase is supported by UV-induced wounding, burns, and erythema that cause cell damage and stimulate regenerative proliferation processes. This includes production of inflammation mediators derived from arachidonic acid (Fig. 7) and involves the occurrence of clastogenic active oxygen species (lipoxygenase reaction). The UVA part of the light (320–400 nm) is only a weak mutagen, but still causes erythema and inflammation. It also stimulates phospholipase A2 and PKC, triggering similar reactions in human skin as phorbol esters in mouse skin. UVA might therefore be a promoter component of UV light.

Psoralene and furocoumarine are plant constituents that have been combined with UVA irradiation for the therapy of psoriasis (psoralen-UVA therapy, or PUVA). Psoralen intercalates in the DNA helix. If exposed to UV light, singlet oxygen is generated and cross-links the DNA strands. At the dose used, this massive damage is cytotoxic and stimulates regenerative proliferation that can be promoting. In experimental animals, PUVA is carcinogenic. Epidemiologic studies showed increased skin cancer risk in patients who had received several cycles of PUVA treatment. The tumors were squamous cell carcinomas and keratoacanthomas, with low malignancy that can successfully be treated locally. After extended treatment, melanomas have been observed. Many affected patients had previous treatments with carcinogens like tar or UVB. PUVA treatment might have acted as the promoter for cells initiated by these treatments. However no data are available to determine whether PUVA represents a complete carcinogen or a tumor promoter.

Liver

Experimental Models

Peraino found that prolonged application of phenobarbital greatly enhanced carcinogenesis in the liver of rats previously subjected to a brief treatment with acetylaminofluorene. Since then, numerous compounds have been tested for initiating and promoting activity in the liver, usually of rats or mice. As endpoints phenotypically altered (putative preneoplastic) cell foci or tumors are used.

For initiation, hepatocarcinogens are given once at high dosage or repeatedly at lower doses. Most hepatocarcinogens are hepatotoxic, leading to cell death and subsequently to (regenerative) cell replication, which is required for initiation. Single low doses of complete hepatocarcinogens or incomplete carcinogens must be combined with a proliferation stimulus such as partial hepatectomy or CCl_4 in order to cause initiation. Effective initiation is shown by subsequent promoter treatment. Virtually all genotoxic hepatocarcinogens and many other genotoxic agents were identified as tumor initiators in the liver. Ethionine, which inhibits endogenous methylation of DNA but is not a genotoxin, also initiated hepatocarcinogenesis after treatment for several weeks.

Promoters administered after initiation will lead to significant enlargement of altered foci within several weeks and to appearance of adenomas and carcinomas within several months. In some models the period required for promotion can be shortened by additional growth stimuli; Solt and Farber described how the promoting effect of acetylaminofluorene was enhanced by partial hepatectomy or CCl_4, resulting in extremely enlarged cell foci within 2 weeks. This was explained by the assumption that acetylaminofluorene inhibits regenerative growth of normal hepatocytes but not of focus cells, which thereby get a selective growth advantage.

Phenobarbital before or simultaneously with genotoxic carcinogens mostly *decreased* initiating activity, probably by enzyme induction and accelerated detoxification of the carcinogen in the liver (anti-initiation or anticarcinogenesis). This illustrates the fact that the same agent can inhibit or promote carcinogenesis, depending on the stage at which it interferes.

Promoting Agents and the Effects on Normal Liver

Numerous foreign and endogenous compounds were found to promote tumor formation in the liver of experimental animals. Furthermore, nutritional imbalance, such as a deficiency in methyl groups from

TABLE 9 Some Liver Tumor Promoters and Their Early Hepatic Effects

Agent, treatment	Growth	Increase of: Enzyme, other protein	Increase of: Organelle	Cytotoxicity
Phenobarbital,[a] DDT, HCH, HCB, some PCB, PBB, etc.[b]	+	Phase I and II enzymes; CYP II B, C	Smooth endoplasmic reticulum	
TCDD[b], some PCB	+	CYP I A		(+)
Some progestins, progesterone	+	CYP III, phase II enzymes	Smooth endoplasmic reticulum	
Some estrogens (estradiol ester, ethinylestradiol)	+	Clotting factors, angiotensinogen, etc.		
Some peroxisome proliferators (clofibrate, nafenopin, diethylhexylphthalate, di- and trichloroacetic acid, other bulky acids)	+	CYP IV, peroxisomal fatty acid oxidizing enzymes	Peroxisomes	
Ethanol	?	CYP II E1		+
Methapyrilene	+		Mitochondria	+
Thioacetamide, thiobenzamide	+	phase II enzymes		++
CCl_4	+			+++
Choline methionine-deficient diet	+			++

[a]Some benzodiazepines and many other drugs; only one (imporant) family inducible by the agent is indicated.
[b]HCH, hexachlorocyclohexane; HCB, hexachlorobenzene; PCB, polychlorinated biphenyls; PBB, polybrominated biphenyls, TCDD, 2, 3, 7, 8-tetrachlorodibenzodioxine.

diets low in choline and methionine, may promote hepatocarcinogenesis (Table 9). An early effect of promoting chemicals or regimens in the liver is the induction of growth, which can be assigned to one of two types. The first one is exerted by *primary* hepatomitogens, without significant toxic damage. It is associated with the stimulation of specific hepatic functions, such as drug metabolism or peroxisomal fatty acid oxidation (Table 9). These changes probably reflect adaptive responses to increased functional load. To cope with enhanced functional load, the liver possesses genetically controlled adaptive programs, which include enhanced synthesis of specific enzymes, induction of growth, and proliferation of specific organelles such as smooth endoplasmic reticulum or peroxisomes (Table 9). Some agents are known to exert these effects via binding to specific receptor molecules within the hepatocytes; activated receptors bind to specific genes and alter their transcription rates, for example, TCDD via the Ah receptor (AhR), peroxisome proliferators via the peroxisome proliferator-activated receptor (PPAR) (Fig. 13), and estrogens via the estrogen receptor (ER). For phenobarbital and many other agents, the mechanisms of action have not been elucidated.

As an alternative explanation of the action of peroxisome proliferators, the oxidative stress hypothesis has been proposed. It assumes that the agents induce the activity of peroxisomal H_2O_2-generating enzymes without a concomitant increase in the H_2O_2-scavenging enzyme catalase. The resulting increase in H_2O_2 causes damage to lipids, DNA, and other cellular molecules, which eventually might result in tumor formation. However, increases of indicators of oxidative stress, such as lipid peroxidation or oxidative damage of DNA, after peroxisome proliferator treatment *in vivo* have not been consistently demonstrated.

The second type of growth is induced by cytotoxic tumor promoters (Table 9). Their acute or chronic application results in cell losses; the ensuing regenerative growth is a *secondary* response to the agent. Likewise choline-methionine deficiency has a cytotoxic effect (fatty liver and cell death). Repeated partial hepatectomies also promote tumor development. Some compounds have both enzyme-inducing and cytotoxic effects (Table 9).

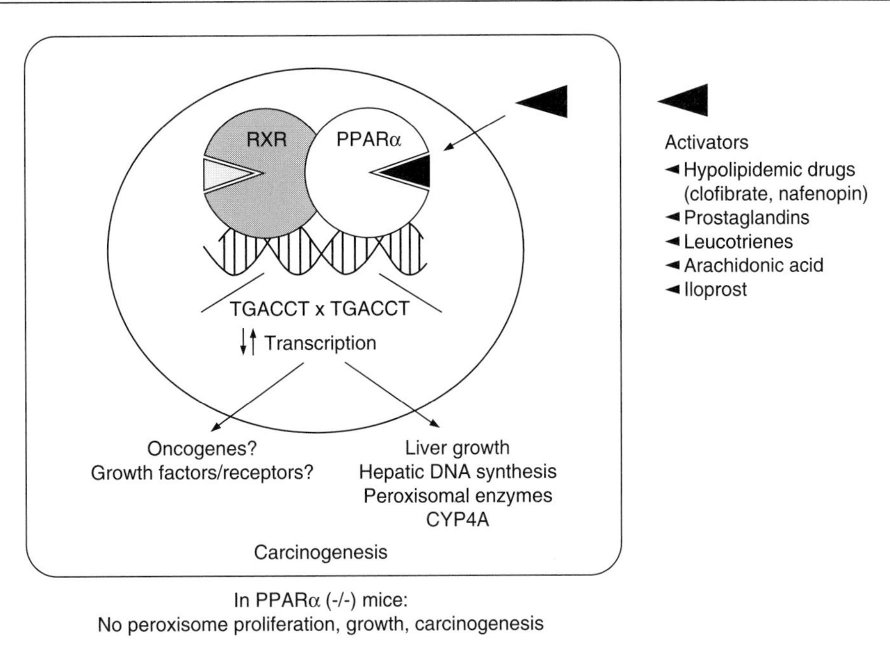

FIGURE 13 Mediation of hepatic effects of peroxisome proliferators via the peroxisome proliferator activated receptor α (PPARα). The PPAR is a member of the steroid nuclear receptor superfamily. It forms heterodimers with the retinoic acid binding receptor "X" (RXR). Peroxisome proliferators diffuse passively into cells, and bind to the PPAR either directly or enhance binding of natural ligands (long-chain fatty acids and some leukotrienes and prostaglandins). Binding activates the PPAR to act as transcription factor, which recognizes specific genes involved in lipid metabolism and growth. Mice lacking PPARα by genetic modulation ("knockout" of PPARα gene) do not show peroxisomal enzyme induction, growth, and tumor development after peroxisome proliferator treatment.

TABLE 10 Properties of Phenotypically Altered, Putative Preneoplastic Cell Foci in the Liver and Effects of Tumor Promoters

Foci appear after administration of all hepatocarcinogens investigated, not after noncarcinogenic hepatotoxins[a]
Tumor formation is always preceded by appearance of foci
Foci (as population) persist throughout life
Foci have an altered ("new") state of differentation; some of the new properties appear also in tumors
Expression of the "new" phenotype in many foci is incomplete and unstable
Tumor promoters have two important effects on foci: they enhance the expression of the "new" phenotype; and they accelerate focus growth selectivity (increase of cell replication and survival)
After promoter withdrawal the enhanced expression of the altered phenotype is lost; enhanced apoptosis may reduce cell number in foci

[a] In aged animals, foci may appear "spontaneously."

Prestages of Cancer in the Liver

Why do tumor promoters lead to selective growth of initiated cells? The liver offers a useful model to study this key question. In this organ, putative initiated cells and their progeny can be detected by histological techniques. They were first observed in 1956 by Weiler as differently stained "islands" in histological sections from rat liver and are designated as foci of altered cells (Table 10).

Initiation probably occurs in normal hepatocytes, which thus are the origin of altered foci. An alternative hypothesis regards "oval cells" as precursors of foci and tumors. Oval cells are derived from liver stem cells located at the canals of Hering in bile ductular areas. Oval cells strongly proliferate after some carcinogens (aromatic amines; choline deficient diet); they may be the origin for neoplasia in some but not all models of hepatocarcinogenesis.

Numerous alterations in foci have been described, providing information on the functional changes associated with the initiated–preneoplastic phenotype. On the basis of morphological characteristics, altered

TABLE 11 Phenotypically Altered Cell Foci in the Rodent Liver and Their Response to Tumor Promoters[a]

	Focus type[b]	
	Clear and/or eosinophilic	Weakly basophilic
Marker		
GGT	+	−
GST-P	+	−
G-6-Pase	−	
Characteristic functional changes		
Glycogen storage	+	
Phase II enzymes	+	
SER	+	
mdr	+	
Peroxisomal enzymes	−	+
Cell replication	+	+
Apoptoses	+	+
Response to tumor promoters		
phenobarbital	+	−
nafenopin	−	+

[a]Abbreviations: +, enhanced response as compared to normal liver; −, no or decreased response compared to normal liver; GGT, γ-glutamyltransferase; GST-P, placental glutathione transferase (=GST 7-7); G-6-Pase, glucose-6-phosphatase; SER, smooth endoplasmic reticulum; mdr, multi-drug-resistance protein.

[b]Appearance of cytoplasm in HE-stained tissue section.

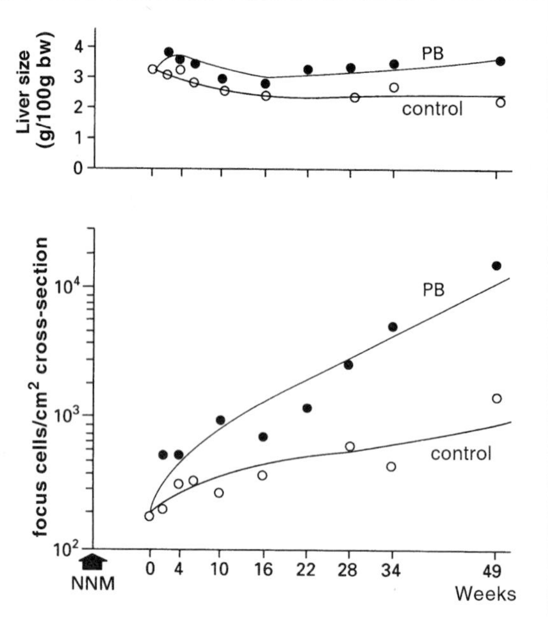

FIGURE 14 Growth of the liver and of phenotypically altered foci during promoting treatment with phenobarbital (PB). PB was administered from 0 to 49 weeks. Note the steady growth of foci on the logarithmic scale. Abbreviation: NNM, *N*-nitrosomorpholine. From R. Schulte-Hermann *et al.* (1990).

foci were assigned to different classes (Table 11). The clear cell and eosinophilic type shows pronounced storage of glycogen, which persists during fasting and may reflect the beginning of regulatory autonomy. Another property of this type of foci is the increase of drug-metabolizing enzymes, particularly of phase-II enzymes, of smooth endoplasmic reticulum, and of the membrane carrier protein mdr, which extrudes multiple lipophilic agents. Enzymes expressed include the placental type of glutathione *S*-transferase (GSTP), which is not found in normal rat liver and therefore is extremely useful for detection of altered foci and even single, presumably initiated, cells. Other focus types show different characteristics (Table 11). Cell proliferation in foci is generally higher than in normal liver, but cell death by apoptosis is also enhanced and largely counterbalances cell replication. The different phenotypic alterations in foci probably reflect a new state of differentiation in which cells are overexpressing specific genes.

Some foci seem to give rise to adenomas that are still benign and show phenotypic characteristics similar to those of foci but are larger and compress the surrounding normal liver parenchyma. They may be precursors of carcinoma. The number of adenomas and carcinomas found is always much smaller than the number of foci.

Effect of Tumor Promoters on Cancer Prestages

Tumor promoters also enhance the expression of the altered phenotype of foci and provide a growth advantage (selective growth) over normal liver cells (Fig. 14). The accelerated growth results from enhanced cell replication and from inhibition of apoptosis in foci. Phenobarbital and some other tumor promoters were shown to act as survival factors rescuing preneoplastic cells from death.

Numerous tumor promoters, such as phenobarbital, TCDD, estrogens, cytotoxic agents or choline-methionine-deficient diet, promote growth of eosinophilic GSTP-positive foci. Peroxisome proliferators have little effect on these foci but strongly enhance growth of weakly basophilic foci. Apparently, different types of initiated cells exist in the liver, which are promotable by different classes of promoters (Table 11).

It is widely assumed that the mechanism of tumor promotion is related to the acute effects on the liver, although this is not scientifically proven. Subsequently, two concepts will be briefly described. The first concept holds that cells in foci show qualitatively similar responses to promoters as normal hepatocytes, such as increased drug metabolism and cell multiplication in eosinophilic foci. Quantitatively, the responses in foci are more pronounced and cell proliferation continuously exceeds cell death. Therefore an *overexpression of adaptive programs* by initiated cells may occur in response to promoters and result in selective growth (Fig. 15).

The second concept is the *resistant cell hypothesis,* which may be particularly relevant for cytotoxic tumor promoters. According to this hypothesis, promoters inhibit mitosis in normal cells while initiated cells are resistant to mitoinhibition. Therefore initiated cells have a growth advantage and may proliferate excessively in situations where cells are lost by cytotoxic events. Enhanced resistance of focus cells to a variety of cytotoxic agents has been shown and may be due to expression of the "resistent phenotype" characterized by increased content of phase-II enzymes, mdr protein, and so on, which accelerate inactivation and/or extrusion of toxic compounds (Fig. 15).

Several molecular mechanisms have been suggested to explain why normal and initiated liver cells respond differently to tumor promoters. Continuous treatment with promoters resulted in decrease of epidermal growth factor (EGF) receptors in normal liver but not in foci. These receptors mediate growth stimulation by EGF. Furthermore, foci may show enhanced production of stimulatory growth factors such as TGF-α, hypothetically leading to autocrine or paraacrine stimulation. TGF-α is also strongly expressed in about 50% of human liver tumors. Transgenic mice

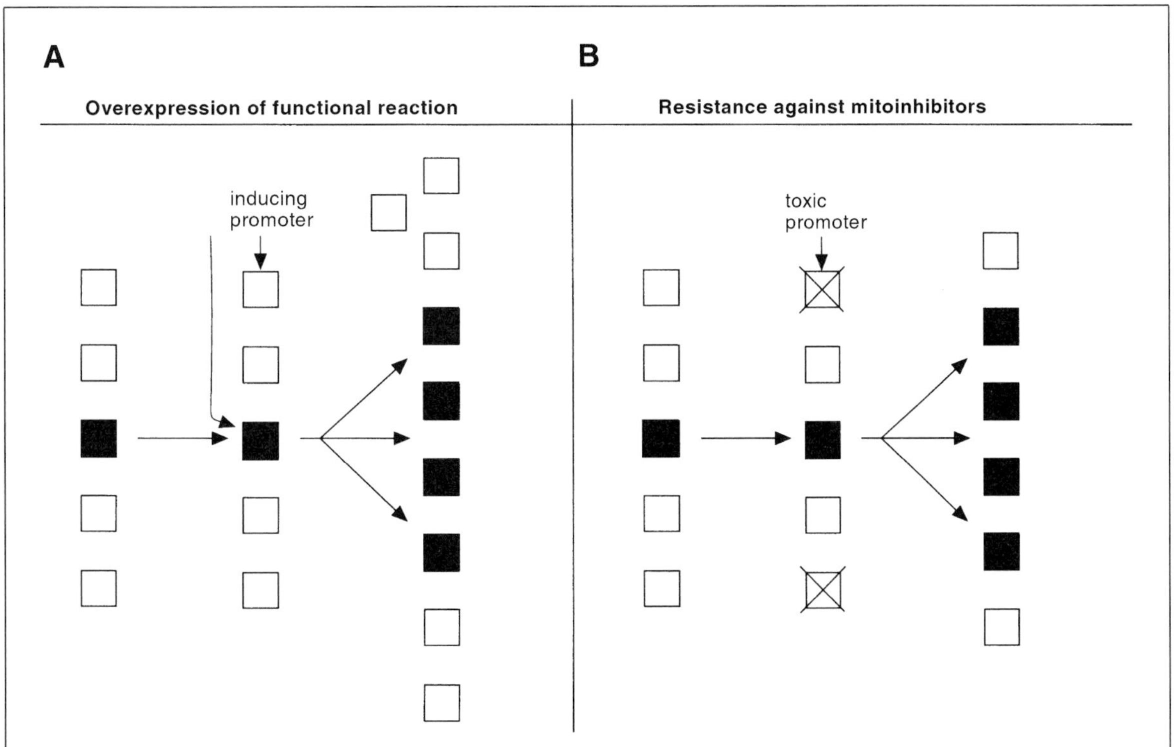

FIGURE 15 Selective advantage of initiated cells. (A) Overexpression hypothesis: In this model, the promoter stimulates function and growth in the target organ. The initiated cell is over-responsive to the stimulatory effect, resulting in preferential multiplication. (B) Resistent cell hypothesis: In this model, the promoter is cytotoxic and cytolethal and inhibits cell replication. The initiated cell is resistant to these effects and can respond to the regeneration signal that follows cell losses.

overexpressing TGF-α rapidly developed liver foci, suggesting that TGF-α is a promoter and nongenotoxic hepatocarcinogen. On the other hand, initiated and neoplastic cells in the liver may show reduced responsiveness to negative growth signals, such as the inhibitory cytokine TGF-β1, possibly by a reduction of TGF-β receptors. This may lead to paracrine inhibition of normal hepatocytes, while cells within the lesions are resistent (Fig. 3).

At the genetic level, mutations of some oncogenes and tumor suppressor genes, such as *ras* in mice or p53 in rats, were found occasionally in altered foci and adenomas. Phenobarbital appeared to promote a focus subpopulation *not* expressing the mutated *ras.* Enhanced expression of immediate-early genes such as *myc* or *fos* was also observed. However, a consistent pattern of molecular changes during initiation has not emerged.

Much of the effect of tumor promotion in the liver is reversible. After withdrawal of promoters, phenotypic alterations in foci become less pronounced, cell proliferation declines, and apoptosis is further enhanced. The majority of foci and adenomas depend on the continuous presence of a promoter for survival of their cells. As a result, after promoter withdrawal lesions stop growing and may even completely disappear ("selective regression") (Table 10). Some foci, however, may show promoter-independent growth and survival or gain such properties during the course of promotion. These lesions will not regress ("persistent foci") and may progress to cancer.

There are pronounced species and strain differences in the response to liver tumor promoters. Hamster liver did not respond to tumor promotion by phenobarbital, although eosinophilic lesions similar to those in mouse and rat liver were found after initiation. Guinea pigs and hamsters showed little or no tumorigenic response to peroxisome proliferators and low increases of peroxisomal enzymes and liver enlargement. Different mouse strains may show dramatic differences in spontaneous incidence of hepatocarcinoma and in response to chemical genotoxic and nongenotoxic carcinogens. C3H mice exhibit high and C57Bl mice low liver tumor incidence; hybrids (B6C3Fl) have intermediate sensitivity—the last are used in the NTP program of carcinogenicity testing. Foci in C3H mice show much higher growth rates than those in C57Bl mice. Available evidence indicates that the high liver tumor sensitivity of C3H mice results from enhanced sensitivity to endogenous and exogenous promoters. The mechanisms have not been identified.

Relevance for Humans

Liver cancer is number 8 among cancer death causes worldwide. Its incidence is very high in less developed countries of Africa and Asia. In the United States and Europe, liver cancer contributes only one or a few percent to overall cancer rates. Most important etiological factors in underdeveloped countries are hepatitis B virus infections and the mycotoxin aflatoxin B_1. These two factors have a strong synergistic effect on liver cancer. Conceivably, each might act as initiator and/or as promoter by means of cytotoxic and inflammatory activity (hepatitis). In view of the presumed role of the tumor suppressor gene p53 for tumor progression, it is important that a mutation in codon 249 of p53 has been found in 30–50% of human liver cancer from areas where humans are exposed to aflatoxin via their diet; this mutation is attributed specifically to aflatoxin B_1, but it is very rarely found in liver cancer in the United States and Europe.

Further factors known or suspected etiological for liver cancer are ethanol, hepatitis C virus, tobacco smoke, hormones, and nutrition. In the United States and Europe, high use of ethanol is the most important known risk factor. The appearance of HCC in alcoholics is usually associated with liver cirrhosis. In some but not all animal experiments, promotion of hepatocarcinogenesis by ethanol has been observed (Table 9); a similar effect in humans is supported by limited epidemiological data. The hepatitis C virus is an important additional risk factor in the United States, Europe, and Japan. Estrogens and anabolic–androgenic steroids may be causal factors for the rare liver adenomas in humans. These steroids appear to be nongenotoxic agents and are tumor promoters in animals. Therefore a promotional effect on spontaneously formed initiated cells in humans is a possible explanation that is supported by a number of observations in which liver adenomas disappeared after the stopping of treatment with the steroid hormones. Independent of the etiology, liver cancer is two to three times more frequent in men than in women, which is consistent with a promoting effect of (endogenous) androgens.

No epidemiological evidence is available to support the possibility that rodent liver tumor promoters other than ethanol and steroids are active in humans. Phenobarbital did not increase tumor incidence in the liver of epileptic subjects treated for many years with relatively high doses that are sufficiently high to induce drug-metabolizing enzymes in human liver. The same doses in rats clearly have tumor-promoting activity. Likewise, sustained treatment with hypolipidemic drugs such as clofibrate or prolonged exposure to diethylhexylphthalate did not produce epidemiological evidence of enhanced liver tumor incidence. Induction of peroxisomes or peroxisomal enzymes by peroxisome proliferators was not detected in human liver or in human hepatocytes in culture. Recent molecular studies suggest that the peroxisome proliferator-activated receptor (PPAR) may be less expressed and/or less responsive to these agents in human liver. Taken together, these findings suggest that the sensitivity of human liver to these specific promoters may be lower than that of rat liver. Occupational exposure to high doses of TCDD or similarly acting agents provided a trend for enhanced tumor incidence in some other organs, but not in the liver.

Oral Cavity, Esophagus, Stomach

Tumors of the oral cavity, the pharynx, and the tongue (head and neck cancers) of humans are usually related to tobacco and ethanol consumption. Both factors act in a synergistic manner. While alcohol and smoking alone increase the risk about 7-fold each, the combined risk may be 40-fold or even more. It is difficult, however, to assign initiating and promoting activities. Tobacco smoke contains mutagenic (initiating) and promoting components. On the one hand, ethanol can act as cocarcinogen via induction of cytochrome P450-IIE1, a microsomal enzyme that activates procarcinogens (e.g., nitrosamines from tobacco smoke). On the other hand, ethanol has been shown to induce proliferation in the mucosa and support tumor promotion in some, but not all experimental models. At concentrations that can certainly be reached in the oral cavity and the esophagus, ethanol causes cell damage and might induce regenerative proliferation and thereby promote.

Introducing 4–5% ethanol into the drinking water of mice or rats after and concomitant with nitrosamine treatment enhances tumor development in the esophagus. Prior to tumor development, premalignant lesions can be detected, including hyperplasia, metaplasia, and papillomas. Ethanol increases proliferation and metaplasia in the esophagus, an effect increased by vitamin A deficiency. Zinc deficiency is another factor in carcinogenesis in the esophagus, enhancing tumor promotion. Human esophageal carcinomas occur at high rates in specific geographic areas. In parts of China, India, Iran, and the former USSR, as well as in Brittany (France), they constitute up to 42% of all gastrointestinal cancers. Extensive studies in the high-risk areas support the assumption that dietary factors are involved in the process of carcinogenesis; patients have lower serum levels of vitamin A, folic acid, and Zn^{2+}, and frequently a low consumption of these micronutrients as well. Abuse of tobacco, betel, and alcohol is also related to increased risk. On the Caribean island of Curacao, the consumption of Welensali tea extracted from croton plants may be related to the high incidence of esophageal tumors. These plants contain considerable amounts of phorbol esters closely related to TPA, which hypothetically promoted development of esophageal tumors. In other regions (e.g., China) the frequent consumption of very hot liquids may cause cellular damage, regenerative proliferation, and promotion. Specific initiators were not obvious in these epidemiologic studies.

Risk of stomach cancer is also related to dietary influences. Nitrate and nitrite from drinking water and food react with dietary amines (amino acids) to form carcinogenic nitrosamines. Ethanol is an additional risk factor, as are high concentrations of salt. Both may be cocarcinogenic as well as tumor promoting. In rats, ethanol and high-salt diets has been shown to promote stomach tumor development, initiated by methylnitronitrosoguanidine or methylchinolin oxide.

Long-term treatment with histamine H_2-receptor blockers is associated with the development of enterochromaffin-like (ECL) cell carcinoids in rat stomach. H2 blockers cause persistent hypergastrinemia, which in turn is considered the cause for ECL hyperplasia and carcinoid development. In humans no evidence has been found so far for induction of hypergastrinemia at therapeutic doses of H_2 blockers. Therefore, no ECL carcinoid risk has to be expected.

Colon

Experimental Models

Initiation of colonic tumors is usually achieved by azo-compounds (azoxymethane) or hydrazines (dimethylhydrazine). More recently, heterocyclic amines have been used, although higher doses were required. In rats and mice these carcinogens cause mainly adenocarcinomas of the colon after 40–50 weeks. Tumors of the small intestine are rarely observed.

The colorectal mucosa is a constantly renewing tissue and a site of high cell proliferation. It consists of one layer of epithelial cells that are folded into crypts. Within each crypt, proliferation is tightly controlled. Stem cells are situated at the very bottom of the colonic crypts and continually produce daughter cells that still possess some proliferation capacity. While they undergo 3–4 transitional divisions they migrate

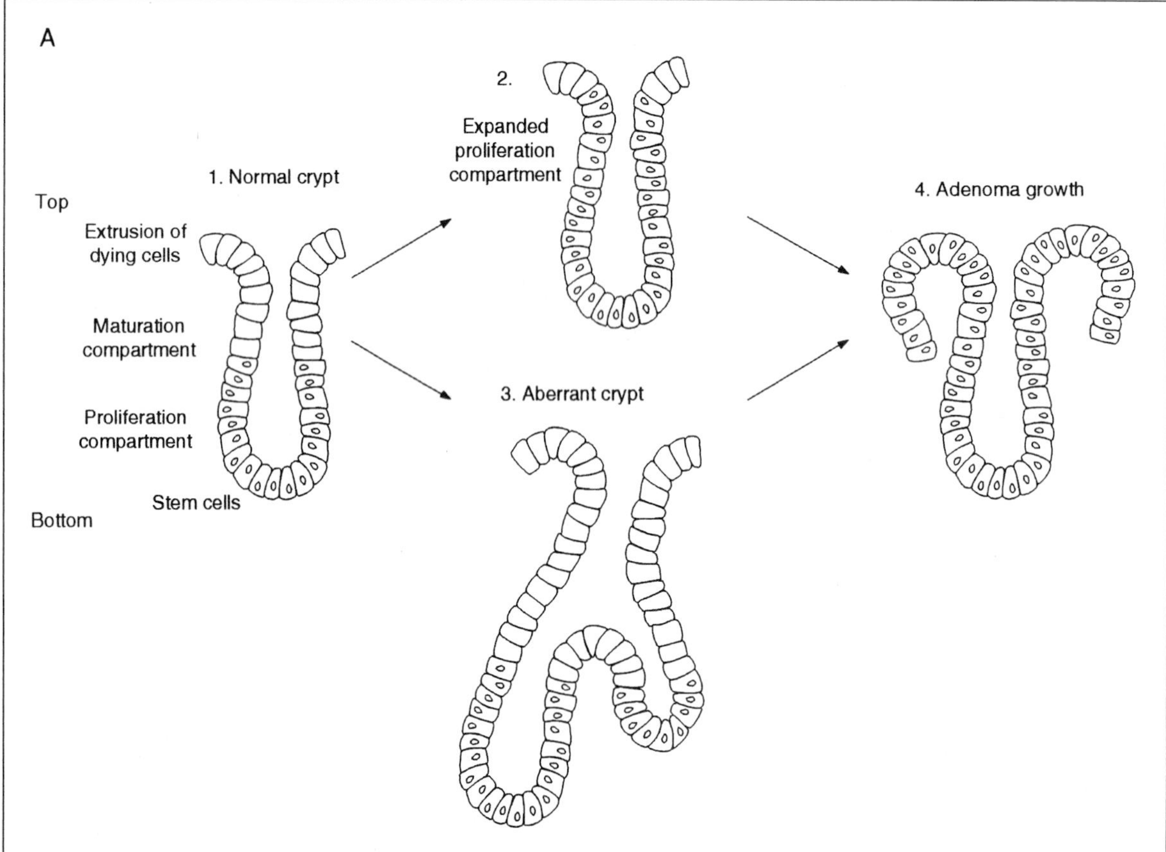

FIGURE 16A Premalignant development in the colon and rectum. (1) Schematic presentation of a colonic crypt. Stem cells are situated at the bottom of the crypt; proliferating cells that synthesize DNA are restricted to the lower half of the normal crypts (proliferation compartment, marked ○) The upper half of the crypts comprises resting terminally differentiated cells (maturation compartment). These cells are determined to undergo active cell death. Early response to carcinogen treatment consists of either (2) focal hyperproliferation with expansion of the growth compartment and delay of differentiation and cell death or (3) the formation of aberrant hyperplastic crypts. These have larger glandular lumina, contain more cells and are often branched. Expanded growth compartments can be observed in patients with a hereditary polyposis coli and may be due to an initiating mutation in the APC gene. (4) shows the schematic concept of polyp growth caused by the enlarged growth fraction and delayed cell death (Deschner and Lipkin, 1975).

up the crypt, terminate proliferation, and enter a resting state. Finally, they initiate active cell death and are extruded into the colonic lumen.

Stem cells are probably the target cells of genotoxic carcinogens. Colon stem cells express bcl-2, a protein that protects from damage-induced cell death, so that survival of initiated stem cells is enhanced compared with the small intestine. The earliest effect of carcinogen treatment is focal hyperproliferation that can be observed after 5–8 weeks of treatment. It consists of expansion of the proliferation compartments and delay in terminal differentiation and cell death. Alternatively, foci of aberrant crypts (AC) are observed that have enlarged lumina, contain more cells, and have different staining characteristics with methylene blue. It is assumed that these crypts arise from initiated stem cells and represent the earliest premalignant lesions. Even though their proliferation compartments are still normal, aberrant crypts have a higher proliferation index than normal crypts and overexpress regulatory proteins. Their appearance is dose-dependent. Hypothetically, premalignant tumors (adenomas) can develop from such foci by specific growth stimulation (Fig. 16A).

Adenomas grow very slowly, probably due to a high level of active cell death, and they slowly develop increased dysplasia over a large fraction of their life span. Carcinomas frequently arise within adenomas, arguing for the occurrence of a progression stage in colorectal carcinogenesis (Fig. 16B). Even though there are some species- and strain-specific variations in the relative importance of the stages, the sequence

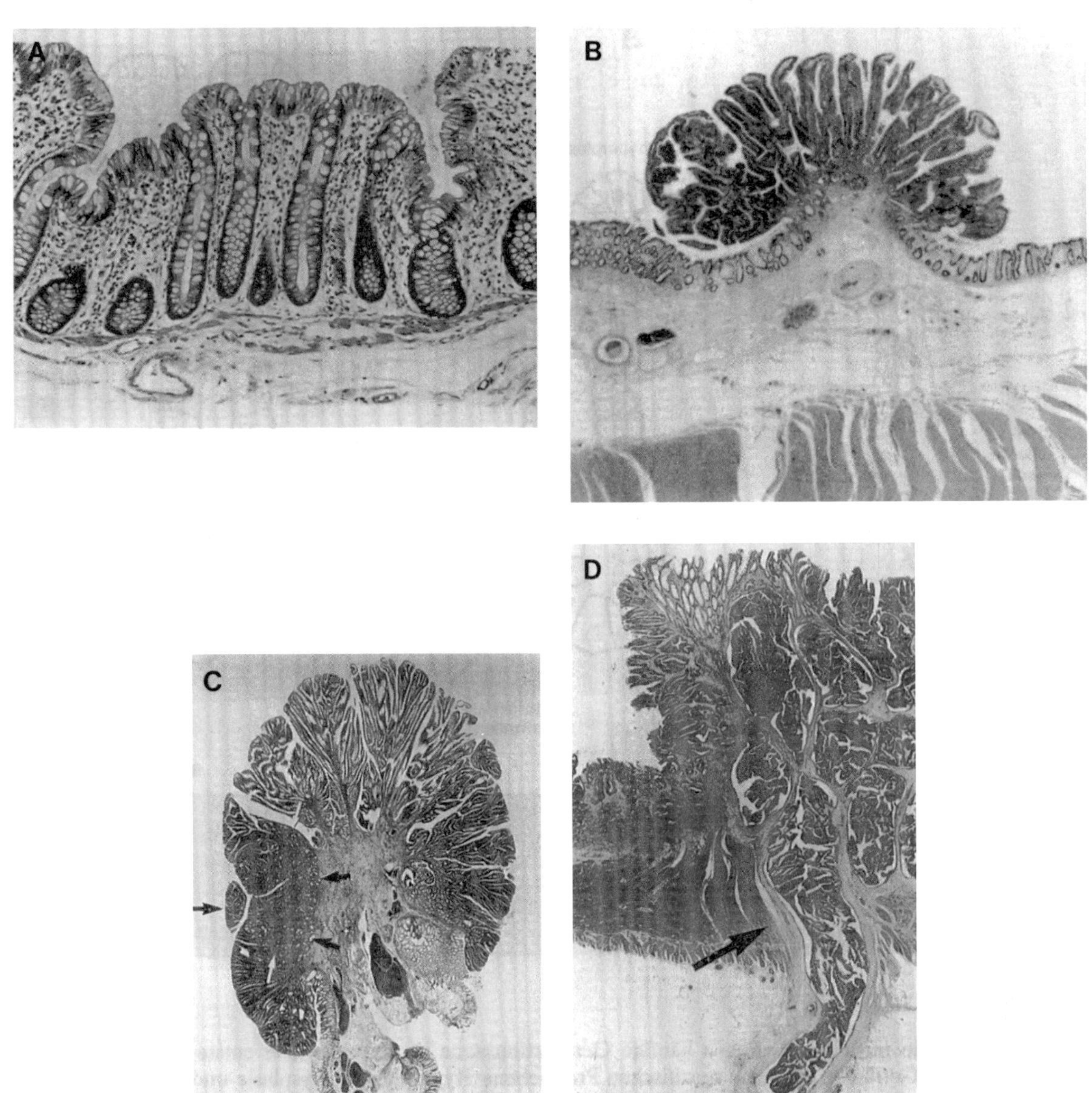

FIGURE 16B Histological presentation. (A) Normal colorectal mucosa consists of one layer of epithelium that is folded to form crypts and separated from the underlying connective tissue by a continuous basement membrane. (B) Adenomatous polyps are premalignant lesions in the gut. (C) The majority of carcinomas arises within such adenomas, from where they spread to displace the surrounding tissue and finally destroy the basement membrane to allow for metastasis (D). Reproduced from Jass *et al.* (1989).

of hyperproliferation > adenomas > carcinomas is well established both in experimental animals and in humans. Proliferative response and, more recently, the appearance of aberrant crypts have been widely used as early indicators of tumor development.

In contrast to human colorectal tumors, the genetic characteristics (Fig. 16c) in experimental mouse and rat tumors have not been thoroughly studied and initiating mutations after carcinogen treatment have not been identified. However, a strain of mice has been found that spontanously develop *m*ultiple *i*ntestinal *n*eoplasms (min-mouse), affecting not only the large bowel but also the small intestine. The mouse strain carries the same germ-line mutation in one allele of the APC gene (adenomatous polyposis coli) that causes the human hereditary cancer syndrome famil-

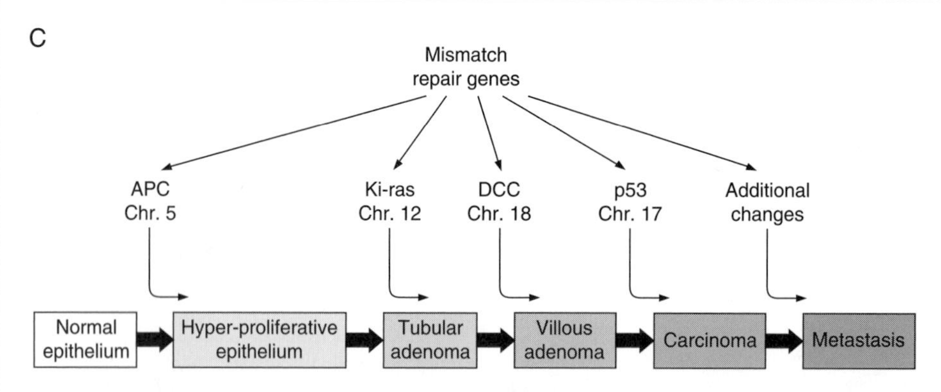

FIGURE 16C Associated genetic defects. As colorectal tumors develop and progress, the tumor cells accumulate genetic defects in their DNA in a preferential sequence as shown. Mutations and loss of the normal genes affect the tumor-suppressor genes APC (responsible for the hereditary predisposition adenomatous Polyposis coli), DCC (deleted in colon cancer), and p53. In addition, the oncogene Ki-*ras* is mutated in about 50% of all tumors (Fearon and Vogelstein, 1990, © Cell Press, with permission). Defects in the mismatch repair genes that cause the hereditary cancer syndrome HNPCC can enhance induction of mutation at all stages and accelerate malignant progression. The process of tumor promotion comprises the growth of premaligant adenomas from initiated cells.

ial polyposis coli. APC is a tumor-suppressor gene and has been named the gatekeeper of colorectal carcinogenesis. Its mutation may be the initation step in colonic tumors. The animals have a hyperplastic mucosa and develop multiple adenomatous polyps, and consequently carcinomas of the colon and the small intestine, about 20 weeks after birth. Min-mice, as well as mouse strains in which the APC gene has been inactivated (APC knock-out strains), are frequently used in studies of tumorigenesis and chemoprevention.

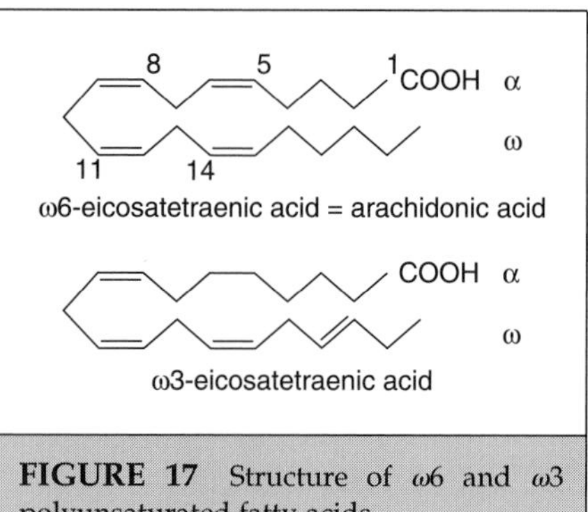

FIGURE 17 Structure of ω6 and ω3 polyunsaturated fatty acids.

Promoting Agents

Dietary factors modulate proliferation response as well as adenoma and carcinoma yield, but often experiments have not been designed with a clear two-stage protocol, so that the number of clearly identified tumor promoters is small. The strongest influence has been observed for nutritional fat; increasing the fat content of the diet from 5% to 20% enhances tumor incidence as well as tumor yield four- to five fold. From the available data, it cannot be determined whether saturated and unsaturated fatty acids differ in their effects. However, fish oils containing ω3-polyunsaturated fatty acids (PUFA) have a tumor protective effect in the colon. The structure of ω3-PUFA differs from that of ω6-PUFA present in most vegetable oils by the positioning of the double bonds (Fig. 17).

Secondary bile acids (lithocholic acid, desoxycholic acid) support tumor promotion in the colon if instilled rectally. Their production and secretion are induced by fat consumption and they may be mediators of the promotional activity of nutritional fat. A promotional activity of ethanol is discussed (Table 12).

Mediators and Mechanisms of Tumor Promotion by Nutritional Fat

The promoting effect of fat may be due to a combination of specific and unspecific effects. Fat is the main energy source in the diet and high calorie uptake favors growth in many organs. Caloric restriction has been shown to decrease tumor incidence and

TABLE 12 Colorectal Tumor Promoters

Promoter	Potency
Nutritional fat	++++
Caloric intake	?/+
Bile acids	
Desoxycholic acid	++++
Lithocholic acid	++++
Cholic acid	++
Chenodesoxycholic acid	++
Ethanol	+/?

yield. High calorie uptake may also be involved in colon tumor promotion. However, the protective effect of fish oils (ω3-PUFA) argues that this unspecific growth promotion is not the only reason why nutritional fat promotes colon tumorigenesis. Additional, more specific mechanisms may include bile acids, 1,2-diglycerides, and prostaglandins.

Bile acid secretion and formation of the promoting secondary bile acids by intestinal bacteria (Fig. 18) are increased by high fat consumption. In contrast, a high-fiber diet counteracts this effect and inhibits colorectal carcinogenesis. Similarly, high Ca^{2+} consumption has been shown to inhibit tumor development, possibly by reduction of bile acid bioavailability. Instillation of secondary bile acids increases cell proliferation in the mucosa and expands the proliferative compartment. Desoxycholic acid paradoxically decreases the number of aberrant crypts in the mucosa; it seems to select a resistant subpopulation of aberrant crypts able to undergo further tumor development. Bile acids stimulate ornithine decarboxylase and induce the expression of proliferation-related genes. They also activate protein kinase C (PKC) by

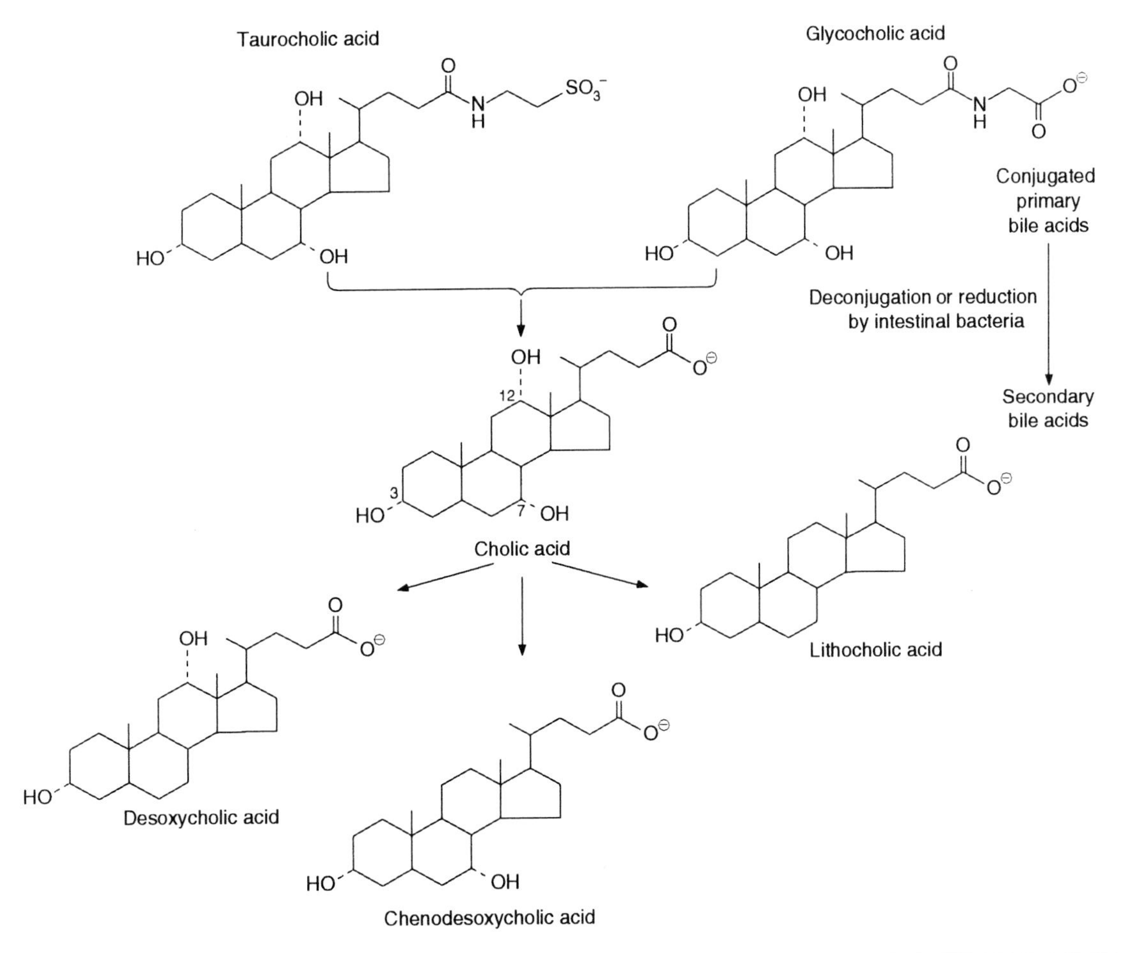

FIGURE 18 Production of bile acids promoting colon tumorigenesis.

an indirect mechanism inducing signaling pathways similar to those of phorbol esters in skin.

1,2-Diglycerides (1,2-DG) containing myristic or palmitic acid are present in the colon at micromolar concentrations. They may be produced from nutritional fat by incomplete digestion in the small intestine or they may be synthesized by intestinal bacteria. No promotional activity in the colon has been experimentally demonstrated, possibly because of their short half-life. Similar 1,2-DG have promoting activity in the skin. In primary cultures of human colonic epithelial cells, they are selective mitogens for initiated premalignant cells, an effect that within the tissue can cause a growth advantage for initiated cells and support adenoma growth. At the molecular level, they stimulate PKC.

The inhibitory effect of ω3-PUFA on tumor development in the colon was one of the earliest indications that arachidonic acid metabolites may be involved in colon carcinogenesis. ω3-PUFA are incorporated into membrane lipids, competing with arachidonic acid. There they reduce levels of arachidonic acid, the substrate of cyclooxygenases, and lower prostglandin (PG) synthesis (Fig. 11).

The involvement of PG in colorectal tumor development is also supported by the observed elevation of PG levels (PGE2) in the mucosa of mice lacking APC function (min-mice). Furthermore, in both adenomas and carcinomas PG levels are enhanced due to overexpression of the inducible cyclooxygenase-2 isoenzyme COX-2. Cyclooxygenase inhibitors normalize mucosal morphology as well as the PG levels, and they can prevent polyp growth. They also inhibit tumor development in carcinogen-treated mice and rats, especially when a high-fat diet is used to promote tumors. Together, these observations argue for a role of PG and specifically (COX-2) products in colorectal tumor promotion. (see Fig. 11 and the previous section on Tumor Prevention Skin).

Dietary Factors Protecting from Colorectal Tumors

Feeding high-fiber diets inhibits tumor development in the colon, but as fiber is a chemically ill-defined agent, it is difficult to identify the mechanisms involved. In addition, different kinds of fiber differ widely in their individual effects and analysis is further complicated by the complex mixture present in any diet. In spite of these difficulties, several possible mechanisms of action have been identified that are effective in different combinations for different fibers. (1) Fecal bulk is increased, causing a dilution effect and stimulation of motility, which, in turn, reduce exposure times to any toxic substance in the colonic lumen. (2) Adsorption processes can bind bile acids as well as carcinogens to biologically inactive forms. (3) Fiber consumption also counteracts the effect of fat on the amount of bile acids in the gut and on the composition of the bile acid mixture by affecting intestinal bacteria. (4) Some fibers can be partially digested by intestinal bacteria producing short-chain fatty acids. The resulting decrease of fecal pH can, in turn, reduce the solubility of bile acids and 1,2-DG. One of the acids, butyrate, directly inhibits proliferation and induces active cell death (apoptosis) in colonic tumor cells *in vitro*.

Relevance for Humans

Human colorectal carcinomas are among the most frequent tumors in western Europe and the United States. In humans tumors are usually localized in the distal colon and the rectum. As in rodents, carcinomas of the small intestine are extremely rare. The human tumors develop through the same series of premalignant lesions—hyperplasia, aberrant crypts > adenoma > carcinoma (Fig. 16A–16B). In addition, sequential accumulation of mutations during tumor development has been demonstrated. The earliest genetic defect is a mutation in the APC tumor, suppressor gene, followed by activation of the Ki-*ras* oncogene that may interact with PKC-activating tumor promoters. Both mutations can already be demonstrated in aberrant crypts. Mutations of the tumor suppressor genes DCC (deleted in colon cancer) and p53 are later events (Fig. 16C).

About 10% of all patients suffer from hereditary predispositions caused either by a germ-line mutation in the APC gene on chromosome 5 or by mutations in genes involved in DNA mismatch repair (HNPCC). The former represents a genetically transmitted initiation event that dramatically accelerates tumor formation as described above for the corresponding animal model (min-mouse, APC knock out strains). The latter reduces the accuracy of DNA replication in a way that enhances the accumulation of genetic defects in tumor cells and consequently tumor progression (similar to mutations in p53).

For sporadic (i.e., nonhereditary) colon cancers, epidemiological studies have identified consumption of meat and fat as the main risk factors. Heterocyclic amines in broiled or grilled meat may act as initiators of human colorectal tumors and fat seems to be the main promoting agent in human diet. Protective effects have been observed from fruits and vegetables, probably based on their content of vitamins and fiber.

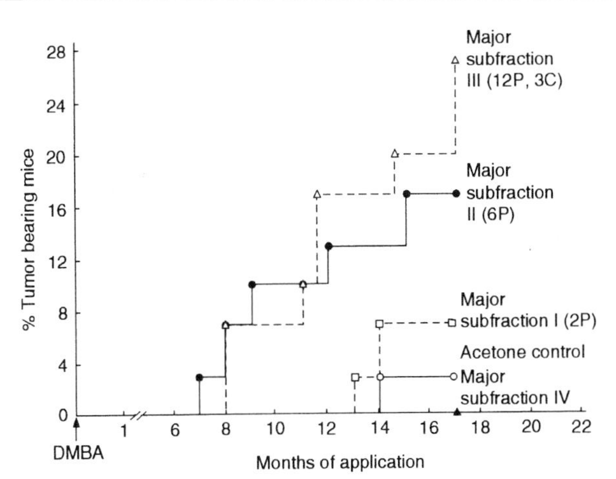

FIGURE 19 Tumor-promoting activity of tobacco-smoke condensates on mouse skin. Tobacco smoke condensates were subfractionated by differential solubility followed by chromatographic separation procedures. The carcinogenic and/or tumor-promoting activity of individual fractions was assayed using tumor induction on mouse skin (see Fig. 8). The "weakly acidic" fraction of the smoke condensate was the major promoting fraction. It contained cyclopentenone derivatives, catechols, hydrochinone, pyridine derivatives, and fatty acids. The "neutral" and "standard tar" fractions had complete carcinogenic activity (Hecht *et al.*, 1975).

ω3-PUFA and antiinflammatory drugs are also protective, indicating an involvement of prostaglandins in tumor promotion.

As in experimental systems, COX-2 is overexpressed in human premalignant as well as malignant tumors and antiinflammatory drugs inhibiting the enzyme also inhibit tumorigenesis. This implies that tumor promotion in humans is caused by the same mediators and mechanisms as in experimental carcinogenesis.

Respiratory Tract

Bronchial cancers are among the most common cancers in humans and epidemiological observations have unequivocally identified tobacco abuse as the main risk factor. Tobacco smoke as a complex carcinogen supports complete carcinogenesis. Evidence for a promoting component mainly stems from epidemiological data; cessation of smoking reduces risk with time, indicating a reversible factor in tumor development.

Furthermore, as with other tumors, respiratory tract cancer develops along a series of premalignant changes—tracheobronchial hyperplasia and metaplasia—that display distinct genetic and regulatory alterations, including upregulation of c-*jun* and activation of EGF- and IGF-related growth pathways. The bioactive peptides gastrin-releasing peptide and bombesin seem to be involved in growth of some lesions. These findings support the occurrence of promotion-like growth processes. Sequential accumulation of genetic defects in tumor cells (mutation of p53 and allelic loss of chromosomes 3 and 9; mutations in Ki-*ras* at late stages) indicate tumor progression.

In experimental models, tumor promotion in the respiratory tract has rarely been demonstrated. Rats and hamsters are relatively resistant to induction of respiratory tract tumors; only mice are more sensitive. There are, however, large strain-specific variations, with strain A mice being most sensitive. Usually tumors develop in the alveolar regions and display different histological types compared with humans.

Investigation of tobacco-smoke condensates for initiating and promoting activities was performed on the mouse skin model. The studies revealed that different fractions obtained from the condensates had either promoting or initiating–complete carcinogenic activity (Fig. 19; Table 6).

Asbestos in combination with cigarette smoke enhances bronchial cancer, while it mostly induces mesotheliomas after sole exposure in humans. Experimental evidence for tumor promotion by asbestos was obtained after implantation of a dimethylbenzanthracene pellet into the tracheal epithelium of rats. The spent pellets were removed and then asbestos fibers were instilled into the tracheal lumen, where they enhanced the appearance of tumors.

Butylated hydroxytoluene (BHT) acts as lung tumor promoter in mice when applied by ip injection. It causes death of alveolar type II cells, regenerative proliferation, and—after repeated treatment—growth of lung adenomas, as well as of few carcinomas that are not histologically related to human tumors. An involvement of radicals is suggested by the observation that BHT supports lung tumor promotion only after activation to BHT-MeOH, BHT-BuOH, or methinquinone via radical semichinone intermediates. In mice as well as in rats polychlorinated biphenyls show the same activity.

The mechanisms of tumor promotion in the respiratory tract are not sufficiently understood. However, there are indications that cell damage and inflammatory reactions play an important role. Intratracheal instillation of tobacco smoke condensates, tar deposits, and asbestos fibers induce injury, inflammatory reactions, and regenerative proliferation followed by tumor growth.

After instillation or inhalation of asbestos fibers, cell proliferation has been observed in the tracheal and bronchial epithelium and in the mesothelium, with mesothelial reactions being more persistent. *In vitro* asbestos fibers cause both altered growth characteristics and aneuploidy in mesothelial cells but only growth stimulation in tracheobronchial epithelial cells. In addition, exposure of mesothelial cell cultures to fibers caused selective cytotoxicity that provided the survival of mutated cells. These observations suggest that asbestos may be a complete carcinogen in the mesothelium, but only a tumor promoter in bronchial epithelia. Hypothetically, cooperation of tumor-promoting asbestos with initiation by genotoxic tobacco-smoke constituents can explain why lung tumors are rare in nonsmoking, but frequent in smoking, asbestos workers.

TABLE 13 Some Tumor-Promoting and Nongenotoxic Carcinogens Acting on Thyroid Gland

Substance or noxious condition	Primary effect[a]
Methyl-, propylthiouracil, aminotriazole, methylmethimazole	Inhibition of thyroid peroxidase
Perchlorate	Inhibition of iodine uptake into thyroid gland
Iodine deficiency precursor	Inhibition of synthesis of T_4
Phenobarbital	Induction of glucuronyl transferase in the liver, accelerated inactivation of T_4

[a]T_4, thyroxine

Thyroid Gland

Animal experiments revealed several different nitrosamines, nitrosamides, and aromatic amines as initiating carcinogens in the thyroid. Furthermore, ionizing radiation has initiating activity. ^{131}I, a radioactive isotope of iodine emitting beta and gamma radiation, is accumulated as efficiently by the thyroid as inactive iodine and incorporated into thyroid hormones. Its physical half-life is 8 days. It is genotoxic and, at higher doses, carcinogenic. Recent epidemiologic studies revealed a pronounced increase of thyroid cancer in children in areas exposed to ^{131}I fallout after the nuclear accident at Tschernobyl. The minimal lag phase between exposure and increase in thyroid cancer incidence was remarkably short (approximately 4 years). These observations suggest that children are much more sensitive to ^{131}I-induced thyroid carcinogenesis than adults. External X rays also have initiating and tumorigenic effects in the thyroid.

Tumor-promoting activities in animal thyroid were found with a number of different agents inhibiting thyroid hormone synthesis (Table 13). Although not genotoxic, these agents produced carcinomas in rats and mice. Examples for experimental animals are some derivatives of thiourea such as propylthiouracil, which is used in human therapy as an antithyroid drug. The inhibitory action of thiourea compounds was first discovered in cattle consuming certain brassica plants (e.g., cabbage, mustard, radish); rats developed thyroid adenoma after feeding on these vegetables. Glucobrassicin, a thioglucoside in cabbage, has been associated with struma formation in humans in certain areas. The same is true for dietary deficiency in iodine. In animals, low-iodine diets lead to thyroid hyperplasia, struma, and carcinomas. After preceding initiation by genotoxins, iodine deficieny promoted tumor development. Likewise, the herbicides amino triazole or perchlorate, which inhibit thyroid function, produce tumors.

Surprisingly, phenobarbital and some other inducers of drug-metabolizing enzymes in the liver also have tumor-promoting and carcinogenic effects in rodent thyroid. These agents do not appear to affect the thyroid directly. However, they enhance degradation of thyroid hormones in the liver (Table 13). Thus, the common denominator of the various tumor promoters and nongenotoxic carcinogens acting on the thyroid is a reduction of circulating levels of thyroid hormones. This in turn will lead to increased thyroid-stimulating hormone (TSH) secretion by the pituitary gland. TSH stimulates hormone synthesis and hyperplasia in the thyroid. It is considered the ultimate effector of tumor promotion in the thyroid gland. Hypophysectomy or treatment with thyroxine blocks the (enhanced) secretion of TSH and prevents promoting and carcinogenic effects of thyroid inhibitors and phenobarbital. In conclusion, this group of agents appears to promote indirectly, via creating a hormonal imbalance.

TSH initially leads to enhanced cell replication and hyperplasia in the thyroid. Cell proliferation returns to normal even if TSH levels are continuously enhanced, while the hyperplasia persists. Apparently thyroid cells have become less sensitive to the mitogenic effect of TSH, although still showing enhanced functional activity (hormone synthesis). Hypothetically, initiated cells lack this desensitization towards the mitogenic action of TSH, possibly as a result of autocrine production of growth factors such as insulin-like growth factor (IGF1) by initiated cells.

In humans, tumor-promoting and carcinogenic effects of TSH are clearly less pronounced than in rats and mice. As in animals, thyroid carcinomas may result from nodular hyperplasia (struma) but are quite rare. After therapeutic application of thyroid inhibitors, enhanced appearance of adenoma or carcinoma in the thyroid has not been documented. Likewise, after therapeutic application of ^{131}I to adults, thyroid carcinoma has not convincingly been demonstrated.

Mammary Gland

Experimental Models

Charles Huggins, at the end of the 1950s, discovered that carcinoma in the mammary gland can be induced by a single dose of a carcinogen. These experiments provided the possibility of investigating tumor initiation and promotion in this organ. Most studies are performed with female rats or mice. A single application of initiating carcinogens such as dimethylbenzanthracene (DMBA), 3-methylcholanthrene (MCA) or *N*-methyl-*N*-nitrosourea (MNU) results in mammary tumor formation within 8 to 21 weeks in almost 100% of the rats; the chemicals are effective after intragastric, subcutaneous, or intravenous application. A "window of sensitivity" to initiating carcinogens exist at a certain age of the animals. Tumor incidence is highest after treating rats at the ages of 40–65 days, but about 10 times lower when 100-day-old animals are treated. Male rats do not develop mammary carcinoma after the same treatment. Many polycyclic aromatic hydrocarbons and aromatic amines were found to be carcinogenic in mammary gland; MCA, DMBA, and MNU are most frequently used for experimental purposes. Many of these compounds act as initiators in liver, skin, stomach, and other organs as well. Their seemingly selective carcinogenic activity on mammary gland is most likely due to the strong promoting effect of female sex hormones. Pregnancy shortly before or after initiation provides a protective effect against breast cancer formation. Likewise, protection results from treatment of animals with estradiol, progesterone, or prolactin before initiation; under this biological condition these hormones act as anticarcinogens. The same hormones enhance tumorigenesis after initiation.

At the genetic level, the exchange of guanosine by adenosine (G → A transition) in codon 12 of the Ha-*ras*-1 gene, which causes its activation, has been suggested to be a conditional oncogenic mutation. The G → A transition occurs during normal development of the mammary gland in rats (Fischer 344) and the mutant cells acquire about a fivefold growth advantage compared to nonmutant epithelial cells. However, the manifestation of the oncogenic potential of this mutation requires additional alterations. A single dose of MNU results in selective outgrowth of preexisting Ha-*ras*-1 mutant cells; this is not achieved by DMBA. Furthermore, this mutation can be detected in most but not all MNU-induced tumors of rats, indicating that there may be alternative oncogenic mutations during initiation.

In mice, Bittner found in 1936 the *m*ouse *m*ammary *t*umor *v*irus (MMTV virus), an initiator that can be transmitted by milk. He also found that genetic factors are involved in the development of breast tumors. Later, mammotropic hormones were identified as important factors for the MMTV-virus-induced carcinogenesis. So far, the significance of the MMTV virus for mammary gland carcinogenesis has been shown unequivocally for mice only.

Endogenous and Exogenous Promoters

Early observations on chemically induced mammary carcinogenesis showed that hypophysectomy inhibits tumor development. Later studies revealed prolactin, a pituitary hormone, to be essential for the manifestation of mammary neoplasia after initiation. Prolactin promotes breast cancer development in male rats and also in females after surgical removal of ovaries, adrenal glands, and hypophysis. Thus, prolactin acts as a tumor promoter in the mammary gland.

Steroid hormones affect mammary tumorigenesis as well. Estrogens promote, whereas androgens inhibit, the carcinogen-induced formation as well as the growth of tumors. The growth stimulatory effect of estrogens on mammary epithelium *in vivo* is mediated by three mechanisms. Directly by (1) the estrogen–receptor-mediated stimulation of epithelial cell proliferation and inhibition of active cell death; and indirectly by (2) stimulation of stromal cells to produce trophic factors and (3) increasing pituitary prolactin secretion. Prolactin appears to be most important during early stages of tumor development, whereas prolonged growth of mammary neoplasia requires estrogen. Tumors may regress upon ovarectomy (Fig. 20). Retreatment with estrogens causes regrowth of tumors. Apparently, survival and growth of mammary tumor cells may depend on the presence of hormones. Tumor regrowth after prolonged estrogen withdrawal indicates progression to estrogen-independent growth (Fig. 20).

In mice, growth of MMTV-virus-positive preneoplastic lesions (hyperplastic alveolar nodules) and development of tumors is accelerated by estrogens and prolactin. The MMTV virus causes an insertion muta-

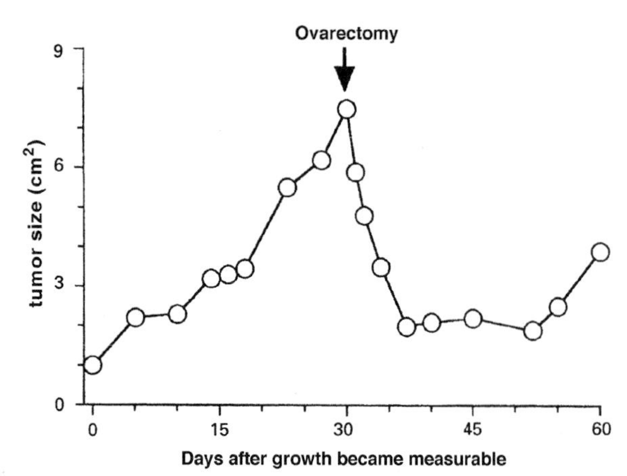

FIGURE 20 Regression of mammary gland tumors upon ovarectomy. Tumors of mammary glands in rats were induced by a single dose of DMBA; the growth of a repesentative tumor is shown. Once a tumor became palpable, its area (longest × shortest diameter) was determined; measurements began on day 0. Note the regrowth of the tumor in later stage of the experiment after prolonged estrogen withdrawal. According to Gullino *et al.* (1972), *J. Natl. Cancer Inst.* **49**, 1333–1348, by permission of Oxford University Press.

tion in *int* genes; steroid hormones lead to their activation. The *int* genes code for growth factors and are activated during sexual maturation. This provides an interesting example of how initiating and promoting factors may cooperate at the molecular level.

In summary, tumor promotion in the mammary gland can be brought about by endogenous factors (hormones). This explains why a single dose of a carcinogen without further treatment can lead to tumor formation. This notion is important in view of cancer-risk assessment because in these experimental models strong *endogenous* promotion may mask a potential tumor-promoting action of *exogenous* factors. Chronic treatment of rats and mice with estrogens or prolactin, without previous administration of an initiating carcinogen, can also result in mamma tumor formation. These hormones can therefore be classified as nongenotoxic carcinogens. Their effect may be explained by promotion of "spontaneous" lesions (see previous sections).

Prolactin levels may be modulated by exogenous factors with neuroendocrine activity. Thus, stress, dopamine, and dopaminergic drugs cause a reduction, whereas neuroleptic drugs (dopamine receptor blockers) increase the prolactin level. Accordingly, chronic treatment of rats and mice may cause either antipromotion or promotion of mammary tumors (Table 3). Dogs may develop mammary cancer in response to progestins or the combination of progestin with estrogen. Progestins do not exhibit a direct stimulatory activity on dog mammary gland but increase plasma levels of somatotropic hormone. Like prolactin in rats and in dogs, somatotropic hormone exhibits a strong stimulatory action on breast growth and lactation and may promote carcinogenesis from spontaneous initiation.

Nutrition is a further important factor for breast cancer development in animal experiments. High fat content facilitates tumor development, which is reversible after changing the diet. Polyunsaturated fatty acids are probably most important for tumor promotion. However, fatty acids may differ extremely in their action. The ω6-fatty acids promote and, in contrast, ω-3 fatty acids inhibit mammary tumorigenesis. The underlying mechanisms are not fully understood; they may be similar as in colon. Caloric restriction lowers mammary tumor incidence. In mice, caloric restriction can block the MMTV-induced *int1, int2,* and *ras* expression.

Cancer Prestages and Effects of Promoters

The postnatal development of the breast provides a basis for understanding the dependency of carcinogenesis on age and hormones. Development starts with the germination of milk ducts, formation of terminal end buds, and their subsequent differentiation into alveoli (sites of milk production). While passing through these developmental stages, cells are considered targets for initiation; they are most sensitive during active growth. Breast development is controlled by a complex interaction of hormones of the hypothalamic–hypophysis axis and the reproductive organs. Pregnancy accelerates differentiation of end bud cells and may protect from initiation by reducing the number of sensitive (undifferentiated) cells. Prolactin, estradiol, and some dopamine receptor blockers exert similar actions. Initiated cells subsequently develop into ductal atypical hyperplasia, ductal *in situ* carcinoma, and finally into infiltrating carcinoma. In rats, cells of atypic hyperplasia and in mice cells of the "hyperplastic alveolar nodule" are considered the target for tumor-promoting factors. In mouse strains with high spontaneous tumor incidence, most of the breast carcinomas derive from hyperplastic nodules, although only a minority of the nodules eventually develop into tumors. Treatment of rats with dimethylbenzanthracene also results in morphological manifestation of hyperplastic alveolar nodules; their tumorigenic potential, however, is low.

The action of promoting hormones on their target cells is mediated by specific receptor–signal transduction pathways, which can be modulated by hormone antagonists. In the multistage concept of carcinogenesis, hormone antagonists (e.g., tamoxifen) can be classified as antipromoters. As to the underlying mechanisms, it is known that hormone withdrawal and treatment with hormone antagonists result in inhibition of cell proliferation; this action has been extensively used to select for effective drugs. Both measures also induce active cell death (apoptosis) in tumors of the breast and other endocrine organs, such as the prostate.

Relevance for Humans

Neoplasia of the female breast belongs to the most frequent cancers in Western countries. It accounts for about one-fourth of all newly diagnosed cancers per year and for about one-fifth of cancer deaths. Epidemiological studies revealed a window of high susceptibility of humans to initiating noxes in the environment. Thus, women exposed at infancy or adolescence to the radiation after the atomic bomb explosions at Hiroshima and Nagasaki had an enhanced mammary tumor risk. Furthermore, commencing tobacco smoking before 14 years of age is suspected of increasing breast cancer risk. In addition, genetic factors such as mutations in the *BCRA1* gene on chromosome 17 and the *BCRA2* gene on chromosome 13 determine the susceptibility of women to breast cancer ("cancer families").

Hormones clearly affect the development of tumors in endocrine organs of humans. Thus, cancers of the breast, endometrium, and ovary are less frequent in women with an early pregnancy than in nullipara. Apparently, accelerated differentiation of breast cells following pregnancy provides some protection from initiating noxes. In contrast, early menarche, late first pregnancy, and late menopause increase breast cancer risk, which may be explained by a long period of promotion by estrogens. Contraceptive steroids do not generally affect breast cancer incidence; only if they are taken from adolescence on may breast cancer risk increase. There is no evidence that dopamine antagonists or other drugs with neuroendocrine activity enhance mammary cancer incidence in humans. The most convincing evidence for a role of hormones in mammary gland carcinogenesis in humans is provided by its sex difference; the breast cancer risk of men is about 100 times lower than that of women.

An increase of breast cancer risk by lifestyle factors (low consumption of fiber, and high consumption of red meat, fat, and alcohol; in general, being overweight) is most probable. As to the fatty acid composition of the diet, there is an inverse relationship between the incidence of breast cancer and the amount of fish consumption, suggesting a protective effect of ω-3 fatty acids also in humans. However, epidemiological studies on the significance of individual risk factors revealed contradictory results.

Understanding the mechanisms of action of hormones on (pre)neoplasia of the breast provides a basis for prevention and therapy. Experimental as well as human tumors often are hormone-dependent and regress upon chemical antagonization of hormones or surgical removal of hormone-secreting organs (ovary) (Fig. 20). The antiestrogen tamoxifen, which binds to but does not activate the estrogen receptor in mammary gland, has proven effective in adjuvant therapy of breast carcinoma. Currently, tamoxifen is being tested as a possible chemopreventive (antipromoting) agent in women with high risk for breast cancer development.

Other Sexual Organs

Prostate

In rats, prostate tumors can be induced by genotoxic carcinogens such as *N*-nitroso-(bis)(2-oxopropyl)amine, methylnitrosourea, or dimethylbenzanthracene. Androgens (testosterone, dihydrotestosterone) are growth-stimulating factors for the normal prostate and also stimulate the growth of prostate tumors. Withdrawal of androgens by castration or treatment with androgen antagonists (cyproterone acetate, flutamide) cause regression of prostate tumors in experimental animals and humans. Regrowth of tumors can be induced by an increase in androgen levels; thus, androgens act as endogenous promoters on which tumor cells seem to depend for proliferation and survival.

The etiology of the human prostate carcinoma is not clear. In about 95% of the cases, prostate carcinoma develops in the epithelium of the peripheral zone of the gland in which focal hyperplasia ("youthful epithelium") may be considered the target cell population for tumor-promoting factors. The cells of the periphery and focal hyperplasia depend on testosterone.

Endometrium

In animals and humans, the incidence of endometrial carcinoma is increased by estrogens and reduced by progestins. Prolonged application of estrogens ("unopposed estrogen replacement therapy") to postmenopausal women resulted in endometrial cancers. Depending on the duration of use, the risk of cancer development may decline upon discontinuation of estrogen treatment. This supports a promotional mechanism of action. Additional doses of progestins prevent tumor formation by estrogens. Tamoxifen also seems to induce endometrial tumors in humans. This may result from some estrogenic activity on endometrium that tamoxifen exerts in addition to its antiestrogenicity. Infiltrating carcinoma of the endometrium develops via a sequence of stages including adenomatous hyperplasia of progressive severity, which gradually lose the ability to involute, and *in situ* carcinoma. The opposite action of estrogen and progesterone may be considered as promotion and antipromotion, because estrogen stimulates whereas progesterone inhibits cell proliferation in animal and human endometrium.

Vagina—Diethylstilbestrol

Diethylstilbestrol (DES) is a synthetic compound that binds to and activates the estrogen receptor. It is a potent estrogen. Since the mid-1940s, diethylstilbestrol was used to prevent abortion, although its carcinogenic potential was already known from animal experiments. Carcinogenic effects of DES in humans were recognized at the end of the 1960s. Daughters of DES-treated mothers developed vaginal carcinoma after puberty (Fig. 21); up to 1985 about 500 cases were registered, most of them in the United States. Of these cases, 60% could be attributed to DES exposure *in utero* (Table 14). In male descendants, anomalies of the gonads, testicular hypoplasia, microphallus, kryptorchism, and other abnormalities were observed. Kryptorchism strongly enhances risk of testicular cancer. The DES-induced carcinoma of the vagina demonstrates the relevance of three important principles of chemical carcinogenesis in humans, namely: (1) transplacentar carcinogenesis, (2) hormonal carcinogenesis, and (3) separation of the stages of initiation and promotion. These observations have been confirmed in animal experiments. Thus, prenatal exposure of mice, rats, and hamsters causes tumors of hormone-dependent tissues such as vagina, cervix, uterus, ovary, mammary gland, and testis.

TABLE 14 Carcinoma of the Vagina and Cervix as Dependent on Maternal Medication[a]

Medication	Cases (%)
Diethylstilbestrol	60
Other hormone or unknown medication	12
No hormones, no medication	23
Medication unknown	5
Total (n = 519)	100

[a] According to Melnick *et al.* (1987).

Transplacentar initiation by DES ensues during the first trimenon of pregnancy. During organogenesis, the sexual anlagen of both genders are formed. During later stages of organogenesis, parts of the Müllerian duct in females differentiate into tubes, uterus, and upper vagina; and in males into pedunculated hydatid (appendix testis) and prostatic utricle (Utriculus prostaticus); while other parts regress by active (programmed) cell death. The primary damage by DES in both sexes is attributed to inhibition of this regression. In fact, abnormal cell populations appear in certain areas of the vagina and in other sexual organs in almost all of DES-exposed daughters, which derive from persistent embryonal Müllerian duct tissue. The mechanism of initiation is unclear. Genotoxic activity of DES was observed *in vitro* but only at extremely high concentrations; it is probably not relevant for humans. Alternatively, nongenotoxic initiation is conceiveable and may be related to abnormal imprinting. Hormonal imprinting occurs during normal embryonal development and leads to a specific expression pattern of hormone receptors. DES may alter physiological imprinting patterns. Thus, prenatal exposure of mice to DES resulted in atypical expression of estrogen receptors in seminal vesicles with a pattern normally found in uterine tissue. Furthermore, DES inhibits active cell death in estrogen-dependent tissues and this may result in the persistance of Müllerian duct cells that physiologically would regress. Surviving embryonal cells, that may be imprinted abnormally are most probably the target for promotion by sex hormones. The time course of the manifestation of the carcinoma suggests that sex hormones act as promoters when secreted at high levels with the onset of puberty (Fig. 21).

Environmental Contaminants with Hormonal Activity and Cancer Risk

A number of environmental contaminants (Table 15) have been hypothesized to mimic or to antagonize the action of hormones ("endocrine disruptors"). Exposure of humans to these compounds has been associated with the increase in breast, endometrial, prostate, and testis cancer. According to the multistage concept of carcinogenesis, at least two ways of action are conceivable; (1) transplacentar imprinting and initiation as found with DES; and (2) tumor promotion during adolescence and adulthood. However, no conclusive experimental or epidemiological data are available to support a significant role of "endocrine disruptors" for human carcinogenesis. Never-

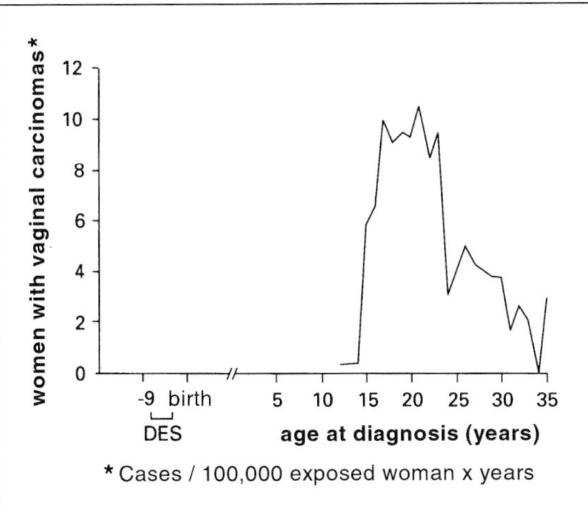

FIGURE 21 Age dependency of the manifestation of vaginal carcinoma after *in utero* exposure to diethylstilbestrol. Cases adjusted to 100,000 women × years (according to Melnick *et al.*, 1987; Copyright 1987 Massachusetts Medical Society. All rights reserved).

theless, although increases in endocrine-dependent tumors are currently believed to result from changes in lifestyle (high-calorie–protein diets) further studies on endocrine active chemicals are required for adequate risk assessments.

TESTING AND RISK ASSESSMENT OF TUMOR PROMOTERS

Growth is a necessary but not sufficient condition for tumor promotion. All tumor promoters directly or indirectly stimulate growth in their target organ. The mechanisms can be attributed broadly either to cytotoxicity and regeneration or to hormonal or hormone-like effects, including interaction with specific receptors. Agents interfering with hormonal feedback circuits frequently induce tumors at sites different from the primary target organ of the agent (Tables 3 and 13). Growth stimulation frequently is a secondary effect of tumor promoters. The primary mechanisms by which tumor promoters stimulate growth are multiple and heterogenous.

Every stimulation of growth is not necessarily associated with tumor-promoting action; additional properties are required for tumor promotion. These are determined by the specific phenotype of the initiated cells. Initiated cells are specifically promotable only by certain promoters; even in the same organ different types of initiated cells may exist that are promotable by different classes of agents. There appears to exist a locker–key relation between initiated cell and promoter. The same principle applies to trophic hormones, which stimulate growth and function only in specifically determined target cells. In conclusion, a generally valid mechanism-based system for testing and risk evaluation of potential tumor promoters is not available.

TABLE 15 Some Environmental Contaminants with Endocrine Activity

Activity	Compounds
Estrogenic	Chemicals: *o,p*-DDT, aldrin, atrazine, dieldrin, methoxychlor, endosulfane, heptachlor, mirex, phosmet, toxaphene, chlordecone, alkylphenoles, bisphenol A, phthalates, polychlorinated biphenyls, benzophenone, phenol red; the mycotoxin zearalenone
Antiestrogenic	Polychlorinated biphenyls (coplanar congeners), polycyclic aromatic hydrocarbons, polychlorinated dibenzodioxines and dibenzofuranes
Androgenic	Tributyltin
Antiandrogenic	*p,p*-DDT, 3,4-dichloroaniline, vincloziline

Testing for Tumor-Promoting Activity

Protocols for carcinogenicity testing of chemicals in long-term animal experiments will detect tumor promoters only if initiated cells are present in the target organ. Therefore, these protocols have limited value in detecting tumor-promoting activities. Reliable testing for tumor promotion requires the application of two-stage protocols *in vivo* (Fig. 1). In these protocols, initiation is achieved in the presumed target organs of the test compound; subsequently the test compound is applied for a prolonged period of time. As endpoints, phenotypically altered cell foci in the liver and other organs, papillomas in skin and bladder, aberrant crypts and polyps in colon, adenomas, and malignant tumors can be used. Use of preneoplastic foci and other early lesions is advantageous because they require relatively short experimental periods for manifestation (medium-term test). The test with liver foci has currently the widest application. It allows the detection of initiating and promoting properties of compounds separately. Hints of a possible tumor-promoting potential are also provided by appearance of organ enlargement, induction of gene programs such as of drug metabolizing enzymes in the liver, cytotoxic effects, or interference with hormonal feedback circuits (Table 16).

Validated *in vitro* tests for tumor promotion are not available. To cover the diversity of mechanisms of action of tumor promoters, the development of test batteries is necessary. Such test batteries should account for organ specificity and allow quantification of promoting effects that play a key role in risk assessment. Endpoints useful *in vitro* include induction of DNA synthesis, inhibition of apoptosis, induction of enzymes, hormonal activity, and cytotoxicity (Table 16). Tests on cultured preneoplastic cells, preferably of human origin, would be particularly valuable; such cells may become available.

Inhibition of gap-junctional intercellular communication *in vitro* has found great interest in the past as a potential test system for tumor promoters. Many but not all tumor promoters identified first *in vivo* were also detected in the communication test *in vitro*. However, target organ and effective doses *in vivo* usually are not predictable from this test.

In conclusion, current *in vitro* tests on promoting activity have very limited reliability. Positive results should be taken to indicate the need for appropriate investigation *in vivo*. Negative results can not exclude promoting action *in vivo*.

TABLE 16 Indicators and Tests for Promoting Effects

	Endpoint
in vivo	Organ enlargement, hyperplasia, DNA increase
	Acceleration of tumor development
	Growth and enhancecd phenotypic expression of preneoplastic foci
in vivo or *in vitro*	Induction of DNA synthesis
	Induction of mitoses
	Inhibition of apoptoses
	Induction of ornithine decarboxylase
	Functional alterations: induction of gene programs, e.g., induction of drug metabolizing or peroxisomal enzymes
	Induction of altered differentiation
	Hormonal effects
	Induction of hormonal imbalance
	Cytotoxicity
in vitro	Inhibition of gap junctional intercellular communication (GJIC)
	Two-stage cell transformation
	Binding to receptors involved in promotion (protein kinase C, PPAR, dioxin receptor, etc.)

Relevance and Risk Assessment of Tumor Promoters

The formation of initiated cells probably is a frequent event. This is suggested by the ubiquitous occurrence of genotoxic chemicals and radiation in the environment. Furthermore, inborn mutations predisposing to cancer and genetic errors during cell replication may cause an initiation-like phenotype of cells. Mutation spectra in tumors suggest the possibility that some mutations initiating the cancer process result from spontaneous events. Thus deamination of 5-methylcytidine yields a G-T mismatch and subsequently may lead to G-A transition. In the presence of (spontaneous) initiated cells, promoters may produce tumors and appear as (complete) carcinogens. Promoting factors of endogenous or exogenous origin therefore are major determinants of human cancer. The large fraction of human cancers associated with unbalanced nutrition and hormones points to the great importance of promoting factors.

Risk assessment of tumor promoters requires epidemiological data, as well as results from animal experiments and *in vitro* tests. Since epidemiological data frequently are not available and since *in vitro* data in general are unreliable with respect to tumor-promoting activity, animal experiments in many cases are the only source of information for risk estimation. The difficulties with extrapolation from animal experiments to humans have to be kept in mind. Remarkably, animal and human experience with tumor promoters is quite concordant on some organs such as colon, mamma, endometrium, prostate, liver (contraceptive steroids), and B lymphocytes. However, human liver seems to be less susceptible than rodent liver to promotion by phenobarbital or peroxisome proliferators, human thyroid seems less susceptible to thyreostatic drugs, and human skin less susceptible to phorbol esters. Since the sensitivity of human tissues to tumor promoters can not be anticipated à priori, promoters identified in animal experiments invariably have to be considered carefully as risk factors for human carcinogenesis.

There are important differences in risk assessment for genotoxic (complete) carcinogens and tumor promoters. This does not mean that tumor promoters generally can be considered less harmful then genotoxic carcinogens. The following principles apply to the assessment of tumor promoters. They resemble those used for the evaluation of nongenotoxic carcinogens.

1. The possibility that the compound to be evaluated has initiating and genotoxic activity needs to be carefully investigated and, as far as feasible, be excluded.

2. Promotion can be considered reversible on the

basis of available experimental data. This reversibility applies to early stages before progression occurs.

3. Available information on mechanisms of promoting actions strongly supports the existence of a dose threshold below which tumor promotion does not occur. Therefore, for risk evaluation of individual compounds mechanistic information is needed. With promoters whose primary action is a cytotoxic effect, a certain dose or number of molecules will be required for cell damage. Below the threshold of cytotoxicity, no regenerative cell replication and no promotion will occur. A similar reasoning may hold for promoters that primarily inhibit specific enzymes or that cause hormonal imbalance. Likewise, reactions primarily mediated by receptors should require a certain number of promoter molecules, which may, however, be very low. In fact, receptor-mediated tumor promotion can be effected by very low doses (e.g., hormones or TCDD). Furthermore, the sigmoid shape of the dose–response relationship of tumor promoters supports the existence of a threshold. To assess this shape, with each individual agent a sufficient number of different dose levels has to be studied. Where a threshold of action exists, the estimation of risk at low exposures by linear extrapolation, as used for genotoxic carcinogens, is not applicable.

4. Quantitative information on the potency of a tumor-promoting effect from dose–response studies is of utmost importance for risk estimation. Doses active in animal experiments (lowest-observed-effect levels, or LOEL), as well as no-observed-effect levels (NOEL), are compared with human exposure. To define acceptable exposures or limit values, frequently NOEL from animal studies are divided by safety (or uncertainty) factors.

5. Elucidation of the mechanisms of tumor promotion in animal experiments is important in applying points 2 and 3. Furthermore, it should be assessed whether the same (primary) mechanisms effecting tumor promotion in animals will possibly hold true in humans. Thereby the relevance of the promoting effect for human health can be judged.

Bibliography

Boutwell, R. K. (1964). Some biological aspects of skin carcinogenesis. *Prog. Exp. Tumor Res.* **4,** 207–250.

Burns, F. J., Vanderlaan, M., Snyder, E., and Albert, R. E. (1978). Induction and progression of mouse skin papillomas. *In* "Carcinogenesis: A comprehensive survey, Vol. 2. Mechanisms of Tumor Promotion and Cocarcinogenesis" (T. J. Slaga *et al.*, eds.), pp. 91–96. Raven Press, New York.

Columbano, A., and Shinozuka, H. (1996) Liver regeneration versus direct hyperplasia. *FASEB J.* **10,** 1118–1128.

Doll, R., and Peto, R. (1981). The causes of cancer: quantitative estimates of avoidable risks of cancer in the United States today. *J. Natl. Cancer Inst.* **66,** 1191–1308.

Farber, E. (1996). Foundations in cancer research: The step-by-step development of epithelial cancer, from phenotype to genotype. *Adv. Cancer Res.* **70,** 21–48.

Farber, E., and Cameron, R. (1980). The sequential analysis of cancer development. *Adv. Cancer Res.* **31,** 125.

Fearon, E. R., and Vogelstein, B. (1990). A genetic model for colorectal tumorigenesis. *Cell* **61,** 163.

Friedman, E., Urmacher, C., and Winawer, S. (1984). A model for human colon carcinoma evolution based on the differential response of cultured preneoplastic, premalignant, and malignant cells to 12-O-tetradecanoylphorbol-13-acetate. *Cancer Res.* **44,** 1568–1578.

Hecker, E., Fusenig, N. E., Kunz, W., Marks, F., and Thielman, H. W. (1982). "Carcinogenesis: A comprehensive survey, Vol. 7. Cocarcinogenesis and Biological Effects of Tumor Promoters." Raven Press, New York.

Ito, N., Hasegawa, R., Imaida, K., Hirose, M., Asamoto, M., and Shirai, T. (1995). Concepts in multistage carcinogenesis. *Crit. Rev. Oncol. and Hematol.* **21,** 105–133.

Jass, J. R., Shepard, N. A., and Maybee, J. D. (1989). Atlas of surgical pathology of the colon, rectum and anus. Churchill Livingston, London.

Leffell, D. J., and Brash, D. E. (1996). Sunlight and skin cancer. *Sci. American* **275,** 38–49.

Luebeck, E. G., and Moolgavkar, S. H. (1996). Biologically based cancer modeling. *Drug Chem. Toxicol.* **19,** 221–243.

Mayer, M. P., and Poste, G. H. (1990). "Colon Cancer Cells." Academic Press, San Diego, CA.

Pitot, H. C. (1990). Altered hepatic foci: Their role in murine hepatocarcinogenesis. *Annu. Rev. Pharmacol. Toxicol.* **30,** 465.

Russo, J. *et al.* (1990). Biology of disease, comparative study of human and rat mammary tumorigenesis. *Lab. Invest.* **62,** 244.

Schulte-Hermann, R. (1985). Tumor promotion in the liver. *Arch. Toxicol.* **57,** 147–158.

Schulte-Hermann, R., Bursch, W., and Grasl-Kraupp, B. (1995). Active cell death (apoptosis) in liver biology and disease. *In* "Progress in Liver Disease" (J. L. Boyer and R. K. Ockner, eds.), vol. 13, pp. 1–35. W. B. Saunders Comp. Philadelphia.

Slaga, T. J. (1984). "Mechanisms of Tumor Promotion." CRC Press, Boca Raton, FL.

Weisburger, J. H., Reddy, B. S., Barnes, W. S., and Wynder, E. L. (1983). Bile acids, but not neutral sterols, are tumor promoters in the colon in man and in rodents. *Environ. Health Perspect.* **50,** 101–107.

Welsch, C. W. (1985). Host factors affecting the growth of carcinogen-induced rat mammary carcinomas: A review and tribute to Charles Brenton Huggins. *Cancer Res.* **45,** 3415.

Whysner, J., Ross, P. M., and Williams, G. M. (1996). Phenobarbital mechanistic data and risk assessment: Enzyme induction, enhanced cell proliferation, and tumor promotion. *Pharmacol. Ther.* **71,** 153–191.

CHAPTER

9

Transgenic Rodent Models

KENNETH R. TINDALL, RAYMOND W. TENNANT

Laboratory of Environmental Carcinogenesis and Mutagenesis, National Institute of Environmental Health Sciences, Research Triangle Park, North Carolina

INTRODUCTION

Rodent species have played many important roles in the field of toxicology from their use as tools to study mechanisms of toxic injury to that of surrogates in the assessment of toxic potential for humans. They have found such diverse applications because they can be reared and propagated easily under a variety of laboratory conditions. They are relatively inexpensive to breed and maintain. They are fecund, providing large litters in short periods of time, and their lifespan is short, permitting studies of the effects of chronic exposures.

Rodents have played a critical role in the efforts that have led to our understanding of the mammalian genome and of the genetic mechanisms by which the genome functions in replication, in DNA repair, and in the processes central to the reproductive transmission of genetic information to progeny. The Human Genome Project will ultimately result in defining the complete coding sequence of the human genome. While this will be the first complete sequence of any mammalian genome, prior genetic studies in rodents have provided basic information that have helped to make the Human Genome Project possible. Most notably, studies in rodents showed that the sequence of genes or loci on specific chromosomes could be mapped and a plethora of mutations have been defined and assigned to linkage maps.

While the study of conserved genes has been important and productive, they are only a part of the genome. Rodents are not humans and there are many genes that differ among mammalian species and account for their individuality. Many genes that determine individuality both among and within species differ from the conserved genes in the degree of variation. Individual genes may show a high degree of similarity, but the differences in base sequence may have profound effects in the amino acid sequence, tertiary structure, and functions of the encoded protein. Such variations between similar genes are termed "polymorphisms," and they can be seen in a variety of ways. Differences in eye color, hair thickness, bone length, enzyme substrate specificity, and so on, are but a few obvious examples of gene polymorphisms. More complex are polymorphisms in genes that are involved in the metabolism of xenobiotics, drugs, environmental chemicals, and combustion by-products. Such polymorphisms can account for many interindividual and interspecies differences in responses to xenobiotics. For example, polymorphisms associated with the CYP450 superfamily of enzymes influence many tissue-specific to species-specific reactions. Thus, while the conserved genes provide for similarities between rodents and humans, polymorphic genes provide for dissimilarities and, therefore, render the species imperfect surrogates of each other.

Rodents used in experimental toxicology and in toxicological testing differ from humans in an important way. Virtually all commercial rodent lines are inbred; that is, they have undergone successive generations of brother-to-sister matings in order to achieve genotypic and phenotypic homogeneity. The reduction of interindividual variation is important in reducing experimental variation and improving the reproducibility of experiments. It also reduces the group size needed in experiments in order to be able to observe meaningful results. Therefore, it is of a practical and economic advantage to use inbred rodents (and other species such as dogs). However, there are also important biological consequences attendant to the use of inbred strains. That is, inbreeding changes the frequency with which alleles of polymorphic genes occur within the inbred population. With subsequent cycles of inbreeding, fewer polymorphisms are retained in each generation. The progeny become less representative of *all* of the individuals in the species and become most representative of the genotype of a particular individual within the population. Under these circumstances, there may be uncertainty whether the responses to a particular chemical or drug or other toxic exposure is representative of the response of the species or specific to the response of an inbred strain. One principle that appears to prevail is that if similar responses are observed in two different species (e.g., rats and mice), it is less likely that the effects of the agents are strain-specific. Conversely, if under similar conditions of exposure (i.e., comparable doses and duration) effects occur in only one strain, it may be a strain- or a species-specific response. Understanding the nature of such responses requires extensive experimental effort in order to define the mechanisms and to identity the gene(s) involved. For example, it has been observed that several chemicals induced tumors only in the kidneys of male rats in long-term (2-year) carcinogenicity bioassays in which both mice and rats were used. Extensive studies have shown an association of the tumors with altered expression of an $\alpha_{2\mu}$-globulin protein, which is thought to be expressed only in the kidney epithelial cells of male rats. It has required years of experimental effort to identify this association and the issue remains open to controversy. It is difficult to envision how much effort will be required to define the basis of other species- or strain-specific effects. However, the rapid development of molecular genetics over the past two decades has raised the possibility of new ways with which to deal with some of the complexities of toxicological assessments.

Development of the methodologies for cloning genes and for the reintroduction of genes into the genome of many species produced a profound effect on the biological sciences. Coupled with the development of methods for germ-line insertion of cloned genes, or conversely the inactivation of specific genes, these methods have provided new ways of identifying developmentally important genes (i.e., those that code for critical events during the development of organisms) and have provided models with which the complex and intricate functions of genes can be better studied and understood. The efforts of John Gordon and his colleagues in 1987 made it possible to selectively introduce genes into the mouse genome and to select for animals that acquire the genes as a germline insertion, thus allowing for the *trans*ferred *gene* (transgene) to be faithfully transmitted to all of the progeny of recipient animal. This methodology has also opened important new lines of investigation in toxicology. This chapter focuses on the application of transgenic models, specifically to problems of interest and importance in toxicology. Many of the models that will be discussed will have important roles to play in understanding many biological processes; however, it is the applications that relate specifically to toxicology that will be the focus of this chapter. It should be recognized that new transgenic models are continually being developed and it is difficult to anticipate which new models can aid in solving problems in toxicology. Therefore, the reader is directed to databases that are now currently assessable on the World Wide Web. Many of these sites cross reference one another. Nevertheless, those listed in Table 1 represent well-designed websites with numerous links to other important and interesting sites.

These sites provide a means of assessing the new models as they become available. The remainder of the chapter will focus on a brief discussion of the methods by which transgenic animals are developed and a discussion of available models as they relate to problems in mutagenesis, carcinogenesis, and other specific areas of toxicology.

GENERAL METHODS FOR DEVELOPMENT OF TRANSGENIC MODEL SYSTEMS

The production of transgenic animals depends upon the success of a series of several complex technical experimental manipulations (Figs. 1 and 2). Even under the best of circumstances, the success of these manipulations can be somewhat variable, depending upon the genetic background of the host or of the recipient cells as well as upon the biological consequences of gene or DNA-sequence modification. Nevertheless, the construction of transgenic animals is available as a resource in most research settings, thus allowing for the systematic *in vivo* evaluation of the consequences of deleting, altering, or overexpressing a single gene or DNA sequence of interest. While both transgenic rats and mice useful for toxicological stud-

TABLE 1 Selected Transgenic Mouse and Rat Web Sites

Internet Resources for Transgenic and Targeted Mutation Research	http://www.bis.med.jhmi.edu/Dan/tbase/docs/dblist.html
TBASE (The Transgenic/Targeted Mutation Database)	http://www.bis.med.jhmi.edu/Dan/tbase/tbase.html
The Big Blue Website (transgenic systems for mutation analysis)	http://darwin.ceh.uvic.ca/bigblue/bigblue.htm
The Jackson Laboratory—Induced Mutant Resource Categorical List (available mutant strains)	http://www.jax.org/pub-cgi/imrpub.sh?objtype = catidx
The Whole Mouse Catalog	http://www.rodentia.com/wmc/
The Genome Web	http://www.hgmp.mrc.ac.uk/GenomeWeb
Genetic and Physical Maps of the Mouse Genome	http://www.genome.wi.mit.edu/cgi-bin/mouse/index
Ratmap (The rat genome database)	http://ratmap.gen.gu.se/
Transgenic Model Studies at NIEHS	http://ntp-server.niehs.nih.gov/Main_Pages/transgen/TransgenicPage.html

ies have been generated, thus far most efforts have focused on the generation of transgenic mouse model systems. As such, our presentation in this chapter will focus on the manipulations necessary to generate a transgenic mouse.

There are essentially two approaches to the generation of a transgenic mouse. First, DNA can be randomly integrated into the genome. Random genomic integration is sometimes termed "nontargeted" integration. Alternatively, a gene or DNA sequence of interest can be integrated into a specific genomic site. This latter approach is termed "targeted" integration. In turn, either nontargeted or targeted integration can result in either the disruption of gene function or in the expression of a gene in normal or altered form. Likewise, either approach may also be used to "tag" the genome with a marker such as the *lacZ* (β-galactosidase) or the *GFP* (green fluorescent protein) genes. Both the nontargeted and targeted integration approaches to generating transgenic animals have advantages and disadvantages; the choice depends upon the experimental question.

Nontargeted Integration

Transgenic mice were first generated in the early 1980s using nontargeted integration as an experimental approach to genome modification. Nontargeted integration is usually achieved by "pronuclear microinjection" (Fig. 1). This is a relatively straightforward approach to delivering DNA to a developing embryo and is a highly efficient means of generating transgenic animals. In short, single-cell, pronuclear embryos are isolated from a superovulated female mouse shortly after fertilization. Before the single-cell embryos undergo nuclear fusion they are microinjected with a few hundred to a few thousand molecules of a DNA. The larger male pronucleus is usually the target for microinjection, although either the male or the female pronucleus can be used. The microinjected DNA integrates randomly, often at a single site within the genome, to yield an integration complex of one to hundreds of copies of the exogenous DNA. Multiple copies usually integrate as a head-to-tail concatemers. Following microinjection, the embryo is implanted into the uterus of a pseudo-pregnant female and the resulting pup is a transgenic animal. Because genomic integration is random, each of the microinjected embryos will result in a different "founder" animal and various founders or their progeny can be further studied depending upon the phenotype of interest. Ideally, pronuclear microinjection results in an animal that carries the integrated transgene in all cells. Therefore, the percentage of founder animals that transmit the transgene to F1 progeny is quite high, often on the order of 90% or more. One distinct advantage of this technique is that transgenic animals of interest can be generated relatively quickly. Within 6 months from the time of microinjection, one can be characterizing transgenic F1 progeny. Nontargeted integration can be useful in marking or tagging the genome with a gene or DNA sequence of interest, in disrupting gene function, or in providing gene function.

Targeted Integration

Alternatively, targeted integration provides an approach for the specific alteration of a gene in its normal chromosomal environment. By using a clone of the gene of interest that includes flanking DNA that is homologous to the genomic sequence, one can select for transgene integration that has occurred by

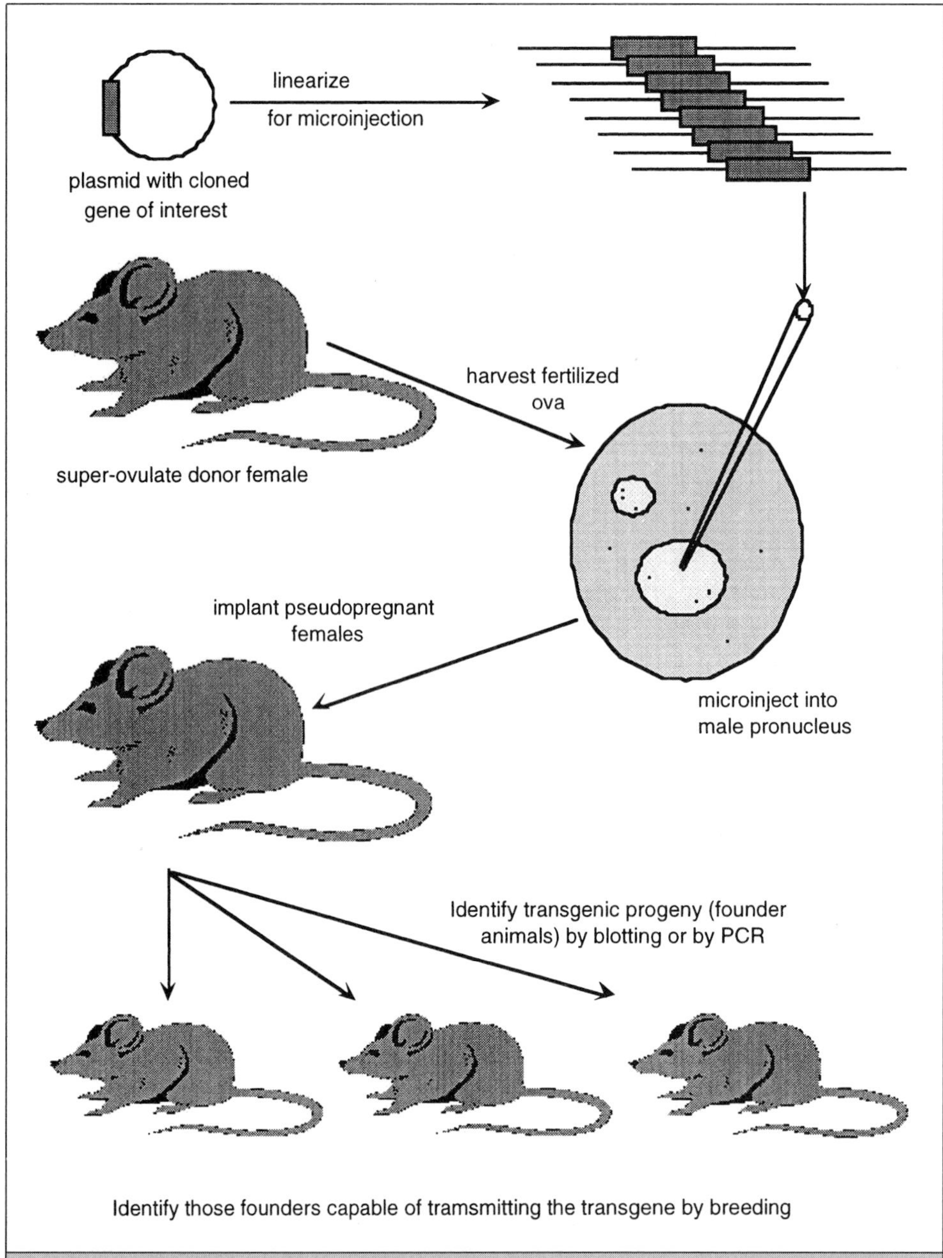

FIGURE 1 Generation of a nontargeted transgenic mouse line. The gene of interest (▭), cloned in a plasmid vector, is linearized and microinjected into the male pronucleus of an isolated fertilized ova. The ova is then implanted into a pseudo-pregnant female and allowed to develop. The transgene is randomly integrated into the genome and the progeny usually carry multiple copies at one or more genomic sites. Most transgenic progeny generated in this fashion are capable of transmitting the transgene to subsequent generations.

targeted homologous recombination (Fig. 2). DNA is introduced, usually by electroporation, to a totipotent embryonic stem (ES) cell, most often derived from the 129 mouse strain. Homologous recombination between flanking regions of the transgene and the ES cell genome results in the replacement of the parental genomic sequence with the incoming transgene sequence. Only the sequence at the sites of recombination needs to be perfectly homologous. Modified genes and/or selectable markers can be added between the regions of precise homology resulting in targeted transgene integration. Such an approach re-

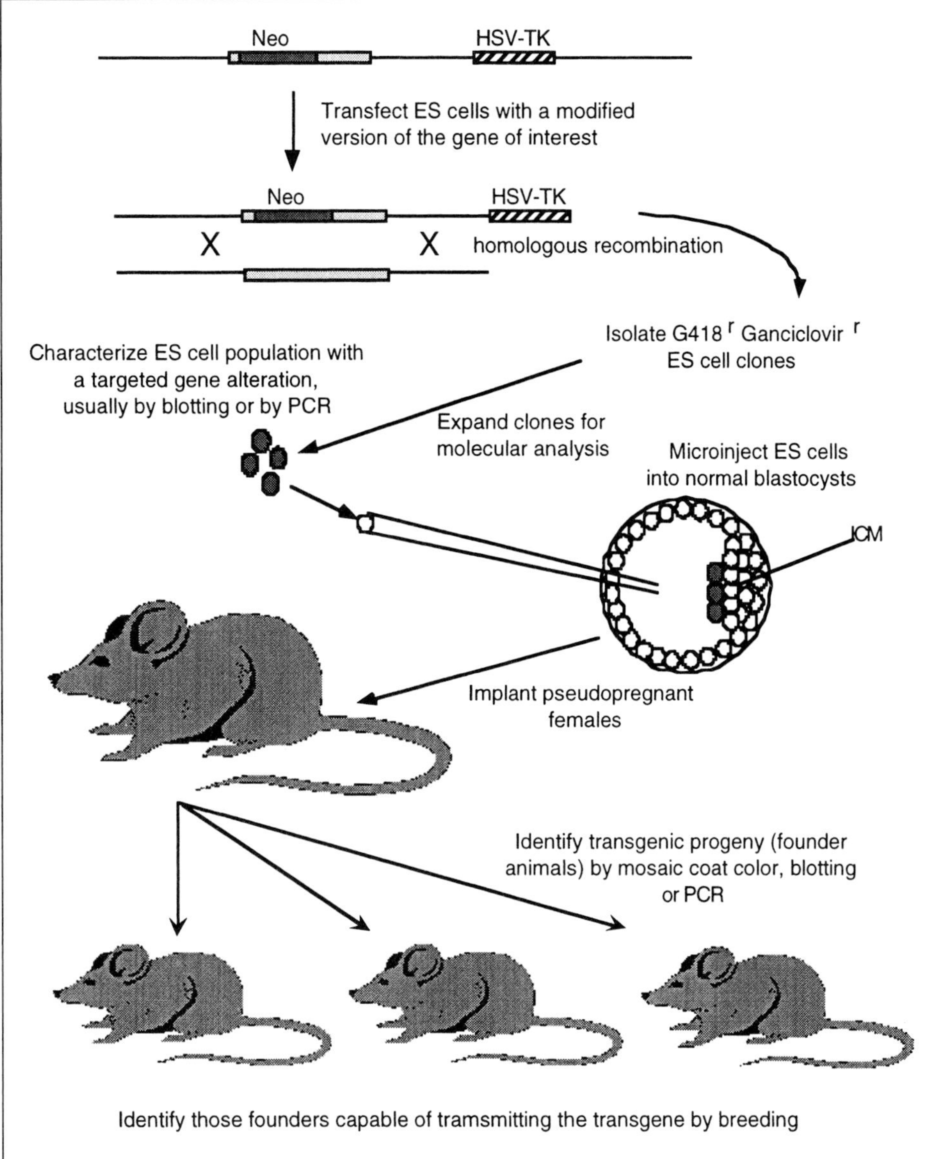

FIGURE 2 Generation of a targeted transgenic mouse line. A plasmid carrying a *Neo*-modified gene of interest ( ) and the HSV-*TK* gene ( ) is transfected into totipotent embryonic stem (ES) cells. Site-specific recombination, as illustrated here, results in replacement of the gene of interest ( ) with a *Neo*-modified version of the gene. Site-specific recombination results in the genomic integration of the *Neo* gene, which confers G418 resistance (G418^r) with the associated loss of the HSV-*TK* gene, thus rendering the cells resistant to the drug Ganciclovir (Ganciclovir^r). ES cells carrying the targeted gene alteration ( ) are microinjected into a normal developing blastocysts, which are, in turn, implanted into pseudo-pregnant female and allowed to develop. Transgenic (chimeric) progeny are often identified by the presence of mosaic coat color or using molecular techniques. Subsequent breeding studies are necessary in order to identify those progeny in which the ES cells have populated the germ-line, allowing for the transmission of the transgene to subsequent generations.

sults in a region of the genome that has been precisely reengineered. Quite often gene function will be disrupted by deleting an essential exon from the gene of interest. Such a deletion has been termed a transgenic "knockout." Note that the recombination represented in Fig. 2 results in a replacement of the gene of interest with a modified version of the gene. Likewise, there are other strategies for targeting a gene disruption, including disruption by insertion, yielding a direct repeat of some of the gene target sequences. Finally, there are a variety of strategies emerging for generating site-specific recombination within a gene of interest (Wei, 1997).

Of course, not all electroporated ES cells give rise to precise homologous recombination events. Rather, about 1/10,000 to 1/100,000 (and sometimes fewer) electroporated cells carry the appropriate genomic recombination mediated alteration. Mostly, clones arise that have undergone nontargeted integration. Thus, one must be able to efficiently identify those clones that carry the transferred gene integrated in the appropriate genomic site. This process has been simplified by the use of a vector that is constructed to allow for the positive selection of clones that have undergone recombination and a negative selection for clones that have integrated vector DNA randomly in the genome. This positive–negative selection technique (Fig. 2) detects site-specific recombination using a drug-resistance gene such as *NEO,* which confers resistance to Geneticin (G418), while selecting against nontargeted integrations using the drug, Ganciclorvir. Ganciclorvir selects against the herpes simplex viral (HSV) thymidine kinase *(tk)* gene carried by the vector construct. Clones that are G418- and Ganciclovir-resistant are candidates for further molecular analysis of the site of transgene integration (Fig. 2). Such a targeted integration has most often been used to "knock out" gene function, usually by deletion of one or more exons. This approach has been used to recombine a specific gene modification into the genome in order to evaluate the genetic effect of a defined mutation. That is, a gene of interest can be replaced by a modified, yet still functional, form of the gene in order to assess various aspects of gene–protein function. This sort of targeted transgene modification has been termed a "knock in" mutation.

Once embryonic stem (ES) cells that have undergone precise homologous recombination have been identified (usually by PCR or by Southern blotting) they are expanded by growth in tissue culture and a few of these cells are injected into a developing blastocyst. Usually, a blastocyst is used that is derived from a different genetic strain of mouse. Thus, following microinjection the blastocyst is genetically chimeric and can be implanted into the uterus of a pseudo-pregnant female. Usually, several blastocysts are constructed and implanted into several females with the hope that some of the modified ES cells will be incorporated into various developing tissues in the pup. The process of identifying chimeric pups is often made simple by using a blastocyst from a mouse with a dark coat color, which will include patches of white fur derived from parental 129 ES cells. Finally, the resulting chimeric progeny are bred to determine if any of the transgene-modified 129 cells were recruited to populate cells in the developing germ-line. The progeny of a founder transgenic mouse will be heterozygous for the transgene modification. Further breeding between male and female heterozygotes allows for the assessment of the effects of homozygosity for the transgenic modification.

TRANSGENIC MODELS FOR MUTAGENESIS

Studies of mutagenesis have long been important in the evaluation of drug or chemical safety. Indeed, mutagenesis studies in bacterial systems such as *Salmonella typhimurium* or using *in vitro* mammalian cell culture systems provide an important initial measure of the genetic activity of chemical and physical agents. The development of transgenic mutation assay systems provides a means of quantifying both mutant frequencies and identifying specific types of mutational events through the generation of "mutation spectra" *in vivo.* In addition to the application of *in vivo* gene mutation assays to drug–chemical-safety evaluations, such systems provide an important experimental tool for mechanistic studies designed to assess the role of induced gene mutations as an etiologic event in the process of carcinogenesis. Until recently, *in vivo* mutagenesis studies in humans or in mice used the X-linked hypoxanthine–guanine phosphoribosyltransferase *(Hprt)* gene. This purine salvage pathway enzyme has a rich history of use in somatic-mutation studies. Unfortunately, the use of *Hprt* as a marker for *in vivo* mutagenesis studies is essentially limited to the T-cell lymphocyte population. Therefore, several transgenic mice have been generated that allow for the efficient recovery of a transgene, thereby providing a relatively simple genetic system for the assessment of mutations in virtually any tissue. To date, there are several systems that were generated by the random genomic integration of a recoverable vector that is easily manipulated in *E. coli.* In addition, there are two systems that have been designed to assess mutations at an endogenous autosomal locus (Table 2).

Most of the nontargeted vector systems (Table 2) are designed to recover a mutated transgene that is carried by a bacteriophage lambda (λ) molecule that has been randomly integrated into the mammalian genome. Briefly, high-molecular-weight genomic DNA

TABLE 2 ***In Vivo* Transgenic Mouse Gene Mutation Assays**

Target gene	Integration	Vector	Mutant selection	Source
Eam3	Random	ϕX174	Plaque formation on *E. coli*	Burkhart et al. (1993)
supF	Random	Lambda	Plaque formation on *E. coli*	Leach et al. (1996)
gpt	Random	Lambda	*E. coli* colony growth	Nhomi et al. (1996)
spi	Random	Lambda	Plaque formation on *E. coli*	Nhomi et al. (1996)
lacZ	Random	Lambda	Plaque formation on *E. coli* plus color selection[a]	Gossen et al. (1989)
lacZ	Random	Lambda	*E. coli* colony growth	Gossen et al. (1992)
lacI	Random	Lambda	Plaque formation on *E. coli* plus color selection[b]	Kohler et al. (1991)
lacI	Random	Lambda	*E. coli* colony growth	Lundberg et al. (1993)
cII	Random	Lambda	Plaque formation on *E. coli*	Jakubczak et al. (1996)
$Aprt^{+/-}$	Targeted knockout	None	T-cell lymphocyte colony growth	Stambrook et al. (1996)
$Tk^{+/-}$	Targeted knockout	None	T-cell lymphocyte colony growth	Dobrovolsky et al. (1996)

[a]Mutants are colorless and wild-type phage plaques are blue in the presence of X-gal [5-bromo-4-chloro-3-indolyl-β-D-galactopyranoside].
[b]Mutants are blue and wild-type phage plaques are colorless in the presence of X-gal.

can be isolated from a tissue of interest and intact phage can be recovered from the mammalian genome using an *in vitro* λ-phage packaging system. Upon infection of *E. coli,* phage with mutations in the marker gene (e.g., *supF, lacZ, lacI, cII*) can be quantified by scoring the fraction of mutated to wild-type phage recovered. If mechanistic implications are of interest, then mutants can be isolated and sequenced to generate a mutational spectrum.

There are limitations to the types of mutations that many of these systems can detect. All of the systems except the ϕX174 reversion assay are designed to assess "forward" mutations (i.e., any sort of mutation that disrupts gene–protein function.) The reversion assay is very specific for detecting only those mutations that revert an amber mutation *(am3)* in *Gene E* of ϕX174. In fact, most of the shuttle–vector systems are useful for detecting point mutations and relatively small deletions or insertions (i.e., ± a few kilobases). Deletions or insertions that significantly effect the size of the phage cannot be packaged. Thus, phage smaller than about 40 kb or larger than about 53 kb will not be packaged into infectious phage particles and will not be recovered for scoring. Nevertheless, smaller insertions or deletions can be scored as mutants. Furthermore, the *spi* selection system is specifically designed to detect deletions. Still, by chromosomal standards these are relatively small deletions; and it is not clear that the mechanisms that lead to smaller deletions (i.e., a few kb) are the same as the mechanisms that lead to much larger deletions (i.e., 1–1000 MB).

In addition, the genomic site of integration may influence the frequency and type of mutations observed. While careful quantitative studies of the effect of integration site on mutant frequency (MF) or mutational spectrum have not been performed, it seems reasonable to assume that the genomic site of transgene integration may have some effect on the efficiency of DNA replication and/or repair. These are not necessarily limitations of the *in vivo* mutational assay systems, as such differences may be extremely useful in providing mechanistic insights into these fundamental processes.

There are data available, however, that suggest that expressing-versus-nonexpressing genes may be differentially sensitive to induced mutagenesis. In studies comparing the mutant frequencies induced at either the *lacI* transgene or the endogenous *Hprt* gene in mouse splenic T-cells, the induced mutant frequency at the two genes is comparable following treatment with the alkylating agent *N*-ethyl-*N*-nitrosourea (ENU). However, the mutant frequency at *lacI* is significantly elevated as compared to *Hprt* following treatment with benzo[*a*]pyrene (B[*a*]P). One possible explanation for these observations may be that as a housekeeping gene, *Hprt* is expressed and, therefore, is subject to transcription-coupled DNA repair (TCR). The *lacI* transgene insertion in Big Blue mice is transcriptionally silent and not subject to TCR. Since ENU adducts are not subject to TCR, comparable induced MFs are observed at *lacI* and *Hprt.* However, B[*a*]P adducts are repaired by the TCR pathway. Therefore, the number of premutagenic lesions present in the *Hprt* gene is reduced as a result of TCR and a lower B[*a*]P-induced MF is observed at *Hprt* than at *lacI*.

As for the use of endogenous loci as markers for *in vivo* mutagenesis studies, at least two transgenic systems have been developed. Both the *Aprt* and the *Tk* genes are autosomal and hemizygous knockout mice have been developed. Since one allele has been deleted as a result of the construction of the knockout, the other allele can serve as a target for forward mutagenesis studies. In addition to point mutations, these systems can potentially detect large-scale genomic rearrangements, intrachromosomal deletions, mitotic recombination, gene conversion, and aneuploidy. Unfortunately, as in the *in vivo Hprt* assay, these systems are essentially limited to detecting mutations in T-cells. Nevertheless, since the gene target is the normally expressed allele of *Aprt* or *Tk* functioning in its normal chromosomal environment, these systems provide an important alternative experimental model to the shuttle–vector systems.

TRANSGENIC MODELS IN THE IDENTIFICATION OF CARCINOGENS

Chemicals, drugs, and other environmental agents that are known to or believed to be associated with the induction of cancer in humans have been codified by the International Agency for Research on Cancer (IARC) and by the U.S. National Toxicology Program in its Report on Carcinogens. Agents with the highest degree of certainty of potential for human carcinogenicity are those for which substantial epidemiological or clinical data exist. A high proportion of agents identified as "known to be associated with carcinogenicity in humans" show characteristic mutagenic or genotoxic potential and the majority that have been adequately tested have shown the capacity to induce tumors in mice, rats and other species. The next category of risk for humans includes agents for which there is sufficient evidence from studies in animals where the induction of tumors can be related to exposure. The third category includes agents for which there are insufficient data from animal studies, but there is some suspicion of carcinogenic potential based upon either chemical structure, mutagenic, or genotoxic potential, or other related factors. Therefore, in the absence of epidemiological or clinical data, results from animal studies play a pivotal role in identifying agents that are generally recognized as potential carcinogens for humans. The methodology that has been used almost exclusively for the past two decades to identify carcinogenic potential in animals are long-term bioassays, generally involving both rats and mice. Both sexes of each species are exposed to substances for 2 years, which accounts for over 60% of the life-span of conventional laboratory rodents. This approach is used in order to ensure that relatively weak carcinogenic potential will not be missed due to relatively small numbers of animals (i.e., 50 animals/sex/species/group/dose). Also, it is conventional to use minimally toxic doses (MTD). Such doses are selected, as nearly as possible, based upon effects such as reduction in weight gain or organ–tissue-specific toxicity derived from subchronic (90-day) exposures. The results of the studies are generally not known until the assay is terminated and the animals have undergone complete post-mortem and histopathological evaluation. Evidence of tumorigenicity is based upon comparison of the treated animals to the concurrent (solvent) controls and to historical control data where they are available. A judgment is reached based upon statistical analyses of all of the available data.

Long-term carcinogenicity bioassays, therefore, are very arduous experiments and because of their complexity and costs they cannot be easily repeated. Extensive efforts are made under rules of good laboratory practice to insure the quality of the experiments, which also add to the costs and complexity of the study. The interpretation of the results of the bioassays is not straightforward. As mentioned, potential chemical effects must be judged in relationship to results seen in concurrent controls and, where possible, in comparison to a strain-specific historical tumor incidence database. The reason for this is the high incidence of spontaneous tumors at a variety of tissue sites that occur in various rodent strains. Virtually all rodent strains show characteristic patterns of spontaneous tumors. The incidence of specific tumors may vary from experiment to experiment and from generation to generation, but a characteristic pattern of tumors is seen through many generations demonstrating that the tumors are of genetic origin. This is one of the consequences of inbreeding and attendant allelic enrichment. The spontaneous tumors are age-dependent in development, and therefore are often seen at the time that the long-term bioassays are terminated. Significant judgment must be applied to distinguish between random modulation of the spontaneous diseases or effects that may represent a clear induction of tumors by the chemical or other agent to which the animals have been exposed. A second important factor is whether the responses are the result of other susceptibility genes in the strain that are not related to the background tumor incidence. Thus, it is important to recognize responses that are potentially strain- or species-specific. The latter are generally manifested by the highly tissue-site-specific and sex–strain-specific induction of tumors, such as the $\alpha_{2\mu}$-globulin-associated renal tumors referred to earlier. All of these factors must be taken into account in the search for alternative methods of identifying potential carcinogens based upon induced tumors as the endpoint.

The factors cited above suggest some characteristics of an ideal short-term carcinogenicity bioassay that would include the following. The system or model should be highly sensitive so that the chemicals or agents that have true carcinogenic potential and risk to human health would not be missed. Conversely, the assays should have a high degree of specificity and not respond to exposures to substances that either lack intrinsic carcinogenic potential or have failed to demonstrate carcinogenic activity in other bioassays. The issue of specificity is important also because it provides confidence in the value of negative responses in the model. Since it is important to be able to distinguish between agents that have carcinogenic potential and those that do not, the ideal assay system should minimize the influence of strain- or species-specific influences; that is, it should reduce the complications associated with high incidence of background or spontaneous tumors and of strain-specific responses related to unique mechanisms of tumor induction. Given the polymorphic nature of genes related to chemical and drug metabolism, it is highly unlikely that any model system can ever be developed that will mimic the allelic diversity seen in the human population, but it will be important to be able to identify potentially important deficiencies or differences in the capacity of the model to metabolize chemicals differently than would be anticipated in the majority of the human population. The ideal assay would be of much shorter duration, thereby reducing costs and complexity and allowing for multiple tests or additional experimentation on agents that show dichotomous or ambiguous initial results. Achieving concordance with even many of the above ideal characteristics should result in a significant improvement in the capacity to efficiently recognize chemicals with intrinsic carcinogenic potential.

The advances in molecular biology and genetics over the past two decades in identifying important genes that are involved in the multistep–multigene pathways of tumor development have provided also a means of focusing on genes that may play critical roles in the tumor-induction process. When a chemical or drug is administered to an animal, there are estimated to be between 80 and 100,000 genes whose action may affect or be affected by exposure to the chemical, but not all of the genes are equally important in the process of neoplasia. Among the genes that have been shown to be most important in the induction of tumors are those that are identified as proto-oncogenes or as tumor-suppressor genes. Through mutation, deletion, or alteration in the function of one or more of these critical genes, the process of neoplasia can be "initiated." It is likely that various tissue- and cell-specific pathways of neoplasia involve different patterns of critical gene inactivation; but for a high proportion of tumors, both in rodents and in humans, a few specific genes have been shown to play critical roles in the development of a number of different types of tumors. For example, the frequency with which mutations have been observed in the *p53* tumor suppressor gene or the *ras* proto-oncogene in tumors, clearly indicates that these genes play a critical role in the development of many types of tumors regardless of species. If these genes are directly or indirectly inactivated or modified during neoplastic progression, then models using these genes as principal targets can potentially meet many of the characteristics of the ideal alternative carcinogenicity bioassay.

Proto-oncogene Models

Over 50 genes have been identified as having at least some properties sufficient to classify them as proto-oncogenes. However, many have only been characterized in highly specific types of tumors or using *in vitro* assay systems. Thus, their potential general significance in the induction of cancer is not yet understood. Of these, approximately 30 different genes have been utilized in developing transgenic models. The goals of most of the studies are related to analyzing the specific function of the gene by inserting multiple copies that are integrated at sites other than the endogenous locus of the gene, or by altering, in a variety of ways, the signals that regulate the expression of the gene. This can be accomplished by altering the nature of the transcriptional promoter for the gene by introducing regulatory mutations or by splicing into the promoter-altered regulatory signals. An abundant literature has developed in which the results of such studies have been reported.

Among the first oncogene-based models to be evaluated for responses to chemicals were three transgenic lines derived from oncogene constructs (*ras, myc, neu*) that had been placed under the control of the transcriptional regulatory sequences derived from the mouse mammary tumor virus (MMTV). The phenotype of the derived transgenic animals each involved the development of mammary tumors and while the tumors were histologically similar at the cellular level, there were differences in the time to onset of the tumors, multiplicity of tumors induced, and in changes in other tissues. The initial construct utilizing the v-Ha-*ras* oncogene and the MMTV promoter sequence also utilized a polyadenylation sequence derived from the SV40 DNA tumor virus. The animals derived from pronuclear injection of this construct were termed "Oncomouse" and the model was subsequently patented. The three MMTV-promoter-driven oncogene transgenic lines were evaluated for responses to chemical carcinogens. While some acceleration of tumorigenesis could be seen, it became clear that the high incidence of background tumors, apparently related to the constitutive expression of the transgene, made the problem of resolving between chemically induced and chemically modulated tumor incidence very similar to the problem encountered with conventional long-term bioassays. Similar results were noted with another transgenic line utilizing the *Pim-l* oncogene under the control of the E_{μ}-promoter derived from the promoter or enhancer of an immunoglobulin gene. These conditions resulted in a high incidence of transgene expression and of tumorigenesis in the hematopoietic system. However, when the *v-Ha-ras* gene from the oncomouse construct mentioned above was placed under the regulatory control of the fetal zeta (ζ)-globin gene promoter, one of five founder animals, derived by pronuclear injection, demonstrated a phenotype that appeared to have utility in identifying potential carcinogens. This line, designated Tg.AC, differed from most other oncogene-based transgenic systems in that the transgene was not constitutively expressed at the primary site of tumorigenesis. Early on in the use of this mouse line, it was noted that male Tg.AC mice that were group housed developed papillomas at the sites of bite-inflicted wounds. Subsequently, Tg.AC mice were shown to be responsive (i.e., to yield papillomas) following treatment with the well-known tumor-promoter TPA (phorbol myristate acetate). These data are consistent with the concept that Tg.AC animals are "genetically initiated." That is, within the framework of the two-stage initiation–promotion model, treatment with a subcarcinogenic dose of a known electrophilic carcinogen results in "initiation" of the skin and tumor development can be elicited by treatment with a chemical that has been characterized as a tumor promoter. It was subsequently recognized that the initiation involved the induction of mutations in the endogenous c-Ha-*ras* gene. Thus, the Tg.AC line carries the initiating mutation in all of its cells; however, the v-Ha-*ras* is not initially expressed. Expression is associated with papilloma formation. The reason for the specific expression of the v-Ha-*ras* transgene in the skin of Tg.AC has yet to be determined; but preliminary evidence suggests that expression is related to two factors. First, the site of integration of the transgene is undoubtedly important since only one of the five founders derived from the use of the same plasmid construct developed the specific Tg.AC phenotype. The transgene has been subsequently localized to the centromere-proximal region of chromosome 11 and the locus consists of multiple copies of the construct. A second important factor is that the ζ-globin promoter utilizes the GATA-3 transcription factor. The GATA family of transcription factors are principally expressed in lymphoid or hematopoietic tissues; but they have also been identified in the skin and their expression appears to play a role in the phenotype of the Tg.AC model. The utility of the model for identifying potential carcinogens has been evaluated utilizing chemicals for which data are available from long-term conventional bioassays. The results of these studies indicate that the Tg.AC line can be induced to develop skin papillomas by both mutagenic and nonmutagenic carcinogens, as well as by tumor promoters. While the database for noncarcinogens is limited, the model has shown few false-positive responses. In this model, the induction of skin papillomas is considered to be a "reporter phenotype." It does not fully characterize a carcinogen but rather identifies the *carcinogenic potential* of a chemical.

An entirely different construct that also employs a *ras* protooncogene is a transgenic mouse line termed, *rasH2*. The development of this line utilized the endogenous c-Ha-*ras* gene derived from human cells under the control of the endogenous promoter; and the gene is constitutively overexpressed in many tissues of the mouse. This model has undergone extensive development and testing in Japan; and initial studies of tumors induced in the *rasH2* line indicate that tumors carry mutations in the c-Ha-*ras* transgene. These data suggest that this model might also be useful in identifying potential mutagenic carcinogens.

Tumor-Suppressor Gene Models

A third model that has also been evaluated for use in transgenic bioassays was derived from the gene knock-out approach in which a *Neo* gene, thus conferring resistance to G418, was inserted into the endogenous *p53* gene using homologous recombination in a similar fashion to the approach illustrated in Fig. 2. The *p53* gene was identified as a tumor-suppressor gene because the absence of its expression was associated with tumor induction; that is, mutation of the gene resulted in development of a neoplastic phenotype. Mutations of other genes that suppress tumor development have been identified in a variety of tumors, but the *p53* gene has been most widely implicated in carcinogenesis.

The *p53* gene is associated with the regulation of cell proliferation and it plays a role in preventing cells that have experienced DNA damage from entering into the cell cycle. These attributes have led *p53* to be called "the guardian of the genome." Thus, the development of transgenic *p53* knock-out animals was followed with great interest by the scientific community. Other tumor-suppressor genes have resulted in embryonic lethality when knocked out, indicating that they play an important role in development. Therefore, it was somewhat of a surprise that viable nullizygous (i.e., $p53^{-/-}$) progeny could be obtained. However, these $p53^{-/-}$ mice develop various types of tumors, including lymphomas and osteosarcomas within a few months of birth. By six months of age, the majority of the animals succumb to tumors. Animals that retain one functional allele (i.e., $p53^{+/-}$) are phenotypically normal for over a year of life. Many tumors that developed later in these *p53* heterozygotes have been shown to have lost the wild-type allele. Therefore, it is plausible that this model could be utilized to detect potential carcinogens based upon their capacity to accelerate the inactivation of the wild-type *p53* allele. Once again, within the context of the multistage carcinogenesis, these animals also appear to be genetically initiated. Experiments have subsequently confirmed that tumors can be induced within a limited exposure period of approximately 6 months; and in some cases it has been possible to demonstrate loss of heterozygosity or inactivation of the wild-type *p53* allele in the induced tumors. Experiments indicate that the model is preferentially sensitive to mutagenic carcinogens. The associated loss of the functional *p53* allele is consistent with this observation. However, there have been reports of tumors in which the wild-type *p53* allele was retained even though the tumors were of the same histotype as others that have lost the functional allele. Therefore, it may be that the expression of the *p53* gene is altered via mutations induced in another gene that regulates the expression of *p53* or by some other mechanism that results in a functional inactivation of the wild-type allele. Despite these uncertainties the *p53* transgenic mouse model appears to be particularly useful for carcinogenicity studies since tumors can be induced in a time frame when the development of spontaneous tumors is minimal. The tumors can be used for subsequent molecular analysis to define the mechanism or mode of action of the chemical. Also, the ability to utilize smaller numbers of animals and smaller exposure periods allows for extended studies of dosimetry.

Other transgenic mouse models such as the *Xpa* knockout can also be useful for the identification of potential carcinogens. The xeroderma pigmentosum (*Xpa*) gene in humans and in mice is involved in the excision repair of DNA damage. Animals with an inactivated *Xpa* gene have been shown to be more susceptible to tumorigenesis following exposure to mutagenic carcinogens. Therefore, it is plausible that other models will be developed in the near future that may also provide additional useful tools in efforts to identify potential cancer hazards for the human population. However, the process of evaluation and validation of these new models requires the development of sufficient experience with any system such that these models can be used with confidence in other laboratories.

Finally, there are concerns expressed by some investigators that the potential "supersensitivity" of such genetically engineered animals may lead to a higher incidence of chemicals being identified as carcinogens (i.e., as false positives); or that the use of animals with specific genes that are targets for the carcinogen may result in the lack of detection of potential carcinogens that may act through other genetic pathways (i.e., false negatives). Such concerns can only be addressed through additional studies, particularly those carried out in a variety of laboratories utilizing different chemicals and different transgenic systems.

TRANSGENIC MODELS TO ADDRESS OTHER ISSUES IN TOXICOLOGY

Development of various other transgenic mouse models have tended to focus on very specific issues related to the expression of individual genes. For example, it has been possible to identify genes involved in development by their selective inactivation. Other models have been developed to address specific pharmacological problems in the cardiovascular, endocrine, and nervous systems. Any gene that is believed to be a target for drug action or that is thought to be involved in other aspects of drug efficacy can be studied through transgenesis. Transgenic models may also be utilized in the evaluation of therapeutic strategies. Other informative models with specific toxicological applications include the inactivation of the arylhydrocarbon-receptor gene to study the mechanism of dioxin toxicity; the development of an estrogen-receptor knockout model to evaluate the pleomorphic role of the estrogen receptor; and knockouts of the cyclooxygenase enzyme isoforms, COX-1 and COX-2, to evaluate the role of prostaglandin synthetase in inflammatory processes and in the mechanism of action of nonsteroidal antiinflammatory drugs. Likewise, a knockout of the peroxisome proliferator receptor has provided insights into the mechanism of action of drugs that induce peroxisome proliferation.

The models described above are a few of the most prominent applications of transgenesis in toxicology and pharmacology. They are presented to provide insight into the many ways in which transgenic models can be used to provide new and informative approaches to solving major problems in toxicology.

FUTURE DIRECTIONS

The transgenic models that are described in this chapter represent only the initial application of transgenic systems to studies of toxicology. Indeed, these systems provide excellent experimental models for the evaluation of gene-specific interactions in studies of metabolism, pharmacology, and carcinogenesis. However, the number of genes important in assessing the mammalian response to exposures to a wide variety of xenobiotics is potentially enormous. Clearly, the application of transgenic systems in toxicology is just beginning. Nevertheless, there are some obvious questions worth posing as the number of different transgenic animals increases.

First, the breeding of different knockout mice has already begun to generate second-generation mice with more than one modified transgene. Such studies provide an opportunity to assess variability of specific gene responses *in vivo,* although accounting for differences in the genetic background of different transgenic strains can be problematic. Nevertheless, the breeding and propagation of two or more modified transgenes within a single animal has the potential of providing significant insights into protein–protein interactions, as well as regarding the redundancy of specific biological-response pathways.

Second, as the development of transgenic models moves from the construction of knock-out animals (i.e., disruption of gene function) to the propagation of various knock-in constructs (i.e., generation of specific gene–protein modifications), one can expect more sophisticated insights regarding the biological role of a given transgene. Many proteins have multiple functions. The ability to study the loss of one activity without disrupting other activities is particularly important in studies of toxicology. Potentially, specifically modified transgenic animals will be generated that allow for a limited response to a toxic agent, thereby better defining the role of a specific gene product in the cellular or organism response pathway. Of course, crossing modified genes into a single animal as suggested above provides for an even more refined assessment of gene function.

Finally, it should be recognized that while transgenic models represent an important interface between toxicology and molecular biology, the models described in this chapter represent a limited sampling of the first-generation systems. In addition to the development of new and more elaborate transgenic models, one can expect to see an increasing number of applications of molecular biology in studies of toxicology in the future. The use of molecular techniques to address seemingly intractable questions in toxicology has resulted in important mechanistic insights regarding the mammalian response to xenobiotic exposures. No doubt future efforts will also take advantage of data being generated by the human and mouse genome projects. Almost certainly, insights derived from these developing initiatives will be applied to future transgenic model systems. The use of transgenic rodent model systems is no longer limited to a few labs. These systems are now widely available and it is clear that transgenic models will continue to be an increasingly important tool in the arsenal of the toxicologist for the foreseeable future.

Bibliography

Adams, J. M., and Cory, S. (1991). Transgenic models of tumor development. *Science* **254,** 1161–1167.

Boutwell, R. K. (1964). Some biological aspects of skin carcinogenesis. *Prog. Exp. Tumor Res.* **4,** 207–250.

Burkhart, J. G., Burkhart, B. A., Sampson, K. S., and Malling H. V. (1993). ENU-induced mutagenesis at a single A:T base pair in transgenic mice containing phi X174. *Mutat. Res.* **292,** 69–81.

Charreau, B., Tesson, L., Soulillou, J-P., Pourcel, C., and Anegon, I. (1996). Transgenesis in rats: Technical aspects and models. *Transgenic Res.* **5,** 223–234.

Dobrovolsky, V. N., Casciano, D. A., and Heflich, R. H. (1996). Development of a novel mouse $tk^{+/-}$ embryonic stem cell line for use in mutagenicity studies. *Environ. Mol. Mutagen.* **28,** 483–489.

Gordon, J. W., Scangos, G. A., Plotkin, D. J., Barbosa, J. A., and Ruddle, F. H. (1980). Genetic transformation of mouse embryos by microinjection of purified DNA. *Proc. Natl. Acad. Sci. USA* **77,** 7380–7384

Gossen, J. A., DeLeeuw, W. J., Tan, C. H., Zwarthoff, E. C., Berends, F., Lohman, P. H., Knook, D. L., and Vijg, J. (1989). Efficient rescue of integrated shuttle vectors from transgenic mice: A model for studying mutations *in vivo. Proc. Natl. Acad. Sci. USA* **86,** 7971–7975.

Gossen, J. A., Molijn, A. C., Douglas, G. R., and Vijg, J. (1992). Application of galactose-sensitive E. coli strains as selective hosts for *lac*Z-plasmids. *Nucl. Acids Rese.* **20,** 3254.

Jakubczak, J. L., Merlino, G., French, J. E., Muller, W. J., Paul, B., Adhya, S., and Garges, S. (1996). Analysis of genetic instability during mammary tumor progression using a novel selection-based assay for in vivo mutations in a bacteriophage lambda transgene target. *Proc. Natl. Acad. Sci. USA* **93,** 9073–9078.

Kohler, S. W., Provost, G. S., Fieck, A., Kretz, P. L., Bullock, W. O., Putman, D. L., Sorge, J. A., and Short, J. M. (1991). Analysis of spontaneous and induced mutations in transgenic mice using a lambda ZAP/lacI shuttle vector. *Environ. Mol. Mutagen.* **18,** 316–321.

Leder, A., Kuo, A., Cardiff, R. D., Sinn, E., and Leder, P. (1990). v-Ha-ras transgene abrogates the initiation step in mouse skin tumorigenesis: effects of phorbol esters and retinoic acid. *Proc. Natl. Acad. Sci. USA* **87,** 9178–9182.

Lundberg, K. S., Kretz, P. L., Provost, G. S., and Short, J. M. (1993). The use of selection in recovery of transgenic targets for mutation analysis. *Mutat. Res.* **301,** 99–105.

Leach, E. G., Narayanan, L., Havre, P. A., Gunther, E. J., Yeasky, T. M., and Glazer, P. M. (1996). Tissue specificity of spontaneous point mutations in lambda-supF transgenic mice. *Environ. Mol. Mutagen.* **28,** 459–464.

Mirsalis, J. C., Monforte, J. A., and Winegar, R. A. (1995). Transgenic animal models for detection of *in vivo* mutations. *Annu. Rev. Pharmacol. Toxicol.* **35,** 145–164.

Nohmi, T., Katoh, M., Susuki, H., Matsui, M., Yamada, M., Watanabe, M., Suzuki, M., Horiya, M., Ueda, N., Shibuya, T., Ikeda H., and Sufini, T. (1996). A new transgenic mouse mutagenesis test system using Spi- and 6-thioguanine selections. *Environ. Mole. Mutagen.* **28,** 465–470.

Piegorsch, W. W., Margolin, B. H., Shelby, M. D., Johnson, A., French, J. E., Tennant, R. W., and Tindall, K. R. (1995). Study design and sample sizes for a *lacI* transgenic mouse mutation assay. *Environ. Mol. Mutagen.* **25,** 231–245.

Rosenberg, M. P. (1993). Transgenic mouse models of oncogenes. *In* "The Molecular Basis of Human Cancer" (B. Neel and R. Kumar, eds.), pp. 379–433. Futura Scientific, New York.

Saitoh, A., Kimura, M., Takahashi, R., Yokoyama, M., Nomura, T. Izawa, M., Sekiya, T., Nishimura, S., and Katsuki, M. (1990). Most tumors in transgenic mice with human *c-Haras* contain somatically activated transgenes. *Oncogene* **5,** 1195–1200.

Simpson, E. M., Linder, C. C., Sargent, E. E., Davisson, M. T., Mobraaten, L. E., and Sharp, J. J. (1997). Genetic variation among 129 substrains and its importance for targeted mutagenesis in mice. *Nature Genet.* **16,** 19–27.

Skopek T. R., Kort, K. L., Marino, D. R., Mittal, L. V., Umbenhauer, D. R., Laws, G. M., and Adams, S. P. (1996). Mutagenic response of the endogenous *hprt* gene and *lacI* transgene in benzo[a]pyrene-treated Big Blue® B6C3F1 mice. *Environ. Mol. Mutagen.* **28,** 376–384.

Stambrook, P. J., Shao, C., Stockelman, M., Boivin, G., Engle, S. J., and Tischfield, J. A. (1996). APRT: A versatile *in vivo* resident reporter of local mutation and loss of heterozygosity. *Environ. Mol. Mutagen.* **28,** 471–482.

Viney, J. L. (1995). Transgenic and gene knock-out mice in cancer research. *Cancer-Metastasis Rev.* **14,** 77–90.

Tennant, R. W., French, J. E., and Spalding, J. W. (1995). Identifying chemical carcinogens and assessing potential risk in short-term bioassays using transgenic mouse models. *Environ. Health Perspect.* **103,** 942–950.

Wei, L-N. (1997). Transgenic animals as new approaches in pharmacological studies. *Ann. Rev. Pharmacol. Toxicol.* **37,** 119–141.

CHAPTER

10

Receptor Toxicology

MARTIN GÖTTLICHER

Karlsruhe Research Center, Institute of Genetics, Karlsruhe, Germany

TRANSCRIPTION FACTORS AS THE CELLULAR TARGETS OF TOXINS

Some toxins act by unspecific destruction of an organism or its constituting cells, but many chemicals are toxic without inflicting primary and obvious damage. Such chemicals, rather, elicit a specific reaction of a biological system that alters physiological balances in the organism; if such changes interfere with the health of the organism, they are called toxins. A specific response of the organism to the challenge by a chemical requires that the toxic agent be specifically recognized by the organism and that the organism have a pre-existing pathway to respond if a chemical is recognized. Usually the cell is the unit in the organism that can specifically respond to chemical signals. The nature of chemical signals to a cell may be of several types, such as physiologic hormonal compounds, pharmaceutically used drugs with an intended therapeutic activity, or unwanted toxic chemicals. However, the cell can not primarily discriminate between these sources. Rather, the cell has to use its preexisting pathways to sense chemicals and respond according to the cell's state of specialized differentiation and function within the organism. Thus, answers to the question how an exogenous chemical like a drug or a toxic contaminant affects a cell and in consequence the physiology of the organism either in an intended therapeutic way or unwanted toxic response need first to know the primary sensors of the cell for an exogenous chemical (or physical) challenge (Fig. 1). Of equal importance is the knowledge of the specific cellular program that is triggered by the compound. Usually this responsive program is cell-specific and genetically defined by a network of gene regulation with increased expression of some genes and repression of others. The final steps toward understanding the biological response to a chemical challenge are the signaling pathways that link the primary recognition of a chemical to a specific genetic program.

The goal of this chapter is to discuss some of the major cellular pathways of chemical signal recognition and subsequent regulation of cellular responses. Important questions to be addressed after an introduction to the pathways are why activation of signaling pathways and genetic programs in one type of settings are essential to the health of an organism and in other cases trigger adverse responses with symptoms of toxicity. The question will arise why evolution has maintained specific pathways leading to obviously adverse symptoms of toxicity at all. To put forward a working hypothesis at the beginning of the chapter, it appears that evolution has maintained response pathways to chemicals because these pathways are required in certain steps of development, physiological adult life, or proper response to the environment. The action of a toxin could appear as the activation (or inhibition) of such pre-existing pathways in the wrong type of cell and/or at the wrong time of life.

CONDITIONAL CELLULAR RESPONSE TO A CHALLENGE BY A TOXIN

A chemical (or physical) challenge, such as mutagens or radiation, can damage a cell without killing it.

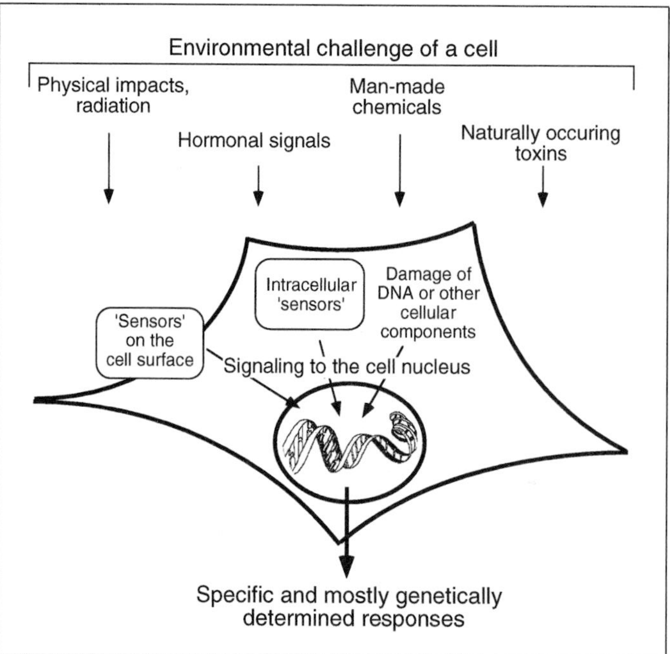

FIGURE 1 Toxins generate signals and induce specific response programs. The specific response of an organism or a cell to toxic chemicals, physical stress, or even damage that has already occurred requires that each impact be specifically recognized by a sensor (e.g., an intracellular or membrane-bound receptor), that the recognition process generate a signal that can be transduced and interpreted in the cell, and that the signal initiate a specific cellular response, which is mostly the activation of a genetic program.

At first glance, damage by radiation or mutagenic chemicals is a stochastic event leading to covalent modifications of DNA in the cell nucleus or covalent modification of cellular proteins. Even though the primary damage is stochastic, the response (and defense) of the cell involves specific pathways. A major example of such a specific response is the stabilization of the p53 tumor-suppressor gene product (p53 protein) by ionizing γ-radiation. The accumulated p53 protein can itself bind to regulatory sequences in the genome and act as a transcription factor. In this way p53 regulates gene expression and triggers a specific response, part of which is the increased expression of the cell-cycle-arrest gene $p21^{Cip/WAF}$. Such an arrest of cell proliferation could serve a protective role by giving the cell the chance to repair damage before entering a new round of replication that could be fatal if replication occurred on a damaged genome. Also mutagenic chemicals like methyl methanesulfonate (MMS) can trigger specific responses by triggering a stress response that involves the activation of specific protein kinases, the "stress-activated protein kinases (SAPKs) (see the following). Activation of SAPKs again leads to activation of specific, though distinct from the radiation-induced, genetic programs, which, for example, serve a protective role by increased synthesis of the cell's antioxidant glutathion. A major unsolved question is whether it is the damage to the cell and particularly to the DNA per se or to a yet-unidentified different target, possibly outside the cell nucleus, that primarily senses the presence of the potentially damaging agent and triggers the specific cellular response. Experimental evidence for either alternative has been provided and possibly both pathways exist.

Among toxic compounds, many do not inflict any detectable damage to cells and yet trigger specific responses. For these nondamaging toxins, a primary sensor in the cell has to exist. Improved molecular understanding of the cellular signaling pathways has revealed the mechanism of action of many toxic compounds, though there are still many for which the mode of action or the 'primary sensor' in the cell is not yet known. Extremely toxic compounds have been developed during evolution of the biosphere as microbial, plant, or animal toxins. Their potency and efficiency at very low doses depend on the fact that they efficiently target the organism's signaling systems or elicit false signals. Also, anthropogenic compounds can affect cellular signaling specifically and be of relevance because of relatively high and/or ubiquitous exposure.

Ligand-Dependent Transcription Factors

Probably the most direct way for a low-molecular-weight signaling molecule or toxin to regulate the genetic program of a cell is for the chemical to directly modulate the activity of transcription factors that govern the activity of a certain target gene (Fig. 2). Such transcription factors are bifunctional proteins. Through one domain of the protein, the DNA-binding domain, they bind to recognition sequences in the regulatory promoter regions of their target genes. Through a second domain, the transactivating domain, transcription factors usually increase the activity of a gene, for example, by facilitating the recruitment of basal transcription factors and the RNA polymerase II complex to the specific target gene. Specificity with respect to the choice of target genes by a given transcription factor is established by the recognition of specific DNA target elements in regulatory gene promoter regions. Such DNA elements are usually composed of 5 to 15 nucleotides and, obviously are different for each transcription factor. For two examples discussed in the following, the consensus recognition element of the Ah (dioxin) receptor comprises seven nucleotides of the sequence TNGCGTG, in which the second position (N) allows for any nucleotide, whereas an idealized element responsive to the peroxisome proliferator-activated receptor (PPAR) reads AGGTCA N AGGTCA. The assembly of many recognition elements in the regulatory region of a certain target gene determines the multitude of transcription factors that contribute to regulation of this particular gene and defines the network of regulatory signals. Almost any gene of an organism has a different regulatory region composed of binding sites for various transcription factors. This combinatorial complexity provides the basis for specific expression of each of the genes in response to complex regulatory networks with cell-type-specific and inducible elements.

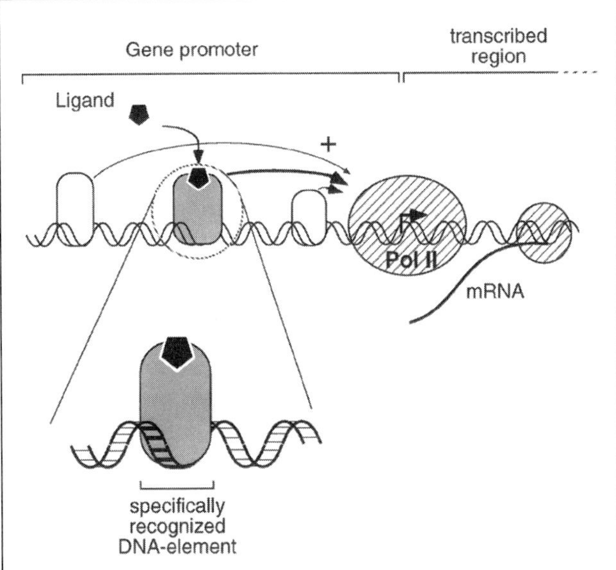

FIGURE 2 Ligand-dependent transcription factors. Ligand-dependent transcription factors (gray rounded rectangle), such as the intracellular steroid or dioxin receptors, serve a dual function in that they can through one domain of the receptor bind their cognate ligands and through a second domain specifically recognize DNA motifs in the regulatory regions of target genes (gene promoters). Ligand-dependent transcription factors usually act in concert with other, mostly constitutively active, transcription factors (white rectangles), which each recognize their individual DNA-recognition motifs in the same promoter. Proper assembly of transcription factors on the gene promoter enhances recruitment of the RNA polymerase II (Pol II, hatched oval) complex to the target gene and transcription of the gene into a messenger RNA (mRNA). The arrow indicates the transcriptional start site within the target gene. The close up schematically indicates that each transcription factor usually recognizes a precise and specific sequence of nucleotides within a short stretch of gene promoter DNA, which rarely comprises more than two helical turns.

Some transcription factors, once bound to their target genes, are ready and activated to enhance gene expression. Many other factors, however, require additional signals to become activated (e.g., conditionally active). Direct binding of a low-molecular-weight ligand, such as a hormone or a toxin, to the transcription factor provides an obvious pathway to conditionally regulate the activity of the ligand-dependent transcription factors. The prime example for this type of ligand-dependent transcription factors or intracellular (nuclear) receptors is provided by the receptors for the classical steroid hormones like glucocorticoids, estrogens, gestagens, and mineralocorticoids, as well as a structurally distinct toxin receptor, the Ah receptor for polyhalogenated dibenzo-*p*-dioxins ("dioxins"). In these receptors, the ligand instructs the receptor to be active as a transcription factor in two ways (Fig. 3). First, in the absence of ligand, the classical steroid receptors (class I) reside in a cytosolic inactive complex with chaperoning proteins like the heat-shock protein 90. Engagement of a ligand triggers the release of the chaperones and allows translocation to the cell nucleus. Though necessary, this activity of the

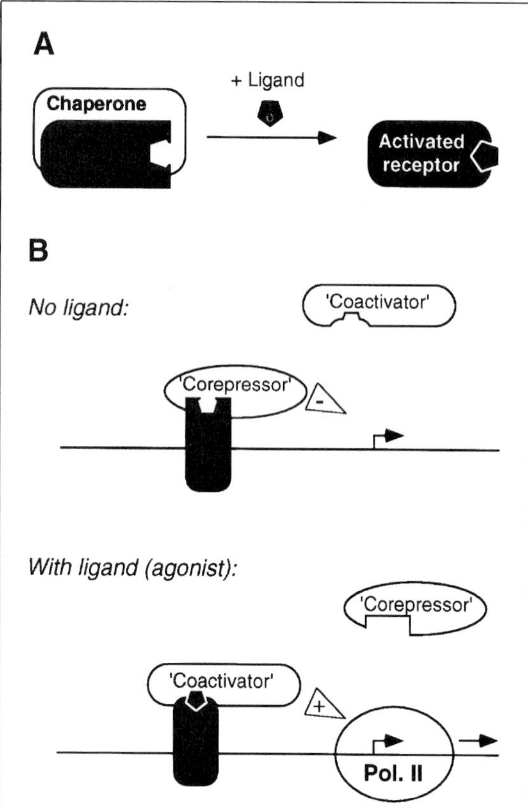

FIGURE 3 Ligands conditionally regulate structure and activity of intracellular receptors. Ligands can determine the activity of their receptors by two modes. (A) Some receptors, such as those for the classical steroid hormones or for dioxins, reside in the absence of ligand in a cytosolic and inactive complex with chaperoning proteins like heat-shock protein 90. Engagement of a ligand triggers the release of the chaperones and enables the receptors to translocate to the cell nucleus. (B) A DNA-bound receptor does not necessarily activate transcription of its target gene and can in some cases even actively repress gene transcription. The binding of an appropriate ligand is required to induce a conformational change in the receptor, which causes the release of transcription-repressing molecules (transcriptional "corepressors") and the recruitment of the necessary protein cofactors (transcriptional "coactivators") for active gene transcription.

ligand seems not to be sufficient, since derivatives of ligands (e.g., "antihormones") are known that allow the release of the chaperones and translocation to the nucleus but do not allow the receptor to enhance gene transcription because additional activities of the receptor are not enabled by the antihormomes. In biochemical terms, the role of the ligand is based on the finding that the DNA-bound receptor occurs as a complex with other proteins. Some of these proteins, called corepressors, inhibit activity of a gene. Other proteins, called coactivators, are required for gene activation by a receptor. The role of the ligand is to instruct the receptor protein to release corepressing molecules and to enable recruitment of coactivators. The bound coactivator appears to serve as a crystallization point, which recruits a complex network of additional cofactors that serve several roles in the regulation of gene expression, including direct interactions with the basal transcription machinery, chromatin organization, and acetylation of histone proteins in the chromatin.

Molecular events and changes in protein structure that occur when a ligand instructs a receptor to be active as a transcription factor have been studied particularly carefully in two cases, the estrogen receptor and the receptors for retinoic acid, the biological active form of vitamin A. The X-ray crystal structure of the ligand-binding domains of these receptors discloses a globular folding with three layers of α-helices arranged almost like the shells of an onion leaving a central space for two β-sheets and the ligand-binding pocket. Binding of an agonistic ligand into this central pocket directs major rearrangements in the whole assembly of the ligand-binding domain, including the repositioning of at least one α-helix and formation of new intramolecular amino acid interactions. This rearranged structure of the ligand-binding domain appears to be capable of recruiting coactivators and possibly establishing other protein–protein interactions required for transcriptional activity that can not be achieved by the ligand-binding domain in the absence of ligand. In the case of binding of an antagonistic ligand, some structural changes are likely to occur and, importantly, the ligand-binding pocket is filled, not leaving access to a second ligand. However, the antagonistic ligand (e.g, an antiestrogen) cannot direct the proper conformational changes, leaving the receptor with the antagonistic ligand in a transcriptionally inactive, though possibly DNA-bound, state.

The estrogen receptor and the retinoic acid receptors are members of a larger receptor family that includes all steroid hormone receptors and also the receptors for vitamin D or thyroid hormones, as well as the peroxisome proliferator activated receptors (PPARs) for peroxisome proliferators like clofibric acid, prostaglandin derivatives, and fatty-acid-derived compounds. All these receptor share a common architecture with the DNA-binding domain containing two zinc-finger motifs in the center of the protein (Fig. 4). The carboxy terminus contains the ligand-binding and transcriptional activation domain, which contains elements conserved among all members of the steroid receptor family. The amino-terminal do-

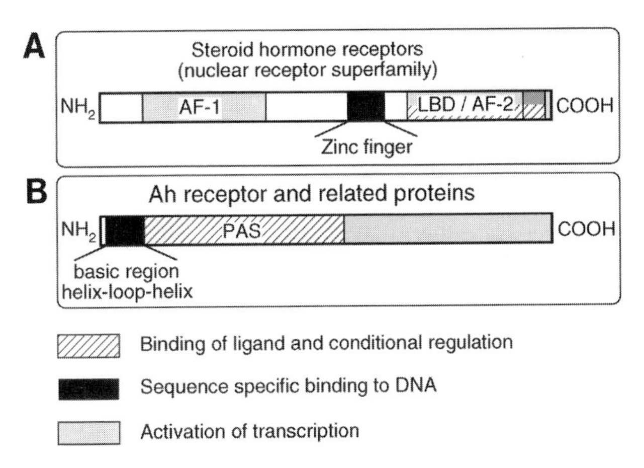

FIGURE 4 Domain structure of intracellular receptors. The functional requirements of a ligand-dependent transcription factor (e.g., binding of cognate ligands, sequence-specific binding to DNA promoter elements, and activation of target gene transcription) are implemented in two types of proteins. (A) The general structure of the large family of steroid hormone receptors as well as the retinoid–thyroid hormone and vitamin D receptors. (B) The domain structure of the Ah (dioxin) receptor. The black rectangles indicate the DNA-binding domains, which in the steroid receptors is a two-zinc-finger structure but a basic-region helix–loop–helix motif in the Ah receptor. AF-1 and AF-2 in the steroid receptor structure depict two domains, which both can activate gene transcription independent of each other. The AF-2 in the steroid hormone receptors is intrinsically linked to the ligand-binding domain (LBD). The darker gray rectangle in AF-2 depicts a core motif that is strictly conserved among all members of this receptor family. In the structure of the Ah (dioxin) receptor, PAS indicates a domain that is homologous to similar domains in the related Per Arnt and Sim proteins. In the Ah receptor the ligand-binding domain is distinct from the transcriptional-activation domain in the carboxyl-terminal part of the protein.

main is less conserved among the members of the receptors, but mostly also carries an additional transcriptional activation domain. The members of the steroid-receptor family may be subdivided in two classes. Class I includes the receptors for the classical steroid hormones associated with heat-shock protein 90 in the unliganded state. Once activated by ligand class I, receptors bind to their responsive DNA elements in regulatory gene-promoter regions as homodimers. The class II receptors appear not to interact with the heat-shock protein 90 and are not kept in the cytosol in their inactive state. Most of them bind to DNA as a heterodimer with one specific retinoid receptor, the retinoid X receptor.

The modes of ligand-dependent activation and ligand-induced conformational changes discussed here appear to be valid for the whole family of receptors because the sequences required for these modes of regulation are conserved among all members of the receptor family. Despite a conserved general mode of regulation, a fine-tuned signaling system demands specificity with respect to the activating signal or ligand and to the target genes that are regulated. This is obviously achieved by the differences in the ligand-binding domains since all the members recognize their respective ligands specifically. Specificity with respect to the regulated target genes is ensured by the binding of different receptors to distinct DNA motifs in the regulatory promoter regions of different target genes.

However, knowledge of the steroid–nuclear-receptor family appears to be just the tip of an iceberg. Hence, the fact that many structural elements are conserved among the known members of the steroid–nuclear receptor family has fueled a DNA-sequence-based search for potential novel members in this family and this search has revealed several dozens of genes, that by sequence homology are likely to code for receptors. Yet for most of them, a physiological role is not known and natural or anthropogenic ligands have not been found for these orphan receptors. Certainly, they may hide the molecular key to the activity of some toxic chemicals; orphan receptors and putative ligands or activators have not been matched very successfully yet.

Example of Intracellular Toxin-Activated Receptors

A number of toxic chemicals act by the activation of intracellular receptors (Table 1).

The Ah Receptor

The model case for such toxins is the class of coplanar polyhalogenated aromatic hydrocarbons derived from the dibenzo-*p*-dioxin, dibenzofurane, or biphenyl backbone. One of the most potent compounds in this group is 2,3,7,8-tetrachlorodibenzo-*p*-dioxin. Coplanar dioxins bind to and activate the intracellular receptor for *a*romatic *h*ydrocarbons and dioxins, the Ah (dioxin) receptor (Fig. 3). The Ah receptor has become a model case for several reasons: genetic evidence clearly indicates that this receptor mediates dioxin toxicity, the high affinity of some dioxins in the subnanomolar range to the Ah receptor is the reason for their toxicity at remarkably low concentrations, and 2,3,7,8-tetrachlorodibenzo-*p*-dioxin has no major biological activities other than activation of the Ah receptor.

Though distinct in biochemical structure, functionally the Ah receptor acts much like a classical steroid hormone receptor. In the absence of ligand, the receptor resides in a cytosolic inactive complex with the heat-shock protein 90 chaperone. Binding of ligands such as dioxins releases the chaperone and enables the receptor to translocate to the cell nucleus and bind to specific DNA-recognition motifs in the upstream regulatory regions of the target gene promoters. In contrast to the classical steroid receptors, this translocation and binding to DNA requires dimerization with a partner, the Arnt protein. Genes that are known to be regulated by the Ah receptor mostly comprise genes coding for enzymes of xenobiotica metabolism like members of the cytochrome P450 monooxygenase families 1A and 1B, glutathione S-transferase and glucuronyltransferase. These genes, however, are not very likely to explain the toxic symptoms elicited by dioxins. Other Ah receptor-regulated genes that have been discovered are involved in cellular signaling and growth control, such as the c-*jun* proto-oncogene, cyclooxygenases, cytokines and their receptors, and components of the basic cell-cycle machinery. With this, the stage appears to be set for understanding the toxicity of dioxins in mechanistic terms. Further investigations in genetically engineered mice that lack certain target genes of the dioxin (Ah) receptor should be performed to prove which of the dioxin-regulated genes is responsible for which phenotype of dioxin toxicity.

TABLE 1 Intracellular Receptors Activated by Toxic Chemicals

	Activators and/or ligands	
Receptor	**Toxin**	**Endogenous or physiological**
Ah (dioxin) receptor	Dioxins, aromatic hydrocarbons	?
Estrogen receptor	Phytoestrogens, xenoestrogens	Estradiol
Retinoid receptors	Retinoids, vitamin A	Retinoic acid
Peroxisome proliferator-activated receptors (PPARs)	Peroxisome proliferators (fibrates ?, phthalates, phenoxy herbizides)	Fatty acids, eiconsanoids

The Estrogen Receptor

In contrast to the Ah receptor, for which no endogenous ligand synthesized in the organism is known, the estrogen receptor primarily serves a prominent role in the physiological function of endogenous estrogenic steroid hormones. The estrogen receptor can also bind a number of exogenous compounds either originating from plant components (phytoestrogens) or introduced as human-made contaminants into the environment and the food chain (xenoestrogens). The major concern about these potential toxic compounds is that they disrupt the homeostasis in naturally hormone-sensitive tissues like the mammary gland or uterine tissues by interfering with the physiological hormonal signals. As a worst case, interference with hormonal regulation is thought to enhance the development of cancer in hormone-sensitive tissues in which proper regulation of cell proliferation and differentiation also depends on appropriate hormonal stimulation under physiological conditions. Endogenous and exogenous estrogenic compounds bind to the same binding pocket at the estrogen receptor, leaving different fractions of the receptor loaded with one of the ligands. A major fraction of the receptor is not carrying a ligand at all. The relevance of a phyto- or xenoestrogen in the body now depends on whether it can bind to a fraction of receptor that is not negligible compared to that carrying a ligand from an endogenous or intended exogenous source (e.g., contraceptive drugs). First, such a comparison must take into account that the binding of a ligand to a receptor follows Michaelis–Menten kinetics with the K_M value corresponding to the concentration required for half-maximum loading of the receptor. For example, subnanomolar concentrations of estradiol are required for efficient binding to the estrogen receptor. The characterized phyto- or xenoestrogens usually have much lower affinities requiring micromolar or millimolar concentrations. At first, it seems unlikely that such high concentrations can be reached only by food uptake. However, a careful analysis is not so simple. The potential accumulation in the body must be taken into account and it must be considered that the loading of the receptor with an endogenous ligand may vary with target tissues or physiological conditions. Finally, binding of an exogenous compound to the receptor does not necessarily lead to activation of the receptor but could also antagonize the activity of an endogenous ligand by occupying the binding site but not triggering the required activating conformational changes of the receptor. Competition of the antagonistic ligand with the (natural) agonist can occur on two levels. The antagonist can limit the number of receptor molecules that are available for binding of an agonist. This, however, can occur only if a major fraction of the receptor population is loaded with either ligand and the numbers of free receptors become limiting. On a second level, a receptor carrying an agonistic ligand may compete with an antagonist-loaded receptor for a binding site on a target gene promoter. In this case, the relative numbers of agonist-carrying vs antagonist-carrying receptors will define the outcome with respect to gene expression.

The Retinoid Receptors

The intricate balance between the physiological need for activation of intracellular receptors and the detrimental outcome of inappropriate stimulation by toxic doses or derivatives of receptor ligands is very clearly exemplified in the case of the retinoid receptors for vitamin A and its metabolite retinoic acid. Retinoid receptors are class II nuclear receptors of the steroid receptor family and are found in two types, *r*etinoic *a*cid *r*eceptors (RARs) and *r*etinoid X *r*eceptors (RXRs), for which three isoforms each are known (α, β, γ). The lack of vitamin A in the nutrition leads, on the one hand, to a syndrome of hypovitaminosis with atrophic symptoms and defects in embryonic development (e.g., the heart and the major blood vessels). On the other hand, an excess of vitamin A causes teratogenicity. Yet the symptoms of vitamin A teratogenicity differ from those of hypovitaminosis in that an excess of retinoids, for example, induces defects in the axial skeleton (homeotic transformations) and disturbs proper closure of the neural tube. Proof that retinoid receptors mediate the occurrence of such defects has been generated in genetically engineered mice lacking certain retinoid receptors (RAR or RXR "knockout mice"). Some of the knockout mice show the defects also found in vitamin A hypovitaminosis and, moreover, specific knockout mice are resistant to the teratogenicity of an excess of retinoic acid.

Peroxisome Proliferator-Activated-Receptors (PPARs)

The genes for this group of class II receptors of the steroid receptor family had initially been identified as orphan receptors without a known ligand or role in physiology. Only later, screening approaches identified peroxisome proliferators as activators of these receptors. Peroxisome proliferators are a heterogeneous class of compounds including lipid-lowering drugs like clofibrate, more recently developed fibrates, phenoxy herbizides, and plastizisers of the phthalate ester type. They all are characterized by their biological activity on cell organelles in the rodent liver, for example, the increase in size and number of peroxisomes that carry large supplies in catalase and a complete fatty acid β-oxidation system in addition to that in the mitochondria. Three isoforms of PPARs (α, β/δ, γ) are known and are to various degrees activated by peroxisome proliferators. Physiologically occurring activators of PPARs are fatty acids like arachidonic acid, linoleic, and oleic acid; saturated medium-chain or long-chain fatty acids like myristic acid also efficiently activate PPARs. Also certain leukotrienes and antidiabetic thiazolidines activate individual PPAR isoforms. Hence, the paradigm of specific recognition of structurally very closely related ligands by one and the same receptor appears not to hold true for PPARs. However, most if not all peroxisome proliferators or their metabolites carry a carboxylic group that usually becomes conjugated to coenzyme A. It could be the ester with coenzyme A that is recognized by the PPARs. The large coenzyme A moiety linked to a hydrophobic carboxylate may provide the common structure that is recognized by PPARs.

Different PPARs serve distinct physiological functions. PPARα, for example, mediates the induction of the fatty-acid-metabolizing enzymes of the peroxisomal β-oxidation, as well as members of the cytochrome P450 4 family, which are fatty acid ω-hydroxylating enzymes. PPARγ plays a role in the differentiation of adipocytes, whereas a specific role of PPARβ/δ is not known yet. Peroxisome proliferators are incriminated as toxins because they promote carcinogenesis in the rodent liver and few are teratogenic in rodents. The key question with respect to toxicity of peroxisome proliferators in humans and a possible role of PPARs in this toxicity is two-fold. The first part addresses whether PPARs mediate toxicity in rodents, and this seems to be the case since PPARα knockout mice are resistant to peroxisome proliferator-induced hepatomas. The answer to the second part of the question is complicated because peroxisome proliferators used as lipid-lowering drugs do not obviously induce liver cancer in humans, though they are biologically active in lowering blood lipid levels. The PPARs as sensors for peroxisome proliferators are conserved in humans. Yet, the presence of the receptors alone does not mean that the whole receptor-dependent genetic program is conserved. Obviously that part of the PPAR-induced genetic program leading to the proliferation of cell organelles is not conserved, whereas other parts (e.g., some of those that affect blood lipid levels) are well conserved. It is speculation whether there exists (a part of) a PPAR-dependent genetic program that might support the development of cancer even outside the liver.

Approaches to the Receptor-Induced Genetic Programs for Toxicity

The examples discussed show strong evidence, for example, from receptor-deficient mutant mice or from structure–activity relationships comparing different receptor ligands, that a certain receptor mediates toxicity. Yet, the reason that receptor activation leads to a toxic phenotype, for example, the development of cancer, birth defects, or immune toxicity, is poorly understood. In most cases the target genes of the receptors that lead to toxicity are not known. Moreover, many genes that are relevant for the physiological role of a receptor are not identified yet, which leaves the question why a receptor in one case is required for physiology and in other cases ectopic activation by exogenous chemicals leads to toxicity.

Analysis of cultured cells or of the developing embryo has revealed relevant receptor target genes of the retinoid or dioxin receptors in the *Hox* gene cluster, in cell-cycle regulation, and among cytokine genes. Activation of these genes at the wrong location or the wrong time could well explain some of the receptor ligands' toxicity. However, knowledge of receptor-dependent genetic programs is far from being complete.

The advance of the genome projects in human and rodents and the development of powerful techniques to analyze close to complete sets of genes that are up- or down-regulated, for example, by activation of a signaling pathway, will dramatically change how we look at the activity of an exogenous chemical in the organism. It is possible to determine close to complete patterns of regulated target genes, and such patterns may be valuable in estimating the biologically activity of a given compound even prior to understanding detailed signaling chains and mechanisms of action.

Signal Transduction Cascades Originating at the Cell Membrane

Many signaling molecules and particularly peptide hormones bind to receptors on the cell membrane that must pass on the signal toward the inner side of the cell membrane and further into the cell nucleus to transcription factors, finally regulating gene expression. This is in some cases achieved by the release of second-messenger molecules such as, cyclic AMP or Ca^{2+} ions. In other cases protein chains transduce the signal by protein–protein interactions and covalent modifications (e.g., phosphorylation or targeted degradation). Besides the signaling pathways leading to the activation of NF-κB and the STAT transcription factors, a prominent pathway of intracellular signal transduction is established by the mitogen- or stress-activated protein kinases (MAPKs and SAPKs), which among other targets regulate the activity of the activator protein-1 (AP-1) transcription factor.

The Cascades of Mitogen- or Stress-Activated Protein Kinases (MAPKs and SAPKs)

MAPKs and SAPKs exist in three known parallel pathways, Erk 1 and 2, Jun-N-terminal kinases (JNKs), and the p38 (HOG) kinase. The MAPK–SAPK pathways play an essential role in the activation of transcription factors, for example, members of the AP-1 family like c-Jun, ATF-2, or the CREB (cyclic AMP-responsive element binding protein), upon stimulation of a cell by mitogens, growth factors, or cellular stress. Conditional activation of these transcription factors does not require the binding of ligands but

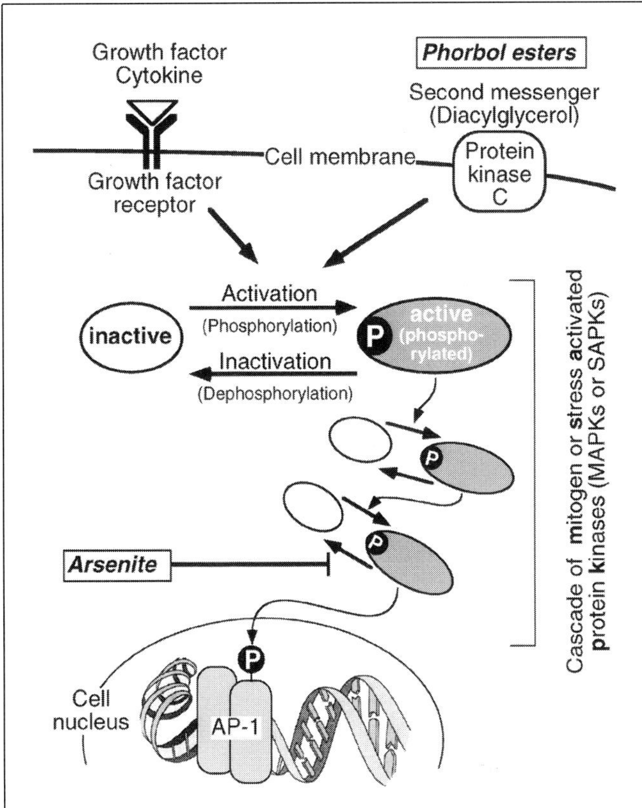

FIGURE 5 Mitogen- or stress-activated protein kinase (MAPK; SAPK) cascades transduce signals from the cell membrane to regulation of gene expression in the cell nucleus. Cascades of MAPKs are activated by signals recognized on the cell membrane, that is, by tyrosine kinase receptor for growth factors, cytokine receptors, or receptors triggering the generation of the diacylglycerol second-messenger molecule. MAPKs and SAPKs are activated by phosphorylation. The activated forms themselves carry a protein kinase activity to phosphorylate other MAPKs/SAPKs on the next lower hierarchical level or to activate target transcription factors, such as the c-Jun proto-oncogene product as part of the AP-1 complex (gray rounded rectangles in the cell nucleus) by phosphorylation. This signaling pathway is susceptible to two types of toxin action (italic lettering in rectangular boxes). Phorbol esters mimic the activity of an endogenous molecule, the diacylglycerol second messenger, and thereby inadequately activate MAPK signaling. Arsenite acts primarily by inhibition of a phosphatase that is required to revert the activation of MAPKs by removal of the activating phosphate. This primarily inhibitory activity results in net activation of MAPK–SAPK signaling because a basal activation is not balanced anymore by inactivating dephosphorylation.

occurs through activating phosphorylation of these factors on serine or threonine residues by MAPKs and SAPKs. Also expression of AP-1 subunits like the proto-oncogene c-*fos* is controlled by the MAP kinases since the predominant transcription factor determining c-*fos* transcription, the Elk protein, is regulated by MAPK (Erk)-dependent phosphorylation. MAPKs and SAPKs in nonstimulated cells exist in an inactive form and become activated themselves by phosphorylation upon appropriate stimulation of a cell (Fig. 5). The protein kinases responsible for this phosphorylation are to some extent specific for either of the three MAP–SAP kinase pathways and they are called the MAP kinase kinases (MAPK kinases). They in turn are activated by a third level of kinases, the MAPKK kinases. The MAPKKKs appear to serve some kind of integrating function and receive activation through several signaling pathways, including small GTP-binding proteins like Rac and Rho, from protein kinase C, the Ras proto-oncogene product, and from tyrosine protein kinase growth-factor receptors through intermediary molecules Shc, Grb2, and Sos. It is difficult to understand how such a fine-tuned network of signaling molecules could be susceptible to low-molecular-weight molecules, such as most toxins. A prominent example of MAPK–SAPK activation by a toxin is the active compound in the croton oil, the phorbol ester phorbol myristoyl acetate (PMA = tetradecanoyl phorbol actetate, TPA), which mimics the activity of the physiological second-messenger diacylglycerol and activates protein kinase C (PKC). PKC in turn activates, among other activities, MAPK cascades and thus falsely induces a state of signaling that, at least in part, is normally induced by growth factors. Hence, PMA triggers, for example, an inflammatory and proliferative response in the skin (Fig. 5).

Ectopic Activation of Signaling by Interference with Negative Regulatory Elements

The examples of toxin-induced activation by gain of function are sparse and alternative routes of activation appear to be followed by exogenous toxins or physical stress. These alternate pathways depend on the fact that many activation events in signal transduction cascades, including the initial tyrosine phosphorylation of growth factor receptors, occur apparently spontaneously at a low rate and that this activation is countered by inactivating principles, mostly phosphatases (Fig. 5). Inhibition of these inactivating phosphatases can lead to a net activation of the signaling pathway and this observation was made first in the case of MAP kinase activation by ultraviolet radiation. Inhibition of dephosphorylation of tyrosine residues in growth factor receptors is the key to a net activation of growth factor receptor signaling by UV irradiation. Also H_2O_2, as well as organo-metal antifouling agents (e.g., tributyl tin), appears to induce specific signaling by net growth factor receptor phosphorylation because of inactivation of their phosphatases.

A second toxin-sensitive inhibitory phosphatase has been found to act on a specific member of the MAPK–SAPK cascades, the Jun N-terminal kinases (JNKs). JNKs and other MAPKs or SAPKs require termination of signaling. This is, as in the case of the receptor tyrosine kinases, achieved preferentially by removal of the activating phosphates by protein phosphatases. The phosphatase(s) acting on the JNKs is inhibited by the arsenite anion, which leads to an arsenite-induced net increase of JNK activity. Accumulation of activating phosphorylation on JNKs and catalytic phosphorylation and activation of their substrates such as the c-Jun proto-oncogene product, are the consequences. This activation of the c-Jun–AP-1 transcription factor has been proposed as being involved in the carcinogenicity of arsenite.

One may assume that the requirements for a xenobiotic destroying a catalytic activity such as a phosphatase are much less stringent than the requirements for eliciting a specific gain of function (e.g., by activation of protein kinase C). If this is true, then a compound is much more likely to exhibit toxicity by interference with inhibitory components than by the specific activation of signaling pathways.

The Nuclear Factor κB (NF-κB) Transcription Factor

A third type of transcription factor conditionally regulated by extracellular challenges is the family of nuclear factor κB (NF-κB) proteins. They were first identified as factors governing the expression of the immunoglobulin κ chain in B cells, but many genes mostly relevant in the inflammatory and immune response or viral promoters are now known to be regulated by NF-κB transcription factors. The NF-κB family in mammalian cells comprises the proteins NF-κB p50, NF-κB p52, NF-κB p65, c-Rel, and RelB. The p50 and the p52 proteins are generated by proteolytic cleavage of the precursors NF-κB p105 and NF-κB p100, repectively. All NF-κB proteins contain a Rel-homology domain in the amino terminus. Transactivation domains are only found in p65, c-rel, and RelB, whereas the other members serve a role in dimerizing with the transactivating members and in forming the DNA-binding complexes. The mode of conditional regulation of NF-κB involves an additional family of inhibitory proteins the IκB proteins. They form complexes with NF-κB complexes, which do not have a high affinity to the cell nucleus and cannot bind to DNA. Activation of NF-κB signaling, for example, by cytokines, phorbol esters, antigens in immune cells, and viral infections, occurs through targeted degradation of IκB. This degradation is initiated by phosphorylation of two serine residues in the amino terminus of IκB and followed by a rapid ATP-dependent degradation by the ubiquitin–proteasome pathway. Degradation of IκB releases the NF-κB proteins, which bind to their specific recognition elements in target gene promoters and activate transcription without the need for any further modifications. NF-κB is activated by reactive oxygen and UV, as well as by ionizing radiation, and is thought to mediate the biological response (e.g., an inflammatory reaction). These adverse stimuli also act through the induced degradation of IκB, but there are apparently other modes for tagging IκB for degradation, in addition to the aminoterminal phosphorylation.

CONSEQUENCES OF TOXIN-INDUCED CELLULAR SIGNALING

Biomarkers of Exposure or Toxicity

It is puzzling why evolution has developed signaling systems that are triggered by exogenous nonphysiological chemicals (or physical impacts). Such pathways appear useful when they implement defense pathways. An example is the irradiation-induced cell-cycle arrest through the p53 tumor suppressor gene product, which could serve a role in halting the onset of genome replication until potential damage could be repaired. In a second example, the activation of the Ah (dioxin) receptor by dioxins, polycyclic aromatic hydrocarbons, or heterocyclic food mutagens may serve an important physiological role by activating enzyme systems that facilitate elimination of most of the inducers before they can damage cellular components. The system of the Ah (dioxin) receptor can, however, become part of a toxic program in two ways. First, dioxins activate the receptor over a prolonged time but are poor substrates for the induced enzymes. It might take the prolonged activation and the induction of target genes other than the xenobiotic-metabolizing enzymes to elicit the specific signs of dioxin toxicity that are not prominent after exposure of metabolizable short-lived other ligands to the Ah (dioxin) receptor. Second, benzo[*a*]pyrene activates the Ah receptor and is readily metabolized, but it is the induced cytochrome P450 monooxygenase activity that metabolically activates benzo[*a*]pyrene to the DNA-adduct-forming and mutagenic intermediate. In general, however, the activation of defense pathways may support overall fitness of an organism in an environment, which inevitably holds potentially damage-inducing physical or chemical challenges.

A second type of specific responses of an organism to a toxic chemical involves pathways that are not supposed to respond to the xenobiotic but rather are required for an essential activity of the endogenous activation or receptor ligand in certain stages of life. Examples are the estrogen receptor, protein kinase C, and the peroxisome proliferator-activated receptors (PPARs), activated by physiologically occurring pathways or ligands as well as being targets of xenobiotics.

Irrespective of whether there exists an endogenous activator for a pathway, the activation of a given pathway by an exogenous compound indicates biologically relevant exposure to this compound. In many cases, there are reasonably simple approaches to monitoring such a biologically relevant exposure, for example, when ingredients of cigarette smoke suffice to induce the activity of the Ah receptor target gene cytochrome P450 IA1 in blood leukocytes. This does not, however, necessarily mean that the observed marker indicates toxicity. First, there is the qualitative problem whether the detected marker (or more specifically, the measured target gene) plays a role in the pathological process of toxicity at all or reflects at least reliably activation of the toxic program. Furthermore, the judgment of toxicity based on activation of intracellular receptors or other signaling pathways is a quantitative problem.

Dose–Response Considerations

The prime character of receptor activation by a ligand such as an exogenous toxin is not stochastic. In cases of stochastic events, such as radiation-induced DNA mutations or mutagenicity of chemicals, any single hit may be the one that causes a relevant damage enabling a cell to develop into cancer. At low-dose impact in a simplified concept, only many more cells have to be looked at before one with the relevant hit is found. Nonetheless, the consequence for a single cell is of dichotomic nature (e.g., whether or not the specific mutation has occurred). Activators of signaling pathways, in contrast, have many target molecules (e.g. receptors) in the cell. The extent of their activation follows in a first approximation the laws of mass action. The binding of a ligand to the singular binding site of an intracellular receptor is not distinct from the interaction of an enzyme with its substrate. It can be, in idealized terms, described by a dose–response relationship following Michaelis–Menten kinetics. This means that increasing concentrations of ligand lead to increased occupation and presumably activation of an intracellular receptor. At low concentrations, the relationship is simply proportional and the slope is steepest; for example, a defined increment in ligand concentration can be expected to lead to the largest change in receptor occupancy (Figs. 6A and 6B, Case A), in absolute terms. The relative change in receptor occupancy by a small amount of an exoge-

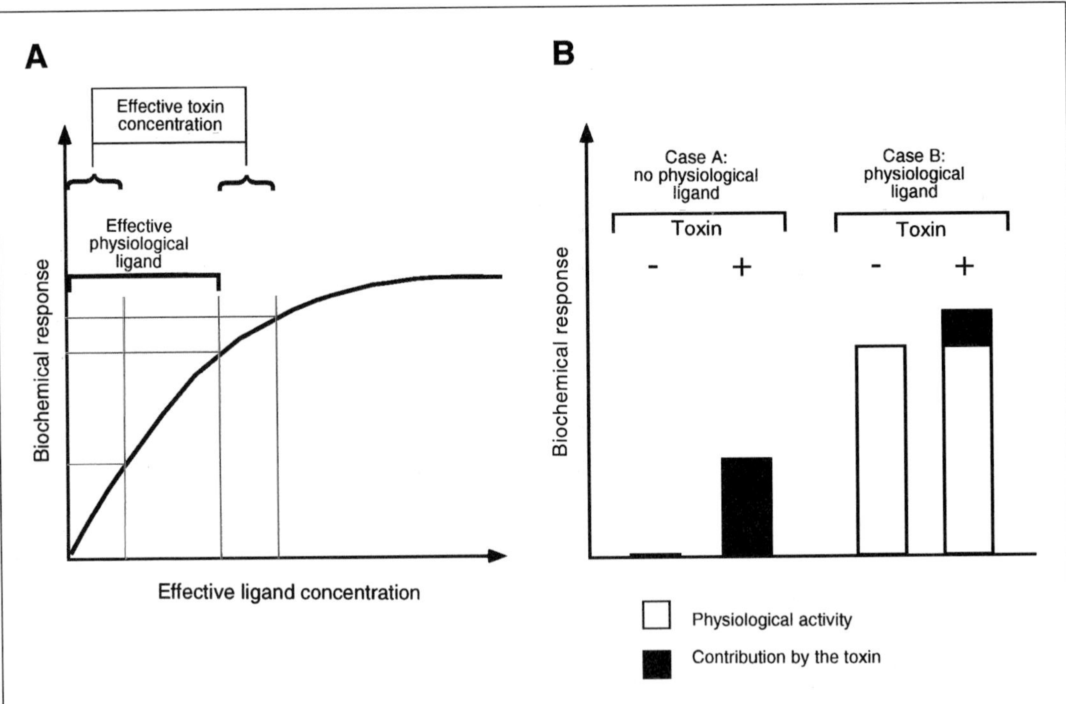

FIGURE 6 Theoretical dose–response consideration for the activation of a cellular receptor by a toxin. The primary interaction of a ligand with a receptor (A) follows the laws of mass action; for example, the relationship between effective ligand concentration and receptor occupancy ('biological response') may be described by Michaelis–Menten kinetics. A simplified view of the primary binding of a toxin to a receptor, disregarding further threshold or nonthreshold downstream events, implies predictions on the activity of low levels of toxins. (B) If there is no endogenous ligand or activator for a receptor present (case A), any small load by a toxin will trigger an, albeit small, activation of a receptor. The primary activation of the receptor follows a nonthreshold, dose–response relationship, though subsequent events in activation of gene expression and ultimately toxic responses may well require activation above a threshold. If there are also endogenous ligands present for the same receptor (case B), the biological efficiency of a small toxin load decreases absolutely and, particularly, relative to the prevailing endogenous activation. Such comparison to endogenous activation may well define a toxin load that becomes irrelevant over the background of physiologic activation of a certain receptor pathway.

nous ligand, compared to the preexisting occupancy, is much less if a receptor is already partially activated by an endogenous ligand (Fig. 6B, Case B). Such considerations again put into focus that one and the same pathway can serve, on one hand, an essential physiological role while mediating, on the other, the toxicity of an exogenous chemical. This means that it cannot be the response triggered by a signaling pathway per se that constitutes the toxic response. It appears instead to be the activation (or inactivation) of a preexisting signaling pathway and its dependent genetic and cellular programs by the xenobiotic at the wrong time and/or the wrong place that twists an otherwise normal program toward induction of pathological symptoms and toxicity. Hence, the question whether a certain dose of a receptor-activating toxin poses a risk to health is intrinsically linked to the question whether the contribution by the exogenous compound changes by any significant means the level of activation of the relevant receptor over activation by preexisting ligands. For example, low levels of xenoestrogens may not play a relevant role in humans, in contrast to endogenous hormone levels. In this specific case, the answer seems to be straightforward, but it may be very complicated in many other cases when all potential target tissues and states of physiology or development have to be considered.

Consequences and Applications

The first and obvious conclusion from knowing that a suspected toxin or environmental contaminant is capable of triggering specific signaling in the cell should lead to avoiding exposure to such a compound unless the observed signaling is intrinsically linked to an intended activity (e.g., of a needed drug). However, if exposure is unavoidable, exposure and even induction of signaling do not necessarily mean toxicity and a risk to health. In the latter case, a careful judgment must be made about the dose–response relationships in comparison to endogenous activators with respect to those organ systems, cellular processes, and target genes that are relevant for the toxic response. Such an analysis indeed requires detailed knowledge of the cellular and molecular biology of the pathway affected by the toxin.

The knowledge of the signaling pathway by a certain toxin or class of toxins provides powerful screening systems even if the mechanisms of action leading from pathway or receptor activation to the toxic response are not fully understood. Usually appropriate cellular-screening systems can be designed by a suitable choice of cell lines or genetically engineered cells that report the activation of a specific receptor or signaling pathway as a simple activation of easily detectable enzymatic activities. Such activities may be endogenous target genes of a pathway, such as the cytochrome P450 IA1 being activated by the Ah (dioxin) receptor or synthetic reporter genes. For example, cell lines expressing the firefly luciferase under the genetic control of an estrogen-receptor- or Ah (dioxin)-receptor-responsive gene promoter provide bioassays for the analysis of various sample materials from the environment. Moreover, they allow simple comparison of individual compounds in a class of related chemicals. A prime example for this use is the comparison of the dioxin-like activities of polyhalogenated aromatic hydrocarbons with that of 2,3,7,8-tetrachlorodibenzo-*p*-dioxin. A battery of target genes or indicator cell lines may also be used for profiling a predicted biological activity of a compound, for example, prior to more thorough toxicity testing of new compounds *in vivo* or during design of pharmaceutically useful compounds.

Bibliography

Baeuerle, P. A., and Henkel, T. (1994). Function and activation of NF-κB in the immune system. *Annu. Rev. Immunol.* **12,** 141–179.

Denison, M. S., and Helferich, W. G. (eds.) (1998). "Toxicant-Receptor Interactions." Taylor and Francis, Philadelphia.

Greenblatt, J. (1997). RNA polymerase II holoenzyme and transcriptional regulation. *Curr. Opin. Cell. Biol.* **9,** 310–319.

Kadonaga, J. T. (1998). Eukaryotic transcription: An interlaced network of transcription factors and chromatin-modifying machines. *Cell* **92,** 307–313.

Mangelsdorf, D. J., Thummel, C., Beato, M., Herrlich, P., Schütz, G., Umesono, K., Blumberg, B., Kastner, P., Mark, M., Chambon, P. *et al.* (1995). The nuclear receptor superfamily: The second decade. *Cell* **83,** 835–839.

Pahl, H. L., and Baeuerle, P. A. (1994). Oxygen and the control of gene expression. *Bioessays* **16,** 497–502.

Papavassiliou, A. G. (ed.) (1997). "Transcription Factors in Eucaryotes." Landes Bioscience.

Sauer, F., and Tjian, R. (1997). Mechanisms of transcriptional activation: Differences and similarities between yeast, Drosophila, and man. *Curr. Opin. Genet. Dev.* **7,** 176–181.

Schmidt, J. V., and Bradfield, C. A. (1996). Ah receptor signaling pathways. *Annu. Rev. Cell. Dev. Biol.* **12,** 55–89.

Sewall, C. H., and Lucier, G. W. (1995). Receptor-mediated events and the evaluation of the Environmental Protection Agency (EPA) of dioxin risks. *Mutat. Res.* **333,** 111–122.

Treisman, R. (1996). Regulation of transcription by MAP kinase cascades. *Curr. Opin. Cell. Biol.* **8,** 205–215.

Whitmarsh, A. J., and Davis, R. J. (1996). Transcription factor AP-1 regulation by mitogenactivated protein kinase signal transduction pathways. *J. Mol. Med.* **74,** 589–607.

CHAPTER

11

Mechanisms of Toxicity

Programmed Cell Death (Apoptosis)

DOROTHEE CHARLOTTE DARTSCH

Department of Toxicology and Environmental Medicine of the Fraunhofer Society, Hamburg, Germany, and Department of Toxicology, Hamburg University Medical School, Hamburg, Germany

INTRODUCTION

Toxicology describes adverse and, in the worst case, lethal effects of substances on tissues, organs, organisms, and even on systems of higher complexity. However, these effects are the outcome of damage to single cells, which results in loss of the cell's specific function for a particular tissue, organ, and system. In many if not in most cases, cell death plays the central role in this process. Obviously, the cell is not a passive victim of a toxic insult but is able to initiate well-defined reactions in response to damage. This can contribute greatly to the characteristic properties of toxic substances, such as organ selectivity. An understanding of the intracellular regulation of cell death is therefore imperative. The existence of regulators implies that there must be different pathways after toxic injury, and research during the past two decades has established that the issues are not only to die or not to die but that there are multiple ways leading to death. Consequently, a confusing wealth of different names and descriptions for the different modes of cell death has been suggested. In a simplified view, we can distinguish between necrotic and apoptotic death, which are characterised by different morphological appearance (see the section Morphology and Biochemistry). Usually, necrotic death is considered a process that is accidental and that cannot be influenced by the cell, whereas apoptotic death is the result of an active and precisely regulated sequence of intracellular signals. Thus, it is the latter form of cell death that can influence the outcome of exposure to toxic substances, and, therefore this chapter is predominantly dedicated to this type of cellular demise. It should be emphasised that there is still a controversial discussion about the nomenclature of this cell death. As the term "apoptosis" was originally used exclusively for the morphological changes of cells in developing tissues and, as it would be strange to speak of "physiological cell death" in the context of toxicology, I prefer the term "programmed cell death," to indicate that a cellular death program exists and can be triggered by a variety of different stimuli. (However, the original definition of this term referred exclusively to cells that are "programmed" to die at precisely defined times and locations in developing tissues or during metamorphosis.)

DISCOVERY OF PROGRAMMED CELL DEATH

In the recent years, the research activities concerning programmed cell death have been increasing tremendously, leading to a flood of publications in this field. However, the phenomenon was first described in 1842 by Carl Vogt, who observed a physiological form of cell death during the development of a toad species. A century later, in 1964, Lockshin and Williams were the first to use the term "programmed cell death." It took another couple of years until, in 1972, Kerr, Wyllie, and Currie described the morphology of cells undergoing physiological cell death and coined the term "apoptosis," a Greek term referring to the falling off of leaves from a tree or petals from a flower, for this process. Only 1 year later, there was first evidence that this form of cell death might have a role in cancer and therefore also in toxicology. Nevertheless, the real burst of apoptosis research did not occur until the beginning of the 1980s, when it became obvious that programmed cell death was an active and genetically controlled process. At the time, a variety of laboratories started their cell death studies using the organism *Caenorhabditis elegans*, a nematode that consists of a precisely defined number of cells, an equally defined number of which die by programmed cell death during development. Soon, three genes that are responsible for the control of the death process were identified: *ced*-3, *ced*-4, and *ced*-9. The first two genes are essential to the process, whereas the third is able to block it, thereby preventing excessive death. Similar genes were discovered in the human species, starting with *bcl*-2 and continuing through what is a whole family of proteins today. When the sequence homology between *ced*-9 and *bcl*-2 was shown in 1994, it became evident that programmed cell death is a highly conserved and hence an important process. Other factors turned out to be essentially implicated in this type of cell death as well (e.g., TNF, CD95/Fas/APO-1, p53, and inhibitor of apoptosis proteins (IAP)). Concomitantly, the number of physiological processes, as well as the number of diseases, that were suspected to be based on a disregulation of physiological cell death increased steadily and is ever-increasing. In 1992, discovery of interleukin-1β-converting enzyme (ICE), a cysteine protease with pro-apoptotic properties, and its sequence homology with *ced*-3, which was reported in 1993, kindled interest in proteases related to programmed cell death. Ten members of the ICE family of cysteine proteases have now been characterized and named caspases 1 to 10. A mammalian homolog to *ced*-4 has been described and named apoptosis protease activating factor 1 (Apaf-1). The tremendous advances in apoptosis research in recent years has led to the expectation that we would soon come to a complete understanding of programmed cell death, including the benefits that it could have for therapeutic strategies in many diseases. However, this turned out to be an illusion; the process becomes more and more complex, complicated, and confusing as more pieces of the puzzle are discovered and put together. Therefore, we probably have a long way to go until we fully unravel the mechanisms of death inducers, signal transduction pathways, and the contributions of programmed cell death to physiological and pathological processes.

PROGRAMMED CELL DEATH IN PHYSIOLOGICAL AND PATHOLOGICAL PROCESSES

The statement that death is essential for the life of an organism certainly seems contradictory, but programmed cell death is absolutely required to balance cell division and thus to maintain cellular homeostasis within the organism. Therefore, most normal cells have a limited life span, and senescent or damaged cells commit an "altruistic suicide," which is controlled cell death, for the benefit of the whole organism. During embryonic development, programmed cell death occurs in a highly focal and specific way, being responsible for the formation of lumina of tubular structures, limbs, interdigital clefts, and the involution of phylogenetic vestiges. Obviously, this is a very sensitive regulation that can be disturbed by a variety of factors. Indeed, a number of teratogenic agents can disturb the balance between cell death and proliferation at their sites of action by various mechanisms (e.g., direct cytotoxicity or alteration of the sensitivity to regulatory signals). But the occurrence of programmed cell death has also been described for many mature healthy tissues (e.g., intestinal epithelia, lymphoid germinal centers, adrenal cortex, thymic cortex, liver, and tissues depending upon endocrine hormones, like prostate and involuting corpus luteum). Programmed cell death also has a vital role in the control of the immune system, as self-reactive clones of immune-competent cells are deleted by induction of apoptotic death.

In addition to these physiological processes, many pathological disorders have been related to a disregulation of programmed cell death. Malignant neoplasms were among the first of these diseases. Histological analyses revealed that apoptotic bodies can frequently be found in certain tumors. While these are normally taken up by phagocytic cells, in malignant neoplasms the majority are engulfed by tumor cells. Although the finding of apoptotic bodies indicates that programmed cell death does occur, in a variety of neoplasms the susceptibility of the tumor cells to undergoing programmed cell death seems to be decreased compared with normal cells. Therefore, tumorigenesis is the result not only of an increased proliferation but also of a decreased mortality of the cells. This finding implies that induction of programmed cell death might be involved in tumor regression following antineoplastic treatment, and indeed, it has been shown that a number of chemotherapeutic agents, as well as radiation therapy, induce cell death by apoptosis rather than by necrosis.

Autoimmune diseases represent another form of deficient programmed cell death, as they result from an insufficient deletion of self-reactive T-cells. Therefore, this is a primary deficiency of programmed cell death that subsequently leads to inappropriate and excessive death of target cells. In the case of autoimmune diabetes, the target are pancreatic β-cells; in the case of the autoimmune lymphoproliferative syndrome (ALPS), there are multiple target cells, leading to a variety of different symptoms. Also, virally infected cells are able to multiply and encourage infection because some viral proteins inhibit apoptotic signaling within the infected cell that would otherwise undergo programmed death.

On the other hand, not only deficient but also excessive cell death can have a devastating impact on organ functions. For example, there are a number of neurodegenerative disorders that may be related to an increased susceptibility to cell death, such as Alzheimer and Parkinson diseases, amyotrophic lateral sclerosis, and spinal muscular atrophy. In addition, augmented programmed cell death has been reported in certain ischemic heart failures, as well as in acquired immunodeficiency (AIDS), where the viral protein gp 120 was reported to prime $CD4^+$ T cells for activation-induced apoptosis. Excessive cell death within the bone marrow may account for a number of hematological diseases, like myelodysplastic syndromes, aplastic anemia, and chronic neutropenia.

Other diseases that have been connected with disregulated cell death are polycystic kidney disease and liver diseases induced by toxic agents or viruses; and the process of aging might also result from an altered equilibrium between cellular life and death (Table 1).

In the field of toxicology, there are surprisingly few descriptions of intoxication-induced programmed cell death. Instead, most toxic cell death is related to necrosis. However, this may be because the significance of programmed cell death gained acceptance rather slowly in experimental toxicology. Thymic involution, for example, is a common finding in rodent toxicology studies using maximally tolerated doses, although immunotoxicity is not a major effect. The reason might be a toxic stress-induced secretion of glucocorticoid hormones, which are well known to induce programmed cell death in thymocytes. The liver is another prominent object of toxicological studies. The classical hepatotoxicant is carbon tetrachloride, which produces coagulative necrosis of rodent centrilobular hepatocytes. Nevertheless, there is recent evidence that programmed cell death and necrosis are induced sequentially in this case.

TABLE 1 Programmed Cell Death in Embryonal and Adult Tissues[a]

	Physiology	Pathology
Embryo	Lumina of tubular structures, limb formation, formation of interdigital clefts, involution of phylogenetic vestiges	Teratogenic effects
Adult	Cellular homeostasis in intestinal epithelia, lymphoid germinal centers, adrenal cortex, thymic cortex, liver, tissues depending on endocrine hormones, aging	Neoplastic diseases, autoimmune diseases, viral infections, neurodegenerative disorders, AIDS, hematological diseases, polycystic kidney disease

[a] A number of physiological and pathological conditions have been related to programmed cell death. These processes are not limited to a certain stage of development, but occur equally in immature and mature tissues.

These examples of how disruption of the homeostasis between physiological cell death and proliferation can lead to severe disregulation of organ functions show clearly that both death and proliferation, and especially the balance between the two, are essential for the life of any multicellular organism. According to this observation, manipulation of programmed cell death should prove to be a valuable concept in the treatment of the diseases described above. Indeed, this mechanism has already been described for a variety of therapeutic drugs. On the other hand, manipulation of programmed cell death is the basis of toxicity of many toxic substances (Table 2).

MORPHOLOGY AND BIOCHEMISTRY OF PROGRAMMED CELL DEATH

Apoptosis (i.e., the final stage of programmed cell death with characteristic morphological changes) can be subdivided into two phases: According to electron microscopic analyses, the first phase begins with a detachment of the moribund cell from its neighbors. Concomitant intracellular changes are a condensation of the chromatin and the cytoplasm followed by fragmentation of the nucleus and formation of blebs protruding from the plasma membrane. These are then

TABLE 2 A Selection of Toxic Chemicals and Therapeutic Agents That Are Discussed in Relation with Programmed Cell Death

	Toxic Agents	Drugs
Inhibitors of programmed cell death	Dichloroacetic acid	Anti-oxidants, growth factors, cyproterone acetate, nafenopin
Inducers of programmed cell death	Isothiocyanates, dimethylbenzanthracene, carbon tetrachloride?, triorgano-tin?, benzene, methylmercury, polychlorinated biphenyls, 2,3,7,8-tetrachloro-*p*-dibenzodioxine, cadmium, arsenic, indium, furan, dimethylnitrosamine, ethanol, acrolein, certain snake venom-enzymes	Mitomycin c, etoposide, camptothecin, *cis*-platinum, methotrexate, anthracyclines, ara-C, tamoxifen, retinoic acid, 5-azacytidine, cidofovir, chloramphenicol, glucocorticoids, salicylate, paracetamol, sulindac, naproxen, indomethacin, piroxicam, methamphetamine, cocaine, MDMA (ecstasy)

released from the rest of the cell and form compact membrane-bound apoptotic bodies containing those cellular structures that happened to be adjacent to this part of the membrane. Although they may be condensed, the organelles apparently remain structurally and chemically intact, as does the membrane of the apoptotic body, thereby preventing intracellular molecules from getting into the extracellular space where they would otherwise cause inflammatory reactions. The second phase of apoptosis is characterised by the uptake of apoptotic bodies by neighboring cells, subsequent degradation, and reutilization of the cellular components, which makes this recycling form of cell death a very economical process.

In contrast to apoptosis (see Table 3), very different morphological changes are observed during accidental cell death: In necrosis the entire cell—including nucleus, endoplasmic reticulum, and mitochondria—swells due to the loss of membrane integrity, until finally the complete rupture of nuclear, organelle, and plasma membranes occurs. This leads to a release of cellular debris and enzymes into the extracellular space and subsequently to an inflammatory reaction. The histologic remnant of a necrotic cell is a faintly stained "shadow" with an indistinct boundary (Fig. 1).

Biochemical changes in the course of programmed cell death affect the structure of the membrane and the DNA, as well as the intracellular distribution of certain proteins and other molecules. Any of these changes can be used for analysis of the mode of cell death. However, the results must be interpreted with caution, as not all criteria must occur simultaneously in a cell, and not all cells in a culture must die from the same type of death nor at the same time! There are various pitfalls in the qualitative and especially in the quantitative analysis of programmed cell death that have to be considered in planning experiments and also in comparing the results of different methods. Changes in the membrane structure obviously

TABLE 3 Biochemical and Morphological Hallmarks of Apoptosis and Necrosis[a]

Parameter	Apoptosis, programmed cell death	Necrosis, accidental cell death
Regulation	Cellular control	No cellular control
Characterization	Intended	Catastrophic
Cell shape	Shrinkage	Swelling
Membrane	Intact	Ruptured
Organelles	Intact	Swollen
Nucleus	Fragmentation	Karyolysis
Chromatin	Condensed	Compact but heterogeneous
DNA	Oligonucleosomal cleavage	Random cleavage
Energy	ATP required	No ATP required

[a]Programmed and accidental cell death can be distinguished by a variety of characteristic changes.

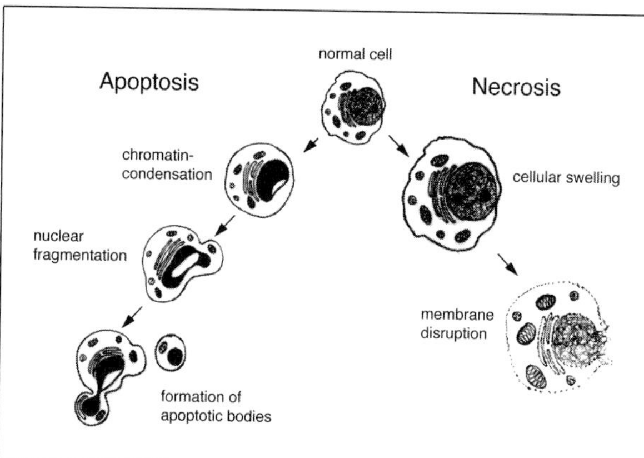

FIGURE 1 Schematic illustration of the typical morphological changes occurring in apoptosis and necrosis. Induction of programmed cell death leads to chromatin condensation, nuclear fragmentation, and formation of apoptotic bodies, whereas induction of accidental cell death results in cellular swelling and membrane disruption.

provide the most reliable parameter of discrimination between programmed cell death and necrosis, as this is definitely a functional difference, in terms of the induction or avoidance of inflammation. As described above, apoptotic cells preserve their membrane integrity for a very long time, while loss of this function is one of the first steps in necrosis. Therefore, apoptotic cells are able to exclude vital dyes, like trypan blue or propidium iodide, in contrast to necrotic cells. An early marker of apoptosis is the externalization of phosphatidylserine to the extracellular leaflet of the membrane, whereas in nonapoptotic viable cells, the majority is present in the intracellular leaflet. Surface exposure of phosphatidylserine may account for phagocyte recognition. A further hallmark of apoptosis is the characteristic degradation of DNA, first to fragments of 50,000–300,000 bp, and consecutively to oligonucleosome-sized fragments, giving rise to characteristic ladder-like patterns after electrophoresis. In necrotic cells, degradation of both DNA and histones takes place, leading to a random, instead of oligonucleosomal, fragmentation. Therefore, electrophoresis does not produce the distinct ladder, but a continuous smear. It should be stressed, however, that in cell cultures where no phagocytic cells are present, DNA from apoptotic cells is finally degraded to random fragments, as during necrosis. There may be two "reasons" for the degradation of DNA in programmed cell death. First, intact and unpackaged chromatin would fill a huge space and it would be difficult for neighboring cells to cope with this situation. Second, DNA of dying cells is taken up by viable cells, and it would therefore be possible that their genome be altered by integration of the incorporated DNA. The cytoplasmic pH is assumed to shift to more acidic values during apoptosis, but there is discussion about this topic in the literature indicating that this might not be necessary for the process. Another discussion is related to intracellular calcium levels. In some systems, the induction of programmed cell death is accompanied by an increase of intracellular free calcium, which may be relevant for the activation of a variety of enzymes. However, induction of an increase in $[Ca^{2+}]_i$ is not sufficient in all systems to elicit apoptosis. A decisive parameter for the mode of cell death seems to be the intracellular energy supply, as it has been shown that the ATP level can determine whether the cell undergoes apoptotic or necrotic death. In some systems, depletion of ATP can inhibit apoptosis and trigger necrosis, even if the stimulus is originally an inducer of programmed cell death under normal energy conditions. Finally, a variety of proteins are affected throughout the process of controlled death, and their cleavage can be used as a criterion for the type of death as well. The role of these proteins will be discussed later, because their analysis is used to gain insight into mechanistic processes rather than to distinguish between apoptosis and necrosis.

INTRACELLULAR APOPTOSIS PATHWAYS

The intracellular events leading to apoptotic cell death can be subdivided into different levels with different cellular elements participating in each one of these levels (Fig. 2). The earliest event is the recognition of an apoptosis signal during the initiation phase. This signal is then modulated by a set of proteins and the intracellular energy supply belonging to the decision level. Once the decision to die is made, the elements of the effector phase are activated, subsequently leading to the biochemical and morphological outcome of apoptosis during the degradation period.

Elements of the Initiation Level

Cellular Sensors for Stress and Damage

A number of sensors or receptors are able to initiate a cell's response to a toxic stimulus. The final response of the cell, in both quality and quantity, depends on the whole orchestra of these receptors and their downstream messengers. Examples of such receptors are heat-shock proteins that are triggered by protein damage or proteins like GADD45, whose expression is induced upon DNA damage. The growth arrest

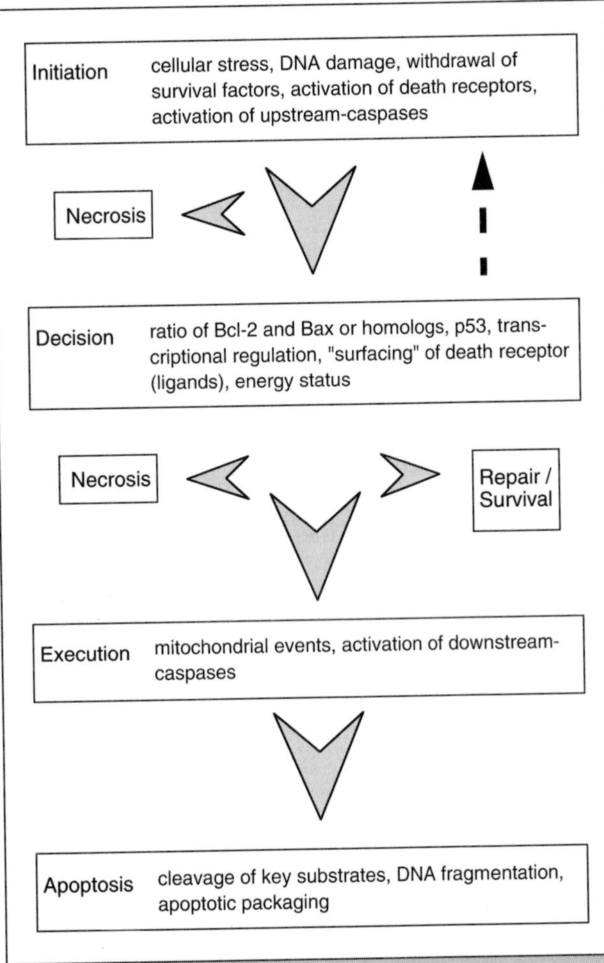

FIGURE 2 The stages of cell death. Each stage contains an orchestra of cellular elements that mediates and modulates death signals.

initiated by GADD45 may provide the necessary timeout for repair of the damage or else for the decision to commit suicide if the damage is too severe. However, another possible response of the cell to injury is an increase in the expression of growth factor receptors or of transcription factors, providing a survival advantage. Clearly, the composition of this orchestra is critical for the cellular reaction and susceptibility to toxic agents and, consequently, for the toxicological outcome.

Receptors for Growth Factors

Receptors for growth factors are membrane-bound proteins with an extracellular domain specifically interacting with the ligand and an intracellular domain accounting for the ignition of signal transduction. Growth factors are indispensable proteins responsible for the control of growth, differentiation, death, and function of target cells. Hematopoietic cells are regulated by an ever-growing number of interleukins, interferons, colony-stimulating factors, and erythropoietin. Their signals are transduced by the JAK–STAT system, the Ras–Raf proteins, the MAPK cascade, c-*fos*, c-*jun*, c-*myc*, and others. Nonhematopoietic cells are regulated by stem cell factor, epidermal growth factor, platelet-derived growth factor, fibroblast growth factor, and nerve growth factor, among others. In their signal transduction pathways, there is probably also a role for c-*myc* and the Ras and MAPK system. Many cells and cell lines depend on the presence of a defined set of growth factors for survival, and withdrawal of these proteins was among the first triggers of programmed cell death to be described.

CD95/Fas- and Tumor Necrosis Factor Receptors (FasR, TNFR1)

These were the first receptors that were discovered to have a unique intracellular "death domain." As this region is able to self-associate, several cytoplasmic proteins also containing a death domain can interact with the receptors (Fig. 3). For example, FasR, which forms a homotrimeric complex as soon as it is activated by its ligand, binds FADD—MORT1 (FasR-associated protein with death domain), whereas TNFR1 recruits TRADD (TNFR1-associated protein with death domain) and FADD. Besides the death domain, FADD and TRADD contain a second conserved do-

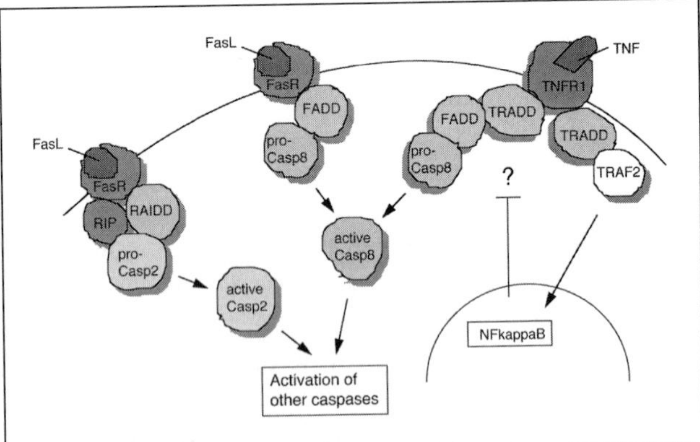

FIGURE 3 Interaction of Fas and tumor necrosis factor receptors with associated proteins. Receptor-associated proteins mediate Fas and TNF signals. Abbreviations: Casp, Caspase; FADD, Fas receptor associated protein with death domain; FasR, Fas receptor; FasL, Fas ligand; NFkappaB, nuclear factor kappaB; RAIDD, RIP-associated ICH-1 homologous protein with death domain; RIP, receptor-interacting protein; TNFR1, tumor necrosis factor receptor 1; TRADD, TNFR1-associated protein with death domain; TRAF, TNFR-associated factor 2.

main, which seems to signal apoptosis, the "death effector domain." This region is able to interact with other proteins, such as pro-FLICE–MACH (FADD-like ICE; now caspase 8), the pro-form of a cysteine protease that binds to FADD and the first enzyme in the signal cascade. Another signaling complex is FasR/RIP (receptor-interacting protein)/RAIDD (RIP-associated ICH-1 homologous protein with death domain)/CRADD (caspase and RIP adapter with death domain)/Caspase-2. FADD and caspase-8 are essential for both Fas- and TNF-induced cell death as dominant negative mutants of one or the other protein are resistant to Fas and TNF. However, FADD cannot bind directly to TNFR1, but it can be linked to the receptor via death effector domain interaction with TRADD. The number of receptors containing death domains is still growing. Examples of newly recognized members of this family are death receptors 3,4, and 5. A wide variety of cells are equipped with one or more of these death receptors. Up- or down-regulation of their number, of course, is of great importance for the cells' susceptibility to death, but the expression of the ligands can also be regulated. In this respect, Fas and tumor necrosis factor are involved not only in the initiation level but also in the decision level because cells can react to a completely different stimulus with the surfacing of either receptor or ligand molecules, thereby facilitating their own death or inducing death of neighboring cells.

Elements of the Decision Level

The Bcl-2 Family of Proteins

The proto-oncogene *bcl*-2 was first discovered in patients with B cell-lymphoma whose tumor cells harbor a translocation placing the *bcl*-2-coding region from chromosome 18 under control of the 5′-IgH gene enhancer on chromosome 14, which results in an overexpression of wild-type Bcl-2 protein. The biological function of Bcl-2 was discovered a few years later, when it was demonstrated that interleukin-3-dependent hematopoietic cell lines with enforced expression of Bcl-2 survived in the absence of the growth factor. Further research confirmed that Bcl-2 inhibits programmed cell death triggered by a broad range of cytotoxic stimuli instead of inducing proliferation, in contrast to all other known oncogenes. In addition, there is recent evidence that besides the inhibition of programmed cell death, Bcl-2 might be involved in cell-cycle control, retarding reentry of quiescent G_0 cells into the cell cycle and promoting exit of proliferating cells into G_0 under conditions of stress. So far, the physiological impact of this property has not been clarified. The physiological role of Bcl-2 has been investigated using *bcl*-$2^{-/-}$ mice, which exhibit inappropriate death of peripheral lymphocytes and of renal cells, leading to progressive immunodeficiency, renal hypoplasia, polycystic kidney disease, and finally to renal failure at about 3–5 weeks of age. From this, it can be concluded that Bcl-2 is indispensable for the maintenance of viability in certain vital tissues or cells. Additionally, a vital role for Bcl-2 can be concluded from the fact that the protein is evolutionarily conserved because Bcl-2 and the cell-death-inhibiting protein Ced-9 from the nematode *C. elegans* show structural and functional homology, and because a number of other homologs have been found in mammals, birds, amphibians, and viruses. Meanwhile, these homologs form a family of proteins that can be divided into two groups, one with antiapoptotic and the other with proapoptotic properties. The first group includes Bcl-2, Ced-9, Bcl-x_L, Bcl-w, Mcl-l, and a variety of viral proteins, whereas the second group consists of Bax, Bcl-x_s (a splice variant of Bcl-x_L), Bak, Bad, Bik, Bid, and Hara-kiri. Some of these proteins are able to form homo- and heterodimeric complexes, which seems to be essential for their biological action. For the Bcl-2/Bax pair, it has been suggested that the amount of either protein is a determinant for death susceptibility, in that with an exceeding amount of Bcl-2, the resulting homodimers block death, whereas with an exceeding amount of Bax, death is facilitated by the Bax homodimers. As for the biochemical mechanism of Bcl-2, considerable research activity has brought up a number of hypotheses, one of which was the idea that Bcl-2 functions in an antioxidant pathway. However, cell death can be blocked by Bcl-2 under low oxygen conditions, as well. As Bcl-2 is localized in the membranes of the endoplasmic reticulum, as well as in the outer membranes of the nucleus and of mitochondria, these localizations probably are of functional significance. Bcl-2 might be responsible for transport processes, regulation of gradients, or other membrane phenomena. It has been proposed that the structure of Bcl-2 allows a pore- or channel-like conformation, but the definitive mechanism of Bcl-2 is still uncertain. Recently, it has been demonstrated that Bcl-2 blocks the efflux of cytochrome c from the mitochondria into the cytosol, and that it binds procaspases via apaf-1, thereby preventing their activation. These processes will be described in the section "Elements of the Effector Level." If cytochrome c is indeed proven to be a central component of the apoptosis pathway, this might represent the universal mechanism of Bcl-2 to block programmed death induced by multiple different stimuli. However, further research is required to elucidate the biochemical roles of Bcl-2 and cytochrome c. Although the Bcl-2 family seem to be important regulators of death and survival, the clinical relevance is not established. First, overexpression of Bcl-2 alone is not sufficient to transform cells. Therefore, additional mutations are necessary to induce tumor formation. For example, the synergy between Bcl-2 and the oncogene c-*myc* has been frequently described. Second, the value of the Bcl-2 level in tumor cells as predictor of prognosis or outcome of chemotherapy is equivocal because, on one hand, several clinical studies have demonstrated a correlation between a high level of Bcl-2 and poor response to chemotherapy in chronic myelogeneous leukemia, small-cell lung carcinoma, and neuroblastoma. Also, the colon—where Bcl-2 is expressed in the crypt epithelia—is much more susceptible to the development of cancer than the small intestine, which does not express Bcl-2. On the other hand, an opposite correlation was described for breast cancer. The toxicological relevance of Bcl-2-like proteins apart from neoplastic diseases has not been well established. Nevertheless, there seems to be an attenuating effect of Bcl-2 overexpression on neuronal toxicity of hypoxia and agents with neurotoxic potential. Also, it has been described that the expression of Bax and Bcl-x_L can be regulated in response to toxic conditions. Yet, it should be stressed that overexpression of antiapoptotic Bcl-2-like proteins is not a guarantee of reduced sensitivity towards toxic insults. Rather, Bcl-2 may delay the onset of cell death, resulting in increased survival only if time was sufficient to repair the intrinsically lethal damage.

Tumor Suppressor p53

In a variety of human cancers, the p53 gene is the most frequently altered locus, one allele being deleted or rearranged, the other one exhibiting a missense mutation in certain mutational hot spots, resulting in the expression of only mutant p53. Wild-type p53 is a sequence-specific DNA-binding protein able to activate or repress target genes (e.g., mdm2, GADD45, $p21^{WAF1/CIP1}$, bax, and epidermal-growth-factor receptor). Interestingly, MDM2 protein inhibits p53, thus forming a regulatory feedback loop to prevent sustained and inappropriate p53 activity. Moreover, p53 functions as a checkpoint, driving the cell either into G_0 cell cycle arrest or into growth arrest with subsequent programmed cell death. Activation of p53 occurs in response to DNA damage (e.g. following UV or ionizing irradiation, or treatment with agents like mitomycin c or etoposide). The result of p53 activation seems to be dependent upon the cell type and thus upon the context of other cell cycle and apoptosis regulators. Also, not all cell types and not all death inducers require p53 to initiate programmed cell death. Low-dose γ-irradiation-induced death of thymocytes, B lymphocytes, and intestinal epithelial cells is dependent on p53, in contrast to glucocorticoid or calcium-ionophore-induced death of thymocytes and pre-B cells. The mechanism of p53 has not yet been established with certainty. In some cells, p53 action may be related to transcriptional activation of target genes, as inhibitors of protein synthesis or transcription block p53-induced cell death. However, in other cell systems, p53 can initiate death in the presence of these inhibitors. Thus, p53 is a very important modulator of a cell's reaction to toxic insult, but the molecular nature of its action is still obscure.

Energy Status

The level of intracellular ATP is an important determinant of the mode of cell death. As induction of ATP depletion leads to cell death by necrosis, this type of death obviously does not require ATP. In contrast, inhibition of both glycolysis and mitochondrial ATP production completely blocks the induction of programmed cell death by Fas, etoposide, dexamethasone, and calcium ionophore, and renewed ATP supply reconstitutes the death pathway. There is evidence that the mode of cell death induced by certain toxicants can switch from apoptosis to necrosis under conditions of insufficient energy supply. In addition, some forms of necrosis (e.g., after treatment with cyanide) are inhibited by overexpression of Bcl-2 or caspase inhibitors (see section "Elements of the Effector Level"). Both these findings indicate that apoptosis and necrosis are not totally distinct pathways but that they share common mediators, and that intracellular conditions can influence or even determine the mode of cell death.

Elements of the Effector Level

Caspases

A number of different types of proteases (e.g., serine proteases, calpains, and proteasomes), have been related to programmed cell death, but certainly, the ICE-like cysteine proteases are considered most important. In order to avoid the confusing diversity of names for the different enzymes, it was recently suggested that the name "caspases," be used, deduced from the biochemical properties they have in common; all these enzymes contain an essential active site cysteine residue and they require an aspartate residue in the P1 position of the substrate. Thus, they are cysteine containing aspartases. The ignition of caspase research in the field of apoptosis came when it was discovered that the human interleukin-1β-converting enzyme (ICE, now caspase-1) exhibits a wide homology to the cell-death-promoting Ced-3 protein of *C. elegans* and that overexpression of caspase-1 could induce programmed cell death. Since then, nine further homologs with different, although partly overlapping, substrate specificity have been characterized (Table 4). The function of this multiplicity is still being discussed. Redundancy might be required as margin of safety in case the function of one of the enzymes is lost. Another reason may be a tissue or intracellular compartment-specific distribution. Indeed, not all caspases are required to induce programmed cell death. The enzymes are synthesized as proenzymes that have to be cleaved at Asp sites to give rise to p10 and p20 fragments that form a $(p10)_2(p20)_2$ tetramer, which is the active enzyme. As many caspases are able to activate other pro-caspases, it seems probable that a caspase cascade functions as signal amplifier and transducer, but the definitive order has not yet been established. An impressive multiplicity of caspase substrates has been described (Table 5), for some of which a possible role in the apoptosis process can be assumed (see "The Degradation Level"). The caspases can be blocked by a variety of inhibitors. First, oligopeptides resembling the cleavage sites and containing an aldehyde or fluoromethyl ketone structure have been synthesized, which are useful inhibitors in the analysis of caspase functions. Second, there are two serpin-like viral proteins that inhibit caspase function by binding to the active site, crmA (a cowpox virus protein) and p35 (a baculovirus protein). Third, Bcl-2 and homologous antiapoptotic proteins can block caspase activation, probably in connection with mitochondrial phenomena, indicating that members of the Bcl-2 family act upstream of caspases. There remain many questions, for example, concerning the order of the cascade or the purpose of the redundant enzymes, but the vital role of caspases for programmed cell death is beyond any doubt.

Mitochondria and Cytochrome c

For a long time, one essential criterion for distinguishing between apoptosis and necrosis was the absence of mitochondrial changes during programmed cell death. This notion now has to be restricted to morphological appearance, as it becomes clear that biochemical interactions between mitochondria and

TABLE 4 Cysteine Proteases in Programmed Cell Death[a]

Caspase	Other names	Subfamily	Substrates	Remarks
Caspase-1	Interleukin-converting enzyme (ICE)	ICE	Pro-Interleukin-1β	
Caspase-2	ICH-1/Nedd2	Ced-3	?	
Caspase-3	CPP32/Yama/Apopain	Ced-3	Poly(ADP-ribose) polymerase (PARP), 70kDaU1 small nuclear riboprotein, DNA protein kinase, protein kinase Cδ, Retinoblastoma tumor-suppressor protein, pro-caspases 6 and 9	"Key executioner"
Caspase-4	$ICE_{rel}II$/TX/ICH-2	ICE	Pro-caspase-1?	
Caspase-5	$ICE_{rel}III$/TY	ICE	?	
Caspase-6	Mch2	Ced-3	Lamin A, pro-caspase-3?	
Caspase-7	Mch3/ICE-LAP3/CMH-1	Ced-3	PARP	Effector of cytotoxic T-cell-induced cell killing?
Caspase-8	MACH/FLICE/Mch5	Ced-3	PARP, pro-caspases 3, 4, 7 and 9	Part of the "death inducing signaling complex" of the Fas receptor
Caspase-9	ICE-LAP6/Mch6	Ced-3	?	
Caspase-10	Mch4	Ced-3	All pro-caspases?	Role in Fas and tumor necrosis factor-induced apoptosis?

[a]The 10 caspases originally carried names that were proposed by the laboratories that first described the protein. Therefore, if different groups had described the same enzyme, it carried different names. The caspases structurally belong to either the ICE or Ced-3 subfamily, and they show different substrate preferences, the function of which has not yet been fully elucidated. It is assumed, however, that the caspases participate in an amplifying cascade, as some are capable of auto-activation and activation of other (pro-) caspases.

TABLE 5 Caspase Substrates in Programmed Cell Death[a]

Effect of cleavage	Substrates
Activation	Pro-caspases, protein kinase Cδ, p21-activated kinase 2, cytosolic phospholipase A2, sterol regulatory element binding proteins, 45kDa DNA fragmentation factor
Inactivation	Poly(ADP-ribose) polymerase, DNA protein kinase, retinoblastoma tumor suppressor protein, GDP-dissociation inhibitor type D4
Alteration of polymerization or depolymerization	Nuclear lamins A and B, Gas2, fodrin, actin
Unknown	70kDa U1small nuclear ribonucleoprotein, huntingtin, Mdm2

[a]The cleavage of caspase substrates can result in an activation or inactivation of the substrate. Especially, cleavage of structure proteins alters their polymerization and depolymerization abilities. However, the consequence of cleavage of other proteins is not yet known.

the cytosol have a pivotal part in programmed cell death. First, mitochondria can directly trigger programmed cell death by generating and liberating reactive oxygen species, like superoxide anion and hydroxyl radical. These molecules are physiological signaling messengers of cell death and also in the activation of transcription factors for the regulation of genes associated with inflammatory and immune responses. Reactive oxygen species may be produced by electron chain transport, and a major place of generation could be the ubiquinone site in complex III. Second, the mitochondrion is turning out to be the primary site where Bcl-2 and its relatives enter the stage. There are two hypotheses concerning how Bcl-2 could influence biochemical properties of mitochondria. The first one suggests that Bcl-2 is able to anchor procaspases to the membrane via Apaf-1, a molecule that shares a central domain of 320 residues with the death protein Ced-4, thereby preventing their processing and activation. In an expansion of this model, the role of Bax and relatives would be to dissociate this complex, thus permitting activation of the enzymes, a concept that is supported by the finding that Bax and Bik can disrupt the association between Ced-9 (the Bcl-2 homolog) and Ced-4 (the Apaf-1 homolog). The second hypothesis proposes that Bcl-2 prevents the release of certain caspase-activating factors, cytochrome c and apoptosis inducing factor (AIF), that are normally sequestered in the space between the inner and outer membranes of the mitochondrion. This idea has already been verified in that Bcl-2 can block the release of cytochrome c following an otherwise lethal stimulus, but the function of cytochrome c still has to be demonstrated.

DNA Endonuclease(s)

Several candidate enzymes with different properties have been related to the DNA fragmentation observed in cells dying by programmed cell death, leading to the conclusion that multiple and redundant endonucleases could mediate this effect. Another finding does not necessarily rule out other endonucleases but suggests that a pair of proteins is responsible for DNA degradation exclusively in cells undergoing apoptosis. One of the proteins is a hitherto unknown nuclease with a nuclear localization signal that is usually sequestered in the cytoplasm by the second protein, which binds to and stabilizes it. Because the nuclease is activated by caspase-3, it was called caspase-activated DNase (CAD) and its binding partner inhibitor of CAD (ICAD), although it is ICAD that contains the cleavage motif for the caspase, instead of CAD, and is therefore rather a caspase-inactivated inhibitor. CAD and ICAD are murine proteins, but ICAD is a homolog of the human DNA fragmentation factor (DFF45) that is cleaved and permits endonuclease activation in programmed cell death.

The Degradation Level

The activation of effector-level enzymes, proteases, and endonucleases determines the final outcome and the characteristics of cell death. Depending upon which target structures are degraded during the last phase of death, typical morphological changes are induced. For example, cleavage of DNA and/or nuclear proteins is thought to be involved in the condensation of chromatin, and proteolysis of actin and lamins might be responsible for membrane blebbing, the fragmentation of nuclei, and finally of the cell. However, little is known about the significance of many other target structures that are degraded in the dying cell. Either they might contribute to a fine tuning of metabolism during the process of programmed cell death, or they might be merely incidentally in the way of aggressive effector molecules. Further experimental effort is needed to bring some light into these mechanisms.

CONCLUDING REMARKS

Some years ago, the conclusion of a chapter about this topic might have been that most toxic substances interfere with the cellular death program and that anything that inhibits apoptosis would protect cells from toxic injury, whereas anything that promotes apoptosis would do the opposite. However, different modes of cell death have been described, and apoptosis and necrosis are but two of the morphologically distinguishable forms of death. It must be emphasised that cells exposed to the same toxic agent do not necessarily have to choose the same type of cell death. Even one cell is able to express characteristics of both apoptosis and necrosis, and most toxic substances can induce both types, depending on the dosage anyway. In addition, inhibition of programmed cell death is not automatically accompanied by protection from toxic damage. For example, clonogenic survival was not increased after cytostatic treatment of HeLa cells protected by Bcl-2 overexpression. Thus, it is not sufficient to choose apoptosis as the endpoint of toxicological experiments and to conclude that the absence or presence of apoptosis means absence or presence of toxicity. The real value of investigating programmed cell death rather is the recognition that the genes and proteins that control this kind of death have an enormous influence on the outcome of exposure to toxic substances. Cells that exhibit the same amount of, for example, DNA damage can react differently, depending on their individual set of death and survival mechanisms. Thus, the quality and quantity of an effect, that is, the target tissue and the dose–response curve, are not solely dependent upon the concentration of a toxic agent at its receptor but also upon the cell's reaction.

Consequently, analysis of the elements of this reaction, and especially of the cellular death program, can contribute greatly to the understanding of molecular mechanisms of toxicity.

Bibliography

Adams, J. M., and Cory, S. (1998). The Bcl-2 protein family: Arbiters of cell survival. *Science* **281,** 1322–1326.

Ashkenazi, A., and Dixit, V. M. (1998). Death receptors: Signaling and modulation. *Science* **281,** 1305–1308.

Cohen, G. M. (1997). Caspases: The executioners of apoptosis. *Biochem. J.* **326,** 1–16.

Evan, G., and Littlewood, T. (1998). A matter of life and cell death. *Science* **281,** 1317–1322.

Green, D. R., and Martin S. J. (1995). The killer and the executioner: How apoptosis controls malignancy. *Curr. Opin. Immunol.* **7,** 694–703.

Green, D. R., and Reed, J. C. (1998). Mitochondria and apoptosis. *Science* **281,** 1309–1312.

Häcker, G., and Vaux, D. L. (1997). A chronology of cell death. *Apoptosis* **2,** 247–256.

Hetts, S. W. (1998). To die or not to die: An overview of apoptosis and its role in disease. *JAMA* **279,** 300–307.

Hickman, J. A., and Boyle, C. C. (1997). Apoptosis and cytotoxins. *Br. Med. Bull.* **53,** 632–643.

Kerr, J. F. R., Wyllie, A. H., and Currie, A. R. (1972). Apoptosis: A basic biological phenomenon with wide-ranging implications in tissue kinetics. *Br. J. Cancer* **26,** 239–257.

Kroemer, G., Petit, P., Zamzami, N., Vayssière, J. L., and Mignotte, B. (1995). The biochemistry of programmed cell death. *FASEB J.* **9,** 1277–1287.

Levin, S. (1995). A toxicologic pathologist's view of apoptosis or I used to call it necrobiosis, but now I'm singing the apoptosis blues. *Toxicol. Pathol.* **23,** 533–539.

Mignotte, B., and Vayssière, J. L. (1998). Mitochondria and apoptosis. *Eur. J. Biochem.* **252,** 1–15.

Patel, T., Gores, G. J., and Kaufmann, S. H. (1996). The role of proteases during apoptosis. *FASEB J.* **10,** 587–597.

Potten, C. S. (1996). What is an apoptotic index measuring? A commentary. *Br. J. Cancer* **74,** 1743–1748.

Raffray, M., and Cohen, G. M. (1997). Apoptosis and necrosis in toxicology: A continuum or distinct modes of cell death? *Pharmacol. Ther.* **75,** 153–177.

Strasser, A., Huang, D. C. S., and Vaux, D. L. (1997). The role of the *bcl-2/ced-9* gene family in cancer and general implications of defects in cell death control for tumourigenesis and resistance to chemotherapy. *Biochim. Biophys. Acta* **1333,** F151–F178.

Thornberry, N. A., and Lazebnik, Y. (1998). Caspases: Enemies within. *Science* **281,** 1312–1316.

Tsujimoto, Y. (1997). Apoptosis and necrosis: Intracellular ATP level as a determinant for cell death modes. *Cell Death Differ.* **4,** 429–434.

Villa, P., Kaufmann, S. H., and Earnshaw, W. C. (1997). Caspases and caspase inhibitors. *Trends Biochem. Sci.* **22,** 388–393.

White, E. (1996). Life, death, and pursuit of apoptosis. *Genes Dev.* **10,** 1–15.

Wyllie, A. H., Kerr, J. F. R., and Currie, A. R. (1980). Cell death: The significance of apoptosis. *Int. Rev. Cytol.* **68,** 251–306.

Zakeri, Z. F., and Ahuja, H. S. (1997). Cell death/apoptosis: Normal, chemically induced, and teratogenic effect. *Mutation Res.* **396,** 149–161.

C H A P T E R

12

Mixtures

JOHN P. GROTEN,* FLEMMING R. CASSEE,† PETER J. VAN BLADEREN,* CHRIS DE ROSA,‡ VICTOR J. FERON*

**TNO Nutrition and Food Research Institute, Zeist, The Netherlands*
†National Institute of Public Health and the Environment, Bilthoven, The Netherlands
‡Agency for Toxic Substances and Disease Registry, Atlanta, Georgia

Chemical mixtures are characteristic of life. Moreover, humans are exposed concurrently or sequentially to large numbers of chemicals from a variety of sources, such as food (several hundred thousands of chemicals!), indoor and outdoor air, drinking water, beverages, soil, and consumer products. Thus, exposure to chemical mixtures is a reality that dictates the necessity—in our efforts to protect public health from adverse effects of chemicals—to pay a great deal of attention to hazard identification, exposure assessment, and risk characterization of mixtures. However, in contrast to this environmental reality, the toxicological reality is that until recently about 95% of the resources in toxicology were devoted to studies on single chemicals. Fortunately, the interest of scientists and regulators in the toxicology and potential risks of combined exposures is growing. In the meantime it is widely recognized that consideration of adverse effects caused by exposure to chemical mixtures must be an integral part of protecting public health (Fig. 1).

Recognizing the legitimacy of the growing public concern regarding exposure to chemical mixtures and attracted to this challenging vanguard of toxicology, research programs on the toxicology and risk assessment of chemical mixtures have been initiated (e.g., TNO in The Netherlands, ATSDR and EPA in the United States). The major aims of these programs are to explore ways to predict and identify hazardous combinations of chemicals relevant to humans and to introduce the concepts of combination toxicology in procedures for hazard identification and risk assessment of *complex* chemical mixtures.

The state of the art of hazard identification and risk assessment of chemical mixtures will be discussed. Basic concepts of combined and interactive effects of chemicals and terminology will be briefly covered. More attention will be given to methodologies for testing simple (defined) or complex mixtures, including the application of efficient statistical designs. To illustrate the complexity of mixture toxicology at the one hand and to offer pragmatic approaches for dealing with safety aspects of mixtures at the other hand, a number of real life examples will be discussed in some detail.

BASIC CONCEPTS OF COMBINED ACTION OF CHEMICALS

The study of combined action or interaction of chemicals involves the challenge of how to characterize antagonistic, additive, or synergistic action. It is therefore of crucial importance to understand the terminology that describes the combined or interactive effect of agents in terms of the mechanisms of action. Half a century ago, three basic concepts of joint action or interaction of combination of chemicals were defined that are still valid.

Simple Similar Action

Simple similar action, also known as "simple joint action" or "dose addition." This is a noninteractive process and each of the chemicals in the mixture act in the same way, by the same mechanisms, and differ only in their potencies (Fig. 2). Similar joint action allows the description of additive effects mathematically using the summation of the doses of the individ-

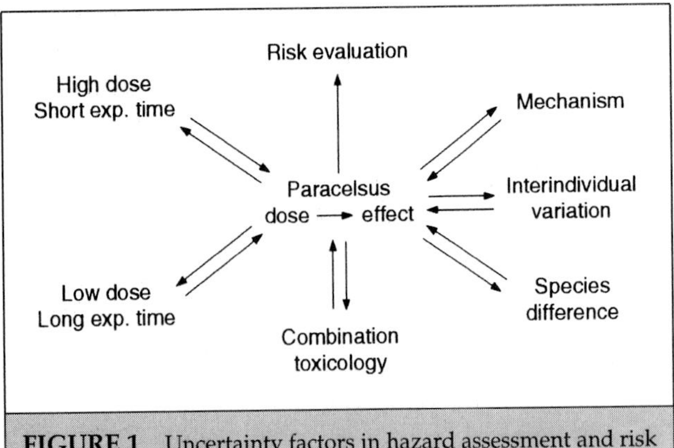

FIGURE 1 Uncertainty factors in hazard assessment and risk evaluation.

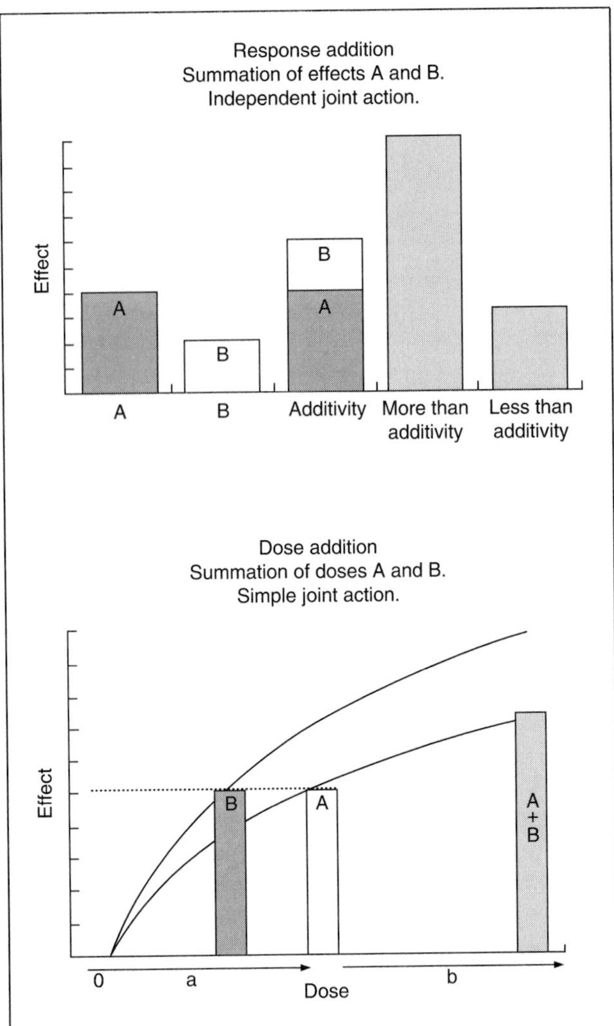

FIGURE 2 Response addition (independent joint action) vs dose addition (simple joint action). In the case of dose addition for chemical B, an equieffective dose of A (= b) must be added to the dose of chemical A.

ual compounds in a mixture after adjustment for the differences in potencies (i.e., two chemicals A and B contribute both to the toxicity of the mixture in proportion to their doses). This form of action also serves as the basis for the use of "toxic equivalency factors" used to describe the combined toxicity of isomers or structural analogs (e.g., PCBs and dioxins).

Simple Dissimilar Action

Simple dissimilar action, also referred to as "simple independent action," "independent joint action," or "response or effect addition." In this event, the chemicals of a mixture do not affect each other's toxic effect. The modes of action and possibly, but not necessarily, the nature and site of the effect differ among the chemicals in the mixture (Fig. 2). Effect addition is the additive effect determined by the summation of the responses to each compound in the mixture. The terms "response" and "effect" are generally used as synonyms and can be applied to effects within or between individuals. However, the term "response addition" should be used more specifically to describe the "number of responders" in a population. This holds true if each individual of the population has a certain tolerance to the chemicals of the mixture and the individual will only exhibit a response to a toxicant if the concentration exceeds the tolerance dose. In this case, the number of responders will be given rather than the average effect of a mixture on a group of individuals.

Interaction

The term "interaction" describes the combined effect between two chemicals resulting in a stronger effect (synergism, potentiation, supra-additivity) or weaker effect (antagonism, subadditivity, inhibition) than expected on the basis of additivity. The term "interaction" should not be viewed in the physiogical sense as describing biological interference for a target or receptor, but as an empirical description to characterize departure from additivity. The mechanism behind the "interactions" may be of physiochemical and/or biological nature and an interaction might occur in the toxicokinetic phase or/and in the toxicodynamic phase.

The most obvious cases for more or less than additive effects in the toxicokinetic phase are enzyme induction and/or inhibition, since metabolism is an important determinant of toxicity (either reactive intermediates are formed—activation—or the toxic agent is removed—detoxification). Compounds that influence the amount of biotransformation enzymes can have large effects on the toxicity of other chemicals. Of course, uptake and excretion processes may also be active processes. For a mixture of compounds with the same target receptor (i.e., the same transport pumps or the same biotransformation enzymes) but with (different) nonlinear dose–effect relatioships, mathematical or physiological modeling can be applied to describe the combined action. In case the joint action between two chemicals can be described by Michealis–Menten kinetics, generally this will result in a phenomenon called "competitive agonism" and the ultimate combined effect will be less than expected on the basis of effect-addition because of the competition for the same receptor. In fact this type of interaction can also be considered as a special case of similar joint action (dose-addition).

All three basic principles of joint action are theoretical. In reality, however, one will most likely have to deal with these concepts at the same time, especially when mixtures consist of more than two compounds and when the targets are more complex.

The first educated guess predicting whether compounds behave in a dose- or response-additive way will be based on the (toxicological) knowledge of the individual compounds or classes of compounds. From this starting point, one might speculate how the compounds will behave in a mixture in acute single-dose experiments. However, the more realistic the mixture study is designed (i.e., repeated doses at low exposure levels), the more complex the list of toxicokinetic and toxicodynamic end-points one has to account for, and as a result the prediction will be very speculative. The only way for the combination toxicologist to describe the combined action of the components in the mixture is to perform experimental studies comparing the effect of the mixture to the effect of the individual compounds.

EXPERIMENTAL APPROACHES FOR MIXTURE STUDIES

Many experimental setups can be used to achieve toxicological knowledge about mixtures with a restricted number of test groups. The study plan will mainly depend on the number of compounds of a mixture and on the question whether it is desirable to assess possible existing interactions between chemicals in a mixture. Preferably a mixture should be tested both at high (effective) concentrations and at low (realistic) concentrations. Interactive effects of compounds in mixtures with more than three compounds can be best ascertained with the help of statistical designs such as (fractionated) factorial designs, ray designs, or dose–effect surface analysis.

Whole Mixtures

The simplest way to study effects of mixtures is to compare the effect of a mixture with the effects of all its constituents at comparable concentrations and duration of exposure at one dose level without testing all possible combinations of chemicals. Although this approach requires a minimum number of experimental groups ($n + 1$, the number of compounds in a mixture plus the mixture itself) and the design of these studies were chosen to reflect the net effect of all compounds in the mixture, it will not be possible to describe the effect of the mixture in terms of synergism, potentiation, and antagonism if there are no dose–effect curves of each single compound. For example, if two chemicals have dose–effect relationships with different slopes (A > B) and agent A inhibits the action of agent B, one can understand that the effect of agent B at low dose levels cannot be predicted from the information about the effect at high dose levels.

Thus, toxicity studies with whole mixtures are mostly chosen to limit the number of test groups. Identification of possible interactive effects of the chemicals in relation to the effects of individual chemicals is not or cannot be taken into account. This strategy has been used to assess the combined toxicity of undefined mixtures (drinking water, coke-oven emission, cigarette smoke) and defined chemical mixtures (aldehydes, halogenated alkenes, pesticides, food additives, and fertilizers). The question whether high-to-low-dose extrapolation is allowed remains to be resolved.

Interactive Effects between Small Numbers of Compounds

To study interactive effects between two or three compounds, physiologically based toxicokinetic modeling, isobolographic, or dose–effect surface analysis is used. Physiologically based toxicokinetic modeling would be especially useful for interactions in the toxicokinetic phase (note that despite similar biotransformation pathways, the mechanism to activate toxins might be quite different or toxins might be influencing each other's biotransformation through induction or inhibition). In the risk assessment of xenobiotics, adequate human data are often not available. The current practice is to extrapolate the risk for humans using animal studies combined with arbitrary safety factors.

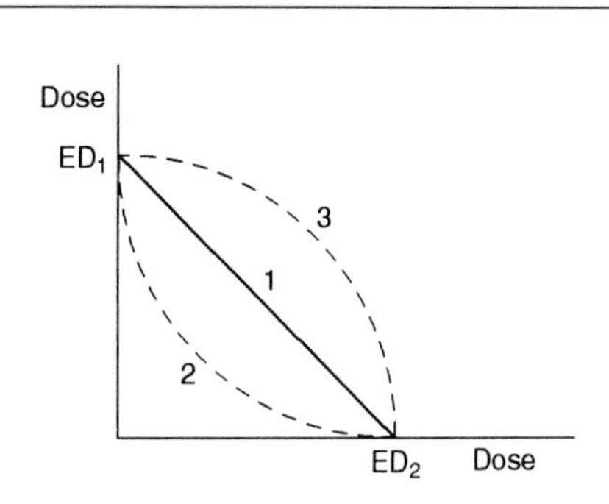

FIGURE 3 An isobologram is a graphical representation of the dosages of two chemicals. The doses of chemical 1 (ED_1) necessary to cause an effect is espressed as a function of the doses of chemical 2 (ED_2). The straight line drawn in the middle represents the contours of equal response (isoeffect line) in the case of dose additivity. Line 2 represents cases of synergism; line 3 represents antagonism.

However, for many compounds, metabolism is the major determinant of the risk and for several hazardous substances considerable insight into the role of metabolism in toxic reactions has become available from laboratory experiments. In principle, the *in vivo* human metabolism can be predicted using *in vitro* enzyme kinetics and thus may be compared with *in vitro* and *in vivo* data from animal studies. In several cases, experiments with microsomal fractions and hepatocytes have been shown to predict accurately the *in vivo* velocity of metabolism for a single metabolic pathway. Such data may be applied in "physiologically based toxicokinetic modeling." At present, several physiologically based toxicokinetic models are available and they offer the possibility of incorporating the interferences between two compounds in the same metabolic pathways.

Isobolographic and dose–effect surface analyses are mathematical models in which the statistical significance of interactions can be determined. The models are most suitable for situations where the target is the same for a limited number of compounds, thus where possible interaction takes place in the toxicodynamic phase. An isobole, originally developed by Loewe and Muischnek in 1926, is a contour line that represents equieffective quantities of two agents or their mixtures. The theoretical line of additivity is the straight line connecting the individual doses of each of the single agents that produce the fixed effect alone. The method is used for a graphical representation to establish if two chemicals act according to the dose-additivity criterion (similar mode of action). It requires tedious experimental determinations of the effects of a number of mixtures. When all equieffect concentrations are connected by a downward concave line, the effect of the combinations is more than additive, and a concave upward curve less than additive (Fig. 3). Such conclusions rely strongly on the exactness of estimated intercepts of the theoretical isobole with the axis (representing the dose of one of the chemicals of the mixture inducing the preferred effect level).

Conceptually less easy to interpret, but much easier to perform, are response-surface analyses. The response or effect surface methodology will yield a statistically based mathematical relationship between the doses of each of the agents of a mixture and the effect parameter. In this design the number of experimental groups is manageable. The mathematical equation is obtained by multiple (log)linear regression. An example of an equation for a three-compound mixture is

$$E = \alpha + \beta_1 \cdot d_1 + \beta_2 \cdot d_2 + \beta_3 \cdot d_3 + \gamma_1 d_1 d_2 + \gamma_2 d_1 d_3 + \gamma_3 d_2 d_3 + \delta_1 d_1 d_2 d_3,$$

where E represents the effect in the presence of a three-compound mixture, d_n the dose of a chemical in the mixture, β_x the magnitude associated with the effect of the chemical, α the effect indicating the background, γ_x, the contribution two-factor interactions, and δ_y the contribution of the interaction between three chemicals. By means of a t test and the standard error of a coefficient, the p value for each regression coefficient can be estimated. For instance, in a study describing the cytotoxicity in nasal epithelial cells exposed to mixtures of aldehydes (formaldehyde, acroleine, and crotonaldehyde) the effect surface analyses revealed that two- and three-factor interactions were significantly different from zero, although the magnitude of the interactions was relatively low compared to the effect of the single compounds. Thus the β term was much higher than the γ and δ terms. It has been shown that effect surface analysis is a rapid statistically sound method for screening of main effects and interactive effects of mixtures of chemicals in doses ranging from none to minimum effect levels of the single compounds.

Interactive Effects between Large Numbers of Compounds

Any time a mixture consists of more than two compounds, two- or three-factor interactions are likely. If all these factors are carefully considered in an experimental setup, the number of possible test combinations increases exponentially with increasing numbers of compounds in a mixture. Likewise, the number of experimental groups will also increase with the number of doses of each compound. Both ethical and practical reasons force researchers to lower the number of experimental groups.

A number of statistical designs are available to evaluate the effects of mixtures compared to their constituents. A common way to detect interactive effects (i.e., nonadditive effects) between more than two chemicals in a chemical mixture is to use factorial designs. The use of factorial designs, in which n chemicals are studied at x dose levels (x^n-treatment groups) has been suggested as one of the valuable statistical approaches to risk assessment of chemical mixtures. Very recently a 2^5 study was presented to describe interactions between the carcinogenic activity of five polycyclic aromatic hydrocarbons at two dose levels and a 5^3 study has been used to identify nonadditive effects of three compounds on developmental toxicity at five dose levels. Full factorial designs, however, lead to very costly experiments, and even if only two dose levels are used, it is already virtually impossible to perform complete conventional toxicity tests using $2^n - 1$ test groups to identify interactions among all chemicals of interest. One way to deal with this problem is the use of fractionated factorial designs. Fractionated designs still identify most of the interactions between the compounds and determine which compounds are important in causing effects and have the advantage that the number of test groups is manageable. Fractional factorial designs have been shown to be an efficient (i.e., cost effective) approach to identifying interactive effects between trace elements and the cadmium accumulation in the body, to determining structure–activity relationships for halogenated aliphatic hydrocarbons, and to determining interactions between drugs and contaminants in food.

If the risk assessor does not attempt to model the complete dose–response surface of the mixture, another approach might be followed in which the interest is focused on departure from the additivity of the mixture as a whole, rather than on the identification of specific interactions. This approach, suggested by Berenbaum (1981), utilizes single chemical dose–response information in addition to the observed responses induced by the particular combinations of interest. The advantage offered by such an approach becomes apparent when the number of experimental groups employed in its application is compared to that required by the use of factorial designs. Apart from this limitation, the strength of the (fractionated) factorial approach is the possibility of formulating a more accurate hypothesis as to most of the relevant or critical interactions and to show which compounds are important in the particular mixture in terms of hazard identification.

When whole reponse surfaces are to be studied for several chemicals at the the same time, factorial designs are too complex in structure. In these cases, other designs (e.g., Box-Behnken or central composite designs) can be used to study deviations from additivity as a first start. These designs should be applied to determine an optimum effect and to perform in a cost-effective way response surface analyses. As a follow-up after this first screening, a factorial design can be applied to verify interactions between selected compounds.

EXAMPLES FROM THE ENVIRONMENT

Complex versus Defined Chemical Mixtures

To successfully study the toxicology of mixtures and to properly assess their potential health risks, it is essential to understand the basic concepts of combined action and interaction of chemicals and to distinguish between whole-mixture analysis (top-down approach) and component interaction analysis (bottom-up approach). In our view, it is equally important to make a clear distinction between simple and complex chemical mixtures. A *simple* mixture is defined as a mixture that consists of a relatively small number of chemicals, say 10 or less, and the composition of which is qualitatively and quantitatively known; examples are a cocktail of pesticides, a combination of medicines, and a group of irritating aldehydes. A *complex* mixture is defined as a mixture that consists of tens, hundreds, or thousands of chemicals and the composition of which is qualitatively and quantitatively not fully known; examples are welding fumes, a workplace atmosphere, environmental tobacco smoke, drinking water, and a new food product. It is self-evident that a bottom-up approach to studying the toxicology of complex mixtures is virtually impossible. For some complex mixtures, the top-down approach may be appropriate; for others, such as the atmosphere at a hazardous waste site or a workplace atmosphere, whole mixture analysis seems to be impracticable and meaningless.

Air Pollutants

Air pollution is a variable complex mixture of chemicals that consists of gases, vapors, and aerosols. Exposure to these chemicals is difficult to avoid. The diversity of environments where exposure might occur and the number of pollutants that may be present pose a challenge in investigating the health effects of air pollutants. The toxicity of these mixtures is determined not only by the adverse effects of the single compounds but also by interactions between two or more chemicals of the mixture. Air pollution is a continuously varying complex mixture with numerous possible combined actions.

Mixtures of Aerosols and Gases

By studying chemical–chemical interactions in the toxicology of air pollutants, it was shown that the untoward effects of certain oxidants may be enhanced in the presence of other aerosols. Damage to the alveolar zone by the antioxidant butylated hydroxytoluene (BHT) can be greatly enhanced by subsequent exposure to oxygen concentrations that otherwise would have little if any demonstrable effect. The synergistic interaction between BHT and oxygen results in interstitial pulmonary fibrosis. Synergistic interactions between either ozone or nitrogen dioxide and relatively high levels of aerosols of sulfuric acid or ammonium bisulfate have been reported and were seen as an increase of alveolar macrophages and fibroblast, increased collagen synthesis and total protein contents in lavage fluid, and a more-than-additive increase in lipid peroxidation in the lung. In most of these cases, exposure levels that exceeded reality were used and whether these additive and synergistic effects found at high levels are predictive of joint action at about the no-observed-adverse-effect level (NOAEL) has not yet been sufficiently studied.

Considerable attention has been paid to the joint action of aldehydes. Aldehydes constitute a group of relatively reactive organic compounds that are omnipresent in the environment as a result of incomplete combustion or pyrolysis of organic materials such as fuels, polymers, food, and tobacco. Combined exposure of rats to formaldehyde and acrolein has been reported to result in higher yields of DNA–protein cross-links in nasal epithelium than exposure to formaldehyde alone, most probably because of inhibition of the oxidative metabolism of formaldehyde due to glutathione depletion by acrolein. Toxicity studies with mixtures of aldehydes showed that histopathological changes and cell proliferation of the nasal epithelium by mixtures of formaldehyde, acetaldehyde, and acrolein appeared to be more severe and more extensive, in both the respiratory and the olfactory epithelium, than those observed after exposure to the individual aldehydes at comparable exposure levels. However, the prediction of joint action of these aldehydes at NOAELs of the individual chemicals did not seem to be possible. Therefore, overall these studies indicate that combined exposure to aldehydes with the same target organ (nose) and excerting the same type of adverse effect (nasal irritation), but with partly different target sites, is not associated with increased nose irritation as compared to exposure to the individual chemicals.

Besides irritation of the nasal epithelium, aldehydes are also known to be potent sensory irritants. Sensory irritation can be measured by a decrease in breathing frequency and is a result of the binding of the aldehydes to the trigeminal nerve receptor. The fact that these aldehydes act on a common binding site at the trigeminal nerve (through a mechanism called "competitive agonism") points in the direction of a similar mode of action and probably allows for the use of a dose-addition model to describe the combined effects of aldehydes. Indeed, exposure to aldehydes at relevant (i.e., low) dose levels has been shown to result in additive effects with respect to sensory irritation. Thus, aldehydes in a mixture show joint action and the effect of mixed exposure is more pronounced than the effect after single exposure. This indicates that in the hazard assessment of mixtures of aldehydes, the joint sensory irritation has to be taken into account.

Particulate Matter

Particulate matter (PM) is a very vague term for a complex mixture with a high diversity in size, composition, and shape. Airborne suspended particulate matter can be either primary or secondary in nature. Primary particles are emitted directly into the atmosphere either by natural or anthropogenic processes, whereas secondary particles have a predominantly human-made origin and are formed in the atmosphere from the oxidation of sulfur dioxide, nitrogen oxides, and volatile organic compounds. In most European countries, industrialization and high volumes of traffic mean that anthropogenic sources predominate, especially in urban areas, and sources of anthropogenic particles are similar throughout Europe. The most significant of these are traffic, power plants, combustion sources (industrial and residential), industrial fugitive dust, loading and unloading of bulk goods, mining activities, human-started forest fires, and, in some local cases, noncombustion sources such as building construction and quarrying. The main natural sources of airborne particulates in Europe are sea spray and soil resuspension by the wind. In addition, in the Mediterranean basin, Saharan dust, volcano emissions, and bioorganic material can also be important natural sources of particulates.

Recent epidemiological studies have associated PM10 (particular matter with a mean aerodynamic diameter of 10 μm) with health effects like increased daily mortality and hospital admissions, exacerbation of asthma, increase of respiratory symptoms, and lung function decline. The levels of PM10 at which these effects are observed are significantly lower than those previously thought to protect human health. Since PM10 is a complex mixture and the current standards are to a large extent based on information from studies using single-chemical aerosols, joint action of chemicals in the mixture of PM10 cannot be excluded. However, at present there is scanty toxicological information on particulate matter. Several approaches have been put forward to test the toxicity of PM mixtures. One way to is to identify the critical chemicals in these complex mixtures by performing toxicity studies with artificially generated aerosols. Another way to test the toxicity of particulate matter mixtures is make use of real-world aerosols from locations dominated by different emission sources (like rural versus urban versus industrialized areas). This is useful to identify those aerosols that are causally related to the observed adverse health effects. A complicating factor is that different exposure parameters such as the size, the number, and the surface area of the particles are considered to be important factors that determine disposition and reactivity in the lung tissue. In this context dosimetry models might be valuable tools to establish the dose at the target site.

Large safety factors have been applied to set exposure limits for especially indoor air pollutants. However, for particulate matter, aldehydes, and ozone, these margins of safety are small and special attention should be paid to the tracing of hazardous combinations within particulate matter (PM) but also between particulate matter and other air pollutants. Due to epidemiological studies in which serious health effects were associated with PM without a sound toxicological explanation, much effort is put into elucidating the toxicological mechanisms underlying these effects. The complexity of PM forces investigators to use study designs that can identify possible interactions of critical components of these mixtures or with gaseous compounds of air pollution.

Threshold levels for combined or interactive effects of chemicals and the underlying mechanisms described in experimental animals are not clearly defined, so that their relevance to humans chronically exposed to low levels of these chemicals remains unclear. As to how far the results of animal studies at high dose levels predict the potential health hazard in humans exposed to lower (no effect) concentrations of the individual chemicals is not clear. Undoubtedly studies on combinations of air pollutants using more realistic concentrations, including levels around the no-observed-effect level (NOEL), are needed.

Food

Food is an extremely complex and variable chemical mixture estimated to consist of several hundred thousands of chemicals. In principle food chemicals may exhibit joint similar or joint dissimilar action, leading to noninteractive combined effects, and may also interact with one another, altering the degree and maybe also the nature of the potential toxic effects of individual food chemicals.

Are such potential combined or interactive adverse effects from exposure to food chemicals likely or unlikely to occur in humans? To answer this question, let's first consider food components in some detail. Generally, food chemicals are classified into four groups: nutrients, nonnutritive naturally occurring components, human-made contaminants, and additives. Extensive toxicological studies and evaluations are required for additives and human-made chemicals that may contaminate food such as pesticides, veterinary drugs, and chemicals from food-packaging materials. Regular toxicology limit values are recommended by national and international committees, usually applying large safety factors of 100 or more. Thus, these chemicals have large margins of safety, in particular in comparison with nutrients with their often small margin between recommended daily allowances (RDAs) and the minimum toxic dose (e.g., 18 for iron, 15 for vitamin A, 10 for zinc, 9 for potassium, 5 for sodium, 5 for vitamin D, 2 for manganese, and 1.4 for fat). Our knowledge about the toxicity of the vast majority of natural food chemicals is characterized by gaps.

As a rule exposure to mixtures of chemicals at (low) nontoxic doses of the individual chemicals in the mixture is of no health concern, and the probability of increased health hazard due to additivity or potentiating interaction seems to be very small, since the dose of chemicals to which humans are exposed is *generally* much lower than the no-observed-adverse-effect level. Exceptions to these rules may be mixtures of chemicals with a similar mode of action or with evidence of potentiating interaction, and mixtures with no or very small safety margins, such as the outdoor air (a mixture with as major constituents

PM2.5, ozone, nitrogen dioxide, and sulfur dioxide). To trace such exceptional mixtures is one of the priorities of the toxicology of mixtures. Do we encounter such exceptional mixtures in food, and if so, how are we dealing with them in food safety evaluation? For food chemicals with similar mode of actions, group ADIs (acceptable daily intakes) are recommended. The use of toxic equivalence factors (e.g., for mixtures of polychlorinated dibenzodioxins, polychlorinated dibenzofurans, and polychlorinated biphenyls occurring in, for example, mother's milk) is another way to deal with mixtures of food chemicals with similar modes of action. Potentiating interaction is expected to be only of minor importance in view of the low-intake levels of nonnutritive food components. An interesting exception is the poisoning (flushing, hypotension, headache, nausea, and vomiting) following consumption of the edible Inky cap mushroom (*Coprinus atramentarius*) in combination with alcoholic beverages. The fungicide thiram is also known to cause alcohol intolerance. This leads us to the category of food chemicals of highest health concern, viz. (essential) nutrients with their relatively small safety margins. Nutritional imbalance may result in deficiencies but also in exceeding the safety margin. As the "drugs of life," nutrients are reactive body-oriented chemicals (in contrast to additives, which are food-oriented and preferably as inert as possible towards the body), which may explain their relatively small margin of safety. For the mixture toxicologist, the priority category of food chemicals would seem to be the nutrients with their body orientation and small safety margins. However, the mixture of nutrients is necessary for growth, maintenance, and reproduction of humans, and when in balance the mixture as such is a prerequisite rather than a threat to human health; in fact, a balanced mixture of nutrients (a balanced diet) is the preeminent medicine of life. On the other hand, because of the importance of nutrients for life, the nutritionist has to be on the alert for interactions of nonnutritive and even nonfood chemicals with nutrients, leading to nutritional deficiencies, while the food toxicologist should always consider the possibility of potentiating interactions between nonnutritive or nonfood chemicals (e.g., drugs) and nutrients.

Finally, the mixture of nutrients is an excellent example illustrating that application of the dose-addition concept for assessing the health risks of mixtures of chemicals that act by mechanisms for which the additivity assumptions are invalid would often greatly overestimate their health risks: it can easily be calculated that simultaneous consumption of nutrients (with their small margins between RDA and lowest toxic dose) at their recommended intake levels turns out to be a rather unhealthy habit when the risk of this mixture is assessed on the basis of dose additivity.

Endocrine Activity of Environmental Pollutants

Accumulating evidence indicates that environmental toxicants may disrupt endocrine function in animal and human populations. This evidence is derived from the findings of wildlife biologists, epidemiologic studies, and toxicologic data. In aggregate these findings may have significant implications for human and environmental health. These implications may have even greater significance based on the potential for joint toxic action based on common mechanisms of action and/or interactions among functionally interrelated mechanisms related to reproduction and development.

Endocrine-disrupting chemicals may interact with a range of physiological processes, including the production, release, transport, metabolism, action, and/or elimination of endogenous hormones. As a consequence of such interaction, a range of effects on reproduction, development, and homeostasis may result.

Mechanism(s) of Action and Interaction

Xenobiotic modulators of endocrine function exert their effect(s) both individually and in combination regarding receptor-mediated mechanism(s) of action of steroidal hormones. Thyroid hormones also function via a receptor-mediated network analogous to that of steroidal hormones. These receptor-mediated networks activate genomic sequences that ultimately control cellular activities. Another example is the relationship between dioxin and the Ah receptor. While not a hormonal receptor per se, the Ah receptor resembles steroid hormone receptors in both structure and mode of action. Figure 4 depicts steroidal hormone molecules that, after entry into the cell, can bind to specific receptor proteins in the cytoplasm or in the nucleus. Once a receptor–ligand complex has been formed, it translocates to the nucleus of the cell. There, the complex interacts with the genome. The subsequent series of events may result in the up-regulation or down-regulation of specific genes, corresponding to altered patterns of protein synthesis that account for phenotypic expression at cellular (biochemical), functional (physiological), and organismal (morphological) levels. Because of this, the system is vulnerable to materials that are structurally, and

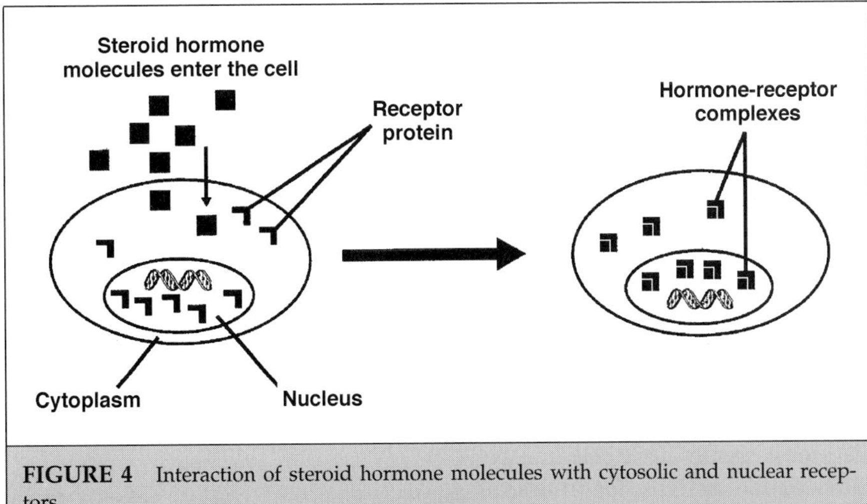

FIGURE 4 Interaction of steroid hormone molecules with cytosolic and nuclear receptors.

therefore functionally, analogous to normal endogenous agents.

Two possible mechanisms of endocrine disruption are described here (Fig. 5). In the first, toxicant A acts as an agonist or promoter of hormonal response by binding to the receptor and initiating the same sequence of events elicited by the endogenous ligand. Alternatively, the material can act as an antagonist, as shown for toxicant B. In this instance, interaction of the toxicant with the receptor prevents access of naturally occurring ligands to the binding site, thereby resulting in failure of hormones to elicit their expected effects.

Other potential mechanisms by which endocrine function can be disrupted include a change in the number of receptors that are elaborated in different germ tissues during development. Organs with hormonal receptors include, but are not limited to, the male and female genitalia, the brain, thyroid, liver, kidney, and those of the immune system. Each of these target organs has a characteristic "population ecology of specific receptor types," as their abundance is defined during development as a function of circulating hormone levels. For example, the number of receptors on the liver available to bind the hormone thyroxine is a function of the levels of circulating thyroxine during fetal development. Exposure to materials other than hormones during development can disrupt this population ecology of receptor types. Other means of disrupting endocrine function include interference with protein synthesis and direct interaction of the toxicants with the hormone, thereby altering its activity.

Moreover, chemicals may affect the developing endocrine system directly or may interfere with a component of the regulating axis controlled by the pituitary, hypothalamus, or other parts of the brain. This results in the complex alteration of multiple endocrine endpoints, known to occur following exposure to endocrine modulators. Developmental processes governed by hormonal factors are complex, interrelated, and multifactorial. The interrelationships of these factors and processes has been termed "combinational complexity"; accordingly, endocrine-mediated processes are vulnerable to imbalances as a result of either endogenous or exogenous factors. For example, the developmental fate of the embryonic urogenital system is determined by the ratio of testosterone and estrogen that the developing fetus is exposed to *in utero*.

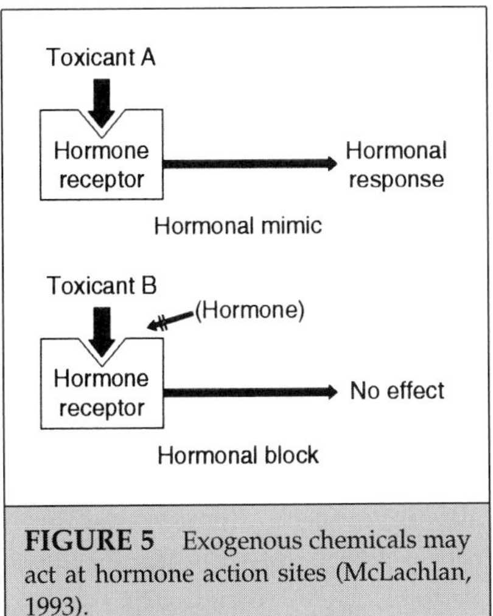

FIGURE 5 Exogenous chemicals may act at hormone action sites (McLachlan, 1993).

In Vitro and In Vivo Studies

Given the ubiquity of chemicals and chemical classes that have been implicated as endocrine disruptors, environmental exposures to combinations of such agents are likely. While the potential for joint toxic action exists, the actual nature of interaction, antagonism, potentiation, synergism, and so on, will vary as a function of actual agents and their impact on one or more physiologic processes.

Preliminary insights into the potential for joint toxic action among endocrine-disrupting chemicals have emerged from some *in vitro* screening bioassays. For example, the E-screen test uses the MCF_7 cell line derived from human breast tissue. This cell line requires estrogen or estrogen-like activity for proliferation and therefore can be used to assess the estrogenicity of chemicals, both individually and in combination. Using this bioassay, it was found that organochlorine pesticides, including toxaphene, dieldrin, and endosulfan had estrogen-like effects similar to those of DDT and chlordecone pesticides with demonstrated estrogenic activity in rodent assays. To assess the potential for joint toxic action or a cumulative effect associated with simultaneous exposure, a mixture of 10 estrogenic compounds was administered to MCF_7 cells as a concentration one-tenth of that required to produce an estrogenic response alone. This combination elicited an estrogenic response that would not be expected, based on estrogenic assays of the compound tested individually.

While these data derived from *in vitro* studies are significant, they are not sufficient to confirm the chemicals being tested as estrogen mimics *in vivo*. The same is true of the results of *in vitro* studies intended to assess the potential for joint toxic action of mixtures. Data that indicate chemical agents eliciting estrogenic effects *in vitro*, either singly or in combination, should be supported by data derived from *in vivo* studies. It should be further noted that some agents may elicit significant estrogenic or other endocrine properties *in vivo* in absence of significant activity revealed by *in vitro* screens.

For the reasons outlined above, *in vivo* data indicating both estrogenic effects and the potential for joint toxic action are critical. Recently the effect of PCB compounds on the developmental fate of reptilian eggs (in this case, turtles) was examined. Turtles and other reptiles exhibit temperature-dependent sex determination. For example, turtle eggs incubated at 31°C typically develop into females, while those incubated at 26°C develop into males. However, at temperature of 26°C, PCB-treated eggs developed into females. Synergistic effects were observed when PCB compounds were applied in combination for the same total dose. Interactions are not always synergistic and may be also antagonistic, as is the case of dioxins and furans. Coadministration of 2,2′,4,4′,5,5′-hexachlorobiphenyl or Aroclor 1254 with TCDD resulted in antagonism of TCDD-mediated teratogenicity and immunotoxicity in mice. These examples indicate the complexity of issues associated with interactions of these chemicals.

While the preponderance of data to date involves interactions of estrogenic compounds with the estrogen receptor, broader patterns of endocrine disruption reflect interactions of hormonally active xenobiotics with multiple receptors. The ability of commercial pesticides to bind to the estrogen receptor (aER) and progesterone receptor (aPR) has been found in an *in vitro* screen derived from the oviduct of the alligator. In competition binding assays with 17β-estradiol, DDT metabolites inhibited 17β-estradiol from binding to a ER in an additive manner.

Public Health Implications

A growing body of experimental data implicates a large number of diverse compounds as endocrine disruptors, thereby accounting for their presumed impact on reproductive and developmental parameters in animals and humans. Given the demonstrated ability of these compounds to interact under laboratory conditions, possibly via similar mechanisms of action, the implications for public health deserve our attention and more precise assessments are necessary, especially for those populations vulnerable by virtue of their exposure (e.g., occupational exposure, suckling infants, high consumption of contaminated fish) or intrinsic physiological susceptibility (e.g., developing organisms, implantation through sexual maturity).

RISK ASSESSMENT OF CHEMICAL MIXTURES

There are all sorts of problems with risk assessment of chemical mixtures. Testing of all kinds of mixtures of chemicals existing in the real world or of all possible combinations of chemicals of a simple defined mixture at different dose levels is virtually impossible. Moreover, even if toxicity data on individual compounds are available, we are still facing the immense problem of extrapolation of findings obtained at relatively high exposure concentration in laboratory animals to humans being exposed to much lower concentrations. This problem has recently been recognized as one of the key issues in the assessment of possible health risks from disinfection by-products in drinking water. Indeed, what is the predictive value of combined or interactive adverse effects occurring (in laboratory animals) at relatively high exposure concentrations for humans being exposed to much lower concentrations of the chemical mixture?

Combinations of Chemicals with Different Target Organs and/or Different Modes of Action

Toxicity studies with mixture of chemicals with different target organs (liver, kidney, haemopoeitic system) or with similar target organs but with different modes of action (nose or kidney) have shown that at the lowest-observed-adverse-effect level (LOAEL) of the mixture, both more and less severe effects were seen than at the LOAEL of each of the individual compounds, indicating additive or interactive effects at this dose level. No effects unambiguously related to treatment were found at the NOAEL of the mixture. Therefore, combined action of the chemicals in these studies very closely, if not fully, meets the criteria of the basic concept "simple dissimilar action" (i.e., independent joint action). The results of the studies allow the conclusion that simultaneous administration of these chemicals with different working mechanisms did not constitute a clearly increased hazard, provided the administered dose of each of the toxicants is a NOAEL. Thus in this case the NOAEL of the mixture is determined by the NOAEL of the chemical with the smallest margin between its actual level in the mixture and its true toxic-effect level, assuming that the actual level of each of the compounds in the mixture is lower than its true no-effect level. In terms of health risks, the risk of the mixtures is thus determined by the risk associated with the risk of the "most risky chemical" (which equals the chemical with the highest risk quotient) of the mixture. A safety factor of "normal" size applied to the NOAEL would establish an acceptable exposure limit for such a mixture.

The studies in which dissimilarly acting chemicals were tested in combination have also indicated that the type of combined action or interaction found at clearly toxic-effect levels is not very helpful in predicting what will happen at no-toxic-effect levels, including levels only slightly lower than the LOAEL. However, precisely what happens at no-toxic-effect levels (including exposure levels only slightly lower than the LOAEL) is what counts in assessing the potential health risk of humans exposed to mixtures of these chemicals. Obviously, as soon as the exposure levels of the chemicals in the mixture acting dissimilarly are in the range of NOAELs, no additivity and no potentiating interaction were found.

Combinations of Chemicals with the Same Mode of Action

When the compounds in mixture act according to the same mode of action, the dose-additivity rule can be applied. For instance, the sensory irritation of mixtures of aldehydes can be explained by using a dose-additivity model. Also, to explain the joint binding of environmental pollutants to the estradiol receptor the dose-addition model seemed to be valid. Dose additivity was also observed in the kidney in a 4-week oral toxicity study in female rats with mixtures of halogen alkenes, hexachlorobutadiene, tetrachloroethylene, trichloroethylene, and 1,1,2-trichloro-3,3,3-trifluoropropene. The nephrotoxicity of these chemicals results from initial conjugation to glutathione in the liver and cysteine conjugate (lyase-)mediated formation of reactive metabolites in the proximal tubular epithelial cells. Relative kidney weight was increased following exposure to the individual compounds at their individual NOAEL (1/4 of LOAEL). It is concluded that the renal toxicity, as assessed by the effect on kidney weight, of a mixture of similarly acting nephrotoxicants at levels slightly below the LOAEL of the individual compounds corresponded to the effect expected on the basis of the additivity assumption.

It is evident that for the previous chemicals the dose-addition model (simple similar action or similar joint action) represents the basic concept to be used for risk assessment of similarly acting compounds. In contrast to the response-additivity model, this model is applicable over the whole range of exposure levels from low nontoxic levels to NOAELs (the highest level of each chemical at which no adverse effect was observed). The dose-addition concept is the most common approach to risk assessment of mixtures. However, its use is justifiable from a scientific point of view only when all chemicals in the mixture act in the same way, by the same mechanism, and thus differ only in their toxic potencies. Of course, in reality the existence of mixtures that meet such conditions is the exception rather than the rule. As evidenced by the other examples described, application of the dose-addition model to mixtures of chemicals that act by mechanisms for which the additivity assumptions are invalid would greatly overestimate the risk.

The Hazard Index (HI)

The hazard index as put forward in the U.S. EPA mixture guidelines should be regarded as an approximation of the risk posed by exposure to the mixture. In this approach the hazard quotients are calculated for individual compounds and the quotients for each compound in the mixture are then added. The hazard index (HI) can be calculated from the equation

$$\mathrm{HI} = \sum_{1}^{n} \frac{\mathrm{Dose}}{\mathrm{RfD}} = \frac{D1}{\mathrm{RfD1}} + \frac{D2}{\mathrm{RfD2}} + \cdots + \frac{Dn}{\mathrm{RfD}n},$$

where D is the level of exposure and RfD is some defined limit exposure value (the reference dose). If the equation exceeds unity, the concern is the same as if an individual chemical exposure exceeded its acceptable level by the same proportion. In case of independent joint action, the hazard index will be that of the agent with the highest quotient. Thus, in a three-compound mixture ABC with exposure levels $A = 1$, $B = 0.5$, and $C = 75$ and a DLs of $A = 10$, $B = 1$, and $C = 100$ the HIs are 0.2, 0.3, and 0.5 for the individual chemicals, repectively. In the case of dissimilar joint action, the HI of the mixture ABC will be 0.75, whereas with similar joint action the HI of the mixture will be 1.35. If the hazard index is greater than 1, there might be an increased risk of exposure to this mixture. The hazard index method is based on the assumption of dose additivity (similar joint action) and is thus valid only under the condition that the compounds in the mixture induce the same toxic effect, via the same mode of action. It will often be impossible to obtain sufficient and adequate toxicological information on each of the compounds of a mixture to make these calculations.

Thus, data on interaction are not included in the HI approach and in several cases the risk of joint action will be overestimated. A different approach, published by Mumtaz and Durkin (1994), takes into account both synergistic and antagonistic interations in the derivation of the HI. In this approach a weight-of-evidence (WOE) classification is followed to estimate the joint actions (additivity, antagonism, and synergism) for binary mixtures of chemicals based on information about the individual compounds.

$$\mathrm{HI} = \mathrm{HI} = \mathrm{HI.\ UF}^{\mathrm{WOE}}$$

$$\mathrm{WOE} = \Sigma\ \mathrm{IF}\ (-1, 1)$$

Here, UF is the uncertainty factor and WOE the interaction factor (additivity = 0, synergism = +, antagonism = −), based on the weight of evidence. In the WOE, several weighing factors are taken into account in the final classification, such as the mechanistic understanding of the binary interactions, the demonstration of toxicity, and additional uncertainty factors (i.e., modifiers of interactions), such as route of exposure and *in vitro* data. The better the data set on the individual compounds, the more precisely the joint action can be predicted. The hazard index method can be regarded as a general first assessment of the risk of joint action. The WOE method should be used as a follow-up in those cases where priority mixture has been established.

Complex Chemical Mixtures

As appears from the previous sections, there are several ways to identify the hazard and to assess the potential health risk of complex chemical mixtures. Different types of complex mixtures call for different approaches. Moreover, the usefulness of a certain approach depends on the context in which one is confronted with the mixture and on the amount, type, and quality of the information that is available on the chemistry and the toxicity of the mixture.

Figure 6 depicts the development of a decision tree for risk evaluation of complex mixtures and it presents a practical guide for hazard identification and risk assessment of complex mixtures. After showing that chemical mixtures should be divided into simple and complex mixtures, the scheme continues with a dichotomy of complex mixtures into mixtures readily available and mixtures virtually unavailable for testing in their entirety. Examples of the former are drinking water, diesel exhaust, welding fumes, tobacco smoke, and new food products; examples of the latter are workplace atmospheres, coke-oven emissions, and atmospheres at a waste sites. To study successfully the toxicology of mixtures and to properly assess their potential health risks, it is essential to understand the basic concepts of combined action and interaction of chemicals, to distinguish between whole mixture analysis (top-down approach) and component-interaction analysis (bottom-up approach), and to distinguish between simple and complex mixtures.

There are various ways to deal with hazard identification and risk assessment of complex chemical mixtures. Different types of complex mixtures call for different approaches to evaluate their safety, and the usefulness of a certain approach depends on the context in which one is confronted with the mixture and also on the amount, type, and quality of the available data on the chemistry and toxicity of the mixture. A conspicuous element of the scheme presented for the safety evaluation of complex mixtures is the dichotomy between mixtures that are virtually unavailable and mixtures that are readily available for testing in their entirety. Moreover, the inclusion in the scheme of the top-10 and pseudo-top-10 approaches (in essence, selection of the 10 most risky chemicals or pseudo-components to be dealt with as a simple mixture) is regarded as another characteristic aspect of the scheme. The scheme aims at stimulating progress

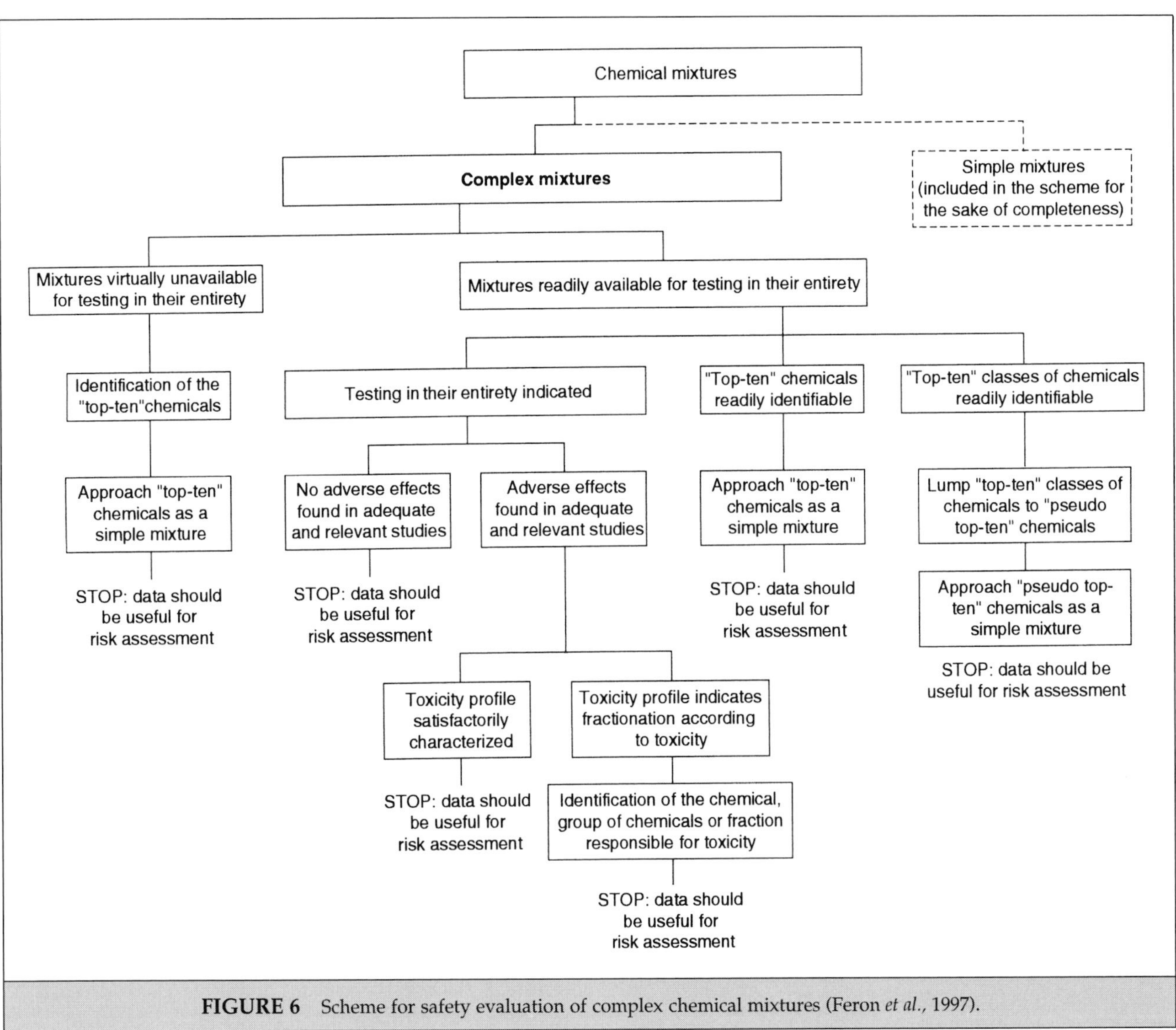

FIGURE 6 Scheme for safety evaluation of complex chemical mixtures (Feron *et al.*, 1997).

in hazard identification and risk assessment of complex chemical mixtures, bringing together and effectively using all available relevant information, methods, technologies, expertise, and experience.

CONCLUSION

From a public health point of view, it is most relevant to answer the question whether chemicals in a mixture interact in a way that results in a reduced or increased overall response, compared to the sum of the responses of the individual chemicals in the mixture, or indeed in an effect that is simply a summation of the expected effects. Approaches to dealing with risk assessment of mixtures rely heavily on some form of additivity model unless data are adequate for a direct risk assessment of the mixture of concern. Although the previously described additivity models are mathematically simple, they require assumptions about the mode of action. The number of mixtures to which direct risk assessment or risk assessment using the relative-potency method have been devoted is limited. The theoretical considerations in risk assessment of chemical mixtures should be verified by simple case studies.

Bibliography

Ashby, J, LeFevre, P. A., Odum, J., Harris, C. A., Routledge, E. J., and Sumpter, J. P. (1997). Synergy between synthetic estrogens? *Nature* **385,** 494.

Bannister, R., Davis, D., Zacharewski, T., Tizard, I., and Safe, S. (1987). Aroclor 1245 as a 2,3,7,8-tetrachlorodibenzo-p-dioxin antagonist: Effects on enzyme induction and immunotoxicity. *Toxicology* **46,** 29–42.

Berenbaum, M. C. (1981). Criteria for analyzing interactions between biologically active agents. *Adv. Cancer Res.* **35,** 269–335.

Bergeron, J. M., Crews, D., and McLachlan, J. A. (1994). PCBs as environmental estrogens: Turtle sex determination as a biomarker of environmental contamination. *Environ. Health Perspec.,* **102,** 780–781.

Birnbaum, L. S. (1995). Developmental effects of dioxins and other endocrine disrupting chemicals(abstract). International Congress of Toxicology, 79-S-5.

Bliss, C. I. (1939). The toxicity of poisons applied jointly. *Ann. Appl. Biol.* **26,** 585–615.

Calabrese, E. J. (ed.) (1991). "Multiple Chemical Interactions." Lewis Publishers, Chelsea, MI.

Cassee, F. R., Arts, J. H. E., Groten, J. P., Schoen, E. D., and Feron, V. J. (1996). Sensory irritation to mixtures of formaldehyde, acrolein and acetaldehyde in rats. *Arch. Toxicol.* **70,** 329–337.

Cassee, F. R., Groten, J. P., and Feron, V. J. (1996). Changes in the nasal epithelium of rats exposed by inhalation to mixtures of formaldehyde, acetaldehyde and acrolein. *Fund. Appl. Toxicol.* **29,** 208–218.

Cassee, F. R., Groten, J. P., Van Bladeren, P. J., and Feron, V. J. (1998). Toxicological evaluation and risk assessment of chemical mixtures. *Crit. Rev. Toxicol.,* in press.

Colborn, T., vom Saal, F. S., and Soto, A. M. (1993). Developmental effects of endocrine-disrupting chemicals in wildlife and humans. *Environ. Health Perspect.* **101,** 378–384.

De Rosa, C. T., Richter, P., Pohl, H., and Jones, D. E. (1997). Environmental exposures that affect the endocrine system: Public health implications. *J. Toxicol. Environ. Health,* in press.

Feron, V. J. (1997). Introduction to adverse effects of food and nutrition. *In* "Food Safety and Toxicity" (J. de Vries, ed.), pp. 111–120. CRC Press, Boca Raton, FL.

Feron, V. J., and Bolt, H. M. (1996). Combination toxicology. *Fund. Chem. Toxicol* **34,** (I–IV), 1025–1185.

Feron, V. J., Groten, J. P., Jonker, D., Cassee, F. R., and Van Bladeren, P. J. (1995a). Risk assessment of simple (defined) mixtures of chemicals. *In* "Toxicology & Air Pollution: Risk Assessment" (V. Burgat-Sacaze *et al.,* eds.), pp. 31–42. Faculté de Médicine et de Pharmacie, Université de Bourgogne, Dijon.

Feron, V. J., Groten, J. P., Jonker, D., Cassee, F. R., and Van Bladeren, P. J. (1995b). Toxicology of chemical mixtures: Challenges for today and the future. *Toxicology* **105,** 415–428.

Feron, V. J., Groten, J. P., and Van Bladeren, P. J. (1997). Exposure of humans to complex chemical mixtures: Hazard identification and risk assessment. *Arch. Toxicol. Suppl.* **20,** 363–373.

Feskens, E. J. M. (1997). Introduction to risk assessment. *In* "Food Safety and Toxicity" (J. de Vries, ed.). pp. 215–228 CRC Press, Boca Raton, FL.

Finey, D. J. (1942). The analysis of toxicity tests on mixtures of poisons. *Ann. Appl. Biol.* **29,** 82–94.

Groten, J. P., Schoen, E. D., and Feron, V. J. (1996). Use of factorial designs in combination toxicity studies. *Fd. Chem. Toxicol.* **34,** 1083–1091.

Groten, J. P., Sinkeldam, E. J., Muys, T., Luten, J. B., and van Bladeren, P. J. (1991). Interaction of dietary Ca, P, Mg, Mn, Cu, Fe, Zn, and Se with the accumulation and oral toxicity of cadmium in rats. *Fd. Chem. Toxicol.,* **29,** 249–258.

Groten, J. P., Stenhuis, W. S., van Bladeren, P. J., and Feron, V. J. (1997). Subacute toxicity of a combination of nine chemicals in rats: Detecting interactive effects with a fractionated two level factorial design. *Fund. Appl. Toxicol.* **36,** 15–30.

Henschler D., Bolt, H. M., Jonker D., Pieters, M. N., and Groten, J. P. (1996). Experimental designs and risk assessment in combination toxicology. *Fd. Chem. Toxicol.* **34,** 1183–1187.

Ito, N., Hasegawa, K., Imaida K., Kurat, Y., Hagiwara, A., and Shirai, T. (1995). Effect of ingestion of 20 pesticides in combination at acceptable daily intake levels on rat liver carconogenesis. *Fd. Chem. Toxicol.* **33,** 159–163.

Jonker, D., Woutersen, R. A., and Feron, V. J. (1996). Toxicity of mixtures of nephrotoxicants with similar or dissimilar mode of action. *Fund. Chem. Toxicol.* **34,** 1075–1083.

Jonker, D., Woutersen, R. A., van Bladeren, P. J., Til, H. P., and Feron, V. J. (1993). Subacute (4-wk) oral toxicity of a combination of four nephrotoxins in rats: Comparison with the toxicity of the individual compounds. *Fd. Chem. Toxicol.* **31,** 125–136.

Kim, C. S., and Kang, T. C. (1997). Comparative measurement of lung deposition of inhaled fine particles in normal subjects and patients with obstructive airway disease. *Am. J. Respir. Crit. Care. Med.* **155,** ISS 3, P899–905

Miller, F. J., Anjilvel, S., Ménache, M. G., Asgharian, B., and Gerrity, T. R. (1995). Dosimetric issues relating to particle toxicity. *Inhal. Toxicol.* **7,** 615–632.

McLachlan J. A. (1993). Functional toxicology: A new approach to detect biologically active xenobiotics. *Environ. Health Perspect.* **101,** 386–387.

Mumtaz, M. M., DeRosa, C. T., and Durkin, P. R. (1994). Approaches and challenges in risk assessments of chemical mixtures. *In* "Toxicology of Chemical Mixtures" (R. S. H. Yang, ed.), pp. 565–598. Academic Press, San Diego, CA.

Mumtaz, M. M., Sipes, I. G., Clewell, H. J., and Yang, R. S. H. (1993). Risk assessment of chemical mixtures: Biologic and toxicologic issues. *Fund. Appl. Toxicol.* **21,** 258–269.

Narotsky, M. G., Weller, E. A., Chinchilli, V. M., and Kevlock, R. J. (1995). Non-additive developmental toxicity of mixtures of trichloroethylene, (di(2-ethyl-hexyl)phtalate, and heptachlor in a 5×5×5 design. *Fund. Appl. Toxicol.* **27,** 203–216.

NRC (1996) "Carcinogens and Anticarcinogens in the Diet." National Research Council, National Academy Press, Washington, D.C.

Sexton, K. Beck, B. D., Bingham, E., Brain, J. D., DeMarini, D. M., Hertzberg, R.C., O'Flaherty, E. J., and Pounds, J. G. (1995). Chemical mixtures from a public health perspective: The importance of research for informed decision making. *Toxicology* **105,** 429–441.

Simmons, J. E. (1995). Chemical mixtures: Challenge for toxicology and risk assessment. *Toxicol.* **105,** 111–119.

Soto, A. M., Chung K. L., and Sonnenschein, C. 1994. Thepesticides endosulfan, toxaphene and dieldrin have estrogenic effects on human estrogen-sensitive cells. *Environ. Health Perspect.* **102,** 380–383.

US EPA (1986). Guidelines for the health risk assessment of chemical mixtures. *Fed. Regist.* **51**(185), 34014–34025.

Van Genderen, H. (1997). Toxicology of mixtures in the light of food safety. *In* "Food Safety and Toxicity" (J. de Vries, ed.), pp. 177–182. CRC Press, Boca Raton, FL.

Vonier, P. M., Crain, D. A., McLachlan, J. A., Guillette L. J., Jr., and Arnold, S. F. (1996). Interaction of environmental chemicals with the estrogen and progesterone receptor from the oviduct of the American alligator. *Environ. Health Perspect.* **104,** 1318–1322.

Yang, R. S. H. (1994). "Toxicology of Chemical Mixtures." Academic Press, San Diego, CA.

PART

II

ORGAN TOXICITY

CHAPTER

13

The Liver

REGINE KAHL

Institute of Toxicology, University of Düsseldorf, Düsseldorf, Germany

MORPHOLOGY AND FUNCTION OF THE LIVER

Macroscopic Anatomy and Histology

The liver is the first organ that comes into contact with enterally absorbed nutrients and xenobiotics via the portal blood. Substances not extracted from the portal blood during the first pass or entering the body through other pathways, as well as metabolites, proteins, and lipoproteins, reach the liver by the hepatic artery, which supplies the liver with oxygenated blood (Fig. 1A). Liver blood flow, at a rate of approximately 1.5 liters/min, comes mainly through the portal vein (about 75%).

The terminal branches of portal vein and hepatic artery run parallel to one another. After confluence of the arterial and portal vessels, the blood flows into the liver capillaries, known as sinusoids, and passes the parenchymal cells (hepatocytes), which are arranged in plates one-cell thick (Fig. 1B). The exchange of substances takes place through the fenestrated endothelium of the sinusoids. The average diameter of 100 nm of the fenestrae allows molecules with a molecular mass of <250 kDa to cross into the interstitial (Disse) space between the endothelium, which does not have a basal membrane, and the hepatocytes (Fig. 1C). Each hepatocyte comes into contact with plasma from at least two sinusoids. Transport of substances takes place by various mechanisms (Table 1).

In addition to the endothelial cells there are three further types of sinusoidal cells (Fig. 1C). Kupffer cells are macrophages that phagocytize bacterial components and secrete inflammatory mediators. Pit cells are lymphocyte-type cells with antitumor cell activity. Ito cells store vitamin A and fat and form collagen that plays a role in the development of liver fibrosis and cirrhosis.

The venous blood is drained from the sinusoids into the terminal branches of the hepatic vein that flow into the inferior vena cava (Fig. 1A). The bile produced in the hepatocytes builds up in intercellular spaces, the bile capillaries. These unite in the bile ducts neighboring the terminal branches of the portal vein and liver artery (Fig. 1B). The topographical unit portal vein–hepatic artery–bile duct is known as the portal triad. The fine architecture of the liver described above corresponds to the microcirculatory concept of the liver acinus, which sees the hepatocytes as being located around the portal triad like a berry (Fig. 2A). The parenchyma is divided into three zones according to proximity to the portal triad. The zones differ in oxygen saturation and in the concentration of different enzymes. In zone 1, where high oxygen saturation exists, high activities of cytochrome oxidase and succinate dehydrogenase, two enzymes important for cell respiration, are found. The peripheral zone 3, where little oxygen is available, shows high concentrations of lactate dehydrogenase, indicating that glycolytic energy production takes place here at a high rate. Cytochromes P450, a class of enzymes responsible for metabolizing many xenobiotics, are predominantly located in zone 3.

The acinar model is opposed to the older concept of the hexagonal lobule, which was based on the microscopic appearance. The hexagonal lobule is seen to arrange itself around the central vein, the terminal branching of the hepatic vein. The periportal fields

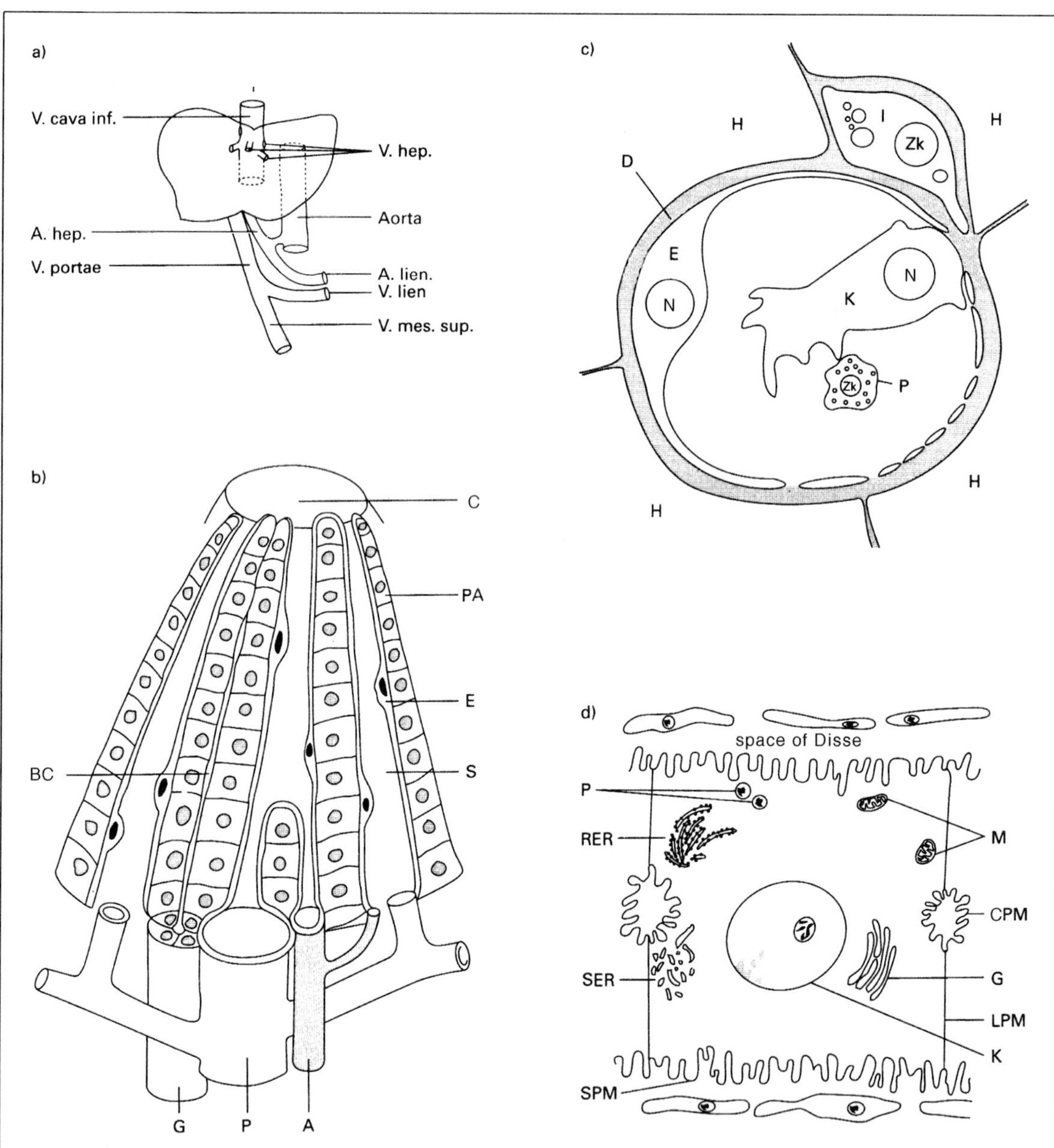

FIGURE 1 Morphology of the liver. (a) The liver's blood supply. Abbreviations: V cava inf., vena cava inferior; A. hep., arteria hepatica; V. portae. vena portae; V. mes. sup., vena mesenterica superior; V. lien., vena lienalis; A. lien., arteria lienalis; V. hep., vena hepatica. (b) Terminal branching of blood vessels and bile ducts. Abbreviations: C, central vein; PA, plate of parenchymal liver cells; E, endothel; S, sinusoid; A, branch of the liver artery; P, branch of the portal vein; G, bile duct; BC, bile capillary. (c) Sinusoidal cells. Abbreviations: D, space of Disse (interstitial space), shaded grey; E, endothelial cell with cell nucleus and offshoots, partly fenestrated; H, hepatocyte; I, Ito cell (fat-storage cell) with fat drops; K, Kupffer cell; P, pit cell with granules; N, nucleus. (d) Architecture of the hepatocyte. Abbreviations: G, Golgi apparatus; SER, smooth endoplasmic reticulum; N, nucleus; CPM, canalicular plasma membrane; LPM, lateral plasma membrane; M, mitochondria; P, peroxisomes; RER, rough endoplasmic reticulum with ribosomes; SPM, sinusoidal plasma membrane.

TABLE 1 Mechanisms of Substance Transport between Plasma and Hepatocytes

Mechanism	Examples
Passive diffusion through the lipid phase of the plasma membrane	Lipophilic drugs
Passive diffusion through water pores	Urea
Pinocytosis	Monosaccharides
Receptor-assisted endocytosis	Proteins
Carrier-assisted facilitated diffusion	Bile acids, fatty acids, amino acids, disaccharides
Carrier-assisted active transport	Na^+/K^+ exchange

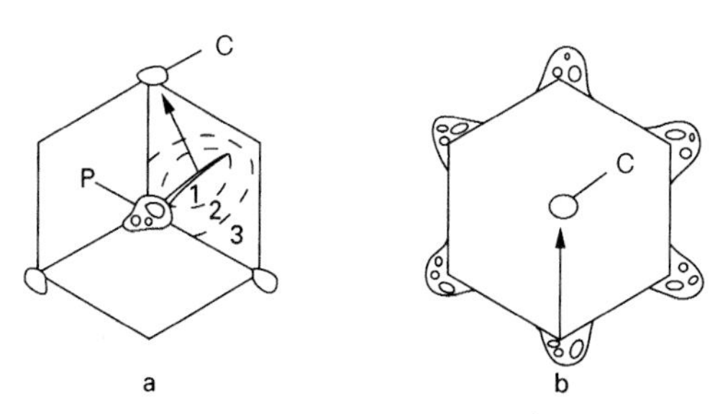

FIGURE 2 Acinar model and lobular model of the liver. (a) Acinar model. The parenchyma is seen to surround the branch of the portal vein in three zones with decreasing supply of oxygen. (b) Classical lobule model. The parenchyma is seen to surround the central vein concentrically; the perivenal area corresponds approximately to zone 3 of the acinus. Abbreviations: C, Central vein; P, portal trias comprising portal vein branch, branch of the liver artery, and bile duct; →, direction of the blood flow in the sinusoids.

with portal vein, hepatic artery, and bile duct can be seen in the corners of the hexagon (Fig. 2B). The lobular model still plays an important role in toxicology today. Liver damage is often not homogeneous, but zone-specific, and is then described in terms of the lobule model, for instance, as "centrilobular." Centrilobular necrosis is the most common form of toxic zonal liver damage. The reason for this is that many xenobiotics first have to be metabolically activated to the ultimate hepatotoxins. This is usually mediated by cytochrome P450 enzymes, which are abundant in the centrilobular region. Cytochrome P450 is subject to zonal induction; after the administration of the enzyme inducer phenobarbital, the newly formed cytochrome P450 is almost always centrilobular. In addition to being the site of metabolic activation, the center of the lobule is poorly supplied with glutathione, an important substance for the protection against liver toxins. The liver contains approximately 200 billion hepatocytes, which account for 80% of its total mass. In adults, these cells very rarely divide; one mitosis is to be found per 1000–10,000 cells. A human hepatocyte has a life expectancy of approximately 30 years. Approximately 30% of hepatocytes have two nuclei and a four-fold chromosome set. Seventy percent of the cell surface borders on the sinusoids or the space of Disse (sinusoidal plasma membrane), 15% lines the bile vessels (canalicular plasma membrane), and 15% forms the border to neighboring hepatocytes (lateral plasma membrane) (Fig. 1D). The cell organelles correspond to those of other cells—the rough endoplasmic reticulum and the Golgi apparatus, which synthesize proteins; the smooth endoplasmic reticulum, particularly prevalent centrilobularly, the location of cytochrome P450; the mitochondria, particularly numerous in periportal cells where aerobic energy production occurs and fatty acids are oxidized; and the peroxisomes in which fatty acids are oxidized concomitantly with the formation of H_2O_2. The biochemical functions of the liver are manifold (Table 2), but with the exception of urea synthesis are not organ-specific. Most of the reactions take place in other tissues as well, although far more slowly than in the liver. After a few days, an experimental animal whose liver has been removed shows all the typical symptoms of ammonia intoxication and dies in a hepatic coma.

Methods for the Detection of Liver Injury

Most clinical tests of liver function can be inferred from the biochemical functions of the liver (Table 2). A test battery is used for the screening routine. Along with testing the integrity of the sinusoidal plasma membrane (release of liver enzymes into the blood) and the biosynthetic capacity of the liver (decrease of albumin in the serum protein electrophoresis), the battery tests for biliary excretion (increase in the serum of bilirubin and liver enzymes to be eliminated via the bile). None of these parameters are even absolutely specific to the liver. Aspartate aminotransferase (AST) can increase after a heart attack, a fall in serum albumin can result from renal or enteral loss of protein, and an increase in bilirubin can be caused by a hemorrhage. If several of these liver function tests fall outside the normal range, a hepatic cause of these changes is indeed likely. In addition to biochemical

TABLE 2 Functions of the Liver and Clinical Tests of Liver Function

Function	Liver function test
Carbohydrate metabolism	
Regulation of blood glucose level	
Glycogen synthesis–glycogenolysis	
Gluconeogenesis–glycolysis	
Conversion of fructose and galactose	Galactose elimination capacity
Protein metabolism	Serum albumin[a]
Synthesis of liver-specific plasma proteins	Concentration of coagulation factors II, VII, IX, X in serum Serum cholinesterase
Conversion and breakdown of amino acids and proteins	
Synthesis of urea (ammonia detoxification)	Ammonia levels in blood
Lipid metabolism	
Formation of fatty acids from glucose	
Synthesis of triglycerides and lipoproteins	
Synthesis and esterification of cholesterol	Decrease of the quotient cholesterol ester/cholesterol in serum
Synthesis of bile acids	
Breakdown of triglycerides, breakdown of fatty acids	
Porphyrin metabolism	
Heme synthesis	Coproporphorin in urine
Glucuronidation of bilirubin	Direct (conjugated) serum bilirubin
Biotransformation of xenobiotics	Amidopyrine breath test
Transport of compounds between cells and extracellular space	Enzyme release through damaged plasma membrane: Aspartate aminotransferase (AST)[a] Alanine aminotransferase (ALT)[a] Lactate dehydrogenase (Isoenzyme LD5) Glutamate dehydrogenase (GlDH) Sorbitol dehydrogenase (SDH) Ornithine transferase (OCT)
Biliary excretion	Serum bilirubin[a] Serum concentration of enzymes excreted with bile: Alkaline phosphatase[a] γ-Glutamyltranspeptidase[a] Bile acid concentration in blood Bromosulfalein test

[a]Belong to the standard tests of liver function.

testing, a histological examination of material obtained by means of a liver biopsy contributes to the diagnosis. Among the clinical symptoms pointing to liver injury are enlargement of the liver, jaundice (icterus) with dark urine due to the increased levels of bilirubin in the blood, and discoloring of excreta due to reduced secretion of bilirubin in the bile. Itching can be attributed to the increased concentration of bile acids in the blood, ascites to hypertension in the portal vein, and hypoglycemia to a decrease in the production of glucose in the liver. Bleeding is due to a decrease in the production of hepatic clotting factors and loss of central nervous functions (hepatic encephalopathy) is due to an increase of ammonia contents in the blood. Methods of testing liver toxicity in animal experiments are listed in Table 3. The histological assessment is indispensable for demonstrating that a hepatotoxic effect is present; the biochemical techniques serve to identify the mechanisms that bring about this effect.

CLASSIFICATION OF HEPATOTOXIC SUBSTANCES

Over 600 drugs, plant extracts, toxins from insects and scorpions, and numerous industrial chemicals and natural substances can cause damage to the liver. It is common practice to distinguish between obligatory and facultative hepatotoxic substances. Few drugs are found in the group of obligatory liver toxins; the use of these drugs that intrinsically lead to liver damage is accepted only under particular circumstances, such as chemotherapy for cancer (methotrexate) or when the lesion only occurs above therapeutic dose levels (e.g., acetaminophen). Almost all of the hepatotoxic drugs belong to the group of facultative liver toxins. Treatment with these drugs leads to clinical symptoms in only a few cases (1:50 to 1:100,000 of patients treated). In other words, symptoms result from host idiosyncracy (i.e., the inability of single individuals to tolerate the compound). There can be two reasons for this.

1. Hypersensitivity phenomena. In such cases the disease is often seen only after the second exposure and is accompanied by clinical symptoms as eosinophilia, fever, arthralgia, and exanthema. Reduced latency of symptoms after repeated administration of the drug is a typical feature (Fig. 3). Acute cholestatic hepatitis may occur, for example, after the administration of sulfasalazine, a molecular combination of sulfapyridine and 5-aminosalicylic acid, in which the sulfonamide is probably the sensitizing component.

TABLE 3 Methods of Experimental Liver Toxicology

Detection of the hepatotoxic effect

In vivo
- Liver function tests (see Table 2)
- Lethality

Ex vivo
- Enlargement of the liver at autopsy
- Histological findings

Examination of the hepatotoxic mechanism

Functional tests in living animals
- Exhalation of ethane and pentane (lipid peroxidation)
- Increase of oxidized glutathione in the blood (oxidative damage)

Tissue examination *ex vivo*
- Qualitative composition of fats (malfunctioning of lipoprotein synthesis)
- Glucose-6-phosphatase (damage to the endoplasmic reticulum)
- Glutathione levels (oxidative damage)
- Pattern of cytochromes P450 (enzyme induction)
- Malondialdehyde and conjugated dienes (lipid peroxidation)
- Preneoplastic lesions (carcinogenic effect)
- Covalent binding of radioactively labeled substances to nucleic acids (carcinogenic effect)

Functional tests in the isolated liver and in isolated hepatocytes
- Oxygen consumption, NAD(P)H/NAD(P) quotient
- Synthesis reactions (leucine incorporation, secretion of lipoproteins)
- Metabolism of xenobiotics
- Cytotoxicity (enzyme leakage into the medium)
- Excretory functions of the isolated organ (bile flow, dye secretion)
- Mutagenicity and malignant transformation in cell culture

Electron microscopy
- Proliferation of endoplasmic reticulum
- Proliferation of peroxisomes
- Lysosomal damage

Studies with subcellular preparations
- DNA strand breaks in cell nuclei
- Inhibition of the respiratory chain in mitochondria
- H_2O_2 production in peroxisomes
- Lipid peroxidation in microsomes

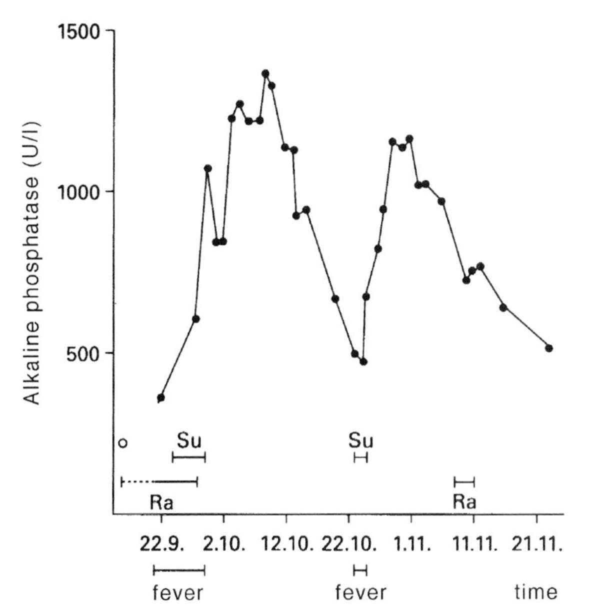

FIGURE 3 Case report of a cholestatic hepatitis in a patient receiving sulfasalazine and ranitidine. A 42-year-old patient was hospitalized for treatment of a severe rheumatic illness with a glucorticoid. Because at the time of her admission a slight increase to 240 U/liter in the level of alkaline phosphatase (AP) was observed, liver function tests were carried out more frequently. On September 22, the AP level was 381 U/liter; on Sept. 28 the level was 608 U/liter. The patient developed fever on September 23. At this point in time she had been administered ranitidine (Ra) to protect the stomach; as of September 24, the antiphlogistic therapy with the glucocorticoid was supplemented by sulfasalazine (Su). Because it was assumed that there was liver damage due to medication, therapy with ranitidine was discontinued on September 28 and sulfasalazine was discontinued on September 29. Nevertheless the AP level continued to rise, reaching a new peak of 1333 U/liter on October 9, after which it fell gradually. The control test on October 23 showed an AP level of 511 U/liter. A liver biopsy carried out on October 15 showed cholestatic acinocentral liver damage. Reexposure to sulfasalazine on October 23 and 24 led to a recurrent bout of fever and a rise of AP again to levels exceeding 1000 U/liter. On November 3 a level of 1025 U/liter was recorded. Reexposure to ranitidine for 3 days only marginally delayed the normalization of the AP levels. Therefore, it must be concluded that there was a causal link between the use of sulfasalazine and the cholestatic hepatitis; it cannot be excluded that ranitidine may also have contributed in part (personal observation).

2. Genetic polymorphism in the metabolism of compounds. Persons affected are either not able to detoxify the parent compound sufficiently or there is an accumulation of toxic metabolites. Such a mechanism has long been presumed to apply in the case of the tuberculostatic isoniazid (INH), but the relation between the metabolic defect and the incidence of liver injury has only been revealed recently. Therapy with isoniazid leads in 10–20% of patients to a moderate elevation of transaminases during the first weeks of therapy. A small percentage of these patients develop clinically manifest liver injury with icterus. The incidence depends on age; it is 0.3% in the age group under 35 years, 1.2% in the age group 35–50 years, and 2.3% in those over 50 years. In most cases there are no indications of an allergic reaction. Isoniazid is acetylated in an initial metabolic step (Fig. 4). This process is subject to a genetic polymorphism. In the white and black populations, approximately 40% are rapid acetylators. In the Japanese population, in contrast, over 90% are rapid acetylators. Acetylisoni-

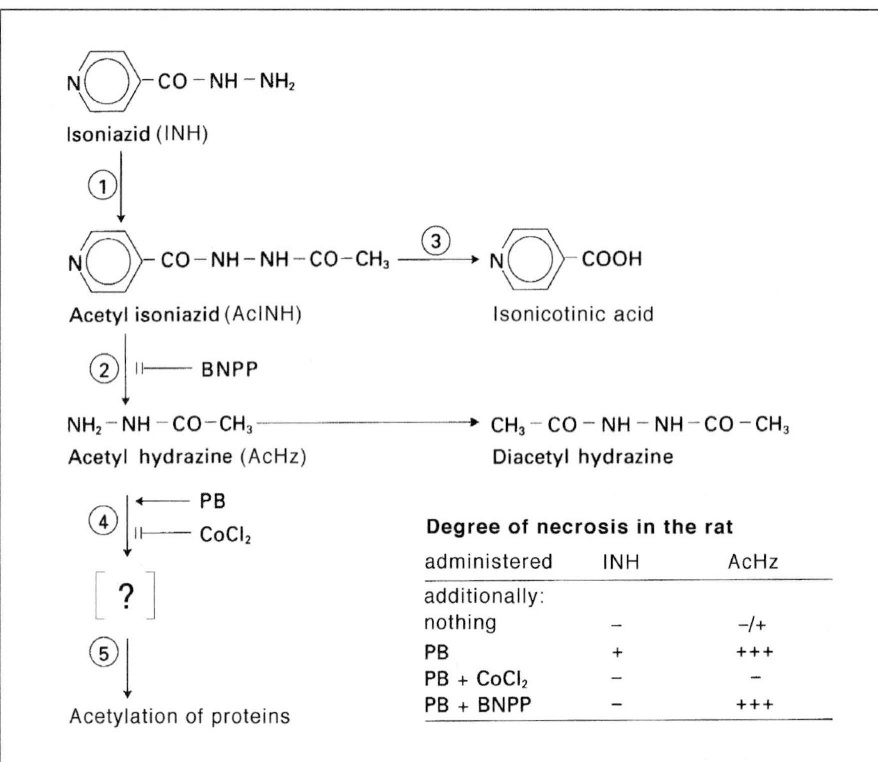

Degree of necrosis in the rat

administered additionally:	INH	AcHz
nothing	–	–/+
PB	+	+++
PB + $CoCl_2$	–	–
PB + BNPP	–	+++

FIGURE 4 Metabolic activation of isoniazid to a hepatotoxic metabolite. (1) Acetylation of isoniazid; (2) and (3) hydrolysis of acetyl isoniazid, which can be inhibited by bis-*p*-nitrophenyl phosphate (BNPP); (4) formation of a protein-acetylating hepatotoxic metabolite from acetylhydrazine by cytochrome P450, whose synthesis is induced in animal experiments by phenobarbital (PB) and can be inhibited by cobalt chloride ($CoCl_2$); (5) acetylation of acetylhydrazine to diacetylhydrazine. Both acetylating steps 1 and 5 are subject to genetic polymorphism. The first step in metabolic activation and the detoxification of the proximate reactive metabolite proceed more rapidly than in slow acetylators. Table: In the rat, isoniazid alone causes liver necrosis after induction of cytochrome P450. The concomitant administration of $CoCl_2$ prevents the induction. If the hydrolysis of acetylisoniazid is inhibited by bis-*p*-nitrophenyl phosphate (BNPP), the step depending on cytochrome P450 cannot take place, and the induction process has no consequences. If the immediate precursor of the ultimate toxic metabolite, acetylhydrazine, is administered instead of isoniazid, the effects of induction in promoting toxicity are considerably more marked—BNPP does not prevent them because hydrolysis was bypassed.

azid is split into monoacetylhydrazine and isonicotinic acid by cytochrome P450. Monoacetylhydrazine is converted into a reactive metabolite that becomes covalently bound to macromolecules. Therefore one could assume that rapid acetylators have a higher risk of developing liver damage because the toxic metabolite is formed more rapidly. However, this is far from having been confirmed by epidemiological studies. Indeed, recent results indicate that, on the contrary, slow acetylators are at higher risk of developing liver injury after treatment with isoniazid. The mechanism is envisaged as follows. Monoacetylhydrazine undergoes further acetylation and the ensuing product, diacetylhydrazine, is no longer able to form hepatotoxic metabolites. The rapid acetylators are thus more rapid to develop the precursor of the hepatotoxic metabolites, but they are also more rapid in rendering it inactive. Given this complex situation, it is hardly surprising that the effects of acetylator type on the incidence of isoniazid hepatitis are not uniform. It is also not surprising that the acetylator state is not closely linked to the incidence of subclinical functional disturbances of the liver.

Idiosyncrasy that is due to genetic polymorphism of a chemical's metabolism is, on closer analysis, not facultative because it is possible to predict whether the patient belongs to the high risk group or not. In

TABLE 4 Manifestations of Toxic Liver Damage

Symptoms	Examples of substances
Primarily cytotoxic manifestation	
Acute liver cell necrosis	Tetrachloromethane, acetaminophen, α-amanitin
Acute hepatocellular hepatitis	Isoniazid, halothane, α-methyldopa
Macrovacuolar steatosis	Methotrexate, ethanol, l-asparaginase
Microvesicular steatosis	Valproate, tetracycline, white phosphorus
Chronic-active hepatitis	α-Methyldopa, oxyphenisatin, nitrofurantoin
Phospholipoidosis	Perhexiline, amiodarone, 4,4-diethyl-aminoethoxyhexestrol
Fatty liver	Ethanol, 1,2-dimethylformamide
Cirrhosis	Ethanol, tetrachloromethane, arsenic
Primarily cholestatic symptoms	
Acute cholestatic or mixed hepatitis	Chlorpromazine, sulfonamides, methylene dianiline
Acute cholestasis	Estrogens, anabolic steroids
Cholangitis and cholangiolitis	Chlorpromazine, carbamazepine, ajmalin
Chronic cholestasis	Chlorpromazine, ajmalin, arsenic
Sclerosizing cholangitis	Floxuridine (administered regionally)
Attack to vascular system	
Noncirrhotic portal hypertension	Vinyl chloride, vitamin A, arsenic
Peliosis hepatis	Anabolic steroids, vinyl chloride
Veno-occlusive disease	Pyrrolizidine alkaloids, azathioprine
Liver vein thrombosis	Hormonal contraceptives, dacarbazine
Liver tumors	
Liver adenoma	Hormonal contraceptives, anabolic steroids
Hepatocellular carcinoma	Arsenic, aflatoxin B_1, thorium dioxide
Cholangiocarcinoma	Thorium dioxide
Hemangiosarcoma	Vinyl chloride, copper sulfate

such cases a dose dependency also has to be reckoned with. Animal models can be designed in which deviating metabolic rates are mimicked in the experimental animal by means of enzyme induction or enzyme inhibition (Fig. 4). Allergy-related idiosyncrasies can also be linked to metabolic deficiencies. In halothane hepatitis, the occurrence of subclinical biochemical changes points to an additional disposition due to the increased production of toxic metabolites or to their insufficient detoxification.

MANIFESTATIONS OF LIVER INJURY

The morphological picture of toxic liver injury is not such that it is possible to trace the damage back to a specific agent or to categorically rule out that the damage may have been of nontoxic origin. In histological classification, three actions of the toxin should be distinguished: the cytotoxic effect on the hepatocytes, the reduced production and secretion of bile, and, less frequently, an attack on the vascular system (Table 4).

Acute Cytotoxic Liver Injury

Necrosis

Toxic damage to the liver parenchymal cells presents histologically as degenerative alterations of the cell (necrosis) or as abnormal storage, usually of fat (steatosis), often accompanying one another (e.g., tetrachloromethane); however, many chemicals lead to necrosis without steatosis (e.g., acetaminophen) or to steatosis without necrosis (e.g., tetracycline). Cell death in liver injury may be of two types; it can be either programmed cell death (apoptosis), an energy-dependent genetically encoded self-destruction of the cell characterized by early DNA fragmentation, or necrosis, a toxic lysis of the cell. The residual apoptotic bodies after the process of programmed cell death are taken up by other cells via phagocytosis. Therefore, apoptosis is probably often overlooked or even undetectable by conventional microscopy. The damage, according to its localization in the liver lobule, is further subdivided as diffuse, focal, or zonal. The spectrum of symptoms stretches from clinically silent elevations of transaminases to outright liver failure with icterus, severe clotting disturbances, and liver coma. Increases in serum transaminases of at least factor 2, but often of 10- to 100-fold in the absence of or with only a small increase in alkaline phosphatase, point to cytotoxic damage. The border between acute and chronic damage cannot be clearly delineated; often it is claimed to be 3 months. With the help of three typical examples, the principal mechanisms of toxic cell necrosis will be described.

Lipid Peroxidation

Tetrachloromethane (carbon tetrachloride, CCl_4) is the prototype of a liver toxin for which lipid peroxidation is seen as a primary mechanism in causing the injury. Therefore, the mechanism of toxicity of CCl_4 is used as a well-investigated example to describe the principles of xenobiotic-induced lipid peroxidation. CCl_4 initiates lipid peroxidation in experimental animals within a few minutes of being administered. The effect is held to be a primary toxic lesion because lipid peroxidation precedes other morphological and functional changes following CCl_4 administration. CCl_4 is found in use as a commercial solvent for cleaning machines. In the past it was available as a stain-removing agent in dry cleaning and for household use. It led to intoxications in persons cleaning large upholstered furniture and carpet surfaces without opening the windows. In 1985, statistics from Great Britain record 19 CCl_4 intoxications, 6 of which involved children, resulting from private use. In the first half of the 1900s, the chemical was also used as a medicinal drug, first as a general anaesthetic and later as a vermicide; even its use as a hair shampoo led to intoxications.

Liver injury becomes apparent after a latency period of 1–3 days. The liver is enlarged and painful upon pressure, the urine is dark in color, and there are icterus, a massive elevation of transaminases, and coagulation disturbances. The effects on the central nervous system of the solvent manifest themselves particularly if the poison has been inhaled. The patients complain of headaches, become somnolent, and finally lose consciousness. Gastrointestinal signs of intoxication with nausea, vomiting, abdominal pain, and diarrhea can occur in the early phase after oral or transdermal uptake. Apart from the liver, the kidney is usually also affected by the cytotoxic effect of CCl_4, more frequently after inhalation than after oral ingestion. Renal failure due to damage to the proximal tubules can dominate the clinical symptoms and lead to death in uremic coma. An evaluation of 128 cases of intoxication between 1953 and 1965 showed a renal contribution in 94% of the patients. The mortality rate was 17%; 60% of the deaths were attributed to liver failure. No therapy for the CCl_4-induced liver damage has been established; in case of renal failure, hemodialysis or peritoneal dialysis is carried out and can save the patient's life. Occasionally, cardiac symptoms can predominate; much like other halogen-substituted compounds, CCl_4 can lead to a sensitization of the myocardium for noradrenaline (norepinephrine) and adrenaline (epinephrine) and can therefore provoke arrhythmia.

CCl_4 belongs to the liver toxins that are biologically active only after having been metabolized (Fig. 5). CCl_4 is metabolically activated by cytochrome P450 to the primary toxic metabolite, the trichloromethyl radical, $CCl_3\cdot$. By contrast to most reactions mediated by cytochrome P450, $CCl_3\cdot$ radical formation does not proceed via monooxygenation but by reduction. The reaction is therefore more rapid under nitrogen than in the presence of oxygen. Early indications of cytochrome P450 dependency in the formation of $CCl_3\cdot$ were shown when it was found that CCl_4 intoxication in experimental animals was intensified by pretreatment with the enzyme inducer phenobarbital. Pretreatment with synthesis inhibitors (cobaltous salts) or with inhibitors of the enzymatic activity (dibenamine) of cytochrome P450 lessened the extent of the intoxication. Because cytochrome P450 is present at a higher concentration in the perivenous areas of the liver lobule than in the periportal areas, centrilobular injury is prevalent. In experiments in which the individual components of the cytochrome P450 enzyme system (cytochrome P450, NADPH–cytochrome P450 reductase, and a phospholipid) were mixed in a test tube to form a reconstituted system, it could be seen that cytochrome P450 IIB1, inducible by phenobarbital, and cytochrome P450 IIE1, inducible by ethanol, can catalyze the bioactivation. This is a possible explanation for the potentiation of the toxicity by ethanol. In experimental animals, the effects of CCl_4 are increased by acute ethanol administration, and there are indications that this holds true also for humans.

CCl_3 sets off a lipid peroxidation in the endoplasmic reticulum by abstracting a hydrogen atom from unsaturated fatty acids from a methylene bridge beside a double bond (H abstraction). In this process, the trichloromethyl radical $CCl_3\cdot$ is reduced to chloroform, a major metabolite of CCl_4 that retains its hepatotoxic properties. In the carbon-centered lipid radicals produced by H abstraction, resonance leads to the formation of conjugated double bonds. The dienes that are thus produced have a characteristic absorption of 233 nm, which is used to test for lipid peroxidation in tissue.

In the presence of oxygen, the peroxyl radical $CCl_3OO\cdot$ is formed. This also contributes to the H abstraction from the unsaturated fatty acids, and, in fact, does this more effectively, than $CCl_3\cdot$. Lipid peroxyl radicals are then formed from the carbon-centered fatty acid radicals by the addition of oxygen. The lipid peroxyl radicals start a new radical chain reaction by attacking intact chains of fatty acids, which are converted into hydroperoxides in this process. Radical chain-breaking antioxidants, such as vitamin E, can curb this process and therefore act preventively in animals; a therapeutic effect for antioxidants in humans after the onset of intoxication has

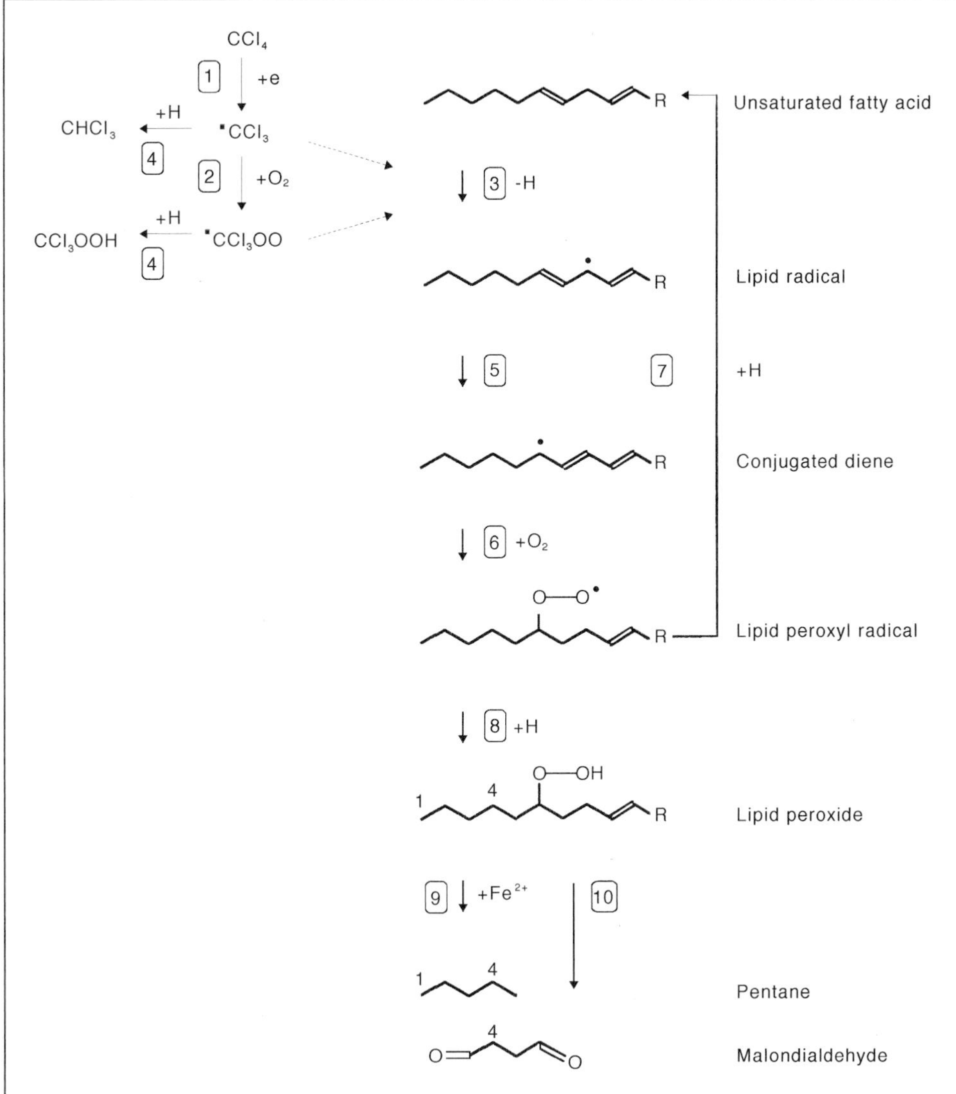

FIGURE 5 Metabolic activation and hepatotoxic mechanisms of tetrachloromethane. (1) Cytochrome P450-dependent reduction to the trichloromethyl radical, $CCl_3\cdot$. (2) Formation of the trichloromethylperoxyl radical, $CCl_3OO\cdot$, by reaction with molecular oxygen. (3) Both can induce a H abstraction from unsaturated fatty acids. (4). In this process, they become saturated by the formation of chloroform or trichloromethyl hydroperoxide. (5) Conversion of the carbon-centered lipid radical to a conjugated diene. (6) Formation of lipid peroxyl radicals by reaction with molecular oxygen. (7) Induction of a radical chain reaction by the lipid peroxyl radical's attack on an as-yet-intact unsaturated fatty acid. (8) In this process the lipid peroxyl radical saturates to lipid hydroperoxide. (9) In a further process with several stages not described in detail, pentane or ethane are formed from the lipid hydroperoxides in the presence of Fe^{2+}. (10) After the formation of an endoperoxide and intramolecular rearrangement, malondialdehyde is formed from lipid hydroperoxides in the presence of Fe^{2+}. Conjugated dienes, lipid hydroperoxides, pentane, ethane, and malondialdehyde can be measured to monitor lipid peroxidation.

not, however, been established. Hydroperoxides are unstable end products of lipid peroxidation. In the presence of iron ions in the biological material, they produce the volatile alkanes ethane and pentane. These are exhaled and can be used as parameters that lipid peroxidation has taken place. A further mechanism of hydroperoxide breakdown yields malondialdehyde. The detection of malondialdehyde after reaction with thiobarbituric acid is the most widely used method of detecting lipid peroxidation. However, the reaction does not rule out other sources of malondialdehyde (deoxyribose). Moreover, in its simplified spectrophotometric form without high-pressure liquid chromatography, the method is not specific for malondialdehyde. Therefore, the reaction product is cautiously named "thiobarbituric acid-reactive substances" (TBARS) instead of "malondialdehyde" by most authors.

Parallel to the lipid peroxidation, other damaging processes take place in the endoplasmic reticulum.

1. The destruction of cytochrome P450; the production of the $CCl_3\cdot$ radicals can be seen as a suicide reaction of the enzyme.
2. Loss of glucose-6-phosphatase activity, which serves as a marker enzyme for the endoplasmic reticulum.
3. Inhibition of protein synthesis, which is shown by electron microscopy as decrease of the ribosome set in the rough endoplasmic reticulum.
4. Damage to the Ca^{2+} pump that mediates the sequestering of Ca^{2+} ions into the endoplasmic reticulum. This leads to an increase in the free cytosolic concentration of Ca^{2+}.

The endoplasmic reticulum is the location of the primary toxic lesion due to CCl_4. The damage later spreads to other compartments of the liver cell. Malfunctioning occurs in the mitochondria with subsequent loss of intracellular ATP content; damage to the plasma membrane leading to the excretion of enzymes and K^+ and the accumulation of triglycerides in the cell occur. The disturbed intracellular distribution of Ca^{2+} plays a major role in the propagation of the damage beyond the endoplasmic reticulum to other cell organelles, an increase in free Ca^{2+} leading to the activation of numerous catabolic enzymes. The accumulation of triglycerides is a characteristic histological finding. It does not result from increased triglyceride synthesis or from a malfunctioning in the breakdown of fatty acids, as in the case of ethanol, but it is instead linked to decreased secretion of very-low-density lipoproteins (VLDL). This is due to a dysfunctioning of the synthesis of the VLDL apolipoprotein. Furthermore, it is thought that the coupling of fat and protein components is disrupted.

The biochemical alterations described above could be consequences of the lipid peroxidation. However, they also could have come about in a different way. The reactive metabolite does not only lead to H abstraction from fatty acids; it also irreversibly becomes bound to lipids and proteins (and to a lesser extent also to DNA). Some signs of damage, such as loss of activity in cytochrome P450 and the inhibition of protein synthesis, cannot be antagonized by antioxidants. There is an ongoing debate whether the lipid peroxidation or the haloalkylation plays the greater role in the hepatotoxicity of CCl_4.

Although hepatocytes are the primary target of CCl_4, nonparenchymal liver cells contribute to the course of the liver injury. Destruction of Kupffer cells by gadolinium chloride greatly attenuates the symptoms in CCl_4-intoxicated animals, indicating that inflammatory mediators released from these macrophages play a role in CCl_4-induced hepatocyte necrosis.

Several other halogenated hydrocarbons lead to hepatotoxic intoxication symptoms equally severe as those of CCl_4. Among these are monochloromethane (methyl chloride), chloroform, bromotrichloromethane, 1,2-dichloroethane, 1,2-dibromoethane, 1,1,2-trichloroethane, 1,1,2,2-tetrachloroethane, and pentachloroethane. Other halogenated solvents are considered to be only moderately hepatotoxic (trichloroethylene, tetra-(per)chloroethylene) or hardly hepatotoxic at all (1,1,1-trichloroethane, dichloromethane) compared to these compounds. Solvents from other chemical classes can also cause liver damage, including 2-nitropropane, dimethyl formamide, ethylene glycol, diethylene glycol, styrol, and toluol. The question of whether exposure to low levels of solvent concentrations causes liver injury is very important in industrial medicine. A causal connection can only be ascertained in careful case control studies. Here confounding factors, such as alcohol consumption and simultaneous exposure to other chemicals in the workplace, must be taken into account.

Covalent Binding to Cellular Macromolecules

Acetaminophen is an example of a hepatotoxic agent acting both by covalent binding of a reactive metabolite to cellular macromolecules and by oxidative stress leading to lipid peroxidation. It is also claimed that protein arylation is the primary lesion, while lipid peroxidation is the result rather than the cause of the necrosis. However, covalent binding may not be sufficient to explain the liver injury because antioxidants can prevent cell death. The protein-arylating metabolite is *N*-acetyl benzoquinonimine (NABQI) (Fig. 6). In the case of acetaminophen intoxication, as with CCl_4 intoxication, the necrosis is centrilobular. This is due to the dependency on cytochrome P450 for bioactivation to NABQI. Enzyme inducers increase toxicity, while inhibitors of cytochrome P450 decrease toxicity in animal experiments. Pretreatment with drugs such as phenytoin, phenobarbital, and carbamazapine (anticonvulsives) can lead to a potentiation of the toxic symptoms because they act as enzyme inducers. While various cyto-

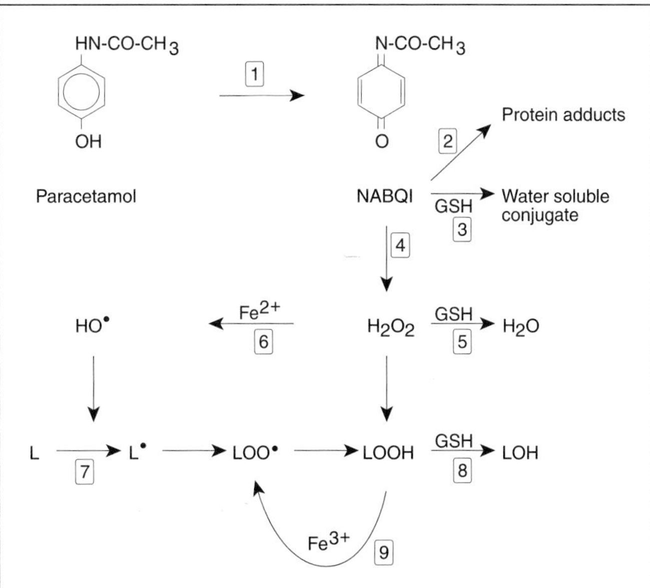

FIGURE 6 Metabolic activation and hepatotoxic mechanisms of acetaminophen. (1) Formation of *N*-acetylbenzoquinonimine (NABQI) by cytochrome P450; (2) covalent binding to proteins; (3) detoxification by production of a water-soluble conjugate with glutathione (GSH), leading to GSH consumption; (4) formation of H_2O_2 via a redox cycle of NABQI; (5) requirement of GSH for the detoxification of H_2O_2 (6) formation of hydroxyl radicals from nondetoxified H_2O_2; (7) induction of lipid peroxidation; (8) requirement of GSH for the detoxification of lipid peroxides (LOOH); (9) formation of lipid peroxide radicals (LOO$^{\cdot}$) from nondetoxified lipid peroxides. Lipid peroxide radicals cause a radical chain reaction forming carbon-centered lipid radicals (L$^{\cdot}$) due to the H abstraction from unsaturated fatty acids (L).

chromes P450 contribute to NABQI formation, cytochrome P450 IIE1 plays a prominent role. In a CYPIIE1 knockout mouse, in which the CYPIIE1 gene is not expressed due to homologous recombination in embryonic stem cells, acetaminophen is considerably less hepatotoxic than in the wild-type mouse. Cytochrome P450 IIE1 can be induced by ethanol, which explains the increased danger of liver failure in alcoholics. However, this effect may be counteracted during acute alcohol intake, where there is competition of ethanol and acetaminophen at cytochrome P450 IIE1.

NABQI forms a water-soluble glutathione conjugate; massive binding to cell proteins arises only when this detoxifying process has been exhausted. Sensitivity to acetaminophen is increased by preceding glutathione depletion in animal experiments. The degree of necrosis correlates closely with covalent binding. Many arylated proteins have been detected in mouse liver mitochondria, nuclei, plasma membrane, cytosol, and microsomes. However, the critical target molecules of the reactive metabolite have not yet been ascertained. In animal experiments, a decrease in protein synthesis can be observed within the first 3 h, followed by a loss of activity in microsomal enzymes. The fully developed intoxication is similar to CCl_4 intoxication with respect to the characteristic massive disturbance of Ca^{2+} distribution in the hepatocytes. DNA fragmentation is observed and indicates the occurrence of apoptosis in advance of massive necrosis of hepatocytes.

Lipid peroxidation was shown, by alkane exhalation and malondialdehyde formation, to have taken place in experimental animals at the latest after 3–4 h. The mechanism causing the lipid peroxidation is associated with the glutathione depletion; glutathione is essential for detoxification of hydrogen peroxide and lipid hydroperoxide (Fig. 6). If hydrogen peroxide can no longer be sufficiently inactivated to water, hydroxyl radicals are formed, and can induce lipid peroxidation; insufficiently detoxified lipid hydroperoxides can be converted under iron catalysis to lipid peroxyl radicals and then return into the radical chain

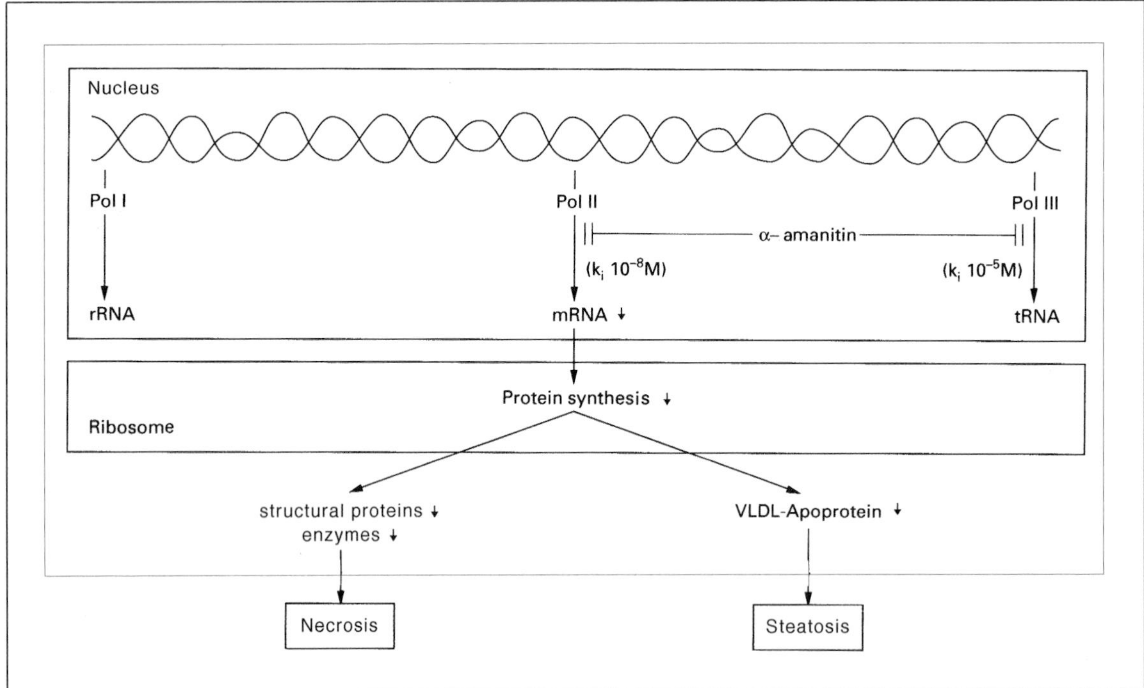

FIGURE 7 Hepatotoxic mechanism of α-amanitin. α-Amanitin inhibits RNA polymerase II, which is responsible for the production of the mRNA resulting in an inhibition of protein synthesis; a deficiency of specific enzyme proteins and structural proteins leads to liver necrosis; the lack of VLDL apoproteins causes a disturbance in the secretion of lipoproteins, leading to steatosis. If there is a higher concentration of α-amanitin, RNA polymerase III, responsible for production of the tRNA as well as the 5S ribosomal RNA, is also inhibited.

reaction. The depletion of the cellular reserves of glutathione for detoxification of the hepatotoxic metabolite can thus put the cell under "oxidative stress." As with CCl_4 hepatotoxicity, activation of Kupffer cells occurs. Immigration of phagocytic cells from the circulation is observed. Necrotic hepatocytes release a neutrophil chemoattractant. Inflammatory mediators and reactive oxygen species from these phagocytes may contribute to the development of the liver injury.

The clinical course of acetaminophen intoxication also shows similarities to CCl_4 intoxication. Liver damage usually manifests only after a latency period, which can be accompanied by nausea and vomiting. The transaminases increase after 12–24 h and are maximal after not more than 3 or more days. Liver enlargement and icterus usually manifest after 2–4 days. Acute kidney failure may complicate the clinical situation in the case of acetaminophen intoxication; however, this occurs less frequently than in CCl_4 intoxication, only in approximately 10% of all cases.

Acetaminophen at a therapeutic dosage of 0.5–3 g per day is a safe analgesic. At doses of 4–10 g per day, some cases of intoxication have been observed in predisposed persons (e.g., with glutathione deficiency), due to chronic alcohol abuse or malnutrition. In healthy adults, the toxic dose is 10–15 g. On a mg/kg basis, the hepatotoxic dose is similar or only slightly higher for children. It is important to note that intoxication in children may occur due to multiple miscalculated overdoses given by parents, especially if preparations for adults are administered instead of adapted pediatric preparations. The decisive role of glutathione status in acetaminophen intoxication has led the way to an effective therapy. The administering of *N*-acetylcysteine provides cysteine for the *de novo* synthesis of glutathione.

Inhibition of Protein Synthesis

Mushroom intoxication due to the ingestion of the green or white *Amanita* species causes severe liver necrosis due to the inhibition of protein synthesis. Two types of poison are present in the *Amanita* species, amatoxins and phallotoxins, and both are hepatotoxic. However, the amatoxins are 10 to 20 times more potent and are assumed to play a critical role in the induction of liver injury. The injury is histologically characterized by changes in the nucleus, glycogen loss, steatosis, and centrilobular necrosis. The prototype of the amatoxins is α-amanitin. Amatoxins inhibit protein synthesis. As outlined in the preceding discussion, this is also the case with other hepatotoxins. However, for most of them the inhibition of protein synthesis is assumed to be a secondary effect. In contrast, the attack of α-amanitin is primary and specific (Fig. 7). This compound is a potent inhibitor of RNA polymerase II with a K_i of about 10^{-8} M. The toxin forms a 1:1 complex with an enzyme subunit. RNA polymerase II is required for the synthesis of mRNA. At concentrations of about 10^{-5} M, RNA polymerase III (the enzyme mediating the synthesis of tRNA) is also inhibited. As a consequence of the inhibition of mRNA synthesis, inhibition of protein synthesis occurs. According to differences in the half-lives of the mRNA species, inhibition manifests with different time courses but will finally lead to the loss of enzymes, structural proteins, and apoproteins for lipoprotein synthesis, resulting in fat accumulation and necrosis.

In a mouse model, it has been shown that tumor necrosis factor α (TNF-α), a cytokine secreted by inflammatory cells including Kupffer cells, is required for α-amanitin toxicity at least under conditions of incomplete transcriptional block. A TNF receptor-1 knockout mouse lacking expression of the 55-kDa TNF-α receptor gene was not susceptible to a dose of α-amanitin, which caused marked enzyme release in the wild-type mouse. The type of cell death in these experiments was apoptosis rather than necrosis, as indicated by the occurrence of DNA fragmentation in advance of membrane leakage.

As little as 30 g of the fresh mushroom can be lethal. After the ingestion of the mushroom, a latency period between 6 and 48 h is observed, after which a gastrointestinal stage ensues that can lead to fatalities with cholera-like symptoms. After 1 to 4 days the liver injury is obvious. Massive coagulation disturbances and hepatic encephalopathy characterize the final stage of the intoxication. Toxicity occurs in all tissues, including the kidney and the pancreas, however, its consequences are most dramatic in the liver because of the high rate of hepatic protein synthesis and also because α-amanitin is subject to enterohepatic circulation and thus repeatedly enters the liver.

Allergic Drug-Induced Hepatitis with Liver Cell Necrosis

A condition generally recognized histologically and clinically as being cytotoxic with additional allergic symptoms can be produced by a range of drugs. One example is halothane hepatitis. In patients who received a general anaesthesia with halothane (2-bromo-2-chloro-1,1,1-trifluoroethane), an often severe liver injury with a massive elevation of serum transaminases and serum bilirubin develops with an incidence of 1:10,000 to 1:100,000. A hepatitis of this type can also occur among medical personnel working in the operating theatre. Biopsy or autopsy shows a centrilobular, sometimes also a diffuse, necrosis accompanied by inflammatory cell infiltrations in the portal regions and in the liver lobule. The mortality rate is up to 70%. The following observations show that halothane hepatitis results from a sensitization.

1. The illness occurs less frequently after first exposure than after repeated exposure. In a study, 24 of 26 patients had received previous doses of halothane, usually just days or weeks beforehand.
2. The latency period between the anaesthesia and the appearance of the hepatitis decreases after repeated exposure. One study estimates the mean latency period after the first exposure to be 11 days, decreasing to 4 days after the fourth exposure.
3. Symptoms of hypersensitivity, such as fever, shivering, leukocytosis, eosinophilia, arthralgia, and exanthema, are almost always present.
4. In a number of patients, antibodies found in the serum reacted specifically with halothane-induced neoantigens from the endoplasmic reticulum and the cell membranes of hepatocytes of rabbits that had been treated with halothane.
5. The severity of injury to the liver and the rate of mortality increase with the frequency of exposure. One study showed the lethality rate to be 35% after the first exposure and 52% after the fourth exposure.

According to the criteria, halothane is apparently a facultative liver toxin. However, if minimal disturbances in liver function are looked for, up to 20% of exposed people show irregularities. Furthermore, a halothane-induced necrosis can be produced in animal experiments. Therefore, halothane must be classified as an obligatory liver toxin. It is not certain, but can be assumed, that there is a mechanistic link between the liver injury seen in the animal experiment, the mild functional disturbances of the liver recorded in 20% of those exposed to halothane, and the extremely rare dramatic form of hepatitis. Similar to CCl_4, halothane is metabolized by reduction to a radical metabolite, the trifluorochloroethyl radical, that covalently binds to proteins and can also cause lipid peroxidation. Furthermore, an oxidative metabolism is described, in the course of which the trifluoroacetyl group binds covalently to microsomal proteins, such as cytochrome P450, and to the plasma membrane. The trifluoroacetyl group is thought to develop antigen properties while binding to proteins. In patients, serum antibodies appear against microsomal polypeptide neoantigens, including protein disulfide isomerase, microsomal carboxylesterase, and calreticulin. A further antibody from the patients' serum binds to the surface of rabbit hepatocytes. The fact that most exposed persons do not respond with a hypersensitivity reaction may be due to tolerance induced by self-peptides with properties similar to the trifluoroacetyl adducts.

Steatosis

The acute abnormal fat storage in liver cells—steatosis—occurs in two forms. In the macrovesicular form, a large drop of fat encompasses almost the entire liver cell, pressing the nucleus to the edge of the cell. This form of steatosis usually stems from a secretion disturbance of the lipoproteins, which is the consequence of an inhibition of apolipoprotein synthesis. It occurs in connection with different cytotoxic mechanisms and is therefore usually accompanied by necrosis. If not accompanied by necrosis, the condition is relatively harmless. In microvesicular steatosis, numerous fine drops of fat are found in the cell; necrosis may be present, but even without necrosis, the condition can be very serious, as described in the following example. In therapy with the anticonvulsant valproate, many patients show an increase in transaminases without any clinical symptoms. However, critical injury to the liver may also develop. Between 1978 and 1984, 37 deaths due to liver failure were reported in the United States in patients treated with valproate. Of these patients, 27 were children 0–10 years old. The illness arises 1–4 months after the commencement of treatment and resembles Reye syndrome, which occasionally develops in the aftermath of a viral infection. After an initial phase with nausea, apathy, and deteriorating convulsion control, an icterus sets in, sometimes with ascites. Clotting disturbances and hypoglycemia make the disturbance of the liver function obvious, although the elevation of transaminases is usually low. Due to an increasing ammonia concentration in the blood, hepatic encephalopathy develops and death occurs in liver coma. There are no signs of allergy or infection. Histological examination often reveals signs of necrosis and/or cholestasis along with the microvesicular steatosis.

Valproate also leads to a microvesicular steatosis in animal experiments. Analysis of valproate metabolism gave some hints as to the mechanisms of steatosis and necrosis.

1. Valproate is oxidized in the mitochondria by β-oxidation to its anticonvulsive metabolite 2-*n*-propyl-2-pentenoate and thereby interferes with the oxidation of fatty acids and mitochondrial oxygen uptake.

2. In the peroxisomes β-oxidation also takes place. In the peroxisomes, fatty acids are oxidized by an enzyme system, which at the same time reduces molecular oxygen to hydrogen peroxide. Under treatment with valproate in the animal experiment, a proliferation of peroxisome arises with increased H_2O_2 production; an "oxidative stress" can result.

3. Due to β-1-oxidation valproate produces 2-*n*-propyl-4-pentenoate in small amounts. Cytochrome P450 activates this metabolite in the endoplasmic reticulum to several toxic metabolites that are finally responsible for the necrosis that often accompanies the steatosis, as well as for the clinically silent increase in transaminases in many patients. In the animal experiment, the induction of cytochrome P450 by phenobarbital exacerbates the symptoms. In humans, previous enzyme induction possibly also plays a role. Most cases occurred in combination with other enzyme-inducing anticonvulsives. Valproate itself induces cytochrome P450 IIB1 and may thus contribute to its own hepatotoxicity.

Also after the intake of tetracyclines, usually in pregnant women but sometimes also in other patients, death due to microvesicular steatosis has occasionally been observed. This can be imitated in animal experiments and traced to an inhibition of the β-oxidation of fatty acids. The clinical symptoms are similar to those of valproate steatosis. Factors leading to a predisposition are, apart from pregnancy, high dosage of valproate, intravenous administration, and renal failure. The more modern tetracyclines, minocycline and doxycycline, are rarely, if ever, associated with these symptoms. An explanation could be that the development of steatosis is dependent on the absolute amount administered—this has been proven not only in animal experiments but also in a 1960 study carried out on pregnant women (!)—and doxycycline and minocycline are applied in considerably smaller doses than the older tetracyclines.

Phospholipoidosis is a particular form of fat storage in the liver cells. It arises due to the inhibition of the lysosomal phospholipases with the consequential accumulation of phospholipids. Clinical symptoms are usually mild.

Chronic Cytotoxic Liver Injury

Acute cytotoxic liver injury that does not develop into hepatic coma usually has a good prognosis; a *restitutio ad integrum,* a complete recovery from morphological and functional disturbances, can be expected. In the case of repeated or prolonged exposure, however, chronic morphological alterations can take place. This can be during drug therapy if the liver injury has not been diagnosed and the drug is further administered or if the therapy is resumed before complete recovery from the liver injury. In the work place, a prolonged exposure to small quantities of hepatotoxic substances can cause damage to the liver. The consequences are a subacute or chronic active hepatitis or liver cirrhosis. The abuse of alcohol equally causes permanent damage to the liver.

Chronic Active Hepatitis

A compound that can cause a subacute or chronic hepatitis and sometimes also cirrhosis is the antihypertensive α-methyldopa. This drug—similar to halothane and valproate—leads in a number of patients to clinically silent elevation of transaminases that are linked to a reactive metabolite. A subacute or chronic hepatitis occurs with a frequency of <1:1000 after a long period of treatment. In the chronic active form, the biopsy shows a "piecemeal" necrosis with periportal cell destruction, periportal fibrosis, and lymphocyte infiltrations along with lobular necrosis. Immunological processes play a part in chronic active α-methyldopa hepatitis. In approximately half of patients, antinuclear antibodies are found, as in systemic lupus erythemathosus, and in about a third there are antibodies against smooth muscle. Half of the patients had a positive Coombs test; some developed hemolysis. α-Methyldopa is thought to inhibit the function of T-suppressor cells and therefore may stimulate uncontrolled production of autoantibodies in the B cells.

Fatty Liver and Liver Cirrhosis

Ethanol is the quantitatively most important cause of chronic toxic liver injury. The frequency of fatty degeneration and cirrhosis of the liver correlates to the daily alcohol intake and the length of the period of alcohol abuse. An intake of 40–60 g per day increases the risk of cirrhosis to six times the risk incurred by an intake of 20 g per day. A daily intake of 210 g (equivalent to a bottle of spirits; see Table 5) over 25 years led to cirrhosis in 50% of cases. Women are more sensitive; a study showed the daily alcohol intake of female cirrhosis patients to average at 52 g, whereas male patients consumed on average 132 g. The reason for this is the smaller volume of distribution in women. A further reason could be that the alcohol dehydrogenase in the stomach, which controls the bioavailability of ethanol, is less active in women. With regard to prevention, one should proceed on the assumption that women who have an alcohol intake in excess of 20 g per day over years and men whose intake exceeds 50 g per day over years run the risk of alcoholic liver cirrhosis.

TABLE 5 Ethanol Content of Alcoholic Drinks

	Vol % (g/liter)	Amount of alcohol per glass
Beer	4–5	1.3–1.6 g/0.4 liter
Wine	10–12	1.6–2.0 g/0.2 liter
Spirits	35–40	Approx 6 g/2 cl

The steatosis, which is in general macrovesicular, usually causes no symptoms and is discovered by chance due to enlargement of the liver or an increase in γ-glutamyltranspeptidase and perhaps aspartate aminotransferase in the serum. The increase in γ-glutamyltranspeptidase is thought not to be the result of cholestasis in this instance but to be due to microsomal enzyme induction. Apart from the steatosis, an injury to the microtubular apparatus in the hepatocytes and a disturbance of protein secretion are thought to be responsible for the enlargement of the liver cells. If the patient abstains from alcohol, the fatty liver reverses within 2–6 weeks. If the patient continues to drink, progressive liver damage may develop. Alcoholic hepatitis with liver cell necrosis and pericellular fibrosis can ensue and is in some cases a precursor to cirrhosis. In other cases, cirrhosis develops in the absence of the stage of alcoholic hepatitis. Alcoholic hepatitis is a steatonecrosis characterized by liver cell necrosis and pericellular fibrosis. It can be chronic and accompanied by mild clinical symptoms, or it may lead to liver failure and death. Abstinence from alcohol after alcoholic hepatitis does not entirely rule out the development of cirrhosis, although the likelihood is reduced. Of patients who continue to drink, 40% develop cirrhosis.

The transition from fatty liver and alcoholic hepatitis to cirrhosis takes place by progressive proliferation of connective tissue. This fibrosis eventually leads to the destruction of the lobule structure. The fibrosis is often initially found around the central veins. If such a perivenous fibrosis is found as early as in the stage of fatty liver, this is viewed as a prognostically bad sign with regard to the development of liver cirrhosis. Eventually, septae of connective tissue form between the central vein and the portal field (Fig. 8). Nodular structures are formed by regenerative processes that can be diagnosed by palpation. The liver has a tough consistency. Clear clinical symptoms may be absent for a long time, and this is referred to as

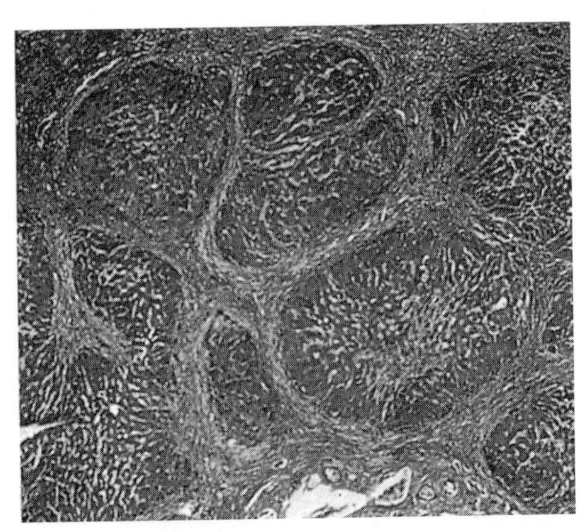

FIGURE 8 Histological picture of alcoholic liver cirrhosis. Micronodular cirrhosis. (From Eder and Gedigk, 1990.)

compensated cirrhosis. Decompensation expresses itself on the one hand in the development of hepatic encephalopathy and on the other hand in signs of portal hypertension.

1. Pressure rises in the sinusoids due to fibrosis in the liver lobule and fluid is forced into the interstitial (Disse) space between endothelium and liver cell plates. Most of this is drained out along the lymph passage, but a part does reach the surface of the liver as transsudate and enters the peritoneal cavity. Ascites (abdominal dropsy) is the result of this.
2. The accumulating blood flows into the collaterals that lead past the liver to the upper or lower vena cava. These overburdoned collateral vessels become widened and visible as "Caput Medusae" on the abdomen. The veins in the wall of the esophagus are also widened; ruptures of these esophageal varices that are manifested as hematemesis (vomiting of blood) are a highly dangerous complication of cirrhosis.
3. A backward flow of blood in the spleen vein leads to splenomegaly. Often skin changes, such as vascular spiders (spider naevi) and reddening of the palms of the hands (palmar erythema), are present; however, they are neither proof of liver injury nor specific to its alcoholic genesis.

The prognosis of alcoholic liver cirrhosis depends on whether decompensation has already occurred and whether the patient has permanently abstained from alcohol (Table 6). Abstinence is thought to be less successful in women, but in both sexes successful recovery is rare after gastrointestinal bleeding. There is no established medical treatment, although there are indications that colchicine, propylthiouracil, glucagon, and antioxidants are beneficial. In up to 15% of surviving patients, hepatocellular carcinoma develops on the base of the cirrhosis, even in the case of abstinence from alcohol. The mechanisms responsible for the development of alcoholic liver injury are almost invariably linked to ethanol metabolism (Fig. 9), with the exception of the direct effects of ethanol on membrane fluidity. As discussed for CCl_4 and acetaminophen, mediators released from inflammatory cell such as Kupffer cells and immigrating neutrophils are assumed to be involved in the development of the liver injury.

TABLE 6 Prognosis of Alcoholic Liver Cirrhosis[a]

	Abstinent	Nonabstinent
Compensated cirrhosis	89%	68%
Decompensated cirrhosis	60%	34%

[a]Patients surviving 5 years after diagnosis of alcoholic liver cirrhosis.

Cholestatic Liver Injury

Cholestatic Hepatitis

Intrahepatic cholestasis due to a disturbance of the biochemical processes in the production of bile in the liver (in contrast to mechanical drainage problems in the extrahepatic bile ducts) is predominantly linked to facultative hepatotoxins. Over 100 compounds are known to be able to cause cholestatic or mixed hepatocellular–cholestatic hepatitis. A prototypical example is the neuroleptic chlorpromazine, which has been withdrawn from the market. In chlorpromazine hepatitis, allergic and toxic mechanisms are involved, as with halothane. Of the obligatory hepatotoxins, only a minority regularly cause cholestasis. One of these is α-naphthylisocyanate, which is used experimentally to induce cholestasis. One example from epidemiology of a toxic hepatitis with mixed morphological symptoms is Epping jaundice. This afflicted 84 inhabitants of the British town Epping after they had eaten bread made from flour that was contaminated with methylene dianiline. Methylene dianiline is used in industry as an epoxy resin hardener in the preparation of isocyanates, in the production of polyurethane and polychloroprene, and as an antioxidant in latex rubber. Consequently, intoxications have also been

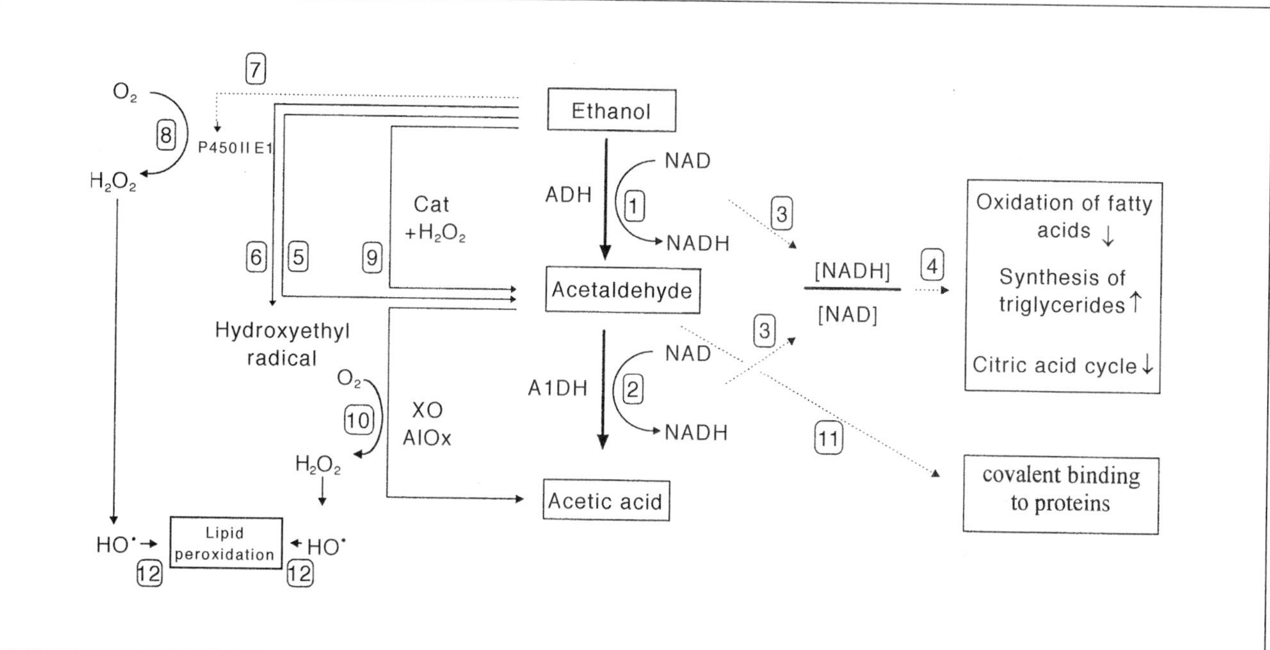

FIGURE 9 Metabolism and hepatotoxic mechanisms of ethanol. The main pathway of metabolism leads through the sequential oxidation to acetaldehyde by means of alcohol dehydrogenase (ADH) (1) and further to acetic acid by means of aldehyde dehydrogenase (AIDH) (2). Alcohol dehydrogenase is localized in the cytosol; the reaction velocity is determined by the provision of the cofactor NAD through mitochondrial NADH oxidation. The lack of the mitochondrial aldehyde dehydrogenase isoenzyme aldehyde dehydrogenase I due to a genetic polymorphism in the Japanese and Mongoloid populations leads to symptoms of acetaldehyde intoxication, but this is thought to concur with a reduced risk of alcoholic liver disease. After chronic alcohol abuse, the acetaldehyde concentration in the serum is increased due to accelerated oxidation of ethanol and slowing of acetaldehyde oxidation. The increase of the NADH/NAD quotient (3) through the alcohol dehydrogenase reaction and the aldehyde dehydrogenase reaction causes massive changes in the intermediary metabolism (4). Approximately 3% of the ethanol metabolism to acetaldehyde take place in the endoplasmic reticulum, primarily due to cytochrome P450 IIE1 (microsomal ethanol oxidizing system, MEOS) (5). This system operates with higher ethanol concentrations than alcohol dehydrogenase (K_M 10–15 mM compared to 0.2–2 mM). In ESR studies, the formation of the hydroxyethyl radical by this system has been shown (6). Cytochrome P450 IIE1 can be induced by ethanol (7). It can produce hydrogen peroxide even more efficiently than other cytochromes P450 (8); this process is supported by ethanol induction. The primarily centrilobular character of the alcoholic liver disease has been linked to the predominantly centrilobular localization of cytochrome P450 IIE1, but there are other explanations (e.g., a synergistic effect of the relative hypoxia in this area, which is further increased by an ethanol-related hypermetabolic status with increased oxygen consumption). In the white population, there is a genetic polymorphism for cytochrome P450 IIE1 that could be related to the individually differing sensitivities to alcoholic liver disease. A further metabolic process to acetaldehyde is mediated by the peroxidizing activity of catalase (Cat) in the peroxisomes (9). The contribution of this metabolic route depends on the extent of hydrogen peroxide production in the peroxisomes and amounts *in vivo,* usually up to approximately 2% of the ethanol metabolism. An alternative metabolic route, which is only active at very high acetaldehyde concentrations, is by means of the cytosolic enzymes xanthine oxidase (XO) and aldehyde oxidase (AlOx) (10); thus, superoxide and hydrogen peroxide are formed. Nondetoxified acetaldehyde can covalently bind to proteins (11). The hydrogen peroxide formed in (8) and (10) can induce lipid peroxidation via the reduction to the hydroxyl radical HO˙ (12). Hydroxyl radicals will also be formed in the aldehyde dehydrogenase and alcohol dehydrogenase reaction. The hydroxyethyl radical formed in (6) is also assumed to induce lipid peroxidation (13); proteins can also be alkylated.

observed in these industries, usually when the agent was used as an epoxy resin hardener.

The cholestasis can be seen microscopically in the form of intracellular bile deposits, as a yellow-brown discoloring of the hepatocytes, or as deposits in the bile capillaries between the individual hepatocytes. The electron microscope shows a flattening and loss of the microvilli on the walls of the bile capillaries. Bile retention is usually accompanied by damage to the liver parenchymal cells leading to a mixture of cytotoxic and cholestatic symptoms, often with an inflammatory component. Sometimes the small bile vessels between the hepatocytes and/or the interlobular bile vessels in the portal field are inflamed (cholangiolitis or cholangitis). There is an increase in alkaline phosphatase (Fig. 3), while the elevation of transaminases is less than in cytotoxic liver injury, usually not exceeding 5- to 10-fold. There is also an elevation of γ-glutamyl transpeptidase in serum. The clinical symptoms of cholestasis are jaundice, itching, dark urine, and discolored excreta. However, there are also anicteric forms. Occasionally the jaundice persists for over 6 months after discontinuation of the drug; this is called chronic cholestasis. In this stage it is possible histologically to record a decrease in interlobular bile vessels. The prognosis for chronic cholestasis is generally good, but the healing process is slow and can take years.

The following mechanisms may underly an intrahepatic cholestasis induced by foreign substance.

1. A Mg^{2+}-ATPase in the canalicular plasma membrane, which plays a part in bile secretion, can be inhibited. This is the case with chlorpromazine and a dihydroxylated chlorpromazine metabolite.
2. Mg^{+}-ATPase is functionally connected to the pericanalicular microfilament system. The mushroom poison phalloidin causes cholestasis because it induces polymerization of actin and thus disturbs the function of the microfilament apparatus.
3. A reduction of membrane fluidity influences the permeability of the canalicular plasma membrane, as shown with estrogens and anabolic steroids.
4. Na^{+},K^{+}-ATPase in the sinusoidal plasma membrane is also inhibited, although the relation to bile secretion is uncertain. Its activity is closely linked to the fluidity of the membrane.
5. Chlorpromazine forms insoluble complexes with bile acids. This interferes with the micelle formation in the bile vessels and could affect bile transport by damaging the bile vessels, inhibit the processes of secretion, or mechanically block the lumen of the bile vessels.

Acute Cholestasis

Some sex hormones can cause a "bland" cholestasis without there being any signs of hepatitis. The physiological androgens and gestagens do not cause a cholestasis of this type. The high levels of estrogen during pregnancy, however, are considered to be the cause of pregnancy jaundice. In hormonal contraceptives, the estrogen component is responsible for the occurrence of cholestasis. The incidence of this was estimated to be between 1:4000 and 1:10,000 in 1972; this number is expected to have fallen in recent years due to the lowering of the estrogen dose in the "pill." Predisposing factors are previous liver disease and genetic components. The jaundice usually occurs between the first and second cycle and takes a mild form. Cholestasis has only very occasionally been observed in relation to synthetic gestagens, and even then only in the cases of 19-demethylated, 17-ethinylated gestagens, which can be metabolized to compounds with estrogen activity. 17-Alkylated androgens used as anabolics are more frequently linked to cholestasis, probably because they are applied in far higher dosage in the treatment of wasting diseases. In one study, half the patients developed a slight increase in alkaline phosphatase without clinical symptoms, but only very few developed jaundice. Another study does, however, show that 18% of a group of patients treated for aplastic anamia with anabolic steroids over 10–20 months developed icterus.

Both estrogens and 17-alkylated androgens cause an inhibition of bromosulfalein secretion in animal experiments. Experiments dealing with the mechanisms of cholestasis have indicated that changes in the constitution of lipids in the plasma membrane, such as the cholesterin–phospholipid relationship, resulted in a change of the fluidity of the plasma membrane, causing the secretion of bile to be reduced.

Vascular Liver Injury

Portal Hypertension

Vinyl chloride, the monomer of the plastic material polyvinyl chloride (PVC), causes diverse injury to the blood vessels of the liver. Portal hypertension is one component of "vinyl chloride disease." It leads to clinical consequences similar to those of portal hypertension caused by liver cirrhosis; bleeding from the varices of the esophagus can be the first and often fatal symptom. Often the liver and spleen are enlarged, but the liver function tests need not necessarily be pathological. On peritoneoscopy, conspicuous focal capsular fibrosis of the liver is found. Biopsy specimens reveal enlargement and thickening of the branchs of the portal veins, intralobular perisinusoidal fibrosis, and collagen deposits in the sinusoidal walls. Degenerative alterations of hepatocytes and a few single-cell necroses indicate a cytotoxic component of the disease.

Vitamin A, taken in high doses over years, can cause portal hypertension. This is due to a massive accumulation of vitamin A in the sinusoidal Ito cells. There is hyperplasia and activation of the Ito cells, which then form large quantities of collagen. Perisinusoidal fibrosis ensues; the obstruction of the sinusoids is the pathophysiological basis of portal hypertension. Periportal fibrosis and cirrhosis can be the consequences of Ito cell activation. The serum concentration of vitamin A is usually, although not always, high, and other signs of hypervitaminosis A, such as hair loss and signs of intracranial hypertension, are frequently present. Jaundice is not one of the symptoms; a yellow discoloring of the skin is attributed to the high concentration of vitamin A.

Peliosis Hepatis

A second vascular lesion induced by vinyl chloride, peliosis hepatis, is characterized by massively enlarged, blood-filled sinusoids. These "lacunae" are induced by the destruction of sinusoidal supporting membranes; the condition is frequently accompanied by hepatocyte injury. Hyperplasia of the hepatocytes leads to the formation of trabeculae invading the lacunae. Beginning clinical symptoms are often lacking; liver function tests can be normal. Later, liver enlargement, signs of portal hypertension, and the biochemical correlates of hepatocellular injury will occur, and the patient may die from liver failure. Peliosis hepatis is assumed to be a precursor of hepatocellular carcinoma.

Veno-occlusive Disease

Pyrrolizidine alkaloids are plant toxins from more than 100 genera. Some of them are metabolically activated to mono- or bifunctional alkylating agents, which can bind to DNA bases. It is assumed that these induce liver tumors and bladder tumors in humans. Hepatotoxic activity has especially been ascribed to the alkaloids from *Crotolaria, Senecio,* and *Heliotropium* species, which are widely used as herbal folk medicine in certain parts of the world (e.g., in African countries and Jamaica). The pyrrolizidine alkaloids lead to a narrowing and eventually to an occlusion of the veins in the center of the lobule. This condition is called veno-occlusive disease. It is at present unclear whether and how the occlusion of the central vein is mechanistically related to the alkylating properties of the drugs. Clinically, veno-occlusive disease leads to hepatomegaly and ascites. On the abdomen, venous collaterales develop, into which the blood is drained. Patients suffer from vomiting and severe abdominal pain. Jaundice is not typical for the disease. Liver function tests are abnormal, indicating damage to parenchymal cells. Histologically, a concentric nonthrombotic narrowing of the central vein is detected concomitantly with hemorrhagic centrilobular necrosis. This acute stage can proceed to a chronic liver injury characterized by a fibrosis, which proceeds from the centrilobular region to the portal area. Epidemic outbreaks of the intoxication have been observed in cases where contaminated flour has been ingested or as a consequence of the intake of bush tea containing pyrrolizidine alkaloids. The prognosis is not favorable. In a group of 64 persons who had ingested contaminated bush tea in 1951, only 50% recovered completely; 25% died in the acute stage and 10% developed liver cirrhosis. In another outbreak in 1975–1977 in India, the 5-year survival was only 50%.

Liver Tumors

Chemically induced liver tumors can arise from the hepatocyte (liver adenoma and primary hepatocellular carcinoma), from the vasculature (hemangiosarcoma), and rarely, from the bile vessels (cholangiosarcoma).

Liver Adenoma

A liver adenoma is a benign tumor consisting of a circumscribed area of normal hepatocytes without portal fields and generally localized on the surface of the liver. It is well supplied with thin-walled blood vessels. Although the adenoma in itself causes no symptoms, there is a danger that these vessels may rupture, with bleeding into the peritoneal cavity. This complication is critical.

The incidence of liver adenoma increased with the introduction of hormonal contraceptives, and a causal relationship is highly probable. This depends on the estrogen dosage and duration of use. If the hormone treatment is discontinued, the tumor usually regresses. The average age of patients is under 30 years for women who have used the pill, and noticeably older for women who have not used the pill. In some instances, liver adenomata have been attributed to treatment with androgens. In animal experiments, estrogens produce malignant liver tumors, and for humans the development of hepatocellular carcinoma due to hormonal contraceptives has been a matter of discussion but has not been proven.

Hepatocellular Carcinoma

In laboratory rodents, many substances have produced liver cell carcinoma. However, an application of this evidence to humans is extremely problematical because mice show a high spontaneous incidence of liver cancer, and certain strains of mice and rats, the B6C3F1 mouse and the Fischer F344 rat, react very sensitively to numerous chemicals, developing liver tumors. In humans, it is highly likely that there is a link between hepatocellular carcinoma and aflatoxin B_1. Arsenicals have also led to hepatocellular carcinoma on the basis of a cirrhosis, as found in a high percentage of Moselle vintners in previous decades who had used pesticides containing arsenicals to protect plants and had consumed the last pressing of the grapes, containing the highest concentration of pesticides, as a "house drink."

Contamination of food with aflatoxin B_1 is rare in the United States and Europe. The contamination is usually in peanuts, chopped almonds, pistachios, and brazil nuts. Exposure does occur in the food production industry, such as the occurrence in Denmark, where workers in this field inhaled 170 ng aflatoxin B_1 daily and incurred a 2–3 times greater risk of developing liver cancer. In geographic regions where the damp heat of a tropical climate favors the growth of mold, humans can have an intake of far higher quantities of aflatoxin than were carcinogenic in animal experiments. There is no definitive proof that aflatoxin B_1 is carcinogenic in humans, but epidemiological data from a range of tropical countries indicate a close correspondence between daily aflatoxin B_1 intake, urinary excretion of the DNA adduct, and incidence of primary hepatocellular carcinoma. However, this evidence cannot be regarded separately from other factors, in particular the high incidence of hepatitis B infections in the tropics. Studies carried out in China, Mexico, and South Africa have shown that in the DNA of hepatocellular carcinoma in a defined position, that is, codon 249 of the p53 tumor suppressor gene, there is frequently a substitution of guanine for thymine—a G-T transversion. This point mutation causes a substitution of arginine by serine. It has been shown that metabolically activated aflatoxin B_1 leads to the occurrence of this transversion also in cell culture. The codon 249 mutation correlates with aflatoxin B_1 exposure also in persons who have not developed hepatocellular carcinoma. The p53 gene is the most frequently mutated gene in human cancers; the mutation leads to the loss of growth and transformation control and inhibits apoptosis. There is, however, an unsettled debate whether p53 mutation is sufficient to explain the carcinogenic action of chemicals or whether it is a epiphenomenon in the carcinogenic process.

The N^7-guanine adduct (Fig. 10) is excreted by the kidneys, can be detected in human urine, and is used in the biomonitoring of aflatoxin B_1 exposure. Among the inhabitants of the Murang'a district, a region of Kenya with a high degree of food contamination by aflatoxin B_1 and a high incidence of hepatocellular carcinoma, the adduct was found in the urine. The determination of aflatoxin B_1 metabolites in the urine has also been used for biomonitoring. In a prospective study of the inhabitants of the Chinese city Shanghai, it was found that in patients who had developed hepatocellular carcinoma the probability of increased metabolite concentrations in the urine was four times higher than normal. The appearance of aflatoxin B_1 albumin adducts in the peripheral blood can be used to monitor exposure; adducts of this nature were found in inhabitants of Thailand and Gambia, countries with a high incidence of liver cancer, but not in France. In Kenya, also a country with a high risk for liver cancer, antibodies against an aflatoxin B_1 epitope were found in the serum. The role of detoxicating enzymes in protecting humans from aflatoxin B_1 hepatocarcinogenicity is illustrated by the finding that genetic polymorphism of epoxide hydrolase and glutathione transferase M1 plays a role in the sensitivity to the carcinogen. Slow metabolizers were more sensitive for both the p53 mutation and for the development of hepatocellular carcinoma.

Occupational fields that show a higher incidence of hepatocellular carcinoma than other sections of the population include laundry and dry cleaning, non electrical machinery, primary-metals industry, farming, work involving contact with pesticides, nickel industry, and plastics industry. There are indications of a carcinogenic potential for humans of polychlorinated biphenyls, which cause liver cancer in experimental animals. In the Yusho affair, the ingestion of contaminated rice oil caused the exposure of nearly 2000 persons to polychlorinated biphenyls and polychlorinated dibenzofurans. A follow-up mortality study of this population has shown that the risk of liver cancer may have been increased. For males, nine liver cancers were observed, whereas only 1.6 were expected. The chemically and toxicologically related 2,3,7,8-tetrachlorodibenzo-*p*-dioxin causes hepatocellular carcinoma in rats and mice. In epidemiological studies of exposed workers, no increased incidence of liver tumors was found, although there was an increased general incidence of malignant tumors. However, a statistically significant increase of hepatic and biliary tumors was found in inhabitants of the Seveso region contaminated in an industrial accident in 1976. This was not based on genotoxic properties but on tumor promotion.

Hemangiosarcoma

Vinyl chloride causes an exceptionally rare liver tumor in humans, a hemangiosarcoma (i.e., a tumor developing from the endothelial cells of the sinusoid). Its occurrence among PVC workers was particularly noticeable because of the low spontaneous incidence of this tumor. The tumor developed especially in those workers who were exposed to high concentrations of the monomer during the cleaning of the autoclave vessels used for the polymerization process. However, angiosarcomata have also been described in persons employed in PVC processing because resid-

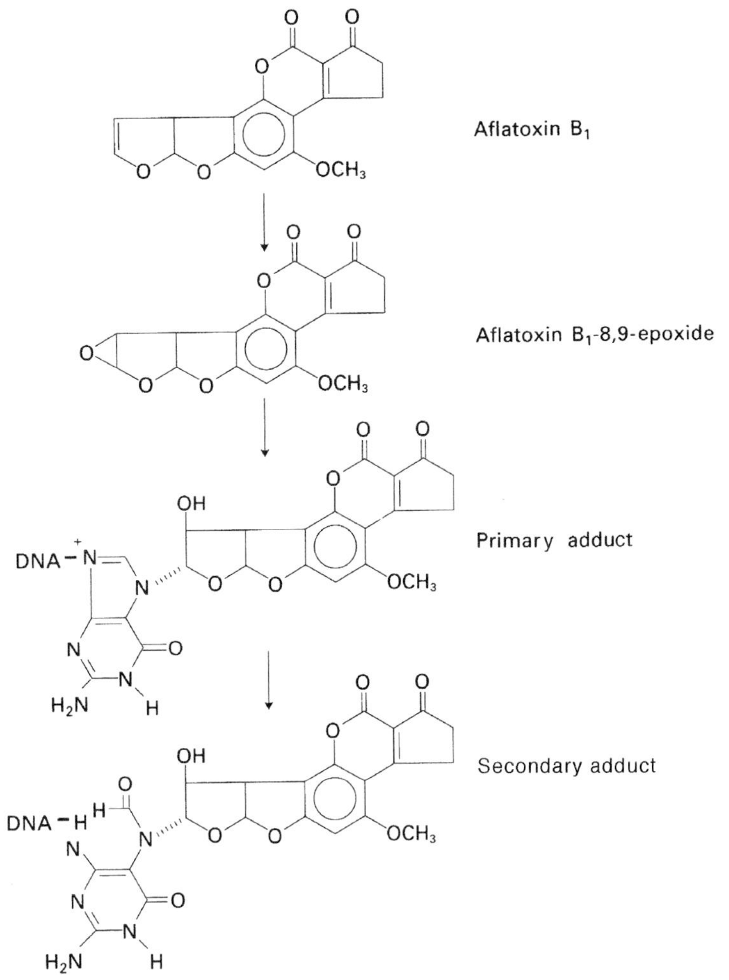

FIGURE 10 Metabolic activation of aflatoxin B_1 and formation of adducts with guanine. Aflatoxin B_1 is metabolized to 8,9-epoxide, which forms an adduct with guanine-N^7. The cytochromes of the CYPIIIA family play a part in the metabolic activation. Other cytochromes P450s (IA2, IIA3, IIB7), however, can contribute to the bioactivation, as shown by experiments with human cytochromes P450 expressed in hepatoma cells. The primary DNA adduct (half-life 7.5 h) is converted in part into the secondary adduct when the imidazole ring opens. The secondary adduct has a far longer half-life in the DNA; it remains at constant levels for at least 3 days. The secondary adduct was seen to be present in the livers of patients with hepatocellular carcinoma.

ual monomer concentrations were frequently very high during these operations.

The carcinogenic potential of vinyl chloride became obvious in 1974 after about 30 years of extensive PVC production. The health hazards of vinyl chloride were known, but most of the attention was paid to vinyl chloride-induced osteolysis. In 1985, 118 cases of hemangiosarcoma were recorded in a central European register. Although the discovery of the causal relationship led to a sharp reduction of vinyl concentrations in the work place, new cases can still be expected due to the long latency period of the tumor's development.

The development of the vinyl chloride lesion in the livers of adult laboratory rodent proceeds via a hyperplasia of liver parenchyma cells and endothelial cells, a dilation of the sinusoids and overgrowing of the dilated areas by clusters of hepatocytes and angiosarcoma cells, to the manifest tumor. The process is thought to be similar in humans. Death is caused ei-

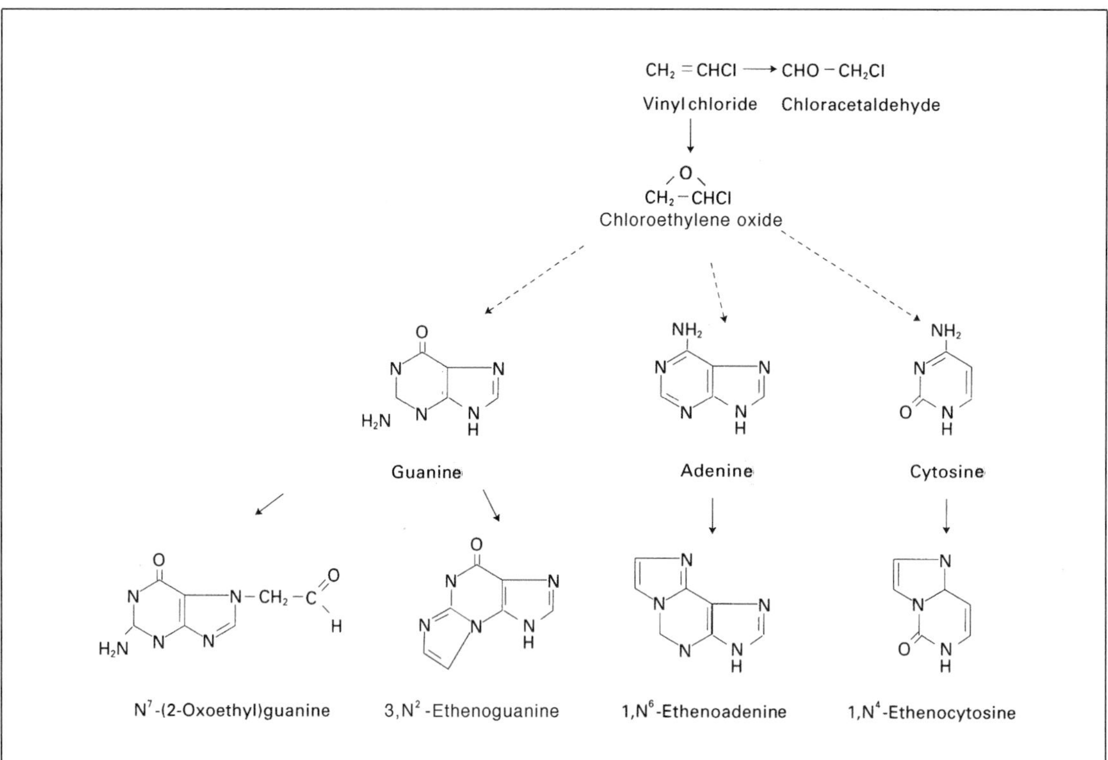

FIGURE 11 Metabolic activation of vinyl chloride and formation of adducts with DNA and RNA bases. The product of the reaction of the epoxide (chloroethylene oxide) with the N^7 of the guanine of the DNA—the *N^7-(2-oxoethyl)guanine*—*in vivo* is most prevalent; the etheno adducts are found *in vitro* and appear also *in vivo* in the DNA and RNA, though at a lower rate. Chloroacetaldehyde, which is formed by the rearrangement of chloroethylenoxide, is also reactive. The site where the reactive metabolite is formed is the liver parenchymal cell. In contrast, only minimal metabolic activation takes place in the target cells, the endothelial cells of the sinusoids. Whether and how the metabolites formed in the hepatocytes enter the endothelial cells have not been clarified.

ther by liver failure or bleeding into the peritoneum after rupture of the tumor. Vinyl chloride forms active metabolites and reacts with nucleic acids (Fig. 11). In a few human vinyl chloride-related angisarcomas, p53 tumor suppressor gene mutations, consisting of A:T to T:A transitions, were detected. Activation of the *k-ras2* protooncogene to an oncogene by a G:C to A:T transition at codon 13 was also found in human hemangiosarcomas associated with occupational exposure to vinyl chloride. The mutant *k-ras2* gene product p21 lacks growth-control properties inherent in the wild-type p21 protein. It has been detected in the serum of exposed persons and may thus be used as a surrogate for *k-ras* oncogene expression at the tissue level.

Bibliography

Arias, I. M., Boyer, F., Jacoby, W. B., Schachter, D., and Schafritz, D. A. (1994). "The Liver, Biology and Pathobiology," 3rd ed. Ravens Press, New York.

Autrup, J. L., Schmidt, J., and Autrup, H. (1993). Exposure to aflatoxin B1 in animal-feed production plant workers. *Environ. Health Perspect.* **99,** 195–197.

Bird, G. L. A., and Williams, R. (1992). Anaesthesia-related liver disease. *In* "Allergic Reactions to Anaesthetics Clinical and Basic Aspects" (E. Assem, ed.), pp. 174–191. Karger Verlag, Basel.

Brotodihardjo, A. E., Batey, R. G., Farrell, G. C., and Byth, K. (1992). Hepatotoxicity from acetaminophen self-poisoning in western Sydney: A continuing challenge. *Med. J. Aust.* **157,** 382–385.

Bulera, S. J., Cohen, S. D., and Khairallah, E. A. (1996). Acetaminophen-arylated proteins are detected in hepatic subcellular fractions and numerous extra-hepatic tissues in CD-1 and C57B1/6J mice. *Toxicology* **109,** 85–99.

Cadenas, E. (1994). One- and two-electron activation of quinonoid compounds. Oxidant and antioxidant aspects. *In* "Free Radicals in the Environment, Medicine, and Toxicology" (H. Nohl *et al.,* eds), pp. 119–135. Richelieu Press, London.

Dianzani, M. U. (1987). The role of free radicals in liver damage. *Proc. Nutr. Soc.* **46,** 43–52.

Dreifuss, F. E., Santilli, N., Langer, D. H., Sweeney, K. P., Moline, K. A., and Menander, K. B. (1987). Valproic acid hepatic fatalities: A retrospective review. *Neurology* **37,** 379–385.

Eder, M., and Gedigk, P. (1990). "Allgemeine Pathologie und Pathologische Anatomie." Springer Verlag, Berlin.

Essigmann, J. M., Croy, R. G., Bennett, R. A., and Wogan, G. N. (1982). Metabolic activation of aflatoxin B1: Patterns of DNA adduct formation, removal, and excretion in relation to carcinogenesis. *Drug Metab. Rev.* **13,** 581–602.

Feuer, G., and DiFonzo, C. J. (1992). Intrahepatic cholestasis: A review of biochemical-pathological mechanisms. *Drug Metab. Drug Interact.* **10,** 1–161.

Goldsworthy, T. L., Hanigan, M. L., and Pitot, H. C. (1986). Models of hepatocarcinogenesis in the rat: Contrasts and comparisons. *Crit. Rev. Toxicol.* **17,** 61–89.

Groopman, J. D., Zhu, J., Donahue, P. R., Pikul, A., Zhang, L.-S., and Wogan, G. N. (1992). Molecular dosimetry of urinary aflatoxin DNA adducts in people living in Guangxi Autonomous Region, People's Republic of China. *Cancer Res.* **52,** 45–51.

Gut, J., Christen, U., and Huwyler, J. (1993). Mechanisms of halothane toxicity: Novel insights. *Pharmacol. Ther.* **58,** 133–135.

Hall, A. J., Harrington, J. M., and Waterhouse, J. A. (1992). The Epping jaundice outbreak: A 24 year follow up. *J. Epidemiol. Community Health* **46,** 327–328.

Harris, C. C. (1995). 1995 Deichmann Lecture—p53 tumor suppressor gene: At the crossroads of molecular carcinogenesis, molecular epidemiology and cancer risk assessment. *Toxicol. Lett.* **82/83,** 1–7.

Hollstein, M., Marion, M.-J., Lehman, T., Welsh, J., Harris, C. C., Martel-Planche, G., Kuster, I., and Montesano, R. (1994). p53 mutation at A:T base pairs in angiosarcomas of vinyl chloride-exposed factory workers. *Carcinogenesis* **15,** 1–3.

Horbach, M., Gerber, E., and Kahl, R. (1997). Influence of acetaminophen treatment and hydrogen peroxide treatment on the release of a CINC-related protein and TNF-α from rat hepatocyte cultures. *Toxicology* **121,** 117–126.

Ishak, K. G., Zimmermann, J., and Ray, M. B. (1991). Alcoholic liver disease: Pathologic, pathogenetic and clinical aspects. *Alcohol. Clin. Exp. Res.* **15,** 45–66.

Laib, R. J. (1982). Specific covalent binding and toxicity of aliphatic halogenated xenobiotics. *Rev. Drug Metab. Drug Interact.* **IV,** 1–48.

Laskin, D. L., and Pilaro, A. M. (1986). Potential role of activated macrophages in acetaminophen hepatotoxicity. *Toxicol. Appl. Pharmacol.* **86,** 204–215.

Lee, S. S. T., Buters, J. T. M., Pineau, T., Fernandez-Salguero, P., and Gonzalez, F. J. (1996). Role of CYP2E1 in the hepatotoxicity of acetaminophen. *J. Biol. Chem.* **271,** 12063–12067.

Leist, M., Gantner, F., Naumann, H., Bluethmann, H., Vogt, K., Brigelius-Flohé, R., Nicotera, P., Volk, H.-D., and Wendel, A. (1997). Tumor necrosis factor-induced apoptosis during poisoning of mice with hepatotoxins. *Gastroenterology* **112,** 924–935.

Lieber, C. S. (1991). Hepatic, metabolic and toxic effects of ethanol: 1991 update. Alcohol. *Clin. Exp. Res.* **15,** 573–592.

Marion, M. J., Froment, O., and Trepo, C. (1991). Activation of Ki-*ras* gene by point mutation in human liver angiosarcoma associated with vinyl chloride exposure. *Mol. Carcinog.* **4,** 450–454.

Marsteller, H. J., Lelbach, W. K., Müller, R., and Gedigk, P. (1975). Unusual splenomegalic liver disease as evidenced by peritoneoscopy and guided liver biopsy among polyvinyl chloride production workers. *Ann. NY Acad. Sci.* **246,** 95–134.

McGlynn, K. A., Rosvold, E. A., Lustbades, E. D., Hu, Y., Clapper, M. L., Thou, T., Wild, C. P., Yia, X.-L., Baffoe-Bonnie, A., Ofori-Adjei, D., Chen, G.-C., London, W. T., Shen, F.-M., and Buetow, K. H. (1995). Susceptibility to hepatocellular carcinoma is associated with genetic variation in the enzymatic detoxification of aflatoxin B1. *Proc. Natl. Acad. Sci. USA* **92,** 2384–2387.

McIntyre, N., Benhamou, J.-P., Bircher, J., Rizzetto, M., and Rodes, J. (1997). "Oxford Textbook of Clinical Hepatology," 2nd ed. Oxford University Press, Oxford.

McLean, M., and Dutton, M. F. (1995). Cellular interactions and metabolism of aflatoxin: An update. *Pharmacol. Ther.* **65,** 163–192.

Mehendale, H. M., Roth, R. A., Gandolfi, A. J., Klaunig, J. E., Lemasters, J. J., and Curtis, L. R. (1994). Novel mechanisms in chemically induced hepatotoxicity. *FASEB J.* **8,** 1285–1295.

Métreaux, J. M., Dhumeaux, D., and Berthelot, P. (1972). Oral contraceptives and the liver. *Gut* **7,** 318–335.

Newberne, P. M. (1984). Chemical carcinogenesis: mycotoxins and other chemicals to which humans are exposed. *Semin. Liver Dis.* **4,** 122–135.

Olsen, J. H., Dragstedt, L., and Autrup, H. (1988). Cancer risk and occupational exposure to aflatoxins in Denmark. *Br. J. Cancer* **58,** 392–396.

Orrenius, S. (1993). Mechanisms of oxidative cell damage. *In* "Free Radicals, from Basic Science to Medicine" (G. Poli *et al.*, eds.), pp. 47–64. Birkhäuser Verlag, Basel.

Plaa, G. L., and Charbonneau, M. (1994). Detection and evaluation of chemically induced liver injury. *In* "Principles and Methods of Toxicology" (A. W. Hayes, ed.), pp. 839–870. Raven Press, New York.

Purchase, I. F. H., Stafford, J., and Paddle, G. M. (1987). Vinyl chloride: An assessment of the risk of occupational exposure. *Food Chem. Toxicol.* **25,** 187–202.

Reichen, J. (1993). Mechanisms of cholestasis. *In* "Hepatic Transport and Bile Secretion. Physiology and Pathophysiology" (N. Travoloni and P. G. Berk, eds), pp. 665–672. Raven Press, New York.

Rivera-Penera, T., Gugig, R., Davis, J., McDiarmid, S., Vargas, J., Rosenthal, P., Berquist, W., Heyman, M. B., and Ament, M. E. (1997). Outcome of acetaminophen overdose in pediatric patients and factors contributing to hepatotoxicity. *J. Pediatr.* **11,** 2–6.

Romero, G. (1994). Protective effects of calcium channel blockers in carbon tetrachloride-induced liver injury. *Life Sci.* **55,** 981–990.

Rosser, B. G., and Gores, G. J. (1995). Liver cell necrosis: Cellular mechanisms and clinical implications. *Gastroenterology* **108,** 252–275.

Satoh, H., Gillette, J. R., Davies, H. W., Schulick, R. D., and Pohl, L. R. (1985). Immunochemical evidence of trifluoroacetylated cytochrome P-450 in the liver of halothane-treated rats. *Mol. Pharmacol.* **28,** 468–474.

Smith, M. T., Evans, C. G., Thor, H., and Orrenius, S. (1985). Quinone-induced oxidative injury to cells and tissues. *In* "Oxidative Stress" (H. Sies, ed.), pp. 91–113. Academic Press, London.

Soini, Y., Chia, S. C., Bennett, W. P., Groopman, J. D., Wang, J.-S., DeBenedetti, V. M. G., Cawley, H., Welsh, J. A., Hansen, C., Bergasa, N. V., Jones, E. A., DiBisceglie, A. M., Trivers, G. E., Sandoval, C. A., Calderon, I. E., Munoz Espinosa, L. E. M., and Harris, C. C. (1996). An aflatoxin-associated mutational hotspot at codon 249 in the p53 tumor suppressor gene occurs in hepatocellular carcinomas from Mexico. *Carcinogenesis* **17,** 1007–1012.

Srivastava, S. P., Chen, N. Q., and Holtzman, J. L. (1990). The in vitro NADPH-dependent inhibition by CCl_4 of the ATP-dependent calcium uptake of hepatic microsomes from male rats. Studies on the mechanism of the inactivation of the hepatic microsomal calcium pump by the $CCl_3\cdot$ radical. *J. Biol. Chem.* **265,** 8392–8399.

Swenberg, J. A., Fedtke, N., Ciroussel, F., Barbin, A., and Bartsch, H. (1992). Etheno adducts formed in DNA of vinyl chloride-exposed rats are highly persistent in liver. *Carcinogenesis* **13,** 727–729.

Schulte-Hermann, R., Bursch, W., Grasl-Kraupp, E., Müllauer, L., and Ruttkay-Nedecky, B. (1995). Apoptosis and multistage carcinogenesis in rat liver. *Mutat. Res.* **333,** 81–87.

Tamburro, C. H. (1984). Relationship of vinyl monomers and liver cancers: Angiosarcoma and hepatocellular carcinoma. *Semin. Liver Dis.* **4,** 158–169.

Treinen Moslen, M. (1996). Toxic responses of the liver. *In* "Casarett and Doull's Toxicology" (J. Doull *et al.*, eds.), pp. 403–416. Macmillan, New York.

Vermeulen, N. P. E., Bessems, J. G. M., and Van de Straat, R. (1992). Molecular aspects of acetaminophen-induced hepatotoxicity and its mechanism-based prevention. *Drug Metab. Rev.* **24,** 367–407.

Williams, A. T., and Burk, R. F. (1990). Carbon tetrachloride hepatotoxicity: An example of free-radical-mediated injury. *Semin. Liver Dis.* **1,** 279–284.

Zimmerman, H. J. (1982). Chemical hepatic injury and its detection. *In* "Toxicology of the Liver" (G. Plaa and W. R. Hewitt, eds), pp. 1–45. Raven Press, New York.

Zimmerman, H. J. (1993). Hepatotoxicity. *Disease-A-Month-Series* **39,** 675–787.

Zimmerman, H. J., and Lewis, J. H. (1987). Drug-induced cholestasis. *Med. Toxicol.* **2,** 112–160.

C H A P T E R

14

The Kidney

CONSTANTIN COJOCEL*, EDWARD A. LOCK†

*Hoechst Marion Roussel, Bad Soden am Taunus, Germany

†ZENECA, Central Toxicology Laboratory, Macclesfield, Cheshire, England

The kidney plays a key role in the body by functioning as an integrating and regulatory organ that maintains the homeostasis of the extracellular fluid and the pH of blood in the normal physiological range. The high excretory capacity of the kidney requires a large blood flow a total of 20–25% of the cardiac output flows through the kidneys, 90% of which passes through the renal cortex. The kidneys continuously eliminate substances such as creatinine, urea, and absorbed xenobiotics (drugs and chemicals) and their metabolites in the urine. At the same time, normal renal function is crucial for retaining valuable blood components, such as glucose and amino acids. As an endocrine organ, the kidney is the site of synthesis for mediating factors, such as renin, erythropoietin, prostaglandins, cytokines, and kinins. The release of renin and kinins from the kidney is of great importance in controlling the volume of extracellular fluid and arterial blood pressure.

The nephron is the morphological and functional unit of the kidney (Fig. 1). Nephrons are constantly exposed to physiological metabolites, environmental chemicals, and drugs. The human kidney consists of 1–1.25 million nephrons. The nephron consists of the glomerulus (the renal corpuscle) and the renal tubule. The tubule in turn can be divided into the proximal tubule (pars convoluta and pars recta), Henle's loop, and the distal tubule. The nephron excludes the collecting duct, as its embryological origin differs from that of the remainder of the tubule. Under normal conditions, glomerular hydrostatic pressure drives water, solutes, and small proteins across the capillary wall into the capsular space of Bowman. This ultrafiltrate of plasma (primary urine) then undergoes modification in the subsequent segments of the renal tubule via sensitively regulated active and passive transport and secretion processes so that vital substances and water are conserved, but unnecessary or harmful substances are excreted.

Thus any alterations in structure and function of glomerular or tubular membranes can result in reversible or irreversible glomerular and/or tubular injury. Xenobiotics may cause various nephropathies that are barely distinguishable from other kidney diseases. The etiology of most renal damage remains unknown, often because the toxic compound and duration of exposure are unknown. Its identification and differentiation may also be impeded by an accompanying disease, such as diabetes.

The normal structure and function of the nephron will now be described in some detail.

GLOMERULAR STRUCTURE

The renal corpuscle (Malpighian corpuscle) consists of the glomerulus and Bowman's capsule. The renal corpuscles of the human kidney have an average diameter of 100 μm and, when engorged with blood, are visible to the naked eye. Properly, the term "glomerulus" refers only to the capillary tuft. However, it is often used interchangeably with renal corpuscle to include the capillary tuft and Bowman's capsule. The glomerulus is a capillary network that is interposed between the afferent (vas afferens) and efferent (vas efferens) arterioles (Fig. 1). Unlike most other organs, the kidney has two capillary networks, one following

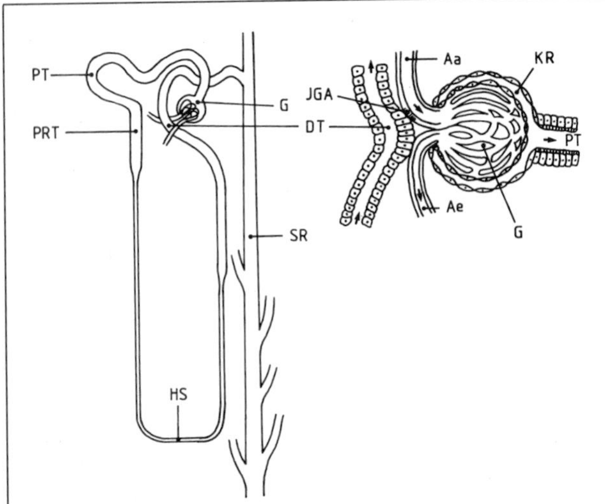

FIGURE 1 Graphic representation of the various segments of a nephron. Abbreviations: G, glomerulus; PT, proximal convoluted tubule; PRT, proximal straight tubule; HS, Henle's loop; DT, distal tubule; SR, collecting tubule; JGA, juxtaglomerular apparatus; Aa, afferent arteriole; Ae, efferent arteriole; KR, urinary space.

the other; one lies inside the renal corpuscle and the other is wrapped around the tubule.

Blood flowing through these capillary networks supply the tubule cells with oxygen and nutrients and exchanges substances with the tubule lumen via absorption and secretion mechanisms. Bowman's capsule consists of an outer (parietal) and an inner (visceral) layer that closely adheres to and completely covers the glomerular capillaries. Between these two layers lies the urinary space into which the primary urine is pressed as an ultrafiltrate of the plasma (Fig. 1). Subsequently, the primary urine passes from the urinary space into the renal tubule system. Blood enters the kidney by the renal artery and flows through the afferent arterioles into the glomeruli to undergo filtration. The blood, which is still rich in oxygen, leaves the glomeruli through the efferent arterioles. Two types of differentiated glomeruli are present in the renal cortex, glomeruli located in the superficial cortex (cortical glomeruli) and glomeruli located in the deep cortex at the junction between the cortex and the medulla (juxtamedullary glomeruli).

The glomerulus almost fills the Bowman's capsule where it is not just a coiled capillary but rather a network of capillaries inserted into the surrounding capsule. The fine structure of the glomerulus under the electron microscope shows three cell types, endothelial, epithelial, and mesangial cells. The basement membrane and mesangial cell matrix play a major role in maintaining the spatial structure and function of the glomerulus.

The glomerular filtration barrier consists of three layers, the capillary endothelial layer, the glomerular basement membrane, and the visceral layer of Bowman's capsule. The fenestrated endothelium of the glomerular capillaries contains pores (500–1000 Å), which are polygonal in shape (Fig. 2). Podocytes, which are specialized cells that constitute the visceral layer, cover the outside of the glomerular capillary basement membrane against the urinary space (Fig. 3). Terminal podocyte extensions, called pedicells, are foot-like in shape and interdigitate with those of an adjacent cell. The underlying surface of foot processes or pedicels is in contact with the basal membrane of glomerular capillary, and the spaces (pores) between pedicels are called filtration slits (25 nm). Each filtration slit is spanned by a 6-nm-thick diaphragm. The filtration slits form the last barrier to the passage of substances eliminated with the urine.

The glomerular basement membrane (GBM), which is approximately 300 nm thick, consists of three layers, the lamina densa, (flanked on either side by two layers), lamina rara interna, and lamina rara externa. The lamina rara interna of the GBM is in direct contact with the blood stream through the endothelial fenestrae, while lamina rara externa is in contact with the urinary space through the filtration slits. The function of the GBM is determined by its complex biochemical composition. The lamina densa contains type IV collagen, whereas heparin sulphate has been identified in the electron-lucent laminae rara. Other substances, such as glycoproteins and proteoglycans, are also found in the glomerular basement membrane. The GBM has a structural support function and is a component of the filtration barrier.

The capillary endothelium, basement membrane, and podocyte foot processes constitute the filtration barrier through which small molecules, electrolytes, and water must pass as they are forced into the capsular space. The ultrafiltrate, which is formed from each of the glomerular capillary tufts, drains from the capsular space through the urinary pole into the beginning of the proximal tubule. During the continuous filtration process, plasma is forced through the filtration barrier and a build up of trapped proteins forms within the GBM. "Unclogging" of the filter is apparently accomplished by mesangial cells that are in contact with lamina rara interna.

The mesangium is composed of the mesangial cells (modified smooth muscle cells) and the mesangial matrix (Fig. 4). The mesangium is located within the

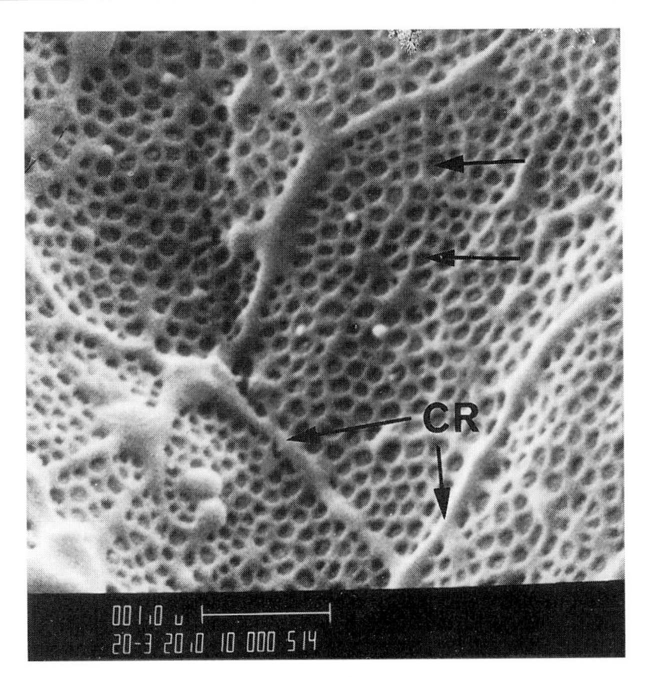

FIGURE 2 Scanning electron micrograph of the endothelial fenestrations of a glomerular capillary from a control rat. Abbreviations: (→) endothelial fenestrae; CR, cytoplasmic ridges (× 18660).

central portion of the glomerular tuft between capillary loops. Mesangial matrix and GBM are the two extracellular matrices in the glomerulus.

The mesangial cells are connected by gap junctions with each other, as well as with the lacis cells of the extraglomerular mesangium and the myoepithelioid cells of the juxtaglomerular apparatus. The mesangial cells and the mesangial matrix are separated from capillary lumen by a fenestrated endothelium (Fig. 4). The mesangial cells are continuously perfused by plasma through the fenestrations of the endothelium and exposed to various immune complexes and circulating or locally released hormones and mediators. The glomerular mesangial cells have the properties of both muscle cells (contractility) and macrophages (phagocytosis). Mesangial cell contraction and relaxation potentially modify glomerular haemodynamics by regulating the surface area available for filtration.

Mesangial cells synthesize the mesangial matrix and are probably involved in the turnover of the GBM, as they phagocytose the GBM and the accumulated proteinaceous debris within it. The mesangial matrix is a dynamic structure and is made up of type IV collagen, glycoproteins, proteoglycans, amyloid-P component, and actomyosin. The mesangial matrix fills the extracellular space between adjacent mesangial cells, between the endothelial and mesangial cells, and between mesangial cells and GBM. The mesangial matrix is also involved in maintaining the flexible spatial structure of the capillary tuft and the glomerular filtration of macromolecules. Both alterations in glomerular haemodynamics and increased accumulation of macromolecules in the mesangium have been implicated in the pathogenesis of the glomerular injury. Under normal conditions, the turnover of mesangial cells in the glomeruli is tightly regulated and quite slow. In the disease conditions, however, the turnover of mesangial cells is increased.

The juxtaglomerular apparatus is formed by the macula densa and the polkissen (myoepithelioid cells). It lies at the vascular pole of the renal corpuscle, is crucially important for the autoregulation of renal function, and at the same time serves to regulate extrarenal (systemic) physiological processes. The myoepithelioid cells of the afferent arteriole form the vasoactive enzyme renin, which is released mainly into the blood, but is also released also into the lymph tract. Therefore, renin has both a local and a systemic regulatory action on the blood vessels and thus on the circulation. The macula densa denotes the point at

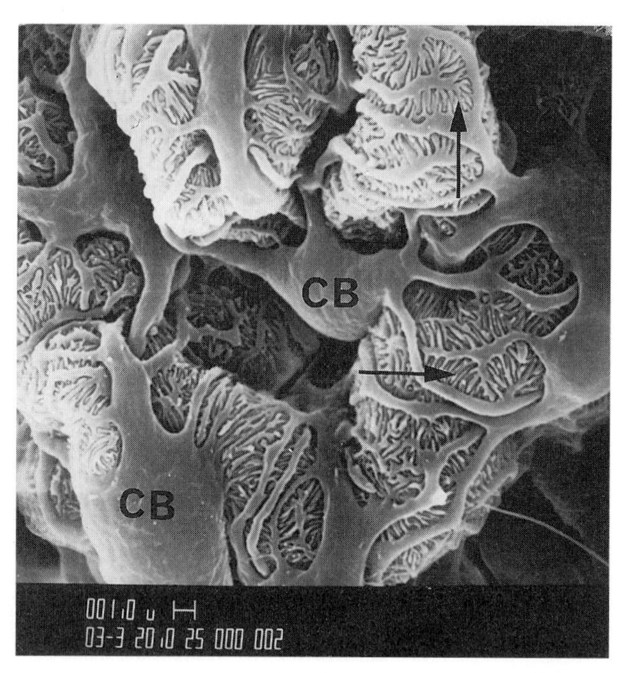

FIGURE 3 Surface morphology of the visceral layer of Bowman's capsule in the rat kidney. The cell body (CB) of the podocytes and their cytoplasmic foot processes (→)(× 4285).

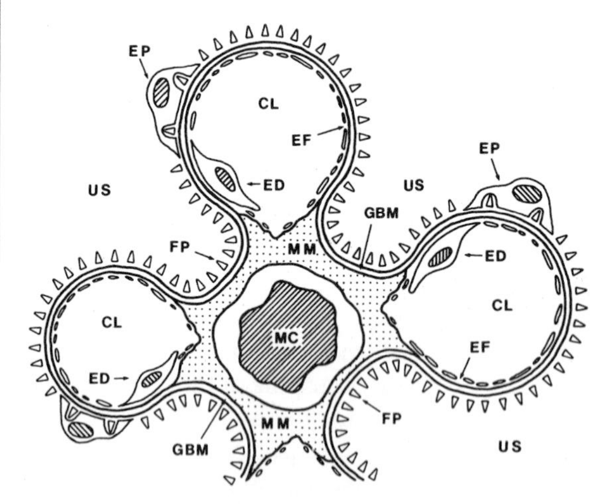

FIGURE 4 Schematic representation of the mesangium. Abbreviations: MC, mesangial cell; MM, mesangial matrix; ED, endothelial cells; EF, endothelial fenestrae; CL, capillary lumen; GBM, glomerular basement membrane; EP, epithelial cells (podocytes); US, urinary space.

which, at the fork between the afferent and efferent arterioles, the distal convoluted renal tubule touches the afferent arteriole of its renal corpuscle (Fig. 1). Thus the juxtaglomerular apparatus is involved in monitoring the changes in sodium concentration in the tubular urine.

A rise in the sodium concentration triggers the release of renin, which leads to a reduction in the blood flow to the glomerulus. The released renin in turn activates the renin-angiotensin-aldosterone mechanism, which counteracts a fall in blood pressure and increases the volume of the extracellular fluid.

RENAL TUBULE STRUCTURE

The proximal tubule starts with the convoluted part (pars convoluta), which is followed by a straight part (pars recta) that descends into the renal medulla and becomes the thin limb of Henle's loop. The loops of the cortical nephrons extend into the outer and in some cases into the inner medulla; the loops of the juxtamedullary nephrons, in contrast, extend into the papillary apices and thus form an important component in the countercurrent system (Fig. 1).

A morphological configuration of this kind is important for the concentration of urine along the final segment of the nephron. The loop of Henle connects the proximal to the distal tubule. The thick, ascending straight part of the distal tubule runs back to the glomerulus where, at the vascular pole, it touches the afferent arteriole of the associated glomerulus and thus with it forms the juxtaglomerular apparatus. The straight part of the distal tubule has attached to it a relatively short, convoluted part of the distal tubule, which becomes an initial collecting tube. Several collecting tubes merge to form urinary vessels with ever larger lumens that open into the calyces of the renal pelvis at the papillary apex (Fig. 1).

The cells of the proximal tubule show on the lumen side a broad and regular brush border (Fig. 5). Between the brush border processes, vesicles of varying sizes are formed (pinocytosis). Through pinocytosis, glomerularly filtered proteins are absorbed from the tubular lumen and brought through the pinocytotic vesicles to the lysosomes where they are degraded into amino acids. The cells of the distal tubule are very similar to the cells of the proximal convoluted tubule. However, the lumen side of the distal tubular cells generally has only individual short microvilli, no brush border.

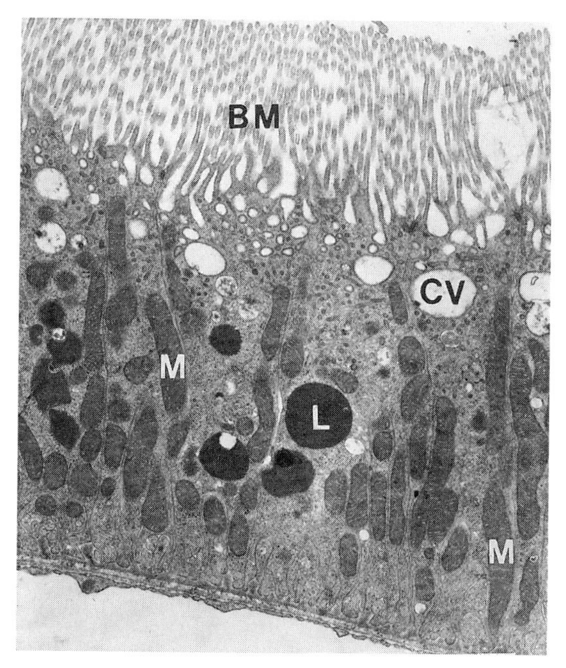

FIGURE 5 Transmission electron micrograph of the tubular cells of a rat kidney. Abbreviations: CV, cytoplasmic vesicles; BM, brush-border microvilli; L, lysosomes; M, mitochondria (× 9320).

GLOMERULAR FUNCTION

The glomerular filtration of a molecule is a very complex process in which an important role is played by molecule size, shape, load, quaternary structure, and hemodynamic factors. Because of the fixed negative charge of the components of the filtration barrier, positively charged macromolecules are filtered better than neutral or negatively charged substances of the same molecular weight.

The volume of fluid filtered by the glomeruli per unit of time (ml/min), known as the glomerular filtration rate (GFR), can be determined by means of the inulin clearance (C_{in}) or the creatinine clearance (C_{cr}). Under physiological conditions, filtration is largely independent of the blood pressure because the renal vascular system is subject to autoregulation.

Inulin is an exogenous substance (fructose polysaccharide) that is freely filtered (molecular mass 5500 Da), is not bound to plasma proteins, undergoes neither tubular absorption nor secretion, and is not metabolized. It may therefore be assumed that the quantity of inulin filtered corresponds to the quantity of inulin excreted, and the following equation applies,

$$U_{in} \cdot V = P_{in} \cdot \mathrm{GFR},$$

where U_{in} is the inulin concentration in the urine, P_{in} is the inulin concentration in the plasma, and V is the urine flow in ml/min. The following thus applies:

$$\mathrm{GFR} = U_{in} \cdot V/P_{in}.$$

Inulin is therefore particularly suitable for measurement of the glomerular filtration rate. However, endogenous creatinine can also be used for determination of the GFR, with certain limitations. Creatinine is formed as a degradation product of creatine and creatine phosphate present in muscle, and undergoes free glomerular filtration. The quantity of creatinine, and thus the level of the plasma concentration, is dependent on muscle mass and is thus slightly higher in men than in women; it does, however, remain relatively constant in the individual, and decreases with age. In dogs, creatinine clearance corresponds to the inulin clearance, whereas in humans it is slightly higher than the GFR. Although endogenous creatinine clearance is not as reliable as inulin clearance, it is adequate for clinical purposes. GFR decreases with age to about 50% of normal at 70–80 years of age;

there is, however, considerable interindividual variation.

The clearance of a given substance (C_s) is calculated using the ratio $U_s \cdot V/P_s$. C_s is often defined as the plasma volume that is completely cleared of the given substance per minute. If the ratio C_s/C_{in} equals 1, the substance is neither absorbed nor secreted, and the quantity excreted corresponds to the glomerular filtration rate. If a substance undergoes glomerular filtration and tubular absorption, C_s/C_{in} is less than 1 (e.g., glucose, amino acids, and lysozyme). Where C_s/C_{in} is greater than 1, the substance is filtered at the glomerulus and secreted into the tubule (e.g., uric acid, and potassium).

Renal plasma flow (RPF) corresponds to the *p*-aminohippuric acid (PAH) clearance to within about 8–10%. The extraction of PAH in one passage through the kidney of a healthy man is about 90%; the PAH extraction declines with damage to the renal cortex. Because the hematocrit is normally about 45%, this means that the RPF accounts for about 55% of the renal blood flow (about 650 ml/min) in a person weighing 70 kg.

GFR is an important parameter for assessing renal function after exposure to xenobiotics. Because of the proportional relationship between the decrease in the glomerular filtration rate and the rise in plasma creatinine, the extent and progression of renal failure can be estimated from the concentration and rate of increase in plasma creatinine.

The glomerular filtration rate of an single nephron (SNGFR) can be measured in animal experiments by the micropuncture technique. Micropipettes can be used to withdraw fluid from inside Bowman's capsule; the inulin concentration of the ultrafiltrate and the blood can then be determined and the SNGFR ascertained using a known rate of ultrafiltrate flow.

The volume of fluid pressed through the filtration barrier is, among other things, a function of the ultrafiltration coefficient (K_f). The ultrafiltration coefficient is an expression of the fluid permeability of the GBM and can be calculated as the product of the hydraulic permeability and the surface area available for filtration. Thus, decrease of K_f may represent a primary alteration in the glomerular filtration barrier or a secondary response to the tubular injury. However, in naive rats K_f may be decreased by as much as 50% without altering SNGFR.

Various drugs, such as cyclosporin A, can increase the resistance of the glomerular arterioles. Changes in the renal vascular resistance can lead to altered renal blood flow and thus to altered glomerular filtration rate and other glomerular functions. Changes in GFR, SNGFR, and K_f may indicate either primary damage to the glomerular filtration barrier or tubular damage.

TUBULE FUNCTION

The glomerular ultrafiltrate undergoes dramatic changes in composition in the various segments of the tubule. Tubular absorption, degradation, biotransformation, and secretion processes determine the excretion of filtered substances and thus the composition of the urine. On the one hand, absorption, secretion, and metabolism influence the elimination of xenobiotics and their metabolic end products; on the other hand, drugs and chemicals may alter the structure and function of the tubule.

Most of the soluble constituents of the primary urine and 99% of the water are reabsorbed and returned to the blood in the peritubular capillaries. After glomerular filtration, water, glucose, amino acid, sodium, chloride, potassium, and phosphate are reabsorbed from the tubular fluid. Many xenobiotics are reabsorbed, while others may undergo enzymatic degradation in the tubular lumen prior to excretion. A few substances are actively secreted from peritubular capillaries (organic acids) or tubular cells (in which they can produce H^+ and ammonia) into the tubular fluid. In the distal convoluted tubule sodium, chloride and water are reabsorbed and potassium is secreted. The tubular proximal reabsorption of water is virtually constant and independent of diuresis, while the urine concentration is dependent on medullary blood flow that occurs in the countercurrent system of the renal medulla according to the hairpin-countercurrent principle. The reabsorption of water, and thus the final concentration of urine, is also under the influence of the antidiuretic hormone in the distal convoluted tubules and in the collecting tubules.

Under normal conditions, only tiny amounts of protein are excreted with the urine (<150 mg/24 h). These are plasma proteins such as albumin (<25 mg/24 h), lysozyme (muramidase), β_2-microglobulin or Tamm-Horsfall mucoprotein synthesized in the ascending thick limb of the Henle loop. Proteins filtered at the glomerulus undergo almost complete absorption in the proximal tubule by pinocytosis and are digested in the lysosomes to amino acids. Pathologically increased protein excretion may have a glomerular and/or tubular cause. The determination in urine of specific marker enzymes and other proteins originating in the nephron serves to elucidate the pathophysiological background to various forms of renal disease. The cell types of different nephron segments have varying vulnerability to inflammatory, ischemic, and toxic injuries.

Increased enzymuria is found in primary and secondary glomerulonephritis, in pathological nephropathy, arterial hypertension, after renal transplantation, after exposure to nephrotoxic xenobiotics such as aminoglycosides and cytostatics (cisplatin), after the injection of radiocontrast media, and in the work place following exposure to certain heavy metals.

The tubular transport rate of a substance is the quantity of substance transported through the cell membrane of the tubular cells per unit of time. In the case of substances with unrestricted filtration and tubular absorption, the transport rate (T_{res}) is calculated from the difference between the quantities of substance filtered and excreted per unit of time:

$$T_{res} = \text{GFR} \cdot P_s - U_s \cdot V \text{ (mg/min)}.$$

In the case of substances with restricted glomerular filtration and tubular absorption, the glomerular sieving coefficient is required to calculate the quantity of substance filtered. Lysozyme undergoes glomerular filtration to a great extent on account of its low molecular mass (14,000 Da) and is almost completely reabsorbed (>99%) in the proximal tubules. With normal GFR, an increase in the renal excretion of proteins such as lysozyme indicates toxic damage to tubular cells by drugs and chemicals. Thus, the lysozyme transport rate (T_{ly}) is calculated from

$$T_{ly} = \text{GFR} \cdot 0.8 \cdot P_{ly} - U_{ly} \cdot V,$$

where 0.8 corresponds to the glomerular sieving coefficient for lysozyme. For substances that are filtered and secreted, the transport rate of secretion (T_{secr}) is calculated from the difference between the quantities of substance excreted and filtered per unit of time:

$$T_{secr} = U_s \cdot V - \text{GFR} \cdot P_s.$$

The measured value for inulin or creatinine clearance is used as the value for GFR.

PATHOPHYSIOLOGY

Drugs and chemicals may lead to functional and morphological damage in the kidney. A substance may cause glomerular, tubular, interstitial, or vascular lesions via toxic or immunological pathomechanisms. Important clinical symptoms are acute renal failure, chronic renal insufficiency, nephrotic syndrome, and tubulointerstitial kidney diseases.

Parenchymal cell loss leading to renal atrophy is characteristic of many chronic progressive renal diseases, while, in contrast, tubular cell loss is the main characteristic of acute tubular necrosis. The mechanism of cell death or loss may occur via either apoptosis, necrosis or a combination of both. Other nephropathies, such as mesangial hypercellularity in proliferative glomerulonephritis and the increased number of fibroblasts observed in renal fibrosis, are defined by an abnormal accumulation of renal cells.

Acute Renal Failure

Acute renal failure (ARF) is often a reversible insufficiency of the glomerular and tubular excretion functions, which may be triggered by renal and extrarenal mechanisms. It may be the result of toxic, hypoxic (circulatory shock), or immunologically induced damage. Renal causes of ARF are due to parenchymal changes resulting from disease or nephrotoxic agents that induce renal disease.

Ischemia and nephrotoxins are the most common causes of ARF. Disease of the renal parenchyma other than ischemia accounts for about 25% of all cases of ARF. These include lesions, such as glomerular injury to the glomerular membrane (acute glomerulonephritis), papillary necrosis, vasculitides, malignant hypertension, acute tubular necrosis, intratubular obstructions, and acute pyelonephritis or necrotizing papillitis. On account of the large renal blood flow, nephrotoxic substances can rapidly reach both kidneys, where they are filtered and enter the tubular lumen. There they are concentrated and may have a damaging effects, frequently in the region of the proximal tubular cells. Moreover, concentration of the urine by the countercurrent mechanism results in an accumulation of the nephrotoxins in the tubular lumen. Metabolism by tubular cells may also further increase their nephrotoxic action.

The harmful substances may be exogenous or endogenous in origin: drugs (e.g., aminoglycosides, cephalosporins, radiocontrast media, salicylates, cisplatin, methotrexate, cyclosporin A, and dextran), poisons (e.g., fungal toxins and snake venom), chemical substances (e.g., heavy metals and organic solvents), and endogenously released substances (e.g., hemoglobin and myoglobin). The clinical picture of toxic nephropathy is similar to that of shock kidney; in most cases, ARF starts with nausea, vomiting, and restlessness. If the damage is severe, dehydration, hypotension, and oliguria soon occur.

The urine produced in the first few days contains moderate quantities of protein, epithelial cells, leukocytes, and occasionally erythrocytes; finally, total anuria of variable duration occurs. Milder, nonanuric cases are sometimes dominated by certain tubular symptoms: glucosuria (ferricyanide intoxication), hyperchloremic acidosis (amphotericin B and sulfonamides), diabetes insipidus (amphotericin B), and Fanconi's syndrome. The multifactorial pathogenesis of ARF includes a disturbance of glomerular microcirculation (afferent and perhaps mesangial constriction, and inadequate efferent dilation) and a disturbance of medullary microcirculation (medullary capillary congestion) attributed to a combination of endothelial damage and tubular dilatation. Tubule cell injuries, which in humans justify the term "acute tubular necrosis," promote the back-leak of glomerular filtrate and shedding of brush-border vesicles. Brush-border components and Tamm-Horsfall protein lead to cast formation and tubular obstruction. Experimental therapeutic approaches focus on the restitution of microcirculation (endothelial receptor antagonists) interference with cast formation (integrin receptor blockers), and on the promotion of the repair and recovery processes by growth factors.

Chronic Renal Failure

Chronic renal failure (CRF) is characterised by progressive and generally irreversible decrease in GFR. A large number of diseases can lead to chronic renal insufficiency. The most common causes of CRF are, however, glomerular diseases such as glomerulonephritis and diabetic glomerulosclerosis (diabetic nephropathy), urological diseases, ischemic nephropathy, and tubulointerstitial kidney diseases (including analgesic nephropathy); CRF may also occur as a result of treatment with cyclosporin A. Diabetes and hypertension are recognized as the leading causes of CRF in the United States. In CRF, impairment of renal function is slow in onset, irreversible, and usually progresses over months or years; it is caused by the loss of functioning nephrons. CRF culminates in end-stage renal disease when about 90% of the nephrons are damaged.

The clinical signs and symptoms of end-stage renal failure is known as the "uremic syndrome." CRF is characterized by reduced renal parenchyma (arteriosclerotic kidney), a probably irreversible reduction in the GFR, excretion of virtually iso-osmolar urine, the chronic retention of substances usually eliminated with the urine, and the chronic disturbance of endocrine functions. The deficit in function is caused by the extent of the loss of functioning nephrons and is largely independent of the nature of the original damage. The build-up of substances usually eliminated with the urine ultimately leads to uremia and terminal encephalopathy (uremic coma). These processes may stop (stationary chronic renal insufficiency) or have a slowly progressive course. A protein-rich diet and hypertension contribute to the progression, which may also occur at the end of diabetes mellitus. Histologically, the progression of chronic renal insufficiency is characterized by the appearance of glomerulosclerotic scars. Glomerulosclerosis may be the result of direct capillary damage caused by glomerular hypertension or by mesangial overload with filtered proteins.

Nephrotic Syndrome

Nephrotic syndrome is a group of signs and symptoms commonly seen in patients with glomerular diseases that are characterized by a significant increase in capillary-wall permeability to serum, either alone or sometimes in addition to glomerular inflammatory changes. The causes of the nephrotic syndrome are often primary glomerular diseases, such as minimal-change lesions, mesangial proliferative glomerulonephritis, focal segmental glomerulosclerosis, membranous glomerulonephritis, and mesangiocapillary glomerulonephritis.

Other possible causes are the consequences of other diseases, such as infections, intoxication (e.g., from gold and mercury compounds), malignancy, systemic diseases (e.g., amyloidosis), or diabetes mellitus. Nephrotic syndrome is characterized by pronounced proteinuria (>3.5 g/liter, 73 m^2/day) in adults, which can be explained as a diffuse disturbance in the permeability of the glomerular capillaries. Nephrotic syndrome also leads to hypoproteinemia, dysproteinemia, generalized edema, hyperlipoproteinemia, lipiduria, and an increased tendency to arterial and venous thrombosis (increased blood clotting). Depending on the type of damage to the glomerular filtration barrier, either mainly micromolecular proteins may pass the filter (selective proteinuria) and/or with severe changes the proportion of macromolecular proteins in the urine increases (nonselective proteinuria).

Tubulointerstitial Kidney Diseases

With tubulointerstitial kidney diseases there are many morphological and functional consequences. Tubular disturbances are the main feature. Morphologically, a tubulointerstitial kidney disease is characterized by more or less diffuse infiltration of the renal interstices with lymphocytes, sometimes eosinophilic leukocytes, tubular atrophy, thickening of the tubular basement membrane, and interstitial edema. Changes in medullary blood vessels are a further cause of damage to the tissue (ischemic necrosis) in the medullary/papillary region. Functionally, a tubulointerstitial kidney disease manifests itself through discrete proteinuria (<1 g/100 ml), mild hematuria, and an early decrease in the renal concentration capacity. Other typical features are diminished production of NH_3, and thus disturbance of H^+ secretion and of HCO_3 absorption, plus reduced formation of calcitriol and erythropoietin.

In chronic interstitial nephritis, there is sterile leucocyturia, more or less pronounced renal insufficiency, and, finally, fibrosis and necrosis (papillary necrosis). This is usually attributable to long-term loading with substances such as lead, cadmium, and lithium and/or the ingestion of combination drugs containing phenacetin or acetylsalicylic acid (analgesic nephropathy).

BIOTRANSFORMATION AND NEPHROTOXICITY

It is now well recognized that the biotransformation of xenobiotics leads not only to the detoxification of the reactive chemical but can also contribute to the production of metabolites that are more cytotoxic than the parent compound.

Although the importance of renal metabolism has in the past usually been ignored or underestimated, more recent studies revealed the contribution of renal metabolism in the development of xenobiotic nephrotoxicity. As in the liver, renal biotransformation of drugs and chemicals occurs in two phases. The cytochrome P450 mixed-function oxidases, localized in the endoplasmic reticulum of the renal cells, catalyze phase I reactions of xenobiotic metabolism, including oxidation, reduction, and hydrolysis, to produce polar substances with better water solubility. Phase II reactions (mainly conjugation reactions) also result in the production of more water-soluble compounds that can be more readily excreted via the kidneys.

Although phase I and II reactions are generally considered as detoxification reactions, it appears that either type of reaction can produce metabolites that are more cytotoxic than the parent compound. For example, the toxicity of industrial solvents, such as chloroform, and drugs, such as acetaminophen, require oxidative metabolism (phase I) to produce cell injury. Similarly, conjugation products of phase II reactions, such as sulfate, glucuronide, and glutathione conjugates, have been shown to mediate the toxicity of 1,2-dichloroethane and hexachloro-1:3-butadiene.

In addition to cytochrome(s), other drug-metabolizing enzymes are active in the kidney, including prostaglandin H synthase, glutathione *S*-transferase, γ-glutamyltranspeptidase, aminopeptidase, *N*-acetyltransferase, sulfotransferase, and uridine diphosphate glucuronosyltransferase. The renal metabolism of xenobiotics can also lead to the formation of highly reactive free radicals, many of which react with cellular macromolecules and produce cytotoxicity. Free radicals may be formed either enzymatically or nonenzymatically and are most frequently generated by oxidation or reduction reactions. The reactive compounds formed as a result of the renal xenobiotic biotransformation may cause renal damage, either directly or after intrarenal activation to toxic intermediate products.

There are at least four possible mechanisms of action for xenobiotic-induced renal damage. First, xenobiotics may enter renal cells and, without being metabolized, react directly with cellular macromolecules and interfere with cell function. Second, after absorption into the renal cells, the xenobiotic may undergo redox cycling to produce superoxide anion, hydrogen peroxide, singlet oxygen, or hydroxyl radicals. These reactive oxygen species can then react with cellular macromolecules and induce cytotoxicity. Third, xenobiotics may enter renal cells, where they are metabolized to form a reactive metabolite. If the reactive metabolite is not detoxified at this stage it can (e.g., through covalent binding to macromolecules or by lipid peroxidation) lead to renal damage. Finally, xenobiotics may undergo extrarenal metabolism to produce a stable metabolite that will be delivered to the kidney and enter renal cells; here it may cause direct damage to renal cells or require further intrarenal metabolic activation to produce damage. Reactive metabolites are generally electrophilic in nature and readily react with nucleophiles such as glutathione, cellular proteins, lipids, and nucleic acids and may result in carcinogenesis, apoptosis, or cellular necrosis.

The nephrotoxic potential of a xenobiotic is strongly related to its ability to interfere with normal biochemical processes and function of the kidney cells.

Most lipophilic compounds are only excreted in the urine only after undergoing biotransformation, while ionized and hydrophilic substances are often excreted directly. Excretion of unchanged xenobiotics and biotransformation may run in parallel, with one of the processes dominant. Unlike in the liver, renal drug-metabolizing enzymes are not uniformly distributed and display a corticomedullary gradient. The morphological and functional differentiation along the nephron corresponds to a certain metabolic heterogeneity of different regions of the nephron. Cytochrome(s)

P450 and many of the renal drug-metabolizing enzymes appear to be primarily concentrated in the pars convoluta and pars recta region of the proximal tubule.

NEPHROTOXIC COMPOUNDS

Anti-infectious Agents

Aminoglycosides

Aminoglycoside antibiotics have an antibactericidal action and are basic substances with several strongly polar groups that behave in the body like lipophobic substances. They belong to the group of antibacterial substances that inhibit ribosomal protein synthesis by binding to the 30S ribosomal subunit and interfere with translation of mRNA after active uptake into bacteria. Aminoglycosides consist, for the most part, of a central 2-deoxystreptamine molecule with glycosidic linkages to two or more amino-sugars. Aminoglycosides react basically ($pK_a \geq 8$), are highly water-soluble, have low lipid solubility, and have a low capacity to penetrate membranes. The number of amino groups per aminoglycoside molecule, and their cationic structure, appears to be correlated to the nephrotoxic potential. Because of their ototoxicity and nephrotoxicity, they are used for treatment in indications where other antibiotics have failed or are not sufficiently effective alone. In rare instances, these antibiotics may trigger intolerance reactions, such as reversible neuromuscular, allergic, hepatic, and hematological reactions.

The incidence and severity of clinically manifest nephrotoxicity during aminoglycoside therapy depends on the total repeated unit dose, the duration of treatment, hypotension, hypovolemia, shock, prolonged endotoxemia, the patient's individual predisposition, age, gender, obesity, previous and concomitant diseases, the quality of treatment monitoring, former aminoglycoside treatments, the toxic potential of the selected compound, and the concurrent administration of other drugs such as loop diuretics, cephalosporins, or vancomycin. The overall incidence of aminoglycoside-induced nephrotoxicity in large patient populations has been estimated to be 5–10%. Even when the plasma concentrations are maintained within the recommended ranges, 10–15% of treated patients showed clinically detectable decreases in renal function. Plasma protein binding is low, and they are excreted unmetabolized. The elimination half-life depends on the GFR, for example, for gentamicin and tobramycin it is 1.8–2.2 h and for amikacin and netilmicin 2.2–2.6 h.

Aminoglycosides accumulate in the renal cortex, mainly in the cells of the proximal tubule after uptake via pinocytosis from the tubular lumen. The renal transport and accumulation follow saturation kinetics. During chronic administration, the rate of accumulation in the renal cortex depends on the dose, the dosage interval, and the length of the treatment period. A threshold concentration of 200 μg/g kidney leads to the development of nephrotoxicity and this is reached in both humans and rats after 4 days of treatment with gentamicin. A steady-state concentration of 400 μg/g kidney is reached after about 7 days of gentamicin treatment and remains unchanged over 14, 21, or 28 days of continuous treatment in rats. Subdividing the daily dose into three portions results in faster achievement of the maximal concentration in the renal cortex.

Whereas individual differences in the grade of nephrotoxic potency of aminoglycosides can reproducibly be detected in animal studies, the differences found clinically are less pronounced. While tobramycin produces slightly less renal accumulation than gentamicin in patients with normal renal function, it shows greater cortical accumulation than gentamicin in patients with kidney disease. Netilmicin, despite similar renal cortex concentrations and the same number of amino groups per molecule, is less nephrotoxic than gentamicin. It should, however, be emphasized that increased tissue concentrations, especially in the renal cortex, are not synonymous with increased toxicity.

A number of studies show that aminoglycosides exert differential nephrotoxic injuries at different sites along the nephron depending on their acute or chronic mode of administration. The acute administration of gentamicin leads to high serum concentrations that are often accompanied by nephrotoxicity.

In rats, a single dose of gentamicin (80 mg/kg body weight) induces, after only 80 min, ultrastructural changes in the proximal tubular cells, such as loss of the brush border, proliferation and multimembranous restructuring of lysosomes, formation of myeloid bodies, distension of the endoplasmic reticulum, and swelling of the mitochondria. The renal damage induced after a single dose may be completely reversible.

Aminoglycoside nephrotoxicity is often associated with a decreased tubular transport of electrolytes, calcium, and magnesium; glucose reabsorption and alterations of tubular protein; and organic anion transport. The presence of strongly cationic substances in the distal tubule lumen may promote increased potassium excretion. Intravenous infusion of cations, such as aminoglycosides or lysozyme, cause increased sodium and potassium excretion. The mechanisms by which they affect amino acid and fatty acid transport into proximal tubule have not been elucidated.

Acute iv infusion of gentamicin in rats resulted in the displacement of the low-molecular-weight protein lysozyme from its binding sites on the proximal tubule, leading to an almost total inhibition of tubular protein reabsorption, measured in case of lysozyme as the quotient C_{LY}/GFR, which rose from 0.23 (control) to 1.0 after 20 min of gentamicin infusion. The gentamicin-induced reduction in GFR was accompanied by an increase in lysozyme clearance in the intact animal. GFR decrease may in part explain the increase in glomerular sieving coefficient of lysozyme from 0.8 to 1.0.

Various polycations are able to interact with glomerular basement membrane anionic sites and have been shown to induce alterations in glomerular permselectivity. Therefore, it is likely that the iv administration to rats of the polycationic gentamicin prior to the cationic lysozyme enabled the occupation of glomerular anionic binding sites by gentamicin, resulting in a loss of the glomerulus ability to regulate the renal fate of lysozyme.

There is growing evidence that not only the renal tubules but also the glomerulus may be the target of chronic aminoglycoside nephrotoxicity. In the early stage of nephrotoxicity, the initial appearance of brush-border and lysosomal enzymes in the urine and granular casts in the urinary sediment is followed by the development of polyuria and nephrogenic diabetes insipidus. A subsequent decline in GFR is associated with a rise in both blood urea nitrogen and plasma creatinine concentration. Kidney damage is already clinically manifest after 24 h and could be measured by phospholipiduria accompanied by increased excretion in the urine of brush border and/or lysosomal marker enzymes, such as alanine aminopeptidase and *N*-acetyl-β-glucosaminidase. Increased excretion of low-molecular-weight proteins, such as β_2-microglobulin and lysozyme (muramidase), was also observed after 3–5 days.

The results of a number of studies indicated little or no morphological change to the glomerulus following aminoglycoside treatment. However, aminoglycoside treatment of rats (30 mg/kg/day for 7, 14, or 21 days) resulted in injury of the glomerular capillary endothelium, of the myoepitheloid cells of the juxtamedullary apparatus, and in alterations of the glomerular permeability. After 7 days of treatment in rats, gentamicin and tobramycin induce a reduction in the number and diameter of the endothelial fenestrae (Figs. 6 and 7), and lead to partial or complete depletion of cytoplasmic granules from the myoepitheloid cells. However, the glomerular epithelial cells of the visceral layer, including the slit diaphragm between podocytic foot processes, were free of any remarkable injuries. Similarly, no changes of the mesangial cells or of the basement membrane were observed. After 7 days of gentamicin treatment, the decrease in the concentrating capability of the kidney, measured as a decrease in urinary osmolality and increasing proximal tubule cell necrosis is paralleled by a significant increase in sodium and potassium excretion. There are also clear reductions in GFR, GSC_{ly}, (Table 1), and renal lysozyme reabsorption (Fig. 8) and degradation. A correlation appears to exist between the lowering of the glomerular filtration area (and consequent decrease in K_f) and the reduction in both the GFR and glomerular protein filtration (Table 1).

When gentamicin therapy is prolonged to 14–28 days, the serum creatinine concentration increases, whereas proximal tubule cell necrosis shows a clear decrease. The pathophysiological renal injuries are reversible after both low and higher doses (Table 1).

The relationship between molecular structure and the nephrotoxic effects of aminoglycosides has yet to be settled. Aminoglycoside-induced phospholipidosis has been proposed as a possible mechanism. According to this hypothesis, the disruption of normal lysosomal digestive function leads to cellular depletion of important substrates necessary for cell membrane regeneration and the maintenance of various metabolic processes and of the function of the various cell organelles. The binding of cationic aminoglycosides to the anionic binding sites of the phosphatidylinositol molecule is electrostatic and is regarded as the first stage in the cellular uptake. Subsequent endocytosis and accumulation in the lysosomes inhibits phospholipid and protein degradation processes. The reduction in lysosomal phospholipid cleavage leads to the intralysosomal accumulation of undigested phospholipids and to the formation of myeloid bodies (phospholipidosis).

The elimination of myeloid bodies and necrotic cells that then occurs leads to the formation of tubular casts, the obstruction of the tubular lumen, and the failure of renal function. Intratubular obstruction appears to be one of the major mechanisms leading to a decline in GFR in both ischemic and nephrotoxic acute renal failure (ARF). Micropuncture studies of ARF revealed evidence of reestablishment of normal single-nephron GFR when microperfusion of the tubule dislodged the obstructing casts or debris.

Polycationic aminoglycosides have an effect on lysosomal structure and function. Their intralysosomal accumulation leads to a decrease in the enzymatic activity of phospholipases and proteases, such as ca-

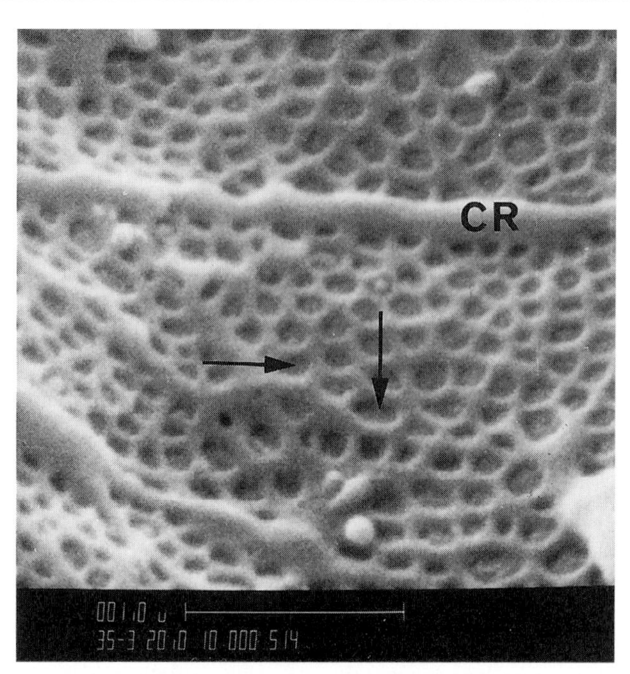

FIGURE 6 Scanning electron micrograph of the luminal surface of a glomerular capillary from a control rat. Abbreviations: (→), endothelial fenestrae; CR, cytoplasmic ridges.

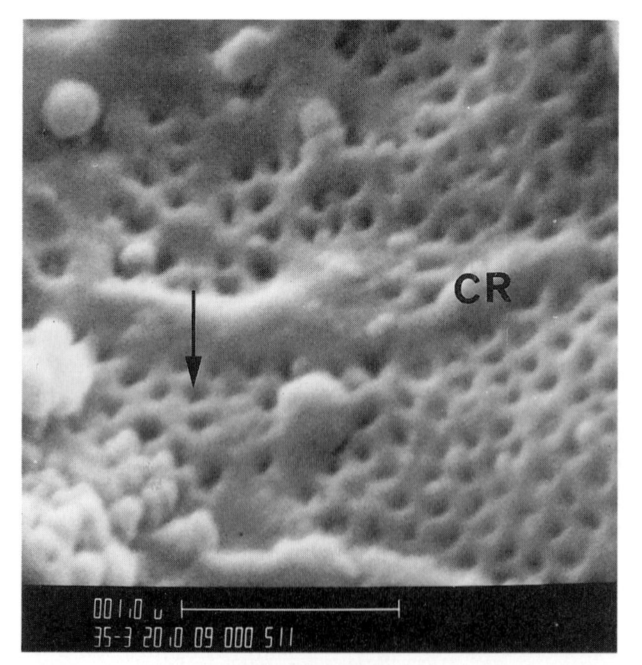

FIGURE 7 Scanning electron micrograph of the luminal surface of a glomerular capillary from a rat treated with 30 mg/kg/day tobramycin for 7 days. Abbreviations: (→), endothelial fenestrae; CR, cytoplasmic ridges.

TABLE 1 Glomerular Filtration Rate (GFR) and Glomerular Sieving Coefficient of Lysozyme (GSC_{ly}) after Chronic Treatment of Rats with Various Aminoglycosides[a]

	Duration of treatment			
	7 days		14 days	21 days
	GSC_{ly}	GFR	GFR	GFR
Control	0.80	0.95	1.02	0.96
Netilmicin	0.78	0.51[b]	0.78[b]	0.80[b]
Kanamycin	0.70[b]	0.43[b]	0.56[b]	0.64[b]
Gentamicin	0.60[b]	0.45[b]	0.42[b]	0.48[b]

[a]After aminoglycoside treatment in rats (30 mg/kg/day) for 7, 14, or 21 days, GFR was measured in intact rats as inulin clearance. GSC_{ly} was measured in the isolated perfused rat kidney after complete inhibition of tubular reabsorption of lysozyme with sodium iodoacetate.

[b]Results are given as mean value. Statistically significantly different from control ($p < 0.05$).

thepsins, resulting in accumulation of phospholipids and formation of myeloid bodies in the renal cortex. Aminoglycosides alter not only the plasma membrane and lysosomes, but also the mitochondria; for example, the swelling of mitochondria can be found in rats, while gentamicin-induced inhibition of mitochondrial oxidative phosphorylation has been observed *in vitro*. Because pinocytosis and intracellular protein cleavage are energy-consuming processes, impairment of mitochondrial respiration could lead to a decrease in pinocytotic protein reabsorption and intralysosomal protein cleavage. However, no correlation has been found between the inhibition of mitochondrial respiration *in vitro* and clinical nephrotoxicity. The results of a number of studies suggest that aminoglycoside-induced lipid peroxidation in the kidney tissue is a consequence and not a pivotal mechanism in the pathogenesis of aminoglycoside nephrotoxicity. Whether nephrotoxicity is exerted via a free-radical mechanism is controversial. Aminoglycoside are considered to be redox-inactive compounds and it is suggested that conversion to a redox-active form may require transition metals such as iron.

The results of a recent *in vitro* study indicate that gentamicin promotes the oxidation of arachidonic acid in the presence of iron salts in a manner similar to that of bleomycin. The results of experiments with scavengers of reactive oxygen species indicate that gentamicin-induced iron release from the mitochondria is mediated by hydrogen peroxide. Thus, beside ferritin, mitochondria should be considered as a potential source of iron for the generation of more reacting oxygen species. Gentamicin nephrotoxicity is increased after concomitant treatment of rats with gentamicin and a specific inhibitor (N^G-nitro-L-argi-

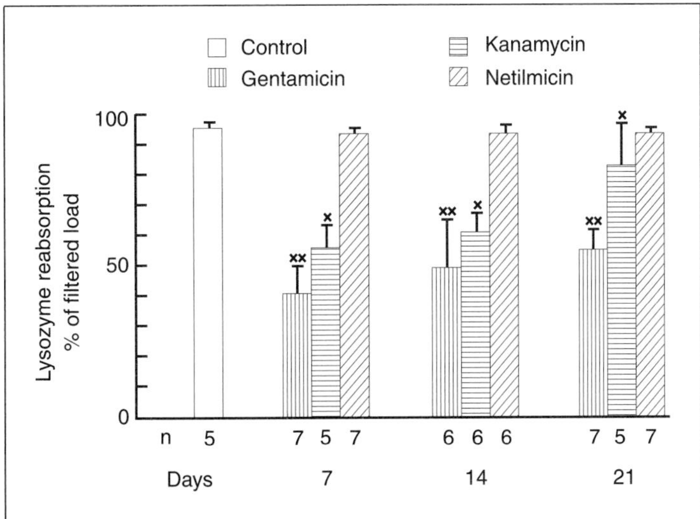

FIGURE 8 Effect of aminoglycosides treatment (30 mg/kg/day) of rats on renal lysozyme reabsorption (n = number of rats). Renal reabsorption of lysozyme was calculated as the difference between the filtered load ($P_{ly} \times GSC_{ly} \times GFR$) and excretion of lysozyme ($U_{ly} \cdot V$) ($p <$ 0.05).

nine methyl ester) of nitric oxide (NO) synthesis. Gentamicin treatment increases glomerular NO synthesis in the kidney. Increased gentamicin nephrotoxicity following the inhibition of NO synthesis suggests that endogenously released NO plays a protective role in gentamicin nephrotoxicity. This protective role of NO may be due, on the one hand, to its vasodilation effect and participation in the regulation of the renin release, and, on the other hand, to its involvement in the defense against cellular damage induced by reactive oxygen species.

Based on the available data, it is unlikely that any of the individual mechanisms of cellular toxicity discussed here is solely responsible for nephrotoxicity, which is more likely to arise through the combined effect of several biochemical and metabolic alterations caused by aminoglycosides.

An increasing number of experimental and clinical studies show that single daily dosing regimens are as effective as multiple-daily doses and have a lower incidence of nephrotoxicity or a longer period of time to the development of nephrotoxicity. It has been shown that poly-L-aspartic acid prevents gentamicin nephrotoxicity in spite of renal-cortical gentamicin accumulation, which is greater in poly-L-aspartic acid-treated rats than in control rats. Combining poly-L-aspartic acid and large gentamicin doses with a less-frequent dosing schedules (once daily) would increase bacterial efficacy while minimizing nephrotoxicity. There is evidence that the protection conferred by poly-L-aspartic acid is related to its ability to serve as an anionic substrate for the cationic aminoglycosides, thereby preventing an interaction with membrane anionic phospholipids.

Patients receiving aminoglycoside should be well hydrated to avoid volume depletion, and should be potassium and magnesium replete. If GFR declines, one should consider replacement by another equally efficacious antibiotic. Aminoglycoside-induced renal injury can progress to acute renal failure, even if treatment is discontinued at the time the serum creatinine begins to rise. Because even a small decrease in GFR can be a signal of progressive renal injury, recognizing incipient renal damage is essential.

Vancomycin

Vancomycin, another potentially nephrotoxic drug, causes renal injury in less than 5% of treated patients. A number of studies, however, suggest that as many as 35% of patients treated with the combination of vancomycin and aminoglycosides will experience nephrotoxicity, confirming animal data. The risk of nephrotoxicity in patients treated with both drugs is influenced by various factors, such as increased age, male sex, liver disease, concurrent amphotericin therapy, neutropenia, and peritonitis. Length of therapy and serum concentrations of these drugs are also associated with increased nephrotoxicity. An investigation of the effect of vancomycin on tobramycin binding to rat renal brush-border membrane showed that binding of tobramycin to the brush-border membrane was enhanced by preincubation with vancomycin because of the increase in the number of the negatively charged binding sites on the membrane surface.

β-Lactams

β-Lactam antibiotics, such as penicillins (penams), cephalosporins (cephems), and derivatives of thienamycin (carbapenems), are a complex group of compounds featuring the β-lactam ring. This molecule core, variably influenced by a series of side-chain substituents, is important to the antibacterial action, renal tubular transport/secretion, and nephrotoxicity of these antibiotics. Other β-lactams, such as clavulanic acid (clavams), moxalactam (oxacephems), and aztreonam (monobactams), which are neither penams nor cephems, proved to be of clinical significance.

Nephrotoxic β-lactams produce distinct ultrastructural damage as early as 5 h after dosing to rats and proximal tubular necrosis by 24 h. While penicillins have little or no direct nephrotoxicity, a number of cephalosporins and carbapenems, such as imipenem, cause ultrastructural and functional injuries of the tubule cells leading to impairment of renal function.

Cephalosporins, chemically related to the penicillins, are a therapeutically important group within the β-lactam antibiotics. They are semisynthetic antibiotics derived from 7-aminocephalosporanic acid, also called the cephalosporin nucleus. The numerous semisynthetic derivatives vary in their antibacterial activity, pharmacokinetics, and metabolic and toxic properties. Cephalosporins are bactericidal and inhibit the cell-wall biosynthesis of proliferating organisms. Because most of the cephalosporins used therapeutically are poorly absorbed following oral administration, they must be administered parenterally. Exceptions are cefaclor, cefadroxil, cefuroxime axetil, cephalexin, and cephradine, because they show relative good intestinal absorption. Plasma protein binding varies from 6–15% (cephalexin) and 58–97% (ceftriaxone). With most cephalosporins, the plasma half-life in adults with normal kidney function is 0.5–2.5 h. Higher values are shown by ceforanid (2.6–3.3 h), cefonicid (3.5–5.8 h), and ceftriaxone (5.4–10.9 h). Antibacterially active deacetylated metabolites are

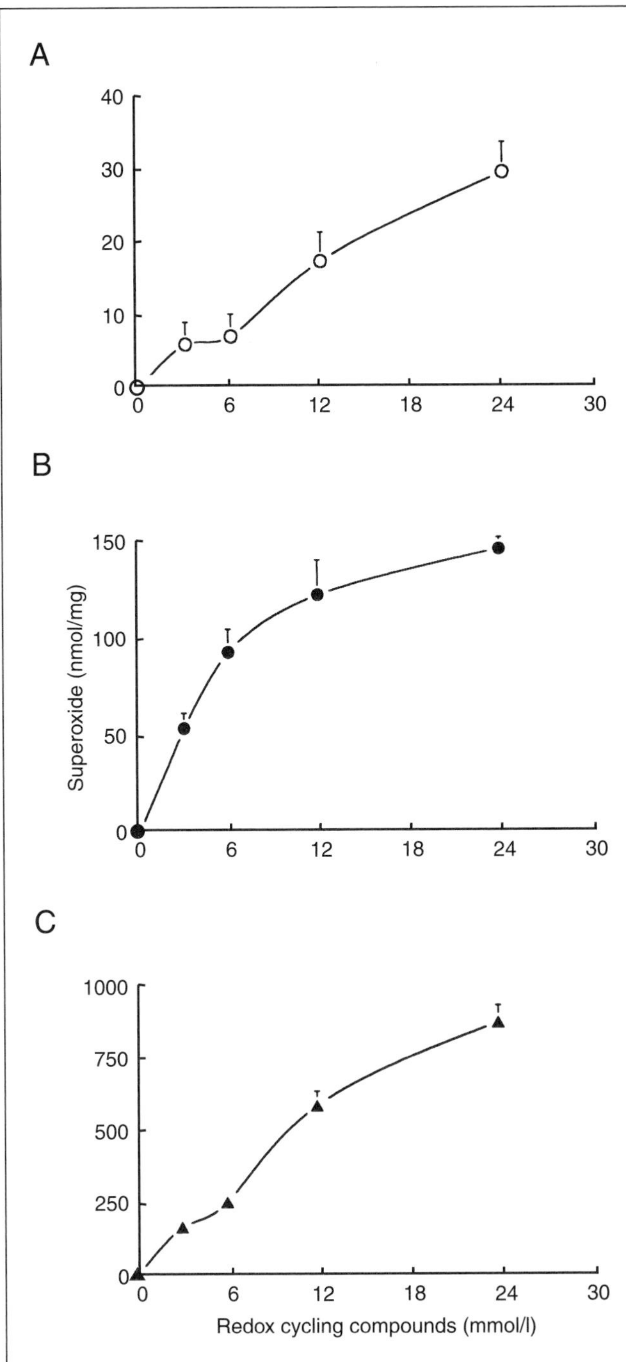

FIGURE 9 Concentration-dependent formation of superoxide after incubation of renal cortex microsomes for 15 min at 37°C with paraquat (C), cephaloridine (B), and cefsulodin (A).

formed after partial hepatic and renal metabolism of cephalothin, cefotaxime, and cephapirin. The other cephalosporins are metabolically stable or undergo only slight metabolism. Apart from ceftriaxone and cefoperazone they are excreted mainly by glomerular filtration, some also by tubular secretion (50–95% after 24 h).

In cephalosporin treatment, allergic reactions, such as urticaria and dermatitis (2–4%) or gastrointestinal disturbances, local incompatibilities, transient elevation of transaminases and alkaline phosphatase, hemorrhages and alcohol intolerance, may occur to varying degrees. Nephrotoxicity is the most important clinical side effect. Cephalosporins have little or no influence on the structure and/or function of the glomerular cells, depending on chemical structure, dose, pharmacokinetic and metabolic properties, period of administration, species, and sex. With impaired renal function and the concomitant administration of aminoglycosides, nephrotoxicity may occur.

To elucidate the mechanism of cephalosporin nephrotoxicity, cephaloridine and cephloglycin (no longer on the market) have been studied as prototypes. Cephaloridine-induced renal lesions are manifested clinically as acute oliguric renal insufficiency with cylinduria and proteinuria as a result of acute tubular necrosis. Despite numerous advances, the mechanism of cephaloridine nephrotoxicity is not fully established. Several mechanisms have been proposed for cephaloridine nephrotoxicity. Results of earlier studies suggested the formation of a reactive intermediate by epoxidation of thiophene ring catalyzed by cytochrome P450, leading to acylation of tubular proteins and inhibition of mitochondrial respiration. Recent experimental findings indicate that, like paraquat and diquat, cephaloridine can also undergoes cyclic oxidation–reduction reactions. An electron from reduced cephaloridine is transferred to oxygen, leading to the formation of reactive oxygen species, such as superoxide anion (Fig. 9). In the renal cells, these oxygen species may cause a loss of cytochrome P450, an increase in oxidized glutathione (GSSG), the peroxidation of membrane lipids leading to formation of malondialdehyde, and a reduction in the transmembrane uptake of organic ions, glucose, and amino acids (Fig. 10). Alterations of other biochemical processes, such as renal protein degradation or renal cortical gluconeogenesis, have been also observed. *In vitro* studies showed that cephaloridine-induced reactive oxygen species readily oxidize porphyrinogens to porphyrin. Cephaloridine treatment in rats caused a dose–dependent increase in renal excretion of the total porphyrin, indicating the formation of reactive oxygen species *in vivo*. This finding was supported by an increase in the concentration of GSSG in the plasma and bile.

The presence of the pyridine ring in a cephalospo-

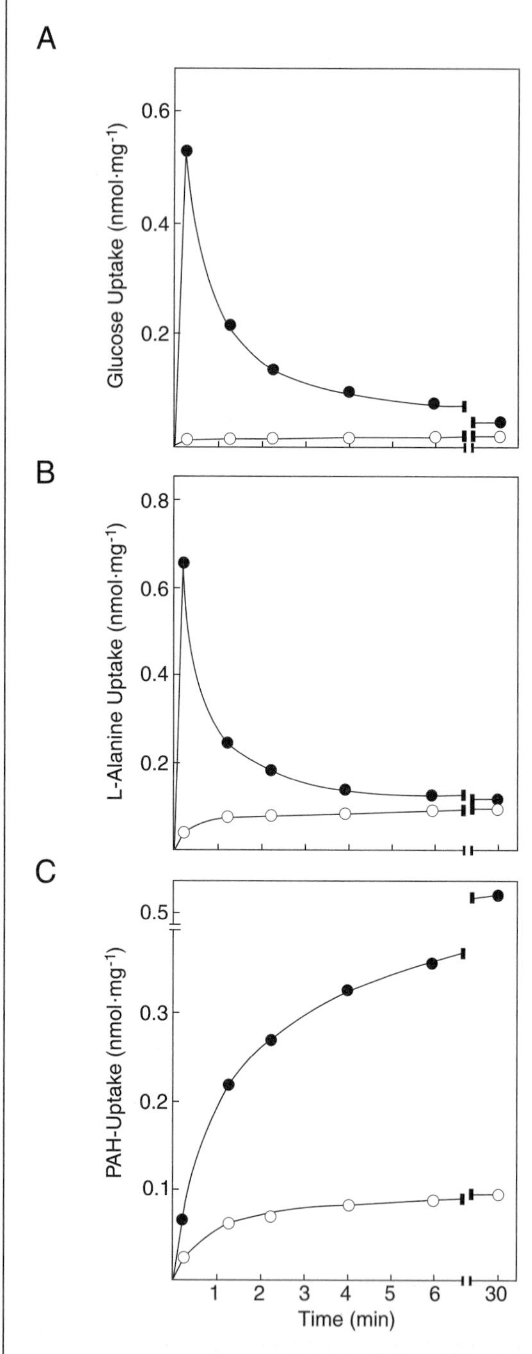

FIGURE 10 Influence of cephaloridine treatment (1200 mg/kg/d for 3d) on the uptake of (A) D-glucose (B) L-alanine, and (C) *p*-aminohippuric acid (PAH) into renal brush border membrane vesicles (BBMV). Abbreviations: •, BBMV from control rats; o, BBMV from cephaloridine-treated rats.

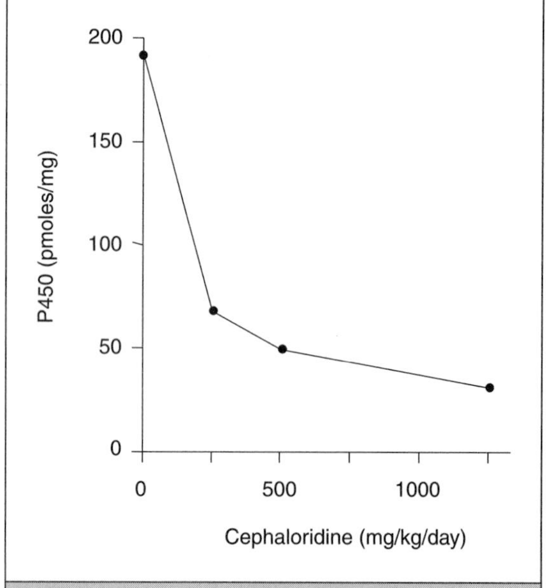

FIGURE 11 Dose-dependent decrease in total microsomal cytochrome P450 from renal cortex after treatment of rats with cephaloridine for 3 days.

rin molecule may give the structure some potential for undergoing cyclic redox processes and the formation of reactive oxygen species, which trigger the oxidative stress. The capacity of a specific β-lactam to generate superoxide, hydrogen peroxide, and other more reactive oxygen species is dependent on its molecular structure. Pyridinium-ring-containing cephalosporins (such as cephaloridine, cefsulodine, and ceftazidime) and other β-lactams (such as mezlocilin and aztreonam, which contain no pyridinium ring) cause superoxide production.

The ranking order of the magnitude of superoxide production by β-lactams *in vitro* is cephaloridine > cefsulodine > mezlocillin > aztreonam > ceftazidime > cefotaxime.

After treatment of rats with cephaloridine there were significant alterations of the polypeptide pattern in the microsomal fraction, whereas no relevant changes occurred in the lysosomal and cytosolic fractions. The *in vivo* depletion of renal cortical cytochrome P450 by cephaloridine was dose-dependent (Fig. 11). More interestingly, the time course of the cephaloridine-induced decrease in renal content of cytochrome P450 indicates that a significant depletion occurred as early as 3 h after a single dose of 1200 mg/kg. An almost complete depletion of cytochrome P450 was measured at 12 and 24 h after administration. A slow recovery of the cytochrome P450 oc-

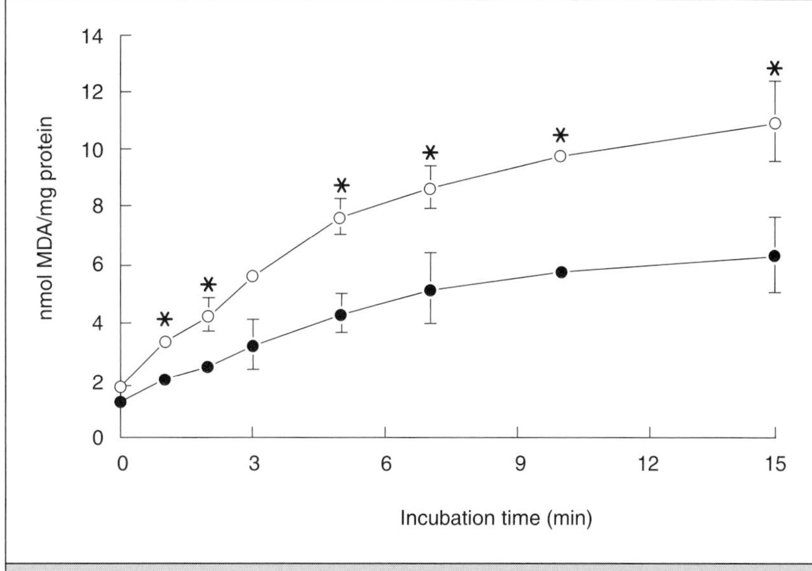

FIGURE 12 Effect of reduced glutathione (GSH) on cephaloridine-induced lipid peroxidation measured as malondialdehyde (MDA). Renal cortical microsomes were incubated with cephaloridine (24 mM) in the absence of GSH (o) ($p < 0.05$) or in the presence of 0.1 mM GSH (•).

curred after 48 and 72 h, despite the continuation of cephaloridine treatment. Measurement of malondialdehyde content in the renal cortex and microsomes of the same experiment showed that a significant increase in cephaloridine-induced lipid peroxidation occurred 24 h after the administration of cephaloridine. Radical scavengers and antioxidants, such as vitamin E, cianidanol (a naturally occurring flavonoid), *N,N'*-diphenyl-*p*-phenylenediamine, and GSH (Fig. 12), are capable of inhibiting the formation of lipid peroxidation products. The results of induction experiments showed a time- and dose-dependent increase in the amount of the 44,000 molecular weight polypeptide that was accompanied by the simultaneous depletion of the 50–53,000 molecular weight polypeptide from the cytochrome P450 region (Fig. 12). These results suggest that 44,000 renal microsomal polypeptide is not a cytochrome P450 isoenzyme but rather an enzyme of the endoplasmic reticulum involved in the detoxification of the reactive species.

Imipenem is a semisynthetic β-lactam antibiotic and is the *N*-formidyl derivative of thienamycin. The penam ring of thienamycin has been altered by replacing the sulfur atom by a carbon atom. Imipenem has been proven to cause proximal acute tubular necrosis in monkeys and rabbits, similar to those produced by cephaloridine. Both the impairment of mitochondrial respiration and oxidative injury appear to be involved in imipenem nephrotoxicity. Panipenem has similar nephrotoxicity to imipenem.

Amphotericin

Amphotericin B is an antimycotic with a broad spectrum of action covering virtually all fungi pathogenic to humans. Much like nystatin and pimaricin, it is isolated from *Streptomyces nodosus* and consists of a macrocyclic lactone with seven conjugated double bonds in an all-*trans* configuration.

After oral administration, amphotericin B is very poorly absorbed, only about 3% of the dose being bioavailable. Amphotericin B binds to plasma lipoproteins and then is slowly eliminated, with a plasma half-life of 18–24 h, which can increase to about 48 h with pronounced impairment of kidney function. Its metabolism is largely unknown and is not influenced by kidney or liver failure or hemodialysis. Elimination occurs in two phases, an initial half-life of 24 to 48 h and a terminal one of about 15 days. Amphotericin B can still be detected in the plasma 7–8 weeks after treatment, and for up to 12 months in liver and kidney tissue. The severity of the side effects of amphotericin B, such as fever, chills, azotaemia, anaemia, distal tubular acidosis, hypokalaemia, nausea, anorexia, weight loss, and phlebitis, depends on the dose and the duration of treatment.

Nephrotoxicity is one of its most important side effects and the limiting factor for clinical use. The incidence of nephrotoxicity may reach 80%. Amphotericin B nephrotoxicity is mainly characterized by alterations of glomerular haemodynamics. It is assumed that the low pH characteristic of the distal tubule lumen renders the renal epithelial cells vulnerable to its toxic action; therefore, alkalinization ameliorates amphotericin B nephrotoxicity in rats. If the blood pressure remains constant, the amphotericin B-induced increase in renal vascular resistance leads to a drop of about 35–40% in RPF and GFR. The results of the glomerular micropuncture studies of single nephrons have shown that amphotericin B causes a significant increase in pre- and postglomerular capillary resistance and a reduction in the plasma flow, SNGFR, and K_f.

Normal renal function is gradually restored after the withdrawal of the therapy. Lasting damage, however, is also occasionally observed. Nephrotoxicity is increased when amphotericin B treatment is combined with aminoglycoside or cephalosporin antibiotics. Salt depletion enhances the development of nephrotoxicity, while salt loading of the patient before the administration of amphotericin B protects against the deterioration of renal function without influencing the potassium loss. Amphotericin B-induced tubular damage cannot therefore be regarded as a consequence of altered glomerular function or of ischemia. These observations suggest involvement of intrarenal regulatory mechanism of the tubuloglomerular feedback.

The mechanism of the nephrotoxic action of amphotericin B is not well understood, but it may be related to the interaction with membrane-bound cholesterol to form aqueous channels, increased permeability to small solutes, and decreased electrical resistance at the cellular level. Additionally, amphotericin B nephrotoxicity may be associated with its stimulatory effect on macrophages and their production of the tumor necrosis factor α and interleukin-1.

The improvement in renal function allows treatment to be continued with the full dose of the immunosuppressive agent cyclosporin A and amphotericin B. Treatment with theophylline also alleviates the amphotericin B-induced deterioration in renal function.

Antiviral Agents

During the last decade, an increasing number of antiviral agents were introduced for the treatment of human immunodeficiency virus (HIV) infections and severe systemic infections in immuno-compromised patients. Whereas most of the antiviral agents do not cause nephrotoxicity, some of these agents have been associated with the development of acute renal failure and specific fluid and electrolyte changes. Acyclovir is a cyclic analog of deoxyguanosine that is active against herpes viruses. The administration of large parenteral acyclovir doses resulted in the development of acute renal failure in 10–48% of patients treated. Acyclovir-induced acute renal failure is likely to be due to obstructive nephropathy from intratubular precipitation of acyclovir or a toxic, immunologic, or hypersensitivity reaction. Alteration of the renal function may be detected within the first few days of therapy. Ganciclovir, an acyclic nucleoside analog of guanine, is structurally similar to acyclovir but has no significant nephrotoxicity. Foscarnet is an inorganic pyrophosphate analog that has antiviral activity against herpes viruses and HIV. Foscarnet-induced acute renal failure has been reported in two-thirds of treated patients. Despite the reduction of the dose or discontinuation, azotemia persists and progresses for a few days before resolving. Foscarnet nephrotoxicity is usually associated with mild proteinuria (<1 g/day).

Foscarnet-induced acute renal failure is usually reversible, although recovery may be slow and persist for several months after discontinuation of foscarnet. Foscarnet therapy also causes a number of fluid and electrolyte disturbances, such as polyuria, hypo- and hypercalcemia, hypo- and hyperphosphatemia, and hypermagnesemia.

Immunosuppressive Drugs

Cyclosporin A

Immunosuppressants are indispensable for combating the rejection of transplanted organs and for the treatment of autoimmune diseases. Alkylating agents (cyclophosphamide), anti-metabolites (methotrexate), azathioprine, and cyclosporin A are most commonly used for the suppression of the immune response to bacteria, fungi, and malignant tumors. Cyclosporin A, a cyclic lipophilic peptide (11 amino acids; molecular weight 1202) with a strong immunosuppressive action, was isolated from a soil fungus (*Tolypocladium inflatum*). It is used in autoimmune diseases, in juvenile type I diabetes or in chronic inflammatory intestinal diseases, and for immunosuppressive therapy in heart, lung, or kidney transplants. It is usually used in combination therapy (e.g., cyclosporin A with azathioprine, steroids, and an antilymphocytic antibody), although cyclosporin A plays the key role. It inhibits the release of interleukin-1 from macrophages and reduces the secretion of interleukin-2 from activated T-helper cells. After it has been taken up by the cells, cyclosporin A is bound to cyclophilin and calmodulin. It is thought that the cyclosporin A–cyclophilin complex binds to the promoter region of the lymphokinin gene and inhibits the gene transcription of lymphokinins. It is not certain whether cyclosporin A also blocks the synthesis of interleukin-2 receptors.

After oral administration, between 20 and 60% of the dose is absorbed. In patients with existing liver damage, cyclosporin A absorption is further reduced (bioavailability < 10%) because cyclosporin A, as a strongly lipophilic substance, is very poorly absorbed by patients with liver disease. Cyclosporin A undergoes metabolism via hepatic cytochrome P450, and both hydroxylated and demethylated metabolites are formed and excreted via the bile. The cyclosporin A that is not metabolized in the liver can be taken up into the renal proximal tubule cells, especially in the S3 segment, where it is metabolized by renal cytochrome P450. The elimination half-life for cyclosporin A is 6–8 h and for its metabolites 8–9 h. Because of the extensive metabolism, only metabolites and their conjugates are excreted.

Among the side effects of cyclosporin A (hepatotoxicity, nephrotoxicity, systemic hypertension, and CNS toxicity), the most important is nephrotoxicity. Hyperkalemia with metabolic acidosis and hypomagnesemia are consequences of nephrotoxicity that accompany cyclosporin treatment. The lipophilic properties of cyclosporin A are likely to be responsible for the alterations in the membrane structure and function of kidney cells and the resulting toxic effects.

Both acute and chronic nephrotoxicity occur following cyclosporin A treatment. Under experimental conditions, dose-dependent changes occur with the acute infusion of cyclosporin A, such as an increase in renal vascular resistance, a reduction in the RPF, the SNGFR and in the K_f, with increasing blood pressure. Because these functional changes are not attributable to morphological lesions in the kidney tissue, they are completely reversible on the cessation of treatment. By contrast, chronic cyclosporin A nephrotoxicity is characterized by the persistence of the elevated renal vascular resistance, a marked reduction in the RPF and in the SNGFR, and a reduction in the blood pressure, while the K_f remains constant. This form of nephrotoxicity is not reversible, can progress, and is manifested histologically as arteriolopathy (thickening of the arteriole walls), striated interstitial fibrosis, and glomerular changes (glomerulosclerosis). It is striking that obliterative arteriolopathy develops only in humans and solely in the distal segment of the afferent arterioles.

The mechanism of action of the acute hemodynamic effects of cyclosporin A has not been established for certain. Many experimental findings point to increased renal vascular resistance as the cause of the reduction in the RPF, the GFR and the K_f. In experimental animals, cyclosporin A leads to hyperplasia of the juxtaglomerular apparatus and increases the renin content of the renal cortex, especially in the afferent arterioles. Because cyclosporin A causes both systemic and renal vasoconstriction, it seems at least plausible that the renin–angiotensin system is involved in this and in the development of renal-vascular resistance. The cause may be disturbed equilibrium of local vasoactive substances, such as platelet-activating factor, prostaglandin E, prostacyclin, endothelin, or angiotensin II. Endothelin synthesis may be stimulated by cyclosporin A in the mesangial cells. The vasoconstrictive properties of endothelin cause contraction of the mesangial cells, and it thus intervenes in the regulation of various glomerular functions.

Various drugs, such as phenobarbital, phenytoin, carbamazepine, rifampicin and probably isoniazid, may induce cyclosporin A metabolism resulting in a reduction in the plasma concentration and the resulting nephrotoxicity. Other substances, such as erythromycin, fluconazole, ketoconazole, cimetidine, and verapamil, in contrast, inhibit its metabolism and increase plasma concentration and nephrotoxicity. Aminoglycoside and amphotericin B potentiate or increase nephrotoxicity, whereas platelet-activating-factor antagonists and pentoxifylline show protective effects.

Tacrolismus, a new immunosupressant, has been developed to replace cyclosporin A in human transplantation. Tacrolismus is a carbocyclic lactone-lactam belonging to the class of macrolide lactones with an oral bioavailability of about 27%. Tacrolismus induces renal injury similar to cyclosporin A, such as renal structural alterations, generalized vasoconstriction, impairment of renal function and some increase in systemic blood pressure. Sirolismus, which is still undergoing clinical investigation, has not caused alterations of the renal structure and function similar to those observed with cyclosporin A and tacrolismus.

Anticancer Drug Nephrotoxicity

Cisplatin

Cisplatin (*cis*-diamminedichloroplatinum) is a cytostatic used intensively in the treatment of tumors in

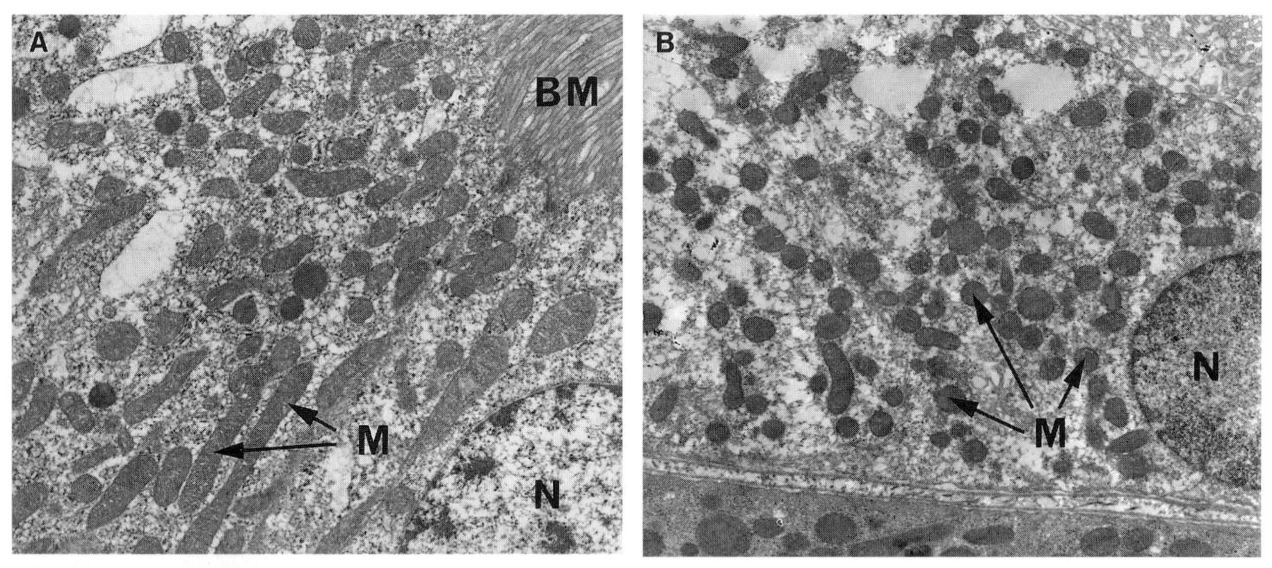

FIGURE 13 Transmission electron micrograph of the S3 segment of the proximal tubule of rats after cisplatin treatment. (A) Control; (B) 3 days after treatment of the rats (5 mg/kg, i.p.). Severe damage to the mitochondria is evident. Abbreviations: BM, brush border; M, mitochondria; N, cell nucleus (× 16,300).

testicular and ovarian cancer; cancer of the bladder, lungs and bones; and tumors in the head and neck region. The antitumor mechanism of action of cisplatin is similar to that of bifunctional alkylating agents, in that the platinum complex and DNA form an irreversible bond that inhibits cell division, especially in the S phase.

Plasma protein binding increases over time after the in travenous administration of cisplatin, reaching 88–90% after just a few hours. Cisplatin is excreted mainly via the kidneys; it undergoes glomerular filtration and is secreted into the tubular cells via the cationic transport system. About 50% of the administered dose is excreted within 24 h, and 76% within 48 h. The elimination half-life for whole platinum is between 30.5 and 107 h with normal kidney function.

Cisplatin accumulates in the tumor tissue, but also in other tissues such as liver and kidneys; high cisplatin concentrations can still be found in the kidneys 2–4 weeks after cessation of the treatment.

Little is known about cisplatin metabolism. It is metabolized to a less toxic, nonmutgenic metabolite, but also to a reactive intermediate that may react with cellular macromolecules. Cisplatin has a high level of antitumor efficacy and, at the same time, a highly toxic action that manifests itself as hematotoxicity, neurotoxicity, ototoxicity, and nephrotoxicity. Among the side effects, dose-limiting nephrotoxicity plays a major role in the treatment of tumors. Its main features are azotaemia, polyuria, and acute renal failure.

In cisplatin nephrotoxicity, the increase in urea and creatinine in the blood, hypomagnesemia, hypokalemia, and hypocalcemia are accompanied by increased excretion of sodium, potassium, glucose, total protein, and the enzymes *N*-acetyl-β-D-glucosaminidase, γ-glutamyltranspeptidase, and alanine aminopeptidase. The incidence of nephrotoxicity is 15–30% of the patients treated. The nephrotoxic action is characterized by both glomerular and tubular damage. With unchanged systemic blood pressure it causes a clear increase in renal vascular resistance and a significant reduction in the GFR and RPF. As micropuncture studies in individual nephrons have shown, in comparison to controls it produces an increase in renal vascular resistance in the afferent and efferent arterioles, reductions of 46% in the glomerular plasma flow, of 10% in the glomerular ultrafiltration pressure, and of 45% in the SNGFR, while K_f remained unchanged. These changes are accompanied by glomerular proteinuria and morphological changes in the structure and function of glomeruli (thickening of the glomerular basement membrane and glomerular proteinuria). Other typical features are degenerative and necrotic damage to the proximal and distal tubular segments, and especially to the S3 segment and the collecting tubule. Under the electron microscope, the cells of the S3 segment show damage, such as loss of the brush border, cell enlargement, cytoplasmic vacuoles, globular mitochondria (Fig. 13), and an increase in the number and size of pinocytotic vesicles and lysosomes. In chronic cisplatin treatment, interstitial fibrosis, cyst formation, and thickening of the tubular basement membrane may also occur. These cisplatin-induced functional and structural alterations appear to be more pronounced in the juxtaglomerular than the cortical nephrons.

The mechanism of cisplatin nephrotoxicity is not fully understood. Cisplatin accumulates in the mitochondria, causing them to swell and producing ultrastructural changes (Fig. 13) plus a reduction in oxygen consumption. The disturbance of mitochondrial respiration is crucially important for the active energy-consuming tubular transport processes and for the development of nephrotoxicity in the early stages of acute renal failure. The results of recent studies suggest that lipid peroxidation is also involved in the development of cisplatin nephrotoxicity. Although a number of antioxidants (such as procaine) and radical scavengers inhibit the formation of lipid peroxides, they offer little or no protection against nephrotoxicity.

Recovery from acute renal failure is accomplished by increased DNA synthesis in renal epithelial cells. Increased thymidine incorporation in DNA occurs simultaneously with the decrease in GFR and polyuria. This temporal relationship, which is also characteristic of mercury chloride-, folic acid-, and gentamicin-induced acute renal failure, could be a causal relationship between cell necrosis, repair, and regeneration and the functional and structural injuries leading to acute renal failure.

Ifosfamide

The alkylating agent ifosfamide, an analog of cyclophosphamide, is a an oxazaphospharine that is very effective in the treatment of a variety of malignant diseases. Liver metabolism of ifosfamide leads to formation of the 4-hydroxy metabolite, which undergoes subsequent metabolism to form an alkylating mustard derivative and acrolein. ARF may occur after one or several courses of therapy and is characterized by a variety of tubular disorders, including mixed proximal and distal tubular acidosis. Impairment of proximal tubule function is most common and usually is present as Franconi's syndrome. The incidence of nephrotoxicity appears to be 10–20% and is more likely to occur in patients previously exposed to or having concomitant cisplatin therapy. The molecular mechanism of nephrotoxicity has not been fully elucidated. Ifosfamide-induced, nephrotoxicity is not prevented by mesna, a synthetic thiol compound, but appears to be reversible in many cases. Ifosfamide is rapidly removed by hemodialysis.

Methotrexate

Methotrexate is an antimetabolite used in the therapy of malignant tumors, such as choriocarcinoma and other trophoblastic tumors. Methotrexate is a dihydrofolate reductase inhibitor. Methotrexate is the drug of choice for the maintenance therapy of acute lymphocytic leukemia. Methotrexate is used in combination therapy with other cytostatics for the treatment of other tumors, such as breast carcinoma, small-cell lung carcinoma, and ovarian tumors.

Methotrexate is well absorbed and concentrates in the liver and biliary tract. Liver metabolism of methotrexate leads to formation of methotrexate–polyglutamates, which can be converted back to methotrexate by hydrolases. These methotrexate–polyglutamates act as inhibitors of dihydrofolate reductase and thymidylate synthetase. Methotrexate is also metabolized to 7-hydroxymethotrexate, which can accumulate in significant amounts when large doses of methotrexate are used. The metabolism is characterized by a considerable enterohepatic recycling and is partially metabolized by intestinal flora after oral administration. Renal excretion is the primary route of elimination and the terminal half-lfe is 8–15 h.

High dosages have been associated with nephrotoxicity, even in the presence of leucovorin, a reduced folate that is co-administered to decrease side effects. Most of the administered dose is protein bound (70%) and is excreted unchanged by the kidney. Methotrexate nephrotoxicity can lead to delayed elimination of the drug and the development of life-threatening toxicity.

Methotrexate is fully ionized at physiological pH, but its solubility is reduced in the acidic environment of the urine. Nephrotoxicity may be due primarily to the intrarenal obstructive nephropathy caused by the precipitation of methotrexate and 7-hydroxymethotrexate, mainly in the distal renal tubule. However, direct glomerular and tubular cell toxicity has been proposed as a mechanism for methotrexate and/or its 7-OH metabolite because decreases in GFR and marked necrosis of the convoluted tubule, without evidence of methotrexate precipitation, have been reported. Close monitoring of the creatinine levels, the hydration state, urine alkalinization, and measurement of plasma methotrexate may help identify those patients at high risk. In preclinical studies, carboxypeptidase-G_2 has been shown to rapidly hydrolyze methotrexate to nontoxic metabolites. Co-administration of carboxypeptidase-G_2, thymidine, and leukovorin was highly effective in reducing nephrotoxicity in patients receiving large doses.

Doxorubicin

Doxorubicin, also known as adriamycin, is a daunorubicin derivative with antitumor properties and belongs to the anthracycline group of antibiotics. The antineoplastic action of doxorubicin is based on intercalation in both of the DNA strands and the formation of an doxorubicin–DNA complex, which leads to the inhibition of DNA, RNA, and protein synthesis for the duration of the entire cell cycle. It is widely used clinically for the treatment of breast tumors, carcinomas of the head and neck, thyroid carcinoma, bladder and bronchial tumors, malignant lymphoma, leukemia, and a large number of sarcomas and carcinomas of the endometrium, the testes, prostate, and cervix. After intravenous administration, the drug quickly reaches the heart, liver, lungs, spleen, and kidneys; but it does not cross the blood–brain barrier. It is metabolized in the liver and other organs to several metabolites; the main metabolite doxorubicinol also has an antineoplastic action, whereas other metabolites, such as doxorubicinone, aglycones, and conjugates, have no therapeutic efficacy.

Doxorubicin is eliminated in several stages. The initial half-life for doxorubicin is 0.6 h, while some metabolites are eliminated with half-lives of 3.3 h, 16.7, and 31.7 h. The fraction bound to plasma protein is eliminated very slowly (half-life 40 h). Only 4–5% of the administered dose appears in the urine unchanged after 5 days.

Doxorubucin's clinical use is limited by its toxic properties, especially its cardiotoxicity. In rats, rabbits, and pigs, doxorubicin leads to a nephrotic syndrome that manifests itself in rats as severe proteinuria, hypoalbuminemia and severe hyperlipidemia. Results of several studies point to glomerular damage as the primary cause of doxorubicin nephrotoxicity. Alterations of tubular structure and function, such as the formation of protein casts and tubular atrophy, are seen more as a direct consequence of the glomerular changes. Chronic treatment results in the development of a progressive nephrotic syndrome, which is characterized by focal and segmental glomerular sclerosis. Glomerular changes affect mainly the juxtamedullary nephrons and involve a progressive lowering of the GFR, accompanied by a reduction in the filtration rate of single nephrons and in the ultrafiltration coefficient.

These changes may be the result of morphological lesions, which reduce the glomerular filtration area. As with puromycin-aminonucleoside nephrosis, the doxorubicin-induced changes to the glomerular capillaries correspond to the typical features of "minimal change" disease in humans, which is characterized by the fusion of epithelial foot processes and subendothelial deposits. Chronic treatment of rats with doxorubicin leads to selective accumulation of the drug in the glomerular epithelial cells, where it causes morphological and physiological changes. The striking feature is that the fusion of the podocyte foot processes occurs before the appearance of proteinuria.

The mechanism of doxorubicin-induced nephrotoxicity has not so far been adequately established. It has numerous toxic effects on various types of cell. It can interfere with protein synthesis in the glomerular endothelial cells and reduce oxygen uptake in the liver mitochondria. Microsomal-metabolizing enzymes, such as cytochrome P450 reductase, can reduce doxorubicin to semiquinone radicals that may trigger the production of reactive oxygen species. The biochemical mechanisms contributing to the development of cardiotoxicity, nephrotoxicity, and nephrocarcinogenicity are considered to be the formation of reactive oxygen species and the production of DNA strand breaks. It has also been suggested that platelet-activating factor and thromboxane B_2 may be involved. Various substances, such as the ACE inhibitor enalapril, inhibitors of 5-lipoxygenase, and platelet-activating-factor antagonists, alleviate or protect against doxorubicin-induced nephrotic syndrome. In patients, cardiotoxicity limits the dose, so that nephrotoxicity is usually not seen.

Analgesics

Ingestion of large amounts of some pain-relieving drugs over long periods of time has been shown to be associated with the development of analgesic nephropathy and eventually kidney failure. Large doses of analgesics, including acetylsalicylate, phenacetin, and combination of these, cause papillary necrosis. Certain evidence suggests that heavy and sustained use of some analgesic mixtures predispose to cancer of the urinary tract, particularly transitional cell carcinoma of the renal pelvis.

Phenacetin

Phenacetin, which was taken off the market years ago, led to interstitial nephritis with papillary necrosis after the chronic ingestion of a cumulative dose of more than 3 kg. Ultimately, infectious destructive pyelonephritis developed and possibly also renal pelvis carcinoma. In the overwhelming majority of cases of "phenacetin kidney," papillary necrosis, and interstitial nephritis were connected with analgesic abuse.

Acetylsalicylate

In many cases analgesic nephropathy was reported when analgesic mixtures containing acetylsalicylate, phenacetin, and caffeine were taken. In clinical studies, phenacetin is thought to be responsible for the renal nephropathy, whereas experimental data in rats implicate acetylsalicylate as the major nephrotoxin, causing the development of renal papillary necrosis. However, acute reversible effects of acetylsalicylate on renal function have been demonstrated in patients with active lupus nephritis. Chronic treatment with aspirin (120–230 mg/kg/day) of female Fischer 344 rats caused renal papillary necrosis and a decrease in urinary-concentrating ability. Aspirin produced injuries to interstitial cells and their matrix, particularly in the mid-papillary region, followed by changes to the thin limbs of the loop of Henle and medullary capillary endothelium. Several prospective clinical studies have been unable to identify a significant risk of chronic renal failure in patients using aspirin alone in therapeutic doses.

Acetaminophen (Paracetamol)

Acetaminophen is used for the treatment of pain and fever. It is an aniline derivative that has an analgesic and antipyretic action, but a weak anti-inflammatory activity. The mechanism of its analgesic action is not fully understood. Acetaminophen inhibits cerebral prostaglandin synthesis more strongly than acetylsalicylic acid, but has less influence on peripheral prostaglandin synthesis. After treatment with high doses, humans and animals may develop acute necrosis of the proximal tubules. Acetaminophen is rapidly and almost completely absorbed from the gastrointestinal tract, maximal plasma concentration being reached within 0.5 to 2 h. Plasma protein binding reaches about 25%, whereas its plasma half-life is between 1 and 3 h. Following overdosage, the plasma half-life of subjects with liver-cell necrosis is over 4 h, and for those in hepatic coma over 12 h.

Acetaminophen undergoes metabolism primarily in the liver although biotransformation also occurs in the kidneys. Acetaminophen metabolites are excreted in the urine as glucuronides, sulfates, or cysteine conjugates. Cytochrome P450, possibly with the involvement of prostaglandin H synthase, metabolizes the drug in the liver and kidneys to reactive metabolites, which are considered responsible for hepatotoxicity and nephrotoxicity. The cytotoxicity is believed to be mediated by formation of the reactive metabolite *N*-acetyl-*p*-benzoquinonimine in renal tubular cells. In addition, acetaminophen can be metabolized in the inner renal medulla by prostaglandin H synthase to *N*-acetyl-*p*-benzoquinonimine.

In this way, acetaminophen (in concentrations 10 times higher in the papillary apices than in the renal cortex) could cause direct damage to the straight arterioles of the kidneys, resulting in ischemia, necrosis, fibrosis, and calcification of the papillae (papillary necrosis).

Renal deacetylation of acetaminophen to produce *p*-aminophenol and its other reactive intermediates may lead to acute tubular cell injury in experimental animals (Fig. 14). *p*-Aminophenol causes necrosis of the pars recta of the proximal tubules in rats. The precise mechanism of this selective toxicity is not known, but it can undergo oxidation to produce a *p*-aminophenoxy free radical. Oxidation or disapropriation of this radical will form 1,4-benzoquinonimine, which can covalently bind to renal tubular macromolecules. It is also known that certain benzoquinol–glutathione conjugates such as 4-amino-3-*S*-glutathionylphenol and 4-amino-2,5-bis-*S*-glutathionylphenol caused renal necrosis that is very similar to that produced by *p*-aminophenol. The dose- and time-dependent loss of cell viability in rat kidney cortical cells induced by these toxic glutathione conjugates was significantly decreased by acivicin, an inhibitor of γ-glutamyltranspeptidase activity. Thus there are a number of routes of metabolism of acetaminophen that can lead to nephrotoxicity.

Radiocontrast Medium Nephropathy

Diagnostic and intervention procedures using radiocontrast media are carried out with growing frequency in elderly patients or in patients with comorbid conditions. Consequently, the contribution of radiocontrast nephropathy to all hospital-acquired acute renal failure has increased to above 30% in recent years. The incidence depends on various factors, such as renal insufficiency, diabetes, congestive heart failure, volume depletion, and the dose of contrast agent. Despite the high frequency of recovery of renal function, the consequences of radiocontrast medium nephropathy are not negligible. Radiocontrast medium nephropathy can result in increased hospital stay and occasional need for dialysis and is likely to increase mortality in patients with preexisting comorbid conditions. In a retrospective analysis of 183 hos-

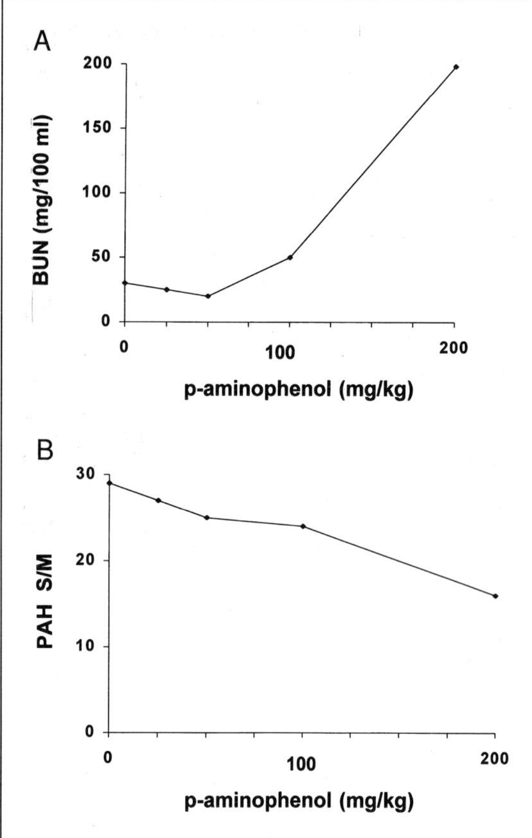

FIGURE 14 Influence of *p*-aminophenol (A) on the concentration of blood urea nitrogen (BUN) and (B) on *p*-aminohippuric acid (PAH) accumulation in renal cortical slices. After 24-h treatment of rats with *p*-aminophenol (s.c.), there is a concentration-dependent increase in BUN (A) and a decrease in PAH accumulation in the renal cortex (B). PAH accumulation is shown as the slice-to-medium ratio (S/M).

pitalized patients, the mortality rate was 34% in patients with radiocontrast medium nephropathy versus 7% in those without.

Serum creatinine concentrations generally peak 4–5 days following exposure to radiocontrast medium and return to normal about 7–10 days after treatment. The radiocontrast medium nephropathy is nonoliguric in most patients. The examination of the urine sediment from these patients reveals granular casts devoid of cellular elements and minimal proteinuria. Following radiocontrast medium exposure, a variety of proximal tubule enzymes, such as the lysosomal enzyme *N*-acetyl-β-D-glucosaminidase, the brush-border enzyme alanine aminopeptidase, and low-molecular-weight proteins (such as α_1-microglobulin and β_2-microglobulin), are excreted into the urine. Tubular obstruction may also play a role in the pathogenesis in some patients. Contrast medium increases urate excretion during the first hours after exposure.

Generally, an immediate decrease in renal blood flow does not occur in well-hydrated patients undergoing exposure to radiocontrast medium. However, changes in renal blood flow can follow after a lag period. Results of various studies indicate that high-osmolality contrast medium decrease renal blood flow and GFR to a greater extent than low-osmolality medium. The decrease in blood flow and oxygen tension leading to medullary ischemia caused necrosis of the medullary thick ascending limbs and was associated with a rise in serum creatinine concentration. Captopril given 20 min prior to contrast medium exposure reduced the decrease in renal blood flow and GFR measured 2 h later. Endothelin, a vasoconstrictor peptide, is normally degraded after filtration by the proximal tubule brush-border enzymes. Urinary endothelin increases following exposure to the contrast medium. Increased urinary excretion of endothelin reflects contrast medium-induced injury to the proximal tubule. Infusion of an antagonist of the endothelin receptor prior to administration of a contrast medium prevents the decrease in renal blood flow seen in the absence of the antagonist.

Immune-Mediated Nephropathy

The kidney can become involved in immune-induced nephropathies through three mechanisms. It can be the primary target of antibody-mediated injury (Good Pasture syndrome), it can be damaged by immune complexes (IgA nephropathies), or it can be injured by immune responses initiated in other organs. Immune complex formation is perhaps the most common form of primary chronic glomerulonephritis and a major cause of end-stage renal failure. The precise mechanism responsible for the IgA nephropathies (Berger's disease) is not known.

There is growing evidence that this type of nephropathy is caused by glomerular depositions of circulating immune complexes containing IgA as the major antibody component in the mesangium. In the majority of cases, the antigens of the circulating immune complexes causing the nephropathy are not of glomerular origin. It is thought that the glomerular mesangium is centrally involved in the pathogenesis of immune-mediated glomerular disease.

Membranous glomerulonephritis associated with gold or penicillamine therapy of rheumatoid arthritis are characterized by the presence of mesangial immune complex deposits, in addition to the basement membrane deposits. Prominent deposition of IgA is associated with proliferative alterations in the mesangium cells and increase in the mesangial matrix. Binding of immune complexes to the mesangial cell may alter cell structure and function in a manner that contributes to the morphological, biochemical, and hemodynamic changes characteristic of glomerular immune injury. The electrostatic charge of the antigen can have an impact on its catabolic rate and affect the distribution of immune deposits in the glomerulus and the potential for immune complex nephropathy.

Heavy Metals

The nephrotoxic effect of metals has been known for many years. The mechanisms whereby these metals produce cellular injury in the kidney varies as a function of the dose, duration of exposure, the chemical species formed, and the intracellular target. Several heavy metals are nephrotoxic because they concentrate in proximal tubular cells to a sufficient degree that they can inhibit essential metabolic processes.

However, there are several mechanisms whereby a renal cell can protect itself, for example by sequestering the metal by means of high-affinity metal-binding proteins, such as metallothionein, or compartmentalization of the metal into lysosomes. The precise mechanism of metal transport into proximal renal tubular cells is not fully understood. Metals can enter by endocytosis following the binding of the metal itself or a metalloprotein complex such as Cd^{2+}-metallothionein to the brush-border membrane. Recent studies have indicated that some metals can enter renal cells as glutathione-derived conjugates by specific transport systems located on both the brush-border and basolateral membranes. Once inside the cell, the metal can be released from the protein by lysosomal degradation. The distribution of the released metal will then depend on the presence of various high-affinity binding sites or sinks in the cell.

After relative high exposure to some heavy metals, the histological pattern of injury is of necrotic proximal tubules with dilatation of the tubular lumen and the presence of proteinaceous casts. The necrosis is thought to be due to a combination of the direct cytotoxic action of the heavy metal, there being a good correlation between the site of localization of the heavy metal and site of morphological damage, and ischemia secondary to vasoconstriction. Chronic salt loading of rats to deplete intrarenal renin, and thereby reduce activation of angiotensin, a potent vasoconstrictor, prior to administration of the heavy metal can protect against the functional impairment but not the extent of necrosis. Thus the nephrotoxicity of heavy metals involves two distinct mechanisms, a vascular component mediated through the release of renin and proximal tubular necrosis, which is due to the accumulation of the metal in cells to a high enough concentration.

Lead

The use of tetraethyllead as an antiknock agent in gasoline engines is decreasing rapidly, although for a long time it was the most important source of accumulating inorganic lead in major cities and alongside motorways. Lead is probably the most abundant nephrotoxic metal. The principal route of exposure is food, but because of industrial exposure (e.g., mining and smelting) and historical exposure in the home (e.g., lead plumbing), there is considerable clinical data.

Lead is ingested in food or by breathing in lead-containing dust, which is absorbed through the gastrointestinal tract. Over 90% of all lead retained in the body accumulates in the bone, where it is released very slowly from these deposits. Lead present in blood is excreted predominantly via the kidneys, with a half-life of about 4 weeks.

Lead-induced nephrotoxicity is characterized morphologically by the presence of lead intranuclear inclusion bodies, karyomegaly, cytomegaly, and ultrastructural changes in mitochondria primarily to the pars recta region of the proximal tubule. Prolonged high-dose exposure leads to a Fanconi-like syndrome with functional changes in glucose, amino acid, and phosphate reabsorption. The majority of lead present in the blood is located in the red cell. Studies in male rats have shown that lead is bound to the protein α2u-globulin, which is synthesized in the liver and transported to the kidney where a proportion is taken up into renal proximal tubular cells. A lead-binding protein in the human kidney has recently been identified as diazapine-binding inhibitor, which has similar properties to α2u-globulin but is not a member of the same gene family. Thus, as with other metals, lead may enter the renal tubular cells by endocytosis and then be released, presumably from secondary lysosomes (Fig. 15).

Once inside the cell, any free metal will initially bind to certain high-affinity lead-binding proteins; two of the main proteins in the kidney are soluble proteins with estimated molecular masses of 11,500 and 63,000 Da, the former having been identified as α2u-globulin. These proteins are thought to carry lead into the nucleus, where *de novo* synthesis of an acidic protein with an approximate molecular mass of 32,000 Da is associated with the lead intranuclear bodies. All of these lead-binding proteins are acidic in nature, possess a high content of aspartate and glutamate res-

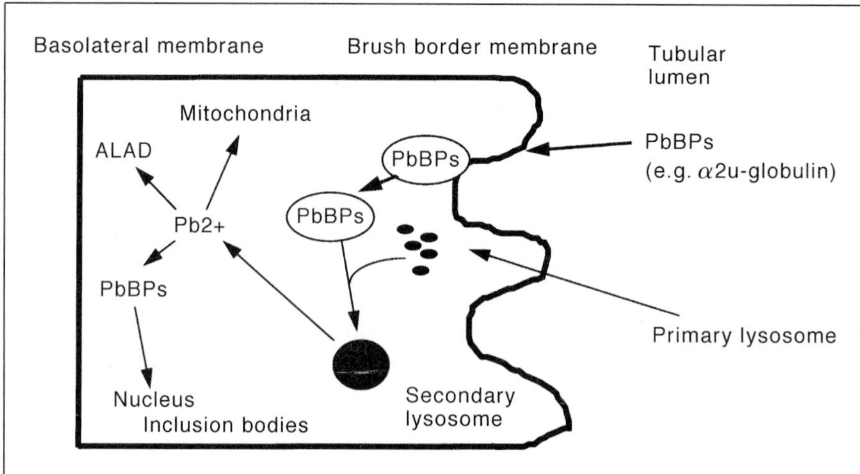

FIGURE 15 Absorption and processing of lead in renal proximal tubular cells. Abbreviations: ALAD, delta-aminolevulinic acid dehydratase; PbPBs, lead-binding protein.

idues, and have K_d values for lead of the order of 10^{-8} M. The lead-binding proteins may make lead bioavailable to lead-sensitive proteins and certain enzymes involved in heme biosynthesis, such as δ-aminolaevulinic acid dehydratase.

The molecular mechanism underlying renal tumor formation in rodents is not well understood. At high doses, lead administration will increase renal proximal tubular cell turnover; however, at doses that did not increase cell turnover, the specific effects of lead have been detected on regulation of the cell cycle. There is some evidence of an apparent increased rate of renal adenocarcinoma in lead-exposed smelter workers.

Whereas chelation therapy effectively reverses acute lead nephropathy, there is no evidence that such therapy reverses established lead-induced interstitial nephritis. Chelation therapy with EDTA should be carried out with caution, especially in patients with serum creatinine levels above 3 mg/dl because it has been reported that $CaNa_2EDTA$ therapy caused alteration of renal function in treated patients.

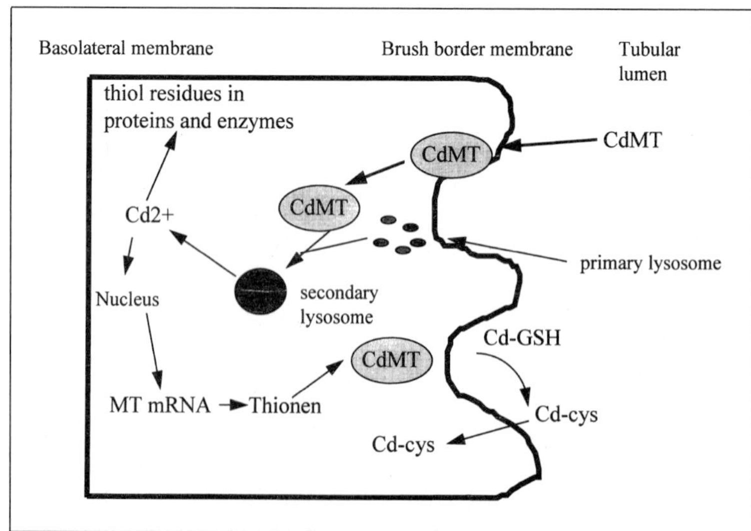

FIGURE 16 Absorption and processing of cadmium in renal proximal tubular cells. Abbreviations: CdMT, cadmium–metallothionein; Cd-GSH, cadmium–glutathione; Cd–cys, cadmium–cysteine.

Cadmium

Damage to proximal renal tubules is a characteristic feature of long-term, but not acute, cadmium exposure in both humans and experimental animals. The primary reason for the long tissue half-life of this metal is its strong binding to the protein metallothionein. The Cd^{2+}–metallothionein complex is then thought to be gradually released from the liver and taken up by the kidney via endocytosis into renal proximal tubular cells, where free Cd^{2+} can be generated due to lysosomal degradation of the complex (Fig. 16). Proximal tubular cells can synthesize metallothionein in response to an intracellular increase in Cd^{2+} concentration and the onset of renal injury may reflect a saturation of all available binding sites in the cell. The kidney is able to accumulate large concentrations of Cd^{2+}–metallothionein without obvious damage until a critical concentration of about 100–200 μg/g renal cortex is attained, at which time renal damage starts to appear. The toxic species that precipitates the renal injury is almost certainly free cadmium. The administration of Cd^{2+}–metallothionein to rats produces a marked nephrotoxicity at much lower doses than does Cd^{2+}, per se. Similarly, administration of Cd^{2+} bound to either GSH or cysteine produced very selective toxicity to the pars recta of the proximal tubule, suggesting that the metal complexed in this form may be actively transported into renal tubular cells. In these more acute models, considerably more Cd^{2+} is delivered to the kidney than in low-level chronic exposures, so that the defense mechanisms such as induction of metallothionein may not be adequate to afford protection.

Severe microproteinuria occurs in cadmium workers when urinary Cd^{2+} concentration exceeds 20 μg Cd^{2+}/g creatinine. When exposure of cadmium workers was reduced below 20 μg Cd^{2+}/g creatinine, microproteinuria was substantially decreased. Results of recent animal studies have shown that *meso*-2,3-dimercaptosuccinic acid can increase biliary excretion of cadmium, while high doses of ascorbic acid can be effective in protection against cadmium-induced nephrotoxicity.

Mercury

The kidneys contain the highest concentration of mercury following exposure to inorganic salts of mercury and mercury vapor, while organic mercury has a greater affinity for the brain.

The nephrotoxicity produced by inorganic mercury salts such as $HgCl_2$ has been extensively studied in experimental animals as a model of acute renal failure. Functional impairment probably results from both vasoconstriction, mediated through the release of renin, and a direct cytotoxic effect of the metal. Small acute doses of $HgCl_2$ in the rat produces a distinct band of necrosis to the pars recta of the proximal tubules extending into the medullary rays. The location of the lesion along the nephron correlates to the localization of the metal. As the dose of $HgCl_2$ is increased, the lesion spreads to the pars convoluta in line with the localization of the mercury along the nephron.

Chronic low-level exposure to mercury will also produce renal injury; however, the total dose of Hg^{2+} accumulated in the kidney is much higher than after an acute nephrotoxic dose. The precise biochemical mechanism whereby $HgCl_2$ produces renal damage is unclear. Mercury will readily react with thiol residues in proteins and enzymes, analogous to Cd^{2+}, and thereby inhibits cellular function.

After acute exposure, metallothionein will avidly bind Hg^{2+} and seems to have little protective effect against the toxicity; but after chronic exposure induction of this protein in the liver will probably contribute to the delivery of the complex from the liver to the kidney and play a role in protecting the proximal tubular cell against injury by inducing its synthesis (Fig. 17). Recent studies have suggested that GSH conjugation of inorganic mercury plays an important role in delivering the chemical to brush-border membrane following filtration at the glomerulus. In the tubular lumen, the Hg–GSH conjugate undergoes sequential metabolism to afford the Hg–cysteinylglycine and Hg–cysteine conjugate, which can then enter renal proximal tubular cells via a neutral amino acid transport system. Support for this mechanism comes from studies where acivicin, a potent inhibitor of γ-glutamyltransferase located on the brush-border membrane of proximal tubular cells, significantly reduces the amount of mercury accumulated by the renal cortex.

In addition, there is evidence to indicate that Hg–GSH or one of its metabolites (Hg–SR) can enter renal tubular cells via an organic anion transport system (*p*-aminohippuric acid-sensitive) located on the basolateral membrane of the proximal renal tubular cell (Fig. 17).

The earliest pathological changes following $HgCl_2$ are loss of brush-border membranes, dispersion of ribosomes, and clumping of smooth endoplasmic reticulum membranes in the cytoplasm. These are followed by the appearance of vacuoles in the cytoplasm and clumping of nuclear chromatin; mitochondrial changes appear to be a late event in the necrotic process. Studies with isolated brush-border membrane vesicles have shown that $HgCl_2$ will inhibit glucose

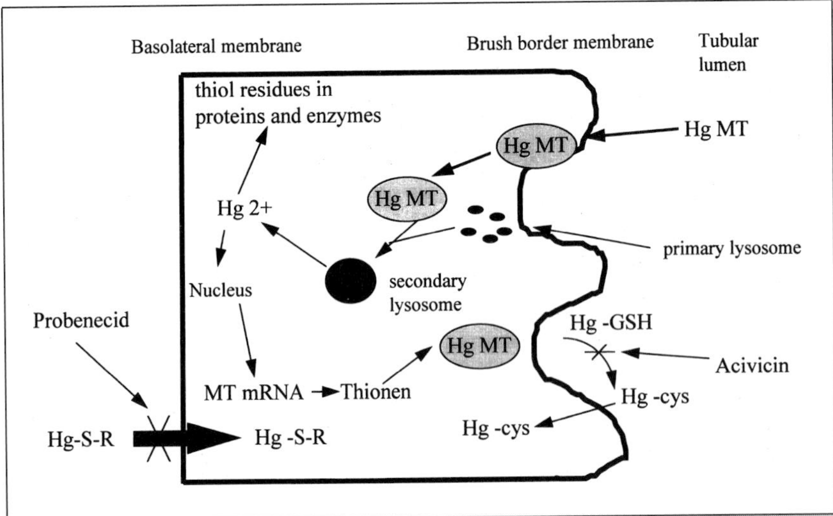

FIGURE 17 Absorption and processing of mercury in renal proximal tubular cells. Abbreviations: HgMT, mercury–metallothionein; Hg-GSH, mercury–glutathione; Hg-cys, mercury–cysteine; Hg-S-R, metabolite of Hg-GSH.

transport by these membranes at a time when no effects are seen on basolateral membrane vesicle function.

Organomercurials

The primary action of organomercurials is on the nervous system; however, they can undergo decomposition, albeit quite slowly, to form Hg^{2+} and produce renal injury. For example, in the methylmercury epidemic in Iraq, polyuria, oliguria with urinary casts, and excretion of albumin were reported, whereas in the more extensive epidemic with methylmercury the kidneys were spared even in the severely affected patients. Nevertheless chronic exposure of rodents to methylmercury will result in renal injury, the location of the lesion being similar to that produced by a single does of inorganic mercury.

Mercury-Induced Glomerulonephritis

Mercury has been reported to produce an immunologically mediated glomerulonephritis in both humans and experimental animals. Studies in rats have shown that the chemical form of mercury does not influence the outcome. The autoimmune response is under genetic control, the Brown Norway rat being the strain most studied. The administration of $HgCl_2$ to this strain of rat produces an increase of circulating IgE, IgG and antiglomerular basement membrane antibodies. These latter antibodies can be found deposited along the glomerular capillary wall and their occurrence is associated with proteinuria and the nephrotic syndrome. The cause of this glomerulonephritis is not well understood.

Glomerular lesions can be produced in other strains of rat; however, the immune response is different from that seen with the Brown Norway rat, being characterized as an immune-complex-type glomerulonephritis with the presence of antinuclear antibodies.

Petroleum Hydrocarbons

Exposure to unleaded gasoline, a variety of light hydrocarbons present in gasoline and some unrelated chemicals, such as *d*-limonene, have been shown to produce a nephropathy in male rats. Following acute exposure, the nephropathy is seen as an excessive accumulation of protein droplets in epithelial cells of the proximal tubule above that normally seen in the male rat kidney, with a concomitant accumulation of tubular casts at the corticomedullary junction and evidence of increased mitotic figures in the proximal convoluted tubule. This response is only observed in male rats; female rats and mice, dogs, and monkeys of either sex do not show this nephropathy. Chronic exposure of male rats to unleaded gasoline, a number of jet fuels, certain industrial chemicals (e.g., 1,4-dichlorobenzene, isophorone, and perchloroethylene), and natural products (*d*-limonene) results in an accelerated increase in the normal chronic progressive nephropathy seen in older male rats, increased foci of atypical hyperplasia, and an increased incidence of late onset renal tumors.

Studies on the mechanism of pathogenesis have shown that the protein that accumulates in the proximal tubular cells is α2u-globulin, a low-molecular-weight protein that is primarily synthesized in the liver of adult male rats, freely filtered at the glomerulus, and only partially reabsorbed by proximal tubular cells. Female rats excrete less than 1% of the amount of α2u-globulin excreted by males; this is due to the repression of synthesis by estrogen. The basis for the accumulation of this protein is due to the reversible binding of the chemical or a metabolite to the protein. This ligand–protein interaction will survive tissue homogenization and centrifugation, and equilibrium-binding studies have shown K_d values for the binding of metabolites of 2,2,4-trimethylpentane and *d*-limonene to α2u-globulin of about 5×10^{-7} M. It is this complex that is taken up into renal tubular cells, primarily in the pars convoluta by endocytosis. These ligand–protein complexes appear to be very resistant to lysosomal degradation and accumulate in phagolysosomes, which on chronic exposure develop into polyangular droplets.

The precise mechanism of cell death is not fully understood; it may be secondary to the release of lysosomal enzymes from the engorged lysosomes or due to a build up of the chemical liberated from the protein complex. However, with increasing dose and time, cell death occurs and this is followed by repair and regeneration. The presence of high concentrations of α2u-globulin is a necessary component in the toxic process. The nephropathy can be produced in transgenic male mice, which have be engineered to express α2u-globulin. In initiation–promotion studies, it was shown that both unleaded gasoline and *d*-limonene act as promotors of *N*-ethyl-*N*-hydroxyethylnitrosamine-initiated renal tumors. However, *d*-limonene does not promote renal tumor formation in the α2u-globulin-deficient rat.

Humans do not synthesize α2u-globulin and by inference would not be expected to be at risk. Detailed studies have shown that human members of the lipocalin family do not bind chemicals that cause the α2u-globulin nephropathy, and further that the human proteins are more rapidly excreted and degraded by the kidney. Recent detailed X-ray crystallographic studies of the binding site or pocket on α2u-globulin have enabled comparisons to be made with other proteins in the superfamily, which show that α2u-globulin has a unique shape and nature for its ligand binding site. Overall, these mechanistic studies have provided clear evidence that this form of renal injury and carcinogenicity seen in strains of male rats that express high levels of α2u-globulin is not relevant to humans.

Hydrocarbon-Induced Glomerulonephritis

A casual association between hydrocarbon exposure and development of glomerulonephritis has been suggested from case reports and from case control studies, and many of the cases exhibited linear IgG deposits and circulating antiglomerular basement membrane antibodies. However, many of the major case control studies conducted to examine hydrocarbons as a possible etiological factor in chronic renal disease have not provided any consistent evidence to definitively implicate hydrocarbons as a cause of chronic renal disease.

Halogenated Hydrocarbons

Halogenated hydrocarbons represent a large group of both aliphatic and aromatic haloalkanes and haloalkenes with diverse applications in industry, agriculture, medicine, and public health. These chemicals may be used as anesthetics, industrial solvents, pesticides, starting products, or by-products formed in the manufacture of other chemicals. The major routes of exposure in the work place tends to be via inhalation or dermal contact; however, the public may be exposed in certain situations when these chemicals are released into the environment or detected in drinking water. Most of the chlorinated compounds are chemically stable and require renal biotransformation to afford metabolites that are directly toxic. Alternatively, metabolites may be formed in the liver and then delivered to the kidney, where they can undergo further metabolism to chemically reactive species.

Two main mechanisms of toxicity will be discussed, one where the chemical undergoes metabolism by cytochrome P450 in the proximal renal tubular cells to produce toxicity and the second where the chemical undergoes extrarenal conjugation with GSH and is then delivered to the kidney where it undergoes activation.

Haloalkanes

Chloroform

Chloroform was once used as an anesthetic but now is used as an industrial solvent and as an intermediate in the manufacture of certain polymers. Low

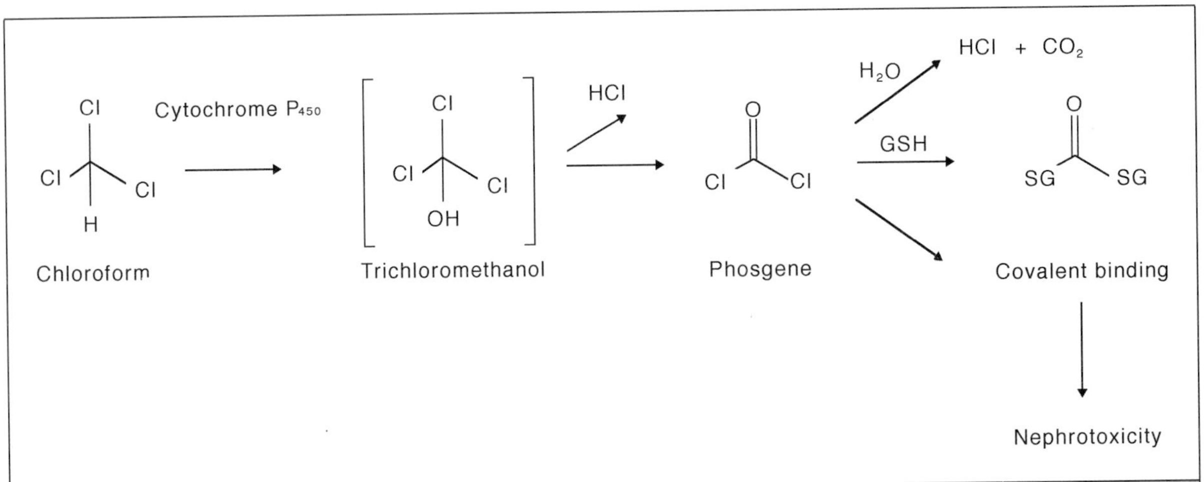

FIGURE 18 Oxidative metabolism of chloroform leading to renal injury.

levels have also been detected in drinking water following chlorination. Chloroform is both hepatotoxic and nephrotoxic in most mammalian species, including humans. The acute nephrotoxicity of chloroform is species, strain, and sex dependent, which is particularly marked in mice. For example, male mice of the ICR strain are susceptible to chloroform-induced renal injury while females are resistant.

Human exposure to chloroform has been associated with oliguria, proteinuria, elevated blood urea nitrogen, and proximal tubular necrosis. A similar response is seen in experimental animals.

Chloroform undergoes metabolism via cytochrome P450 2E1 (and perhaps other isoforms) to CO_2 in humans and experimental animals following oral administration, and it is the formation of phosgene, which can degrade to CO_2, that is believed to be the toxic species (Fig. 18). Renal cortical slices from rats, rabbits, and male (but not female) mice can metabolize $^{14}CHCl_3$ to $^{14}CO_2$. Evidence that this metabolism is cytochrome(s) P450-dependent is that it requires NADPH and O_2, that it can be inhibited by carbon monoxide and metyrapone, and that $^{14}CDCl_3$ is metabolized more slowly and is less nephrotoxic than chloroform itself. Thus, in the kidney chloroform can undergo oxidative dechlorination catalyzed by cytochrome P450 to give phosgene. This reactive metabolite may then react with GSH and thereby become inactivated or react with critical cellular macromolecules in proximal tubular cells to cause cellular injury.

The marked sex and strain differences in chloroform-induced nephrotoxicity in the mouse appears to be due to the relative rates of cytochrome P450-dependent metabolism. Male mice have about a fivefold higher concentration of renal cytochrome P450 than female mice. Modulation of the renal content of cytochrome P450 by hormonal treatment can modulate the nephrotoxicity; for example, testosterone treatment of female mice can alter the renal cytochrome P450 profile to a more male-like pattern and thus render them susceptible to chloroform-induced nephrotoxicity.

In many species, the primary target organ for chloroform toxicity is the liver. This is presumably due to the higher concentration of hepatic cytochrome P450 2E1, and hence its ability to form the chemically reactive metabolite at higher concentrations in hepatocytes. However, following chronic low-level exposure to chloroform, an increased incidence of renal tumors in male rats and in one study female mice has been reported. The precise mechanism of carcinogenicity is not fully understood, but the formation of toxic metabolites in renal proximal tubular cells does result in an increased cell turnover that may be an important factor in the carcinogenic process.

1,2-Dichloroethane (Ethylene Dibromide)

1,2-Dichloroethane is used mainly as an intermediate in the production of vinyl chloride and a number of other industrial chemicals. Exposure in the work place is mainly by inhalation. Cases of human exposure resulting in renal injury have been reported, with oliguria, albuminuria, and elevation in blood urea nitrogen. Renal tubular degeneration appeared to be localized to the proximal tubule. Acute or subacute inhalation exposure to a number of species of experimental animal results in renal injury, although when given in the drinking water the extent of renal injury is much less.

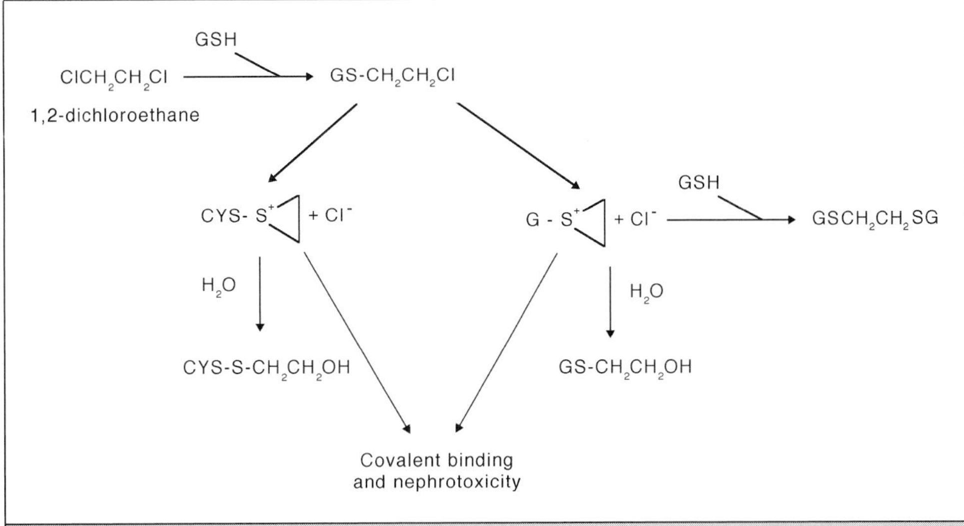

FIGURE 19 Glutathione *S*-transferase-dependent metabolism of 1,2-dichloroethane, leading to renal injury.

There are two main pathways of metabolism for 1,2-dichloroethane, oxidation by cytochrome P450 2E1 and conjugation with GSH. Both pathways may occur in the kidney, but it is currently thought that formation of the GSH conjugate, which can rearrange to form a reactive episulphonium ion (Fig. 19) is the pathway resulting in toxicity. The GSH conjugate may be formed in the liver and then delivered to the kidney, where it can undergo further metabolism to the cysteine conjugate (*S*-2-chloroethylcysteine), which can concentrate in proximal renal tubular cells and also rearrange to form a reactive episulphonium ion and lead to cytotoxicity.

Haloalkenes

Several haloalkenes have wide industrial use, such as trichloroethylene, tetrachloroethylene, and tetrafluoroethylene, or are by-products of their synthesis, such as heaxachloro-1,3-butadiene. All these compounds and several other structurally related analogs have been shown to produce renal injury in experimental animals. Some of the early observations arose when soybean meal was extracted with hot trichloroethylene, which led to the formation of *S*-(1,2-dichlorovinyl)-L-cysteine, which in turn produced aplastic anemia and nephrotoxicity when fed to young cattle. Subsequent studies in rats showed that *S*(1,2-dichlorovinyl)-L-cysteine is nephrotoxic, a single dose producing necrosis to the proximal tubules and altered renal function. The mechanism was shown to involve metabolism of this compound by the enzyme cysteine conjugate β-lyase, resulting in cleavage of the C-S bond and transfer of the sulfur to the haloalkene moiety, which rearranges to form a chemically reactive species (Fig. 20). Subsequent studies with hexachloro-1,3-butadiene have shown that this chemical, which in the rat produces selective necrosis to the pars recta of the proximal tubules, undergoes conjugation with GSH primarily in the liver and is then transported to the kidney.

Delivery to the kidney involves a complex series of steps involving enterohepatic circulation. The GSH conjugate may be filtered at the glomerulus and undergo further metabolism by enzymes located on the brush-border membrane to form the cysteine conjugate that may then enter the proximal renal tubular cell via an amino acid transport system. The conjugate can also be delivered to the kidney via the basolateral membrane, probably as the *N*-acetylcysteine conjugate, where it can enter the renal tubular cell via a probenecid-sensitive transport system. Once concentrated within cells of the proximal tubule, the mercapturic acid can undergo de-acetylation to afford the cysteine conjugate, which is a substrate for cysteine conjugate β-lyase, leading to the formation of an electrophilic chlorothioketene metabolite. Much of the chemical evidence to support this hypothesis has been established using rodent liver or kidney subcellular fractions, isolated cells or slices, and perfused organs and selective inhibitors. These include acivicin, which inhibits γ-glutamyltransferase and hence the processing of GSH-derived conjugates; amino(oxy)acetic acid, which inhibits the pyridoxal phosphate-dependent

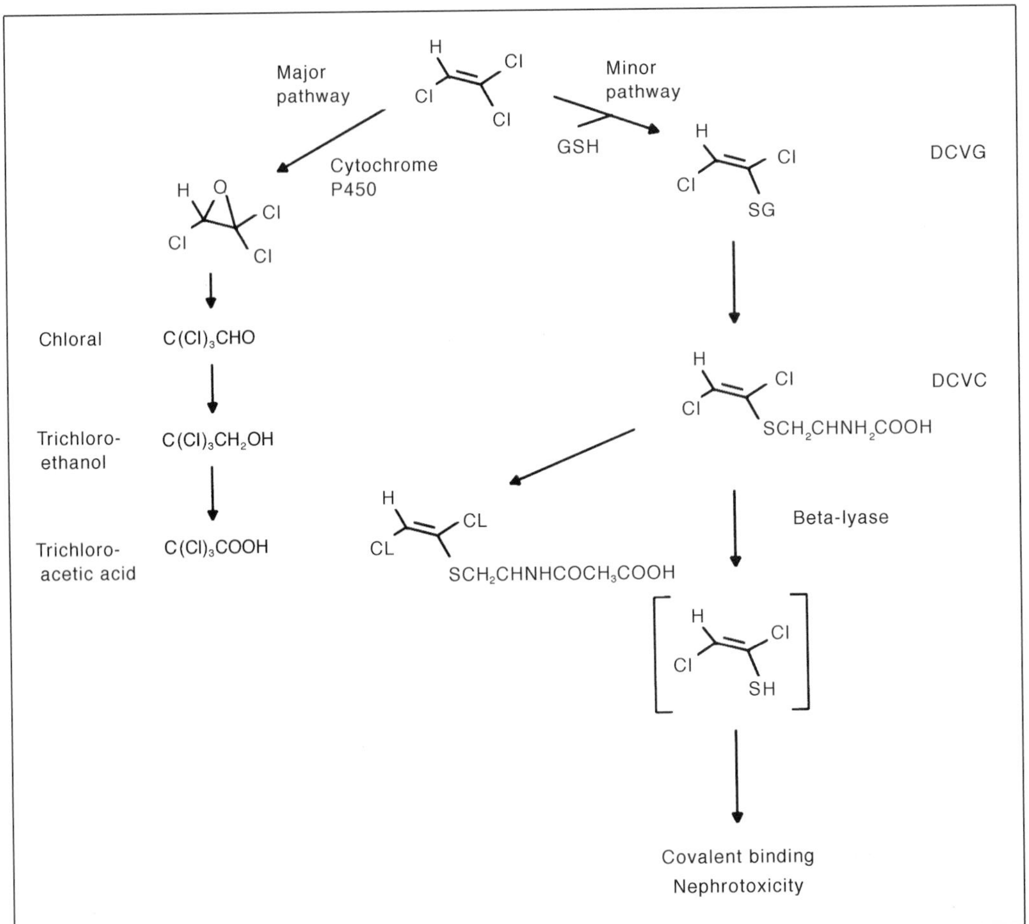

FIGURE 20 Glutathione *S*-transferase-dependent metabolism of trichloroethylene.

enzyme cysteine conjugate β-lyase and hence the formation of the chemically reactive species; and probenecid, an inhibitor of the renal organic anion transport system, which blocks the accumulation of the chemical into the renal cell.

The mechanism of cell death is believed to be due to inhibition of mitochondrial energy metabolism, and it is the intramitochondrial localization of cysteine conjugate β-lyase, which appears to be a different isoform from that located in the cytosol, that is responsible for the local generation of the reactive metabolite. Mechanistic studies have reported a series of findings in the cascade of events that leads to cell death, such as increases in transcription of certain genes such as *Hsp70*, c-fos, and c-myc, loss of mitochondrial membrane potential, changes in intracellular Ca^{2+}, loss of ATP, and lipid peroxidation.

Some of the reactive metabolites formed will also react with DNA and are mutagenic in *in vitro* assays, such as the Ames bacterial mutagenesis assay. Many of these chemicals have also been reported to cause a small increase in the incidence of renal tumors in rodents. The precise basis for the formation of these tumors is not fully understood. One mechanism may involve the formation of GSH conjugates of these chemicals *in vivo*. However, their rate of formation is often very low, relative to other pathways of metabolism, such as by cytochrome P450. Thus, the formation of reactive genotoxic metabolites will be very small and they may be rapidly detoxified. Another mechanism may be related to a chemically induced increase in the rate of degeneration and regeneration of proximal tubular cells, which may lead to the promotion of initiated cells and the formation of preneoplastic foci. Some of these chemicals have also been reported under certain conditions to cause the accumulation in male rats of the protein α2u-globulin, which has been linked to renal tumor formation (see the section on petroleum hydrocarbons). It may be a combination of these various pathways or a new, as yet undiscovered mechanism.

Acute nephrotoxicity in humans due to these chemicals is very rare. It is chronic low-level exposure that has been of concern. However, many occupational-exposure studies of workers exposed to tri or tetrachloroethylene have provided only very limited evidence of an increased incidence of nephropathy or an increased incidence of renal cancer. All of the metabolic pathways described above are present in humans, but their overall rate of metabolism relative to rodents is much lower.

Haloaromatic Compounds

One of the best studied compounds in this class is bromobenzene, which is toxic to the liver, lung, and kidneys of both mice and rats. The metabolism of bromobenzene is extensive with multiple reactive metabolites being formed. The hepatotoxicity is thought to be due to the formation of bromobenzene-3,4-oxide. This metabolite is not, however, formed by the kidney, and, although bromobenzene-3,4-oxide formed in the liver can enter the bloodstream and be delivered to the kidney, it has been suggested that renal GSH-transferases will rapidly detoxify the epoxide and thereby protect the kidney from injury. Subsequent studies have shown that the pathway of metabolism responsible for the renal injury is via *o*-bromophenol and 2-bromohydroquinone and its conjugation with GSH.

2-Bromohydroquinone is readily oxidized to the corresponding 1,4-benzoquinone and in the presence of GSH gives rise to a series of mono- and di-substituted conjugates. One of these conjugates, 2-bromo-bis(glutathion-*S*-yl) hydroquinone, is a very potent nephrotoxic metabolite, producing a lesion to the pars recta of the proximal tubules in the rat identical to that seen with bromobenzene, but at about one-thousandth of the dose.

Conjugation of 2-bromohydroquinone with GSH ultimately leads to the conjugate being delivered to the kidney, where it can be further metabolized by γ-glutamyltransferase to afford the cysteine conjugate and then enter renal tubular cells. The subsequent metabolism does not appear to involve cysteine conjugate β-lyase; as inhibition of this enzyme with amino(oxy)acetic acid afforded no protection against 2-bromo-bis(cystein-*S*-yl) hydroquinone-induced nephrotoxicity. The formation of the cysteine conjugate (2-bromo-bis(cystein-*S*-yl) hydroquinone) does, however, lead to a chemical that is more readily oxidized than either 2-bromohydroquinone, itself, or the GSH conjugates. The precise mechanism of cellular injury has not been fully elucidated, but studies *in vitro* with isolated renal proximal tubular cells or with renal cell lines have shown that the di-substituted GSH conjugate causes DNA strand breaks and it has been suggested that this may reflect the formation of quinone-thioether-derived hydroxyl radicals.

A role for reactive oxygen species in 2-bromo-bis(glutathion-*S*-yl) hydroquinone-mediated cytotoxicity and DNA single-strand breaks is supported by findings that the treatment of cells with catalase or deferoxamine affords protection. Thus in isolated renal cells, the cytotoxicity of the bis-GSH conjugate of bromobenzene seems to be linked to the generation of hydrogen peroxide and the subsequent iron-mediated formation of hydroxyl radicals, resulting in DNA strand breaks. Covalent binding of reactive metabolites to renal proteins and mitochondrial injury have been observed, but they do not appear to be early events in the toxicity.

In summary, certain nephrotoxic halogenated hydrocarbons appear to mediate their toxicity following conjugation with GSH. This then leads to either non-enzymatic or enzymatic formation of a metabolite that is chemically more reactive than the parent compound.

Bibliography

Anders, M. W., Dekant, W., Henschler, D., Oberleithner, H., and Silbernagl, S. (eds.) (1993). "Renal Disposition and Nephrotoxicity of Xenobiotics." Academic Press, San Diego.

Bennett, W. M. (1996). Insights into chronic cyclosporin nephrotoxicity. *Int. J. Clin. Pharmacol. Ther.* **34,** 515–519.

Bennett, W. M. (1997) Drug nephrotoxicity: an overview. *Renal Failure* **19,** 221–224.

Choudhury, D. and Alzmed, Z. (1997). Drug-induced nephrotoxicity. *Med. Clin. N. Am.* **81,** 705–717.

Cojocel, C., Dociu, N., Maita, K., Pasino, D. A., Kuo C.-H., and Hook, J. B. (1983). Metabolic heterogeneity of the proximal and distal kidney tubules. *Life Sci.* **33,** 855–861.

Cojocel, C., Dociu, N., Maita, K., Sleight, S. D., and Hook, J. B. (1983) Effects of aminoglycosides on glomerular permeability, tubular reabsorption, and intracellular catabolism of the cationic low-molecular-weight protein lysozyme. *Toxicol. Appl. Pharmacol.* **68,** 96–109.

Cojocel, C., Hannemann, J., and Baumann, K. (1985) Cephaloridine-induced lipid peroxidation initiated by reactive oxygen species as a possible mechanism of cephaloridine nephrotoxicity. *Biochim. Biophys. Acta* **834,** 402–410.

Commandeur, J. N. M, and Vermeulen, N. P. E. (1990). Molecular and biochemical mechanisms of chemically-induced nephrotoxicity: A review. *Chem. Res. Toxicol.* **3,** 171–194.

DeBroe, M. E., Porter, G. A., Bennett, W. M., and Verpooten, G. A. (1998) "Clinical Nephrotoxins." Kluwer Academic Publishers B.V., Dordrecht, The Netherlands.

Dekant, W. and Vamvakus, S. (1996). Biotransformation and membrane transport in nephrotoxicity. *Crit. Rev. Toxicol.* **26,** 309–334.

Fowler, L. M., Moore, R. B., and Lock, E. A. (1991). Nephrotoxicity of 4-aminophenol glutathione conjugate. *Hum. Exp. Toxicol.* **10,** 451–459.

Goldstein, R. S. (ed.) (1997). "Comphrensive Toxicology, Vol. 7, Renal Toxicology." Pergamon Press, New York.

Goyer, R. A. (1991). Toxic effects of metals. *In* "Casarett and Doull s Toxicology" (M. O. Amdur et al., eds.), 4th ed. pp. 623–680. McGraw-Hill, New York.

Hard, G. C., and Whysner, J. (1994). Risk assessment of *d*-limonene: An example of male rat-specific renal tumourigens. *Crit. Rev. Toxicol.* **24,** 231–254.

Hook, J. B., and Goldstein, R. S. (eds.) (1993). "Toxicology of the Kidney," 2nd ed. Raven Press, New York.

IPCS CEC (1991). "Environmental Health Criteria 119. Principles and Methods for the Assessment of Nephrotoxicity Associated with Exposure to Chemicals." World Health Organisation, Geneva

Kaloyanides, G. J. (1991). Metabolic interactions between drugs and renal tubulointerstitial cells: Role in nephrotoxicity. *Kidney Int.* **39,** 531–540.

Kanwar, R. G. (1984). Biology of disease: Biophysiology of glomerular filtration and proteinuria. *Lab. Invest.* **51,** 7–21.

Kessel, R. G., and Kardon, R. H. (1979). "Tissues and Organs: A Text-Atlas of Scanning Electron Microscopy." W. H. Freeman and Company, San Francisco.

Kramer, W., Cojocel, C., and Mayer, D. (1988). Specific alterations of rat renal microsomal proteins induced by cephaloridine. *Biochem. Pharmacol.* **37,** 4135–4140.

Lau, S. S. (1995) Quinone-thioether-mediated nephrotoxicity. *Drug Metab. Rev.* **27,** 125–141.

Lauwerys, R. R. (1991). Occupational toxicology. *In* "Casarett and Doull's Toxicology" (M. O. Amdur et al., eds.), pp. 947–969, 4th ed., McGraw-Hill, New York.

Lock, E. A., and Reed, C. J. (1998). Xenobiotic metabolizing enzymes of the kidney. *Toxicol. Pathol.* **26,** 18–25.

Marquardt, H., and Schäfer, S. G. (eds.) (1994) "Lehrbuch der Toxikologie." BI-Wiss.-Verlag, Mannheim.

Miano-Mason, T. M. (1997). Mechanisms and management of amphotericin B-induced nephrotoxicity. *Cancer Pract.* **5,** 176–181.

Monks, T. J. and Lau, S. S. (1992). Toxicology of quinone thioethers. *Crit. Rev. Toxicol.* **22,** 243–270.

Pits, R. F. (1976). "Physiology of the Kidney and Body Fluids." Year Book Medical Publishers Inc., Chicago.

Rush, R. F., Smith, J. H., Newton, J. F., and Hook, J. B. (1984). Chemically induced nephrotoxicity: Role of metabolic activation. *CRC Crit. Rev. Toxicol.* **13,** 99–160.

Smith, J. H. (1986). Role of renal metabolism in chloroform nephrotoxicity. *Comments on Toxicology* **1,** 125–144.

Tune B. M., Hsu, C. Y., and Fravert, D. (1996). Cephalosporin and carbacephem nephrotoxicity. Role of tubular cell uptake and acylating potential. *Biochem. Pharmacol.* **51,** 557–561.

Ullrich, K. J., Rumrich, G., and Fritzsch, G. (1992). Substrate specificity of the organic anion and cation transport systems in the proximal renal tubule. *In* "Progress in Cell Research" (E. Bamberg and H. Passow, eds.), Vol. 2, Elsevier, Amsterdam/New York.

CHAPTER

15

Respiratory Tract

HARTWIG MUHLE*, ROGER O. MCCLELLAN†

*Fraunhofer Institute of Toxicology and Aerosol Research, Hannover, Germany

†Chemical Industry Institute of Toxicology, Research Triangle Park, North Carolina

THE LUNG AS A TARGET ORGAN FOR INHALED TOXIC MATERIALS

The lung is the organ where the exchange of oxygen and carbon dioxide between the air and the vascular system takes place. The inhaled air is transported via the conductive airways to the pulmonary region (see Fig. 1), which has a huge inner surface area. This large surface area is favorable to the gas exchange, but is also a point of entry for "toxic" substances suspended in the inhaled air.

Humans are absolutely dependent on the quality of the surrounding air, as they can stop breathing for only a short time. For the assessment of the health-affecting potential of the inhaled pollutants, for example, in hazardous situations (chemical accidents, fires), the concentration and the toxicological properties of the airborne substances have to be known.

Inhalative uptake is of importance for both occupational and environment exposures. On average, a human breathes daily about 15,000 liters of air. This figure, however, varies depending on body weight and activity. Dust particles can enter the body together with inhaled air and, depending on their physicochemical properties, can have a long residence time in the lung. Typical examples are quartz and coal particles, which have been found in the lungs of miners many years after exposure. For a toxicological assessment of occupational diseases, the consideration of inhalation exposure is important. The lung is usually the target organ for inhaled toxicants, but it can also be the target organ for toxic effects by other routes of administration. This pattern of effect is termed "lung toxicity." The lung can also serve as a portal of entry for toxicants reaching other organs. For example, exposures to high levels of benzene produce leukemia and high levels of vinyl chloride result in liver cancer.

Beyond the essential involvement in gas exchange and delivery, the respiratory tract carries out other vital functions. These functions include its role as an elaborate biochemical system that aids in olfaction and in detoxification (decreasing toxic acitivity) or activation (increasing toxic activity) of inhaled chemicals. The respiratory tract also has immunological capabilities, serves as a blood reservoir, and plays a key role in acid–base balance. Each of these vital functions capabilities may be altered by inhaled materials, including particulate matter.

Inhalation toxicology covers the following aspects:

- Physical and chemical characteristics of airborne materials.
- Anatomy and physiology of the respiratory tract.
- Dosimetry of inhaled materials.
- Pathobiology of the respiratory tract.

This chapter on the respiratory tract is organized according to this sequence. The major elements of inhalation toxicology are depicted schematically in Fig. 1, with mechanistic linkages between sources, exposure, dose, and response for airborne materials. The understanding of the mechanistic linkages provides a basis for the evaluation of the potential health risks of airborne materials, as well as for the identification of related research needs. These concepts are also critical to the design, conduct, and interpretation of specific experiments. A further aspect covered in this chapter

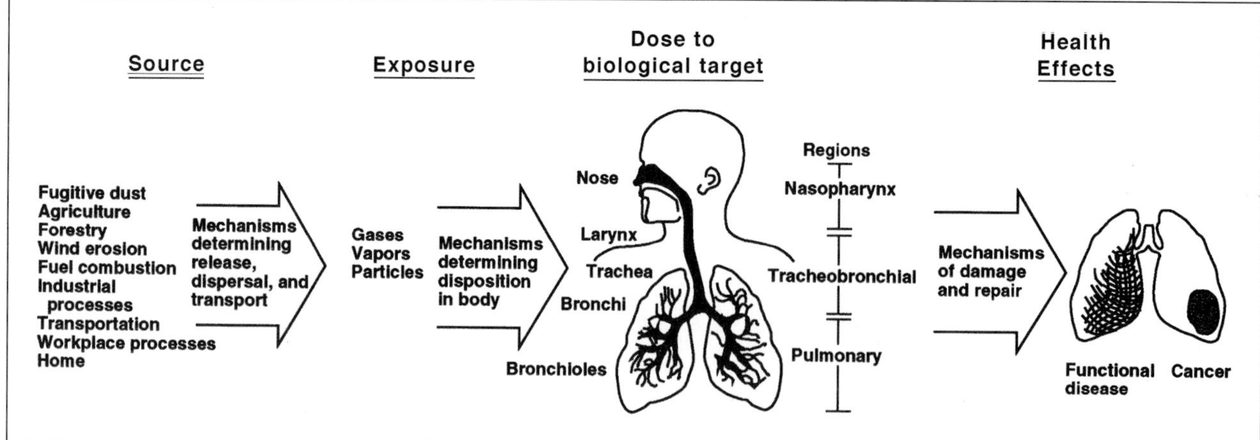

FIGURE 1 Schematic representation of the major elements of inhalation toxicology oriented toward understanding the toxicity of airborne materials. From *Concepts in Inhalation Toxicology*, pp. 3–21, McClellan. Taylor & Francis, Washington, DC. Reproduced with permission. All rights reserved.

is the experimental setup of animal exposure systems and test strategies.

One of the ultimate goals of inhalation toxicology is the assessment of risk to humans exposed to airborne materials. According to the National Research Council of the United States (1983) the following steps have to be addressed:

- Hazard identification.
- Exposure assessment.
- Exposure → dose → response assessment.
- Risk characterization.

Approaches to answering some of these issues include epidemiological studies, investigations using

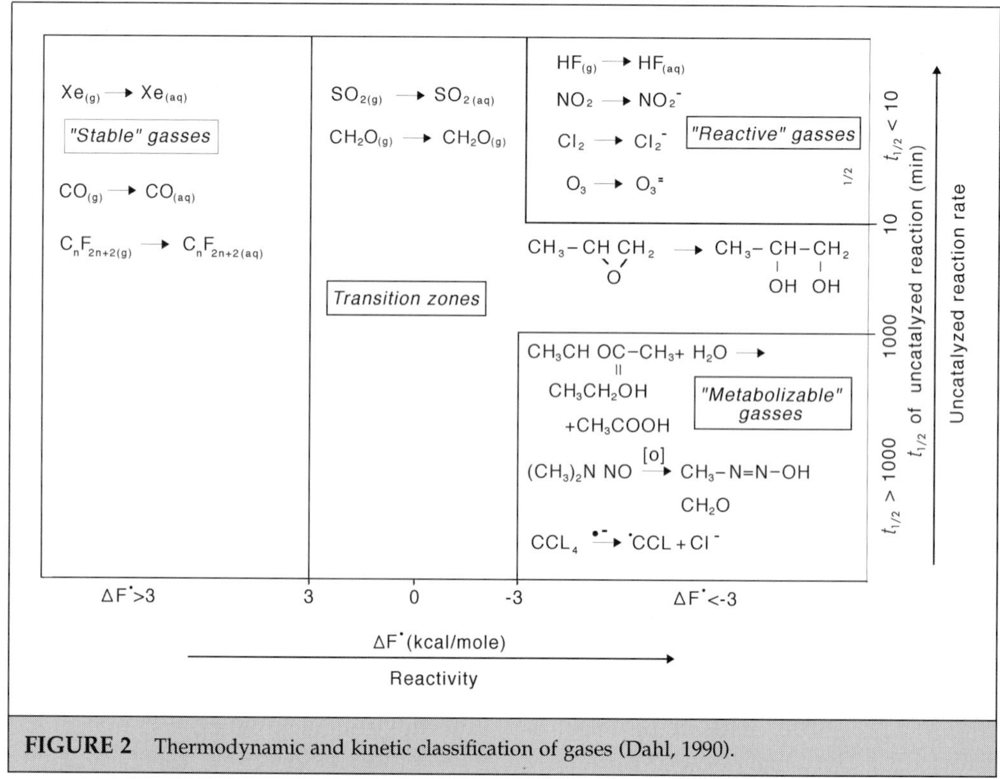

FIGURE 2 Thermodynamic and kinetic classification of gases (Dahl, 1990).

experimental animals, and research using cell and tissue cultures.

Toxicity databases for chemical substances are being developed to try to understand and ultimately prevent adverse health effects. Data from the direct study of humans are preferred when such data are available. However, when human data are not available on airborne materials, animal studies are the next best alternative. This is the case because the unique aspects of inhalation exposure cannot be directly reproduced in cell culture and tissue culture systems and exposure–response relationships applicable to the respiratory tract cannot be obtained from the *in vitro* systems. Extrapolation to humans is in many cases not an easy task and is one of the challenges in toxicology.

PHYSICAL AND CHEMICAL CHARACTERIZATION OF AIRBORNE MATERIALS

Hazardous substances that can enter the body via inhalation are divided into two broad categories. (1) gases and vapors and (2) aerosols, which are suspensions of liquid or solid particles in air.

Gases and Vapors

One usually distinguishes between gases and vapors. Gases are substances that are completely suspended in air on a molecular scale, whereas vapors are special gases that are in equilibrium with the corresponding liquid or solid phase at room temperature. Generally a high substance pressure of a toxic substance increases the hazard. The concentration, the duration of exposure, the water solubility of gases, and their reactivity with biological components govern the location and amount of uptake in the respiratory tract. For example, formaldehyde is primarily resorbed in the upper airways due to high water solubility, whereas ozone reaches the deep parts of the lung.

The solubility of gases in liquids is characterized by Henry's law, which relates the equilibrium vapor pressure, $p_{a'}$, of a gas above a liquid surface and the molar concentration, x_a, of the substance dissolved in the liquid phase:

$$p_a = Hx_a \cdot \tag{1}$$

The Henry constant H for the solubility of a gas in water for SO_2 is, for example, about 100 larger than the value for ozone.

In addition to water solubility, thermodynamic characteristics in biological media and reactivity govern the effects of gases in the respiratory tract. According to Dahl (1990) the free energy of the reaction, ΔF, and the half-times of the uncatalyzed chemical reaction in physiological systems can be used for classification of the reactivity of gases in the respiratory tract (Fig. 2). In this scheme the gases are called thermodynamically stable when $\Delta F > 3$ kcal/mol. Examples of stable gases are xenon, CO_2, and saturated fluorohydrocarbons (Fig. 2). Their effect (narcosis) is not dependent on their reactivity but on their solubility in the fluids and membranes of the body.

Gases characterized by $\Delta F < -3$ kcal/mol and by a fast uncatalyzed reaction ($t_{1/2} < 10$ min) are called reactive according to this scheme. In this case no enzymes need to be involved. Examples are HF, NO_2, Cl_2, and O_3.

Gases are called metabolizable if enzymes are needed. Typically, the $t_{1/2}$ for metabolizable gases is >1000 min. Examples are CCl_4, dimethylnitrosamine, and ethyl acetate (Fig. 2).

Aerosols

Single aerosol particles are characterized by their size, shape, and density. The morphology of particles is a very important parameter, as it may influence deposition, retention, and the mechanisms of lung damage. An example is the role of the shape of fibers such as asbestos. The transportation and deposition of particles in the respiratory tract are strongly influenced by the aerodynamic behavior of particles in flowing gases. The aerodynamic properties of particles are characterized by the concept of the "aerodynamic diameter," d_{ae}, and density. This quantity is defined by the diameter of a unit density sphere ($\rho_o = 1$ g/cm^3), which settles in air at the same velocity as the particle under consideration. For spherical particles larger than 2 μm the relationship between the aerodynamic diameter, d_{ae}, and the geometric diameter, d_g, is given by

$$d_{ae} = d_g \sqrt{\frac{\rho_g}{\rho_o}}, \tag{2}$$

where ρ_g is the material density of the aerosol particles and ρ_o the unit density of 1. For particles between 0.5 and 2 μm the Cunningham slip correction factor $C(d)$, which is a function of the diameter, is applied, which takes into account the thermal diffusion of the particles (Brownian motion). The more general formula is

$$d_{ae} = d_g \left[\frac{\rho_g C(d_g)}{\rho_o C(d_{ae})} \right]^{05}. \tag{3}$$

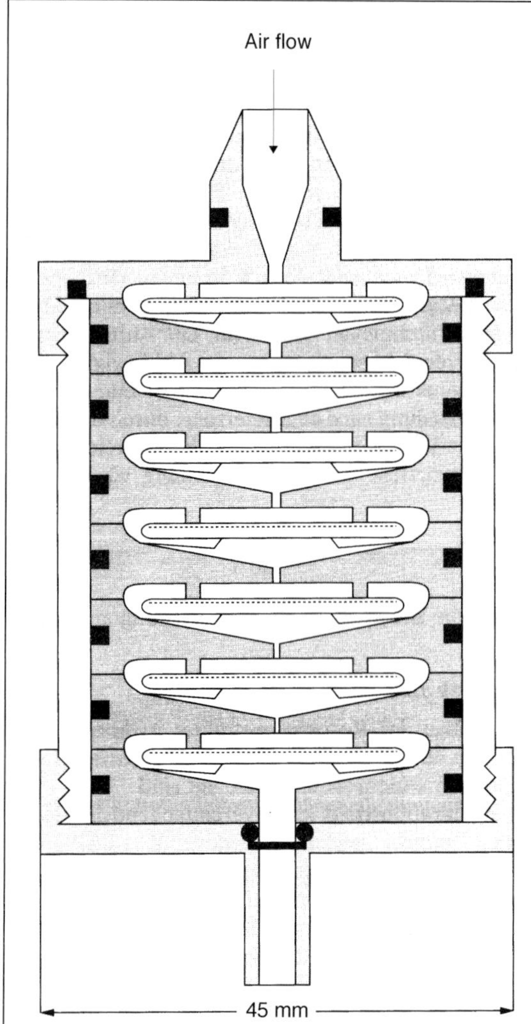

FIGURE 3 Cascade impactor used for the analysis of the aerodynamic diameter. An aerosol is pulled through a system of nozzles that become smaller stepwise. The particulates are deposited depending on their sizes on plates that are below the nozzles. Reprinted from *J. Aerosol. Sci.* **1**, Mercer *et al.*, A multi-stage, low flow rate cascade impacter, pp. 9–15, with kind permission from Elsevier Science Ltd., The Boulevard, Langford Lane, Kidlington OX5 1GB, UK.

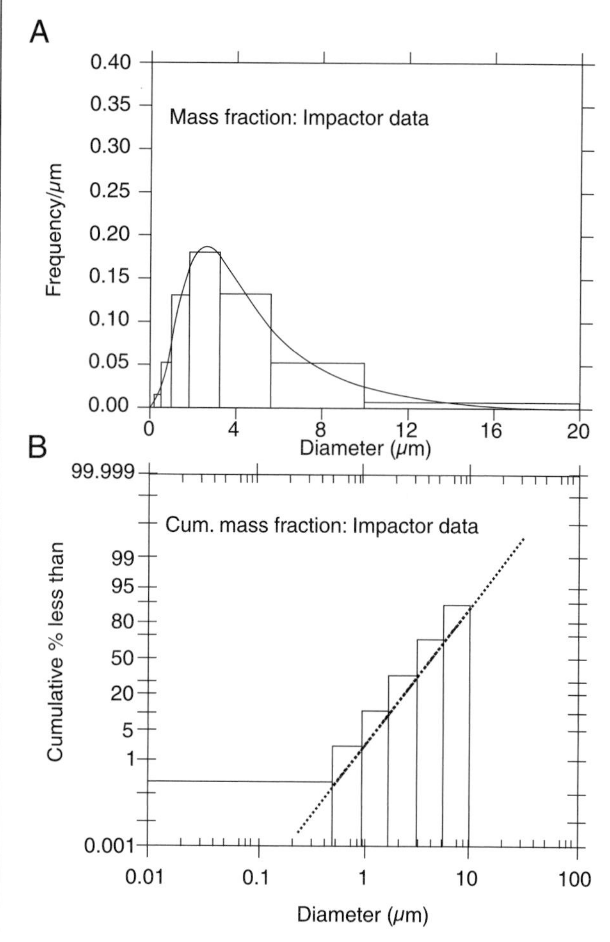

FIGURE 4 Characteriziation of an aerosol by cascade-impactor measurements. (A) Sampled mass fraction in dependence on the particle diameter. (B) Cumulative mass fraction depending on the logarithm of the diameter. The 50% volume represents the mass medium aerodynamic diameter. From *Concepts in Inhalation Toxicology*, pp. 91–128, Moss and Cheng. Taylor & Francis, Washington, DC. Reproduced with permission.

For the purpose of inhalation toxicology, the most important data that quantify the population of aerosol particles in air are the mass concentration and the particle size distribution of the suspended phase. The most widely used method of determining the mass is gravimetric analysis. This is done usually by filtration of the aerosol and weighing the filter. Special sampling devices have been developed to distinguish between different size fractions of the suspended dust. Important fractions are the inhalable particulates, defined as particles with a size that allows them to potential enter the respiratory tract, and the respirable fraction, particles with a size that allows them to potential reach the gas-exchange region of the lung. The definitions of these fractions are described in the context with threshold limit values (TLV) in the booklet of the American Conference of Governmental Industrial Hygienists (1996). However, it is important to recognize that the inhalable- and respirable-size fractions for laboratory animals are different from those for humans.

Usually, the particulates are not monodisperse; that is, they do not have all the same diameter. Very often the diameters of the particles can be quite well described by a log normal function. A standard apparatus for measuring the mass distribution of an aerosol as a function of the aerosol diameter is the cascade impactor (Fig. 3). The principle of this device is to draw an aerosol through a system of nozzles that become stepwise smaller. The flow hits plates below the nozzles. The impaction surfaces are treated with sticky materials serving as dust collectors. The flow velocity increases from stage to stage in the cascade impactor. The size classification is determined by the competition between inertial and friction forces acting on the particles. The larger particles cannot follow the stream of the gas flow and are impacted on the plates. By this principle, the largest particles impact on the first stage and the smaller particles are captured on the later ones. By weighing the plates, the deposited mass is determined.

Figure 4 shows an example for a size distribution extracted from an impactor measurement. The upper part is the density distribution, that is, the mass fraction per size unit as a function of the aerodynamic diameter. The cumulative distribution is presented in the lower part of the figure as a function of the logarithm of the aerodynamic diameter. Here, the y axis is transformed according to the Gaussian probability function. For a log normal distribution, a straight line is obtained for this kind of representation. The distribution is characterized by the median and the geometric standard deviation δ_g.

The geometric standard deviation is calculated from the 50% and 84.1% values of the distribution:

$$\delta_g = \frac{84.1\%}{50\%}. \tag{4}$$

This quantity gives information on the width of the size distribution of the aerosol.

ANATOMY OF THE RESPIRATORY TRACT

According to a proposal of the International Standards Organisation (ISO), the three main compartments are the extrathoracic (E), tracheobronchial (B), and alveolar (A) compartments.

- The extrathoracic compartment (sometimes referred to as nasopharyngeal) comprises the nose, mouth, nasopharynx, oropharynx, and larynx.
- The tracheobronchial compartment comprises the trachea, bronchi, and terminal bronchioles.
- The alveolar compartment (sometimes referred to as pulmonary) comprises the respiratory bronchioles, alveolar ducts, alveolar sacs, and alveoli.

In humans the right lung is slightly larger than the left lung and is divided into three lobes; the left lung has two lobes. Rats have only one lobe in the left lung and four lobes in the right lung. The structure of the respiratory tract is complex, involving over 40 different cell types.

Extrathoracic Compartment

Species differences exist in the size and volume of the nasal cavity, in the luminal surface area, and in the size and complexity of turbinate structures. The percentage of the area covered by the olfactory epithelium in rats, mice, rabbits, and dogs is much higher than that in humans. This difference might be important for the interpretation of inhalation toxicity studies. In rats the respiratory epithelium contains ciliated cells, goblet cells, basal cells, cuboidal cells, nonciliated columnar cells, and brush cells. The physiological functions of the nose include warming up and humidifying inhaled air and filtering coarse particles. The fraction of deposition of coarse particles is significantly higher in the rat nose than in the human nose. As the relative surface area of the nose in rats is higher than that in humans, resorption of water-soluble gases is greater in this animal species.

Tracheobronchial Compartment

A schematic drawing of the anatomy of the tracheobronchial compartment is presented in Fig. 5. The trachea divides into two main bronchi and these continue to divide up to 16–20 times in humans. The inner lining of the bronchi is covered by epithelial cells; among them are ciliated cells, mucus-secreting goblet cells, serous cells, basal cells, and nonciliated bronchiolar epithelial cells (Clara cells). Brush cells and neuroendocrine cells are found to a lesser extent. The synchronization of the ciliary beat is essential to the unidirectional movement of the mucus, which is transported by ciliary activity toward the pharynx. By this mechanism, deposed particles can be removed from the tracheobronchial compartment and leave the body after swallowing via the GI tract ("ciliary clearance"). The tracheobronchial compartment of rodents shows some characteristic structural differences from that of humans. Whereas in humans symmetrical divisions into smaller bronchi exist, in rodents a highly asymmetric branching is seen. The number of generations of branching in rats is lower than that in humans.

Alveolar Compartment

This part of the lung is also shown in Fig. 5. The terminal airways consist of the respiratory bronchioles, alveolar ducts, and alveoli, with a dramatic increase in the cumulative surface. The extent of transi-

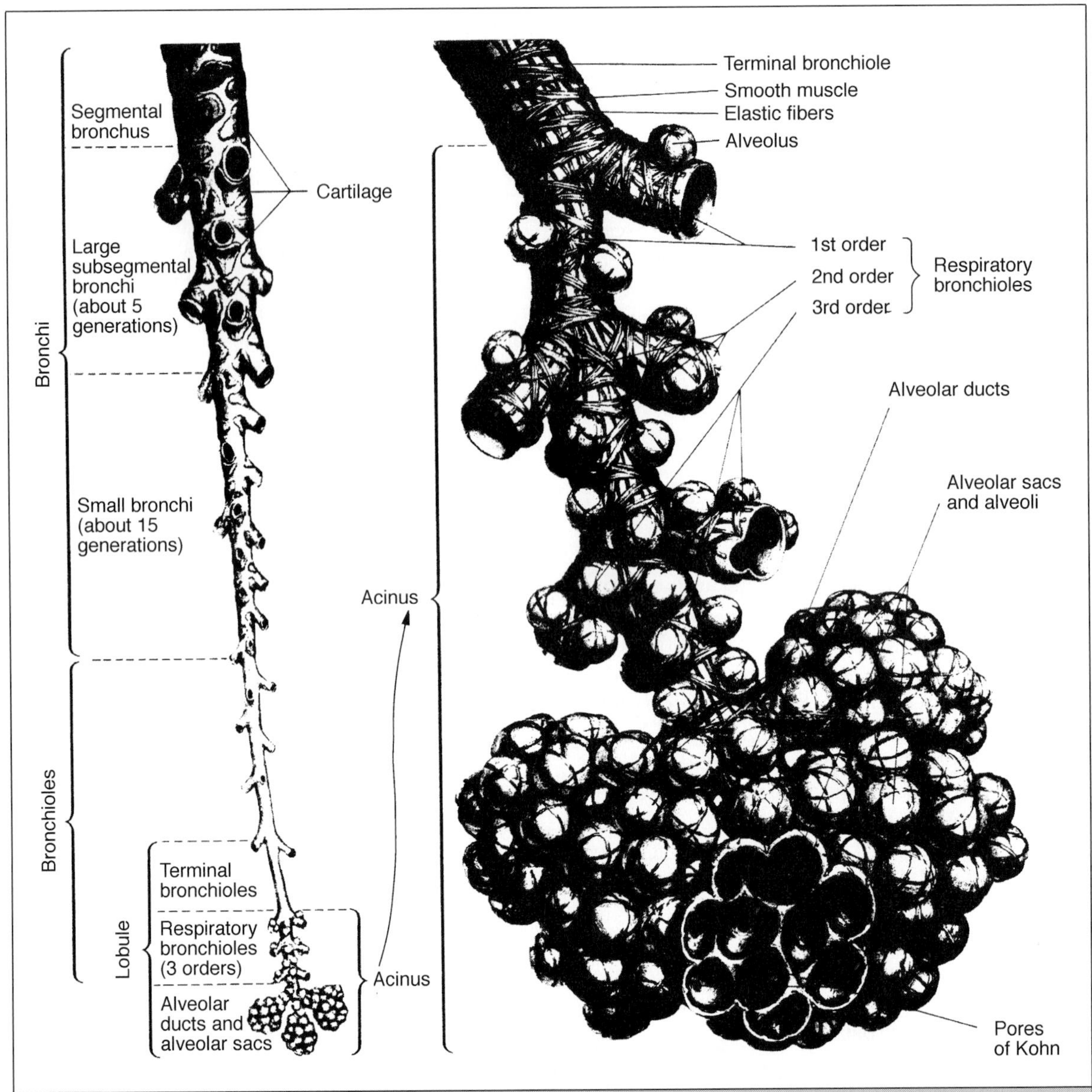

FIGURE 5 Bronchi, bronchioles, alveolar ducts, and alveoles. Bronchi divide about 20 times to the bronchioles. (Copyright 1979. Novartis. Reprinted with permission from *The Netter Collection of Medical Illustrations, Vol. 7,* illustrated by Frank H. Netter, M.D. All rights reserved.)

tional or respiratory bronchioles varies significantly in different species. Whereas in humans and dogs this transitional zone is well developed, it is only poorly developed in the lungs of rodents. In humans the respiratory bronchioles are a significant location of airway diseases. The respiratory bronchioles lead to more than 10 million alveolar ducts, which in turn lead to more than 500 million alveoli.

The diameter of a single human alveolus is 200–300 μm. The total area of gas exchange is about 100 m^2, which is roughly 50 times more than the surface of the skin. The gas exchange takes place primarily in the alveoli, which are separated by very thin septae containing the blood capillares (Fig. 6). For the diffusion of gases, the surfactant, the alveolar epithelium, basement membranes, and the vascular endothelium have to be passed. The diameter of this layer is about 0.4–2.5 μm.

The surface of the alveoli is covered by two epithelial cell types, which are called alveolar type I and alveolar type II cells. The alveolar type I cells are very thin, have a smooth surface, and cover about 90% of

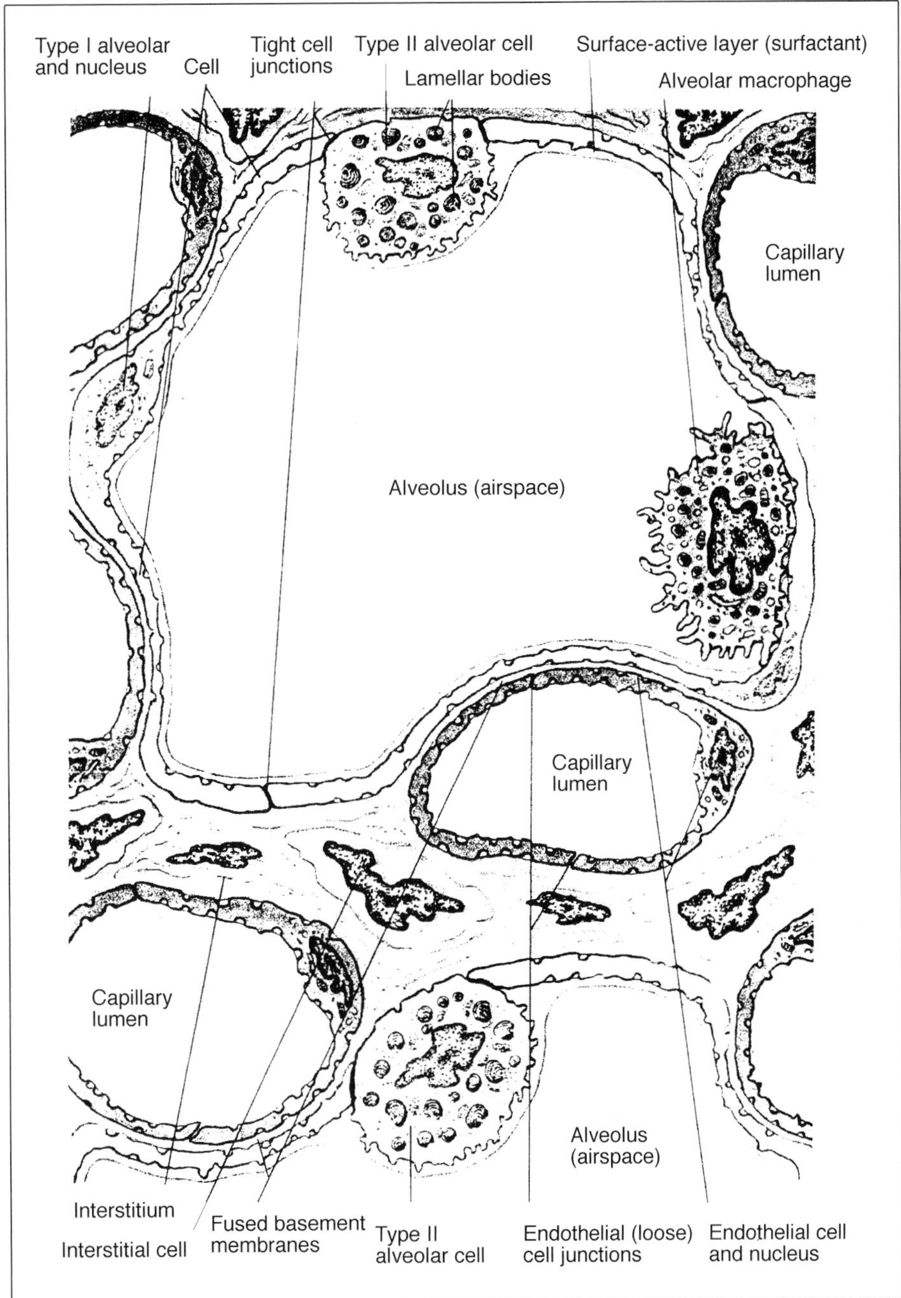

FIGURE 6 Ultrastructure of pulmonary alveoli and capillaries. (Copyright 1979. Novartis. Reprinted with permission from *The Netter Collection of Medical Illustrations, Vol. 7*, illustrated by Frank H. Netter, M.D. All rights reserved.)

the surface of the alveoli. Alveolar type II cells are cuboidal and are more numerous, but they cover only about 10% of the surface of alveoli. These cells contain granules that form the surfactant lining film after secretion. The surfactant reduces significantly the surface tension of the alveoli and is therefore important for the pulmonary mechanics. Because of their large surface area, type I cells are vulnerable to noxious agents; they can be replaced by type II cells, which then differentiate to type I cells.

The alveolar macrophage is a cell type that phagocytoses inhaled particles and that can migrate from the alveolar region to the ciliated airways. A dominant role of the macrophage is taking up and killing infectious agents. This cell type plays a central role in the immune response and inflammatory reactions in the lung (e.g., by secreting cytokine).

LUNG FUNCTION TESTS AND BRONCHOALVEOLAR LAVAGE

Lung Function Tests

Pulmonary function tests allow nondestructive measurements to assess the functional impact of inhaled noxious agents. These types of tests, together with histopathological evaluations, allow an integrated assessment of structure and function. One unique value of nondestructive functional tests relates to the opportunity to make serial temporal observations of the progression of disease in individual subjects. Principal measurements include respiratory frequency, lung volume changes during ventilation, airway compliance and resistance, forced expiration, nitrogen washout test (uniformity of distribution of ventilation), and the efficiency of the gas exchange process (see Table 1). The extended lung function tests especially, using involuntary pulmonary maneuvers, provide endpoints with higher sensitivity than measurements of spontaneous respiration because changes are detected at maximum attainable flow rates and lung volumes. These lung function measurements can be made in humans as well as in experimental animals. Methods for measuring these parameters in laboratory animals are described by Costa and Tepper (1988), Mauderly (1995), and Hoymann and Heinrich (1997). Some reference values of different species are presented in Table 2.

In an obstructive airway disease, the expiratory flow is reduced, for example, by a temporal or persistent decrease of the diameter of the airways. With restrictive disorders, lung inflation is restricted, for example, by an increase of the "stiffness" of the lung, as in fibrosis. A diffusion disorder can be caused by the loss of surface area, thickening of the diffusion path by fluid accumulation, cellular infiltration, and membrane thickening. Inhomogeneity of ventilation is observed in regional uneven distributed airway obstruction (e.g., fibrosis).

The basic ventilatory characteristics as defined in Table 1 can be changed for example, by sensory irritation or impairment in gas exchange.

TABLE 1 Physiological Endpoints Used in Toxicity Studies

Term	Definition
Basic ventilatory characteristics	
Tidal volume (V_T)	Volume of inhaled or exhaled air per breath
Respiratory frequency	Number of breaths per minute
Minute volume	Volume of air exchanged per minute
Lung volumes and capacities	
Vital capacity (VC)	Volume of air that can be exhaled after maximum inspiration
Residual volume (RV)	Volume remaining in lungs after maximum inspiration
Functional residual capacity (FRG)	Volume of air remaining in lungs at the end of a tidal volume
Total lung capacity (TLC)	Total volume of air in the lungs after maximal inspiration
Respiratory mechanics	
Lung resistance	Transpulmonary pressure difference divided by the flow rate difference
Dynamic compliance	Volume difference divided by transpulmonary pressure difference
(Quasistatic) compliance (C, C_{qs})	Elasticity of the lung measured by volume–pressure curves $C = \Delta v/\Delta p$
Forced expiratory volume in 1 second (FEV_1)	Maximum exhaled volume in 1 second
Forced expiratory flow at 10 to 75% of FVC ($FEF_{10...75}$)	Maximum expiratory flow at different lung volumes
Blood gas analysis and diffusion tests	Information on gas-exchange impairment
Nitrogen washout test	Information on inhomogeneity of distribution of ventilation

Bronchoalveolar Lavage

The analysis of fluid obtained by lavage of the lungs of experimental animals has been found to be a very useful procedure in studies that examine the effects of inhaled pollutants on lung structure and function. Both nasal and bronchoalveolar lavage are frequently used as diagnostic procedures in human clinical medicine and have also been used in animal investigations. In rodents, the procedure is usually performed in excised lungs. Measured parameters are protein content and differential cell count (alveolar macrophages, polymorphonuclear leukocytes, and lymphocytes). Indicators of cytotoxicity in the respiratory tract are enzymes such as lactate dehydrogenase, acid phosphatase, and glutathione reductase. The protein content of the lavage fluid is a very sensitive indicator of pulmonary edema.

TABLE 2 Breathing Characteristics of Commonly Studied Species[a]

Species	Body weight (g)	Frequency (breaths/min)	Tidal volume (ml)	Minute ventilation (ml)
Human				
Rest	70,000	12	750	9000
Light exercise		17	1700	28,900
Dog	10,000	20	200	3600
Monkey	3000	40	21	840
Guinea pig	500	90	2.0	180
Rat	350	160	1.4	240
Mouse	30	180	0.25	45

[a]From Kennedy and Valentine (1994), with permission.

UPTAKE AND ELIMINATION OF XENOBIOTICS

Definition of Dose

Dose ideally describes the time integral of the effective concentration of a material present at the effector site. In inhalation toxicology, a determination of the dose according to this definition is difficult. The amount of deposited dose depends on respiratory parameters, such as the tidal volume, breathing frequency, and physicochemical characteristics of the inhaled material. Numerous factors can influence the rate of clearance (and of the converse, retention) of deposited materials. The retained dose in the target organ is in many cases not directly proportional to the exposure concentration. Thus, studies of the kinetics of inhaled materials should always include an exposure concentration that is as close as possible to the concentrations likely to be experienced by people.

Deposition of Particles

The principal mechanisms of deposition of inhaled PM are impaction, sedimentation, interception, and diffusion (Figs. 7–8). The first three of these processes are strongly influenced by the aerodynamic characteristics of particulate matter (PM). Impaction is the process by which particles suspended in the air travel along their original path due to inertia and impact on a surface rather than following the airflow around a bend, as might occur near an airway bifurcation. Sedimentation (settling out) of particles predominates when air flow is low. The rate of sedimentation is determined by the terminal velocity of particles. For particles 0.5 μm in diameter, the sedimentation rate is about 0.001 μm per second, or the same as the diffusional displacement. As particles increase in aerodynamic diameter, the terminal velocity increases markedly such that sedimentation has a greater role in the deposition of larger aerodynamic diameter particles.

Interception is a process that is most significant for fibers because their length increases the probability that the ends of the fiber will intercept the walls of the airways. Fibers are a special class of particles with a length that is at least three times greater than the diameter.

Diffusion is the major process governing deposition of particles less than 0.5 μm in diameter. As particle size decreases, the diffusional displacement motion increases, and it will thereby come into contact with the surfaces of airways. Diffusional deposition is highest when the particles have just entered the naso-

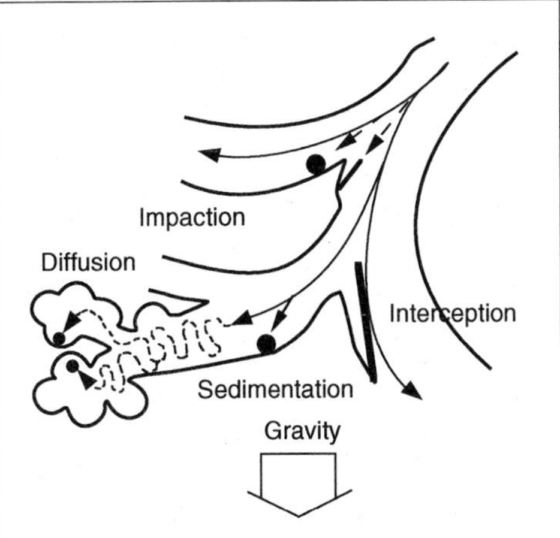

FIGURE 7 Primary mechanisms of deposition of inhaled particles in the respiratory tract. Streamline is indicated by solid lines; particle and fiber trajectory are indicated by dashed lines.

Air flow					
Directional changes	Velocity	Segment	Cross-sectional area	Residence time	Dominant deposition mechanisms
Slight	High	Nasopharynx	Few cm^3	Brief	Diffusion, impaction
Minimal	Medium	Trachea	Few cm^3	Brief	Impaction
Marked	Low	Bronchioles	> 10 cm^3	Brief	Impaction, interception
Limited	Low or none	Pulmonary	> 10 cm^3	Long	Sedimentation, diffusion

FIGURE 8 Dominant deposition mechanisms of particles in the respiratory tract.

pharynx and is also high in the pulmonary region, where the air flow is low.

Due to the morphology of the respiratory tract, an inspired aerosol flows through the upper airways at high velocity and remains for only a short period of time in these regions. Consequently, in the extrathoracic and upper bronchial region, particle deposition is determined by inertial particle transport (Fig. 8). Impaction takes place when the airborne particles do not follow the air flow after directional changes but hit the wall of the airways. This effect is of primary importance for particles >5 μm. Impaction of particles occurs after sharp directional changes (e.g., in the nose and at bifurcatios of ciliated airways). In the deeper region of the ciliated airways, the distances in the airways become smaller; the velocity of an inspired aerosol is much lower and its residence time longer than in the upper airways. In this area, deposition caused by sedimentation becomes more important. This is primarily due to particles in the range of 1–5 μm. In the alveolar region, deposition by diffusion processes for particles <1 μm plays a dominant role.

In summary, depending on the particle size, three domains of particles transport can be considered: a thermodynamic, an intermediate, and an aerodynamic domain (Fig. 9). In the thermodynamic domain, particle deposition is solely due to diffusional particle transport onto airway and airspace surfaces. The total deposition decreases with increasing particle diameter. It is independent of particle density and aerosol flow rate and increases with increasing breathing cycle period. In the intermediate domain, particle deposition is due to simultaneous diffusional and gravitational particle transport onto airway and airspace surfaces. In this domain, the total deposition reaches a minimum when diffusional and gravitational particle losses in the respiratory tract are equal. In the aerodynamic domain, particle deposition is due to gravitational and inertial particle transport and increases with increasing particle diameter, particle density, aerosol flow rate, and breathing-cycle period. An example of regional aerosol deposition in the respiratory tract is shown in Fig. 10.

Clearance of Particles

Clearance describes the removal of deposited particles from the respiratory tract. The retention of particles is determined by the amount deposited minus the amount cleared. A schematic overview is given in Fig. 11.

Particles can be cleared from the respiratory tract by a variety of mechanisms. Among these are

1. Direct clearance via the mucociliary apparatus.
2. Clearance via macrophage ingestion and removal via the mucociliary apparatus.
3. Ingestion by macrophages and dissolution.
4. Ingestion by macrophages and transport into the interstitial tissue of the lung.
5. Ingestion by macrophages and transport via the lymphatic vessels or regional lymph nodes.
6. Dissolution directly into surrounding fluids or tissue.

Materials deposited in the nasopharynx are cleared rapidly by being moved forward on the mucociliary blanket through sneezing and nose blowing or by be-

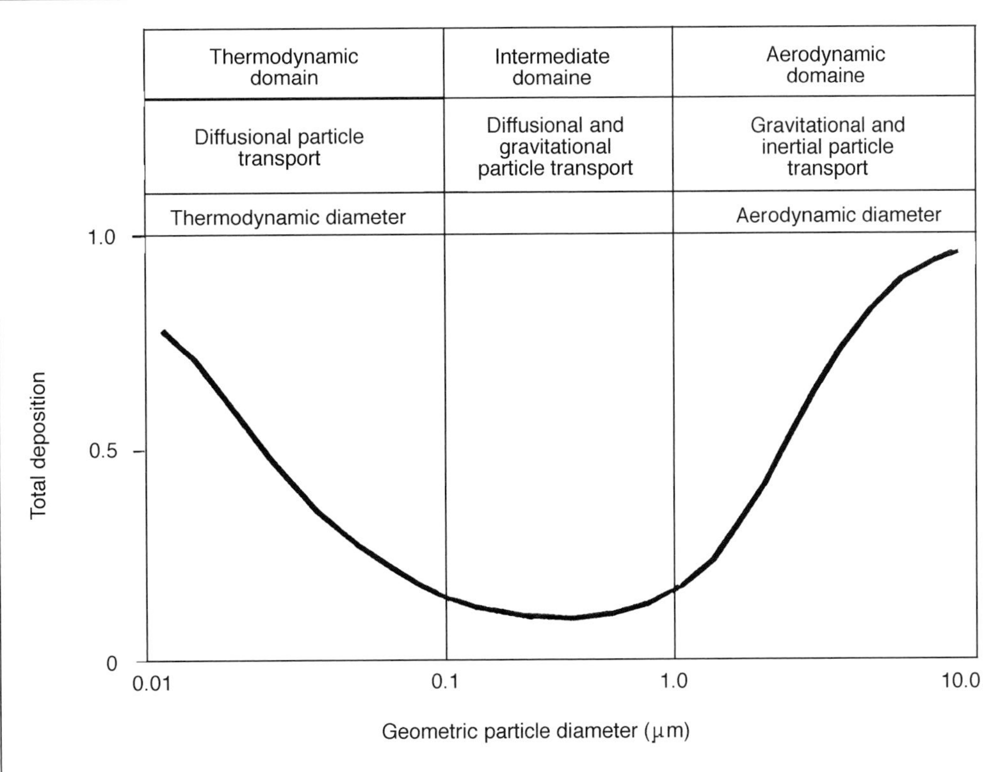

FIGURE 9 Domains of particle transport onto human airway and airspace surfaces (calculated according to Heyder *et al.*, 1986).

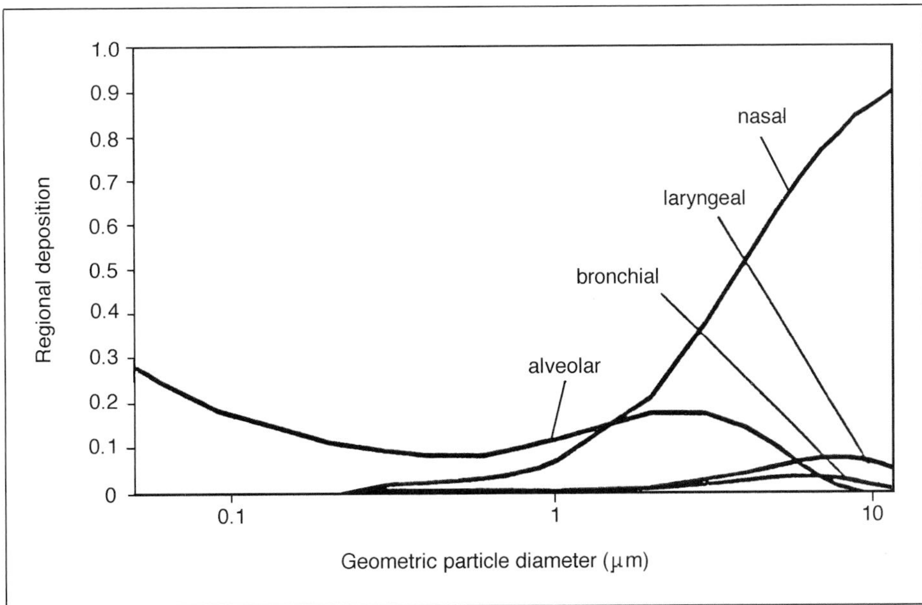

FIGURE 10 Deposition of unit density spheres in the human respiratory tract during nasal breathing with a tidal volume of 390 cm^3 and a breathing cycle period of 3.75 (calculated according Heyder *et al.*, 1986).

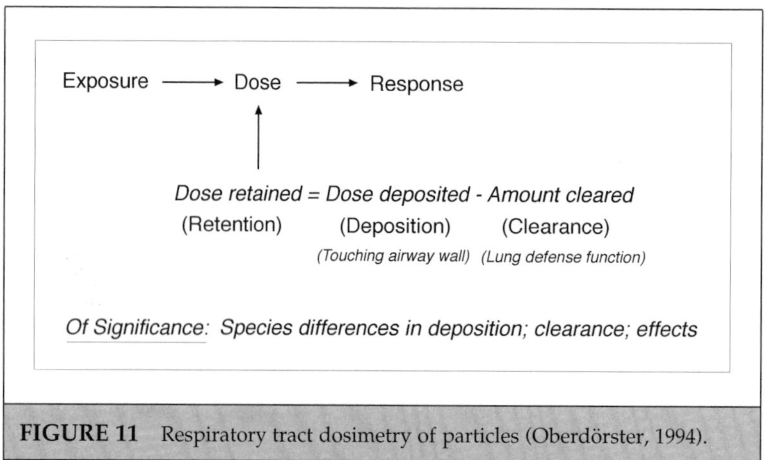

FIGURE 11 Respiratory tract dosimetry of particles (Oberdörster, 1994).

ing moved posteriorly through mucociliary action to the mouth, where the material is swallowed or expectorated. A schematic of deposition and clearance is presented in Fig. 12. Materials deposited in the tracheobronchial region are also cleared rapidly (in a matter of hours). Movement up the bronchioles and trachea on the mucociliary escalator occurs, with material frequently contained within macrophages. The clearance mechanisms that remove particles also serve to remove bacteria and viruses, thereby helping to protect the respiratory tract from infectious agents. However, Stahlhofen *et al.* (1994) have reported a slow phase clearance in the ciliated airways of humans. The significance of a slow tracheobronchial clearance phase for the toxicity of solid particles is not fully understood.

In the alveolar region, where cilia are not present, macrophage-mediated clearance is the predominant mechanism of removing particles. This process is, in general, much slower than ciliated clearance; therefore an impairment of this defence mechanism is of particular relevance. In humans half-times are in the range of 400 days. Particles may migrate also into the interstition and be cleared via the lymphatic system to lung-associated lymph nodes (Fig. 12).

The specific principles of the toxicokinetics of poorly soluble particles are presented here because long-term retention in the respiratory tract is of major concern in occupational dust exposure; for example, there are reports of an accumulation of up to 20 g dust in the lungs of miners. While the clearance of particles from the lungs is important because it represents an essential defense mechanism for the respiratory system, the failure to clear particles leads to their accumulation. This phenomenon is called "dust overloading of lungs." In the F-344 rat, lung overloading is generally reached in the range of 0.5–1.5 mg or approximately 1 mg of material/g of lung tissue. Studies of lung overloading provided evidence of macrophage accumulation, epithelial cell proliferation, inflammatory reactions, and increased dust presence in the interstitium. Dust overloading of the lungs is characterized by immobility and dysfunction of macrophages resulting from an excessive uptake of materials. This phenomenon represents a serious confounding complication in toxicologic assessment, one in which the intrinsic toxicity of the test material is either masked or modified by the nonspecific effects of dusts on macrophage transport.

For human risk assessment, it must be taken into account that the clearance retardation induced by a high burden of particles with low toxicity in the lung will also affect the clearance of more toxic particles, which could be inhaled at very low concentrations.

PATHOBIOLOGY OF THE RESPIRATORY TRACT

This section can give only a very rough survey of the complex pathological reactions following inhalation exposure. For more detail, see the Bibliography.

The respiratory tract is a complex organ and, not surprisingly, exhibits a wide range of alterations, extending from physiological adaptation to mild dysfunction to serious life-threatening disease. Many of these disease responses can be produced by inhaled toxicants, including particulate matter. In addition to responses involving the respiratory system alone, the close integration of pulmonary and cardiac function raises the possibility of combined cardiopulmonary effects.

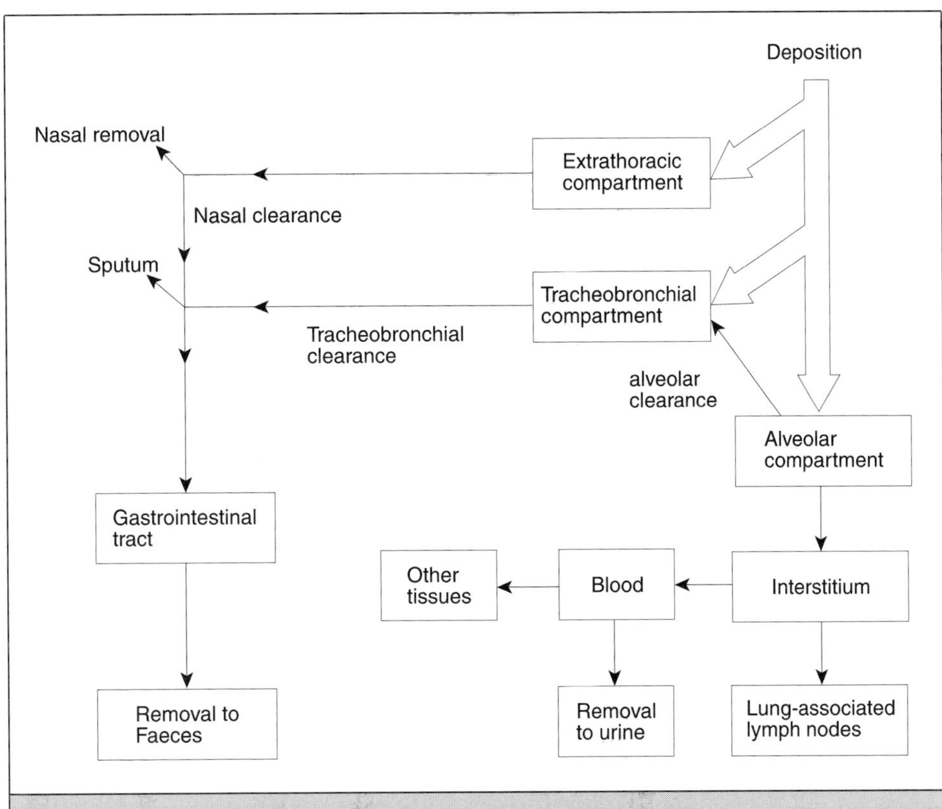

FIGURE 12 Scheme of deposition (thick arrows) and clearance of inhaled insoluble particles. Transportation inside the body is marked by thin arrows.

In addition to serving as a target organ, the respiratory tract serves as a portal of entry for some inhaled pollutants that cause disease in other organs or systems. For example, long-term exposure to sufficiently high levels of vinyl chloride increases the risk of liver cancer, inhaled lead affects the bone marrow and nervous system, and inhaled carbon monoxide impairs oxygen transport, which in turn, affects the heart and central nervous system.

Particulate matter deposited in the respiratory tract may elicit a wide range of responses by a variety of mechanisms. Particles may interact with neurogenic receptors at different loctions in the respiratory tract to alter breathing frequency and depth. Some of these receptors are located in the nose, while other are in the upper portions of the tracheobronchial region. Sensory nerves that trigger coughing extend from the larynx to the segmental bronchi. Coughing can be triggered by a wide range of inhaled agents, from distilled water and hypertonic saline to chemical irritants and dusts.

Some respiratory tract responses involve the ingestion of particles by macrophages, which are located throughout the respiratory tract but are predominantly found in the alveolar region. Other respiratory tract responses arise primarily from direct interactions between particles and other respiratory tract cells. Macrophages are both the first line of defense against particulate matter and a potential intermediary for producing injury. As noted earlier, macrophages play a key role in clearing particles from the respiratory tract. In the process of phagocytosis (ingestion) of particles, however, macrophages become activated and release a wide spectrum of mediators. These mediators include oxygen radicals such as superoxide anion and hydrogen peroxide, which can directly injure respiratory tract cells. Other mediators (cytokines) serve to stimulate the proliferation of respiratory tract cells. Some mediators are also involved in the recruitment of inflammatory cells such as neutrophils. Macrophages are generally believed to play a key role in lung injury from particulate matter.

Because of the close integration of respiratory and cardiovascular function, changes in the respiratory tract can readily have a cascading effect on cardiac function, for example, through disturbances in blood flow. Individuals with preexisting respiratory disease, such as chronic obstructive pulmonary disease or heart disease, are especially vulnerable to a breakdown in normal function following respiratory tract injury.

The physiologic and pathologic processes just described are not unique to particulate matter. Other insults to the respiratory tract, including infectious agents, can produce similar effects. And a major portion of respiratory and heart disease is well known to be directly related to cigarette smoking. In our opinion, the overwhelming influence of cigarette smoking makes identifying the potential effect of a surrogate index like particulate matter very difficult because it is, at best, a low potency risk factor compared with cigarette smoking.

General Reactions to Inhaled Toxicants

Common responses of the respiratory tract to toxic materials are inflammatory and proliferative reactions.

Inflammation

Inflammatory events belong to the first reactions of the respiratory tract to inhaled toxicants. After acute injury, an intraluminal exudation frequently is observed and is composed of cellular and glandular secretions and detritus from dead epithelial cells. Together with these reactions, a broad variety of cellular and humoral markers of inflammation are induced, among them cytokines. Bronchoalveolar lavage, which collects the epithelial lining fluid and cellular components, has been proven to be a powerful method of studying the sequence of events.

Proliferative Reactions

The death of epithelial cells and inflammatory processes after inhalative exposure commonly lead to the proliferation of epithelial cells (alveolar type II cells, and Clara cells) as a repair mechanism. In the hierarchy of sensitivity to direct-acting toxicants, alveolar type I cells and ciliated cells are most sensitive to damage, secretory bronchiolar (Clara) cells are of intermediate sensitivity, and mucous cells and type II alveolar cells are the most resistant. A method frequently applied to measure the proliferation of cells is the use of the thymidine analog bromodeoxyuridine (BrdU) to label the newly synthesized DNA. BrdU incorporated in DNA can be recognized by specific staining methods.

The chronic proliferative response of epithelial cells may lead to the formation of squamous metaplasia or hyperplasia. With chronic inflammation, centriacinar regions sometimes become lined by bronchiolar epithelium, which is called "alveolar bronchiolization." This is generally believed to be the result of the peripheral extension of bronchiolar cells, presumably because they have a selective advantage for survival over type II cells.

Fibrosis

Pulmonary fibrosis may be defined by the presence of an increased amount of newly formed collagen fibers. The formation of connective tissue is a complex process. There is a growing database associating specific macrophage secreted cytokines with the pathogenes of fibrosis. Tumor necrosis factor α (TNFα) can stimulate fibroblasts to produce collagen. Other cytokines involved are fibronectin and various growth factors, such as transforming growth factor β (TGFβ).

Fibrosis can be induced after the chronic inhalation of inorganic dusts, such as silica and asbestos, but also after high exposure to a variety of low-soluble dusts. Virtually all chronic lung injuries that are capable of sustaining chronic inflammation can lead to fibrosis.

Tumors

Although chemical carcinogenesis is treated in a separate chapter, some specific perspectives are presented here. By far the dominant factor for the induction of lung cancer in humans is tobacco smoking. In major developed countries approximately 90% of the lung cancers are attributable to cigarette smoking. Among the other substances that cause lung tumors in humans are asbestos, bichloromethyl ether, nickel-containing fumes, and pyrolysis products from organic material, which contain specific polycyclic aromatic hydrocarbons. Annually updated lists of carcinogens are published by the TLV committee in the United States and by the German MAC commission. The International Agency for Research on Cancer publishes a series of monographs describing the carcinogenicity at individual chemicals and occupational activities.

In humans, about 90% of lung tumors are found in the bronchial region; in rodents tumors usually appear in the deeper airways. The tumor types observed in humans and rodents are somewhat different. Small-cell carcinomas, which are frequent in humans, are not found in rodents. On the other hand, cystic keratinizing squamous cell tumors are observed in rats, but are extremely rare in humans. This latter types of tumor is frequently observed in rats after chronic exposure to particles that are poorly soluble, such as diesel particulates, carbon black, or TiO_2 dust under dust-overload conditions. The significance of these results to humans is a point of controversy. The mechanism of inducing these tumor types in rats may be different for humans at lower concentrations (McClellan, 1996; Mauderly, 1996).

Toxic Effects in Different Compartments of the Respiratory Tract

Nose

Depending on the physicochemical behavior of the inhaled materials, resorption differs in each of the compartments of the respiratory tract. The nasal mucosa responds, for example to gases with high water solubility (e.g., formaldehyde) or to coarse aerosols (wood dust). Inflammatory reactions can be induced by irritant gases or allergens.

The retained dose per area may be considerably higher in the nose than in other parts of the respiratory tract. This is especially true in rodents, in which the nose serves as a very effective filtering system.

Tracheobronchial Compartment

Reactions to toxicants in this area include airway constriction leading to an increase of the airway resistance, hypersecretion of mucus, and swelling of bronchial walls. For example, an airway constriction is observed after exposure to SO_2, NH_3, and sulfuric acid mists. Further types of reaction are allergic or pseudoallergic responses, giving rise to asthma and pulmonary eosinophilia.

Asthma

Asthma is characterized clinically by intermittent symptoms of wheezing, dyspnea, and cough. Typically, airflow limitation is observed due to reversible narrowing of the airways (bronchoconstriction), with edema, mucosal inflammation, and mucus secretion. Most asthmatic patients, even in periods without any symptoms, have some degree of persistent airflow obstruction.

The pathogenic processes in asthma have been recognized as including disregulation of inflammation. Cytokines play an important role in the initiation and resolution of the inflammatory response.

The role of environmental factors is controversial. Epidemiological findings have identified a possible role for ozone in adult-onset asthma. Other environmental factors, such as sulfate and NO_2 exposure, may alter the composition and fate of aeroallergens.

Occupationally induced asthma has been described after exposure to diisocyanate, formaldehyde, to chromium and nickel salts, and to a large variety of naturally occurring dusts, such as flour and grain dusts, and some specific wood dusts, such as Canadian Red Cedar.

Chronic Bronchitis

Chronic bronchitis is defined clinically as the presence of a chronic productive cough for more than half the time over a period of 2 years. About 90% of all cases occur in smokers. Epidemiological studies have shown a correlation between chronic bronchitis and high dust and SO_2 concentrations. In coal mining and in foundries, an increased incidence of chronic bronchitis has been reported.

Alveolar Compartment

Edema

Pulmonary edema represents an acute exudative phase of lung injury and generally reflects an alteration in the permeability of the epithelium and/or the endothelium of the gas-exchanging regions of the lung. The gas-exchanging function of the lung is hindered by edema fluid, which alters the ventilation–perfusion relationships and limits the diffusive transfer of O_2 and CO_2. When damage becomes more severe, the edema fluid can no longer be removed by the lymphatic vessels because these are compressed. Finally, a leakage of protein-rich fluid into the alveolar spaces may lead to the formation of hyaline membranes. These further prevent the gas exchange and commonly cause death. An example of a toxic agent acting by this mechanism is phosgene.

Emphysema

Emphysema is defined as irreversible enlargement of airspaces distal to the terminal bronchioles, accompanied by destruction of the alveolar walls without significant fibrosis. This disease can be viewed as the opposite of fibrosis; rather than becoming smaller and stiffer, the lungs become larger and too compliant. The destruction of gas-exchanging tissue results in a distended, hyperinflated lung that no longer effectively exchanges oxygen and carbon dioxide. The major cause of emphysema is tobacco smoking.

In toxicant-induced emphysema inflammation is observed, especially alveolitis with the release of proteolytic enzymes by participating leukocytes. Normally proteolytic enzymes are counterbalanced by antiproteolytic components (e.g., α_1-antitrypsin). This balance can be disturbed, for example, when the elastolytic activity predominates over the anti-elastolytic mechanisms leading to destruction of the lung parenchyma. Increased numbers of neutrophils, which contain serine elastase and other proteases, are found in the bronchoalveolar lavage of smokers. Frequently emphysema and chronic bronchitis are observed together.

Sensitive Populations

The epidemiological results point to several subpopulations as being at special risk for particulate matter exposures: children, individuals with respiratory diseases (e.g., chronic obstructive pulmonary disease, acute bronchitis, asthma, and pneumonia) and cardiovascular disease (e.g., pneumonia), and the elderly. As previously noted, a significant portion of the adults at special risk, such as those with chronic obstructive pulmonary disease, chronic bronchitits, and cardiovascular disease, suffer from these diseases because of cigarette smoking. This emphasizes the importance of understanding the interactions of multiple risk factors in evaluating the risks of low-level environmental exposures to particles and other pollutants.

EXPOSURE TECHNIQUES

The conduct of toxicity studies of airborne materials requires that special attention be given to generating and delivering well-characterized atmospheres of test materials to the breathing zone of test subjects. These can include human subjects in controlled human-exposure studies, as well as a wide range of laboratory animal investigations. The principal elements of an exposure system are the generation of test atmosphere, the exposure chamber, the monitoring of the exposure, and the exhaust clean up. The reader is referred to Cheng and Moss (1995).

SUMMARY

In this chapter we have briefly reviewed key concepts of how the respiratory tract responds to airborne materials. The toxicity of airborne materials is markedly influenced by their physical and chemical properties; thus, considerable attention has been given to describing how differences in these properties influence the deposition of inhaled materials and their subsequent kinetics within the body. For some toxicants, the respiratory tract serves both as the portal of entry for a toxicant and as the target organ (i.e., airborne dusts, such as coal dust, quartz, and nickel fumes). In other cases, the respiratory tract is the portal of entry and the target organ is another tissue, such as an benzene going to hematopatetic tissue and lead to the nervous system and bone.

The respiratory tract poses a unique target for both inhaled toxicant and toxic agents, such as paraquat, that may reach the respiratory system via the systemic circulation. The uniqueness of the respiratory tract relates to its physical dimensions and vital functions, which are sustained by over 40 different cell types. The key vital function can be compromised by changes in function, especially in how gases are delivered to and removed from the lungs and in gases exchange between the alveolar spaces and blood. In addition, the respiratory tract is a common site of cancers produced by inhaled material. The prevalence of lung cancers attributable to cigarette smoking serves as a constant reminder of the importance of being accurate in identifying potential respiratory tract carcinogens.

Probably more than for any other toxicological specialty, inhalation toxicology requires that extraordinary attention be given to the methods used for the conduct of inhalation toxicity studies and to how toxic agents are delivered to experimental subjects. The success of any study using airborne materials is dependent upon: (a) framing a defined experimental hypothesis, (b) delivery of an appropriately characterized material to the breathing zone of the subject, (c) use of appropirate well-defined subjects (either healthy animals or animals that have specific well-characterized diseases), and (d) use of appropriate experimental techniques for studying the dispositional kinetics of the test material (and its metabolites) and the molecular, biochemical, physiocological, and pathological responses induced by the test material. The complexities result in the need for multidisciplinary teams to evaluate the toxicity and human health risks of airborne materials.

Bibliography

American Conference of Governmental Industrial Hygienists (1998). "Threshold Limit Values for Chemical Substances and Physical Agents Biological Exposure Indices (TLVs and BEls)." ACGIH, Cincinnati.

Bergmann, I., and Casswell, C. (1972). Lung dust and lung iron contents of coal workers in different coalfields in Great Britain. *Br. J. Indust. Med.* **29,** 160.

Cheng, Y.-S., and Moss, O. R. (1995). Inhalation exposure systems. *In* "Concepts in Inhalation Toxicology" (R. O. McClellan and R. F. Handerson, eds.), pp. 25–66. Taylor and Francis, Washington, D.C.

Dahl, A. R. (1990). Contemporary issues in toxicology. Dose concepts for inhaled vapors and gases. *Toxicol. Appl. Pharmacol.* **103,** 185–197.

Deutsche Forschungsgemeinschaft (1998). "List of MAK and BAT values—Maximum Concentrations and Biological Tolerance Values at the Workplace." Wiley–VCH, Weinheim, Germany.

Driscoll, K. E. (1995). Role of cytokines in pulmonary inflammation and fibrosis. *In* "Concepts in Inhalation Toxicology" (R. O. Mc-

Clellan and R. F. Henderson, eds.), pp. 471–503. Taylor and Francis, Washington, D.C.

Dungworth, D. L., Hahn, F. F., and Nikula, K. J. (1995). Non-carcinogenic responses of the respiratory tract to inhaled toxicants. *In* "Concepts in Inhalation Toxicology" (R. O. McClellan and R. F. Handerson, eds.), pp. 533–576. Taylor and Francis, Washington, D.C.

Gardner, D. E., Crapo, J. D., and McClellan, R. O. (1999). "Toxicology of the Lung." Taylor and Francis, Washington, DC.

Hebel, R., and Stromberg, M. W. (1986). "Anatomy and Embryology of the Laboratory Rat." BioMed Verlag, Wörthsee, Germany.

Henderson, R. F. (1989). Bronchoalveolar lavage: A tool for assessing the health status of the lung. *In* "Concepts in Inhalation Toxicology" (R. O. McClellan and R. F. Henderson, eds.), pp. 415–444. Hemisphere Publishing Corp., New York.

Heyder, J., Gebhart, J., Rudolf, G., Schiller, C. F., and Stahlhofen, W. (1986). Deposition of particles in the human respiratory tract in the size range 0.005–15 μm. *J. Aerosol Sci.* **17,** 811–825.

Heyder, J., Gebhart, J., and Scheuch, G. (1985). Interaction of diffusional and gravitational particle transport in aerosols. *Aerosol. Sci. Technol.* **4,** 315–326.

Heyder, J., and Scheuch, G. (1983). Diffusional transport of nonspherical particles. *Aerosol. Sci. Technol.* **2,** 41–44.

Kennedy, G. L., and Valentine, R. (1994). Inhalation toxicology. *In* "Principles and Methods of Toxicology" (A. W. Hayes, ed.), 3rd ed., pp. 805–837. Raven Press, New York.

Koren, H. S., and Utell, M. J. (1997). Asthma and the environment. *Environ. Health Perspect.* **105,** 534–537.

Mauderly, J. (1995). Assessment of pulmonary function and the effects of inhaled toxicants. *In* "Concepts in Inhalation Toxicology" (R. O. McClellan and R. F. Henderson, eds.), pp. 355–412. Taylor and Francis, Washington, DC.

Mauderly, J. (1996). Lung overload: The dilemma and opportunities for resolution. *In* "Particle Overload in the Rat Lung and Lung Cancer. Implications for a Human Risk Assessment" (J. L. Mauderly and R. J. McCunney, eds.), pp. 1–28. Taylor and Francis, Washington, DC.

McClellan, R. O. (1995). An introduction to inhalation toxicology. *In* "Concepts in Inhalation Toxicology" (R. O. McClellan and R. F. Henderson, eds.), pp. 3–21. Taylor and Francis, Washington, DC.

McClellan, R. O. (1996). Lung cancer in rats from prolonged exposure to high concentrations of carbonaceous particles: Implications for human risk assessment. *In* "Particle Overload in the Rat Lung and Lung Cancer. Implications for a Human Risk Assessment" (J. L. Mauderly and R. J. McCunney, eds.), pp. 193–226. Taylor and Francis, Washington, DC.

Mercer, T. T., Tillery, T. T., and Newton, G. J. (1970). A multi-stage, low flow rate cascade impactor. *J. Aerosol. Sci.* **1,** 9–15.

Morrow, P. E. (1988). Possible mechanisms to explain dust overloading of the lungs. *Fundam. Appl. Toxicol.* **10,** 369–384.

Morrow, P. E., and Mermelstein, R. (1988). Chronic inhalation toxicity studies: Protocols and pitfalls. *In* "Inhalation Toxicology—The Design and Interpretation of Inhalation Studies and Their Use in Risk Assessment" (U. Mohr, ed.), pp. 103–117. Springer-Verlag, New York.

Moss, O. R., and Cheng, Y.-S. (1995). Generation and characterization of test atmospheres: Particles and droplets. *In* "Concepts in Inhalation Toxicology" (R. O. McClellan and R. F. Henderson, eds.) pp. 91–128. Taylor and Francis, Washington, DC.

Muhle, H., Bellmann, B., Creutzenberg, O., Heinrich, U., and Mermelstein, R. (1990). Dust overloading of lungs: Investigations of various materials, species differences and irreversibility of effects. *J. Aerosol Med.* **3,** S111–S128.

National Academy of Sciences (1983). "Risk Assessment in the Federal Government: Managing the Process." National Research Council, Committee on the Institutional Means for Assessment of Risks to Public Health, National Academy Press, Washington, DC.

Oberdörster, G. (1994). Respiratory tract dosimetry of particles: Implications for setting of exposure concentrations and extrapolation modelling. *In* "Respiratory Toxicology and Risk Assessment" (P. G. Jenkins *et al.,* eds.), pp. 83–110. Wissenschaftliche Verlagsgesellschaft, Stuttgart, Germany.

Schlesinger, R. B. (1995). Deposition and clearance of inhaled particles. *In* "Concepts in Inhalation Toxicology" (R. O. McClellan and R. F. Henderson, eds.) pp. 191–224. Taylor and Francis, Washington, DC.

Snider, G. L., Lucey, E. C., and Stone, P. J. (1986). Animal models of emphysema. *Am. Rev. Respir. Dis.* **133,** 146–169.

Stahlhofen, W., Scheuch, G., and Bailey, M. R. (1994). Measurement of the tracheobronchial clearance of particles after aerosol bolus inhalation. *Ann. Occup. Hyg.* **38** (Suppl. 1), 189–196.

CHAPTER

16

Blood and Blood-Forming Organs

PETER EYER, REINHARD KLIMMEK

Walther Straub Institute of Pharmacology and Toxicology, Ludwig Maximilians University, Munich, Germany

INTRODUCTION

Constituting approximately 8% of human body weight, blood is one of the largest organs and the main means of transport for the exchange of substances between the organs. Blood plays an important role in the defense and repair processes of the body. Less known is its significant contribution to the biotransformation of foreign substances.

Erythrocytes, granulocytes, and monocytes are equipped with enzyme systems that are able to perform a variety of oxidations. In this second defense chain, foreign compounds that have not been completely disposed of in the liver can be transformed to harmless ones before more sensitive target organs are affected. Frequently, the cells are directly damaged by the reactive compounds they have generated. Methemoglobinemia, hemolysis, and leukopenia are especially obvious signs of harmful actions. The sacrifice made by these cells to protect the rest of the cell society often has no further consequences. The damage is repaired or entails the destruction of easily replaceable mature cells in the bloodstream. A genetic damage is not transmitted because the mature blood cells are no longer capable of undergoing cell partitions. This makes them especially useful in a defensive function.

Nevertheless, the danger exists that blood cells may become antigenic due to the covalent binding of reactive compounds to the cell membrane, thus initiating immunological reactions with the possibility of intact cells being attacked too. Agranulocytosis, hemolytic anemia, and thrombocytopenia may be the sequelae. Unforseeable differences in the individual sensitivity to drugs and other foreign substances, mostly concerning only a small portion of the population, are observed. In the past, complete ignorance about the pathological mechanisms underlying these nonimmunological events led clinicians to call such a toxic manifestation an "idiosyncrasy" (from idios, Greek for "individual", and syncrasia, Greek for "mixture"). The obscure meaning of this term has become increasingly clear in recent years. The term now generally implies an abnormal, genetically determined, extremely intense or extremely weak responsiveness to a drug or any other chemical that is based on a metabolic polymorphism and unrelated to an antigen–antibody reaction. Correspondingly, metabolic processes also must be taken into account more extensively than in the past when describing toxic actions on the blood and its stem cells.

FUNDAMENTALS OF HEMATOPOIESIS

Ontogenesis

In the course of human embryonic development, several organs participate in hematopoiesis. Beginning in the yolk sac some 20 days after impregnation, hematopoiesis is demonstrable in the liver at the fifth week, then in the spleen, and eventually in the bone marrow at about the 20th week. The bone marrow does not take a leading role in hematopoiesis until the last trimester, but it is finally the main site of hematopoiesis at the time of birth. However, in chronic hypoxia the production of red blood cells can be reactivated in liver and spleen up to the age of 4 years, later only in exceptional cases. In neonates, the total bone marrow contributes to hematopoiesis. In the young child, fat cells already occupy the space of the long tubular bones, and in the adult hematopoiesis is mainly limited to the marrow of the central skeleton (the vertebrae, ribs, pelvis, shoulder blade, and skull). In the case of increased blood formation, it can still revive in the fatty marrow.

Differentiation of Stem Cells

Extended genetic analyses have revealed that the blood cells (e.g., erythrocytes, granulocytes, monocytes, macrophages, platelets, and lymphocytes) originate from a single pluripotent stem cell. The stem cells are present in the circulating blood, but differentiate only in the intact bone marrow. The differentiation of stem cells into precursors of mature blood cells is controlled by colony-stimulating factors that reach the bone marrow with the blood. In conjunction with macrophages and T-helper cells, the precursor cells of the megaloblast type appear to further differentiate in the presence of hormones (poietins). Thus, proerythroblasts arise from erythroid precursor cells by means of erythropoietin, and megakaryocytes from megakaryocyte precursor cells under the influence of thrombopoietin.

Erythropoietin is the best investigated of the poietin family. It is a glycoprotein that is predominantly formed in the kidney and, in the fetal period, also in the liver. The synthesis of erythropoietin is promoted under hypoxic conditions. The expression of erythropoietin is indirectly initiated by cobalt salts, which may explain the occurrence of polycythemia upon chronic exposure to cobaltous compounds.

Erythropoiesis

Following several divisions, the large proerythroblast matures in the bone marrow to the (polychromatic) basophilic normoblast with a concomitant increase in the synthesis of hemoglobin, and eventually to the (orthochromatic) normoblast with a higher hemoglobin content. The normoblast enters the bloodstream through the fenestrated thin-walled sinus endothelium of the vessel as a cytoplasmatic protrusion, leaving behind the ligatured nucleus whose material is submitted to phagocytosis. The nucleus-free reticulocyte thus originating still possesses basophilic ribosomes (stained with brilliant cresyl blue) that get lost in the circulation within 1–2 days. The now mature erythrocyte is no longer able to synthesize proteins and has lost the enzyme systems of the aerobic metabolism. The normal reticulocyte count is 2% in adults and 6% in children, with the life span of the mature erythrocyte averaging 120 days.

An increase in reticulocyte count (reticulocytosis) indicates an elevated erythropoiesis due to hemolysis, hypoxia, or profuse blood loss. Immature elements (blast cells) are found when the nucleic acid synthesis (supply of C_1 bodies for purine synthesis) is impaired by vitamin B_{12} and folic acid deficiencies.

Granulocytopoiesis

Following several cell divisions, the myeloblast, which can hardly be distinguished from the proerythroblast, turns to the promyelocyte by developing granules. During maturation, the promyelocyte further differentiates to a neutrophilic, eosinophilic, or basophilic myelocyte. Polymorphonuclear leukocytes and monocytes formed by nuclear condensation are delivered into the bloodstream. The maturation needs about a week, and the average half-life of the mature cells is 7 h.

Development of Lymphocytes

Unlike the B-lymphocytes and granulocytes evolving from the stem cell in a similar way, the maturation of T-lymphocytes seems to follow a separate path in a very early stage. T-lymphocytes are often spared from genetic aberrations, whereas all the other blood cells are usually affected in a uniform manner.

The bone marrow stem cell is the exclusive site of T-lymphocyte formation only at the beginning of ontogenesis; later, most T-lymphocytes are formed in the thymus from prethymocytes. B- and T-lymphocytes are of decisive importance for the immune response; B-lymphocytes are activated to antibody-producing plasma cells and T-lymphocytes are responsible for cell-mediated immunity. T-lymphocytes differentiate into cytotoxic T-cells as well as into regulatory helper and suppressor cells.

Development of Thrombocytes

Megakaryocytes originating from the stem cell under the influence of thrombopoietin release many anucleate thrombocytes, the rest (chromatin) being phagocytized. The circulation time of thrombocytes in blood is 7–10 days.

TOXIC ACTIONS ON THE BONE MARROW

Damage to Stem Cells

Because only about 10% of the pluripotent stem cells are active in a reproductive state, losses of the stem cells can be compensated for at first. However, pancytopenia develops when their number decreases below 10% of normal. Acute toxic diminution of these cells results in pancytopenia in the peripheral blood with a latency period corresponding to the average lifetime of the individual blood cells. Granulocytopenia develops within days and thrombocytopenia within 1–2 weeks, while the loss of erythrocytes needs months to become clinically manifest. The erythrocyte count reveals 0.8% loss per day, on average, following the complete stop of red blood cell formation. Aplastic anemia, diagnosed by bone marrow punction, develops due to complete destruction of the stem cells.

The causes of damage to stem cells are multiple: ionizing radiation, antimetabolites, alkylating agents (e.g., mustard gas), chloramphenicol, hydantoin derivatives, pyrazolones, gold salts, benzene, trinitrotoluene, arsenic compounds, phenothiazines, thiamazol, and sulfonamides.

Disturbances of Maturation

Toxic events also may have an impact on later stages of bone marrow cell development. Occasionally, the cell picture of the marrow punctate is largely normal in aplastic anemia, as only few cells are affected by defective differentiation. The maturation of erythroblasts is impaired by folic acid antagonists (e.g., methotrexate in tumor treatment; pyrimethamine and proguanil against malaria; and trimethoprim in conjunction with sulfamethoxazol) and upon folic acid and vitamin B_{12} deficiencies. This results in oversized oval erythrocytes in the peripheral blood and in an accumulation of megaloblasts in the bone marrow (megaloblastic anemia). Drugs, as phenylbutazone, may be capable of disturbing the granulocytopoiesis, probably by defective maturation of myelocytes. Maturation is impaired due to disturbances of DNA synthesis in the bone marrow.

Mechanisms of Bone Marrow Toxicity

The mechanisms of bone marrow toxicity are unknown for a variety of foreign compounds. However, our knowledge about some compounds has grown in recent years and it is worth describing them in more detail.

Benzene

The dose-dependent toxicity of benzene in the bone marrow is well known. In addition, it can cause leukemia. Both actions may be due to the formation of reactive metabolites covalently binding to DNA, RNA, and proteins (Fig. 1). The oxidation products of benzene are mainly generated in the liver (e.g., benzene epoxide, *trans-trans*-muconaldehyde, phenol, hydroquinone, and catechol), but partially also in the bone marrow. These cells possess cytochrome P450, myeloperoxidases, and prostaglandin synthetases, which are able to activate benzene and its metabolites by oxidation. Semiquinones, quinones, and muconaldehyde are considered the ultimate reactive electrophiles. According to the present state of knowledge, several benzene metabolites are involved at different points of attack.

Chloramphenicol

The antibiotic effect of chloramphenicol (Fig. 2) comes about by inhibition of bacterial protein synthesis. It binds to 50 S subunits of bacterial 70 S ribosomes and is assumed to interact there with a peptidyltransferase. The similarity of bacterial 70 S ribosomes and mitochondrial ribosomes of eukaryotes suggests that chloramphenicol also acts on the mitochondria of mammalian cells. Moreover, the mitochondrial ferrochelatase is inhibited by chloramphenicol, resulting in a reduced synthesis of heme. The particular sensitivity of erythroid precursor cells to chloramphenicol thus finds an explanation. The toxicity is dose-dependent and becomes apparent definitely at plasma concentrations of more than 10 mg/liter. Newborns, who metabolize chloramphenicol much more slowly than adults, are affected if the dosage intervals are not adjusted to this age. Thereby, gray-baby syndrome may be produced with respiratory insufficiency, reduced myocardial function, acidosis, cyanosis, and hypothermia. Mitochondrial dysfunction is likely to be involved in the development of these reversible symptoms.

Aplastic anemia (incidence 1:10,000 to 1:200,000) is another untoward response to chloramphenicol. This toxic reaction appears to be independent of the dose of chloramphenicol and the duration of treatment. Its occurrence in identical twins points to a genetic predisposition. Nitrosochloramphenicol (Fig. 2), a reduction product of chloramphenicol, is by two orders of magnitude more toxic than the parent compound. In-

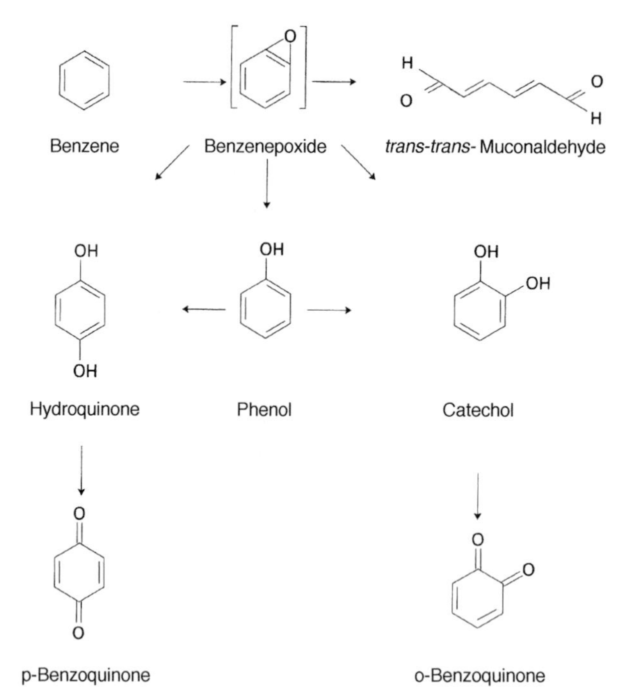

Benzene
Benzenepoxide
trans-trans- Muconaldehyde
Hydroquinone
Phenol
Catechol
p-Benzoquinone
o-Benzoquinone

FIGURE 1 Metabolic activation of benzene to metabolites potentially toxic to the bone marrow. Presumably, benzene is oxygenized to an intermediary epoxide. This is either transformed to phenol or to the unstable benzene dihydrodiol (not shown) by means of an epoxide hydrolase, followed by oxidation to catechol. The latter also may be formed by phenol hydroxylation in the same manner as hydroquinone. Hydroquinone and catechol autoxidize via semiquinones to the corresponding benzoquinones. There are some indications that phenol may directly arise from benzene by an OH radical attack. The mechanism of oxidative ring opening with formation of *trans-trans*-muconaldehyde has not been fully elucidated.

testinal bacteria reducing the nitro group to nitroso were assumed to produce the metabolite, which is toxic to the bone marrow. The differences in sensitivity among various populations were thought to come about by different habits in nutrition and corresponding variations in the intestinal flora. Moreover, the incidence of aplastic anemia seemed to be greater upon oral administration of chloramphenicol.

This conception is no longer tenable because it has been shown that nitrosochloramphenicol is too reactive to survive the liver passage and the transport in blood. It disappears in the blood within seconds, due to an extremely rapid reaction with the red blood cell glutathione. Another metabolite of chloramphenicol is dehydrochloramphenicol (Fig. 2), which, in contrast to the parent compound, can be reduced to the corresponding nitrosodehydrochloramphenicol (Fig. 2) by the bone marrow cells themselves. Its toxicity resembles that of nitrosochloramphenicol.

Leukemias Due to Foreign Compounds

The action of ionizing radiation on the development of leukemia has been studied in great detail. Our knowledge about the toxic mechanisms underlying the induction of leukemia by foreign substances, however, is small because appropriate animal models are lacking. The stem cell in its various stages of maturation is assumed to be the starting point of leukosis.

Myeloic leukemias induced by foreign compounds were first found in workers exposed to benzene. This acutely occurring disease is usually preceded by ane-

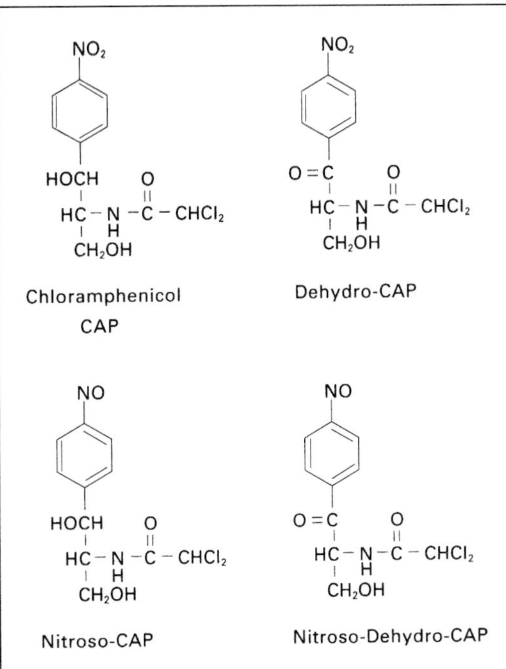

FIGURE 2 Chloramphenicol metabolites potentially toxic to the bone marrow. Intestinal bacteria are able to reduce chloramphenicol to nitrosochloramphenicol or to oxidize it to dehydrochloramphenicol. The latter may be converted to nitroso dehydrochloramphenicol by reduction of the nitro group.

mia, neutropenia, and thrombocytopenia for several months, indicating a dysfunction of the bone marrow. Frequently, mostly irreversible chromosomal aberrations with preference for chromosomes 5 and 7 are observed in lymphocytes and bone marrow cells.

In addition, 1,3-butadiene, styrol, ethylene oxide, and vinyl chloride are suspected of causing acute leukemia. Cases of leukemia associated with the occupational use of solvents could not be assigned to a single agent, but the solvents usually contained benzene.

Among the drugs used in tumor therapy, alkylating agents (e.g., chlorambucil and melphalan) are related to the occurrence of leukemia. The dose and the duration of administration seem to be decisive for the development of leukemia. Other cytostatic compounds intervening in the DNA synthesis of stem cells (cisplatin, daunorubicin, doxorubicin) likewise appear to be leukemigenic with a latency period of 4–6 years.

Acute myeloic leukemias associated with damage to chromosomes 5 and 7 are surprisingly resistant to therapy. Interestingly, the genes coding for growth factors (M-CSF, GM-CSF, PDGF, CD 14) are all localized on chromosome 5.

TOXIC ACTIONS ON GRANULOCYTES

The counts and the physiological function of granulocytes may be reduced due to toxic actions of foreign compounds. The clinical state with <500 granulocytes/μl of blood is referred to as agranulocytosis. This disease is nearly always caused by drugs. In contrast, only 50% of the aplastic anemias is associated with the administration of drugs. The mortality is much more pronounced in aplastic anemia than in agranulocytosis, and the recovery period is markedly longer. Because the polymorphonuclear leukocytes mainly consist of neutrophilic granulocytes, a diminution in the count of these cells is of utmost importance. The bone marrow smear can show different pictures in the agranulocytosis of peripheral blood:

- Reduced count of all granulocytic cells.
- Normal or elevated counts of white precursor cells with absence of mature granulocytes ("maturation block").
- Normal or even elevated counts of mature granulocytes.

In the last case, the toxic action mainly affects the granulocytes of the bloodstream; a more detailed account of this aspect will be given. Remember that the toxic actions of an agent may become manifest in stem cells and precursor cells, as well as in mature granulocytes. Many notions about toxic mechanisms remain quite hypothetical.

In most cases, there is generally no doubt that the reaction is largely determined immunologically. Recent findings indicate that hapten (antigen) formation results from a primary toxic reaction followed by an immunological response varying markedly between the individuals.

The function of the polymorphonuclear (neutrophilic) granulocytes is roughly characterized by a migration process and by destructive activity. Induced by chemotactic stimuli, the granulocytes are marginated from the circulating blood to the vessel wall, to which they are attached before permeating through the wall towards the target tissue. Once recognizing the target cells, the granulocytes bind to and envelop them, thereby forming the phagosome. During this process, an NADPH oxidase of the outer cell membrane is activated with concomitant massive generation of superoxide radicals that eventually are converted to hydrogen peroxide and oxygen by enzymatic dismutation. Furthermore, a myeloperoxidase is activated, forming a compound I complex with hydrogen peroxide and oxidizing chloride to hypochlorite (i.e., the active principle of chlorinated lime). This oxidant is extraordinarily bactericidal and virucidal. Finally, the phagosome is digested by proteases. The sudden onset of oxygen consumption and the "oxygen burst" can be induced experimentally, for example, by phorbol esters.

Agranulocytosis Mediated by Xenobiotics

Stimulated granulocytes can activate a number of foreign compounds by the oxidative way. Thereby, aromatic amines are either N-oxygenated or converted by means of hypochlorite to reactive chloramines, eventually giving rise to the generation of radical compounds.

The formation of *N*-hydroxyarylamines by activated granulocytes has been described for procainamide, dapsone, sulfadiazine, sulfamethoxazole, and diclofenac. The formation of radical cations from tertiary amines is likely to occur with aminopyrine (= aminophenazone; withdrawn) and phenothiazines, chlorpromazine, and clozapine. Phenylbutazone and benzene are hydroxylated by activated granulocytes. Phenolic compounds generated thereby are able to produce reactive phenoxy radicals. Quinonimines can be formed by activated granulocytes and myeloperoxidase and hydrogen peroxide from amodiaquine, paracetamol (acetaminophen), and vesnarinone.

Hydrazine derivatives such as hydralazine and isoniazid, are converted by stimulated granulocytes to reactive intermediates covalently binding to proteins. Covalent binding is also observed during activation of phenytoin and carbamazepin. Drugs containing a thiol group (propylthiouracil, D-penicillamine, captopril) are possibly activated via sulfenyl chlorides in activated granulocytes to form disulfides and thioethers. The pertinent metabolic studies indicate that foreign compounds can be activated in stimulated granulocytes to covalently bind to macromolecules. The altered macromolecules may gain antigenicity with the potential of inducing toxic agranulocytosis of the immunological type (Table 1).

Sera obtained in the acute phase of patients sensitized in this way are able to agglutinize the granulocytes of nonsensitized healthy donors. Owing to their special metabolism, granulocytes may serve to illustrate the selective sensitivity of target cells to toxic influences ("target toxicity"). Certainly one cannot exclude the possibility that granulocytes may also be affected by reactive metabolites produced in other organs (e.g., liver) or become the victims of an immunological process.

TABLE 1 Xenobiotics Inducing Toxic Agranulocytosis of the Immunological Type

Aminopyrine, paracetamol (acetaminophen), phenylbutazone, diclofenac, mefenamic acid, *p*-aminosalicylic acid, sulfasalazine (analgesics, antipyretics, anti-inflammatory agents)
Mianserin (antidepressant)
Chlorpromazine, clozapine (neuroleptics)
Carbamazepine (anticonvulsant)
Captopril (antihypertensive)
Vesnarinone (positive inotropic)
D-Penicillamine (metal antidote)
Methimazole = thiamazole, propylthiouracil (antithyroids)
Metoclopramide (antiemetic)
Aminoglutethimide (inhibitor of cortisol and aldosterone synthesis)
Sulfamethoxazole, sulfapyridine, sulfadiazine (antimicrobials)
Dapsone (antileprotic)

TOXIC ACTIONS ON ERYTHROCYTES

Due to their longevity (120 days) and to the extraordinarily high oxygen concentration (about 25 mM in terms of oxyhemoglobin) compared to other cells and the body fluid (<0.2 mM), mature erythrocytes are exposed to oxidative processes in a particular manner. Under standard conditions, a sudden release of the whole oxygen bound to hemoglobin iron would result in an oxygen pressure of more than 20 bars. From an evolutionary point of view, these specialized cells were prone to develop very effective systems to control oxygen binding and dissociation and to prevent or at least repair the damage from oxidation reactions.

It is surprising that the hemoglobin iron does not "rust" quickly in the electrolyte solution. Embedding the iron–oxygen complex in the porphyrin structure alone would not prevent the flow of electrons from iron to oxygen. Only the hydrophobic protein matrix of the hemoprotein complex shields the iron from valency instability, in particular owing to the tetrameric structure. Nevertheless, even under normal conditions a certain amount of autoxidation takes place continuously, with 0.5 to 1% of the hemoglobin (Fe^{2+}) being converted to ferrihemoglobin (Fe^{3+}). Ferrihemoglobin is no longer able to bind oxygen and therefore becomes useless for the oxygen transport. A number of hemoglobin variants with a changed amino acid sequence are much more prone to autoxidation. These M hemoglobins (M for methemoglobin, which is ferrihemoglobin) are also partially unstable in another respect, manifested by the formation of hemichrome precipitates in the erythrocytes. Individuals carrying these hemoglobin variants have ferrihemoglobin contents of several percent as compared to normal, and their heme iron is usually more susceptible to ferrihemoglobin producing substances.

The dissociation of the hemoglobin–oxygen complex normally yields deoxyhemoglobin (Fe^{2+}) and molecular oxygen in the peripheral tissue, thus maintaining the physiological oxygen partial pressure. However, the oxygen polarized in the iron bond may quit the hemoglobin molecule also as a superoxide radical anion ($O_2^{\bullet-}$), leaving behind Fe^{3+}. By dismutation of two superoxide radical anions, oxygen and hydrogen peroxide arise, the latter forming ferrihemoglobin very rapidly. The initial autoxidation is not favored thermodynamically because ferrihemoglobin with a redox potential of some +130 mV ($HbFe^{3+}/HbFe^{2+}$) is reduced by superoxide ($O_2/O_2^{\bullet-}$ = −179 mV) under physiological conditions. The autoxidation process, however, may be remarkably increased by many xenobiotics with co-oxidation of the iron and the reducing agent, resulting in a formal reduction of oxygen to hydrogen peroxide. The details of the mechanisms will be dealt with later on. In advance, it may be mentioned that reactive compounds are formed by most of the reducing agents via radical intermediates upon co-oxidation, exposing the erythrocytes to great oxidative stress.

Protective Systems against Oxidative Stress

Being a transport cell for oxygen, carbon dioxide, and protons, the erythrocyte is provided with a highly specialized metabolism. The modules responsible for reproduction, protein synthesis, and oxidative phosphorylation are absent. Thus, the mature erythrocyte lacks the cell nucleus, ribosomes, mitochondria, and endoplasmatic reticulum. In turn, the hemoglobin constitutes up to 90% of the cellular dry mass. Beside the complete enzyme setting for glycolysis, the red blood cell is richly equipped with the enzymes of the pentose phosphate pathway and displays high activities of superoxide dismutase and catalase. Both enzymes cooperate in eliminating the reactive oxygen species, superoxide radical, and hydrogen peroxide, without expenditure of energy. This exemplary disposal also prevents the secondary formation of aggressive oxygen species as singlet oxygen and OH radicals. Singlet oxygen arises from spontaneous dismutation of superoxide radicals but not during the reaction catalyzed by superoxide dismutase. OH radicals, characterized by a redox potential of some +2 V, are preferentially produced by the reaction of complexed divalent iron ions with hydrogen peroxide. They react extremely rapidly (diffusion-controlled) with nearly all organic molecules. In turn, the trivalent iron ion arising during this reaction can be reduced again.

$$Fe^{2+}\text{ Complex} + H_2O_2 \longrightarrow Fe^{3+}\text{ Complex} + {}^{\bullet}OH + OH^-$$

$$Fe^{3+}\text{ Complex} + O_2^{\bullet-} \longrightarrow Fe^{2+}\text{ Complex} + O_2$$

In this way, iron ions catalyze OH radical formation from superoxide and hydrogen peroxide (Fenton reaction). The survival of the cells is completely dependent on a tuned degradation of both oxygen species in a medium of iron ions.

In addition to catalase, the red blood cell contains glutathione peroxidase to metabolize hydrogen peroxide and organic hydroperoxides by means of glutathione (GSH). This enzyme reduces hydrogen peroxide to water with the formation of glutathione disulfide (GSSG). For this kind of hydrogen peroxide disposal, substantially more energy is used up than for the catalase reaction, but it has the advantage of high efficiency even at low hydrogen peroxide concentrations (K_m of H_2O_2 about 1 to 10 μM). The GSSG thereby produced is usually rapidly reduced to GSH by glutathione reductase and NADPH. If GSSG results in large amounts, mixed disulfides with protein SH groups that affect the intermediary metabolism may be formed. A thiol transferase isolated only recently is able to split the mixed disulfides by means of GSH. The formation of reactive oxygen species and the most important enzyme systems protecting the red blood cells from oxidative damage are illustrated in Fig. 3. Other oxidizing agents, such as radicals and quinoid compounds, are reduced by α-tocopherol (vitamin E) and ascorbic acid. The lipophilic vitamin E acts predominantly in the hydrophobic regions of proteins and membranes. The vitamin E radical that arises is reduced again by ascorbic acid. Oxidized ascorbic acid, in turn, is redox related to NADPH, in association with GSH and ascorbate reductase. In addition, ferrohemoglobin is also able to reduce the radicals and quinoids, yielding ferrihemoglobin, which in turn is reduced by cytochrome b_5. The latter is regenerated by an NADH-dependent "diaphorase" (methemoglobin reductase). The NAD^+ formed is reduced again by glyceraldehyde phosphate dehydrogenase

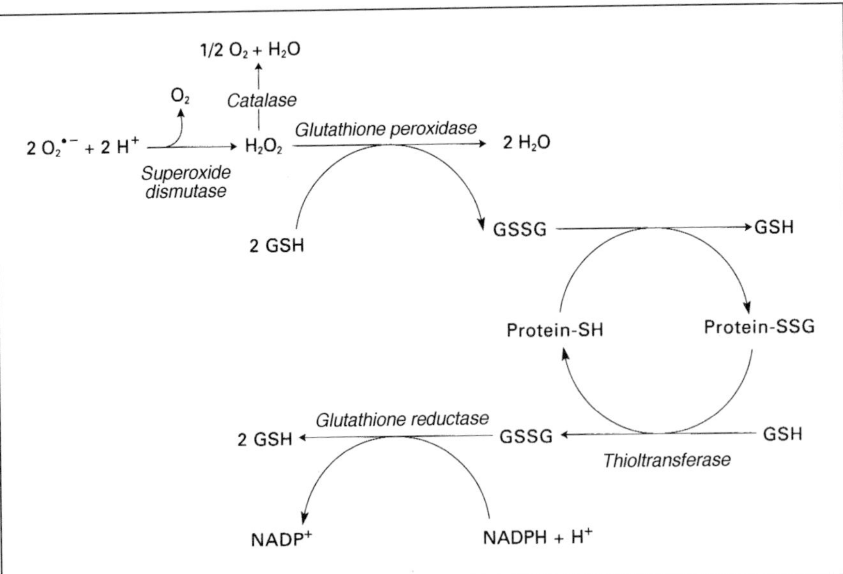

FIGURE 3 Enzyme systems protecting the erythrocyte from oxidative damage. The concentrations of reactive oxygen compounds ($O_2^{\bullet -}$ and H_2O_2) are normally kept very low by superoxide dismutase, catalase, and glutathione peroxidase. Glutathione disulfide is rapidly reduced by glutathione reductase and NADPH. A thiol transferase is capable of regenerating mixed protein–glutathione disulfides.

during glycolysis (GAPDH; Fig. 4). The final products of red blood cell glycolysis, lactate and pyruvate, are released to the plasma. The supply with glucose and the disposal of pyruvate and lactate are taken over mainly by the liver.

Apart from the cytochrome b_5/NADH-dependent methemoglobin reductase, an NADPH-dependent diaphorase functions as a methemoglobin reductase in the presence of unphysiological redox mediators, (e.g., dyes, such as methylene blue and toluidine blue). They are reduced by the flavin-containing diaphorase to leuko dyes, which reduce ferrihemoglobin in a direct reaction. These dyes can be therapeutically life saving in dangerous methemoglobinemia. The prerequisites for this are an intact enzyme system and the availability of NAD(P)H in erythrocytes (Fig. 4). The ramification rate of glucose-6-phosphate via glycolysis or pentose phosphate pathway may vary largely upon elevated oxidative stress. The rate may be switched from normally 9:1 (glycolysis/pentose phosphate pathway) to maximally 3:97.

Genetic Enzyme Defects

Methemoglobin Reductase

Methemoglobin reductase deficiency, with up to 50% of the hemoglobin being in the oxidized form, is not a rare finding. From 1 g of ferrihemoglobin/100 ml of blood onward, the brown pigment produces a pale gray discoloration, especially of the mucous membranes. The absolute content of ferrihemoglobin determines its diagnosability from the complexion. In anemia, methemoglobinemia is recognized only at a higher percentage of ferrihemoglobin. Such a discoloration is often misinterpreted as an "hypoxic cyanosis" with an elevated content of deoxyhemoglobin in the circulating blood and referred to a congenital cardiac defect. In one case, for example, congenital cyanosis was assumed to be due to an atrial septum defect. When the female patient was an adult she suffered from Crohn's disease and was therefore treated with sulfasalazine. This resulted in a massive change in her complexion, prompting the diagnosis of a methemoglobin reductase deficiency for the first time. Such a deficiency is usually only of cosmetic relevance and generally is compensated for by increased erythropoiesis. Even when the methemoglobin reductase is completely absent and autoxidation takes place continuously, there is a balance between ferrohemoglobin and ferrihemoglobin, indicating that some other mechanism of ferrihemoglobin reduction may exist, possibly by means of ascorbic acid. People affected by this enzyme deficiency are very sensitive to ferrihemoglobin-forming substances. Newborns show a diminished methemoglobin reductase activity. Moreover, the fetal hemoglobin is more readily oxi-

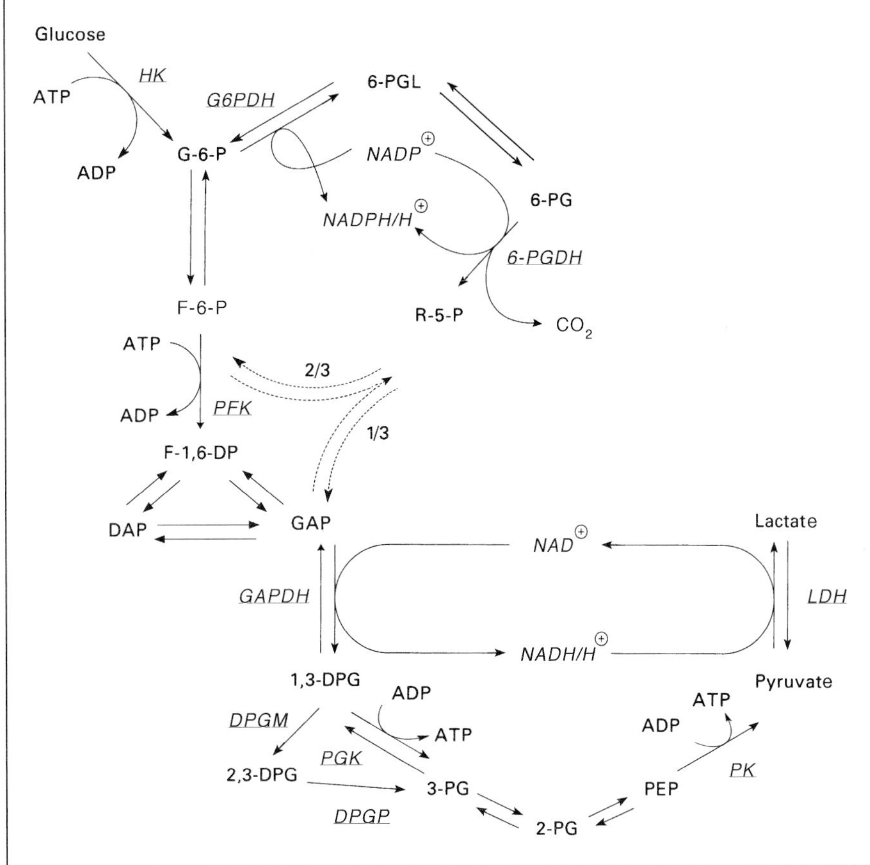

FIGURE 4 Supply of NAD(P)H in the erythrocyte. NADPH is regenerated by G6PDH and 6-PGDH in two steps of the pentose phosphate pathway. NADH is mainly made available by the GAPDH reaction. However, part of NADH is used up for pyruvate reduction. Abbreviations: DPGM, diphosphoglycerate mutase; DPGP, diphosphoglycerate phosphatase; GAPDH, glyceraldehyde-3-phosphate dehydrogenase; G6PDH, glucose-6-phosphate dehydrogenase; HK, hexokinase; LDH, lactate dehydrogenase; 6-PGDH, 6-phosphogluconate dehydrogenase; PGK, 3-phosphoglycerate kinase; PFK, phosphofructokinase; PK, pyruvate kinase.

dized. Therefore, neonates react with a markedly higher sensitivity to the methemoglobin-forming nitrite, which arises by reduction of nitrate through the intestinal bacteria. For this reason, well water with a nitrate content of >100 mg/liter should not be used to prepare baby food.

Catalase

In humans, a complete lack of catalase is a rare finding. Acatalasia was observed first in Japan. The cleaning of a wound with hydrogen peroxide did not produce the foaming usually seen upon release of oxygen but a brown-blackish discoloration of the tissues, pointing to the formation of ferrihemoglobin and ferrimyoglobin. This autosomal recessive hereditary disease of the Japanese type is often associated with ulcerative stomatitis, whereas another variant, the Swiss type, which was detected accidentally during a medical examination of recruits, is asymptomatic. The prognosis is generally benign because hydrogen peroxide can be normally scavenged by the glutathione peroxidase system.

Glutathione Reductase and Glutathione Peroxidase

Complete glutathione reductase deficiency occurs infrequently; the residual activity mostly amounts to some 50% of normal. The content of this flavin-containing enzyme may also be diminished due to a lack of riboflavin. Patients with considerable glutathione reductase deficiency react to xenobiotics that expose

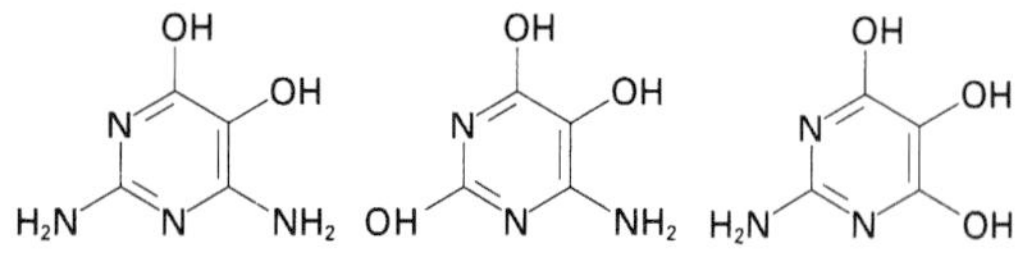

Divicine (DH_2) Uramil Isouramil

$$DH_2 + O_2 \longrightarrow {}^{\bullet}DH + O_2^{\bullet -} + H^+ \quad (1)$$

$$DH_2 + O_2^{\bullet -} + H^+ \rightleftharpoons {}^{\bullet}DH + H_2O_2 \quad (2)$$

$$^{\bullet}DH + O_2 \rightleftharpoons D\,(Quinone) + O_2^{\bullet -} + H^+ \quad (3)$$

$$DH_2 + D \rightleftharpoons 2\,{}^{\bullet}DH \quad (4)$$

$$D + 2\,GSH \longrightarrow DH_2 + GSSG \quad (5)$$

$$2\,O_2^{\bullet -} + 2\,H^+ \xrightarrow{SOD} O_2 + H_2O_2 \quad (6)$$

$$H_2O_2 + 2\,GSH \xrightarrow{GPx} GSSG + 2\,H_2O \quad (7)$$

FIGURE 5 Important reactions of substances contained in broad beans upon oxidative stress of erythrocytes. Initially, divicine and uramil autoxidize very slowly, forming a divicine radical (•DH) and a superoxide radical anion (1). After an induction period, the kinetics of divicine autoxidation are accelerated autocatalytically by reactions (2), (3), and (4). Two radicals arise in the comproportionation reaction (4), with the velocity of divicine consumption increasing quadratically. The autoxidation is decelerated by superoxide dismutase (SOD) in reaction (6) as reaction (2) does not take place. In reaction (5), GSH is much more effective due to suppression of reaction (4). If GSH regeneration is absent (e.g., in G6PDH deficiency), the autocatalytic processes of reactions (3) and (4) are no longer prevented, resulting in massive production of hydrogen peroxide via reactions (2) and (6) with concomitant additional consumption by glutathione peroxidase (GPx) of GSH in reaction (7). (According to Winterbourn, 1989.)

the red blood cells to an oxidative stress with increased hemolysis, similar to the response found in glucose-6-phosphate dehydrogenase deficiency.

Appreciable deficiency in selenium-containing glutathione peroxidase likewise is seldom found. Because glutathione peroxidase, in contrast to catalase, is also able to reduce organic hydroperoxides to the corresponding alcohols, a lack of glutathione peroxidase in cases of oxidative stress will be more serious. A selenium-free glutathione peroxidase exists, in particular in the liver; it appears to be identical to a subtype of glutathione *S*-transferase. The activity of this enzyme with regard to hydroperoxides is, however, marginal in erythrocytes.

Glucose-6-phosphate Dehydrogenase Anomalies

The most frequent enzymopathy encountered in erythrocytes affects the glucose-6-phosphate dehydrogenase (G6PDH). This recessive X-chromosome-bound heredopathy occurs in particular in populations of the Mediterranean area and the Middle East and in African groups. More than 100 million humans are estimated to have a G6PDH anomaly. So far, more than 50 G6PDH mutants, differing by pH optima and Michaelis constants, have been detected. Corresponding to the X-chromosomal coding for the enzyme, pronounced G6PDH deficiency is 10 times more frequent in males than in females. In Caucasians with the G6PDH anomaly, the enzyme activity is reduced to <3% of normal in the whole body. In African groups, the activity rarely falls below 10% in erythrocytes, while it is almost normal in other cells. The expressed enzyme is relatively unstable in these cases, appearing as an "enzyme deficiency" in the long-lived erythrocytes.

In carriers of unstable red blood cell G6PDH exposed to an oxidative stress, the content of reduced glutathione decreases at first in the older erythrocytes, entailing Heinz body formation, which indicates a damage to hemoglobin, and hemolysis due to cell membrane injury. If these individuals are continously given the same dose of an oxidative agent (e.g., the antimalarial primaquine) only a low-degree hemolysis is observed because the younger erythrocytes are relatively insensitive. The average lifetime of the red blood cells is shortened and the formation of new cells is increased (reticulocytosis). The latter may help compensate for the impending anemia.

Favism

Hemolytic anemias are observed in individuals with G6PDH deficiency after eating Vicia fava beans (broad beans). This species of beans is an important staple food in the Mediterranean countries. The substances responsible for the hemolytic crisis are the glycosidically bound divicine and isouramil, which are released by the enzyme β-glucosidase. They are extraordinarily autoxidizable pyrimidines, leading to the formation of ferrihemoglobin and hydrogen peroxide and to glutathione oxidation. The elucidation of the underlying reactions illustrates impressively the significance of an "operation in concert" between several antioxidative protective systems (Fig. 5).

In contrast to the structurally related aminophenols and phenylenediamines, the fully substituted hydroxypyrimidines do not allow 1,4-reductive addition reactions to the unsaturated double bonds (Michael

TABLE 2 Compounds Oxidizing Ferrohemoglobin Directly

Ferricyanide	Nitrite, NO, NO_2, sodium nitroprusside
Copper(II) salts	Nitrogen trifluoride
Hydrogen peroxide	Tetranitromethane
Chlorate	Quinones, quinone(di)imines, quinoid dyes (menadione, Bindschedler's green, toluidine blue, methylene blue)
Chromate	
Hydroxylamine	

type) and are therefore not eliminated. Hence, cellular antioxidants (e.g., ascorbic acid, GSH, and ferrohemoglobin) may be overstrained. Upon insufficient provision of NADPH (i.e., in case of G6PDH anomaly) methemoglobinemia and hemolysis occur. However, not all persons with the G6PDH anomaly show the symptoms of favism. An additional immunologic factor is assumed to be involved, as incomplete antibodies were detected in the serum of these patients (positive direct and indirect Coombs test) after sensitization with bean pollen. Obviously, the full manifestation of this disease requires a G6PDH anomaly and a previous sensitization.

Interestingly, the genetic defects exposing the erythrocytes to an increased oxidative stress (e.g., sickle cell anemia, thalassemia, M-type hemoglobin, persistent fetal hemoglobin, and G6PDH deficiency) are found quite often in areas where tropic malaria prevails. In the red blood cells affected by any of these defects, the development of the various forms of *Plasmodium falciparum,* which are extremely sensitive to oxidative stress, is inhibited by a hostile medium. This creates a selective advantage to the carriers of these anomalies in areas with tropic malaria. Moreover, broad beans are a main food in such areas, exposing the erythrocytes to an additional oxidative stress. It is striking that such a stress is also produced by most of the antimalarials used, suggesting that oxidative stress also may play a role in their therapeutic action.

Methemoglobinemia

Because many substances that oxidize the red dye of the blood are simultaneously also able to damage other erythrocyte constituents oxidatively and to elicit hemolysis, methemoglobinemia is often associated with an increase in the plasma ferrihemoglobin concentration. The dissociation of the heme from the protein matrix is markedly greater in the trivalent oxidation state than in the divalent state. For this reason, ferriheme bound to albumin (methemalbumin) is also sometimes found together with methemoglobinemia and concomitant hemolysis.

Apart from the hemoglobin anomalies mentioned, most methemoglobinemias are caused by foreign compounds that produce ferrihemoglobin at rates exceeding those of enzymatic reduction. Principally, three types of foreign compounds may be differentiated.

1. Compounds oxidizing ferrohemoglobin directly.
2. Compounds forming ferrihemoglobin in the presence of oxygen.
3. Compounds producing ferrihemoglobin after biotransformation.

Compounds Oxidizing Ferrohemoglobin Directly

Compounds of this type (see Table 2) oxidize deoxyhemoglobin much more rapidly than oxyhemoglobin. Purified deoxyhemoglobin, for example, is oxidized by potassium hexacyanoferrate(III), hydrogen peroxide, or benzoquinone at a rate 30 times higher than oxyhemoglobin is. Therefore, the directly oxidizing agent is assumed to attack the unliganded ferrohemoglobin, but not the liganded oxyhemoglobin, which makes up 97% of the hemoglobin at normal oxygen partial pressure. This conception is corroborated by experiments with carbon monoxide hemoglobin. In the presence of CO–hemoglobin, the rate for direct oxidation of ferrohemoglobin is reduced due to the retarded dissociation of CO from hemoglobin.

Potassium Hexacyanoferrate(III)

Potassium hexacyanoferrate(III) is often used in the laboratory because it is relatively selective in forming ferrihemoglobin directly. It does not permeate the erythrocyte membrane, so that methemoglobinemia is not caused *in vivo.* Potassium hexacyanoferrate(III) produces stoichiometric quantities of ferrihemoglobin with concomitant stoichiometric release of oxygen from oxyhemoglobin.

Hydrogen Peroxide

Hydrogen peroxide forms ferrihemoglobin and greenish oxidation products from hemoglobin, which are therefore also called verdoglobin or choleglobin. These compounds bear a likeness to sulfhemoglobin, which is formed in the presence of H_2S. They are oxidation products of the porphyrin structure and vicinal amino acid residues, probably due to formation of OH radicals. Hemoglobin altered in this way can no longer be repaired and forms poorly soluble green precipitates combining with the cell membrane. These precipitates can be stained with crystal violet and are called Heinz bodies, after their discoverer. Heinz bodies tend towards forming mixed disulfides with SH groups of the membrane. In this way, the deformability of the red blood cell membrane is hampered, resulting in intravasal hemolysis under certain conditions. In normally metabolizing, intact erythrocytes, hydrogen peroxide is metabolized very efficiently, thus scarcely producing ferrihemoglobin.

Chlorate

Chlorate forms ferrihemoglobin *in vivo* and *in vitro.* The reaction proceeds autocatalytically because it is accelerated by the ferrihemoglobin formed.

Nitrite

Nitrite which is used as a meat salt, has occasionally been mistaken for table salt with subsequent severe methemoglobinemia. Especially in neonates, life-threatening methemoglobinemia also may be elicited by the excessive ingestion of nitrate, which is reduced to nitrite by intestinal bacteria. In addition to contaminated well water, green vegetables from strongly fertilized soil, in particular hot-house vegetables in the winter season, may contain considerable amounts of nitrate.

The mechanism of ferrihemoglobin formation by nitrite varies, depending on the presence and absence of oxygen. Under strictly anerobic conditions, 1 mol of ferrihemoglobin is formed by 1 mol of nitrite according to a second-order reaction with generation of nitrosyl ferrohemoglobin (HbNO). The affinity of NO for ferrohemoglobin is by some three orders of magnitude greater than that of carbon monoxide. In addition, nitrite ferrihemoglobin is formed with an excess of nitrite, which is a weak ligand of ferrihemoglobin.

In the presence of oxygen, the ferrihemoglobin production by nitrite is much more complex. Following an induction period (lag phase) differing between the hemoglobins of various animal species, a quasi-autocatalytic course of ferrihemoglobin formation is observed. Several observations characterize this process. Nitrate is produced at concentrations that depend on the initial concentrations of both reactants. With a twofold excess of nitrite over HbO_2, nitrate is only a minor product. At a ratio $[NO_2^-]/[HbO_2] > 8$ nitrate approaches the limiting 1:1 stoichiometry. While methemoglobin alone has no definite effect on the time course of the reaction, adding H_2O_2 shortens the induction period, and the combination of methemoglobin and H_2O_2 eliminates the lag phase completely. The autocatalytic reaction phase, in turn, is suppressed when free methemoglobin and H_2O_2 are quenched by cyanide and catalase, respectively. Hence, a reaction product of methemoglobin and hydrogen peroxide appears to be involved in the propagation phase. In fact, a ferrylhemoglobin radical species, $^{\bullet}HbFe^{IV}{=}O$, resembling the compound I complex of peroxidases, can be detected. Its concentration is highest just before the autocatalytic process begins. $^{\bullet}HbFe^{IV}{=}O$ can be reduced by another nitrite molecule under formation of the nonradical ferryl species, $HbFe^{IV}{=}O$, which ultimately is reduced by a third nitrite molecule to give methemoglobin. The expected NO_2 has been detected as an intermediate. Last, compounds scavenging NO_2 or reducing ferrylhemoglobin have been shown to eliminate the autocatalytic reaction phase. Therefore, the following reactions have been proposed:

$$HbFe^{II}O_2 + NO_2^- + H^+ \rightarrow HbFe^{III}{-}OOH + NO_2 \quad (1)$$

$$HbFe^{III}{-}OOH + H^+ \rightleftarrows HbFe^{III} + H_2O_2 \quad (2)$$

$$HbFe^{III}{-}OOH \rightarrow {}^{\bullet}HbFe^{IV}{=}O + H_2O \quad (3)$$

$$^{\bullet}HbFe^{IV}{=}O + NO_2^- + H^+ \rightarrow HbFe^{IV}{=}O + NO_2 \quad (4)$$

$$HbFe^{IV}{=}O + NO_2^- + H^+ \rightarrow HbFe^{III} + NO_2 + OH^- \quad (5)$$

$$HbFe^{II}O_2 + NO_2 \rightarrow HbFe^{III} + O_2 + NO_2^-. \quad (6)$$

While reaction (1) is expected to be rate-limiting, reactions (4) and (5) are thought to be responsible for the fast propagation phase due to NO_2 formation. Nitrate formation may occur from the dimerization of nitrogen dioxide, followed by disproportionation of N_2O_4.

No true catalyst of methemoglobin formation is involved because nitrite only forms stoichiometric amounts of methemoglobin. Rather, the acceleration phase may be due to the shift of equilibrium (2) to the left during ferrihemoglobin formation, thereby enhancing formation of the ferryl species that produces the rapidly acting NO_2.

Several intracellular reductants may compete with nitrite for the strongly oxidizing ferryl species, thereby initiating a variety of radical chain reactions in which superoxide radical anions, NO, and peroxynitrite may be involved. The complexity found *in vitro* suggests that the action of nitrite on oxyhemoglobin might be even more intricate *in vivo.*

Nitrite is also formed *in vivo* from esters of nitrous acid and nitric acid. The latter is converted enzymatically in the presence of glutathione and a variety of "nitrous acid ester reductases," apparently identical to isozymes of glutathione *S*-transferase. Correspondingly, the ferrihemoglobin production by glyceryl trinitrate or glycol dinitrate, as observed in workers of the explosives industry, has been related to the liberation of nitrite. Amyl nitrite and butyl nitrite, which are extremely volatile, are sniffed by homosexuals for an aphrodisiac effect. Excessive inhalation may be followed by severe methemoglobinemia. After therapeutic dosing of amyl nitrite, glyceryl trinitrate, or isosorbide nitrates in angina pectoris, methemoglobinemia of toxicological significance has not been observed as yet.

Quinones and Quinoid Dyes

Quinones and quinoid dyes are potent producers of ferrihemoglobin. According to their one-electron redox potential, ferrihemoglobin is formed either directly or by semiquinone radicals following one-electron reduction. A quinone of greatest therapeutic significance is menadione (vitamin K_3 or 2-methyl-1,4-naphthoquinone). An overdose of this drug has led to methemoglobinemia and hemolysis.

In this context, it may be mentioned that the rate of ferrohemoglobin oxidation by the radicals arising (redox potential >240 mV) is considerably higher than that of the total reaction. This points to a limitation by the initial reaction. Moreover, reduction of the portion of deoxyhemoglobin by increasing the oxygen partial pressure results in a retarded reaction. Maximal rates are seen at a pO_2 of 40 mmHg with 90% O_2 saturation of hemoglobin.

Compounds Forming Ferrihemoglobin Only in the Presence of Oxygen

As already discussed for nitrite, compounds of this class are co-oxidized with the heme iron by the polarized heme-bound dioxygen. The primary reaction products are a xenobiotic radical species and an intermediate methemoglobin–hydrogen peroxide complex, $HbFe^{III}{-}OOH$. With its trivalent iron, this complex is detectable only at low temperatures. It either decays into methemoglobin and hydrogen peroxide or rearranges, with transfer of the oxidizing equivalents from the ligand to both the heme iron and the globin moiety. The resulting ferryl species, $^\bullet HbFe^{IV}{=}O$, resembles the compound I complexes of catalase and peroxidases. The mechanism and site of globin radical formation are not entirely known, but the available data suggest a tyrosine phenoxy radical most likely to be involved. Compound I is a strongly oxidizing species, capable of one-electron abstraction from another xenobiotic molecule. Thereby, the globin radical disappears in favor of a compound II type species, $HbFe^{IV}{=}O$, in analogy to the behavior of peroxidases. Finally, compound II can be reduced by a third xenobiotic molecule with formation of methemoglobin, $HbFe^{III}$, a hydroxide ion, and a xenobiotic radical.

Such a sequence has also been proposed for the ferrihemoglobin formation by aminophenols. 4-Dimethylaminophenol (RX^-), belonging to this class of compounds, has taken a special place because it is able to form ferrihemoglobin in a quasi-catalytic reaction. This property is made use of to induce methemoglobin formation for the treatment of cyanide poisoning. The reactions may proceed as follows:

$$HbFe^{II}O_2 + RX^- + H^+ \rightarrow HbFe^{III}{-}OOH + RX^\bullet \quad (1)$$

$$HbFe^{III}{-}OOH + H^+ \rightleftarrows HbFe^{III} + H_2O_2 \quad (2)$$

$$HbFe^{III}{-}OOH \rightarrow {}^\bullet HbFe^{IV}{=}O + H_2O \quad (3)$$

$$^\bullet HbFe^{IV}{-}O + RX^- + H^+ \rightarrow HbFe^{IV}{-}O + RX^\bullet \quad (4)$$

$$HbFe^{IV}{-}O + RX^- + H^+ \rightarrow HbFe^{III} + RX^\bullet + OH^- \quad (5)$$

$$HbFe^{II} + RX^\bullet \rightarrow HbFe^{III} + RX^- \quad (6)$$

In these reactions, the oxygen is "neatly" reduced to the oxidation step of water without the liberation of free hydrogen peroxide. Accordingly, superoxide dismutase and catalase do not exert an effect on the kinetics of ferrihemoglobin formation. Reactions (3) and (4) are much faster than Reaction (2). The three phenoxy radicals ($RX^\bullet$), in turn, oxidize ferrohemoglobin to ferrihemoglobin, simultaneously being reduced again to 4-dimethylaminophenol in Reaction (6). Thus, the catalytic cycle is closed.

Another reaction type is observed with the analog *N,N*-dimethyl-*p*-phenylenediamine. In this case, the addition of catalase diminishes the rate of ferrihemoglobin formation by one-third. Therefore, it is suggested that Reaction (2), with liberation of free H_2O_2 and ferrihemoglobin, is faster than Reactions (3) and (4) and that only one aminyl radical ($RX^\bullet$) is formed in Reaction (1) and reduced to the parent compound in Reaction (6). Two molecules of ferrihemoglobin are formed in the catalytic cycle, while a third molecule of ferrihemoglobin is generated by H_2O_2, in accordance with a reduction by one-third of the reaction rate in the presence of catalase.

A third reaction type is observed with phenylhydroxylamine. Upon co-oxidation, a phenylnitroxide radical is formed which, however, is unable to oxidize ferrohemoglobin because of its low redox potential.

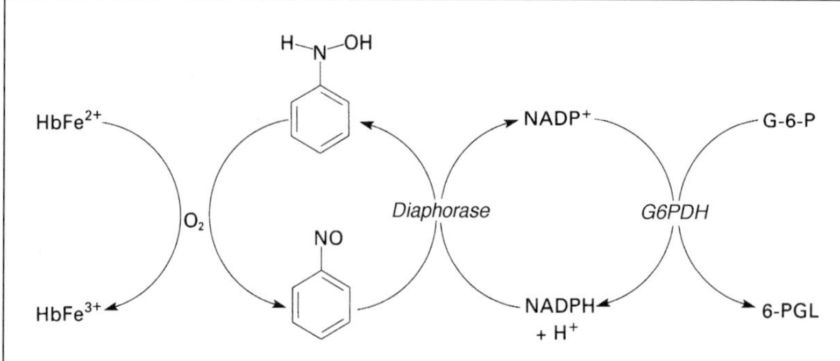

FIGURE 6 Ferrihemoglobin formation by phenylhydroxylamine (Kiese cycle). Nitrosobenzene produced by co-oxidation of ferrohemoglobin and phenylhydroxylamine is reduced to phenylhydroxylamine by an NADPH-dependent diaphorase. Thus, catalytic amounts of phenylhydroxylamine or nitrosobenzene are able to produce many equivalents of ferrihemoglobin. $NADP^+$ is then reduced via the pentose phosphate pathway. (For abbreviations see Fig. 4.)

The radical is rather oxidized at once to nitrosobenzene. Phenylhydroxylamine has been shown to produce only one equivalent of ferrihemoglobin with the formation of about stoichiometric amounts of nitrosobenzene. In this co-oxidation, two electrons are taken from phenylhydroxylamine and one electron from the hemoglobin iron. Correspondingly, the hemoglobin-bound oxygen may be formally reduced to OH^- and •OH. However, until now no hints to a destructive action of •OH have been found.

While its reaction with purified hemoglobin only yields stoichiometric amounts of ferrihemoglobin, a quasi-catalytic ferrihemoglobin formation by phenylhydroxylamine is observed in red blood cells with normal metabolism. In erythrocytes starved to become glucose-free, this "catalytic" effect is lost. Lactate cannot replace glucose. An NADPH-dependent diaphorase reducing nitrosobenzene to phenylhydroxylamine is responsible for the "catalysis." This Kiese cycle (Fig. 6), as it is called after its discoverer, makes phenylhydroxylamine and nitroso derivatives the most potent ferrihemoglobin producers *in vivo*. The diaphorase is also able to reduce ferrihemoglobin in the presence of an appropriate redox mediator.

The closely related phenylhydroxamic acids are likewise potent ferrihemoglobin producers, presenting a nearly catalytic reaction with purified hemoglobin. The redox potential of the nitroxide radical amounts to several hundred millivolts, sufficient to rapidly oxidize ferrohemoglobin. Thus, the mechanism of ferrihemoglobin formation resembles that of the aminophenols. (See Table 3.)

TABLE 3 Compounds Forming Ferrihemoglobin Only in the Presence of Oxygen

Aminophenols: *p*-aminophenol from paracetamol (acetaminophen); 2-hydroxyphenetidine from phenacetin; 4-methylaminophenol (developer); 4-dimethylaminophenol (cyanide antidote); 5-aminosalicylic acid (anti-inflammatory)
Arylhydroxylamine and hydroxamic acids
Phenylenediamines (hair dyes)
Hydroxyurea derivatives (herbicides)
Arsines and phosphines
Hydrazine derivatives (alkyl and arylhydrazines, e.g., in rocket fuels)

Compounds Forming Ferrihemoglobin After Biotransformation

Aromatic amines

Ferrihemoglobin production by the parent compounds is insignificant, except for arylamines carrying electron donating substituents (e.g., *p*-NR_2 or *p*-O-R). Aromatic amines (Table 4) are bioactivated by oxygenation, especially in the liver. Aminophenols arise from C-oxygenation, and *N*-hydroxyarylamines and hydroxamic acids from N-oxygenation in microsomal, cytochrome P450-dependent reactions, the products being able to produce many equivalents of ferrihemoglobin. The parent compound determines which of the oxygenation products plays the main role in ferrihemoglobin formation. Moreover, these reactions differ widely among the animal species. However, before leaving the liver the major part of the proximate

TABLE 4 Compounds Forming Ferrihemoglobin after Biotransformation
Industrial chemicals
Aniline, chloroaniline, nitroaniline, toluidine, xylidine, anisidine, benzidine
Naphthylamines
Azo dyes
Nitrobenzene derivatives in nitro lacquers, diluents, and explosives (trinitrotoluene, tetranitromethylaniline)
Drugs
Acetanilide, phenacetin, paracetamol (analgesics)
Primaquine (antimalarial)
Procaine, benzocaine, prilocaine, carticaine, lidocaine (local anesthetics)
Phenazopyridine (local anesthetic in urinary tract)
Dapsone, sulfanilamide, sulfapyridine, nitrofurantoin (antimicrobials)
Metoclopramide (antiemetic)

oxygenated compounds is already inactivated, thus preventing ferrihemoglobin formation in the blood.

Aminophenols, for example, are rapidly conjugated to glucuronides and sulfates. *N*-Hydroxyarylamines can be reduced again or, furthermore, be oxidized to nitroso derivatives. These can react extremely rapidly with thiols, especially with glutathione, so that only a minor part will arrive in the systemic circulation. In addition, *N*-hydroxyarylamines are also able to undergo NO conjugation, resulting in metastable intermediates splitting off reactive nitrenium ions in a weakly acid medium. So, phenetidine *N,O*-glucuronides and *N,O*-sulfates are regarded as causes of uroepithelial tumors, which were occasionally observed in the abuse of phenacetin (withdrawn). *N*-Hydroxyarylamines are also N-acylated, yielding hydroxamic acids, which in turn are able to form ferrihemoglobin (Fig. 7). Hydroxamic acids can also arise by N-oxygenation of the corresponding *N*-acylarylamines. In the attempt to convert lipophilic xenobiotics into water-soluble compounds excretable by the kidneys, reactive potentially dangerous compounds are generated by the organism in phase I metabolism (Fig. 7). Upon exceeding the capacity of the phase II reactions, phase I metabolites escaping from the liver may damage other organs. The damage is especially conspicuous in case of methemoglobinemia. Activated metabolites of aniline derivatives with electron-attracting substituents (e.g., *p*-chloroaniline and 3,4-dichloroaniline (degradation products of the herbicides linuron and propanil), *p*-aminoacetophenone, *p*-aminopropiophenone, *p*-nitroaniline, and *p*-aminobiphenyl), form ferrihemoglobin very efficiently.

Methemoglobinemia was described following injection of local anesthetics of the aniline type, comprising procaine, benzocaine, prilocaine, carticaine and lidocaine. *p*-Sulfoaniline derivatives, such as dapsone, and also sulfanilamides, such as sulfadiazine and sulfapyridine arising from salazopyridine, may lead to methemoglobinemia. Metoclopramide, phenacetin and, to a lesser extent, paracetamol (acetaminophen) may also produce ferrihemoglobin. Polycyclic arylamines, such as naphthylamines, aminofluorenes, 4-aminobiphenyl, 4-aminoazobenzene, and benzidine, are strong ferrihemoglobin producers. Their toxicological interest is, however, determined more by their carcinogenic potential.

Aminoquinoline derivatives

Among these derivatives, the antimalarial primaquine is of particular significance. Which metabolites are responsible for the methemoglobin formation has not been clarified. Chloroquine, hydroxychloroquine, and mefloquine may cause hemolysis upon G6PDH deficiency, while methemoglobinemia is clinically insignificant.

Azo compounds

The reductive splitting of the azo bridge, especially by intestinal bacteria, releases ferrihemoglobin-forming arylamines. In this respect, chrysoidine sulfonamide, phenazopyridine (a local anesthetic for the urinary tract), and salazopyridine are to be pointed out. Salazopyridine is degraded to sulfapyridine, which is capable of producing ferrihemoglobin indirectly, and to 5-aminosalicylic acid, whose potential of forming ferrihemoglobin directly is comparably small.

Nitroaromatics

The reduction of the nitro group, especially by intestinal bacteria, results in a variety of ferrihemoglobin-forming products, as mentioned here. The ferrihemoglobin-producing potential of the products is comparable to that of their arylamine analogs. The high lipophilicity and volatility of the nitro derivatives permit an efficient absorption via skin and lungs.

Correspondingly, nitrobenzene (mirbane oil, a surrogate of bitter almond oil) and similar compounds that are widely used in the chemical industry for syntheses and as solvents (e.g., nitro lacquers and nitro diluents) are able to produce ferrihemoglobin not only after oral but also after cutaneous and inhalative uptake. Occasional methemoglobinemia has been observed in workers at ammunition factories in conjunction with trinitrotoluene. The property of ferrihemoglobin formation is not inherent to all nitro-

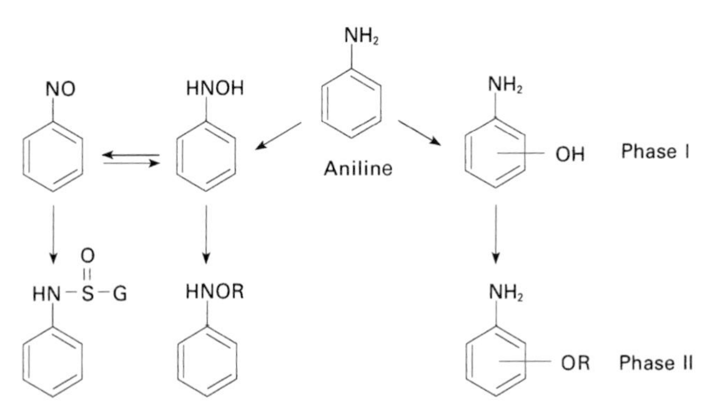

FIGURE 7 Hepatic activation and inactivation reactions for aniline. The reactive metabolites arising in phase I are rapidly conjugated to polar compounds that are excreted by the kidneys. The residue R (phase II) may represent glucuronides or sulfates. G indicates glutathione residue.

benzene derivatives. Methemoglobinemia has not been found following the ingestion of the drugs chloramphenicol and nifedipine, but it has been found after the ingestion of nitrofurantoin, a nitrofuran derivative. The metabolites responsible for ferrihemoglobin formation by nitrofurantoin have not been identified as yet. The most important occupational and medical ferrihemoglobin producers are compiled in Table 4.

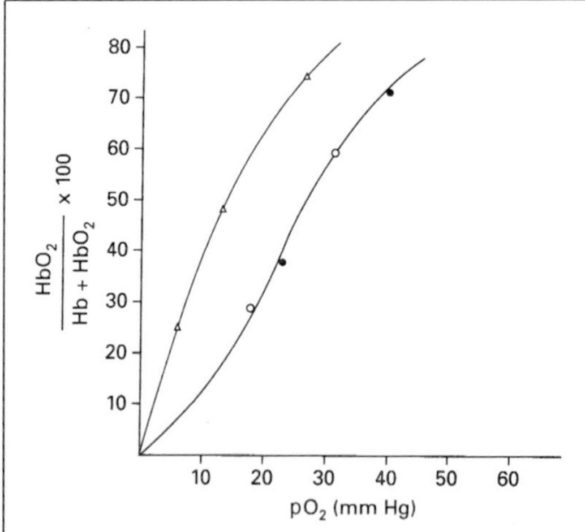

FIGURE 8 Influence of the ferrihemoglobin content on the oxygen dissociation curve of canine blood. After i.v. injection of sodium nitrite in a dog, 69% ferrihemoglobin has been formed. The oxygen dissociation curve of this blood (△) is plotted along with the curves obtained before (●) and 23 h after nitrite injection (○). The oxygen affinity of the partially oxidized hemoglobin is elevated in comparison to normal blood; half-saturation = 15 mm Hg, versus 27 mm Hg. At pO_2 27 mm Hg, normal oxyhemoglobin releases 50% of its oxygen, while only 25% of the oxygen can dissociate with 70% of the hemoglobin existing in the trivalent state. (According to Darling and Roughton, 1942, with permission.)

Symptoms of Methemoglobinemia

Methemoglobinemia is characterized by oxygen transport deficiency of the blood and reduced liberation of oxygen to the tissue. In this respect, methemoglobinemia resembles the effects of CO poisoning and is thus more threatening than a corresponding transport-deficiency anemia. These relations were first described by Darling and Roughton in 1942. Partially oxidized hemoglobin exhibits an elevated oxygen affinity (Fig. 8) due to a decrease in the allosteric cooperativity of tetrameric hemoglobin. Similar to hemoglobin partially loaded with carbon monoxide, partially oxidized hemoglobin exists to a greater extent in the oxy-conformation. Thereby, the oxygen affinity of hemoglobin increases and the oxygen dissociation curve loses its sigmoid shape.

Ferrihemoglobin fractions of up to 20% are largely tolerated at normal total hemoglobin, besides a pale gray complexion and some restriction on physical fitness. Sudden onset of methemoglobinemia (≥30% ferrihemoglobin) is associated with headache, tiredness, yawning, and poor concentration. Light physical exercise leads to dyspnea and tachycardia. Ferrihemoglobin contents of more than 50% are life-threatening, and the chance of surviving 80% ferrihemoglobin is low.

Intense methemoglobinemia is usually manifested by lactacidosis due to tissue hypoxia. A decrease in blood pH reduces the oxygen affinity of hemoglobin

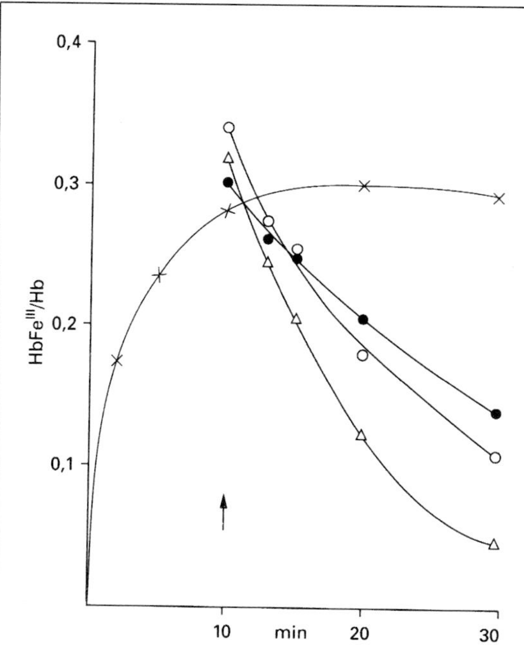

FIGURE 9 Influence of methylene and toluidine blue on methemoglobin reduction in humans. About 30% methemoglobin was produced by injection of 4-dimethylaminophenol HCl, 3.25 mg/kg i.v. Ten minutes later (arrow) methylene blue (●), 2 mg/kg i.v., or toluidine blue (○), 2 mg/kg or (△) 4 mg/kg i.v., was injected, resulting in a remarkable acceleration of methemoglobin reduction compared to spontaneous reduction (X). (From Kiese *et al.* (1972), *Eur. J. Clin. Pharmacol.* **4**, 115–118; copyright Springer-Verlag, with permission.)

and facilitates the release of oxygen to the tissue (Bohr effect). The acidosis requires a rapid correction, because otherwise even the anerobic glycolysis may cease. Severe methemoglobinemia will nearly always induce hemolysis and the formation of Heinz bodies as manifestations of additional oxidative damage to the erythrocytes. With many ferrihemoglobin-forming substances, methemoglobinemia is not to the fore. Many solvents exhibit central symptoms, and vasodilator actions are predominant with nitrous and nitric acid esters.

Therapy of Methemoglobinemia

A special treatment is unnecessary below 30% ferrihemoglobin. High oral doses of ascorbic acid (1–2 g) are indicated in individuals with congenital methemoglobin reductase deficiency or M-hemoglobinopathy. Redox dyes (e.g., methylene blue and toluidine blue) enable the NADPH-dependent diaphorase to transfer reducing equivalents from the pentose-phosphate pathway to ferrihemoglobin (Fig. 4). They should be used in cases with intense methemoglobinemia. Toluidine blue is more effective in reducing ferrihemoglobin (Fig. 9) and apparently better tolerated. The injection of these dyes is also effective in case of methemoglobin reductase deficiency, but not of G6PDH deficiency, as NADPH cannot be made available. It is to be pointed out that the "cyanotic" complexion appearing upon injection of methylene blue or toluidine blue is not a manifestation of hypoxia but directly related to the dye injected. Still, emergency physicians unaware of this fact often call the poison centers. If in doubt, blood gas analyses will help clarify it.

Extreme methemoglobinemia is treated with hyperbaric oxygen, resulting in sufficient amounts of oxygen physically dissolved in the plasma to meet the oxygen demand of the tissue. Because massive hemolysis is also observed upon extreme methemoglobinemia, a fractional exchange transfusion of whole blood is recommended to remove the nephrotoxic amounts of free hemoglobin and to make available intact red blood cells.

Therapeutic Methemoglobinemia

Ferrihemoglobin is produced therapeutically for binding toxic ligands to ferrihemoglobin. The main indication for such a measure is cyanide poisoning. Sometimes, ferrihemoglobin formation has also been advocated for azide and hydrogen sulfide poisoning.

Sodium nitrite (about 4 mg/kg iv in a 3% solution over 4 min in adults; final methemoglobin concentration some 20%) and, with doubtful success, amyl nitrite (inhaled from broken ampuls) are used to induce therapeutic methemoglobinemia. A more rapid and safer way to produce therapeutic methemoglobinemia is the iv injection of 4-dimethylaminophenol hydrochloride (4-DMAP, 3.25 mg/kg). At this dose, a ferrihemoglobin maximum of 30% is reached within 15 min with $t_{1/2}$ being <1 min. This can detoxify five lethal doses of cyanide (cf. Chapter 33, "Gases").

Toxic Hemolysis

Oxidative Stress

Oxidative damage to the erythrocytes manifests itself not only as ferrihemoglobin formation. Reactive oxidants are able to further oxidize ferrihemoglobin, attacking the iron–porphyrin complex and the globin matrix with the generation of several green pigments. These chemically ill-defined hemochromes have some features in common, such as poor water solubility, precipitation, and attachment to the cell membrane (Heinz bodies). Also quinoid compounds originating from ferrihemoglobin producers (e.g., hydroquinones, aminophenols, and phenylenediamines) and nitrosobenzene intermediates are able to covalently bind to SH groups of red blood cell membrane constituents, enzymes, and hemoglobin, with subsequent functional impairment. The membrane fluidity and the plasticity of the erythrocytes are reduced, thus hampering their easy passage through the capillaries. While passing through spleen, liver, and bone marrow, these cells are "culled out" from the blood by means of the reticuloendothelial cells, comparable to the elimination of red blood cells at the end of their lifetime.

A decrease in cell fluidity also results from direct oxidative damage to the cell membrane due to lipid peroxidation or to cross-linking via disulfide bridges in the membrane proteins. Moreover, essential ion pumps may be affected. Disturbances in ion and water transport generally lead to cell swelling with subsequent sequestration in the spleen or direct intravasal hemolysis. If the antioxidative defense and repair systems are deficient, hemolysis and Heinz bodies are already produced by these potentially harmful agents at concentrations usually well tolerated. In case of G6PDH deficiency, for example, nearly all the compounds able to induce methemoglobinemia also produce hemolysis with or without Heinz bodies. Some compounds characterized by hemolysis rather than by methemoglobinemia shall be mentioned here.

Arsine

Arsine (arsenic hydride, AsH_3), arising in some industrial processes, elicits a massive intravasal hemolysis with mostly only slight methemoglobinemia. Probably due to a reaction of arsine with SH groups of membranes and enzymes, the intoxication manifests itself by hemoglobinuria, jaundice, and severe anemia. An inhibition of catalase and peroxidative damage to the red blood cell membrane are also discussed.

TABLE 5 Compounds Causing Hemolysis and Heinz Body Formation by Oxidative Stress

Industrial chemicals
Phenylhydrazine, acetylphenylhydrazine, aniline, nitrobenzene, trinitrotoluene, chlorate, lead salts, copper salts, arsine
Drugs
Acetanilide, phenacetin (analgesics)
Phenazopyridine (local anesthetic in urinary tract)
Nomifensine (antidepressant)
Niridazole (anthelmintic)
Primaquine (antimalarial)
Dapsone, nalidixic acid, nitrofurantoin, sulfasalazine, sulfonamides (antimicrobials)
D-Penicillamine (chelator)

Copper

Free copper ions, which are known to be excessive in the plasma of patients suffering from Wilson's disease, cause hemolytic anemias. The autoxidation of thiols is considerably accelerated by catalytic amounts of copper ions, resulting in disulfide formation in membrane proteins with release of hydrogen peroxide. The copper ions undergo a valency change with equal toxicity of Cu^{+} and Cu^{2+}. Increased hemolysis in hemodialysis patients was put down to copper-containing devices.

Lead

In poisoning with lead salts, the biosynthesis of heme is disturbed at various stages. Moreover, the lifetime of the erythrocytes is shortened. Due to inhibition of pyrimidine-5′ nucleotidase, the mature erythrocytes retain a ribonucleotide that is believed to be responsible for the basophilic stippling observed. Lead anemia is therefore a sequela of disturbed hemoglobin synthesis and increased degradation of red blood cells. Patients with thalassemia react with a special susceptibility.

Chlorate

Chlorate, which has been used as a weed-killer, induces severe hemolysis besides methemoglobinemia.

Snake Venom

Snake venoms may contain enzymes converting lecithin to lysolecithin, which exhibits hemolytic activity. Still, hemorrhage instead of hemolysis determines the clinical picture following snakebites. Detergents and saponines are well-known for their hemolytic activity. In the past, they were notorious for this action when used in soap abortions with their tragic outcomes.

The most significant compounds with regard to Heinz body formation and hemolysis, in particular in G6PDH deficiency, are compiled in Table 5.

Immunologic Hemolytic Anemias Induced by Xenobiotics

Following the attachment of immunoproteins, erythrocytes can be phagocytized during the passage through spleen, liver, and bone marrow, or they can be lysed by IgM antibodies and complement. This type of hemolysis is mostly found upon blood group incompatibility (e.g., during blood transfusion), but occasionally lysis may also be elicited by foreign compounds. Distinct mechanisms are responsible for this phenomenon.

Formation of Immunological Complexes

IgM antibodies against xenobiotics or their protein adducts form immunological complexes docking with red blood cells that are lyzed following complement binding. In these cases, the xenobiotic is not chemically bound to the cell membrane nor is the antibody directed against the red blood cell. The erythrocyte acts as an "innocent bystander" hit by the immunological complex. This phenomenon has been described for stibophen (anthelmintic), quinine (antimalarial), quinidine (antiarrhythmic), chlorpropamide (hypoglycemic), rifampicin (antimicrobial), antazoline (antihistamine), and methotrexate (cytostatic).

Binding of Xenobiotics to the Erythrocyte Membrane

Stable complexes recognizable to IgM antibodies are formed on the outer membrane of the red blood cell, eventually initiating hemolysis. This type of hemolysis is encountered with penicillin, cephalosporins, tetracyclines (antimicrobials), and carbromal (sedative-hypnotic). In contrast, hemolytic anemias induced by α-methyl-dopa (antihypertensive), L-dopa (antiparkinsonian), or mefenamic acid (anti-inflammatory) appear to be associated with the formation of antibodies against a preexisting erythrocytic antigen, which is related to the rhesus complex. It has been proposed that hemolysis may also come about by an action of these compounds on T-lymphocytes, thereby abolishing their suppressor function.

TOXIC ACTIONS ON THROMBOCYTES

The thrombocytes of the circulating blood contain a variety of vasoactive substances that are readily made available to initiate the reactions that stop bleeding (hemostasis). Endothelial lesions, antigen–antibody complexes, acidosis, and hemolysis stimulate the formation of pseudopodia and membrane alterations fostering the coagulation. ADP and thromboxane A_2, an arachidonic acid metabolite, are released, which promotes the aggregation of thrombocytes and their secretion. In parallel the plasmatic clotting system is activated. Due to this positive feedback mechanism, the thrombocytes are able to exert their hemostatic function very rapidly. This vital task can be impaired by many toxic influences.

Inhibition of Thrombocytic Functions

Inhibition of Membrane Functions

The receptor-mediated aggregation of thrombocytes by ADP and thromboxane A_2 is inhibited by a few β-lactam antibiotics (e.g., by high doses of carbenicillin, penicillin G, oxycillin, and cephalotin). The effect sets in rapidly, depending on the concentration, and is reversible. A similar effect is observed with calcium antagonists of the verapamil type (e.g., ticlopidine). *In vitro* studies indicate that membrane-stabilizing drugs that act by hampering the signal transduction also may inhibit thrombocyte functions. Among them are local anesthetics (e.g., dibucaine and tetracaine), tricyclic antidepressants (e.g., imipramine, amitriptyline, and nortriptyline), and phenothiazine neuroleptics (e.g., chlorpromazine, promethazine, and trifluperazine). Obviously, this is clinically insignificant because confirmative case reports are missing, probably because the plasma concentrations of these drugs are far below those required to impair platelet aggregation. Moreover, heparin and higher-molecular-weight dextran are able to reduce the responsiveness of thrombocytes to physiological agonists, possibly by coating the membrane receptors.

The count of functioning platelets is often found to be diminished upon antiarrhythmic treatment with quinidine and occasionally also occurs with amiodarone. The reduction in the counts and the responsiveness of platelets is attributed to antigen–antibody complexes. A similar mechanism is also discussed for diuretics (e.g., thiazides and furosemide), antimicrobials (e.g., sulfonamides, streptomycin, and rifampicin), quinine (also in beverages), and anti-inflammatory (e.g., phenylbutazone) or analgesic and antipyretic drugs (e.g., phenacetin).

Inhibition of Eicosanoid Formation

The inhibition of thrombocyte cyclooxygenase by nonsteroidal anti-inflammatory drugs results in reduced thromboxane A_2 synthesis with the subsequent impairment of platelet aggregation. Cyclooxygenase is irreversibly inhibited by acetylsalicylic acid. Because the platelets have lost the ability to synthesize new cyclooxygenase, the platelet aggregation defect is likewise irreversible. With other nonsteroidal anti-inflammatory drugs, the cyclooxygenase inhibition is reversible, correlating with the plasma concentration.

Ethanol reduces thromboxane A_2 formation and therefore increases the inhibitory effect of acetylsalicylic acid if taken along with this drug. Conversely, alcohol withdrawal may be associated with increased thromboxane A_2 synthesis and platelet aggregation.

Alcohol is likely to act at various sites. The impairment of the inositol triphosphate-dependent intracellular calcium release as induced by agonists is discussed. Epidemiological studies suggest that a moderate consumption of alcohol (<50 g per day) may give protection from ischemic heart disease. Such an effect also may be accounted for by a reduced reactivity of the platelets due to inhibition of the adrenaline-induced ADP release. This might also explain the fact that the tendency to bleed increases in alcohol intoxication despite an intact plasmatic clotting system. The platelet aggregation is also hampered by increased c-GMP concentrations. This may account for the inhibition of aggregation by drugs forming NO (e.g., glyceryl trinitrate and sodium nitroprusside), thereby activating the soluble guanylate cyclase of the platelet. Similar actions are known for the azides and hydroxylamine, which are also able to release NO.

Activation of Thrombocytic Functions

Fibrinolytics, which are used in recent myocardiac infarction, are capable of stimulating the formation of thromboxane A_2 with concomitant increase in platelet aggregation. This may result in partial resistance to therapy with anticoagulants. Cyclosporine A, which is increasingly used to prevent graft rejection reactions, may increase platelet aggregation with subsequent thrombotic complications.

TOXIC ACTIONS ON HEMOSTASIS

Increased Hemorrhagic Tendency

The primary hemostasis is impaired in bone marrow suppression and in immunological reactions reducing the platelet count and inhibiting their normal function. The platelet plug cannot be strained mechanically beyond a certain limit, requiring a fibrin network with the inclusion of other cellular elements for solidification. Disturbances in the stopping of bleeding are to be reckoned with when the synthesis of clotting factors has been impaired, in particular in the liver. In addition to specific inhibitors of the synthesis of these factors (e.g., the vitamin K antagonist coumarin), any more severe liver damage by xenobiotics also entails the reduced synthesis of the clotting factors (Table 6).

TABLE 6 Potentially Hepatotoxic Compounds Reducing the Synthesis of Clotting Factors

Industrial chemicals and toxins
Antimony, arsenic, lead, phosphorus, selenium, thallium
Benzene, dioxane, phenylhydrazine, resorcinol
Chlorinated hydrocarbons (e.g., chloroform, carbon tetrachloride, dichloroethane)
Death cap toxins *(Amanita phalloides)*
Drugs
Acetazolamide (carbonic anhydrase inhibitor)
Cycloserine, iproniazid, viomycin (tuberculostatics)
Sulfonamides (antimicrobials)
Paracetamol (acetaminophen; overdose) (analgesic)
Gold compounds (antirheumatic)
Chlorpromazine (neuroleptic)
Halothane (inhalation anesthetic)
MAO inhibitors
Vitamin A

Disseminated Intravasal Coagulopathy

Substances acting like thromboplastin and inducing coagulation can elicit disseminated intravasal clotting while entering the bloodstream. This may happen following extensive erosion of the mucosa or cellular necrosis in parenchymatous organs by acids, lyes, $HgCl_2$, death cap toxins, and chlorinated hydrocarbons, such as CCl_4 and dichloroethane. Clotting is also promoted by acidosis that frequently occurs in severe poisoning with methanol, formic acid, carbon monoxide, cholinesterase inhibitors, and biguanide hypoglycemics. Snake venoms are able to initiate disseminated intravasal clotting by a proteolytic attack at the prefactors of clotting. The generalized activation of the coagulation system and fibrinolysis entail an unrestricted turnover of clotting factors that is manifested clinically as a consumptive coagulopathy with severe bleeding due to the consumption of clotting factors and by thromboses in the terminal vessels with consumption of thrombocytes.

Bibliography

Buettner, G. R. (1993). The pecking order of free radicals and antioxidants: Lipid peroxidation, α-tocopherol, and ascorbate. *Arch. Biochem. Biophys.* **300,** 535–543.

Bunn, H. F., and Forget, B. G. (1986). "Hemoglobin: Molecular, Genetic and Clinical Aspects." W. B. Saunders, Philadelphia, PA.

Casarett L. J., Klaassen, C. D., Amdur, M. O., and Doull, J. (1996). "Casarett and Doull's Toxicology: The Basic Science of Poisons," 5th ed. McGrawHill, New York.

Castro, C. E. (1980). Mechanisms of reaction of hemoproteins with oxygen and hydrogen peroxide in the oxidation of organic substrates. *Pharmacol. Ther.* **10,** 171–189.

Clark, I. A., and Cowden, W. B. (1985). Antimalarials. In "Oxidative Stress" (H. Sies, ed.), pp. 131–149. Academic Press, San Diego, CA.

Darling, R. C., and Roughton, F. J. W. (1942). The effect of methemoglobin on the equilibrium between oxygen and hemoglobin. *Am. J. Physiol.* **137,** 56–68.

Dukes, M. N. G. (1996). "Meyler's Side Effects of Drugs," 13th ed. Elsevier, Amsterdam.

Ellenhorn, M. J., Schonwald, S., Ordog, G., and Wasserberger J. (1996). "Ellenhorn's Medical Toxicology: Diagnosis and Treatment of Human Poisoning," 2nd ed. Williams & Wilkins, Baltimore, MD.

Elstner, E. F. (1990). "Der Sauerstoff: Biochemie, Biologie, Medizin." B.I. Wissenschaftsverlag, Mannheim.

Eyer, P. (1991). Activation of aromatic amines by oxyhemoglobin. *In* "N-Oxidation of Drugs, Biochemistry, Pharmacology and Toxicology" (P. Hlavica and L. A. Damani, eds.), pp. 371–391. Chapman & Hall, London.

Eyer, P. (1994). The role of erythrocytes in the biotransformation of xenobiotics. *In* "Metabolic Aspects of Cell Toxicity" (P. Eyer, ed.), pp. 149–165. B.I. Wissenschaftsverlag, Mannheim.

Eyer, P., Lierheimer, E., and Schneller, M. (1984). Reactions of nitrosochloramphenicol in blood. *Biochem. Pharmacol.* **33,** 2299–2308.

Fisher, J. W. (1992). Handbook of Experimental Pharmacology, Vol. 101, "Biochemical Pharmacology of Blood and Bloodforming Organs." Springer-Verlag, Berlin.

Forth, W., Henschler, D., Rummel, W., and Starke, K. (1996). "Pharmakologie und Toxikologie," 7th ed. Spektrum Akademischer Verlag GmbH, Heidelberg.

Hardisty, R. M., and Weatherall, D. J. (1982). "Blood and Its Disorders," 2nd ed. Blackwell Scientific Publications, Oxford.

Hardman, J. G., Limbird, L. E., Molinoff, P. B., Ruddon, R. W., and Goodman Gilman, A. (1996). "Goodman & Gilman's The Pharmacological Basis of Therapeutics," 9th ed. McGraw-Hill, New York.

Heimpel, H. (1988). Drug-induced agranulocytosis. *Med. Toxicol.* **3,** 449–462.

Irons, R. D. (1985). "Toxicology of the Blood and Bone Marrow." Target Organ Toxicology Series. Raven Press, New York.

Jacobs, A. (1989) Benzene hematotoxicity and leukemia. *In* "Assessment of Inhalation Hazards" (U. Mohr, ed.), pp. 223–231. ILSI Monographs. Springer-Verlag, Berlin.

Jollow, D. J., Bradshaw, T. P., and McMillan, D. C. (1995). Dapsone-induced hemolytic anemia. *Drug Metab. Rev.* **27,** 107–124.

Keller, D. F. (1971). "G-6-PD Deficiency." CRC Press, Butterworth, London.

Kiese, M. (1974). "Methemoglobinemia: A Comprehensive Treatise." CRC Press, Cleveland, OH.

Kiese, M., Lörcher, W., Weger, N., and Zierer, A. (1972). Comparative studies on the effects of toluidine blue and methylene blue on the reduction of ferrihemoglobin in man and dog. *Eur. J. Clin. Pharmacol.* **4,** 115–118.

Klimmek, R., Krettek, C., and Werner, H. W. (1988). Ferrihemoglobin formation by amyl nitrite and sodium nitrite in different species in vivo and in vitro. *Arch. Toxicol.* **62,** 152–160.

Klöcking, H.-P., and Güttner, J. (1992). "Toxische Einflüsse auf die Hämostase." Ullstein Mosby GmbH & Co. KG, Berlin.

Kosaka, H., and Tyuma, I. (1987). Mechanism of autocatalytic oxidation of oxyhemoglobin by nitrite. *Environ. Health Perspect.* **73,** 147–151.

Matanoski, G. M., Santos-Burgoa, C., Zeger, S. L., and Schwartz, L. (1989). Epidemiological data related to health effects of 1,3-butadiene. *In* "Assessment of Inhalation Hazards" (U. Mohr, ed.), pp. 202–214. ILSI Monographs. Springer-Verlag, Berlin.

Moeschlin, S. (1986). "Klinik und Therapie der Vergiftungen," 7th ed. Georg Thieme, Stuttgart.

Niesink, R. J. M., de Vries, J., and Hollinger, M. A. (1996). "Toxicology: Principles and Applications." CRC Press, Boca Raton, FL.

Ortiz de Montellano, P. R. (1992). Catalytic sites of hemoprotein peroxidases. *Annu. Rev. Pharmacol. Toxicol.* **32,** 89–107.

Rice-Evans, C. (1987). "Free Radicals, Oxidant Stress and Drug Action." Richelieu Press, London.

Schrör, K. (1991). Toxic influences on platelet function. *Arch. Toxicol. Suppl.* **14,** 147–152.

Sies, H. (1985). "Oxidative Stress." Academic Press, London.

Stolze, K., and Nohl, H. (1995). Reactions of reducing xenobiotics with oxymyoglobin, formation of metmyoglobin, ferryl myoglobin and free radicals: An electron spin resonance and chemiluminescence study. *Biochem. Pharmacol.* **49,** 1261–1267.

Szorady, I. (1991). "Klinische Pharmakogenetik." Ernst Reinhardt Verlag, München.

Uetrecht, J. P. (1992). The role of leucocyte-generated reactive metabolites in the pathogenesis of idiosyncratic drug reactions. *Drug Metab. Rev.* **24,** 299–366.

von Bruchhausen, F., and Walter, U. (1997). Handbook of Experimental Pharmacology, Vol. **101**, "Platelets and Their Factors." Springer-Verlag, Berlin.

Williams, W. J., Beutler, E., Erslev, A. J., and Lichtman, M. A. (1990). "Hematology," 4th ed. McGraw-Hill, New York.

Winterbourn, C. C. (1989). Inhibition of autoxidation of divicine and isouramil by the combination of superoxide dismutase and reduced glutathione. *Arch. Biochem. Biophys.* **271,** 447–455.

Yunis, A. A. (1988). Chloramphenicol: Relation of structure to activity and toxicity. *Ann. Rev. Pharmacol. Toxicol.* **28,** 83–100.

C H A P T E R

17

Immune System

REINHARD NEUBERT*, DIETHER NEUBERT†

*Dept. of Neurology–Neurosurgery, Scientific and Medical Association for Research and Technology, Annecy, France
†Institute of Clinical Pharmacology and Toxicology, Benjamin Franklin Medical Center, Free University of Berlin, Berlin, Germany

INTRODUCTION

Analysis of adverse effects of xenobiotics and physical factors on components and functions of the immune system is a relatively new field in toxicology and pharmacology. About 25 years ago effects of chemicals on certain immunological variables were studied in experimental animals for the first time. These early attempts are intimately connected with the names of Vos, Moore, Dean, and a few others.

Within the past two decades, knowledge of immunology has increased and is unmatched by hardly any other field of biology or medicine. This is due to the development of new techniques and experimental approaches, such as the production and use of monoclonal antibodies (mAbs), flow cytometry, and culture techniques, thus enhancing the possibilities of performing applied research in toxicology and pharmacology. In tandem with the advance of immunological research, adverse effects on the immune system, especially sensitizing reactions, were reported to have increased during the past decades in the populations of industrialized countries. This has been attributed to exposure to new consumer products, such as cosmetics, cleaning products, food additives, and "pollution." In addition, the reduction in infectious diseases and the resulting shifts within the immune system, for example, from Th1- to Th2-type cells, may be contributory.

The interest in assessing the possible significance of adverse effects on the human immune system has increased considerably in recent years. However, in contrast to other fields of toxicology, the assessment of possible adverse effects on the immune system has been impaired by the lack of universally accepted experimental testing strategies. Although a number of suggestions have been made during the past 15 years, guidelines are absent, and no battery of testing procedures has received general acceptance. Risk assessment, as well as evaluation of the significance of experimental findings for the situation in humans, is also hampered by the fact that the effects of only a few substances have been the subject of studies in reliable human trials. Even on extensively employed therapeutic substances or environmental agents, the information is largely lacking. Considerable differences in the immune systems of rodents and primates are known. In studies, typically performed in rodents, it is difficult or impossible to assess the toxicological significance for the majority of the biological endpoints, and extrapolations to the situation in humans is virtually impossible.

The field of immunotoxicology is still under much discussion. Even the term is difficult to define. New developments must be expected within the next decade. Systematic basic research must be increased before a meaningful toxicological testing strategy may emerge. This includes studies on nonhuman primates. Unfortunately, funding is this area has so far been negligible. It is easy to predict that with the present approach substances with pronounced effects on the immune system may not be detected before human clinical trials are performed. With the clinical studies currently conducted, most effects on the immune system will also be revealed by chance.

Definition of Immunotoxicology and Immunopharmacology

It is impossible to clearly distinguish between immunotoxicology and immunopharmacology, as it is generally difficult to distinguish between pharmacological and toxic effects. Most often only the applicability determines this difference, as exemplified by cyclosporin A. This substance has become an almost essential agent in transplantation surgery, and it is classified as a pharmacological agent. If cyclosporin A were an environmental chemical (which it technically is, because it is produced by a fungus), it would be designated as an extremely immunotoxic agent.

With respect to chemically induced alterations on the immune system, it is especially difficult to define what "toxic" is. In this context, all adverse immunological alterations that obey the laws of toxicology, especially with regard to dose–response relationships, should be included in this definition. Allergic reactions, which are largely unrelated to dose, would be excluded. Therefore, it appears prudent to avoid confusion with the use of the term "immunotoxic." It is preferable to refer to "alterations in immunological components and functions," a designation that would include allergic reactions.

The physiologic function of the immune system is to respond and to adapt to environmental challenges. Reactions (e.g., to infections or to tumor cells) must not be considered "pathologic." Rather, such responses are essential for the survival of the higher organisms. However, from a medical point of view an exaggerated response may become "adverse." Examples are excessive inflammation as it occurs in the leprosy reaction (erythema nodosum leprosum), or allergic reactions triggered by atopic disposition, or autoimmune diseases (e.g., rheumatoid arthritis and diabetes type I). Alterations within the immune system are bound to occur *unspecifically* in highly intoxicated individuals, as in many other fields of toxicology. These examples indicate the difficulties encountered in defining immunotoxicology. They explain *a priori* the high variability in the reference values and emphasize the need for controlling the numerous confounding factors when attempting to draw conclusions regarding cause-and-effect relationships of chemical-induced effects.

One can state with confidence that it will be virtually impossible to assess specific or xenobiotic-induced alterations in immunological components and functions in patients with poor health status.

Features of the Immune System with Relevance to Perturbations

The immune system must not be considered as separate entity. Although having its own specificity, this complex system is embedded within many organs and it interacts with many other systems. The bone marrow has many other functions, aside from being a dominant source of immune cells. The blood is not just a major transport system for immune cells, just as the spleen is not limited to immunological functions, as are the lung, the intestine, or the skin.

Intimate interconnections exist between the immune and the inflammatory system. For example, several cell types, such as macrophages, have key functions in both inflammatory and immunological reactions. Mutual interactions exist between the immune reactions and the nervous and the hormonal system.

Differentiation between Immunotoxic and Allergic Reactions

Toxic effects on the immune system and allergic effects must be distinguished from one another. One of the main reasons is that we expect a clear-cut dose–response relationship in the case of a toxic effect, but there is no obvious dose relationship in allergic responses, although a certain dose seems to be required. This distinction is important because chemically induced allergic reactions by far predominate over clearly toxic effects on the immune system. When considering the likelihood of adverse effects, the recognition of a possible sensitizing potential of a substance is at least as relevant or even more important than revealing a "toxic" potency. It is unlikely that the present techniques in animal experimentation for revealing the allergic potential of chemicals with relevance for humans are satisfactory, and tests in humans are still essential. "Idiosyncratic" allergic reactions are peculiar to many substances, and in this condition only a few susceptible persons are affected. Idiosyncratic reactions, occurring at a frequency of 1: 1000 or even less in humans, cannot be recognized in animal tests.

Differentiation between Immunologic and Inflammatory Reactions

In spite of many similarities, such as involvement of the same or similar cell types, an acute inflammatory reaction must be distinguished from an immune

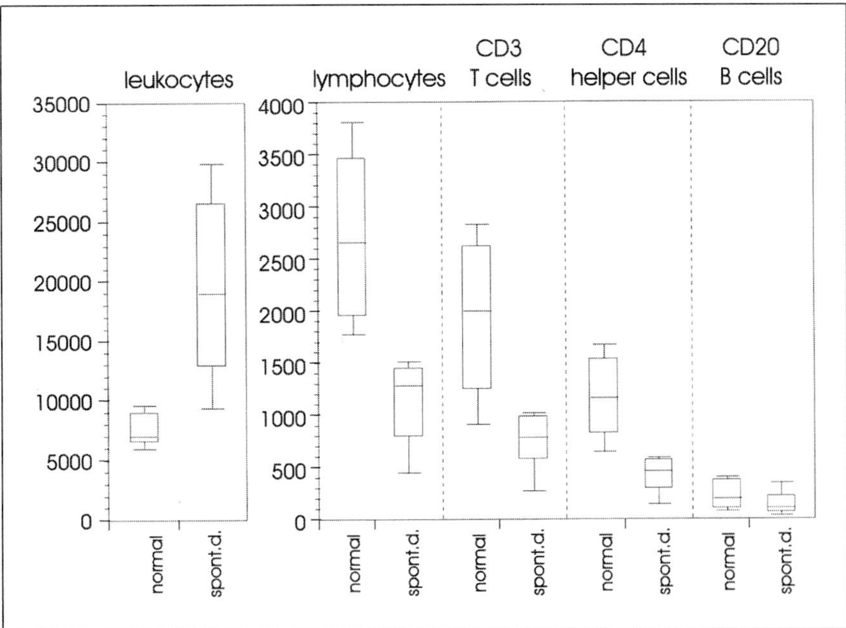

FIGURE 1 Hematological changes during a physiological stress situation (spontaneous delivery of a baby [spont.d.]), in comparison with healthy age-matched women. The pronounced leukocytosis is accompanied by a drastic decrease in the number of lymphocytes and lymphocyte subfractions, total T cells ($CD3^+$), T-helper cells ($CD4^+$), as well as B-cells ($CD20^+$). The effect is reversible within 24–48 h.

response. Inflammation is a symptom of many allergic reactions; however, chronic inflammatory responses most often proceed without any participation of the immune system.

Multiple causes may trigger an acute inflammatory reaction. The most important, yet not exclusive, initiators are various types of infections. Inflammatory cells (e.g., granulocytes, macrophages, and NK cells) are the first line of attack against invading microorganisms. This unspecific defense can be mobilized rapidly, while specific immunological responses require some time. However, infections are not the only cause of acute inflammations, and there are also "sterile" inflammations, such as gout, skin irritation caused by UV sunlight, or even arthrosis.

Neutrophil leukocytes (polymorphnuclear neutrophils, PMN) by themselves are not part of the immune system proper. However, in the context of inflammation and defense, some types of lymphocytes play a role, together with inflammatory cells (neutrophils), monocytes and macrophages, and mast cells. Close contact of leukocytes and lymphocytes with cells of blood vessels (high endothelial venules) is required to direct the blood cells to the extravasal location of inflammation.

Interactions of the Immune System with Other Systems

The interactive connections of the immune system with the endocrine system and the central nervous system (CNS) are highly relevant. Although only fragmentarily understood, the influences of the human psyche on immunological reactions are highly likely, and identical cytokines may be used for modulating interactions between the immune system and the CNS.

Physiological stress (e.g., the spontaneous delivery of a baby or Marathon running), with its changes in hormones, such as glucocorticoids and various transmitter substances, drastically changes the number of leukocytes, as well as various subpopulations of lymphocytes in peripheral blood (Fig. 1).

With respect to links of the immune and the CN systems, a number of mediators are known to be formed by cells of both systems, and they may exert effects on both the systems and interlink them. Endogenous and exogenous *opioids* modulate pain perception, and simultaneously induce important effects on opioid receptor-containing immune cells. Opioid peptides exhibit numerous functions on the immune system, among them the facilitation of chemotaxis, stimulation of the release of various cytokines, and induction of changes in immunocytes, which may be considered to be cell activation. Interestingly, proenkephalin present in immunocytes may rapidly be processed to [Met]enkephalin and enkelytin. While the former substance may stimulate immunological functions, the latter component exhibits antibacterial properties. These new concepts suggest much more pronounced interactions than were previously known between different systems of the complex organism. It is quite feasible that substances acting on the CNS may also interfere with functions of the immune system, and this field requires much future research.

Is has long been known that CNS and the immune system interact at the level of the hypothalamic–pituitary–adrenal axis. In addition to cortisol and certain opioids (e.g., β-endorphin), it is now known that "classical" transmitters, such as norepinephrine, and a number of cytokines, such as IL-6 and TNF-α, are recognized and bound by receptors on the immune cells and have functional significance. This neuronal regulation was observed in splenic nerves, but it may have a broader significance within the immune system. The presence of other neurotransmitters, such as acetylcholine, calcitonine gene-related peptide, somatostatin, substance P, vasoactive intestinal peptide, and neuropeptide Y, has been demonstrated in certain lymphoid organs. The functions, however, have not been completely elucidated. The response seems to vary considerably with respect to the environmental conditions and the microenvironment (e.g., whether or not bacteria are present) (Table 1). The findings of direct nervous influences imply the possibility that immunologic components and functions may be modulated at either the CNS level by psychopharmacological drugs or by transmitter agonists and antagonists at autonomic nervous system synapses. Furthermore, it has been suggested that macrophage-derived IL-6, regulated via nerve impulses, may polarize native T cells to become effector Th2 cells, thus possibly providing an essential control mechanism in determining the type of immune response.

TABLE 1 Suggestion of a Dialog between CNS and Nerve Terminal-Macrophage Contact Sites in the Spleen[a]

Condition: Cortisol present	Condition: Bacteria present	Receptor involved	Effect[b] on splenic IL-6 secretion microenvironment
Ø	Ø	β-adrenergic	=
+	Ø		↓
Ø	+		↑
+	+		↓↓
Ø	Ø	α2-adrenergic	↓
+	Ø		↑
Ø	+		↓
Ø	Ø	μ-opoidergic	↓
+	Ø		↑

[a]Modified from Straub *et al.* (1998).
[b]Abbreviations: =, no effect; ↓, inhibition; ↑, stimulation.

Similar to its function in the CNS as an important factor in maintaining the homeostasis of behavioral, cognitive, and neuroendocrine functions, β-endorphin has been suggested as playing a similar role in the immune system, maintaining homeostasis through the balancing of Th1/Th2 responses. While some diseases known to be associated with a Th2-situation, like HIV infection, were found to be associated with increased β-endorphin concentrations, decreased concentrations of this peptide were reported in the cases of other diseases (e.g., multiple sclerosis, rheumatoid arthritis, and Crohn's disease) that are believed to be associated with a Th1-type response.

Possible Role of Cannabinoids on Immune Reactions

Another clue regarding the connections between the immune system and the CNS comes from studies with marihuana cannabinoids, which are both psychoactive and active on the immune system. The main psychoactive constituent, Δ-tetrahydrocannabinol, also binds to receptors of immune cells. Even more potent derivatives have been synthesized. Two receptors are involved in the binding of cannabinoids, of which CB1 is mostly located within the brain, while CB2 is predominantly expressed in the periphery, especially on cells of the immune system. Both single-chain receptor proteins of 360 and 472 amino acids, respectively, exhibit the typical features of a G-protein-coupled receptor (with 7-transmembrane α helices). Interestingly, an endogenous ligand, anandamide (arachidonylethanolamide), was also found. Several additional ligands have now been described; their exact functions in the CNS and the immune system are largely unknown.

The effects of marihuana smoking on the immune functions have been reported since the 1970s. Observations of an increased incidence of viral infections and also of allergic reactions in marihuana users were subsequently supported by animals studies, which revealed a suppression of host resistance against a variety of microorganisms. In recent years, results have been published that indicate there are effects of cannabinoids on T cells, B cells, NK cells, and macrophages. It has been proposed that cannabinoids alter the Th1/Th2 ratio, and redirect the cytokine pattern from cell mediated immunity (i.e., from the Th1-type response) to humoral immunity and predominant production of IL-4 and other Th2-type cytokines. This may explain the reduced host resistance to viruses, parasites, and certain intracellular bacteria, which is a characteristic Th1-type response. This is an active area of research, and many details have eluded investigators. The accumulated evidence indicates that it is highly likely that cannabinoids regulate the immune system, and the possibility of pharmacological interferences can be predicted.

BASIC FUNCTIONS OF THE IMMUNE SYSTEM

It is not the purpose of this chapter to give an extensive review of immunology. Therefore, only the essential general characteristics of the systems necessary to understand adverse effects will be covered.

One of the most important evolutionary developments is the emergence of protective mechanisms that enable mammalian organisms to defend themselves against the invasion of exogenous organisms, such as bacteria, viruses, and disease-causing parasites. Such mechanisms serve two independent functions, the detection or recognition of an invader and its efficient elimination. These tasks are performed by the immune system, the foremost function of which is to guarantee the homeostasis integrity of the organism (Fig. 2). *Immunity* is the ability of an organism to resist foreign substances called antigens.

Postnatally the immune system needs the continuous challenge from the infections for which evolution has adapted it, and the proper cytokine balance and fine-tuned T-cell regulation must be maintained. Modern vaccination fulfills only part of this task by providing immunity against certain diseases, but it does not induce the long-lasting unspecific systemic changes connected with natural recovery from infections. Recovery (e.g., from natural measles infection) reduced the incidence of atopy and of allergic reactions to the house dust mite to half the incidence seen in vaccinated children. This seems to be due to a systemic long-lasting nonspecific switch to the Th1-type reactivity. Vaccination against diphtheria, tetanus, and pertussis does not affect atopic diseases. It was speculated that these vaccinations may induce the

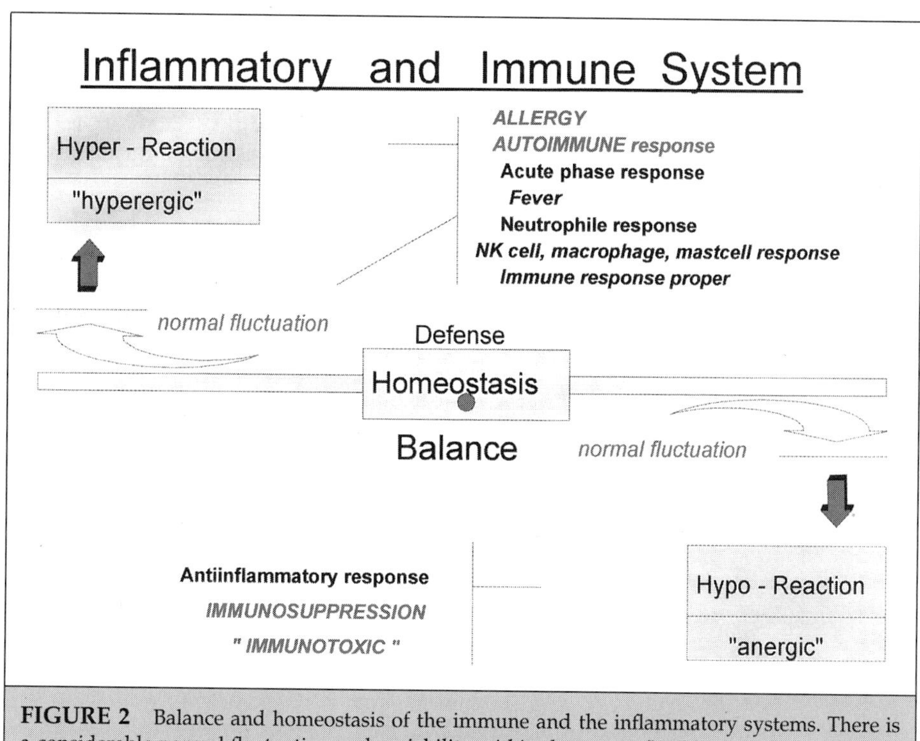

FIGURE 2 Balance and homeostasis of the immune and the inflammatory systems. There is a considerable normal fluctuation and variability within these very flexible systems. Only excessive alterations in both directions (hyper and hypo) or abnormally long-lasting effects may be considered as pathological.

Th2-type status, but this was contradicted. The findings suggest that vaccination is not the whole story, and attempts are being made to better mimic the overall immunologic changes associated with recovery from some infectious diseases.

Antigens and Their Function

The most important reaction of the immune system, save autoimmune disorders, is the response against exogenous or endogenous antigens. All antigens were once considered *anti*body-*gen*erating molecules. It is now known that not all antigens induce antibody production. The term is employed in a broader sense and describes molecules being recognized by the acquired immune system. Antigens eliciting antibody production are designated as immunogens. Haptens are substances with low molecular mass (<300 Da) that must be linked to protein carriers in order to induce an immune response. Hapten-carrier complexes play an important role in drug-induced hypersensitivity.

Antigens can be divided into particular (e.g., bacterial, viral, and fungal) and soluble (e.g., proteins, polysaccharides, lipids, and nucleic acids) antigen structures.

Innate and Adaptive Immunity

The mammalian immune system is part of a two-component defense system:

1. The phylogenetically older innate, nonadaptive responses.
2. The phylogenetically newer adaptive reactions, which are characterized by specificity and memory.

As defined, in innate immune responses, the organism is not required to learn these responses, and they constitute the generally unspecific reaction of the first line of defense. Closely connected to these are the responses of the inflammatory system.

Adaptive immune reactions are more complex and the organism must react to the environment. These specific immune reactions require recognition of what is "self" and what is "foreign." The process of acquiring specificity is correlated with "memory" by very persistent "memory cells," qualifying the immune system to recall the previous recognition of an undesirable antigen.

Defects in this defense system will have clinical implications. An inborn or acquired defect, evident as an immunodefect syndrome, may not allow sufficient defense against infections. Hyperreactions may manifest themselves as inflammation or allergy, possible even as neoplastic transformation such as lymphoma. The failure to recognize the organism's own structures as self will cause self-destructive autoimmune diseases.

The Immune Response

Pragmatic and didactic reasons have previously prompted a division of the immune system into cel-

TABLE 2 Unspecific (Innate) and Specific (Adaptive) Cellular and Humoral Components of the Mammalian Defense System

System	Defense system	
	Cellular	Humoral
Unspecific ("innate")	Granulocytes Monocytes Macrophages NK cells	Complement system Cytokines Properdin system
Specific ("adaptive")	T-lymphocytes: Helper (CD4$^+$) cells Suppressor (CD8$^+$) cells	Immunoglobulins: IgA 1–2 IgD IgE
	B lymphocytes: B (CD20$^+$) cells	IgG 1–4 IgM
	Antigen-presenting cells Epithelial cells of the thymus	
	Antibody-dependent cellular cytotoxicity (ADCC)	

lular and humoral compartments (Table 2). This distinction is arbitrary because the humoral defense system, which is involved in the formation of antibodies, critically depends on cellular reactions (Fig. 3.).

Immune responses can be further classified as

(1) Primary (the first contact with a given antigen) or secondary (renewed contact with the same antigen) (Fig. 4).
(2) Active (acquired through contact with antigen) or passive (acquired by transfer of antibodies or sensitized lymphocytes).

Furthermore, the interplay between cellular immunological components cannot be understood without considering the autocrine and paracrine influences of cytokines on these cells. Some of these cytokines are formed and released by cells from other than immunological tissues.

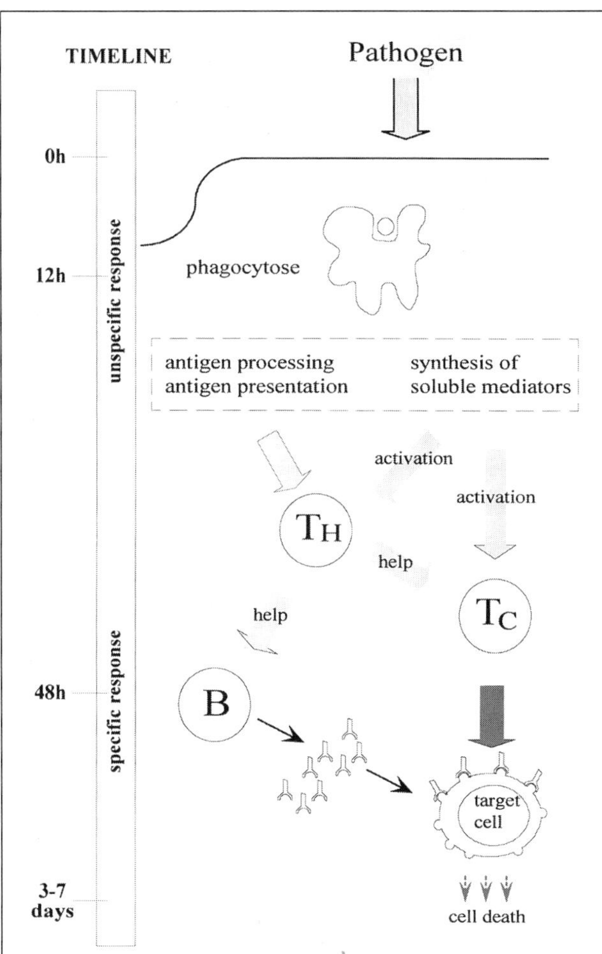

FIGURE 3 Main components and interactions of the adaptive immune system during an immune response. The timeline given is the approximate sequence of the initiation of the corresponding cellular response. The total time can exceed 7 days in severe and especially in chronic reactions.

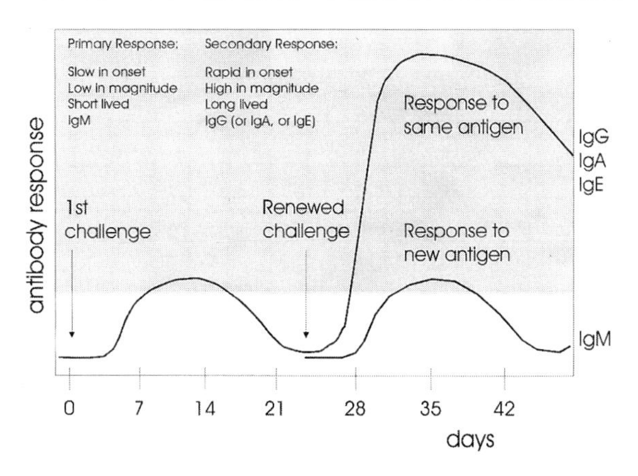

FIGURE 4 Primary and secondary immune responses differ in time course and amplitude of the response, as well as the type of humoral immune responses. During the primary responses against an unknown antigen, primarily IgM is formed. In secondary immune reactions, relying on the immunologic memory of the participants, mainly specific IgG is produced.

The immune system consists of three distinct morphologic components.

- Lymphatic organs proper (thymus, lymphnodes, and spleen).
- Additional lymphatic tissue in several other organs (e.g., intestine, lung, and skin).
- Lymphatic cells in the periphery, in the blood, and at the site of their function.

The immune system is involved in the following functions.

- Response and defense against infections (e.g., viruses, bacteria, and parasites).
- Response and defense against tumors.
- Transplant rejections.
- Allergic reactions.
- Autoimmune diseases.

Components of the Immune System

Numerous components of the immune system provide ample points of attack. Only a few of the possibilities of interfering with immunological components and functions have been elucidated, but toxicologists must be aware of these sites of possible interactions.

Primary and Secondary Lymphoid Organs

The primary lymphoid organs in mammals are the thymus and bone marrow. In the mammalian embryo, hematopoiesis first occurs in the extra-embryonic yolk sac before being taken over by the fetal liver. Throughout post-natal life, hematopoiesis occurs within the bone marrow, the source of pluripotent stem cells (PSC), from which all blood cells arise. Stem cells proliferate in the appropriate microenvironment and in the presence of various colony-stimulating factors (CSF). Thus cells differentiate into erythroid, myeloid, or lymphoid lineage derivatives. The primary lymphoid organs control the further selection of lymphocytes. The thymus provides the appropriate microenvironment and essential hormones for the maturation and primary differentiation of thymic (T) lymphocytes. This organ, which has a cortex as well as a medulla, is located in the mediastinal and originates in part from epithelial cells of the endoderm of the third pharyngeal pouch. The bone marrow is the site of B-cell differentiation, accompanied by immunoglobulin (Ig) gene rearrangements and subsequent Ig class switching. The secondary lymphoid organs (e.g., lymphnodes, spleen, and intestine) are the sites of secondary differentiation, triggered by the encounter with a processed antigen.

Cells of the Adaptive Immune System

Phagocytic cells made mainly up by macrophages (stationary and blood-borne) and neutrophil granulocytes (microphages) are the body's first defense line against an antigen. The phagocytes respond by ingesting and breaking up the encountered antigen and by releasing soluble signaling molecules. Those mediators (e.g., interleukin 1) mobilize the next line of defense via the cellular immune response. This specific response involves two types of lymphocytes, the T- and the B-cells. The number of these cells is quite different at various locations of the organism.

Antigen Recognition

How does the human body recognize an antigen? The complexity of the human organism is such that it is capable of forming antibodies against virtually any molecule or epitope (reactive part of a molecule) that the body encounters.

The principle of antigen recognition is based on trial and error. It relies on the almost unlimited diversity of structures found on the surface of lymphocytes. The assumption is that sooner or later a lymphocyte will "tag along," bearing a receptor for just the required antigen. The generation of molecular diversity is brought about by pairs of protein chains, chemically linked to form these complex structures, the receptors. Each of the chains is divided into a constant and a variable domain. The constant or invariant domain is responsible for the receptors signaling and effector mechanisms and is physically linked to other membrane complexes. The variable domain is responsible for the recognition of antigen. T- and B-cells, triggered via antigen binding to their receptors, respond by proliferation and differentiation to mature stages, the effector stages. For this, the assistance of auxiliary signaling molecules is obligatory. Due to the differing numbers of segments available for recombination, the formation of receptors is slightly divergent in T- and B-cells.

Clonal Selection and Deletion How does the immune system distinguish a foreign molecule from one produced by its own organism? The answer is still incomplete. The organism selects and eliminates cells reacting with autologous structures before they are released into the periphery. This is called clonal selection and deletion. While there is good evidence for the mechanism in T-cells, the mechanism of selection and deletion of autoreactive B-cells is unknown. For T-cells it appears that during the developmental phase the thymus actively "selects" the nonaggressive functional cells released into the rest of the immune system, retaining only those cells with autoreactivity. This selection process results in the death (apoptosis) of more than 90% of the initially formed T-cells. The importance of the elimination of autoreactive cells can be appreciated in autoimmune disorders, such as myasthenia gravis, a neurological condition involving the production of soluble auto-antibodies directed against the α chain of the nicotinic acetylcholine receptor of neuromuscular junctions on skeletal muscle cells. The antibody causes a block in neuromuscular transmission and leads to progressive muscular weakness and ultimately death.

In young organisms, T-lymphocytes are typically formed within the thymus, but this organ regresses after childhood. It is speculated that in the adult organism, most of the T-lymphocytes are formed in the lymph nodes. Whereas the absence or loss of the thymus has a clearly observable effect in young children (e.g., DiGeorge syndrome), thymidectomy in adult humans has only a transient influence on the pattern of circulating T-lymphocytes. The original number of the T-cells in peripheral blood is quickly restored after removal of the thymus.

The Major Histocompatibility Complex The recognition of autoreactivity, and therefore of the mechanism of selection, is intimately linked to a group of

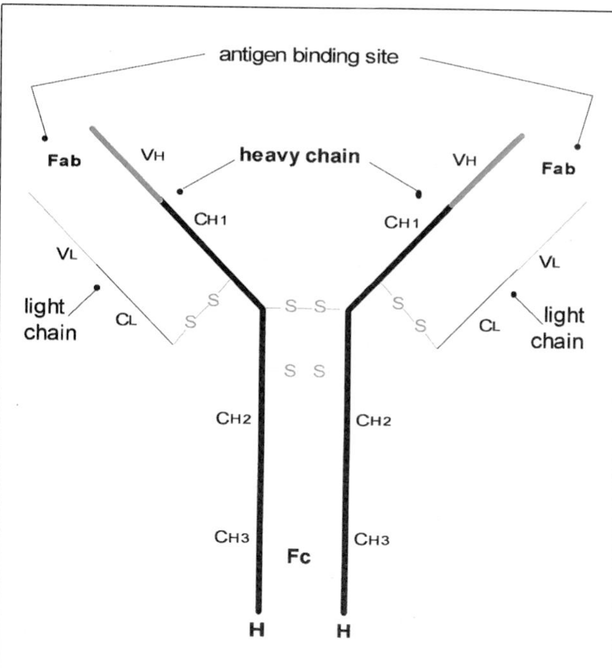

FIGURE 5 Structure of the immunoglobulin G1 (IgG1). The number of disulfide bonds between H chains varies greatly within the IgG subclasses (see Table 16).

gene products involved in antigen presentation. These are coded for by a gene complex, referred to as major histocompatibility complex (MHC). In humans, the whole complex has been mapped to chromosome 6 and codes for three different classes of glycoproteins. Two of those act as antigens and receptors and are located on the cell surface of somatic cells. Class I molecules are found on the cell surfaces of all nucleated cells with the exception of erythrocyte precursors and choriotrophoblasts. They are individually specific and, because they are responsible for graft rejection, they are referred to as "transplantation antigens." Class II molecules are found on macrophages and other antigen-presenting cells (e.g., dendritic cells and Langerhans cells), epithelial cells in the thymus, and B-lymphocytes; they provide the self-recognition essential for the interaction with other immunocompetent cells. The most common of the Class II molecules is called immune–response associated, Ia. These Class II molecules are not expressed on cell surfaces, but are rather a subset of serum proteins involved in the complement system.

Formation and Function of B-Lymphocytes

One of the peculiarities of B-cells is their dual function in antigen presentation and antibody production. A second phenomenon is the extreme specificity of the individual B-cell, expressing immunoglobulin for only a single antigen (monoclonal antibodies). The gene rearrangement begins in the fetal liver and continues postnatally and throughout life in the bone marrow. New naive B-cells, bearing highly diverse surface immunoglobulin molecules, are continuously released into the periphery. These surface immunoglobulins act as highly specific receptors for antigens. The basis of this specificity is dependent on the trial-and-error principle. Highly diverse immature B-cells are produced, but only those encountering "their" specific antigen undergo differentiation and clonal expansion.

B-Cell Differentiation and Maturation The B-cell receptor for soluble or surface bound antigens is a membrane-bound immunoglobulin (Ig). The structure of the elementary Ig (primarily monomeric IgM but also IgD) is programmed by gene rearrangement of small coding segments during B-cell maturation. This rearrangement is the basis of lymphocyte diversity within the human immune system. It is essential for the individual recognition of a practically unlimited number of specific antigens, against which approximately one trillion lymphocytes are on guard.

The development of B-lymphocytes consists of two independent stages. First, there is the antigen-independent stage in which recombination of the genetic information, with respect to heavy and light Ig chains, is achieved. The pluripotent stem cell differentiates initially to a pro-B-cell, then to a pre-B-cell, and ultimately to mature naive B-cell, expressing IgM as well as IgD on the cell surface. Second, the antigen-dependent stage binding of an encountered antigen leads to activation and clonal expansion. Further activation of the B-cells is dependent on the nature of the encountered antigen. If this antigen is a protein, endocytosis is induced and the internal processing with the subsequent expression of the ensuing peptides as a complex in combination with MHC II molecules performed. If the antigen is not a protein (e.g., saccharides and lipids), the secretion of soluble IgM is induced through alternative RNA processing.

In both cases, further B-cell development is T-cell dependent. The following T-cell–B-cell interaction leads to isotype switching and differentiation to IgG (Fig. 5), IgE, or IgA producing plasma cells,[1] or alternatively to the acquisition of "memory" (B-memory

[1] Plasma cells produce a single antibody only ("monoclonal antibody"). The antibody type may be IgM, IgG, IgD, IgA, or IgE. Cells typically express, for example, the CD20 receptor. They are derived from antigen-specific B-cells and are rich in rough endoplasmic reticulum.

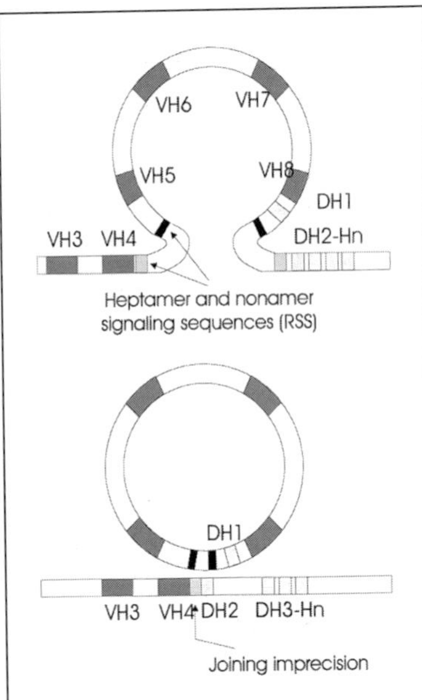

FIGURE 6 Example of heavy chain recombination. The three segments (V, D, J) contained in the heavy chain locus combine to produce the exon coding for the VH domain and the functional V-D-J gene. Each of several hundred V genes can combine with each of 30 D segments and one of six J segments creating one of the thousands rearrangements responsible for the genetic diversity of B cell genes.

cell). It is on this acquisition of memory that the secondary immune response is based.

T-cell–B-cell cooperation relies essentially on two mechanisms: cytokine presence and receptor–ligand interaction of the cell surface molecules. Although it is probable that many other cytokines, known and unknown, may produce an effect on T-cell–B-cell interaction, IL-2 and IL-4 are well known for this effect. Among the receptor–ligand interactions, it is important to mention CD40 and CD40L. The combination of CD40L and IL-4 is thought to be the synergizing force for driving the clonal expansion that precedes antibody production. IL-4 is secreted by the T-helper (Th2) cell and therewith acts directly on the antigen-specific target cell.

Genetic Basis for Antibody Variability Each individual responds to an estimated 10^9 different antibody molecules and hence to the same number of distinct B-cell clones. All genetic information concerning antibody proteins is found on a mere three genes on three chromosomes. Two of these genes code for the light chains κ and λ (on chromosomes 2 and 22, respectively); the third codes for the heavy chain and is situated on chromosome 14. This gene defines the five heavy-chain segments identifying the immunoglobulin type, μ for IgM, δ for IgD, γ for IgG, α for IgA, and ϵ for IgE. The proper rearrangement of exons is achieved by looping out intervening DNA (Fig. 6). This is done in the following precise order.

1. Rearrangement of the heavy chain.
   a. D is joined to J.
   b. V is joined to DJ.

If, through this initial rearrangement, a functional heavy chain results, the light chains again rearrange.

2. Rearrangement of the light chains
   a. First κ, then (if κ is unproductive or cannot pair with the heavy chain) λ is rearranged.
3. Vl is joined to J.

The expression of one heavy chain prevents rearrangement on the other chromosome. This process is called allelic exclusion and is designed to prevent the simultaneous expression of two antibodies by the same B-cell. In this process, several enzymes are involved, such as lymphocyte-specific recombinases recognizing conserved heptamer and nonamer sequences found adjacent to the V, D, and J exons, exonucleases, and ligases. In addition, RAG1 and RAG2, two recombination-activating genes, have been shown to affect the rearrangement of Ig as well as the T-cell receptor genes.

Formation and Function of T-Lymphocytes

The acquisition of receptors for the restricted major histocompatibility complex of either type I or II (MHC I and MHC II) is the primary role of maturation in the thymus. This system constitutes the major recognition mechanism of self and nonself on a cellular basis. T-cells can recognize an antigen only in the form of small peptide fragments bound to the MHC and expressed on a cell surface.

During development in the thymus, contact with antigen will result in death of cells (apoptosis) before they have reached the mature single-positive CD4[2] or CD8 stage. There is evidence that the type of fetal or neonatal antigen-presenting cells (APCs) influence the decision of the, certainly rather few, T-cells to respond

[2] CD means "cluster differentiation." The characterization of surface receptors is by international nomenclature. Specific receptors on white blood cells are identified by the reaction with specific mAb to this receptor, but several mAb may react to various epitopes of this surface protein.

or not. Although predominantly occurring during the perinatal and neonatal period, tolerance can be created at any stage of life, depending on the APC's guidance on the T-cell responses, giving either signals leading to death (apoptosis) or to functioning immunocytes.

The T-Cell Receptor The receptor recognizing antigen is the T-cell receptor (TCR). Its recognition mechanism is dependent on two auxiliary surface receptors, CD8 (in combination with MHC I), and CD4 (in combination with MHC II). The TCR consists of two peptide chains, of which four different types are known: α, β, γ, and δ. The gene locations for the TCR chains are situated on two human chromosomes, chromosomes 7 and 14. Approximately 95% of all peripheral T-cells bear the TCR α/β receptor. The remaining T cells express TCR γ/δ. All T-cells expressing the TCR α/β are of either the $CD4^+CD8^-$ or $CD4^-CD8^+$ phenotype. Cells with the γ/δ receptor are generally of the $CD4^-CD8^-$ phenotype, with only a few exceptions. TCR α/β is always associated with a group of surface molecules called the CD3 complex. This complex, made up of four other chains, join with the TCR heterodimer and transports it to the cell surface. Along with a homodimer of ξ chains, the CD3 complex is responsible for signaling to the cell's interior that antigen binding has occurred. The cytoplasmic domains of the CD3 complex contain protein sequences that permit it to join with cytosolic protein tyrosine kinases to achieving this signaling.

Whereas the recognition of MHC antigen, in conjunction with the auxiliary molecules CD4 or CD8, is in principle for all TCR α/β-bearing T-cells, no such restriction appears to apply to TCR γ/δ T-cells. The functional mechanism of the cells is called "antibody-dependent cell-mediated cytotoxicity" (ADCC). It has been shown that, although TCR γ/δ T-cells are rather rare in peripheral blood, their number is quite important in epithelial tissues, such as the epidermis, the small intestine, and the genitourinary tract.

Selective Processes and MHC Restriction Once the antigen-receptor genes are rearranged and the surface receptor is expressed, the formation and maturation of T lymphocytes within the thymus proceed as a sequence of events destined primarily for selecting self-tolerant cells and eliminating the others. The screening is performed by two independent processes known as positive selection (selection for self-MHC restriction) and negative selection (elimination of cells coding for self-reactivity). Most of the different steps can be recognized by characteristic changes in the pattern of the surface receptors on these lymphocytes (Fig. 7). At the end of these processes, typical naive helper ($CD4^+$) and cytotoxic–suppressor ($CD8^+$) T-cells are released into the periphery.

Antigen Presentation

T-cells are incapable of autonomously recognizing an antigen. In order to initiate a T-cell reaction, the intervention of another cell type, the antigen-presenting cell (APC), is essential. Typical APCs are macrophages, dendritic cells, von Kupffer cells, Langerhans cells, and even B-cells (IgM and IgD). Within minutes after an exogenous immune challenge, the antigen is taken up by phago- or endocytosis and digested after fusion with lysosomes. In the case of endogenous challenge (e.g., viral infection), this reaction is slightly different. The processing of antigen into peptides is performed in intracellular organelles (endosomes, phagolysosomes, and proteasomes). The resulting peptides must have a minimal length (13–17 amino acids for MHC II and 8–10 amino acids for MHC I), as well as a defined amino acid sequence to be recognized by the MHC. If this sequence is even slightly altered, binding to the MHC cannot take place. This conditional binding indicates that only a very small proportion of the ingested antigen (<1%) actively participates in the immune response. The remaining antigen is reduced to unbound, nonimmunogenic peptides and amino acids and is effectively eliminated.

Thus joined to the APC's MHC complex, the peptides are returned to the cell surface by exocytosis. Depending on the type of challenge, the processed peptides are expressed with either MHC II (exogenous antigens) or MHC I (endogenous antigens). The peptide–MHC I or II complexes on the cell surface can now be recognized by the T-cell receptors on cytotoxic or helper cells, respectively (Fig. 8).

One exception must be mentioned with respect to the binding of peptides to the peptide-binding groove of MHC class II because of the often-disastrous consequences. Special peptides produced by bacteria, viruses, and mycoplasmas, called superantigens, have the capacity of binding directly to MHC molecules without being previously preprocessed. Instead of binding to the groove of the MHC molecule, superantigens link to the outer surface of the MHC II molecule and the $V\beta$ region of the TCR. This enables them to stimulate very large numbers of T-cells, causing the massive production of cytokines by T-helper cells, ultimately leading to systemic toxicity and suppression of the adaptive immune response. Well-known bacterial superantigens are the staphylococcal enterotoxins regularly responsible for common food poisoning and the dreaded toxic shock syndrome (toxin-1 and TSST-1).

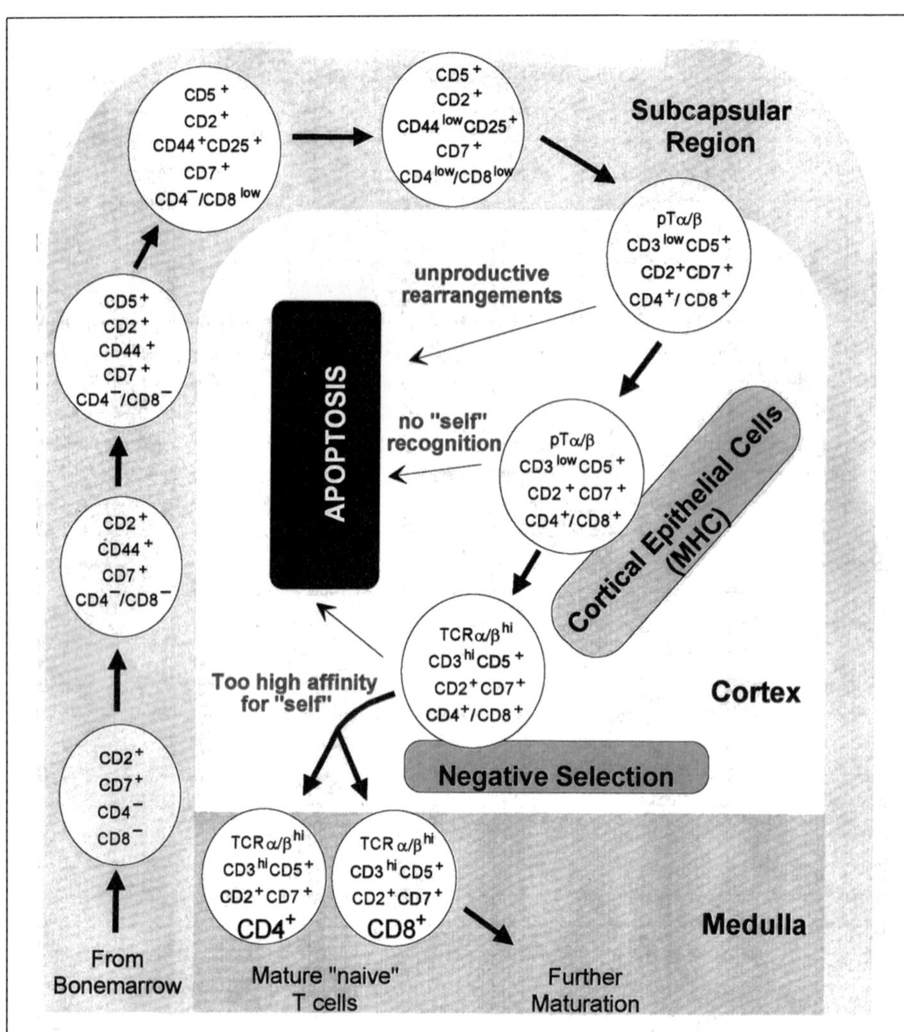

FIGURE 7 Differentiation and selection in the thymic microenvironment. Prethymic cells enter the subcapsular region of the thymus and proliferate, giving rise to a large pool of cells further differentiating and migrating to the thymic medullary region. The differentiation processes are accompanied by changes in the surface receptor expression. Two selection processes in which the pre-TCR (pre-T-cell receptor) must recognize autologous MHC in contact with cortical thymic epithelial cells and differentiate self are eliminatory mechanisms for the deletion of autoreactive cells. This clonal selection of nonautoaggressive cells leads to the development of mutually exclusive expression of either CD4 or CD8 surface receptors, defining the future function of the naive T-cell as helper or the cytotoxic lymphocyte.

Activation and Surface Receptors

Lymphocytes are not a homogeneous population but a quite heterogeneous group of cells with a variety of functions. The divergent reactivity is achieved through a multitude of surface receptors, giving rise to many subpopulations with distinct surface receptor pattern. This pattern is also used to characterize the various lymphocyte subtypes, using monoclonal antibodies and flow cytometry (Table 3).

T-lymphocytes are released from the thymus to the peripheral blood system without having come into contact with antigens. After this, these cells circulate in the blood and migrate into peripheral lymphoid tissues until they encounter antigens. These types of T-cells generally are designated "naive" cells and are characterized by expressing the CD45RA surface receptor. T-cells encounter their specific antigen especially in the cortex of the lymphnodes. When antigen

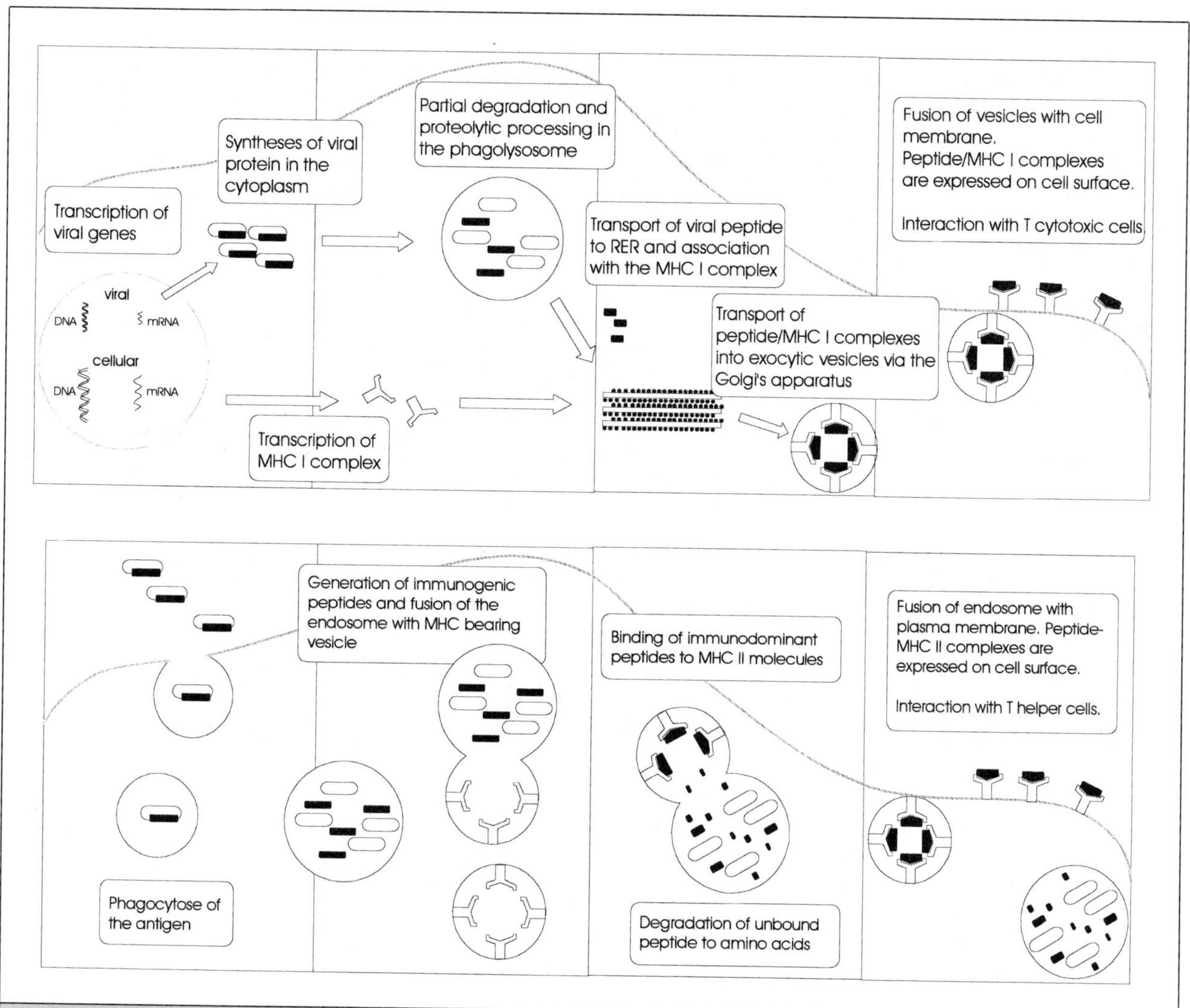

FIGURE 8 Antigen processing and presentation of MHC I and MHC II expressing cells. Such cells, also designated as professional antigen presenting cells (APC), are mainly dendritic cells or macrophages, although B cells can also function as APC.

contact is made, the naive cells are induced to proliferate and differentiate into effector cells. Depending on the type of peptides and the origin of the pathogen encountered on APC, effector cells belong to one of three functional categories. Peptides presented by MHC I complexes and originating from pathogens multiplying in the cytoplasm of the APC are recognized by CD8 cells. These differentiate into cytotoxic effector cells, whose function is the killing of the infected target cells. Peptides presented by MHC II complexes and originating from pathogens, such as viruses that multiply in intracellular vesicles, as well as peptide antigens derived from ingested toxins and bacteria, are presented to T-cells carrying the CD4 receptor.

$CD4^+$ cells can differentiate into two different types of T-helper cells, the Th1 and Th2 cells, differing in function as well as cytokine pattern, they secrete or respond to

- Th1 cells produce IFN-γ and TNF-β, which activate macrophages and are involved in delayed-type hypersensitivity reactions. These T-cells typically express the surface activation marker lymphocyte activation gene 3 (LAG-3), a member of the immunoglobulin superfamily. The cells are especially aimed at protecting against intracellular parasites (viruses).
- Th2 cells produce IL-4, IL-5, IL-10, and IL-13, which are responsible for strong antibody responses, in-

TABLE 3 Examples of Important Subpopulations of White Blood Cells of Primates and Surface Receptors Characterized by Monoclonal Antibodies (mAbs)

Surface receptor pattern	Designation of cell population[a]
$CD2^+$	Cell with erythrocyte-rosetting receptor (pan T-cell)
$CD3^+$	Pan **T**-cell (practically all $CD2^+$)
$CD3^+HLA\text{-}DR^+$	Activated T-cell
$CD3^+CD25^+$	Activated T-cell (IL-2 receptor)
$CD4^+CD3^+$	Pan helper T-cell (practically all $CD2^+$)
$CD4^+CD45R0^+CD45RA^-$	Helper-inducer ("memory") cell
$CD4^+CD45R0^+CD45RA^-CD29^{[high]}$	Memory cell, activated (with β-chain of $\beta1$ integrin)
$CD4^+CD45RA^{[high]}CD45R0^-$	Suppressor-inducer ("naive") cell
$CD4^+CD56^+$	Cytotoxic/killer effector cell
$CD8^+CD3^+$	Pan suppressor/cytotoxic T-cell
$CD8^+CD56^-$	Suppressor cell
$CD8^+CD56^+$	Cytotoxic cell, NCAM-expressing
$CD3^-CD8^-CD4^-CD56^+$	Natural killer cell subset
$CD3^-CD8^-CD4^-CD16^+$	Natural killer cell subset
$CD20^+$	Pan **B** cells
$CD14^+$	Monocytes
Adhesion receptors	
$CD11a^+/CD18^+$	Cell with LFA-1 ($\beta2$-integrin) receptor (both chains)
$CD11b^+CD18^+$	Cell with Mac-1 ($\beta2$-integrin) receptor (both chains)
$CD11c^+CD18^+$	Cell with p150,95 ($\beta2$-integrin) receptor (both chains)
$CD49b^+CD29^+$	Cell with VLA-2 ($\beta1$-integrin) receptor (both chains)
$CD49d^+CD29^+$	Cell with VLA-4 ($\beta1$-integrin) receptor (both chains)
$CD54^+$	Cell with ICAM-1 receptor
$CD44^+$	Cell with "homing" receptor
$CD62L^+$	Cell with L-selectin receptor

[a] Abbreviations: NCAM, neural cell adhesion molecule; LFA, lymphocyte function-associated molecule; VLA, very late activation antigen; ICAM, intercellular adhesion molecule; CD2 is also an adhesion receptor.

cluding IgE production, and inhibit several macrophage functions. These T-cells typically express the surface activation marker CD30, a member of the TNF receptor family. Protection against metazoan parasites is apparently provided by the Th2 responses.

T-helper cells expressing cytokines of both patterns have been designated Th0 cells. The factors influencing the decision whether a proliferating CD4 cell will differentiate into a Th1 or a Th2 cell are not yet fully understood. It appears that this differentiation is due to the type of pathogen peptide presented, as well as the predominating cytokine present at the time of differentiation. The early presence of IFN-γ and IL-12 and pathogens accumulating inside macrophage vesicles seem to stimulate differentiation into Th1 cells. The early presence of IL-4 and extracellular antigen apparently are the most potent stimulus for Th2 polarization (Fig. 9).

Th1 cells are crucial in the activation of the microbicidal properties of macrophages and induce B-cell production of IgG antibodies, particularly effective at opsonizing extracellular pathogen for uptake by phagocytes. Th2 cells are extremely efficient in stimulating the humoral response, especially in primary responses, by activating the naive antigen-specific B-cells into those producing IgM antibodies, as well as the formation of IgA, and especially IgE. The two subsets are capable of regulating each other by secreting mutually inhibiting cytokines. Hence, interferon-γ produced by Th1 cells prevents the activation of Th2 cells, whereas IL-10 produced by Th2 cells indirectly inhibits the development of Th1 cells by acting on the APCs. Once one subset becomes predominant, a shift to the other subset is difficult. However, it should be accepted that Th1 and TH2 represent the extremes of many possible intermediate situations, not identical even in different tissues of the same organism at a given time or in different species under similar con-

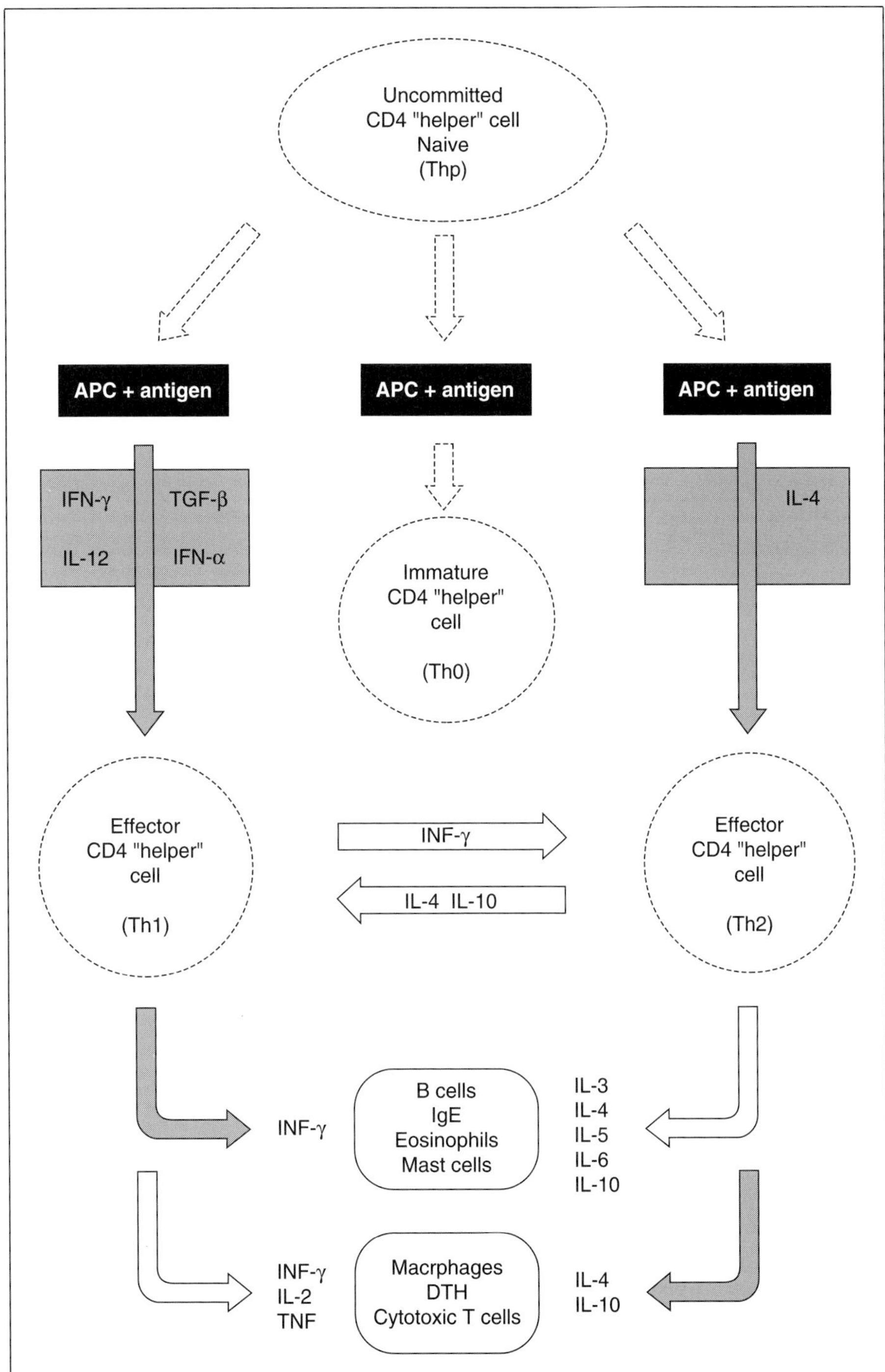

FIGURE 9 Differentiation of T-helper cells (TH0, TH1 and TH2) from an uncommitted (naive) helper cell precursor cell (Thp). In this hypothetical model the interaction of the major differentiation factors (mediators) is indicated as stimulatory (shaded arrows) or inhibitory (white arrows). TH0 cells may allow a switching between TH1 and TH2 cytokine pattern. Th1 and Th2 may represent extremes of many possible cytokine pattern.

ditions. They should not be considered to be mutual exclusive and responses in a sequence seems to be a common phenomenon.

After contact with the appropriate antigen, the naive ("helper-suppressor") cells differentiate to the corresponding memory cells, also designated "helper-inducer" cells. This transition is correlated with the loss of the CD45RA and the acquisition of the CD45R0 and other surface receptors such as adhesion molecules.

From recent evidence it has been hypothesized that Th2-type reactivity is favorable for mammalian pregnancy, and progesterone was suggested as promoting the development of human Th2-type cells and of factors suppressing mitogen-induced lymphocyte proliferation and NK cell activity. IL10, a typical Th2-type cytokine, was reported to prevent murine fetal wastage and the corresponding antibodies increased fetal loss. A Th1 situation and the associated cytokine pattern (e.g., during a viral infection) may then bear a risk of pregnancy failure, and parasitic infections should be compatible with pregnancy. The possible consequences for pregnancy outcome of such an assumption, also with respect to Th1–Th2 alterations induced by chemicals, are still obscure. Interestingly, neonatal T cells are biased towards the Th2 profile.

Intercellular Interactions

Basically two types of cellular interactions can be distinguished: interaction by direct cell–cell contact, and communication by indirect contact via the secretion of mediators (cytokines).

Cell–Cell Interactions Many interactions in the immune system require physical cell–cell contact. There are at least three critical cell–cell contact events among immune cells:

- Antigen-presenting cells (APC) reacting with the naive T-cells.
- Activated T-cells reacting with an antigen-specific B-cells.
- Activated B-cells and follicular dendritic cells (FDC) presenting the antigen.

Additionally, there are a number of cell–cell interactions involving one immune cell and another cell type, namely contact of:

- Cytotoxic T or NK cells with their target cell (infected or tumor cell, or transplant).
- Immunocompetent cells with endothelial cells (e.g., during "rolling" and "homing").

The initial contact of a naive T-cell with its specific antigen is an obligate cell-contact event because of the requirement for MHC presentation. The critical antigen-presenting cell is the dendritic cell. However, the MHC peptide–TCR interaction is insufficient for signaling and other nonantigen-specific membrane-bound ligand–receptor pairs (the auxiliary signaling molecules) are necessary for the dendritic cell–T-cell interaction. The most important connection of the CD28 molecule on the T-cell with the dendritic cell is through one of the two ligands, B7.1 (CD80) or B7.2 (CD86). The CD28 molecule delivers an essential second signal, without which the activation of the T-cell is not achieved and it becomes unresponsive.

For the antibody response to most antigens, T-cell help is an absolute requirement. It is delivered by both cytokines and cell–cell contact and is thus designated T-cell dependent. B-cells bind specific antigens via their surface Ig and subsequently endocytose, process, and present the processed antigen on their class II MHC molecules. Presentation of the MHC II peptide enables the B-cells to be recognized by specific T-helper cells. Although this cell–cell interaction also requires CD28 binding to B7 on the B-cell, the activation of the T-cell has induced expression of a molecule called CD40 ligand or CD40L. This molecule binds to its specific counterpart, CD40, on the B cells. CD40L is a T-cell surface molecule belonging to the tumor necrosis factor (TNF) family. This cross-linking of CD40 promotes B-cell proliferation and immunoglobulin isotype switching, and prevents the apoptosis of germinal-center B-cells. When the CD40–CD40L interaction is blocked by mAbs specific for CD40L, B-cell proliferation and Ig production in response to T-cells are inhibited. The CD28–B7 and CD40–CD40L receptor–ligand interactions are both essential for the dialog between B- and T-cells that results in their mutual activation (Fig. 10).

Activated B-cells that have migrated into the germinal centers of the lymphoid organs are specifically bound to follicular dendritic cells (FDC). These are specialized stromal cells capable of holding intact (i.e., unprocessed) antigens on their surface in the form of stable immune complexes. FDC express CD23, which binds to germinal center B-cells via their complement (CR2) receptor and initiates the differentiation into antibody-producing plasma cells.

Adhesion Receptors and Their Significance Concurrent with the acquisition of the CD45R0 marker on the memory T-helper cells, several other surface receptors are expressed. Among these, the heterogeneous group of adhesion receptors is of considerable interest. The occurrence of such receptors is by no means restricted to the immune system. These components are also expressed on inflammatory cells (e.g., neutrophiles), and their participation and impor-

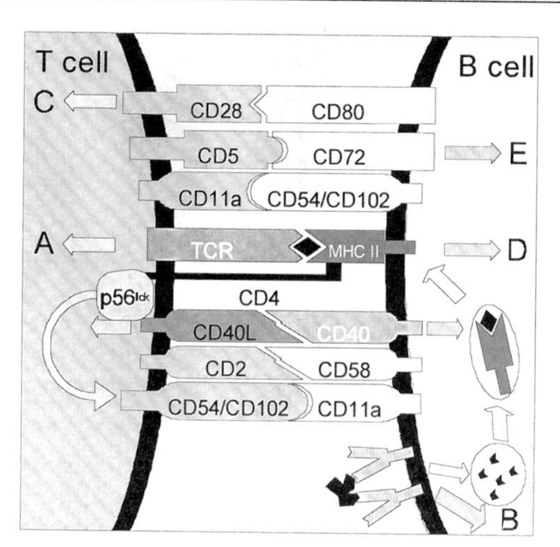

FIGURE 10 Surface receptors interacting in T-cell–B-cell recognition. The shaded arrows indicate the signals necessary for the initiation of blast cell transformation. A and B are signals inducing the signal transduction via thyrosine phosphorylation and PIP2 breakdown. The antigen receptors also regulate the expression of preformed adhesion receptors (e.g., CD11a → CD54/CD102). The auxiliary signals by CD28 and CD40L/CD40 are indicated, as well as a supplementary signal by CD72 in the B-cell. The interactions of mediators are not shown.

tance in morphogenetic differentiation and migration processes during embryonic development is increasingly revealed. With respect to inflammatory and immune responses, these receptors are involved in the numerous "docking" phenomena essential in many immunological functions. Typically, the reaction takes place between a defined pair of different receptors, from which one is localized on one cell and the counterpart on the other (Fig. 11). Interactions only occur between these two specific components, according to the lock and key principle.

- Reactions between antigen-presenting cells and T-helper cells.
- "Help" of the activated T-helper cells for B-cells.
- "Docking" of cytotoxic ($CD8^+$) T-cells on, for example, tumor cells or allografts.
- "Rolling" and transfer of lymphocytes from the blood into affected tissue.
- Reactions between a cell and components of the extracellular matrix.

The importance of adhesion molecules in many types of cellular and extracellular activities has been fully recognized. In the initial phases of maturation and migration from the bone marrow to the thymus, the influence of CD44 (hyaluronic acid receptor) is now recognized as of utmost importance. CD44 is expressed as one of the earliest markers in thymocyte-dependent T-cell differentiation and has been termed the "homing receptor" because of its importance in early tissue migration, as well as in the migration of memory T-cells.

All antigen-unspecific binding of the cellular surface of immune cells to other cells, tissues, or other structures of the extracellular matrix is closely controlled by adhesion molecules. The main classes of adhesion receptors involved in the interaction of immune cells are the integrins, the selectins, the immunoglobulin superfamily, and the addressins.

Tissue migration through the high endothelial venules (leukocyte rolling) is regulated by the selectin family of receptors. Members of this receptor family can be found on leukocytes (L-selectin, CD62L) or on vascular endothelium (E-selectin, CD62E or P-selectin, CD62P). L-selectin is expressed on naive T-cells and binds to the carbohydrate moiety of either of two vascular addressins, CD34 and GlyCam-1, found on high endothelial venules in lymph nodes. Another of the vascular addressins, MAdCAM-1, is expressed on endothelium in mucosa and is responsible for lymphocyte migration into the mucosal lymphoid tissue, such as that of the gut.

The regulatory mechanism between selectins and addressins is responsible for the homing of naive cells to lymphoid organs. The binding, however, is not sufficient to enable the cells to cross the endothelial barrier without the help of two other families of adhesion molecules, the integrins and the immunoglobulin superfamily.

Integrins comprise three families of surface proteins capable of mediating adhesion within cells, as well as between cells and the extracellular matrix in inflammatory and immune responses. The heterodimeric integrins[3] are structurally alike and consist of a large α chain noncovalently attached to a smaller β chain, which defines the relationship to the $\beta1$, $\beta2$, or $\beta3$ integrin subfamily. All T-cells express a leukocyte integrin believed to be the most important adhesion molecule for lymphocyte activation, the lymphocyte function-associated antigen-1 (LFA-1 or CD11a/CD18). The importance of this molecule has been demonstrated in numerous experiments, showing that antibodies directed against this surface structure inhibit the activation of both naive and effector T-cells.

[3] Integrins are heterodimers consisting of a common β chain (e.g., $\beta1$ = CD18, $\beta2$ = CD29, $\beta3$ = CD61) and a variable α chain. Expressed on most immune cells, but also on many other cells of the mammalian organism, they react as specific ligand pairs.

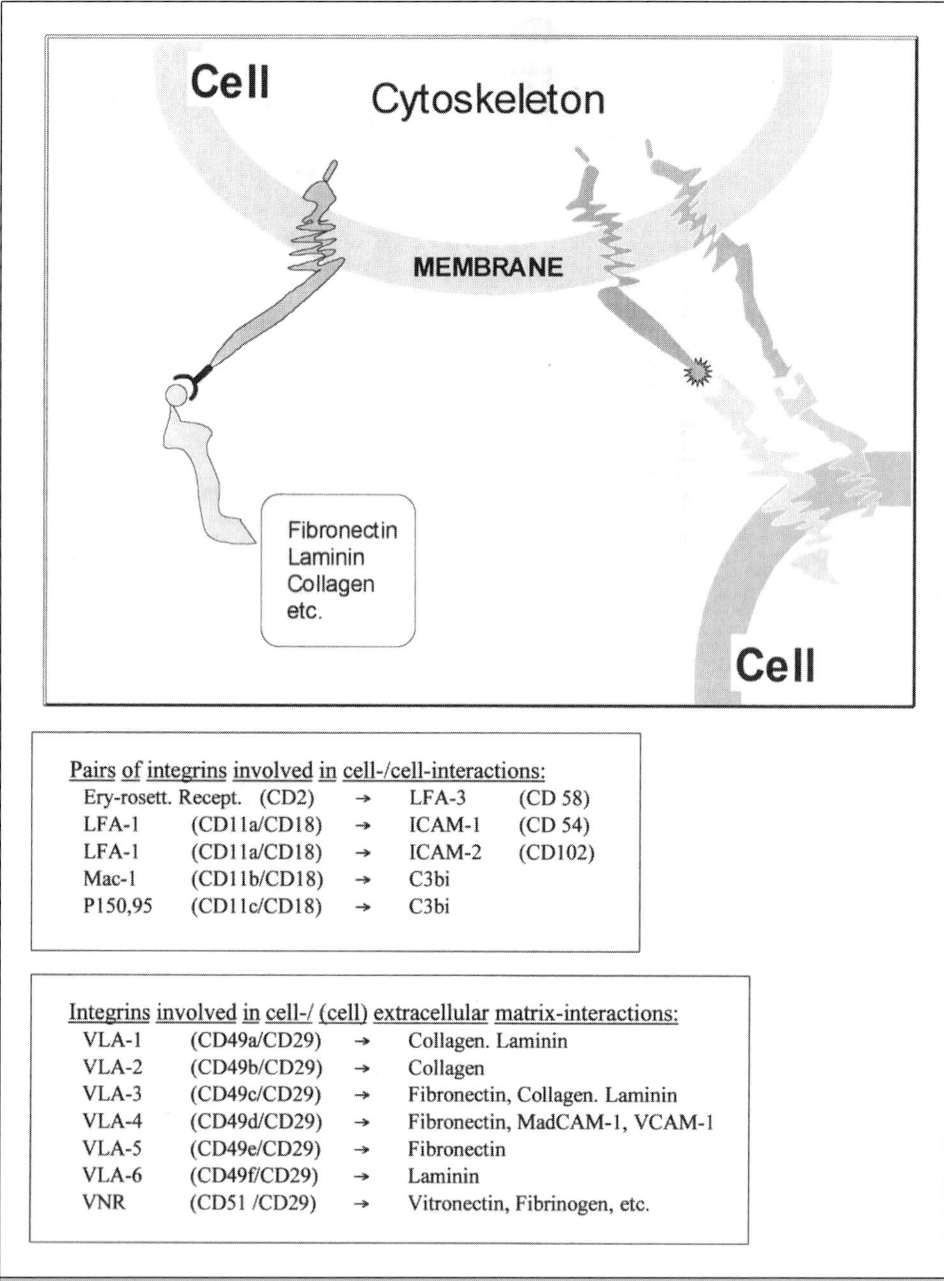

Pairs of integrins involved in cell-/cell-interactions:

Ery-rosett. Recept.	(CD2)	→	LFA-3	(CD 58)
LFA-1	(CD11a/CD18)	→	ICAM-1	(CD 54)
LFA-1	(CD11a/CD18)	→	ICAM-2	(CD102)
Mac-1	(CD11b/CD18)	→	C3bi	
P150,95	(CD11c/CD18)	→	C3bi	

Integrins involved in cell-/ (cell) extracellular matrix-interactions:

VLA-1	(CD49a/CD29)	→	Collagen. Laminin
VLA-2	(CD49b/CD29)	→	Collagen
VLA-3	(CD49c/CD29)	→	Fibronectin, Collagen. Laminin
VLA-4	(CD49d/CD29)	→	Fibronectin, MadCAM-1, VCAM-1
VLA-5	(CD49e/CD29)	→	Fibronectin
VLA-6	(CD49f/CD29)	→	Laminin
VNR	(CD51 /CD29)	→	Vitronectin, Fibrinogen, etc.

FIGURE 11 Diagram of the biological effects of integrins. The receptor symbol represents a heterodimer. Pairs of specific adhesion receptors of two cells can interact with each other, or the $\beta 1$-integrin of one cell can react with specific binding sites of the extracellular matrix. The intracellular domain of the receptor is linked to the cytoskeleton, thus transducing signals into the cell. Examples for pairs of adhesion receptors that specifically react with each other are shown.

Clinically, the importance is recognized in the hereditary leukocyte adhesion-deficiency syndrome. This results from a defect in the synthesis of the α, β, or both integrin chains, resulting in the impairment of immunity to extracellular bacteria due to the defective macrophage and neutrophile function.

The largest group of adhesion receptors probably belongs to the immunoglobulin superfamily. This group of adhesion receptors includes the antigen receptors of T and B-cells; auxiliary CD4, CD8, and CD19 receptors; and the invariant domains of the MHC complexes. However, by far the most important members of this family are the intracellular adhesion molecules ICAM-1, ICAM-2, and ICAM-3, the T-cell-expressed CD2, and the more universally expressed CD58 (LFA-3). Whereas ICAM-1 and ICAM-2 (CD54 and CD102) are expressed on the endothelium as well as on antigen-presenting cells enabling tissue migration, ICAM-3 is found only on leukocytes and is thus thought to play a decisive role in the adhesion between T-cells and APCs.

Cytokines and Their Function

Cytokines are small soluble short-lived cell-signaling molecules, acting at very low concentrations (typically 10^{-10}–10^{-15} M). These permit the exchange of basic information over a certain distance. Cytokines may be regarded as having a dual function, chemotactic (calling other cells to an area of inflammation) and regulatory (directing the "orchestra" of cellular reactions in one or the other direction). Cytokines are immune-specific polypeptides and the products of many different cells, not only of immune cells. Their main effects are to a great extent on the immune cells. Similar to hormones, cytokines exert their effects indirectly by binding to specific receptors on the cell surface, which, in turn, signal to their target cells. Cytokines produced by lymphocytes are often referred to as lymphokines.

Two aspects are characteristic for the action of cytokines: pleiotropism and redundancy. Pleiotropism is the capacity to induce different functional effects, either on different cell types or on the same cell. Practically, this means that blocking or genetically ablating ("knockout") a particular cytokine must not result in widespread or dramatic effects. Conversely, exogenous administration or overexpression of a single cytokine generally has a variety of diverse effects. Redundancy means that the function of each cytokine can also be performed by other cytokines (e.g., many different cytokines have the capacity to initiate cell division in activated immune cells). Cytokines can act systemically (endocrine) or locally, either on other cell types close by (paracrine) or on the same cell (autocrine).

Functionally, three basic categories of cytokines can be distinguished: growth factors, inflammation mediators, and immune modulators (interleukins). However, this distinction is not exclusive and some cytokines may be classified in several groups.

Growth Factors

Growth factors are mainly produced by bone marrow stromal cells, endothelial cells, and fibroblasts. Common members of this group are SFC (stem cell factor), GM-CSF (granulocyte and macrophage colony-stimulating factor), IL-3 and IL-7 (growth factors with a very wide spectrum of cell targets—myeloid, and T-cells and B-cells, respectively). Many of these factors can also be produced by T-cells to permit up-regulation of hemopoietic cell production or activation of mature cells at local sites of inflammation.

Inflammation Mediators

The production of inflammation mediators is stimulated non-specifically by viruses or microbial pathogens. The most common members are:

Type I interferon (IFN-α, IFN-β), produced by lymphocytes and fibroblasts in response to viral infection and stimulating the intrinsic defense against virus infection in a wide range of cell types.

Tumor necrosis factor (TNF-α), primarily produced by macrophages stimulated by bacteria with a very wide range of biological effects including the activation of neutrophils, up-regulation of adhesion molecules, and stimulation of IL-1 production (monocytes) and acute phase proteins. Overproduction of TNF causes toxic shock and death.

Interleukin-1 (IL-1α, IL-1β), primarily produced by activated macrophages in response to lipopolysaccharide (LPS) and TNF. It stimulates the IL-6 production by macrophages. IL-1 is an endogenous pyrogen and stimulates acute-phase response (in concert with IL-6 and TNF).

Interleukin-6 (IL-6), produced by macrophages plays an essential role in inducing acute-phase protein response by liver.

Immune Modulating Cytokines

There are 18 known or recognized interleukins, with new members waiting for homologation. Additional members are discovered on an almost yearly basis.

The most important interleukins are:

IL-2. The primary T-cell growth factor (autocrine) and main factor in the activation and differentiation of T-cells, as well as inducer of B-cell growth.

IL-4. Main T-cell differentiation factor and important B-cell growth factor. Required for IgE synthesis. Mast cells are a major source of IL-4 in acute inflammation.

IL-5. Principal role in eosinophil activation and maturation, for example, in response to helminths.

IL-6. A major growth factor for differentiated B-cells and preplasma cells. IL-6 also has important systemic effects.

IL-10. Acts on macrophages in an inhibitory fashion, antagonistic to IFN-γ.

IFN-γ. A potent activator of macrophages, stimulating secondary release of TNF-α, IL-1, and so on. Critical in inducing secondary killing mechanisms vital to eliminating intracellular pathogens. Has a wide variety of other effects, including being antiviral potent, up-regulating MHC class I, and inducing class II on a wide range of cell (e.g., monocytes, endothelial cells and epithelial cells). Major differentiation factor for T- and B-cells (antagonizes IL-4), critical role in CTL maturation, and activates NK cells. NK cells are an important *in vivo* source, certainly in response to viruses and possibly in general (perhaps stimulated by IL-12).

TGF-α. Inhibitory role, an important anti-inflammatory cytokine, little understood.

RANTES. A chemokine for $CD4^+$ T cells.

IL-12. Produced by macrophages. Acts on T-cells and NK cells. Regulatory role in T-cell differentiation.

Signaling and Signal Transduction

Following the binding of MHC-peptide to TCR α/β, activation signals are sent into the cell, mainly via the homeodimer ξ chains associated with the CD3 complex. The early cellular events are complex and only a grossly simplified overview is presented here. Subsequent to the triggering of the TCR–CD3 complex, a rise in intracellular Ca^{2+}, an efflux of K^+, an increased turnover of phosphoinositol, activation of protein kinase C, and a rise of intracellular pH are observed in the activated cells. The initial rise in Ca^{2+} from intracellular stores appears to be transient, while sustained high Ca^{2+} levels are produced by influx from extracellular medium. T-cell activation mediated by TCR–CD3 results in an activation of the phosphatidylinositol pathway. Here phosphatidylinositol biphosphate (PIP2) is converted to inositol triphosphate (IP3) and diacylglycerol (DAG) by phospholipase C. The coupling of phospholipase to TCR–CD3 is probably mediated by G proteins, the GTP-binding proteins. DAG can activate protein kinase C, which is crucial to signal transduction and cell proliferation, while IP3 mobilizes Ca^{2+} from intracellular stores. It appears that the release of this Ca^{2+} leads to IP3 phosphorylation to IP4 (inositol tetraphosphate), which has been shown to be involved in the opening of Ca^{2+} channels. At some stage during activation, phosphorylation of some of the CD3 chains occurs at one (serine 126) or two (serine 123 and 126) sites. Phosphorylated forms of CD3 molecules are constitutively endocytosed, indicating internalization and receptor recycling in TCR–CD3-mediated activation.

An alternative activation pathway exists involving the binding of CD2 receptor (demonstrated using CD2 specific mAbs) to its natural ligand LFA-3, a receptor found on all somatic cells. Functionally, all these T-cell receptors can be thought of as working together.

Formation and Function of Natural Killer (NK) Cells

In contrast to similarly functioning cytotoxic T-cells, natural killer cells express neither the TCR and CD3 complex nor any other known antigen-specific receptor. As such, NK cells constitute a unique third lymphocyte (or lymphocyte-derived) population, called large granular lymphocytes (LGL), representing 5–15% of the total blood lymphocytes. NK cells mature in the bone marrow and show prominent intracellular granules. First discovered because of their ability to "kill" some neoplastic cells, it is recognized today that NK cells play an important role in innate immunity. In some respects these cells, expressing very low epitope density CD8, strong expression of Fcγ-R III (CD16) receptors and NKH-1 (CD56) markers to various degrees, may be considered a link between the immune and the inflammatory systems. Target cell recognition by NK cells is achieved by the recognition of the IgG1 and IgG3 antibody coating of these cells, and cytotoxic attack is triggered. The encounter with IgG antibodies increases the cytotoxic potential by a factor of 10–20. The destructive mechanism employed closely resembles those encountered in the cytotoxic T-cells, ADCC. It involves the release of cytoplasmic granules containing perforin and granzymes independent of an interaction with MHC molecules (MHC nonrestricted). In contrast to the highly specific and efficient killer T-cells (belonging to the CD8 group), the cytotoxic potential of NK cells can be induced within minutes.

Helper Cells and Their Functions

Obviously, the primary function of the helper cell is to provide assistance to B-cells, via cytokine release, mainly "helping" them to produce antibodies in response to an antigenic challenge. However, as usual in immunology, the function of CD4 cells is not restricted to this unique action. Helper cells act on a multitude of adaptive immune processes. These range from the activation of macrophages, inducing accelerated lysosomic fusion (e.g., in bacterial infection), to chemotaxis for phagocytes and neutrophils, the induction of alternative recognition and signaling mechanisms of T-cell subsets, and the activation of humoral responses. Possibly, we may realize that each individual helper cell has its own unique function and distinct cytokine pattern, and that many immune reactions rely on the complicated interaction of diverse cells and multiple cytokine patterns to explain the highly specific and individually divergent immune reactions, grossly simplified today. The maturation of helper cells has been extensively studied and a model of *in vitro* differentiation has been proposed recently. Because the receptor expression of naive and memory helper cells differs significantly, one distinction is possible on the basis of this receptor expression. It has been argued that two crucial components of memory, rapid recall and long life, belong to two distinct $CD4^+$ subsets differing in their CD45 receptor complexes. It is suggested that only the $CD4^+$ $CD45R0^+$ subpopulation depends on persisting antigen.

Cytotoxic and Suppressor T-Cells and Their Functions

Much is known about the cytotoxic reactions (Tc cells) and the mechanisms of the cytotoxic–cytolytic T-killer mechanisms. Little is known about the supposed suppressor activity (Ts cells). The most direct CD8 cell actions are Tc actions. The mechanism is comparatively simple. It includes the recognition of altered (nonself) surface structures, activation and "capturing" of the target cell via adhesion mechanisms, concentration of granzyme–perforin–fragmentin–lysin-bearing granules at the contact site, and degranulation in the direction of the target cell. This induces apoptosis[4] or membrane dissolution and death of the target cell. After detachment from the target cell and "reloading" of the cellular components (granules), there may be a continued search for nonself targets.

The second subfraction of CD8 cells is the still mysterious suppressor T-cells (Ts). This type of cells is characterized only from *in vitro* assays, where such cells are capable of suppressing not only the naive and effector mechanisms of the helper, but also to some extent of the cytotoxic, T-cells. The transfer of such suppressor cells induces tolerance in several animal models, for example, skin graft rejection in neonatal rats and transfer of this tolerance to adult rats. The suppressor subset of CD8 positive cells is probably extremely heterogeneous. A number of unique characteristics have been revealed. The CD8 receptor is generally expressed at a higher epitope density, the cells do not express several surface markers that are considered typical for the cytotoxic capacity (e.g., CD56, CD57, and CD94), but they do express co-stimulatory molecules such as CD28. Such noncytotoxic cells can be found in approximately 50–70% of the total CD8 cells. If, and which, cytokines are produced by these cells is unknown.

[4] Apoptosis means programmed cell death. This may be physiologic (e.g., occurring during embryonic development), or induced during pathological reactions. Several molecular–biological mechanisms are known to induce this process.

Complement System

The complement system was originally discovered from its bactericidal capacity. There are two pathways by which complement activity is initiated. The *classical pathway* is activated by antibody–antigen complexes. The *alternative pathway* is initiated when a previously activated complement component (C3b) binds to the surface of a pathogen, where it is protected. The complement system is a complex system of serum proteins found in the plasma and other body fluids, which, upon activation, interact in a cascade. Many of the early components are serine proteases activating each other sequentially. Altogether, 20 known proteins; the complement components C1–C9; the complement factors D, B, I, and H; and properdin participate in the various reactions.

The classical activation pathway is triggered when a molecule of C1 binds an antibody–antigen complex. The alternate pathway of activation is initiated when a previously activated complement component (C3b) binds to the surface of a pathogen (e.g., the bacterial cell membrane). Both activation mechanisms, although initiated differently, have a common "terminal reaction sequence."

Classical Complement Pathway

The classical pathway of complement activation requires the presence of antigen–antibody complexes. It cannot be initiated by soluble antigen alone. The Fc receptor of the complexed antibody constitutes the binding site for the first complement component C1. This first complement component is a complex of five subunits (one C1q, two C1r, and two C1s); C1q has six binding sites for IgFc. The affinity of a single C1q binding site for one Fc is low, so that at least two sites are required for the stable binding of C1q and subsequent activation of C1r. This requires two juxtaposed IgGs or a distorted IgM. Free IgG and IgM do not activate complement. Activated C1r cleaves C1s to generate the active C1s protease, which in turn cleaves C4 (to C4a and the unstable C4b). After C2 has bound C4b, C1s protease cleaves C2 into C2a and C2b. C4b, in conjunction with C2a, generates C4bC2a, the classical C3 convertase.

C4b contains a highly reactive (but unstable) thiol–ester bond, which can attach to nearby proteins and carbohydrates on immune complexes and cell and bacterial surfaces by covalent binding.

Alternative Complement Pathway

The alternative pathway (AP) is initiated independently from immune complexes and participation of C1, C4, and C2. This activation pathway is based on two initiating complement factors B and D, two down-regulating factors H and I, as well as properdin (as stabilizing factor), and relies on the prior generation of activated C3.

Water reacts with the thiol–ester bond in C3 in solution, generating an activated form, C3(H_2O), which is equivalent to C3b. This process proceeds spontaneously at a slow rate and is called "C3 tick-over." Because C3b is also supplied by the classical pathway, the alternative pathway can be considered a positive feedback mechanism for the classical activation of complement. Surface-bound C3b binds factor B, which, once bound to C3b, is cleaved to Ba and Bb by another serum protein, factor D. The resulting C3bBb is the alternative C3 convertase. This complex is unstable, but is can be stabilized on certain microbial surfaces by the binding of the serum factor properdin (P). The alternative C3 convertase is inactive on self-cells because it is inactivated by regulatory proteins.

Common Terminal Sequence of the Classical and Alternative Pathways

The early phases of the classic and alternative pathways generate the key players in complement activation C3 convertases. The C3 convertases are powerful amplifiers of complement activation, up to 1000 C3 molecules are cleaved to C3b by each molecule of active C3 convertase (Fig. 12).

The result of the classic and the alternative pathway and the ultimate enzymatic step in the complement cascade is the cleavage of C5 into C5a and C5b. In all subsequent steps, intact proteins are bound or polymerized. Each C3 convertase can be converted into a C5 convertase by the binding of a C3b molecule, splitting C5 into C5b and C5a. In the following, C5b binds C6, C7, and C8. Finally one or more C9 molecules are bound, building the terminal complement complex (TCC), often also designated membrane attack complex (MAC).

The small cleavage fragments C3a, C4a, and especially C5a act on specific receptors and produce localized inflammatory responses. They are also frequently referred to as anaphylatoxins.

Biological Effects of Complement

The functions of the produced complement factors are

1. Chemotaxis. Mainly the attraction of neutrophil granulocytes.
2. Bactericidal action. Direct damage of microorganisms.
3. Inflammation. Induction of inflammatory reaction at the site of complement activation. The C5a, and the less potent C4a and C3a, fragments are important inflammatory activators inducing smooth muscle contraction, vascular permeability, recruitment, and activation of phagocytes, contributing to the initiation of the adaptive immune response.
4. Opsonization. Facilitating adherence and phagocytosis of pathogens (microorganisms and particulate antigens) by activated complement or antibody complexes. C3b and, to a lesser degree, C4b molecules are such opsonins, binding to the pathogens. Through such opsonization the invader becomes "recognizable" to the defense system.
5. Lysis. C5b recruits and binds C6 and C7 to target surfaces. C7 and subsequently C8 change conformation to expose hydrophobic domains, which insert into the lipid bilayer. The C5b678 complex catalyzes the polymerisation of the final component C9, which creates a transmembrane pore of 100 Å in diameter, causing lysis of the cell.
6. Immune complex clearance. The complement has a very important role in solubilizing and causing the immune complexes to be removed from the circulation.

Regulation of Complement Activation

The potential damage through illicit complement activation is tightly regulated. The regulatory mechanisms act primarily at three points.

1. The first reactant C1 is regulated by the C1 inhibitor (C1-INH), acting in two ways, the binding of free C1 in serum ([C1-INH] > [C1]) and the inhibition of the activation of C4 and C2 by binding and inhibiting the C1r and C1s proteases.
2. The life time of C3 convertase is regulated by two distinct but related mechanisms.
   a. CR1 and C4 binding protein (C4bp) promote the dissociation of the C3 convertase by binding to the covalently bound component (C4b or C3b), displacing the associated cofactor (decay accelerating factor, (DAF).

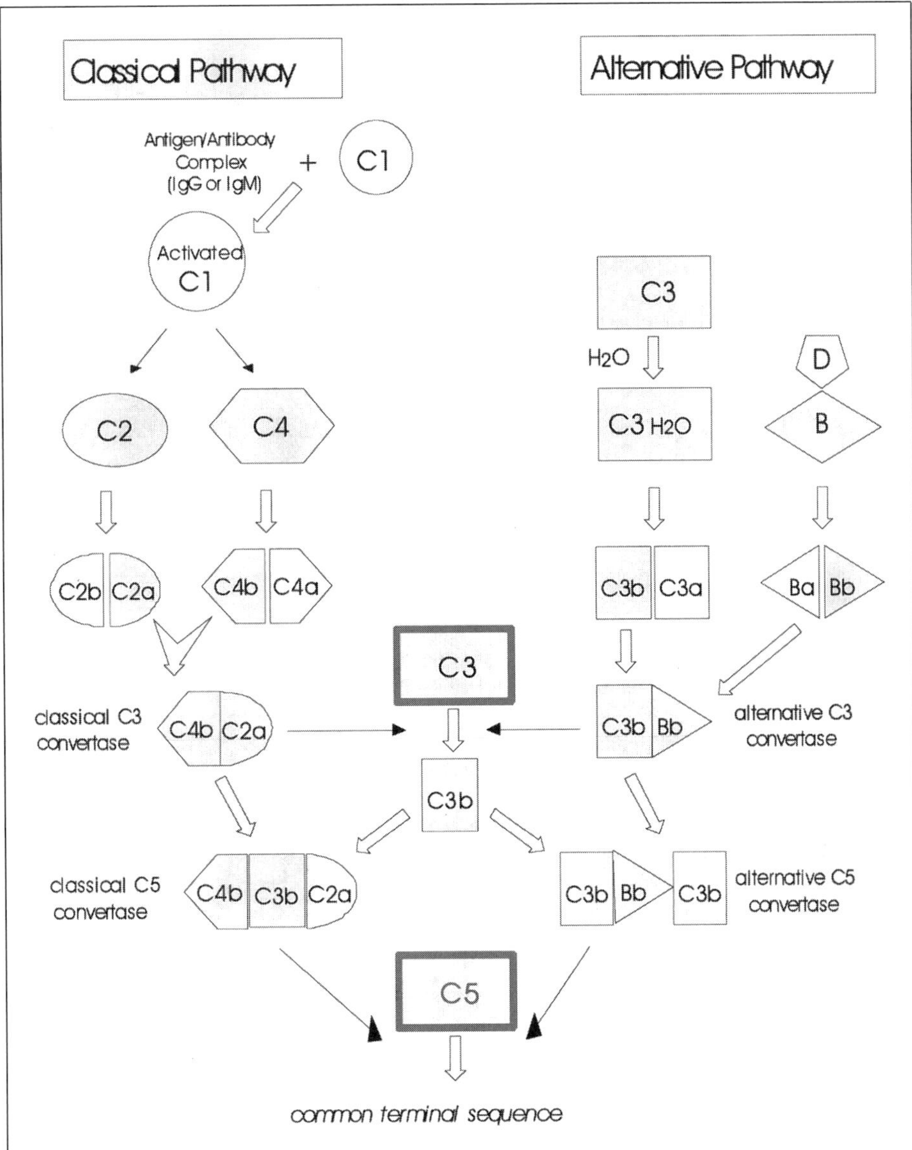

FIGURE 12 Classic and alternative pathways of complement activation to C5 convertase. In the classical pathway C1 is activated by antigen–antibody complexes to split C2 and C4 convertase into fragments. The smaller fragments (gray) are lost and the remaining larger fragments combine to classical C3 convertase.

b. C4bp, factor H, CR1, and another protein (membrane cofactor protein, MCP) catalyze the permanent inactivation of C3b and C4b through proteolytic cleavage by factor I (generating, e.g., iC3b).

3. The activity of the TCC (or MAC) is also regulated by cell surface proteins; the best known is protectin or CD59.

Complement Receptors

CR1 binds C3b and C4b. CR1 is found on erythrocytes, where it plays a vital role in removing immune complexes from circulation. It is also found on macrophages and neutrophils and can trigger phagocytosis, but only after the activation of cells by other mediators, including C5a. CR1 also has a regulatory role.

CR2 binds iC3b and is found on B-cells, where it plays an important role in activating class switching and memory formation.

CR3 and CR4 are related receptors that bind iC3b and are found on monocytes/macrophages and neutrophils. They trigger phagocytosis of opsonized particles, either in concert with Fc receptors or independently. Phagocytosis of microorganisms via CR3, and via CR1+FcR, is the major defense mechanism against bacterial and fungal infection.

Interference with Complement Functions

The pronounced pathological consequences (i.e., greatly increased susceptibility to bacterial infections) of an inherited deficiency of the important components of the complement system is well established. Chemically induced alterations of the complement system have rarely been reported. However, such changes apparently were seldom investigated.

Examples of alterations in the complement system are an increased level of C3 and C4 in some TCDD-exposed persons, and a suppression of mouse complement activity after treatment with cobra venom or with high doses of technical-grade pentachlorophenol.

Hypersensitivity Reactions (Allergy)

When adverse health effects induced by chemicals on immunological variables are considered, hypersensitivity (allergic) manifestations by far outweigh possible toxic effects. Allergic reactions are idiosyncrasies; that is, they require a certain special susceptibility for their manifestation. "Strong" allergens will affect many people (e.g., dinitrochlorobenzene [DNCB] affects almost all humans), while weak allergens will affect only very few.

It is obvious that the foremost functions of the immune response are the humoral and cellular recognition and the expedient elimination of infectious agents and other foreign antigens. An exaggerated ("hypersensitive") response to an antigen (allergen) may be triggered after reexposure to the same antigen by a previously sensitized individual. The immunological reactions are associated with inflammation, tissue damage, or cardiovascular responses. The most severe consequences are shock or death.

The allergic reaction differs from immunization in which, generally, no adverse effect results. Although there are various mechanisms of inducing allergic reactions, the final manifestations are monotonous, and they may also be induced by nonantigenic means. This holds true for symptoms such as exanthema or erythema, urticaria, dermatitis, asthma, rhinitis, and shock.

Typically, allergens are 10- to 55-kDa proteins of plant or animal origin, relatively inert, and not self-multiplying or, by themselves, cytopathic.

Allergic reactions require a second exposure for their manifestation. Generally about a week is needed for the formation of a sufficient amount of antibodies. Allergic reactions can manifest themselves in various organ systems:

- Skin, as the main target tissue (e.g., exanthema, urticaria, eczema, contact dermatitis, and purpura).
- Mucous membranes (e.g., rhinitis, conjunctivitis, and sinusitis).
- Lung (e.g., asthma and eosinopohilic [Löffler's] pneumonia).
- Vascular system (e.g., anaphylactic[5] shock, vasculitis, and angiitis).
- Skeletal system (e.g., arthritis).

Classically, hypersensitivity reactions are classified into four types with respect to their mechanisms of action. Types I through III are antibody-dependent; type IV is (T) cell-dependent. However, there are no sharp boundaries between the types of reaction. An agent may well induce more than one type of response.

Type I (Anaphylaxis or Immediate Response Reaction)

Type I hypersensitivity reactions are generally IgE-mediated (only in very rare cases are they IgG-mediated) and are caused by mast cell–basophil-mediated release of inflammatory cytokines. The antibody is cytophillic. Individuals who respond to such antigens suffer from atopy. Reexposure to the antigen elicits an immediate response. If this response is systemic, it is called anaphylaxis. This immediate response (e.g., to pollen, mite or animal antigens, and food antigens) is mediated by histamine and other mediators released by the degranulation of previously primed mast cells and basophils. The response has several stages:

1. During sensitization (i.e., upon the primary exposure to a defined antigen) specific **IgE** is produced by B-cells, newly differentiating into plasma cells. This differentiation and the subsequent switching to IgE production of the plasma cell are strongly Th2-dependent because the necessary IL-4 is primarily produced by this cellular subset.
2. The subsequent step is marked by the linking of the available IgE to the high-affinity $Fc_{\epsilon}RI$ receptors on mast cells and basophils. The cells are now primed and possess a highly allergen specific receptor on their cell surface.
3. Subsequent contact with the specific allergen induces instant recognition by the specific receptor and

[5] Anaphylaxis is a systemic immediate immunological reaction after reexposure of a previously sensitized individual. The manifestation may concern blood pressure (anaphylactic shock), bronchoconstriction, and so on. See the section on Type I allergy.

induction of the immediate response. However, to be effective, an allergen must cross-link at least two IgE molecules on the cell membrane of the mast cell or basophil, causing an increase of intracellular Ca^{2+}, in turn triggering release of preformed primary mediators (histamine and proteases) and secondary, newly formed mediators (leukotrienes, prostaglandins, and platelet-activating factors). The ensuing degranulation is massive, and the resulting common reactions are the contraction of smooth muscles and dilation of capillaries. The degree of the response varies from mild symptoms to sudden death. The manifestations are urticaria, eczema, asthma, hay fever, and even anaphylactic shock. Susceptibility to this adverse reaction is designated as an atopic disease.

4. The immediate response is often (e.g., as in asthma) followed by a late-phase reaction. This begins about 2–6h after the initial allergen contact and persists up to several days (generally 1–3). This reaction is an inflammatory response induced by secondary chemotactic activity for other cells (mainly eosinophils, monocytes, macrophages, and T-cells). These cells infiltrate the inflammatory tissues, the polymorphnuclear cell first and the mononuclear cells later, being attracted in turn by the secretions of the former. As a result, late-phase lesions typically contain 30% each of lymphocytes, neutrophils, and eosinophils, and 10% of monocytes and macrophages, including isolated basophils.

5. In the absence of continued exposure to the allergen, the reaction typically disappears. Prolonged or chronic exposure to the allergen leads to permanent damage of the infiltrated tissues.

Anaphylaxis is the extreme endpoint of the type I reaction, when the otherwise locally confined reaction becomes systemic, for example, by the administration of a medical substance or insect bite. The ensuing general reactions of vasodilation and plasma loss through exudation into tissue induce generalized hypotension and shock. The previously described effects further enhance these primary effects. Without immediate treatment, such anaphylactic shock can easily be life threatening.

For example, although the exact figures are lacking, it is estimated that at least 4 of 100,000 patients treated by the systemic application of penicillin experience anaphylactoid reactions; about 10% of these people die (100 to 500 yearly deaths in the United States).

Atopic diseases include neurodermatitis, allergic urticaria, and allergic asthma, triggered by various antigens, including animal constituents and excretions, pollen, and food components. In industrialized countries, an impressive proportion of the population (8–15%) shows a genetic predisposition to this type of allergic reaction. It is commonly admitted that this disposition is mainly acquired through multifactorial autosomal inheritance. Recently it has been found that women are approximately twice as exposed to anaphylaxis as men.

Type II (Antibody-Dependent Cytotoxic Response)

Type II hypersensitivity reactions are very closely related to the "normal" immune responses observed in reactions to multicellular parasites and other microorganisms. The mechanism is also referred to as cytotoxicity. The principle is the recognition of antibodies directed against cellular structures or tissue antigens and the subsequent linkage of these antibodies to effector cells or complement via their Fc domains. In both cases, the destruction of the cell is preprogrammed. In type II hypersensitivity, the antibodies are produced during an immune response to recognize and bind antigens, which are structural components of the cell surface, the extracellular matrix, or other tissue components. The antigen can be intrinsic (part of the host tissues) or extrinsic (absorbed onto host tissue surfaces). In contrast to type I hypersensitivity, IgG and IgM antibodies are bound to these antigens. The typical effector mechanisms related to these immunoglobulins are induced, leukocyte activation via Fc receptors, phagocytosis, and complement activation. The activation of C1 of the classic complement pathway, inducing C3 and generating mediators of acute inflammation (degranulation of neutrophils after defective phagocytosis) is an especially typical mechanism of hypersensitivity type II. The result is the complement-mediated lytic damage of the target cell or the creation of a membrane defect by the deposit of C5b-9 membrane attack complex (MAC) on the cell surface, also leading to cell lysis and cell death.

Examples of antibody-mediated–complement-dependent reactions are transfusion reactions, reactions to certain drugs, and autoimmune hemolytic anemia. The hyperacute rejection observed by allogenic[6] transplantation is often a type II reaction against preformed antibodies. These are already resident in the host before transplantation and, after binding to the transplanted tissue, initiate the immediate rejection process.

[6] Allogenic refers to different genotypes of the same species. Autogenic refers to components of the same individual. Isogenic refers to the same genotypes in two individuals of the same species (e.g., monozygotic twins). Xenogenic refers to different genotypes in individuals of different species; this is important in organ transplantation.

Often the formation of the immune complexes does not lead to the activation of the complement system. In such circumstances the binding of the antibodies to cell surfaces still leads to cell injury; this is called antibody-dependent cell-mediated cytotoxicity (ADCC).

In a third possibility of deregulation, the specific antibodies bind to cell surface receptors and prevent or mimic the occupancy of the physiologic ligand. This is the case in for example, myasthenia gravis, where antiacetylcholine receptor antibodies block neuromuscular transmission, resulting in extreme muscular weakness.

Type III (Immune-Complex Reaction)

Very similar to the type II reaction in the spectrum of the response, type III hypersensitivity differs essentially by the reaction against soluble antigen complexes. The formation of such soluble immune complexes is a "normal" reaction every time antibody encounters antigen. Immune complexes form in the circulation and deposit in various tissues, where they may trigger the classic pathway of complement activation. Mediators of acute inflammation are generated at the sites of immune complex deposition. These complexes are then phagocytosed and eliminated via the reticuloendothelial system. In type III hypersensitivity, two general types of complexing elude the recognition mechanisms of phagocytic cells.

1. Tissue-trapped complexes. When antibody and antigen encounters are tissue located, such as in skin perforations, the resulting immune complexes activate the complement, leading to the generation of C3a and C5a, the anaphylatoxins. The same immune complexes induce macrophages to cytokine release (mainly tumor necrosis factor, TNF, and IL-1). The complement fragments C3a and C5a induce the degranulation of mast cells and attract neutrophils into the tissue. The attracted polymorph cells attempt phagocytosis of the complexes, but small tissue-trapped complexes are difficult to ingest and the cells concerned degranulate ("frustrated degranulation"), initiating a localized inflammatory reaction. A typical example is the Arthus reaction, for example, alveolitis and interstitial nephritis. A typical disease is farmers' lung.

2. Membrane-trapped complexes. The formation of immune complexes in the blood or serous systems may lead to membranous attachment. The inflammatory reaction is then either localized at the attachment point or systemic due to the distribution of the immune complexes throughout the concerned system. Typical examples for localized manifestations are vasculitis (e.g., glomerulonephritis or pleuritis) and, for general manifestations, the systemic lupus erythematosus.

Type IV (Cell-Mediated or Delayed-Type Hypersensitivity)

Delayed-type hypersensitivity is a collective appellation for all hypersensitivity reactions requiring more than 12 h to develop (excluding IgE-dependent reactions). These involve cell-mediated, rather than humoral, immune reactions.

Type IV hypersensitivity is closely CD4 (TH1-helper cell) related, but can, in a few cases, also be initiated by CD8 cytotoxic T-cells (type IVb). CD4 T-helper cells recognize either intracellular or extracellular synthesized antigen when it is complexed with class II MHC molecules. The ensuing liberation of pro-inflammatory cytokines causes plasma exudation through increased vascular permeability. Through secretion of chemotactic factors, adhesion molecules on endothelial cells are activated and induce a cellular infiltration consisting essentially of T-cells and macrophages. The macrophages act as antigen-presenting cells and release interleukin-1, which promotes the proliferation of T-helper cells. T-helper cells release interferon-γ and interleukin-2, which together regulate delayed hypersensitivity reactions. The attracted activated cytotoxic T cells destroy target cells, such as allografts, on contact. Natural killer cells can kill target cells directly, in the absence of prior immunization and without MHC restriction, as well as by antibody-dependent cellular cytotoxicity (ADCC). Activated macrophages express increased phagocytic, bactericidal, and cytocidal activity.

The typical clinical affection of type IV hypersensitivity is contact dermatitis, triggered by inorganic agents such as chromate or nickel, organic agents such as picric acid, or the ingredients in poison ivy or oak. Contact dermatitis requires between 24 and 72 h until full development of the lesions. For this reason this type of allergy is referred to as delayed-type hypersensitivity. The contact-induced allergy can be triggered by a multitude of allergens, among them cosmetics, detergents, medical substances, and environmental and household agents (e.g., cement and jewelry). It is recognized today that genetic causes influence the susceptibility to type IV hypersensitivity.

The cascade of events that results in contact dermatitis and the precise contribution of T-cells is not well understood. It is agreed upon that a sensitizing phase may be distinguished from an elicitation stage.

During sensitization, epicutaneously applied hapten is taken up by the Langerhans and possibly by other antigen-processing cells and processed to antigen, while these cells convert from a resting to an activated state, induced by cytokines (IL-1β, IL-6, chemokines, TNF-α, etc.) secreted by keratinocytes or Langerhans cells due to a hapten stimulus. Activated Langerhans cells migrate to the regional lymph node, where the antigen is presented to naive T cells (mostly MHC class I-restricted $CD8^+$ cells), transforming those to hypersensitivity effector cells. Sensitization is generally asymptomatic.

Apparently, elicitation of contact dermatitis (i.e., the clinical manifestation on recontact) initially requires some type of pro-inflammatory stimulus besides the hapten-specific immunologic recognition. Although the earliest histopathological findings are mast cell degranulation, vasodilatation, and influx of neutrophils, contact dermatitis is clearly T-cell dependent. Haptens seem to be capable of directly and nonimmunologically inducing pro-inflammatory stimuli on epidermal and endothelial cells, with enhanced expression of adhesion molecules and cytokine secretion without requiring antigen-specific recognition. Apparently, most of these haptens are capable of reacting as irritants. Interestingly, this pro-inflammatory effect is clearly dose-dependent (which is unusual in allergic reactions!) and requires much higher doses of the hapten than is necessary for sensitization. The nonspecific pro-inflammatory reaction of leukocyte chemo-attraction, adhesion, and activation seems to enhance the probability for sensitized T-cells to meet their antigen, and thereby amplify the immune response proper, which needs only very small doses of hapten.

It should be remembered that the distinction between these four types of allergy is not always clear-cut.

Possible Role of Th1 and Th2 in Atopic Diseases

The pathogenesis of atopic inflammatory manifestations involves a complex interplay of genetic, environmental, psychological, and pharmacological factors. It has been hypothesized from existing evidence that the symptoms of atopic dermatitis result from sequential activation of T-helper cells of type 2 (Th2) and type 1 (Th1). Thus it is assumed that Th2- and Th1-type responses are not mutually exclusive but that both types of cells may act simultaneously in different organs or sequentially in the same disease. These types of reactions are interlinked by IL-12, formed from skin-invading macrophages, and eosinophils, leading to activation of allergen-specific and nonspecific Th1 and Th0 cells. The chronic state is believed to be caused by the predominance of IFN-γ-producing T-helper cells. The characteristic pattern of cytokines plays an essential role in these types of T-helper cell reactions, as revealed in studies with animal and human cells. The Th1 type, mostly involved in cell-mediated immune response, is characterized by the predominant release of IFN-γ and IL-2 (the latter specifically only in mice), whereas the Th2 type is mostly involved in humoral response (e.g., IgE synthesis) and proceeds with the release of IL-4, IL-5, and IL10 (the latter specifically only in mice). Interfering with the action of such cytokines may be a future strategy for therapeutic intervention. However, this distinction should not be taken too seriously. Recent research has shown that the functions of helper cells greatly exceed these fixed categories, and it appears obvious that several other helper cell subfractions, Th3–Th*n* are bound to exist. The diversity of helper cells may be as great as the diversity of B-cells.

This model of the two T-helper cell types may also provide an explanation for the frequent observations that within a population with frequent infectious diseases, either viral or parasitic, allergic reactions are rare events. Preventing such diseases, as is the case in industrialized countries, will largely enhance the frequency of allergic responsiveness within such a population. This could provide an explanation for the increase in allergic diseases in many highly industrialized countries.

EXAMPLES OF ALTERATIONS OF IMMUNOLOGICAL COMPONENTS AND FUNCTIONS

Substances altering components and functions of the immune system may be divided into two groups, those depressing and those stimulating the system. Overall, four different situations may arise:

- Enhancement of immune functions (immunomodulation).
- Depression of immune functions (immunosuppression).
- Overreaction of the immune system (allergic reactions).
- Failure to recognize self (autoimmune reactions).

Theoretically, members of all classes of chemicals should be able to induce the last three types of effects. However, there are clear-cut focal points. Immunosuppressants have mostly been medicinal drugs designed and therapeutically used for this purpose. Although there are also many drugs initiating allergic reactions, the majority of the responsible agents come from nature (e.g., pollen, animal antigens, and plants) or from components of daily life (e.g., cosmetics and detergent). Autoimmune reactions increasingly gain

TABLE 4 Compilation of Important Components and Functions of the Immune System That May Be Modified by Chemical Substances

Specific variations in *components* of the immune system
- Morphological changes in specific tissue (thymus, lymph nodes, spleen, etc.)
- Changes in the composition and pattern of white blood and tissue cells (lymphocytes, neutrophiles, monocytes, macrophages, etc.)
- Alterations of important surface receptors and their specific ligands
- Changes in the overall concentration of immunoglobulins
- Changes in the concentration and pattern of cytokines and other (e.g., growth) factors
- Changes in the composition of the complement system
- Other changes of relevant components, (e.g., lymphatic cells in special tissues)

Specific variations in the *function* of the immune system
- Reduced complex functions of the immune system
  - Reduced host resistance against infections (by bacteria, viruses, parasites, etc.), and against tumors
  - Reduced interactions of cellular and extracellular components, homing and migration of blood cells into tissue
  - Reduced transplant rejection
  - Reduced antibody formation to specific antigens
- Increased complex functions of the immune system
  - Hypersensitivity reactions, auto immune reactions, etc.
  - "Immunostimulation" as an increased defense against infections and tumors
- Altered functions of circumscript systems (e.g., functions of neutrophils and macrophages, interactions between lymphocytes and other cells, cell proliferation and differentiation, and formation of specific mediator substances)

Indirect and unspecific variations in the immune system
- Modifications through hormonal actions
- Modifications through actions on the CNS
- Modifications through "stress"
- Secondary alterations of immune reactions through general toxicity

importance; in addition to infections, medicinal drugs may play a role.

Important components and functions of the immune system that may be modified by chemical substances are compiled in Table 4. Most of such pathological manifestations have been revealed in animal studies, but an increasing number of endpoints can also be evaluated in humans.

Knowledge of the immune functions is very recent, and many of the interactions are either incompletely understood or not yet explainable. With few exceptions, therapeutic attempts on specific modulations are generally immunesuppressive. During the last decade, several important mechanisms concerning the suppression of rather precise phases of immune reactions have been recognized and are currently exploited, for example, immunosuppression with cyclosporin A or tacrolimus.

Immune-enhancing mechanisms are largely confined to the administration of soluble mediators (active immunomodulation), with the limitations known, or immunoglobulins (passive immunomodulation). During clinical application, many of such immune-modulating substances (e.g., cytokines) exhibit massive and often uncontrollable adverse effects. However, certain mediators, such as G-CSF (granulocyte colony-stimulating factor), GM-CSF (granulocyte–macrophage colony-stimulating factor) and IL-3, are currently used in the therapy of infections with leukozytopenic origin, just as IL-2 has a limited use in some cancer diseases.

Immunosuppressive Agents Affecting the Human Immune System

The mode of action of these immunosuppressive agents is quite heterogeneous. All of them typically exhibit more than one effect on the immune system. For this reason, it is not always easy to decide which of the properties of a given agent is responsible for a defined therapeutic or toxic effect.

Although many of these components are of natural origin, most of them have been selected and designed for medical purposes. They are predominantly used therapeutically in transplantation surgery, but they are also used to counteract inflammatory and immune reactions in allergic and autoimmune diseases. Although there are hints for the immunosuppressive effects of "environmental chemicals" from animal studies (e.g., organotin compounds), at present none has been verified in humans.

Because it has so far not been possible to achieve allograft transplantation without effective immunosuppression, the use of substances preventing transplant rejection is an integral part of transplantation surgery. Immunosuppressive agents are now widely used not only for preventing transplant rejection, but attempts have also been made to use them to treat a variety of diseases, preferentially of the autoimmune type. Their therapeutic action is aimed at preventing or reducing overshooting or unfavorable effects of the immune system. Generally the therapeutic success rate is not as high as that achieved against transplantation rejection.

The possible mechanisms of action of immunosuppressive agents are compiled in Fig. 13. Not all of them are usable for therapeutic interventions.

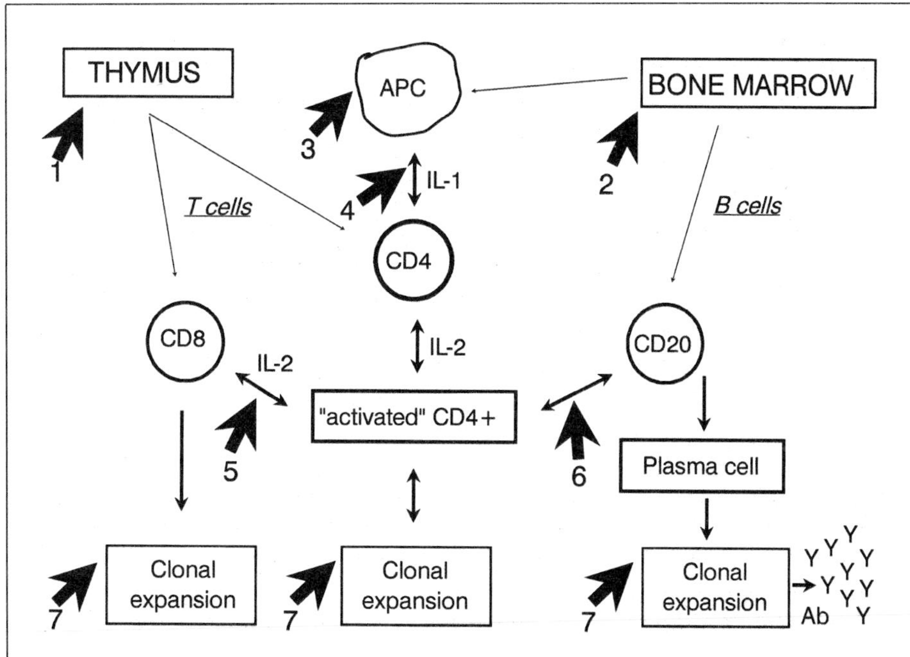

FIGURE 13 Possible points of attack of immunosuppressive agents on the immune response at various levels. Lymphocyte-forming organs (e.g., involution of the thymus), interference with antigen processing and presentation, the functions of B- and T-cells, and proliferation processes (clonal expansion).

- Interference with immunocyte development in thymus and bone marrow (toxic effects).
- Interference with antigen-presentation mechanisms.
- Interference with T-cell function; inhibition of signal transduction or receptor actions (e.g., monoclonal antibodies, cyclosporin, tacrolimus, and thalidomide).
- Interference with B-cell function.
- Interference with proliferation; clonal expansion (e.g., azathioprine, 6-mercaptopurine, cyclophosphamide, and methotrexate).

Immunosuppressive agents illustrate the double-edged situation in immunopharmacology and -toxicology. While of considerable therapeutic benefit, the effects of all these agents would be considered highly toxic when exhibited by an environmental agent. As expected, the biological profile is not confined to interference with the immune system. There is not perfect organotropy, but the immune system is a preferred target.

Cyclosporin A and Similar Substances

The naturally occurring substance cyclosporin, derived from the fungus *Tolypocladium inflatum,* has become the prototype of an immunosuppressive agent. The unique cyclic polypeptide (11 amino acids) contains an unusual and a D-amino acid, the amide nitrogen of seven amino acids is methylated and four of the amide groups are interlinked by hydrogen bonds. Cyclosporin A and the structurally quite different but similarly acting (and about 100 times more potent) macrolide antibiotic tacrolimus derived from *Streptomyces tsukubaensis,* have become, often combined with a glucocorticoid, the preferred drugs for the prevention and treatment of allograft rejection in organ transplantations.

The effects of cyclosporin on numerous systems and reactions can be demonstrated, depending on the test system and the concentration (dose) used. It is difficult to decide which of the numerous actions is responsible for beneficial and adverse effects in humans at therapeutic doses or overdoses.

Evidence accumulated suggests that the inhibition of activation and proliferation of T-cells and the block in the interleukin-2 (IL-2) expression certainly are key mechanisms. It is important to note that cyclosporin is not lymphotoxic. The mechanisms of action of cyclosporin and tacrolimus on the signal transduction in T-helper lymphocytes are almost identical, suggesting that the two molecules, with unrelated chemical structures, act on a common or very similar molecular

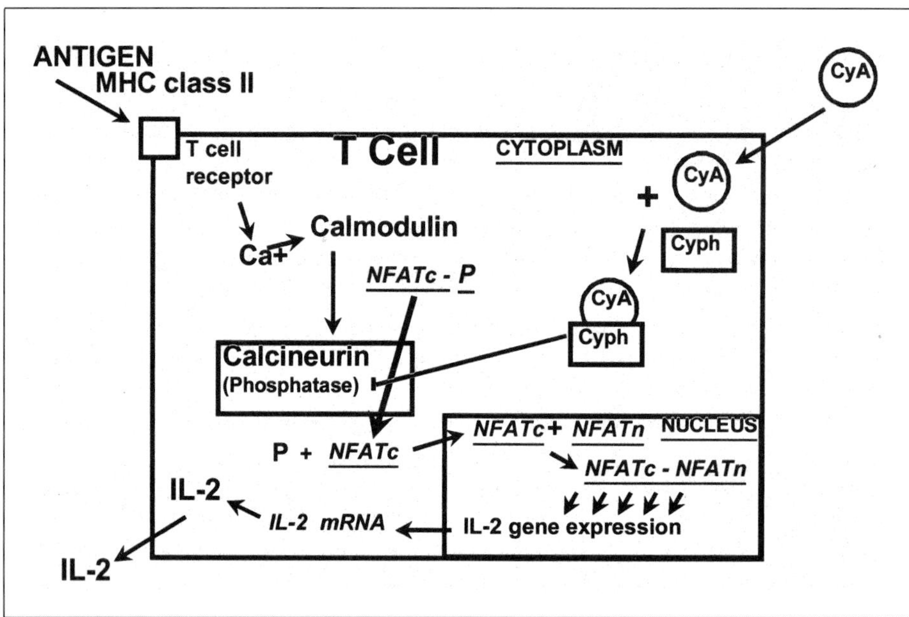

FIGURE 14 Interference by cyclosporin (and similarly by tacrolimus) with an important metabolic pathway involved in the immune response. The action of cyclosporin occurs within the cytoplasm and is not directly associated with the reactions in the cell nucleus. As a result, the formation of IL-2 is reduced.

targets. Both drugs are potent inhibitors of T-cell activation. In the course of one of the typical and apparently most important modes of action (Fig. 14) the substances are each bound to a cytoplasmic receptor protein (cyclophilin and FKBP, respectively) within the T-helper cells. The complex inhibits the serine-threonine phosphatase calcineurin, which catalyzes the dephosphorylation of a cytoplasmic protein (NFATc), which, after being transferred to the cell nucleus, combines with its nuclear subunit (NFATn). The resulting transcription factor triggers the enhanced transcription of a number of cytokines, especially interleukin-2 (IL-2). The overall result of the inhibition of this sequence of events is a reduced formation of IL-2 by the T-helper ($CD4^+$) cells. The lack of stimulation by this cytokine is thought to subsequently reduce the attack of cytotoxic ($CD8^+$) T-cells on the transplant.

Inhibition of cyclosporin on the calcium-dependent pathway in T-lymphocytes is not located on the first steps of the sequence, the antigen-induced increase in cytoplasmic Ca^{2+} concentration. The increase in intracellular Ca^{2+} following antigen stimulation is not altered, and mitogenesis directly induced by calcium ionophore is also inhibited by cyclosporin. However, phorbol ester (TPA)-induced cell stimulation and IL-2 receptor formation via protein kinase C are relatively resistant to cyclosporin.

Besides this reaction mechanism, the two antibiotics induce a number of further effects on the immune system. Both attenuate IL-2 production via an additional mechanism in which an increased expression of transforming growth factor β is involved. TGF-β is an inhibitor of IL-2-stimulated T-cell proliferation and the generation of antigen-specific cytotoxic T-lymphocytes. Thus, these two mechanisms exaggerate an effect on IL-2.

Certainly the inhibitory effect of both antibiotics on the expression of IL-2 and its receptor is an important mode of action. However, interference with the expression of this interleukin is not the only result. The formation of many other cytokines, such as IL-3, IL-4, granulocyte–macrophage colony-stimulating factor, and interferon-γ is also affected. The consequences of the action of these antibiotics are not limited to T-cells, but the Ca^{2+}-dependent stimulation of B-cells is involved as well, providing a rather complex picture of interactions.

The action of cyclosporin seems to critically depend on its chemical structure. Attempts to develop derivatives, especially those with reduced nephrotoxicity, have not been successful. However, immunosuppressants with structural similarity to tacrolimus, for example, rapamycin (Sirolimussymbol 226), have been found to similarly bind to FKBP but interact differently on intracellular signal transduction processes.

This again underscores the multiplicity of actions of this class of antibiotics.

As outlined, cyclosporin and tacrolimus bind to structures within the cells that may be designated as immunophilins. The two antibiotics do not cross-react with respect to the binding to their respective receptor molecules. These proteins are ubiquitous structures, highly preserved during phylogenesis, and common not only in almost all mammalian cells, but also found in many lower organism. Although they exhibit rotamase activity (i.e., catalyzing the *cis–trans* isomerization of peptyl–prolyl bonds) and thereby are possibly of significance for protein folding, the functions of these proteins are only partly understood. A functional similarity to heat-shock proteins is feasible. Because many of the immunosuppressants are antibiotics, primary actions on organisms not possessing an immune system are likely.

Although they act within the immune system selectively on T-lymphocytes, both cyclosporin and tacrolimus exhibit adverse effects on other organs, such as nephrotoxicity, hepatotoxicity, neurotoxicity, hypertension, and other adverse reactions at appropriately high dose levels. First-year survival of cadaveric renal allografts was greatly improved after the introduction of cyclosporin in the early 1980s, but the frequency of chronic rejection was not much altered. Insufficient immunosuppression by too low doses of this suppressant were considered responsible for this unfavorable outcome. Nephrotoxicity of cyclosporin limits the use of higher doses. Histopathological lesions of chronic cyclosporin toxicity share similarities with those of chronic renal rejection—interstitial fibrosis, tubular atrophy, and vascular changes. Such toxic effects have been associated with the induction of growth factors, especially TGF-β. While the induction of several TGF-β isoforms within the transplant may contribute to the favorable immunosuppressive action of cyclosporin and tacrolimus soon after transplantation, prolonged expression of these types of cytokines seems to participate in the pathogenesis of chronic allograft nephropathy and toxic manifestations of these agents. To circumvent the use of higher doses of cyclosporin, its use in combination with other immunosuppressants exhibiting other toxicologic profiles will be the therapeutic solution.

Mycophenolic acid, the active metabolite of mycophenolate mofetil, suppresses the *de novo* DNA synthesis and thereby proliferation of T- and B-cells by inhibiting inosine monophosphate dehydrogenase. Lymphocytes critically depend on this pathway for purine synthesis rather than on the salvage pathway. This immunosuppressant has experimentally and clinically been shown to prevent allograft rejection. In contrast to cyclosporin, mycophenolate was shown to inhibit TGF-β production.

Pentoxifylline and 15-Deoxyspergualine

Pentoxifylline, a derivative of methylxanthine and an inhibitor of phosphodiesterase, was originally used in the therapy of peripheral arterial occlusions. More recent studies have demonstrated the potential of this substance to modify production and function of certain cytokines, such as IL-2, IFN-γ, or TNF-α, as well as functions of polymorphonuclear leukocytes and natural killer cells. The effect of pentoxifylline appears to be mediated through up-regulation of cAMP. Pentoxifylline was shown to inhibit the inflammatory action of IL-1 and TNF-α, diminish endothelial inflammation, and clinically reduce mortality in patients with septic syndromes. Oral pentoxifylline treatment in humans (400 mg) resulted in a reduced superoxide anion production at concentrations as low as 0.6 mg/liter, and it was effective in reducing the neutrophil respiratory burst. A reduced activation of immature NK cells and an increase of chemotaxis was also reported.

15-Deoxyspergualin (gusperimus, DSP) is a 15-deoxy analog of the antineoplastic antibiotic spergualine and a potent immunosuppressant, currently used in clinical trials on the treatment of graft rejection in renal transplantation. The mechanism of action is not yet completely elucidated. First believed to be similar to the action of rapamycin, it appears that this drug possesses a novel mechanism of pharmacological immunosuppression, primarily displayed at the level of autoreactive B-cells and monocytes. Its binding to a heat-shock protein (hsp 70) was reported and this was suggested as a possible mechanism of action. Clinical tests have shown that in healthy subjects the secretion of polyclonal immunoglobulin (Ig) M and G from the B-lymphocytes was diminished by 15-deoxyspergualin. Neither the proliferative response of normal T- and B-cells to mitogenic stimulation nor the cytokine secretory capacities of these cells (e.g., IL-2, IL-4, IL-6, and interferon-γ) and of monocytes (e.g., IL-1β and IL-6) were affected by the drug. In mononuclear cells obtained from patients suffering from lupus erythematosus, 15-deoxyspergualin inhibited the spontaneous production of polyclonal and anti-DNA IgG antibodies and suppressed the IL-1β secretion from the monocytes. The drug did not alter other functional responses of T-cells, B-cells, and monocytes in such patients, including mitogenic activation and cytokine secretion. Other experimental studies demonstrated a clear influence of the substance on the differentiation of T-cells in the thymus. The thymic differentiation was blocked at the $CD4^-CD8^-$ to $CD4^+CD8^+$ transition, depending on the expression of the pre-TCR complex including the variable TCRβ chain, but not TCRα chain. Later transitions displaying conventional α and β TCR complexes appeared to be unaffected, as did activation of mature T-cells both *in vitro* and *in vivo*. The pre-B-cell differentiation in the bone marrow was blocked at a precisely equivalent point—the A-C to C′ transition, controlled by the expression of a prereceptor complex containing the Ig heavy, but not light, chain. Mature B-cells appeared to be unperturbed by these changes. These findings suggest interference of DSP with common signaling pathways in early lymphocyte differentiation, clearly distinct from those found in mature cells. During rejection episodes, DSP specifically reduced B-cell expansion, antibody production, and blast cell generation, without influencing the suppressor-T-cell mechanisms. In the clinical studies, a retarded immune response as well as a suppression of graft-versus-host response was observed. Additive effects in combination with cyclosporin A and methylprednisolone were also observed.

Glucocorticoids

Glucocorticoids represent the second important class of immunosuppressants. Again, this group of natural and semisynthetic compounds is characterized by a multitude of biological actions. The effects on the mammalian organism are not confined to immunosuppression; pronounced actions on acute and chronic inflammatory processes are well known. Furthermore, such diverse systems as bone structure and mood are affected and receptor-mediated actions of several substances are exaggerated. Glucocorticoids are typically substances inducing various gene expressions via a specific cytoplasmic receptor.

While some effects of natural glucocorticoids may be observed within the physiological range (e.g., stress reactions), many other therapeutic actions are induced at pharmacologic, highly unphysiological doses.

Although the immunosuppressive action is used in preventing transplant rejection, always in combination with other immunosuppressive agents, the main therapeutic indications are conditions associated with inflammations, allergic reactions, and autoimmune diseases. In fact, glucocorticoids are the most potent antiallergic substances.

It has been known for many decades that glucocorticoids rapidly alter the composition of white blood cells in peripheral blood. The number of polymorphonuclear[7] leukocytes is increased within a few hours after a single application, and the number of lymphocytes is decreased. This phenomenon is due to an altered distribution away from the periphery in the case of lymphocytes and an opposite effect on neutrophils (i.e., increased release from the bone marrow). However, increased destruction of lymphocytes may also occur under certain conditions, induced by increased apoptosis triggered by these hormones via activated transcription of target genes. This effect of high doses is therapeutically used in the treatment of acute lymphatic leukemia in pediatrics.

Alteration of gene expression is the common and predominant mechanism believed to be responsible for most of the actions of glucocorticoids. Because there are many glucocorticoid-responsive elements within the DNA, a multiplicity of actions will result. The process of induced formation of specific proteins is the same as that typically known for such inducing agents altering gene expression (e.g., steroid sex hormones, vitamin D). Briefly; the hormones are bound in target tissue to a specific cytoplasmic glucocorticoid receptor, replacing some heat-shock proteins. The complex is translocated into the cell nucleus and binds to the various glucocorticoid-responsive elements of DNA, initiating an increased gene transcription. By processing and splicing, more mRNA is formed, leading to increased translation of specific proteins. Of course, this sequence of processes requires some time. Recently, as a mechanism of some immediate effects of these agents, nongenomic actions (e.g., actions via membrane-bound receptors) were also discussed.

With respect to actions on white blood cells, most of the effects of glucocorticoids were assumed to be induced by direct action of the glucocorticoid–receptor complex on the corresponding responsive DNA elements.

Because some of the genes for cytokines were found not to contain such glucocorticoidresponsive elements, more indirect mechanisms were explored to explain the action of these hormones. A new overall mechanism was proposed recently (Fig. 15). The central role in this reaction sequence is played by a transcription factor (NF-κB) capable of inducing a number of important immunoregulatory genes. This interest-

[7] Polymorphonuclear cells are white blood cells of the inflammatory (and immune) system with a lobulous nucleus, e.g. leukocytes (granulocytes: neutrophils, basophils, eosinophils). In contrast to mononuclear cells (e.g., lymphocytes, NK cells, monocytes/macrophages).

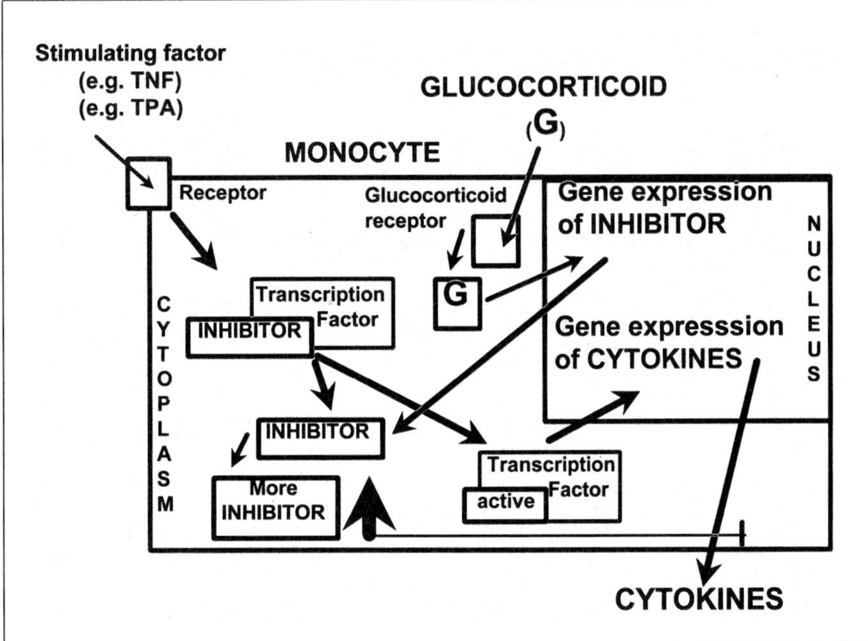

FIGURE 15 Action of glucocorticoids on formation and release of various cytokines from immunocytes (e.g., monocytes) without directly interfering with the gene expression of these cytokines. This may be a major mechanism of the anti-inflammatory and immunosuppressive effects. Certain stimuli (e.g., TNF-α, IL-1, TPA) induce the formation of a transcription factor (NF-κB), which after nuclear translocation plays a central role in the regulation of a large number of genes encoding many cytokines. Normal activation occurs by degradation of a short-lived inhibitory protein (IκBα) bound to NF-κB, and subsequent release of the active transcription factor. Glucocorticoids enhance the expression of the inhibitor (IκBα), resulting in an increased binding and reduced action of the transcription factor.

ing mechanism permits the regulation of genes to which the hormone has no direct access. Cytokines and factors encoded by such genes include IL-1, IL-2, IL-6, TNF-α, IFN-γ, granulocyte–macrophage colony-stimulating factor, and endothelial leukocyte adhesion receptor. In its inactive form, the transcription factor NF-κB is complexed in the cytoplasm with a short-lived inhibitor (κBα), from which NF-κB is released by cell-activating stimuli (e.g., from TNF-α, IL-1, or TPA). Glucocorticoids interfere with this sequence of events by inducing the transcription and translation of the inhibiting protein IκBα. When there is an excess of this inhibitor IκBα, most of the NF-κB is bound (NF-κB–IκBα complex) and prevented from nuclear translocation in its active form. Glucocorticoids act indirectly as inhibitor of the transcription factor NF-κB.

The well-established adverse effects of high doses of glucocorticoids after long-term treatment on the defense of certain infections, on bone structures, and or the chance of developing Cushing's syndrome limit the chronic application of these substances.

Antimetabolites and Alkylating Agents

In many reactions of the immune system rapid proliferation processes are mandatory. These include the immense daily replacement of immunocytes, as well as the clonal expansion of lymphocytes. For this reason several antimetabolites and alkylating agents exhibit immunosuppressive properties. Because the cells of the immune system are not the only rapidly proliferating cells of the organism, no selective organotropy can be expected with these drugs.

With respect to the susceptibility of the immune system, it is favorable that lymphocytes lack the capacity for extensive nucleotide synthesis via the salvage pathway. Therefore, interfering with the reactions of DNA and RNA precursor synthesis, for example, by purine or pyrimidine antimetabolites (see the section on Mycophenolate Mofetil) or folic acid antagonists, provides some degree of specificity. Alkylating agents, such as cyclophosphamide, were formerly used therapeutically as immunosuppressants, but these chemicals, having a cancerogenic potential, are no longer needed for this indication. Nevertheless, these substances might induce adverse or toxic effects on the immune system when persons are exposed during therapy.

Because of its effect on lymphocyte formation, methotrexate has been successfully applied in the management of acute lymphoblastic leukemia in children. When the substance is used, for example, to treat colon cancer, bone marrow toxicity is the most serious adverse effect. The intestinal epithelium and hair follicles, liver, and kidneys may be the targets of further adverse drug reactions of methotrexate.

More recently, this folic acid antagonist has increasingly been used outside cancer therapy. In addition to its use for severe psoriasis, the treatment has been recommended for diseases with presumed autoimmune causes, such as rheumatoid arthritis.

Because tetrahydrofolic acid (FH4) is a co-factor involved in numerous reactions of the intermediary cell metabolism concerned with DNA replication and cell proliferation, it is hardly justified to expect a single mechanism of action. There are several FH4 cofactors with bound C_1 fragments (Fig. 16), apparently with some specificity for defined enzymatic reactions. These components, with methyl, methylene, methenyl, formyl, and formimino groups attached, are converted by enzymatic reactions and may represent different pools. For this reason it seems simplistic to confine the analyses of pharmacological or toxicological evaluations to the total folic acid content.

Several FH4 components are involved in the *de novo* synthesis of DNA precursors such as purine and thymidine nucleotides. Especially significant is the coupling of thymidylate synthetase with dihydrofolate reductase activity (Fig. 17). Because the tetrahydrofolate coenzyme serves both as methyl and as hydrogen donor in thymidylate synthetase, the end product is TMP and dihydrofolate. Thus, the continuous reduction to FH4 is mandatory and inhibition of dihydrofolate reductase by methotrexate effectively blocks the formation of TMP and thereby DNA synthesis in the corresponding cells.

N^5-Methyltetrahydrofolate (N^5-methyl-FH4) is the methyl donor in the remethylation cycle, salvaging homocysteine by accepting a methyl group to form

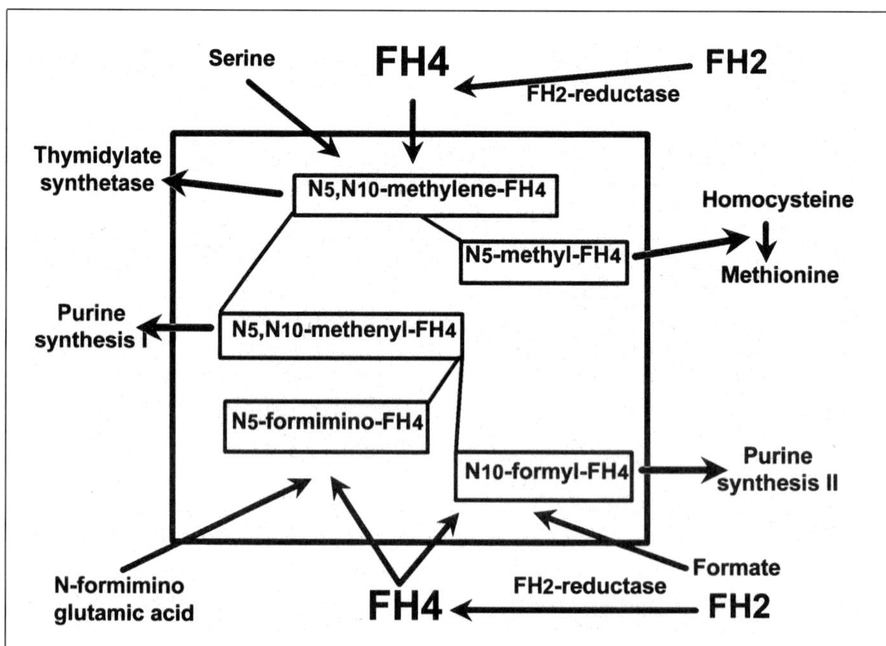

FIGURE 16 Pool of different (FH4) folic acid cofactors, apparently involved in C1-transfer reactions. Because C1 transfer is an essential reaction in many metabolic pathways, inhibition of dihydrofolic acid reductase affects the proliferation and differentiation reactions of susceptible cells.

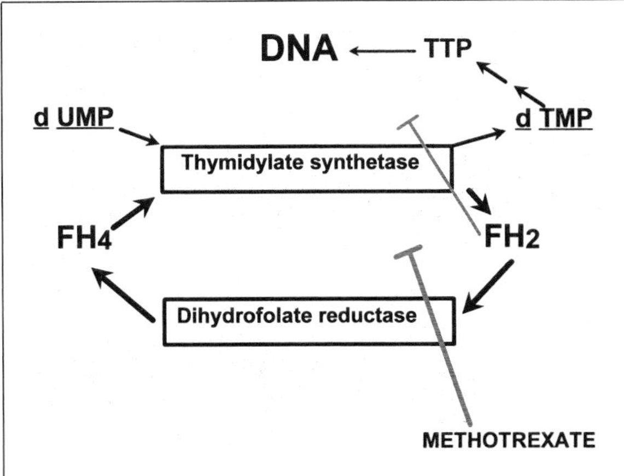

FIGURE 17 Folic acid antagonists inhibit the formation of TMP, an essential DNA precursor. After dihydrofolic acid (FH2) has been formed during the thymidylate synthetase reaction, tetrahydrofolic acid (FH4) must be regenerated from the FH2, catalyzed by dihydrofolate reductase. This reduction is inhibited by the folic acid antagonists. Accumulation of FH2 further inhibits the reductase reaction.

methionine. Using vitamin B_{12} and N^5-methyl-FH4 (Fig. 15) as cofactors, the reaction is catalyzed by the N^5,N^{10}-methylentetrahydrofolate reductase. Lack of N^5-methyl-FH4 results in elevated plasma homocysteine levels, which have been associated with the increased risk of endothelial dysfunctions, atherosclerotic vascular disease, and venous thromboembolism. A dose of 1 to 5 mg folate per day rapidly decreases the elevated homocysteine plasma concentrations.

Thalidomide

A few years after thalidomide had been taken off the market as a tranquilizer because of the malformations induced in thousands of children and because of the polyneuropathy induced, anti-inflammatory (antiphlogistic) and possibly also immunosuppressive properties were discovered in studies on humans. Thalidomide is used today as the primary substance in the treatment of erythema nodosum in leprosy. Meanwhile, it has been successfully administered to ten thousands of leprosy patients, and a therapeutic success has also been described in a variety of dermatological diseases and urogenital ulcerations, including those associated with AIDS. There have also been favorable experimental and clinical effects on the graft versus host reaction after bone marrow transplantations. This example illustrates that even in humans very important and conspicuous pharmacological effects may never be discovered or may be discovered only at a very late stage upon extensive clinical efficacy evaluations.

Two effects of the drug have been found and have been suggested as being the mechanisms responsible for these anti-inflammatory actions:

1. The expression of adhesion molecules on the surface of white blood cells is changed. Lymphocytes as well as monocytes and granulocytes are involved. This effect, first observed in nonhuman primates, could be completely confirmed in healthy human volunteers. The effect is fully reversible. There is a very similar response in nonhuman primates and humans (Table 5).
2. The formation and release of tumor necrosis factor alpha (TNF-α) is inhibited in *in vitro* systems. However, this *in vitro* effect has not been reproduced in other laboratories. Diametrical results have been obtained with different test systems. Also nonteratogenic (and possibly noninflammatory) derivatives may exhibit such actions. Although this effect was quite doubtful *in vivo,* thalidomide has been used hastily in trials for the treatment of cachectic conditions (tuberculosis and AIDS) in the United States. Thalidomide derivatives that are devoid of teratogenicity and much more potent inhibitors of TNF-α will certainly be much better suited for attempts in this direction.

The large and still increasing group of adhesion receptors is one of the most interesting and universal receptors in biology. These receptors, belonging to quite different superfamilies, are involved in cell–cell interactions, as well as in contacts between cells and the extracellular matrix. Integrins have turned out to be especially interesting and versatile in this respect. These heterodimer adhesion receptors, which frequently react in pairs, not only are involved in cell–cell and cell–extracellular matrix interactions but are connected with the cytoskeleton in the cell and may thereby transmit extracellular signals to these structures (Fig. 11). Therefore, the suggestion that an interference with the expression of such receptors is associated with the anti-inflammatory properties of agents such as thalidomide is justified. By elucidating this effect of thalidomide on adhesion molecules, the door has been opened to an interesting new research area. Many other substances may exhibit similar effects.

It may be worth mentioning that thalidomide has also been found to inhibit angiogenesis. Although this mechanism will not explain the teratogenicity and may have little impact on the effects on the immune

TABLE 5 Comparison of the Effects Induced by Thalidomide in Marmosets and in Humans[a]

Surface receptor		Effect on Marmosets	Effect on Humans
$CD3^+$	Pan T-cell receptor		Ø
$CD4^+$	"Helper" cells	Ø	Ø
$\Sigma\ CD8^+$	"Suppressor + cytotoxic" cells	Ø	Ø
$CD8^+CD56^-$	"Suppressor" cells	↑	↑
$CD8^+CD56^+$	"Cytotoxic" cells	↓	↓
$CD2^+$	"Rosetting" receptor	↓	Ø
$CD18^+$	β2-integrin, β-chain	↓	↓
$CD11a^+$	LFA-1, α-chain	↓	↓
$CD58^+$	LFA-3, α-chain	↓	↓
$CD4^+CD54^+$	Helper cells with ICAM-1 receptor	↓	↓
$CD8^+CD54^+$	Supp/cyt cells with ICAM-1 receptor	↑	↑
$CD44^+$	"Homing" receptor	↓	↓
$CD14^+CD11b^+$	Monocyte with Mac-1 receptor		↓

[a]Data from Neubert *et al.* (1992c, 1993); Nogueira *et al.* (1994).

[b]Abbreviations: ↓, decrease of expression of surface receptor; ↑, increase of expression of surface receptor; Ø, no change when compared with control values.

system, it is in accord with the trend of developing anticancer agents.

Ultraviolet Light

Many people have experienced an exacerbation of their herpes labialis after extensive exposure to sunlight. The systemic immunosuppressive effect of UV light has been revealed in many experimental studies as well as in human trials. In addition to increased susceptibility to (mostly viral) infections, experimental contact hypersensitivity of the skin (e.g., against dinitrochlorobenzene, DNCB) is dose-dependently inhibited by UVB in humans and in susceptible mouse strains. Apparently, this UV susceptibility is genetically controlled. It may also be a risk factor for skin cancer. Pronounced effects have been observed with doses higher than the individual minimal erythema dose. Urocanic acid seems to be involved in the mechanism of the immunosuppressive action of UV light. Although the effects mentioned are predominantly caused by UVB, some effects on immunological components (e.g., on NK cells) may also be induced by the UVA fraction. UV light may also be therapeutically beneficial, as seen in certain infections (e.g., erysipelas and herpes zoster) or in psoriasis.

Dioxins

The incorrect name "dioxins" is the trivial expression for polyhalogenated dibenzo-*p*-dioxins and dibenzofurans (PHDD; PHDF), the halogen substitution predominantly being chlorine (PCDD; PCDF). The best known of these substances is 2,3,7,8-tetrachlorodibenzo-*p*-dioxin (TCDD), the Seveso dioxin that became notorious after an explosion of a chemical factory in Seveso, Italy, in 1976.

Studies performed in nonhuman primates (see the section on animal tests) provided the basis for evaluating whether the human immune system is equally susceptible to these pollutants as that of the New World monkey (*Callithrix jacchus*). Because of the cross-reactivity of antihuman monoclonal antibodies (mAb) against epitopes on white blood cells of *Callithrix*, it is possible to perform human trials with exactly the same technique as in the previous animal studies. Clear-cut hypotheses could be formulated before initiating the trials.

Because the most sensitive and reproducible endpoint was a reduction of a certain T-cell subset ($CD4^+$ $CD45RO^+$) and of B-cells ($CD20^+$) in *Callithrix*, these variables were systematically investigated in human volunteers with extremely high TCDD body burdens. As a result of the study of more than a hundred exposed volunteers as well as reference persons, including highly TCDD-exposed residents of the Seveso area, it may be stated that, with respect to the endpoints studied, the human immune system is much less susceptible to the action of this pollutant than that of a nonhuman primate. This is a clear-cut example of a case where even very extensive animal studies only provide clues or suspicions, but tell us little about a real health risk for humans. At present there is no evidence that even high body burdens of PCDD and PCDF are associated with diseases of the immune system in humans. There is some evidence that kinetic causes (differences in fat content) may be responsible.

Some immunological markers may deviate from the range of a reference population in a few of highly PCDD- and PCDF-exposed persons, but the values for the majority of volunteers remain within the reference range. Deviations observed in humans are decreased $CD4^+CD45RA^+CD45R0^-$ (naive) cells and increased in $CD4^+CD45RA^-CD45R0^+$ (memory) cells. This is the opposite finding from that observed in monkeys at high TCDD exposures.

Because of the high variability of the individual data, the effects may be verifiable statistically, but they are not impressive from a medical point of view (Fig. 18). The regression coefficient of the trend is always <15%, although statistically significant. The result is typical for many effects induced on the immune system. The deviations in the T-cell subpopulations cannot be associated with diseases of the immune system. Interestingly, multiregression analyses reveal much stronger influences by confounders, such as smoking and age, underscoring the importance of controlling such confounders in clinical trials. In contrast to the results of animal studies, there is no effect on B-cells in humans.

Another finding with respect to TCDD is of interest. Recently it was found that in persons highly exposed to TCDD, as were children in Seveso, the proliferative response of lymphocytes, as well as the level of specific antibodies in plasma, persisted *longer* after a tetanus vaccination in subjects with a high TCDD body burden than in volunteers of the reference group. There are neither clues on the mechanism nor the possible significance of this finding, but it certainly cannot be regarded as an adverse effect (Fig. 19).

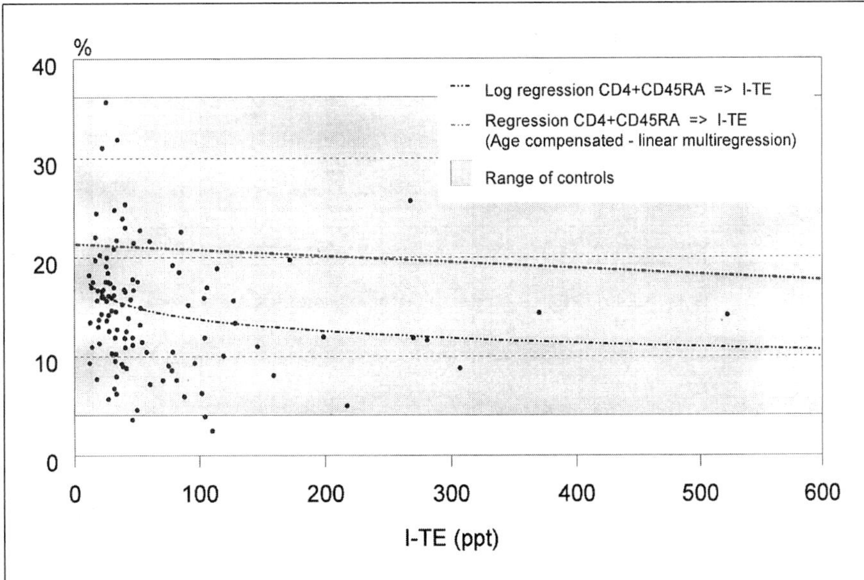

FIGURE 18 Effect of exposure of workers to PCDD and PCDF (polychlorinated dibenzo-*p*-dioxins and dibenzofurans). The data cloud of the percentage of naive-type T-lymphocytes ($CD4^+$ $CD45RA^+CD45R0^-$) in the blood of the volunteers is indicated. PCDD and PCDF were quantified as International (TCDD) Toxicity Equivalents (I-TE). The result of the regression depends on the type of model applied analysis (black line in the log model):

Linear model:	CD45RA = 15.81 − 0.011 * I-TE,	r^2 = 2%, P = 0.120
Exponential model:	CD45RA = exp (2.68 − 0.00082 * I-TE),	r^2 = 2%, P = 0.129
Logarithmic model:	CD45RA = 21.62 − 1.71 * 1n I-TE,	r^2 = 5%, P = 0.016

Multiregression analysis (top line) indicates a pronounced influence of the confounder: age (P = 0.006). Compared with smoking, the influence of the exposure is only about 1/20 (y = 20.81 − 0.12 [age] − 0.0057 * [I-TE]). Overall, there is no medically relevant effect of the exposure; almost all values are within the (large) reference range.

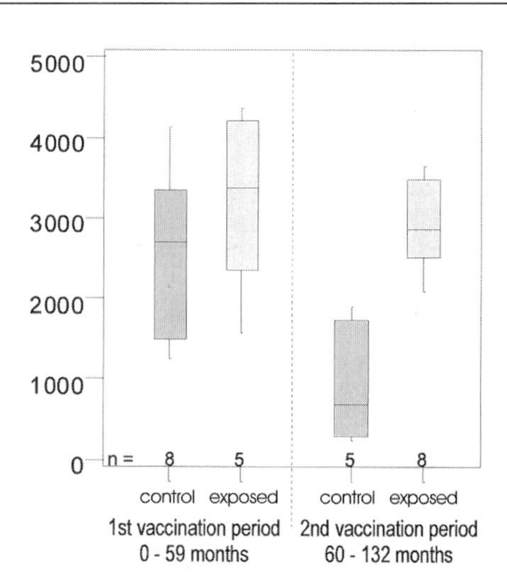

FIGURE 19 Proliferative response of lymphocytes to stimulation with tetanus toxoid as recall-antigen. Lymphocytes of male volunteers, exposed as children to TCDD in Seveso (Italy), were cultured *ex vivo* in the presence of the recall-antigen (proliferative response measured with [^{3}H]-thymidine as Δcpm). The box plots indicate medians, 25%–75% quartiles, and ranges. Data are shown for two post-vaccination periods (0–59 and 60–132 months after the last booster). While the response to the recall-antigen decreases within this period in the reference persons, it remains longer at the increased level in the exposed persons. Similar results were obtained when the serum tetanus antibody titers were measured.

Heavy Metals

A limited number of immunological variables were investigated in a few reports, mostly prior to 1990, of workers occupationally exposed to relatively high levels of lead or mercury. The variables studied included serum immunoglobulins and the proliferative capacity of lymphocytes *ex vivo* after stimulation with mitogens. Occupational exposure levels reached at those times are avoided today in industrialized countries. Corresponding body burdens may only be reached during accidents or by carelessness.

In contrast to the extensive literature regarding toxic effects of heavy metals on immunological variables in experimental animals, data on highly exposed humans are scarce. There is no evidence that effects reported after occupational exposure to lead or mercury are of relevance with respect to the prevailing exposure of the general population to these metals. However, allergic reactions to these and other heavy metals are known.

Role of Selenium in a Properly Functioning Immune System

Selenium deficiency generally depresses various functions of immune cells. Supplementation with Se has been shown in animal studies as well as in humans to improve several immune functions. About a dozen selenoproteins have been characterized, among the best known redox enzymes are glutathione peroxidase and thioredoxin reductase. Adequate selenium intake (60–100 μg/day) was found to protect the immune system from oxidative damage (the selenium content of local food depends critically on the Se concentration in soil). Such protection appears necessary because oxidative stress and free radicals are generated by neutrophiles and macrophages during inflammatory processes to clear infectious agents and damaged tissue. Furthermore, highly reactive oxygen species are formed during metabolic processes within cells and after UV radiation of the skin.

Subsequent to a selenium-deficient state, supplementation with selenium up-regulates the expression of the high-affinity IL-2 receptor on the T-cells, enhancing T-cell responses. Furthermore, IgG and IgM titers are increased in humans, which may be the result of a facilitated T-helper function.

A number of human diseases have been associated with selenium deficiency. These include endemic cardiomyopathy (Keshan disease) and deforming arthritis (Kashin-Beck disease), observed in Se-deficient areas in China. Reduced immunity against certain viral infections induced by selenium deficiency has been suggested as a cause of these diseases, as well as of other diseases, such as hepatitis B-induced hepatoma.

Of interest is the report that coxsacki B virus can mutate to a virulent cardiotoxic form when it passes through selenium-deficient mice with weakened immune systems. Subsequently, such a mechanism has been suggested as possible cause of viruses, such as HIV, crossing the species barrier in selenium-deficient areas, with relevance for humans.

Role of Zinc in a Properly Functioning Immune System

The essential trace element zinc is required for a variety of immune functions. As with many essential exogenous components, physiological levels (about 10–15 1 μM) greatly enhance monocyte and lymphocyte functions, and overdoses (i.e., 5–10 times this physiological concentration) are T-cell immunosuppressive. Thus, a delicate balance of the concentration of this component of many metalloenzymes is essential for homeostasis in the immune system.

Is It Useful to "Stimulate" the Immune System?

The prospect of enhancing the ability of the immune system to prevent disease is very tempting. However, stimulation of the immune system may be achieved only via the cytokine-signaling network. Except for very special situations (clearly pathologic), an overall "stimulation" of the immune system cannot be desirable. The chance of inducing a hypersensitivity reaction or of inducing autoimmune diseases is real and cannot be estimated or prevented with our actual knowledge of immunology.

A number of preparations, mostly of undefined composition, have been propagated as claiming to "stimulate" the immune system (e.g., extracts of echinacea), and many people expect from these beneficial effects on their health. This raises the two questions: whether such an effect is desirable and whether it can be achieved with these preparations. From our, admittedly insufficient, knowledge, both questions must be answered, no. Fortunately, most of the propagated "immunostimulants" do not hold up to the claims made. They are probably ineffective in this respect.

Immunosuppressive Effects as Revealed in Animal Studies

There is a vast body of literature on the effects of a multitude of chemicals on certain components and functions of the immune system. The majority of these studies were performed quite unsystematically, using systems that were simply at hand, most often with an overdosing of the substances. Because the general toxicity was rarely documented adequately, it is impossible to put the observed results about the components and functions of the immune system into perspective as regards other toxic manifestations. Kinetic data were also almost never evaluated simultaneously. For these reasons the animal data are largely descriptive and not suitable for any type of evaluation with respect to humans. Therefore, these kinds of data are not extensively discussed here. There are compilations on this subject, for example, Decotes (1988).

Only two examples will be discussed here as typical of the problems in many respects:

- Studies performed with organotin substances.
- Studies with "dioxins."

Effects of Organotin Compounds on Animals

Various organotin compounds, especially bis(tri-*n*-butyltin) oxide (TBTO), and di-*n*-butyltin or -octyltin dichloride are a group of chemicals that were studied extensively in rodents at an early stage of the recognition of the importance of immunotoxicology in the 1970s. These chemicals were widely used as molluscocides and as softeners in plastics.

The biologically active derivatives of this group induce a dose-dependent rapid reduction of thymus weight in rats. Cell populations in the thymus and spleen, but not in bone marrow, were found to be decreased. In rats treated with TBTO, reduced host resistance to infections with *Trichinella spiralis* and *Listeria monocytogenes* was reported, as were a suppressed delayed-type hypersensitivity response to ovalbumin and tuberculin and a suppressed IgG response to challenge with sheep erythrocytes. The effects on the thymus were apparently caused via an inhibition of thymoblast proliferation and a depletion of all types of thymocytes. These effects could be induced with doses devoid of general toxicity. Monobutyltin and tetrabutyltin compounds seem to lack the general and the specific toxicity of the di- and trialkyl derivatives.

No data on humans are available. Whether humans are exposed to significant level of these substances is not known.

Effects of TCDD Exposure in Animals

2,3,7,8-Tetrachlorodibenzo-*p*-dioxin is among the few agents whose effects on various facets of the immune system were extensively studied in animal models. In contrast to those of the rat, the immunological functions of the mouse proved to be highly susceptible to the action of TCDD. Thus, there are already differences in the response between rats and mice. A single dose of 10 ng TCDD/kg body weight was reported to reduce the host resistance against a certain virus in mice. Unfortunately, many of the other studies were performed with overdoses, which induced general toxicity. Therefore, the data of the numerous studies on immunotoxicity are difficult to comparatively evaluate. Dose–response relationships can seldom be assessed, kinetic data are lacking, other relevant types of toxicity are not documented, and important results could not be confirmed in other laboratories. The situation in the case of TCDD is somewhat more favorable because kinetic data in animals and humans, as well as information on the possible molecular mode of action of this type of substances, are available in the literature. This would provide the basis for a hazard minimization, that is, an attempt to extrapolate from animal data to humans.

Studies with TCDD in a monkey (*Callithrix jacchus*) have revealed four results:

- Single doses as low as 10 ng TCDD/kg body weight are able to alter the ratio of memory to naive T-helper cells ($CD4^+CD45R0^+$ or $CD4^+CD29^+$ versus $CD4^+CD45RA^+$ cells). Simultaneously, the number of B cells ($CD20^+$) in peripheral blood was dose-dependently greatly reduced.
- All the effects of TCDD observed in animals tests (e.g., size and morphology of the thymus, and effects on surface receptors and lymphocyte subsets) have been shown to be reversible. The same holds true for the involution of the thymus observed after the application of organotin compounds.
- Following a booster after vaccination with tetanus toxoid, a prolonged capacity for lymphocyte proliferation in response to the recall-antigen was observed.
- During long-term treatment with weekly doses of either 300 pg TCDD/kg body weight or somewhat higher exposures (1.5 ng/kg body weight), a biphasic alteration of $CD4^+CD45R0^+$ cells was observed. The lower doses increased the percentage and absolute number of these memory-type T-helper cells in young animals. Higher exposure levels reduced these cells dose-dependently (Fig. 20).

Thus, pronounced alterations in the peripheral white blood cells were induced by extremely low doses of TCDD in this nonhuman primate. The body burdens (TCDD in adipose tissue) resulting from this single dose were much lower than levels measured in people after the accident in Seveso, Italy. These findings in monkeys formed the basis for performing corresponding trials and assessing the susceptibility in humans (with well-known TCDD body burdens) with exactly the same technique.

Orientating comparative studies with 2,3,7,8-substituted tetradioxins with other halogen substitution indicated similar effects, but none of the congeners was more potent than TCDD in the animal studies.

The response to a recall antigen, which is routinely used in humans, is also provided by information from animal studies that can be directly confirmed or rejected by corresponding human trials. It is interesting that in the monkeys also no immunosuppression resulted after treatment with TCDD but rather a stimulation of the immunological functions occurred (Table 6). This casts doubts on the assumption that TCDD, especially at low dose levels, can be considered a depressor of the immune system.

The biphasic effect observed on the immunologic component ($CD4^+CD29^+$), as well as similar results obtained in TCDD-induced pre-carcinogenic hepatic lesions, cast serious doubts on the validity of attempts to even in the same species extrapolate experimental data obtained at high doses (more or less linearly) to effects postulated to occur at very low exposures.

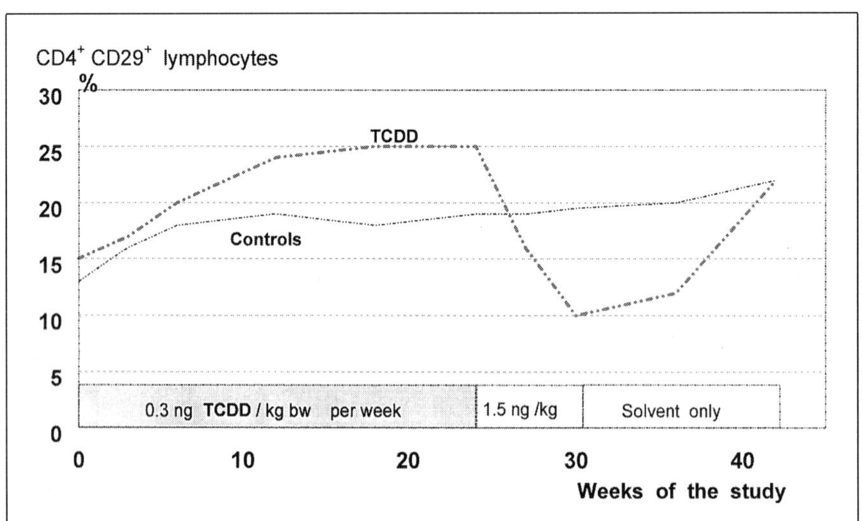

FIGURE 20 Biphasic dose response of the effect of TCDD on helper-inducer T-cells ($CD4^+$ $CD29^+$) in young New World monkeys (*Callithrix jacchus*). During treatment with an extremely small dose (300 pg TCDD/kg body weight per week) the expression of this surface receptors was increased (or the physiological change exaggerated). When the dose was increased to 1.5 ng/kg body weight per week, a rapid reduction in the percentage of this lymphocyte subpopulation occurred. The effect is slowly but completely reversible after discontinuation of the treatment.

TABLE 6 Proliferative Capacity of Lymphocytes after Inoculation of Marmosets with Tetanus Toxoid and Effect of TCDD Treatment Together with the Second Booster[a]

		[^{3}H]Thymidine incorporation (cpm)			
Marmoset No.	Before inoculation	Tetanus inoculation	1st booster	2nd booster + TCDD	Difference 2nd − 1st booster
Controls					
1	406	1639	8053	8971	918
2	345	1441	3479	4245	766
3	305	2827	5122	5157	35
4	390	1479	4934	4254	0
5	271	2522	10,666	11,405	739
6	215	1696	3885	4760	875
7	315	3189	7318	8021	703
8	356	5819	17,304	20,847	3543
Median		2109	6220	6589	753
TCDD					
5	287	3103	5664	9032	3368
6	323	2119	10,271	14,488	4217
7	475	1419	4327	6799	2472
8	303	1374	9709	10,910	1201
Median		1769	7686	9971	2920
P^b =		0.89	0.80	0.27	0.034

[a]Data from Neubert *et al.* (1995). Marmosets were inoculated intramuscularly with tetanus toxoid, and they were boostered after 3 months and after 1 year with the same dose. [^{3}H]Thymidine incorporation was measured *in vitro* during stimulation with tetanus toxoid in the culture medium. TCDD was given subcutaneously as a single dose of 100 ng/kg body weight together with a second booster.

[b]Mann–Whitney test.

Typical Agents Inducing Hypersensitivity Reactions in Humans (Allergy)

The complex immune system is capable of reacting to exogenous challenges with several responses:

1. As with all other organ systems of the mammalian organism, toxic effects can be induced. This includes the possibility of carcinogenic effects in the various tissues of the immune system (e.g., thymoma, lymphoma, and lymphatic leukemia). Immunosuppression and cytotoxicity of various immunologic components, but also chemically or physically induced inhibition of host resistance, belong in this first category.
2. Many statistically significant alterations of immunologic components and functions induced by chemical or physical agents may be designated as phenomena. They are not associated with a disease.
3. Allergic reactions may be induced, with a humoral as well as a cellular response, which do not obey the simple laws of toxicology (e.g., dose–response).

Almost any chemical may induce allergic reactions, some at a higher incidence than others. Some examples of typical allergens are compiled in Table 7.

When typical effects of chemicals on well-established allergic reactions are being compiled, it must be remembered that, on the one hand, a substance may induce, simultaneously or under different circumstances (e.g., different routes of application), more than one of the classic four types of allergies (Table 8). On the other hand, reactions may not be easily classifiable according to these four categories, and mixed reactions and overlapping types are quite feasible.

Dose Response in Allergic Reactions

The main aspect of assessing an allergic potential is that a qualitative evaluation is asked for. Most often, information on dose response is not required, and kinetic variables must not be taken into account. However, metabolic activation of a substance and possible species differences in this respect remain of

TABLE 7 Examples of Natural and Human-Made Allergens

Natural sources
Pollen from weeds, trees, and grass
House dust mites: Dermatophagoides,
Domestic animals and insects: cats, dogs, guinea pigs, hamsters, horses, rodents, bees, and wasps,
Fungi and spores: Penicillin, aspergillus, fusarium, and cephalosporum
Food allergies: Milk, egg white, sea food, legume, nuts, fruit, and vegetables[a]
Human-made sources
Medicinal drugs: antibiotics (penicillins, cephalosporins, tetracyclines, sulfonamides); other pharmaceutical (α-methyldopa, cimetidine; cosmetics, hair dyes, deodorants
Chemicals in household preparations, such as washing powders, softeners, cleaners, and disinfectants
Occupational chemicals, such as metals (e.g., platinum) and their fumes and salts (also chromium, cobalt, nickel),[b] various amines, and various anhydrides

[a]These are often not truly IgE-associated reactions.
[b]These often also cause type IV reactions.

utmost significance. Highly reactive intermediates are more likely to act as, for example, haptens than inert substances. The major problem of allergy is that it mostly concerns only a small percentage of exposed individuals. Individual susceptibility can rarely be predicted beforehand. Furthermore, allergy may develop after exposure was well-tolerated for many years.

However, we would be wrong to assume that there is no dose response at all in allergic reactions. For most allergens, a critical extent of exposure is required, and there are dose ranges in which no response occurs. Due to the numerous mechanisms and manifestations of allergic reactions, it is impossible to make general statements. However, dose responses have clearly been demonstrated in animal studies. As in toxicology in general, two different aspects must be considered:

- The dose response with respect to the incidence of allergies within a population.
- The dose response for an allergic reaction with respect to a susceptible individual.

The first problem is easier to solve. There is a good chance that with increasing amounts of an allergen in the environment more people will be affected; for example, with a higher amount of pollens around, more persons will suffer from hay fever. The reasons may be that more individuals become exposed at the higher concentrations, and for more people, a the critical dose for triggering a response is reached. There are also numerous reports from animal studies in which a higher incidence was found with increasing doses.

It is more difficult to address the second problem. Individual threshold ranges, below which a response

TABLE 8 Characteristics of the "Classic" Types of Hypersensitivity

Coombs & Gel →	Type I	Type II	Type III	Type IVa	Type IVb
Name	Immediate type	Cytotoxic	Immune complex	Delayed type	
Alias	Anaphylaxis	Ab dependent		Cell mediated	
Antigen/allergen	Soluble	Cell bound	Soluble	Cell bound	
Time	<15 min	1–24 h	4–6 (24) h	>24 h	
Response	IgE	IgG, IgM	IgG (IgM)	CD4 T cells	CTL
Mediators	Histamine, LTC4	CDC, ADCC	C3a, C5a, neutrophil proteases	Lymphokines, monokines	CTL-mediated cytotoxicity
Pathology	Mast cell degranulation, accumulation of neutrophils; eosinophils	Antibody deposition, phagocytosis, lysis of target cells, tissue damage	Neutrophil accumulation, lytic lysosomal enzyme release	Lymphocyte and macrophage infiltrate, granuloma	CTL infiltrate, tissue damage
Clinical examples	Anaphylaxis, allergic rhinitis, hay fever, bronchial asthma, atopic dermatitis, urticaria	Transfusion reaction, hemolytic disease (newborn), myasthenia gravis, autoimmune hemolytic anemia, Graves disease	Serum sickness, SBE, SLE (nephritis, vasculitis), ICGN	Contact dermatitis, allograft rejection, granulomatous disease, Hashimoto's thyroiditis, insulin-dependent diabetes mellitus	

becomes unlikely, also seem to exist for allergic reactions. However, this range may vary considerably among susceptible individuals. Many additional factors greatly modify the response. For this reason, clear-cut dose–response relationships cannot be established for most allergic reactions. However, there are a number of examples for dose–responses. When guinea pigs were exposed via inhalation to toluene diisocyanate, a substance inducing occupational asthma in humans, there was a strict dose-dependency in the increase of serum IgG1 among the groups treated with doses of 0.02 to 1 ppm (0.02 ppm was a NOEL). Interestingly, all the animals did not react simultaneously with a pulmonary response, but the number of responders and the severity of the reaction increased dose-dependently (Table 9).

A special dose-dependent response is triggered during chronic hyposensitization (immunotherapy) of IgE-dependent allergies with injections containing increasing doses of the allergen. Multiple changes result from such a treatment—a decrease in serum IgE, a reduced sensitivity of basophils, a decrease in the number of eosinophils and $CD4^+$ cells in the mucosa, and a switch from Th2 to Th1. The anti-allergic action certainly is the result of several changes. The induction of specific IgG antibodies, IgG1 and especially IgG4, is of special interest. These IgG molecules are capable of neutralizing circulating antigens, and they may thus exhibit an anti-IgE effect. However, a close correlation of IgG serum levels and the clinical success of hyposensitization has not been established.

TABLE 9 Dose Dependency of the Immune Response to Toluene Diisocyanate (TDC) in Guinea Pigs

Endpoint	Response[b]	Toluene diisocyanate (ptt) 0	0.02	0.2	0.6	1.0
Pulmonary Response[c]	0	6	6	2	3	2
	+	—	—	4	3	1
	++	—	—	—	—	3
Serum IgG1 Titer[d]	0	6	6	2	1	—
	+	—	—	3	2	1
	++	—	—	1	3	5
Histamine Response[e]	0	6	6	2	3	2
	+	—	—	4	3	2
	++	—	—	—	—	2

[a]Modified from Huang *et al.* (1993). Number of animals responding (out of 6 per group).

[b]Abbreviations: 0, no response; +, moderate response; ++, pronounced response.

[c]Pulmonary response was measured plethysmographically.

[d]Serum IgG titers were against TDC.

[e]Histamine release was measured in isolated lung mast cells after stimulation with a TCD–guinea pig serum albumin conjugate.

Reactions Belonging into the Allergy Category Type I

Allergic reactions of the immediate response type I are triggered by an IgE-mediated release of inflammatory mediators from mast cells. Although identical in the response to the allergen, from a pragmatic point of view two situations may be distinguished:

- Atopic diseases, in which a pronounced genetic background plays an important role.
- Other type I reactions, in which the genetic disposition is less clear.

Although responding to a number of fairly typical allergens, atopic persons do not react to many other allergens that cause the typical IgE-mediated response in other persons. Why atopic diseases exist and why some persons respond with allergy to certain chemicals and others never do have so far eluded investigators.

Allergens are widespread in nature. Compared with natural allergens human-made substances play a minor overall role in allergic reactions. However, there is almost no chemical against which an allergic response is not possible. Some components are more likely to be allergenic than others, and these are commonly designated as "the allergens."

It must be stressed that designating a product as "natural" cannot be considered favorable with respect to its capability of inducing allergies. Substances and, even more often, mixtures with unproven therapeutic properties are not harmless, because they may well induce undesired allergic reactions. This is quite evident from the official compilation of side effects of these "remedies." Consuming such preparations without clear-cut benefit is associated with an unnecessary health risk for susceptible persons.

Allergens involved in IgE-mediated responses react within the mucous membrane with the corresponding IgE species on the local mast cells. This signal causes the rapid release of inflammatory mediators (early-phase response), such as histamine, leukotrienes, and prostaglandins. In a second step, longer-lasting hyperirritability and congestion (late-phase response) result from the exudate following the chemotactic action initiated during the early-phase response. This hyperirritability may sensitize the mucous membranes and the bronchi against further concurrent but otherwise subthreshold stimuli, such as temperature, sunlight, dust particles, and irritating gases (e.g., SO_2 and ozone). Some drugs (e.g., acetylsalicylic acid, other NSAIDs, and sulfite) may also trigger a response, thus exaggerating and considerably prolonging the allergic reaction.

Very often the allergic response is not confined to a single defined allergen. Cross-allergy against several exogenous components is a common phenomenon. Such a hypersensitivity to several allergens inducing typical type I allergy reactions (IgE-dependent), seems to be predominantly due to similarities in the protein structure of the corresponding responsible proteins. A well-known example is the cross-allergy of tree pollen allergens (e.g., birch, alder, and hazel) with the ingestion of nuts, kiwi, and stone or pome fruit. Recent investigations have found that a homolog of the main birch allergen (Bet v 1) is also present in several bell pepper strains. Another birch allergen (profilin) was also detected in many other plants (including bell peppers). The N-terminal amino acid sequence of the protein P23 detected in some bell pepper strains turned out to be identical with a corresponding P23 protein of tomatoes.

Of special medical interest is the widespread allergy to natural latex proteins (e.g., present in surgical gloves and numerous other medicinal products). The responsible allergic component again exhibits a pronounced cross-allergy with numerous other allergens. These type I allergies are especially acquired by surgery patients and medical personnel. In nursing care, 6 to 11% of the people employed were reported to be sensitized against natural latex. About 60% of these exhibit hypersensitivity reactions. The main allergen from natural latex, hevein, has been isolated from a number of other allergenic latex proteins (e.g., rubber elongation factor [Hev b1]). It is among the first clinically important allergens to be thoroughly characterized. Containing two helical and one β-pleated sheet sequence, it is a protein (43 amino acids, including 4 cystine-S-S-bridges), apparently split off a larger precursor protein (prohevein, 20 kDa). The structure of hevein exhibits similarity to the C-domain of wheat germ agglutinin ("closely spaced disulfide linkages"), characteristic of the class of chitin-binding plant-defense proteins, such as lectin. The allergenic property is linked to the tertiary structure, and the allergenic capacity is abolished by the splitting of the disulfide bonds. IgE binding to the total latex allergens is blocked by hevein from 65 to 100% in various sera of latex-allergic patients, thus illustrating the dominant role of this protein in latex allergy. This IgE-mediated allergy seems to be significantly associated with the HLA alleles DRB1*04 and DB1*0302, both coding for defined MHC-II molecules expressed on cells presenting the antigen-epitopes to the T-cell receptor.

The situation seems to be even more complicated because increasing body temperature (e.g., by excessive exercising) was reported to sensitize mast cells and to trigger subsequent allergic reactions. In the extreme, allergic shock may be induced under the influence of allergens that, otherwise, alone are incapable of inducing pronounced clinical reactions.

Drugs are generally too small to act directly as allergens. Therefore, for a drug allergy to be produced, the chemical must be coupled, most often covalently, to a larger molecule, preferentially a protein. Thus the drug–macromolecule complex becomes the immunogenic component. The drug participating in this process is called a hapten. The resulting immune reaction may be IgE-mediated or not. It may induce a T-cell- or a B-cell-mediated response. On the other hand, several cytokines are polypeptides large enough for an immunologic reaction in another species. This may have consequences when testing, for example, recombinant human peptides in animal experiments. Several drugs may induce the formation of IgG antibodies in many treated persons. Only in some cases does a clinical immunologic response manifest itself.

Antibodies to medicinal drugs may act in one of two ways:

- They may induce an immunologic clinical response (e.g., IgE-mediated or T-cell-mediated).
- They may neutralize the drug and thus inhibit the pharmacologic (or toxic) response (neutralizing antibodies).

Studies on patients with an allergy to penicillin or sulfonamides revealed that only a few responded to the original drug. In the majority of persons, metabolites or hydrolysis products were responsible for the allergic reaction. A similar situation exists for halothane-induced hepatitis. This must be taken into account when using skin tests for IgE-mediated responses, patch tests to reveal contact allergy, or when using *in vitro* procedures (e.g., lymphocyte proliferation) to verify the nature of the allergen. In the case of penicillin, 6-aminopenicillanic acid and other cleavage products were identified as predominating allergens.

There are three aspects governing the immunologic response of a chemical agent:

- The immunogenic potential of the substance.
- The route of administration of the chemical.
- The genetic background and therefore susceptibility of the individual.

Some agents are more immunogenic than others. Dermal exposure often leads to a clear-cut immunologic reaction, while oral or parenteral application does not. Some persons are very susceptible to allergic reactions, while others are not at all.

A chemical can serve as a hapten in several ways:

- Antibodies may be formed against the substance or its metabolites or hydrolysis products within the hapten–protein complex. This is used in ELISA[8] assays, for example, to measure the plasma concentration of a drug during therapy.
- Antibodies may be formed to the drug–protein complex only. When this protein is not present, no antigen–antibody complexes are formed (e.g., conjugates with other proteins).
- The drug induces a conformational change of the protein, and antibodies are formed against this new protein structure. This may result in drug-induced autoimmunity if the antibodies should not only recognize the altered but also the native protein. Autoimmunity caused by hydralazine seems to be induced by such a mechanism.

Allergy to penicillin and cross-reactivity with similar chemicals has been studied extensively. In most patients skin reactions predominate, but many cases of fatal anaphylactic shock are reported in the literature. Although the incidence of this severe adverse health effect appears to be extremely rare and does not keep physicians from generously prescribing the drug, hundreds of millions of persons must have been exposed to this substance with the result of hundreds of fatal outcomes worldwide.

Because the penicillin G-type allergy in different patients is not directed against the same epitope, the prediction of cross-reactivity with other penicillin derivatives and the related groups of other β-lactam chemotherapeutic agents is still a gamble. One must presume a cross-allergy to other penicillins in a patient allergic to penicillin G-type. However, not all skin reactions observed during therapy with, for example, amoxicillin are allergic. More difficult is the prediction of cross-allergy of a penicillin-allergic person exposed to cephalosporins. While such a cross-reactivity seems to be rather high, as in the case of the first-generation cephalosporins, this incidence seems to be smaller with the newer drugs of this class. However, a few cases of fatal anaphylactic shock have also been reported for these medicinal drugs.

Anaphylactoid Reactions

Because the mammalian organism has only a limited repertoire of pathological responses at its disposal, it is not surprising that the same reactions observed in allergic diseases may also be caused by nonallergic processes, that is, those without the association with IgE and allergens. Such reactions are often designated "anaphylactoid" responses or "pseudo-allergic" reactions. Inflammatory mediators, such as histamine, are released from the mast cells by other than allergic means. This response does not require a previous sensitization, but may actually occur at the first exposure. It is sometimes rather difficult to decide whether a chemically induced response is allergic or anaphylactoid because the clinical picture is identical. The manifestation may be skin rash, urticaria, asthmatic reaction, irritation of mucosal membranes, or even circulatory failure (shock).

Several drugs and chemicals capable of initiating allergic responses can also cause anaphylactoid reactions (Table 10). Some of these have long been known as "histamine liberators" (e.g., morphine and its derivative).

Pseudo-allergic idiosyncrasy[9] or intolerance,[10] characterized by a sensitivity to very small doses, has often been associated with food intolerance or idiosyncrasy to food additives and preservatives. Sulfite, *p*-hydroxybenzoic esters, antioxidants (e.g., butylhydroxyanisole), and some natural and artificial dyes are a few examples.

A further complication is the fact that even without direct chemical exposure such manifestations (e.g., hives or other phenomena) may arise after extensive exercise, as the result of emotional stress, or from exposure to sunlight or cold. As is well known from atopic diseases, psychic factors may play an important role also in pseudo-allergic responses. Placebo-controlled tests may be required for the diagnosis, and

TABLE 10 Examples of Substances Capable of Inducing Anaphylactoid Reactions
Ionic iodinated contrast media
Highly charged agents, such as polymyxin B
Nonsteroidal anti-inflammatory drugs (NSAIDs) (e.g., acetylsalicylic acid)
Morphine and derivatives
Curare and derivatives
Plasma expanders (dextrans and mannitol)

[8] ELISA stands for *e*nzyme-*l*inked *i*mmunosorbent *a*ssay. This is a frequently used assay system in which a specific antigen–(monoclonal) antibody complex is coupled with an enzyme to amplify the reaction and facilitate the measurement.

[9] Idiosyncrasy is the exaggerated sensitivity to simple chemicals or complex noxae, not necessarily associated with allergic reaction.

[10] Intolerance is the pharmacologic description of a higher sensitivity to defined chemicals when compared to the general population. It is often due to pharmacogenetics (e.g., polymorphism). Lactose intolerance is an example.

psychological or psychiatric help may be indicated in such patients.

Chemically Induced Immune Hemolytic Anemia and Thrombocytopenia

There are several causes of hemolytic anemia. Some types of this disease have been associated with chemical exposure (Table 11). However, not all of these originate from immunologic mechanisms. Well known is the chloroquine-induced hemolysis due to hereditary glucose-6-dehydrogenase deficiency, which is not a immunological reaction. The mechanism involved in immune hemolytic anemia is also by no means uniform in these chemically induced diseases. Two types of mechanism appear to be established in connection with specific chemicals. Substances of the first group form circulating complexes with the corresponding antibodies. This immune complex sensitizes the erythrocytes for hemolysis. Probably the complement system is involved. Substances of the second group bind directly to the erythrocytes. This subsequently attracts the corresponding, mostly IgG, antibodies, and hemolysis results.

Thrombocytopenic purpura is mostly "idiopathic" and associated with viral infections. However, numerous drugs have been recognized as haptens probably inducing this disease (Table 11). Again drug–antibody complexes seem to bind to the platelet membrane, and thus the half-life of the platelets (4 to 5 days) is greatly shortened. The complement system is apparently involved. Recently, heparin treatment for the prevention of thrombosis has been associated with an increasing number of deaths. As the mechanism, heparin-induced IgG antibodies are assumed to increase thromboxane synthesis and to facilitate aggregation of platelets.

Allergic Contact Dermatitis

The allergic contact dermatitis formerly designated "delayed hypersensitivity" is a typical T-cell hypersensitivity, mediated by specifically sensitized T-cells. Haptogenic chemicals play a major role in the initiation of this disease. The classical procedure used in humans and animals for the confirmation of this type IV allergic reaction is the patch test.

TABLE 11 Examples of Substances Inducing Immune Responses in Various Organs

Substances capable of inducing immune hemolytic anemia
Immune complex formation
Quinine, quinidine, phenacetin
Hapten binding to erythrocyte membranes
Penicillins, cephalosporins
Substances capable of inducing immune thrombocytopenia
Sulfonamides, quinidine, thiazide diuretics, acetazolamide, carbamazepine, phenytoin, spironolactone, thioguanine, gold salts, heparin, propranolol, atenolol

Although many chemicals can induce this hypersensitivity reaction, some metals and a number of typical organic molecules are the best-known examples (Table 12). This type of dermatitis and eczema must be distinguished from the largely identical lesions observed in atopic neurodermatitis, an IgE-mediated process. The allergen is processed by an antigen-presenting cell within the skin at the site of contact. T-cells are activated and the long-lasting process is generalized within the body.

Somewhat special are chemicals requiting photoactivation to induce contact dermatitis. The mechanisms and clinical pictures are identical to those of the previously mentioned agents, accept for the need to form the reactive species from the corresponding pro-drug.

Contact dermatitis may be caused by numerous agents at various incidences within a given population (Table 13). This type of allergic reaction certainly belongs to the most frequent manifestations. Besides the disposition, the duration and frequency of exposure may play a role. Therefore, the frequencies of dermal hypersensitivity reactions may be higher in occupationally exposed persons than when the same chemical is tested once in selected volunteers.

All types of chemical structures are included in chemicals related to contact dermatitis, including medicinal drugs, occupational chemicals, and cosmetics. Allergens include many naturally occurring agents. In addition to these agents causing contact dermatitis at a relatively high incidence, numerous agents are suspected to induce such effects at a low frequency. Interestingly, physiological and anti-inflammatory substances, such as hydrocortisone, can also trigger such skin reactions in a few susceptible persons. A frequency of 0.3% has been reported from tests in volunteers and about 2% has been recorded during topic glucocorticoid therapy.

Contact dermatitis is also well known to be caused by many biological mixtures. Some ingredients from such mixtures have been isolated and analyzed (Table 14). While some of the ingredients induce contact allergy in all of the persons susceptible to the mixture, other components cause such skin reactions only in a certain percentage of these volunteers, thus illustrating the complexity of the situation.

Hypersensitivity Pneumonitis

Pulmonary hypersensitivity disorders are predominantly caused by inhaled occupational allergens from

TABLE 12 Examples of Substances Inducing Contact Dermatitis (Type IV Allergy)

Metals	Organic chemicals	Natural products
	Contact dermatitis	
Nickel and salts	*p*-**Phenylenediamine**	**Poison ivy**
Potassium **dichromate**	**Formaldehyde**	**Poison oak**
Chromium and salts	**Epoxy resin**	Oil of laurel
Cobalt and salts	**2,4-Dinitrochlorobenzene**	Peruvian balsam
Cadmium sulfate	**Neomycin sulfate**	
Gold	**Benzocaine**	
	Thiuram	
	Photoallergic contact dermatitis	
Drugs		
Sulfonamides		
Phenothiazines,		
	Sunscreen agents	
Benzophenones		
p-Aminobenzoate esters		
	Soap ingredients	
Salicylanilides		

microorganisms (e.g., bacteria and fungi [farmers' lung]) or insects and their constituents. However, exposure to certain chemicals has for a long time also been recognized as possible cause of this disease.

After a long debate, it is now generally agreed that this allergic disease, with an inflammation of the alveoli and the interstitium, is a result of complex immunologic phenomena. However, local cellular reactions by T-lymphocytes seem to dominate. Although the role of B-cells and mucosal IgA is not fully understood, IgA but not IgG is found to be increased in bronchoalveolar lavage fluid. There is no evidence that IgE is involved in hypersensitivity pneumonitis.

Chronic berylliosis is the prototype of a type IV pulmonal hypersensitivity disorder. Characteristic is the discrepancy of the small alterations found in peripheral blood and the pronounced immunologic changes in bronchoalveolar lavage fluid. The results of patch tests were generally disappointing and, using beryllium sulfate exposure *in vitro,* the lymphocyte stimulation index in patients with chronic berylliosis was found to be about 100 for bronchoalveolar lavage lymphocytes, but only 5 when peripheral blood lymphocytes were used. Proliferating cells were predominantly $CD4^+$ cells and to a much lesser extent $CD8^+$ cells.

Another typical type IV hypersensitivity disorder of the lung is silicosis, which is mostly caused by chronic exposure to alpha quartz. Although this exposure was not studied as well as berylliosis, increased numbers of cells and increased levels of immunoglobulins (especially IgA and IgG) were reported in bronchoalveolar lavage fluids. Into this category also belongs asbestosis to some extent, in which the number of neutrophil and eosinophil cells is increased three- to five)-fold in the bronchoalveolar lavage fluid compared with controls.

With respect to organic chemicals, isocyanates used in various industrial processes have been reported to induce occupational hypersensitivity reactions in workers' lungs. Chemical hypersensitivity pneumonitis has also been associated with inhalative exposure to metals and metal fumes (e.g., cadmium, manganese, zinc, vanadium, and osmium).

Autoantibodies and Autoimmune Diseases

Autoimmune diseases occur when specific responses of the adaptive immune system are directed against self antigens. As the body's defense mechanisms attempt to eliminate the recognized (self) antigen, cellular reactions are very similar to those encountered in protective immune reactions and allergy. A major difference is that in the case of reactions against self, the antigen is impossible to eliminate completely. This leads to a situation in which the employed effector pathways of immunity induce chronic inflammation and recurring or permanent injury to body tissues. This situation may well prove to be lethal.

In the human body, autoimmune reactions generally occur spontaneously. How the autoimmune reaction is initiated and which factors are necessary to

TABLE 13 Various Chemicals Capable of Inducing Contact Dermatitis in Humans[a]

Substance	Overall frequency		Susceptible groups	Application[b]
Aminoazobenzene	2–11%	12%	Shoe eczema	o,x,c
Aminodiethylaniline		56%	Occupation: photo industry	o,x
Ampicillin		60%	Occupation: production	d
Amalgam		18%	Occupation: stomatology	o,x
Aniline	5–13%	3%	Occupational eczema	o,x
Benzoyl peroxide	5%	2–56%	Under therapy	d,o,x
Bisphenol A–diglycidylether	2%	16%	Occupational exposure	o
Citral	2%	3–33%	Cosmetics dermatitis	c,o,x
Cloxacillin		42%	Occupation: medicine/pharmacy	d,o
Diaminotoluene		46%	Occupation: hairdresser	o
Dibutylphthalate		10–17%	Occupational exposure	o,c
Diphenhydramine	2–10%			d
Disperse red 1		29–70%	Textile dermatitis	o,x
Dithiomorpholene	6%	11%	Occupation: rubber industry	o
Dodecyl mercaptan		3–33%	Shoe eczema	b
Ethylenediamine	1–13%			d,c,o,x
Gentamyin	4%			d
Gold cyanide		63–80%	Occupational exposure	o
Isoeugenol	2%	3–12%	Photodermatosis	d,c,x
Lauryl gallate	0.2–21%	40%	Occupational exposure	c,o,x
Mercaptobenzothiazole	1–8%	18%	Shoe eczema	o,x
Metoprolol		38%	Reaction to ophthalmica	d
Nitrodimethylaniline		33–69%	Occupational exposure	o
Octyl gallate	17%			x
Pentachlorophenole		26%	Occupation: placarding	o,c
Phenol	0.2–10%			o,d,c
Phenolformaldehyde resin	0.2–4%	100%	Occupation: shoe production	o
Phenylbutazone	7%	27%	Rheuma ointments	d
p-Phenylenediamine	1–10%	45%	Occupation: hairdresser	o,c
Streptomycin		5–94%	Occupation: nursing care	d
Turpentine	0.6–22%			o,d,c,x
Tetracyclin		29%	Occupation: medicine/pharmacy	d
Toluylenediamine	1–22%	8%	Occupation: hairdresser	o,c

[a]Overall frequencies of the reaction (included are only incidences of >3%) were tested in about 100 persons. Substances inducing contact dermatitis within special exposure groups are only included when the incidence was >15%. Examples extracted from the compilation of Klaschka and Voßmann (1994).
[b]Application: d, drug therapy; o, occupational exposure; c, used as cosmetic; x, other.

induce such a reaction against self elude our understanding. From research, it is possible to assert that a rather strong association exists between infections and the occurrence of autoimmune reactions. This suggests that infections (or infectious agents) play a critical role in the development of such processes. Current investigations of several autoimmune diseases are focused on the concept of molecular mimicry. This term implies that viral, bacterial, or other foreign antigens bearing antigenic epitopes with amino acid-sequence homology to epitopes on a normal host protein elicit the production of antibodies. Activated T-cells that react with the host protein as well as with the foreign protein in responsive individuals initiate the pathological response.

From our knowledge, autoimmune diseases, other than those induced by substances, are closely associated with hereditary susceptibility genes. The most consistent association in this respect has been with the MHC genotype. This association of autoimmune disease and MHC genotype is not surprising, as all autoimmune responses heavily rely on T-cell responses, and this ability is closely dependent on MHC. Unfortunately, the MHC genotype alone does not determine whether a person will develop an autoimmune disease. Studies performed mostly in patients suffering from autoimmune diabetes have shown that there are certainly several disease-susceptibility loci in addition to MHC, as well as other important factors. The main additional factor in disease susceptibility that

TABLE 14 Special Allergies to Biological Mixtures and Cross-Reactivity of Contact Dermatitis to Defined Chemicals Present in These Mixtures[a]

Allergy to biological mixture	Contact dermatitis induced by chemically defined ingredients of the mixture
Colophony	Abietol (75%), dehydroabietic acid (40%), ambietic acid (70%)
Costusroot oil	Alantolactone (100%), ambrosin (46%), arbusculin A and C (60–70%), conchosin A (77%), confertin (64%), cronopilin (27%), costunolid (96%), cumambrin A (0–10%), deoxycumambrin B (80%), helenalin (36%), parthenolid (100%), tamaulipin A/B (100%)
Garlic	Allicin (50–60%), allylmercaptan (100%), Allylpropyl disulfide (100%), diallyl disulfide (78%)
Peruvian balsam	Benzylbenzoate (7%), benzyl cinnamate (8%), cinnamic acid (18%), vanillin (6%)
Epoxide resin	Butylglycidylether (50%), cresylglycidylether (50%), diethylenetriamine (21%)
Woolwax alcohol	Ethylene glycol (8%), glyceryl monostearate (2%), isopropyl myristate (22%), lauryl alcohol (43%), sorbit monostearate (4%), stearyl alcohol (14%)

[a]Percentage of responders in parenthesis. Examples extracted from the compilation of Klaschka and Voßmann (1994).

has been discovered appears to be the hormonal status of the patient. This leads to the fact that many autoimmune diseases show a strong gender bias. Other contributory factors include host factors (weakness of immunoregulatory controls, defects in suppressor T-cells, and polyclonal stimulation of B-cells resistant to controls), environmental factors (certain microbial infections), and antigen-driven mechanisms (sequestered antigen, cross-reacting exogenous antigen, and molecular mimicry) that may bypass self tolerance in a nominally normal immune system.

Assumptions on the Mechanisms of Autoimmune Reactions

The mechanisms of autoimmune response can be classified in a manner very similar to hypersensitivity reactions. In contrast to hypersensitivity reactions, where type I and type IV reactions prevail, autoimmune responses are more often of the immune complex types II and III. Autoimmune diseases can be classified into two broad groups: organ-specific and systemic responses.

In the first type, local injury, inflammation, or dysfunction is produced by autoantibody- or cell-mediated reactions to a specific target antigen located in a specialized cell, tissue, or organ. Clinical examples include autoimmune hemolytic anemia (erythrocyte autoantibodies); Hashimoto's thyroiditis (thyroid autoantibodies and autoreactive T-cells); myasthenia gravis (acetylcholine receptor autoantibodies); Grave's disease, characterized by diffuse goiter and hyperthyroidism (thyrotropin receptor autoantibodies); Goodpasture's syndrome, comprising anti-GBM nephritis and pulmonary intraalveolar hemorrhage (anti-GBM autoantibodies); and type I (insulin-dependent) diabetes (pancreatic β-cell autoreactive T-cells and autoantibodies).

In a systemic autoimmune disease, tissue injury and inflammation occur at multiple sites. They are usually initiated by the vascular leakage and tissue deposition of circulating autologous immune complexes. These immune complexes are formed by autoantibody responses to ubiquitous soluble cellular antigens of nuclear or cytoplasmic origin. The chronic inflammatory disease of systemic lupus erythematosus (SLE), with alternating exacerbation and remissions and a multiple organ involvement (joints and muscles, skin, kidneys, lungs, heart, nervous system, and vascular system, etc.) is characterized by the production of multiple antinuclear antibodies, including those against DNA. SLE is the classic example of an immune-complex-mediated systemic autoimmune disease.

The presence of autoantibodies is by no means sufficient to induce autoimmune disease. In fact, autoantibodies of the IgM type are common even in healthy, normal subjects. For autoantibodies to lead to autoimmune diseases, the autoantibody must be of high affinity and, especially, autoantigen must be available for binding.

Typical Substances Inducing Autoantibodies

While most autoimmune diseases have been associated with previous infections or cell damage, in a number of cases exposure to chemicals was assumed or verified as the cause of such diseases. A drug-

TABLE 15 Examples of Medicinal Drugs Inducing an Erythematosus-like Syndrome[a]

Hydralazine*	Trimethadione	(Phenylbutazone)
Procainamide*	Propylthiouracil	(Methyldopa)
Penicillamine	Quinidine	(Phenytoin)
Chlorpromazine	(Spironolactone)	
Ethosuximide	(Phenobarbital)	
Isoniazid	(Carbamazepine)	

[a]**Bold,** Occurs as a frequent event; *, in >20% of patients; ( ), occurs as a very rare event only.

induced SLE-like syndrome has been associated with such a chemical exposure (Table 15). Antinuclear antibodies predominantly found in patients with drug-induced SLE are to single-stranded DNA and histones.

The best studied drug-induced responses of this kind are those to hydralazine and procainamide. With respect to hydralazine, it is assumed that the drug binds to a tissue component or protein, altering the structure at a site different from the binding. This altered body component is then recognized as "foreign" by the organism, and antibodies or cellular responses against it are initiated. In contrast to the persistent essential SLE, the drug-induced SLE-like adverse effects mostly disappear when the drug exposure is discontinued.

Opposite Capabilities of Some Substances

It would be a one-sided description to only refer to the adverse effects of chemicals with respect to inducing allergies. Many medicinal drugs are simultaneously powerful tools for the effective prevention and the treatment of immunologic diseases. For example, although penicillin is a well-established allergen in a few percent of exposed persons, because of its antibiotic property it is primarily a highly effective drug in the prevention of immunologic complications subsequent to β-hemolytic streptococcal infections. On the other hand, antihistamines with pronounced properties against some allergic diseases may themselves induce allergies in some susceptible persons.

METHODS FOR ASSESSING EFFECTS ON THE IMMUNE SYSTEM

For human risk assessment, human data are essential. Extrapolation from animal or *in vitro* data is still extremely difficult in the field of immunotoxicity. Therefore, only qualitative hazard minimization may be attempted, with little relevance to the real situation in humans. Furthermore, not a single agent has been recognized until now that adversely alters the immune system in a selective manner. All chemicals affecting immunological components and functions have also profound effects on other organ systems, often at lower dose levels.

Observations in Humans

For a long time, the assessment of certain immunological variables in exposed humans, has been attempted using often-unreliable methodology. In most instances, only selected endpoints have been investigated and no evaluation of an overall immunological status has been attempted. Many such publications were extended case reports, with all known limitations; or (too) small groups of exposed persons were studied. Often interlaboratory reference ranges exhibited larger differences than the "effects" attributed to the exposure. Important confounders were not considered and multimorbid people were studied, obfuscating cause and effect. With respect to the possible effects on immunological variables, surprisingly little information is available even on extensively used therapeutic drugs. All in all, the data pool on the possible effects of chemical or physical agents on immunological variables in humans is meager. For this there are a number of explanations:

- The immune system exhibits an unusual flexibility and a huge adaptability. In fact, this ability to respond is the main purpose of this system.
- Certain deviations in immunological components and functions (e.g., alterations in surface receptors, minor deviations in white blood cell components, and changes in the proliferative capacity after stimulation with mitogens, cytokines, or recall antigens) are not necessarily correlated with clinically relevant insufficiencies and diseases of the immune system. It is largely unknown to what extent such variables must be altered before pathological situations arise.
- Only few exposure scenarios have been investigated.
- Many confounders modify the response of the immune system and have not been taken into account.
- For many variables, no agreed-upon reference ranges have been established.

Immunological Variables Accessible in Humans

It is obvious that only a selection of immunological variables can be assessed in human studies when compared with animal experiments. In the intact organism we can only look into the immune system through small windows. This is predominantly the blood, with its various cellular and humoral components. Many hypersensitivity reactions manifest themselves at the skin level, but almost any other organ may be involved, for example, as in autoimmune disease.

Progress in immunology has greatly increased the possibilities of studying normal and abnormal situations in the immune system. The first achievement is the use of monoclonal antibodies (mAb) in enzyme-linked immunosorbent assay (ELISA) and similar setups, as well as in combination with modern flow cytometry. This allows the measurement of concentrations of numerous cytokines essential for many immunological reactions, as well as the quantitative analysis of a vast number of receptors on the surface of white blood cell subpopulations and of other immunocompetent cells.

Another group of suitable methods are *ex vivo* studies on the functional capacities of cells (preferentially blood cells, but also cells from bronchoalveolar lavage, etc.) isolated from patients or volunteers after chemical exposure. A procedure well established for many decades is the testing of the proliferative capacity of lymphocytes in culture after stimulation with mitogens, such as phytohemagglutinin (PHA), concanavalin A (ConA), pokeweed mitogen (PWM), and lipopolysaccharides (LPS). While PWM acts more uniformly on the lymphocytes, PHA shows some preference for T-cells, ConA for Tc cells, and LPS for B-cells. Traditionally, proliferation was assessed from [^{3}H]thymidine incorporation rates. However, with the tools available, changes in surface receptor expression can also be analyzed.

It is quite possible to monitor immunological functions after routine vaccination. This is a variable that can be investigated in a large number of volunteers, including those specially exposed. Either the proliferative capacity to recall antigen or the antibody titers in blood can be measured. This has been done using a vaccination with tetanus toxoid, but the approach has not been used on very large scales. As a complicating factor, it must be taken into account that these variables decline after vaccination or boostering (Fig. 21).

Certainly a limitation is the inability to satisfactorily monitor the host resistance against microorganisms and tumors in humans. The evaluation of possible reduced resistance to infections in humans is extremely difficult and the results are unreliable when deduced from patient specifications. Most of such infections occur epidemically. Especially in children, up to seven infections per year is considered "normal." Furthermore, an established higher susceptibility to respiratory tract infections, for example, may be due to many reasons, exogenous factors being the least probable ones. A few research attempts have been made on this topic in persons with increased TCDD body burdens. No difference, or a minor one, was found when the data were retrospectively compared to a reference group at risk for upper respiratory tract infections, influenza, pneumonia, chronic bronchitis or chronic obstructive pulmonary disease, ventilatory function, and thorax and lung abnormalities. Clear-cut reduced host resistance to influenza virus infections had been previously reported in mice.

Extensive studies were performed on the exaggeration of asthma or bronchitis in connection with air pollution (SO_2, NO_2, ozone, dust particles). Data are controversial, especially due to simultaneous exposure to many other components and factors.

Analysis of Serum Immunoglobulins

It also may be helpful to measure the serum levels of immunoglobulins. Using specific antibodies, an exact analysis of immunoglobulin subclasses with either ELISA or nephelometric methods is possible.

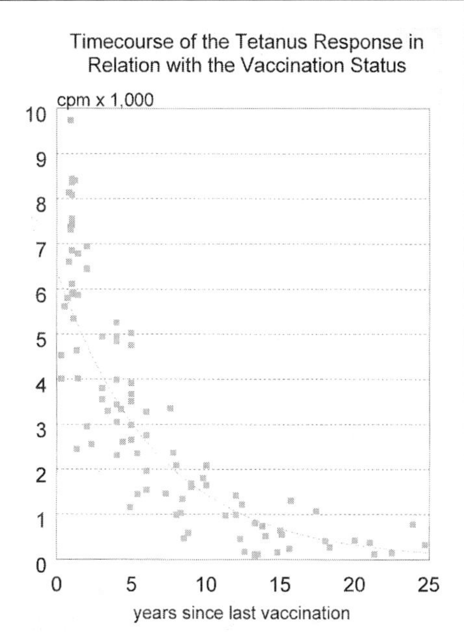

FIGURE 21 Time course of the proliferative response of lymphocytes to a recall-antigen (tetanus toxoid) in normal volunteers. Serum tetanus antibody titers exhibit a very similar time-dependency.

Serum concentrations of immunoglobulins (Ig) may be evaluated in several ways:

- Total serum Ig characterized as the main classes, such as IgA*, IgD, IgE, IgG, and IgM (IgA mainly occurs in mucosa and secretions), may be measured.
- Subfractions of the immunoglobulin classes (e.g., IgG1, IgG2, IgG3, and IgG4) may be analyzed.
- Immunoglobulins to specific antigens (e.g., tetanus antibody titer) may be studied.

In the adult human, IgG contributes most to the immunoglobulins (about three-quarters) in circulating blood. However, as may be expected, the individual variability is considerable, critically depending on the type and number of antigen exposures. IgG is the most important long-term protective antibody of the secondary immune response. It is the only type of immunoglobulin easily crossing the placenta, and the concentration in the newborn is similar to that of the mother. With this supply, the newborn must make do until the own IgG synthesis takes over at about 4 months of age. During at this period the child has the lowest antibody titers, and it takes about 6 to 10 years before adult values are reached again (Table 16).

IgG is not uniform, but consists of four subfractions with differing properties and functions (Table 16). IgG1, the largest subclass, is mainly formed in response to protein antigens, and it can activate complement. IgG2 is predominantly formed in response to polysaccharide antigens (e.g., capsulated bacteria). The most efficient complement activator is IgG3, also found as many autoantibodies. IgG4 is found after chronic allergen stimulation, and it may block an IgE response.

Decreased or increased serum concentrations of IgG subclasses may occur under certain pathological conditions. The total IgG serum level may not change considerably under such circumstances. Besides inborn errors and infections, certain additional conditions (e.g., chemotherapy, radiation, and high doses of glucocorticoids) may decrease IgG levels. IgG serum concentrations may be increased in atopic disease and allergy. For these reasons, it is justified to include the analysis of IgG subclasses in immunological investigations of possible changes induced by chemical exposures.

Surface Receptors on White Blood Cells

As established by using the techniques of flow cytometry and monoclonal antibodies (mAb), all white blood cells express numerous receptor proteins on their surface. This pattern of receptors, typical for various cell types, largely characterizes the functional capabilities of these specific cells. These data have provided the picture of lymphocytes not representing a uniform entity but being composed of numerous different subsets. These lymphocyte subpopulations not only represent the different functional states (e.g., "precursor," "activated," "naive," and "memory"), but are also involved in specific, although different, functions. Such functions include, among others, adhesions between cells and between cells and components of the extracellular matrix, the capability of cytotoxic responses, and the ability to produce and liberate spe-

TABLE 16 Exemplified Characteristics of Human IgG Subclasses[a]

	IgG1	IgG2	IgG3	IgG4
Serum concentrations (g/liter)				
Adult	4–7–13	1–3–6	0.2–**0.7**–2	0.05–**0.6**–2
Newborn	2–11	1–4	0.1–0.6	0.05–0.6
Five months old	2–7	0.3–2	0.2–0.8	0.03–0.4
Heavy chain	$\gamma 1$	$\gamma 2$	$\gamma 3$	$\gamma 4$
Molecular weight	146,000	146,000	170,000	146,000
Interchain disulfide bridges	2	4	11–15	2
κ/λ ratio	2.4	1.1	1.4	8
Half-life in serum (days)	21	12–21	7–8	11–21
Complement activation	++	+	+++	—
Fc receptor binding to macrophages	++	—	++	+
mast cells	—	—	—	+

[a]From Behring Diagnostik Information (2/95).

cific cytokines. Flow cytometry and the use of highly specific mAb form the basis for characterizing the normal pattern of such cell subfractions and for recognizing deviations from a defined reference range.

As may be expected, such surface receptors are not identical among animal species. Defined functions may be performed by different receptors in various species. The largest pool of mAb available exists for human surface epitopes. It has been shown that many of these antihuman mAb cross-react with surface receptors on white blood cells of nonhuman primates (e.g., marmoset and rhesus). Of more than 100 antihuman mAb tested, about 50% cross-reacted with epitopes in marmoset white blood cells. In comparisons of rhesus and *Callithrix jacchus*, Old World monkeys did not perform better in this respect than the New World monkey (Table 17).

Analysis of Surface Receptors in Pharmacologic and Toxicologic Studies

Flow cytometry is an elegant technique for elucidating deviations from a defined reference range that have been induced by chemical or physical agents. A large selection of antihuman mAb is commercially available. Additionally, a sufficient number of commercial mAb are available to perform such analyses on rodents (mice and rats). However, studies are best performed directly on humans exposed to such noxae. A few trials have been performed after the exposure of humans to special xenobiotics.

Analysis of Hyperreactivity Reactions

Because allergies play a major role as adverse effects on the human immune system, extensive testing in this area is essential. Prick and patch tests are well established methods. These tests are used every day in medical practice. Test in humans are vastly superior to attempts to recognize such properties in animal studies.

Confounding Factors in Human Trials

In attempts to assess chemically or physically induced immunosuppression as revealed in components and functions, many confounding factors must be taken into account. Without such a multiregression analysis, no causal relationship can be established. We must accept that often the confounding factors are stronger than the immunotoxicological aspects. This is not surprising because the function of the immune system is to respond to many exogenous forces.

Acute infections will cause complex changes within the immune system. Such infections are an exclusion factor in immunotoxicological studies. This is not easy because typical changes in the immunological components are already observable before the clinical symptoms occur. Some chronic diseases affecting the immune system and some drug medications may also complicate the interpretation of immunological data.

Two strong confounding factors are age and cigarette smoking. Without controlling for these factors,

TABLE 17 Cross-Reactivity of Anti-Human mAbs against Surface Receptors of White Blood Cells of Rhesus and Marmoset Monkeys[a]

mAb	Rhesus	Marmoset	mAb	Rhesus	Marmoset	mAb	Rhesus	Marmoset	mAb	Rhesus	Marmoset
CD1	–	–	CD16	(+)	+	CD32	(+)	?	CD54	(–)	+
CD2	+	+	CD17	(+)	?	CD33	(+)	–	CD56	?	+
CD3	(+)	–	CD18	?	+	CD34	(–)	+	CD57	?	?
CD4	+	+	CD19	(+)	–	CD35	(+)	?	CD58	?	+
CD5	(+)	?	CD20	+	+	CD38	(–)	+	CD64	(+)	?
CD6	+	?	CD22	?	–	CD44	(–)	+	CD66	(+)	?
CD8	+	+	CD23	?	+	CD45	(–)	–	CD69	?	+
CD9	+	–	CD24	(+)	–	CD45RA	+	+	CD71	(–)	+
CD10	(+)	–	CD25	+	+	CD45R0	?	+			
CD11a	(–)	+	CD26	(–)	+	CD49b	?	+			
CD11b	(+)	+	CD27	(+)	?	CD49c	?	+			
CD11c	(–)	+	CD28	+	+	CD49d	?	+			
CD14	(+)	+	CD29	+	+	CD49e	?	+			
CD15	–	–	CD31	(+)	?	CD49f	?	+			

[a]Data on Rhesus from Jonker *et al.* (1989), Neubert *et al.* (1995), and unpublished data..
Abbreviations: +, same clone positive; (+), other clone positive; –, same clone negative; ?, same clone not tested in other species.

immunotoxicological studies are almost worthless. Age-dependent changes are especially pronounced in children, and comparable changes can also be observed in young animals. The immune system of newborns is immature in many respects, and the immunological tackling with components of the environment is an integral part of normal development. Age-dependent changes in memory-type and naive-type T-helper lymphocytes are shown in Fig. 22.

For these reasons, immunological studies of the possible adverse effects of interacting chemical or physical agents must be carefully planned. This is not easy to accomplish because many confounding aspects must be considered. Another difficulty is to recruit an appropriate reference group. It is more difficult to convince healthy persons to participate in a trial than volunteers with excessive exogenous exposures.

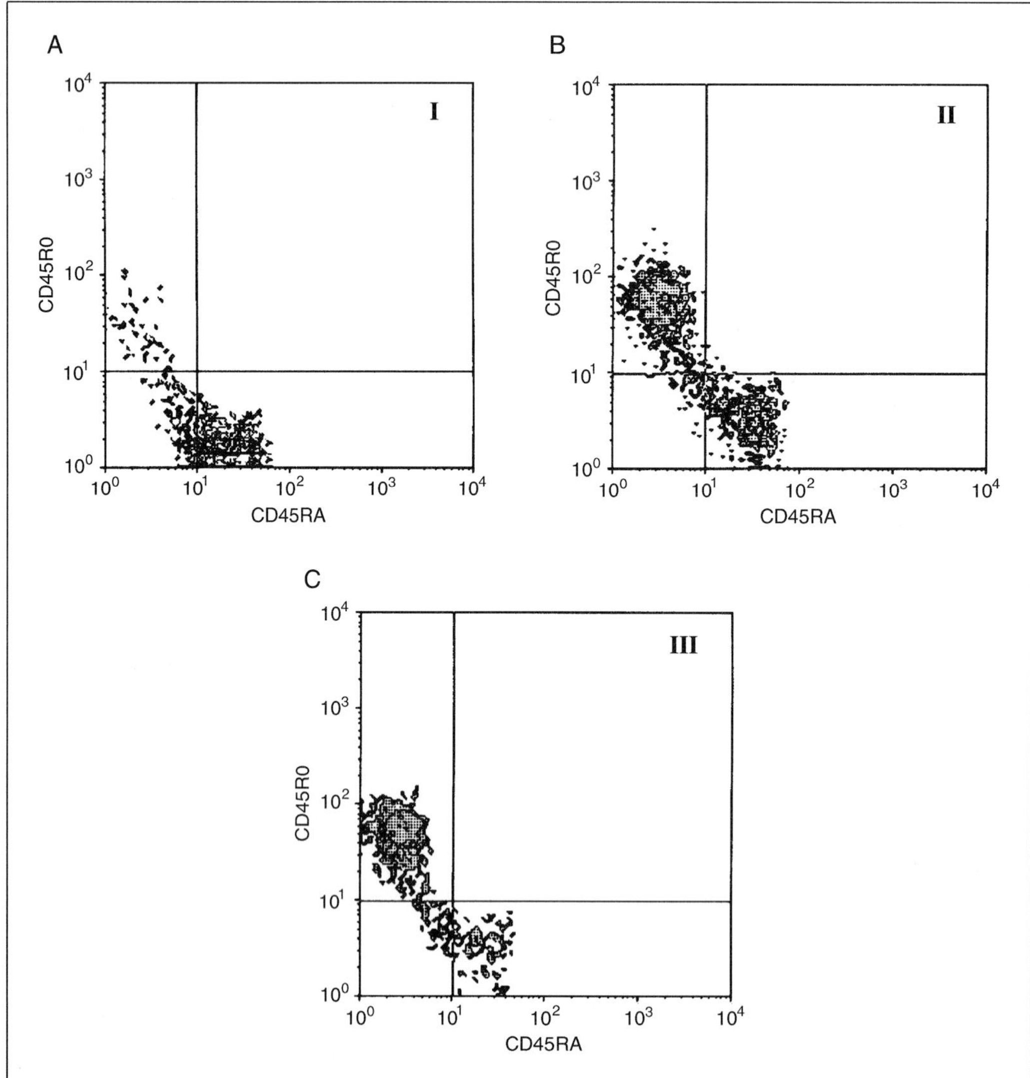

FIGURE 22 Age-dependent changes in some human lymphocyte subpopulations. Differences with respect to the CD45 receptors are shown. (A) The data of a 1-year-old child, (B) data of a 26-year-old, and (C) data of a 72-year-old male volunteer. Original FACScan graphs. Exemplified is the pronounced transition from naive-($CD4^+CD45RA^+CD45R0^-$ to memory type ($CD4^+CD45RA^-CD45R0^+$) T-helper cells. While $CD4^+CD45R0^+$ memory -type cells are nearly absent in the child, these cells are abundant in the 72-year-old volunteer.

Geography and the "Sunshine" Factor

It is impossible to conduct an immunological and even more so an immunotoxicological investigation without taking in account the geographic location and the ethnic origin of the participants. The geographic location, as well as the season of the year in which a study is performed, has clear consequences on the cellular distribution of leukocytes in the body (e.g., there are fewer respiratory infections in summer, there are more frequent allergic reactions in spring, and in the fall there is the famous "flu season"). None of the studies performed have considered such influences. The shifts can alone cause a highly increased number of associations falsely attributable to possible chemical exposures. Studies in northern and southern Germany, northern Italy, and southern Spain have shown that the reference values were slightly different at similar time, during the same year of investigation. Such fluctuations and "sunshine" factors, including increased exposure to the sun (UV light), higher temperature, different patterns of opportunistic infections, different nutritional factors, and possibly psychological factors, should be considered confounding factors.

Other important factors are the ethnic origin of the participants, the homogeneity of the study population, and a similar ethnic distribution in the exposed and reference groups. Variations in some endpoints due to ethnic origins have been found in multinational studies. These range from simple shifts of the leukocyte fractions to absent subfractions or unusual surface markers (such as the CD4 surface structure recognized by the Okt4a monoclonal antibody, found only in Asians) and differences in receptor densities. Clear differences in the cellular components of the peripheral blood are also found in countries where tropical infectious diseases are frequent and immunity to parasites, for example, is endemic.

As outlined in the next paragraph, quantitative (and often even qualitative) extrapolation from animal experiments to the situation presumed to exist in humans is difficult, if not impossible. This calls for many more well controlled studies in humans, agreed-upon protocols, and large databases of reference data.

Animal Studies of Immunological Variables

The aim of animal studies in medical research is to obtain information helpful to improving our understanding of normal and pathological findings in humans. The prerequisites for this strategy are the similarities in physiology and in pathological responses between laboratory animals and the special animal, humans.

While the basic features of physiology and biochemistry may be very similar among mammals, there are also pronounced species differences. In pharmacology and medical toxicology differences among species are of utmost concern. It is largely impossible to quantitatively extrapolate data from one species to another. What, then, are the value and limitations of animal studies in toxicology? These are:

- To obtain hints on adverse reactions, as revealed in experimental animals, as a basis for conclusions with relevance to humans.
- Because considerable species differences cannot be excluded, data from animal tests must be confirmed or rejected on the basis of subsequent human data. The animal data may not be relevant for the situation in humans under defined exposure conditions. If no human data will become available, we will never truly know whether an adverse effect observed in animal studies will ever occur in humans at realistic circumstances.
- Because of the species differences, humans may suffer from adverse effects not revealed in animal studies. There is no all-inclusive safety!

The advantage of animal studies is threefold:

1. Immunological variables are evaluated that cannot or that can only with considerable difficulties be studied in humans.
2. The extent, route, and period of exposure can be exactly controlled; well-defined animal strains can be used for the studies.
3. Clues to the mechanism of action of defined agents are obtained, improving our understanding of adverse reactions in humans.

Intrinsic to these advantages are also the disadvantages, because exposures in humans may be highly variable (e.g., to environmental chemicals) and ill defined. Thus it is difficult to make predictions from animal tests. In addition, humans are genetically heterogeneous.

Immunological Variables in Animals

Because the methodology will be different, it is advisable to distinguish with respect to recognizing adverse effects on the immune system between (Table 18):

- Reduction of normal responses (immunosuppressive actions of agents).
- Enhancement of normal responses (hyperreactivity against foreign or self).

TABLE 18 Variables That May Be Studied with Experimental Animals, and Suitability of Monkeys as Compared with Rodents

Variable to be considered	Studies with rodents are possible	Primates are better suited than rodents
Morphology of specific tissue	Yes	Possibly
Changes in white blood cells in blood and tissues	Yes	Yes
Alterations in surface receptors	Yes	Yes
Changes in immunoglobulins	Yes	Yes
Changes in cytokines	Yes	Possibly
Changes in the complement system	Yes	Possibly
Changes in other relevant components	Feasible	Possibly
Host resistance against parasites	Yes	Possibly
Host resistance against bacteria	Yes	Probably not[a]
Host resistance against viruses	Yes	Probably not[a]
Host resistance against tumors	Yes	Probably not[a]
Homing and migration	Possibly	Questionable
Transplant rejection	Yes	Possibly
Antibody formation to specific antigens	Yes	Possibly
Hypersensitivity, autoimmunity	Problematic	Possibly
"Immunostimulation"	Problematic	Possibly
Functions of circumscript systems	Yes	Yes[b]
Hormonal influences	Problematic	Possibly
Influences of the CNS	Problematic	Probably
Influence of "stress"	Little information	Not evaluated
Alterations by general toxicity	Yes	Probably

[a]For ethical reasons.
[b]If this is not studied with human components; comparative studies are possible.

Analysis of Immunosuppressive Effects

While some of the endpoints are well known from human and veterinary pathology, such as evaluations of organ toxicity (e.g., of the thymus, bone marrow, lymph nodes, and spleen) and hematology, others are unique to the immune system and not assessed in routine toxicological examinations. Important responses that are relatively easy to study in animal experiments but hard to assess in humans are host resistance to microorganisms and tumors.

Methods using monoclonal antibodies (mAb) for analyzing concentrations of cytokines and surface receptors on white blood and other (e.g., thymus, lymph node, and spleen) cells may be applied. A variety of mAb specific to mice and rats are now commercially available. The proliferative capacity of lymphocytes can also be measured *ex vivo*.

Assessment of Host Resistance These tests represent an important part of animal testing because similar endpoints can only be studied in humans with difficulty or not at all. However, the problem exists of how data from such experiments are to be interpreted with relevance to humans. So far, no satisfactory strategy has been developed. The direct risk assessment for humans certainly is not possible from such animal data alone. Nevertheless, these studies may provide important information for preventive hazard minimization. Ultimately, it is again a matter of the dose.

Host Resistance to Microorganisms Various animal tests, using a multiplicity of microorganisms, have been described in the literature and the effects of a number of chemicals have been evaluated. Generally rodents are used for these tests. The general test design is always similar—groups of animals (mostly mice) pretreated with the test substance are inoculated with just under the lethal number of the corresponding infectious microorganism (mostly bacteria or viruses), and the increase in *mortality* caused by the pretreatment is used as an endpoint.

A frequent result of such tests is that reduced host resistance is found to some bacteria or viruses, but not against others. Because, for obvious reasons, microorganisms not pathogenic to humans are used, generalizations from such data with respect to species similarities are extremely daring and unreliable.

In a modification of this procedure, animals are infected (e.g., with the parasite *Trichinella spiralis*) and the spreading of the larvae within typical muscle tissue and the formation of specific antibodies are chosen as criteria. This test system has been used to study some organotin substances, as well as TCDD.

Host Resistance to Tumors The test design for evaluating the interference of the immunological resistance of an organism to tumors is similar to that used for microorganisms. After pretreatment with the test substance, a tumor is transplanted into the animals, and tumor growth or death are used as endpoints for the evaluation. Although of theoretical interest, this test design has only infrequently been used for the evaluation of possible chemically induced immunotoxic effects. The interpretation of the results from such studies is even more difficult, and its significance for human hazard minimization is really doubtful because human tumor disease and tumor immunology are extremely complex issues.

From studies of patients with long-term immunosuppression (e.g., after organ transplantation), it is well established that the growth of certain tumors within the transplanted tissue, and of certain tumors of the immune system, may be facilitated. At present there is no evidence that the overall incidence of tumor diseases in general is increased by immunosuppression, although such an assumption might not be absurd.

Analysis of the Proliferative Capacity of Lymphocytes Measuring the proliferative capacity of mononucleated blood cells, mostly assessed as incorporation of [^{3}H]thymidine in the presence of mitogens, has been widely used as a test system. Various types of T- or B-lymphocytes respond somewhat differently to the stimuli. As an advantage, the test can also be performed with human blood samples *in vitro* or *ex vivo*. However, the test is rather unspecific and not too sensitive. For this reason, this approach is no longer included in the test battery of the NTP animal testing program. However, such a decision may be premature because the test protocol can be greatly improved by incorporating the analyses of surface receptors and by using recall-antigens (e.g., tetanus toxoid) as stimuli. This provides an excellent means of comparing data from experimental animals to results obtained in humans, and it may become one of the most valuable approaches.

Another modification of the proliferation tests is the mixed lymphocyte essay. Lymphocytes of a responder are co-cultured with allogenic stimulator cells with a different histocompatibility (either MHC I or MHC II) complex. Responder T-cells recognize the stimulator cells as foreign and respond to the cellular antigen. This experimental design can be used with cells of both experimental animals and humans. In human trials, the test is difficult to use and may be prone to misinterpretations because of the genetic heterogeneity of humans and the necessity of using cells from donors with many MHC variants. A considerable variation is known to occur within the reference group, and this must be taken into account by studying large groups of both exposed and unexposed volunteers.

Analysis of Cytotoxicity Reactions Cytotoxicity to tumor cells and virus-infected cells, mediated by cytotoxic T-cells or NK cells, is an important function of the unspecific as well as the specific mammalian defense system. Appropriate test systems have been designed and extensively used. In addition to the possibilities of recognizing alterations in these cell populations by monitoring typical surface receptors (e.g., with triple-labeling techniques), functional tests have been used for a long time. For this purpose, tumor cells or virus-infected cells are labeled with ^{51}Cr, or target cells are labeled with dyes. After incubation of the cell suspension *in vitro*, release of radioactivity or of the color or fluorescence from the altered or killed target cells is measured. While extensive tests with animals were conducted, only few studies with blood of humans exposed to chemicals have been performed.

Analysis of Macrophage Activity Assays have been used in rodents to assess the phagocytotic activities of macrophages or other phagocytoting cells. *In vitro*, the uptake of fluorescent latex particles, ^{51}Cr-labeled chicken erythrocytes, or radioactively labeled bacteria may be taken as an indicator of the non-immune-mediated macrophage function. Some of the tests (e.g., iv. injection of ^{51}Cr-labeled sheep erythrocytes and measuring the tissue distribution in mice) may also be conducted *in vivo*. No assays have been suggested and used routinely to test the most important function of macrophages, the processing and presenting of antigens.

Analysis of Antibody Response to Sheep Red Blood Cells A simple test widely used in experimental research is the response in rodents of T-cell-dependent antibody formation to the red blood cells of sheep. As endpoints, the "plaque-forming" cell assays with spleen cells *in vitro* are chosen or the measurements of antibody titers. Each plaque within the agar is formed from one IgM-producing plasma cell. Generally, this type of test is believed to have a high predictive value with respect to immunotoxicity, especially when used in combination with assessing NK cell activity or with analyzing the expression of surface receptors.

The approach has also its limitations. It has so far only been validated for spleen cells. Alternatively, serum titers of IgM, IgG, and IgA to sheep red blood cells may be measured in rats (e.g., with ELISA methods). However, the predictive value with respect to the relevance for humans is obscure. The test was applied because it was available in immunological research, not because of toxicologic considerations.

Analysis of Hypersensitivity Reactions

Because chemically induced hypersensitivity reactions are of the highest significance for humans, revealing such a potential of chemicals in animals tests should be of utmost importance. However, the prediction of such a property from animals studies is still unsatisfactory. The reasons include:

- Many of these reactions are idiosyncrasies and thereby rare events in humans. This can rarely be revealed in animal studies.
- There are several endpoints at which allergic reactions may manifest themselves (e.g., the skin, mucous membranes, lung, and vascular system). It is difficult to evaluate possible effects on all these organ systems.
- Susceptibility in humans is often coupled with a special genetic background (e.g., atopic diseases).
- Allergic reactions are often provoked not by the original substance but by the metabolites.
- Only substances with a strong antigenic potential may be expected to be recognized in animal tests. On the other hand, experimental test systems should not be oversensitive.

There are a number of test systems for revealing pronounced delayed-type hypersensitivity. IgE-mediated effects can rarely be predicted from animal studies.

Therefore, evaluation in humans will remain important for revealing the potential and potency of chemically induced allergic reactions. Prick tests for IgE-mediated reactions and patch tests for delayed-type allergy (contact dermatitis) are still the methods of choice.

Skin Hypersensitivity Tests in Guinea Pigs Patch tests with guinea pigs seem to be capable of predicting agents with a high potential for contact dermatitis. For detecting the potential of skin sensitization (i.e., delayed-type hypersensitivity), a number of animal tests have been suggested and widely used by industry laboratories. All these tests mimic the two levels of the immune response, the induction and proliferation of immunocompetent cells (sensitization), and the challenge to reveal the situation of hypersensitivity (provocation). During the first stage, the test substance is applied either intracutaneously or epidermally (patch test), once or repeatedly. The simultaneous application of Freund's adjuvant[11] increases the sensitivity of the procedure, the maximizing test (Magnusson-Klingman). In another version (the optimizing test), the test substance is applied on the skin for both sensitization and challenging, without Freund's adjuvant (Buehler). While the latter test procedure is less sensitive, it may be more similar to the situation of human exposure.

There are always two sides of the coin. On the one hand, the animal test may be too sensitive to predict the possible effects in humans; on the other hand, all conditions under which sensitization occurs in humans cannot be mimicked in such tests. However, the situation is also complex when testing humans because an allergy may not manifest itself until after many years of exposure (this is typical for allergies to pet animals). As in the entire field of toxicology, the issue is different for medicinal drugs and industrial chemicals. In the first case, the evaluation in humans is quite feasible and achieved for most of the substances; animal tests are of minor importance. In the latter case, the results of animal tests will be required for preventive measures, that is, to minimize the contact of people with substances exhibiting a strong sensitizing potential.

Ear-Swelling Test in Mice A noninvasive mouse ear-swelling test, using topical sensitization on the abdomen first and later a topical challenge of the ears, was reported to detect contact sensitizers, and it may also be conveniently used for testing dyes or undefined mixtures (e.g., in cosmetics).

Lymph node Tests in Rodents Simple tests for revealing an immune response are investigations in which an antigen is injected into an animal and the

[11] Complete Freund's adjuvant is a suspension of mycobacteria in mineral oil, used to exaggerate immune responses.

cellular response, predominantly a T-cell response, of the regional lymph nodes is studied.

There are three types of design:

- Injection of a substance and directly measuring the lymph node response.
- Injection of an antigen and attempting to modify (mostly inhibit) the response by systematic treatment with a chemical.
- Injection of cells from an immunized animal into a recipient together with the antigen and monitoring the specific lymph node response in the recipient.

Regional lymph nodes used for the purpose of tests were the auricular and the popliteal nodes; the ear and foot pad were the locations of the exposure. For example, the injection of human erythrocytes into the foot pad of rats or mice induces an increase in size and cellularity of the ipsilateral popliteal lymph node, and this experimental design has been suggested for testing T-cell-dependent immunosuppressive effects of systemically applied substances. A similar increase in the size of and number of cells in the lymph node may be induced by injecting streptozotocin into the foot pad. Strong immunosuppressants, such as cyclophosphamide and cyclosporin, effectively blocked this reaction. However, TCDD, which profoundly affects the immune system of rodents, was inactive in this test at reasonable dose levels in rats.

A similar test, evaluating the auricular lymph node, was used to reveal agents capable of inducing a T-cell response (e.g., involved in contact dermatitis). The sensitivity of such a test system was greatly increased when the sensitization was by intradermal injection into the abdominal skin, preferentially with the use of Freund's adjuvant.

Lymph node tests in rodents seem to be superior to the classic patch tests in guinea pigs for several reasons:

- They are more versatile than the patch tests, and the applicability extends over skin sensitization. Several modifications of the experimental design are possible.
- Cell-mediated hypersensitivity reactions may be evaluated, as well as immunosuppressive effects and possibly also autoimmune reactions.
- The test species, rodents, are commonly used in toxicology. It is feasible to integrate the test design into a general toxicity testing (e.g., a 28-day toxicity test). However, this has not been attempted.
- The endpoints are quantitatively evaluated, and several endpoints may be chosen (e.g., weight of lymph nodes, number and type of T cells, and [^{3}H]thymidine incorporation).
- The test agent may be irritating, colored, or a mixture.
- Some information on the mechanism of action may be obtained.

Disadvantages are that the experimental animals must be killed, and a considerable number of animals are required when a moderate effect is evaluated.

Choice of Experimental Animals

Specific test systems have mostly been established for one animal species only. Most immunological studies have been performed in the mouse. For sensitizing reactions, often the guinea pig is used (patch test). However, for toxicological studies, usually rats and dogs are preferred. With respect to the dog, only data on the pathology of immunological organs and on hematology are available.

Recently, SCID mice have been grafted with human immune cells (either fetal lymphoid tissue or peripheral lymphocytes). These animals may become interesting additional tools for research. Whether such hybrid animals are suitable models for hazard minimization remains to be established.

Primates versus Rodents as Models

However, there are more similarities between nonhuman primates and humans than between humans and rodents. This especially holds true with respect to variables of the immune system. Although in toxicological research (and especially immunology) nonhuman primates would be better models than the usually used rodent species, there are considerable drawbacks and limitations in the usability of such species. These include:

- Some of the nonhuman primates are endangered species and the research is considered by many as to be more delicate than experiments using rats and mice.
- Generally only few animals are used per experimental group, hampering statistical evaluations.
- Nonhuman primates are genetically heterogeneous, necessitating the use of a larger number of experimental animals.
- Old World monkeys are large, requiring a considerable amount of the test substance in a longer-term study. These monkeys also are expensive and need large housing facilities.
- Primates in general are more susceptible to stress. For immunotoxicological studies this supposes particular housing and breeding conditions, not easily maintained.

However, there are also a considerable number of advantages to using certain nonhuman primates (Table 18). When New World monkeys are used, there is no problem of conservation because they can be bred in large numbers in laboratory colonies. They are small, easy to handle, and their immune system has been well investigated.

With the experience available, it appears that a combination of studies using rodents and nonhuman primates is essential for any serious attempt to reveal the adverse effects on the immune system using animal studies. With both species, emphasis should be laid on endpoints that can be evaluated, preferably with the identical technique, in humans (Table 19).

Verifying the results of animal data in humans is essential because even such simple endpoints as hematological variables are not identical in nonhuman primates and humans (Table 20). The incorporation of nonhuman primates into the test protocol will give an approach to toxicology that has the possibility of obtaining data that have more relevance for humans.

TABLE 19 Immunological Variables That Can Be Studied in Humans

Hematology
Absolute number of total white blood cells (WBC) (cells/μl)
Relative and absolute number of neutrophiles (% of total WBC, cells/μl)
Relative and absolute number of total lymphocytes (% of total WBC, cells/μl)
Relative and absolute number of monocytes (% of total WBC, cells/μl)
Absolute number of thrombocytes (cells/μl)
Analysis of lymphocyte subpopulations (preferentially with triple labeling technique)
Relative and absolute number of main populations: CD3, CD4, CD8, CD20
Relative and absolute number of special CD4 subsets: CD45R0. CD45RA, CD25, HLA-DR adhesion receptors
Relative and absolute number of special CD8 subsets: CD56,CD57 CD45RA, CD25
Relative and absolute number of special CD20 subsets: CD19, CD23
Relative and absolute number of special NK cell subsets: CD16, CD56
Proliferative capacity of lymphocytes ([^{3}H]-thymidine incorporation *ex vivo*)
Proliferative response to PWM, Con A, PHA, LPS, IL-2
Proliferative response to tetanus toxoid
Analyses of immunoglobulins (preferentially with ELISA)
Serum concentrations of IgG, IgM, IgA (?), IgE
Serum titers after vaccination to tetanus toxoid
Concentration in saliva: IgA
Analyses of serum antibody concentrations
Serum concentrations of anti: nuclear, -DNA, -mitochondrial
Analyses of serum cytokine concentrations (not yet well established)
Serum concentrations of IL-2, IL-6, IL-10, TNF-α, INFγ, etc.
Tests for antigen response and hypersensitivity
Tests for Type I hypersensitivity: prick tests
Tests for delayed-type hypersensitivity: patch tests
Tests for unspecific inflammatory diseases
Acute phase proteins: e.g., C-reactive protein
Tests for special immune diseases (only to be evaluated in humans)
Lung function tests in asthma
Tests for different allergic diseases
Tests for rheumatic diseases

Value of *In Vitro* Systems

As in other areas of toxicology, *in vitro* tests will be of little use for "primary-stage" testing, that is, to recognize an unknown risk for humans. However, such *in vitro* test systems may be applicable for revealing a mode of action, as well as to screen a series of chemicals for a defined effect on immunological variables.

Culturing blood cells or macrophages is a well-established standard technique that can be performed with the blood of several species, including humans. Established lymphocyte (tumor) cell lines have been widely used for basic research in immunology. While *in vitro* studies with white blood cells had been confined to proliferation assays, the availability of mAb and flow cytometry has extended this possibility to monitoring changes in numerous surface receptors and the synthesis of numerous cytokines. Using cord blood for culturing greatly increases these experimental possibilities. Even when human white blood cells are used, it remains difficult to extrapolate from the *in vitro* to the *in vivo* situation because many effects will not be initiated at the level of the peripheral blood.

A number of organ culture systems have been developed and may be used for studying the special effects of chemicals. Culturing fetal rat or mouse thymus lobes provides a convenient technique for studying substance-induced effects on thymus development. The size of the explant increases about 10-fold in culture and the differentiation of lymphocytes takes place within the correct microenvironment. The effects of a number of substances, including virustatic agents (Table 21), have been investigated with such an system.

It should be remembered that the results of *in vitro* systems alone are almost useless for drawing quantitative conclusions with respect to toxicity in humans because all kinetic and metabolic variables cannot be taken into account.

TABLE 20 Comparative Reference Values for Some Major Surface Receptors of Lymphocytes of Adult New World Monkeys and Humans[a]

Cell type[b]		Humans (n = 62) Min	Median	Max	Marmosets (n = 426) Min	Median	Max
White blood cells	cells/μl	3400	**6200**	13,500	2900	**9200**	30,900
Lymphocytes	cells/μl	800	**2050**	4900	800	**5450**	22,600
$CD4^+$	%	27.8	**39.5**	56.8	24.6	**35.6**	59.6
	cells/μl	316	**801**	2,102	472	**2207**	7932
$CD4^+CD29^{high}$	%	12.7	**19.6**	33.1	10.3	**16.4**	34.7
	cells/μl	197	**421**	996	276	**988**	10,590
$CD8^+$	%	20.0	**31.2**	50.0	3.9	**25.3**	47.3
	cells/μl	218	**652**	1,575	165	**1492**	6344
$CD8^+CD56^-/57^-$	%	1.7	**5.3**	22.0	3.3	**13.6**	37.5
	cells/μl	27	**110**	616	134	**962**	3839
$CD8^+CD56^+$	%	7.1	**23.3**	36.8	2.8	**8.5**	34.7
	cells/μl	163	**494**	1,214	145	**605**	2438
$CD20^+$	%	3.1	**11.9**	22.2	9.8	**27.7**	58.0
	cells/μl	62	**232**	701	275	**1713**	7200

[a]Unpublished data from the authors' laboratory.
[b]%, percentage of subpopulation from total lymphocytes; cells/μl, absolute number of cells (number of cells/μl blood).

Recommended Test Batteries and Guidelines

From the 1970s on, recommendations have been made for test batteries and for testing guidelines, but so far they have not gained universal acceptance. There are no generally accepted test batteries or guidelines recommended for human studies.

Recommended Batteries for Animal Testing

There are two ways to assess the possible effects of chemicals on the immune system, and both have advantages and limitations:

- To attempt to integrate immunological evaluations into the existing longer-term toxicity studies (e.g., 28-day or 13-week studies with rats).
- To perform immunological evaluations as separate entities along with the classic toxicity studies.

The subchronic or chronic toxicity studies are performed at present with rats and dogs; for immunological studies mice were preferentially used. While data from a variety of previous studies of immunological variables with rats are available, there are virtually no data for dogs. The possibility of integrating immunological endpoints into the protocol of general toxicity

TABLE 21 Development of the Fetal Rat Thymus in Organ Culture[a]

Concentration in culture medium after culturing	Number of mobile cells per thymic lobe (× 10^4 cells/lobe) Zidovudine	Aciclovir	Ganciclovir	2'3'-Dideoxycytidine
10 μM	90 ± 11	67 ± 15	74 ± 6	47 ± 4
100 μM	67 ± 8	21 ± 2	16 ± 6	11 ± 2

[a]Examples of effects of virustatic nucleoside analogs. Data modified from Foerster *et al.* (1992).
Controls: Before culturing: **7** ± 2 × 10^4 cells/lobe;
After culturing: **101** ± 12 × 10^4 cells/lobe.
Thymic lobes of fetuses (day 17 of gestation) were cultured in the presence of the drugs indicated (five doses each) for 7 days using a Trowell-type technique. Additionally, surface receptors of the T lymphocytes and precursors were characterized. Zidovudine is less toxic in this system than the other nucleoside analogs. This is in accord with *in vivo* studies.

testing is limited; for example, host resistance tests can rarely be incorporated. With such an integrated but limited approach it is likely that, on one hand, important effects on the immune system may be missed. On the other hand, the induction of general toxicity, a purpose of this type of investigation, will induce unspecific effects on the immune system that are irrelevant to humans.

While some evidence was presented suggesting that supplementation of a carefully performed 4-week safety study with immunological variables is not necessary, there were strong suggestions, for example, in the U.S. (National Toxicology Program, NTP), for performing separate immunological tests (e.g., in mice). The statement that such data obtained in mice should also be representative for rats, the species predominantly used in toxicology, is open to criticism, especially if a quantitative evaluation is attempted. When the strategy of performing separate studies on immunology is chosen, appropriate dose levels could be carefully selected, and the main variables of interest could be evaluated in a umber of parallel studies. The disadvantage is that additional animals are needed for this type of testing.

In 1992, the results of the U.S. NTP program were published. About 50 compounds had been included in the screening, but the data set was not complete for all the substances. Furthermore, there was a considerable selection bias with respect to the substances tested, limiting the general conclusions. The authors' summary was that, from all the tests evaluated, only those analyzing certain surface markers or using the splenic antibody plaque-forming cell response were good predictors for immunotoxicity in rodents. However, only major surface markers were evaluated in this NTP study, and the CD4/CD8 ratio, suggested as the best predictor for rodent immunotoxicity, certainly is a poor and quite insufficient marker for chemically induced alterations in the immune system of primates (including humans).

Taken together, the data published from the NTP program would argue against separate studies on immunology rather than for it, because either one of the recommended tests (the evaluation of surface markers or the plaque test) could easily be incorporated at the end of a 4-week safety study in rats.

Routine Testing According to a Tiered Approach

Most suggestions for routine animal testing on immunotoxicity recommended the use of a tiered approach; subsequent to a limited tier-1 examination, a more elaborate test should be performed at the tier 2 level (Table 22). Although it may be popular, such an approach is dangerous from a toxicological point of view. The strategy is useful and pragmatic only when it is agreed that if tier 1 has negative results, no further studies are necessary. This would require that the "screen" of tier 1 is fine-meshed enough to guarantee health safety, which is difficult to achieve. On the other hand, when immunotoxicity was established at tier 1, why are further studies required? This would only make sense when endpoints are evaluated that can also be tested in humans.

At present, no binding international guidelines have been agreed upon and published. This is wise, because hasty recommendations for elaborate rodent studies will lead to many useless data and unnecessary animal studies.

Validation of Tests to Reveal Immunotoxicity

The crucial aspect of all toxicological tests is the predictive value for humans. This implies that tests should be validated. At present such a validation has not been performed for any of the suggested test sys-

TABLE 22 Tiered Approach for Animal Testing[a]

Tier I (screen)
Immunopathology
Weights: body, spleen, thymus, kidney, liver
Hematology: leukocyte count
Cellularity: spleen, bone marrow
Histology of lymph organs: spleen, thymus, lymph nodes
Humoral immunity
IgM antibody plaque-forming assay
Cell-mediated immunity
Lymphocyte blastogenesis: PHA, Con A, mixed leukocyte response, LPS
Nonspecific immunity
NK cell activity
Tier II (conprehensive testing)
Immunopathology
Quantitation of T and B cells: CD4, CD8, CD3, CD20
Humoral immunity
Enumeration of IgG antibody response to sheep red blood cells
Cell-mediated immunity
CTL cytolysis, delayed hypersensitivity response
Host-resistance models
Resistance to syngenic tumor cells (PYB6 sarcoma; B16F10 melanoma)
Resistance to bacteria (*Listeria monocytogenes, Streptococcus* species)
Resistance to viruses (*Influenza*)
Resistance to parasites (*Plasmodium yoelii, Trichinella spiralis*)

[a]US-NTP program as an example. Experimental animals were mice. Modified from Luster *et al.* (1988).

tems. When attempting a validation, two aspects must be considered:

- Validation against what?
- Selection of substances to be used for the validation.

A meaningful validation can only be against humans, the species of primary interest. Such a validation has, to date, been performed for no substance. However, there are a number of cases in which data from animals and from humans may be compared. While there was good agreement in one case (see the section on Thalidomide), there was a poor association in others (see the section on "Dioxins"). There is no evidence that the effects of chemicals on the immune system, as revealed in animal studies, have relevance for humans under realistic exposure conditions.

The difficulties associated with attempts at validation have been discussed (see Chapter 21 on Reproduction). There has been no selection of suitable reference chemicals or, even better, pairs of positive and negative candidate substances to be used for such an approach. It has not even been established in comparative studies whether rats and mice respond in an identical, or at least similar, way. There is some evidence from studies with dioxins that this may not be the case.

A few ring studies have been performed to test the interlaboratory reproducibility, a prerequisite for any routine testing and the chance of detecting adverse effects on the immune system. They have not reached the standard of a validation.

To reach the goal of designing comparative studies between animal species and humans, the endpoints to be assessed in both species should be comparable. It is surprising that sensitization of rodents against sheep red blood cells continues to be recommended when this is an impractical procedure in humans. Vaccination against tetanus toxoid, or other vaccinations routinely performed in humans, would be a much better choice. It is clear that the mutual understanding between scientists interested in animal testing and clinical pharmacologists and toxicologists must be improved considerably.

PREDICTIVE POWER OF ANIMAL DATA FOR ASSESSING RISK

In discussions of the predictive power of animal data for the situation possibly existing in humans, the distinction made in this chapter between immunotoxicity and allergy must be taken into account. The number of publications on immunological issues has exploded in the last decades of the 20th century, and the need to assess the alterations in immune components and functions induced by medicinal drugs and other chemicals has been discussed upon numerous occasions since the 1970s. However, immunotoxicological evaluations with relevance for humans are still *"in statu nascendi."*

For the vast majority of medicinal drugs there is almost no database of observations in humans, and human risk assessment is impossible for almost all substances. This is barely understandable because the methodology for such investigations is certainly available. Preventive hazard minimization must rely solely on data from rodent studies, with all the limitations intrinsic to such an approach, especially in the field of immunology.

There is a danger in hastily suggesting and introducing guidelines for routine animal tests in order to attempt to reveal the adverse effects on components and functions of the immune system of newly developed chemicals. It should be realized that part of such investigations are already included in the routinely performed toxicity studies, for example, in assessing toxicity on organs of the immune system and the analyses of blood cells. The pitfalls associated with guidelines on extended animal studies of immunological aspects are obvious. There is the danger of accumulating a multitude of data, whose significance for humans must remain obscure. There are a number of reasons for this:

- There are considerable differences in the immunological reactions and responses of rodents and primates, especially humans. Even more than with respect to the toxicity on other organs, it must be doubted that animal data, which most often are obtained with overdosing, are relevant to the actual situation in humans.
- Many simple baseline data (such as the number of white blood cells; relative size and persistence of the thymus; and percentage, absolute number, and biological functions of surface receptors on white blood cells) are different in rodents and humans. This hampers an evaluation of the significance of animal data for the situation in humans.
- There are considerable species and strain differences among rodent species (e.g., rats versus mice). Such conflicting results cannot be meaningfully extrapolated to humans. While the mouse is a species preferred by immunologists, it is unsuited for many toxicological studies.

- The significance of many routinely used experimental models systems (e.g., host resistance tests with bacteria or viruses and challenging rats with sheep red blood cells) designed for immunological but not toxicological purposes is questionable for assessing possible adverse effects on humans. One should at least attempt to use test systems that are directly comparable to situations in humans (e.g., response to vaccination).
- The kinetics and tissue distribution of many substances are very different in rodents and humans.

The only logical consequence would be for medicinal substances to be used in extensive trials on components and functions of the immune system in humans. This would not only provide the necessary information on the actual substance itself, but also make it possible to produce a baseline for reference data and their variability, which is known to be considerable in this area. The methods of using monoclonal antibodies and flow cytometry, as well as many other test systems, are available for such studies in humans, and there is no need to speculate on the possible human hazards from animal data.

As in the entire area of toxicology, the situation is much less favorable in the case of environmental chemicals. For the majority of these substances the human database is meager, and it probably will remain so in the next future (or forever?). This requires that our efforts be confined to performing animal tests, although we know that their predictive value is quite limited with respect to possible effects on the human immune system.

The distinction between medicinal drugs and environmental chemicals is also helpful in assessing the potential of hypersensitivity reactions. Information on an allergic potential of medicinal drugs is again best obtained from clinical observations. With respect to environmental chemicals, the situation is somewhat more favorable than for the immunotoxic effects. In the case of hypersensitivity responses, we will be satisfied with a largely qualitative evaluation (i.e., yes or no). Thus kinetic species differences and the need for quantitative extrapolations will be of minor significance. For this reason, data from carefully selected animal studies are helpful for preventive hazard minimization with respect to hypersensitivity.

Bibliography

Abbas, A. K., Lichtman, A. H., and Pober, J. S. (1991). "Cellular and Molecular Immunology." W. B. Saunders, Philadelphia, PA

Ader, R., Felten, D., and Cohen, N. (1990). Interactions between the brain and the immune system. *Annu. Rev. Pharmacol. Toxicol.* **30,** 561–602.

Adorni, L (ed.) (1990). The molecular basis of antigen presentation to T lymphocytes: Novel possibilities for immunointervention. *Int. Rev. Immunol.* **6,** 1–88.

Alomran, A. H., and Shleamoon, M. N. (1988). The influence of chronic lead exposure on lymphocyte proliferative response and immunoglobulin levels in storage battery workers. *J. Biol. Sci. Res.* **19,** 575–585.

Anneroth, G., Ericson, T., Johannson, I., Mornstad, H., Ryberg, M., Skoglund, A., and Stegmayr, B. (1992). Comprehensive medical examination of a group of patients with alleged adverse effects from dental amalgam. *Acta Odontol. Scand.* **50,** 101–107.

Auphan, N., DiDonato, J. A., Rosette, C., Helmberg, A., and Karin, M. (1995) Immunosuppression by glucocorticoids: Inhibition of NF-(B activity through induction of I(B synthesis. *Science* **270,** 286–290.

Basketter, D. A., Bremmer, J. N., Kammüller, M. E., Kawabata, T., Kimber, I., Loveless, S. E., Magda, S., Pal, T. H. M., Stringer, D. A., and Vohr, H. W. (1994). The identification of chemicals with sensitizing and immunosuppressive properties in routine toxicology. *Food Chem. Toxicol.* **32,** 289–296.

Bencko, V., Wagner, V., Wagnerova, M., and Ondrejcak, K. (1990). Immunological profiles in workers occupationally exposed to inorganic mercury. *J. Hyg. Epidemiol. Microbiol. Immunol.* **34,** 9–14.

Bernier, J., Brousseau, P., Krzystyniak, K., Typhonas, H., and Fournier, M. (1995) Immunotoxicity of heavy metals in relation to Great Lakes. *Env. Health Perspect.* **103,** Suppl. 9, 23–34.

Buehler, E. V. (1994). Occlusive patch method for skin sensitization in guinea pigs: The Buehler method. *Food Chem. Toxicol.* **32,** 97–101.

Burleson, G. R., Lebrec, H., Yang, Y. G., Ibanes, J. D., Pennington, K. N., and Birnbaum, I. S. (1996). Effect of 2,3,7,8-tetrachlorodibenzo-p-dioxin (TCDD) on influenza viral host resistance in mice. *Fund. Appl. Toxicol.* **29,** 40–47.

Coombs, R. R. A., and Gell, P. G. H. (1975). Classification of allergic reactions responsible for clinical hypersensitivity and disease. In "Clinical Aspects of Immunology," 3rd edition (Gell, P. G. H., Coombs, R. R. A., Lachmann, P. J., eds.), pp. 761–781. Blackwell Scientific, Oxford.

Dean, J. H., Luster, M. I., Munson, A. E., and Kimber, I. (1994). "Immunotoxicology and Immunopharmacology," 2nd ed. Raven Press, New York.

Delgado, I., Neubert, R. and Dudenhausen, J. W. (1994). Changes in white blood cells during parturition in mothers and newborn. *Gynecol. Obstet. Invest.* **38,** 227–235.

Dencker, L., Hassoun, E., d'Argy, R., and Alm, G. (1985). Fetal thymus organ culture as an in vitro model for the toxicity of 2,3,7,8-tetrachlorodibenzo-*p*-dioxin and its congeners. *Mol. Pharmacol.* **27,** 133–140.

Descotes, J. (1988). "Immunotoxicology of Drugs and Chemicals," 2nd ed. Elsevier Science, Amsterdam.

Descotes, G., Pinard, D., Gallas, I.-F., Penacchio, E., Blot, C., and Moreau, C. (1996). Extension of the 4-week safety study for detecting immune system impairment appears not necessary: Example of cyclosporin A in rats. *Toxicology* **112,** 245–256.

Ewers, U., Stiller-Winkler, R., and Idel, H. (1982). Serum immunoglobulin, complement C3, and salivary IgA levels in lead workers. *Environ. Res.* **29,** 351–357.

Foerster, M., Delgado, I., Abraham, K., Gerstmayer, S., and Neubert, R. (1997). Comparative study on age-dependent development of surface receptors on peripheral blood lymphocytes in children and young nonhuman primates (marmosets). *Life Sci.* **60,** 773–785.

Foerster, M., Kastner, U., and Neubert, R. (1992). Effect of six virustatic nucleoside analogues on the development of fetal rat thymus in organ culture. *Arch. Toxicol.* **66,** 688–699.

Frank, M. M., Austen, K. F., Claman, H. N., and Unanue, E. R. (1995). "Samter's Immunologic Diseases," 5th ed. Churchill Livingstone, Philadelphia.

Garcia Ortiz, J. C., Moyano, J. C., Alvarez, M., and Bellido, J. (1998). Latex allergy in fruit-allergic patients. *Allergy* **53,** 532–536.

Geyer, H. J., Scheuntert, I., Rapp, K., Kettrup, A., Korte, F., Greim, H., and Rozman, K. (1990). Correlation between acute toxicity of 2,3,7,8-tetrachlorodibenzo-*p*-dioxin (TCDD) and total body fat content in mammals. *Toxicology* **65,** 97–107.

Gleichmann, E., Kimber, I., and Purchase, I. (1989). Immunotoxicology: Suppressive and stimulatory effects of drugs and environmental chemicals on the immune system. A. Discussion. *Arch. Toxicol.* **63,** 257–273.

Grabbe, S., and Schwarz, T. (1998). Immunoregulatory mechanisms involved in elicitation of allergic contact hypersensitivity. *Immunol. Today* **19,** 37–44.

Grewe, M., Bruijnzeel-Koomen, C. A. F. M., Schöpf, E., Thepen, T., Langeveld-Wildschut, A. G., Ruzicka, T., and Krutmann, J. (1998). A role for Th1 and Th2 cells in the immunopathogenesis of atopic dermatitis. *Immunol. Today* **19,** 359–361.

Harding, M. W., Galat, A., Uehling, D. E., and Schreiber, S. L. (1989). A receptor for the immunosuppressant FK506 is a *cis-trans* peptidyl-prolyl isomerase. *Nature* **341,** 758–760.

Heagy, W., Crumpacker, C., Lopez, P. A., and Finberg, R. W. (1995). Inhibition of immune functions by antiviral drugs. *J. Clin. Invest.* **87,** 1916–1924.

Hess, A. D., Esa, A. H., and Colombani, P. M. (1988). Mechanism of action of cyclosporine: effects on cells of the immune system and on subcellular events in T cell activation. *Transplantation Proc.* **20,** 29–40.

Holsapple, M. P., Snyder, N. K., Wood, S. C., and Morris, D. L. (1991). A review of 2,3,7,8-tetrachlorodibenzo-*p*-dioxin-induced changes in immunocompetence: 1991 update. *Toxicology* **69,** 219–255.

Huang, J., Aoyama, K., and Ueda, A. (1993). Experimental study on respiratory sensitivity to inhaled toluene diisocyanate. *Arch. Toxicol.* **67,** 373–378.

Ikarashi, Y., Tsuchiya, T., and Nakamura, A. (1993). A sensitive mouse lymph node assay with two application phases for detection of contact allergens. *Arch. Toxicol.* **67,** 629–636.

Janeway, C. A., Jr., and Travers, P. (1997). "Immunobiology, the Immune System in Health and Disease," 3rd ed. Current Biology Ltd./Garland Publishing, New York.

Jensen-Jarolim *et al.* (1998). Bell peppers (Capsicum annuum) expresses allergens (profilin, pathogenesis-related protein P23 and Bet v 1) depending on the horticultural strain. *Int. Arch. Allergy Immunol.* **116,** 103–109.

Kimber, I., Stonard, M. D., Gidlow, D. A., and Niewola, Z. (1986). Influence of chronic low-level exposure to lead on plasma immunoglobulin concentration and cellular immune function in man. *Int. Arch. Occup. Environ. Health* **57,** 117–125.

Kimber, I., and Weisenberger, C. (1989). A murine local lymph node assay for the identification of contact allergens. *Arch. Toxicol.* **63,** 274–282.

Klaschka, F., and Voβmann, D. (1994). "Kontaktallergene, Chemische, Klinische und Experimentelle Daten (Allergenliste)." Erich Schmidt Verlag, Berlin.

Klein, T. W., Newton, C., and Friedman, H. (1998). Cannabinoid receptors and immunity. *Immunol. Today* **19,** 373–381.

Krensky, A. M., Weiss, A., Crabtree, G., Davis, M. M., and Parham, P. (1990). T-lymphocyte-antigen interactions in transplant rejection. *N. Engl. J. Med.* **322,** 510–517.

Luster, M. I., Munson, A. E., Thomas, P. T., Holsapple, M. P., Fenters, J. D., White, K. L., Lauer, L. D., Germolec, D. R., Rosenthal, G. J., and Dean, J. H. (1988). Development of a testing battery to assess chemical-induced immunotoxicity: National Toxicology Program's guidelines for immunotoxicity evaluation in mice. *Fundam. Appl. Toxicol.* **10,** 2–19.

Luster, M. I., Portier, C. Pait, D. G., White, K. L., Gennings, C., Munson, A. E., and Rosenthal, G. J. (1992). Risk assessment in immunotoxicology. 1. Sensitivity and predictability of immune tests. *Fundam. Appl. Toxicol.* **18,** 200–210.

Magnusson, B., and Klingman, A. M. (1969). The identification of contact allergens by animal assay. The guinea pig maximization test. *J. Invest. Dermatol.* **52,** 268–276.

Marx, J. (1995). How the glucocorticoids suppress immunity. *Science* **270,** 232–233.

McKenzie, R. C., Rafferty, T. S., and Beckett, G. J. (1998). Selenium: An essential element for immune function. *Immunol. Today* **19,** 342–345.

Moszczynski, P., Lisiewicz, J., Bartus, R., and Bem, S. (1990). The serum immunoglobulins in workers after prolonged occupational exposure to the mercury vapors. *Rev. Roum. Méd. Int.* **28,** 25–30.

Neubert, R., Golor, G., Maskow, L., Helge, H., and Neubert, D. (1994). Evaluation of possible effects of 2,3,7,8-tetrachlorodibenzo-*p*-dioxin and other congeners on lymphocyte receptors in Callithrix jacchus and man. *Exp. Clin. Immunogenet.* **11,** 119–127.

Neubert, R., Foerster, M., Nogueira, A. C., and Helge, H. (1995). Cross-reactivity of antihuman monoclonal antibodies with cell surface receptors in the common marmoset. *Life Sciences* **58,** 317–324.

Neubert, R., Golor, G., Stahlmann, R., Helge, H., and Neubert, D. (1992a). Polyhalogenated dibenzo-*p*-dioxins and dibenzofurans and the immune system. 4. Effects of multiple-dose treatment with 2,3,7,8-tetrachlorodibenzo-*p*-dioxin (TCDD) on peripheral lymphocyte subpopulations of a non-human primate (Callithrix jacchus). *Arch. Toxicol.* **66,** 250–259.

Neubert, R., Helge, H., and Neubert, D. (1995). Proliferative capacity of marmoset lymphocytes after tetanus vaccination and lack and 2,3,7,8-tetrachlorodibenzo-*p*-dioxin to reduce a booster effects. *Life Science* **56,** 437–444.

Neubert, R., Maskow, L., Webb, J., Jacob-Müller, U., Nogueira, A. C., Delgado, I., Helge, H., and Neubert, D. (1993). Chlorinated dibenzo-*p*-dioxins and dibenzofurans and the human immune system. 1. Blood cell receptors in volunteers with moderately increased body burdens. *Life Sci.* **53,** 2007–2018.

Neubert, R., and Neubert, D. (1996). Nonhuman primates as models for evaluating substance-induced changes in the immune system with relevance for man. *In* "Experimental Immunotoxicology" (R. J. Smialowicz and M. P. Holsapple, eds.), pp. 63–98. CRC Press, Boca Raton, FL.

Neubert, R., and Neubert, D. (1997). Peculiarities and possible mode of the action of thalidomide. *In* Handbook of Experimental Pharmacology, 124 II, "Drug Toxicity in Embryonic Development II" (R. J. Kavlock and G. P. Daston, eds.), pp. 44–119. Springer Verlag, Berlin.

Neubert, R., Nogueira, A. C., Helge, H., Stahlmann, R., and Neubert, D. (1992b). Feasibility of studying effects on the immune system in non-human primates. *In* "Risk Assessment of Prenatally-Induced Adverse Health Effects" (D. Neubert *et al.*, eds.) pp. 313–346. Springer Verlag, Berlin.

Neubert, R., Nogueira, A. C., and Neubert, D. (1992c). Thalidomide and the immune system. 2. Changes in receptors on blood cells of a healthy volunteer. *Life Sci.* **51,** 2107–2117.

Neubert, R., Nogueira, A. C., and Neubert, D. (1993). Thalidomide derivatives and the immune system. I. Changes in the pattern of integrin receptors and other surface markers on T lymphocyte subpopulations of marmoset blood. *Arch. Toxicol.* **67,** 1–17.

Neubert, R., Stahlmann, R., Korte, M., van Loveren, H., Vos, J. G., Golor, G., Webb, J. R., Helge, H., and Neubert, D. (1993). Effects of small doses of dioxins on the immune system of marmosets and rats. *Ann. NY Acad. Sci.* **685,** 662–686.

Newcombe, D. S., Rose, N. R., and Bloom, J. C. (eds.) (1992). "Clinical Immunotoxicology." Raven Press, New York.

Newcombe, D. S., and Terry, P. B. (1992). Bronchoalveolar lavage and bronchial reactivity in humans associated with environmental chemical exposure. *In* "Clinical Immunotoxicology" (D. S. Newcombe *et al.* eds.), pp. 277–337. Raven Press, New York.

Nogueira, A. C., Neubert, R., Helge, H., and Neubert, D. (1994). Thalidomide and the immune system. 3. Simultaneous up- and down-regulation of different integrin receptors on human white blood cells. *Life Sci.* **55,** 77–92.

Panerai, A. E., and Sacerdote, P. (1997). β-Endorphin in the immune system: A role at last? *Immunol. Today* **19,** 317–319.

Pascual, M., Swinford, R. D., Ingelfinger, J. R., Williams, W. W., Cosimi, A. B., and Tolkoff-Rubin, N. (1998). Chronic rejection and chronic cyclosporin toxicity in renal allografts. *Immunol. Today* **19,** 514–519.

Paul, W. E. (1993). "Fundamental Immunology," 3rd ed. Raven Press, New York.

Raghupathy, R. (1997). Th1-type immunity is incompatible with successful pregnancy. *Immunol. Today* **18,** 478–482.

Roitt, I. M., Brostoff, J, and Male, D. K. (1993). "Immunology," 3rd ed. Mosby-Year Book Europe Limited, London.

Romagnani, S. (1997). The Th1/Th2 paradigm. *Immunol. Today* **18,** 263–266.

Rook, G. A. W., and Stanford, J. L. (1998). Give us this day our daily germs. *Immunol. Today* **19,** 113–116.

Sampaio, E. P., Sarno, E. N., Galilli, R., Cohn, Z. A., and Kaplan, G. (1991). Thalidomide selectively inhibits tumor necrosis factor α production by stimulated human monocytes. *J. Exp. Med.* **173,** 699–703.

Sapin, C., Mandet, C., Druet, E., Günther, G., and Druet, P. (1981). Immune complex type disease induced by HgCl2: Genetic control of susceptibility. *Transplantation Proc.* **13,** 1404–1406.

Scheinman, R. I., Cogswell, P. C., Lofquist, A. K., and Baldwin, A. S. (1995). Role of transcriptional activation of I(B in mediation of immunosuppression by glucocorticoids. *Science* **270,** 283–286.

Schlossman, S. F., Boumsell, L., Guks, W., Harlan, J. M., Kishimoto, T., Morimoto, C., Ritz, J. R., Shaw, S., Silverstein, R., Springer, T., Tedder, T. F., and Todd, R. F., eds. (1993). "Leukocyte Typing V, White Cell Differentiation Antigens." Oxford University Press, Oxford.

Shannon, E. J., and Sandoval, F. (1996). Thalidomide can be either agonistic or antagonistic to LPS evoked synthesis of TNF-alpha by mononuclear cells. *Immunopharmacol. Immunotoxicol.* **18,** 59–72.

Sheskin, J. (1965). Thalidomide in the treatment of lepra reaction. *Clin. Pharmacol. Ther.* **6,** 303–306.

Siekierka, J. J., Hung, S. H. Y., Poe, M., Lin, C. S., and Sigal, N. H. (1989). A cytosolic protein for immunosuppressant FK506 has peptidyl-prolyl isomerase activity but is distinct from cyclophilin. *Nature* **341,** 755–757.

Smialowicz, R. J., and Holsapple, M. P. (eds.) (1996). "Experimental Immunotoxicology." CRC Press, Boca Raton, FL.

Smialowicz RJ, Riddle MM, Rogers RR, Leubke RW, Copeland CB, Ernest GG (1990) Immune alterations in rats following subacute exposure to tributyltin oxide. Toxicology 64:169–178.

Smialowicz, R. J., Riddle, M. M., Williams, W. C., and Diliberto, J. J. (1994). Effects of 2, 3, 7, 8-tetrachlorodibenzo-p-dioxin (TCDD) on humoral immunity and lymphocyte subpopulations: Differences between mice and rats. *Toxicol. Appl. Pharmacol.* **124,** 248–256.

Spiekermann, K., Emmendoerfer, A., Elsner, J., Raeder, E., Lohmann-Matthes, M. L., Prahst, A., Link, H., Freund, M., Welte, K., and Roesler, J. (1994). Altered surface marker expression and function of G-CSF induced neutrophils from test subjects and patients under chemotherapy. *Br. J. Haematol.* **87,** 31–38.

Springer, T. A. (1990). Adhesion receptors of the immune system. *Nature* **346,** 425–434.

Stahlmann, R., Korte, M., Van Loveren, H., Vos, J. G., Thiel, R., and Neubert, D. (1992). Abnormal thymus development and impaired function of the immune system in rats after prenatal exposure to aciclovir. *Arch. Toxicol.* **66,** 551–559.

Stefano, G. B., Salzet, B., and Fricchione, G. L. (1998). Enkelytin and opioid peptide association in invertebrates and vertebrates: Immune activation and pain. *Immunol. Today.* **19,** 265–268.

Straub, R. H., Westermann, J., Schölmerich, J., and Falk, W. (1998). Dialogue between the CNS and the immune system in lymphoid organs. *Immunol. Today* **19,** 409–413.

Taylor, J. R., Schmieder, G. F., Shimizu, T., Tier, C., and Streilin, J. W. (1994). Interrelationship between ultraviolet light and recurrent herpes simplex infections in man. *J. Dermatol. Sci.* **8,** 224–232.

Thorne, P. S., Hawk, C., Kaliszewski, S. D., and Guiney, P. D. (1991). The noninvasive mouse ear swelling test. *Fundam. Appl. Toxicol.* **17,** 790–820.

Tucker, A. N., Vore, S. J., and Luster, M. I. (1986). Suppression of B cell differentiation by 2,3,7,8-tetrachlorodibenzo-*p*-dioxin. *Mol. Pharmacol.* **29,** 372–377.

Van Loveren, H., Schuurman, H.-J., Kampinga, J., and Vos, J. G. (1991). Reversibility of thymic atrophy induced by 2,3,7,8-tetrachlorodibenzo-*p*-dioxin (TCDD) and bis(tri-*n*-butyltin)oxide (TBTO). *Int. J. Immunopharmacol.* **13,** 369–377.

Van Loveren, H., Timmerman, H., Dortant, P., and De Waal, E. (1993). "Validation of a Screening Battery for Immunotoxicity of Drugs within a 28 Day Oral Toxicity Study, Using Cyclosporin as a Model Compound." RIVM Report 312 620 001. National Institute of Public Health, Environmental Protection, Bilthoven.

Von Mutius, E., Fritzsch, C., Weiland, S. K., Roll, G., and Magnussen, H. (1992). Prevalence of asthma and allergic disorders among children in united Germany. *Br. Med. J.* **305,** 1395–1399.

Vos, J. G., (1977). Immune suppression as related to toxicology. *CRC Crit. Rev. Toxicol.* **5,** 67–101.

Vos, J. G. (1980). Immunotoxicity assessment: Screening and function studies. *Arch. Toxicol.* **4 (Suppl),** 95–108.

Vos, J. G., DeKlerk, A., Krajnc, E. I., Van Loveren, H., and Rozing, J. (1990). Immunotoxicity of bis(tri-*n*-butyltin)oxide in the rat: Effects on thymus-dependent immunity and non-specific resistance following long-term exposure in young versus aged rats. *Toxicol. Appl. Pharmacol.* **105,** 144–155.

Vos, J. G., Van Loveren, H., and Schuurman, H.-J. (1991). Immunotoxicity of dioxins: Immune function and host resistance in laboratory animals and humans. *Banbury Report* **35,** 79–88.

Weir, D. M., and Stewart, J. (1995). "Immunology," 5th ed. Churchill Livingstone, Philadelphia.

Wellinghausen, N., Kirchner, H., and Rink, L. (1997). The immunobiology of zinc. *Immunol. Today* **18,** 519–521.

White, K. L., Gennings, C., Murray, M. J., and Dean, J. H. (1994). Summary of international methods. Validation study, carried out in nine laboratories, on immunological assessment of cyclosporin A in the rat. *In Vitro Toxicity* **8,** 957–961.

WHO (1996). "Principles and Methods for Assessing Direct Immunotoxicity Associated with Exposure to Chemicals." Environmental Health Criteria (IPCS) No. 180, WHO, Geneva.

Wiederrecht, G., and Etzkorn, F. (1994). The immunophilins. *Perspect. Drug Discov. Design* **2,** 57–84.

Zober, M. A., Ott, M. G., Päpke, O., Senft, K., and Germann, C. (1992). Morbidity study of extruder personnel with potential exposure to brominated dioxins and furans. I. Results of blood monitoring and immunological tests. *Br. J. Industr. Med.* **49,** 532–544.

Zwick, H., Popp, W., Wagner, C., Reiser, K., Schmoger, J., Bock, A., Herkner, K., and Radunsky, K. (1991). Effects of ozone on the respiratory health, allergic sensitization, and cellular immune system in children. *Annu. Rev. Respir. Dis.* **144,** 1075–1079.

CHAPTER

18

Skin

NANCY A. MONTEIRO-RIVIERE, JIM E. RIVIERE

Center for Cutaneous Toxicology and Residue Pharmacology, North Carolina State University, Raleigh, North Carolina

INTRODUCTION

This chapter on dermatotoxicology depicts how anatomical structures within the skin can contribute to and influence barrier function by providing an overview of the structure and function of the skin, viewed from a multifaceted perspective. The primary function of the skin is to act as a barrier to the external environment. There has also been a surge of interest in the skin as a target organ, due in part to the fact that it is experimentally accessible, directly interfaces with the environment, and is an important route of entry for a myriad of environmental toxins. Recent developments in percutaneous absorption and dermal toxicology have considered how anatomical factors may affect the barrier function, thereby altering the rate of absorption. It is the purpose of this chapter to provide an overview of general principles of percutaneous penetration, metabolism, and cutaneous responses to specific chemicals. In addition, the mechanisms of direct irritation and sensitization will be discussed to provide a basis for selecting appropriate biomarkers for evaluating dermal toxicity. This overview will present basic principles and illustrate the field's complexity while provoking scientific curiosity as to the wide range of interactions seen when chemicals come in contact with the skin.

Dermatotoxicology is the branch of toxicology that involves assessing the skin responses to specific toxicants. This field has expanded its horizons in recent years. There is a flourishing interest in dermal toxicology because of environmental and occupational exposures and the development of novel transdermal drug delivery systems. Skin is one of the largest organs of the body and is the primary barrier to absorption from the environment. Because of its accessibility and continuous exposure to a myriad of chemicals, both accidentally and deliberately (e.g., cosmetics), it is a common target for toxic chemicals. This requires that substantial testing occur to assess the dermatotoxic potential of chemicals. The animal rights movement has had a major impact on the type of testing that it done by researchers. In response, new *in vitro* testing methods have been developed to study irritation, absorption, corrosion, and toxicity. However, before data from these tests can be interpreted, these surrogate models must be analyzed from the perspective of their capability of mimicking the wide range of responses seen in intact skin.

The two properties of a chemical that relate to its propensity to cause dermatotoxicity are its ability to penetrate the skin and its subsequent interactions with the biological components of skin that could elicit a toxicological response. This chapter will review the basic anatomical factors that may effect both of these processes (absorption and potential targets for toxicity), discuss the barrier properties of skin that determine whether a compound can be absorbed, and then overview the nature of the toxicological responses that could be elicited.

RELEVANT ANATOMY AND PHYSIOLOGY

Epidermis

The integument or skin consists of an outer epidermis and an inner dermis (Fig. 1). One of the primary functions of the skin is to act as a barrier between the well-regulated *milieu interieur* and the outside environment. However, the skin is a complex, integrated, dynamic organ that has several functions that go far beyond its role as a barrier to the environment. Several of these functions are listed in (Table 1). Skin is a very nonhomogeneous organ that anatomically comprises two distinct principal components: a stratified, avascular outer cellular epidermis and an underlying dermis consisting of connective tissue with numerous cell types and special adnexial structures.

The epidermis consists of a keratinized stratified squamous epithelium derived from ectoderm. It undergoes an orderly pattern of proliferation, differentiation, and keratinization. Various skin appendages, such as the hair, sweat and sebaceous glands, digital organs (e.g., hoof, claw, and nail), feathers, horn, and glandular structures, are specializations of the epidermis. Two primary cell types, the keratinocytes (stratum basale, stratum spinosum, stratum granulosum, stratum lucidum, and stratum corneum) and the nonkeratinocytes (melanocytes, Merkel cells, and Langerhans cells), are present. The keratinocytes are organized in layers above the basement membrane, reaching to the outer surface—stratum basale (basal layer; stratum germinativum), stratum spinosum (spinous or prickle layer), stratum granulosum (granular layer), stratum lucidum (clear layer), and stratum corneum (horny layer).

The stratum basale is a single layer of columnar or cuboidal cells that are attached to the underlying irregular basement membrane by hemidesmosomes and laterally to each other and to the overlying stratum spinosum cells by desmosomes. The basal cells are constantly undergoing mitosis, causing the daughter cells to be displaced outward to keep the epidermis replenished as the stratum corneum cells are con-

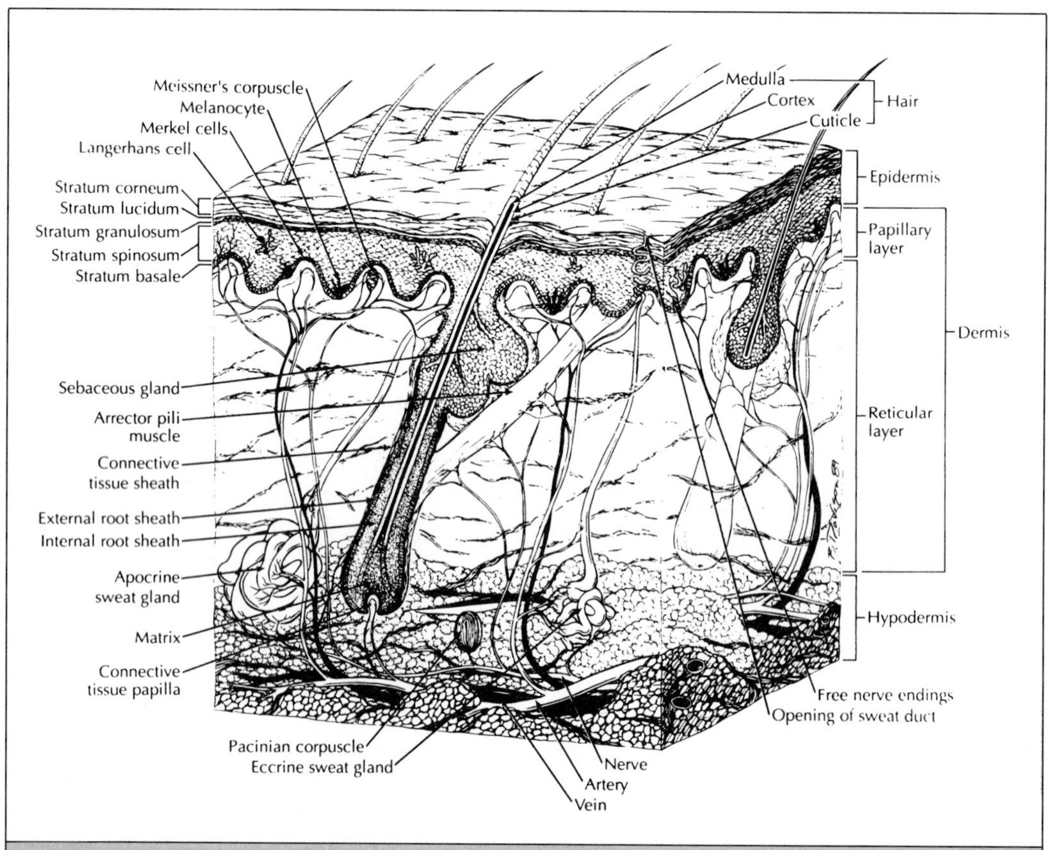

FIGURE 1 Schematic of skin illustrating the complexity of mammalian skin found in various regions of the body. (Reprinted from Monteiro-Riviere, 1991).

TABLE 1 Functions of Skin[a]

Environmental barrier
Diffusion barrier
Metabolic barrier
Temperature regulation
Regulation of blood flow
Hair and fur
Sweating
Immunological affector and effector axis
Mechanical support
Neurosensory reception
Endocrine (e.g., vitamin D)
Apocrine/eccrine/sebaceous glandular secretion
Metabolism
Keratin
Collagen
Melanin
Lipid
Carbohydrate
Respiration
Biotransformation of xenobiotics

[a]Monteiro-Riviere, N.A. (1991). Comparative anatomy, physiology, and biochemistry of Mammalian Skin. *In* "Dermal and Ocular Toxicology: Fundamentals and Methods" (D.W. Hobson, Ed.). Chapt. 1, pp. 3–71. CRC Press, Inc., New York.

stantly being sloughed from the surface epidermis. This process of cell turnover and self-replacement in normal human skin is thought to take approximately 45–75 days, depending on the region of the body, age, disease states, and other modulating factors. Chemical carcinogens that transform basal keratinocytes may result in squamous cell carcinomas.

The succeeding outer layer is the stratum spinosum, or "prickle cell layer," which consists of several layers of irregular polyhedral cells that become flattened as they reach the surface. These cells are connected to the adjacent stratum spinosum cells and to the stratum basale cells below by desmosomes and contain the same complement of organelles as the stratum basale cells. The presence of numerous tonofilaments differentiates them morphologically from the other cell layers. The uppermost layers of the stratum spinosum contain small membrane-bound organelles known as lamellar granules.

The third layer is the stratum granulosum, which consists of several layers of flattened cells lying parallel to the epidermal–dermal junction. This layer contains irregularly shaped, nonmembrane-bound, electron-dense keratohyalin granules. These granules contain profilaggrin, a structural protein and a precursor of filaggrin, and are thought to play a role in keratinization and barrier function. Another characteristic feature is the presence of lipid-containing lamellar granules (Odland bodies, lamellated bodies, or membrane-coating granules). These granules are smaller than mitochondria and are found near the Golgi complex and smooth endoplasmic reticulum (SER). In the upper epidermis, the lamellar granules increase in number and size, move toward the cell membrane, and release their lipid contents by exocytosis into the intercellular space between the stratum granulosum and stratum corneum, thereby coating the cell membrane of the stratum corneum cells. The major components are lipids, including the ceramides, cholesterol, fatty acids, and small amounts of cholesteryl esters; and hydrolytic enzymes, such as acid phosphates, proteases, lipases, and glycosidases. The content and mixture of lipids can vary among species and are considered to function as the primary component of the permeability barrier. Toxicants that target the formation or function of these granules or alter the activity of their constitutive enzymes may be manifested in impaired barrier function.

The stratum lucidum is a thin, translucent, homogeneous layer between the stratum granulosum and the stratum corneum. It is found only in distinct anatomical areas of exceptionally thick skin and in hairless regions (e.g., plantar and palmar surfaces). It consists of several layers of fully keratinized, closely compacted, dense cells devoid of nuclei and cytoplasmic organelles. Their cytoplasm contains protein-bound phospholipids and a keratin-like protein, eleidin.

The outermost layer of the epidermis is the stratum corneum, consisting of several layers of completely keratinized dead cells, which are constantly being shed. This layer appears clear, anucleated, and lacking in cytoplasmic organelles. The most superficial layers of the stratum corneum that undergo constant desquamation are referred to as the stratum disjunctum. The stratum corneum cell layers vary in thickness depending on the area (i.e., abdomen versus back) of the body and on the species. The stratum corneum cells are highly organized and are stacked on one another to form vertical interlocking columns having a flattened tetrakaidecahedron shape. This 14-sided polygonal provides a minimum surface:volume ratio, which allows for space to be filled by packing without interstices. This spatial arrangement helps facilitate the maintenance of the skin's efficient barrier function. The intercellular lipids derived from the lamellar granules of the stratum granulosum are located between the stratum corneum cells and form the intercellular lipid component of the complex stratum corneum barrier. This prevents both the penetration of

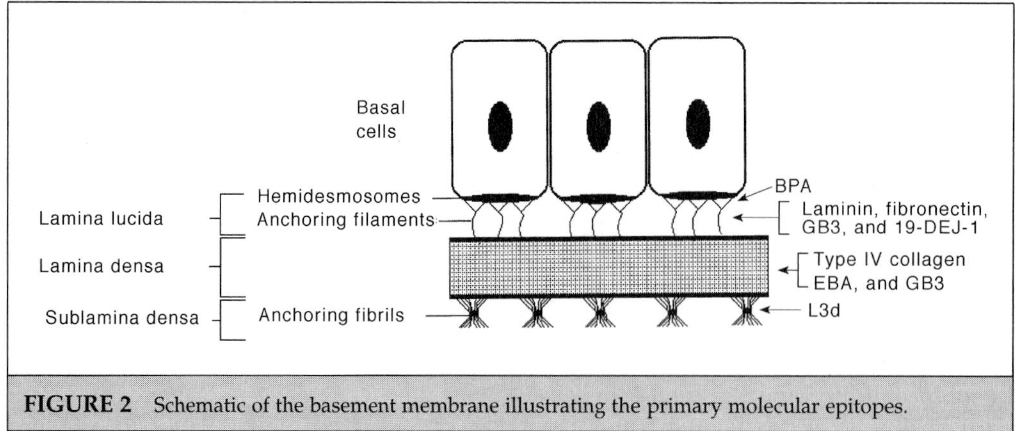

FIGURE 2 Schematic of the basement membrane illustrating the primary molecular epitopes.

substances from the environment and the insensible loss of body water by surface evaporation. These cells are surrounded by a plasma membrane and a thick submembranous layer that contains the protein involucrin. This protein is synthesized in the stratum spinosum and cross-linked in the stratum granulosum by an enzyme that makes it highly stable. Involucrin provides structural support to the cell, allowing the cell to resist invasion by microorganisms and destruction by environmental agents, but does not appear to play a role in barrier permeability.

Nonkeratinocytes

Melanocytes are derivatives of the neural crest and are located in the basal layer of the epidermis. Melanocytes have several dendritic processes that extend between adjacent keratinocytes or run parallel to the dermal surface. The cytoplasm is clear except for pigment-containing membrane bound ovoid granules, referred to as melanosomes, that impart color to skin and hair. Melanosomes are transferred to keratinocytes, where they are randomly distributed within the keratinocyte's cytoplasm. They often become localized over the nucleus to form a cap-like structure that protects the sensitive genetic material from ultraviolet radiation. Skin color is determined by several factors, including the number, size, distribution, and degree of melanization of melanosomes. In chemical carcinogenesis, chemicals that transform melanocytes may result in malignant melanomas.

Merkel cells are located in the basal region of the epidermis. Their long axis is parallel to the surface of the skin and, thus, perpendicular to the columnar basal epithelial cells above. These cells contain spherical electron-dense granules and are connected to adjacent keratinocytes by desmosomes. When these cells are associated with axons they are referred to as a Merkel cell–neurite complex. Specialized areas containing these complexes are known as Haarscheiben (hair discs, tactile hair discs, or tylotrich pads). The axon associated with a Merkel cell arises from a myelinated nerve, but as it approaches the epidermis it loses its myelin sheath and terminates as a flat meniscus on the basal aspect of the cell. Merkel cells are thought to function as slow-adapting mechanoreceptors for touch.

Langerhans cells are most commonly found in the upper spinous layer of the epidermis, yet have been identified in other stratified squamous epithelium. Ultrastructurally, Langerhans cells have an indented nucleus and contain common organelles, but lack tonofilaments and desmosomes. A unique feature of this cell is the presence of a distinctive rod- or racket-shaped granules known as Langerhans (Birbeck) cell granules. Langerhans cells have long dendritic processes that traverse the intercellular space up to the granular cell layer. Langerhans cells are derived from bone marrow and are functionally and immunologically related to the monocyte–macrophage series. They play a major role in the skin immune response because they are capable of presenting antigen to lymphocytes and transporting them to the lymph nodes for lymphocyte activation. They are considered to be the initial receptor for initiating a cutaneous immune response (delayed-type hypersensitivity) to certain contact allergens and thus play an initiating role in some forms of immune-mediated dermatologic reactions.

All of these cell layers are situated above the basement membrane zone or epidermal–dermal junction, which provides mechanical support to the epidermis. Ultrastructurally, this junction consists of four components: (1) the cell membrane of the basal epithelial cell, which includes the hemidesmosomes; (2) the lamina lucida (lamina rara); (3) the lamina densa (basal lamina); and (4) the sub-basal lamina (reticular lamina), which contains a variety of fibrous structures (anchoring fibrils, dermal microfibril bundles and microthread-like filaments). The basement membrane has a complex molecular architecture with numerous components that play a key role in the adhesion of the epidermis to the dermis (Fig. 2). The basement membrane components, which are ubiquitous components of all basement membranes, include type IV collagen, laminin, entactin and nidogen, and heparan sulfate proteoglycans. Other basement membrane components, such as bullous pemphigoid antigen (BPA), epidermolysis bullosa acquisita (EBA), fibronectin, GB3, L3d, and 19DEJ-1, are limited to skin. The basal cell membrane of the epidermal–dermal junction is undulating and irregular, forming finger-like projections into the dermis. Several functions have been attributed to the basement membrane—maintaining epidermal–dermal adhesion, acting as a selective barrier between the epidermis and dermis by restricting some molecules and permitting the passage of others, influencing cell behavior and wound healing, and serving as a target for both immunologic and nonimmunologic injury. The basement membrane is the target for vesicating chemical agents, which cause blister formation after topical exposure.

Dermis

The dermis or corium is of mesodermal origin and consists of dense irregular connective tissue that extends to the hypodermis or subcutaneous tissue. The matrix of this connective tissue is composed of collagen, and elastic and reticular fibers embedded in an amorphous ground substance of mucopolysaccharides. The cell inhabitants of the dermis are fibroblasts, mast cells, and macrophages. Plasma cells, chromatophores, fat cells, and extravasated leukocytes are often found along with blood vessels, nerves, and lymphatics. In addition, adnexial appendages, such as sweat glands, sebaceous glands, hair follicles, and arrector pili muscles, are anchored within the dermis. The dermis can be arbitrarily divided into a superficial papillary layer that blends into a deep reticular layer. The papillary layer is thin and consists of loose connective tissue, which is in contact with the epidermis and conforms to the contour of the basal epithelial ridges and grooves. It can protrude into the epidermis, giving rise to the dermal papilla. When the epidermis invaginates into the dermis, epidermal pegs are formed. The reticular layer is thicker and constitutes irregular dense connective tissue with fewer cells and more fibers. A major component of the dermis is the extensive network of capillaries that function to regulate body temperature. Blood flow through the skin can vary by 100-fold depending on environmental conditions, making it one of the most highly perfused organs in the body.

There is considerable variations in skin thickness, both among species and within the same species in various regions of the body. Over the dorsal and lateral surfaces of limbs, the skin is thick, and on the ventral and medial surfaces of limbs, the skin is thinner. In hairy areas, the epidermis is thin, while in nonhairy skin, such as the mucocutaneous junctions, the epidermis is thicker. The stratum corneum is thickest on the palmar and plantar surfaces, where considerable abrasive action occurs.

ADNEXIAL APPENDAGES

Hair

Hairs are keratinized structures derived from epidermal invaginations and are found almost everywhere on the body surface except for specific body sites, which include the palms, soles, and mucocutaneous junctions.

The hair follicle is embedded at an angle in the dermis, with the bulb sometimes extending as deep as the hypodermis. This fundamental anatomical arrangement is often ignored when dermatomed skin sections or epidermal membranes are employed in *in vitro* diffusion cell systems. In these preparations, holes appear where the hair shafts once were. The hair follicle consists of four major components: (1) internal root sheath, (2) external root sheath, (3) dermal papilla, and (4) hair matrix. The cells covering the dermal papilla and composing most of the hair bulb are the hair matrix cells. These are comparable to stratum basale cells of regular epidermis, except for being more lipid deficient and producing harder keratin than their epidermal counterparts.

Hair growth varies from species to species and according to body site and age of an individual. The process of keratinization is continuous in the surface epidermis, while in the hair follicle the matrix cells undergo periods of quiescence during which no mitotic activity occurs. Cyclic activity of the hair bulb accounts for the seasonal change in the hair coat of domestic animals. The hair cycle in which the cells of the hair bulb are mitotically active and growth occurs is called anagen. When the follicles go through a regressive stage and metabolic activity slows down, it is referred to as catagen. In this phase, the base of the follicle migrates upward in the skin toward the epidermal surface. The hair follicle then enters telogen, a resting or quiescent phase, in which growth stops and the base of the bulb is at the level of the sebaceous canal. Following this phase, mitotic activity and keratinization start over again and a new hair is formed. As the new hair grows beneath the telogen follicle, it gradually pushes the old follicle upward toward the surface, where it is eventually shed. This intermittent mitotic activity and keratinization of the hair matrix cells constitute the hair cycle, which is controlled by several factors, including the length of daily periods of light, ambient temperature, nutrition, and hormones, particularly estrogen, testosterone, adrenal steroids, and thyroid hormone. Of particular significance to toxicology is that a chemical whose mechanism of action requires interaction with an active metabolic process may exert toxicity only when hair growth is in an active growth phase. Exposure at other times may not elicit any response. Many cytotoxic chemicals (e.g., cancer chemotherapeutic drugs and immunosuppressants, such as cyclophosphamide) whose mechanism of action is to kill dividing cells will produce hair loss (alopecia) as an unwanted side effect of mainly nonselective activity (e.g., thallium).

Associated with most hair follicles are bundles of smooth muscle fibers that make up the arrector pili muscle. This muscle attaches to the connective tissue sheath of the hair follicle and extends toward the epidermis, where it connects to the papillary layer of the dermis. It is innervated by the autonomic nerve fibers. The arrector pili muscles are especially well developed in humans and when they contract during cold weather they elevate the hairs, forming "goose pimples." The contraction of this muscle may also play a role in emptying the sebaceous glands.

Sebaceous Glands

The sebaceous glands secrete lipid and consist of a single layer of low cuboidal cells. These cells move inward through mitotic activity and accumulate lipid droplets to release their secretory product, sebum, by the holocrine mode of secretion. Sebum, which is derived from the disintegration of these cells, contains antimicrobial lipids. The major lipids in the human sebaceous gland are squalene, cholesterol, cholesterol esters, wax esters, and triglycerides. In lower mammals, the sebaceous glands can become specialized and are often associated with a pheromone-secreting role. Human sebum plays a major role during early adolescence in acne vulgaris, and thus its production is involved in the evaluation of anti-acne drug candidates. Toxicants that interact with sebaceous gland function and induce an acne-like response or comedons induce a condition termed chloracne. Several chloracnegens, including chloronaphthalenes, polychlorinated biphenyls, tetrachloroazoxybenzene, tetrachloroazobenzene, polychlorinated dibenzodioxins, polychlorinated dibenzofurans, and polychlorinated biphenyls have been identified as eliciting responses in humans. Most of these chloracnegens induce a cytochrome P450-mediated microsomal monoxygenase response.

Eccrine Sweat Glands

Sweat glands can be classified into apocrine or eccrine (merocrine) based on their morphologic and functional characteristics. In domestic animals, the apocrine gland is extensively developed and found throughout most of the skin. In humans, the eccrine (merocrine) glands are found over the entire body surface, except for the lips, external ear canal, clitoris, and labia minora. They are simple tubular glands that open directly onto the skin surface. Myoepithelial cells are found in the secretory portion and are specialized smooth muscle cells, which, upon contraction, aid in moving the secretions toward the duct. The duct of the eccrine sweat glands comprises two layers of cuboidal epithelium resting on the basal lamina and opens in a straight path onto the epidermal surface. Some workers postulate that the duct of these glands provide an alternate pathway for polar molecules, normally excluded by the stratum corneum, to be absorbed through skin.

This exocrine gland whose principal function is thermoregulation, is one of the major cutaneous appendages and is functionally very active in humans. Sweating in humans refers to a distinct physiological function of excreting body fluids to the surface of the skin. This is necessary for fluid and electrolyte homeostasis. Physiologically stressed individuals can excrete 2 liters/h to support evaporative heat loss. Only the higher primates have a built-in mechanism that can accommodate this large volume loss without circulatory collapse. The secretory portion secretes isotonic fluid that is low in protein and similar to plasma in ionic composition and osmolarity. On its passage down the duct portion, it becomes hypotonic and the reabsorption of sodium chloride, bicarbonate, lactate, and a small amount of water occurs. Abnormality in this fluid and electrolyte transport system leads to cystic fibrosis. In fact, the analysis of this secretion is a prime diagnostic tool for this disease.

Apocrine Sweat Glands

In humans, the apocrine sweat glands are limited to the axillary, pubic, areolae, and perianal regions. They can be simple sacular or tubular, having a coiled secretory portion and a straight duct. The secretory portion is usually found in the lower reticular dermis and hypodermis. Depending on the stage of secretory activity, the epithelium may be simple columnar or cuboidal. The acini portion of the sweat gland contains two types of secretory cells, a clear cell and a dark seromucous cell. Myoepithelial cells are present between the basal lamina and the secretory cells to aid in cell secretion. The duct has a narrow lumen consisting of two layers of cuboidal cells and is found adjacent to the hair follicle. The duct runs parallel to the follicle, penetrates the epidermis of the follicle, and opens alongside the follicle at the surface. Based on physiologic and evolutionary development, the axillary apocrine sweat glands and possibly other apocrine glands function as scent glands in humans.

Impact of Anatomy on Toxicology

As can be appreciated from this brief anatomical overview of the skin, a number of cell types may be targets for chemical toxicants. The toxicological response of these cells (primarily keratinocytes, melanocytes, and Langerhans cells), structures (stratum corneum and basement membrane) or adnexial appendages (hair follicles and sebaceous and sweat glands) will define the nature of the dermatotoxicity produced. Two of these cells, the keratinocytes and melanocytes, are the target cells that undergo transformation in the process of chemical carcinogenesis and produce the squamous cell carcinomas and melanomas observed in "skin painting" carcinogenicity bioassays. When these epidermal cells are affected by exogenous chemicals independent of etiology, the dermis often reacts to their damage in a process mediated by cytokines of epidermal origin. The dermis, being primarily a vascular organ, responds by increasing the blood flow to remove the offending toxicant and brings in cellular components of the immune system to effect repair. This dermal reaction is macroscopically observed as erythema and edema, the two hallmarks of cutaneous toxicity.

If a chemical is capable of interacting with one of these cutaneous cell types, the potential for dermatotoxicity exists. However, the chemical must be able to reach the target cell to affect its action. The barrier properties of the stratum corneum thus must be overcome for this potential toxicity to be expressed. The nature of this unique barrier will now be presented.

PERCUTANEOUS ABSORPTION AND PENETRATION

The ability of a toxicant to enter skin is a primary determinant of its dermatotoxic potential. The quantitative prediction of the rate and extent of percutaneous penetration (into skin) and absorption (through skin) of topically applied chemicals is complicated by the biological variability inherent in skin. The many and varied biological roles lead to functional and structural adaptations that impact on the skin's barrier properties and thus the rate and extent of percutaneous absorption.

The skin is generally considered to be an efficient barrier preventing absorption (and thus systemic exposure) of most topically administered compounds. It is a membrane that is relatively impermeable to aqueous solutions and most ions. It is, however, permeable in varying degrees to a large number of lipophilic solid, liquid, and gaseous xenobiotics or specific matrices, making the concept of barrier inappropriate for these substances. Although one tends to think of most cases of poisoning as occurring through the oral or, less frequently, the respiratory route, the widespread use of organic chemicals has produced many toxicants that can easily penetrate the epidermal barrier. An example is the large number of agricultural workers who have experienced acute dermal poisoning from their direct exposure to pesticides such as parathion during application or from more casual exposure such as worker contact with vegetation previously treated with such insecticides.

Compared to most routes of drug absorption, the skin is by far the most diverse across species (e.g., sheep versus pig) and body sites (e.g., human forearm compared to scalp). The stratum corneum appears to afford the greatest deterrent to absorption. This outer barrier is formed from continuous maturation of the basal epidermal cell layer. The end result in the stratum corneum is the dead proteinaceous keratinocytes embedded in an extracellular lipid matrix composed primarily of sterols, other neutral lipids, and ceramides, a structure referred to by Elias (1983) as the "Brick and Mortar" model (Fig. 3). The intercellular lipids composition is not homogeneous in all layers of the epidermis, making the lipid topography complex. Species differences are also evident. Although highly

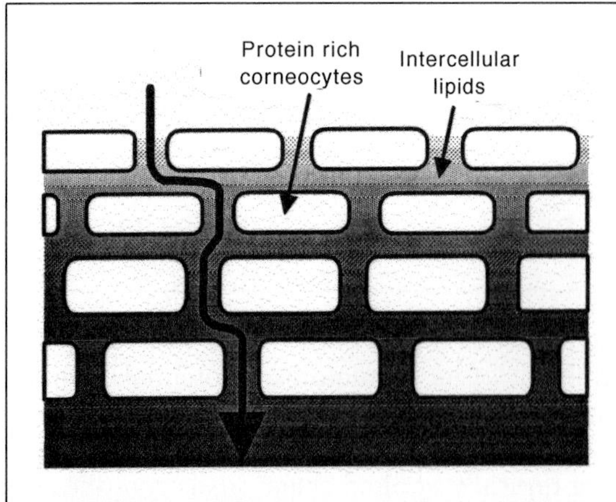

FIGURE 3 Idealized representation of the barrier property of skin composed of proteinaceous cells (bricks) embedded in a lipid extracellular matrix (mortar). (Reprinted from Riviere, 1994.)

water retarding, the dead keratinized cells are highly water absorbent (hydrophilic), a property that keeps the skin supple and soft as they absorb water on its way to being evaporated from the surface. A natural oil covering the skin, the sebum, appears to maintain the water-holding capacity of the epidermis but has no appreciable role in retarding the penetration of xenobiotics.

A number of investigations have shown that disruption of the stratum corneum removes all but a superficial deterrent to penetration. One line of evidence uses "stripping" experiments, in which an adhesive (cellophane tape) is placed on the skin repeatedly, removing progressive sections of the corneum. At some critical point, the skin loses its ability to retard penetration and compound flux increases greatly. This can be noninvasively assessed by measuring the skin's ability to prevent insensible evaporative water loss from the body to the environment and thus uses water as a marker of molecular transport across the cutaneous barrier. This is performed by measuring transepidermal water loss (TEWL) with an instrument called an evaporimeter. TEWL increases greatly when the stratum corneum is either stripped, removed by extracting the intercellular barrier lipids, or damaged in response to cutaneous toxicants, making TEWL a sensitive noninvasive biomarker of cutaneous toxicity.

For many compounds, the stratum corneum has been calculated to afford 1000 times the diffusional resistance to chemical penetration as the layers beneath it. Exceptions to this rule are extremely lipid soluble compounds with tissue–water partition coefficients greater than 400. As in most other epithelial tissues, the two other layers of the skin (dermis and subcutaneous tissue) generally offer little resistance to penetration, and once a substance has penetrated the outer epithelium, these tissues are rapidly traversed. For the highly lipid soluble compounds, this may not be true and the dermis may function as an additional barrier, preventing a chemical that has penetrated the epidermis from being absorbed into the blood.

Dermatopharmacokinetics

The rate of diffusion of a topically applied chemical across the rate-limiting stratum corneum is directly proportional to the concentration gradient across the membrane, the lipid–water partition coefficient of the drug, and the diffusion coefficient for the compound being studied. This can be summarized by Fick's law of diffusion in the equation

$$\text{Rate of diffusion (mg/s)} = \frac{D(\text{cm/s})P}{h(\text{cm})}(\Delta X)(\text{mg}),$$

where D is the diffusion coefficient for the specific penetrant in the membrane being studied, P is the partition coefficient for the penetrant between the membrane and the external medium, h is the thickness or actual length of the path by which the drug diffuses through the membrane, and ΔX is the concentration gradient across the membrane. The diffusional coefficient for the drug is a function of the molecular size, the molecular conformation and solubility in the membrane milieu, and the degree of ionization. It should be noted that if the compound is dosed in an organic vehicle, the vehicle itself may penetrate into the intercellular lipids of the stratum corneum and change the estimated diffusional coefficient. The partition coefficient reflects the ability of the penetrant to gain access to the lipid membrane. Depending on the membrane, there is a functional molecular size–weight cutoff that prevents very large molecules from being passively absorbed across any membrane. When the rate of this process is dependent upon a rate constant such as DP/h and a concentration gradient, a linear or first-order kinetic process will be operative. The total flux of drug across a membrane is dependent upon the area of membrane exposed and thus usually expressed in terms of cm^2. This relationship, which works well in an *in vitro* experiment, is only an approximation *in vivo* since penetration may be slow and a long period of time required to achieve steady state. When steady state is not achieved, Fick's second law of diffusion may be used to estimate instantaneous fluxes, a discussion of which is beyond the scope of the present chapter. Finally, if the applied dose saturates the absorptive capacity of skin, zero-order or nonlinear absorption kinetics will be observed.

If the lipid water partition coefficient is too great, the compound may be sequestered in the membrane rather than traverse it, and thus some fraction of X will actually not be available for diffusion through the system. However, in general, passage through the skin correlates with various lipid–water partition coefficients. The systems most often used are octanol/water, and olive oil/water. In some cases where the specific lipid composition of the membrane is known (e.g., the stratum corneum from a specific species), the slurry of the actual lipids may be employed. This is becoming more sophisticated with the advent of advanced organ culture techniques in which, for example, in skin, lipid membranes are very similar in composition, structure, and function to the *in vivo* and can be prepared in culture and used to study drug transport.

From the perspective of pharmacokinetic models of transdermal and topical drug delivery systems, there are significant differences from other routes of administration (e.g., oral and intravenous) as to what constitutes a dose. For most exposures, the amount applied to the surface of the skin exceeds the absorption capacity, making the rate of absorption constant or zero-order. Thus, the application of higher doses results in a decreased fraction of dose being absorbed but an increase in actual drug flux. However, for therapeutic transdermal patches with a fixed concentration of drug and rate-controlled release properties, it is the contact surface area that more accurately reflects the dose, and thus dose is expressed not in mg/kg, but mg/cm^2 of dosing area. This surface area dependence also holds for any topical application, even if absorption capacity is superseded. This is particularly important in dermatotoxicology where the area of skin exposed to a toxicant is the primary determinant of dose. This explains why infants, with a relatively small ratio of skin surface area to body mass, are particularly prone to systemic toxicity from topical poisons when large areas of skin are exposed. This is further potentiated in neonates who do not have a fully developed cutaneous barrier.

Another source of nonlinearity results secondary to the effects of occlusive (water-impermeable) drug vehicle or patches. As the skin hydrates, a threshold is reached where transdermal flux dramatically increases (approximately 80% relative humidity). When the skin becomes completely hydrated under completely occlusive conditions, flux can be dramatically increased. This occlusion effect must be accounted for when extrapolating toxicology studies conducted under occlusive conditions to field scenarios where the ambient environmental conditions are present. Therefore, dose alone is often not a sufficient metric to describe topical doses, with application method and surface area becoming the controlling factors. Dose should properly be expressed as mg/cm^2 of exposed skin.

Hydration may also markedly affect the pH of the skin, which varies between 4.2 and 7.3. For drugs or chemicals with pK_a's in this range, the principles embedded in the Henderson–Hasselbach equation become important. The unionized fraction may change as a function of skin pH, thereby further modulating percutaneous absorption.

The dermis is a highly vascular area, providing direct access for distribution once the epithelial barrier has been passed. The blood supply in the dermis is under complex interacting neural and local humoral influences, whose temperature-regulating function can have an effect on distribution by altering blood supply to this area. This function of mammalian skin is different from other epithelial tissues discussed and offers another variable for predicting systemic toxin exposure. The absorption of a chemical possessing vasoactive properties would be affected through its action on the dermal vasculature; vasoconstriction would retard absorption and increase the size of a dermal depot, while vasodilation may enhance absorption and minimize any local dermal depot formation. For a systemic toxicant, vasodilation would potentiate activity while a vasoconstriction might blunt the response. However, if the chemical is directly toxic to the skin, the reverse effect occurs with vasoconstriction, preventing removal of drug to the systemic circulation away from cutaneous toxic sites, thereby potentiating local effects.

Routes of Absorption and Penetration

The appendages of the skin are found in the dermis and extend through the epidermis, as previously mentioned. Because these structures extend to the outer surface, they may play a role in the penetration of certain compounds and may be selective targets after topical exposure. Anatomically, percutaneous absorption might occur through several routes. The current consensus is that the majority of nonionized, lipid-soluble toxicants appear to move through the intercellular lipid pathway between the cells of the stratum corneum, the rate-limiting barrier of the skin. Previously, it was thought that the primary route was transcellular (through the cells), but more recent work has discredited this view. A third possible route is through the appendages such as hair follicles or sweat ducts. Very small and/or polar molecules appear to have more favorable penetration through appendages or other diffusion shunts, but only a small fraction of drugs are represented by these molecules. Initial penetration particularly may be aided by the appendages. In addition, the epidermal surface area is 100–1000 times the surface area of the skin appendages, depending on species. The only exceptions to this rule are particulate exposures (microspheres and liposomes) that may lodge in the opening to hair follicles and provide a unique access to the dermal circulation. Passage through the skin is passive, there being no evidence for active transport.

Polar substances, in addition to movement through shunts, may diffuse through the outer surface of the protein filaments of the hydrated stratum corneum, while nonpolar molecules dissolve in and diffuse through the nonaqueous lipid matrix between the protein filaments. The rate of percutaneous absorption through this intercellular lipid pathway is correlated to the partition coefficient of the penetrant. This has resulted in numerous studies correlating the extent of percutaneous absorption with the drug's lipid/water partition coefficient. Some investigators further correlated skin penetration to molecular size and other indices of potential interaction between the penetrating molecule and the skin (e.g., hydrogen bonding), which is not reflected in the partition coefficient. For most purposes, dermal penetration is often correlated to partition coefficient. If lipid solubility increases too much, then the compounds that penetrate the stratum corneum may remain there and form a reservoir, evidenced by a plateauing in absorption versus partition coefficient plots. Alternatively, penetrated compounds may also form a reservoir in the dermis. For such compounds, much like in the scenario of cutaneous vasoconstriction described above, slow release from these depots may result in a prolonged absorption half-life and potentiate systemic toxicity. Conditions that alter the composition of the lipid (e.g., harsh delipidizing solvents, dietary lipid restrictions, and disease) may alter the rate of compound penetration by changing its partitioning behavior.

Recent studies have demonstrated that the skin may be responsible for metabolizing topically applied compounds. Both phase I and II metabolic pathways have been identified. For some compounds, the extent of cutaneous metabolism influences the overall fraction of a topically applied compound that is absorbed, making this process function as an alternate absorption pathway. Cutaneous biotransformation is used to promote the absorption of some topical drugs that normally would not penetrate the skin. By modifying these drugs to more lipid-soluble ester analogs, the drug penetrates the stratum corneum and the free drug is liberated through the action of cutaneous esterases. Cutaneous metabolism may also be important for certain aspects of skin toxicology when nontoxic compounds are bioactivated within the epidermis (e.g., benzo[*a*]pyrene).

Penetration of drugs through different body regions varies. In humans, it is generally accepted that for most nonionized toxicants, the rate of penetration is in the following order: scrotal > forehead > axilla = scalp > back = abdomen > palm and plantar. The palm and plantar regions are highly cornified and their much greater thickness (100–400 times that of other regions) introduces an overall lag time in diffusion. In addition to thickness, differences in stratum corneum cell size and hair follicle density may also effect the absorption of some molecules. The scalp should thus be considered in a different light than the rest of the body. Finally, differences in cutaneous blood flow have been documented in different body regions and may be an additional variable to consider in predicting the rate of percutaneous absorption. These factors are equally applicable in animals.

Factors and Chemicals That Affect Percutaneous Absorption

Soaps and detergents are perhaps the most damaging substances routinely applied to skin. Whereas organic solvents must be applied in high concentrations to damage skin, 1% aqueous solutions of detergents and many other surfactants (e.g., sodium lauryl sulfate) increase the penetration of the solute through the human epidermis. Alteration of the stratum corneum from their surfactant effects appears to be the cause of increased penetration.

Organic solvents can be divided into damaging and nondamaging categories, relative to their effects on the barrier properties of skin. The damaging category includes methanol, acetone, ether, hexane, and mixed solvents such as chloroform:methanol or ether: ethanol. These solvents and mixtures are able to extract lipids and proteolipids from tissues and would be expected to alter permeability for this reason. Another mechanism for explaining this solvent effect is that the solvents themselves may partition into the intercellular lipid pathway, changing its lipophilicity and barrier property, which results in an increased diffusion coefficient. The use of more polar or amphoteric solvents may enhance the penetration of the polar molecules in some cases by forming "ion pairs," which have a greater ability to penetrate the lipid domain. In contrast, solvents such as higher alcohols, esters, and olive oil do not appear to damage skin appreciably. However, the penetration rate of solutes dissolved in them is often reduced. This is best explained by partitioning of the penetrant into the nonabsorbed solvent, preventing release of the chemical into the stratum corneum. This is very similar to the strategies used to formulate injectable depot preparations. Thus, one can appreciate that for a specific chemical, the rate of penetration can be drastically modified by the solvent system used.

These phenomena bring into question the wisdom of using organic solvents to decontaminate skin after exposure to lipophilic toxicants because they will be easily absorbed into the skin and may enhance toxicant absorption through their interaction with intercellular lipids. Not surprisingly, it has been found that lipid-soluble toxicants may be markedly resistant to washing within a short time after application, due to subsequent depot formation. For example, 15 min after application, a substantial portion of parathion cannot be removed from the exposed skin by soap and water. This practice should be strongly discouraged.

In environmental exposures, the chemical may come into contact with the skin as a mixture or in contaminated soil. In mixtures, other components may function as solvents and modulate the rate of absorption. This may be a determining factor in the toxicity of a complex chemical mixture. Our laboratory has extended this concept to classify chemical mixtures based on how components (mixtures of defined solvents, surfactants, reducing agents, and vasoactive compounds) may modulate the absorption or direct cutaneous toxicity of suspected toxicants, using a classification paradigm termed Mechanistically Defined Chemical Mixtures (MDCM). This approach would allow complex environmental mixtures to be assesssed for the presence of such modulating compounds in order to triage them according to toxic potential. In soil, a large fraction of the toxicant may remain bound to soil constituents, thereby reducing the fraction absorbed.

Electrically Assisted Transdermal Drug Delivery

In the pharmaceutical arena, the final strategy for transdermal delivery is to overcome the cutaneous barrier by using electrical (iontophoresis, electroosmosis, and electroporation) or even ultrasonic (phonophoreses) energy, rather than the concentration gradient in diffusion, to drive drug penetration. These techniques hold the most promise for delivering large hydrophilic peptides and oligonucleotide (antisense) drugs that are produced by the ever-expanding biotechnology industry and that can be administered only by injection. In these cases, dose is based on the surface area of application and the amount of energy required to actively deliver the drug across the skin. In iontophoresis, this amounts to a dose expressed in $\mu A/cm^2$. The formulation factors are also very different because many of the excipients used are also delivered by the applied electrical current in molar proportion to the active drug. Finally, a recent but related strategy is to use very short-duration high-voltage electrical pulses (electroporation) to reversibly breakdown the stratum corneum barrier, allowing larger peptides and possibly even small proteins to be systemically delivered.

The toxicological potentials of iontophoresis and electroporation have been investigated as modes of transdermal drug delivery. Using *in vivo* and *in vitro* porcine skin, we demonstrated a pattern of morphological changes induced by lidocaine hydrochloride iontophoresis that suggests that epidermal alterations occur at focal areas and are only occasionally associated with hair follicles. Similar changes were not noted after passive (diffusion-based) lidocaine exposure or after iontophoresing other molecules such as LHRH or arbutamine. The lidocaine changes appeared immediately after the iontophoretic episode and spontaneously resolved in 5 to 7 days. This change was characterized by the appearance of flattened dark basophilic-staining nuclei oriented parallel to the stratum corneum in the stratum granulosum and spinosum layers. In severe cases, these changes extended down to the stratum basale. The stratum corneum was not affected. Transmission electron microscopy showed specific alterations in the tonofilaments of the epidermal cells, where they had lost their characteristic structure and appeared as an amorphous matrix. An immunological etiology could be ruled out because they occurred both *in vivo* and in the *in vitro* perfused skin flap, which lacks a functional immune system.

This observation led to studies assessing the potential targets in the skin accessible to drugs penetrating the skin under the influence of an electrical field. The anatomical pathway through which a compound traverses the stratum corneum has not been precisely defined. Mercuric chloride was iontophoresed in pig skin and visualized by precipitating the mercury to mercuric sulfide after exposure to ammonium sulfide. These studies unequivocally showed that iontophoresis of mercuric chloride occurs via an intercellular pathway in *in vivo* porcine skin, a finding in agreement with *in vitro* human skin studies. It must be stressed that this technique of mercury precipitation to localize the pathway of transdermal delivery does not measure the active flux of the absorbed ion; rather, it only locates precipitated mercury that has remained after 60 min of iontophoretic administration. However, it is axiomatic that the precipitate reflects mercury that has traversed this pathway. The localization of this precipitate in the deep epidermal and dermal regions by TEM after iontophoresis confirms the potential for transdermal delivery by iontophoresis. The results of passive mercury delivery are essentially identical to those previously reported in human skin and in the nude mouse. This intercellular pathway for the delivery of mercuric chloride by iontophoresis may also provide an anatomical basis for interpreting potential size restrictions on defining the putative "pores" in mathematical models of iontophoresis that assume an intercellular pathway. The maximal diameter correlates better with the width of the intercellular space and not that of a hair follicle shaft or sweat duct.

EXPERIMENTAL TECHNIQUES USED TO ASSESS ABSORPTION

Although generalizations are tenuous at best, human skin appears to be more impermeable than the skin of the cat, dog, rat, mouse, or guinea pig. The skin of pigs and that of some primates serve as useful approximations to human skin, but only after a comparison has been made for each specific substance. The major determinants of species differences are keratinocyte thickness, cell size, hair density, lipid composition, and cutaneous blood flow.

Whole animal *in vivo* studies generally assess the fraction of the applied dose that is absorbed into the body using classic pharmacokinetic techniques, where the absorbed chemical is measured in the blood, urine, feces, and tissues with mass balance calculations. Recently, techniques have been applied to assess absorption by the amount of chemical that has been absorbed into the stratum corneum, assuming that because diffusion is the driving force, the amount in the stratum corneum correlates to the amount of drug finally absorbed into the body. In routine techniques, cellophane tape strips are collected at 30 min after chemical exposure and the amount of drug assayed in these strips is correlated to the amount absorbed using urinary excretion endpoints. If the focus of the research is to determine the amount of chemical that has penetrated the skin, core biopsies may be collected and serially sectioned, and a profile of the chemical as a function of skin depth may be obtained.

There are many *in vitro* approaches to assess topical penetration. Most employ diffusion cell systems, which sandwich skin of various thickness between a donor and a receiver reservoir. The chemical is placed in the donor side (epidermis), and the appearance of compound in the receiver (dermal) is monitored over time. This system can use a variety of "skin" sources, ranging from full-thickness specimens (epidermis and dermis) to epidermis alone to various "artificial" membranes, such as lipid layers. In most skin studies, the donor reservoir is left open to the ambient environment. This basic diffusion cell in which the receiver solution is a fixed volume is called a static cell. If instead, the receiver solution is continuously pumped through the dermal reservoir of the cell, a "flow-through" system results, which mimics the *in vivo* setting where blood continuously removes absorbed compound. Various cell and organ culture approaches that assess the absorption across cultured epidermal and/or dermal membranes have also been developed. The rate of steady state flux can directly be used to calculate a permeability constant (cm^2/s) for the chemical under study.

In vitro studies should be conducted at 35°C to mimic skin surface temperature. Debate exists as to which receptor fluid to use. In pharmaceutical studies involving relatively hydrophilic drugs, saline is often the receptor of choice. In contrast, toxicological investigations generally involve the assessment of lipophilic compounds, which require a receptor fluid in which the penetrant is soluble (e.g., albumin-based buffers and solvent/saline mixtures). These systems have been used to assess cutaneous metabolism, although maintenance of viability using oxygenated perfusate and glucose-containing receptor fluid is then required.

The next level of *in vitro* systems is the use of isolated perfused skin flap (IPSF) preparations, which employ surgically prepared vascularized skin flaps harvested from animals and then transferred to an isolated organ perfusion chamber. This model allows the absorption to be assessed in skin that is viable and anatomically intact and has a functional microcirculation.

Numerous studies have been conducted to assess the percutaneous absorption of drugs and pesticides in the IPSF and then compared to human studies. In all of these studies reported, the correlation between the IPSF and human *in vivo* total absorption was generally high.

Possible Responses of Skin to Chemicals

If a cytotoxic chemical is capable of traversing the stratum corneum, it may have a high probability of causing toxicity to the skin. The clearest approach to assessing chemical-induced damage to skin is to assess what abnormalities occur when the specific anatomical structures discussed previously are perturbed after exposure to topical compounds.

A large number of cutaneous irritants specifically damage the barrier properties of skin, which results in an irritation response. These include organic solvents that extract the intercellular lipid and perturb the skin's barrier, as assessed by increasing TEWL. Some chemicals destroy or digest the stratum corneum and underlying epidermis. These are properly termed corrosives. These compounds cause chemical burns and include strong acids, alkalis, and phenolics. They essentially attack the epidermal barrier and chemically destroy the underlying viable cell layers. The best treatment in these cases is to dilute and remove the offending agents by flushing with water. The exception is CaO (quicklime), which reacts violently with water and generates heat, which causes further thermal damage, and metallic (e.g., tin and titanium) tetrachloride compounds, which hydrolize to hydrochloric acid, causing further damage. These types of reactions are easy to assess using *in vitro* models such as the Corrositex system, which detects macromolecular damage to a collagen matrix resulting in a chemical color change in an associated detector system.

In other cases, epidermal cells are affected, which may then initiate other sequelae. If a penetrating compound is capable of interacting with the immune system, the manifestations seen will be dependent upon the type of immunologic response elicited (e.g., cellular versus humoral and acute hypersensitivity). It should be stressed that immune cells (e.g., Langerhans cells, lymphocytes, and mast cells) may modulate the reaction or the keratinocytes themselves may initiate the response. In fact, keratinocytes were once thought to produce only keratin and mucopolysaccharides, but studies have shown that they can produce growth factors, chemotactic factors, and adhesion molecules. Keratinocytes may act as the key immunocyte in the pathophysiology of allergic contact and irritant contact dermatitis. Figure 4 illustrates the potential pathways that may trigger the production of pro-inflammatory cytokines when skin comes in contact with irritants. Direct irritation of the keratinocytes by toxic chemicals may also initiate this cytokine cascade without the involvement of the immune system, blurring the distinction between direct and indirect cutaneous irritants. The interested reader should consult dermal immunology texts for further details on the broad range of immunological manifestations possible.

It must be stressed that the primary mechanism of many topical irritants (e.g., organic solvents and corrosives) is the impairment to the stratum corneum barrier properties discussed earlier, reflected by an

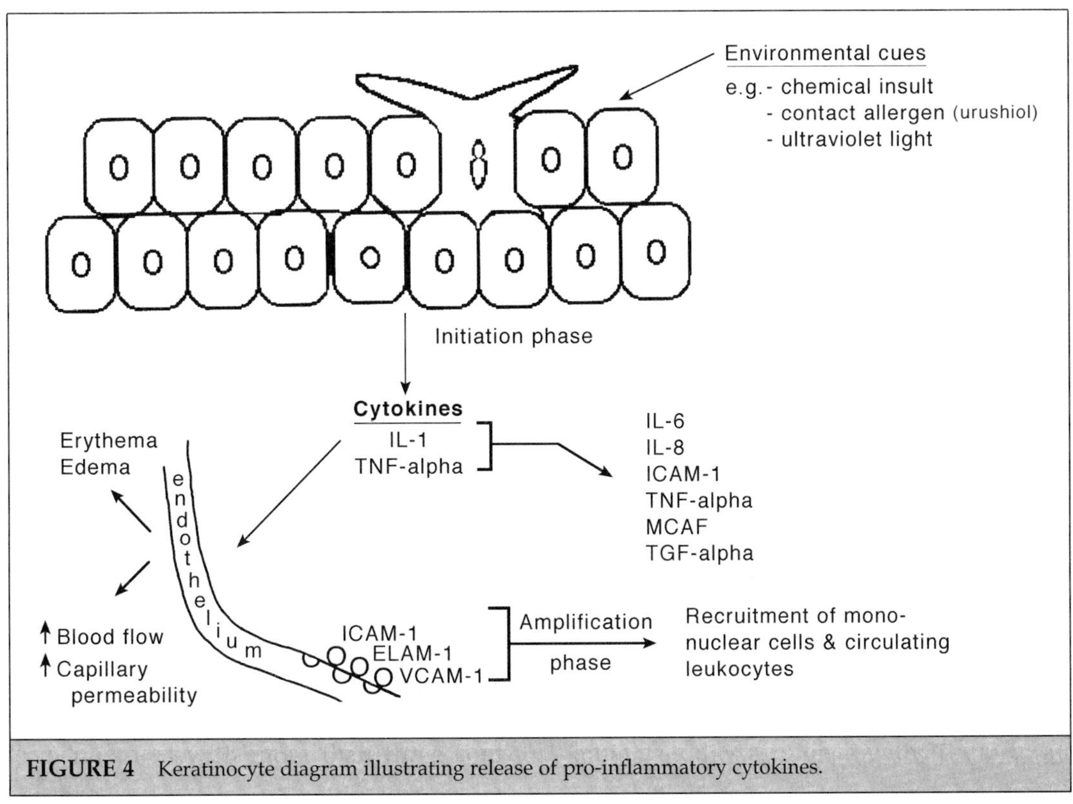

FIGURE 4 Keratinocyte diagram illustrating release of pro-inflammatory cytokines.

TABLE 2 Draize Skin Reaction Assessment Scores

Score	Erythema	Score	Edema
0	No significant change	0	No significant change
1	Very slight (barely perceptible)	1	Very slight (barely perceptible)
2	Well-defined; pale red	2	Slight; edges show definite raising
3	Moderate to severe; definite red; area well defined	3	Moderate; edges raised 1 mm
4	Severe; beet or crimson red	4	Severe; raised more than 1 mm and extending beyond area of exposure

increase in TEWL. If the stratum corneum barrier is perturbed, a feedback response may be initiated whereby the regeneration of the barrier occurs. This reaction is mediated by cytokines (TNF-α) originating locally within the epidermis. However, additional responses to these inflammatory mediators may in themselves launch an irritation response mediated by the keratinocytes. Thus, regardless of the initiating mechanism, the sequelae to many irritants is the same.

Direct Irritation

Direct irritation may be defined as an adverse effect of compounds directly applied topically to the skin, but not involving prior sensitization and thus initiation by an immune mechanism. Several types of adverse effects and chemical interactions may be manifested when a compound is placed upon the skin surface. Irritation is usually assessed by a local inflammatory response characterized by erythema and/or edema. Other responses that do not elicit inflammation, such as an increase in thickness, may be present. Irritant reactions may be classified by many characteristics, including acute, cumulative, traumatic, and pustular; however, two classifications are generally studied by toxicologists. Acute irritation is a local response of the skin usually caused by a single agent that induces a reversible inflammatory response. Cumulative irritation occurs after repeated exposures to the same compound and is the most common type of irritant dermatitis seen. The mechanisms of irritation are thus very complex and are still being characterized since they involve the interaction of inflammatory cytokines with subsequent involvement of the immune system.

Several types of irritancy testing protocols are performed to comply with federal and international safety regulations. The most common test, developed in 1944, is the Draize test to measure acute primary irritation. The test compound is applied in an occluded fashion to a clipped area of abraded and intact skin of at least six albino rabbits and evaluated after 24 h when the patches are removed. The exposed areas are reevaluated at 24 h and 72 h and scored (Table 2). Many modifications have been made to this scoring system over the years, and most cosmetic and pharmaceutical companies have their own modified Draize test. Because these tests are conducted occluded, the irritancy is potentiated due to hydration reducing the skin barrier. The Draize test may be modified to assess sensitization by preexposing animals to a sensitizing dose of the study chemical and then rechallenging the animals at a later date to elicit the immune-mediated response.

Markers of *in vivo* irritancy more sensitive than gross examination have been developed. Many studies have correlated the Draize scores with biophysical estimates of cutaneous barrier function and erythema (the hallmark of skin irritation). As mentioned in the section on absorption, a sensitive indicator of barrier function is TEWL, which increases with irritation. Erythema may be assessed using a myriad of different color-measuring instruments that attempt to objectively quantitate on a continuous scale the subjective categorical assessment inherent to human scoring systems. These systems are based on reflectance principles and operate by irradiating skin with specific light wavelengths and measuring the color of the reflected light. These systems can also detect toxin reactions that alter the melanization process and produces altered skin pigmetation. Erythema, which results from increased blood flow, may be directly assessed using noninvasive laser Doppler velocimetry, which directly measures dermal blood flow.

A great deal of research has been conducted to develop humane alternatives to the Draize test. The majority of these use a skin organ culture approach, which attempts to provide the stratum corneum barrier and viable epidermal cells that can react to penetrated compounds. Because these are essentially organ culture systems, cell viability may be assessed by sampling the bathing culture medium. Glucose utilization is easily assayed. Neutral red (3-amino-7-dimethyl amino-2-methylphenazine hydrochloride) can be used to probe lysosomal integrity, while thiazol blue (MTT), a mitochondrial enzyme substrate, that can be used to assess whether these organelles are metabolically viable. Leakage enzymes, such as lactate dehydrogenase (LDH), can be assayed to detect cell membrane damage. Reactive products (e.g., cytokines and prostaglandins) produced by the keratinocytes may be detected in the culture medium. Alternatively, histochemistry can be performed on the tissue samples and specific enzymes examined that more closely reflect the mechanism of the offending chemical. The IPPSF described previously has also been validated as a useful model for the assessment of direct chemical toxicity in the skin using studies with acids and bases, paraquat, bis (2-chloroethyl sulfide), chlorovinylarsine dichloride, and irritants such as sodium lauryl sulfate.

Phototoxicity

Sunlight that reaches Earth is essential to the survival of most living organisms; however, the skin is continuously exposed and often is adversely affected. Ultraviolet (UV) radiation encompasses shortwave UVC (200–290 nm), midwave UVB (290–320 nm), and longwave UVA (320–400 nm). With the recently identified increase in UVB exposure in certain geographical regions, apparently secondary to ozone depletion, this topic is becoming increasingly important. Although the ozone layer surrounding Earth filters out all UVC radiation, enough UVB and UVA reach Earth's surface to pose chronic and acute health hazards. Most known biological effects, including sunburn and skin cancer, may be attributed to UVB exposure. Sunburn, the excessive cutaneous exposure to UVB radiation, is the most frequent and familiar phototoxic reaction. Phototoxicity is a nonimmunological UV-induced response. The effects on the skin are similar to a typical sunburn, characterized by erythema, edema, vesication, increased skin temperature, and pruritis followed by hyperpigmentation.

Irradiated skin injury is manifested not only grossly by erythema and edema, but also histologically. The most characteristic feature is the presence of sunburn cells, usually found in the stratum basale layer of the epidermis. These cells are dyskeratotic with a bright eosinophilic cytoplasm and a pyknotic nucleus in H&E-stained tissue. Ultrastructurally, they possess cytoplasmic vacuoles and condensed filament masses mixed with remnants of other cytoplasmic organelles. Phototoxicity (UVA and UVB) has been studied with *in vitro* models, which include *Candida albicans*, photohemolysis of red blood cells, tissue culture, and isolated normal human fibroblasts. Such ethical models lack the complexity of living skin systems and are often unreliable. *In vivo* models using guinea pigs, rabbits, mice, and opossum have studied sunburn cells (SBC) in the epidermis following UV radiation. However, the skin of most animal models is not anatomically comparable to human skin, sometimes resulting in false positive or false negative results. Studies have shown that UVB-induced erythema and SBC expression in miniature pigs are comparable to those in humans. These results are not surprising because pig skin has been described as being morphologically and histochemically similar to human skin. Also, epidermal turnover time and the size, orientation, and distribution of vessels in the skin are comparable. Thus the pig is an accepted animal model for studying UV-induced phototoxicity.

The optimal *in vitro* cutaneous model should possess viable cells and structures similar to intact skin, as well as a functional vasculature. This would allow all manifestations of the pathogenesis of UVB exposure to be investigated. The previously described IPPSF was used to study UV phototoxicity using these endpoints. In addition to morphologically assessing the dose-dependent formation of SBCs, decreased glucose utilization was observed accompanied by increased vascular resistance and cell proliferation, decreased by assaying proliferating cell nuclear antigen (PCNA). Levels of prostaglandin E_2 in the perfusate from UVB-exposed skin flaps also increased in a dose-dependent manner, reflecting the cutaneous irritation response. The utility of this model was demonstrated because the morphological, biochemical, and physiological changes could be experimentally monitored and evaluated in the same preparation. Because the absorption of chemicals is similar to *in vivo*, the model has also been used to assess topical therapies that may modulate UVB-induced phototoxicity.

Humans are exposed to a plethora of environmental insults and phototoxic chemicals that may be encountered. In addition to the direct effects of UV light on the skin, some chemicals may be photoactivated to toxic intermediates, which then cause skin toxicity. Exogenous phototoxic chemicals can be found in therapeutic, cosmetic, industrial, or agricultural formulations (Table 3). Phototoxicity may also be caused by endogenous substances resulting from disorders of intermediates of heme biosynthesis, such as porphyrins, which is caused by an inherited or acquired enzymatic defects. Two types of phototoxic events may occur: oxygen-dependent and non-oxygen-dependent. When a reaction involves oxygen, the molecules can absorb the photons and transfer the energy to oxygen

TABLE 3 Phototoxic Compounds

Antiinfectives	Furocoumarins
Nalidixic acid	Angelicin
Sulfanilamide	5 Methoxypsoralen (bergapten)
Tetracyclines	8-Methoxypsoralen (xanthotoxin)
Demethylchlortetracycline	Trimethoxypsoralen
Chemotherapeutics	Nonsteroidal antiinflammatories
Decarbazine	Benoxaprofen
Fluorouracil	Naproxen
Vinblastine	Piroxicam metabolite
Diuretics	Plant products
Hydrochlorothizide	Celery
Furosimide	Figs
Drugs	Limes
Amiodarone	Hogweed
Chlorpromazine	Parsnips
Chloroquin	Fennel
Tolbutamide	Dill
	Polycyclic aromatic hydrocarbons
Dyes	(coal-tar derivatives)
Anthraquinone	Anthracene
Disperse blue 35	Fluoranthene
Eosin	Acridine
Methylene blue	Phenanthrene
Acridine orange	Benzopyrene
Toluidine blue	Creosote
Cadmium sulfide	Pitch
Fragrances	Pyridine
Bergamot oil	Prophrins derivatives
	Hematoporphyrin

molecules thereby generating singlet oxygen, superoxide anions, and hydroxyl radicals that cause damage to the skin. This is what happens to protoprophyrins when they are irradiated. A photochemical reaction involves the absorbance of photons by the chemical, resulting in an excited state that will react with the target molecules to form photoproducts. A good example of this type of reaction is 8-methoxypsoralen (xanthotoxin), which reacts with specific sites on DNA by forming covalent bonds between the pyrimidine base and the furocoumarin. This phototoxic reaction, which may be restricted to areas of the skin exposed to UV light, has been used as a therapeutic technique to treat accessible skin tumors and psoriasis. With other compounds like chlorpromazine and protriptyline, the molecules absorb photons to form stable photoproducts, which then induce cutaneous toxicity.

Vesication

Another mode of chemical-induced damage to the skin involves agents that cause blisters, called chemical vesicants. There are two histological classes of blisters, which implicate different mechanisms of vesication. Intraepidermal blisters are usually formed due to the loss of intercellular attachment caused by cytotoxicity or cell death, while defects in the basement membrane components contribute to the blisters that occur within the epidermal–dermal junction (EDJ). The classic chemical that has been used to define this type of toxicity is the chemical warfare agent sulfur mustard (bis-2-chloroethyl sulfide, HD). HD is a bifunctional alkylating agent that is highly reactive with many biological macromolecules, especially those containing nucleophilic groups, such as DNA and proteins. HD is known for its severe cutaneous damage and systemic toxicity.

The HD-induced dermal lesion is characterized by vesication and slow wound healing. Epidermal–dermal separation associated with vesication occurs in the upper lamina lucida of the basement membrane after HD-induced dermal injury in the IPPSF. It was once thought that alkylation of DNA with subsequent DNA cross-links or breaks was the primary and initial event responsible for HD cutaneous toxicity. Thus, a hypothesis regarding DNA alkylation, metabolic disruption, and proteolytic activity has been proposed. In this scenario after HD exposure, DNA-repair processes are induced, including the activation of poly(ADP-ribose) polymerase, which uses NAD^+ as a substrate. As repair continues, NAD^+ is depleted, which decreases epidermal glycolysis and stimulates activation of the $NADP^+$ dependent hexose monophosphate shunt, resulting in protease release. Extracellular proteases attack the dermal tissue, causing cell death, inflammation, and blister formation. However, results from several laboratories have failed to support this hypothesis. Inhibitors of NAD^+ synthesis did not cause vesication. Additionally, when nicotinamide was used to increase NAD^+ levels, there were normal levels of glycolysis, although cell death and microblister formation still occurred.

Studies using the IPSF have shown that gross blisters and microvesicles, with separation occurring at the upper lamina lucida of the basement membrane, were present at 5 h after HD exposure. This suggests that a basement membrane component is the target of HD alkylation. Other DNA-alkylating agents do not cause vesication and the other pathological changes characterized by HD. Therefore, based on all of these considerations, it is reasonable to think that cell death may not be directly related to HD-induced vesication, although they may occur at the same time. Alkylation of DNA may not be a primary biochemical event in acute cutaneous injury of HD leading to vesication. In fact, HD may have unique protein targets in the cutaneous basement membrane, which leads to diminished stability of the epidermal–dermal junction in the process of dermal toxicity and vesication. HD exposure may be accompanied by apoptosis, which is initiated in the population of epidermal cells in the proper phase of their cell cycle. However, it is unlikely that this would be the primary pathogenic event because all cells must be in the same phase to undergo this form of cell death. Thus, the inflammation, necrosis, and even apoptosis that accompany HD vesication may not be sufficient or specific enough to explain all aspects of this phenomenon.

The jury is still out on the primary mechanism responsible for chemical vesication: DNA alkylation or direct alkylation of basement membrane components. In all probability it is a combination of these processes. The mechanism is important because if alkylation of laminin occurs, it would be expected that wound healing would be delayed, requiring therapeutic strategies that must remove this damaged laminin scaffolding before normal skin regeneration could occur.

CONCLUSION

As can be appreciated from this overview, the field of dermatotoxicology is a complex interaction between unique aspects of dermal anatomy and immunology, properties of the cutaneous barrier, and mechanism of action of cytotoxic agents. The principles apply equally to studies of the effects of exposure to occupational chemicals (e.g., solvents, and corrosives), environmental pollutants (e.g., pesticides and other organics), vesicant agents, cosmetics or dermatologics, and transdermal drugs that are designed to cross the epidermal barrier. To properly study the dermatotoxicity of these chemicals, their ability to penetrate the stratum corneum barrier must be assessed. The target cells or structures in skin must then be defined, the potential cytotoxic response classified, and the ubiquitous cutaneous immune response taken into account. The proper surrogate *in vitro* or *in vivo* models that are capable of characterizing all of these events must be selected to adequately study the nature of the response seen after human exposure.

Bibliography

Baynes, R. E., Brownie, C., Freeman, H., and Riviere, J. E. (1996). *In vitro* percutaneous absorption of benzidine in complex mechanistically defined chemical mixtures. *Toxicol. Appl. Pharmacol.* **141,** 497–506.

Bergstresser, P. R., and Taylor, J. R. (1977). Epidermal "turnover time" a new examination. *Br. J. Dermatol.* **96,** 503–509.

Bijman, J. (1987). Transport processes in the eccrine sweat gland. *Kidney Int.* **32,** S109–Sl12.

Bodde, H. E., de Haan, F. H. N., Kornet, L., Craane-van Hinsberg, W. H. M., and Salomons, M. A. (1991a). Transdermal iontophoresis of mercuric chloride *in vitro*: Electron microscopic visualization of pathways. *Proc. Int. Symp. Control. Rel. Bioact. Mater.* **18,** 301–302.

Bodde, H. E., van den Brink, I., Koerten, H. K., and de Haan F. H. N. J. (1991b). Visualization of *in vitro* percutaneous penetration of mercuric chloride: Transport through intercellular space versus cellular uptake through desmosomes. *Control Rel.* **15,** 227–236.

Bowman, K. F., Monteiro-Riviere, N. A., and Riviere, J. E. (1991). Development of surgical techniques for preparation of *in vitro* isolated perfused porcine skin flaps for percutaneous absorption studies. *Am. J. Vet. Res.* **52,** 75–82.

Crow, K. D., and Puhvel, M. (1977). Chloracne. *In* "Dermatotoxicology" F. N. Marzulli and H. I. Maibach, eds.), 3rd ed., pp. 515–534. Hemisphere Publishing, Washington D. C.

Daniels, Jr. F., (1965). A simple microbiological method for demonstrating phototoxic compounds. *J. Invest. Dermatol.* **44,** 259–263.

Danno, K., and Horio, T. (1980). Histochemical staining of sunburn cells for sulphhydryl and disulphide groups: A time course study. *Br. J. Dermatol.* **102,** 535–539.

Danno, K., and Horio, T. (1982). Formation of UV-induced apoptosis relates to the cell cycle. *Br. J. Dermatol.* **107,** 423–428.

Draize, J. H., Woodard, G., and Calvery, H. O. (1944). Methods for the study of irritation and toxicity of substances applied topically to the skin and mucous membranes. *J. Pharmacol. Exp. Ther.* **82,** 377–390.

Ebling, F. J. G. (1989). Aprocine glands in health and disorder. *Int. J. Dermatol.* **28,** 508–511.

Elias, P. M. (1983). Epidermal lipids, barrier function, and desquamation. *J. Invest. Dermatol.* **80,** 44–49.

Fleisher, A. S., Harber, L. C., Cook, J. S., and Baer, R. L. (1966). Mechanism of in vitro photohemolysis in erythropeoietic protoporphyria (EPP). *J. Invest. Dermatol.* **46,** 505–509.

Forbes, P. D., Urbach, F., and Davies, R. E. (1977). Phototoxicity testing of fragrance raw materials. *Food Cos. Toxicol.* **15,** 55–60.

Freeman, R. G., Murtishaw, W., and Knox, J. M. (1970). Tissue culture techniques in the study of cell photobiology and phototoxicity. *J. Invest. Dermatol.* **54,** 164–169.

Grissom, R. E., Monteiro-Riviere, N. A., and Guthrie, F. E. (1987). A method for preparing mouse skin for assessing *in vitro* dermal penetration of xenobiotics. *Toxicol. Lett.* **36,** 251–258.

Guy, R. H., and Hadgraft, J. (1989). Mathematical models of percutaneous absorption. *In* "Percutaneous Absorption: Mechanisms, Methodology and Drug Delivery" (R. L. Bronaugh and H. I. Maibach, eds.), 2nd ed., pp. 13–26. Dekker, New York.

Halprin, K. M. (1972). Epidermal 'turnover time' a reexamination. *Br. J. Dermatol.* **86,** 14–19.

King, J. R., Riviere, J. E., and Monteiro-Riviere, N. A. (1992). Characterization of lewisite toxicity in isolated perfused skin. *Toxicol. Appl. Pharmacol.* **116,** 189–201.

Lasarow, R. M., Isseroff, R. R., and Gomez, E. C. (1992). Quantitative in vitro assessment of phototoxicity by a fibroblast-neutral red assay. *J. Invest. Dermatol.* **98,** 725–729.

Lavker, R. M., Dong, G., Zheng, P., and Murphy, G. F. (1991). Hairless micropig skin: A novel model for studies of cutaneous biology. *Amer. J. Pathol.* **138,** 687–697.

Ley, R. D., and Applegate, L. A. (1985). Ultraviolet radiation-induced histopathologic changes in the skin of the marsupial *Monodelphis domestica.* II. Quantitative studies of the photoreactivation of induced hyperplasia and sunburn cell formation. *J. Invest. Dermatol.* **85,** 365–367.

Marzulli, F. N., and Maibach, H. I. (1996). Photoirritation (phototoxicity, phototoxic dermatitis). *In* "Dermatotoxicology" (F. N. Marzulli and H. I. Maibach, eds.), 5th ed., pp. 231–237.

Meyer, W., Schwartz, R., and Neurand, K. (1978). The skin of domestic mammals as a model for the human skin, with special reference to the domestic pig. *Curr. Probl. Dermatol.* **7,** 39–52.

Montagna, W., and Yun, J. S. (1964). The skin of the domestic pig. *J. Invest. Dermatol.* **43,** 11–21.

Monteiro-Riviere, N. A. (1986). Ultrastructural evaluation of the porcine integument. *In* "Swine in Biomedical Research" (M. E. Tumbleson, ed.) Vol. 1, pp. 641–655. Plenum Press, New York.

Monteiro-Riviere, N. A. (1990a). Altered epidermal morphology secondary to lidocaine iontophoresis: *In vivo* and *in vitro* studies in porcine skin. *Fundam. Appl. Toxicol.* **15,** 174–185.

Monteiro-Riviere, N. A. (1990b). Specialized technique: Isolated perfused porcine skin flap. *In* "Methods for Skin Absorption" (B. W. Kemppainen and W. G. Reifenrath, eds.), pp. 175–189. CRC Press, Boca Raton FL.

Monteiro-Riviere, N. A. (1991). Comparative anatomy, physiology, and biochemistry of mammalian skin. *In* "Dermal and Ocular Toxicology: Fundamentals and Methods" (D. W. Hobson, ed.). pp. 3–71. CRC Press, New York.

Monteiro-Riviere, N. A., Bristol, D. G., Manning, T. O., and Riviere, J. E. (1990). Interspecies and interegional analysis of the comparative histological thickness and laser Doppler blood flow measurements at five cutaneous sites in nine species. *J. Invest. Dermatol.* **95,** 582–586.

Monteiro-Riviere N. A. and Inman, A. O. (1997). Ultrastructural characterization of sulfur mustard-induced vesication in isolated perfused porcine skin. *Micros. Res. Tech.* **37,** 229–241.

Monteiro-Riviere, N. A., Inman, A. O., and Riviere, J. E. (1994). Development and characterization of a novel skin model for cutaneous phototoxicology. *Photodermatol. Photoimmuno. Photomed.* **10,** 235–243.

Monteiro-Riviere, N. A., Inman, A. O., and Riviere, J. E. (1994). Identification of the pathway of transdermal iontophoretic drug delivery: Light and ultrastructural studies using mercuric chloride in pigs. *Pharm. Res.* **11,** 251–256.

Monteiro-Riviere, N. A., King, J. R., and Riviere, J. E. (1991). Mustard induced vesication in isolated perfused skin: biochemical, physiological, and morphological studies. *In* "Proceedings of the Medical Defense Bioscience Review" pp. 159–162. U.S. Army Medical Research Institute of Chemical Defense, Aberdeen Proving Ground, MD.

Monteiro-Riviere, N. A., and Riviere, J. E. (1991). Cutaneous toxicity of mustard and lewisite on the isolated perfused porcine skin flap. DAMD17-87-C-7139; *NTIS,* ADA229922. pp. 1–144.

Monteiro-Riviere, N. A., Stinson, A. W., and Calhoun, H. L. (1992). The integument. *In* "Textbook of Veterinary Histology" (H. Dieter-Dellman, ed.), pp. 285–312. Lea and Febiger, Malvern, PA.

Monteiro-Riviere, N. A., and Stromberg, M. W. (1985). Ultrastructure of the integument of the domestic pig (*Sus scrofa*) from one through fourteen weeks of age. *Anat. Histol. Embryol.* **14,** 97–115.

Nickoloff, B. J. (1993). "Dermal Immune System." CRC Press, Boca Raton, FL.

Papirmeister, B., Feister, A. J., Robinson, S. I., and Ford, R. D. (1991). "Medical Defense Against Mustard Gas: Toxic Mechanisms and Pharmacological Implications." CRC Press, Boca Raton, FL.

Qiao, G. L., Brooks, J. D., Baynes, R. E., Monteiro-Riviere, N. A., Williams, P. L., and Riviere, J. E. (1996). The use of mechanistically defined chemical mixtures (MDCM) to assess component effects on the percutaneous absorption and cutaneous disposition of topically exposed chemicals. I. Studies with parathion mixtures in isolated perfused porcine skin. *Toxicol. Appl. Pharmacol.* **141,** 473–486.

Quinton, P. M., and Reddy, M. M. (1989). Cl^- conductance and acid secretion in the human sweat duct. *Ann. NY Acad. Sci.* **574,** 438–446.

Riviere, J. E. (1994). Absorption and distribution. *In* "Introduction to Biochemical Toxicology" (E. Hodgson and P. E. Levi, eds.), pp. 11–48. Appleton and Lange, East Norwalk.

Riviere, J. E. (1999). "Comparative Pharmacokinetics: Principles, Techniques and Applications." Iowa State University Press, Ames (in press).

Riviere, J. E., and Heit, M. C. (1997). Electrically-assisted transdermal drug delivery. *Pharm. Res.* **14,** 687–697.

Riviere, J. E., Monteiro-Riviere N. A., and Williams, P. L. (1995). Isolated perfused porcine skin flap as an *in vitro* model for predicting transdermal pharmacokinetics. *Eur. J. Biopharm.* **41,** 152–162.

Sambuco, C. P. (1985). Miniature swine as an animal model in photodermatology: Factors influencing sunburn cell formation. *Photodermatol. Photoimmunol. Photomed.* **2,** 144–150.

Sharata, H. H., and Burnette, R. R. (1988). Effect of dipolar aprotic permeability enhancers on the basal stratum corneum. *J. Pharm. Sci.* **77,** 27–32.

Spoo, J. W., Rogers, R. A., and Monteiro-Riviere, N. A. (1993). Effects of formaldehyde, DMSO, benzoyl peroxide, and sodium lauryl sulfate on isolated perfused porcine skin, *In Vitro Toxicol.* **5,** 251–260.

Srikrishna, V., and Monteiro-Riviere, N. A. (1991). The effects of sodium hydroxide and hydrochloric acid on isolated perfused skin. *In Vitro Toxicol.* **4,** 207–215.

Srikrishna, V., Riviere, J. E., and Monteiro-Riviere, N. A. (1992). Cutaneous toxicity and absorption of paraquat in porcine skin. *Toxicol. Appl. Pharmacol.* **115,** 89–97.

Stewart, M. E. (1992). Sebaceous gland lipids. *Seminars in Dermatol.* **11,** 100–105.

Williams, P. L., Thompson, D., Qiao, G. L., Monteiro-Riviere, N. A., and Riviere, J. E. (1996). The use of mechanistically defined chemical mixtures (MDCM) to assess mixture component effects on the percutaneous absorption and cutaneous disposition of topically exposed chemicals. II. Development of a general dermatopharmacokinetic model for use in risk assessment. *Toxicol. Appl. Pharmacol.* **141,** 487–496.

Woodcock, A., and Magnus, I. A. (1976). The sunburn cell in mouse skin: Preliminary quantitative studies on its production. *Br. J. Dermatol.* **95,** 459–468.

Zhang, Z., Peters, B. P., and Monteiro-Riviere, N. A. (1995a). Assessment of sulfur mustard interaction with basement membrane components. *Cell Biol. Toxicol.* **11,** 89–101.

Zhang, Z., Riviere, J. E., and Monteiro-Riviere, N. A. (1995b). Topical sulfur mustard induces changes in prostaglandins and interleukin-1α in isolated perfused porcine skin. *In Vitro Toxicol.* **8,** 149–157.

CHAPTER

19

The Eye

D. A. SCHWINDT, H. F. MERK

Department of Dermatology and Allergology, University Clinic, Aachen, Germany

In the early 1930s, the use of artificial eyelashes containing *p*-phenylenediamine caused severe eye injury with necrosis, ulceration, blindness, and even death. A toxicological assay was therefore necessary that would predict and, ideally, prevent such eye damage. Intense research resulted in the introduction of the Draize test. This test serves in its modified version as a standard for the evaluation of acute toxic eye injury.

ANATOMY OF THE EYEBALL

The eyeball is made up of three layers, the fibrous layer comprising the cornea and sclera; the vascular layer or uveal tract, comprising the iris, ciliary body, and choroid; and the nervous layer, or retina, comprising sensory and neural epithelium. These layers build the anterior eye chamber, a site often chosen for toxicological testing. The angles of the anterior chambers are essential for the drainage of the aqueous humor. Bowman's and Descemet's membranes, together the vitreous membrane, ensure a high water content of up to 75% of the cornea. Thus, despite the high inner-eye pressure of about 15 to 20 mm Hg, tissue elasticity is provided (turgescence). Descemet's membrane, which is 5 to 10 μm thick, represents the basal membrane of the endothelium and has especially high ATPase activity. This enzyme maintains the electrolytic flow and thus cornea hydration. In the posterior chamber is the ciliary body, whose epithelium produces the aqueous humor. The inner eye chamber contains the jelly-like vitreous humor.

ACUTE TOXICITY

Studies on acute toxicity in the eye have been primarily descriptive, and only a few investigations report on pathomechamisms. For ideal vision, the optic system, the photoreceptors, and the conducting nerves have to perform and interact at optimum. A layer of tears (lacrima) protects the eye from dryness and infection. Acute toxicity, when accompanied by reduced lacrima production, can result in ulceration and even total loss of the cornea and vision. The causative agent may have contaminated the eye directly or may have been taken in orally. Repeated intake of chloroquine, an antimalarial drug, in doses of 250–500 mg/day can, for example, cause keratopathy. Therefore, toxicological investigation and assessment are often needed. Eye inflammation, frequently accompanied by conjunctival hyperemia, is a reversible reaction of the eye and its mucous membranes. Toxicological testing must evaluate an appropriate time period (21 days), as some substances might cause pain but no signs of inflammation, or lead not only to acute but also to delayed reactions. Alkali may cause severe

TABLE 1 Drugs with Definite or Presumable Risk of Cataractogenesis[a]

Cataractogenic[b]	Potentially cataractogenic[b]
Corticosteroids	Benzodiazepins
Phenothiazines	Phenytoin
Miotic agents	Methoxsalen
Metals	Allopurinol
Alkylating agents	Amiodarone
Locally anesthetic eye drops	Oral Contraceptives

[a]From Herbst and Maibach (1991), *Contact Dermatitis* **25,** 305–321, © 1991 Munksgaard International Publishers Ltd. Copenhagen, Denmark.
[b]Cataract = clouding of the lenses.

injury—corneal edema, loss of corneal glycoaminoglycanes, vascularization, cicatrices, severe conjunctivitis, and uveitis have been described. Damage of the lens and retina can occur. Acids usually result in mild damage, superficial erosions, and swelling and hemorrhage of the conjunctiva; stronger acids, however, might cause necrosis. (See Table 1.)

Detergents

Another group of potentially eye-damaging substances is detergents. Their toxic potency differs depending on their charge, either anionic, cationic, or neutral. Cationic detergents are mainly quartenary ammonium salts, such as benzalkoniumchloride. Although it is only slightly toxic, and is even a component of eye drops at lower concentration, higher concentrations of benzalkonium chloride might cause severe eye injury. Anionic detergents are mainly sodium or potassium salts with long-chain fatty acids (soaps), which are of lower toxicity. Neutral detergents, such as fatty acids, fatty alcohols with polyoxyethylene, and sorbitol, have the lowest eye toxicity. Some local anesthetics deserve special attention. (See Table 2.)

TABLE 2 Commercially Available Drugs That Disturb the Electroretinogram[a]

Pharmacological group	International trade name
Tranquilizer	
Thioxanthen derivatives	Chlorprothixene
Butyrophenone derivatives	Metixene Haloperidol Spiroperidol[b] Trifluperidol
Alkaloids	Reserpine Meprobamate Diazepam Chlordiazepoxide
Antidepressants	
Dibenzazepine	Imipramine Desipramine
Antiepileptics	
Oxazolin derivatives	Trimethadione

[a]Clinically no retinal damage demonstrated, 1993.
[b]Not distributed in Germany.

Organic Solvents

Occupational or domestic contamination of the eye may occur with neutral organic solvents, such as ethanol, ethyl ether, acetone, ethyl acetate, hexane, or benzene. As all these substances are lipid solvents, they induce pain; severe exposure may cause cloudiness, which has been attributed to a partial loss of epithelial cells. The irritation of the sensitive nerve endings of the cornea seems to be responsible for the pain reaction. Injury is reversible, though, when contamination occurs at room temperature (approximately 20°C), as all these substances are volatile. Severe injury has been reported after contamination with hot solvents, where thermal damage contributes considerably to the overall damage. For example, the use of trichlorosilane ($HSiCl_3$), used in the electronic industry for microchip cleaning, bears a high risk. When mixed with air, this substance is explosive and then decomposes, evolving HCl vapor, which might be irritating to the eye.

Methanol

Methanol is a well known cause of ocular toxicity, neurological symptoms, metabolic acidosis, and vasodilatation, leading to blindness and even death. As a common industrial solvent, it is used, for example, as antifreeze fluid and as a component of paint removers. Methanol intoxication was common during Prohibition and World War II because of its use as an adulterant. Methanol is rapidly absorbed by inhalation, oral, and topical exposure. In primates, metabolism by an alcohol dehydrogenase system occurs rapidly and yields the toxic intermediates formaldehyde and formic acid. Whereas formaldehyde is rapidly oxidized to formic acid, with a half-life of about 1.5 min, formic acid is only slowly metabolized to CO_2, and therefore accumulates in the tissues, including the eye. A severe metabolic acidosis results, which precedes the most distinct aspect of methanol intoxica-

TABLE 3 Scoring of Eye Lesions

Cornea	
Severity of corneal cloudiness (*A*)	
None	0
Diffuse, iris clearly visible	1
Moderate loss of transparency, iris little adhesive,	2
Loss of transparency, details of the iris barely visible	3
Loss of transparency, iris not visible	4
Area of involved cornea (*B*)	
Less than 1/4, but not 0	1
More than 1/4, but less than 1/2	2
More than 1/2, but less than 3/4	3
More than 3/4 to complete	4
Iris (*A*)	
Normal	0
Edema, displacement, reaction to light	1
No reaction to light, hemorrhage, destruction	2
Conjunctiva	
Vascularization (*A*)	
Normal vessels	0
Vascularization	1
Diffuse vascularization, individual vessels can not be differentiated	2
Edema, closure of eyelids incomplete (half)	3
Edema, closure of eyelids incomplete (less than half)	4
Contracture (*B*)	
No contracture	0
Different from normal	1
Contracture of lid and lashes (esp. in contact zone)	2
Contracture of lid, lashes and lid margin	3

tion, visual impairment. In a first phase, after approximately 3 days, the pupils are dilated and unreactive, and the vision is blurred due to retinal edema. The second phase may be observed after intake of even small amounts (15 mg) of methanol; loss of the ganglion cells and optic atrophy often result in permanent blindness. It is generally accepted that not formaldehyde, but formic acid plays the predominant role in methanol toxicity. For example, ocular toxicity essentially identical to that produced in methanol poisoning has been described after formate treatment. As formic acid is an inhibitor of mitochondrial cytochrome oxidase, it causes decreased intracellular ATP and histotoxic hypoxia. Thus, formate accumulation accounts for metabolic acidosis, either directly by delivering protons or indirectly as a result of hypoxic metabolism. Methanol itself appears to be essentially nontoxic. Recent investigations, however, have demonstrated its direct contractile effect on canine cerebral arteries. An intracellular release of calcium seems to be required for these methanol-induced contractions; moreover, magnesium deficiency seems to potentiate the observed effects. Spasms of the major cerebral blood vessels could result in severe deficits in cerebral blood flow and may account for the CNS and possibly the eye disturbances.

Studies on the kinetics of methanol metabolism revealed species-specific differences. In rodents, the reaction of formic acid to CO_2 occurs faster, and formic acid does not accumulate to the degree observed in primates. Thus, the results of methanol toxicity studies in rodents cannot predict its toxicity in primates.

Treatment aims at combating acidosis and preventing methanol oxidation. Ethanol, which competes for alcohol dehydrogenase, should be administered to block the formate, and folic acid should be administered to enhance formate oxidation to carbon dioxide. Dialysis for the elimination of formic acid should be prolonged to compensate for a deranged cellular proton excretion mechanism.

EYE IRRITANTS

A great number of substances may cause tearing at low concentrations. Besides natural substances (e.g., onions), some substances are specially used to cause tearing, the tear gases. The most widely used substances are α-chloroacetophenone, α-bromobenzyle cyanide, and ethyl iodoacetate. These substances cause strong tearing. At very high concentrations, as might be the case when they are sprayed from a short distance, they can result in permanent cloudiness.

The mechanism of action seems to be related to the inhibition of sulfhydryl-containing enzymes, a characteristic that all of these substances have in common. On the other hand, not all the compounds that bind to SH groups cause tearing (i.e., iodoacetate and British Anti-Lewisite (BAL)). Heavy summer smog can also result in tearing; compounds that develop from car emissions under UV light are held responsible, for example, ozone, nitrous oxides (NO_x), olefins, aromates, and aliphatic carbohydrates. Peroxyalkyl nitrates have some effect on the induction of tearing. Thus, they are presumably the cause of the irritation.

Draize Test

To test eye inflammation, the substance to be tested is applied to the conjunctival sac and fixed over a set time period. Eye reactions are evaluated over 21 days. The contralateral eye serves as control. The reaction is scored and analyzed as to the involvement of cornea, iris, and conjunctiva. Various test systems use different score units, complicating a comparison between the scoring systems. (See Table 3.)

TABLE 4 Frequent Sensitizers in Eye Cosmetics

Preservatives	**Epoxides**	**Antibiotics**	**Local anesthetics**
Parabens	Colophony	Bacitracin	Benzocaine
Phenyl mercuric acetate	Dihydroabietyl	Chloamphenicol	Procaine
Imidazolidinyl urea	Alcohol	Gentamicin sulfate	Oxybuprocaine
Quarternium-15	Ointment bases	Kanamycin	Proxymetacaine
Benzalkoniumchloride	Lanolin	Neomycine sulfate	**Enzymatic contact lens cleaners**
Chlorhexidinegluconate	Propylene glycol	Polymyxin-B-sulfate	Papain
Cetalkoniumchloride	**Beta-blocking agents**	Thiamphenicol	Tegobetain
Na-EDTA	Befunolol	**Antiviral agents**	**Miotic agents**
Sorbic acid	Levubenulol	Ido(deso)xuridine	Pilocarpine
Thiomersal	Metipranolol	Trifluridine	Tolazoline
Antioxidants	Timolol	**Antihistamines**	ε-Aminocaproic acid
Butylated hydroxyanisole	**Mydriatric agents**	Chlorphenoxamine maleate	
Butylated hydroxytoluene	Atropine sulfate	Sodium cromoglycate	
Propyl gallate	Scopolamine		
Di-*tert*-butyl-hydroquinone	Hydrobromide		

Alternatives to the Draize test for testing eye irritancy are needed; in, particular, the applicability to the human eye as a test is questionable. Various test systems, done *in vitro* and *in vivo,* and differing in their endpoint definitions, have not yet replaced the Draize test because of their lack of safety. However, they are used as screening tests, reducing the large number of Draize-tested animals. The more important tests are performed on *in vitro* cell systems. They are derived either directly from eye tissue or from easily accessible cells, such as fibroblasts or keratinocytes, that can be obtained from hair follicles, thus not requiring biopsies. Concerning *in vivo* tests, the hen's egg test deserves mention; this is regarded as an animal experiment in several countries. Varying endpoint definitions have been tested in *in vitro* cell systems to determine cytotoxicity, DNA or RNA content, protein content, expression of shock proteins, enzyme deliberation, and dye uptake or release.

Periorbital Eczema

The very sensitive periorbital skin is especially prone to irritant reactions, often affecting patients with atopic dermatitis. Direct or indirect sensitizing can cause periorbital allergic contact dermatitis. Especially those sensitizers that are part of the standard series for patch testing play a role (Table 4).

Bibliography

Bruner, L. H. (1992). Ocular irritation. *In* "In Vitro Toxicity Testing" (J. M. Frazier, ed.), pp. 149–190. Marcel Dekker, New York.

Chan, P. K., and Hayes, A. W. (1989). Principles and methods for acute toxicity and eye irritancy. *In* Hayes, A. W. (ed.): "Principles and Methods of Toxicology" (A. W. Hayes, ed.), 2nd ed., pp. 169–220. Raven Press, New York.

Draelos, Z. K. (1991). Eye cosmetics. *Dermatol. Clinics* **9,** 1–7.

Franzier, J. M. (1991). Alternatives to acute ocular and dermal toxicity tests in animals. *In* Marzulli, F.N.; Maibach, H.I.: "Dermatotoxicology" (F. N. Marzulli and H. I. Maibach, eds.), 4th ed., pp. 814–833. Hemisphere Publishing Corp., New York.

Frankenberg, S., Jugert, F., and Merk, H. (1993). Multiple cytochrome P450 isoenzymes present in human hair follicle derived keratinocytes. *J. Invest. Dermatol.* **100,** 518.

Herbst, R. A., and Maibach, H. I. (1991). Contact dermatitis caused by allergy to ophthalmic drugs and contact lens solutions. *Contact Dermatitis* **25,** 305–321.

Luepke, N. P. (1986). The hen's egg test (HET)—An alternative toxicity test. *Br. J. Dermatol.* **115,** 133–135.

Li, W., Altura, B. T., and Altura, B. M. (1998). Methanol-induced contraction of canine cerebral artery and its possible mechanism of action. *Toxicol. Appl. Pharmacol.* **150,** 361–368.

MacMartin, K. E., Ambre, J. J., and Tephly, T. R. (1980). Methanol poisoning in human subjects. *Am. J. Med.* **67,** 804–807.

Liesivuori, J., and Savolainen, H. (1991). Methanol and formic acid toxicity: Biochemical mechanisms. *Pharmacol. Toxicol.* **69,** 157–163.

CHAPTER

20

Nervous System

K. ANDREAS*, D. E. RAY[†]
[†]Neurotox Section, MRC Toxicology Laboratory, University Leicester, Leicester, England
*Institute of Pharmacology and Toxicology, Technical University, Dresden, Germany

Neurotoxicology is a relatively young speciality within toxicology and has developed much since the 1960s. Neurotoxic agents have been recognized since the earliest times, natural products such as strychnine, nicotine, tetrodotoxin, curare, arsenic and mercury, being used as poisons both legally and illegally. Socrates was executed by being made to drink the juice of the hemlock (*Conium maculatum*), which contains the neurotoxic alkaloid conine. The neurotoxicity of inorganic lead has been known since Roman times and became a major problem in Europe with industrial development in the 19th century. However, it was perhaps the need to understand the action of neurotoxic organophosphorous compounds in the 1940s that first stimulated the development of the academic discipline of neurotoxicology.

Much of our basic knowledge of the organization and function of the nervous system comes from experimental work with selectively neurotoxic substances such as curare, strychnine, and tetrodotoxin. In this way the use of neurotoxic agents has contributed greatly to neuroscience. With industrialization and increased human exposure to neurotoxicants in the workplace and environment, neurotoxicology has also become a practical concern, but has continued to benefit from basic neuroscience for the understanding of mechanisms. Hence a general appreciation of the principles of morphological and functional neuroscience, as well as knowledge of the basic toxicology, is necessary for an understanding of neurotoxicity. Factors such as the blood–brain barrier, neuronal energy requirements, the role of myelin, synaptic transmission, and the limited regenerative ability of neurons are all important features that need to be understood before one can study the response of the nervous system to toxic agents. The very specialized measures needed to detect neurotoxicity also present a challenge to the beginner in this area. An outline of the major approaches is given in this chapter.

FUNCTIONS OF THE NERVOUS SYSTEM

The nervous system is an extraordinarily complex network of cellular connections. It forms the structural basis of recognition, perception, memory, speech, locomotion, and feeling, as well as unconscious hormonal and autonomic functions. The brain and spinal cord are the principal components of the central nervous system. The peripheral nervous system is subdivided into somatic and autonomic components. The somatic parts are the cranial nerves, the spinal nerve roots, the dorsal root ganglia, and the peripheral nervous pathways with their motor and sensory terminals and their special receptors. Because the retina contains the cell bodies of the optic (or second cranial) nerve and the retina and optic nerve are both protected by blood–tissue barriers in the same way as the brain, it is useful to class the retina with the central nervous system. The peripheral autonomic system consists of the parasympathetic pathways of the cranial and sacral nerves with their associated ganglia and the sympathetic system with its paravertebral ganglionic chain and associated ganglia. All parts of the central and peripheral nervous systems are potential targets of toxic effects.

Neurons are the primary functional cell type of the nervous system and show marked cellular differentiation, with long processes termed dendrites and axons. The dendrites are multiple and are ramified and densely interconnected with axonal processes to receive, integrate, and conduct neuronal signals. The structure of the neuronal network is the basis for interneuronal communication, coordination, and the functional integration of the nervous system. The axon is single (although sometimes bifurcated), and is an exceptionally long process in cellular terms. A single motor axon can extend as far as from the sacrolumbar cord to the foot muscles. Central axons can span from the dorsal tracts of the spinal cord to the somatosensory neocortex, where touch, vibration, proprioception, and pain are perceived.

Each region of the neuron has a special function. The dendrites and the membrane surface of the cell body are the basis of the transduction and integration of incoming synaptic signals. The molecular constituents of the cytoskeleton and cell membrane and transmitters used in the axon terminals are synthesized in the cell body. Materials produced in the cell body pass through the axonal cytoplasm by active transport, while the axonal membrane conducts the information encoded by the action potentials. Chemical communication at the synapse requires both presynaptic and post-synaptic receptors. Any local defect within neurons produces specific injuries. Thus, for example, specific effects are seen following damage to the myelin sheath, as signal transmission and conduction velocity depend on the integrity of the myelin.

Other cell types have distinct functions and can also be targets for neurotoxic chemicals. In the central nervous system, astrocytes control development during early life and maintain vascular, ionic, and metabolic homeostasis. It is the chemical environment created by astrocytes that limits neuronal regrowth within the adult central nervous system. Oligodendrocytes are responsible for myelination of central axons. Microglial cells are responsible for immune surveillance in the central nervous system and show a characteristic reaction to damage (gliosis). The endothelial cells of brain blood vessels are specialized to form tight junctions, which give rise to the blood–brain barrier. In the peripheral nervous system, Schwann cells are responsible for the myelination of axons. Part of the extracellular space of the central nervous system forms a series of linked ventricles, which are filled with cerebrospinal fluid. This is secreted by the choroid plexi and has a highly regulated composition similar to plasma, but much lower in protein. The ventricles are lined by ciliated ependymal cells.

THE NERVOUS SYSTEM AS A TARGET FOR TOXIC CHEMICALS

The nervous system presents a target to toxic chemicals that is very variable, across both region and cell type, and also with time. Different cell types and anatomical regions show different degrees of vulnerability. Consequently, few if any agents are general neurotoxicants—most are selective in their action. This causes neurotoxicologists problems in diagnosis and the design of test systems, as there is no one "typical" neurotoxic agent or vulnerable neuron. Although the number of basic cell types is no larger than in other tissues, the chemical and morphological differentiation within these cell types is extreme, and this leads to differential vulnerability to toxic agents (Table 1).

Vulnerability

Adult brain neurons are terminally differentiated and thus incapable of replacement by cell division. To ensure the reliable transmission of action potentials from one neuron to another, very high densities of ion channels are expressed, which, if activated in a prolonged manner (as by a neurotransmitter analog such as the algal neurotoxin kainic acid), can lead to uncontrollable and ultimately cytotoxic transmembrane ion and water fluxes. The need to maintain ion gradients in the face of even normal ion channel activity requires continuous ion pumping, and this results in the brain having an obligate resting glycolytic demand as high as the demand of maximally exercising skeletal muscle. If this activity is not maintained, toxicant-induced loss of function can lead to the death of the whole organism as a result of respiratory failure or other maladaptive behavior. Neurons with long ax-

TABLE 1 Examples of Mechanisms in Selective Neurotoxicity

Target distribution
Kainate (ligand-gated ion channels)
Pyrethroids (voltage-gated ion channels)
Carbamates (ligand inactivation systems)
Bioactivation
Phenytoin (by P450 in cerebellar motor nuclei)
MPTP (to MPP^+)
Access
Cysteine (in areas with poor blood–brain barrier)
Uptake
$MPTP^+$ uptake by mitochondria; flurocitrate (into astrocytes)
Sequestration
Lead (neuronal toxicity reduced by cerebral astrocytes)

onal processes are particularly specialized, processes of at least one meter in length being supported by the cell body. This requires highly efficient intracellular transport and communication processes and makes long neurons particularly vulnerable to any agents that disrupt the cytoskeleton or interfere with energy supply.

Vulnerability may vary with time or functional state, as well as with cell type. This can lead to unexpected interactions, as illustrated in controlled experiments on rats in which an increase in sound input to just one ear during intoxication with metronidazole or dinitrobenzene produces a correspondingly increased severity of the lesions caused by these agents in the auditory pathway on the stimulated side. Similarly, if motor activity is increased during dinitrobenzene poisoning, greater lesion severity is seen in brain-stem motor areas; and the ototoxicity produced by carbon monoxide or by aminoglycoside antibiotics is enhanced by moderate auditory stimulation. Such lesions may be termed use-dependent, and similar effects have occasionally been described in humans, although it is obviously much more difficult to be sure of exactly what the functional state is during chronic poisoning. However, it has been noted that lead or thallium neuropathies occur more frequently in the dominant arm, and that the ototoxicity produced by toluene or carbon disulfide is enhanced in noisy working environments.

Resistance

Opposing these vulnerability factors are others conferring resistance on the nervous system. These also vary with cell type or with functional state.

The remarkable degree of flexibility of brain function is very important. Few higher brain functions can be localized to a specific area and, even when they are so localized, often other areas are capable of taking over their specific functions if they are damaged. Thus relatively large forebrain lesions (if they are symmetrical, as most chemically induced lesions are) produce only small deficits in function once time is allowed for recovery. In the case of slowly developing lesions, loss of function may not even be noticed unless it is unmasked by the effects of aging. A further source of resistance is the strong homeostatic protection of the brain environment by the equally specialized brain vasculature. The blood–brain barrier formed by endothelial cell tight junctions prevents most hydrophobic chemicals with unwanted neuroactivity from reaching the brain. This barrier protection is achieved, however, at the energy cost of requiring active transport of all nutrients across the barrier. Brain homeostasis is maintained even in the face of large changes in blood pressure, oxygen supply, and ionic balance. Glial support cells (astrocytes, oligodendrocytes, and microglia) have taken over many specialized functions, such as the maintenance of ion balance, myelin synthesis, and immune surveillance.

Selective Toxicity

Selective toxicity is often seen, even where the target appears at first sight to be uniform, as with agents that selectively attack either central or peripheral myelin (cuprizone and tellurium, respectively). Sometimes it is possible to relate this selective toxicity to specific aspects of the extreme specialization of the nervous system (Table 1). Selective neurotoxicity can usefully be considered to be a consequence of

1. The need to transfer excitation rapidly and completely from a small synapse to a large cell body or dendritic tree. In excess this leads to excitotoxicity.
2. The need to sustain and control long axonal processes distant from the cell body. If disrupted, this leads to axonopathy.
3. The need to maintain a highly specialized electrically insulating layer about the myelinated axons. Damage to this is termed myelinopathy.
4. The need to maintain transmembrane ion gradients in the face of ion channel activity, which necessitates a very high rate of glycolysis. Interference with this leads to energy depletion neurotoxicity.
5. The highly ordered sequence of developmental events needed to produce the adult nervous system. This leads to the highly specific time windows of vulnerability that are seen in developmental neurotoxicity.

The component cells of the nervous system are, of course, also vulnerable to modes of toxicity common to all cells and are killed by extremes of pH, low oxygen tension, and deprivation of energy. However, the intact nervous system occupies a uniquely privileged place with regard to homeostatic control, being for example the last tissue to lose weight during adult or developmental malnutrition. Hence, although neurotoxicity may occassionally be the result of gross systemic disturbance, as in hepatic encephalopathy or carbon monoxide poisoning, neurotoxicity generally arises from an attack on a specific property of the nervous system.

Blood–Brain Barrier

The central nervous system is protected against external influences by a morphologically defined barrier. Paul Ehrlich observed as early as 1885 that intravenously injected acidic vital dyes fail to reach the brain and the spinal cord, even though other organs are stained. He came to the conclusion that a barrier exists, later called the "blood–brain barrier." It was subsequently realized that the barrier was to the large protein molecules that bound these dyes, rather than to the dyes themselves.

The morphological basis of the barrier (Fig. 1) in mammals is the tight junction (zonula occludens) between the cells of the capillary endothelium in the central nervous system. The trophic influence of the perivascular end feet of astrocytes contributes to the maintenance of this barrier. The tight junctions between endothelial cells prevent molecules from passing between them. Hence, those molecules that cannot pass through the cell membranes cannot enter the extracellular space within brain tissue. This barrier excludes those water-soluble molecules that do not have specific transport systems, but allows lipophilic molecules to pass. In addition to the morphological barrier, there are also a chemical barrier, with much of the phase-I and phase-II xenobiotic metabolizing capacity of brain tissue, and a multidrug resistance transporter, which is concentrated in the endothelium and astrocytes. The blood–brain barrier has gaps at the margins of the central nervous system, in the dorsal root ganglia and autonomic ganglia, and also in those brain areas that need to maintain direct contact with the blood, such as the median eminence, the area postrema, the subfornical organ, and the neurohypophysis. The cerebrospinal fluid (CSF) is protected from anything that might enter through these few open barrier areas by tight ependymal junctions, which prevent drainage from them into the CSF. There is no ependymal diffusion barrier in other brain areas, the extracellular space of which is in passive equilibrium with the CSF.

Toxic agents can damage the blood–brain barrier directly or indirectly. High blood pressure (mean arterial pressure in excess of 180 mm Hg) or extreme vasodilatation produced by hypercapnia can cause a breakdown of the barrier as a result of increased vessel wall tension. Toxic chemicals that cause prolonged seizures can therefore produce secondary barrier breakdown. Other chemicals act directly on the barrier. Barrier breakdown may lead to edema and entry of plasma proteins or, in more severe cases, to petechial hemorrhage. Inorganic lead can cause barrier breakdown in neonates, as can nitropropionate, dinitrobenzene, and metronidazole in adults. Hepatic encephalopathy can also lead to barrier breakdown, as can strongly hyperosmolar intravascular injections. The latter have been exploited therapeutically, and the barrier has been opened in this way to enable antibiotics and anticancer drugs to gain access to the brain.

The blood–brain barrier is incomplete at the time of birth. Hence the immature brain is more sensitive to substances normally excluded by the barrier, for example, protein-bound inorganic lead or unbound bilirubin associated with liver damage.

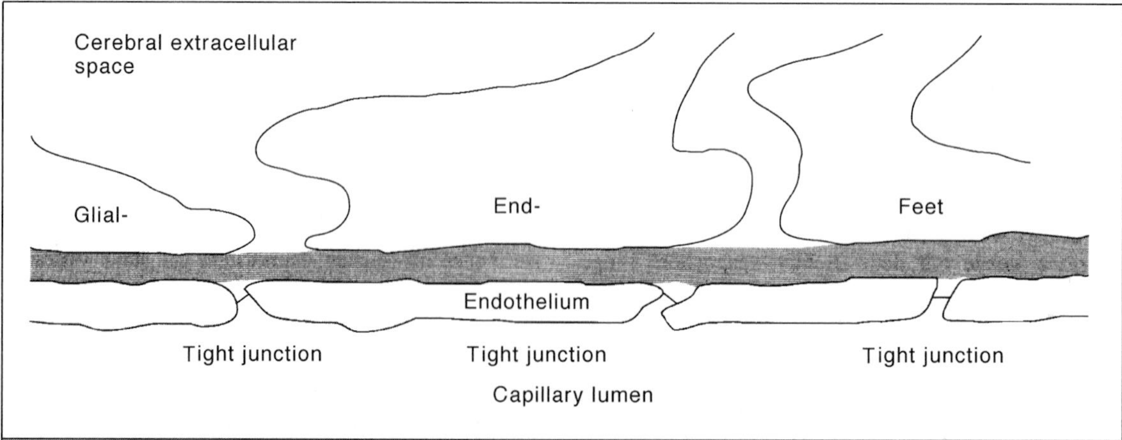

FIGURE 1 Blood–brain barrier, schematic representation. Endothelial cells are tightly connected by Zonulae occludentes (tight junctions). Astrocytic end feet cover the capillaries.

ACUTE AND CHRONIC NEUROTOXIC EFFECTS

Some neurotoxic agents produce effects that are purely acute and reversible, such as the narcosis produced by anesthetics or most organic solvents. For such agents, only chronic exposure can produce a chronic effect, and this effect will disappear once exposure ceases. In contrast, other agents can produce a chronic effect from just a single acute exposure. Such chronic effects last much longer than the duration of exposure and may even be irreversible. Thus, acrylamide can produce a persisting neuropathy, even though acrylamide itself disappears from the body with a half-life of a few hours. Other agents produce a mixture of both acute and chronic effects, and this can lead to complex situations. Thus, some organophosphates produce both an acute reversible toxicity via inhibition of acetylcholinesterase and a poorly reversible chronic axonopathy. Similarly, *n*-hexane produces both an acute reversible narcosis and a lasting degeneration of peripheral nerves. In both of these cases, the agents produce their acute and their chronic effects by completely different mechanisms, but many neurotoxic agents are found to have more than one mechanism of action.

It is therefore important to distinguish clearly between acute or chronic exposures and acute or chronic effects. Sometimes an apparently chronic effect may not be so, due to a failure to recognize that some lipophilic agents can have surprisingly long half-lives and still be present in the body after exposure has ceased. Thus white spirits (a solvent) have a major body half-life of about 180 h. Reversibility of action is a key feature in determining the severity of neurotoxicity; reversible changes are generally less significant. However, acute reversible effects can be equally important in some contexts. For example, substituted hydrocarbons are used as both industrial solvents and anesthetics. The molecular events leading to the stabilization of membranes and inhibition of ion fluxes are the same for both uses, as are the consequences they produce in the brain: impaired alertness, uncoordination, sedation, anesthesia, and respiratory depression. Such effects are fully reversible on discontinued exposure and cause no problems in the context of controlled surgical anesthesia. However, if a spray painter fell from his ladder due to being overcome by solvent vapor, the inherent reversibility of the effect would probably afford him little consolation. A final complication of this example is that it has been suggested that even the relatively simple mild narcotic effect of some organic solvents might also be associated with long-term consequences, chronic effects. Epidemiological studies have shown an association between combined solvent and alcohol use and neuropsychiatric problems, and some experimental studies with nonneuropathic solvents have shown incomplete recovery from neurochemical changes some weeks after exposure. This is a contentious area in neurotoxicology, some countries recognizing a chronic solvent-induced "psycho-organic syndrome" and others not.

Human and *in vivo* experimental neuropathology is very frequently the study of end-stage phenomena, the "tombstones" of what were evolving pathological processes. It is rarely possible to discover from these studies how many neurons may have been affected by (but have recovered from) a toxic agent. Consequently, such studies tend to underestimate the reversible toxic effects. To see these requires a time course study, which is impossible in humans. The same can also be said of much routine toxicity testing in animals, because the nervous system is usually examined either after death has been caused by the toxic agent or at the end of a 90-day experimental period during which toxicity has time either to develop or to resolve. Where more thorough experimental studies have followed the time course of functional or morphological damage, it has often proved possible to see that a wider range of cells show acute precytotoxic responses that are not followed by death. An example of this is the dramatic cerebellar stellate and basket cell vacuolation produced by the mycotoxin penitrem A, which is, however, fully reversible at moderate doses, and no evidence of it is seen if animals are allowed to survive more than 24 h.

FUNCTIONAL EFFECTS

Functional neurotoxicity can occur in a number of ways (Table 2). The simplest is essentially overdose pharmacology, as when ethanol leads to decreased alertness. This effect is essentially reversible, unless it is severe enough to cause systemic toxicity. There are many other instances of such functional toxicity, such as the hyperexcitation produced by pyrethroid insecticides (which act on the nerve membrane sodium channel) or strychnine (which acts by antagonizing the action of the inhibitory neurotransmitter glycine). In both cases, there are no chronic effects and no direct structural injuries—even in lethal poisonings—and there is no cytotoxicity *in vitro*.

More difficult to understand are the acute reactive

TABLE 2 Different Manifestations and Mechanisms of Neurotoxicity
Functional toxicity
Overdose pharmacology (ethanol → decreased alertness); reversible.
Acute reactive changes (cessation of triazolam → rebound agitation); reversible.
Chronic reactive changes (chlorpromazine → tardive dyskinesia); sometimes reversible.
Cytotoxicity
Selective cytotoxicity (adriamycin → dorsal root ganglion cells); usually irreversible.
Secondary cytotoxicity (*m*-dinitrobenzene → astrocyte death → neuronal death); irreversible.
Tertiary cytotoxicity (ethanol → thiamine deficiency → astrocyte death → neuronal death); irreversible.

changes, where exposure to a neuroactive substance leads to changes in receptor regulation. In the case of the benzodiazepine triazolam, the rapid removal of the drug can uncover receptors that had up-regulated in an attempt to restore excitability suppressed by the drug. On abrupt withdrawal of the drug, these new receptors are no longer needed and can produce rebound agitation and suicidal behavior, but only until the receptors down-regulate. In other cases, reactive changes in both pre- and post-synaptic receptors can lead to the development of tolerance to toxic effects, as with nicotine or organophosphorous esters, which inhibit acetylcholinesterase. Such changes are ultimately reversible in the adult. However, if they are produced in neonatal animals during the brain growth spurt (when the patterns of adult neurotransmitter balance are not yet established), then the normal recovery process may fail and chronic changes in receptor density may be seen. Instances of this are seen following perinatal exposure of rodents to haloperidol or diazepam, and the phenomenon has been termed "chemical imprinting." Similar doses given to normal adults fail to produce chronic effects, presumably because the pattern of neurotransmission is already fixed and the system is able eventually to return to its normal set point.

STRUCTURAL INJURIES

Xenobiotics can damage many cellular components (Table 3): the neuronal cell body (e.g., mercury), the dendrite (e.g., glutamate), the axon (e.g., *n*-hexane), and myelin (e.g., hexachlorophene). Many agents (e.g., lead) impair more than one structure, however. Such a classification of injuries by morphological target is relatively simple and points to the sensitivity of specific structures and targets (Fig. 2), but a full understanding of this selectivity requires a mechanistic explanation.

Neuronopathy

Several substances damage neurons, and if the damage progresses to cell death the resulting neuronal loss is irreversible in the adult brain. Though many substances have the potential to damage neurons, very few if any damage all types of neurons due to their differential neuronal sensitivities. In other cases, the expression of cellular injury may be a diffuse encephalopathy with global dysfunction. Neuronopathies may be divided into cytoplasmic, nuclear, and postsynaptic neuronopathies (Table 3).

TABLE 3 Main Structural Targets of Neurotoxic Chemicals

Type of injury	Injured structure		Substance
Neuronopathy	Neuronal cell body	Cytoplasm	Methylmercury, aluminum
		Nucleus	Doxorubicin
		Postsynaptic membrane	Glutamate
Axonopathy	Axon	Proximal	β, β'-Iminodipropionitrile
		Distal	Acrylamide, carbon disulfide, tri-ortho-cresyl phosphate, *n*-hexane
Myelinopathy	Myelin cells	Schwann cells (PNS), oligodendrocytes, myelin sheath	Diphtheria toxin, cuprizone, triethyl tin, hexachlorophene, acetylethyltetramethyltetralin
Neurovasculopathy	Neuronal vasculature		*m*-Dinitrobenzene, lead

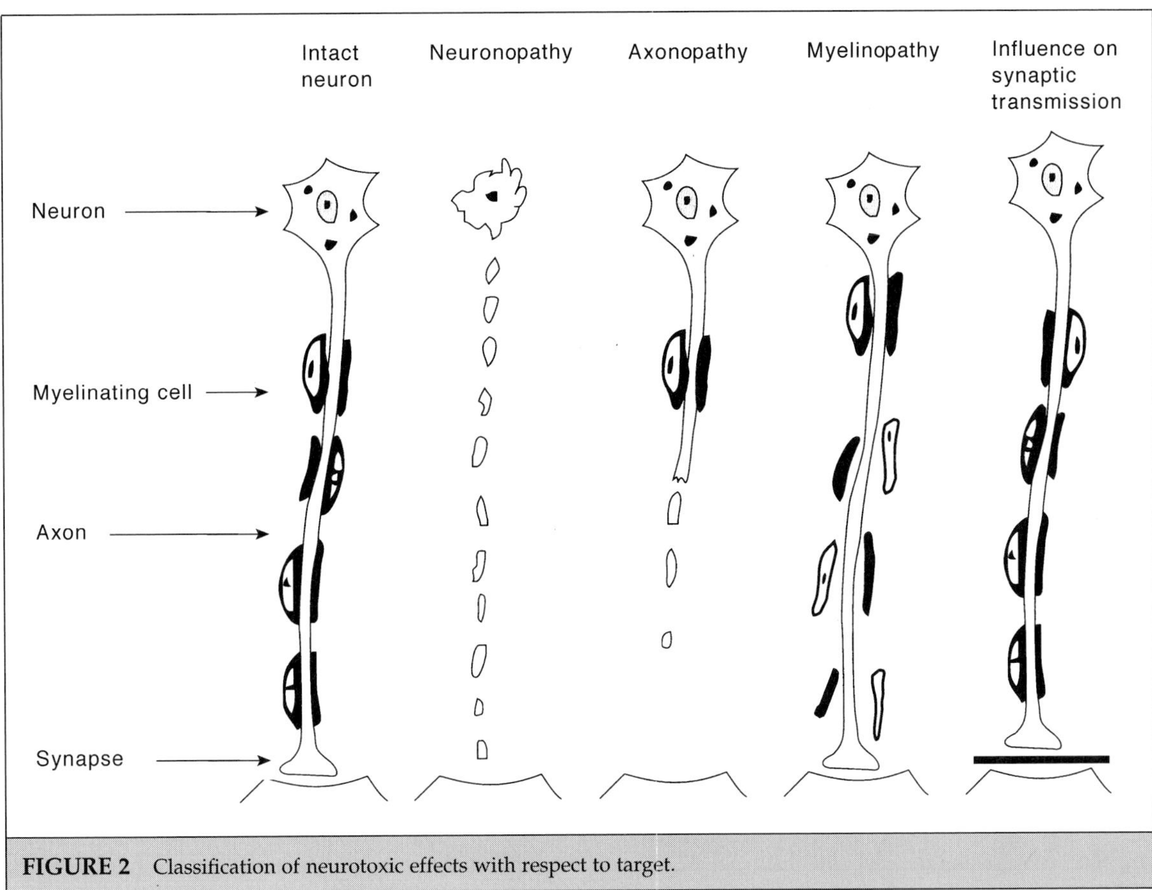

FIGURE 2 Classification of neurotoxic effects with respect to target.

Primary damage to the nerve body (neuronopathy) rapidly causes the secondary breakdown of the axonal and dendritic processes and the ensheathing myelin (Fig. 2), due to the near-total metabolic dependence upon the cell body and the loss of trophic links between the axon and the myelinating cell. While the loss of neurons is irreversible, the surviving cells can recover and reinnervate by sprouting peripheral (but not central) axon collaterals. Such sprouting and reinnervation may be sufficient to prevent gross muscle atrophy, as in mild acrylamide neuronopathy.

Axonopathy

This is a selective loss of the axon, without neuronal death. A common pattern of axonopathy is distal retrograde axonal degeneration (distal or "dying-back" axonopathy). The pathological alterations begin at the nerve terminals, and hence the main symptom of sensory axonopathy is paresthesia in the hands and feet, with a glove or stocking distribution. The loss of the sensation of vibration is associated with the denervation of the Pacinian corpuscles and the distal degeneration of their long central processes. Axonopathy can be either proximal or distal.

Motor axonopathies result in the denervation of muscle fibers and in weakness and a flaccid paralysis with muscle atrophy, often affecting the long axons before the short ones. Recovery by axonal regrowth takes several months and advances from the proximal to distal muscles.

Within the sensory pathways of the CNS, the longer gracile tract (tractus gracilis), innervating the legs, is often more sensitive than the cuneiform tract (tractus cuneiformis), innervating the arms. Degeneration results in the loss of vibration sensitivity in hands and feet. Severe degeneration of the sensory spinocerebellar or motor corticospinal tracts produces persistent spasticity or ataxia. Recovery from central neuropathy is seen only as a result of functional plasticity, because the mature CNS environment does not permit axonal sprouting. Recovery from a mixed central and peripheral neuropathy is associated with progression from flaccid to spastic paralysis, as the upper motor neuron function does not recover and therefore

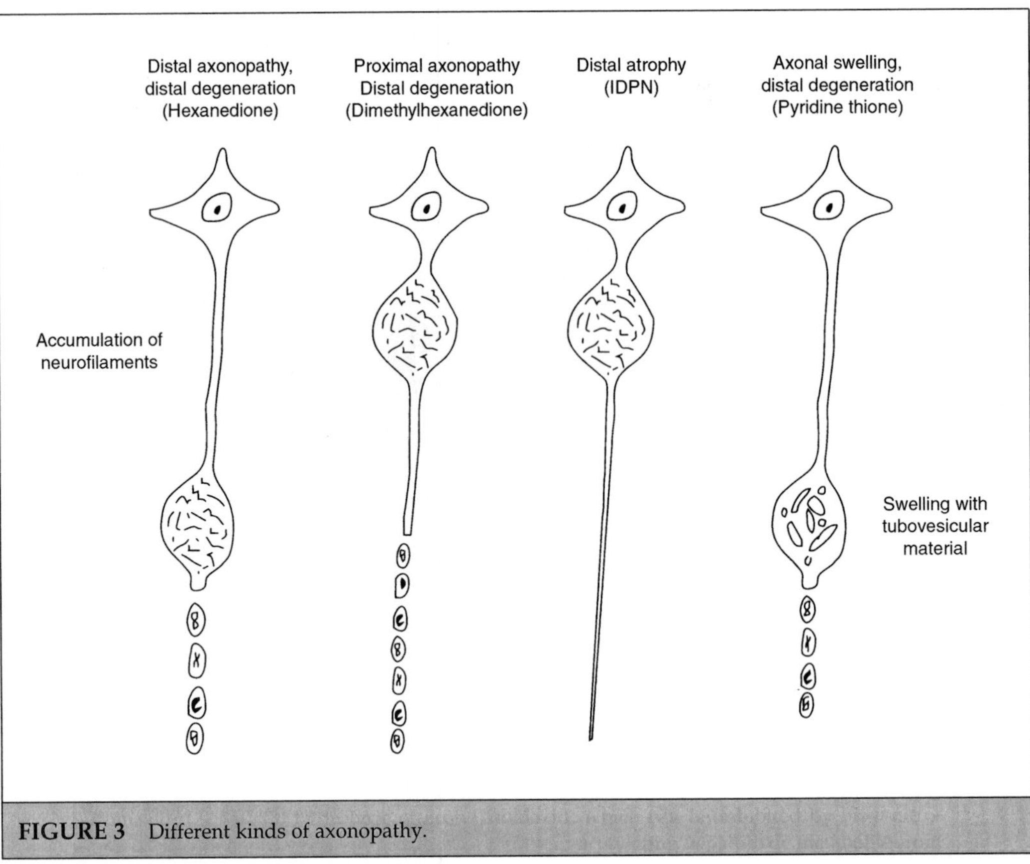

FIGURE 3 Different kinds of axonopathy.

fails to exert normal inhibitory control over the recovering lower (spinal) motor neurons (Fig. 3).

MECHANISMS OF NEUROTOXICITY

Myelin Damage

The formation of myelin takes place in the central nervous system by oligodendrocytes and in the peripheral nervous system by Schwann cells. Both types of cells form myelin in concentric layers (whorls) around the axon. Each Schwann cell myelinates one internode of one axon, more layers being produced around thicker fibers, but always with a characteristic periodicity of 12 nm. In contrast, each oligodendrocyte myelinates several, often functionally unrelated, central axons found within 5 to 40 μm of the cell body. The periodicity between myelin layers is 10.6 nm. During myelination by either cell type, the extracellular space is reduced by the fusion of the cytoplasmic faces of the myelin whorls, a process known as myelin compaction. Because the lipid environment of myelin has a high electrical resistance, this compaction greatly increases the transverse electrical resistance across the axonal membrane, increasing the electrical space constant of the axon, which causes the longitudinal current to spread much further along the axon, and thereby increases the conduction velocity. Myelin damage is therefore associated with disorders of nerve conduction. Mild or focal damage leads to a slowing of conduction velocity, a diagnostic feature of which is the enhanced temperature dependence of the conduction velocity. A more severe loss of myelin may lead to the failure of conduction. Sodium channels are found only at a very low density in those parts of the axon normally covered by myelin. Hence where the axon is newly exposed by demyelination, there may not be enough sodium channels present to generate an action potential and not enough myelin left to enable the action potential to spread far enough to bridge the gap between undamaged sections. With intermediate degrees of demyelination, conduction may be good for low frequencies but fail at higher frequencies.

Three kinds of myelin damage may be seen, intramyelinic edema (myelin swelling), primary demyelination (myelin breakdown), and secondary demyelination. Examples of chemicals causing these will be found in the section on myelin-damaging substances.

Myelin Swelling

A disturbance of myelin homeostasis or a metabolic insult to the myelinating cell can lead to the formation of intramyelinic edema. This may be focal or generalized, usually involves the splitting of the interperiod line between the former extracellular faces of the myelin whorls, and is usually reversible over a period of days or hours. The functional consequences are, however, similar to those of demyelination, with the disruption of nerve conduction and an increase in tissue water content. There is, however, no loss or breakdown of myelin associated with myelin swelling per se, and no myelin constituents, such as myelin basic protein, are liberated into the extracellular space. In some severe cases, myelin swelling may progress to primary demyelination.

Primary Demyelination

This is seen when an agent either directly attacks myelin or the myelinating cell causing the loss of myelin content or myelin breakdown. A number of toxic agents produce primary demyelination, as does diphtheria toxin. Demyelination is associated with the liberation of myelin basic protein and other markers into the extracellular space. Damage can be restricted to the area of the nodes of Ranvier (paranodal demyelination) or may be more generalized (segmental demyelination). There is no primary involvement of the axon itself, although if demyelination is very severe and leads to brain swelling, axonal loss secondary to local ischemia or hypoxia may then be seen. Within a week or so of damage, remyelination begins after surviving myelinating cells divide. This process resembles that seen in normal development, but is less effective in the central than in the peripheral nervous system. Repaired myelin shows shorter internodal distances and is often thinner and less effective.

Secondary Demyelination

Secondary demyelination is an active process that follows irreparable damage to the axon. The Wallerian degeneration seen after traumatic injury and primary toxic axonopathies are both followed by a macrophage digestion of the associated myelin.

Disturbances of Axonal Transport

In addition to hormonal transmission of information via the bloodstream, the nervous system has a highly specific intracellular communication system acting with a relatively high velocity over large distances by transport along axons. These axonal processes are 100,000 times longer than the diameters of the cells. The volumes of the longer axons are therefore much larger than those of their cell bodies, even though the axons have small diameters. Essential protein synthesis takes place in what light microscopists describe as the Nissl substance, which consists of ribosomal clusters. The Nissl substance is found only in the cell body of neurons, which imposes a need for effective transport to the periphery. This transport may be divided into fast anterograde, fast retrograde, and slow. All of the transport processes depend on microtubules, ATP, the activity of a calcium–magnesium-dependent ATPase, and calmodulin. The "motor proteins" kinesin and dynein are involved in the fast systems, and dynamin in the slow system.

The fast anterograde system runs from the cell body out to the periphery and carries predominantly membrane-bound materials, such as enzymes, neurotransmitters, calcium, and amino acids. In peripheral nerve it has a velocity of 410 mm per day, but in optic nerve it is 250 mm per day. The transport of mitochondria has a slower velocity of 34 to 68 mm per day. Fast retrograde transport is needed for recycling materials from the axon terminals, usually in the form of lysosomes, and also for carrying back information from the periphery, probably in the form of trophic factors. The volume of retrograde transport is about half of that of anterograde transport (in terms of protein). Slow transport at 0.2 to 8 mm per day carries by far the greatest bulk of material, mainly metabolic enzymes and structural protein.

Due to the essential nature of these transport processes, any lasting interruption of axonal transport results in the degeneration of the axon.

Disturbances of Synaptic Transmission

Intercellular communication is realized by chemical transduction at the synapse or motor end plate. A neurotransmitter released from the afferent axon terminal acts as a first messenger. The binding of the transmitter to postsynaptic receptors then results in the activation of either a transmembrane ion flux or the activation of a second-messenger system in the postsynaptic cell. The normal function of synaptic transmission requires several steps, all of which can be disrupted by neurotoxic chemicals. These steps are transmitter synthesis, storage in vesicles located in the axon terminals, signal- and ion-dependent release of the transmitter into the synaptic cleft, its binding to the receptor, and its inactivation by neuronal or astrocytic re-uptake or metabolism. For all transmitters, synthesis takes place in the nerve terminals (amines and amino acids) or in the cell body (peptides), followed by axonal transport. Feedback mechanisms via the presynaptic autoreceptors, co-transmitters, and the plasticity of the receptors all modulate synaptic transmission. The most important neurotransmitters are acetylcholine; the amines, dopamine, noradrenalin (norepinephrine), adrenalin (epinephrine), 5-hydroxytryptamine, and histamine; the amino acids, glutamic acid, γ-aminobutyric acid, and glycine; and the peptides, tachykinin and opioids. In addition, neurotransmission is modulated by agents such as nitric oxide. Neurons may release more than one transmitter, but all the terminals of any one neuron release the same substances. Some neurotoxic substances that act by disturbing neurotransmission are 6-hydroxydopamine (dopaminergic), 6-hydroxydopa (noradrenergic), strychnine (glyceinergic), picrotoxin (GABAergic), kainic acid (glutamatergic), and soman (cholinergic).

The Immature Nervous System and Species Differences

The developing nervous system shows many differences from that of the adult, and several of these differences lead to heightened vulnerability to neurotoxic agents. During brain development, neurons divide, migrate, and develop synaptic contacts. Following the establishment of the adult pattern of connections, excess neurons (roughly 50% of the total) then die by apoptosis, and excess synapses are removed (synaptic trimming). The processes of migration, apoptosis, and trimming back are all conducted under the influence of growth factors and in close relation to astrocytes and the Bergmann glia. Once the adult pattern is established, neuronal cell division in the central nervous system ceases and the glia play a more conservative role, limiting further neuronal growth or regrowth. This pattern of growth is not uniform across all brain areas, some maturing relatively early, such as the brain-stem, and others relatively late, such as the cerebellar cortex. The brains of different species mature at different rates, with the brain growth spurt (the time of peak brain growth and vulnerability) occurring at 10 days post natal in the case of rats and mice, but at the time of birth in humans. The growth phase is associated with increased metabolic rate and biosynthetic demand, compared to the adult state. In addition to the gross changes shown in terms of brain weight, other measures, such as the expression of ion channels and receptors, synaptogenesis, and myelination, peak at different times in different brain areas.

Where toxic agents interfere with supply—as in the case of *n*-hexane, which interferes with axonal transport–toxicity can be enhanced in both growing and regrowing axons. The immature nervous system has some advantages, however, in that it has a greater resistance to hypoxia, and a greater capacity for repair and regeneration. It is thought that this is why young animals are relatively resistant to the effects of neuropathic organophosphates.

The lack of a blood–brain barrier during early development can lead to vulnerability of the central nervous system to agents, such as protein-bound lead or bilirubin, which would not normally reach the adult brain. This can be particularly unfortunate, as young children are more prone to accidental poisoning than other age groups, due to their undiscriminating ingestion of foreign bodies. Lead poisoning from old paint or contaminated soil is an important example of this particular problem. Damage to neuronal division, migration, connectivity (by interference with dendritic arborization and synaptogenesis), and myelination can be produced during early development, and these can cause lasting functional deficiencies and diminished weight of the brain. Substances ineffective in adults can produce such effects if given during gestation. Methylazoxymethanol administered to pregnant rats induces microencephaly in the offspring, but is not neurotoxic in adults, even after direct injection into the cerebrospinal fluid.

ASSESSMENT OF NEUROTOXICITY

The methodological approaches described here should all be considered to be complementary to each other, as each has strong and weak points, and can best be interpreted in the context of data from other methods. An integrated multidisciplinary approach is best and can save time as well. For example, while the histopathological study of the cochlea to verify ototoxicity is very difficult, audiometry by means of evoked potentials is quick and easy. Another difficulty inherent both in neuropathology and in post mortem biochemistry is that lesion progression or recovery can only be inferred by comparison between individuals with different survival times. This causes problems, as there is often a great deal of individual variability, but functional monitoring can often give a useful monitor of the individual time course and is therefore of particular value for such studies. Functional measures alone, however, can be difficult to interpret without morphological information.

Behavioral Toxicology

Studies of behavior have greatly expanded since the 1970s, with development of both individual tests and also batteries of tests designed to act as screens for neurotoxicity. Some animal behavioral tests have been specifically designed to be compatible with human behavioral measures.

Because behavior is the final output of the nervous system, and the only one determinable in animals, it provides the most meaningful endpoint for studies of toxicant-induced dysfunction. If an agent does not modify behavior or sensitize the subject to other agents that do so, then it must be considered to be non-neurotoxic at that dose. Analogous statements could not be made concerning neurochemical or morphological endpoints. Because behavior is the end product of a wide range of biochemical and electrophysiological functions carried out in many morphological structures, it is capable of revealing all possible toxicological effects. In addition, behavioral measures are often very sensitive to toxic agents. Thus behavioral tests are very sensitive to the prenarcotic effects of solvents in humans and in rats. However, untangling the many individual functional components that generate behavior in order to determine which component has been damaged is a very difficult process. Indeed, it can be impossible to determine mechanism of action from purely behavioral data, or even to discriminate between neurotoxicity and generalized systemic effects. Broader but less mechanistically interpretable behavioral tests, such as social or open-field behavior, are useful, but are more suited to preliminary screens or to the determination of threshold dose levels, where an understanding of mechanism is less important.

In clinical and epidemiological tests of behavior, particular attention needs to paid to the study design because social background, ethnicity, and language have strong influences on neurobehavioural test scores and may confound any toxicant-induced effects if they vary across exposure groups. Performance in behavioral tests is a matter of learned as well as of innate skills, and hence the matching of subjects in terms of educational level and other social factors is very important. Some measure of individual premorbid ability must also be included, and where it is impossible to obtain such data, a surrogate measure that is relatively resistant to toxic agents can be used (such as vocabulary size). In animal tests, responses are often variable between individual animals, and between laboratories. Factors such as ambient light, noise, animal handling practices, and time of day can make large differences to the response in behavioral tests.

Relatively small structural or neurochemical injuries to critical structures, such as the brainstem nuclei, spinal cord, or peripheral nerve, where there is less flexibility of functional organization than in higher centers, can produce disproportionate behavioral effects. Conversely, adaptive processes in the higher centers can produce remarkable functional compensation, especially for slowly developing lesions. In all but the higher cognitive functions, animal studies have often proved good predictors of effects in humans. Thus methyl mercury, lead, acrylamide, and phenytoin produce similar neuropathological and behavioral findings in humans, monkeys, and rodents. The narcotic and anesthetic action of organic solvents is also quite remarkably constant across a very wide range of species from fish to humans.

Sensory Disturbances

In many ways sensory disturbances are the easiest to characterize because a wide range of methods are available. However, in simple experimental screening studies they can be very difficult to detect unless one is very familiar with animal behavior. Thus blindness or deafness can easily be missed in rodents, whose behavior is dominated by tactile and olfactory cues. The disturbance of the sensory pathways by demyelination and peripheral neuropathies can cause visual and auditory disorders, alterations in sensitivity to temperature, touch, and pain, and paresthesias. Selective neuronal loss in specific brain sensory regions can produce loss of sensation (e.g., cortical blindness), even when sense organs and sensory pathways are intact. Examples are lead encephalopathy and the visual cortical damage produced by methyl mercury intoxication in children. Usually paresthesias accompany the destructive phase of sensory neuropathies. When sensory disturbances involve muscle spindles (as in organophosphate-induced polyneuropathy), the loss of proprioceptive feedback can lead to incoordination and ataxia.

Methods such as operant conditioning linked to a suitable sensory stimulus can be used to determine threshold sensitivity to light or sound in animal experiments and are sensitive enough to recognize minor functional disturbances. Direct functional examination of sensory pathways can be made by electrophysiological methods, such as the recording of visual-evoked potentials from the retina or at the surface of the neocortex. These are often somewhat less sensitive than behavioral measures, but are capable of examining the whole range of stimulus intensities, not just thresholds.

Motor Disturbances

Damage to the neurons and demyelination can lead to motor dysfunction. The determination of grip strength, the observation of spontaneous locomotion, and the observation of ability to maintain balance on an accelerating rotating rod (Rota-rod test) are common motor–behavioral tests and have proved useful for *n*-hexane and acrylamide. Integrated sensory–motor coordination can be measured by the examination of gait, the mid-air righting reflex, and foot splay on landing. In humans the anticancer agents vincristine, cisplatin, and taxol can cause marked motor weakness as a dose-limiting side effect of therapy.

Cognitive Disturbances

The main application of neurobehavioral tests is in the detection of disorders of cognition or affect (mood) or (in humans) specific mental disorders such as anxiety and depression. Test methods for the evaluation of functional ability in animal experiments are the shuttle-box conditioned avoidance test and reward-based learning for lever pressing or maze learning.

Disturbances of learning and memory can be seen at dosages not producing any other neurotoxic effects, but it is important to recognize that defects in sensory–motor and motivational factors can generate false positive results in most cognitive measures. Neurotoxic substances which produce effects on the limbic system, such as lead and trimethyltin, have a strong effect on learning and memory.

Behavioral Toxicological Test Batteries

Several clinical test batteries have been designed primarily for toxicological use and a reasonable number of data showing normal and abnormal responses have been obtained. Most recent tests are computer administered, which removes some of the variability introduced by subject–investigator interactions. The use of computers also allows a wider range of tests and can provide feedback, which gives better motivation than written tests. Most are based on tests originally developed by cognitive psychologists for diagnostic purposes and contain elements designed to test factors such as mood, attention span, reaction time, and linguistic and spatial reasoning. Many cognitive tests are based on subsets of the Wechsler Adult Intelligence Scale—Revised (WAIS-R), which can be used to estimate verbal and nonverbal skills. Commonly used test batteries are the automated Neurobehavioural Evaluation System (NES) and the Milan Automated Testing System (MANS). Versions are available for use in several languages.

For animal work, a good start for behavioral screening is the simple observation of the animals in their home cages. Such monitoring should not, however, be a substitute for a full interactive evaluation. This should be modeled on a clinical neurological evaluation and involve simple tests designed to provoke abnormal reactions. An example is the Functional Observational Test Battery (FOB). This should evaluate the state of alertness, reflex coordination (startle, eye blink, and mid-air righting reflexes), muscle tone, motor performance (gait, grip strength, and balance), basic sensory performance (auditory startle, edge avoidance, and pinch response), general condition, and a search for specific abnormal signs (tremor, partial or generalized seizure activity, lacrymation, urinary or fecal incontinence, poor grooming, fearfulness, or aggression). It should be remembered that some signs may not be easy to detect when animals are in their sleep phase. In general, problems of coordination or balance are only visible on active examination because the affected animals avoid unnecessary movement. Inexperienced observers have confused the rapid but poorly coordinated righting responses seen in such animals with seizure activity.

Several of the more sophisticated behavioral tests demand previous training, especially studies of learning and memory. Examples are the Skinner box system for conditioned avoidance of an electric shock and various maze tests such as the Morris water maze. Such tests pose problems in experimental design, as it is impossible to obtain the same results on re-test due to the time- and sequence-dependent nature of learning.

Electrophysiological Parameters

A wide range of electrophysiological measures are available to both the clinical and the experimental scientist (Table 4). The applicability of most of these tests to both animals and humans is a great aid in their interpretation. The most common measures allow the evaluation of sensory and motor nerve conduction, neuromuscular function, central sensory projections, and the electroencephalogram (EEG).

Peripheral nerve conduction can be assessed by conduction velocity or amplitude. Both are sensitive to fiber or myelin damage, but amplitude measures are very dependent on exact electrode placement and generally show wide intersubject and interexperiment variability. Hence, although amplitude measures are usually more sensitive, conduction velocity is usually the better index, because it is simple to determine with precision. Because different nerve groups conduct at different rates, a multicomponent waveform is usually seen. This can be analyzed to separate the slower responses of small diameter fibers from the faster responses of larger fibers. All peripheral nerve functions are temperature-sensitive, and it is important to control skin temperature during determinations. The electomyogram can be recorded with simple needle electrodes and used to evaluate basic neuromuscular function. In addition, Fourier analysis can be used to characterize and quantify spontaneous tremor frequency. Muscle microelectrodes can be used to measure single fiber activity, and the increased variability of latency between responses in adjacent fibers in the same motor unit (jitter) provides a sensitive measure of damage to the fine terminal branches of motor nerves.

Sensory function can be assessed by recording auditory, visual, or somatosensory-evoked responses. These usually involve synchronized averaging of the response to a large number of individual stimuli, a process that reduces the contribution of spontaneous activity. Such averaged sensory responses detected by neocortical electrodes consist of a series of waves generated at various identifiable stages in the sensory projection pathways. These can be used to provide highly specific and quantifiable indices of central or peripheral sensory dysfunction. Central motor pathways are more difficult to assess, although in humans it is possible to use focal electromagnetic stimulation of the motor cortex.

The spontaneous EEG provides a valuable measure, largely of the degree of synchronization of brain activity. The normal alert neocortex generates little signal that is detectable by surface electrodes, but it has a tendency to generate local rhythmic electrical activity when not activated by external stimuli. Such local rhythms are enhanced during sleep, with the loss of arousal due to narcotics, and after brain injury. In addition, focal damage can lead to hypersynchronization of neuronal activity, which appears as focal spike and wave discharge similar to those seen during petit mal epilepsy. The interpretation of EEG records is a difficult and specialized task, but Fourier analysis can provide a very useful quantitative index.

Finally, a range of specialized local functions can be evaluated by electrophysiological tests. A good example is long-term potentiation of excitability in the hippocampus, which can provide a measure of learning that has been shown to parallel the cognitive loss seen during neonatal lead poisoning. Recurrent inhibition can be used to evaluate integrated synaptic function, while patch clamp techniques can resolve activity at the single receptor molecule level.

Neuropathological Methods

Morphological and neuropathological methods are indispensable for the detection of long-lasting or irreversible defects. The extreme functional diversity seen within the nervous system and the dramatic regional selectivity of many neurotoxic agents mean that a comprehensive range of tissue samples are needed for exploratory investigations. Thus about five levels of brain sections, several spinal cord sections, and both transverse and longitudinal peripheral nerve sections need to be examined for a general survey. There is no such thing as a single "representative" brain section, in the sense that might be possible with liver or kidney. Functional observations can be very useful in guiding a neuropathological survey to specific areas, such as the sensory or motor nerve.

TABLE 4 Electrophysiological Methods Used in Clinical and Experimental Neurotoxicology

Method	Object	Remarks
Maximum conductance velocity of motor nerves	Function of large diameter motor fibers in peripheral nerves	Frequently used, relatively insensitive, tibial, ulnar nerves
Conduction velocity of slow motor fibers	Function of small diameter motor fibers	Rarely used
Conduction velocity of sensory nerves	Function of sensory nerves	Difficult technique, median, radial, sural nerves
Electromyogram	Neuromuscular function, denervation, damage to distal nerves	Denervation hypersensitivity causes repetitive waves, fine electrodes can evaluate single fibers
H-reflex	Monosynaptic stretch reflex	Test of muscle spindles
EEG (electroencephalogram)	Degree of alertness, brain damage, hyperexcitable states	Can localize lesions
Sensory-evoked potentials	Assess central sensory pathways	Visual, auditory, and somatosensory responses, recorded via EEG electrodes
Electroretinogram	Retinal function	Recorded from conjunctiva

Great care has to be taken either to avoid or to recognize tissue fixation artifacts, such as the dark cell change that occurs if the brain is handled prior to or during fixation and that can be confused with toxicant-induced necrosis. Such artifacts are best avoided by vascular perfusion with fixative *in situ* for experimental studies.

Two aims dominate in neuropathology: the determination of the characteristic lesion topography and the investigation of the cellular nature of the injury. Most agents produce specific topographic patterns of damage that remain relatively constant across species. Although lesions often become more widespread as the dose is increased, there is usually a hierarchy of more and less vulnerable areas. In the investigation of the cellular nature of injury, it is important to look early in the time- course of the response. There are a number of secondary features common to all brain injuries, namely local hypertrophy and hyperplasia of astrocytes and local accumulation of microglia. These develop over 3–10 days and can provide a very useful marker of brain injury, especially when visualized by immunohistochemical markers such as glial fibrillary acidic protein (GFAP), which are up-regulated during the tissue reaction. Such secondary reactions, however, can obscure the nature of the primary lesion if only late-stage material is examined.

Electron microscopy provides the only technique for unambiguous identification of cellular pathology, although immune markers for neurofilaments, synapses, astrocytes, microglia, and myelin provide more convenient measures. Vascular dysfunction can be detected by using tracers that do not normally penetrate the blood–brain barrier, such as protein-bound dyes. Such methods usually require the use of thicker sections than normal because vascular damage may be hard to see in standard 4-μm sections.

Biochemical Methods

The primary action of toxic chemicals is always biochemical. An understanding of toxicological mechanisms is ultimately based on the interaction of xenobiotics with target molecules, although there are many important secondary processes that can modify the consequences of this interaction. The goal of mechanistic toxicology is to identify such interactions. Despite our greatly increased knowledge of fundamental neurochemistry since the 1960s, only a minority of neurotoxic chemicals act by known biochemical mechanisms (Table 1). Sometimes a number of potential candidate processes have been identified, but it is difficult to decide which are relevant to actual exposures.

There are two characteristics that need to be remembered when considering neurochemical mechanisms. First, the brain shows a high degree of metabolic compartmentation, consisting of many very different and highly specialised macro- and microenvironments, not all of which can be resolved by most biochemical methods. Thus, for example, only astrocytes and not neurons show pentose phosphate shunt and glutamine synthetase activity; myelin is produced only by oligodendrocytes or Schwann cells; and protein synthesis occurs only in the cell body, not in nerve terminals. Different neurotransmitters are expressed by neurons in specific pathways, and the expression of neurotransmitter re-uptake systems, even by astrocytes, is not global but varies to match that of the local neuronal population. Not all areas show the high metabolic activity characteristic of the brain as a whole, the rate of glucose phosphorylation in central fiber tracts being at least four times lower than in active brain nuclei. Second, nervous system activity is highly dynamic. Thus local glucose phosphorylation can double after functional activation.

These two characteristics have made it necessary to develop special methods for neurochemistry. Postmortem artifacts can be avoided either by rapid inactivation of enzymes by freezing or microwave inactivation or by *in situ* monitoring via carbon fiber voltametry, microdialysis, or NMR spectroscopy. Turnover studies of variables such as glucose utilization or axonal transport, can be made by introducing a tracer and using its rate of accumulation or disappearance over a limited period to estimate steady-state conditions. The problem of compartmentation can be approached by morphological fractionation. Thus, mitochondrial preparations, myelin fractions, synaptosomes and synaptosomal components such as vesicles, neurotransmitters, and presynaptic and postsynaptic membrane elements can be isolated. Microdissection can be used to separate brain areas. There are, however, difficulties in applying some standard biochemical measures. Thus the far lower incorporation of radiolabeled amino acids into the brain than into other tissues was at first thought to indicate that the brain had a low rate of protein turnover, whereas it is now recognized that this is due to the blood–brain barrier limiting uptake of the tracer amino acids.

Many intracellular functions involve the glutathione system, which forms the basis of antioxidant protection against reactive metabolites of xenobiotics. Ascorbate is another antioxidant found at high concentration in the brain and is maintained in the reduced state by glutathione. Both depend on the mitochondrial generation of reducing equivalents.

Secondary (catabolic) biochemical changes can be used to monitor lesion development in the same way as secondary morphological responses. Thus β-glucuronidase and β-galactosidase provide sensitive indicators of reactive hypertrophy of microglia and astrocytes.

A number of biochemical targets are listed in the section on specific toxic agents, such as neuropathy target esterase, in the case of delayed neurotoxicity of organophosphorus compounds, and the glutamate receptor complex, in the case of kainate.

Pharmacological Mechanisms

The central nervous system shows remarkable temporal plasticity in both function and dysfunction. Although neurons are terminally differentiated in the adult brain, cytoplasmic processes, dendrites, and axons can regenerate to an amazing extent. On average, each of the 10^{10} neurons of the human brain forms synapses with about 10^4 other neurons. This neuronal combination is not static like a wiring diagram but changes with time by growth or regression. Synaptic transmission also varies, the number of postsynaptic receptors increasing or decreasing with use. Hence neurotoxic agents interact with a dynamic system. The normal distinction between reversible and irreversible effects is complicated by this active and reactive nature of brain function. Prolonged exposure to pharmacologically active agents often leads to the induction of such reactive changes to restore function to normal, Thus, repeated or continued exposure to the same dose of acetylcholinesterase inhibitors can lead to diminishing cholinergic signs due to reactive changes in release and receptor systems that gradually compensate to maintain normal function, despite a continuing underlying toxic effect. Another example is the dopamine antagonist haloperidol, which blocks and decreases synaptic transmission. This blockage triggers the formation of new receptors, resulting in supersensitivity. Such processes underlie drug tolerance and withdrawal signs, both via the alteration of receptor number or affinity for the endogenous ligand. The administration of agonists produces down-regulation with right-shifting of the dose–response curve and decreased sensitivity. Antagonists produce up-regulation with left-shifting of the dose–response curve and supersensitivity. However, agonist-induced supersensitivity is also possible. The dopamine agonist apomorphine produces dose-dependent postsynaptic decreased sensitivity but also presynaptic (autoreceptor) supersensitivity. Receptor–binding studies can be used to verify such alterations of synaptic sensitivity. Specific receptor agonists and antagonists are vital for such investigations.

In Vitro Methods

Development of *in vitro* models has been in response to three main requirements: the need to better define the biological and chemical variables contributing to neurotoxicity seen *in vivo;* the desire to reduce animal suffering; and the hope of saving time and money by the use of rapid *in vitro* screening systems. For the first objective, *in vitro* methods have already proved to be successful. Specific questions, such as the definition of the xenobiotic metabolic capacity of specific cell types or the distinction between actions on neurotransmitter release or re-uptake, can often best be answered *in vitro.* More open-ended but vital questions such as "Is this agent safe?", which can be difficult to answer even by clinical trials, become more difficult to answer using animals, and become almost impossible with purely *in vitro* systems. The reason for this is that the increased definition of variables that is obtained *in vitro* comes at the cost of the decreased capacity of the system to show the more complex adverse responses that concern us. It can easily be seen that it would be very difficult to incorporate even those mechanisms common to humans and mice into a practical *in vitro* test system. Despite this limitation, *in vitro* systems have proved successful in answering specific questions about toxic potential (hazard), and have usefully supplemented and reenforced data from animal experiments. Examples of this include the use of cells expressing defined targets, such as glutamate receptors to assess excitotoxicity or human cytochrome P450 isozymes to assess bioactivation.

Many levels of *in vitro* culture systems are used, at varying levels of complexity:

- Organotypic culture (maintenance of tissue fragments or explants).
- Primary cell culture (growth of cells dissociated from tissues).
- Transformed cell culture (growth of tumor cells with enhanced capacity for division).
- Cell-free systems (cell homogenates and specific organelles).

All of these show a number of specific advantages and limitations (Table 5). Common to most is the capacity to define the culture conditions and the toxicant exposure. However, systemic xenobiotic metabolism either is not seen in culture or is represented by rather arbitrary elements, such as microsomal mixes. Also, the important capacity of the nervous system itself for xenobiotic metabolism is very region-specific and can be lost after continued culture. The loss of the capacity for bioactivation will result in underestima-

TABLE 5 *In Vitro* Systems for Neurotoxicology

Type of system	Examples	Advantages	Disadvantages
Cell free	Brain homogenates, synaptosomes, mitochondria	Well defined, retain metabolic capacity	Very limited life *in vitro,* no cell type specificity
Transformed cell	Neuroblastomas, astrocytomas, Schwannomas	Neuronal proliferation large cell yield, no animal use, long life time	Loss of normal phenotype, phenotypic instability with repeated subculturing
Primary cell	Cerebellar granule cells, astrocytes, vascular endothelium	Preservation of normal phenotype, defined co-cultures,	Poor yield, contamination with other proliferating cell types, limited life time
Reaggregate	Micromass spheroids	Large cell yield, can show differentiation, long life time	Poor definition of environment, overgrowth can lead to necrosis in center of aggregates complexity limits end points
Organotypic	Hippocampal slice, nerve-diaphragm	Anatomical preservation, some function maintained, long life time	Technical difficulty, complexity limits end points

tion of toxic potential, while the loss of the capacity for bioinactivation will result in overestimation of toxicity. Many potential neurotoxicants are highly lipophilic and the delivery of these can be difficult *in vitro.*

Transformed (Continuous) Cell Lines

Established cell lines of human and animal neuroblastoma or glioma cells, as well as hybrid cells, are available, although the choice of neuronal lines is limited. These cell lines are effectively "immortal" in culture, although the phenotype often becomes unstable after roughly 50 cell divisions. This can be overcome by freezing the cells from early cultures and reestablishing the line at intervals. Homogenous populations of undifferentiated cells are easy to obtain, but are of limited value. Differentiation introduces desirable target properties that can reproduce many characteristics of primary cells, but this process also introduces phenotypic variability. Commonly used lines are the cholinergic NG-108-15; the sympathetic PC12; the NIE115 mouse and IMR32 or SY5Y human neuroblastomas; and the C6 glioma. Genomic transfections can be used to add specific properties, such as the expression of human target proteins.

Primary Cell Cultures

The use of dissociated cell cultures was introduced in the 1960s, and they are the most widely used method. Embryonic or neonatal tissue is used to provide cells that are still replicating, dissociated by limited proteolytic digestion. These are then fractionated to remove debris and cultured. As most cells are highly substrate-dependent, a collagen or polylysine surface is needed. Specific cell types can be selected by varying brain area and stage of development, fractionation (for capillary endothelial cells), differential adhesion, or growth conditions. Antimitotics are used to inhibit the growth of nonneuronal cells. Reasonably specific cultures of neurons, endothelial cells, astrocytes, oligodendrocytes, microglia, and Schwann cells have been obtained. Specific co-cultures can be used; for example, glial cell substrates can be used to study the role of trophic factors on neurite outgrowth, and astrocyte–endothelial co-cultures can be used to replicate some properties of the blood–brain barrier.

Reaggregate and Suspension Cultures

Reaggregate primary cultures can provide large cell populations and are possible from telencephalon, mesencephalon, diencephalon, and rhombencephalon. The cells are maintained in suspension by a gyratory mixer. Certain areas such as cerebral cortex will form larger aggregates than others, for example, the cerebellum. Cell aggregation is maximal if the tissue is dissociated when cells are actively proliferating and migrating, but larger aggregates tend to develop a necrotic core, which limits their usefulness. Layers of cells with differentiation and alignment resembling that seen *in vivo* can be produced, and these can show synaptogenesis and myelination. Aggregating cell cultures provide models for the investigation of transmitter synthesis, storage, and release, receptor binding, synaptogenesis, and myelination, but their very complexity can make defined investigations difficult.

Organotypic Cultures

Brain slices, ganglia, and neuromuscular explants have long been used in neurotoxicology. Nervous tissue was one of the earliest explant tissue cultures, with embryo frog spinal cord grown in a hanging drop of lymph. Now tissues are normally taken from prenatal or neonatal rodents and the slices are cultured in well-oxygenated systems such as roller tubes. Hippocampal, cerebellar, and locus coeruleus slice cultures have been particularly well characterized. Although a great deal of selective cell death occurs in the first week or so of culture, a remarkable degree of both anatomical preservation and complex functional development (such as synaptic networks and neuromuscular junctions) can be seen. Such systems can be used either to study the effect of agents on tissue slice studies over weeks or months or to replicate the course of normal postnatal development.

Endpoints for In Vitro Neurotoxicity

These represent both an opportunity and a challenge. It is possible to measure many things readily *in vitro* that are either impossible or very difficult to measure *in vivo.* Thus intracellular potential and calcium concentration, neurotransmitter release, axonal transport, and the individual time course of morphological change can all be measured. Cytotoxicity, the usual endpoint for non-nervous-system toxicity *in vitro,* is also widely used. Common indices are vital dye exclusion, leakage of lactate dehydrogenase, and loss of capacity to reduce 3-(4,5-dimethylthiazol-2yl)-2,5-diphenyltetrazolium bromide (MTT). However, cytotoxicity measures are often at least an order of magnitude less sensitive than functional indices, and some potent neurotoxic agents (such as the pyrethroid insecticides) have virtually no cytotoxic potential. The main value of cytotoxic indices is to provide a reference measure against which the more sensitive functional indices can be assessed.

NEUROTOXIC SUBSTANCES

In this section, the neurotoxicities of a number of specific agents are briefly summarized. Further details are provided in specialist works on neurotoxicology, such as Chang and Slikker (1995), Hayes and Laws (1991), Isaacson and Jensen (1992), O'Donoghue (1985), Spencer and Schaumberg (1985), and Vinken and Bruyn (1994). It is impossible to overstate the importance of dose levels in providing a vital context for the interpretation of all forms of toxicity, and hence a neurotoxic (single oral) dose value has been provided whenever possible in order to give a general indication of potency. However, the reader should appreciate that in many cases there is a wide variation in effect between acute and chronic exposure and with route of administration.

Substances Interfering with Energy Metabolism

6-Aminonicotinamide

This is an antimetabolite of nicotinamide, and the production of the 6-aminonicotinamide analogs of NADPH and NADH interferes with the transfer of reducing equivalents. In addition, 6-phosphogluconate dehydrogenase is inhibited. At 10 mg/kg, in addition to a general inhibition of metabolic activity, specific brain lesions are seen closely resembling those produced by chlorosugars, but with greater involvement of petechial hemorrhages.

Azide

At a dose of 10 mg/kg, azide inhibits cytochrome oxidase and induces a marked fall in blood pressure due to a prominent cardiotoxic action. It is predominantly this hypotension that leads to secondary neuronal damage.

Carbon Monoxide

Carbon monoxide has a 200-fold higher affinity for hemoglobin than does oxygen. Thus 1000 ppm carbon monoxide in the air produces 60% saturation of hemoglobin at steady state, although the time needed to reach steady state can be several hours if the pulmonary ventilation rate is not increased by exercise. Carbon monoxide causes primary hypoxia without disturbance of perfusion or energy supply. Because brain has a very high obligate oxygen demand (33 ml/kg/min), the nervous system is a particular target of this hypoxia, together with cardiac muscle. Judgment and visual acuity are impaired at 10% carboxyhemoglobin, and at roughly 50% carboxyhemoglobin impaired cardiac function plus brain hypoxia leads to edema and neuronal necrosis with petechial hemorrhages. The globus pallidus, hippocampus, neocortex, cerebellar Purkinje cells, and substantia nigra are most commonly affected, although fiber tracts are also damaged, probably as a late consequence.

Chlorosugars

A number of chlorinated sugars, such as α-chlorohydrin (a rat poison) and 6-chloro-6-deoxyglucose (a candidate male antifertility agent), inhibit D-glyceraldehyde 3-phosphate dehydrogenase. These chemicals produce both testicular damage and neurotoxicity. The primary targets in the brain are astrocytes and oligodendrocytes within the more metabolically active brain areas, particularly those of the brain stem. Lesions are focal and characterized by glial vacuolation and degeneration. Neurons and blood vessels are only involved at a late stage in the more severe lesions.

Cyanide

The inhibition of cytochrome a_3 during cyanide poisoning leads to a generalized failure of oxidative phosphorylation, and the brain is a prominent target due to its reliance on oxidative metabolism. Death is usually rapid and associated with centrally mediated respiratory failure, but where the dose has been close to the lethal threshold (about 200 ppm) and death has been delayed, damage resembles that which would be expected from a combination of hypoxia and hypotension.

Nitrobenzenes

Trinitrobenzene is an explosive used predominantly as a detonator, while dinitrobenzene and nitrobenzene are bulk chemical intermediates. In experimental animals *m*-dinitrobenzene (30 mg/kg), and to a lesser extent trinitrobenzene and mononitrobenzene (200 mg/kg), is capable of producing focal gliovascular lesions closely resembling those caused by 6-aminonicotinamide. Neuronal involvement is only seen in severe lesions or at a late stage of pathogenesis. It is likely that these agents are bioacativated by brain P450 reductase and then undergo redox cycling with depletion of reducing equivalents and consequent metabolic disruption.

3-Nitropropionic Acid

This is a fungal metabolite that has been responsible for outbreaks of poisoning after the consumption of moldy sugar cane. It produces the irreversible inhibition of succinate dehydrogenase, thereby interfering with oxidative metabolism. At a dose of 30 mg/kg, lesions are seen, primarily involving the caudate, putamen, hippocampus, and thalamus, and are characterized by neuronal and astrocytic swelling, breakdown of the mitochondria, neuronal necrosis, and petechial hemorrhage. Lower doses in experimental animals produce a selective loss of caudate interneurons.

Nitrogen Trichloride

This substance became known in connection with the "dog hysteria" of the 1940s. Running seizures were seen in dogs after the consumption of food containing wheat flour bleached with nitrogen trichloride. The toxicity results from the formation of methionine sulfoximine *in vivo*. Neuronal necrosis is seen in the cerebral cortex, hippocampus, and cerebellar cortex. The pathogenesis is probably complicated by secondary hypoxia following the seizures. The related buthionine sulphoximine is a potent inhibitor of glutathione synthesis, and this also causes a disturbance of the redox balance associated with running fits and neuronal damage.

Myelin-Damaging Substances

Acetyl Ethyl Tetramethyl Tetralin (AETT)

Formerly used as a perfume ingredient, AETT was recognized as myelinotoxic as a result of animal studies and was withdrawn from use before human intoxication occurred. The first change to be seen is myelin swelling, but this is succeeded by progressive primary demyelination in the spinal cord, brain stem, ventral spinal roots, dorsal spinal roots, and peripheral fibers. The threshold toxic dose in rats is 50 mg/kg/day. Remyelination occurs even during the latter phase of demyelination.

Cuprizone

This agent is a potent copper chelator and has been extensively used to produce experimental myelin damage. It has little or no effect on peripheral myelin or Schwann cells, but it is directly toxic to oligodendrocytes and produces widespread myelin swelling and primary demyelination in the CNS. Its mode of action probably relates to chelation of the copper needed by enzymes such as carbonic anhydrase.

Hexachlorophene

Hexachlorophene is a broad-spectrum antibacterial and fungicidal agent, particularly useful for topical treatment of skin. Unfortunately, it is also myelinotoxic and when used at high concentrations (3%) in the 1960s, it was responsible for a number of human fatalities. Babies and young children were particularly susceptible. After absorption through the skin, hexachlorophene distributes rapidly and reaches the central nervous system. There and in the peripheral nervous system it induces myelin swelling with splitting at the intraperiod lines of myelin lamellae. Myelin swelling is the primary effect, with demyelination or axonopathy only occurring as a late complication in severe cases. Larger CNS fibers are most vulnerable, but all central and peripheral myelin may be affected in younger animals or at higher dose levels. Experimental studies of the erythrocyte membrane show that hexachlorophene binds to cell membranes and induces breakdown of the transmembrane ion gradients. Such an effect could lead to myelin edema.

Initially the edema is reversible, but continued intoxication results in segmental demyelination and in brain swelling. The enlargement of the brain causes an increase of intracranial pressure and this compromises circulation, leading to development of secondary ischemic damage, which is the usual cause of death. Hexachlorophene also damages retinal photoreceptors.

Inorganic Lead

In addition to its action on the developing brain, lead also produces a peripheral primary demyelination with focal segmental demyelination and damage to Schwann cells and subsequent endoneural oedema. Demyelination and axonal degeneration are both seen, sometimes separately, but myelin appears to be the more sensitive target. Lead neuropathy primarily affects motor nerves and has long been recognized as a hazard resulting from use of lead-based paints or pottery glazes and lead water pipes. Nerve conduction velocity is decreased at blood lead concentrations in excess of 50 μg/dl. Lead avidly binds to plasma proteins and therefore does not enter the adult CNS.

Tellurium

Used in steel alloys, tellurium salts have produced experimental but not clinical myelinopathy. Young rats are more sensitive than adults, and peripheral myelin is the primary, although not the exclusive, target, despite entry of tellurium into the CNS. Myelin swelling and damage to Schwann cells is followed by primary demyelination, with remyelination occurring even during exposure. Tellurium appears to act by direct inhibition of squalene epoxidase, a key enzyme in cholesterol biosynthesis and hence in myelin production.

Triethyltin

As triethyltin is neurotoxic other alkyltins, such as tributyltin and dibutyltin, are now used in its place as biocides. Triethyltin is a potent myelin-damaging agent, inducing myelin swelling almost exclusively in the CNS at 10 mg/kg; the effects on the peripheral nerve are largely restricted to the spinal nerve roots. It is also directly ototoxic. Oligodendrocytes do not seem to be directly damaged, and demyelination is only seen after very severe intoxication. The myelin swelling is completely reversible if secondary damage does not develop. Spongy degeneration and splitting of the myelin lamellae also occur in the optic nerve. As with hexachlorophene which produces similar effects, there appears to be a direct chemical interaction with the myelin membranes, which leads to an inability of the whorls to remain tightly opposed and to an extracellular edema. Triethyltin is capable of acting as a lipophilic ionophore, facilitating chloride/hydroxide exchange across membranes. In France 290 people were poisoned in 1954 by use of an organotin preparation intended to treat boils, but contaminated by 5% triethyltin. Of these, 110 died. The symptoms were attributable to myelin swelling and the effects of raised intracranial pressure, namely nausea, vertigo, blindness, paraplegia, and convulsions.

Axonopathy-Inducing Substances

Acrylamide

Acrylamide, 2-propenamide, is the monomer of polyacrylamide, which is used as a soil stabilizer and has many other industrial uses. There have been at least 60 cases of human poisoning, usually via the residual monomer leaching into water supplies. Typically, acrylamide induces a "dying-back" pattern of axon degeneration, which affects the deep touch and muscle spindle afferents before motor fibers become involved. In severe cases, all fiber types can be damaged. Only secondary demyelination is seen. Central effects include axonopathy in the longer central tracts and swelling of cerebellar Purkinje cells at the axon hillock. The primary action of acrylamide appears to be the disruption of axonal transport, with both central and peripheral accumulation of neurofilaments at axonal swellings and degeneration. It has been proposed that the inhibition of the retrograde axonal transport of essential growth factors needed by the cell body may be a cause of the axonopathy. The effects of acute exposure can be reversible, but chronic exposure results in poorly reversible sensory disturbance in the extremities, weakness, and ataxia. The neurotoxic dose is aproximately 100 mg/kg and is cumulative even over several weeks.

Arsenic

Arsenic produces a distal polyneuropathy, which develops 10 to 20 days after a single exposure. Sensory signs (paresthesia or numbness) can sometimes be seen in advance of motor signs (weakness), but they are usually seen together. The acute toxicity of arsenic salts varies with bioavailability, but trivalent arsenic oxide is lethal at 2 mg/kg. Due to the natural presence of arsenic in some well waters, arsenical neuropathy is probably the most common chemical neuropathy in humans and is seen if the water concentration is greater than 0.05 ppm arsenic.

Carbon Disulfide

Carbon disulfide is used in tire, rayon, carbon tetrachloride, and cellulose production. Two distinct forms of toxicity are seen: acute mania and peripheral neuropathy. The former is only produced by very high-level exposure and is caused by dithiocarbamate metabolites chelating copper, which is an essential cofactor for dopamine-β-hydroxylase. Exposure at 400 ppm or greater induces a central and peripheral "dying-back" axonopathy with secondary demyelination and also damages the cochlear hair cells, leading to deafness in factory workers. Such exposures are now rare. The mechanism of action is thought to be due to a cross-linking reaction of the metabolites with neurofilaments. Carbon disulfide is also a metabolite of the drug disulfram, which is used to treat alcoholics, and this has sometimes produced a similar neuropathy.

Ethanol

Ethanol is a popular recreational drug owing to its disinhibiting and sedative effects. Acute poisoning (blood ethanol in excess of 4 g/l) results in respiratory failure. Chronic alcoholism results in cerebellar cortical and, to a lesser extent, cerebral cortical necrosis, and also in a distal sensory–motor peripheral neuropathy. The cerebellar lesion is remarkably selective, revolving primarily Purkinje cells in the vermis. In fetal alcohol syndrome, produced by alcoholism during pregnancy, similar but more dramatic cerebral and cerebellar degeneration is seen. Thiamine deficiency is often associated with chronic alcoholism, and plays a role both in the development of alcoholic neuropathy and in the central effects, although these can be seen in the absence of deficiency. Wernicke's encephalopathy (thiamine deficiency) results in brain-stem lesions rather similar to those produced by 6-aminonicotinamide.

n-Hexane and Methyl n-Butyl Ketone

Long-term inhalation of the industrial solvents *n*-hexane or methyl *n*-butyl ketone causes a "dying-back" central and peripheral neuropathy in both humans and animals at concentrations of 300 ppm or more. Although early studies indicated that long large-diameter motor neurons were the primary target, later work has shown that secondary muscle spindle afferents and unmyelinated autonomic fibers are also very sensitive. Axonopathy was first reported in the 1960s and has resulted in at least 600 occupational cases and also a number related to solvent abuse. Both of these agents form γ-diketones (2,5-hexanedione and 3,4-dimethyl-2,5-hexanedione) by hepatic oxidation, and these are the direct toxicants, 2,5-hexanedione being 38 times more potent than *n*-hexane. Other related structures, such as methyl *n*-ethyl ketone, which follows a similar metabolic path but forms a β-diketone, do not produce neuropathy, although they can enhance *n*-hexane neuropathy by influencing its metabolism. The probable targets of γ-diketones are lysyl amino acids of neurofilaments, with which they from pyrrole adducts. This then leads to functional impairment of neurofilament transport, axonal atrophy, and (with continued exposure) to accumulation of ineffective neurofilaments in giant axonal swellings proximal to the narrowing of the axon that accompanies each node of Ranvier. In more severe intoxications, internodal swellings are also seen. The exact way in which pyrrole adducts interfere with neurofilament function is not known. Secondary demyelination follows axonopathy. As the requirement for axonal transport is greatest in growing or regenerating nerves, it is not surprising that these are the most sensitive to hexane. Hexane is also capable of producing ototoxicity at very high exposure levels.

Iminodipropionitrile

β, β'-Iminodipropionitrile is an industrial intermediate that has been used as an experimental neurotoxin. It produces a bizarre hyperactive chorea-like motor syndrome in mice, but only ataxia in other species, at 1 g/kg. Axonopathy in spinal motor neurons, dorsal root ganglia, and brain stem neurons is associated with a proximal axon swelling and accumulation of neurofilaments. In contrast to the "dying back" neuropathies, the distal parts of the axon rarely degenerate.

Organophosphorous Compounds

Certain organophosphates, such as tri-*ortho*-cresyl phosphate (TOCP), leptophos, or mipafox, have the potential to produce serious central-peripheral distal axonopathies. A massive epidemic occurred in the United States after the contamination of the illicit beverage "Ginger Jake" with tri-*o*-cresyl phosphate. The paralysis became known as "Ginger Jake Paralysis." A further mass intoxication in Morocco was caused by the contamination of cooking oil by tri-*o*-cresyl phosphate.

One of the targets of organophosphates is a neuronal, membrane-associated serine esterase, neuropathy target esterase (NTE). Although catalytic inhibition of this protein by a range of agents does not lead to axonopathy, those that are capable of a subsequent covalent reaction leading to charge redistribution within the molecule (the "aging" reaction) initiate an irreversible polyneuropathy. Agents that occupy the catalytic site of NTE but do not undergo the aging reaction protect against coexposure to neuropathic agents. The axonal degeneration shows a characteristic delayed onset; clinical symptoms occur 7 to 10 days after acute exposure. The axonopathy is both sensory and motor, with long and large-diameter fibers, such as those from muscle spindles, being the most severely affected. Young persons and animals are less severely affected. The pattern of degeneration resembles that seen after a physical injury to the axon (Wallerian degeneration), with the cell body and proximal axon being spared. Because the target protein is known, the propensity of a given organophosphate to produce either neuropathy (via NTE) or acute cholinergic signs (via acetylcholinesterase) can be determined by measuring the ratio of inhibition of the two target proteins *in vitro*. This has proved to be a very effective predictor of relative neuropathic potential in humans, and it has been possible to class agents as producing neuropathy at doses that are not acutely toxic (tri-*o*-cresyl phosphate); at doses that are acutely toxic but survivable (mipafox); or at doses that are only survivable with acute cholinergic therapy (trichlorophon and dichlorovos). Other agents have little or no neuropathic potential at any dose (sarin and paraoxon). The first two classes are banned from use as pesticides, but some of the third class have produced neuropathy in persons who have attempted suicide but have survived due to intensive care therapy. It is important to note that unexpected neurotoxicity can be produced by otherwise safe organophosphates containing neuropathic impurities, as has happened with some samples of trichlorophon. Tri-*o*-cresyl phosphate (TOCP) is neuropathic at doses of 500 mg/kg and has produced several large outbreaks of human poisoning, largely from the use of contaminated lubricants.

Thallium

Thallium poisonings are relatively rare, as its use as a rodenticide has declined (rats are relatively resistant compared to other species). It produces a distal and predominantly sensory neuropathy with painful paresthesia and ataxia at 10 mg/kg. The axonopathy is of the "dying-back" type, with a distal pattern of degeneration that preferentially affects longer larger-diameter sensory fibers. Demyelination appears to be a secondary event. Central involvement is restricted to the dorsal (sensory) tracts, but high doses produce a poorly characterized encephalopathy. The effects of thallium closely resemble those of arsenic, and they may share a common mechanism via the inhibition of the pyruvate dehydrogenase complex.

Vinca Alkaloids, Colchicine, Taxol and Cisplatin

Vinca alkaloids, such as vincristine and vinblastine, are used for cancer chemotherapy. Much like colchicine, taxol, and cisplatin, they act as antimitotics by inhibiting the formation of microtubules, but they also act on neurofilaments, thereby causing a peripheral neuropathy. Vincristine can sometimes cause acute encephalopathy in young children, probably as a result of penetration of the incomplete blood–brain barrier.

Zinc Pyridinethione

Zinc pyridinethione is a broad-spectrum antimicrobial used in shampoos. In rats it can produce a primary distal axonopathy, probably via a direct action of the pyridinedithione on axonal transport.

Neuronopathy-Inducing Substances

The loss of neurons is irreversible and includes the degeneration of all cytoplasmatic processes and myelin. Neuronopathy can result in either a diffuse encephalopathy with global dysfunction, or a more specific neuronal loss with a specific syndrome of dysfunction.

Hydroxydopapamine

A major component of the progressive loss of catecholaminergic neurons that is seen with age is attributed to the toxicity of oxidized catecholamines. The oxidation of catecholamines by monoamine oxidase produces cytotoxic active oxygen species such as hydrogen peroxide. The glutathione content of the cells protects against these reactive oxygen species, glutathione peroxidase against hydrogen peroxide, and superoxide dismutase against peroxide anions. Dopamine is the most important catecholamine with regard to oxidative damage.

The dopamine analog 6-hydroxydopamine produces a particularly intensive chemical sympathectomy. This compound does not penetrate the blood–brain barrier but enters nerve terminals by an active catecholamine transport mechanism. The result is a selective destruction of sympathic innervation, with consequent changes in heart rate and hypermotility of the gastrointestinal tract. Local injection into the central nervous system results in selective damage to dopaminergic neurons.

Neonatal rats given 6-hydroxydopamine can be used as a model of dopamine deficiency analogous with Lesch–Nyhan disease. Lesch–Nyhan syndrome is characterized by the deficiency of hypoxanthine phosphoryl transferase and loss of central dopaminergic neurons. The consequence is compulsive self-mutilating behavior. Both Lesch–Nyhan and Parkinson's disease are characterized by dopamine deficiency.

Methyl Mercury

Examples of human methyl mercury poisonings were the (episodes of "Minimata disease," seen in Japan in 1956–1960 and in Iraq in 1972. The earliest symptoms are sensory deficiencies, followed by ataxia and motor incoordination. The small neurons of the visual and cerebellar cortices are lost, cerebellar granule cells being particularly sensitive. Adult rats show a loss of sensory neurons in the spinal ganglia, these showing greater accumulation of methyl mercury, and also a "dying-back" peripheral neuropathy. This peripheral neuropathy may not be produced in humans. The exact mechanism of methyl mercury toxicity is not known, but the inhibition of protein synthesis or oxidative stress are thought to be involved. In the developing brain, marked hypoplasia and interrupted neuronal migration are produced. Methyl mercury is not significantly broken down in the brain, and less than 6% of brain mercury is converted to the metallic form.

Metallic mercury (mercury vapor) causes different syndromes in adults and in children. Chronic exposure in adults leads to a reversible syndrome of irritability, confusion, and coarse tremor. Children given mercurous chloride develop a peripheral neuropathy (pink disease) associated with cold, pink, hypotonic, and anesthetic limbs.

Methylphenyltetrahydropyridine (MPTP)

In 1979, a meperidine analog sold as "synthetic heroin," 1-methyl-4-phenyl-1,2,3,6-tetrahydropyridine (MPTP), produced an irreversible neurodegenerative syndrome that was remarkably similar to Parkinson's disease (e.g., rigidity, tremor, and bradykinesia) within hours or days after intake. MPTP is a nonpolar compound at physiological pH. It penetrates the blood–brain barrier and diffuses into the cells. Monoamine oxidase B in astrocytes oxidizes it to the corresponding methylphenyldihydropyridinium salt ($MPDP^+$) and then to methylphenylpyridinium (MPP^+). MPP^+ is then concentrated into dopaminergic neurons of the substantia nigra by the dopamine uptake system and is accumulated by the mitochondria, where it inhibits electron transport by an action on complex I. Although MPP^+ is not very potent as an inhibitor (10^{-3} M), the successive concentration by the dopamine and mitochondrial uptake systems leads to a potent and highly cell-selective effect (Fig. 4). The specifically Parkinsonian syndrome reflects the extreme selectivity of MPTP to nigral neurons. Primates are more sensitive than rodents.

Lead

High-level exposure to inorganic lead (greater than 100 μg/dl blood) can result in encephalopathy in children, in addition to colic and the peripheral neuropathy described under myelin-damaging agents. The characteristic symptoms of acute lead intoxication are vomiting, ataxia, apathy, convulsions, and coma. Morphological correlates are brain edema, focal neuronal necrosis with a disproportionate astrocytic reaction and proliferation, and swelling of endothelial cells associated with increased vascular permeability. Exposure can occur via ingestion of old lead paint, of soil, or of water standing in lead pipes. Atmospheric lead from combustion of leaded gasoline is another source.

Lower-level chronic exposure during early childhood can lead to developmental effects, such as reduced synaptogenesis, and considerable efforts have been devoted to determining the blood lead levels associated with such effects. Estimates suggest that a concentration above 10 μg/dl may give cause for concern. This is roughly 10 times lower than that causing encephalopathy. It is difficult to assign precise values to the effect produced by low-dose lead exposure because social deprivation is often correlated with lead exposure, and social deprivation alone has a strong effect on intellectual development. However, a meta-analysis of several well-controlled longitudinal and cross-sectional epidemiological studies suggests that an increase in blood concentration from 10 to 20 μg/dl is associated with a drop of roughly 1–2 IQ points. While it is difficult to decide on such threshold effects, there is no doubt as to the adverse effect of higher-level exposures, and animal studies have shown delayed synaptogenesis and impaired learning performance at 25 to 50 μg/dl. These lower lead concentrations do not produce pathological signs or increased vascular permeability, but functional measures (such as long-term potentiation of synaptic transmission following a conditioning stimulus) show changes that parallel the learning defects. The mechanism of this effect is not yet known, but lead has a potent effect on the glutamatergic NMDA receptor, and it substitutes for calcium, producing an effect that is essentially pharmacological but that could last throughout brain development with continued exposure Competition between lead and calcium for intestinal absorption leads to the greater bioavail-

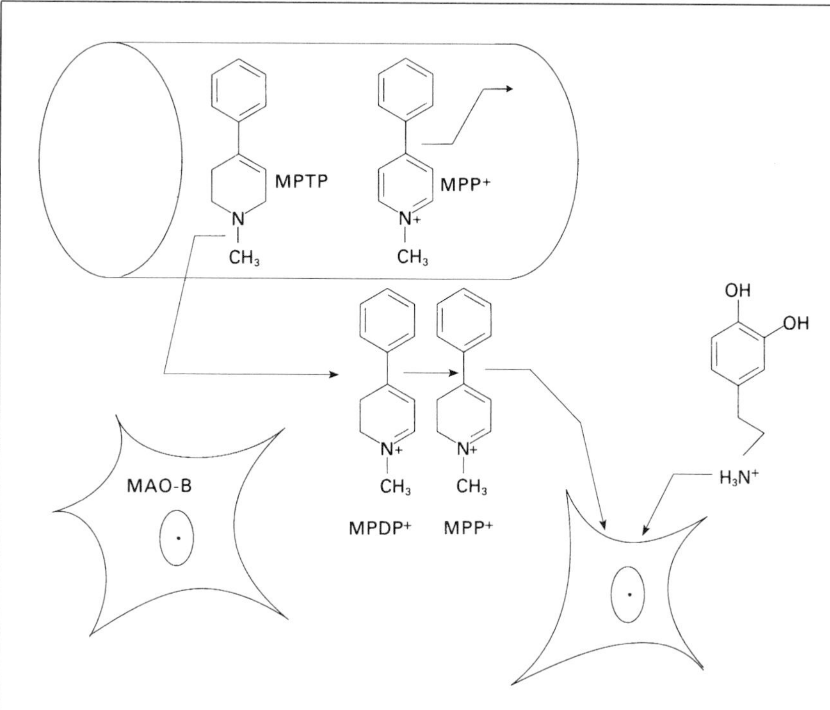

FIGURE 4 Mechanism of action of systemic 1-methyl-4-phenyl-1,2,3,6-tetrahydropyridine (MPTP). The proximal toxin, MPP^+, does not penetrate the blood–brain barrier. However, the lipophylic precursor MPTP does penetrate the barrier and is then oxidized progressively to $MPDP^+$ and then MPP^+ by astrocytic monoamine oxidase B (MAO B). MPP^+ does not pass back out of the blood–brain barrier and is then taken up by monoaminergic neurons in competition with dopamine and further concentrated within their mitochondria, where it inhibits respiration.

ability of lead if there is a lack of calcium in the diet.

Manganese

Manganese exposure, via mining and the production of alloys and batteries, causes "manganese madness," which appears to represent the onset of a selective neuronal loss in the basal ganglia, particularly the globus pallidus, and sometimes the cerebellum. Once this neuronal loss has developed, characteristic motor problems such as rigidity, ataxia, and fine tremor persist. Catecholaminergic neurons appear particularly susceptible, and manganese-catalyzed free-radical oxidative damage is a likely mechanism of pathogenesis. The neuronotoxic effects of manganese appear to be purely central.

Trimethyltin and Triethyllead

These two organometals produce a remarkably similar and selective neuronotoxicity. Trimethyltin is an effective biocide, and triethyllead is produced by hepatic metabolism of tetraethyllead, which is still widely used as a fuel additive. With both agents, damage is mainly restricted to the limbic system. The manufacture of trimethyltin has been associated with eight human poisonings, of which one was fatal. Poisoning with tetraethyllead has been much more common, due to its widespread use in gasoline, resulting in exposure during manufacture, tank cleaning, and solvent abuse by gasoline sniffing. There have been 160 deaths recorded. Signs of poisoning are headache, anxiety, hallucinations, tremor, delirium, and schizophrenia-like episodes. In experimental studies, trimethyltin at 10 mg/kg produces a marked increase in hippocampal neuronal excitability followed by development of dendritic vacuolation and pyramidal neuronal necrosis typical of that produced by excitotoxic agents such as the glutamate analogs. This is accompanied by a chromatolytic change characterized by the swelling of the Golgi apparatus and smooth endoplasmic reticulum, accumulation of secondary lysosomes, and loss of polyribosomes. This chromatolytic effect may be reversible and is not produced by

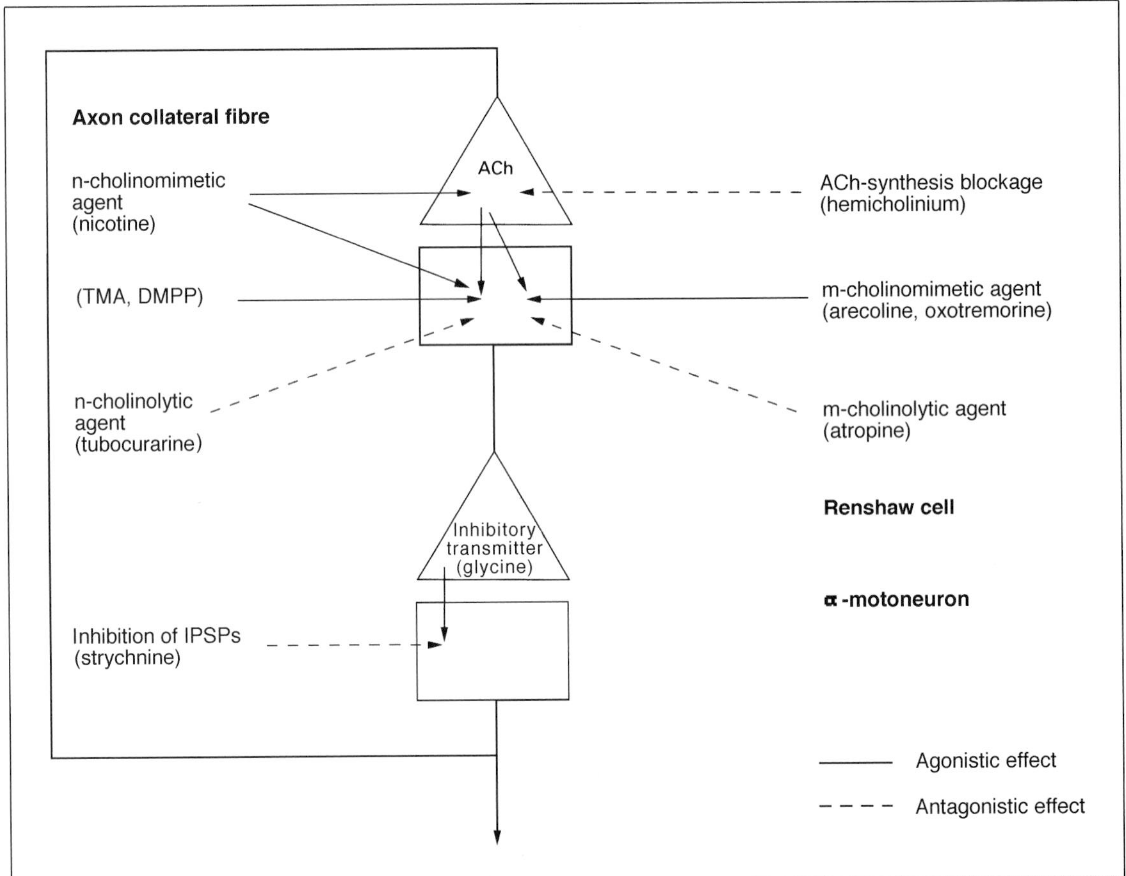

FIGURE 5 The excitation of Renshaw cells is involved in the effects of centrally effective cholinomimetic agents such as arecoline, oxotremorine, and also nicotine. Glycine release inhibits α-motoneurons and consequently limits anti-excitatory capacity.

other excitotoxic agents. Although reversible changes can develop in several different neuronal types, the primary effect is seen in the CA1 and CA3 regions of the dorsal hippocampus and in the pyriform and entorhinal cortices. The myelin edema so characteristic of triethyltin poisoning is not seen, however, possibly because the neuronotoxic effect is so potent that it is not possible to see an effect on myelin at survivable doses. It has been proposed that trimethyltin may be concentrated in vulnerable neurons by their possession of a potent binding protein (stannin), and that this is what confers selective vulnerability.

Substances Affecting Synaptic Transmission

Synapses are particularly sensitive to toxic agents, the relatively nonspecific sedative action of organic solvents being mediated entirely at the synapse. Thus ethylbenzene, xylene, styrene, methyl *n*-ethylketone, tetrachloroethylene, and trichloroethylene all produce sedation and lack of alertness, and this is the basis for setting safe working levels of these agents. Although their action on the membrane may be relatively nonselective, synaptic processes and receptors are particularly sensitive transducers of this action. The synaptic function requires the synthesis, vesicular storage, and release of transmitters, their reaction with receptors, and finally their inactivation. Each of these steps can be influenced by toxic chemicals. Transmitter excess resulting from the inhibition of inactivation produces permanent depolarization and disturbance of synaptic transmission. Alteration of synthesis, storage, or release has also serious consequence. Substances acting as analogs of transmitters can act on receptors as synergists or antagonists and disrupt both excitatory and inhibitory function (Fig. 5). Receptor blockade leads to formation of new postsynaptic receptors and enhanced presynaptic transmitter release.

Anticholinesterase Pesticides

Organophosphates (e.g., malathion and chlorpyrifos) and carbamates (e.g., bendiocarb and carbaryl) act by inhibition of acetylcholinesterase, both in insects and in humans. Like all insecticides they are highly lipophilic and therefore readily penetrate the blood–brain barrier. They are, however, rapidly hydrolyzed by mammalian esterases, and this detoxification process is the basis of their selective toxicity to insects. If the exposure is sufficiently large to overcome metabolic capacity (as in suicide attempts or accidental drenching of the skin with concentrate) or if the metabolic capacity is impaired (as by major coexposure to other organophosphates that inhibit carboxylesterases), poisoning is seen. This takes the form of a complex mixture of central and peripheral muscarinic and nicotinic cholinergic signs due to the accumulation of acetylcholine at the synapse and neuromuscular junction. The principal effects are muscle fasciculations, followed by flaccidity (as the postsynaptic receptor desensitizes), excessive salivation, lachrymation, and bronchial secretion, and seizures. As the effects are predominantly of a pharmacological nature, they regress as the inhibited acetylcholinesterase is either reactivated or resynthesized, usually over hours or days. Two other effects can be seen with some agents, a polyneuropathy (see the section on axonopathy-producing substances), and an "intermediate syndrome." This latter can follow severe acute intoxications and involves a proximal motor weakness with the preservation of distal motor function. It particularly affects the respiratory muscles, lasts for up to 18 days, and may relate to a delayed effect of the massive cholinergic hyperactivity associated with acute poisoning.

Excitatory Amino Acids

Domoic acid (produced by algae and accumulated by mussels), glutamic acid, and kainic acid are excitatory amino acids. Domoic acid sometimes causes headache, confusion, and memory loss in persons poisoned with mussels harvested at the time of algal blooms. Experimental studies with all of these amino acids show that, especially in the neonate where the blood–brain barrier does not exclude them very efficiently, all can produce direct excitotoxicity. Circumventricular cells or cells in the dorsal root ganglia or autonomic ganglia also have a special sensitivity. High oral doses of monosodium glutamate (used as a taste-enhancing ingredient) produce the loss of neurons and dendrites in circumventricular regions and necrosis of retinal neurones.

In addition, the excessively sustained release of endogenous glutamate (as a consequence of brain injury, stroke, or epilepsy) leads to secondary neurodegenerative injury. Neurons are differently sensitive to glutamate; four major receptor types are expressed, showing specific sensitivities. These are the NMDA receptor (*N*-methyl D-aspartate, glutamate), which gives rise to slow calcium influx; two quisqualate receptors (quisqualate, and α-amino-3-hydroxy-5-methyl-4-isoxazolyl propionic acid, AMPA), one of which is inotropic, and another (metabotrophic) receptor, which couples to phosphoinositide hydrolysis via a G protein; and finally the kainate receptor (kainate). The involvement of these different receptor types can be investigated by the use of selective antagonists. NMDA antagonists, such as dizocilpine, have been shown to be effective against experimental excitotoxicity, although the situation is complicated by higher doses of these agents causing a paradoxical excitotoxicity.

The sustained activation of NMDA receptors leads to a calcium and water influx swelling, initially restricted to dendrites but progressing to neuronal vacuolation and chromatin condensation and necrosis. The exhaustion of energy reserves causes this initial exaggeration of normal synaptic transmission to progress to an irreversible alteration of membrane permeability, intracellular Ca^2 excess and consequent oxidative damage to cell membranes, and death by necrosis. If, however, excitotoxicity is more gradual and mitochondrial function is sufficiently preserved, an alternative, apoptotic mode of neuronal death mediated by nitric oxide is produced.

GABA-Receptor Neurotoxins

GABA (γ-aminobutyrate) is the most important inhibitory neurotransmitter in the brains of mammals. There are two types of GABA receptors: $GABA_A$ and $GABA_B$. The $GABA_A$ receptor is a membrane-bound receptor with three binding sites (benzodiazepine, barbiturate and picrotoxin and *t*-butyl bicyclophosphorothionate), which determine the conductance of a Cl^- ion channel component. $GABA_B$ receptors produce a sustained potassium conductance. Bicuculline (found in Fumariaceae) is a potent convulsant and blocks $GABA_A$ receptors. The receptor has binding sites with high and low affinity. Subacute administration of bicuculline produces up-regulation of $GABA_A$ receptors, while the binding site for picrotoxin remains unchanged.

Picrotoxin is nitrogen-free polycyclic lactone, found in plants (Menispermaceae). Picrotoxin is a mixture of two components, picroitoxinin (active) and picrotin (inactive). Picrotoxin blocks the $GABA_A$ receptor.

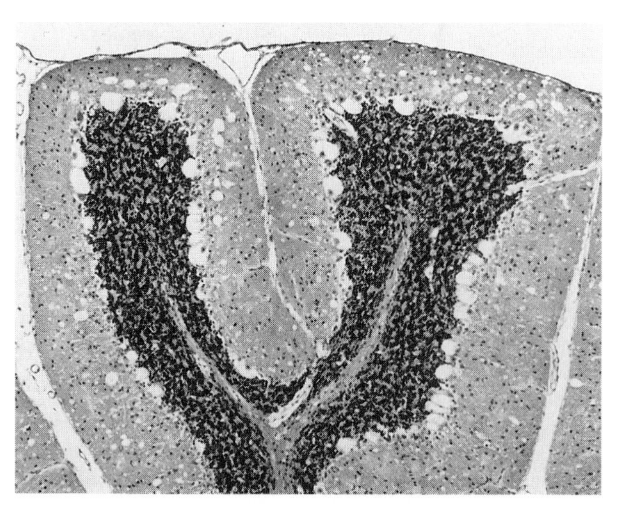

FIGURE 6 Selective destruction of cerebellar Purkinje cells by the fungal tremogen penitrem A. Sagittal section through the cerebellar cortex of a rat 2 days after administration of 3 mg/kg penitrem A. All of the Purkinje cells have been destroyed, and their position is marked by the empty spaces at the junction of the pale-staining molecular layer and the dark-staining granule cell layer. At this dose there is no loss of other cell types.

Anisatin is a convulsion-inducing substance from the Japanese plant *Illicum anissatum* and acts also as a potent GABA antagonist. However, it is a noncompetitive antagonist with binding sites in the Cl^- ion channel. Muscimol, found in fly agaric (*Amanita muscaria*), is a $GABA_A$ agonist. Baclofen acts as a $GABA_B$ agonist.

Glycine-Receptor Neurotoxins

Strychnine is a potent antagonist of the spinal glycine receptor, which is the major inhibitory receptor in the spinal cord. It is used as a rodenticide, and human poisoning is associated with potent spinal hyperexcitation (tonic extensor spasm and rictus).

Insecticides Acting on the GABA Receptor

Cyclodienes, hexachlorocyclohexane, lindane, and toxaphene act as noncompetitive $GABA_A$ receptor antagonists. At high doses they are convulsants in humans, their potency paralleling their capacity to bind to the $GABA_A$ receptor.

Poisons of Animals, Plants, and Microbes

Botulinum toxin binds irreversibly to peripheral cholinergic presynaptic axon terminals and inhibits the release of acetylcholine. Muscles show changes consistent with denervation. The neuron reacts initially with chromatolysis and swelling. The nucleolar and ribosomal RNA increase. During recovery, the neurons sprout again and form new synapses.

Tetanus toxin blocks glycine and GABA synapses.

α-Lactrotoxin (black widow spider toxin), glycerotoxin (from a marine worm), and leptinotoxins (from a beetle) produce transmitter (acetylcholine) depletion.

Agents Acting on Ion Channels

The pyrethroid insecticides (e.g., permethrin and deltamethrin) are synthetic analogs of the natural pyrethrins found in chrysanthemum flowers. Both are potent sodium-channel toxins, prolonging the open channel state, but having little effect on its voltage dependence. This, coupled with an action of some pyrethroids on the voltage-gated chloride channel, leads to a state of sustained neuronal hyperexcitability without depolarization. Pyrethroids are highly lipophilic but, like organophosphates, are rapidly detoxified by ester hydrolysis in mammals. Hence, intoxication has only been seen in humans after deliberate overdose or major dermal contamination with concentrates. The signs of intoxication depend on the degree of prolongation of the open state of the sodium channel, agents causing prolongations of 1–10 ms causing fine tremor and reflex hyperexcitability (type I poisoning), and agents causing longer prolongation producing choreoathetosis and seizures (type II poisoning). Intoxication is reversible once the pyrethroid has been eliminated, and there are no direct long-term effects.

Tetrodotoxin (from pufferfish), saxitoxin (from marine plankton), and μ-conotoxin (from cone-shells) block sodium channels and inhibit action potentials. These produce paralysis. Batrachotoxin (a poison of South American frogs), veratridine (from green hellebores and death camas), aconitine, and grayanotoxin cause persistent activation of sodium-channel permeability, leading to prolonged depolarization.

Inactivation of sodium channels is delayed by scorpion α-toxins, the toxin of sea anemones, and γ-agatoxins (spider toxins). The blockade of calcium-dependent potassium channels is produced by apamin (toxin of the honey bee) and charybdotoxin (toxin of the scorpion). The blockade of calcium uptake and inhibition of transmitter release (ACh) is caused by β-bungarotoxin, crotoxin, notoxin, and taipoxin. Further calcium-channel-blocking toxins are ω-conotoxin, atrotoxin, and ω-agatoxin. α-Bungarotoxin blocks the nicotinergic acetylcholine receptor.

The avermectins (e.g., ivermectin) are used as antihelminthics and act as both voltage- and ligand-gated chloride-channel agonists. They have a very large therapeutic index in mammals, however, because they are effectively excluded from the CNS by the multidrug receptor transporter located in the blood–brain barrier.

The fungal toxin penitrem-A is a potent blocker of high-conductance calcium-activated potassium channels and induces severe tremor, followed by the development of selective cerebellar Purkinje and granule cell death (Fig. 6). It is likely that this is related to an excitotoxic process caused or enhanced by the loss of potassium-channel function. The related mycotoxin lolitrem is responsible for perennial ryegrass staggers in cattle and horses.

Cycad Neurotoxicity

Serious neurodegenerative conditions, resembling a combination of Parkinson's disease and amyotrophic lateral sclerosis (ALS), have been seen in some islands of the West Pacific region. In all these locations ALS is connected with the consumption of flour made from the fruits of cycad plants. Cycads have also been found to produce ataxia and degeneration of the spinocerebellar tracts and dorsal root ganglia of cattle. Although the presumed neurotoxic substance has not been found, two compounds with different neurotoxic properties can be isolated from the seeds of various cycads: β-*N*-methylamino-L-alanine and methylazoxymethanol. Methylazoxymethanol is hepatotoxic, carcinogenic, and neuroteratogenic. It inhibits the mitosis and migration of cerebellar neurons in neonatal rodents. Experimental studies have, however, shown it to have little or no neurotoxic potential at subhepatotoxic doses in adults. β-*N*-Methylamino-L-alanine (BMAA) is a glutamatergic excitotoxin that produces remarkably selective damage to GABA-ergic cerebellar neurons at 4 g/kg in rats, but does not seem to be sufficiently potent to produce the ALS syndrome. Epidemiology, however, suggests a connection between the consumption of cycad flour and these neurodegenerative injuries, and it is possible that amino acid deficiency associated with a high rate of consumption of these plant proteins in some way synergizes the neurotoxicity of these agents.

Bibliography

Baker, D. J., and Sedgwick, E. M. (1996). Single fibre electromyographic changes in man after organophosphate exposure. *Hum. Exper. Toxicol.* **15,** 369–375.

Beal, M. F., Kowall, N. W., Ellison, D. W., Mazurek, M. F., Swartz, K. J., and Martin, J. B. (1993). Neurochemical and histologic characterization of striatal excitotoxic lesions produced by the mitochondrial toxin 3-nitropropionic acid. *J. Neurosci.* **13,** 4181–4192.

Bleecker, M. L., Bolla, K. I., Agnew, J., Scwartz, B. S., and Ford, D. P. (1991). Dose-related subclinical neurobehavioural effects of chronic exposure to low levels of organic solvents. *Amer. J. Ind. Med.* **19,** 715–728.

Bradbury, M. (1992). "Physiology and Pharmacology of the Blood-Brain Barrier." Springer-Verlag, Berlin.

Cattabeni, F., and Abbracchio, M. P. (1988). Behavioral teratology: an inappropriate term for some uninterpretable effects. *T.I.P.S.* **9,** 13–15.

Cavanagh, J. B., Holton, J. L., Nolan, C. C., Ray, D. E., Naik, J. T., and Mantle, P. G. (1998). The effects of the tremorgenic mycotoxin Penitrem A on the rat cerebellum. *Veterinary Pathol.* **35,** 53–63.

Chang, L. W., and Slikker, W. (1995). "Neurotoxicology—Approaches and Methods." Academic Press, San Diego, CA.

Chaudhuri, J., Chakraborti, T. K., Chanda, S., and Pope, C. N. (1993). Differential modulation of organophospate sensitive muscarinic receptors in rat brain by parathion and chlorpyrifos. *J. Biochem. Toxicol.* **8,** 207–216.

Cherry, N. (1993). Neurobehavioural effects of solvents: The role of alcohol. *Environ. Res.* **62,** 155–158.

Crofton, K. M., Howard, J. L., Moser, V. C., Gill, M. W., Reiter, L. W., Tilson, H. A., and MacPhail, R. C. (1991). Interlaboratory comparison of motor activity experiments: Implications for neurotoxicological assessments. *Neurotoxicol. Teratol.* **13,** 599–609.

Ghesi-Egea, J. F., Perrin, R., Leninger-Muller, B., Suleman, G., Seist, G., and Minn, A. (1994). Localisation of drug-metabolising enzyme activities to blood-brain interfaces and circumventricular organs. *J. Neurochem.* **62,** 1089–1096.

Gutowski, M., Altmann, L., Sveinsson, K., and Wiegand, H. (1997). Postnatal development of synaptic plasticity in the CA3 hippocampal region of control and lead-exposed Wistar rats. *Dev. Brain Res.* **98,** 82–90.

Harry, G. J. (1994). "Developmental Neurotoxicology." CRC Press, Boca Raton, FL.

Hayes, W. J., and Laws, E. R. (1991). "Handbook of Pesticide Toxicology." Academic Press, San Diego, CA.

Hu, H.-L., Bennett, N., Lamb, J. H., Ghersi-Egea, J.-F., Schlosshauer, B., and Ray, D. E. (1997). Capacity of rat brain to metabolize *m*-dinitrobenzene: An *in vitro* study. *Neurotoxicology* **18,** 363–370.

Isaacson, R. L., and Jensen, K. F. (1992). "The Vulnerable Brain and Environmental Risks," Vol. 1. Plenum Press, New York.

Kostrzewa, R. M. (1998). "Highly Selective Neurotoxins, Basic and Clinical Applications." Humana Press, Totowa, NJ.

Steensgaard, A., Ostergaard, G., Jensen, C. V., Lam, H. R., Topp, S., Ladefoged, O., ArlienSoborg, P., and Henriksen O. (1996). Effect on the content of n-acetylaspartate, total creatine choline containing compounds, and lactate in the hippocampus of rats exposed to aromatic white spirit for three weeks measured by NMR spectroscopy. *Neurotoxicology* **17,** 785–792.

Leist, M., Volbracht, C., Kuhnle, S., Fava, E., Ferrando-May, E., and Nicotera, P. (1997). Caspase-mediated apoptosis in neuronal excitotoxicity triggered by nitric oxide. *J. Mol. Med.* **3,** 750–764.

Lowndes, H. E. (1987). "Electrophysiology in Neurotoxicology." CRC Press, Boca Raton FL.

O'Donoghue, J. L. (1985). "Neurotoxicity of Industrial and Commercial Chemicals." CRC Press, Boca Raton, FL.

Pryor, G. T., Uyeno, E. T., Tilson, H. A., and Mitchell, C. L. (1983). Assessment of chemicals using a battery of neurobehavioural tests: a comparative study. *Neurobehav. Toxicol. Teratol.* **5,** 91–117.

Ray, D. E. (1992). Hazards from solvents, pesticides and PCB's. *In* "Indoor Air Pollution" (Leslie, G. B. and Lunau, F. W., eds.), pp. 131–159. Cambridge University, Cambridge.

Ray, D. E. (1997). Function in neurotoxicity: Index of effect and also determinant of vulnerability. *Clin. Exp. Pharmacol. Physiol.* **24,** 857–860.

Spencer, P. S., and Schaumberg, H. (1985). "Experimental and Clinical Neurotoxicology" Williams & Wilkins, Baltimore, MD.

Spurgeon, A., Gompertz, D., Harrington, J. M. (1996). Modifiers of non-specific symptoms in occupational and environmental syndromes. *Occupat. Environ. Med.* **53,** 361–366.

Thiel, R., Chahoud, I., Schwabe, R., and Neubert, D. (1989). Device for monitoring locomotor activity of 120 animals: Motility of offspring of dams exposed to haloperidol. *Neurotoxicol.* **10,** 621–628.

Vinken, P. J., and Bruyn, G. W. (1994). "Handbook of Clinical Neurology, Vol. 64, Intoxications of the Nervous System." Elsevier, Amsterdam.

WHO (1986). "Principles and Methods for the Assessment of Neurotoxicity Associated with Exposure to Chemicals." Environmental Health Criteria 60, World Health Organization, Geneva.

Zbinden, G. (1992) "The Brain in Bits and Pieces: In Vitro Techniques in Neurobiology, Neuropharmacology and Neurotoxicology." MTC Verlag, Zollikon, Switzerland.

CHAPTER

21

Reproduction and Development

DIETHER NEUBERT,* BIRGIT JÖDICKE,† FRANK WELSCH‡

*Institute of Clinical Pharmacology and Toxicology, Benjamin Franklin Medical Center, Free University Berlin, Berlin, Germany

†Wetzlar, Germany

‡Chemical Industry Institute of Toxicology, Research Triangle Park, North Carolina

INTRODUCTION

Developmental and reproductive toxicology are comparatively young areas of research. Before the thalidomide disaster (1959–1962), no routine toxicological evaluation of chemically induced adverse effects on reproduction and development was performed. Although malformations were induced experimentally using a selection of substances, this was not done in the frame of safety evaluations of new medicinal products. Therefore, thalidomide had not been tested for possible teratogenic effects before marketing. The disastrous experience with thalidomide has drastically altered the general opinions on drug safety and risk assessment, as well as legislation, in all fields of toxicology. Since the mid-1960s, systematic preclinical studies of the possible adverse effects on reproduction and development are an integral part of the requirements needed for registration of new pharmaceutical products and certain types of environmentally occurring chemicals, such as pesticides.

With respect to the possible number of adverse effects and according to the periods during which such effects can be initiated, reproductive and developmental toxicology represents by far the largest and most complex field in toxicology because the adverse effects may manifest themselves from fertilization until the end of life. This area of research is interlinked with many other fields of toxicology, such as transplacental carcinogenesis, organ toxicity, neurotoxicology, and immunotoxicology. Various aspects of embryology, of cell biology, and more recently also of molecular biology must be taken into account when analyzing abnormal development.

Remarks on Embryology

It is not within the scope of this chapter to review embryology, and the interested reader is referred to excellent textbooks on this subject. Knowledge of the basic principles of normal development and reproduction is essential to the understanding of the possible interference with these processes.

Some milestones of prenatal development are compiled in Table 1. Figure 1 shows the rapid change in size. Somewhat simplified, the first week of gestation may be designated as the preimplantation period. The zygote has no direct contact with the maternal organism, and the blastocyst implants within the uterus at the end of the first and the beginning of the second week. The primitive organs are formed during the second and third gestational week. Organogenesis, the important target developmental stage of teratogenic effects, starts at the end of the second and extends until the end of the 8th to 9th gestational week. At that time, most of the primordia (organ anlagen) have differentiated, and the appearance of the conceptus is human-like. The heart is beating and the circulation functioning.

TABLE 1 Selected Stages of Human Development and Approximate Embryonic Age

Carnegie stage[a]	Organ development	Somite pairs	Days[b]	mm
1	Zygote		1	
2	2- to 16-cell stage		1.5–3	
3	Free blastocyst		4	
4	Attachment of blastocyst within the uterus		5–6	
5	Implantation, two germ layers		7–11	
6	Primitive streak		13	0.2
9	First somites		20	2–3
10	Fusion of neural folds, heart is beating	4–12	22	
11	Fusion of rostral neuroporus	13–20	24	3–5
12	Upper limb bud appears	21–29	26	
13	Four limb buds, ear vesicle	30+	28	4–6
15	Upper limb with hand plate, eye lens	30+	37	8–11
23	Embryo largely developed, contact of palatal shelves		56–63	26–30

[a]Developmental stages for primates expressed as: Carnegie stages 1 to 23, based on embryos of a collection from the Carnegie Institute, U.S. Stages are only defined for the embryonic period.
[b]Only rough estimate possible because of considerable variability at the early stages.

Early developmental stages may correlate only poorly with days of gestation because considerable individual variability exists. If such a correlation is shown in textbooks, it certainly is a didactic simplification.

After the embryonic period, the fetal period of prenatal development begins, during which many of the organ systems mature. Fetogenesis is generally assumed to start at palatal closure (9th or 10th gestational week in humans) and lasts until birth. During this prenatal period, many possibilities for disturbances still exist. Birth is a drastic change for many mammalian organisms, and many adaptation processes must be properly initiated, such as breathing and cardiovascular changes.

The speed of development greatly differs among species (Table 2) and is not identical even in many nonhuman primates and humans. Because the length and extent of fetal development varies considerably in different species, the state of maturity at birth is

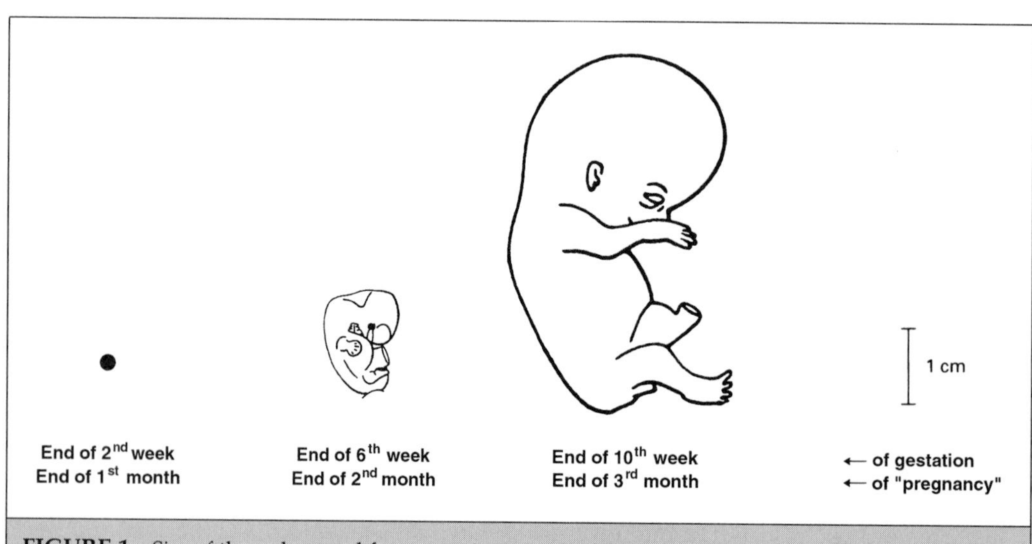

FIGURE 1 Size of the embryo and fetus at various stages of development. Indicated is the original size of the different developmental stages.

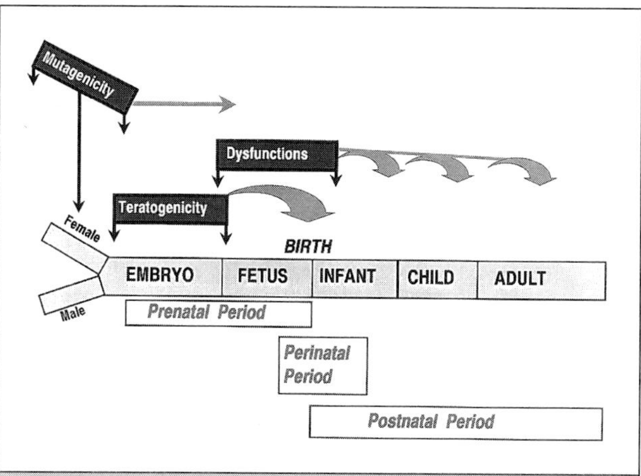

FIGURE 2 Developmental periods and typical stage-specific pathological manifestations.

very different in various mammals. For example, horses or guinea pigs are capable of walking around very soon after birth, but in humans and many other mammals development is by no means complete at birth and the newborn is quite immature in many respects. Such species differences must be taken into account when extrapolating data from an experimental animal model to humans.

With respect to reproduction and fertility, it is important that all oocytes are preformed before birth, while in males spermatogenesis continues during the entire life span. This creates quite different situations with respect to the possibility of disturbances. In both genders, important differentiations take place during the perinatal period (shortly before and a few weeks after birth), many of these processes cannot be made up for during later life. Irreversible lesions result when such differentiation processes are perturbed (see the section on Hormonal Disrupters).

Terminology

The most comprehensive statement of the topic addressed in this chapter on developmental and reproductive toxicology is "toxic (or adverse) effects elicited by chemical substances or physical factors on pre- and postnatal development and the reproductive capacity." It is thus obvious that this specialty area in toxicology must concern itself with the vast multiplicity of all aspects of potential adverse effects induced by naturally occurring and human made chemicals on either the male or the female of the species of interest. In the context of this chapter, developmental and reproductive toxicology will be presented as a science with an anthropocentric orientation. Primary consideration will be given to human aspects and to mammalian studies, with emphasis on extrapolations to situations possibly existing in humans.

In the English scientific literature, it has become customary to distinguish "developmental toxicity" from "reproductive toxicity." Reproduction is largely synonymous with fertility, including the formation and function of male and female germ cells. Development refers predominantly to the prenatal and early postnatal (lactational) periods. Of course, develop-

TABLE 2 Comparison of Developmental Stages in Selected Species

	Estimated gestational age[a]			
Developmental stage	**Human**	**Rabbit**	**Rat**	**Mouse**
Zygote[b]	1	1	1	1
Implantation, two germ layers	7–11	5–6	5–6	6–7
First somites	20		9–10	8–9
Start of heart beat	22–24		10–11	9–10
Upper limb bud appears	26–27	10–11	10–11	9–10
Palate closure	56–70	19–20	16–17	14–16
Total gestational period[c]	255–275	31–34	21–23	19–21

[a]Only rough estimates are possible; values are not identical in different strains of the same species.

[b]Zygote; fertilized egg cell ("one-cell embryo").

[c]Gestational period, also "prenatal period" or time after conception (p.c. = post conceptionem), period from fertilization until birth. In women, always 2 weeks less than the obstetrical designation of pregnancy (defined from the beginning of the last menstruation).

ment continues well into infancy and childhood and in some respects even much further into adult life.

Nomenclature in Reproductive Toxicology

With respect to research activities, reproductive toxicology is divided along gender lines. Most of the methods with a high degree of predictability in human reproductive toxicology require the analysis of both the male and the female partner because information on male fertility can only be obtained from studies on women and their offspring. Male reproductive toxicity in humans is primarily concerned with the potential interference of exogenous agents disturbing the ability of exposed men to father normal healthy children. Information on the components and functions related to male reproductive capacity may be obtained from hormone analyses (serum or urine samples), semen analyses, or testes biopsies. While semen samples may be relatively easily obtained under controlled although rather poorly standardized, conditions, the procedure poses a problem with regard to the invasion of privacy. In women, reproductive toxicity assessments are hampered by the lack of biological samples that can be collected by noninvasive approaches, which are critical to differential diagnosis. Almost all clinical exploration, exclusive of urine samples for hormone excretion analyses, require good cooperation of the volunteers or patients and are challenging to human sensitivities and the desire for privacy. The more recent advances have offered increased avenues for prenatal assessments by advanced diagnostic methods (e.g., ultrasound, amniocentesis, and placental villus sampling) and thereby facilitate the evaluation of abnormal development in humans, though not necessarily aspects of fertility.

Nomenclature in Developmental Toxicology

It is justified to classify developmental toxicity according to the period of exposure to the exogenous agent (Fig. 2) as toxicity due to prenatal exposure (prenatal toxicity), toxicity due to perinatal exposure (perinatal toxicity), and toxicity due to postnatal exposure (toxicity in the neonate, infant, and child).

A considerable amount of research in developmental toxicology is specifically directed towards the pregnant female and her product(s) of conception (the conceptus) and specifically the mammalian embryo and fetus. Several endpoints of the adverse effects on the embryo may be distinguished; "embryotoxic" refers to any kind of toxic effect on the embryo (i.e., the conceptus until the end of the organogenesis period). Such toxic effects include (Fig. 2) embryolethal effects (embryomortality, resorptions in polytocous animals, or abortion in humans), teratogenic effects (gross structural defects), and retarded growth (which is generalized or confined to certain primordia).

Abnormal development may also be induced during the fetal period because the structures and functions of several organs continue to differentiate during this period. All toxic effects induced during this period are designated as "fetotoxic." Examples are the abnormal development of external genitalia (e.g., caused by androgens [masculinization of female fetuses] or anti-androgens [feminization of male fetuses]) and behavioral defects. The mechanisms of induction of such abnormalities, as well as the type of the outcome, are different from those induced during the embryonic phase. Therefore, structural or functional fetotoxic defects should not be designated as "teratogenic" because this a typical embryotoxic effect.

Developmental toxicology extends well into the postnatal period (termed dysfunctions, i.e., effects on functional organ maturation) because development in humans is by no means completed at birth. A few examples are the brain, the hormonal system, and the immune system, which develop to a large extent postnatally and whose development is susceptible to exogenous influences during early postnatal life. Overall, pre-, peri- and postnatally inflicted insults can affect the newborn directly or can have an impact on later postnatal life or even on the next generation.

Advantages and Limitations of Epidemiological Studies

Like the entire field of human medicine, developmental and reproductive toxicology is anthropocentric and thus information obtained in humans has the greatest significance. However, sufficient human data most often are not available, and the significance of this type of human case reports is often overestimated by laymen. For most chemicals it is rarely possible to even attempt a human risk assessment on the basis of human data. While it may be feasible to obtain some information on reproductive and developmental toxicity of medically used drugs, the situation is almost hopeless in the case of chemicals and environmental substances. This rests in the *a priori* limitations of epidemiology; it is a basic rule of epidemiology that the results of single studies cannot provide evidence for causal relationships. Only suspicions may be raised or hypotheses formulated, which must be verified or disproved by further independent studies. This is extremely costly and time consuming, and further studies may not be justifiable from an ethical point of view if a serious suspicion has been raised.

Preventive measures may have to be taken to reduce or even prohibit the exposure to such a potentially dangerous agent before the issue is scientifically clarified. It may be difficult or even impossible to control the numerous confounding factors because nobody is exposed to only one noxious agent, and many of the constituents in mixtures may be unknown. For most manifestations of reproductive or developmental toxicology, spontaneous rates exist, which must be taken into account when evaluating additional adverse effects.

For a risk assessment, quantification of the exposure is essential. This is comparatively easy in the case of medically used drugs, but almost impossible in the case of environmental chemicals. The predictive value of exposure assessment efforts concerned with the latter type of chemical agent is generally low. Mostly it is impossible to establish dose–response relationships, the strongest criterion for a substance-induced effect. At present it is difficult or even impossible to evaluate other than teratogenic endpoints.

Many people feel a curious urge to associate the cause of adverse effects with medical treatment rather than with the underlying diseases. During pregnancy most drugs are given for therapeutic reasons. Therefore, one must ask whether abnormal development may be the result of a disease and not of the medication, and for a number of diseases such a correlation is well established, for example, for convulsive disorders, poorly managed diabetes, and other complications of pregnancy (Table 3). It should be noted that generally only ratios of 1.5 and above can be considered as medically significant. We must keep in mind that in general only pronounced effects can be recognized under realistic study conditions. This holds true for both observations in humans and results of animal studies. Although of minor or no medical significance, possible borderline effects provide the grounds for endless political discussions, which are always useless because no meaningful answer can be expected.

Spontaneous Rates of Malformations and Abortions

It is often assumed that the majority of manifestations of abnormality, such as frank malformations or also tumors, are caused by toxic, that is, environmental or extrinsic, factors. This is increasingly doubted by many experts, and we must take into account the distinct possibility that such adverse reactions may be predominantly caused or are greatly modified because of spontaneous or intrinsic reasons. Knowledge of the extent of such spontaneous rates is essential for any assessment of toxic effects caused by chemical or physical agents because the rate of any toxic effects can only be meaningfully evaluated superimposed upon the spontaneous occurrences.

With regard to human development, we must accept the fact that after implantation a healthy baby is not born in all cases. While prenatal wastage occurs in all species, the rate is especially high in humans and nonhuman primates. The reasons for this are only partly understood.

While no data are available on preimplantation loss, early embryo losses in humans are especially pronounced shortly after implantation, about 35% as deduced from studies measuring β-HCG, and the chance for prenatal mortality becomes smaller as pregnancy advances (Table 4). Some information on this topic is also available from *in vitro* fertilizations.

TABLE 3 Maternal Diseases and Complications of Pregnancy Associated with an Increased Malformation Rate[a]

Disease or complication	Standardized relative risk (srR)[b]	Disease or complication	Standardized relative risk (srR)[b]
Diabetes, >5 years	2.4	Single umbilical artery	4.1
Convulsive disorders	1.7	After three abnormal children	2.9
Altered blood clotting	1.7	Hydramnios	2.4
Hemorrhagic shock	1.6	Maternal age >40	1.5
Vena cava syndrome	1.5	Maternal age <14	1.4
Bleeding within first trimester	1.1	X rays, abdominal	1.1
Hyperemesis gravidarum	1.0	Smoking >30 cigarettes/day	1.0[c]

[a]Data from Heinonen *et al.* (1977).
[b]srR of 2.0 means doubling of the risk compared with the reference group.
[c]Relates only to malformations, not to other complications.
Hydramnios: Pathologically increased amount of amniotic fluid.

TABLE 4 Estimates of the "Spontaneous" Prenatal Mortality at Different Developmental Stages in Humans[a]	
Type of prenatal wasting	**Percentage**
Preimplantation loss	?20
Early postimplantation loss	30–35[b]
Clinically observed abortions	7–10[b]
	10–15[c]
Stillbirths	≈1[c]
Neonatal mortality (within first postnatal week)	≈1[c]
Spontaneous deaths within the first postnatal year	≈1[c]
Sum of wastage until the end of the first postnatal year	≈45–70[b]

[a]The rate is influenced by many factors, such as maternal age, number of previous abortions, and socioeconomic status. (Data from Miller *et al.* (1980). For comparison, maternal mortality (in Germany) is about 0.01%.

[b]Based on implantations.

[c]Based on viable newborn.

The early loss is not associated with typical clinical signs and is often taken as an atypical menstruation.

Clinically obvious spontaneous abortions are observed in numerous countries at a rate of 10 to 15%. The risk is not equally distributed within a population, and it depends on maternal age, socioeconomic status, the number of previous pregnancies and abortions, and other factors. It is now well established from large studies that in a high percentage (at least 50%) of these spontaneous abortions, chromosomal aberrations (mostly nondisjunctions) are present within the embryo. Therefore, attempts to save these conceptuses by various means will be largely unsuccessful and undesirable. It could be shown that in the mouse *all* possible types of trisomies do not survive pregnancy. Although most of these types of chromosomal aberrations will also cause prenatal loss in humans, a few may survive, depending on the type of trisomy (e.g., trisomy 21, Down's syndrome). Maternal age has been found to be one etiologically important factor (Table 5), but some aberrations are of paternal origin.

Spontaneous malformations also occur in all species, but at different percentages. In humans, the over-

TABLE 5 Association between Frequency of Chromosomal Aberrations and Maternal Age and Paternal Age[a]

		Trisomy			
Maternal age	**Number of pregnancies**	**13**	**18**	**21**	**All aberrations**
25–30				<0.1%	
30–34				0.1%	0.3%
35–39	34,076	<0.1%	0.1%	0.7%	1.3%
40–44	18,020	0.1%	0.4%	1.8%	3.0%
45–>46	869	0.1%	0.5%	5.2%	8.1%

	Maternal age, all aberrations			
Paternal age ↓	**35–37**	**%**	**41 to >44**	**%**
≤40	18/1635	1%	15/375	4%
>44	9/244	4%	36/544	7%

[a]Data as percent of cases from prenatal diagnosis. Data from: International Clearinghouse (1991) and Weitzel (1992).

TABLE 6 Example of the Frequency of Abnormal Development in Humans[a]

Type of abnormality	Observed frequency	
	Absolute	Percentage
Stillbirths	798/50282	(1.6%)
Neonatal mortality	806/50282	(1.6%)
Infant mortality (within the 1. postnatal year)	384/50282	(0.8%)
Infant mortality (between 2 and 4 years of age)	239/50282	(0.5%)
Sum of mortality	2227/50282	(4.4%)
Total malformations[b]	2277/50282	(4.5%)
Severe malformations	1393/50282	(2.8%)
Minor malformations	898/50282	(1.8%)
Syndromes	176/50282	(0.4%)
Tumors	164/50282	(0.3%)

[a]Data of a large study from the U.S. (performed 1958–1965). 50,282 mother-/child-pairs were evaluated. Data from Heinonen *et al.* (1977).

[b]The frequency of malformations is based on: stillbirths, viable or decreased children during the first year of postnatal life, and children dying until the end of the 4. year of postnatal life.

all rate of spontaneous severe malformations is about 2–3% among live births (Table 6). Because many of the malformations, such as cardiac defects, are not detected at that time, the rate of malformations is about twice as high at the end of the first year of postnatal life.

Spontaneous rates are not constant but may vary considerably within a certain range with respect to different time periods and the size of the population investigated. Only incidence rates above this background fluctuation are of significance in clinical toxicology. The large numbers of mother–child pairs necessary for assessing a reliable background rate can only be obtained in long-term or multicenter studies.

The difficulty in revealing the exact rate of spontaneously occurring malformations within a given population has simple statistical reasons (see Chapter 51 on risk assessment). The fluctuations within various years will be small if a large number of mother–child pairs is evaluated, but the amplitude will be large when a relatively small population is evaluated. The spontaneous rate of any single malformation is rather small, in the range of <1‰, and large study groups are required to provide reliable frequencies (Table 7).

There is now good evidence that many of the malformed embryos and fetuses die prenatally, thus contributing to the prenatal wastage. In fact it appears that the malformations detectable at birth are only the tip of the iceberg (Table 8). This may be considered as a protective mechanism, and any successful attempt to interfere with this wastage and save the pregnancy is likely to increase the malformation rate observed at birth.

Statistical Considerations

Some basic and simplified information on the statistical power of studies in terato-epidemiology is compiled in Table 9. The spontaneous rates assumed in this compilation correspond to the total frequency of malformations in a human population, the frequency of the sum of malformations at certain organs (e.g., 0.8% cardiac abnormalities), and the frequency of single malformations (assumed to be about 0.05%).

From this calculation, it can be deduced that in a study with 100 children exposed *in utero*, only an 80-fold increase above the spontaneous rate of a single malformation (0.05%) can be recognized (four pathological cases). If only three cases are observed (a 60-fold increase above the spontaneous rate), no significant difference compared to the controls can be deduced. This example indicates the low predictive power of this type of study if negative results are obtained. Because of these limitations, experimental studies are inevitable for preventive hazard minimization.

Statistical limitations, of course, also exist with respect to animal studies. This holds especially true when no malformations occur within the concurrent controls, but single defects are observed among the

TABLE 7 Important Malformations in Humans Detectable at Birth (percent)[a]

Type of malformation[b]	Percent[c] U.S.[d]	Variation[e]
Anencephaly	0.03	(0.008–0.2)
Spina bifida	0.05	(0.02–0.2)
Encephalocele	0.01	(0.003–0.03)
Hydrocephalus	0.05	(0.02–0.09)
Microtia	0.02	(0.001–0.06)
Transposition of great vessels	0.01	(0.001–0.05)
Hypoplastic heart syndrome	0.01	(0.001–0.03)
Cleft palate	0.05	(0.03–0.10)
Complete cleft lip	0.09	(0.05–0.16)
Esophageal atresia	0.02	(0.004–0.04)
Anorectal atresia	0.03	(0.01–0.06)
Kidney agenesis or -dysgenesis	0.02	(0.004–0.04)
Hypospadia	0.1	(0.02–0.30)
Limb reduction defect	0.04	(0.03–0.08)
Diaphragmatic hernia	0.02[f]	(0.006–0.04)
Omphalocele	0.03[f]	(0.01–0.04)

[a]Data from large statistical evaluations within the U.S. (12.8 million births, 1974–1988) and from 23 other centers (worldwide with 0.2 to 9.5 million births each). Data from International Clearinghouse (1991). In contrast to Table 6, only defects detectable at birth are considered.

[b]Agensis: congenital complete missing of an organ anlage. Anencephalia: within the early embryonic period initiated malformation (always lethal within the first week of postnatal life) with defect and largely missing brain, caused by lack of closure of the upper neuroporus, often combined with other malformations. Atresia: congenital lack of opening of a physiological body orifice. Dysgenesis: congenital lack of a special organ function. Encephalocele: malformation with defect of the skull and protrusion of meninx and parts of the brain. Hydrocephalus: "dropsy of head" through enlargement of the liquor cavities. Hypospadia: malformation with urethral orifice below the normal position. Microtia: defect with too small auricle. Omphalocele: congenital umbilical hernia. Spina bifida: malformation with cleft spine (rhachischisis), most often at the lower vertebral column.

[c]Births after >20 gestational weeks, mean values over >10 years

[d]1200 hospitals with about 15% of the birth within the U.S. (Stillbirths at an age of >20 weeks are included in the percentages).

[e]Average frequency (1974–1988) in 23 additional centers.

[f]In this case only percentages of 0.4 million births in Atlanta, GA, are given.

offspring of the treated groups. In such cases, the evaluation of historical control data from the same laboratory is helpful or even essential.

Possible Manifestations in Developmental and Reproductive Toxicology

It is characteristic that toxic effects on development and reproduction can manifest themselves on numerous endpoints and in a multiplicity of developmental stages. In fact, abnormal development may be induced from the time before conception (e.g., mutagenic effects) until well into childhood (Fig. 2). The consequences of interference may appear either shortly after the insult has been initiated (e.g., embryolethal or teratogenic effects) or after a very long latency period, even late in postnatal life (e.g., effects on fertility, behavior and organ dysfunctions).

The development of primates, in particular, is far from complete at birth, and the evaluation of post-

TABLE 8 Estimated Intrauterine Mortality Rate of Human Embryos with Selected Malformations during Defined Gestational Intervals[a]

Gestational interval[b]	Estimated prenatal mortality in embryos and fetuses (%)			
	Neural tube defects	Holoprosencephaly	Cleft lip	Polydactyly
Stages 12–14 (≈week 5)	21%	5%	—	—
Stages 15–17 (≈week 6)	16%	24%	—	—
Stages 18–20 (≈week 7)	11%	20%	39%	42%
Stages 21–23 (≈week 8)	44%	46%	47%	31%
Fetal period (week 9–term)	6%	4%	10%	22%
Total mortality until birth	98%	99%	96%	95%

[a]Evaluated from 7358 specimens of legal abortions. Percentage of malformed specimens observed among nonviable embryos and fetuses after legal abortions in Japan. Data from Shiota (1993).
[b]Carnegie stages.

natally induced lesions is thus an integral part of developmental toxicology. Here the possible route of exposure via breast milk may be of some importance, and the special sensitivity of the developing infant towards certain xenobiotics can also play a role.

Reproduction and development consist of a large sequence of reactions that are repeated in every generation. The transmission of the genetic material from one generation to the next and the creation of new life is collectively called the "reproductive sequence" (Fig. 3). The term reproductive cycle, which is sometimes used, is misleading because it is not a cyclic process.

Many of these actions are interlinked with one another and they may influence each other. This also holds true for the link between reproduction and development. While no development, either normal or abnormal, is possible without intact reproductive functions, the opposite (the reproduction of a malformed organism) is quite feasible.

Not every prenatally induced toxic lesion leads to a pronounced permanent defect. Many, if not most, lesions to the conceptus or offspring are transient and can be repaired fairly quickly or are compensated for during the time span of embryonic development (Fig. 4). This toxicological behavior in chemical teratogenesis is very similar to that in carcinogenesis, induced by chemical or physical agents.

TABLE 9 Minimal Number of Pathological Cases Necessary to Recognize a Chemically Induced Effect and the Minimal Recognizable Risk (in parenthesis)[a]

Size of the exposed group	Spontaneous rate in the normal population		
	0.05%	0.8%[b]	3%[b]
25	3 (240×)	4 (20×)	6 (8×)
50	4 (160×)	5 (13×)	8 (5×)
100	4 (80×)	7 (9×)	11 (4×)
200	4 (40×)	8 (5×)	17 (3×)
400	4 (20×)	13 (4×)	26 (2×)
800	6 (15×)	20 (3×)	44 (2×)

[a]One-sided binominal test at 5% error of type 1 and 2. Calculated by Prof. Dr. R. Meister, Berlin.
[b]If the rate of the normal population is not known very well, even more pathological cases are required to largely exclude an association by chance.

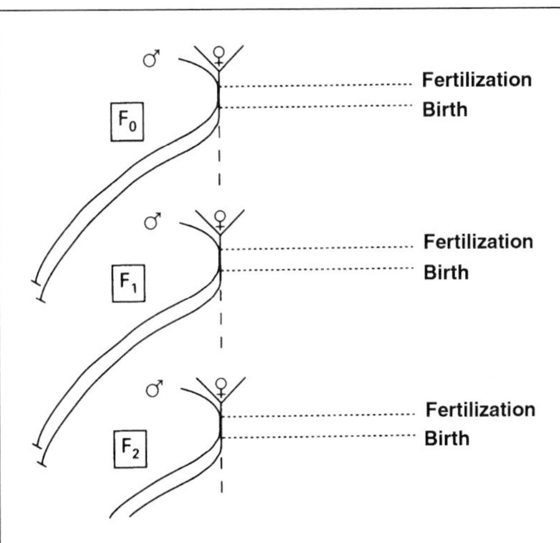

FIGURE 3 Reproductive sequence. A toxic effect may manifest itself late postnatally, possibly as late as the next generation (e.g., adverse effect on fertility).

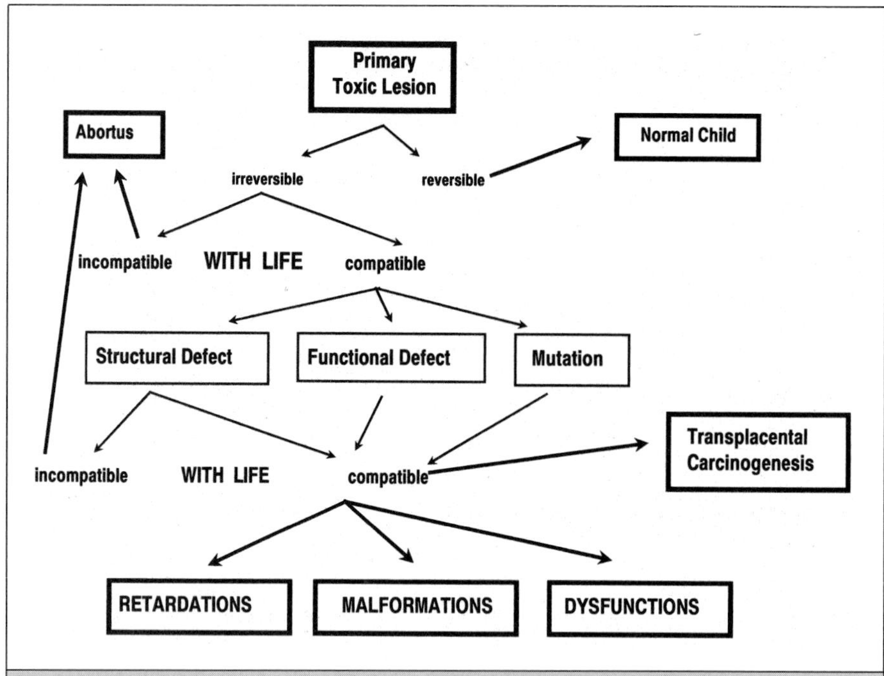

FIGURE 4 Possible manifestations of a prenatally induced lesion. The result of an embryotoxic effect may be either reversible or irreversible and either compatible or incompatible with life.

The crucial issue is whether or not an existing defect is compatible with life. A lethal effect may appear very shortly after the exposure to a noxious insult or only very much later, even late postnatally, once the affected function gains vital importance. This can occur right after birth during the radical adjustment to the new living conditions of respiration, food intake, and confrontation with the environment, or it may occur much later. The reason for many later occurring infant deaths, for example, sudden infant death syndrome (SIDS) with an incidence of 1–3% per live births, is still largely unknown. The prolongation of the QT interval in the ECG of newborns has been found to be strongly correlated with SIDS.

If the lesion is compatible with life, then the question arises whether a complete restitution is possible or whether the insult will lead to a permanent defect in morphology or function (Fig. 4).

The term "congenital malformation" implies that the defect is present at birth; yet, as stated above, it may take time for the congenital malformations to manifest themselves (e.g., cardiovascular defects). Teratogenic effects are considered to be irreversible, unless corrected surgically. However, not all morphological defects initiated *in utero* must be permanent. For example, experimentally induced wavy ribs in rodents or rudimentary additional ribs can be compensated for postnatally and should not be designated as congenital malformation. Rather they may be classified as "transient abnormalities." Persisting lesions may become functionally compensated for, as is known for many defects within the CNS. In this case the success may largely depend on the amount of attention and care devoted to the affected children (e.g., in Down's syndrome or in children born to drug-addicted mothers).

Advantages and Limitations of Experimental Studies

Intrinsic to experimental studies are both advantages and, more importantly, considerable limitations. The tremendous advantage is the possibility of planning and performing studies under well-controlled conditions with well-characterized experimental animals and a wide selection of appropriate dose levels. Many more endpoints may be evaluated than in epidemiological studies, especially when a complete postmortem analysis of the animals is included.

The most profound limitation of all animal studies in toxicological research is the need to extrapolate from the results obtained in animals to the situation assumed to exist in humans. By definition, extrapolations are speculations, and there is no possibility of controlling the validity of these extrapolations. A definite statement with respect to humans based on animal data (i.e., ". . . so many children will be born with malformations . . .") is never possible and is always greatly misleading. While the medical sciences of physiology and biochemistry largely depend on the similarities among species, toxicology is faced with the serious problem of species differences as the main issue.

Another drawback in toxicology, including reproductive and developmental toxicology, is the limitation in the number of animals used per experimental group. This number is commonly <30 per group. There is an attempt in toxicology to compensate for this too small sample size by using exceedingly high doses, up to the maximum tolerable dose (MTD). Such a strategy is *a priori* unsatisfactory and prone to many misinterpretations.

Evaluation of Abnormal Development

Data on abnormal development may be obtained from two quite different sources:

- From observations in humans.
- From animal studies.

Information from both sources must be used for a risk assessment or a preventive hazard minimization, but the applicability of the dissimilar sources of information is fundamentally different. In order to observe adverse effects, humans must have been exposed to the agent. The aim of animal tests performed on agents with unknown properties is to identify potential hazards of a given substance and to avoid human exposure (primary prevention).

Observations in Humans

Information on humans may be compiled from various sources. While the relevance of single-case reports is negligible for risk assessment, multiple-case reports may signal a dangerous situation. The teratogenicity of thalidomide was revealed solely by multiple-case reports, and systematic epidemiological studies were neither performed nor required to reveal the danger. Most epidemiological studies in toxicology are retrospective, with all the advantages (e.g., relatively easy to perform, providing results within a rather short time, and rather inexpensive) and serious limitations. There is the difficulty of verifying the type and time of exposure (due to recall bias or deliberately false information, if financial compensation is possible) and the inability to control important confounding factors. Large and expensive prospective studies have been performed, but some of the data are now rather antiquated (e.g., the U.S. Boston Study and the German DFG Study), and information on newer substances is lacking. Serious attempts to comprehensively monitor the frequency of malformations and to link them to defined exposures are a neglected medical inquiry area all over the world. In the long run, only large-scale monitoring programs extending over several decades will be helpful.

Evaluation of Abnormal Development in Animals

In animal studies there are two possible ways to reveal the presumed adverse effects on reproduction and development, the evaluation of the different phases of reproduction and development in a single-experiment approach (multigenerational study) or the evaluation of the different phases in a segmental approach (several separate study designs).

As is to be expected, both approaches have advantages and disadvantages. For medicinal substances (i.e., agents with great demands for safety by the public), the segmental approach (segments I to III, or modifications) is generally preferred (Fig. 5) because it allows a more sophisticated evaluation. The numerous phases of reproduction and development, extending over more than one generation, are divided into several segments, preferentially with considerable overlaps. If the primary stage testing gives unambiguous results, further studies with unconventional but defined experimental designs (including *in vitro* studies) may be required.

Multigeneration studies are often preferred when assessing the possible toxicity of environmental chemicals. Reproductive toxicity and developmental toxicity are evaluated in a single experiment that extends over a considerable length of time (Fig. 5). This could have the advantage that different adverse effects may be exaggerated and that the most susceptible function becomes rate limiting, increasing the sensitivity of the test. On the other hand, the limitation of the applicable doses to the most sensitive variable may become a certain disadvantage when the effects on a less vulnerable endpoint cannot be detected because of dose limitations. Additionally, the resulting body burden may fluctuate considerably between the various stages, especially in rodents (see section on risk assessment), an effect that is exaggerated when the test substance is mixed into the feed. The interpretation of results obtained with highly lipophilic substances with a long elimination half-life, in particular, may be hampered. Furthermore, it may be difficult to localize the cause of an observed adverse effect (making ad-

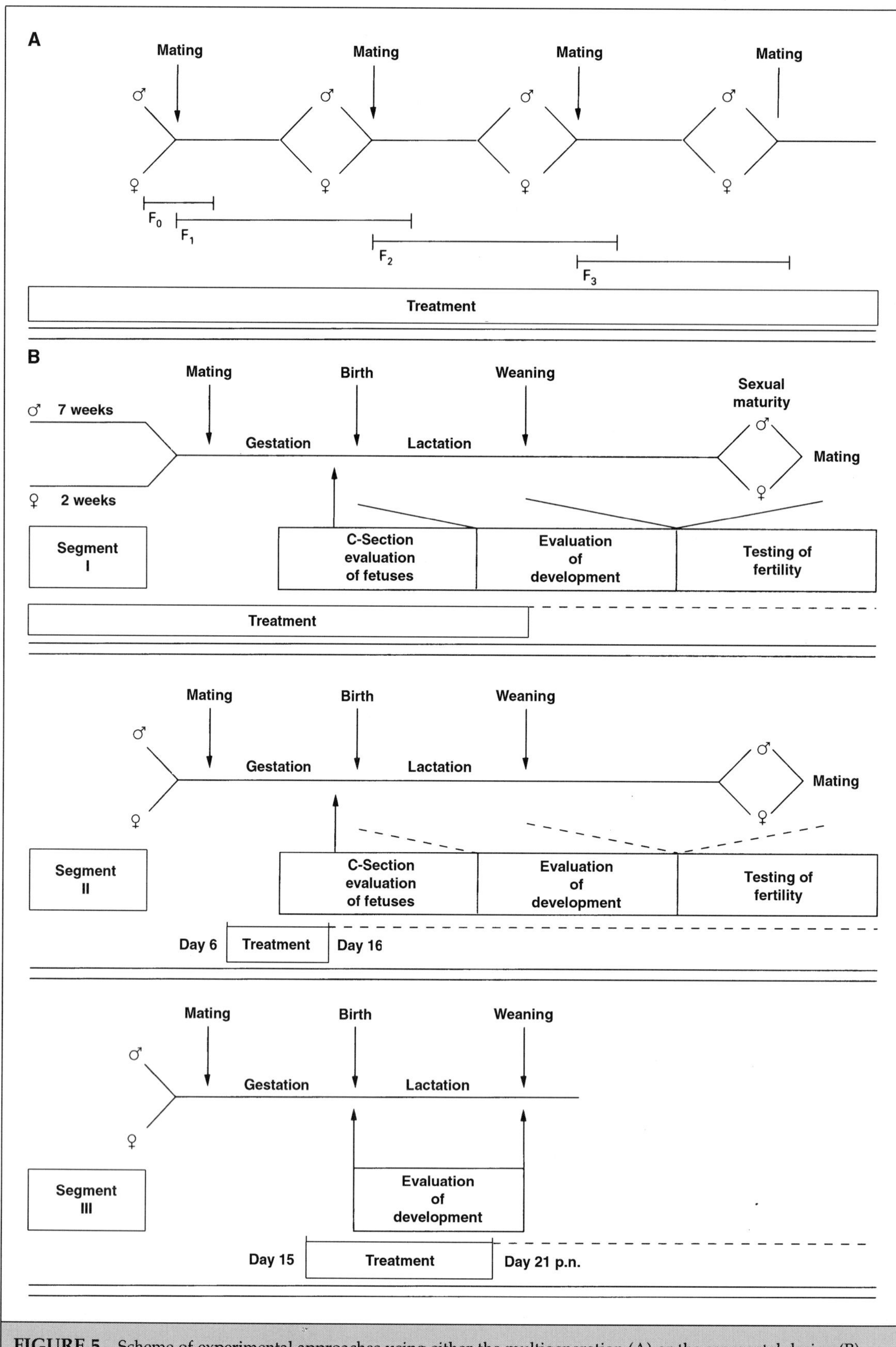

FIGURE 5 Scheme of experimental approaches using either the multigeneration (A) or the segmental design (B).

ditional studies necessary). Some manifestations (e.g., teratogenic effects) may only be recognized indirectly or even not at all. The long duration of the complex experimental design is prone to complications and repeating a study may be time consuming and expensive.

REPRODUCTIVE TOXICITY

Reproductive toxicology is concerned with adverse effects on male and female fertility. The final manifestation of an adverse effect on reproduction is the inability to produce the next generation. There are several situations on the way to this endpoint, which may be considered pathological, but which are still compatible with fertility, unless the subject is affected very severely. Such functions include sperm production, ovulation, and numerous psychological situations.

Sexual functions may be directly impaired by a direct action on certain components of sexual functions or sexual behavior or may be affected indirectly, for example, by disturbing the balance of sexual hormones or by interfering with functions of the nervous system essential for reproduction. While direct adverse effects are almost exclusively confined to the male sex, indirect effects may be of concern for both sexes.

Physiology of Female and Male Gametes

There are fundamental differences in the formation of male and female gametes, and this must also have a considerable impact on pathological situations and the possibilities of inducing adverse effects.

Primary oocytes are formed from oogonia by mitotic division during early fetal life. These oocytes begin their first meiotic division before birth. At birth all oocytes are formed, and they remain in this prophase until puberty. This long duration of the first meiotic division, (i.e., several decades until the end of reproductive life) is believed to be one reason for the susceptibility for chromosomal aberrations (nondisjunctions) increasing with age. The first meiotic division is completed shortly before ovulation, giving rise to only one single secondary oocyte and the second meiosis does not occur before fertilization. Ovulation is a highly selective process; from probably >1,000,000 primary oocytes at birth, many regress and only about 40,000 may remain at puberty, less than 500 of which are released during a woman's reproductive period.

Spermatogonia are formed by mitotic division during the fetal period within the tubuli seminiferi and they continue to be formed during puberty. They convert to primary spermatocytes, which through the first meiotic division are transformed to secondary spermatocytes and through the second meiosis to four haploid spermatids. These spermatids mature to sperm with sustenance by Sertoli cells (spermiogenesis). Spermatogenesis (i.e., the differentiation from the spermatogonium to mature sperm) requires about 9 weeks.

Sperm production involves a tremendous wastage. From usually several hundred million sperm of one ejaculate, most typically only one successfully combines with an oocyte. Selection processes that are presumably involved are largely unknown.

Role of Hormonal and Nervous Systems

Sex hormones are essential for the formation of sperm and of the egg preparing for fertilization. Without these hormonal influences no reproduction is possible. Although all types of sex hormones are found in both genders, it is justified to distinguish male (androgens) and female (estrogens and progesterone) sex hormones.

There are four levels at which sex hormones are formed, regulated, and active, and at all these levels adverse effects on reproduction may be triggered:

- The control of formation and secretion of sex hormones by regulators of the hypothalamo–pituitary axis (FSH, LH, and releasing hormones).
- The metabolic pathways leading to the various hormones.
- The synthesis of sex hormones within and the secretion from the gonads.
- The action of the hormones at receptor sites.

In addition to hormonal regulation, important functions of the central nervous system (CNS) are essential for sexual behavior.

Many of these reactions and the adverse effects induced by interfering agents are complex and influenced by the tuned interplay of a multitude of factors, due to hormones as well as to actions of the central nervous system and various sexual organs (Fig. 6).

Adverse Effects on Fertility

The chemically induced perturbation of fertility is difficult to ascertain in humans, and clear-cut evidence has been revealed for only a few substances. In such incidences occupational exposure predominated.

We must differentiate between the impairment of male and female fertility and the following alterations may be associated with impotence or childlessness.

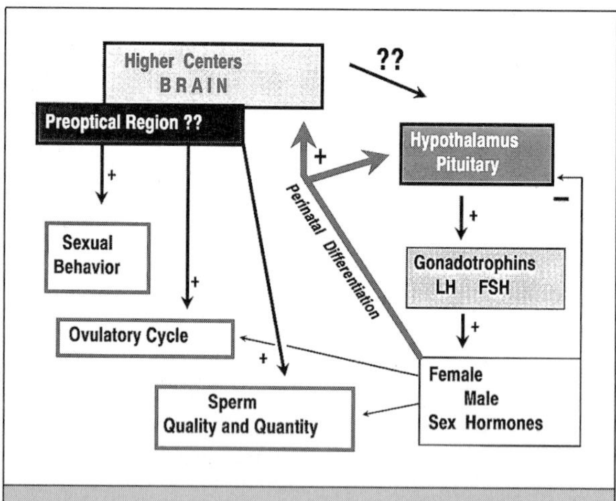

FIGURE 6 Regulatory sequences and circles involved in the homeostasis of reproductive biology.

In males:

- Reduced spermatogenesis.
- Abnormal spermatogenesis.

In females:

- Ovulation cycle disorders.
- Preimplantation loss.
- Impaired implantation.
- Elevated rate of abortions.

In both:

- Reduced libido.

TABLE 10 Influence of 1,2-Dibromo-3-chloropropane (DBCP) on the Number of Sperm in Production Workers and Applicators

	Study	Azoospermia[a]		Oligospermia[b]	
(A)	DBCP-exposed	14/107	(13%)	18/107	(17%)
	Not exposed	1/35	(3%)	2/35	(6%)
(Ba)	DBCP-exposed	5/64	(8%)	14/64	(22%)
	Not exposed	0/20	(<5%)	2/20	(10%)
(Bb)	DBCP-exposed	1/71	(1%)	12/71	(17%)
	Not exposed	0/37	(<3%)	3/37	(8%)
(C)	DBCP-exposed			20/74	(27%)
	Not exposed			1/22	(5%)

[a]Azoospermia: 0–1 million sperm/ml.
[b]Oligospermia: <20 million sperm/ml.
Volunteers with <20 million sperm/ml in reference groups of other studies: 5–15%. (A) DBCP production (Whorton *et al.* 1979); (B) DBCP production in 2 companies (a and b) (Lipshultz *et al.*, 1980); (C) DBCP application during farming.

- Congenital or acquired alterations in sexual organs.

Numerous confounding factors must be considered and excluded when a causal relationship of reduced fertility with chemical exposure is assumed. Because both genders are always involved, the adverse effect responsible may have acted upon the organism either quite recently or a long time before. The possible points of attack include

Male Reproduction

- Impotence, the inability to cohabit (impotentia coeundi) or to reproduce (impotentia generandi).
- Direct impairment of spermatogenesis.
- Indirect impairment of spermatogenesis by hormonal dysregulation.

Female Reproduction

- Psychological factors.
- Infertility because of genital tract infections.
- Hormonal imbalance.
- Congenital abnormalities.
- Mutations at the zygote stage.
- Repeated spontaneous abortions.

Chemically induced impairments of reproduction in humans have only been confirmed by observations in males. We cannot provide an example of a proven effect in the human female, except contraception or induced abortion, but these are clearly examples of a desired change of fertility. Only a few cases of substance-related changes of spermatogenesis, which is not identical with infertility, except for the extreme of azoospermia, have been convincingly documented.

Direct Toxic Effects on Male Reproduction

Interference with the morphology and function of the testes may take place at various levels. In contrast to experimental studies, the exact point of attack is seldom elucidated in humans. The question most important to answer is whether an observed adverse effect is reversible.

Example: 1,2-3-Dibromo-monochloropropane (DBCP)

This compound was produced as a nematocide and was used in agriculture predominantly in North and South America. Several published studies of workers involved in the production of DBCP or with the application of this substance (by spraying) during farming operations reported a reduced number of sperm in the ejaculate (Table 10). No altered libido or impairments of other primary or secondary sexual functions were reported. Biopsies of the testes showed an atrophy of the semen-producing epithelium, but unchanged Sertoli and Leydig cells. In patients with reduced sperm counts, significantly higher plasma levels of FSH and LH were observed, but no changes in the testosterone level.

An exact quantification of the exposure could not be performed in any of the studies, as is common for most studies in occupational medicine. Anyway, exposure was probably quite variable. A clear-cut association of values of <1 million sperm/ml (azoospermia) and the length of occupation could only be detected after at least 3 years of exposure. After up to 3 months of employment, normal values (>40 million sperm/ml) were found. Such scanty exposure data allow no conclusions about a possible dose–effect relationship. The plasma concentrations of FSH and LH were only elevated unequivocally if a considerable impairment of testicular functions existed. Hormonal analysis was not found to be suitable as an early biomarker for identifying a possible impairment by this type of intoxication.

The results of several studies in humans led to the assumption that oligospermia (1–20 million sperm/ml) induced by DBCP was reversible, but azoospermia was usually not, even when monitored over a period of 5 years. The evaluation of the fertility proper of these men with reduced sperm counts was much more difficult. Most of them fathered healthy children, which was reported even for some men classified as azoospermic.

The effect of DBCP on testes morphology and sperm production has also been confirmed in animal studies.

Indirect Effects on Male and Female Reproduction

Indirect interference with the male or female reproductive capacity may be caused by influencing sexual behavior or by inducing hormonal imbalance. While the first aspect is of considerable importance in reproductive medicine, pharmacological and toxic effects are almost exclusively induced by hormonal imbalance. The best example is hormonal contraception, practiced worldwide by millions of women.

While processes depending on the action of sex hormones continue to be important until adult life, some defined periods of development are especially vulnerable to modifications in hormone levels. Often such processes may be altered either directly by certain agents or indirectly by interference with sex hormone actions.

Effects of Hormonal Disrupters on Male and Female Sexual Functions and Behavior

It is now widely accepted by the scientific community that certain environmentally occurring natural chemicals as well as human-made substances have the potential to interact with hormone receptors in many species (xenohormones). With regard to xenobiotics, the issue was first brought to the attention of the public at large by the book *Silent Spring*, published by Rachel Carson in 1962. Early on, the accused substances included numerous liberally used pesticides (DDT in particular, but also lindane and other polychlorinated compounds and organophosphate insecticides and herbicides). In the intervening decades, the list of suspects and proven "bad actors" has grown substantially and includes, among many others, some organotin compounds, PCBs, dioxins and related compounds of the polyhalogenated variety, and plasticizers.

Although this section will focus on human health aspects and risk assessment, this restriction of coverage does by no means belittle the ecotoxicology and wildlife connections. The adverse effects of overdoses of human-made chemicals on wildlife populations of either sex are now well documented. It is thus established that a diverse and large number of xenobiotics has the potential to interfere with endocrine homeostasis in either sex in a wide array of species at appropriate doses, which are very high and most often atypical compared to the anticipated human occupational or environmental exposure levels. For example, in field studies in the United Kingdom, measurable concentrations of estrogenic hormones were found by analytical chemistry in wastewater effluent from sewage treatment plants. Not only were such agents chemically detectable, but their biological effects were measurable in male fish held in cages close to the inflow point of the treated wastewater into natural river waters. Expression of the vitellogenin gene and its protein product, normally found only in female fish, were detectable in male fish. The speculation was thus put forward that naturally occurring materials in the environment with hormone-like activity (ecohormones) or human-made hormones (xenohormones) excreted into the wastewater stream and environment by animals and women, might have an impact on the ecosystem or even on humans. The source identification among the hormones in the water revealed me-

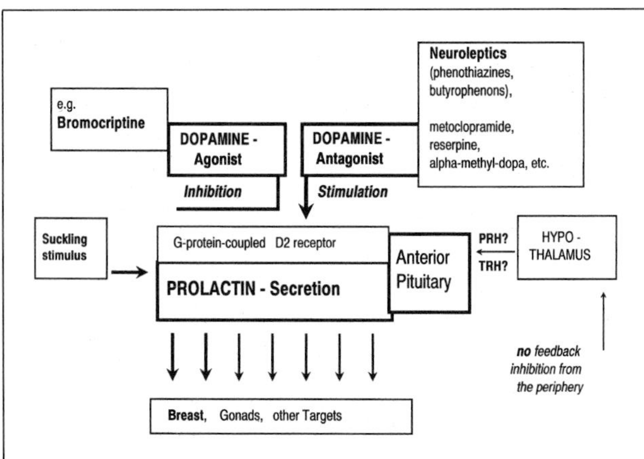

FIGURE 7 Indirect interference with homeostasis of sexual hormones at the level of prolactin formation and action. Interfering agents do not interact with hormone receptors, but affect the regulatory factor dopamine at the anterior pituitary. In this way hormonal effects on target tissue are triggered. Reprinted from Neubert (1997).

tabolites of endogenous mammalian hormones and synthetic hormones used by women as anticonceptional drugs or for other therapeutic indications.

In 1991 (Colburn and Clement, 1992) the substantially misleading, but very catchy, term "endocrine disrupters" surfaced. For chemicals of natural origin, the term "ecohormones" has become popular, and xenohormones are even lumped together with "ecohormones."

Human health concerns for both genders related to endocrine disrupters have prompted an avalanche of opinions. Aside from scholarly writings, all mass media have been involved in this highly visible and audible topic, which has taken on strong political overtones.

Three different classes of hormonally active chemicals with the potential to interfere with reproduction and development (including prenatal carcinogenesis) must be distinguished.

- Natural and synthetic steroidal or nonsteroidal chemicals with well-known hormone agonist (xenohormones) or antagonist actions in experimental animals and humans. For most of these substances, there are extensive databases available from clinical medicine and therapeutic uses in humans.
- Synthetic nonsteroidal environmental chemicals with hormone agonist (xenohormones) or antagonist actions in experimental animals. Many of these substances are pesticides, often organochlorine compounds. While data of *in vivo* and *in vitro* animal tests and reports on adverse effects on wildlife (mostly by heavy contamination) are available, no sufficient data for humans risk assessment have been presented.
- Naturally occurring chemicals (e.g., constituents of food stuffs) may exhibit very low hormone potency in various experimental test systems (often *in vitro*), phytoestrogens (e.g., genistein and daidzain) and mycoestrogens (e.g., zearalone). Little information is available about hormone-like biological activity at reasonable exposure levels in experimental animals. The lack of relevant human data is also quite obvious. The objective of several ongoing studies is to obtain a better characterization of the effects elicited by phytoestrogens alone and in combination with other weak synthetic estrogens.

The initial focus on estrogenic effects is barely justified from a scientific point of view. Almost all hormone systems could be involved, among them the thyroid or components of the hypothalamic–hypophyseal–gonadal axis. The sphere of interest now includes anti-estrogenic, androgenic, and anti-androgenic effects, progestagenic and antiprogestagenic effects, as well as reproductive peptide hormone effects. While these oversimplified designations imply the interactions of the chemical or drug with highly specific receptors, the same hormonally active molecule can exert mixed biological activities on steroid hormone receptors in different target organs of the same organism, from full agonist to partial agonist and to antagonist, depending on the tissue. The perturbation of endocrine homeostasis also may occur by mechanisms other than the direct interaction of chemical with hormone receptors. The increased prolactin secretion induced by neuroleptics and other drugs (Fig. 7), the inhibition of essential steps in hormone synthesis (e.g., by finasteride), and the thyroid hormone-mediated effects on sex hormone-initiated reactions are examples.

Human Database

In the context of endocrine disrupters, most of the emphasis has been put on the exposure of immature males, both during prenatal and early post-natal exposure, as well as the exposure of adult men. However, the potential adverse effects of sex hormone agonists or sex hormone antagonists are not confined to male reproduction. The endogenous hormones at issue are also essential for female reproduction and, to a lesser extent, for female differentiation during perinatal sexual development.

Only speculations on endocrine disruptors in humans are possible, but there is an unusually large database available on very potent pharmaceutical

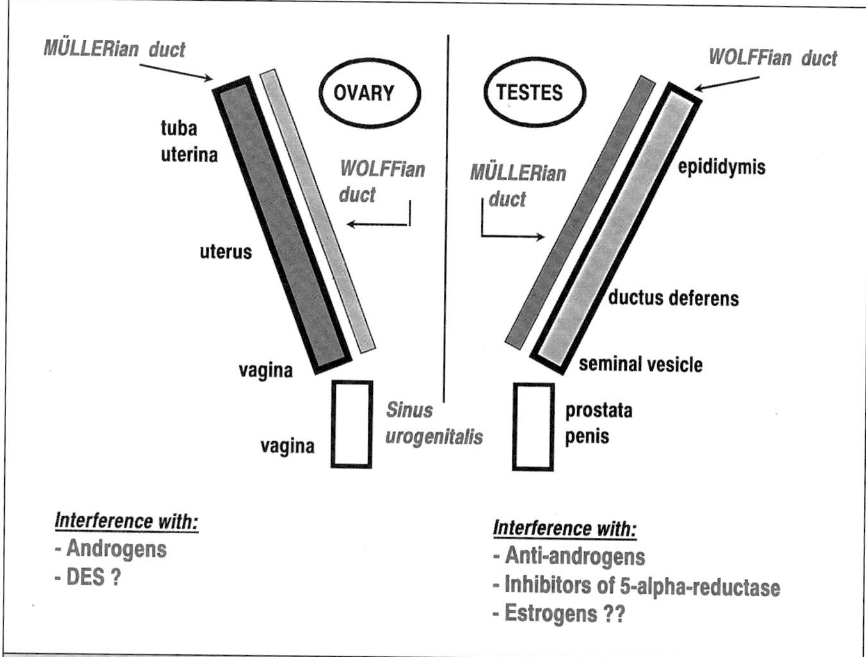

FIGURE 8 Differentiation and regression of the Müllerian and Wolffian ducts in the two genders and possible interferences. In the male, the Müllerian duct regresses and genital organs are formed from the Wolffian duct under the influence of 5α-dihydrotestosterone; interference by inhibitors of 5α-reductase (e.g., finasteride) or anti-androgens (e.g., cyproterone acetate). Female sexual organs are formed from the Müllerian duct; interference by androgens. Reprinted from Neubert (1997).

products that by design and therapeutic targeting act on the steroid hormone receptors in men and women. This vast body of information on estrogens and androgens, as well as on typical antagonists to these sex hormones, may help to evaluate the proposed similar effects by ecohormones on male and female reproduction. In humans, endocrine system side effects have been observed during clinical efficacy trials or may have manifested themselves upon therapeutic use in a large number of patients. Aside from many others, extensive information on DES is available, as discussed elsewhere. Adverse effects on the development of human external genitalia are well established as a result of excess androgens (masculinization of females), or anti-androgens, (feminization of male fetuses), such as cyproterone acetate or finasteride (Fig. 8).

Controversial data on adverse effects of "xenohormones" in the human male have been published. Several epidemiological studies have claimed that worrisome declines in human sperm counts and semen quality have occurred since the 1940s. In several instances, men in sperm donor facilities or those seeking medical advice from fertility clinics in various parts of the world made up the study populations. These reports are rather controversial. Several studies were conducted in countries around the globe to examine present human sperm counts. More recent studies of more diverse male populations in different parts of the world have revealed surprising differences in sperm numbers in various parts of the same country (U.S.) and, overall, no evidence for declining sperm counts. Other reports have described very high sperm counts in a specific region of one country (Odense, Denmark) and stable numbers over many years (Australia). Epidemiological analyses of the same database of human sperm counts have led to diametrically opposite conclusions.

The measurement of a single ejaculate at any given time, as has been performed in all of these studies, is certainly not representative for any given individual (Table 11). Most important, it is well established that sperm counts cannot be directly correlated with fertility, unless an azoospermia is diagnosed. There are many examples of men with very low sperm counts having fathered children. A correlation has been found between the number of sperm in the ejaculate and the *time* required to impregnate a female. Often the inability to have children is due to psychological rather than physiological reasons. This may greatly

TABLE 11 Inter- and Intraindividual Variability of Sperm Counts

	Himalayan rabbit[a]							
	1	2	3	4	5	6	7	8
n^b	8	6	6	6	4	8	7	8
Median[c]	503	645	263	848	735	720	975	960
Min–max	90–1515	255–990	120–570	150–1410	540–1710	60–885	105–4425	225–1950

	Humans[d]						
	1	2	3	4	5	6	7
Number of specimens	61	62	83	80	77	105	205
Sperm concentration (million sperm/ml)[e]	51	78	116	156	128	86	124
(range)	17–176	9–239	28–335	61–376	24–318	23–188	16–317
Ejaculate volume (ml)[e]	2.3	3.9	3.4	2.5	2.0	3.1	2.7
(range)	0.5–4.8	1.5–5.6	1.5–6.2	1.0–4.0	0.4–3.5	0.7–5.5	0.5–5.0
Percentage motility[e]	74%	71%	72%	70%	73%	71%	69%
(range)	45–94	32–88	50–91	52–86	54–90	50–89	37–94

[a]Unpublished data: Chahoud and Neubert.
[b]Number of days with sperm analyses.
[c]Sperm concentration (in million sperm/ml).
[d]Considerable variability of semen quality in normal men. Semen quality was repeatedly measured in 61 to 205 samples per healthy semen donors over a period of 72 to 324 weeks. Data from Mallidis *et al.* (1991).
[e]Mean values.

complicate an evaluation of the chemically induced alteration of fertility. For the reasons mentioned, data from epidemiological studies on the possible effects of chemical exposures on fertility in males, and even moreso in females, must be interpreted with utmost caution, unless they are designed in a sophisticated way that carefully considers not only the physiological or pathological situation of the male, but also the gynecological status of the female partner. It is essential to provide a complete set of data for the cases outside the reference range and on what is special in these volunteers. One should never be satisfied with statistical data only. Nevertheless, the possibility that there might be a gradual reduction in human sperm counts occurring cannot be laid to rest, and more analyses of truly representative populations with highly standardized methods and unequivocal scientific standards are warranted. Such studies are extremely difficult to perform, and it is in the nature of the investigative task at hand that the results will always be strongly criticized.

If there were indeed real alterations over time, many causes and changes in lifestyle over the past several decades must be considered as confounding factors. Hormonal imbalances were just one among many possibilities. Among various possible causes are malformations and mutations, infections, tumors, psychological factors, and temperature. There is good reason to doubt that effects induced by drugs and chemicals (i.e., those therapeutically used as well as environmentally present substances) are responsible for the majority of male fertility problems.

The claim that the frequency of hypospadias has generally increased over time cannot be substantiated from the published birth defects data from many countries. However, there is some suspicion that this type of malformation might have slightly increased after the accident in Seveso, Italy. Although TCDD is not unequivocally classified as an estrogen, low testosterone levels were reported in men occupationally exposed to dioxin in some studies, but not in others. Furthermore, a transient shift in the sex ratio towards female offspring was reported after the Seveso incident.

There are reports pointing to a possible increase in the rate of testicular tumors in young men in some countries, especially in Denmark. The absolute tumor incidence rates are surprisingly different (e.g., in Finland vs Denmark). Comparisons have been made between these two countries focusing on use of DDT and its estrogenic activity. The estrogenic potency of DDT and some of its metabolites is much, much lower than that of DES. Human DDT exposures of the general population and their body burdens since the 1970s were estimated. This was the time when the young men who had the testicular tumors would have been exposed perinatally. The best estimates of the exposure data and the DDT exposure levels in those years did not differ between Finland and Denmark, yet the testicular tumor incidence rates were now higher in Denmark. If there was indeed an increase in the testicular tumor rates, again many reasons may be responsible, including changes in the reporting strategies, which can cause apparent changes in tumor rates. A major risk factor for testicular cancer is cryptorchism, with about 10% of the cases coinciding with this condition. A slight increase in both conditions was found in sons exposed *in utero* to DES, and the weight of the evidence of human prenatal DES exposure suggests an apparent no effect level for the induction of cryptorchism.

When attempting to reveal some general principles from the clinical and experimental studies with medical relevance, the following may be stated. Many of the substances studied do not reveal an effect on a single hormonal system but simultaneously exhibit several effects, for example, estrogenic and anti-androgenic (cyproterone acetate), and progestagenic and androgenic (many components of hormonal contraceptives). Such multiple actions may also be expected for xenohormones, and it would be a grave mistake to concentrate on single receptor effects. Within a given class, several substances exhibit both receptor agonistic and antagonistic effects, with a different organotropy (e.g., the anti-estrogenic effects of tamoxifen on breast cancer, but its agonistic estrogenic effects on bone structure). Such divergent actions may also be expected to occur with xenohormones. Apparent paradoxical reactions may occur with certain substances, for example, the stimulation of ovulation and of spermatogenesis by the synthetic anti-estrogenic substance clomifene, a triphenylethylene derivative.

Another complicating factor for experimental studies is the existence of specific hormone-binding proteins (sex-hormone-binding globulin and albumin in humans; α-fetoprotein in laboratory rodents). These proteins are believed to function in a protective sense as binding sites for endogenously occurring hormones as their levels rise, for example, those of estradiol during human pregnancy. It has been observed that several xenoestrogens bind less intensely to those serum proteins than estradiol does. This difference in binding characteristics may increase their effective free concentration in serum and make them available for placental transfer to the developing conceptus.

These examples indicate that the situation is very complex. Furthermore, the reactions of hormone-responsive target cells may also be modulated by nonhormonal agents acting on additional receptors on the same cell (Fig. 9). This must have consequences for routine testing and create difficulties when attempting extrapolations between species.

Interference with sex hormonal systems should by no means always be considered adverse. On the contrary, millions of women voluntarily take hormones daily to disrupt estrus cyclicity and thus prevent conception. Vast numbers of pre- and postmenopausal women are given estrogens because beneficial health effects are expected. It is quite feasible that possible effects of ecohormones, if they occur in humans, are not always adverse to health. In fact, substantial beneficial health effects are attributed to diets high in soybean-associated phytoestrogens, consumed in certain Asian countries. A lower incidence of a variety of cancers, among them breast cancer, in those populations is claimed as one of the dietary benefits. Systematic well-designed phytoestrogen studies in animals and humans are ongoing.

Experimental Research Activities

Well known in endocrinology is the special vulnerability of sexual differentiation upon exposure to exogenous chemicals during genetically programmed, endogenous hormone-dependent events of late prenatal and early postnatal differentiation of sexual organs, functions, and behavior. Inadvertent exposures might induce irreversible effects and cause lifelong sexual dysfunction and behavioral consequences. Among the anticipated changes could be the capacity for appropriate sexual functions, the development of the regulation of sex hormone concentrations, and the inhibition of the perinatal formation of certain cell types within the testes (e.g., Leydig cells), which cannot be compensated for during later stages of postnatal development. The effects might not grossly manifest themselves at birth or soon thereafter, but may become apparent only at later stages of life. If there is a significance of hormonal disruptors in humans, this would be the most likely period of susceptibility.

Because of the large variety of hormone-dependent processes occurring during late prenatal and early postnatal development and continuing into adult life, numerous possibilities of interference with such hormone-triggered processes and functions must be anticipated. Direct toxicity and altered hormone actions have to be contrasted. There are four possibilities for interfering with fertility, and especially with male fertility.

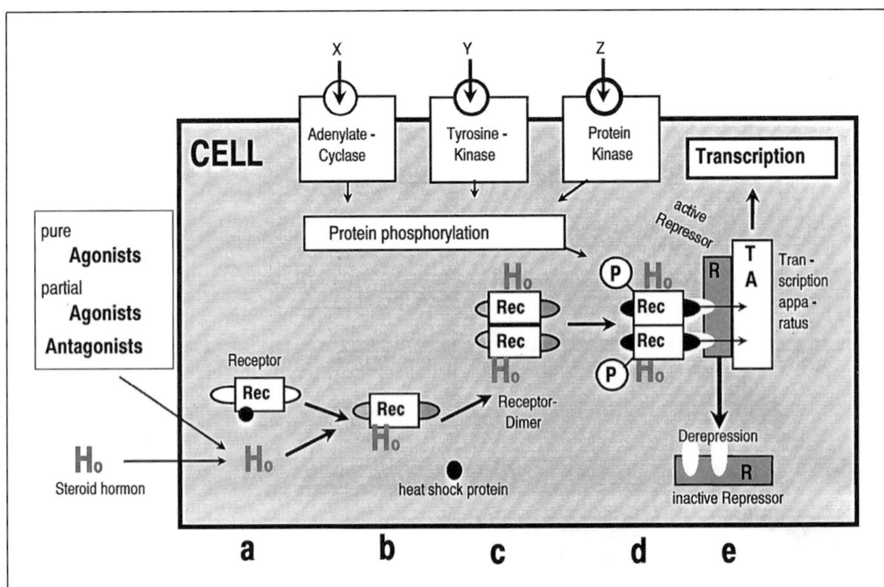

FIGURE 9 Scheme of the action of a steroid hormone on a target cell. After binding [b] of the hormone (Ho) to a cytoplasmic receptor [a] and replacing another component (e.g., heat shock protein) from the receptor, the receptor–hormone dimer complex [c] is phosphory lated [d] and transferred into the cell nucleus where it displaces a repressor from the hormone-responsive DNA element [e], thus inducing transcription and the translation of specific factors. Binding of other nonhormonal substances (x,y,z) to additional receptors of the same cell modifies the hormone-triggered process. Reprinted from Neubert (1997).

- Perturbation of the prenatal development of the gonads.
- Interference with the development of the external genitalia.
- Indirect toxic effects by interference with the development of hormonal regulations.
- Direct toxic effects on the (adult) gonads.

In addition to medicinal drugs, a few agents have been studied rather extensively in animal tests. In almost no case has a database been established satisfying scientists concerned with risk assessment with respect to humans. However, some interesting general principles have emerged, which justifies a discussion.

The effects of 2,3,7,8-tetrachlorodibenzo-*p*-dioxin (TCDD) on the development of male sex organs, sex functions, and sexual behavior have been studied rather extensively in rats. However, many aspects remain obscure, as is the possible significance of the findings for species other than rats, and the significance of the findings for other dioxin congeners. When applied for one day in late pregnancy, a variety of deviations from controls could be observed in male rats. Several of these alterations were irreversible and they included sex organ weights, functions, and behavioral processes presumed to be androgen-dependent, such as anogenital distance, weights of seminal vesicles, prostate and epididymis, daily sperm production and epididymal sperm counts, and copulatory rate. There were unequivocal signs of general prenatal toxicity at the TCDD doses affecting the male sex organs and functions, but in further studies the effects on sperm formation were induced also with very low doses. It is important to note that the reproductive outcome was normal in all the offspring exposed *in utero*, even at the highest dose tested. The authors concluded that TCDD does not induce a generalized inhibition of imprinting, but it seems that the responsiveness of cells to hormones is altered. This would represent a rather novel aspect.

Significance and Outlook for Risk Assessment

When attempting risk assessments for endocrine disrupters and ecohormones, one has to make a clear distinction between effects on ecosystems and possible adverse effects on humans. Ecotoxicological effects appear to be established for some of the chemicals, yet convincing evidence for any cause-and-effect association for the phenomena attributed to adverse endocrine disruptor actions in humans has not been provided. Human exposures are quite different and must generally be assumed to occur to mixtures of chemicals at very low levels. The fact that effects on ecosystems have been demonstrated does not imply at all that humans will be affected. In fact, for the majority of substances adverse endocrine system-mediated effects seem rather unlikely.

The crucial question is whether the body burdens encountered among the general population with respect to very lipophilic and persistent environmental chemicals, mostly stored in adipose tissue, are sufficient to induce adverse effects. This issue can only be answered for specific substances and requires a sufficient pool of human exposure and human health data. Unfortunately, in most cases human exposure assessments under realistic conditions are either unavailable or rather incomplete.

Extrapolations from rodent data to the exposure situation that might possibly exist in humans will be difficult at best in the problem area of endocrine disruptors. It seems rather impossible to create a scientific database that can account for considerable species differences in the endocrine system homeostasis. Considerable interspecies variables may be expected for several parameters, and kinetic data for either the experimental animals or human subjects most often are not available. Solid data from nonhuman primates appear to be indispensable for a scientifically based risk assessment, but such data are not available.

Many experts concur that, in general, the prevailing reproductive toxicity *in vivo* testing methods appear to have been adequate in protecting the human population from such toxicity. However, some additional testing strategies may be indicated to respond to the heightened human health protection concerns. In the United States the endocrine disupters issue is driven by political pressure, and the U.S. EPA has been charged with establishing validated endocrine toxicity test systems. Some scientists have offered historical perspectives from preceding major ambitious prescreening and screening programs (such as carcinogenesis) and cautioned about the complexities of the endocrine system, with profound concerns over the likelihood of success.

Effects Attributed to Chemicals with Hormone-like Activity in the Human Female

There have been numerous reports claiming that the health status of the human female is also threatened by xenohormones. The attention has in particular focused on one disease condition, breast cancer, whose detected incidence is presumably on the rise in several parts of the world. The epidemiological literature tying rising rates of breast cancer to environmental chemical exposures of women, and specifically to xenohormones with estrogenic activity, is as controversial as the cause-and-effect association regarding sperm count declines in men. The results of large epidemiological studies argue against rather than for an association of breast cancer with specific environmental agents, such as DDT, DDE, and PCB, but the shortcomings of these studies were recognized.

The second adverse outcome health issue in women that may be on the rise and that has been claimed to be related to xenohormones in the human habitat is endometriosis. The prevalence of endometriosis in women in the United States has been estimated to be in the range of 1 to 7%. The cause of the condition is thought to be associated with retrograde menstrual flow and endogenous estrogen production; immunological factors have also been invoked. In this painful condition, estrogen-responsive epithelial cells that are normally only situated in the uterine lining (endometrium) are found in locations other than the uterus and may start proliferating in those inappropriate sites. Again, as in the male situation, only additional carefully planned studies with an adequate number of women examined with unequivocal xenohormone exposure histories will be able to shed light on the present controversy over whether the rising incidence of endometriosis may possibly be related to such environmental chemicals.

A third, less publicized, phenomenon revealed by epidemiological studies is that the age of girls at menarche has been declining in recent decades. It has been speculated that the exposure of young girls to environmental chemicals mimicking estrogen's biological activity might be responsible for this observation.

DEVELOPMENTAL TOXICITY

This is the largest area with the greatest number of endpoints to be affected. For almost all the possible levels, adverse effects have been demonstrated in experimental animals and, in many instances, also in humans.

General Aspects of Prenatal Toxicity and Teratogenicity

Prenatally induced toxic effects, and especially the exogenous triggering of malformations, have attracted the most attention for a long time.

Prenatally induced toxicity may manifest itself at various levels.

- Prenatal death.
- Prenatal growth retardation.
- Gross structural abnormalities (malformations).
- Postnatal death.
- Postnatal retardation of growth and physical development.
- Postnatal dysfunctions with respect to various organ systems.

Typically, not all agents induce all these manifestations at a given toxic dose level. While growth retardation and mortality may be considered as rather unspecific toxic manifestations, the induction of teratogenicity and of dysfunctions must be regarded as rather circumscript interference with development.

It is characteristic of embryo fetomortality that it may be triggered at any period of prenatal development, and it may manifest itself soon after the lesion has been set or after a longer lag phase, possibly even postnatally. This heterogeneity results from the multiplicity of causes of prenatal mortality. A lethal effect may be induced as such (i.e., by drastically interfering with cell metabolism), it may be caused by extensive tissue necroses formed over an extended period of time, or it may be the result of malformations or a dysfunction incompatible with further life.

Teratogenicity (i.e., the exogenous induction of gross structural abnormalities or malformations) is a special aspect of embryotoxicity. "Embryotoxicity" is the overall term, including all types of toxic actions affecting the embryo (not confined to embryo mortality). Congenital malformations can be induced

- Endogenously by (spontaneous) dysregulation of normal development or by mutations prior to organogenesis (in the parent generation or before).
- Exogenously by (teratogenic) influences during organogenesis.

Little is known about the possibility that some of the numerous processes involved in morphogenetic differentiation may be error prone and proceed falsely by themselves. Because a vast multitude of processes is necessary for the development of the complex human organism from the zygote, such a possibility cannot be dismissed. Considerable information is available on the possibility of mutation-induced abnormal development. Such a mutation must have taken place within one of the gametes or within the cells at the very early stage of the embryo. The mutated gene often is passed on to the next generations, and the malformation would be heritable. If malformations are induced within a population by a defined mutagenic agent, the generation of a variety of malformations would be expected because mutations hit the genome at random. Because mutations are rare events, the resulting frequency will be low, and no agent has been convincingly shown to act in this way in humans, i.e., to induce heritable defects.

Teratogenic effects result from a direct (or indirect) interference of the agent with specific morphogenetic differentiation processes during embryogenesis. It must be recalled that many of the lesions are repaired, and furthermore that many malformed embryos are aborted in primates. In contrast to malformations induced via mutations, teratogenic effects will occur with a high incidence if the dose is high enough. Experimentally, an almost 100% effect can be induced if high enough doses are used and the conceptuses survive. The manifestation frequently is limited to only a few substance-specific types of malformations.

With respect to a single child with a defined malformation, it is always difficult and often even impossible to decide whether the defect was induced endogenously (i.e., spontaneously via a mutation) or exogenously by an agent with a teratogenic potential.

The Four "Specificities" of Teratogenic Actions

There are four specificities that govern the induction of teratogenic effects:

- Phase specificity. The teratogenic effect may be inducible during a short sensitive period only (see the section on Specific Teratogenic Effects).
- Substance specificity. At a given developmental stage, all chemical substances do not induce the same pattern of malformations.
- Species specificity. The teratogenic effect may be reproducible in some species, but not in others.
- Dose specificity. The predominating defect changes with increasing doses. Certain malformations may be inducible in a narrow dose range only.

Phase specificity implies that the treatment period must cover the entire phase of organogenesis in order to reveal a possible teratogenic effect. Phase specificity is not confined to teratogenic effects, but also relates to embryolethal effects and postnatal manifestations of prenatally induced lesions, and to a certain abnormal outcome induced postnatally on development and reproduction.

Substance specificity is an important specialty of prenatal toxicity. Because many differentiation processes occur during a given period of gestation, it is not surprising that some chemically induced effects are directed against some of these, but not against others. In this way some kind of pattern may be recognized when a given substance is applied for a limited period only. This pattern may also be recognizable after a longer-term exposure, when a rather specific effect is induced by the agent. Typical is the substance specificity of thalidomide, and it was found to be very difficult in animal studies to reproduce the typical pattern with other agents.

Species specificity is well known from other areas of toxicology. Carcinogenic effects are often inducible in one species only, and the same holds true for certain types of organ toxicity. Adverse effects confined to one species pose considerable problems when attempting to extrapolate to the situation assumed to exist in humans. Most often no scientifically based conclusions are possible and worst-case assumptions predominate.

Although dose specificity is a general phenomenon in toxicology (higher doses induce more effects), this phenomenon may cause special problems in developmental toxicology. Although it may be of little significance for a risk assessment if more severe malformations cover up more subtle defects (e.g., amelia obscuring polydactyly), this may hamper studies on dose–response relationships. Furthermore, this phenomenon may cause problems in revealing teratogenic effects if embryomortality occurs in some species but not in others. Thus it has been found to be difficult to recognize the teratogenic potency of very strong teratogens of the thalidomide type in rabbits because of the pronounced embryolethal effects not seen in nonhuman primates.

Types of Teratogenic Effects

It is useful to differentiate between "universal" and "specific" teratogenic effects (Table 12); however, the boundary between these two types is fluid.

Agents with universal teratogenic potency may induce a variety of gross structural defects. Such multiple defects can be triggered over a comparatively long period of time (poor phase specificity). The damaging agent acts relatively unspecifically; that is, it may interfere with a variety of embryonic differentiation processes (e.g., certain antimetabolites, alkylating agents, and extremely high doses of ionizing radiation). Many of such agents with universal teratogenic potential are intrinsically dangerous. Often such agents are simultaneously mutagenic and carcinogenic or exhibit a pronounced organ toxicity.

The second type of agents, those inducing specific teratogenic defects, are the more important ones, and the agents are harder to recognize and evaluate. Such agents induce malformations during a limited phase of development only (pronounced phase specificity), and only one malformation or a typical pattern of few defects results. Experimental examples are the induction of cleft palates in mice by glucocorticoids or TCDD or the malformations induced by thalidomide in humans and nonhuman primates, which are triggered during a small window of 2 weeks in humans and result in a typical defect pattern that never includes the brain. The damaging agent obviously only acts rather specifically upon a limited number of morphological differentiation processes.

Contribution of Maternal Toxicity to Prenatal Toxicity

There is no doubt that embryonic and fetal development may be impaired by maternal toxicity, but the situation is complex. An obligatory appearance of gross structural abnormalities should not be expected

TABLE 12 Characteristics of Embryo and Fetotoxic Effects That Can Be Induced

	Embryo and fetotoxic effects		
	Specific	**Universal**	**Indirect**[a]
Phase specificity	Pronounced	Largely lacking	Largely lacking
Structural defects	One or few, circumscript typical malformations	Multiple typical malformations	Mostly minor abnormalities
Prenatal mortality	Often absent[b]	Often together with teratogenicity	Often together with structural defects
Prenatal retardation	Sometimes together with teratogenicity	Often together with teratogenicity	Often together with structural defects
Postnatal retardation	Mostly absent	Often induced	Often induced
Postnatal mortality	Possible (specific causes)	Possible ("unspecific" causes)	Possible ("unspecific" causes)

[a]For example, via maternal toxicity.
[b]Could be the result of pronounced teratogenicity, but may also be induced specifically without simultaneously occurring malformations.

with any agent at doses that are highly toxic to the mother. Karnofsky's law that any substance is teratogenic in high doses may apply to the chicken embryo, but for mammals this claim certainly is wrong. There are many examples from experimental research in which largely normal offspring were delivered by the survivors of the administration of maternal doses equivalent to LD_{20} to LD_{50}. In humans there are also numerous case reports of severe maternal intoxications (e.g., suicidal) after which healthy children were born.

However, pre- or early postnatally induced effects revealed in experimental studies are particularly relevant when they occur well below maternal toxicity. For humans, this is the only situation of interest. The unspecific triggering of abnormal reactions in the embryo or the child cannot be ruled out completely for any substance at dose levels highly toxic to the mother. Nobody would dare to conclude safety for humans at extremely high doses from negative animal data.

The problem rests in the difficulty of defining "maternal toxicity," which is generally impossible. There is such a large variety of possibilities that they cannot be expected to result in the same outcome. Various types of organ toxicity leading to quite different changes in intermediary metabolism, hormonal imbalance, effects on placental perfusion, and uterine contraction are just a few examples. The outcome with respect to the offspring will depend critically on the type of maternal impairment, which in most conventional testing is not characterized. The exclusive evaluation and reporting of maternal toxicity as "body weight loss" is certainly unsatisfactory, and pronounced alterations in maternal metabolism may occur without any overt signs of toxicity. On the other hand, a 10% loss of body weight in humans induced by a chemical within a few weeks would be considered to be a sign of profound toxicity and from a medical point of view would not be designated mild.

Attempts have been made to correlate developmental toxicity results from animal studies with data from the literature on adult toxicity (e.g., LD_{50} values) in the same species. Such an endeavor is bound to fail because both types of toxicity will vary considerably with respect to animal strains and experimental conditions, and for most substances these variations are much larger than the difference between developmental and adult toxicity. Furthermore, dose–response curves are bound to differ for these two types of toxicity. Therefore, A/D (adult/development) ratios are largely worthless and have not been used for any kind of hazard minimization. A/D values are beyond any reasonable consideration when used to compare data from an *in vitro* test with adult toxicity. Maternal and prenatal toxicity can only be compared on the basis of data from the same or a corresponding test design in the same laboratory and under identical experimental conditions.

Taking into account the different slopes of the dose–response curves for developmental and maternal toxicity, suggestions have been made to use a set of ratios from prenatal and adult data, such as $ED_{10(embryo)}/LD_{10(mother)}$. Rather well-defined dose–response curves are necessary for such an approach, which are not available from most routine safety evaluation studies. Therefore, this approach is not applicable to the data of most preclinical studies. Because corresponding dose–response curves in humans will certainly be different, the predictive value of such ratios is questionable.

Several regulatory agencies specifically require studies with dose levels well into the maternal toxicity range (e.g., inducing 10% weight loss in the dams within a few days). Except for the fact that such a situation would be considered highly dangerous in humans, certain minor embryo- and fetotoxic effects are bound to be observed under such extreme conditions, if the evaluation is performed carefully enough. It would be a more relevant strategy and would greatly facilitate the interpretation of the data to define maternal toxicity in dose-range-finding studies in pregnant animals and to use dose levels clearly below this level in the definitive study.

Possible Modes of Embryo- and Fetotoxic Actions

It is fair to state that the exact molecular mode of action is unknown for virtually all teratogenic effects, but some interesting suggestions for specific interactions have been made. Some general mechanisms have long been recognized, through which abnormal prenatal development can be triggered. There are a number of crucial biological phenomena essential for normal embryological development, and interference with these may induce abnormal development. These processes include:

- Morphogenetic differentiations.
- Cell proliferation.
- Cell migrations.
- Cell–cell interactions.
- Cell–extracellular matrix interactions.
- Apoptosis.

Embryonic tissue in the early phase of organogenesis is the fastest proliferating tissue known. The rate of cell division is much higher than in fast-proliferat-

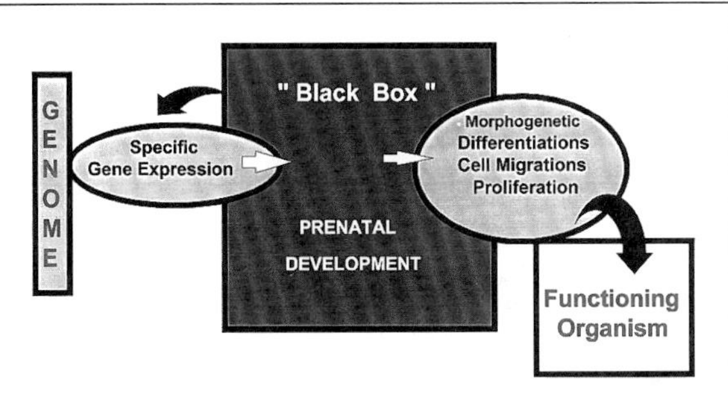

FIGURE 10 Black box of normal and pathological morphogenetic differentiations. While some clues exist on aspects at the genomic level (left) and the endpoints (right) can be well characterized, no information is available on the middle part (i.e., mechanisms acting at the cellular level and being responsible for the morphogenetic differentiations and migration processes). Reprinted from Neubert *et al.* 1980), *Curr. Topics Pathol.* **69**, 241–331, copyright notice of Springer-Verlag.

ing tissues of the adult organism, such as intestinal epithelium, blood-forming organs, or tumors. For this reason, all cytostatic agents and similar substances may exhibit an embryotoxic potential.

The formation of the primordia from the zygote requires countless differentiation processes. During embryonic development these are largely morphogenetic differentiations that are genetically predetermined pattern formations. Molecular biology is just on the verge of understanding a few of these regulatory processes, especially the specific genes expressed at defined stages of development, but the points of attack of teratogenic effects have eluded investigators. While some information on molecular biology may be available, knowledge in cellular biology is largely lacking. This is still a huge black box (Fig. 10). It can be expected that all substances that affect the morphogenetic differentiation processes dramatically (e.g., via altering transcription or translation) may interfere with embryonic development. It must be stressed that this is by no means the only feasible, possibly not even the most common, cause of an exogenously triggered abnormal development (Fig. 11).

Studies of developmental biology have indicated that many morphogenetic differentiation processes require extensive interaction between different cell types. The communication of epithelial cells in the apical ectodermal ridge with the underlying blastema cells during limb development is a typical example. Such specific contacts between cells are now considered to be of special importance in biology, and this is by no means confined to the well-established role in immunology. Maybe it is *the* most important biological phenomenon in the development of multicellular organisms. Apparently a number of specific surface adhesion receptors (e.g., integrins) play a major role in these cell–cell interactions.

Equally important for differentiations during embryonic development are interactions between cells and components of the extracellular matrix (e.g., collagen, fibronectin, and laminin). For example, it has been shown experimentally that the lack of the expression of collagen type I is incompatible with prenatal development. Components of the extracellular matrix also seem to be of major importance for crucial cell migration processes during embryogenesis, such as cell migration from the neural crest or cell migrations essential for the development of the brain areas or the limbs.

Cell death is of particular importance for normal as well as abnormal embryonic development. Without programmed physiological cell death (apoptosis), many steps of organogenesis are impossible; examples are the development of the hand or of the intestinal lumen. A pronounced inhibition of these apoptotic processes must result in abnormal development. On the other hand, exogenously triggered necroses are a common cause of malformations and many agents exhibit their teratogenic effects through this mechanism. If the number of viable cells within a given blastema is reduced beyond a critical value, normal development is no longer possible. There are two ways of inducing malformations, via extensive cell necroses within the target primordium and without necroses. In primates, thalidomide seems to induce limb defects without first causing extensive necroses.

The assumption that all kinds of lesions lead to severe teratogenic impairment is surely wrong. Many of the primary lesions may be repaired prenatally as long as the process involved is still reversible. The ability to repair lesions is especially pronounced in embryonic tissue for two reasons: (1) morphogenetic differentiation during embryogenesis does not depend on a single cell; and (2) dead cells may be rapidly replaced by new ones because of the high proliferation rate.

Paternal Contribution to the Induction of Malformations

There is no doubt that mutations in the male germ cells, as in oocytes, can cause (hereditary) malformations. Because mutations are largely a stochastic process, no accumulation of a single type of malformation is to be expected, but an increase in the sum of all possible abnormal developments may occur and become detectable.

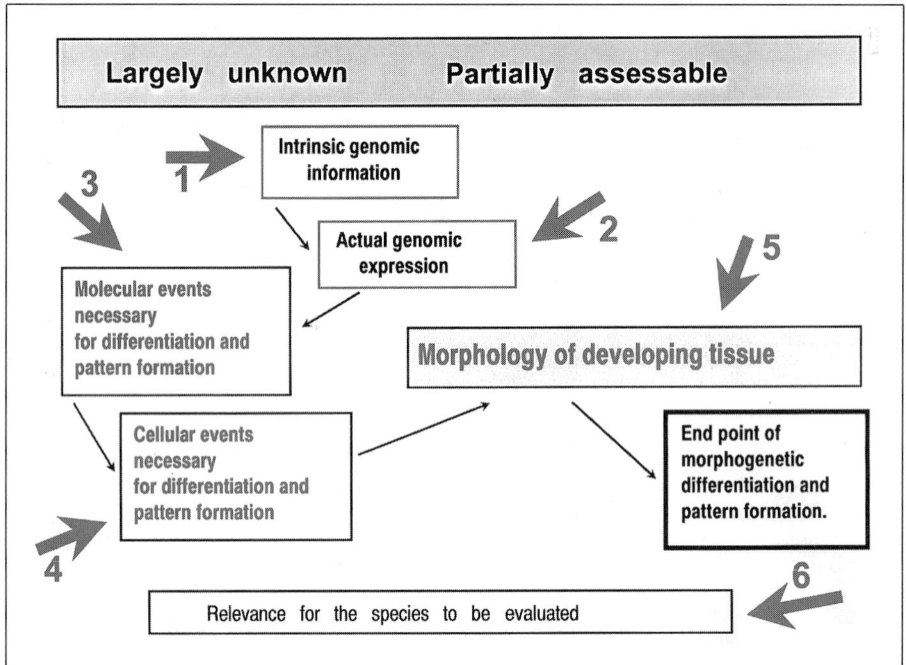

FIGURE 11 Examples of possible points of attack within the sequence of reactions during organogenesis (1) Mutations in the germ cells can induce prenatal death dominant lethal effect or malformations. (2) Interference with the genomic expression essential during organogenesis. (3) and (4) Interference with interactions between cells or with cells and the extracellular matrix. (5) Alterations of the morphology of the developing tissue, e.g., induction of cell necroses. (6) Not all interactions are induced in all species or are of relevance for all species and strains.

Recently, it has been claimed in several publications that the exposure of males to exogenous agents might have resulted in gross structural abnormalities in their children. While such an increase in the overall malformation rate within a group exposed to a strong mutagen is feasible, the incidence would be expected to be very low. This conclusion is based on dominant lethal effects and the low fertilizing capacity of damaged sperm cells. The occurrence of such paternally induced malformations is extremely unlikely for agents without mutagenic properties, and there is no biological rationale for such an effect to occur. Although the epigenetic transfer of some information from one generation to the next has been demonstrated (genetic imprinting), there is no indication that interference with crucial steps of morphogenetic differentiation may occur in this way.

In connection with exposure of U.S. Vietnam War veterans to the herbicide Agent Orange, which contained TCDD as a contaminant of the two phenoxyacetic acid herbicide active ingredients, claims of paternally caused malformations attributed to TCDD were made based on case reports. This supposition was not verified by several epidemiological studies. As was to be expected, massive and close to lethal dosing of male laboratory animals with TCDD failed to induce such an adverse effect in these rat studies.

Heritable transfer of identical defects to the next generation has also been claimed to occur in cases of thalidomide-induced malformations of the father in some publications. Such allegations cannot be taken seriously for a substance devoid of any mutagenic potential. Even if a mutation had occurred, the same defects could not be expected. It is now well established that during the thalidomide epidemic, heritable syndromes had been misdiagnosed as thalidomide embryopathy. Thus, the heritability of limb defects would argue against a thalidomide-induced embryopathy in the first generation.

Kinetic Aspects

Just as for all other pharmacological and toxic effects there are two prerequisites for triggering embryotoxic effects:

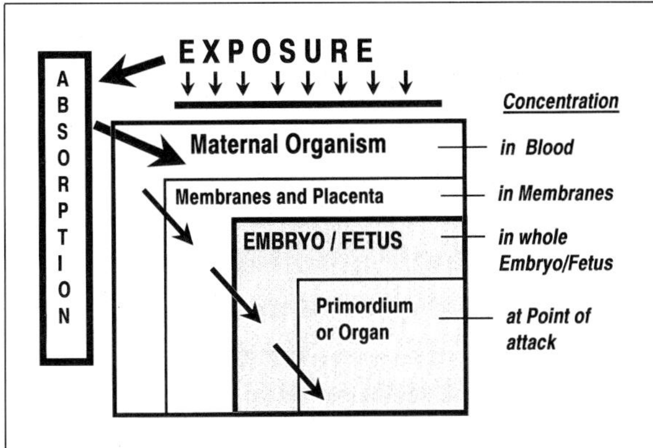

FIGURE 12 Complex kinetics between mother and conceptus. For direct effects on the embryo or fetus, the concentration at the target tissue is crucial as well as the duration of the primary effect. Since target tissue concentrations are almost never accessible, maternal plasma concentration is used as surrogate marker.

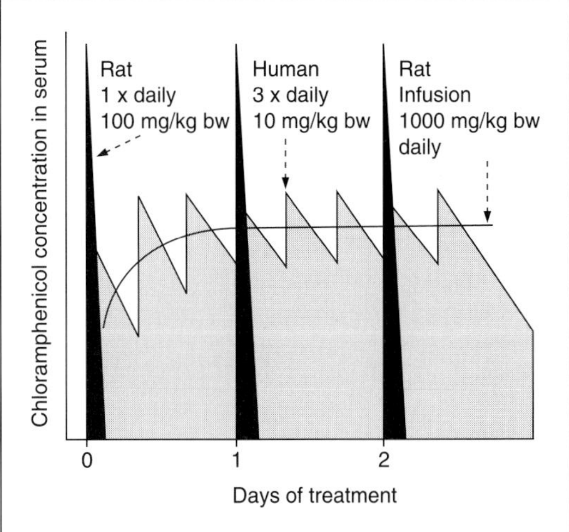

FIGURE 13 Pharmacokinetic problems with substances exhibiting very short elimination half-lives in animals but longer ones in humans. Chloramphenicol serves as an example. The experimental design must be adapted to this situation.

- A sufficiently high concentration of the agent at the target cell.
- A sufficient duration of exposure at the target.

These two factors determine whether an effect remains below a threshold and thus may remain reversible, or whether an irreversible impairment results. Only rarely has extensive information on kinetic variables been gathered in animal studies for agents inducing embryotoxic effects. This is due to the complex situation of the kinetics in the maternal organism versus the kinetics and concentrations in the conceptus (embryo and fetus, including the placenta) (Fig. 12). The transfer rate to the conceptus is not a constant, but may change drastically during the gestational period. Human transfer studies have been usually limited to the end of pregnancy and may not be relevant to the situation at organogenesis.

Kinetic measurements are almost always limited to the maternal organism, and it is usually assumed (most often rightly so) that a corresponding dose–response relationship also holds true for the conceptus. Because there is sufficient evidence that pronounced species differences exist with respect to kinetics, a comparative extrapolation from the experimental species to humans is no longer acceptable on the basis of doses. This requires that (maternal) kinetic data from the animal species and from humans are available, which often is not the case.

For practical purposes it is important to realize that the elimination half-life in rodents for many substances is much shorter than in humans. In animal testing, a single daily application of a substance may not lead to toxic concentrations over a sufficiently long period, and the plasma concentration curve may deviate considerably from that obtained after therapeutic applications in humans (Fig. 13). This problem has been known since the early 1970s and methods have been suggested and applied (e.g., multiple applications per day, continuous infusion, and constant rate infusions from minipumps) in order to achieve kinetics in the experimental animals similar to the situation in humans. An adverse potential may be missed if this kinetic aspect is not considered. The data obtained may not be useful to attempt a quantitative hazard minimization.

There has been some discussion whether embryo- and fetotoxic effects of a number of substances correlate with the maternal peak plasma concentrations. This would have a practical significance because it could be used to attempt to reduce the possible adverse effects of a therapeutic drug by altering the form of application.

Unfortunately, in connection with the characterization of teratogenic effects the pharmacokinetic term AUC (area under the maternal plasma concentration curve) has been brought into the debate. According to basic pharmacological knowledge, this pharmacokinetic variable is designed for defining the bioavailability in the same species. AUC cannot be correlated directly with a rather short-lasting effect. There is no

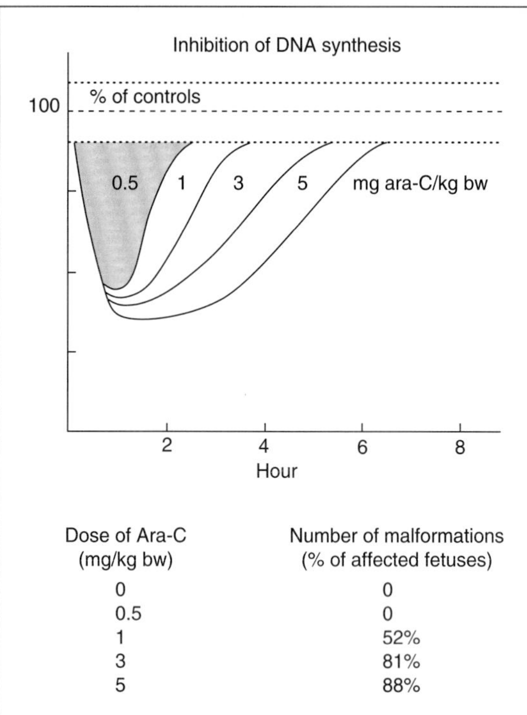

Dose of Ara-C (mg/kg bw)	Number of malformations (% of affected fetuses)
0	0
0.5	0
1	52%
3	81%
5	88%

FIGURE 14 Teratogenic effect of cytosine arabinoside (ara-C) depending on the duration (not the extent) of inhibition of DNA synthesis. Mice were treated iv with ara-C on day 10 of pregnancy, and incorporation of ^{14}C glucose into embryonic DNA was measured (see graph). Biochemical data can be correlated with malformation rates (see table).

need and no significance for an AUC value in the case of very long-lasting effects.

Crucial for the induction of embryotoxic effects is a critical concentration of the substance at the target (e.g., receptor) for a sufficient length of time. This prerequisite is not at all identical with the AUC of the maternal plasma concentration, and a correlation may only exist by chance. In particular, the AUC of the maternal plasma concentration is entirely useless for a correlation with toxic effects if irreversible or pseudo-irreversible effects occur at the target. Examples are the administration of alkylating agents or certain folic acid antagonists, which are potent inducers of embryotoxic effects. With such substances, the induction and extent of the teratogenic effects surely are not a function of the free concentration of the parent substance in the maternal plasma. Rather, the effect on the embryo can and should be correlated with the concentration or, even better, with the primary reaction at the target organ, as has been done in many experimental studies in which metabolic activation of the substance is required.

Evidence that the teratogenic outcome and the length of time required for a defined effect at the primary target are correlated was obtained decades ago. After a single administration of the antimetabolite cytosine arabinoside, teratogenic effects occurred only at a dose of 1 mg/kg body weight or higher. The inhibition of DNA synthesis in the embryos proper was not much more pronounced at that dose than after 0.5 mg/kg body weight, a dose that was ineffective with regard to terata, but the inhibition of DNA synthesis lasted longer after 1 mg/kg (Fig. 14). Apparently, the critical process must be blocked for a certain length of time in order to trigger an irreversible lesion, in this particular case a critical percentage of cell necroses, within the primordium.

A problem confounding the interpretation of the effects and catabolism may arise with substances strongly inducing their own metabolism. Conventional developmental hazard identification studies are always performed with single daily repeated applications of the test chemical. The dosing period is started on day 6 of pregnancy in the rat. If, for instance, the substance induces cleft palate when given acutely and singly on either day 13 or 14 of pregnancy, the concentration achieved in the multiple dosing design might be insufficient at that time to reveal the potential to induce this effect because of metabolism induction. This example illustrates the necessity of having kinetic data available.

Short-lived active metabolites generated by the dam may not reach the conceptus because they react with macromolecules of the maternal organism and are not available for placental transfer.

Drug-metabolizing reactions of phase I and phase II are not expressed in the cells of the embryo, and neither metabolic degradation nor activation of chemicals via these pathways occur in the mammalian embryo. This has the consequence that short-lived active metabolites may not be formed with the embryonic tissue. Therefore, indirectly acting alkylating agents, such as dimethyl-and diethylnitrosamine, are not teratogenic. When the active hydroxylated component can be released within the embryo (e.g., from the ester as is acetoxymethyl-methylnitrosamine by embryonic esterases), malformations are induced.

While in rodents the expression of hepatic drug-metabolizing monooxygenases begins almost exclusively after birth, some of these enzyme activities are already measurable in fetal primates. Thus, distinct metabolic capability differences exist between rodents and primates. Nevertheless, many of these metabolic conversions still proceed at a low rate at birth in humans and nonhuman primates.

It would be wrong to conclude that no metabolic activation can occur in embryonic tissue because there is a high metabolic activation capacity for certain reactions. Nucleic acid synthesis proceeds at a very high rate within the rapidly proliferating tissue, and many antimetabolites (e.g., 6-MP, 5-FU, and ara-C) are easily activated within the embryo and may induce severe malformations.

Dose–Response Relationships

Like all other toxic effects, embryo- and fetotoxic effects are strictly dose–dependent. Because of the dose specificity discussed, certain teratogenic effects can only be evaluated over a limited dose range, for example, if mild effects are overshadowed by another more pronounced effect (such as teratogenicity by embryomortality and defects of the digits by amelia).

Experimental studies have shown that the dose–response curves for embryotoxic and especially for teratogenic effects are usually rather steep. With decreasing doses, the frequency of malformations declines rapidly. For most agents with high teratogenic potency, the ratio between the lowest observable adverse effect level (LOAEL) and the dose needed for inducing almost 100% malformations is less than one order of magnitude (Fig. 15). One gets the impression that the developing mammalian system is, on one hand, rather well protected, but, on the other hand, the system "tips over" at a certain point, which may explain the steep dose–response curve. Often along with severe teratogenicity or at only slightly higher doses, an increase in embryofetomortality is seen. Under such circumstances, a teratogenic effect can only be recognized within a small window of doses. An apparent exception in this respect is thalidomide, which under suitable conditions may induce typical malformations over about three orders of magnitude in nonhuman primates, due to the lack of embryomortality in this dose range. However, the percentage of malformations stays constant over an extended dose interval, and the slope of the increasing part of the dose–response curve is also rather steep (Fig. 16). The almost nonexistent prenatal mortality implies that the embryotoxicity after thalidomide administration is compatible with prenatal life. On the other hand, some of the malformations, such as severe heart defects, can very well lead to postnatal death, as has been observed in humans. The localized appearance of minor defects (e.g., at the outer ear) in humans after thalidomide exposure may not be a result of a low dose, but is explainable by the marked phase specificity of the thalidomide effect.

In experiments with polytocous animals (litters of >1) a pronounced interlitter and even intralitter variability of embryotoxic and teratogenic effects exist, even after very short exposures. While this phenomenon may partly be explained by pharmacokinetic differences (e.g., different kinetics within the individual dams) and unequal distribution of blood to the embryos or fetuses within the uterus, a major reason is the fact that individual embryos of the same litter are at different stages of development. The variability of the toxic reaction for different individuals of the same litter rests in the phase specificity of the induction of malformations (Table 13). This phenomenon applies for inbred as well as for outbred mouse strains, and similar data have been obtained for rats.

A large number of experimental studies have shown that in the range of measurable data good linear relationships in dose–response curves were found if the probit of the effect (teratogenicity) is plotted against the logarithm of the dose. When the slope of the dose–response curve is steep, the type of mathematical transformation (e.g., probit, logit, or Weibull) does not make a difference (Table 14). When attempting a regression analysis, sufficient data points must be available to construct a reliable dose–response curve. In routine studies such data most often are not obtained. However, the steepness of the dose–response curves has been shown not to be identical for various teratologic endpoints. A prerequisite for a comparative evaluation is that the kinetics in the experimental animals and in humans are similar. Most conventional routine animal tests have not been designed to meet this requirement, with the exception of some evaluations of potential pharmaceutical products.

For the reasons mentioned, extrapolations into a dose range that cannot be verified by experimental data are speculative and their predictive value for humans is limited. This holds especially true for extrapolations into exposure ranges far lower than the experimental data (e.g., ED_{01} data or even lower ranges), while extrapolations close to the measured data may provide more reliable values. Extrapolations to incidences of 1:1000 and below (e.g., 1:1 million) in reproductive toxicology are always pure speculation and the results allow only a very vague estimate of the toxicity potency of the substance under investigation. For most preventive hazard minimizations this is sufficient because it serves the purpose of arguing that the probability of a chemically induced effect is very low.

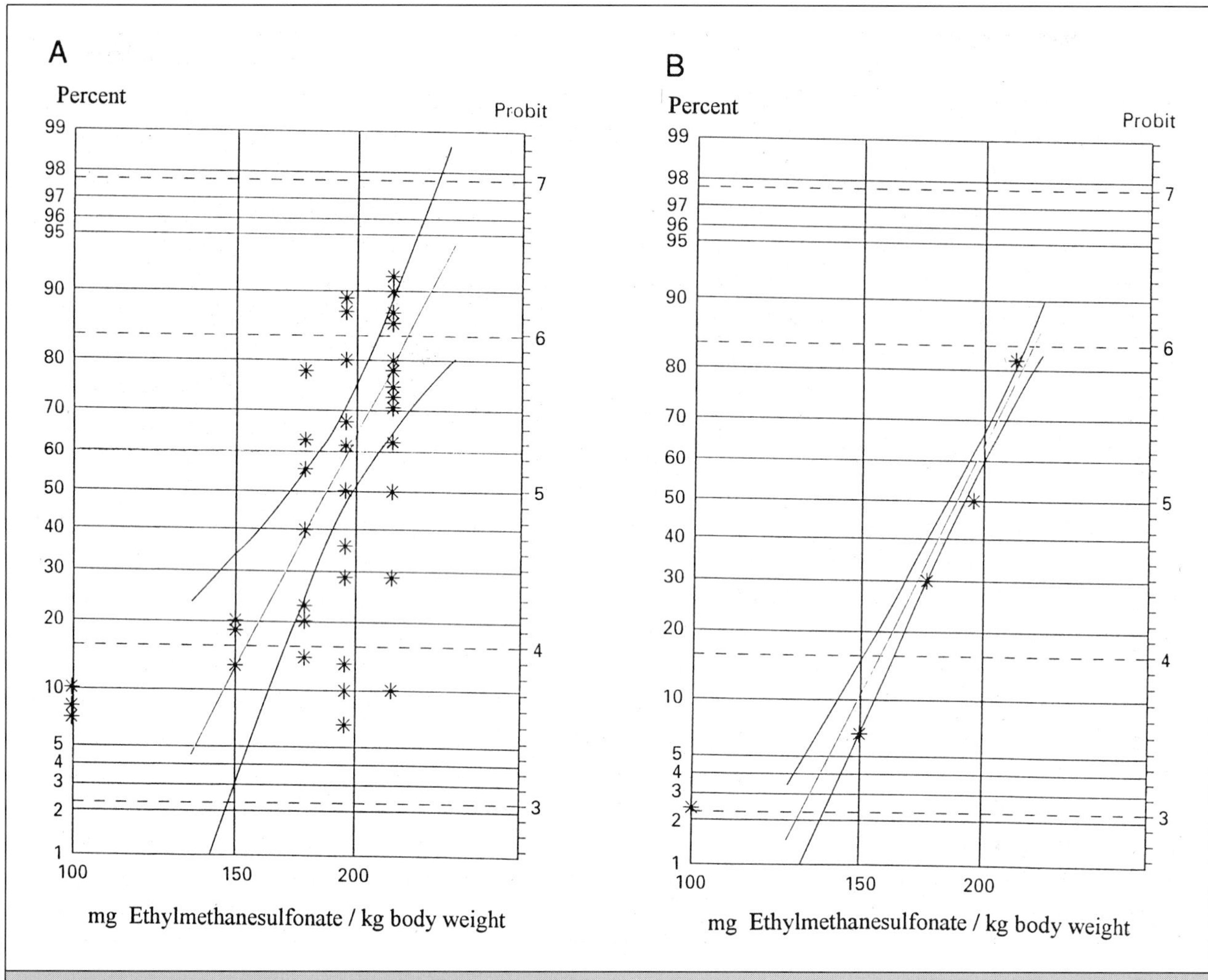

FIGURE 15 Dose–response relatioships of teratogenic effects. Both graphs represent data from the same study, using hydroxyurea in rats. (A) Data points based on the individual litters. (B) Data based on total fetuses per dose group. The slopes of both regression curves are identical, the confidence intervals are quite different.

It is typical for teratogenic effects with steep dose–response relationships that an uncertainty factor of 10 used together with a NOAEL (no observed adverse effect level) is more conservative than a theoretical extrapolation to a possible incidence of 1:1 million (Table 14). The species specificity and the lack of knowledge of whether humans are a susceptible species to the effect under discussion are limiting.

Several attempts have been made to assess whether a threshold limit exists for teratogenic effects. While all scientific facts argue for the existence of an exposure range beyond which the teratogenic potency of an agent is negligible, the absolute negative can never be proven. From a pragmatic point of view, the uncertainty factor approach is acceptable. Linear extrapolations to zero down to extremely low exposure levels lack a scientific basis and are largely political exercises. It is absurd to assume that one molecule of an agent with a teratogenic potential could still induce a teratogenic effect.

Examples of Abnormal Development

In the following section some typical examples of exogenously triggered congenital, persisting abnormalities will be discussed. The exemplified effects will be divided into the following categories:

- Abnormalities detectable at birth after prenatal exposure.
- Postnatal dysfunctions after prenatal exposure.
- Defects induced perinatally with postnatal manifestation.

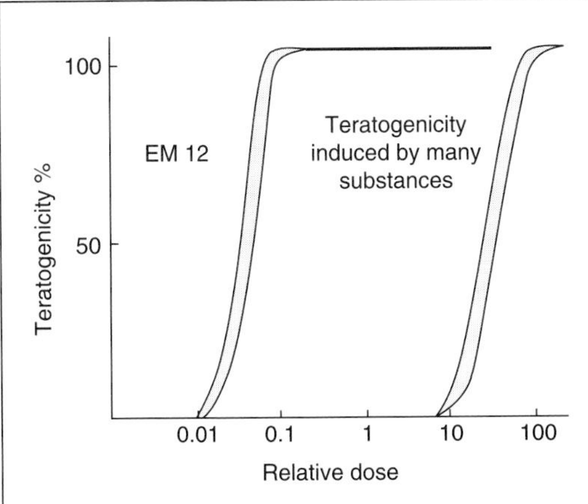

FIGURE 16 Dose–respose of a thalidomide derivative (EM12) and a schematic slope typical for many other agents. The slopes of the curves are similar, but thalidomide induces defects over an extended dose range because there is no clearly increased mortality in primates.

- Defects induced early postnatally.
- Defects induced during infancy.

Abnormalities Detectable at Birth after Prenatal Exposure

For a long time attention has been focussed on gross structural abnormalities. It is now recognized that this is only one manifestation of exogenously induced abnormal development. Although irreversible, a good proportion of the morphological defects can be surgically corrected and a close to normal function obtained.

Example: Thalidomide

Although somewhat antiquated, thalidomide still represents the most notorious teratogenic substance for humans. Because some of the features of this substance are typical for teratogenic agents, and others are quite unique, the aspects of the thalidomide teratogenesis will be described in some detail.

The large-scale application of thalidomide as a sedative and hypnotic started in the late 1950s and lasted for only about 4 years, until 1961–1962. The trade name of the most frequently used over-the-counter preparation was Contergan. This substance showed remarkably little acute toxicity in animal tests and, in contrast to other sedatives and hypnotics used at that time, attempts to commit suicide with thalidomide were entirely unsuccessful. For several reasons the thalidomide disaster undoubtedly belongs to the major catastrophes in medicine:

- Some decades ago it seemed unimaginable that a sedative and hypnotic or a tranquilizer with such a low general toxicity for the adult organism could lead to such severe gross structural malformations at therapeutic doses of about 1–3 mg/kg body weight. This experience entirely changed the attitude toward drug safety, and stringent preclinical testing became mandatory in most industrial countries.
- The malformations, especially of the limbs, were extremely severe (ranging from phocomelia to complete amelia of all four limbs in extreme cases) and they equally intrigued relatives, physicians, and laymen.
- Rough estimates of the number of cases of thalidomide-induced embryopathy, the exact figures are unknown, were about 4000 victims in Germany and worldwide about 7000 malformed children.

Thalidomide has the chemical structure of *N*-phthalimido-glutarimide (Fig. 17) or 2-(2,6-dioxopiperidine-3-yl)-phthalimide. It is very poorly water soluble, and at the same time exhibits poor solubility in oil. It is slowly hydrolyzed *in vitro* and *in vivo* to about a dozen hydrolysis products. The requirements for the chemical structure to be essential for the teratogenic action are largely unknown.

After this terrible experience it was suspected that we might be surrounded by many substances with similar teratogenic potentials. Fortunately, extensive research since the 1960s proved this not to be true.

The epidemic of these otherwise extremely rare limb malformations was first published by the pediatrician Wiedemann in Kiel, Germany, in 1961, and he suggested an exogenous cause. In a joint effort of many investigators, the number of suspected agents was reduced, and thalidomide eventually identified as the causal substance. A considerable number of case reports were compiled only retrospectively, and no true epidemiological studies on the teratogenic effects of thalidomide exist. This fact illustrates two major points of interest regarding chemical teratogenesis. First, without systematic studies only those side effects that are spontaneously very rare and that are quite unusual in their appearance can be easily recognized. Second, when such exotic effects are observed, rising numbers of case reports may be sufficient to provide a strong hint for a cause-and-effect relationship. Even under such extreme conditions, single-case reports are largely useless for this purpose. On the other hand, even a large number of case reports are insufficient for identifying cases of chemically induced abnormalities that already occur spontaneously at a high incidence. Because of these

TABLE 13 Intra- and Interlitter Variability of the Developmental Stages in the Mouse[a]

Litter number	Number of somite pairs: 32	33	34	35	36	37	38	39	40	41	42	43	44	45	46	47	Litter size
1												4	3				(7)
2									3	1	1	2					(7)
3							1	1		1		4	2	1			(10)
4									2		4	4	1	1			(12)
5							2	1		3	1	2		2	1		(12)
6							1		1	1	4	4		1		1	(13)
7									1	1	3	1	4	2	1		(13)
8		1			1			1	1	3	3	2	1				(13)
9	1					1	1	5	4	1	1						(14)
10										2	4	2	3	3			(14)
	1%	1%			1%	1%	4%	7%	10%	11%	18%	22%	12%	9%	2%	1%	($n = 115$)
											40%						
											63%						

[a]The number of somite pairs was taken as convenient measure of the developmental stage. From Neubert *et al.*, 1987, *Arch. Toxicol.* **60,** 238–245, copyright notice of Springer-Verlag, with permission.

TABLE 14 Extrapolation[a] of Methylnitroso Urea (MNU) in the Mouse

Measured or extrapolated frequency	Mathematical transformation (mg MNU/kg body weight): Probit	Logit	Weibull	γ-Multihit
ED_{80}[b]	4.6			
ED_{50}[b]	3.8			
ED_{10}[b]	2.7			
NOAEL[c]	2			
NOAEL/10[d]	0.2			
benchmark $ED_{10}/10$[e]	0.3			
ED_{01}[f]	2.2	2.2	2.2	2.2
ED_{001}[f]	1.9	1.6	1.7	1.8
$ED_{10^{-6}}$[f]	1.3	0.7	0.7	1.1

[a]Using linear regression to a theoretical incidence of 1 : 1 million, and a NOAEL uncertainty factor approach ("safety" factor of 10). The extrapolated values are theoretical assessments only, and the corresponding probability are not postulated to occur either in the experimental animal or in humans. Data from Platzek *et al.* (1987); Platzek *et al.* (1992).

[b]Measured values.

[c]Derived from measured values.

[d]Using a safety factor of 10.

[e]Using a benchmark of ED_{10} and a safety factor of 10.

[f]Extrapolated values using mathematical transformations. Slope of the dose–response curve (tan α): 18 ± 1.

limitations, there is practically no information to answer the question of how many women have delivered healthy babies despite taking thalidomide during the critical phase of pregnancy. All attempts to assess the frequency of malformations after ingesting thalidomide at therapeutic doses must remain speculative, but clues from animal data suggest that this percentage must have been rather high.

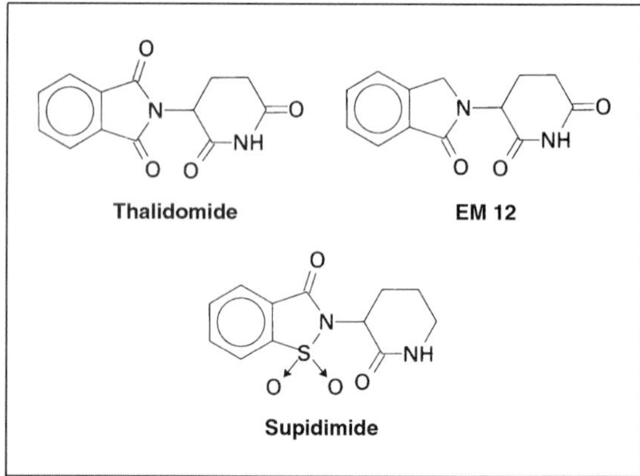

FIGURE 17 Chemical structures of thalidomide and some derivatives.

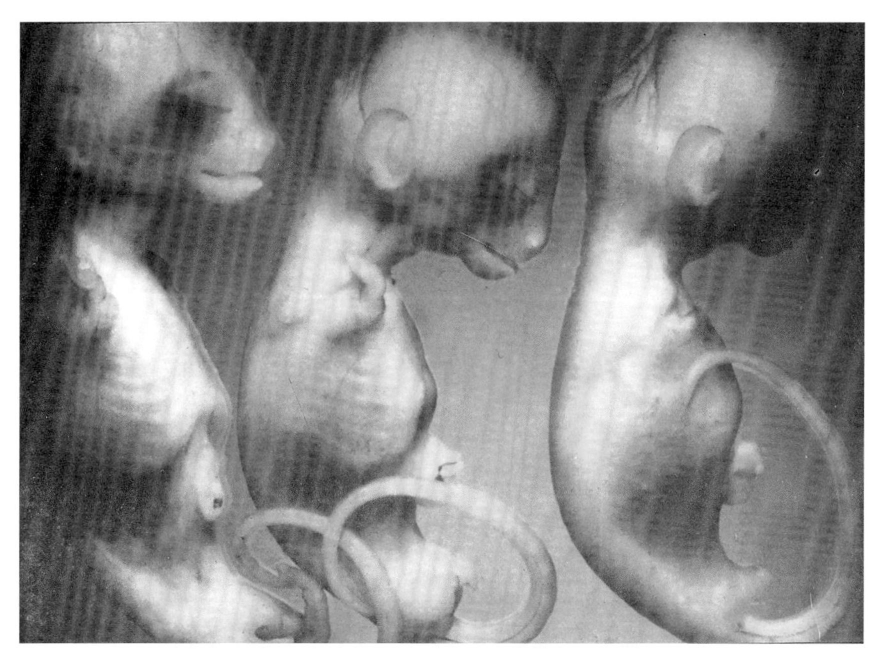

FIGURE 18 Teratogenic effect of the thalidomide derivative EM12 on the primate species *Callithrix jacchus*. Example of one litter. All three offspring show the typical amelia of all four limbs (daily dose: 5 mg/kg body weight). Note the rudimentary upper limbs (without bone structures), the missing pelvic girdle and the absence of the lower limbs.

Just as in human embryos, the teratogenic potential of thalidomide in the primate is not restricted to the induction of limb malformations. The pattern of gross structural abnormalities typical for thalidomide includes heart defects and malformations of the intestinal tract. A considerable percentage of the babies adversely affected by thalidomide died after a few years, surely not because of the limb malformations. Although we know today that the malformation-inducing effect of thalidomide is unusual in many respects, it still remains the most notorious human teratogen. The mystery about this substance's mode of action has lasted for more than 30 years, in spite of an abundance of theories. While none of these hypotheses could be proven by experimental testing, some clues to the possible mode of action have been obtained.

A special feature of the teratogenic effects of thalidomide is its marked species specificity. Even with the highest possible doses, no corresponding malformations can be induced in the commonly used rodent laboratory animals. When treated with comparatively high doses, embryos of certain rabbit strains show a low incidence of malformations with some similarities to those occurring in humans. The typical pattern of defects can reproducibly be triggered with small doses (1–20 mg/kg range) in all primates studied so far (Fig. 18).

The typical pattern of thalidomide-specific malformations in nonhuman primates can only be induced within the short time frame of about 2 weeks (Table 15). No congenital malformations can be induced before or after this critical period. Many retrospective investigations indicate that there is a comparably

TABLE 15 Sensitive Period for the Induction of Typical Limb Malformations with Thalidomide in Primates

Primate species	Thalidomide-sensitive period (approximate gestational age, days)
Rhesus	24?–33
Baboon	26–32
Bushbaby	26–34
Marmoset	46–61
Human	(20) 24–33 (36)

TABLE 16 Differences in the Teratogenic Effects of the $S(-)$- and $R(+)$-Enantiomers of the Thalidomide Derivative EM 12[a]

Malformation	Affected fetuses/total number studied	
	$S(-)$-EM12	$R(+)$-EM12
Upper limbs		
Amelia	7/18	0/11
Phocomelia	6/18	0/11
Humerus, radius		
Deformed	3/18	1/11
Lower limbs		
Amelia	11/18	0/11
Phocomelia	1/18	0/11
Mandibula		
Synostosis	5/18	4/11
Fetuses without malformations	0/18	6/11

[a]These effects were induced and observed in marmosets (0.5–1 mg/kg body weight). *In vivo* some spontaneous reracemization occurs rendering a final evaluation difficult.

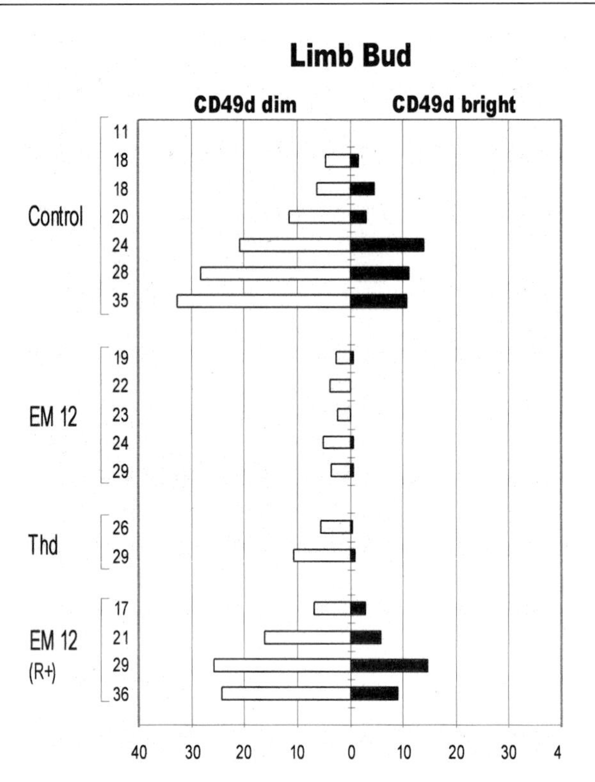

FIGURE 19 Example of changes induced by thalidomide on embryonic surface cell receptors after treatment of marmosets with teratogenic and nonteratogenic thalidomide derivatives during the sensitive period. Expression of the adhesion receptor. CD 49d, a B1-integrin, increases during the developmental period studied. This expression is greatly down-regulated by the teratogenic thalidomide and EM12 (racemate), but not influenced by the "nonteratogenic". R(+)-EM12 enantiomer. Cells of primordia were isolated and surface receptors analyzed with monoclonal antibodies and flow cytometry. Light-colored columns, cells with low receptor density; darker-colored columns, with high density. Each column represents one litter, the small numbers indicate the developmental stage (number of somite pairs).

short sensitive period (from day 20–24 to 33–36 of gestation) in humans.

The sensitive period for thalidomide corresponds, according to studies in nonhuman primates, to a very early stage in the development of the limb buds (Carnegie stage 10–12), well before the onset of chondrogenesis. Furthermore, from the two enantiomers of the highly teratogenic thalidomide derivative EM 12, the S(−)-form is substantially more effective (Table 16) than the corresponding R(+)-enantiomer. Daily doses of less than 100 μg/kg body weight of highly teratogenic thalidomide derivatives are sufficient to induce a marked percentage of typical malformations in nonhuman primates. The teratogenic potential of a few thalidomide derivatives has been studied experimentally in monkeys. EM12 (Fig. 17) with only one carbonyl group in its "phthalimide ring" (which is a phthalimidine ring) is more stable to hydrolysis than thalidomide and forms only two or three hydrolysis products or metabolites. Because studies in rabbits and nonhuman primates have shown this compound to have a still higher teratogenic potency than thalidomide itself, it is especially useful for experimental studies. The teratogenic effect does not correlate with the sedative effect of thalidomide because by only a slight modification of the chemical structure the teratogenic potential is lost, as in supidimide (Fig. 17), while the sedative properties are retained.

After treatment of nonhuman primates or human volunteers with thalidomide, pronounced changes in the expression of surface adhesion receptors were found on the white blood cells. Because interactions between cells and between cells and the extracellular matrix are well known as representing key events during the differentiation and migration processes governing embryonic development, interference with such reactions may also be visualized as a cause of the teratogenic effects of thalidomide. A drastic down-regulation of several adhesion surface receptors of the integrin type was found on limb bud cells of embryos from nonhuman primates (Fig. 18) after treatment with thalidomide or its teratogenic derivative (e.g., EM12 racemate). The effect was confined to the thalid-

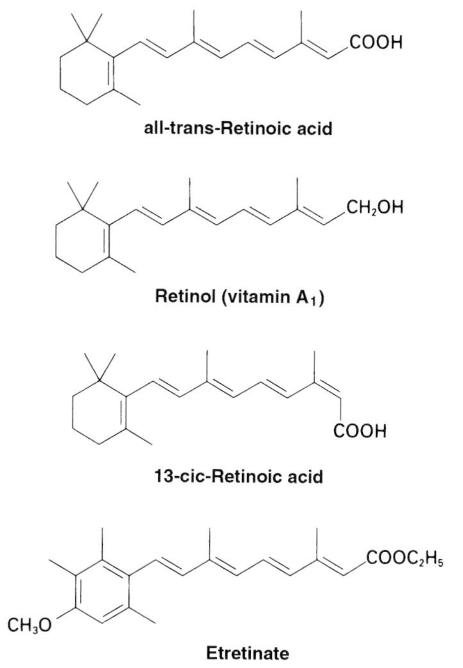

FIGURE 20 Chemical structure of some retinoids.

omide-susceptible primordia (limbs and heart) and did not occur in the primordia not affected by thalidomide (e.g., the brain). The changes in receptor expression were only observed with the teratogenic derivatives and not with the much less teratogenic R(+)-EM12 enantiomer. Thus, at present the hypothesis that the teratogenic effect of thalidomide are associated with a down-regulation of adhesion surface receptors offers the best mechanistic explanation, especially because this mode of action is the only one being proven in primate embryos at the thalidomide-sensitive stage. The exact details of this mechanism of action must be elucidated.

Limitations to the long-term application of thalidomide for the new therapeutic indication of anti-inflammatory effects and immunosuppression are, aside from the teratogenic potential, the occurrence of polyneuropathy, which had already been observed as a rare side effect. This thalidomide neuropathy has often been found to be poorly reversible, and the long-term application of thalidomide without measuring nerve conduction velocity before and during the treatment period must be considered as sin of omission.

Example: Retinoids

As a further example of substances clearly teratogenic in humans, vitamin A is an excellent example of the Janus face of such substances. There is no doubt that in low doses this vitamin is essential for the development of the conceptus (the recommended daily dose is approximately 5000 IE vitamin A during pregnancy). It has long been known that a lack of vitamin A causes abnormal development, and vitamin A deficiency was one of the first manipulations in experimental animals to induce malformations. The standardization of the vitamin is somewhat confusing, because all the metabolites do not have identical potencies at different targets and because of differences in oral absorption. One microgram of all-*trans*-retinol (1 retinol equivalent) was defined as 3.3 IU of vitamin A activity; because of the poorer absorption, this equals 6 μg of dietary β-carotene (or 10 units of dietary vitamin A).

An overdose of vitamin A also is well known to be capable of inducing abnormal development in experimental animals. Such dose-dependent opposite behavior is not uncommon among certain vitamins, hormones, and transmitters. This illustrates the fact that toxicity is a quantitative phenomenon and not an intrinsic property of an agent.

While the provitamins A (e.g., β-carotene) are common and abundantly occurring plant pigments, retinol (vitamin A_1) is present in animals, especially in fish liver, in esterified form. Vitamin A stored in human liver also represents a buffer against hypovitaminosis. The oxidation products of retinol are retinaldehyde and retinoic acid (Fig. 20). All three derivatives exist as isomers (i.e., as the all-*trans* and the -*cis* form). Retinaldehyde, biologically only interesting as 11-*cis*-retinal, is a part of rhodopsin within the rods of the retina, an essential component for the visual cycle. Otherwise vitamin A is essential for the structure and function, especially, of epithelial cells in many organs, such as mucus production and secretion, keratinization, growth, and differentiation. Retinoic acid seems to be the active form for these processes, and it is much more active than retinol.

While the teratogenic effects could not be induced with the carotene provitamins, abnormal development is triggered in many experimental animal species, including nonhuman primates by many of the vitamin A derivatives proper as well as many synthetic retinoids.

All-*trans*-retinoic acid (tretinoin) is in equilibrium with the 13-*cis* form (isotretinoin) within the organism. While the elimination-half-life of all-*trans*-retinoic acid is rather short, that of 13-*cis*-retinoic acid is considerably longer (3–36 h) and is further exceeded by some of the metabolites (e.g., 4-oxo-isotretinoin). Although the predominating active species cannot be revealed, there is evidence for 13-*cis*-retinoic acid be-

TABLE 17 Pattern of Malformations in 21 Newborns with Deformities after *In Utero* Isotretinoin Exposure

Malformations	Frequency	
	Number	Percent[a]
Microtia, anotia	15	(71%)
Micrognathia	6	(29%)
Cleft palates	3	(14%)
Cardiac defects	8	(38%)
Thymus defects	7	(33%)
Defects of retina and optical nerve	4	(19%)
Defects of CNS[b]	18	(86%)

[a]Percentage of the 21 malformed babies.

[b]Forms of hydrocephalus (9), microcephaly (3), cerebellar hypoplasia or agenesis (6), megacisterna magna (3), and focal cortical agenesia.

ing more potent than the all-*trans* form. Subsequent to multiple dosing, the serum concentration of the 13-*cis*-retinoic acid greatly exceeds that of the all-*trans* isomer, while the all-*trans* isomer seems to exhibit a greater affinity to the receptor.

In the early 1980s, isotretinoin was licensed as a medicinal drug for dermatological indications. A number of vitamin A derivatives (retinoids) were synthesized, and very few (Fig. 20) are in use as therapeutics, such as etretinate, which exhibits a high efficacy in specific skin disorders. These two substances have gained great importance in dermatology for the treatment of severe acne and psoriasis, respectively. Even though the teratogenic potency of vitamin A was well known and had also been proven experimentally for the newly synthesized derivatives, a considerable number of malformations in children were seen after their mothers had been treated with these drugs or shared prescriptions with other persons, especially in the United States. Prescription sharing with men suffering from severe acne has turned out to be the source of isotretinoin in severe malformation cases. Even urgent warnings in the package circular had obviously not kept doctors from prescribing these substances without positively excluding pregnancy during the course of therapy.

In humans, the multiple malformations after ingestion of such retinoids manifest themselves (Table 17) as defects of the central nervous system (e.g., hydrocephalus and hypoplasia of the optical nerve), of the cardiovascular system (e.g., interventricular septal defect and alterations of the large vessels), of the ears (e.g., microtia, anotia, and atresia of the auditory canal) and as structural deviations of the skeletal system (e.g., cleft palate and micrognathia). Also behavioral deficits were diagnosed in the affected children. According to a prospective study of 36 isotretinoin-exposed mother–child pairs, 8 (22%) of the pregnancies ended as spontaneous miscarriages, 5 (5/28, 18%) of the newborn showed malformations (one of these children with malformations was stillborn), and 23 (82%) of the children were without pathological findings at delivery. If the five severe malformations of the children >19 gestational weeks old are compared to a large reference group in Atlanta (i.e., 194/27866), a relative risk of 26 (95% confidence interval, 11–58) was calculated. The therapeutically recommended dose range of isotretinoin (0.5 mg/kg body weight) is clearly sufficient to induce teratogenic effects in humans.

Isotretinoin and etretinate differ considerably from all-*trans*-retinoic acid in their pharmacokinetic properties. For this reason, effective contraception should be continued for at least 4 weeks after discontinuing isotretinoin treatment. Etretinate features a special phenomenon, as the substance remains within a deep compartment of the human organism (adipose tissue) for many months. One case of a child with typical malformations was reported after the mother had discontinued using the substance 51 weeks prior to conception. Therefore, as a precautionary measure pregnancy must be avoided for 2 years after the discontinuation of treatment with this substance.

Even though the mode of action for triggering abnormal development during embryogenesis by retinoids is unknown, several indications exist on the general molecular mechanism of action of these substances. Retinoic acid is the only substance for which convincing evidence of an important physiological role in pattern formation during organogenesis was established in animal models, such as development of the vertebral column and the limbs. Although not proven in the mammalian embryo, the substance may be visualized to act via a typical induction within the cell nucleus after binding to specific retinoid receptors. Similar to the receptor-mediated mechanism of steroid hormones (Fig. 9), it can be assumed that the interaction of retinoic acid with its receptor triggers a whole cascade of regulatory processes with the result of activating specific gene groups. According to the classic model of the mode of action of steroid and thyroid hormones, the binding of the ligand to the receptor causes an allosteric change that enables the ligand–receptor complex to bind to the corresponding DNA element in the promoter region of the target gene, causing a modulation in gene expression.

TABLE 18 Symptoms of Alcohol Embryopathy

Typical symptoms	Approximate frequency in affected children
Main symptoms	
Dystrophy (growth retardation)	98%
Statomotoric and mental retardation	89%
Microcephaly	84%
Hyperactivity	68%
Muscular hypotonia	58%
Craniofacial dysmorphy[a]	95%
Frequent other abnormalities	
Cardial defects	29%
Skeletal (limb) malformations	~50%
Changes of palmar lines	69%
Inguinal hernia	12%
Hemangioma	11%

[a]Includes the following symptoms: receding, narrow forehead; deep hairline; epicanthus, ptosis, antimongolian palpebral achsis, strabismus; dysplasia of the ear; shortened dorsum of the nose; longer philtrum, microgenia, retrogenia, hypoplasia of the teeth.

However, the effects of retinoic acid are very versatile and several distinctly different subtypes of receptors for retinoids have been identified, and there are numerous interactions with other inducing substances. The reactive DNA motive, AGGTCA, not only is recognized by the retinoid–receptor complex, but also plays an important role in the interaction with receptors for thyroxin, vitamin D, and estrogens. All in all, more than 50 retinoid-responsive genes are known in different cell types. Among these are the homeobox genes, oncogenes, growth factor, and transcription factors, which can again influence the expression of other genes. As a complex biological result of such modifications in different cell types, either stimulation or inhibition of certain processes occurs. This explains the broad applicability of retinoids in medicine, from the treatment of skin diseases up to treatment of tumor diseases or tumor prophylaxis. Even tumor-inducing effects are being discussed. Aside from the binding to specific receptors, the binding of retinoids to certain carrier and storage proteins (CRBP and CRABP) may be of importance in regulation. By binding to these cytoplasmic proteins, the concentration of free retinoic acid obviously is kept low, resulting in a decreased supply to the nucleus.

Experimental studies in mice have suggested an interaction of retinoic acid with *hox* genes. When sequentially expressed, assisted by retinoic acid, these genes seem to play a major physiological role in the development of the body axis (vertebral column). Delayed or protracted activation of these genes by retinoic acid have been associated with the induction of abnormal development.

It seems paradoxical that vitamin A, which is very important for many cell functions including normal embryonic development, exhibits, experimentally and in humans, such a high teratogenic potency if the proper dose is exceeded. Even though the precise mechanism for abnormal development is still largely unknown, it can be imagined that false regulation processes may be activated if unphysiological doses are applied. In animal studies, glucocorticoids also induce abnormal development (e.g., cleft palate, particularly in mice with high glucocorticoid-receptor expression) when overdoses are used.

Example: Alcohol Embryopathy

Abnormal prenatal development caused by ethanol exposure, as caused by severe chronic alcohol abuse, is not a manifestation of modern times. Yet, the typical picture of fetal alcohol syndrome, or rather the alcohol embryopathy, was first described in France in 1968, followed in 1973 by reports from the United States. Many pediatricians must have seen children with corresponding symptoms, but failed to make cause-and-effect connection. Most often the drinking father was blamed and made responsible. Not all the symptoms are seen in every case, as shown in Tables 18 and 19. Craniofacial dysmorphisms are the major manifestations of this syndrome.

TABLE 19 Classification of Stages in Ethanol Embryopathy[a]

Mild form (1st degree)
Almost normal mental and neurological development
Only few craniofacial or internal malformations

Medium form (2nd degree)
Microcephaly
Mild neurological abnormalities
Moderate mental and statomotoric developmental retardation
Rarely internal malformations

Severe form (3rd degree)
Very typical facial malformations
All or nearly all symptoms in Table 18

[a]Infantilism and reduced body weight are obligatory. The severity of the alcohol embryopathy is assessed according to the number of symptoms present (see Table 18).

TABLE 20 Educational Status at Follow-up of Children with Different Severity Stages of Alcohol Embryopathy at Birth[a]

	Educational status[b]							
	A		B		C		D	
	n	%	*n*	%	*n*	%	*n*	%
Stage 1	(9)	39.1	(12)	52.2	(2)	8.7	(0)	0
Stage 3	(1)	6.7	(8)	53.3	(2)	13.3	(4)	26.7

[a]Stage 1 is mild and stage 3 is severe alcohol embryopathy at birth (see Table 19). Data from Spohr and Steinhausen (1987).
[b]A = normal school or preschool,
B = school for educationally subnormal students,
C = training center,
D = severely subnormal.

The most frequent features of ethanol embryopathy are rather unspecific, such as dystrophy (growth retardation) and multiple minor anomalies. As a consequence, retarded intellectual and psychomotor development may result. It takes long-term follow-up by skilled investigators to unmask these problems.

With the present knowledge it is not difficult to come with the correct diagnosis, if the syndrome is strongly developed, but diagnosis is much more difficult if symptoms are only mild. The exposure to alcohol must be firmly established, and a multitude of the typical symptoms must be observed. Even then, many confounders causing similar symptoms complicate the diagnosis of an alcohol embryopathy, and severe alcohol abuse by the mother does not in every case result in such a syndrome. Furthermore, the evidence for a dose–response relationship is not convincing. Obviously several factors are necessary for the triggering of these malformations.

Typical ethanol embryopathy is defined as the result of severe and chronic alcohol abuse, starting before pregnancy. A chronic disease to begin with is essential, not only the alcohol exposure of the embryo or the fetus during its development. It is difficult to judge how much of the prenatal damage is directly due to alcohol and what role the multiple metabolic changes in the maternal organism associated with chronic and severe alcoholism may play.

The difficulties described for human alcohol embryopathy are also obvious in attempts to devise an animal model for this disease. This is especially difficult because of the rapid ethanol metabolism in rodents. Although there is evidence that in rats and mice extremely high doses of ethanol may induce certain malformations, including those of the head under special experimental conditions, it is doubtful whether they are representative of the human alcohol embryopathy. The animal data also do not allow any conclusions and extrapolations with respect to dose–response relationships.

There is controversy over whether moderate and occasional alcohol consumption during pregnancy may constitute a risk for the developing child. Even though the literature data are not uniform, the risk apparently is minor if the alcohol consumption is confined to an occasional drink.

In a prospective multidisciplinary trial, follow-up examinations revealed that with increasing age dysmorphic signs became less apparent; neurologic performance, psychiatric status and cognitive functions improved; and EEG recordings showed less pathological patterns. However, normalization was incomplete, and hyperactivity was one of the cardinal symptoms. With respect to the persisting handicap, the group as a whole contained a remarkably high proportion of children with poor educational status (Table 20) possibly due to the persisting hyperactivity and distractibility. To some extent, the long-term fate of the children is largely dependent on the attention they receive postnatally. This is obviously quite a problem in many cases of chronic maternal alcoholism. Even though a number of behavioral disorders can be attenuated by appropriate therapy and one-on-one attention, the long-term prognosis in severe cases is unfavorable. This situation is similar to children of opiate-dependent mothers.

Example: Cytostatic Drugs

Cytostatic agents used for tumor chemotherapy interfere with cell proliferation and some inhibit various cell differentiation processes. This group of substances is heterogeneous, including antimetabolites, alkylating agents, and substances interfering with mitosis and DNA replication. Such actions are easy to be suspected as embryotoxic or teratogenic if the chemotherapy is conducted during pregnancy.

Antimetabolites have been among the first substances shown in experimental animals to be embryotoxic and teratogenic. Several of the resulting effects may be classified as universal teratogenic actions.

Purine and Pyrimidine Antimetabolites Antimetabolites, such as 6-mercaptopurine and 5-fluorouracil are well-known model substances for inducing teratogenic effects in experimental animals. Extensive experimental research with 6-mercaptopurine has revealed the phenomenon of dose specificity: 12 mg/kg given to pregnant mice induced a high frequency of polydactyly, 25 mg/kg caused phocomelia, and 50 mg/kg produced amelia. Thus certain malformations (e.g., polydactyly) can only be induced within a restricted dose range.

As an interesting group of antimetabolites, the teratogenic potential of antiviral substances was studied. Acyclovir, a guanine analog, is frequently used in the therapy of herpes infections, while ganciclovir and zidovudine are used for treatment of cytomegaly virus and HIV infections, respectively. These chemically rather similar medicinal drugs were found to exhibit rather different properties with respect to developmental and reproductive toxicity in preclinical studies. While high doses of acyclovir induced a variety of malformations in the rat, including effects on the thymus and the immune system; zidovudine seems to be largely devoid of such a potential. This difference can also be revealed using the rodent whole-embryo culture. Ganciclovir induces pronounced adverse effects on the testes at doses close to those used therapeutically in humans.

On the basis of serum concentrations, there seems to be a sufficient safety margin with respect to oral therapeutic doses of acyclovir in humans and the occurrence of malformations in animal studies. Due to a much better bioavailability, this difference is smaller when intravenous doses (e.g., 10 mg/kg body weight) of acyclovir are applied. After oral administration of some well-absorbed newer prodrugs, the human serum drug levels reached are similar to those of aciclovir after iv administration. Critical concentrations may be reached in humans after high dosing with these prodrugs, such as valacyclovir (readily converted to acyclovir) and famciclovir (converted to penciclovir). Reliable data on humans are lacking.

Folic Acid Antagonists Aminopterin has been used in attempts to induce abortions in women. However, the desired result was not obtained with the antineoplastic drug in all cases, and malformed children were born in a high percentage of these women. This was one of the first examples of the iatrogenic induction of malformations in humans, well before the thalidomide disaster. Therefore, this folic acid antagonist is a proven human teratogenic agent.

Reproducing in experimental animals the teratogenic potential of aminopterin seen in humans is difficult; even studies in monkeys failed to produce clear-cut malformations. Furthermore, it is difficult to induce malformations in experimental animals by folic acid deficiency alone. In most investigations folic acid antagonists have been added to the diet. Either nutritional deprivation of folic acid is insufficient under these conditions, or aminopterine induces effects in addition to folic acid deficiency.

In a number of case reports, treatment with methotrexate during pregnancy was associated with the occurrence of malformations at therapeutic doses. The medical indications have been widened since then, and the drug is not only used as an anticancer agent, but increasingly as an immunosuppressive drug (e.g., in rheumatic diseases). Again, investigators did not readily succeed in inducing teratogenic effects in mice or monkeys with this drug. There is a report of methotrexate being an efficient abortive agent in first trimester of pregnancy, but it was administered together with misoprostol, which makes the contribution of methotrexate difficult to interpret. Details on the mechanism of action of methotrexate are given in Chapter 17.

The complexity of the situation becomes obvious in published attempts to prevent the recurrence of CNS defects in further pregnancies by folic acid supplementation in pregnant women. It is known that women having given birth to a child with neural tube defects have an increased risk of bearing further children with such defects. Five intervention studies have been performed, three randomized and two nonrandomized, three of which showed a statistically significant benefit with the relative risks being between 0.12 and 0.29 (and an upper limit of the 95% confidence interval of <1.0). Although the relative risk in the other two studies was also <1.0, the number of cases was too small for statistical evaluations. In addition, attempts were made to reduce the frequency of neural tube defects in the pregnant population at large. As is expected, the results of five studies were not as convincing as the studies monitoring the selected pregnancies. However, in four of those studies, there were also statistically significant reductions in the incidence of CNS defects reported. In some of the studies multivitamin supplements, containing folic acid, were given.

It is now established and generally accepted that the occurrence of neural tube defects can be prevented by folic acid supplementation, 0.4 to 4 mg daily, in many though not all pregnancies. Because more than one cause can be assumed for CNS defects, as for most malformations, complete protection may not be achievable. The mechanism of action of folic acid supplementation is unknown. In most cases, the overall folic acid concentrations in serum were not profoundly different in the affected and unaffected cases. However, the situation may be more complicated because only total folic acid had been measured and considerable differences within the various folic acid metabolites may be expected, which were not taken into account (see Chapter 17).

In contrast to the folic acid antagonists with high affinity to the mammalian enzyme, an approximately 100,000-fold lower concentration of trimethoprim is required to inhibit the bacterial dihydrofolate reductase compared to the human reductase. In combination with a sulfonamide (sulfamethoxazole), trimethoprim is widely used (co-trimoxazole) as an effective antimicrobial combination drug. While high doses of co-trimoxazole have been reported to induce malformations and embryomortality in rats, several (but rather small) studies in humans have not revealed any evidence for teratogenicity at therapeutic doses. Again, animal data are not indicative for the situation in humans.

TABLE 21 Correlation of the Frequency of Malformations with Alkylation Rates in the Guanine N-7- or O-6 Position in the Embryo's DNA[a]

	N-7[b]		O-6[b]	
Alkylating agent	ED_{10}	ED_{50}	ED_{10}	ED_{50}
Acetoxymethyl methylnitrosamine	39	81	5	10
Methylnitroso urea	46	90	5	11
Ethylmethane sulfonate	98	255	4	10

[a]The teratogenicity correlates in the case of every directly alkylating agent with the rate of alkylation at the O-6 position. Data from Platzek *et al.* (1992). The alkylation rates were intrapolated from accurate dose–response curves for the ED_{10} and ED_{50} values. From this ester the short-lived reactive intermediate of dimethylnitrosamine is formed by esterases present within the embryo.

[b]In pmoles alkylated bases/μmol guanine.

Alkylating Agents Alkylating agents also have been known as experimental teratogens in rodents for several decades. We must recall that these agents will be covalently bound to many cell components, predominantly to proteins. DNA is not the major target, but a very important one.

Cyclophosphamide, a prodrug requiring hepatic metabolic activation, has been among the first cytostatic agents studied extensively in pregnant animals since the 1960s. Although most experiments on the alkylating properties were directed to the carcinogenicity of the substance, a similar mechanism seems to apply to teratogenicity. It has been shown that this multifunctional alkylating agent probably acts via cross-alkylation between DNA strands or between DNA and proteins. There are two ultimate reactive constituents, phosphoramide mustard and acrolein. It is not entirely clear which one is responsible for the embryotoxic and teratogenic action *in vivo* because both have been shown to be capable of inducing abnormal development. Furthermore, there is evidence that some of the open-ring intermediates (e.g., aldophosphamide) will be able to alkylate, and these also may be the ultimate teratogens.

The teratogenicity of directly acting monoalkylating agents was studied systematically in mice. The accumulated evidence indicates that the teratogenic potential is rather specific, because it correlated with the guanine O-6 alkylation and not with the much more unspecific guanine N-7 alkylation responsible for cytotoxicity (Table 21). Teratogenicity occurred at a certain extent of guanine O-6 alkylation in the embryo, and the extent of an embryotoxic effect could be predicted from quantitative DNA alkylation data. The database was used extensively for attempts to assess dose–response relationships and extrapolations (Platzek *et al.*, 1993).

Relevance for Humans Not all antimetabolites and alkylating agents were found to be teratogenic in animal studies, but with such potentially dangerous substances one would not dare to suggest a lack of teratogenicity for humans solely on the basis of negative animal data. There are several early case reports of malformations associated with the application of therapeutic doses of cytostatic agents, such as cyclophosphamide, during pregnancy. However, we must recall that, similar to carcinogenicity, teratogenic effects do not occur in all cases at a suboptimal exposure level, and a number of women under chemotherapy (including cyclophosphamide) were reported to have born healthy children. Interindividual differences in susceptibility may be considerable.

Example: Immunosuppressive Drugs

Immunosuppressive agents are increasingly used to prevent transplant rejection after organ transplantation and for the therapy of autoimmune diseases. This heterogeneous group of drugs includes glucocorticoids, azathioprine, methotrexate, cyclosporine, and similar compounds.

Glucocorticoids The application of high doses of glucocorticoids is a well-established model for inducing cleft palate in mice dose-dependently. There exist striking strain differences in susceptibility, which can be related to glucocorticoid receptor densities in the developing palatal shelves. In this species, an increase in the level of these hormones during stress, as caused by handling, noise, restraint or drug treatment, may already induce this malformation. This is a typical example of a specific teratogenic effect. Cleft palate cannot only be induced in mice, but has also been observed in monkeys with some glucocorticoids, such as triamcinolone. Abnormal development with these substances has also been achieved with appropriate *in vitro* systems of palatal shelve culture in other species (e.g., rats) that respond poorly *in vivo*.

Although it is more difficult to obtain reliable data from clinical observations, a variety of trials have not shown an increased rate of cleft palates in children exposed to glucocorticoids *in utero* stressing the need for reconfirming data from animal studies in pregnant women. However, the number of mother–child pairs exposed during early pregnancy, mostly to prednisone and prednisolone, is still limited and a small risk cannot be excluded because not all glucocorticoids have been studied to the same extent. Insufficient data are available on short-term exposure to very high doses, while the risk for gross structural abnormalities from maintenance therapy seems to be minimal. Hundreds of women with kidney transplants were reported to have delivered healthy babies after being continously treated with a combination of glucocorticoids and azathioprine during pregnancy. It is well known that most often doses inducing Cushing's syndrome were used in the early transplantations.

Glucocorticoids represent another example of compounds exhibiting both essential and possibly adverse effects, depending on the stages of development exposed and the dose levels. This hormone certainly plays an important physiological role in maturation processes during late prenatal development. Glucocorticoids are used therapeutically to promote surfactant production and lung maturation in premature babies, and to facilitate extubation and improve pulmonary compliance in premature infants who cannot be weaned from ventilator support, although the efficacy of such a dexamethasone treatment has been debated. Dexamethasone treatment in these children has been reported to be associated with increased incidence of nosocomial bacteremia and hyperglycemia.

It is important to remember the difference in the placental transfer of natural and synthetic glucocorticoids to the embryo or fetus. The natural hormones, like cortisol, reach the conceptus to a limited degree only, probably because it is metabolized in the placenta, and may be used for treating the mother for bronchial asthma or allergic diseases with minimal effects on the conceptus. While the fetal plasma concentration of prednisone was found to be about 1/10 of the mother's, other synthetic hormones (such as dexamethasone or triamcinolone) readily reach the fetus and are suitable for the treatment of the unborn child. Thus, the glucocorticoids may not be equal with respect to beneficial and potential adverse health effects during the pre- and perinatal periods.

Azathioprine Azathioprine, a derivative of 6-mercaptopurine (6-MP), had been used extensively and often in combination with glucocorticoids to avoid transplant rejection before the immunosuppressive agents became available. The usual daily maintenance dose after kidney transplantation is 1–3 mg azathioprine/kg body weight. Like 6-MP and its ribonucleoside, to which it is converted in the organism, azathioprine was found to be embryotoxic and teratogenic in experimental studies *in vivo* and *in vitro*. Because 6-MP is metabolized to 6-thiouric acid by xanthine oxidase, and this enzyme is inhibited by azathioprine and allopurinol, co-administration of azathioprine with either 6-MP or allopurinol will greatly enhance its toxicity.

When the outcomes of about 200 pregnancies under immunosuppressive azathioprine therapy (in combination with prednisone) after kidney transplantation were evaluated, prematurity apparently was diagnosed in about 40% of the children. The incidence of malformations calculated from pooled data of several reports ($n \approx 200$) was about 5%. Thus the incidence may only be slightly above the normal risk. No clustering of defined abnormalities was noticed, arguing against a clearly teratogenic potency of the multidrug treatment under these conditions. Although there are many confounding factors, the therapeutic use of azathioprine during pregnancy seems to be acceptable at the clinically effective dose level. Azathioprine has mutagenic and clastogenic properties.

Cyclosporine This drug has increasingly replaced azathioprine for the prevention of transplant rejection. According to a number of publications, healthy children have been born to kidney-transplant recipients treated with cyclosporine in combination with prednisone over the entire pregnancy. When the outcomes in 32 offspring, compiled in several reports, were evaluated, prematurity and intrauterine dystrophy were both observed in more than 50% of the children. Because only one malformation was reported in these newborn, the number is too small for a reliable risk assessment. However, the teratogenic risk does not seem to be excessive. The average birth weight after 35 weeks of pregnancy (range, 28 to 40 weeks) was only 1885 g (range, 820 to 3360 g), but this value is not reliable because it was calculated from the data of several reports.

Available data indicate that pregnancy is possible under immunosuppressive therapy with cyclosporine (and prednisone), but it should be considered as risk pregnancy. Maternal complications may be frequent, including those arising from multidrug therapy. There is an increased chance of viral and bacterial infections in the mother and child and intrauterine fetal growth must be carefully monitored. No information is available on possible effects of cyclosporine on the developing immune system and data on postnatal development in general are lacking.

Because cyclosporine is transferred into breast milk and possible adverse effects cannot be excluded, it is prudent to avoid nursing while on cyclosporine therapy.

Example: Antiseizure Drugs

With respect to chemical structure, this also is a very heterogeneous group. All of these substances have been extensively studied in animal experiments, and data from a number of clinical trials are available. A number of peculiarities exist with respect to the therapeutical use. The data from mother–child pairs exposed during pregnancy suggest that a combination therapy exhibits a higher teratogenic risk for the offspring than monotherapy.

Preferentially, medical advise should be given already when planning a pregnancy and the following aspects must be considered:

- Is a drug therapy necessary at all during pregnancy?
- Is it possible to apply a monotherapy? Which is the most appropriate substance?
- What is the lowest effective dose?

When a combination therapy using carbamazepine, phenytoin, and valproate is felt to be necessary in women of child-bearing age, appropriate anticonceptive measures are essential.

Valproic Acid During a birth-defects surveillance in France, an increased odds ratio of posterior neural tube defects (spina bifida aperta) was observed in children exposed *in utero* to valproic acid. Data from this retrospective study were confirmed in other trials, and a risk of about 1% was estimated for a child of acquiring spina bifida from the mother's valproate treatment during pregnancy.

Anterior neural tube defects (exencephaly) can also be induced by valproate in mice, but despite extensive studies, the mode of the teratogenic action of this chemically simple compound remains unknown. The most significant outcome of these experiments is that the anticonvulsive and teratogenic potential does not run parallel within this class of compounds. Thus it may be possible to design a substance with anticonvulsive properties that is devoid of a teratogenic potential. The derivative 2-*en*-valproic acid may be such a candidate.

Although the increase in the odds ratio is substantial (20-fold?), spina bifida is a rare malformation and the additional risk must be evaluated against the total spontaneous malformation rate of 2–4% among the general population in all countries. Furthermore, it is well known that this overall spontaneous risk is roughly doubled in epileptic women, apparently due to the disease and not caused by any treatment. The reason for this increase in the malformation rate in the children of epileptic mothers is unknown. Is cannot be explained by the occurrence of repeated seizures. Compared with the spontaneous risk for having a malformed child, the additional risk from a valproate treatment is small, and many mothers are willing to accept such an additional risk if anticonvulsive treatment with this drug is required during pregnancy and no good alternative exists. This example shows that even with respect to established teratogenic effects in humans a closer benefit assessment is required and hasty decisions would be of little help.

Trimethadione Numerous case reports have associated treatment with trimethadione during pregnancy with the occurrence of a trimethadione syndrome in several of the offspring. Because the substance is rarely given during pregnancy, the frequency of the occurrence of such defects is not well documented. The pattern of malformations included facial abnormalities, cleft palate, cardiac defects. Very high doses of this substance were also capable of inducing malformations in mice.

Phenytoin and Carbamazepine Although much time has been spent to elucidating the possible teratogenic effects of diphenylhydantoin experimentally and in clinical studies, the results are not too convincing and no typical syndrome of gross structural abnormalities has been clearly established with the monotherapy. There are reports associating prenatal exposure to carbamazepine with the occurrence of embryotoxic effects, such as growth retardation and craniofacial defects.

There are reports on minor anomalies occurring more frequently in children exposed *in utero* to phenytoin and possibly also to carbamazepine. These anomalies were even at one time described as diphenylhydantoin syndrome (DPH syndrome) and they include epicanthus, broad nose and mouth, narrow palpebral fissure, dysplasia of the end phalanges, nail hypoplasia, and dysplasia. It is now questioned whether such a syndrome specific for phenytoin exists because these anomalies were also observed after treatment with other substances.

Phenytoin may decrease vitamin K concentrations by increasing the metabolism of the vitamin. Reductions in the concentration of vitamin K-dependent proteins may result, and hemorrhages in the newborn of mothers on phenytoin therapy during pregnancy have been reported. As expected, vitamin K is effective as a prophylactic agent and as an antidote.

It should be taken into account that phenytoin and carbamazepine both are capable of inducing hepatic monooxygenases in humans at therapeutic doses, resulting in lower drug concentrations when given in combination. Carbamazepine is metabolized to the 10, 11-epoxide and the accumulation of this active component apparently is exaggerated by concurrent phenytoin administration. This epoxide has been suggested as playing a role in the teratogenic potency of this drug combination.

Example: Antiemetic Drugs

Because "morning sickness" (nausea and vomiting) is a common symptom in early pregnancy, antiemetic drugs of several classes (e.g., antihistamines and phenothiazines) have been used by probably millions of pregnant women within the last decades. Because of the extensive use of some of these substances, especially of some of the antihistamines, the largest body of information has been accumulated about drug therapy during pregnancy for this specific indication.

Data gathered from many unusually large investigations did not reveal any evidence for a teratogenic potency of doxylamine or cyclizine. In pro- and retrospective studies, more than 10,000 pregnancies were evaluated and compared with more than 100,000 references. Both substances have been found to be teratogenic in animals at high dose levels.

It is questionable whether such an excessive consumption of antiemetics (at one time estimated to be 25% of all pregnant women in the United States) is necessary during pregnancy. Because the discomfort to be treated is caused by the physiological change in sex hormones, these signs are considered an indication of an intact pregnancy, and no adverse pregnancy outcome is to be expected, unless severe alterations in electrolyte and water balance or food intake result. Physicians should educate women and convince them not to complicate a normal pregnancy with the additional consumption of drugs, even if the risk is small or negligible. The symptoms exhibit a high responsiveness against placebo medication.

The Special Case of Bendectin It is difficult to understand why doxylamine in combination with vitamin B6 (marketed as Bendectin in the United States and as Lenotan in some European countries) triggered a furious mass media. Extremely subjective and unbalanced information was provided to the public and tremendous fear was instilled in many pregnant women. After a flood of scientifically completely unjustified law suits, gobbling up enormous amounts of money and resources, the drug's manufacturers finally decided to withdraw the drug from the market.

Three aspects may be important in this respect:

- There is no absolute safety. Even the largest study cannot exclude a very small risk. It is impossible to prove the negative. However, a high degree of safety can be deduced from good studies, and the frequency of the induced pathological condition must exceed the spontaneous rate.
- When a large number of mother–child pairs are investigated or treated with any substance, spontaneous malformations are bound to occur, as in every other large enough group. Because this spontaneous frequency is 2–4% of the live births at the time of delivery, in a group of 1000 mother–child pairs, 20–40 malformed children must be included. If the mother has taken a drug during pregnancy she might be inclined to link this defect causally to the dug intake. This clearly shows that only experts can obtain clues on causal relationships, and this

can never be accomplished in single case reports, when no clue on a specific association exists.

- It is a good and certainly not new policy to prescribe and consume medicinal drugs during pregnancy only when there is a clear-cut medical indication, such as convulsive disorders, diabetes, or hypertension.

Example: Hyperthermia

For several decades, evidence has been presented that increased core temperature (hyperthermia) may induce malformations. Ample evidence has been presented from studies of various experimental animal species, but the significance of these results for the situation in humans is still highly controversial. Although some epidemiological studies were performed on this problem, the issue is complicated because hyperthermia in humans is most often associated with (viral) infections, which will constitute a serious confounding factor.

A wide variety of malformations have been induced in guinea pigs, including neural tube defects, microcephaly, facial defects, micrognathia, microphthalmia and other eye defects (coloboma and cataracts), vertebral column defects, and heart defects. Corresponding malformations have been induced under similar conditions in other experimental species, including rodents, rabbits, sheep, pigs, and monkeys. The CNS seems to be most vulnerable to hyperthermia. Alterations in heat-shock proteins or increased apoptotic cell death have been suggested as a possible cause of the malformations.

There seem to be threshold conditions above which the defects are induced. In rats and mice, an increase in normal temperature by 3.5°C for 10 min is sufficient to induce defects. The time period required for inducing abnormalities was found to be shorter when the temperature was further increased. The critical threshold temperature is not absolute, but depends on the rather variable normal temperature of the species (about 37.5°C for the pig, 38.5°C in the rat, but 39.5°C in guinea pigs). The data compiled suggest that an elevation of 2 to 2.5°C above the normal resting temperature is required to cause the pathological outcome. Extrapolation from these data could suggest a critical temperature of about 39 to 39.5°C for humans.

Three types of conditions were studied in humans, hyperthermia associated with (viral) infections, increased body temperature during excessive physical activity (e.g., marathon running), and hyperthermia from sauna and hot-tub bathing. It is obvious that an interpretation of the results will be difficult because of many confounding factors. It is not surprising that positive as well as negative results were obtained, and the reasons for this have been discussed extensively. The increased frequency of CNS defects was reported in several studies after Asian influenza epidemics, relative risks ranging between 2 and 3, but the viral infection could not be excluded as a causal factor. Most interestingly, in countries where sauna or hot-tub bathing are part of the cultural tradition during pregnancy, such as Finland and Japan, retrospective studies did not reveal an increased rate of CNS malformations in children of mothers frequently using such facilities. Although there is some evidence, it cannot be decided whether hyperthermia is a human teratogen, and, if so, what the critical temperature and duration of exposure are.

From a few observations it may be postulated that the abortion rate could be increased after hyperthermia. Possible causal factors for this high rate are the wastage of embryos with CNS defects and wastage dure to increased myometrial activity.

Example: Smoking

In addition to drinking alcohol, cigarette smoking is a common addiction in many countries, and one-third or more of pregnant women have been reported to smoke during pregnancy. Smoking cigarettes is associated with exposure to an extremely complex mixture of several thousand chemicals. Other than nicotine, carbon monoxide, and chemicals with a mutagenic and carcinogenic potential (e.g., PAH and nitrosamines), the majority of compounds are still unknown. Many chemicals present in cigarette smoke have been shown to easily cross the placenta.

While ample evidence has been presented for the adverse effects on the human conceptus, the evaluation of the possible effects of exposure to cigarette smoke is complicated by a number of facts, which in many respects play a similar role in adults:

- Many women who smoke heavily during pregnancy deliver normal babies, and unequivocally adverse effects are confined to a minority of offspring.
- Most of the deviations associated with smoking occur within the limits or normal data on pregnancy and gestation, and predominantly differences in average values have been published.
- It is unknown which components of cigarette smoke are responsible for defined types of abnormal development.

A number of mechanisms have been proposed as responsible for inducing the possible adverse actions of cigarette smoke on pregnancy and prenatal development:

1. Formation of carboxyhemoglobin in the mother and conceptus by carbon monoxide may induce fetal hypoxia.
2. Catecholamine levels increased by nicotine may decrease uteroplacental blood flow.
3. A higher frequency of degenerative changes have been observed in smoking women's placentas, such as calcification, fibrin patches, or altered umbilical cord vessels. Placentas often are small when standardized on the baby's body weight.

There is some evidence of deviations from a reference range in smoking pregnant women and their children, including:

- Some increases in the frequency of spontaneous abortions, premature births, and perinatal mortality and complications at delivery.
- Some increases in the frequency of abruptio placentae and placenta previa.
- Reduction in average birth weights by 100–300 g, and doubling the number of babies weighing <2500 g. The medical significance of this is unknown because a number of additional factors (e.g., socioeconomic status, other living conditions, and race) are known to affect birth weight. Small infants are not necessarily identical with endangered children.

Numerous reports have also been published regarding the adverse effects of tobacco use on long-term postnatal development in children of mothers smoking during pregnancy and after delivery. The adverse sequelae associated with cigarette smoking include increased postnatal mortality, more frequent hospital stays, higher frequency of SIDS, and deficiencies found in neurological and psychological tests.

Maternal smoking has been shown to increase fetal blood flow velocities in the aorta and umbilical vessels, and reduced synthesis of prostacycline was found in umbilical arteries from the newborns of smoking mothers. Doppler examinations 20 to 42 hours after birth revealed cerebral blood flow velocities significantly higher in 41 infants of smoking mothers than in 59 control infants. No information is available on the possible long-term consequences. Smoking is also known to interfere with placental amino acid transport, an effect that has been linked to small-for-date babies.

Although a higher incidence of childhood tumors has been associated with maternal smoking, the results are not conclusive.

The results of extensive animal data on the effects of nicotine on developmental processes have been compiled. It was found in rats that nicotine affected specific neurotransmitter receptors in the fetal brain, altered cell proliferation and differentiation processes, and influenced synaptic activity. Dose levels were assumed to be similar to those achieved by smokers. Cigarette smoking is chemically much more complex than an exposure to nicotine, and it is oversimplification to reduce the multifaceted problem of smoking during pregnancy to nicotine exposure of the human conceptus. Furthermore, comparisons of the rodent and human brain and their pre- and postnatal development are extremely difficult, especially when quantitative conclusions with respect to toxic effects are attempted. More rewarding and informative with respect to the physiological and functional sequelae of the human offspring than animal studies would be to spend effort and money on the real problem, that is, on large and more extensive long-term follow-up studies in children, if exposure to all ingredients of tobacco smoke *in utero* cannot be avoided in the long run.

It is well established that cigarette smoking during pregnancy induces the activity of some human placental monooxygenases, preferentially reactions catalyzed by cytochrome P450 IA1 (CYPIA1). This effect is pronounced in the placentas of all heavily smoking women and is also demonstrable in the adult human liver, as evaluated with a [^{13}C]caffeine breath test. Apparently, the enzymatic activity of the corresponding hepatic enzyme, CYPIA2, is not increased in the fetus by maternal smoking, although other monooxygenases are inducible prenatally in experimental animals by strong inducers like TCDD. The possible significance of this change in the metabolic capacity of human placental tissue is unknown. CYPIA2-dependent caffeine demethylation is very low in the human newborn and apparently is not induced by maternal smoking of filtered cigarettes.

Example: Polychlorinated Dibenzo-p-dioxins, and Dibenzofurans, and Biphenyls

The possible adverse effects on development and reproduction have also been discussed for a few human-made chemicals that exist as environmental substances and are ingested by organisms every day. The most notorious examples are (Fig. 21) polychlorobiphenyls (PCB), polychlorinated dibenzo-*p*-dioxins (PCDD), and dibenzofurans (PCDF). It is appropriate to discuss these different classes of polyhalogenated polycyclic compounds together because PCDF have appeared as contaminants of PCB, and some representatives overlap in their biological and toxicological activity profiles. Many of the chemicals mentioned are effectively eliminated with the milk (human and cow) from the maternal organism and transferred to the

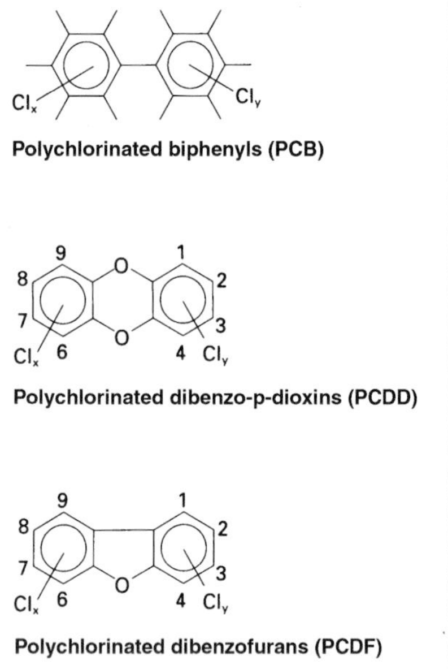

FIGURE 21 Chemical structures of PCB and PCDD, and PCDF.

TABLE 22 Frequency of Malformations in the Population of Seveso (Italy) after the Accidental TCDD Exposure in 1976[a]

	Number of births	Number of malformations: Severe, Isolated	Severe, Total	Mild
Zone A	26	0 (. . .)	0 (. . .)	2 (7.7%)
Zone B	435	10 (2.3%)	13 (3.0%)	12 (2.8%)
Zone R	2439	42 (1.7%)	54 (2.2%)	56 (2.3%)
Non A + B + R	12,391	267 (2.2%)	343 (2.8%)	262 (2.1%)

Abnormalities	Odds ratio[b]: Zones AB	Zones ABR
All isolated defects	0.97 (0.58–1.64)	0.81 (0.63–1.03)
Multiple defects	0.71 (0.14–3.70)	1.12 (0.63–2.02)
Syndromes	1.85 (0.57–6.05)	0.74 (0.33–1.63)
All severe defects	1.02 (0.64–1.61)	0.83 (0.67–1.04)
All minor defects	1.44 (0.92–2.24)	1.14 (0.92–1.42)
All defects	1.20 (0.88–1.64)	0.97 (0.83–1.13)

[a]Data from Mastroiacovo *et al.* (1988).
[b](95% confidence interval.)

newborn. Such chemicals pose a number of special problems:

- There is no convincing evidence that the pollution of the habitat and the exposure of the general population has caused any kind of toxic manifestations.
- A level of exposure causing toxic symptoms did occur in adults occupationally exposed at insufficiently protected work places and during several major accidents. In the latter disaster scenarios, pregnant women ingested or inhaled the chemicals and children were exposed *in utero* or postnatally.
- Several of these classes of substances occur in the environment as mixtures, often of very many congeners. It is impossible to obtain information on all of these congeners, and it is difficult to assess the toxicity of such mixtures.

TCDD For 2,3,7,8-tetrachlorodibenzo-*p*-dioxin (TCDD), the PCDD congener with the highest biological potency, a multitude of experimental data regarding adverse effects on development and reproduction have been published. With respect to prenatal toxicity, TCDD obviously does not exhibit a universal teratogenic potential. Animal experiments performed *in vivo* and *in vitro* during early organogenesis have not revealed any adverse effect on development, but TCDD induces a very specific defect, and this only in one animal species—cleft palate, predominantly in some mouse strains. This effect is strictly dose-dependent, and it can be triggered with a single dose of 10 μg TCDD/kg body weight or with even smaller doses when applied over several days. We must recall that mice are especially susceptible to the induction of cleft palate. The effect of TCDD apparently is linked to a sufficient expression of the *Ah* locus. In susceptible strains of this species, TCDD was also found to reduce hyperkeratosis and the proliferation of the epithelium of the ureter with the subsequent desquamation of debris, causing stenosis with dilatation of the ureter and finally hydronephrosis. This is not a typical teratogenic effect, and it can also be induced postnatally. In nonhuman primates it has not been possible to trigger any malformations, even with high doses of TCDD.

The teratogenic effects observed in mice have focused the attention on the possible malformation-inducing properties of TCDD in humans. So far there is no convincing evidence of teratogenicity of TCDD in humans. As a consequence of a chemical plant explosion in Seveso, Italy, in July 1976, no increase in the rate of severe malformations has been observed in highly exposed mothers (Table 22). The total number of registered malformations in all contaminated regions is either within the normal limits or the data are not significantly different from the references (lower confidence interval always below 1.0; Table 22). The authors concluded that if there is any increased teratogenic risk related to TCDD, the overall risk is unlikely to be large or might be limited to very rare and specific birth defects. Also the limits of detectability of the method was calculated, and a doubling of major malformations within this population could be excluded (only a four to five-fold increase in zone A). Although no increased malformation rate was observed in Seveso, the data are insufficient for evaluating the more subtle effects of TCDD on prenatal development, but they also do not provide any proof of such effects. An increase in the incidence of some minor abnormalities (hemangioma and hypospadia) in specific exposure zones (zones A and B combined) cannot be excluded due to the limitations of the data.

It has been reported that during the years right after the accident in Seveso only girls were born to highly TCDD-exposed couples. Between April 1977 and December 1984, among the 74 total births of residents living in the most contaminated A zone, 26 were boys and 48 girls (χ^2 test, $p < 0.001$). This ratio declined from 1985 to 1994 and was no longer significant (60 males versus 64 females). The authors did not have an explanation for this phenomenon. An interference of TCDD with sex hormone actions might be one possibility, among many others.

Other PCDD and PCDF In animal studies, cleft palates could also be triggered in mice with other congeners of polyhalogenated dibenzo-*p*-dioxins and dibenzofurans, including brominated congeners. It can be concluded that all 2,3,7,8-substituted chlorinated and brominated congeners exhibit this potential in this animal model, within a different and very wide range of potency. Whether International TCDD toxicity equivalencies (I-TEq) are helpful for extrapolating the results from the animal studies to the situation assumed to exist in humans may be doubted because the kinetics and organ distribution of the various congeners are known to be different in mice and humans.

PCB No trustworthy data are available on the possible embryotoxicity of PCB under ambient, noncatastrophic, and nonaccidental exposure conditions. It is likely that this risk also is very small.

It is more difficult to assess a possible risk of very high exposures to PCB on prenatal development. While no indications for teratogenic risks exist, the possibility of postnatal manifestations after prenatal exposure (see the later discussion) cannot be completely excluded.

Yusho and Yu-cheng Diseases Accidents have occurred in Japan (Yusho) and Taiwan (Yu-cheng) involving the exposure of a large number of people to rice oil highly contaminated during the manufacturing process with PCB and PCDF, and also with several other unknown components formed during the heating process.

Among the victims were pregnant women and their offspring, who were exposed during these catastrophic episodes either *in utero* or postnatally. These children attracted attention because of their brownish skin color ("cola-colored babies"), but typical gross malformations were not described. The following symptoms were seen; however, they were not seen in all of these children.

- Reduced birth weight.
- Hyperbilirubinemia.
- Symptoms of the mucous membranes of the eyes (e.g., conjunctivitis).
- Hyperkeratosis and atrophy of the epidermis.
- Hypoplasia of the nails.
- Premature eruption of teeth at birth.

These observations also demonstrate that the embryo- and fetotoxic actions are not limited to teratogenic effects. It is not possible to decide whether the symptoms reported were caused by either PCB or PCDF, a combination of both, or by still unknown factors. Therefore, it is almost impossible to draw firm conclusions with respect to causal relationships due to specific substances from these data. Yusho and Yucheng should be considered as poisoning episodes of their own, and the data should not be taken as evidence for the actions of PCB and PCDF.

Peri- and Postnatal Manifestations

Abnormal development is not limited to gross structural abnormalities (malformations). Furthermore, not all prenatally induced abnormalities are recognizable at birth. This holds true for major malformations, of which only about one-half are diagnosed at birth, excluding most of the cardiac defects.

During fetal developmental, in particular, lesions may be induced that manifest themselves postnatally as functional defects (dysfunctions) during later life. Often such dysfunctions become critical for the organism when the associated functions are required. They can appear, for example, as altered fertility, behavioral disorders, hormonal dysregulation, or abnor-

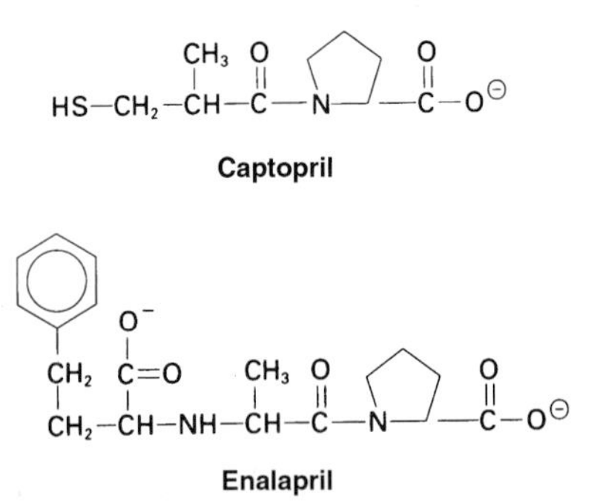

FIGURE 22 Chemical structures of some ACE inhibitors.

mal immune responses. Because the responsible systems develop, particularly during the fetal phase or even after birth, it is obvious that not only the first trimester of pregnancy, during which organogenesis occurs, must be considered as a vulnerable period. For this reason, the evaluation of morphological defects at or shortly after birth is not sufficient for hazard identification, dose–response, and risk assessment regarding developmental toxicity. Abnormal postnatal developmental may be induced pre- or postnatally. In routine preclinical testing of potential pharmaceutical products, this is taken into account by performing segment-I, and -III studies, in addition to the segment-II tests (Fig. 5).

Postnatal Dysfunction after Prenatal Exposure

Experience from experimental research with a variety of substances indicates that abnormal postnatal development after prenatal exposure is not rare at all. Such abnormalities may manifest themselves as increased postnatal mortality or a delayed body weight increase in the animals after prenatal exposure. The postnatal abnormalities may even represent the most sensitive indicators of adverse effects.

Preterm birth is of major concern in obstetrics because it is responsible for about half of neonatal deaths and of congenital neurological defects. Preterm births are due to either premature labor (≈50% of the cases), spontaneous rupture of the membranes (≈30%), or delivery of premature infants (≈20%). Surprisingly, from 1981 to 1994 the rate of preterm births has stayed rather constant, around 10% of live births in the United States. Most neonatal deaths and disorders involve births before 32 weeks of pregnancy (2% of all births). Although the cause of most of these premature births is unknown and may change with time and among different populations, it may be one manifestation of prenatally induced lesions by chemicals, including the use of alcohol and tobacco during pregnancy. Progress in obstetrical and neonatological interventions have reduced mortality during the last 30 years from ≈50% to ≈5% among neonates with birth weights between 1000 and 1500 g, and from ≈95% to ≈20% in those weighing 500–1000 g. Despite considerable advances in neonatology, the few infants (about 1% of all live births) with a birth weight of between 500 and 1000 g still contribute to half of all neonatal deaths. Among the survivors, preterm birth seems to have little functional consequence later in life if an infant does not have any lung or neurological disorders, and does not require prolonged hospitalization.

Some evidence has been accumulated that even major diseases, such as diabetes type I, atopic manifestations, and possibly essential hypertension, may be associated with pre- or early postnatal exposure to certain substances or to certain diseases (e.g., infections). In the following, a few examples are given for postnatal manifestations of toxic effects after prenatal exposure.

Example: ACE Inhibitors

ACE (angiotensin-converting enzyme) inhibitors (Fig. 22) block the conversion of angiotensin I to angiotensin II, which is a very potent endogenous vasoconstrictor. This class of drugs has been on the market since the early 1980s and is an important component in the treatment of high blood pressure and cardiac insufficiency. It is not surprising that these substances were also tried in treatment of pregnancy-associated hypertension.

When ACE inhibitors were used to treat pregnant women in the second or third trimester, an oligohydramnios (decreased amount of amniotic fluid) developed and intrauterine growth retardation of the fetus was observed. Obviously the drugs caused a decrease in blood pressure lasting far into the neonatal period and resulting in reduced renal perfusion and anuria (Table 23). Because the formation of amniotic fluid requires fetal urine, the oligohydramnios can be explained by impairment of fetal urine production by the ACE inhibitor. The increased sensitivity of the unborn as compared to the mother may be explained by the special relevance of the fetal and neonatal renin–angiotensin system because it is well known that renal perfusion is comparatively low during these stages of development.

Apparently the described functional impairment is the result of a corresponding pharmacological effect. Such defects in the newborn have been seen after *in*

TABLE 23 Characteristics of a Fetopathy after Therapeutic Administration of ACE-Inhibitors during Pregnancy

Of 88 *in utero* exposed children 16 newborns developed an ACE-inhibitor fetopathy with the following symptoms:
- Oligohydramnios already in the middle of the pregnancy
- Intrauterine growth retardation
- Long-lasting blood pressure decreases in the newborn and anuria

Further defects
- Pulmonary hypoplasia, dysplasia of the renal tubules, calvarial hypoplasia, persisting ductus arteriosus

Cause
- Presumably drug-induced blood pressure decrease in the fetus followed by a decrease in blood perfusion of the kidneys, lasting into the newborn period

Sensitive period
- Only an exposure during the 2nd or 3rd trimester bears a risk. Accidental treatment during the 1st trimester is only associated with a minor or no risk involved (this medication should be discontinued immediately!)

utero exposure to captopril, enalapril, and lisinopril. Thus the effects seem to be induced through the same mechanism and will be characteristic for the whole group of substances with the same pharmacological effects, if the specific drug reaches the fetus. In contrast, the administration of ACE inhibitors during the first trimester has not caused any adverse effects. This example again illustrates that the conceptus is endangered by foreign substances during organogenesis and that lesions, especially dysfunctions, may also be induced in the second and third trimesters. The kidney dysfunctions induced by ACE inhibitors in humans could not be predicted from the previously done safety evaluations in animals. This is due to the special sensitivity of the animal species used; rabbits are highly sensitive to ACE inhibitors, while the rat is quite insensitive. Nonhuman primates have not been studied.

No data are available of similar effects caused by the angiotensin II receptor blockers (AT_1 receptor antagonists), but such fetotoxic effects are feasible based on the anticipated mode of pharmacological action.

Example: Methyl Mercury

Between the years 1952 and 1960, symptoms of intoxication were noticed in Japan that were described in the literature as Minamata disease caused by the consumption of methyl mercury-contaminated fish from the Minamata bay area (Kyushu, Japan), which was heavily polluted by industrial waste discharges. During these intoxications, 25 cases of fetal and 31 cases of neonatal exposure were recorded, and 13 of these 56 pre-, peri-, postnatally exposed children died. Another intoxication with this specific chemical was reported from Iraq after the consumption of bread made from seed grain containing methyl mercury as a fungicide. In connection with this disaster, about 30 cases of prenatally exposed children have been reported in the literature. Only minor structural abnormalities were seen, such as strabismus and abnormal dental development. However, the CNS was found to be especially vulnerable to methyl mercury, and the exposed children showed pronounced neurological disorders—spastic cerebral palsy with motor deficiencies and behavioral alterations. These defects were seen even if the fetus was exposed as late as the third trimester only. Similar to the sequelae of exposure to ionizing radiation, some cases of microcephaly were seen (in 7/25 cases in Minamata). Usually the concentration of methyl mercury was higher in tissues of the child than in the mother. This supports the experimental data from rats, where methyl mercury apparently is accumulated in the fetal brain.

Because almost all the mothers of children with Minamata disease showed no CNS changes, the functional evidence points to the special vulnerability of the immature brain to alkyl mercury (Table 24). The fetus with an almost completely developed brain architecture seems to be especially vulnerable to these substances. The locations of the lesions seem to be much more diverse than during neonatal exposure or intoxication of the adult organism.

Adverse effects on the postnatal behavior after prenatal exposure can be experimentally reproduced in animals, and methyl mercury has become one of the standard chemical reference material for the demonstration of corresponding congenital behavioral changes in animal tests. Similar to the effect of thalidomide with respect to malformations, the effects of methyl mercury on behavioral patterns seems to be rather exceptional. Extensive experimental studies performed in recent decades have not revealed numerous substances with similar properties.

Embryo- and fetotoxic effects are especially significant when they occur at dose levels that are apparently nontoxic to the adult organism. In the case of methyl mercury, one must conclude that prenatal exposure at maternally nontoxic doses causes behavioral changes that become detectable in the postnatal phase in experimental animals and in humans.

Example: PCB

In some publications, a correlation between moderately increased intrauterine PCB exposure and the disturbed mental development of exposed children is

TABLE 24 Pathological Changes in the Human Brain Observed at Different Developmental Stages during Minamata Disease[a]

Abnormalities	Exposed as		
	Fetus	Infant	Adult
At nerve cells of the cortex	+++	+++	+
At nerve cells of the cerebellum	+	+++	+++
Disturbed development of the cortex	+++	−	−
Reduction of brain weight	+++	++	+

[a]Data from Murakami (1972).

postulated. The clinical data reported are controversial; the number of children studied is small, and quantification of the exposure (different PCB congeners and the specification of the existing additional body burdens such as PCB or heavy metals) was insufficient and not according to standards (in particular the important nonortho congeners have not been analyzed).

In contrast to PCDD and PCDF, the PCB are rather easily transferred to the fetus. The effects that are suggested to occur in the exposed children at 4 years of age included poorer short-term memory function on both verbal and quantitative tests. The adverse effects on the behavior were only observed after prenatal exposure and not subsequent to the even higher exposure to PCB via breast feeding. The adverse effects were not confirmed in other studies in groups of similarly exposed children. Even though the adverse effects reported are not very convincing, this problem could be studied further with more precise analytical methods, if highly exposed populations could still be found at this time. After catastrophic exposures (Yusho), functional CNS alterations in children exposed *in utero* cannot be ruled out. However, it was pointed out before that this polyexposure is not representative of a PCB poisoning.

Example: Exposure to Ionizing Radiation

The classic example for postnatal manifestations of prenatally induced functional lesions is the induction of mental retardation of victims exposed *in utero* following the atomic bombings of Hiroshima and Nagasaki. Fetal microcephaly and idioty due to radiation has been described as early as 1926. The abnormalities, apparently strongly dependent on the radiation dose, show certain similarities to the changes reported after methyl mercury exposure, and they are unusual in many respects:

- An increase in the incidence of gross structural malformations can be induced in animal experiments after exposure to very high doses of radiation. While teratogenic effects following radium therapy for uterine cancer were described in the older literature, in humans no increase of malformations was found after pelvic X-ray irradiation for medical diagnostic purposes (Table 25). Even after the exposure to radiation from the atomic bombs, no increase in gross structural abnormalities induced during organogenesis was reported.
- The fetal period (8–17 weeks p.c.), is sensitive to prenatal induction of defects by ionizing radiation not the embryonic phase (Table 26). This period corresponds to the stage of neuron formation within the developing brain. In Hiroshima and Nagasaki, a high percentage of children exposed *in utero* were reported to exhibit severe mental retardation. The children were institutionalized, unable to communicate or to solve simple mathematical equations, and they were not able to take care of themselves.
- Mental retardation was associated with morphological abnormalities (microcephaly) in cases of high radiation exposure.
- The risk of developing cancer during early adolescence after prenatal exposure to ionizing radiation is apparently increased (transplacental carcinogenesis). After diagnostic X-ray exposure of the pelvis, this otherwise rather low cancer incidence seems to at least double (Table 25).

The data of the prospective Boston Study in the United States were confirmed by retrospective analyses showing that there is an increased frequency of cancer in children after *in utero* radiation exposure. The diagnostic use of pelvic X-rays was rather popular in some countries several decades ago. An association with neoplasms was found in the analysis of data presented in the Oxford Register, a collection of all fatal cancer cases under the age of 16 between the years 1953 and 1979 in England, Scotland, and Wales. For an estimated exposure of 2–5 mGy (200 to 500 mRad) per diagnostic procedure, a mean odds ratio

TABLE 25 Malformations and Tumors in Children after Exposure *In Utero* to X-Rays (Pelvic and Abdominal Diagnosis of the Mother) within the First 4 Months of Pregnancy

	Children with malformations or tumors[c]		
	Not exposed[a]	Exposed[b]	Odds ratio
All malformations	1687	590	(1.2)
Severe malformations	1016	377	(1.3)
CNS malformations	203	63	(1.1)
Cardiovascular malformations	293	111	(1.3)
Neoplasms, benign	90	50	1.9[d]
Neoplasms, malignant	15	9	2.0[d]
Children dying because of tumors, exposure anywhere during pregnancy	294	187	2.1[e]
Children dying because of tumors, OR for 1st trimester vs. OR for 3rd trimester			2.7[f]

[a]Number of unexposed children: 38,882.
[b]Number of exposed children: 11,400.
[c]Data compiled from Heinonen *et al.* (1977).
[d]Statistically significant according to multivariate logistic analysis.
[e]Statistically significant (data only for deaths within 4th and 5th year of postnatal life).
[f]This is not an odds ratio but the quotient of the odds ratios of 1st trimester/3rd trimester.

of 2 was reported, (i.e., one cancer death among 992 *in utero* exposures to obstetric diagnostic irradiation). The authors estimated that about 7% of all childhood neoplasia at that time might have been caused by exposure to radiation *in utero*. This is the first case of a possible correlation of early childhood neoplasia with a well-defined exogenous prenatal exposure. In contrast to the induction of mental retardation, the cancer risk seems to be highest in the first trimester; an exposure to radiation then was suggested to have a 2.7 times higher risk than an exposure during the third trimester, and it was estimated to be six times higher than that for unexposed children. The highest association was found for cancer cases diagnosed at the age of 4–5 years.

TABLE 26 Frequency of Mental Retardation in Children after *In Utero* Exposure to Ionizing Radiation (Atomic Bombs) in Hiroshima and Nagasaki[a]

Exposure (cGy [rad])[b]	Gestational age (weeks) at exposure *in utero*			
	0–7	8–15	16–25	>26
1–9	0/42	2/64 (3%)	2/94 (2%)	0/92
10–49	0/19	3/48 (6%)	1/49 (2%)	0/53
50–99	0/ 2	4/11 (36%)	2/14 (14%)	0/ 7
>100	0/ 1	5/ 8 (63%)	1/ 6 (17%)	1/ 4

[a]Data from Otake and Schull (1984). Reference group: nine cases of mental retardation/1085 children (1%).
[b]Exposed: <2 km from the hypocenter. Reference group: >3 km from the hypocenter (certainly <1 cGy [rad]).

Absolute risk coefficients for the incidence of all cancers over the ages of 0–14 years associated with irradiation *in utero* were calculated as 600 cancer cases/10,000 exposed/ Gy. From the data available, transplacental carcinogenesis seems to be the most sensitive manifestation of adverse effects after prenatal exposure to radiation.

Example: Diethylstilbestrol

From the late 1940s to the 1960s, estrogens had been used worldwide, often in combination with progestins. The drugs were given to prevent the loss of the products of conception (recurrent miscarriage) that occurs in the early stages of pregnancy. Tragically, diethylstilbestrol (DES) turned out to be ineffective for this indication, but it induced profound and long-lasting developmental toxicity in the offspring born from these pregnancies.

In the United States the synthetic estrogen DES (Fig. 23) was very often administered for the indication described. It has been estimated that there have been a vast number of pregnant women (several million) who were prescribed DES from the 1940s until 1971 at surprisingly different doses and for variable lengths of time for the same indication. The administration of female hormones at that time was just as common in Europe, including Germany, as in the United States. According to a study conducted by the German Research Association (Deutsche Forschungs-

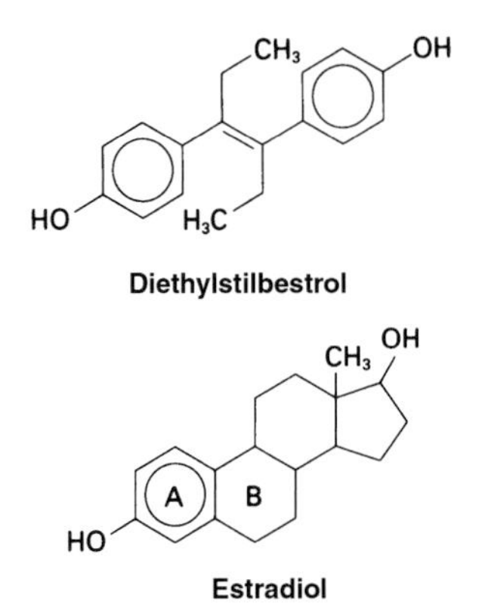

Diethylstilbestrol

Estradiol

FIGURE 23 Chemical structures of some estrogens.

gemeinschaft, DFG) at least 18% of all pregnant women in the former West Germany received female hormones for therapeutic reasons not counting the hormones used for pregnancy diagnostics. However, in Germany natural estrogens were administered almost exclusively. Natural estrogens are metabolized in the placenta and reach the fetus only to a small extent. In contrast, DES apparently passes the placental barrier easily. The human database on DES offers very important perspectives on the debate regarding endocrine disruptors, which have much less estrogenic potency than DES has.

In 1971 an increased occurrence of otherwise rare adenocarcinoma (clear-cell carcinoma) of the vagina or the cervix was observed in young girls. These tumors were soon linked to an exposure of these adolescent women to DES *in utero.* The average latency period was about 20 years, the youngest patient being 7 years old, the oldest 29 years. Around the age of 14 there was a steep increase of the incidence–age curve, with a maximum at 19 years. Because treatment with DES was not limited to the United States, a number of such tumors were subsequently associated with DES exposure in other countries as well (e.g., Australia, Belgium, France, and Mexico).

This was the first example of drug-induced transplacental carcinogenesis in humans. The possibility of

TABLE 27 Follow-up Study of Female and Male Offspring Exposed to DES *In Utero*[a]

	DES-exposed[b]	Placebo[b]	*P* value
Pregnant women in the prospective study	840	806	
Female offspring traced and evaluated	229	136	
Male offspring traced and evaluated	163	168	
Male offspring with sperm analyses	39	25	
Abnormalities			
Female offspring			
Vaginal adenosis	153 (67%)	5 (4%)	<0.005
Vaginal metaplastic cells	140 (61%)	2 (2%)	<0.0005
Vaginal hyperkeratosis	44 (19%)	0	
Vaginal circumferential ridges	(40%)	0	
Pregnancies[c]	18%	33%	<0.005
Live births	13%	23%	
Miscarriages	5%	11%	
Irregular menstrual cycles	18%	10%	<0.005
Male offspring			
Epididymal cysts	22	8	<0.01
Hypotrophic testes	12	2	<0.01
Capsular induration	5	1	
Hypoplastic penis	4	0	
Total patients with some abnormalities	41 (25%)	11 (7%)	<0.0005
Sperm count <20 mio/ml	10/39 (26%)	0/25	<0.01
<40% motile sperm	10/37 (27%)	4/25	NS
Ejaculate volume <1.5 ml	10/39 (26%)	0/25	<0.01

[a]Data from Bibbo *et al.* (1977).
[b]Results in % of the corresponding group.
[c]At the time of the first visit.

TABLE 28 Frequency of Neoplasms Reported in Mothers and Sons after Exposure to DES during Pregnancy[a]

Type of tumor	Number of studies	Mean total dose of DES (g)	Combined Relative Risk[b]
Neoplasms in mothers			
Breast cancer[c]	5	2–16	1.4 ($p = 0.002$)
Neoplasms in sons exposed *in utero* to DES			
Testicular cancer[d]	5	?	2.5 ($p = 0.014$)

[a]From IARC Monograph (1979).
[b]Calculated from all the studies.
[c]Apparently long latency period (15–20 years).
[d]Often associated with cryptorchism, a risk factor for this type of tumor.

inducing tumors prenatally (e.g., with the direct alkylating agent ethylnitrosourea) was known for decades from animal experiments conducted by Druckrey and co-workers. It was only after the observations in humans that systematic experimental studies in laboratory animals were initiated with DES, which have reproduced almost all of the effects observed in the offspring of DES-treated pregnant women.

As in all other carcinogenic effects in humans, the vaginal carcinomas after DES treatment occurred only in a minority of the girls exposed *in utero*. The estimated incidence was about 0.1 to 1:1000 up to the age of 24 years, but it is still unknown whether the risk continues to increase in later years. Although some dose dependency was suggested, this is difficult to verify because the doses and duration of treatment varied considerably. Daily doses varied from 3 to 150 mg, and the applied total quantity from <1 to 47 g; the duration of the treatment varied from 1 to 36 weeks.

Results compiled at the University of Chicago within a frame of an ongoing double-blind, placebo-controlled investigation during 1951–1952 are especially helpful for the assessment of adverse effects induced in adolescents exposed to DES *in utero* (Table 27). In accord with the frequencies found in other studies, none of the 229 female offspring developed tumors within the 24 years of the study. Colposcopic evaluation revealed vaginal adenosis in 67% of the DES-exposed female offspring (4% in the placebo group), 61% showed metaplastic cells in the vagina (2% in the controls), and 40% of the DES-exposed women had circumferential ridges in the vagina (none on the placebo group). Although more of the DES-exposed women had irregular menstrual cycles than offspring of the consol group (10%), 18% of the exposed women had become pregnant at the time of the first visit to the hospital (33% in the control group). The percentage of live birth was 13% in the DES-exposed and 23% in all of the women of the placebo group. The results must be viewed with some caution because individual exposure *in utero* occurred at quite different stages of development, as the mothers were treated at various periods during pregnancy.

Undoubtedly, DES can form reactive metabolites by oxidation, and these metabolites might play a role in the carcinogenesis in the adult organism. However, because of the preferred target organ localization (especially breast cancer) the carcinogenic potential of DES may result from a mechanism similar to that known for the natural estrogenic sex hormones.

For prenatally induced tumors the situation seems to be different because they apparently are the result of abnormal prenatal development. Changes are induced by DES during the phase of the vagina development (first to second trimester). The abnormalities mentioned seem to develop from the Müllerian duct. Additional factors, such as the hormonal changes during puberty, may stimulate these abnormally localized cells and initiate malignant transformation in certain individuals.

A significant increase in neoplasia, in this case mammary carcinoma, has also been reported in the treated mothers (Table 28). The risk for endometrial carcinoma was apparently not increased by the diethylstilbestrol medication.

During the trial performed at the University of Chicago, some abnormalities were also reported in 25% of the male offspring exposed to DES *in utero* (Table 27). The pathological changes observed included epididymal cysts (14% versus 5% in the placebo group), hypotrophic testes (7% versus 1% in the controls), and

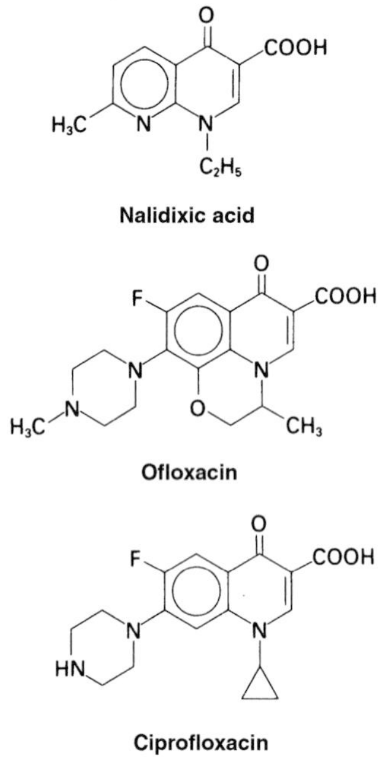

Nalidixic acid

Ofloxacin

Ciprofloxacin

FIGURE 24 Chemical structures of fluoroquinolones.

testicular capsular induration (3% versus 0.6%). More of the offspring DES-exposed *in utero* had ejaculates with low sperm counts of <20 million/ml or a low volume of <1.5 ml (26% versus 0/25 in controls). In the exposed men, 2 of the 25 were azoospermic. Although the number of patients in this group is small, the results are rather representative for this situation.

In several studies performed between 1979 and 1986, an increased tumor incidence was found in the males. The odds ratio of testicular carcinoma was found to have approximately doubled (Table 28). Because cryptorchism, an anomaly known to favor the tumor formation, was found to be increased in boys exposed to DES *in utero*, this could be a factor facilitating the tumor formation.

Abnormal Development due to Postnatal Exposure

The main sources of chemical exposure in infancy, in the neonatal period and early childhood, are medicinal drugs and food (milk). Space does not permit a detailed discussion of the manifold quantitative differences in the sensitivity to drugs known from pediatrics. Only the exposure of nursing infants to xenobiotics via milk will be briefly mentioned because special features can be recognized.

Example: Fluoroquinolones (Gyrase Inhibitors)

A good example of adverse health effects induced postnatally by drugs are fluoroquinolones (Fig. 24), a group of modern antibacterial agents with extremely interesting therapeutic properties. The number of gyrase inhibitors is rapidly increasing. They have been studied thoroughly in prenatal tests, including animal tests, with respect to developmental and reproductive toxicity. Aside from fertility disorders after treatment with high doses, minor findings with regard to conventional prenatal toxicity were reported, but the results of these studies were not impressive.

Following postnatal administration to juvenile animals, a special phenomenon was discovered—all the animal species, such as rat, rabbit, dog, and nonhuman primate, showed an impairment of the joint cartilage, especially of the limbs. Apparently this is an effect characteristic of the quinolones, which can be irreversible and appears at a dose range not much above the therapeutic level. For example, in juvenile dogs this cartilage toxicity appeared after 1 weeks of daily administration of 20 mg ofloxacin/kg body weight.

In experimental animals, clinical symptoms were only observed when weight was put on the joints during standing or walking. With more sensitive methods of evaluation, such as fluorescence or electron microscopy of the joint cartilage, morphological lesions can be detected prior to the onset of clinical symptoms or any macroscopically visible changes (Fig. 25). In comparative studies, the histological changes induced by ofloxacin in juvenile rodents and nonhuman primates were found to be very similar, and identical lesions are also seen after the application of other quinolones. Lesions as revealed by electron microscopic examinations were induced in the animal studies with doses causing about 10 times higher plasma concentrations than those reached in humans after therapeutic doses.

In order to evaluate the significance of chondrotoxic effect, the kinetic characteristics of the quinolones must be considered. According to our knowledge of pharmacology and toxicology, comparative extrapolations from the effects seen in the experimental animal to humans cannot be based on doses, but should be performed taking into account kinetic data (e.g., plasma C_{max} values). The reason for the special vulnerability of the juvenile cartilage may well be that this tissue is a deep compartment, so that high concentrations accumulate after long-term administration.

Available data suggest that all fluoroquinolones

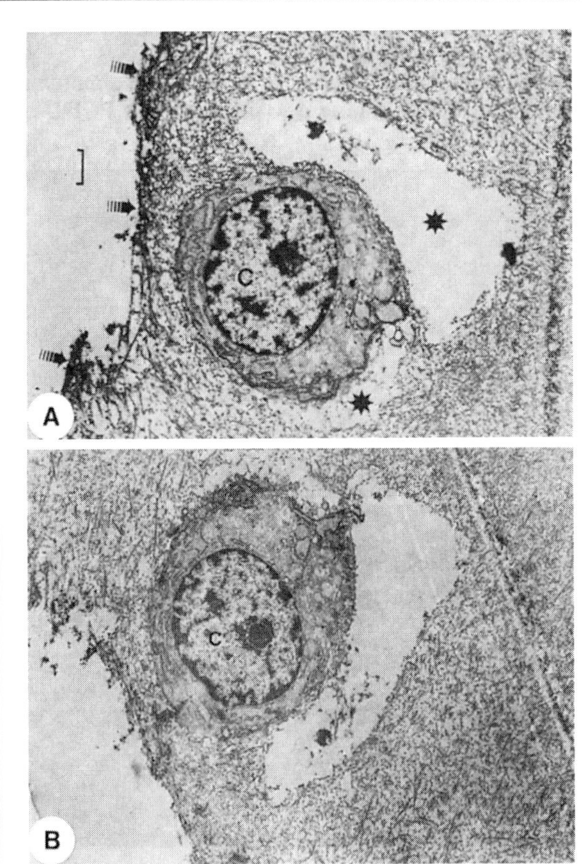

FIGURE 25 Defects in the cartilage of a knee joint of juvenile experimental animals after treatment with ofloxacin. Electron microscopic evaluation. (A) from juvenile rats; (B) from juvenile marmosets. The defects are almost identical. ×16000. (Reprinted from Stahlmann *et al.*, 1990, *Arch. Toxicol.* **64,** 193–204, copyright notice of Springer-Verlag.)

may exhibit this chondrotoxicity. However, the degree of accumulation within the cartilage when compared with active concentrations at the location of the chemotherapeutic action may be different for the various derivatives and critical for the manifestation of chondrotoxicity. Such comparative data are largely lacking. The inhibition of gyrase itself may not be responsible for the chondrotoxic effect, and chelation of magnesium has been proposed as one possible mechanism of action. It is unknown why chondrotoxicity cannot be induced prenatally during development and differentiation of the cartilage.

Some limited data from children chronically treated with ciprofloxacin for mucoviscidosis indicate that chondrotoxicity is not a significant toxic side effect with the usually recommended daily doses.

Exposure of the Newborn via Breast Milk

Because milk is the only nutrient for the infant, he or she will be exposed to all the xenobiotics present in the milk. The possible exposure of human babies to xenobiotics can be from either breast or cow's milk. There are two possible sources for such a contamination:

- Xenobiotics transferred into the milk subsequent to acute exposure of the maternal organism (e.g., from medication or a special diet).
- Compounds stored in maternal adipose tissue, mostly from chronic low-level uptake of persistent (ubiquitously existing) environmental substances that are transferred into the milk fat.

There are only very limited data on the amount of xenobiotics in cow's milk, and such components are not routinely measured. It is commonly assumed that exposure of a few animals (e.g. by drug treatment) will not play a major role because of the high dilution of the pooled milk during processing in dairies. There could be the possibility of an allergic potential of xenobiotics present in the milk because allergic reactions may be triggered by very small amounts. However, more interest is focused on the allergic potential of the natural components of cow's milk and the subsequent occurrence of atopic diseases in infants.

An abundance of data on the concentration of some xenobiotics in breast milk is available. Because humans may be at the end of the food chain, a considerable accumulation of highly persistent environmental substances is possible. For example, the concentration of polychlorodibenzo-*p*-dioxins and dibenzofurans in cow's milk is only about one tenth of the concentration in breast milk.

Environmental Substances in Breast Milk An impressive pool of data on the concentration of xenobiotics in breast milk has been gathered by many national and international agencies. It is now well established that lipophilic substances with a high persistence in the environment and within the mammalian organisms (i.e., with very long elimination half-lives) may accumulate in adipose tissue and remain there for many years. Because of this phenomenon, we all still have clearly detectable amounts of DDT and its metabolites, as well as dieldrin and hexachlorocyclohexane and other pesticides, in our adipose tissue, although these substances have not been used in industrialized and wealthy countries for many years. These compounds have spread out in the environment, remain there for decades, and are over and over again taken up with food. DDT and other pesti-

TABLE 29 Examples of Concentrations of Xenobiotics in Breast Milk[a]

Xenobiotics[b]		(ng/g) Milk fat	
		Median values	Range
PCBs		1,500	500–7,000
α-HCH		30	1–2,000
β-HCH		400	50–9,000
γ-HCH		100	1–1,400
HCB		1,000	250–6,000
p,p′-DDT		300	10–4,000
p,p′-DDE		2,000	500–11,000
PCDDs			
2,3,7,8-	-T4CDD	0.003	0.001–0.01
1,2,3(4)(6),7,8,(9)-H6CDD		0.1	0.008–0.36
	OCDD	0.1	0.02–1.30
PCDFs			
2,3,7,8-	-T4CDF	0.002	<0.001–0.01
3,4,7,8	-P5CDF	0.03	<0.001–0.10
(1),2,3(4)(6),7,8	-H6CDF	0.04	0.005–0.12
Sum PCDDs/PCDFs (I-TEq)		0.029	0.006–0.09

[a]Data from the Federal Republic of Germany. Data from Neubert (1988); Beck *et al.* (1991).

[b]PCBs, polychlorinated biphenyls; PCDDs/PCDFs, polychlorinated dibenzo-*p*-dioxins and dibenzofurans; HCB, hexachlorobenzene, HCH, Hexachlorocyclohexane; I-TEq, International Toxicity Equivalencies (TCDD = 1) according to: NATA/CCMS (1988).

cides are still heavily used in some African and Asian countries, and they are redistributed over the globe from these user countries by atmospheric drift and trade.

For several of these substances, it is well documented that the concentration found in milk fat is nearly equivalent to that within the maternal adipose tissue or maternal blood fat (Table 29). Although there is a considerable interindividual variability in the length of breast feeding, it is interesting to calculate how much of such foreign substances is taken up by the infant over a lactation period of 6 months. It is

TABLE 30 Concentrations of Some PCDD and PCDF Congeners in Two Breastfed and Two Formula-Fed Infants[a]

Congener	Breastfed I		Breastfed II		Formula-fed I		Formula-fed II	
	Mother	Infant[b]	Mother	Infant[b]	Mother	Infant[c]	Mother	Infant[c]
2,3,7,8-TCDD	1.9	3.7	1.8	4.3	2.0	<1	1.8	—
Ratio: infant/mother		2.0		2.4		>0.5		—
2,3,4,7,8-PeCDF	8.6	23.1	7.1	31.5	11.7	1.5	9.7	3.5
Ratio: infant/mother		2.7		4.4		0.1		0.4
I-TEq	12.3	29.2	10.5	37.5	16.9	2.4	13.8	2.6
Ratio: infant/mother		2.4		3.6		0.1		0.2
Ratio: breastfed/formula-fed				≈18				

[a]Data from Abraham *et al.* (1996). In ppt (pg/g fat) in blood fat.
[b]After a 4-month breast-feeding period, the body burdens were measured at the age of 11 months.
[c]After formula-feeding, the body burdens were measured at the age of 11 months.

obvious that breast feeding is an effective elimination mechanism for certain xenobiotics from the human body. By breast feeding for 6 months, 25–30% of the entire body burden of TCDD may be eliminated from the maternal organism. This percentage is much lower than that observed in the common rodent laboratory species.

These findings have led to heated discussions regarding the question of whether breast feeding should be recommended in spite of milk contamination with xenobiotics. It must be stressed that all experts and all national and international agencies have clearly decided in favor of breast feeding because the advantages by far exceed the possible disadvantages.

A common error in the discussion on the high uptake of PCDD and PCDF by nursing infants was the direct comparison of the daily uptake by the infant (approximately 140 pg I-TEq) compared to the adult (approximately 2 pg I-TEq). For substances with extremely long elimination half-lives this kind of information alone is misleading because the duration of the exposure, life long for adults compared to a typical length of 6 months for infants, is the essential factor for the cumulation. Decisive and significant for the medical evaluation is the resulting body burden. A simple calculation showed that the additional amount taken up by the baby could at most reach three fold the maternal body burden (assuming complete absorption and no elimination).

An unknown factor is how much of the xenobiotics are absorbed by the infant. Even though one could assume good absorption of the lipophilic substances, this apparently does not apply for all the xenobiotics mentioned.

It is not easy to measure the absorption of these substances by the infant and the resulting body burdens, and three methods have been applied.

- Constructing a balance sheet from the amount of PCDD and PCDF taken up and the remaining concentration in the stools.
- Measuring tissue concentrations in children deceased from sudden infant death syndrome (SIDS), when some data on breast feeding were available.
- Measuring PCDD and PCDF uptake from breast- and formula feeding and the resulting concentrations within blood fat of the infants.

While the first two approaches provide some preliminary data, the last method gives direct information, although on a limited number of infants.

Studies on the balance indicate that not all PCDD and PCDF congeners are equally well absorbed. While TCDD and its main congener in breast milk (2,3,4,7,8-pentachlorodibenzofuran) are almost completely absorbed from the milk, the higher chlorinated congeners exhibit incomplete absorption. However, they do not contribute much to the I-TEq. It is noteworthy that some of the higher chlorinated substances can be actively secreted into the intestinal lumen. This has been clearly demonstrated experimentally in rodents. Thus under certain conditions and for certain congeners, the infant could eliminate more than it is taking in.

The data of the SIDS children seemed to show markedly lower tissue concentrations than would have been expected from the calculation of the maximally attainable body burdens. There is no explanation for this finding. Newer data from the third-mentioned approach confirmed the calculations. When the TCDD body burdens of two infants breastfed for 4 months were measured at the age of 11 months, the concentrations in blood fat were 2 to 2.5 times higher than in the mothers, and the difference in the I-TEq was 2-to 4-fold (Table 30). However, the concentrations of these congeners in the blood fat of formula-fed infants were ~5–7 times lower than the maternal body burdens (Table 30). Apparently there was a negative balance with respect to these substances, possibly due to excessive excretion. Overall, a 10- to 20-fold lower body burden resulted in the formula-fed infants compared with the breastfed babies. These data demonstrate that extrapolations based solely on uptake estimates and neglecting kinetic factors can lead to the wrong conclusions.

Exposure to Pharmaceutical Drugs via Breast Milk In contrast to prenatal embryo- and fetotoxic risk posed by chemicals, the danger of a considerable impairment of the infant's health by medical drugs excreted in breast milk seems to be low. Transient drug-induced symptoms can occur, but are rarely serious. Nevertheless, the possible risks for the infant through medications taken by the mother should be taken into account. Although no severe pharmacological or toxic symptoms may appear, a certain chance of an early allergic sensitization might exist.

Most substances are transferred by diffusion from the blood to milk and for only a few chemicals was active transport mechanism detected. The concentration in the milk and the amount of xenobiotics taken up by the infant are determined by a number of variables. These may be divided into maternal factors, infant factors, and special characteristics of the substance, itself (Table 31).

The concentration ratio milk/maternal plasma (M/P) is often used as a measure of the transfer into milk. If the M/P ratio is 1, the concentrations are identical; a M/P ratio >1 indicates an accumulation in the milk. Information on these M/P ratios are relatively unreli-

TABLE 31 Some Factors Determining the Dose of a Chemical Substance Taken up by the Infant from Breast Milk

Aspects concerning the mother
Time interval between substance application and breast feeding
Time interval between breast feedings
Amount of body fat of the mother?
Composition of the milk
Fat and protein content
pH value
Characteristics of the substance
Pharmacokinetics of the substance (especially elimination t½)
Solubility of the substance (in fat, water)
Binding to plasma proteins
pK_a value (ionization within plasma and milk)
Molecular weight
Aspects concerning the infant
Amount of milk consumed
Body weight
Percentage of body fat
Pharmacokinetics within the infant (e.g., metabolism)
Enteral absorption (when compared with the adult)
Distribution (e.g., penetration through the blood–brain barrier)
Elimination (e.g., longer persistence than within the mother)

able because often only single-point data were collected. M/P ratios presented in the literature often show considerable variability. Data compiled in the literature can only provide approximate information. Only extensive kinetic data, like AUC data, should be used for calculating the possible total exposures of the infant, but more recent publications also lack these more reliable AUC data. Even with this procedure, only information on one dosing regiment are obtained. For pharmacokinetic studies, a three-component model was introduced and its applicability was studied with a few substances (salicylates and morphine).

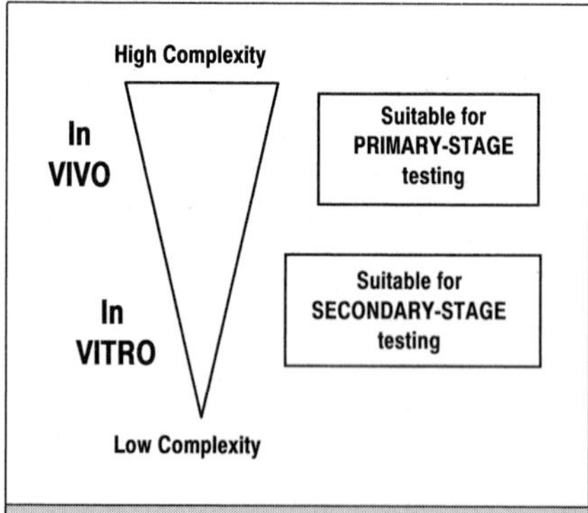

FIGURE 26 Difference biological complexities of *in vivo* and *in vivo* methods, and resulting suitability for answering specific scientific questions. (Modified from Neubert, 1982.)

Elusive Dream of *In Vitro* Teratology

Appropriate methods should always be selected according to scientific questions. Therefore, *in vivo* and *in vitro* methods would be equally suitable if they possessed the same predictive power. According to our knowledge, this does not hold true in prenatal toxicology. The reason is the vast difference in biological complexity of the *in vivo* and the *in vitro* systems (Fig. 26). This degree of complexity is essential for the applicability of the test systems to answer two types of questions regarding prenatal toxicity:

- Does a substance pose a presently unknown toxicity hazard if applied during pregnancy? Evaluations designed to answer this question have been designated "primary-stage testing."
- Can additional information concerning a specific question be obtained for a substance with an already known or a suspected specific toxicity potential? Evaluations designed to resolve this question have been designate "secondary-stage testing."

The first strategy largely excludes a large variety of possible effects; the second one is aimed at obtaining additional very selected information concerning a specific hypothesis and on a defined target.

In recent decades numerous alternative test systems have been suggested for primary- and secondary-stage testing in developmental toxicology. Special emphasis was put on revealing a possible applicability of simple test systems, including in lower organisms (e.g., hydra, xenopus, and fish). It is fair to state that all these simple systems are largely worthless for testing in prenatal toxicology, if conclusions relevant to humans are the goal.

For primary-stage testing, a very complex system is needed that must serve as a model for the complex pharmacokinetic and pharmacodynamic characteristics of the chemical of interest. The model applied must reflect the numerous possibilities of interfering with development and reproduction. This can only be achieved by using the whole pregnant mammalian organism. Attempts to solve primary problems of chemical safety for compounds with unknown biological effects in developmental and reproductive toxicology solely with *in vitro* techniques, including those of mammalian origin, are bound to fail. Past experience has shown that the money spent for this purpose is wasted.

For secondary-stage testing, a carefully selected simple biological model is best suited, in which the specific problem can be studied with as few confounding factors as possible. Such a model can very well be a differentiating *in vitro* system using mammalian tissue, which may be much superior to the complexity of the intact organism.

Culture systems used extensively from the 1970s were from mammalian embryonic tissue, and all of them allowed the evaluation of some type of morphogenetic differentiation. They include (in increasing complexity):

- Rodent organoid cultures, that is, the differentiation of densely packed dispersed cells from different primordia (limb buds, brain primordia and lung).
- Rodent organ culture, that is, of limb buds, of palatal shelves, of tubuli seminiferi, and of many other organs.
- Rodent whole-embryo cultures, that is, the culture of embryos during early organogenesis.

While the whole embryo culture is capable of mimicking development to the same extent as *in vivo* tests, prenatal development in all organ and organoid cultures deviates more or less (mostly drastically), from the situation *in vivo* while allowing the evaluation of important, but always highly selected, morphogenetic differentiations.

As an example, in Fig. 27 two *in vitro* systems are shown, which have been used on a large scale for several years, namely rodent whole-embryo culture and rodent embryo limb-bud culture. In both culture systems, the uniformity of the development is amazing, quite in contrast to the conditions *in vivo*. This uniformity of the differentiation is possible because the initial stages can be standardized and the development thereby synchronized.

In rodent whole-embryo culture (rat and mouse), the culture is only possible for the limited period of about 2 days because then the explant gets too large, and nutrition via a functional chorioallantoic placenta is lacking *in vitro*. Further development of the primordia, for example, the differentiation of the limb buds to full limbs, cannot be achieved with this system. The whole-embryo culture technique cannot serve as an adequate substitute for *in vivo* experiments, which allow the evaluation of the entire embryonic period. In spite of these shortcomings, the whole-embryo culture today is one of the most frequently applied *in vitro* systems.

Organ or organoid cultures, the culture of parts of the embryo or fetus, can be performed with almost any primordium or later developmental stages, and many such systems have been used in research laboratories all over the world. None of these culture systems is representative of the entire embryo, but investigations of essential and well-defined developmental processes in a defined tissue are possible for a limited period of time. It is not feasible to achieve complete simulation of the situation *in vivo* of the respective organs, for instance with respect to the size or all the tissue components involved in development. In the case of the extensively used limb-bud culture (Fig. 27), certain processes of the morphogenetic differentiation of the cartilaginous skeleton (i.e., typical pattern formation) can be studied in detail, but the development of muscles, vessels, and nerves cannot be evaluated *in vitro*. These serious limitations also hold true for all other organ cultures, for example, the culture of palatal shelves, which only allows limited conclusions with respect to the situation *in vivo* because almost no increase in size occurs. A few attempts have also been made to use human embryonic tissue for culturing (e.g., pieces of palatal shelves), but the results have been rather unconvincing.

Examples of normal and abnormal development achieved *in vitro* are shown in Fig. 27 and Tables 32–33. The first drug, valproic acid (VPA), illustrates excellent dose–response relationships with the whole-embryo culture. The *in vitro* as well as *in vivo* slope of the concentration–response curve is very steep.

Some *in vitro* systems are well suited for prescreening a large series of structurally related chemicals, if a suitable model system for the teratogenic effects of the initial substance can be selected from previous *in vivo* and *in vitro* testing. Thus, substances can be selected that do not induce abnormal development *in vitro*. Such screening for hints concerning specific abnormal development among a group of structurally similar chemicals has been used extensively in some laboratories of the pharmaceutical industry, but some papers on this topic have also been published from university institutes. One example is that, in contrast to valproic acid (the reference substance), the derivative 2-*en*-valproic acid shows a much lower potential for the induction of abnormal development in the whole-embryo culture. This result was confirmed *in vivo*.

In each case, those compounds with a negative test result must be subsequently studied with conventional *in vivo* tests because developmental and reproductive toxicity other than that detectable with the special *in vitro* test cannot be excluded. This means that the substance could still exhibit a teratogenic po-

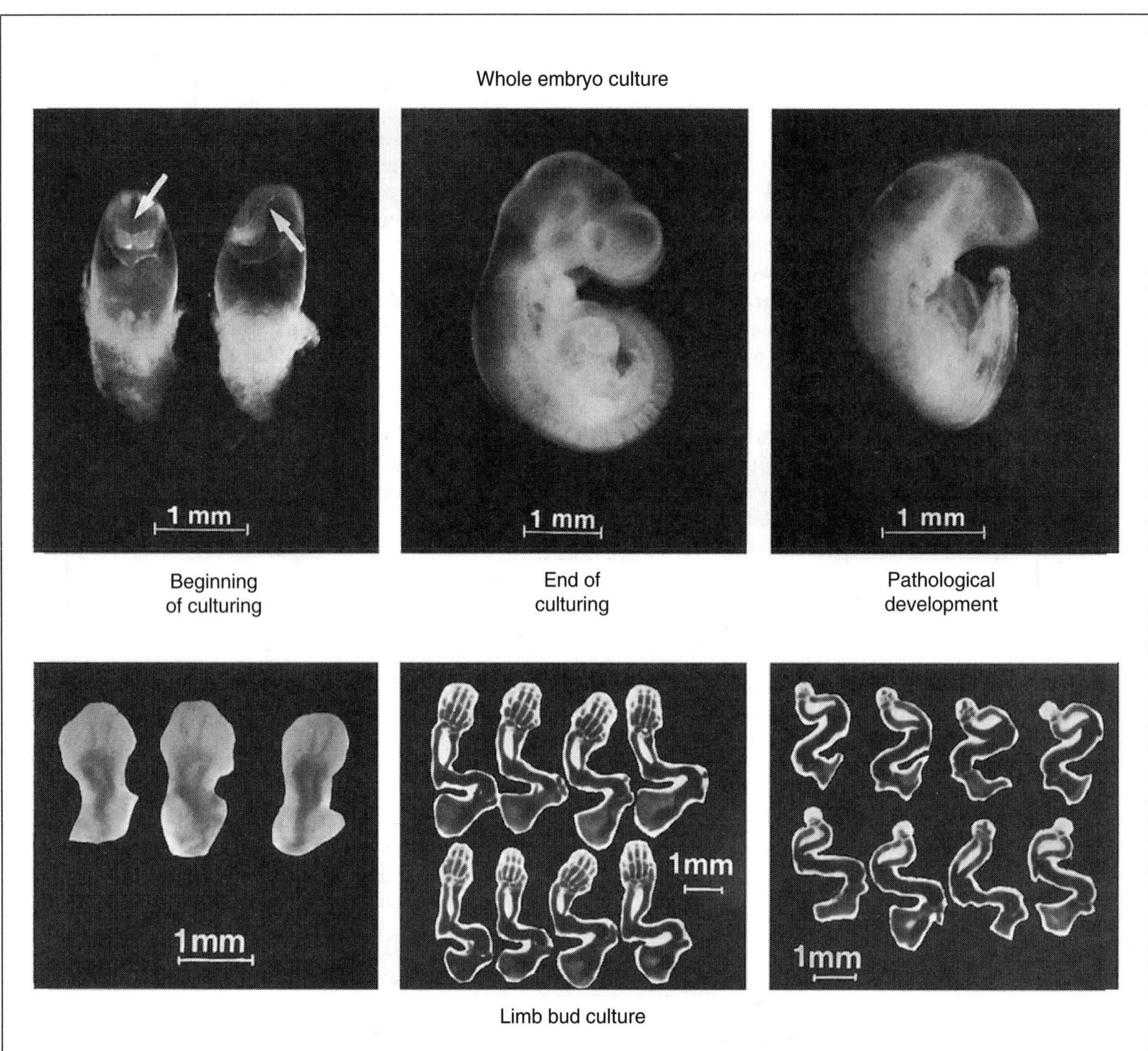

FIGURE 27 Example of two *in vitro* methods with differing biological complexities, and evaluating different developmental periods. *Arrow:* rat embryo within its membranes at the start of culturing (day 9.5 of gestation) and end of whole-embryo culture 48 h later. The dramatic growth and numerous differentiations are obvious. Culturing of mouse limb buds was started at day 11 or 12 of gestation, and it ended 6 days later.

tential (in another organ system), despite a negative result in the *in vitro* test.

The second example (Table 33) shows the first, and so far apparently only, case in which a teratogenic effect was initially found in an *in vitro* system. After abnormal development caused by the well-known virostatic agent acyclovir was elicited *in vitro*, the very marked teratogenic potential was then verified by specific *in vivo* tests. It was again possible to compare other similar antimetabolites for their potential of inducing abnormal development with the same system. In selected cases, a preventive hazard minimization may be attempted when correlating toxicologically effective concentrations from *in vitro* data with plasma concentrations achieved therapeutically in humans. Such calculations have been performed in the case of acyclovir.

Validation of In Vitro Tests

The most difficult problem with respect to the decision of using such *in vitro* tests on a larger scale for human preventive hazard minimization is the assessment of the predictive power of *in vitro* tests, that is, the problem of validation. There are three prerequisites for a meaningful validation:

- A validation can only be attempted against results of *in vivo* tests performed in the same species. Appropriate data must be available.
- Validation must be performed with substances

TABLE 32 Example of a Concentration–Response Relationship for a Substance-Induced Abnormal Development *In Vitro*[a]

Concentration	*n*	Somite pairs	Protein	"Score"	Abnormalities
Control	18	**25** (24–26)	**203** (146–249)	**36** (35–37)	0
0.3 mM VPA	15	**24** (23–26)	**141**[b] (114–166)	**35**[b] (33–36)	0
0.6 mM VPA	19	**21**[b] (18–26)	**132**[b] (77–167)	**33**[b] (25–35)	32%
1.2 mM VPA	17	**19**[b] (16–21)	**80**[b] (49–110)	**15**[b] (12–23)	100%
1.8 mM **2-en**-VPA	15	**26** (23–27)	**136**[b] (122–173)	**36** (35–37)	0

[a]The effect of the antiseizure drug valproic acid (VPA) was evaluated in the whole-embryo culture. The derivative 2-*en*-VPA also exhibits *in vivo* a much smaller teratogenic potency than VPA. **Bold:** median values; in parentheses: (extreme values). From Klug and Neubert (1992), Risk assessment of prenatally induced adverse health effects, copyright notice of Springer-Verlag, with permission.

[b]$p < 0.05$, Man-Whitney test

whose biological activity is largely unknown at the onset of the comparison *in vitro* versus *in vivo.* Validation using highly selected substances with known properties *in vivo* (positives and negatives) is not acceptable because such selections are considerably biased and therefore unreliable. A series of chemically very similar substance pairs, one of which is effective and the other not, may be acceptable. However, a sufficient number of such pairs suitable for a trustworthy validation is not available.

- The pharmacokinetics *in vivo* and *in vitro* must be comparable.

A number of attempts have been made to validate *in vitro* tests for the use in primary-stage testing. Most results of such exercises were quite unreliable because the outcome could be largely predicted even without performing the tests—there were highly reactive substances within the positive group and largely inert ones among the negatives. Furthermore, several outcomes of the *in vivo* studies were equvocal. Therefore, claims regarding sensitivity and specificity of different *in vitro* tests do more to confuse the issue than clarify it. In no case were the results of the proposed *in vitro* tests convincing enough to use the assay for primary hazard minimization. No special validation is required when the *in vitro* tests are used for secondary-stage evaluations.

Conclusions on the Applicability of In Vitro Tests

Extensive work performed in several laboratories has shown that *in vitro* tests have their established place in research on mechanisms of developmental toxicity. If one wants to use these techniques, it is essential to have several test systems available and to select the method most appropriate for solving a specific problem. More complex systems allowing one to monitor special morphogenetic differentiations are generally preferable. These are the whole-embryo culture and a variety of organ and organoid cultures. The strategy of exclusively using *in vitro* test systems is almost worthless for primary-stage testing, except

TABLE 33 Example of a Concentration–Response Relationship for an Abnormal Development *In Vitro*[a]

Concentration	*n*	Somite pairs	Protein	"Score"	Abnormalities
Control	44	**26** (25–27)	**235** (176–284)	**37** (35–38)	0
25 μM acyclovir	19	**26** (25–27)	**237** (209–264)	**37** (35–37)	0
50 μM acyclovir	18	**26** (24–27)	**130**[b] (110–175)	**35**[b] (33–38)	28%
100 μM acyclovir	19	**26** (25–27)	**138**[b] (122–175)	**32**[b] (31–33)	95%

[a]The effect of the antiviral agent acyclovir was evaluated in the whole-embryo culture. The adverse effect was first found *in vitro* and then confirmed *in vivo.* From Klug and Neubert (1992), Risk assessment of prenatally induced adverse health effects, copyright notice of Springer-Verlag, with permission. Bold, median values; in parentheses, extreme values.

[b]$p < 0.05$, Mann-Whitney test

for the special situation of prescreening a large number of similar compounds for inducing circumscript abnormalities.

Past experience teaches us that investigational efforts should not only concentrate on unrealistic ambition of replacing *in vivo* experiments by *in vitro* tests. Supplementation of one study design with the other is much more important and holds promise for solving problems in developmental toxicology. This is the strength and important potential contribution of *in vitro* methods. Therefore, the designation of *in vitro* tests as alternative methods in this very complex field is misleading. Both *in vitro* and *in vivo* systems have their place when problems of prenatal toxic are being studied, but the applicability is quite different.

It must be stressed that *in vitro* systems can only be used for studying limited aspects of prenatal toxicity. No useful *in vitro* tests are available for revealing the postnatal manifestations of prenatally induced lesion, perinatally induced or post-natally triggered adverse effect, or possible adverse effects on fertility. Because all these possibilities of interference must be considered when assessing developmental and reproductive toxicity hazard potential, even a battery of *in vitro* tests is bound to be inadequate and insufficient for this task.

RISK ASSESSMENT AND PREVENTIVE HAZARD MINIMIZATION

The critical concepts of human risk assessment and of preventive hazard minimization are extensively discussed elsewhere. However, some peculiarities in epidemiological research and special attempts to extrapolate the results of animal data to the exposure situation postulated to exist in humans may be unique in reproductive and developmental toxicology.

Because of the great complexity and the variety of possible effects, the evaluation of the data collected in developmental toxicology requires considerable professional expertise. Particularly difficult is the problem of possible species differences, and the ultimate step of extrapolation to a presumed effect in humans. These steps include the analysis of dose–response relationships. Only if a large database is available that includes comparative kinetic data are far-reaching conclusions possible.

Every analysis of possible toxic effects ultimately results in the evaluation of quantitative relationships. Embryo- and fetotoxic effects are dose-dependent. A decrease in the dose delivered to the conceptus reduces the risk as well, and with very small doses the risk will become negligible.

Special Problems in Epidemiological Studies on Developmental Toxicity

There are at least six aspects that greatly hamper epidemiological studies in pregnant women and the outcome of pregnancy.

- Prospective studies are difficult to perform. They require a permanent system (because new chemical substances are continuously used), are expensive, and do not provide answers within a short period. Often multicenter studies are essential. Retrospective studies are easier to perform, but typically suffer from a pronounced recall bias. This shortcoming is especially profound when a malformed child has been born and when financial compensation obtained through litigation may be in sight.
- All types of malformations occur spontaneously. Without taking such rates into account for the population studied, the results are almost worthless, unless extremely pronounced and rather exotic effects occur.
- Children must be examined by an experienced pediatrician soon after birth. Follow-up studies for at least 1 year are required because only about 50% of the gross structural defects are recognized at birth.
- Fortunately, not too many pregnant women take different sorts of medications or are heavily exposed to environmental agents during pregnancy. However, this makes it difficult to compile a large enough and statistical meaningful cohort that has been exposed to single agents that are rarely used by women of child-bearing age.
- In order to reach a sufficiently large number of cases, the evaluated period often is extended beyond the exposure during the susceptible period for the induction of a given adverse effect. This means that all cases are compiled for a medication given within the first trimester of pregnancy. This may substantially dilute the cases exposed during a small window of susceptibility, and it weakens the predictive power of the study.
- It is difficult to exclude or to control the many confounders possibly involved in a prenatally induced adverse health effect.

Even without exposure to living (e.g., rubella virus), chemical (Table 34), or physical (e.g., radiation) noxious agents during pregnancy, a significant spontaneous, probably endogenous, risk for abnormal pre- and postnatal development exists. For a toxicological risk evaluation only additional risks that clearly exceed this spontaneous rate are relevant. Only very few known exogenous insults double this initial risk, and it should be considered that even in such cases a 50% chance exists that in a single case the abnormality

TABLE 34 Tentative Compilation of Xenobiotics with Proven or Presumed Potency to Interfere with Human Development and Reproduction

Substance	Application	Adverse effect in humans
ACE inhibitors	Antihypertensive drug	Kidney lesions in the fetus[a]
Androgenic hormones		Masculinization of female fetuses
Antiepileptic drugs		Multiple defects (combination-therapy![b])
Lead	"Environmental agent"	CNS defect in children have been proposed[c]
Diethylstilbestrol	Synthetic estrogen	Transplacental carcinogenesis.
Ethyl alcohol	Stimulant, mood modifier	Alcohol embryopathy[d]
Folate antagonists	Chemotherapy	Some derivatives are clearly teratogenic[e]
Ionizing radiation	"Diagnostics"	Transplacental carcinogenesis (CNS defects[f])
Methyl mercury	"Environmental agent"	CNS defects[g]
Misoprostol	Antacid	Abortion (high doses[h])
Retinoids	Dermatology	Multiple malformations (therapeutic doses!)
Tetracyclines	Chemotherapy	Dental defects (older substances?[i])
Thalidomide	Antiphlogistic drug	Multiple malformations (therapeutic doses!)
Warfarin	Anticoagulant	Multiple malformations (Warfarin syndrome)

[a]Induced during the fetal and perinatal period. Cause: fetal hypotension.
[b]Monotherapy is recommended. Valproic acid induces a low frequency of spina bifida at therapeutic doses.
[c]Controversially discussed.
[d]Chronic heavy drinking required for the full syndrome.
[e]Evidence was provided for aminopterin and to a lesser extent methotrexate.
[f]No typical malformations at diagnostic doses at organogenesis. Mental retardation with fetal exposure.
[g]At high accidental exposures.
[h]Was successfully used for inducing abortion.
[i]No information available for newer derivatives (e.g., doxycycline).

observed has an endogenous cause. To retrospectively establish a causal relationship for an individual case of a malformation is very difficult and can hardly ever been proven with a sufficiently high probability. Even in the case of doubling the spontaneous risk of major malformations, there is still a >90% chance of delivering a child with no visible defects at birth. Excessive phobia is not appropriate and, because of the reasons indicated, drug administration without the knowledge of an existing pregnancy almost never serves as a medical indication to interrupt a pregnancy. Although the risk may be very small, it is, of course, prudent as a precautionary measure to avoid exposure to drugs, alcohol and tobacco, environmental chemicals, and radiation during pregnancy as much as possible. In Table 34 substances generally accepted as interfering with human development and reproduction are compiled.

Extrapolating Animal Data to a Situation Possibly Existing in Humans

There is a most important prerequisite to detect the potential for eliciting embryo- and fetotoxic effects in humans from the outcome of animal studies. One must assume that such *potential* can be detected by the outcome in routine animal tests. As for all of toxicology and its reliance on animal-testing data, this will be a matter of sensitivity and specificity. "Sensitivity" is defined as ability to detect all relevant agents (all correct positives), missing as few as possible (classifying none as false negatives). "Specificity" is defined as not responding to irrelevant agents (no false positives) but correctly recognizing them as such (to reveal all correct negatives). Generally speaking, the sensitivity of the common pregnant-animal models (e.g., rats, mice, and rabbits) may be considered to be rather high, but the specificity may be rather low, and the special toxic potential may be assessed at the expense of many false positives. This is the principle of a preventive hazard minimization, that is, we would rather be mistaken on the safe side. The situation is not much different from that existing with respect to detecting a carcinogenic potency with relevance for humans.

The following accumulated observations may serve to illustrate the situation. Among more than 4000 chemicals and drugs that have undergone conventional developmental toxicity testing in common laboratory animals, more than 900 have revealed the potential of eliciting such toxicity. However, fewer than 30 agents are recognized as established or strongly suspected human developmental toxicants (or teratogens). The apparently low percentage of recapitulating in humans the positive results from animal tests should not be interpreted to mean that the animal data are irrelevant for hazard minimization in pregnant women. Quite the contrary, the adverse effects in the animal studies often were observed at very high doses with no relevance for the anticipated human exposure levels. Furthermore, in meeting the objectives of hazard minimization studies to provide primary prevention, production and use of many chemicals that have revealed a developmental toxicity potential in laboratory animal testing will not be continued. The suspicion of developmental toxicity activity will lead to the precautionary termination of the production, and the risk for humans will remain unknown forever. Confidence in the philosophy of the present animal testing strategy seems to be justified by more than 3 decades of experience, and as a consequence the likelihood of another major malformation disaster appears remote, short of accidental or catastrophic exposure during human pregnancy. The validity of this assumption could be greatly enhanced by the availability of pharmacokinetic data from the test animal and humans.

It should be considered that the relative duration of certain specific developmental stages is different in various species. This is especially true for the relatively short gestational phase of rodents in contrast to humans (Table 35) and a very long fetal phase in primates. A single dose of a substance with embryotoxic potential may not lead to the same consequences in laboratory animals and humans. Because of the longer duration of some developmental stages in humans, the ability to repair a lesion could be improved.

Quantitative Extrapolation of Animal Data to a Situation Postulated to Exist in Humans

In the course of a preventive hazard minimization for human pregnancy, quantitative extrapolations from animal data are commonly performed. These may be divided into two approaches.

- Extrapolation on the basis of doses, using a safety (uncertainty) factor approach. This is presently done by using a no observed adverse effect level (NOAEL) for the most sensitive endpoint of developmental toxicity in the most sensitive species. The safety factor applied is arbitrarily chosen between 10 and 1000. An alternative is the benchmark dose concept. While for medicinal drugs in Europe an uncertainty factor of 10 is often considered to be sufficient, for environmental chemicals this factor is at least 100 in the United States: a factor of 10 for interindividual differences and 10 for interspecies differences, if a NOAEL is available. If there is no NOAEL, an additional factor of 10 is used, that is, 1000 overall.
- Extrapolation on the basis of comparative kinetic data (from humans and the experimental animal species). Again a NOAEL and safety factor approach, or the benchmark dose concept, may be used.

TABLE 35 Rough Comparison of the Length of Developmental Periods in Rats and Humans[a]

Developmental period	Approximate duration of the developmental period (days) Rat	Humans	Ratio Humans/Rat
Implantation	5 to 6	6 to 10	<2×
Neural plate → closure of neuroporus	9 to 11	18 to 27	3×
Fusion of heart tubes → complete septum	9 to 15	21 to 46	4×
Eye vesicle → complete lens	10 to 12	24 to 35	4×
Limb buds → cartilaginous phalanges	11 to 14	26 to 44	5×
"Embryonic" phase[b]	6 to 16	15 to 63	5×
"Fetal" phase	17 to 22	63 to 266	34×
Total gestational period (days)	22	266	12×

[a]Data from Neubert *et al.* (1987). This complication may only provide a rough overview because of considerable strain differences, etc. From Klug and Neubert (1992).

[b]From the trilaminar embryo to palatal closure.

It must be stressed that the NOAEL is not a dose at which no effect can be observed—it refers to the specific study and the evaluated endpoints only. There are a number of variables that make the NOAEL from a routine study an imprecise value.

- The number of animals used is rather small.
- The dose groups are few and the doses are not chosen sufficiently close together.
- The NOAEL has a confidence limit and is not an exact value.
- There is a statistical error when comparing groups of treated animals with the concurrent controls, especially when variable spontaneous rates exist for the endpoint.
- When repeating a study, which is typically not done, the NOAEL will probably be not completely identical.
- The NOAEL is restricted to the endpoints evaluated.

Extrapolations on the basis of dose–effect data in animal models is quite unsatisfactory because it is well known that large species differences exist with respect to kinetics. It makes little difference whether a NOAEL or the benchmark concept is used because a high safety factor must compensate for the considerable uncertainty. In the benchmark dose attempt, which is a modification of the NOAEL and safety factor approach, some information on the dose–response relationship is incorporated into the hazard minimization, but such data must be available (which is most often not the case). From these dose–response data, a dose with a defined low incidence of a selected adverse outcome endpoint (e.g., ED_5, ED_{10}, or ED_{20}) is selected, and again a safety factor is applied. The improvement obtained with this suggestion should not be overestimated because the low incidence selected cannot be determined with real data from the majority of the studies with sufficient accuracy. The advantage is more theoretical than practical. It remains an administrative regulatory agency proposition and does not become a scientific procedure.

Extrapolations based on comparative kinetic data provide the scientifically best approach that is routinely available. It requires comparative kinetic data from humans and the experimental animal species. In general such data are available for newly developed pharmaceutical products, or the necessary tests can be conducted to provide these data. It is then assessed for example, whether the plasma concentrations required for an effect in animal tests (or at a NOAEL) will be reached at the exposures levels anticipated in humans for therapeutic efficacy.

A few attempts have been made to use biologically based mathematical models for risk assessment. Although this may have a number of advantages in the future, good kinetic data from humans and the animal species are also required, in addition to a great number of physiological data from the two species to be compared. The conventional tests do not provide these data.

Although comparative kinetic data provide the best approach available, this strategy also suffers from a number of inadequacies:

- The elimination half-lives in rodents and humans are typically quite different. Therefore, kinetic studies in the animal species must be performed in a way comparable to human exposures (Fig. 13). This often requires another route and/or mode of application in the animal than in humans. A prerequisite for proper animal experimental design is that data on humans are available at the early stages of animal testing.
- Metabolism in the animal species and in humans should be comparable. Otherwise, the main metabolites from humans will have to be tested in the animal in separate studies. Unfortunately, metabolic profiles often exhibit quite pronounced species differences.
- The kinetic data from humans are seldom available for environmental chemicals, although they could be easily obtained in clinical trials without putting human subjects into unjustifiable danger. The strategy based on kinetic data is impossible to apply without the appropriate information.

Preventive hazard minimization with respect to environmental substances most often ends up as a semiquantitative or even qualitative approach.

Developments Concerning Testing Guidelines and Promising Innovations

There have been considerable changes that affect the design and conduct of safety evaluation studies to detect reproductive hazard potential of chemical and pharmaceutical products.

For quite some time, all such studies have had to comply with the strict quality assurance and record-keeping standards spelled out in great detail in documents that are internationally known as the regulations of "good laboratory practices" (GLP). For many years the design of conventional testing studies was dominated by strict adherence to written test guidelines by both the investigators and the regulators in governmental agencies. The work conducted in experimental biology has brought considerable progress applicable to the science of toxicology. The new insights need to be applied to the scientific issues at hand in toxicology. Revisions of the reproductive and developmental toxicity testing guidelines in Europe and in the United States have granted the investigator more responsibility and freedom in conducting GLP-governed guideline safety evaluation studies. It is now possible for the investigator to adapt the testing procedures to special situations caused by the properties of a specific agent under evaluation. This change will also require the officials in regulatory agencies to change their review approach and be more open to concepts that have emerged from toxicological research and can be defended based on scientific knowledge.

The exposure duration may now be extended into the preimplantation phase and have to cover almost the entire fetogenesis period. For example, partially in response to the high priority attached to the endocrine system-altering activity of chemicals, the exposure duration in developmental toxicity studies now lasts to near term. This is in recognition of the fact that important aspects of prenatal sexual differentiation occur in the late fetal stages of development. Under the old study guidelines, chemical exposure stopped before this period. Furthermore, new endpoints of potential manifestations of toxicity in the ovary and testes need to be examined in reproduction studies.

Another considerable achievement was the harmonization of the diverging test guidelines existing in various countries, especially the United States, the EU, and Japan. The global operations of internationally engaged pharmaceutical and chemical companies and international market developments have made universally agreed-upon guidelines for initial hazard identification studies (primary-stage testing) very desirable. Appropriate methods for further studies must be used if additional tests are necessary based on the outcome of primary testing. The design of appropriate follow-up studies requires a high degree of expertise from both the investigator and the individuals responsible for review in regulatory governmental agencies.

Bibliography

Abraham, K., Knoll, A., Ende, M., Päpke, O., and Helge, H. (1996). Intake, fecal excretion, and body burden of polychlorinated dibenzo-*p*-dioxins and dibenzofurans in breastfed and formula-fed infants. *Pediatr. Res.* **40,** 671–679.

Adami, H. O., Lipworth, L., Titus-Ernstoff, L., Hsieh, C.-C., Hanberg, A., Ahlborg, U., Baron, J., and Trichopoulos, D. (1995). Organochlorine compounds and estrogen-related cancers in women. *Cancer Causes Control* **6,** 551–566.

Ashby, J., Houthoff, E., Kennedy, S. J., Stevens, J., Bars, R., Jekat, F. W., Campbell, P., Miller, J. V., Carpanini, F. M., and Randall, G. L. P. (1977a). The challenge posed by endocrine disrupting chemicals. *Environ. Health Perspect.* **105,** 164–169.

Ashby, J., Odum, J., Tinwell, H., and Lefevre, P. A. (1997b). Assessing the risks of adverse endocrine-mediated effects: Where to from here? *Regulat. Pharmacol. Toxicol.* **26,** 80–93.

Bancroft, J. (1993). Impact of environment, stress, occupational, and other hazards on sexuality and sexual behaviour. *Environ. Health Perspect.* **101 (suppl),** 101–107.

Barlow, S. M., and Sullivan, F. M. (1982). "Reproductive Hazards of Industrial Chemicals." Academic Press, London.

Beck, H., Droβ, A., Ende, M., Fürst, C., Fürst, P., Hille, A., Mathar, W., and Wilmers, K. (1991). Polychlorierte Dibenzofurance und -dioxine in Frauenmilch. *Bundesgesundheitsblatt* **34,** 564–659.

Bibbo, M., Gill, W. B., Azizi, E., Blough, R., Fang, V. S., Rosenfield, R. L., Schumacher, G. F. B., Sleeper, K., Sonek, M. G., and Wied, G. L. (1977). Follow-up study of male and female offspring of DES-exposed mothers. *Obstetr. Gynecol.* **49,** 1–8.

Bjerke, D. L., Sommer, R. J., Moore, R. W., and Peterson, R. E. (1994). Effects of in utero and lactational 2,3,7,8-tetrachlorodibenzo-*p*-dioxin exposure on responsiveness of the male rat reproductive system to testosterone stimulation in adulthood. *Toxicol. Appl. Pharmacol.* **127,** 250–257.

Bouié, J., Philippe, E., Giroud, A., and Bouié, A. (1976). Phenotypic expression of lethal chromosomal anomalies in human abortuses. *Teratology* **14,** 3–20.

Carney, E. W., *et al.* (1997). Estrogen modulation: tiered testing for human hazard evaluation. *Reprod. Toxicol.* **11,** 879–892.

Chahoud, I., Krowke, R., Schimmel, A., Merker, H.-J., and Neubert, D. (1989). Reproductive toxicity and pharmacokinetics of 2,3,7,8-tetrachlorodibenzo-*p*-dioxin: 1. Effects of high doses on the fertility of male rats. *Arch. Toxicol.* **63,** 432–439.

Chambon, P. (1994). The retinoid signaling pathway: molecular and genetic analyses. *Sem. Cell Biol.* **5,** 115–125.

Colburn, T., and Clement, C. (eds.) (1992). "Chemically-Induced Alterations in Sexual and Functional Development." Princeton Scientific.

Daston, G. P., Gooch, J. W., Breslin, W. J., Shuey, D. L., Nikiforov, A. I., Fico, T. A., and Gorsuch, F. W. (1997). Environmental estrogens and reproductive health: A discussion of the human and environmental data. *Reprod. Toxicol.* **11,** 465–481.

Edwards, M. J., Shiota, K., Smith, M. S. R., and Walsh, D. A. (1995). Hyperthermia and birth defects. *Reprod. Toxicol.* **9,** 411–425.

Eto, K. (1997). Pathology of Minamata disease. *Toxicol. Pathol.* **25,** 614–623.

Faqi, A. S., Dalsenter, P. R., Merker, H.-J., and Chahoud, I. (1998). Reproductive toxicity and tissue concentrations of low doses of 2,3,7,8-tetrachlorodibenzo-p-dioxin in male offspring rats exposed throughout pregnancy and lactation. *Toxicol. Appl. Pharmacol.* **150,** 383–392.

German, J., Kowal, A., and Ehlers, K. H. (1970). Trimethadione and human teratogenesis. *Teratology* **3,** 349–361.

Golden, R. J., Noller, K. L., Titus-Ernstoff, L., Kaufman, R. H., Mittendorf, R., Stillman, R., and Reese, E. A. (1998). Environmental endocrine modulators and human health: an assessment of the biological evidence. *Crit. Rev. Toxicol.* **28,** 109–227.

Gray, L. E., Jr. *et al.* (1997). Endocrine screening methods workshop report: detection of estrogenic and androgenic hormonal and antihormonal activity for chemicals that act via receptor or steroidogenic enzyme mechanisms. *Reprod. Toxicol.* **11,** 719–750.

Greco, T. L., Duello, T. M., and Gorski, J. (1993). Estrogen receptors, estradiol, and diethylstilbestrol in early development: the mouse as a model for the study of estrogen receptors and estrogen sensitivity in embryonic development of male and female reproductive tracts. *Endocrine Rev.* **14,** 59–71.

Heger, W., Klug, S., Schmahl, H.-J., Nau, H., Merker, H.-J., and Neubert, D. (1988). Embryotoxic effects of thalidomide derivatives in the non-human primate *Callithrix jacchus:* 3. Teratogenic potency of the EM 12 enantiomers. *Arch. Toxicol.* **62,** 205–208.

Heinonen, O. P., Slone, D., and Shapiro, S. (1977). "Birth Defects and Drugs in Pregnancy." Science Group Inc., Littleton, MA.

Hendrickx, A. G. (1972). A comparison of temporal factors in the embryological development of man, old world monkeys and galagos, and craniofacial malformations induced by thalidomide and triamcinolone. *In* "Medical Primatology" (E. I. Goldsmith and J. Moor-Jankowski, eds.), pp. 259–269. Karger, Basel.

Henkel, L., and Willert, H. E. (1969). Dysmelia. A classification and pattern of malformations in a group of congenital defects of the limbs. *Br. J. Bone Joint Surg.* **51,** 399–414.

Herbst, A. L., Cole, P., Colton, T., Robboy, S. L., and Scully, R. E. (1977). Age-incidence and risk of diethylstilbestrol-related clear cell adenocarcinoma of the vagina and cervix. *Am. J. Obstet. Gynecol.* **128,** 43–48.

Herbst, A. L., Ulfelder, H., and Poskanzer, D. C. (1971). Adenocarcinoma of the vagina. Association of maternal stilbestrol therapy with tumor appearance in young women. *N. Engl. J. Med.* **284,** 878–881.

Holzgreve, W., Carey, J. C., and Hall, B. D. (1976). Warfarin induced fetal abnormalities. *Lancet* **2,** 914–915.

Hunter, D. J., Hankinson, S. E., Laden, F., Colditz, G. A., Manson, J. E., and Willett, W. C., Speizer, F. E., and Wolff, M. S. (1997). Plasma organochlorine levels and the risk of breast cancer. *N Engl. J. Med.* **337,** 1253–1258.

IARC (1979). Sex hormones (II). WHO, Lyon. *IARC Monographs on the Evaluation of the Carcinogenic Risk of Chemicals to Humans* **21,** 11–561.

International Clearinghouse (1991). "Congenital Malformations Worldwide. A Report from the International Clearinghouse for Birth Defects Monitoring Systems." Elsevier Science, Amsterdam.

Jones, K. L., Smith, D. W., Ulleland, C. N., and Streissguth, A. P. (1973). Pattern of malformation in offspring of chronic alcoholic mothers. *Lancet* **1,** 1267–1271; **2,** 999–1001.

Katzenellenbogen, B. S., Montano, M. M., Kraus, W. L., Aronica, S. M., Fujimoto, N., and LeGoff, P. (1995). Estrogen-receptor and antiestrogen-receptor complexes: cell- and promotor-specific effects and interactions with second messenger signaling pathways. *In* "Organ-Selective Actions of Steroid Hormones" (D. T. Baird *et al.*, eds.), pp. 29–50, Ernst Schering Research Foundation Workshop 16. Springer-Verlag, Berlin.

Kavlock, R. J., and Daston, G. P. (1997). "Handbook of Experimental Pharmacology, 124 I and II, Drug Toxicity in Embryonic Development." Springer Verlag, Berlin.

Kavlock, R. J., Daston, G. P., DeRosa, C. Fenner-Crisp, P., Gray, L. E., Kaattari, S., Lucier, G., Luster, M., Maczka, C. *et al.* (1996). Research needs for the risk assessment of health and environmental effects of endocrine disruptors: a report of the U.S. EPA-sponsored workshop. *Environ. Health Perspect.* **104 (suppl. 4),** 715–740.

Klug, S., Lewandowski, C., Wildi, L., and Neubert, D. (1989). All-*trans* retinoic acid and 13-*cis*-retinoic acid in the rat whole-embryo culture: Abnormal development due to the all-*trans* isomer. *Arch. Toxicol.* **63,** 440–444.

Klug, S., and Neubert, D. (1992). Possible contribution of in vitro methods to risk assessment in reproductive and developmental toxicology. *In* "Risk Assessment of Prenatally-induced Adverse Health Effects" (D. Neubert, R. J. Kavlock, H.-J. Merker, and J. Klein, eds.), pp. 449–473. Springer Verlag, Berlin.

Klug, S., and Thiel, R. (eds.) (1997). "Methods in Developmental Toxicology and Biology." Blackwell Science, Berlin.

Kochhar, D. M., and Satre, M. A. (1993). Retinoids and fetal malformations. *In* "Dietary Factors and Birth Defects" (R. P. Sharma, ed.) pp. 134–230. Pacific Division AAAS, San Francisco.

Lamb, D. J. (1997). Hormonal disruptors and male infertility: are men at serious risk? *Regulat. Pharmacol. Toxicol.* **26,** 30–33.

Lammer, E. J., Chen, D. T., Hoar, R. M., Agnish, N. D., Benke, P. J., Brasun, J. T., Curry, C. J., Fernhoff, P. M., Grix, A. W., Lott, I. T., Richard, J. M., and Sun, S. C. (1985). Retinoic acid embryopathy. *N. Engl. J. Med.* **313,** 837–841.

Lemoine, P., Harousseau, H., Boteyru, J. P., and Menuet, J. C. (1968). Les enfants de parents alcooliques: anomalies observées, a propos de 127 cas. *Quest. Med.* **25,** 477.

Lenz, W. (1985). Thalidomide embryopathy in Germany, 1959–1961. *In* "Prevention of Physical and Mental Congenital Defects, Part C: Basic and Medical Science, Education, and Future Strategies" (M. Marois, ed.), pp. 77–83. Alan R. Liss, Inc., NY.

Lipshultz, L. I., Ross, C. E., Ehorton, D., Milby, T., Smith, R., and Joyner, R. E. (1980). Dibromomonochloropropane and its effect on testicular function in man. *J. Urology* **124,** 464–468.

Mallidis, C., Howard, E. J., and Baker, H. W. G. (1991). Variation of semen quality in normal men. *Int. J. Androl.* **14,** 99–107.

Mastroiacovo, P., Spagnolo, A., Marni, E., Meazza, L., Bertoleini, R., and Segni, G. (1988). Birth defects in the Seveso area after TCDD contamination. *JAMA* **259,** 1668–1672.

Merker, H.-J., Heger, W., Sames, K., Stürje, H., and Neubert, D. (1988). Embryotoxic effects of thalidomide-derivatives in the non-human primate *Callithrix jacchus.* I. Effects of 3-(1,3-dihydro-1-oxo-2H-isoindol-2-yl)-2,6-dioxopiperidine (EM 12) on skeletal development. *Arch. Toxicol.* **61,** 165–179.

Miller, J. F., Williamson, E., and Glue, J. (1980). Fetal loss after implantation: a prospective study. *Lancet* **2,** 554–556.

Mocarelli, P. Brambilla, P., Gerthoux, P. M., Patterson, D. G., and Needham, L. L. (1996). Change in sex ratio with exposure to dioxin. Talking points (dioxin changes sex ratio?). *Lancet* **348,** 409.

Moore, K. L. (1982). "The Developing Human, Clinically Oriented Embryology," 3rd ed. Saunders, Philadelphia, PA.

Murakami, U. (1972). The effect of organic mercury on intrauterine life. *Adv. Exp. Med. Biol.* **27,** 301–336.

Murphy, D. P. (1929). The outcome of 625 pregnaancies in women subjected to pelvic radium or roentgen irradiation. *Am J. Obstet. Gynecol.* **18,** 179–187.

Nagel, S. C., vom Saal, E. S., Thayer, K. A., Dhar, M. G., Boechler, M., and Welshons, W. V. (1997). Relative binding affinity-serum modified access (RBA-SMA) assay predicts the relative in vivo bioactivity of the xenoestrogens bisphenol A and octylphenol. *Environ. Health Perspect.* **105,** 70–76.

Nau, H. (1993). Teratogenesis, transplacental pharmacokinetics, and metabolism of some retinoids in the mouse, monkey and human. *In* "Retinoids. Progress in Research and Clinical Applications" (M. A. Livrea and L. Packer, eds.), pp. 599–616. Marcel Dekker, Inc., NY.

Nau, H., Hauk, R.-S., and Ehlers, K. (1991). Valproic acid induced neural tube defects in mouse and humans: Aspects of chirality, alternative drug development, pharmacokinetics and possible mechanisms. *Pharmacol. Toxicol.* **69,** 310–321.

Nau, H., and Scott, W. J. (eds.) (1986). "Pharmocokinetics in Teratogenesis." CRC Press, Boca Raton, FL.

Neubert, D. (1988). Significance of pharmacokinetic variables in reproductive and developmental toxicity. *Xenobiotics* **18,** 45–58.

Neubert, D. (1997). Vulnerability of the endocrine system to xenobiotic influence. *Regulat. Toxicol. Pharmacol.* **26,** 9–29.

Neubert, D., Barrach, H.-J., and Merker, H.-J. (1980). Drug-induced damage to the embryo or fetus (molecular and multilateral approach to prenatal toxicology). *In* E Grundmann (ed) "Current Topics in Pathology" (E. Grundmann, ed.), Vol. 69, pp. 241–331. Springer-Verlag, Berlin.

Neubert, D., Bochert, G., Platzek, T., Chahoud, I., Fischer, B., and Meister, R. (1987). Dose-response relationships in prenatal toxicology. *Cong. Anom.* **27,** 275–302.

Neubert, D., and Chahoud, I. (1985). Significance of species and strain differences in pre- and perinatal toxicology. *Acta Histochem.* **31,** 23–35.

Neubert, D., Chahoud, I., Platzek, T., and Meister, R. (1987). Principles and problems in assessing prenatal toxicity. *Arch Toxicol* **60,** 238–245.

Neubert, D., Heger, W., Merker, H.-J., Sames, K., and Meister, R. (1988). Embryotoxic effects of thalidomide derivatives in the non-human primate *Callithrix jacchuns*. II. Elucidation of the susceptible period and of the variability of embryonic stages. *Arch. Toxicol.* **61,** 180–191.

Neubert, D., Kavlock, R. J., Merker, H.-J. and Klein, J., (eds.) (1992). "Risk Assessment of Prenatally-induced Adverse Health Effects." Springer-Verlag, Berlin.

Neubert, D., and Merker, H.-J. (eds.) (1981). "Culture Techniques. Applicability for Studies on Prenatal Differentiation and Toxicity." de Gruyter, Berlin.

Neubert, D., Merker, H.-J., Hendrickx, A. G., (eds.) (1988). "Non-Human Primates, Developmental Biology and Toxicology." Ueberreuter Wissenschaft, Wien.

Neubert, D., Merker, H.-J., Kwasigroch, T. E., Kreft, R., and Bedürftig, A. (eds.) (1977). "Methods in Prenatal Toxicology." Georg Thieme Verlag, Stuttgart.

Neubert, R., Hiinz, N., and Thiel, R. (1997b). Embryonic development and surface integrin receptors. *In* "Methods in Developmental Toxicology/Biology" (S. Klug and R. Thiel, eds.), pp. 209–226. Blackwell Science, Berlin.

Neubert, R., Hinz, N., Thiel, R., and Neubert, D. (1995). Down-regulation of adhesion receptors on cells of primate embryos as a probable mechanism of the teratogenic action of thalidomide. *Life Sci.* **58,** 295–316.

Neubert, R., and Neubert, D. (1997a). Peculiarities and possible mode of actions of thalidomide. *In* "Handbook of Experimental Pharmacology, 124/II, Drug Toxicity in Embryonic Development" (R. J., Kavlock and G. P., Daston eds.), pp. 41–119. Springer Verlag, Berlin.

O'Rahilly, R., and Müller, F. (1992). "Human Embryology and Teratology." Wiley-Liss Inc, New York.

Otake, M., and Schull, W. J. (1984). In-utero exposure to A-bomb radiation and mental retardation: a reassessment. *Br. J. Radiol.* **57,** 409–414.

Pabelick, C., Kemmer, F., and Koletzko, B. (1991). Befunde bei Neugeborenen nierentransplantierter Mütter. *Monatsschr. Kinderheilk.* **139,** 136–140.

Pauli, R. M. (1997). Anticoagulants. *In* "Handbook of Experimental Pharmacology, 124/II, Drug Toxicity in Embryonic Development II" (R. J. Kavlock and G. P. Daston, eds.), pp. 191–229. Springer Verlag, Berlin.

Pelkonen, O., Jouppila, P., and Kärki, N. T. (1972). Effect of maternal cigarette smoking on 3,4-benzpyrene and N-methyl-aniline metabolism in human fetal liver and placenta. *Toxicol. Appl. Pharmacol.* **23,** 399–407.

Platzek, T., Bochert, G., Meister, R., and Neubert, D. (1992). Prenatal-toxic risk estimation based on dose-response relationships and molecular dosimetry. *In* "Risk Assessment of Prenatally-Induced Adverse Health Effects" (D. Neubert *et al.*, eds.), pp. 245–266. Springer Verlag, Berlin.

Platzek, T., Bochert, G., Meister, R., and Neubert, D. (1993). Embryotoxicity induced by alkylating agents: 7. Low dose prenatal-toxic risk estimation based on NOAEL risk factor approach, Dose-response relationships, and DNA adducts using methylnitrosourea as a model compound. *Teratogen. Carcinogen. Mutagen.* **13,** 101–125.

Platzek, T., Meister, R., Chahoud, I., Bochert, G., Krowke, R., and Neubert, D. (1986). Studies on mechanisms and dose-response relationships of prenatal toxicity. *In* F. Welsch (ed) "Approaches to Elucidate Mechanisms in Teratogenesis" (F. Welsch, ed.), pp. 59–81. Hemisphere, Washington, D.C.

Rama Sastry, B. V. (1995). Chapter 3. "Placental Toxicology," pp. 45–81. CRC Press, Boca Raton, FL.

Regulat. Pharmacol. Toxicol. (1997). **26.**

Rier, S. E., Martin, D. C., Bowman, R. E., Dmowski, W. P., and Becker, J. L. (1993). Endometriosis in rhesus monkeys (*Macaca mulatta*) following chronic exposure to 2,3,7,8-tetrachlorodibenzo-*p*-dioxin. *Fundam. Appl. Toxicol.* **21,** 433–441.

Robert, E., and Guibaud, P. (1982). Maternal valproic acid and congenital neural tube defects. *Lancet* **2,** 937.

Roman, B. L., Sommer, R. J., Shinoyima, K., and Peterson, R. E. (1995). In utero and lactational exposure of the male rat to 2,3,7,8-tetrachlorodibenzo-*p*-dioxin: impaired prostate growth and development without inhibited androgen production. *Toxicol. Appl. Pharmacol.* **134,** 241–250.

Schardein, J. L. (1993). "Chemically Induced Birth Defects," 2nd ed., Dekker, New York.

Schardein, J. L., and Keller, K. A. (1989). Potential human developmental toxicants and the role of animal testing in their identification and characterization. *CRC Crit. Rev. Toxicol.* **19,** 251–338.

Schulz, T., and Neubert, D. (1993). Peculiarities of biotransformation in the pre- and postnatal period. *In* "Frontiers in Biotransformation, 9, Regulation and Control of Complex Biological Processes by Biotransformation" (K. Ruckpaul, H. Rein, ed), pp. 162–214. Akademie Verlag, Berlin.

Shepard, T. H. (1992). "Catalog of Teratogenic Agents," 7th ed. Johns Hopkins University Press, Baltimore, MD.

Shiota, K. (1993). Teratothanasia: Prenatal loss of abnormal conceptuses and the prevalence of various malformations during gestation. *In* "Birth Defects: Original Article Series" (March of Dimes Birth Defects Foundation) **29,** 189–199.

Slotkin, T. A. (1998). Fetal nicotine or cocaine exposure: which one is worse? *J. Pharmacol. Exp. Ther.* **285,** 931–945.

Spohr, H.-L., and Steinhausen, H. C. (1987). Follow-up studies of children with fetal alcohol syndrome. *Neuropediatric* **18,** 13–17.

Springer, T. A. (1990). Adhesion receptors of the immune system. *Nature* **346,** 425–434.

Stahlmann, R., and Klug, S. (1997). Antiviral agents. *In* "Handbook of Experimental Pharmacology, 124/II, Drug Toxicity in Embryonic Development II" (R. J. Kavlock and G. P. Daston, eds.), pp. 231–264. Springer Verlag, Berlin.

Stahlmann, R., Merker, H.-J., Hinz, N., Chahoud, I., Webb, J., Heger, W., and Neubert, D. (1990). Ofloxacin in juvenile non-human primates and rats. Arthropathia and drug plasma concentrations. *Arch. Toxicol.* **64,** 193–204.

Steinberger, E. (1992). Disorders of the male reproductive system. *In* "Principles and Practice of Environmental Medicine" (A. Bezman Tarcher, ed.), pp. 437–457. Plenum Medical, New York.

Stephens, T. D. (1988). Proposed mechanisms of action in thalidomide embryopathy. *Teratology* **38,** 229–239.

Wald, N. (1993). Folic acid and the prevention of neural tube defects. *Ann. NY Acad. Sci.* **678,** 112–129.

Weitzel, H. (1992). "Behinderungen im Kindesalter: Praxis der Vorsage." Umwelt & Medizin Verlagsgesellschaft. Frankfurt/M.

Welsch, F. (1987). "Approaches to Elucidate Mechanisms in Teratogenesis." Hemisphere, Washington, D.C.

Welsch, F. (1990). Short term methods of assessing developmental toxicity hazards. *In* "Issues and Reviews in Teratology," (H. Kalter, ed.), Vol. 5, pp. 1125–1153, Plenum Press, New York.

WHO (1984). "Principles for Evaluating Health Risks to Progeny Associated with Exposure to Chemicals during Pregnancy." Environmental Health Criteria (IPCS) 30, WHO, Geneva.

Whorton, D., Milby, T. H., Krauss, R. M., and Stubbs, H. A. (1979). Testicular function in DBCP exposed pesticide workers. *J. Occup. Med.* **21,** 161–166.

Whorton, M. D., and Milby, T. H. (1980). Recovery of testicular function among DBCP workers. *J. Occup. Med.* **22,** 177–179.

Wilson, J. G., and Fraser, G. C. (1977). "Handbook of Teratology." Plenum Press, New York.

Zappert, J. (1926). Über röntgenogene fetale Microcephalie. *Montsschr. Kinderheilkd.* **34,** 490–493.

C H A P T E R

22

Endocrine System—Adrenal Cortex, Thyroid, and Pancreas

MICHAEL J. THOMAS*, JOHN A. THOMAS†

*Department of Internal Medicine, University of Iowa, Iowa City, Iowa

†Department of Pharmacology, The University of Texas Health Science Center, San Antonio, Texas

INTRODUCTION

Organs or subpopulations of cells in the endocrine system, as well as the fetus and the neonate, can also be affected by drugs and chemicals. Teratogenesis is an important aspect of endocrine aberrations caused by some chemicals or drugs. Furthermore, various chemicals are toxic to the female reproductive system, to male accessory sex organs, and to specific subpopulations of cells within the male gonad. Organs like the thyroid gland, the adrenal gland, and the pancreas can also be affected by certain drugs and chemicals. Drugs and synthetic steroids can alter glandular internal secretions directly or by modifying trophic hormone secretion from the adenohypophysis. Unanticipated effects of drugs on endocrine function and on endocrine function tests can complicate the assessment of diagnostic procedures. The majority of all endocrine toxicities (about 90%) appear in the adrenal gland, the testes, and the thyroid gland (Table 1). Some endocrine target organs, such as the adrenal cortex, appear to be more vulnerable to toxic agents, and this may lead to multiple changes in hormonal balance. Chemically induced modifications in gonadal function can affect the thyroid gland, while chemically induced changes in sex steroids (e.g., estrogens) can affect the secretion of insulin or other organ systems.

Major alterations in endocrine secretion(s) have been recognized for decades, although more recently interest has focused on chemical- or drug-induced changes. Such chemically induced or drug-induced changes, particularly in view of more potent endocrine modulators, have become more prevalent and recognizable. Synthetically derived hormone antagonists or agonists (mimics) have an established presence in clinical endocrinology. Various hormone replacement therapies exhibit fewer adverse events than those hormonal agents that are used in therapeutic conditions involving supraphysiological doses. Classifications of endocrine toxicities have been proposed, some based upon clinical endocrine function and pathology, and some based upon adverse endocrine reactions to xenobiotics that have been observed clinically. The adverse effects of drugs on the endocrine system are nearly all due to normal or exaggerated pharmacological responses. It has been stated that the endocrine system of rats is sensitive to the toxicity of xenobiotics and that the endocrine system of the rat is second only to the liver as the most frequently affected target organ. Outcomes from a large number of potential therapeutic agents screened for their adverse effects on the endocrine system revealed only a small proportion of these compounds as possessing serious side effects. Furthermore, generalized stress can be considered to be a major contributing factor in causing altered endocrine secretions. Such a common etiology would certainly account for changes in adrenal

TABLE 1 Chemically Induced Lesions of the Endocrine System[a]

Frequency	Endocrine organ	
1	Adrenal gland	90% of all lesions
2	Testis	
3	Thyroid gland	
4	Ovary	
5	Pancreas	
6	Pituitary gland	
7	Parathyroid gland	

[a]Modified from Ribelin (1984) and Colby (1988).

gland secretions. However, it should be emphasized that these changes are not attributed to any toxicity.

ENDOCRINE MODULATION

Adenohypophysis

Excluding synthetic progestational agents (e.g., oral contraceptives) and morphine-like drugs, there is generally a paucity of specific studies examining the effects of xenobiotics on the pituitary gland or its secretions. It is possible, in part, that this is due to the relatively low exposure of pituitary cells to xenobiotics because the vascular supply and concentrating ability of the adenohypophysis are much less than those of other major organs of excretion and metabolism. On a molecular weight basis, the blood–brain barrier does not pose a deterrent to xenobiotics because many larger molecules gain entrance to the brain. Relative to certain endocrine target organs such as the gonad, there are far fewer reports describing chemically induced histopathologic lesions in the anterior pituitary gland. Furthermore, if the pituitary gland and/or its secretions are impacted by chemicals or drugs, it is often the blood or a peripheral endocrine target organ (e.g., gonads) that receives investigative attention. Pituitary–target organ relationships are important in predicting toxic manifestations in the endocrine system (Fig. 1). A rudimentary understanding of classical hormonal feedback systems is important in recognizing endocrine–target organ modulations or toxicities. While the measurement of specific hormone levels may not be economically feasible for general toxicological screening protocols, certain bioassays (e.g., gravimetric responses) and histopathological tests (e.g., liver morphology) may be expedient and useful. Ordinarily, chemically induced changes that alter the pituitary–target organ axis are manifest only after the multiple administrations of a toxic agent. Chemicals (e.g., goitrogens and pesticides) that have the potential of exerting deleterious effects on the endocrine system ordinarily require a longer duration of exposure and repeated administration. Although chemically induced stress can provoke a rapid response in catecholamine secretion and an outpouring of glucocorticoids, other hormonal responses would ordinarily not be so immediate. Xenobiotics (e.g., organochlorines and organophosphates) causing the induction of hepatic microsomal enzyme systems that are involved in hormone metabolism may require several days before changes in hormone levels occur.

It is important to understand the basic hormonal relationships between the adenohypophysis and their respective endocrine target organs (Fig. 1). Certain classes of therapeutically active drugs can perturb the release of trophic hormones or interfere with their synthesis (e.g., morphine, reserpine, and bromocriptine). Other toxic agents can exert inhibitory actions on the biosynthesis (e.g., aromatase inhibitors, 5α-reductase inhibitors, and DDD) of target organ hormone secretions. Hence, there are multiple levels of chemical interactions with the adenohypophyseal–target organ feedback systems. These sites of actions may differ in their sensitivity to toxic agents. Target organs such as the gonads are sensitive to toxic substances because rapidly dividing cells are often vulnerable to chemical insult. Environmental stresses can affect the secretory activity of certain hypothalamic-releasing hormones (e.g., corticotropin releasing factor, CRF) and alter pituitary–target organ relationships. Most anterior pituitary trophic hormones have a respective hypothalamic-releasing hormone or inhibitory factor. Trophic hormones can be either proteins or glycoproteins and ordinarily cannot be measured by standard spectrophotometric procedures. These hormones must either be bioassayed or measured by using radioimmunoassays (RIAs). Bioassays, once useful for assessing certain of the adenohypophyseal hormones, have been replaced by newer and more sensitive RIAs. Bioassays might be used when a secondary interest exists in determining whether a particular toxicological agent is affecting trophic hormone secretion or when a RIA is not readily available for certain species. Despite the more complex and involved RIAs methodologies, bioassays are of immense value for measuring different hormones. In contrast, RIAs represent an analytical, highly sensitive approach to measuring hormones. Such techniques have been applied to over 200 biological substances, many of which cannot be assayed by other methodologies. The greater

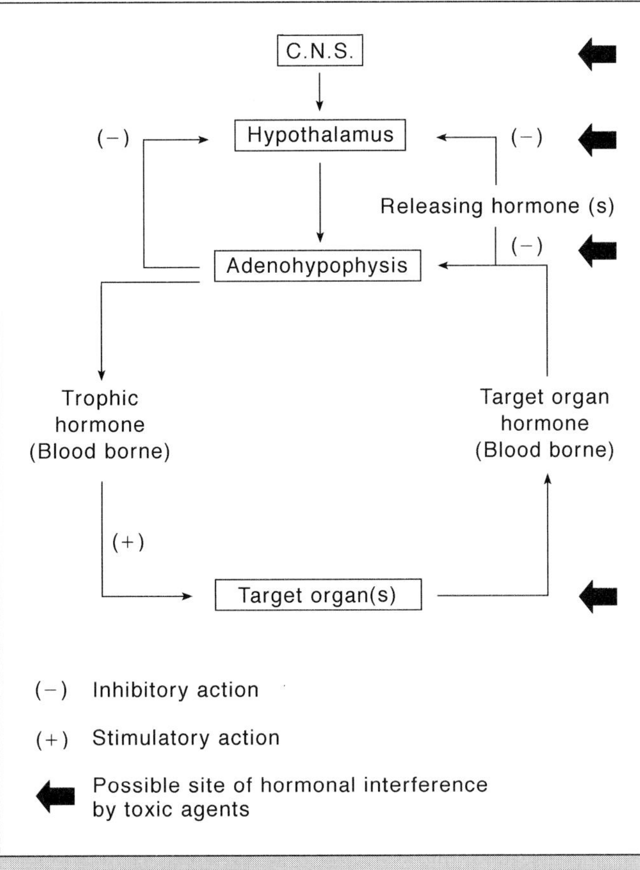

FIGURE 1 Relationship between adenohypophyseal–hypothalamic axis and hormone target organs Arrows indicate possible sites of perturbation. From *Principles and Methods of Toxicology*, pp. 1039–1063, Thomas and Thomas, Taylor & Francis, Washington, DC. Reproduced with permission.

sensitivity of RIAs can be attained using very small samples of biological specimens.

Hormones can be measured by competitive assays either by using an immune system or a nonimmune system. In the immune system assay, the antibody acts as the binding protein (e.g., insulin and ACTH), whereas in the nonimmune assay system the binding reagent is often a naturally occurring protein with a high affinity for the hormone being measured (e.g., cortisol and thyroxine). Monoclonal antibodies are also used in the measurement of hormones.

ADRENAL CORTEX

Physiologic Considerations

The adrenal cortex is a polyfunctional steroidogenic organ. Adrenal failure leads to significant and deleterious changes in electrolytes and carbohydrate metabolism leading to circulatory collapse, hypoglycemic, coma, and death. Steroid hormones of the adrenal cortex act at the level of gene expression to affect fundamental biochemical processes in the cell.

There are three major categories of adrenal steroid hormones mineralocorticoids, whose actions affect the body content of sodium and potassium; glucocorticoids, whose actions affect body fuel metabolism and responses to injury; and androgens, which function as male sex hormones. Mineralocorticoid secretions are controlled by the kidney through the secretion of renin and the consequent production of angiotensin. The secretion of glucocorticoids and androgens is modulated by the anterior pituitary gland through the secretion of corticotropin (ACTH). Members of an additional class of steroids, known as the neuroactive or neural steroids, are synthesized by the central nervous system (CNS) and appear to have specialized functions, but their function is poorly understood. The

TABLE 2 Agents Affecting the Adrenal Gland[a]

Adrenal medulla	
Acrylonitrile	Mannitol
ACTH	MPTP[b]
Alloxan	Neuroleptics
Blocadren	Nicotine
Chlordecone	Pyrazole
o-Chlorobenzylidine malononitrile	Reserpine
Cysteamine	Retionyl acetate
Dichloromethane	Sorbitol
7,12-Dimenthylbenzanthracene	Thiouracil
Estrogens	TSH
Growth hormone	Thyroid hormones
Interleukin-2	1,1,2-Trichloroethane
Lacitol	Xylitol
Lactose	
Malathion	
Adrenal cortex	
Acrylonitrile	Mefloquine
ACTH	Methanol
Aflatoxin	Nitrogen oxides
Aminoglutethimide	Parathion
Aniline	PBBs, PCBs
Carbon tetrachloride	Polyanthosulfonate plus aminocaprionic acid
Chenodeoxycholic acid	Polygulutamic acids
Chloroform	Pyrazole
Chlorphentermine	Spironolactone
Clotrimazole	Sulfated mucopolysaccharides
Cyproterone	Suramin
o′, *p′*-DDD	Tamoxifen
Danazol	Tetrachlorvinphos
Phenytoin (DPH)	Testosterone
7,12-Dimethylbenzanthracene	Thioacetamide
Estrogen	Thioguanine
Ethanol	Toxaphene
Etomidate	Triparanol
Fluphenazine	Urethane
Hexadimethrine bromide	Zimelidine
Iprindole	
Ketoconazole	

[a]Colby and Longhurst (1992); Thomas and Keenan (1986).
[b]Methyl-4-phenyl-1,2,3,6-tetrahydropyridine.

adrenal cortex and the medulla interact as a functional unit and integrate many biochemical changes in the internal or external environment. The adrenal medulla, or inner region, is a component of the sympathetic nervous system and participates in a wide array of regulatory responses that are characteristic of this division of the autonomic nervous system. The adrenal medulla is a neuroendocrine organ consisting of chromaffin cells, which synthesize and secrete epinephrine and norepinephrine in response to sympathetic nerve stimulation. Adrenal medullary tumors composed of neoplastic chromaffin cells are known as pheochromocytomas. Drugs such as reserpine and indolidan can produce pheochromocytomas in certain strains of rats. Many drugs and chemicals can produce lesions in the adrenal medulla (Table 2).

In humans, aldosterone is the principal mineralocorticoid, although deoxycorticosterone exhibits mineralocorticoid activity. Cortisol, the major glucocorticoid produced in humans, also has some mineralocorticoid activity. Aldosterone modulates body electrolytes and promotes the renal reabsorption of sodium in the ascending portion of the loop of Henle, in the distal tubule, and in the collecting tubule. It facilitates the urinary excretion of potassium and hydrogen ions. The excretion of hydrogen ions can produce alkalosis and an increased extracellular content of bicarbonate ions. Mineralocorticoid deficiencies produce a rise in extracellular fluid potassium concentration and reductions in sodium and chloride content that, if not restored, can lead to diminished cardiac output and death.

Cortisol (hydrocortisone), corticosterone, and cortisone all possess varying degees of glucocorticoid activity. Glucocorticoids regulate carbohydrate, protein, and fat metabolism. The glucocorticoids stimulate gluconeogenesis and decrease glucose utilization. Glucocorticoids produce a marked reduction in cellular protein content, although hepatic protein increases, as does the production of plasma protein by the liver. Glucocorticoids appear to interfere with the transport of amino acids into extrahepatic cells and, combined with the continuing protein catabolism in these cells, this results in an increase in plasma amino acids. Increased plasma amino acid levels and their subsequent transport into the liver may promote gluconeogenesis. Glucocorticoids also promote the mobilization of fatty acids from adipose tissue, which elevates plasma fatty acid levels. This effect, plus an increased oxidation of fatty acids in the cells, is probably involved in the switch from glucose utilization to fatty acids.

Corticosteroids bind to plasma proteins. Corticosteroid-binding globulin (CBG) has a high affinity, but a low binding capacity. Conversely, plasma albumin has a low affinity and a relatively high binding capacity. Physiologically, most of the hormone is bound to CBG; pharmacological doses quickly overload the total binding sites on CBG. In some steriodogenic tissues, there are agents (e.g., high doses of salicylates) that have been shown to lead to an increase in the level of steroid hormone biosynthesis. Many compounds (e.g., phenytoin–ACTH and oral contraceptives–FSH/LH) have been shown to inhibit both basal and hormone-stimulated steroid hormone synthesis. In the majority of steroidogenic tissues, these responses often arise from the stimulation by appropriate trophic hormones acting through the cyclic AMP second-messenger signaling pathway. The focus for this acutely regulated step in steroidogenesis appears to be determined by the transfer of the substrate cholesterol to the inner mitochondrial membranes. This family of mitochondrial proteins probably plays an important role in the regulation of acute steroidogenesis. These proteins have been termed steroidogenic acute regulatory (StAR) proteins. The extent to which StARs are affected by acute chemical and drug insult is not clear.

Pharmacological and Toxicological Effects

The adrenal cortex is very susceptible to chemical lesions. Several agents produce morphological or functional lesions in the adrenal gland (Table 2). Such lesions may be localized and in specific anatomical areas of the gland. Chemically induced changes can cause specific biochemical changes. Carbon tetrachloride causes adrenocortical necrosis, but its locus of toxicity is in the zona reticularis. Spironolactone, a mineralocorticoid antagonist, causes functional lesions in the zona fasciulata of the adrenal cortex. DDT metabolites (e.g., 3-methylsulfonyl-DDE) exert their adrenotoxicity by specifically binding to a nonextractable residue in the zona fasciculata. A number of cationic amphiphilic compounds produce adrenal cortical histologic lesions.

A variety of chemicals, such as acrylonitrile, produce adrenal necrosis in experimental animals. The acute adrenocorticolytic effect of acrylonitrile rapidly causes adrenal hemorrhage and necrosis. Cysteamine, a naturally occurring derivative of cysteine, and pyrazole produce lesions qualitatively similar to those produced by acrylonitrile. Repeated injections of DMBA (7,12-dimethylbenz[*a*]anthracene) produce mammary tumors in experimental animals and result in a slow progressive adrenal necrosis. In contrast to the single-dose administration of other adenocorticolytic agents (e.g., acrylonitrile and cysteamine), multiple injections of thioguanine are required to produce hemorrhagic necrosis of the adrenal cortex. Hexadimethrine bromide causes toxic damage to the zona glomerulosa and ischemic necrosis of the zonae fasciculata and reticularis.

Agents may directly or indirectly affect adrenal cortical secretions. The response of the adrenal gland to adrenocorticotropin (ACTH) may be compromised by chemically induced changes on membrane receptors, cyclic nucleotide levels, protein synthesis, and other biochemical processes involved in stimulating steroidogenesis. Changes in biochemical events in adrenal cortical secretions caused by chemicals can be mediated by several mechanisms. The vascularity of the adrenal cortex is excellent, so that the delivery of toxic agents is seldom a limiting factor. It is rich in lipids, and hence fat-soluble toxins are readily assimilated and sequestered in the adrenal gland. Both humans and guinea pigs have adrenal glands that are very adept at metabolizing xenobiotics. The capacity of the adrenal cortex to metabolize foreign substances is due, in part, to its high concentration of cytochrome P450. Xenobiotics undergo detoxification during metabolism, potentially resulting in more toxic intermediates. The production of more active metabolitics, bioactivation metabolites, may actually be associated with intermediates with greater inherent toxicities.

Triaryl phosphates (e.g., tricresyl phosphate, TCP, and butylated triphenyl phosphate, BTP) cause the inhibition of cholesteryl ester hydrolase. Cholesterol acyltransferase inhibitors are also adrenotoxic. Agents that inhibit acyl-CoA:cholesterol acyltransferase (ACAT), an enzyme that catalyzes the esterification of cholesterol, exerts a cytotoxic action on the adrenal gland. Steroidogenic tissues, including the adrenal cortex, are inhibited by triaryl phosphate and the butylated derivative (BTP). Both compounds, unlike aminoglutethimide, which inhibits steroid biosynthesis, do not interfere with the synthesis of corticosterone.

Adrenal activation of xenobiotics contributes to the frequency of chemically induced lesions in the gland. Differences in adrenal metabolism of xenobiotics among species may account for some differential toxicities. Adrenal xenobiotic-metabolizing P450 isozymes may also contribute to the overall toxicological actions of a compound.

THYROID GLAND

Physiological Considerations

In humans, normal thyroid hormone functioning is required to regulate the metabolism of virtually every organ. In all of these processes, thyroid hormone acts as an important modulator and has an indispensable role in growth and development. Normal thyroid function is a prerequisite for the normal development of the nervous system. The thyroid gland is an unusual endocrine gland because it not only is functionally dependent on the dietary intake of a single element, but also is the main epithelial component derived embyologically from the endoderm.

Thyroid or thyroid-like tissue is present in all vertebrates including fish. The human thyroid gland is anatomically situated at the base of the neck and surrounds the trachea. The two large lateral lobes that constitute the majority of the gland lie on either side of the trachea and are connected by a thin isthmus. The follicular cells of the thyroid are arranged in closed epithelial-lined spherical structures known as follicles. They possess a central lumen containing colloidal material. A normal secreting thyroid gland is termed euthyroidism. A hypersecreting thyroid gland leads to a condition called hyperthyroidism (thyrotoxicosis), whereas an undersecreting gland leads to hypothyroidism (myxedema). Congenital hypothyroidism results in cretinism and is characterized by mental retardation. Thyroid hyperplasia (goiters) may result from autoimmune or nutritional deficiency of iodine.

Pharmacological and Toxicological Effects

Understanding thyroid gland biochemistry is important to understanding endocrine toxicity. Thyroxine (T_4) and triiodothyronine (T_3) are biosynthesized in several steps, and toxic agents can inhibit this synthesis at several sites (Table 3). These agents can be categorized by their mechanism of toxic action(s). Still other drugs, such as salicylates, anticoagulants, phenytoin, and other classes of drugs, can alter thyroid function by affecting T_3 uptake, ^{131}I uptake, and thyroid-binding globulin concentrations (Table 4). Propylthiouracil (PTU), a therapeutic drug used in the

TABLE 3 Biochemical Inhibition of Thyroid Secretion[a]

Blockade of iodide trapping	Blockade of iodide oxidation	Mechanism not established
Chlorate	Amphenone	Acetazolamide
Hypochlorite	Carbimazole	Chlorpromazine
Iodate	Cobalt	Chlortrimeton
Nitrates	Methimazole	Thiopental
Perchlorate	*p*-Aminosalicylate	Tolbutamide
Thiocyanate	Phenylbutazone	
	Phenylinadanedione	
	Propylthiouracil	
	Resorcinol	

[a]Modified from Thomas and Keenan (1986). See also Atterwill *et al.* (1992).

TABLE 4 Drugs That Modify Thyroid Activity[a]

Drug or hormone	T_3 uptake	^{131}I uptake	Thyroid-binding globulin concentrations
Aminosalicylic acid	—	↓	—
Anabolic steroids	↑	—	↓
Anticoagulants (dicumarol and heparin)	↑	—	—
Anti-flammatory agents (phenylbutazone)	↑	↓	—
Indocyanine green (cardiogreen)	—	↓	—
Corticosteroids	—	↓	↓
Phenytoin (DPH)	↑	—	—
Oral contraceptives	↓	—	↑
Lithium carbonate	—	↑	—
Phenothiazines	—	↓	↓
Salicylates	↓	—	—
Sulfonamides	—	↓	—

[a]Modified from Thomas and Keenan (1986). See also Barsano and Thomas (1992); Atterwill *et al.* (1992); Gittoes and Franklin, (1995).

treatment of hyperthyroidism, decreases both T_3 and T_4. Phenoxyisobutyrate derivatives, such as clofibrate, produce histological changes in the thyroid gland.

Lithium, a commonly used drug for bipolar affective disorders, can produce hypothyroidism. Various mechanisms have been proposed for lithium's ability to cause thyroid dysfunction. It may act by directly inhibiting the iodine-concentrating capacity and interfering with the biosynthesis of iodotyrosine and iodothyronines. It may also inhibit the secretion of thyroid hormones by stabilizing the follicular cell microtubular systems. Amiodarone, an antiarrhythmic drug, can cause both hyperthyroidism or hypothyroidism. Amiodarone has specific inhibitory effects on agonist-stimulated functions in thyroid cells, perhaps by interfering with thyroid-stimulating hormone (TSH)–receptor interactions. Amiodarone contains large quantities of iodine (over 75% by molecular weight is iodine) and may bear some structural homology with thyroid hormone.

Some agents can affect the binding, distribution, and metabolism of thyroid hormones, but they seldom cause permanent alterations in thyroid function, primarily because of endocrine regulatory mechanisms (Tables 3–4). Prolonged thyroid hormone alterations caused by xenobiotics may lead to follicular-cell carcinogensis. Xenobiotic-induced thyroid tumor function may to be due to increased circulating levels of TSH, perhaps the result of increased metabolism of T_4 via hepatic enzymatic conjugation uridine diphosphate glucuronosyl transferase, (UDPGT). Increases in UGT activity might be a useful biomarker for tumorgenic changes in thyroid hormone levels subsequent to 2,3,7,8-tetrachlorodibenzo-*p*-dioxin (TCDD) exposure.

Natural and synthetic agents can alter thyroid gland function. Several plant toxins are considered natural goitrogens. Vegetables like broccoli, brussel sprouts, cauliflower, horseradish, mustard seed, and turnips contain a chemical class of compounds known as glucosinolates. Glucosinolates can be metabolized into thiocyanates and isothiocyanates, which are potent natural goitrogens. Garlic, onions, and chives contain 5-substituted cysteine sulfoxides, which are also natural goitrogens. Raw soybeans, in the absence of inadequate iodine uptake, may produce simple goiters. Heating the soybean destroys the natural goitrogens. Cassava, a starchy plant, contains considerable amounts of hydrogen cyanide, which produce an increased incidence of goiters.

Certain herbicides—chlorinated phenylureas, biscarbamates, substituted uracils, pyridazinones, and the diphenyl ethers—can produce changes in thyroid gland activity. Nitrofen, a halogenated nitrophenol with selective pre- and postemergence herbicide properties, reduces follicular size and colloidal density in

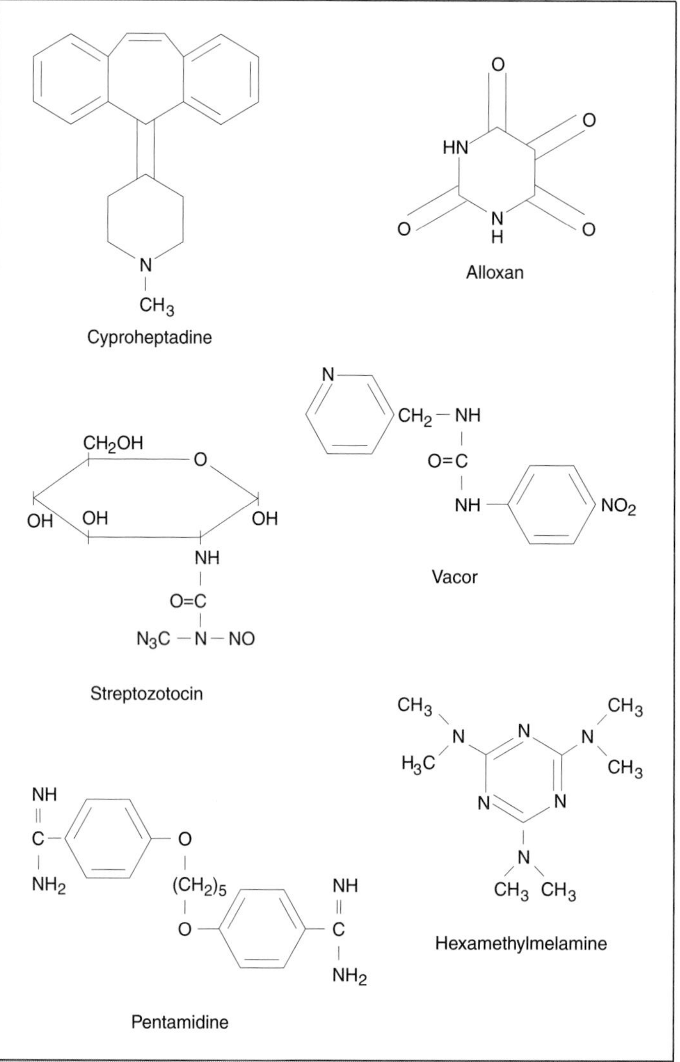

FIGURE 2 Chemical structures of diabetes producing compounds.

the thyroid gland. Triazines are herbicides that also suppress the thyroid. The prolonged feeding of amitrole to animals causes thyroid tumors. Amitrole inhibits thyroid peroxidase, leading to an increase in TSH and goitrogenicity. Aminothiazole has a direct action on the thyroid and acts by inhibiting T_4 synthesis and accelerating its deiodination. The herbicide 2-4-D can decrease serum protein-bound iodine. Fungicides like Nabam, Zineb, and Zuram are capable of inhibiting iodine uptake by the thyroid. Chlorine dioxide, an alternative disinfectant in municipal water supplies, may decrease T_4 concentrations. Thiazopyr, a fluorinated herbicide, causes an increase in thyroid follicular cell tumors in rats by enhancing TSH.

Reviewing the toxic effects of various industrial chemicals on the thyroid gland showed that polyhalogenated biphenyls (polychlorinated biphenyls, PCBs) affect thyroid gland metabolism in a number of animals. Experimental animals fed PCBs and polybrominated biphenyls (PBBs) develop goiters and hypothyroidism. It has been hypothesized that the ability of PCBs to induce hypothyroxinemia in mammals may be related to some aspects of their developmental neurotoxicity. Polyhalogenated dibenzodioxins and dibenzofurans (e.g., TCDD) can reduce serum T_4 concentrations in rats. At present, there is minimal evidence that these compounds produce thyroid dysfunction in humans. *In vitro,* several polyhydroxy-

TABLE 5 Diabetogenic Agents[a]

Agent	Use	Susceptible species
Alloxan	Experimental diabetes	Several
Streptozotocin	Experimental diabetes; anticancer agent	Several
Cyproheptadine	Antihistamine and anti-5-HT drug	Rodents
Hexamethylmelamine	Anticancer drug	Rat
PNU[b]	Rodenticide	Human

[a]Modified from Fischer (1985).
[b]Pyridymethylnitrophenylurea (PNU) (Vacor).

phenols, including resorcinol, catechol, hydroquinone, phloroglucinol, and orcinol, have been shown to inhibit thyroid peroxidase (TPO). These compounds are considerably more potent than propylthiouracil.

Various drugs and chemicals (e.g., thioamide drugs) act directly on the thyroid gland. In addition to the direct-acting antithyroidal agents, some drugs affect liver thyroid hormone-conjugating enzymes. Drugs that induce hepatic microsomal P450, such as phenobarbital and β-naphthoflavone, can cause hepatocellular and thyroid follicular cell hypertrophy. Some drugs that alter thyroid function act via the central nervous system (CNS) or the adenohypophysis. Phenytoin (DPH) results in a 50% decrease in the TSH response to thyrotropin-releasing hormone (TRH) by enhancing the cellular uptake and metabolism of T_4. High doses of aspirin can significantly suppress TSH responsiveness, possibly by the displacement of thyroid hormones from thyroid-binding globulin (TBG). The effects of L-dopa appear similar to those of aspirin. Multiple high doses of glucocorticoids can also impair basal and TRH-stimulated TSH levels.

PANCREAS (ENDOCRINE)

Physiological Considerations

The pancreas exhibits both exocrine and endocrine functions. Insulin and glucagon are hormones synthesized in the islets of Langerhans by β cells (insulin) and α cells (glucagon). The relationship between insulin and carbohydrate, fat, and protein metabolism, can be illustrated by diabetes mellitus (Type I). Insulin is an anabolic hormone that promotes sequestration of carbohydrate, fat, and protein in storage depots throughout the body. Its actions are exerted principally on skeletal muscle, liver, and adipose tissue, whereas those of glucagon are counter-regulatory to insulin, producing gluconeogenesis and glycogen breakdown in the liver. The interplay of these two hormones contributes to homeostasis in glucose concentrations and thus the availability of metabolic energy to all cells. Somatostatin is also an islet cell hormone, but its physiological role in the pancreas is unclear. Another peptide, pancreatic polypeptide, is also poorly understood. Glucagon acts in concert with other fuel-mobilizing hormones to balance the effects of insulin. In diabetes mellitus, hyperglycemia results from an impaired utilization of glucose.

Pharmacological and Toxicological Effects

Many chemicals or drugs can be toxic to pancreatic β cells (Fig. 2). There are few chemical similarities among the various pancreotoxic agents. Alloxan destroys pancreatic β cells and causes experimental diabetes mellitus. Alloxan has an avidity for pancreatic β cells and concentrates in this target organ. Alloxan is rapidly metabolized to dialuric acid, a product that undergoes autoxidation to yield amounts of peroxide, superoxide anion, and free radicals. Another β cell toxin is streptozotocin, whose toxic properties resides in its *N*-methylnitrosourea moiety. Streptozotocin is also an alkylating agent. Both alloxan and streptozotocin damage pancreatic DNA. Exposure to nitroso agents, such as streptozotocin and cycasin, induces long-lasting damage to the β cells.

Agents effective in producing hyperglycemia are referred to as diabetogenic substances (Table 5). Their biologic spectrum may vary, but their common toxicity resides in their ability to cause the destruction of pancreatic β cells. Although alloxan was probably the

TABLE 6 Possible Mechanisms of Drug-Induced Pancreatitis[a]

Mechanism	Drugs implicated
Pancreatic duct construction	Indomethacin
	Salicylates (via prostaglandin inhibition)
	Opiates
Immune suppression	Steroids
	Azathioprine
Cytotoxic effect	Azathioprine
	Colaspase (L-asparaginase)
Arteriolar thromboses	Estrogens
Osmotic effects	Contrast media
Pressure effects	Contrast media
Metabolic effects (ionic changes)	Thiazides
Direct cellular toxicity	Sulfonamides
	Furosemide
	Chlorothiazide
Possible hepatic mechanism (via free radicals)	Paracetamol (acetaminophen)
	Tetracyclines

[a]From Banerjee *et al.* (1989); Runzi and Laver (1996).

first agent used to produce β-cell necrosis, it has largely been replaced by the methylnitrourea analog streptozotocin to produce experimental insulin-dependent diabetes. Cyproheptadine (CHP), pentamidine, and hexamethylmelamine are also capable of suppressing the function and altering the morphology of insulin-secreting cells. Cyproheptadine, an antihistamine–antiserotonin drug, produces a reversible inhibition of insulin synthesis and release. Cyproheptadine and its analogs have a unique and specific action on the endocrine pancreas. Phenytoin (DPH) and diazoxide (proglycem) exert inhibitory effects on insulin secretion. They may also act by preventing the peripheral utilization of glucose. Diazoxide has a dual effect on insulin metabolism—it decreases insulin secretion and increases insulin-receptor binding. Thiazolidinedione and related compounds augment the action of insulin in insulin-resistant states.

Oral hypoglycemia drugs (e.g., sulfonylureas) can stimulate β-cell insulin secretion and are used therapeutically in noninsulin-dependent diabetes mellitus (NIDDM, Type II diabetes). Cyclosporin, a potent immunosuppressant agent, may temporarily ameliorate the requirement for insulin in insulin-dependent diabetes mellitus (IDDM, Type I), but its mechanism of action upon the β cell remains largely unknown. Cholecystokinin (CCK), an endogenous hormone capable of enhancing insulin secretion, can be antagonized by loxiglumide. Cholecystokinin antagonists may reduce the level of metabolic stress on the acinar cells and have been shown to mitigate the severity of acute pancreatitis. The CCK receptors reside in gall bladder and pancreatic membranes. Vanadate can mimic virtually all the biological effect of insulin.

Chemicals such as cobalt can selectively destroy the α cells of the pancreas. There are species differences with regard to α-cell destruction. The injection of cobalt chloride has been shown to produce degranulation and vacuolization of the α cells in rabbits, dogs, and guinea pigs.

While some agents (e.g., alloxan and streptozocin) produce destruction of β cells, leading to diabetogenic states, still others cause pancreatitis. Thus, both the endocrine and exocrine functions of the pancreas are vulnerable to inflammation and chemically induced necrosis. Drugs and chemicals that cause acute pancreatitis seldom produce chronic pancreatitis. Acute pancreatitis is frequently accompanied by increased blood levels of pancreatic enzymes, notably amylase. The mechanism(s) of cellular inflammation in pancreatitis is not understood, but several factors may contribute (Table 6). Drug-related episodes of pancreatitis are uncommon. Only a few drugs, such as tetracyclines, thiazides, salicylates, and vinca alkaloids, are consistently associated with acute pancreatitis. In many instances, preexisting unfavorable conditions in the presence of certain drugs can trigger acute inflammation of this organ. Adverse reactions of drugs have also been associated with causing acute pancreatitis (Table 7). Diuretic-induced changes in electrolytes appear to be correlated with acute pancreatitis, particularly in association with hyperamylasemia. Tetracy-

TABLE 7 Drugs Implicated as Causing Acute Pancreatitis[a]

Definite	Probable	Possible	
Azathiorine	Cimetidine	Bumetanide	ERCP contrast media
	Indomethacin	Anticholinesterase	Ethacrynic acid
Cisplatin	Mefenamic acid	Carbamazepine	Isoniazid
Colaspase (L-asparaginase)	Estrogens	Chlorthalidone	Isotretinoin (13-cis-retinoic acid)
	Opiates	Clonidine	Mercaptopurine
Frusemide (furosemide)	Paracetamol (acetaminophen)	Colchicine	Methyldopa
Tetracycline	Phenformin	Corticosteroids	Metronidazole
	Valproic acid	Cotrimoxazole	Nitrofurantoin
Thiazides	Fonofos	Cyclosporin	Oxphenbutazone
Sulfonamides	Diazinon	Cytarabine (cytosine arabinoside)	Piroxicam
		Diazoxide	Procainamide
		Enalapril	Rifampicin
		Ergotamine	Salicylates
			Sulindac

[a]Modified from Banerjee *et al.* (1989); Runzi and Layer (1996); Wilmink and Frick (1996).

clines may exert a direct pancreotoxicity; azathioprine suppresses the immune system yet also has a direct cytotoxic action. Certain drugs may exert direct cytotoxic action, such a valproic acid and possibly L-asparaginase, whereas allergic reactions are associated with sulfonamides. Although some drugs can cause acute pancreatitis, their mechanism(s) of toxicity is poorly understood. In others, some underlying aspects of the pathobiology of experimental acute pancreatitis are known. Animal models of pancreatic carcinoma have been induced by chemical carcinogens and by transgenic methods. Hence, drugs or chemicals exert short-term inflammatory responses in the pancreas, and their chronic effects may lead to tumorigenesis.

Several agents induce disorders of glucose metabolism (Tables 8 and 9). The effects of a drug on glucose metabolism may be due to a combination of factors involving the secretion and action of insulin as well as counter-regulatory hormones and responses. Table 8 reveals some possible hypoglycemic mechanisms. By far the most important agents causing hypoglycemia are insulin and sulfonylurea drugs. Alternatively, several drugs can produce hyperglycemia (Table 9). The adverse metabolic effects of a drug and their underlying mechanisms may provide important

TABLE 8 Possible Hypoglycemic Mechanisms of Some Commonly Used Drugs[a]

Decreased counterregulatory responses	Increased insulin secretion	Increased insulin sensitivity
ACE inhibitors	β sympathomimetics	ACE inhibitors
β blockers	Aspirin (acetylsalicylic acid)	α blockers
Alcohol (ethanol)	Disopyramide	Recombinant human insulin-like growth factor
Octreotide	Cibenzoline	
	Alcohol	
	Pentamidine	
	Quinine	
	Sulphonylureas	
	Cotrimoxazole (trimethoprim-sulfamethoxazole)	

[a]Chan *et al.* (1996).

TABLE 9 Possible Hyperglycemic Mechanisms of Some Commonly Used Drugs[a]

Increased counterregulatory responses	Reduced insulin secretion	Decreased insulin sensitivity
β sympathomimetics	β blockers	β blockers
Diazoxide	Diazoxide	Diuretics
Growth hormone	Diuretics	Corticosteroids
Corticosteroids	Ocetreotide	

[a]Chan *et al.* (1996).

insights into the control of glucose regulation and its potential for modulation.

Bibliography

Alemzadeh, R., Slonim, A. E., Zdanowicz, M. M., and Maturo J. (1993). Modifications of insulin resistance by diazoxide in obese Zucker rats. *Endocrinology* **133,** 705–712.

Atterwill, C. K., and Flack, J. D. (1992). Introduction to endocrine toxicology. In "Endocrine Toxicology" (C. K. Atterwill and J. D. Flack, eds.), pp. 1–11. Cambridge University Press.

Atterwill, C. K., Jones, C., and Brown, C. G. (1992). Thyroid gland II—Mechanisms of species-dependent thyroid toxicity, hyperplasia and neoplasia induced by xenobiotics. In "Endocrine Toxicology" (C. K. Atterwill and J. D. Flack, eds.), pp. 137–182. Cambridge University Press.

Banerjee, A. K., Patel, K. J., and Grainger, S. L. (1989). Drug-induced acute pancreatitis: A critical review. *Med. Toxicol. Adverse Drug Exp.* **4,** 86–198.

Barsano, C. P., and Thomas, J. A. (1992). Endocrine disorders of occupational and environmental origin. *Occupat. Med.* **7,** 479–502.

Bastomsky, C. H. (1977). Enhanced thyroxine metabolism and high uptake goiters in rats after a single dose of 2,3,7,8-tetrachlorodibenzo-*p*-dioxin. *Endocrinology* **101,** 292–296.

Baylis, P. H., and Tunbridge, W. M. G. (1985). Endocrine disorders. *In* "Texbook of Adverse Drug Reactions" (D. M. Davies, ed.) 3rd ed., pp. 335–351. Oxford Medical Publications.

Capen, C. C., and Martin, S. L. (1989). The effects of xenobiotics on the structure and function of thyroid follicular and C-cells. *Toxicol. Pathol.,* **17,** 266–293.

Chan, J. C. N., Cockram, C. S., and Critchley, J. A. J. H. (1996). Drug-induced disorders of glucose metabolism mechanisms and management. *Drug Safety* **15,** 135–157.

Chatterjee, A. K., Varayotha, V., and Fischer, L. J. (1991). Interactions of diabetogenic compounds: Cyproheptidine and alloxan. *Fundam. Appl. Toxicol.* **16,** 188–197.

Colby, H. D. (1988). Adrenal gland toxicity: Chemically induced dysfunction. *J. Am. Coll. Toxicol.* **7,** 45–69.

Colby, H. D., Huang Y., Jiang, Q., and Voigt, J. M. (1996). Toxicology of the adrenal cortex: Role of metabolic activation. In "Endocrine Toxicology" (J. A. Thomas and H. D. Colby, eds.), 2nd ed., pp. 81–114. Lippincott-Raven, New York.

Colby, H. D., and Longhurst, P. A. (1992). Toxicology of the adrenal gland. In "Endorine Toxicilogy" (C. K. Atterwill and J. D. Flack, eds.), pp. 243–281. Cambridge University Press.

Eizirik, D. L., Spencer, P., and Kisby, G. E. (1996). Potential role of environmental genotoxic agents in diabetes mellitus and neurodegenerative diseases. *Biochem. Pharmacol.* **51,** 1585–1591.

Ewing, L. L. (1992). The Leydig cell. In "Reversibility in Testicular Toxicity Assesment" (A. R. Scialli and E. D. Clegg, eds.), pp. 87–126. CRC Press, Boca Raton, FL.

Fischer, L. J. (1996). Toxic effecs of cyproheptadine and its analogs in insulin-producing cells. In "Endocrine Toxicology" (J. A. Thomas and H. D. Colby, eds.), 2nd ed., pp. 257–286. Lippincott-Raven, New York.

Foote, R. H., and Berndtson, W. E. (1992). The germinal cells. In "Reversibility in Testicular Toxicity Assessment" (A. R. Scialli and E. D. Clegg, eds.), pp. 1–55. CRC Press, Boca Raton, FL.

Foster, P. M. D. (1992). The sertoli cell. In "Reversibility in Testicular Toxicity Assessment" (A. R. Scialli and E. D. Clegg, eds.), pp. 57–86. CRC Press, Boca Raton, FL.

Gittoes, N. J. L., and Franklyn, J. A. (1995). Drug-induced thyroid disorders. *Drug Safety* **13,** 46–55.

Granner, D. K., and O'Brien, R. M. (1992). Molecular physiology and genetics of NIDDM. *Diabetes Care* **15,** 369–395.

Grendell, J. H. (1992). Receptor strategies in pancreatitis. *Yale J. Biol. Med.* **65,** 431–436.

Harvey, P. W. (1996). In "The Adrenal in Toxicology." Taylor & Francis.

Heywood, R. (1984). Prediction of adverse drug reactions from animal safety studies. In "Detection and Prevention of Adverse Drug Reactions" (H. Bostrun and N. Ljungstedt, eds.), pp. 173–189. Almquist and Wiksell Int., Sweden.

Hill, R. N., Erdreich, L. S., Paynter, O. E., Roberts, P. A., Rosenthal, S. L., and Wilkinson, C. F. (1989). Thyroid follicular cell carcinogenesis. *Fundam. App. Toxicol.* **12,** 629–697.

Hotz, K. J., Wilson, A. G. E., Thake, D. C., Roloff, M. V., Capen, C. C., Kronenberg, J. M., and Brewster, D. W. (1997). Mechanism of thiazopyr-induced effects on thyroid hormone homeostasis in male Sprague-Dawley rats. *Toxicol. Appl. Pharmacol.* **142,** 133–142.

Jensen, R. T. (1992). Pancreatic pathology. *Yale J. Biol. Med.* **65,** 465–469.

Kohn, M. C., Sewall, C. H., Lucier, G. W., and Portier, C. J. (1996). A mechanistic model of effects of dioxin on thyroid hormones in the rat. *Toxicol. Appl. Pharmacol.* **165,** 29–48.

Longnecker, D. S., Memoli, V., Pettengill, O. S. (1992). Recent results in animal models of pancreatic carcinoma: Histogenesis of tumors. *Yale J. Biol. Med.* **65,** 457–464.

Matt, D. W., and Borzelleca, J. F. (1995). Toxic effects of the female reproductive system during pregnancy, parturition, and lactation. *In* "Reproductive Toxicology" (R. J. Witorsch, ed.), 2nd ed. pp. 175–193. Raven Press, New York.

Morse, D. C., Wehler, E. K., Wesseling, W., Koeman, J. H., and Brouwer, A. (1996). Alterations in rat brain thyroid hormone status following pre- and postnatal exposure to polychlorinated biphenyls (aroclor 1254). *Toxicol. App. Pharmacol.* **136,** 269–279.

Rani, C. S. S. (1990). Amiodarone effects of thyrotropin receptors and responses stimulated by thyrotropin and carbachol in cultured dog thyroid cells. *Endocrinology* **127,** 2930–2937.

Ribelin, W. E. (1984). The effects of drugs and chemicals upon the structure of the adrenal gland. *Fundam. Appl. Toxicol.* **4,** 105–119.

Runzi, M., and Layer, P. (1996). Drug-associated pancreatitis: Facts and fiction. *Pancreas* **13,** 100–109.

Saltiel, A. R., and Olefsky, J. M. (1996). Thiazolidinediones in the treatment of insulin resistance and type II diabetes. *Diabetes* **45,** 1661–1669.

Steer, M. L. (1989). Classification and pathogenesis of pancreatitis. *Surgical Clinics N. Am.* **69,** 467–480.

Steer, M. L. (1992). Pathobiology of experimental acute pancreatitis. *Yale J. Biol. Med.* **65,** 421–430.

Stevens, J. T., and Sumner, D. D. (1991). Herbicides. *In* "Handbook of Pesticide Toxicology" (W. J. Hayes, Jr. and E. R. Laws, Jr., eds.), pp. 1317–1408. Academic Press, San Diego, CA.

Stocco, D. M., and Clark B. J. (1996). Regulation of the acute production of steroids in steroidogenic cells. *Endocrine Rev.* **17,** 221–244.

Sundaram, K., and Witorsch, R. J. (1995). Toxic effects of the testes. In "Reproductive Toxicology" (R. J. Witorsch, ed.), 2nd ed., pp. 99–121. Raven Press, New York.

Szabo, S., and Sandor, Z. (1996). Chemicaly induced lesions in the adrenal cortex. In "Endocrine Toxicology" (J. A. Thomas and H. D. Colby, eds.), 2nd ed., pp. 115–131. Lippincott-Raven, New York.

Tischler, A. S., Powers, J. F., Downing, J. C., Risenberg, J. C., Shahsavari, M., Ziar, J., and McClain, R. M. (1996). Vitamin D_3, lactose, and xylitol stimulate chromaffin cell proliferation in the rat adrenal medulla. *Toxicol. App. Pharmacol.* **140,** 115–123.

Thomas, G. A., and Williams, E. D. (1992). Thyroid gland I—physiological control and mechanisms of carcinogenesis. *In* "Endocrine Toxicology" (C. K. Atterwill and J. D. Flack, eds.), pp. 117–136. Cambridge University Press.

Thomas, J. A. (1989). Pharmacology and toxicology responses in the neonate. *J. Am. Coll. Toxicol.* **8,** 957–962.

Thomas, J. A. (1996). Action of chemicals and other factors on Leydig cell growth & proliferation. *In* "Endocrine Toxicology" 2nd edit. J. A. Thomas and H. D. Colby, eds.), 2nd ed., pp. 245–256. Taylor & Francis.

Thomas, J. A., and Ballantyne, B. (1990). Occupational reproductive risks: Sources, surveillance, and testing. *J. Occupat. Med.* **32,** 547–554.

Thomas, J. A., and Bell, J. U. (1982). Endocrine toxicology. *In* "Principles and Methods of Toxicology" (A. W. Hayes, ed.), pp. 487–507. Raven Press, New York.

Thomas, J. A., and Keenan, E. J. (1986). *In* "Principles of Endocrine Pharmacology." Plenum Press: New York.

Thomas, M. J., and Thomas, J. A. (1994). Hormone assays and endocrine function. *In* "Principles and Methods of Toxicology" (A. W. Hayes, ed.), 3rd ed., pp. 1039–1063. Raven Press, New York.

Vanderpump, M. P. J., and Turnbridge, W. M. G. (1993). The effects of drugs on endocrine function. *Clin. Endocrinol.* **39,** 389–397.

Walker, R. F., and Cooper, R. L. (1992). Toxic effects of xenobiotics on the pituitary gland. *In* "Endocrine Toxicology" (C. K. Atterwill and J. D. Flack, eds.), pp. 51–82. Cambridge University Press.

Wilmink, T., and Frick, T. W. (1996). Drug-induced pancreatitis. *Drug Safety* **14,** 406–423.

Wilson, A. G. E., Thake, D. C., Heydens, W. E., Brewster, D. W., and Hotz, K. J. (1996). Mode of action of thyroid tumor formation in the male Long-Evans rat administered high doses of alachlor. *Fundam. Appl. Toxicol.* **33,** 16–23.

Wilson, M. J. (1995). Toxicology of the male accessory sex organs and related glands. *In* "Reproductive Toxicology" (R. J. Witorsch, ed.), 2nd ed., pp. 123–139. Raven Press, New York.

CHAPTER

23

Gastrointestinal Tract

KLAUS SCHÜMANN, BERND ELSENHANS, ELMAR RICHTER

Walther-Straub Institute of Pharmacology and Toxicology, Ludwig Maximilians University, Munich, Germany

The small intestine of an adult human is between 5 and 7 meters long. When compared to that of a simple cylinder, its surface is enlarged by Kerckring's folds, villi, and microvilli by a factor of 600 and covers more than 200 m^2 (Fig. 1). Thus, the small intestinal mucosa is one of the largest areas of contact of the human organism with the environment. The intestinal mucosa is almost continuously exposed to potentially harmful xenobiotics in food and other ingested material. However, the gastrointestinal tract is not a major target organ for the noxious contaminants in food and environment. This chapter will focus on the mechanisms that mediate or counteract toxic effects of noxious substances at low concentrations. The induction of carcinoma seems to be the most drastic effect that xenobiotic food contaminants at low concentrations can cause in the gastrointestinal tract; the incidence of cancer is frequent enough for epidemiological consideration. Selected groups of toxic substances that may cause harm to the gastrointestinal tract at low or high concentrations are discussed briefly. Bacterial and viral infection of the intestine and immunological reactions are not addressed.

PHYSIOLOGY

Protective Mechanisms

During evolution, several specific and unspecific mechanisms have evolved to protect the intestine against noxious food constituents.

Pre-epithelial Diffusion Barriers

For many substances, the pre-epithelial water and mucus layers are more difficult to cross than the cell membranes of the intestinal mucosa. The pre-epithelial compartment shields the mucosal surface. It consists of a thin "unstirred water layer" that covers the lipophilic surface of the mucosa. The resistance of this layer to diffusion depends on its thickness (200–600 nm) and is increased, in addition, because it fills the gaps between villi and microvilli and, thus, reduces the accessible surface area for luminal solutes (Fig. 2). The pre-epithelial compartment also contains a mucus layer of comparable thickness that merges with the glycocalix of the underlying brush-border membrane. The absorption of many xenobiotics depends on the diffusion rate through the pre-epithelial mucus layer. The absorption of lipophilic substances (e.g., quinine) is reduced by the physicochemical properties of the preepithelial mucus layer. This relationship has been formed in a mathematical model that regards the mucus gel as a macromolecular network. The diffusion coefficient of a compound depends on its molecular weight and lipophilicity, as well as on the glycoprotein concentration and on the water content of the mucus, which determines the density of the network. In addition, mucus binds iron and keeps it available for absorption under acidic conditions (e.g., in the stomach). The mucus binding of zinc, cobalt, and lead also depends on pH.

Weak acids, such as benzoic acid, or weak bases, such as benzylamine, are best transferred across the lipid membranes of the small intestinal wall in their

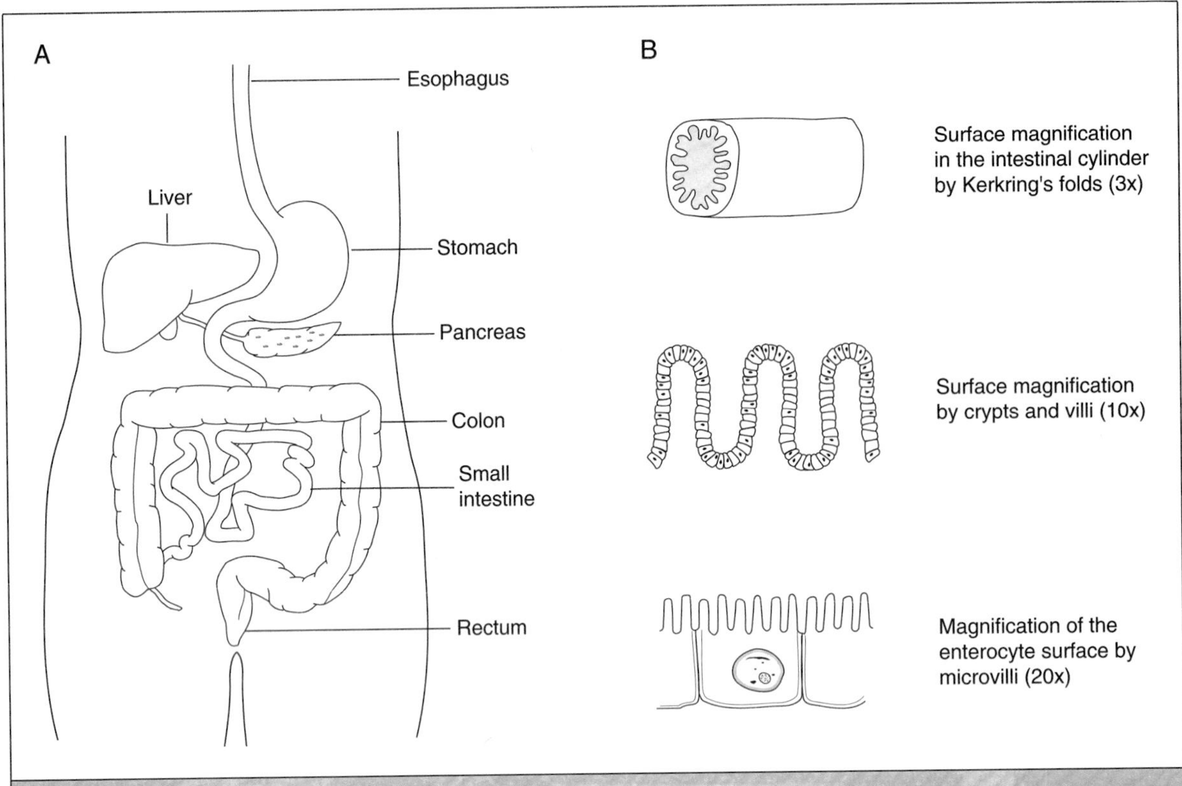

FIGURE 1 The sequence of the different sections of the gastrointestinal tract as shown in (A). The intestinal surface is increased 600-fold by Kerkring's folds, by the villi and crypt structure, and by microvilli at the surface of enterocytes (B).

undissociated form. According to the pH partition theory, the dissociation of a weak electrolyte depends on its p*K* value and on the pH of the medium and can be calculated by the equation of Henderson and Hasselbalch. Between the villi and the crypts, the pH differs substantially from the pH in the luminal medium. These differences can be measured by microelectrodes and show a specific profile, with marked differences along the villus–crypt axis. The differences seem to be caused by the compartmented secretion of acid and base equivalents along the villus–crypt axis. The luminal pH values vary between 4.5 and 9.0, whereas the pH values between the villi vary only between 5.4 and 6.8. Many xenobiotics are weak bases or acids. The extent to which they are absorbed depends on the pH values between the villi.

Regeneration of the Intestinal Mucosa

Having passed the pre-epithelial compartment, substances reach the intestinal mucosa. The turnover of enterocytes is among the highest in the organism; their proliferation, however, is restricted to the lower two-thirds of the crypts (proliferation compartment). Therefore, at this location the enterocytes are protected during their sensitive mitotic phase and can rarely be reached by food contaminants. This may partly explain why malignant diseases are very rare in the small intestine, despite its huge surface.

If the ingesta contain cytotoxic substances, the enterocytes are exfoliated into the intestinal lumen at a higher rate. The structural integrity of the mucosa is maintained by a sensitive balance between the rate of mitosis and the migration rate of enterocytes along the crypt–villus axis, which requires 26 to 72 hours, depending on species, kind of ingested food, and nutritional status. Cytotoxic compounds increase the mitotic activity, the proliferation compartment in the crypts is elongated, and the villi become shorter. The exfoliation zone at the tip of the villi increases. Due to these changes, the period during which the single enterocyte is exposed to cytotoxic food contaminants and during which it serves its functions becomes shorter (hyperregenerative transformation). The absorption of glucose and the enzyme activity in the mucosa decrease, as has been demonstrated by histochemical techniques.

Due to the high cell turnover, the intestinal mucosa regenerates quickly even after substantial damage. As

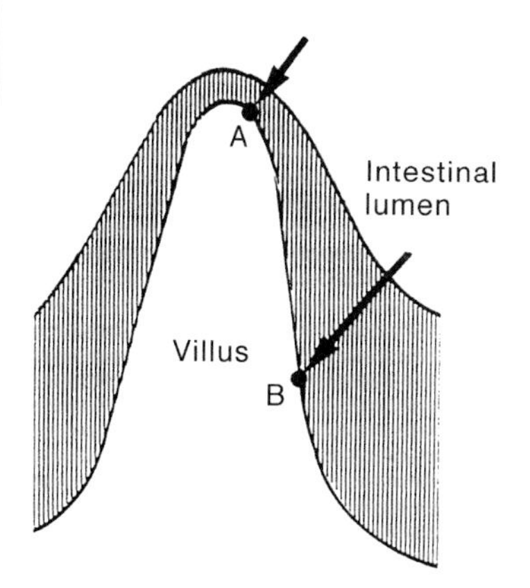

FIGURE 2 The resistance of the unstirred water layer (UWL, shown by vertical stripes) to diffusion increases in proportion to its thickness and decreases in proportion to the surface area of the layer. The surface of the UWL is much smaller than that of the intestine, as it covers villi and microvilli. Therefore, the resistance to solute diffusion is increased. In addition, the UWL is much thinner at the villus tip as compared to the villus base. In consequence, the diffusion of a solute through the UWL is favored at the tip of the villi (A) as compared to deeper areas (B).

early as 24 hours after an experimental interruption of the blood supply, the villi in the dog ileum were covered again with an epithelial layer. The villus tips were most sensitive to hypoxia, although the villi were substantially shortened during the early regeneration period. Later, when enough enterocytes were formed in the proliferation compartment, the villi regained their former length and structure.

Metabolism of Xenobiotics in the Intestinal Mucosa

In addition to these unspecific protective mechanisms, the intestine is equipped with specific detoxification systems. The smooth endoplasmatic reticulum of the enterocytes contains cytochrome P450, which metabolizes nitrosamines (e.g., CYP2E1) and other xenobiotics, such as aflatoxin B1 or heterocyclic arylamines (e.g., CYP1A2). This enzyme system is mainly expressed in the villus tips of the upper small intestine (i.e., where the enterocytes are exposed to the highest concentrations of xenobiotics). In rats, the activity of benzo[*a*]pyrene hydroxylase, *N*-nitroanisol-*O*-demethylase, NADPH–cytochrome P450 reductase, and the contents of cytochrome P450 are three to four times higher at this location than in the crypt cells. The difference in metabolic capacity may be another explanation for the low incidence of neoplasms in the small intestine. Dividing stem cells in the crypts will not produce reactive metabolites (e.g., activated carcinogens) to any significant extent. Activation in nondividing cells at the villus tip can not lead to a genetic lesion.

Because cytochromes contain a heme group, the P450 enzymes depend on a sufficient iron supply. The metabolites of the monooxygenase reaction are glucuronidated and sulfated in adjacent subcellular compartments by phase 2 enzymes and become water soluble, as is demonstrated by the metabolism of benzo[*a*]pyrene in the intestine. After pretreatment with 3-methyl cholanthrene (induction of the P450 system), the concentration of hydroxylated and glucuronidated metabolites increased 1.5-fold and 3-fold, respectively. After the administration of a semisynthetic diet for 7 days, the activity of *N*-glucuronyltransferase in healthy volunteers was unaltered; the activity of the cytochrome P450 system in jejunal biopsies, however, had decreased significantly. These examples show that the mucosal ability to metabolize lipophilic xenobiotics, among others, depends on the food intake.

The organotropy of carcinogenic effects in the organism depends on local differences in the deconjugation (e.g., deglucuronidation) of carcinogens and on an increased affinity of carcinogenic metabolites to a certain organ. As a case in point, the intestine itself not only detoxifies xenobiotics but may also convert them into more toxic forms. *N*-Nitrosodibutylamine, for example, undergoes ω-hydroxylation during jejunal absorption, which produces *N*-nitrosobutyl-3-carboxylpropylamine, a specific bladder carcinogen.

Absorption Mechanisms

The physiology of intestinal absorption is only briefly surveyed. For absorption, a substance should become dissolved in order to optimize its contact with the absorbing surface of the intestine. This is readily achieved with hydrophilic substances. Lipophilic substances, such as fatty acids and their glycerides, can be solubilized by forming mixed bile-salt micelles. Depending on the chemical and physical properties of the compounds, absorption occurs via various mechanisms.

Diffusion

Intestinal uptake by diffusion (Fig. 3) depends mainly on the physicochemical properties (e.g., ki-

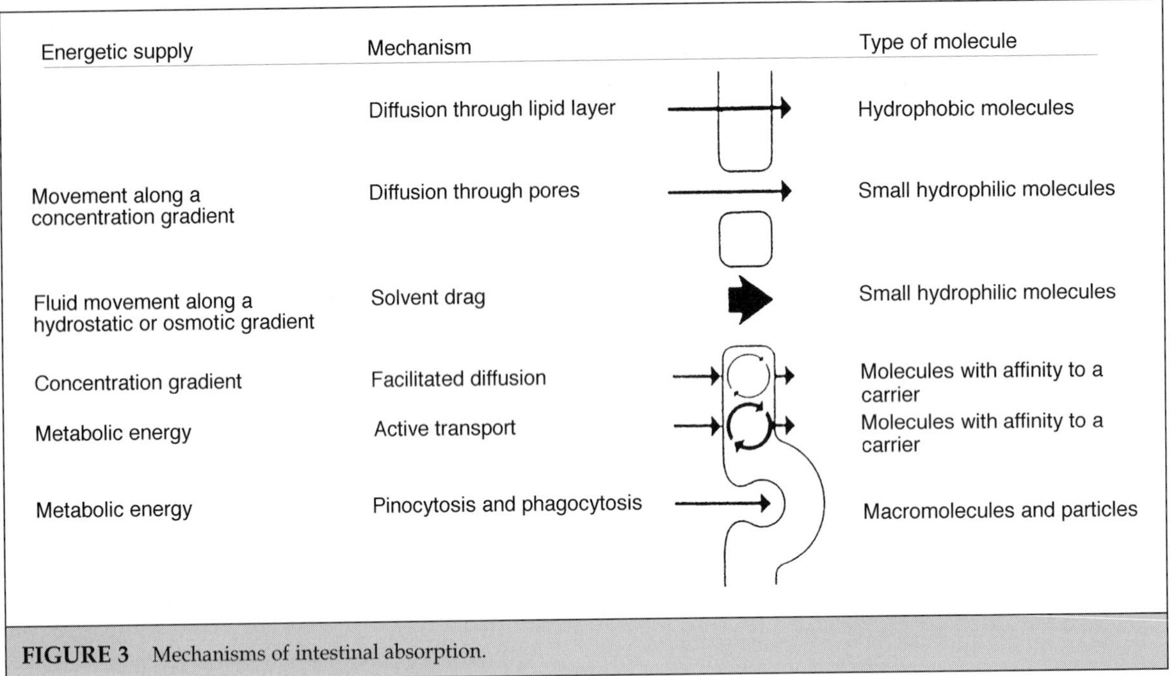

FIGURE 3 Mechanisms of intestinal absorption.

netic energy and electric charge) of the substance and on the electric polarity of the membrane. The diffusion of neutral molecules through mucosal membranes is proportional to the chemical concentration gradient across the membrane. The diffusion of ions is influenced by their electric charge and by the polarity of the membrane. Furthermore, diffusion is influenced by the thickness and by the surface area of the membrane, as well as by the diffusion constant. The latter takes into account the molecular mass of the diffusing substance. The sum of these impacts enters into the permeability constant, according to Fick's law. Depending on lipophilicity, diffusion takes place across lipid membranes or through pores (Fig. 3). The nature of diffusion is exclusively physical and basically independent from the cellular energy. However, the integrity of the cellular and subcellular membranes and compartments depends on cellular energy, so that diffusion is probably not completely independent from cellular metabolism.

Nonionic Diffusion

The lipid membranes are less permeable for ionized than for nonionized compounds of the same molecular mass. Weak electrolytes are partly charged, partly uncharged. Only the uncharged fraction crosses the luminal membrane of the enterocyte by diffusion. However, the mucosa is not equivalent to a single membrane. Depending on the pH and the pK in different subcellular compartments, weak electrolytes may dissociate to various degrees. Therefore, the transport of such compounds across the intestinal mucosa is a complex process.

Thus, nonionic diffusion is neither clearly related to electrochemical potential differences nor clearly coupled to cellular energy. In spite of this somewhat vague characterization, nonionic diffusion is a useful tool for describing the intestinal ion absorption of many xenobiotic contaminants and drugs that are weak electrolytes (e.g., organic acids and amines). For a more complex analysis, a three-compartment model was developed to describe the transport of weak electrolytes across the intestinal mucosa (partition theory). According to this model, the transport process is determined by the different hydrogen ion concentrations in the different mucosal compartments and by the selectivity of the interposed barriers for the ionic and nonionic forms of a compound.

Facilitated Diffusion

The chemical concentration gradient is the driving force for diffusion, as well as for facilitated diffusion (Fig. 3). By means of this mechanism, compounds are transported until the concentration on either side of the membrane is balanced. However, the transport rate is markedly higher than expected for a molecule of a certain size and lipophilicity, according to Fick's law. Transport is facilitated by a limited number of membrane transport proteins (carriers) that show substrate specificity. In contrast to simple diffusion, the transport rate is linear only at low substrate concentrations. At higher concentrations it becomes saturated. This implies that a maximum transport rate will not be exceeded when the luminal substrate concentration is increased. This transport process shows the same kinetic characteristics as an enzymatic reaction. The uptake of substances that are absorbed by facilitated diffusion (e.g., fructose, riboflavin, and choline) can be inhibited by structural analogs.

Active Transport

Transport of a substance against its electrochemical potential difference (e.g., against its concentration gradient), is called "active transport" (Fig. 3). It is not exclusively subject to physical forces, but requires cellular energy. Active transport may either depend directly on cellular energy or it may be coupled to a second energy-dependent transport system. The second scenario has been demonstrated for the transport of monosaccharides and amino acids in the small intestine. In this case, the inwardly directed concentration gradient for sodium ions provides the necessary driving force. The sodium gradient, in turn, is maintained by an ATPase at the basolateral membrane of the enterocyte that consumes metabolic energy. Characteristics of active transport are substrate specificity, saturability, competitive or noncompetitive inhibition, substrate binding, and counter transport. The importance of such specific carrier systems becomes obvious in genetic disorders leading to syndromes like congenital glucose–galactose malabsorption (due to an absent or defective glucose carrier), Hartnup disease (due to a transport defect for neutral amino acids), and Wilson's disease.

Water Tranport and Solvent Drag

There is no active transport mechanism for water. Transmural water transport is a passive phenomenon that follows the osmotic and hydrostatic gradient resulting from the active transport of solutes, such as electrolytes and nonelectrolytes. Water is predominantly transported by paracellular routes, which are located at the tight junctions. The permeability of these pores decreases continuously from duodenum to colon. The underlying mechanism works (simplified) as follows. The active transport of solutes increases the concentration and, thus, the osmotic pressure in the intercellular space. As a result, water is dragged in. This mechanism leads to an increased intercellular hydrostatic pressure, which causes the water to flow into the capillaries. Water transfer from the intestinal lumen through the mucosa in addition causes a concomitant transfer of solutes, called solvent drag. This process is based on two mechanisms. First, dissolved substances are carried through the pores together with the water flow. Second, along with the paracellular water flow, the removal of water from the intestinal lumen increases luminal solute concentration. That process, in turn, increases the chemical or electrochemical gradient and, thus, the transfer of substances by simple diffusion until the potential difference has leveled off.

In general, absorption processes can be differentiated into a transcellular and paracellular component. Solved molecules or particles can be transported transcellularly by pinocytosis or phagocytosis, depending on metabolic energy. After binding to the cell membrane, small vesicles are formed by membrane invaginations, which are transported through the cell (Fig. 3). Intestinal transport of inorganic ions is probably mainly paracellular. The transport of sodium ions by this route indirectly influences active transcellular sodium transport processes.

PATHOPHYSIOLOGICAL IMPACTS ON GASTROINTESTINAL FUNCTIONS

Influences on the Absorption of Xenobiotic Food Contaminants

Usually, environmental contaminants occur at very low concentrations. However, such materials will accumulate in the organism when the rate of excretion is smaller than that of absorption. In this context, active carrier-mediated intestinal uptake processes are of special interest, because they can transfer substances against a concentration gradient and lead to increased concentrations in the organism. During evolution, active intestinal transport mechanisms have developed for substances that are scarce or poorly bioavailable and for which a steady supply is advantageous (e.g., for many trace elements and vitamins, amino acids, peptides, and glucose). Although xenobiotics and food contaminants do not belong to those groups, some of these substances can share these intestinal transport mechanisms because of structural analogy to nutrients. Thus, some amino penicillins are transported by peptide carriers. The intestinal secretion of organic acids and organic bases is also mediated by carriers and there seem to be carriers for the metabolites of carbaryl, a carbamate pesticide that is metabolized in the small intestine. Many of these findings are based on animal experiments, and their applicability for humans is not yet proven. The importance of such mechanisms for the absorption of environmental contaminants is under discussion.

In the intestine, there are no specific transport mechanisms for toxic trace metals. However, toxic trace metals can use the mechanisms of essential trace metals, at least in part. In iron deficiency, for example, intestinal iron absorption is elevated by an increased number of carriers in the brush-border membrane of the human duodenum. Environmental contaminants such as lead, cadmium, nickel, and plutonium, partly share the absorptive routes of iron. Therefore, routine iron supplementation is advocated in children with marginal iron deficiency who live in lead-contaminated areas. Lead and cadmium also seem to interact with the regulated absorption mechanisms for calcium. Specific interactions between aluminum and iron and between zinc and cadmium during intestinal absorption were observed in animal experiments. Intestinal absorption is affected by physiological and pathological influences, such as changes in nutrition, both of which may lead to functional as well as morphological adaptation in the intestine. For example, in rats consuming a protein-rich diet, the absorption of amino acids is increased while that of glucose is decreased. Even inert substances such as kaolin clays lead to a significant adaptation of the villi structure when compared to a diet poor in fibers. Changes in the stomach retention time and in the motility of the small intestine are further examples of unspecific physiological impacts on intestinal absorption.

Gastrointestinal diseases may change the absorption of nutrients and drugs. Such changes are likely to affect xenobiotic food contaminants as well, although this aspect has so far been poorly investigated. However, the same disease may influence intestinal absorption of different compounds in opposite ways. In celiac disease, for instance, the absorption of some antibiotics increases while that of others decreases. Therefore, the extrapolation of predictions should be regarded with care.

In analogy to drugs, which are far better investigated, the chemical structure of a toxic xenobiotic may suggest that it will cross the intestinal mucosa by diffusion or by nonionic diffusion. The lipophilicity of the substance in its uncharged form is responsible for the diffusion rate across lipid membranes. In analogy to dietary fat, very lipophilic poorly water-soluble food contaminants are likely to form mixed micelles with bile salts. The higher absorption of DDT in the presence of fat suggests such mechanisms. The lymphatic transport of poorly water-soluble xenobiotics, such as DDT and polychlorinated biphenyls, after intestinal absorption shows similarities to the absorption of fat, as well.

Age Dependence of Xenobiotic Absorption

Undoubtedly, age influences intestinal absorption. Age-dependent changes in gastrointestinal functions are shown in Table 1. While it may be difficult to distinguish between physiological and pathological influences at advanced age, the maturation of intestinal functions during growth definitely is a physiological event. The absorption of macromolecules is increased during the first days of life and decreases thereafter, a phenomenon sometimes referred to as "intestinal closure." The question of to what extent the decreased absorption of proteins is due to the maturation of the intestinal mucosa or to the increasing activities of proteolytic enzymes in the gastrointestinal lumen is not entirely settled.

The intestinal absorption of toxic trace metals is a good example of age-dependent changes in absorptive capacity. In the first 3 years of their lives, children accumulate approximately one-third of their cumulative life-time body burden of cadmium. Thus, intestinal cadmium absorption is obviously increased in very young children. The bioavailability of cadmium and bivalent mercury ions in milk is increased in suckling rats as compared to adult animals. The mercury concentration in human milk is approximately 5% of that in the mother's blood. Thus, toxic mercury intake via breast feeding must go along with a severe mercury exposure of the mother.

Children absorb approximately 50% of the food lead content, while in adults fractional absorption is reduced to about 10%. In addition, the bioavailability

TABLE 1 Age-Dependent Changes in Gastrointestinal Functions

GI segment	Function	Changes in children	Changes in the aged
Stomach	Production of gastric acid	Decreased	Decreased
	Gastric transit time	Prolonged	Generally longer, reduced at increased pH
Small bowel	Mucosal blood perfusion	Varying	Reduced
	Mucosal surface	Increased	Decreased
Intestinal flora	Slowly increasing from a very low level	Increased	

of lead is influenced by dietary factors. In children between 1 and 12 years old, an increased blood-lead concentration is three times more likely in iron deficiency (transferrin saturation less than 10%) than in children with normal transferrin saturation. The low iron content and the high content of fat promote lead absorption from milk while its high calcium content is inhibitory. In rat milk, lead binds to casein; the lead–casein complexes, however, are not absorbed in the duodenum of the rat pups, as the casein cannot be decomposed in the lumen due to the low production of gastric acid and pepsin in the immature stomach. The lead–casein complexes are taken up into the ileal mucosa, from where only a small fraction reaches the organism at large. The major part returns into the lumen via desquamated enterocytes and is excreted with the feces. These examples illustrate the complexity of the interactions among lead, food ligands, and the maturation of the gastrointestinal tract.

SELECTED GROUPS OF TOXIC SUBSTANCES

A vast variety of substances can cause emetic effects and physical damage to the gastrointestinal mucosa by direct or indirect mechanims. For pharmaceutical agents that cause such damages (e.g., nonsteroid anti-inflammatory drugs, some antibiotics, cyclophosphamide, colchicine, and 5-fluoruracil) the reader is referred to pharmacology textbooks. This leaves us with a wide variety of household agents, industrial and environmental chemicals, and metals. The gastrointestinal effects of selected compounds shall be addressed.

Ulcerogenic Substances

Damage to the gastrointestinal tract can be caused by direct local action of a noxious compound, which may be aggravated by the accumulation of the substance or of its metabolites due to disturbed absorption. In the proximal small intestine, local ulcerogenic events begin at the villus tip and may lead to loss of the villi. Bleeding and perforation of the intestinal wall may be caused by the corrosion of the intestinal blood vessels and the muscular layers of the intestinal wall. Such damage is primarily caused by direct effects of the corrosive agent. Feedback mechanisms mediated by neurotransmitters, such as histamine, GABA, acetylcholine, and dopamine, may aggravate the process by stimulating the production of pepsin and protons in excess of the buffer capacity.

Corrosives like sodium and potassium hydroxides, ammonia, and various carbohydrates or phosphates are locally active agents that may cause vomiting, abdominal pain, and hemorrhagic diarrhea after ingestion. Acidic corrosives and oxidizing agents destroy the mucosa, primarily by precipitating proteins. Alkaline substances, among which are frequently used household cleaning agents, will exert their damage primarily by hydrolysis, leading to a gelatinous appearance of the tissue. Aldehydes, such as formaldehyde and acrolein, are another group of potent local irritants. They can damage the gastrointestinal mucosa by forming permanent cross-links between the functional groups of proteins, such as amido and amino groups, and hydroxyl and sulfhydryl groups. A fourth group of highly corrosive agents are phenols that can cause tissue damage in the mouth, esophagus, stomach, and intestine. Alcohols, alkanes, some aromatic chemicals, and solvents may also show ulcerogenic properties.

At high concentrations, metal ions with oxidative properties, such as iron and mercury, may produce ulcerations and necrosis of the gastrointestinal mucosa. Pharmaceutical iron preparations can induce nausea, heartburn, and epigastric pain because of mucosal irritation. Iron intoxication at excess doses (>180–300 mg/kg) will start with severe ulceration and necrosis in the upper gastrointestinal tract, leading to bloody diarrhea and vomiting. If the victim survives the subsequent systemic symptoms, scarring of the pylorus and other parts of the gastrointestinal tract may require surgical intervention.

Substances with Unspecific Effects

In addition to their ulcerogenic properties, alcohols, alkanes, some aromatic chemicals, and solvents may cause vomiting, abdominal cramps, diarrhea, and constipation. These effects are not related to chemical structures. They can be caused by alcohols, ethers, esters, ketones, and hydrocarbons alike. In analogy to the anesthetic effects of inhaled solvents, it has been proposed that the intestinal effects may be due to unspecific membrane effects and to an inhibition of the Na^+,K^+-ATPase. Detergents, especially polyphosphates, are known to cause emesis.

Acute fluoride toxicity can lead to anorexia and severe vomiting, diarrhea, and abdominal pain, which may go along with inflammation, hemorrhage, and necrosis of the gastrointestinal mucosa. Gastrointestinal symptoms, however, are also observed after subcutaneous administration of fluorides. The systemic effect is related to an inhibition of intestinal fluid transport, which, in turn, may be related to an inhibition of acetylcholinesterase and adenylate cyclase by fluoride, both of which influence intestinal fluid absorption and motility. Chronic fluoride ingestion may induce hypoplasia of the teeth ("mottling").

The carcinogenic effects of aromatic amines, *N*-nitroso compounds, and dimethylhydrazine in the gastrointestinal tract are discussed later. Epoxides, such as dieldrin and endrin, and alkylating agents, such as ethylenimine, cisplatin, and *N*-methyl-*N*-nitrosourea, may lead to nausea, vomiting, diarrhea, and weight loss. These substances show cytostatic and cytotoxic actions that affect tissues with rapidly dividing cells most severely and lead to a marked flattening of the gastrointestinal mucosa. In consequence, intestinal water absorption is impaired, which may explain the frequent appearance of diarrhea. Epoxides can induce stomach cancer.

Halogenated aliphatics may cause hepatic damage associated with intestinal toxicity; they may also cause gastrointestinal neoplasia after metabolic activation. In humans, nausea was observed after small doses of halogenated aliphatics, while higher doses were associated with anorexia, vomiting, diarrhea, abdominal pain, and intestinal hemorrhages. Halogenated aromatic hydrocarbons, such as chlorobenzene or bromobenzene, can also induce hepatic and intestinal damage, such as mucosal hyperplasia, although these effects are highly species specific.

Carbamates and organophosphates inhibit acetylcholinesterase. Some of these compounds are used as pesticides. Therefore, they are widely distributed. Their toxicity is due to increasing concentrations of acetylcholine in the synaptic gap. In the gastrointestinal tract, muscarinic receptors mediate an increased intestinal motility and tone, which leads to spastic contraction, abdominal cramps, and diarrhea. In addition, acetylcholine impairs sodium and water absorption and increases chloride secretion, which aggravates diarrhea. Anorexia, nausea, and vomiting are likely to be induced by central mechanisms, as intrathecal application of physostigmine, neostigmine, and acetylcholine provoke vomiting as well. Specific antidotes to organophosphates and carbamates are atropine (via receptor blockade) and obidoxime (via enzyme reactivation).

Metals

Nonspecific symptoms, such as loss of appetite, nausea, and abdominal pain, are associated with most metal intoxications. This reaction provides a protective effect as the stomach content is discharged and further ingestion of the metal is stopped. $CuSO_4$ induces vomiting at low concentrations (10–15 mg/liter). Some authors described an emetic effect even at 1 mg Cu/liter, which is the maximum permissible concentration for Cu in drinking water, as recommended by the WHO. Usually, drinking water contains less than 0.2 mg Cu/liter. Unspecific gastrointestinal symptoms are also observed as early symptoms of thallium intoxication. The ulcerogenic properties of high iron and mercury concentrations were discussed previously.

Lead colics are common after excessive lead ingestion and go along with nausea, vomiting, and alternating diarrhea and constipation. Chronic lead exposure reduces the intestinal absorption of glucose and sodium in rats, which may explain part of the symptoms. Spasms of the smooth muscles in the gastrointestinal tract (colica pictonum) and in the intestinal blood vessels, as well as impaired function of the sympathic and parasympathic feedback mechanisms, are also discussed as possible modes of action.

After prolonged high dietary cadmium exposure, such as during the itai-itai events in Japan (>1 mg Cd/kg food), atrophic gastritis and mucosal atrophy with shortened ciliated epithelia were observed in the human intestine.

TUMORS IN THE GASTROINTESTINAL TRACT

According to the cause-of-death statistics in 1995 for Germany, 24.7% of all deaths were caused by malignant tumors. Approximately one-fourth of all tumors are found in the intestinal tract, with no significant difference between men (25.9%) and women (25.3%). The distribution between the different segments of the intestinal tract shows gender-specific differences (Fig. 4). Most gastrointestinal tumors are found in the colon and rectum, followed by the stomach. Tumors of the oral cavity and pharynx are much more frequent in men than in women. On the other hand, women have more colon tumors than men. Tumors of the small intestine are neglegibly rare in both sexes.

Since the 1970s, the incidence of stomach tumors has decreased markedly, while colon tumors have become more frequent (Fig. 5). An increasing number of epidemiological studies reveals a marked influence of nutrition and lifestyle on the incidence of tumors in the intestine. In general, the ample intake of fresh fruits and vegetables has been associated with a protective effect, presumably caused by the high content of ascorbic acid and other antioxidants and antimutagens of this type of food. Coffee intake is not a risk factor in oral, pharyngeal, esophageal, and stomach carcinogenesis. For the colon, coffee drinking is, rather, a protective factor against carcinogenesis, presumably because of the decreased bile flow in coffee drinkers.

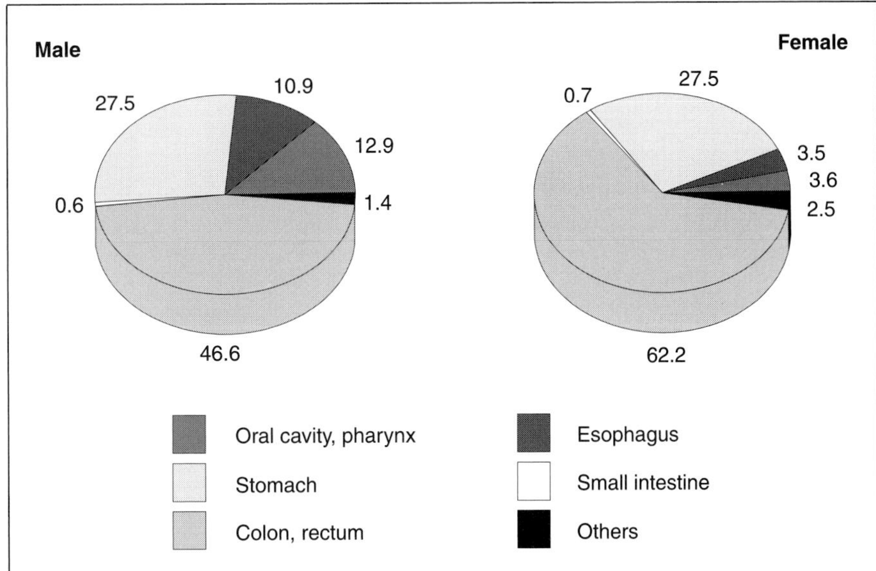

FIGURE 4 Pie chart of percent distribution of cancer mortality in the gastrointestinal tract, Germany 1995. (All GI tumors = 100%; data from the German Federal Office of Statistics, 1995.) Classification of tumors numbered according to International Classification of Diseases: oral cavity and pharynx, 1400 – 99; esophagus, 1500 – 09; stomach, 1510 – 19; small intestine, 1520 – 39; large intestine, 1530 – 39; rectum and anus, 1540 – 49; others, 2101 – 19, 2300 – 09, 2350 – 55, 2390. The incidences of the tumors specified by these numbers were pooled as indicated and used to create Figure 4.

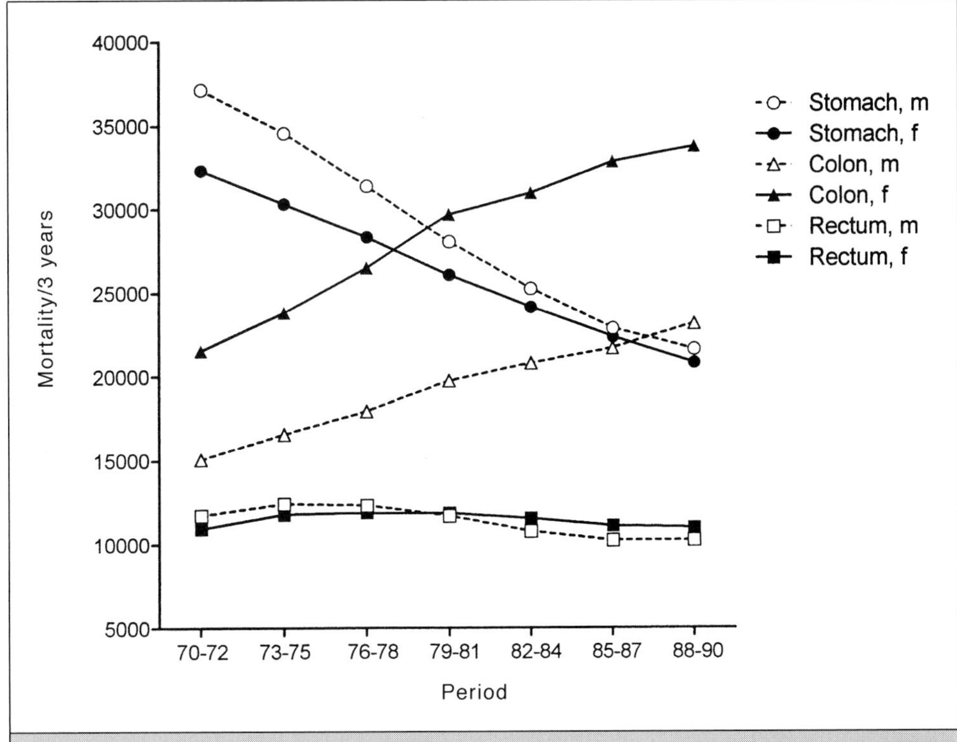

FIGURE 5 Incidence of tumors in the gastrointestinal tract in Germany, 1970–1990 (drawn using data from Geddes *et al.*, 1994.)

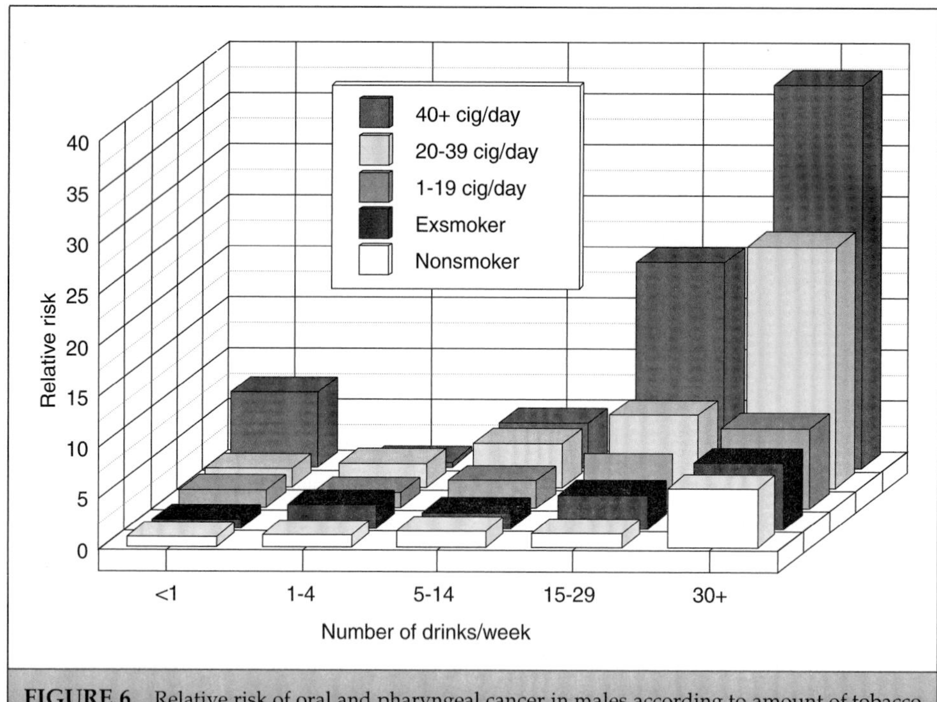

FIGURE 6 Relative risk of oral and pharyngeal cancer in males according to amount of tobacco smoking and alcoholic-beverage drinking (drawn using data from Blot, 1992).

Tumors in the Oral Cavity and Pharynx

The most important factor for oropharyngeal tumors is tobacco consumption, no matter whether by smoking, chewing, or snuff dipping. Alcohol consumption alone is also a clear risk factor. The consumption of both alcohol and tobacco increases the risk synergistically from 4 to 7 times if just one of these risk factors is present, and from 25 to 40 times when both risk factors apply at the same time (Fig. 6). In animal experiments, the risk of oral cancer induced by tobacco consumption could be increased by previous infection with herpes simplex virus. In addition to other tumors, 2,3,7,8-tetrachlorodibenzo-*p*-dioxin (0.001–0.1 μg/kg/day for 2 years) also increased the incidence of tumors in palate and tongue of rats. Little is known about further risk factors in humans.

Tumors of the Esophagus

For esophageal cancer, smoking and alcohol consumption are important risk factors, to which nutritional risk factors are added. In certain regions in China, nitrosamines generated by the mold *Fusarium moniliforme* are held responsible for the increased incidence of esophageal tumors. In animal experiments, the esophagus was shown to be the most important target organ for nitrosamines, independent of the route of application. In almost half (45%) of the 150 rats examined, nitrosamines induced tumors in the esophagus. The mechanism of this organotropy cannot be explained sufficiently. The high esophageal epithelium metabolic activation of nitrosamines, together with a comparatively low DNA repair, probably plays the most important role. In addition, chronic stress factors, which lead to a high stimulation of epithelial turnover, are a pacemaker for malignant progression. In some countries, the traditional consumption of extremely hot drinks lead to constant burns of the esophagus, which increases the risk. Mate, a nonalcoholic brew frequently consumed as tea in Uruguay, appears to be a high risk factor for esophageal cancer.

Stomach Tumors

Changes in nutritional habits probably play an important part in the decreasing incidence of stomach tumors in the past decades. Since the introduction of refrigeration, less food that has been conserved with salt or other food preservatives is consumed. In additions, fresh vegetables and fruits are available all year round. The nitrite intake, the nitrite concentration in the stomach, the pH, and the increased endogenous nitrosation of nutrients in the stomach are discussed as causative factors. A European multicenter study failed to show a correlation between salt intake and the incidence of intestinal metaplasia, which is an early stage of stomach cancer. Such a correlation would have supported the nitrosamine hypothesis. Infections with *Helicobacter pylori* are also under discussion as a risk factor for adenocarcinoma of the distal stomach. The putative mechanism is chronic inflammation, leading to cell proliferation and the production of free radicals and *N*-nitroso compounds. Prospective epidemiological studies revealed an increased risk for stomach cancer of three to six times in the group that was seropositive for *H. pylori.* The cause of the 2.3-fold increased risk of stomach cancer in professional truck drivers in a Swiss study is unexplained. It might be related to an increased exposure to polycyclic aromatic hydrocarbons (PAH) and nitro-PAH in car exhaust. Epidemiological studies show an increased risk in persons lacking a certain isoenzyme of glutathione *S*-transferase (GSTM1). This enzyme plays an important role in the metabolic inactivation of PAH (e.g., benzo[*a*]pyrene), causing stomach tumors in animal experiments. Preneoplastic hyperplasias are caused in animal experiments by polyhalogenated aromatic hydrocarbons. This effect was observed for the first time in monkeys kept in animal housings where the walls were painted with colors containing polychlorinated biphenyls (PCB). Further experiments revealed that the stomachs of monkeys and pigs are much more sensitive to PCB than the stomach of rats. Gastric hyperplasias were observed in accidental mass poisonings with PCB in humans in Japan and Taiwan.

Colon Tumors

The etiology of colorectal tumors is unclear. Model experiments in animals have clearly established hydrazine and azoxymethane as inducers of colon cancer. However, their role in human cancer is not clear. Fecapentaene 12 (FP12) is a fecal, unsaturated, ether-linked lipid, produced by the anerobic microflora of the colon. It is excreted by most human individuals in Western populations, although excretion is modulated by binding to fibers and calcium. FP12 is genotoxic and carcinogenic in newborn mice and it has been suggested as initiating and promoting colon carcinogenesis in humans. These effects seem to be mediated by direct DNA alkylation and by oxygen-radical-induced DNA damage, which can be blocked by nonsteroidal anti-inflamatory agents. Carcinogenicity studies with FP12 in adult rats and mice, however, have been predominantly negative. Thus, the adult rodent and human colons may have adequate biochemical defense mechanisms against low-level exposure to FP12, even at continuous exposure.

The increase in colon tumors in the past decades suggests an influence of nutrition and lifestyle, as both have changed markedly since the Second World War in Germany. An important risk factor is familial polyposis, leading to manifest colon cancer before the age of 40 if not treated. Many genetic changes are associated with the manifestation of colon tumors (multiple hit theory), for example, in familial adenomatous polyposis the loss of the APC gene on chromosome 5 and mutations of oncogenes, especially the *ras* gene on chromosome 12 and tumor-suppressor genes such as p53 on chromosome 17. Point mutations can be induced by chemical carcinogens (e.g., heterocyclic aromatic amines, HAA). These compounds are generated by heating proteins, especially during frying or barbecuing of meat and fish. In rats and mice, HAA produce colon cancer, though the amounts found in food are about 1000 times lower than the effective carcinogenic doses in animal experiments. It has to be kept in mind, however, that different HAA have been shown to act additively, and that not all HAA have been identified and examined for their carcinogenic potency. Epidemiological studies support HAA being an important risk factor for colon cancer because they revealed an increased risk for fast acetylators (*N*-acetyltransferase 2, NAT2) and for extensive N-oxidizers (cytochrome P450 1A2). Both enzymes contribute to the metabolic activation of HAA to their ultimate carcinogenic forms. The first step, N-oxidation, takes place mainly in the liver; the second metabolic step, O-acetylation, mediated by NAT2, of the target tissue, takes place in the colonic mucosa.

Among the endogenous factors, an increased secretion of bile acids, especially of deoxycholeic acid and lithocholic acid, has been identified as increasing the risk for colonic cancer. A special risk factor exclusively for rectal cancer is beer consumption, presumably because of acetaldehyde accumulation leading to DNA adducts.

EFFECTS OF FOOD AND LUMINAL FACTORS

Food Components with Noxious Effect

Vegetable food often contains endogenous toxins that serve as natural pesticides and to reduce the risk of being eaten by animals. The ability of plants to produce substances for their own protection was used to breed a resistant potato species, which, however,

TABLE 2 Selected Compounds and Groups of Compounds That May Damage or Protect the Gastrointestinal Tract

Compounds	Effects
Solanine, chaconine	Teratogenic effects
Acidic and alkaline corrosives, formaldehyde, acrolein, oxidizing agents, phenols, alcohol, iron and mercury (high concentrations)	Ulcerogenic effects
Alcohols, detergents, fluorides (high concentrations)	Emesis
Dieldrin, endrin	Emesis, diarrhea, weight loss
Highly chlorinated aromatic carbohydrates	Mucosal hyperplasia
Halogenated aliphatics	Cancerogenic effect, emesis, anorexia, hemorrhages at high concentrations
Carbamates, organophosphates	Abdominal cramps, diarrhea, emesis
Copper	Emesis
Lead (high concentrations)	Colic
Cadmium (high concentrations)	Mucosal and intestinal atrophia
Tobacco, alcohol, 2,3,7,8-tetrachlorodibenzo-p-dioxin	Oral and pharyngeal cancer risk increased
Nitrosamines, hot beverages (e.g., mate tea)	Esophageal cancer risk increased
Nitrate, nitrite, polycyclic and polychlorinated aromatic carbohydrates	Stomach cancer risk increased
Heterocyclic aromatic amines, nitrosamines	Colon cancer risk increased
Antioxidative vitamins; phenethyl thiocyanate (PEITC), capsaicin, benzyl isothiocyanate, diallyl trisulfide, and related substances	Potentially anticarcinogenic

had to be removed from the market because of high concentrations of teratogenic solanines and chaconines. There was a similar experience with a newly bred celery species that caused dermatitis during handling. Its content of 8-methoxypsoralene and other related psoralenes was 10 times higher than in wild-type celery. Plants also contain endogenous carcinogens in comparatively high quantities. The impact of natural cancerogens ingested in food that is consumed beyond the caloric demand is estimated to have an influence on the total cancer risk that is more than 10 times greater than that of anthropogenic carcinogens.

Food Components with Protective Functions

The Impact of the Intestinal Flora on the Metabolism of Xenobiotics

The intestinal flora influences the absorption and metabolism of xenobiotics in the colon. Promutagens are bound by polysaccharides in the wall of *Lactococcus cremonis* and lactis. Correspondingly, the excretion of mutagenic substances with the urine decreases as the colonic lactobacillus content increases. Many carcinogenic xenobiotics are detoxified by binding to glucuronic acid in the liver (hepatic glucuronidation) before they are excreted with the bile. In the intestinal lumen, glucuronides can be hydrolyzed by bacterial β-glucuronidases with very low substrate specificity. Thus, carcinogenic aglycones are released in the colon. *Escherichia coli* shows a very high β-glucuronidase activity; that in lactobacilli is by far lower. Intake of *L. acidophilus*, as well as of tetracyclines and erythromycin, changes the bacterial flora and reduces the β-glucuronidase activity. Nitrates are reduced to nitrite and further to nitrogen and ammonia by nitrate reductase of the intestinal flora. Nitrite is an intermediate product that can be used to synthesize carcinogenic nitroso compounds. Lactobacilli take up nitrite from the intestinal lumen. In contrast to *E. coli* and many gram-negative enterobacteria, clostridium, and staphylococcus species, however, lactobacilli have no nitrate reductase. They have nitrite-reducing enzymes and detoxify nitrites under anerobic conditions.

Anticarcinogens in the Food

The frequency of tumors in the gastrointestinal tract is influenced by the composition of the diet (Table 2). Many vegetables and fruit juices that are supposed to decrease the cancer risk were shown to reduce the impact of heterocyclic aromatic amines (HAA) in mutagenicity tests *in vitro*. The high fiber content of the food accelerates the passage of the ingesta in colon. Thus, it reduces the exposure to noxious food constituents and decreases the bioavailability of HAA. In addition, the increased filling of the sigma with fibers reduces the exposure of the mucosa to secondary bile acids and mutagens. An increased fiber consumption reduces the risk of colon cancer even in persons with precancerogenic colon polyps.

The cancer risk in the gastrointestinal tract is also influenced by natural anticarcinogens in the food. The frequency of precancerogenic lesions of the esophagus in the Lin-Xian area of China is correlated with the nitrosamine concentrations in the blood of the patients. The lower risk of esophageal carcinoma in a subpopulation was associated with a high intake of fruit and vegetables that contained anti-oxidant vitamins. High intake of onions and garlic, which are rich in sulfhydryl groups, reduced the risk of stomach cancer in the Shanxshi area of China. The low risk for colon cancer in Mediterranean countries could be explained by the widespread use of olive oil, with its high content of unsaturated fatty acids. In this context the term "Mediterranean diet" was coined for a diet with a low cancer risk.

Physical exercise is also assumed to protect against colon cancer. However, neither the necessary extent of the physical training nor the underlying mechanism is known. Animal experiments showed that voluntary exercise in a running wheel decreased the risk for colon cancer, while forced exercise increased the risk, probably due to increased stress.

Anticarcinogenic effects can be mediated by different mechanisms, such as metabolic inactivation and detoxification, binding of carcinogens, and competition for the binding of carcinogens to DNA. Phenethyl isothiocyanate (PEITC), which is found in broccoli and cauliflower, decreases the binding of the nitrosamine 4-methylnitrosamino-1-(3-pyridyl)-1-butanone (NNK) to DNA. Capsaicin, which contains substance P and is found in hot peppers, inhibits *in vitro* the metabolism of benzo[*a*]pyrene and its binding to DNA. Cabbage vegetables increase the activity of benzopyrene hydroxylase in the rat gastrointestinal tract, which seems to inhibit the induction of gastric tumors by benzo[*a*]pyrene in rats. Allyl methyl trisulfide, allyl methyl disulfide, diallyl trisulfide, and diallyl sulfide are found in garlic and onions and stimulate the detoxification of benzo[*a*]pyrene via induction of glutathione *S*-transferase in the forestomach of female AJ mice. A diet rich in antioxidative vitamin E seems to reduce the rate of colon tumors, as was shown in mice after the application of 1,2-dimethylhydrazine.

The results from the different working fields must be carefully reconciled before they are entered into the dietary recommendations. The European Codex for the Control of Cancer recommends ceasing smoking and restricting alcohol consumption. Instead, an ample intake of fresh fruits, vegetables, and fiber-rich cereals is recommended. However, such general dietary recommendations are of limited value as long as the risk populations cannot be spotted. Thus, more than 95% of the general population is not at risk for colon cancer. For the remaining 4–5%, the risk can be reduced approximately by half by dietary manipulations. Such statistical considerations urge the development of genetic test systems to spot risk populations.

Bibliography

Blot, W. J. (1992) Alcohol and cancer. *Cancer Res.* **52,** 2119s–2123s.

Caspary, W. F. (1987). "Structure and Function of the Small Intestine." Excerpta Medica, Amsterdam.

Csaky, T. Z. (1984). Intestinal absorption of xenobiotics. *In* "Handsbook of Pharmacology, Vol. 70/II, Pharmacology of Intestinal Permeation II" (T. Z. Csaky, ed.), pp. 1–30. Springer, Berlin.

Doll, R. (1996). Nature and nurture, possibilities for cancer control. *Carcinogenesis* **17,** 177–184.

Eisenbrand, G., and Tang, W. (1993). Food-borne heterocyclic amines. Chemistry, formation, occurrence and biological activities. A literature review. *Toxicology* **84,** 1–82.

Geddes, M., Balzi, D., and Tomatis, L. (1994). Progress in the fight against cancer in EC countries: Changes in mortality rates, 1970–90. *Eur. J. Cancer Prev.* **3,** 31–44.

Hathcock, J. N. (1982). "Nutritional Toxicology," Vol. I. Academic Press, New York.

Hathcock, J. N. (1987). "Nutritional Toxicology," Vol. II. Academic Press, Orlando, FL.

Hill, M. J. (1995). Diet and cancer: a review of scientific evidence. *Eur. J. Cancer Prev.* **4 (Suppl. 2),** 5–42.

Rozman, K., and Haninen, O. (1986). "Gastrointestinal Toxicology." Elsevier, New York.

Tyler, T. R. (1993). Peroral toxicity. *In* "General and Applied Toxicology" (B. Ballantine *et al.*, eds.), Vol. 1, pp. 413–431. Stockton Press, New York.

CHAPTER

24

Cardiovascular System

PAUL J. BOOR

Laboratory of Cardiovascular Toxicology, Department of Pathology, University of Texas Medical Branch, Galveston, Texas

INTRODUCTION

The cardiovascular system is a complex, interconnected system of blood vessels with greatly varying diameters, pressures, and flow rates. At the center of this system is the heart, a remarkable organ that provides the driving force to distribute blood to meet the needs of peripheral tissues, which is the sole function of the cardiovascular system. The heart and blood vessels are susceptible to injury by toxic compounds, but because of the varied and diffuse nature of the cardiovascular system, its toxicology is complex.

In this chapter, toxic insults to the heart or blood vessels will be reviewed, specific examples of experimentally induced lesions will be defined, and, where possible, the underlying mechanisms of cellular injury to cardiovascular tissue will be summarized. The details of some of typical, or classic, experimental procedures used by investigators to induce pathologic alterations in cardiovascular tissues will be outlined as well. Because each of the toxic injuries addressed is itself a complex topic, this chapter can only scrape the surface of the large body of literature that exists concerning cardiovascular toxicology. An effort will be made, however, to be as organized and as comprehensive as possible with regard to the various types of toxic injury discussed, and to include a rudimentary bibliography, so that readers can go more deeply into areas of their choice.

CARDIAC TOXINS

The heart is a unique organ because of the remarkable ability of the myocardium to do an enormous amount of fluid dynamic work in an automatic synchronous fashion. These properties (i.e., pumping capacity and automaticity) are also potential targets for toxins to exert their deleterious effects. The cardiotoxicity of compounds, therefore, can be divided into broad categories based on the adverse functional effects that result. One large category of cardiac toxins includes those compounds that cause a disturbance of the automatic and extremely regular rhythm of the heart; such disturbances are known as "arrhythmias" or "dysrhythmias." These arrhythmogenic cardiotoxins can result in a severe dysfunction of the heart's pumping action by causing abnormal, inefficient, and even fatal rhythms. A characteristic of these toxins is that, because they act through inducing subtle cell membrane actions that effect the cardiac conduction tissue of the heart, they can cause death with very little or no structural damage.

A second category of cardiac toxins consists of those substances that cause severe irrreversible cell injury, resulting in myocyte death or necrosis. This is a broad category of substances, including chemicals that are directly cytotoxic to myocardial cells and chemicals that induce myocardial necrosis by effects on the coronary circulation, essentially resulting in anoxic or ischemic necrosis. Often, these two mechanisms (direct toxicity vs. indirect action through anoxia) are difficult to separate definitively; nevertheless, myocyte necrosis due to necrotizing toxins is a distinct lesion that can result in eventual heart failure and death of the organism.

A third, somewhat more subtle, category of toxins is that group of substances causing non-necrotizing injury of cardiac myocytes. These toxins, although they may cause little or no overt acute myocardial necrosis, can cause eventual failure of the myocardium to keep up with the demands of peripheral tissues and, thus, result in cardiac failure and death. This category of cardiotoxin might be termed "contractile" toxins because many of these compounds have deleterious actions on the contractile apparatus of the myocyte, causing cardiac dysfunction without causing cell death. It should be noted, however, that a few toxic substances exert more than one type of deleterious effect on the heart.

Arrhythmogenic Cardiotoxins

Pharmacology and Toxicology of Cardiac Glycosides

The largest group of arrhythmogenic cardiotoxic compounds possess chemical structures that are characterized by a complex aglycone, or genin, linked to a variable number of sugars in a glycosidic bond (Fig. 1). A large number of cardiac glycosides and related compounds, isolated from both plant and animal sources, have been found to have both pharmacological and cardiotoxic actions. The most extensive experimental work has focused on plant glycosides that empirically have been used for centuries in the treatment of heart failure. As pharmacology and toxicology developed, however, the mechanisms by which cardiac glycosides both beneficially and adversely affect the heart have been elucidated. The physiological effects of therapeutic doses of digitalis are complex—including an increase in cardiac output, decreased peripheral edema, diuresis, and decreased venous pressure—but most effects can be attributed directly to the remarkably positive effect on cardiac contractility, known as a positive inotropic effect. The basis of the positive inotropism induced by digitalis and other cardiac glycosides is pharmacological inhibition of electrolyte regulatory mechanisms, specifically an Na^+,K^+-ATPase localized in the myocyte sarcolemma. The inhibition of this membrane-bound enzyme results in complex alterations in intracellular electrolyte balance, and a consequent increase in the pools of

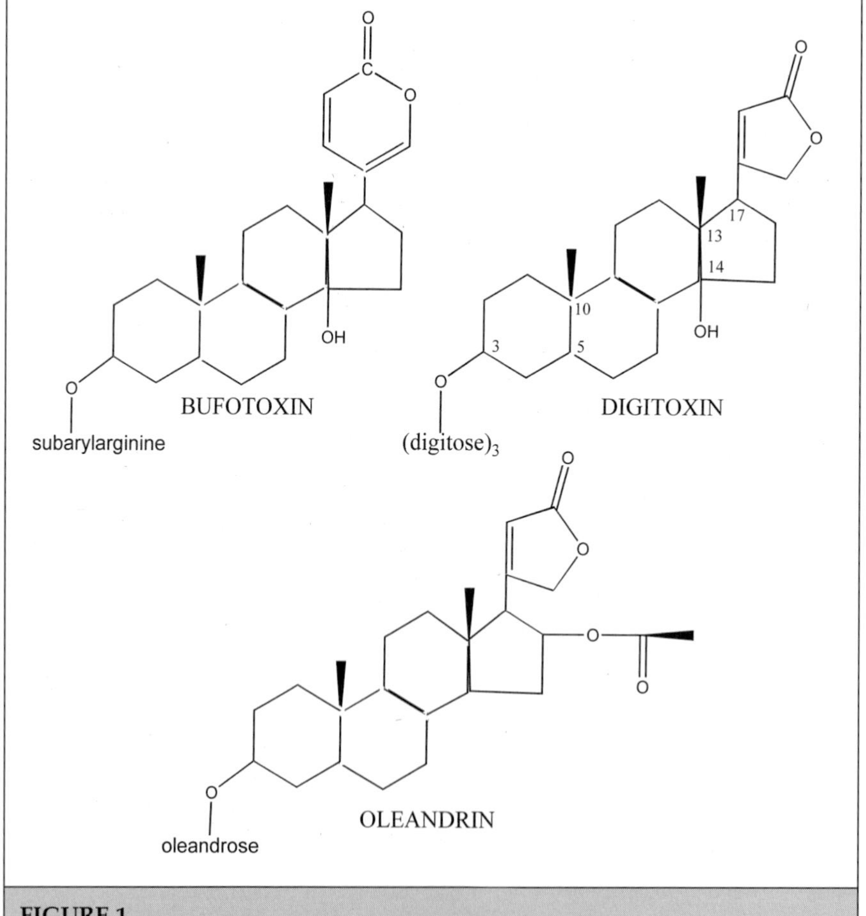

BUFOTOXIN

subarylarginine

DIGITOXIN

$(digitose)_3$

OLEANDRIN

oleandrose

FIGURE 1

intracellular calcium that augment the contractile apparatus, thus resulting in positive inotropism.

Virtually all cardiotoxic glycosides have some degree of potential therapeutic usefulness; however, the basis of their beneficial effect on myocardial contractility is also the basis of their toxicity. Excessive inhibition of cardiac Na^+,K^+-ATPase in the conduction tissue of the heart results in aberrant fluxes of Na^+,K^+, and Ca^{2+} across the cell membrane, with consequent changes in the transmembrane electrical potential leading to abnormal rhythms that eventually prove fatal, generally in a dose-dependent manner.

Digitalis Glycosides

The most extensively studied glycosides are those related to digitalis, a drug derived from the leaves of the foxglove plant (*Digitalis purpurea*) that has been known as a beneficial pharmacological agent for centuries. A large number of synthetic digitalis-like compounds have also been developed. Most of these compounds display some degree of species variability in toxicity, however, and the investigation of digitalis toxicity is complicated by this fact. Digitalis sensitivity also varies dramatically with age, further adding to the complexity of studies of cardiac glycosides.

For example, the laboratory rat is digitalis resistant compared to the human, rabbit, and especially guinea pig, which is quite sensitive. The dog, on the other hand, has a sensititivity to digitalis cardiac toxicity that is very similar to that of the human; this similarity may be due to the analogous structures of the α subunit of dog and human myocardial Na^+,K^+-ATPase, resulting in similar affinity and binding to cardiac glycosides. On the other hand, the extreme resistance of the rat to cardiac glycoside toxicity may be related to structural differences of the rat membrane ionic channels.

Within a species, the immature animal is generally less sensitive than the adult counterpart to the toxic effects of digitalis. In the rat, however, this situation is reversed, with the newborn rat being as much as 40- to 1000-fold more sensitive than the adult rat (Table 1). For example, the LD_{50} dose of digitoxin is 94 mg/kg in the adult rat compared to 0.1 mg/kg in the newborn rat. This great disparity in the glycoside sensitivity of new-born and adult rats may be partially explained by biochemcial variations in the membrane Na^+,K^+-ATPase, but the immaturity of the excretory mechanisms and/or the hepatic metabolism of cardiac glycosides could also play a role. Therefore, the investigation of cardiac glycoside toxicity must of necessity take into account the species being examined and its relevance to the human response.

Other Plant Arrhythmogenic Toxins

A plethora of cardiotoxic substances, most notably glycosides and related cardenolides and genins, have been isolated from a variety of plants. The most well-studied plants include *Cryptostegia* species (including *C. grandiflora* and *C. madagascariensis*) and the common oleander. *Cryptostegia* are climbing shrubs, commonly known as "rubber vine," that are indigenous to Madagascar and Australia; these plants have been imported into the United States where they are used as ornamental shrubs, especially in the state of Florida. Fatalities among cattle grazing on *Cryptostegia* have been reported from Australia, and *Cryptostegia madagascariensis* has been employed as a means of suicide and homocide in Madagascar. The clinical syndrome described for *Cryptostegia* toxicity closely resembles that of digitalis overdose. The potentially cardiotoxic compounds isolated from these plants include three genins, five cardenolides, two rhamnosides, and a glycosidic cardenolide not previously described from any other source (14,16-dianhydrogitoxigenin-3-rhamnoside). Although it is highly likely that these compounds are responsible for the known, presumably arrhythmogenic, cardiotoxicity of these plants, no investigations have specifically tested the toxic properties of these isolates.

The oleanders, a group of evergreen flowering shrubs of the family Apocynaceae, are ubiquitous plants that grow both ferally and as decorative landscaping shrubs worldwide throughout large portions of tropical and subtropical regions. Ingestion of all parts of the oleander, as well as inhalation of the smoke of burning oleander, has been associated with fatalities in livestock, pets, and humans. Although most ingestions and poisonings are inadvertent—as in accidental ingestion by children—the making of tea from the leaves of oleander is one of the most common forms of committing suicide in parts of India and other tropical regions.

Many bioactive constituents have been identified in virtually all tissues of the pink oleander, *Nerium oleander;* two of these constituents are cardiotoxic arrhythmogenic glycosides (oleandrin and folinerin) and a third is a genin (digitoxigenin). The yellow oleander, *Thevetia peruviana,* contains six identified cardiac glycosides (thevetin A and B, thevetoxin, nerifolin, peruviside, and ruvoside). Again, the cardiotonic action of several of these compounds is based on their actions on cardiac sodium–potassium-sensitive membrane-bound enzymes (Na^+,K^+-ATPase), resulting in both pharmacological and toxicological actions that are very similar to those of the digitalis glycosides.

TABLE 1 Cardiovascular Toxins

Compound	Predominant effect	Experimental animals	Dose; Route	References
Digitalis compounds	Arrhythmogenic	Rat, adult	94 mg/kg	
		Rat, newborn	0.1 mg/kg	
		Guinea pig	0.08–.20 mg/kg	
Cryptostegia sp.	Arrhythmogenic	Cat	0.2–0.5 mg/kg (leaf)	Everist (1974); Sanduja *et al.* (1984)
		Horse	0.28 g/kg	
Oleander	Arrhythmogenic	Monkey	3–30 mg/kg	Langford and Boor (1996)
Toad toxins	Arrhythmogenic	Mouse	400 γ (purified)kg	Habermehl (1981); Meyer and Linde (1971)
Hydrocarbons				
Chloroform	Arrhythmogenic	Cat	Anesthesia	Zakhari (1992)
Halothane	Arrhythmogenic	Dog	Anesthesia with 0.5–4%	Zakhari (1992)
Trichloroethylene	Arrhythmogenic	Dog	Anesthesia	Zakhari (1992)
Fluorocarbons	Arrhythmogenic	Cat	Anesthesia with 2–9%	Zakhari (1992)
Catecholamines				
Epinephrine	Myocardial necrotizing	Rat	6.1 mg/kg (LD_{50})	Van Fleet and Ferrans (1986); Waters (1957); Waters and DeSoto-Nagy (1950)
	Vascular/medial	Dog (12 kg)	3–5 cc in 1 h/day × 4 days	
Norepinephrine	Myocardial necrotizing	Rat mesenteric artery	5.9×10^{-7} mol/liter	Joseph *et al.* 1997
	Vascular/medial	Dog	2–5 μg/kg/min × 6 h	Szakacs and Mehlman (1960)
Isoproterenol	Myocardial necrotizing	Rat	0.2–80 mg/kg; LD_{50} = 58 mg/kg	Dhalla *et al.* (1992); Herman and Ferrans (1991)
Allylamine	Myocardial necrotizing	Rat	50–100 mg/kg	
Cocaine	Myocardial necrotizing	Human	Overdose; anesthesia	Boor (1987)
Anthracyclines	Contractile toxin	Mouse	10–30 mg/kg (acute)	Toraason (1991a)
		Dog	18–24 mg/kg (chronic)	
		Pig	2.4 mg/kg × 6 (18 weeks; chronic)	
Ethanol	Contractile toxin	Human	Unknown	
	Arrhythmogenic	Human	Unknown	
Cobalt	Contractile toxin	Rat	20 mg/kg/day	Herman and Ferrans (1991); Toraason (1991b)
Homocysteine/methionine	Vascular/endothelial	Rat	200 mg/kg/day × 7.14 days	Matthias *et al.* (1996)
Methysergide	Vascular/endothelial	Human	4–5 mg/day (3 months–years)	Regan and Poletti; (1968)
Monocrotaline pyrrole	Vascular/endothelial			
Mitomycin C	Vascular/endothelial	Human	75 mg × 5 or 42 mg/m² (body surface area)	McCarthy and Staats (1986)
Methoxamine	Vascular/medial	Rat	30 μg/kg sc	Joseph *et al.* (1997)
		Rat mesenteric artery	10 μg/mg, direct application	
Minoxidil	Myocardial necrosis/hemorrhage	Pig	10 mg/kg/day × 2 days	
	Vascular/medial	Pig	10 mg/kg/day × 2 days	
Fenoldopam	Vascular/medial	Rat	50 μg/kg/min × 23 h, iv	Joseph *et al.* (1997)
Hydralazine	Vascular/medial	Dog	24 mg/kg, bid × 2 days	Mesfin *et al.* (1987)
Ergopeptine alkaloids	Vascular/medial	Cattle	50 ng–5 μg/g grass (grazing)	
Ergotamine	Vascular/medial	Human	10 mg/week (adult)	
β-Aminopropionitrile	Vascular/medial	Rat, weanling	1 g/kg/day × 3–6 weeks	
Allylamine + β-aminopropionitrile	Vascular/medial	Rat, adult	100 mg/kg/day (allylamine) + 1 g/kg/day (β-aminoproprionitrile) × 10 days	

Cardiotoxins Synthesized by Animals

Many cardiotoxins in nature are substances produced by animals, especially amphibians and reptiles, as a protective mechanism. Some of the most potent toxins known to humans are the toad and frog venoms that have been used by primitive peoples as arrow or dart poisons. These amphibian toxins are extractable from skin, skin secretions, or parotid gland of a variety of toxic species, and they consist of several different classes of cardiotoxic substances, including catecholamines and cardiotoxic steroid derivatives, including bufogenins and their conjugates. These structures are very similar to the digitalis-related compounds, except for a differing substitution at C17 and an ester linkage to subarylarginine (as opposed to a variety of sugars) at C3 (Fig. 1). These toxins have powerful pharmacological and arrhythmogenic effects on the heart that are presumably exerted through mechanisms similar to those defined for plant cardioactive glycosides. Few toxicological investigations have addressed the animal toxins, however. Thus, the cardiac glycosides of both plant and animal origin have been quite extensively studied, although it is likely that a host of other such compounds are yet to be discovered in both the plant and animal kingdoms.

Cardiotoxicity of Anesthetics, Solvents, and Propellants

Arrhythmogenic toxicity has been shown for a variety of nonglycoside compounds; the majority of these compounds, however, appear to induce sporadic arrhythmias that do not display a clearly dose-dependent toxic effect. These compounds include xenobiotic or industrial solvents that have a long history of use as anesthetics and other halogenated hydrocarbons that have been widely used as propellants.

In the early days of medical anesthesia, Levy and Lewis discovered that chloroform anesthesia was associated with a high incidence of sudden death in cats. These investigators also demonstrated that death was due to the sensitization of the myocardium to epinephrine-induced arrhythmias. Subsequent studies confirmed that a variety of halogenated hydrocarbon compounds, including those that have enjoyed widespread use as anesthetics and industrial solvents (including carbon tetrachloride, halothane, and trichloroethylene) have this same adverse effect of causing both cathecholamine-induced and spontaneous arrhythmias.

During the 1970s, the inhalation of halogenated compounds extensively used as commercial aerosols was associated with the occurrence of arrhythmias. The toxicity of these very common propellants, along with serious concerns about their damaging effects on the environment, led to the discontinuation of many of their uses and reduced production. These compounds include trichlorofluoromethane, dichlorodifluoromethane, and dichlorotetrafluoromethane (known as FC11, FC12, and FC114, respectively).

Many of these propellants have been implicated in human deaths from the abuse of propellants or other solvents, which on a worldwide basis is one of the most common forms of substance abuse, especially by children and adolescents. Besides propellants, however, a variety of compounds have been implicated in human deaths due to "sniffing" of glues and adhesives (e.g., benzene, zylene, toluene, *n*-hexane, trichloroethylene, and trichloroethane), plastic cement (e.g., methyl ethyl ketone, methyl isobutyl ketone, and ethyl acetate), and dry cleaning agents (e.g., methyl chloroform and methylene chloride).

Finally, at least one instance of the cardiotoxic effects of aerosols not associated with intentional abuse has been documented. Specifically, the occurrence of arrhythmias was documented in pathologists who used propellants to rapidly freeze tissue specimens for the purpose of frozen section diagnosis. Pathologists using propellants typically do so in the confined space of a cryostat, which, upon repeated spraying to freeze a specimen, inadvertently becomes an exposure chamber.

Necrotizing Cardiac Toxins

Vasoactive Amines

It has been known since the early 1900s that the endogenous catecholamines epinephrine and norepinephrine cause acute subendocardial necrosis when given in large doses. The literature also proliferated during the 1950s and 1960s concerning this same cardiotoxic effect of several synthetic catecholamines, especially the drug isoproterenol, a β-adrenergic agonists, which for many years was extensively used in the therapy of acute asthma. The specific scientific literature on isoproterenol is truly voluminous, with literally thousands of publications regarding the acute myocardial necrosis resulting from administration by a variety of routes. Most studies of isoproterenol-induced myocardial necrosis focused on experimental animals such as rat, rabbit, and dog.

The lesions caused by a single dose of isoproterenol given intraperitoneally or subcutaneously are characterized by acute myocardial necrosis, with contraction bands, involving primarily the subendocardium or inner lining of the heart. These myocardial lesions appear to be correlated with the β effect; because the LD_{50} of isoproterenol is generally much less than that of other catecholamines, the myocardial necrotizing effects are most pronounced. Repeated doses of isoproterenol result in severe loss of myocardium, with extensive, even transmural scars. Many experiments have explored both protective and exacerbating cotreatments. Myocardial necrosis was found to be potentiated by hyperthyroidism, cold exposure, and other forms of acute stress, high-fat diet, and obesity. Protection against myocardial necrosis was afforded by β-adrenergic blockade, diabetes, antioxidants such as vitamin E, reduced body weight, exercise, and hypocalcemia. The calcium channel blockers so commonly used in heart therapy today were initially studied for their protective effect in experimental models of isoproterenol-induced cardiotoxicity. Hence, this extensively used experimental model is, in large part, responsible for the foundations of modern cardiac therapy and has added immensely to the experimental focus on the important role played by calcium in myocardial function and injury.

Many other vasoactive drugs used as pressor agents (i.e., as positive inotropic agents that raise the blood pressure during congestive heart failure) also induce myocardial damage, although modern pressor therapy is generally less injurious to the heart. Agents such as dopamine and dobutamine cause less marked physiologic effects on the heart than other catecholamines, although they also are associated with subendocardial necrosis and hemorrhage when used in high prolonged doses for severe myocardial failure.

Allylamine

In addition to the many vasoactive substances already addressed, chemically simpler amines have been shown to induce acute myocardial necrosis. The most notable is allylamine, or 3-aminopropene, which was once extensively used in the vulcanization of rubber and is also used in the manufacture of pharmaceuticals. Allylamine has been given to a variety of species (including rat, rabbit, dog, monkey, and calf) by many routes of administration, with the consistent finding of subendocardial necrosis, which is essentially the same morphological lesion caused by cathecholamines. Although long-term administration of allylamine results in arterial lesions consisting of intimal proliferation of the vascular smooth muscle cells, it has been shown that the acute myocardial necrosis caused by allylamine precedes these structural vascular lesions, which occur only after prolonged administration (weeks to months). Recent studies of these interesting vascular changes caused by allylamine have characterized the phenotypic modulation that smooth muscle cells undergo in rats treated chronically with allylamine, thus providing important insights into the underlying mechanisms by which early atherosclerotic lesions may develop in humans.

Mechanisms of Myocardial Necrosis

The underlying mechanism by which amines cause myocardial necrosis has been extensively debated. One view is that the marked physiological effects of most catecholamines, including the severe hypotension in the case of β-agonists, combined with a positive chronotropic effect on the heart result in a relative hypoxia of the endocardium. This phenomenon has been termed a relative "subendocardial steal"; that is, the blood flow to the last area of myocardium supplied is so reduced that it results in anoxic necrosis. The morphological picture of catecholamine-induced myocardial necrosis is compatible with this theory. Another theory, however, is that amines induce direct biochemical alterations in the cardiac myocyte that are lethal to the more susceptible subendocardial cells. Catecholamine metabolism, especially by some form of monoamine oxidase, has also been implicated in this theory of direct toxic insult, especially in view of the experimental demonstration of protection by monoamine oxidase inhibitors.

Drastic physiologic changes are not caused by amines that are structurally simpler than the catecholamines, such as allylamine. Thus, a direct biochemical injury has been proposed. With specific regard to allylamine-induced myocardial necrosis, it has been clearly shown that metabolism to a highly reactive aldehyde by an enzyme largely localized in the media of blood vessels is necessary for the *in vivo* toxic myocardial damage. Another mechanism has also been proposed—the possibility of amine-induced vasoconstriction of either large or medium coronary arteries, with resultant ischemic necrosis. It is of interest that this pathophysiological mechanism has also been proposed to explain the frequent sudden deaths associated with cocaine abuse. Cocaine abuse has clearly been shown to induce myocardial necrosis in young adults who have little underlying obstructive atherosclerotic coronary vascular disease. A striking example of this capacity for the cardiotoxicity of cocaine is seen in a case report of a myocardial infarction occurring in a young woman undergoing cocaine anesthesia, a form of topical anesthetic commonly used in nasal surgery. The patient was documented to have normal coronary vasculature, strongly implicating vasospasm of the coronary arteries as the etiology of the myocardial necrosis caused by cocaine.

The debate concerning the mechanism of the myocardial necrosis induced by a variety of both vasoactive and nonvasoactive amines illustrates the problems in understanding cardiac injury. The heart is an obligate aerobic organ, easily injured by a short period of anoxia. Hence, any theory to explain myocardial necrotizing injury must weigh the physiologic effects of a toxic compound against the direct toxic actions of the compounds and its metabolites on subcellular components of the myocyte.

Contractile Toxins

Anthracycline Cardiotoxicity

Anthracycline antitumor drugs, including doxorubicin and daunorubicin, are among the most highly successful chemotherapeutic agents ever used against a variety of leukemias and solid malignancies. An unfortunate side effect of these compounds, recognized initially in clinical use of the drugs, is a cumulative dose-dependent cardiotoxic effect characterized by intractable congestive heart failure, also known as a "dilated" type of cardiomyopathy. Because little myocardial cell necrosis occurs with even large doses of anthracyline drugs, the cardiotoxicity is thought to be due to severe dysfunction, or failure, of the contractile apparatus. Aberrations of the intracellular calcium metabolism and especially of the components of the mitochondrial respiratory chain are early changes caused by acute anthracycline administration in a variety of experimental animals, most notably rabbit and mouse. The majority of experimental models of anthracycline cardiotoxicity are chronic models, in order to more closely replicate the chronic contractile failure seen in humans, with repeated doses given over a period of weeks or even months.

The role of free radical injury in cardiac injury is, perhaps, best illustrated in the case of experimental anthracycline toxicity. The importance of the metabolism of the anthracyclines to free radical species was recognized with the work of Myers *et al.* (1971) on the protective effect of free radical scavengers. Subsequent work by these and other investigators demonstrated the importance of iron-linked metabolism of doxorubicin to a semiquinone form, which acts as the highly reactive intermediate to generate reactive oxygen species, thus inducing lipid peroxidation in cellular components, such as mitochondria, contractile apparatus, and other cellular membranes. Although the induction of superoxide dismutase and catalase occurs in the myocardium, apparently it is at a level insufficient to afford protection. Cardiotoxicity, however, is reduced by a 60- or 100-fold overexpression of catalase, induced by a heart-specific promoter in transgenic mice, confirming the potential importance of catalase as an antioxidant defense mechanism.

Although early efforts to counteract doxorubicin cardiotoxicity focused on the intracellular calcium effects, the most recent, remarkably successful means of diminishing these toxic contractile effects have largely focused on altering the iron-linked generation of the semiquinon intermediate and other free radical species by the anthracyclines.

Alcoholic Cardiomyopathy and Cobalt Cardiotoxicity

The occurrence of severe heart failure in chronic alcoholics has long been recognized as a distinct clinical entity; the term "alcoholic cardiomyopathy" has come to be used for this form of contractile toxicity that results in intractable heart failure. The etiology of this entity, and experimental support for a direct toxic effect of alcohol on the contractile apparatus, is not entirely clear, however. Ethanol has an acute negative inotropic effect on the heart, although this effect may be a combination of sympathetic nervous effects, as well as the direct inhibition of contractile function due to the interference with calcium regulation at the level of the contractile apparatus.

A third postulated mechanism through which contractility may be acutely and chronically deranged is by a direct effect of ethanol on membrane fluidity; such physical changes have been associated experimentally with mitochondrial alterations and defects in the electron transport chain. Although these various mechanisms of explaining the occurrence of human alcoholic cardiomyopathy have received much attention in the past and have substantial experimental support, it should be noted that an exact experimental model that reproduces the major clinical findings of the human disorder has not been described. Hence, the development of the full-blown human disorder has been thought to also necessitate some other factor, such as the specific nutritional deficiency of thiamine, extremely long-term exposure to alcohol, concurrent infections, or perhaps some genetic predisposition.

A striking example of a synergistic toxic effect between alcohol and a second toxin was seen in several human epidemic outbreaks of toxic exposure to cobalt that occurred principally in Quebec City (Canada), and subsequently in the United States and Europe as well. A large number of chronic alcoholics, generally heavy beer drinkers, were admitted to hospitals over a period of months because of severe congestive heart failure with a more rapidly progressive clinical course than generally seen in alcoholic cardiomyopathy. This outbreak eventually became known as "cobalt-beer cardiomyopathy" when it was discovered that the outbreak coincided with the recent brewery practice of adding cobalt to draft beer as a foam-stabilizing agent.

Subsequent experimental studies suggested that the cobalt–alcohol toxicity was indeed a synergistic one because cobalt on its own proved to be toxic only at extremely high doses. Furthermore, it was known that patients treated with high doses of cobalt for anemic disorders do not develop cardiac abnormalities. Cobalt has been experimentally shown to specifically block several oxidative steps of the Kreb's cycle by binding to sulfhydryl groups of α-lipoic acid, but the toxic effects on the heart appear to be augmented by concurrent protein deficiency. Thus, it appears that cobalt's effects, in combination with those of alcohol, represent a toxic synergistic interaction, resulting in this striking example of human cardiac toxicity that directly led to strict control of the use of cobalt in manufacturing.

VASCULAR TOXINS

Intimal Injury

Role of the Endothelium

The intima of arterial vessels is a highly reactive tissue component; when damaged by a host of differing agents that injure the single-cell layer of endothelium, proliferative lesions develop that are quite constant in their morphological character. The most evident example of this basic vascular reaction to injury is seen following physical injury. Following single-cell or minor injury, the endothelium rapidly and efficiently reestablishes its integrity through spreading and cell migration. Following more severe injury involving larger areas of endothelium, however, such as experimental balloon catheter denudation, an exuberant circumferential proliferation of the vascular smooth muscle occurs, drastically narrowing the lumen and reducing the blood flow. Severe endothelial injury, no matter the underlying cause, also renders the vessel prone to thrombus formation, which in itself perpetuates the injury through a variety of growth factors released by components of the clot itself, and also by subsequent inflammatory reaction.

Homocysteine and Methionine

Given this reaction of the endothelium to severe injury, it is assumed that any toxin that results in thrombogenesis, or severe injury of large areas of endothelium, will result in proliferative lesions that may become significantly occlusive. An excellent example of such an apparently direct toxic insult to endothelium is that of homocysteine. It has been known for many years that patients with inborn metabolic defects resulting in high serum levels of homocysteine develop severe fatal occlusive and thrombotic vascular disease. Essentially, as children or young adults, such homocystinemic patients develop severe vascular disease resembling accelerated atherosclerosis. More recently, the level of homocysteine in the blood has also been established as an independent risk factor for the development of atherosclerotic vascular disease in humans without clear-cut identifiable metabolic disorders. Thus, even moderate increases in serum methionine appear to predispose humans to vascular injury.

Experimental studies in a variety of species, including rabbits, baboons, rhesus monkeys, pigs, and rats, have indicated that the administration of homocysteine thiolactone results in marked endothelial injury of large blood vessels such as the aorta. Furthermore, the administration of methionine, which is degraded *in vivo* to homocysteine, results in high hyperhomocysteinemia and severe endothelial cell lysis and denudation. In this model, some superficial smooth muscle cell damage is also present in the media. Thus it appears that homocysteine in blood acts as a direct endothelial toxin, possibly related to the generation of oxygen-derived free radicals that target intracellular sites such as DNA and NAD^+.

Methysergide and Monocrotaline

Methysergide is a drug that at one time was used extensively for headache disorders. Methysergide therapy in humans has been associated with focal intimal proliferation in a variety of blood vessels, including small vessels found in the mesentery of the bowel and larger vessels such as carotid artery. In addition, a well-described thickening of the cardiac valves and the inner lining of the heart has been found in patients given methysergide as therapy for headaches. These cardiac lesions have been likened to the fibroblastic lesions of blood vessels and cardiac valve leaflets that occur secondary to endogenously produced histamine in the carcinoid syndrome (i.e., a cardiovascular pathophysiological reaction with structural lesions, secondary to the high concentrations of histamine produced by carcinoid tumors).

Both the cardiac and vascular lesions cause serious dysfunction of heart, lung, bowel, and other organs. Hence, patients receiving methysergide are carefully observed for the development of cardiac or vascular complications, and the dosage regimens are carefully monitored.

A very clear example of endothelial toxicity and vascular injury ocurring secondary to the metabolism of a primary toxin is found in the well-studied alkaloid plant toxin, monocrotaline. The metabolic activation of monocrotaline to the highly reactive toxic pyrrole occurs in the liver, and rapid passage to the lung results in covalent binding to lung macromolecules and subsequent vascular alterations, including the development of pulmonary hypertension (medial thickening of small arteries and right ventricular hypertrophy). The initial target of this toxic injury is thought to be the endothelial cell within the specific target organ (i.e. the lung). Early platelet sequestration and thrombosis has been demonstrated, followed by structural damage of the endothelium of small vessels preceding the increase in pulmonary arterial pressure.

At least one clinically relevant drug, the anticancer agent mitomycin C, may act through similar mechanisms to cause pulmonary injury. Intracapillary fibrin thrombi in the lung, pulmonary hypertension, and pulmonary interstitial infiltrates indicative of lung damage have been documented in human acute toxicity with mitomycin C. In addition, however, a diffuse small-vessel thrombotic process was documented, with resultant renal failure due to vascular damage to the kidney. The activated metabolites of mitomycin C are pyrrole-based bifunctional alkylating agents with structural similarities to monocrotoline pyrrole; hence, it is possible that similar mechanisms operate to induce diffuse systemic endothelial injury in the case of mitomycin C, whereas during experimental monocrotoline intoxication the hepatic metabolites apparently localize to the pulmonary vasculature.

Medial Injury

Medial Smooth Muscle vs Endothelial Injury

All arteries possess a medial layer that is composed predominantly of vascular smooth muscle cells and extracellular matrix. The extracellular component varies in composition from vessel to vessel, with the arteriolar and muscular arterial media consisting predominantly of collagen, whereas the larger elastic arteries contain abundant elastic tissue that is responsible for their elastic properties. The target of toxic injury discussed in this section is primarily the vascular smooth muscle cell of the media; however, associated with cellular injury in the media are alterations in the extracellular matrix and, hence, the structural components of the blood vessel wall, which are also important in these forms of vascular toxicity.

The media's role is most prominent in the distribution and physiological regulation of the blood flow that is the primary function of the muscular arteries, the conductance vessels or arterioles, and the large elastic arteries (the aorta and its immediate branches). Hence, injury to the media can have far-reaching pathological results with regard to blood pressure and the integrity of the vasculature.

Substances that injure the endothelium will also often cause alterations in the media. An example of this is seen in the experimental model of monocrotoline intoxication previously discussed; in that model, small pulmonary vessels undergo extensive remodeling, with prominent medial hypertrophy, following the initial endothelial damage. In this section, however, the focus will be on toxic compounds that injure the smooth muscle component (i.e., the media) of vessels either without extensive endothelial damage or with delayed intimal proliferative lesions that temporally follow the initial endothelial injury.

Vasoactive Substances

Many of the agents that cause acute arterial medial lesions without significant early endothelial damage are vasoactive substances; that is, these compounds induce marked systemic hypertension, directly cause arterial or arteriolar constriction, or may conversely cause hypotension through vasodilatation. Some of these compounds also are among those vasoactive substances discussed above as inducing acute myocardial necrosis. The cardiac lesions caused by these compounds are relatively acute, whereas the vascular injury discussed in this section is more chronic.

It has been known since the early 1900s that large doses of both endogenous and exogenous catecholamines, including adrenaline and norepinephrine, will induce fibrinoid necrosis of small and large arteries acutely and will result in chronic medial calcification. These effects are presumed to be due to the marked systemic hypertension induced by catecholamines; in fact, nonpharmacological induction of hypertension through the rapid infusion of blood or saline results in diffuse medial fibrinoid necrosis with very similar morphological characteristics in both the dog and rat. High doses of vasoconstrictor agents, including vasopressin, 5-hydroxytryptamine, methoxamine, angiotensin II, and dopamine, cause similar medial necrosis of small arteries and arterioles.

In vitro studies of methoxamine and other vasoconstrictors indicate that this form of vascular necrotizing injury is independent of any hypertensive or hypotensive effect that these compounds exhibit. Although the endothelium usually remains intact following methoxamine-induced of segmental vascular medial necrosis, a few studies have shown that subtle alterations in endothelial permeability occur and, when doses are high or vasoactive substances are directedly applied to the vessels, endothelial cells may desquamate, resulting in fibrin and platelet thrombi as a presumably secondary phenomenon. It should be noted, however, that an alternative explanation is suggested by some authors who suggest that diffuse endothelial damage of arterioles is the primary event in systemic hypertension, and the necrotizing arteriopathy of the media is actually secondary to the insudation of plasma components into the medial vascular smooth muscle cells. Although this last theory deserves consideration, the bulk of evidence appears to support the media as the primary target of vascular injury due to vasoactive substances.

Arterial lesions with somewhat different characteristics from those induced by hypertensive and constrictor agents are seen following large doses of vasodilator compounds. Well-studied examples of such substances include minoxidil (which opens plasmalemmal potassium channels), fenoldopam (a dopamine agonist), and phosphdiesterase inhibitors; the pharmacology and toxic effects of these compounds has been recently reviewed by Joseph *et al.* (1997). In general, the small arteries of the splanchnic vasculature are affected by the continuous intravenous infusions of these substances, resulting in medial degeneration, and necrosis and hemorrhage into the media. Endothelial damage occurs only in rare areas of severe vascular necrosis following vasodilator intoxication.

Minoxidil, a long-acting hypotensive agent used in the treatment of severe hypertension, in high doses causes atrial intramyocardial hemorrhages in the dog and vascular lesions in the coronary arteries (a large muscular artery) as well as in larger muscular arteries of the mesentery, pancreas, and elsewhere. These vascular lesions are characterized by marked medial hemorrhage, with focal and transmural medial necrosis. Capillary endothelial injury has been noted ultrastructurally, although endothelial damage or thrombi are not generally thought to be prominent components of the lesion.

Ergot Alkaloids

A most interesting vascular toxin has been known for many years to cause a severe, often fatal syndrome in livestock and also has been proposed to have affected human populations throughout history with sporadic epidemic outbreaks of intoxication. The source of this family of extremely potent vascular toxins are grasses (e.g., rye) that are infested with endophytes of the species *Acremonium,* producing a series of ergopeptine alkaloids known generally as the ergot alkaloids. Included among such vasculotoxic compounds are lysergic acid amide (ergine), ergovaline, ergotamine, the clavine class of alkaloids, and the pyrrolizidine alkaloids, including permine.

Of these compounds, ergotamine has been used for a variety of therapeutic reasons in humans since the late 1800s. It was used in obstetrical practices in the past, and began to be used for migraine headaches in 1925 (following its isolation from ergot extract in 1918). Ergotamine is presently the most common drug prescribed for the treatment of migraine. Although the clinical use of ergotamine is generally safe, excessive use as well as the potentiation of toxicity by the concomittant use of other vasoactive compounds (erythromycin, the anticoagulant heparin, and methysergide) may result in severe arterial vasospasm in a variety of vascular beds, with serious complications including necrosis of bowel and extremities and overt myocardial infarction.

Contamination of livestock grazing grasses has been known for many years to result in severe toxicosis and complications, including gangrene of the distal extremities. Human populations have also been subject to outbreaks of such contamination of rye grasses, with major epidemics presumed to have occurred in Europe throughout recorded history (e.g., Saint Anthony's Fire). Because there are many biologically active compounds produced by contaminating grass endophytes, a variety of central nervous system effects are also described during such outbreaks.

It has been postulated that the witch trials of 1692 in Salem, Massachusetts, represent an outbreak of convulsive ergotism in which bizarre convulsant disorders, as well as gangrene of the extremites, affected a series of young women who were accused of practicing witchcraft. Indeed, it is likely that all the community members, including the judges involved, were themselves suffering central nervous system effects because a whole community would affected by the bread produced from flour made from contaminated grains. Although only a few experimental studies have examined the mechanism by which ergot alkaloids exert their extreme vascular toxic effects, it appears that a complex interplay of direct vasoconstrictive action, central nervous system effects, and inhibitory effects on vascular reflexes exists to result in vasospasm that may affect a variety of peripheral blood vessels.

Lathyrism

The term "lathyrism" was a term originally coined to describe the neurotoxic effects found in humans consuming flour made from the toxic sweetpea, *Lathyrus odoratus.* Although epidemics of this toxic exposure have been known since ancient times (lathyrism was known by Hipppocrates) to occur during times of famine when the sweetpea was used as a source of nutrition, it was not until the early 1900s that experimental workers reproduced some of the toxic manifestations seen in the human disorder. These manifestations include central nervous toxicity, bone and connective tissue abnormalities, and the formation of lethal aneurysms. The subsequent isolation of the toxic component of the sweetpea as β-aminopropiontrile, and extensive work on the mechanism of it action on collagen metabolism has led to a better understanding of the bone, connective tissue, and especially large vessel effects of this toxin.

Since the discovery and characterization of β-aminopropiontrile as the toxic compound found in the toxic sweetpea, a variety of other natural and synthetic compounds have been shown to have similar toxic effects on the blood vessel wall. Several of these toxins are structurally very similar to β-aminopropionitrile, including direct derivatives and aminoacetonitrile. Hydrazine compounds, such as semicarbazide and the antituberculous drug isoniazid also cause vascular injury similar to that seen in classic lathyrism. Several sulfhydryl compounds including cystamine and β-mercaptoethylamine may also have somewhat weaker adverse effects on the vascular media.

The presumed mechanism by which these compounds—including β-aminopropiontrile—act in immature animals is by the inhibition of the enzyme lysyl oxidase, a key enzyme in the cross-linking of collagen from immature protocollagen. It is of interest, therefore, that the toxic effect of β-aminopropiontrile is prominent only when given to immature, or suckling, animals for prolonged periods of time (i.e., weeks to months). This is presumed to be the period of most rapid synthesis of connective tissues, and it is during this period of rapid growth that lathyrogenic toxins have their most pronounced effects.

On the other hand, more recent studies of a synergistic toxicity between the cardiovascular toxin allylamine and β-aminopropiontrile has demonstrated that intoxication with combinations of allylamine and β-aminopropiontrile leads to a more acute degenerative change in the aorta and large vessels of the mature adult rat. The underlying mechanisms of this more acute, necrotizing toxic effect has yet to be elucidated, although it bears a resemblance to degenerative disorders that affect human blood vessels, resulting in aneurysm and death.

TREATMENT AND CONCLUSIONS

With regard to most cardiovascular toxins, few if any antidotes exist, although many modalities have been devised to cope with the clinical situations of intentional or inadvertant overdose. Most arrhythmogenic toxins, such as digitalis compounds or the similar compounds in plants or animals, exert their effects as long as circulating plasma levels remain at toxic levels. Hence, several ingenious clinical methods have been developed to remove or bind free toxin moieties in the plasma of humans having ingested a potentially fatal dose of digitalis, or the glycosides found in the oleander plant. For instance, standard therapy for such exposure consists of using specific antibodies (or fragments of antibodies) that react with the toxic glycoside, inactiviating its toxic arrhythmogenic actions on the membrane of the cardiac myocyte. The dialysis of such glycoside–antibody complexes through hemoperfusion techniques has also been employed to remove the complexes from the blood. With regard to many of the vasoactive toxic compounds, antagonistic drugs may reduce the acute toxicity of the specific compound. For instance, treatment with β-blockers or α-blockers for isoproterenol or epinephrine toxicity, respectively, attenuates toxicity.

The most effective prevention of vasculotoxicity by the compounds discussed here is clearly avoidance of exposure to the toxin. This is especially true in the case of known vasculotoxic or cardiotoxic therapeutic agents, such as daunomycin or ergotamine, where the therapeutic use should be closely confined to appropriate therapeutic regimens, and toxicity should be closely monitored by appropriate techniques. Similarly, limiting the exposure of humans (especially children) or domestic animals to the naturally occurring cardiovascular toxins discussed here (e.g., oleander, amphibian toxins, and ergot alkaloids) is of paramount importance in limiting or minimizing the potential harmful effects.

In conclusion, a vast array of cardiovascular toxins exists in the natural world. Many of these toxins, however, have historically been used as highly useful therapeutic agents and have led to the development of commonly used and highly efficacious cardiovascular drugs.

Bibliography

Akera, T., Hook, J. B., Tobin, T., and Brody, T. M. (1972). Cardiac glycoside sensitivity of ($Na^+ + K^+$)-activated ATPase in newborn rats. *Res. Commun. Chem. Pathol. Pharmacol.* **4,** 699–706.

Akera, T., Yamamoto, S., Chubb, J., McNish, R., and Brody, T. M. (1979). Biochemical basis for the low sensitivity of the rat heart to digitalis. *Naunyn-Schmiedeberg's Arch. Pharmacol.* **308,** 81–88.

Allen, J. C., and Schwartz, A. (1969). A possible biochemical explanation for the insensitivity of the rat to cardiac glycosides. *J. Pharmacol. Exp. Ther.* **168,** 42–46.

Aversano, R. C., and Boor, P. J. (1983). Histochemical alterations of acute and chronic doxorubicin cardiotoxicity. *J. Mol. Cell Cardiol.* **15,** 543–553.

Aviado, D. M. (1975). Toxicity of aerosol propellants in the respiratory and circulatory systems. IX. Summary of the most toxic: trichlorofluoromethane. *Toxicology* **3,** 311–319.

Berman, R. S., and Martin, W. (1993). Arterial endothelial barrier dysfunction: Actions of homocysteine and the hypoxanthine-xanthine oxidase free radical generating system. *Br. J. Pharmacol.* **108,** 920–926.

Blundell, G., Jones, B. G., Rose, F. A., and Tudball, N. (1996). Homocysteine mediated endothelial cell toxicity and its amelioration. *Atherosclerosis* **122,** 163–172.

Boor, P. J. (1987). Amines and the heart. *Arch. Pathol. Lab. Med.* **111,** 930–932.

Boor, P. J., Gotlieb, A. I., Joseph, E. C., Kern, W. D., Roth, R. A., and Tomaszewski, K. E. (1995). Chemical-induced vasculature injury. *Toxicol. Appl. Pharmacol.* **132,** 177–195.

Boor, P. J., and Langford, S. D. (1997). Pathogenesis of chemically induced arterial lesions. *In* Bishop SP, Kerns WD, eds. "Cardiovascular Toxicology" (S. P. Bishop and W. D. Kerns, eds.), pp. 309–332. Pergamon Press, New York.

Boor, P. J., Reynolds, E. S., and Moslen, M. T. (1976). Neurotoxicity of digitoxin in adult and newborn rats: Drug distribution. *Arch. Int. Pharmacodyn.* **224,** 4–12.

Byrom, F. B., and Dodson, L. F. (1948). The causation of acute arterial necrosis in hypertensive disease. *J. Pathol. Bacteriol.* **60,** 357–368.

Chen, K. K., and Robbins, E. B. (1944). Influence of age of rabbits on the toxicity of ouabain. *J. Am. Pharmac. Assoc.* **33,** 61–62.

Dhalla, N. S., Yales, J. C., Naimark, B., Dhalla, K., Beamish, R. E., and Ostadal, B. (1992). Cardiotoxicity of catecholamines and related agents. *In* "Cardiovascular Toxicology" (D. Acosta, Jr., ed.), 2nd ed. pp. 239–282. Raven Press, New York.

Everist, S. L. (1974). Poisonous plants of Australia. *In* pp. 77–84. Angus and Robertson, Sydney.

Habermehl, G. G. (1981). "Venomous Animals and Their Toxins," 2nd ed. Springer-Verlag, Berlin.

Herman, E. H., and Ferrans, V. J. (1991). Overview of morphologic changes induced by the toxic effects of drugs on the cardiovascular system. *In* "Principles of Cardiac Toxicology" (S. I. Baskin, ed.), pp. 607–681. CRC Press, Boca Raton, FL.

Hougen, T. J., Lloyd, B. L., and Smith, T. W. (1979). Effects of inotropic and arrhythmogenic digoxin doses and of digoxin-specific antibody on myocardial monovalent cation transport in the dog. *Circ. Res.* **44,** 23–31.

Joseph, E. C., Mesfin, G., and Kerns, W. D. (1997). Pathogenesis of arterial lesions caused by vasoactive compounds in laboratory animals. *In* "Cardiovascular Toxicology" (S. P. Bishop and W. D. Kerns, eds.), pp. 279–307. Pergamon Press, New York.

Kang, Y. J., Chen, Y., and Epstein, P. N. (1996). Suppression of doxorubicin cardiotoxicity by overexpression of catalase in the heart of transgenic mice. *J. Biol. Chem.* **271,** 12610–12616.

Langer, G. A. (1981). Mechanism of action of the cardiac glycosides on the heart. *Biochem. Pharmacol.* **30,** 3261–3264.

Langford, S. D., and Boor, P. J. (1996). Oleander toxicity: an examination of human and animal toxic exposures. *Toxicology* **109,**1–13.

Levy, A. G., and Lewis, T. (1911). Heart irregularities, resulting from the inhalation of low percentage of chloroform vapour, and their relationship to ventricular fibrillation. *Heart* **12,** 99–111.

Mason, J. W., Billingham, M. E., Friedman, J. P. (1977). Methysergide-induced heart disease. A case of multivalvular and myocardial fibrosis. *Circulation* **56,** 889–890.

Matthias, D., Becker, C. H., Riezler, R., and Kindling, P. H. (1996). Homocysteine induced arteriosclerosis-like alterations of the aorta in normotensive and hypertensive rats following application of high doses of methionine. *Atherosclerosis* **122,** 201–216.

McCarthy, J. T., and Staats, B. A. (1986). Pulmonary hypertension, hemolytic anemia, and renal failure. *Chest* **89,** 608–611.

Mesfin, G. M., Shawaryn, G. G., and Higgins M. J. (1987). Cardiovascular alterations in dogs treated with hydralazine. *Toxicol. Pathol.* **15,** 409–416.

Meyer, K., and Linde, H. (1971). Collection of toad venoms and chemistry of the toad venom steroids. *In* Bucherl W, Buckley E, eds. "Venomous Animals and Their Venoms" (W. Bucherl and E. Buckley, eds.), pp. 521–556. Academic Press, New York.

Morris, L. E., Noltensmeyer, M. H., and White, J. M, Jr. (1953). Epinephrine-induced cardiac irregularities in the dog during anesthesia with trichloroethylene, cyclopropane, ethyl chloride and chloroform. *Anesthesiology* **14,** 153–158.

Okita, G. T. (1967). Species difference in duration of action of cardiac glycosides. *Federation Proc.* **26,** 1125–1130.

Porter, J. K. (1995). Analysis of endophyte toxins: Fescue and other grasses toxic to livestock. *J. Animal Sci.* **73,** 871–880.

Pratt, W. B., and Taylor, P. (1999). "Principles of Drug Action: The Basis of Pharmacology." Churchhill Livingstone, New York.

Regan, J. F., and Poletti, B. J. (1968). Vascular adventitial fibrosis in a patient taking methysergide maleate. *JAMA* **203,** 165–167.

Sanduja, R., Lo, W. Y. R., Euler, K. L., Alam, M., and Morton, J. F. (1984). Cardenolides of *Cryptostegia madagascariensis*. *J. Nat. Prod.* **47,** 260–265.

Saxena, P. R., and de Vlaam-Schluter, G. M. (1974). Role of some biogenic substances in migraine and relevant mechanism in antimigraine action of ergotamine-studies in an experimental model for migraine. *Headache* 142–163.

Schwartz, D. T. (1965). Relation of superior-mesenteric-artery of obstruction to renal hypertension. A review of 46 cases. *NEJM* **272,** 1318–1321.

Scott, W. J., Beliles, R. P., and Silverman, H. I. (1971). The comparative acute toxicity of two cardiac glycosides in adult and newborn rats. *Toxicol. Appl. Pharmacol.* **20,** 599–601.

Silberstein, S. D., and Young, W. B. (1995). Safety and efficacy of ergotamine tartrate and dihydroergotamine in the treatment of migraine and status migrainosus. *Neurology* **45,** 577–584.

Szabuniewicz, M., Schwartz, W. L., and McCrady, J. D. (1972). Experimental oleander poisoning and treatment. *Southwestern Vet.* **25,** 105–114.

Szakacs, J. E., and Mehlman, B. (1960). Pathologic changes induced by 1-norepinephrine. Quantitative aspects. *Am. J. Cardiol.* **5,** 619–627.

Tarkowska, J. A. (1971). Antimitotic action of glycosides of *Nerium oleander*. *L. Hereditas* **67,** 205.

Toraason, M. (1991). Biochemical principles of cardiac toxicology. *In* "Principles of Cardiac Toxicology" (S. I. Baskin, ed.), pp. 39–70. CRC Press, Boca Raton, FL.

Toraason, M. (1991). Overview of morphologic changes induced by the toxic effects of drugs on the cardiovascular system. *In* Baskin SI, ed. "Principles of Cardiac Toxicology" (S. I. Baskin, ed.), pp. 39–70. CRC Press, Boca Raton, FL.

Upchurch, G. R., Jr., Welch, G. N., and Loscalzo, J. (1996). Homocysteine, EDRF, and endothelial function. *J. Nutrition* **126,**1290S–1294S.

Van Fleet, J. F., and Ferrans, V. J. (1986). Myocardial diseases of animals. *Am. J. Pathol.* **124:** 98–178.

Waters, L. L. (1957). Studies on the pathogenesis of vascular disease. The effect of a fatty meal on the course of acute inflammatory lesions of the coronary arteries and aortas of dogs. *Yale J. Biol. Med.* **30,** 101–109.

Waters, L. L., and DeSoto-Nagy, G. I. (1950). Circulatory factors in the pathogenesis of experimental arteriolar necrosis. *Yale J. Biol. Med.* **22,** 751–766.

Waters, L. L., DeSoto-Nagy, G. I. (1950). Lesions of the coronary arteries and great vessels of the dog following injection of adrenalin. Their presentation by dibenzamine. *Science* **111,** 634–635.

Weidner, M. E., Sigurdsson, S. T., and Hopkins, P. B. (1990). Sequence preferences of DNA interstrand cross-linking agents: dG-to-dG cross-linking at 5′-CG by structurally simplified analogues of Mitomycin C. *Biochemistry,* **29,** 9225–9233.

Wollenberger, A. Jehl, J., and Karsh, M. L. (1953). Influence of age on the sensitivity of the guinea pig and its myocardium to ouabain. *J. Pharmacol. Exp. Ther.* **108,** 52–60.

Zakhari, S. (1992). Cardiovascular toxicology of halogenated hydrocarbons and other solvents. *In* "Cardiovascular Toxicology" (D. Acosta, Jr., ed.), 2nd ed., pp. 409–454. Raven Press, New York.

PART III

TOXICOLOGY OF COMPOUNDS

CHAPTER

25

Hydrocarbons

GÜNTER KOSS*,†, IRENE TESSERAUX*

*Department of Labor, Health, and Social Affairs, Hamburg, Germany

†Department of Toxicology, Hamburg University Medical School, Hamburg, Germany

INTRODUCTION

Hydrocarbons are aliphatic (paraffinic), alicyclic (naphthenic) and aromatic, saturated and unsaturated, volatile, liquid and solid compounds. They are recovered from their natural source petroleum (e.g., gasoline, kerosene, mineral spirits, petroleum naphtha, petroleum ether, mineral seal oil), coal tar (benzene, toluene, xylene), and pine wood (turpentine). Volatile compounds (e.g., shorter-chain alkanes) are recovered from natural gas. In some cases, hydrocarbons are products of chemical syntheses (e.g., ethylbenzene, styrene) or produced by distillation of wood or fermentation of biological materials (e.g., alcohols). Another group of hydrocarbons might also be referred to as products because they are generated by incomplete combustion. They are characterized by homocyclic polynuclear aromatic structures. These compounds are called polycyclic aromatic hydrocarbons (PAH). While the latter group of compounds is of toxicological interest only, the other hydrocarbons are widely used industrial and commercial products and as such may contaminate the environment, including the work place. The two most common routes of exposure for hydrocarbons are inhalation and ingestion. In many cases, humans are exposed to mixtures of hydrocarbons. The toxicology of only a few selected commonly occurring and used individual chemicals will be described.

AROMATIC HYDROCARBONS

Benzene

Benzene is contained in mineral oil, natural gas, coal tar, gasoline, and motor-vehicle emissions. Also, it is part of tobacco smoke. Benzene is a chemical intermediate in the synthesis of styrene; alkylated, nitrated, and halogenated benzenes; phenols; aniline; and hexachlorocyclohexane. According to 1972 convention of the International Labour Organization (ILO), the use of benzene is prohibited if suitable substitute products are available. The content is restricted in gasoline. Its biogenic development from substances of biological importance (via decarboxylation of benzoic acid) can be neglected. The amount of production and, even more importantly the emissions from mobile sources, which account for 85% of the total emissions in the United States, lead to ubiquitous contamination, mainly via the air and to a lesser extent via food and drinking water.

Ambient air concentrations in urban areas range from 3 to 18 $\mu g/m^3$ (1–5.7 ppb). The background levels are around 1 $\mu g/m^3$ (0.5 ppb). Indoor residential concentrations in the United States were reported to be between 5 and 10 $\mu g/m^3$ (1.5–3.1 ppb) in the homes of nonsmokers and between 5 and 17 $\mu g/m^3$ (1.6–5.3 ppb) in the homes of smokers. Inhalation is the dominant route of human exposure, accounting for more than 99% of the total daily intake. Estimates reveal that humans have a total daily intake of 250 μg/person. Mainstream tobacco smoke accounts for about 50% of the total U.S. population burden, with environmental tobacco smoke (ETS) contributing 5%.

Absorption, Distribution, Metabolism, and Excretion

Inhalative benzene absorption is characterized by a saturation kinetic determined by the inhalative portion. At the beginning of a benzene exposure, approximately 80% of the benzene is absorbed. In steady state between inhalation and exhalation, the absorption rate ranges between 40 and 50% and depends on ventilation parameters (minute volume of respiration) and the individual's intake capacity (biotransformation, adipose tissue). The odor threshold is about 16 mg/m^3.

Benzene can be absorbed well dermally and orally. Human skin is able to absorb 400 μg/cm^2 per hour after administration of fluid benzene. In rhesus monkeys an absorption rate of 7 μg/cm^2 per hour was determined. After epidermal application of a solution of benzene in other solvents, the absorbed amount of benzene is much lower. After oral intake, benzene is almost completely absorbed from the gastrointestinal tract.

After an oral dose of 1.5 mg/kg of [^{14}C]benzene (analogous to 16 mg/m^3 air, 6 h inhalation) in animals, radioactivity is detected in the liver, kidney, blood, bone marrow, nasal and pharyngeal cavities, and Zymbal, and mammary glands. Increasing the dose to 15 mg/kg (analogous to 160 mg/m^3 air, 6 h inhalation) leads to an accumulation of radioactivity in the Zymbal and mammary glands.

Due to the lipophilic character of benzene, the distribution in the organism is mainly dependent on the lipid amount of organs and tissues (Table 1). Adipose tissue has the highest concentration and storage capacity. A distribution ratio of 2:1 between erythrocytes and plasma appears in the blood. Inhalation studies with rats reveal that the benzene concentration can reach a steady state within 4 h in the blood, within 6 h in adipose tissue, and in less than 2 h in the bone marrow. The distribution of benzene in the organism is largely independent of the species or mode of administration.

Hepatic cytochrome P450-dependent enzymes catalyze the addition of an oxygen atom to the benzene ring. The postulated epoxide is a reactive short-lived intermediary product that changes nonenzymatically into phenol after administration of high benzene doses. A small portion of the epoxide is transformed into dihydrodiol (epoxide hydrase) and into catechol (dehydrogenases). Alternatively the epoxide can be conjugated with GSH in the presence of GSH *S*-transferases. Afterward, the glutathione conjugate is transformed into phenylmercapturic acid, which is able to pass through the kidney (Fig. 1). At lower doses of benzene (5 ppm in the air, analogous to 1.5 mg/kg body weight) the cytochrome P450-dependent enzymes catalyze the formation via ring hydroxylation of phenol, catechol, hydroquinone, and 1,2,4-benzenetriol. Starting from the epoxide and continuing on to the postulated oxacycloheptane or a glycolic intermediary product, as well as to catechol, *trans, trans*-muconaldehyde—after the opening of the ring—can be formed and is transformed into *trans, trans*-muconic acid after further oxidation. In the liver and partly also in the target organ of benzene toxicity, the red bone marrow, the hydroxylated metabolites are transformed into glucuronides and sulfate conjugates.

Nonconjugated metabolites are subject to further oxidation processes after their distribution into the bone marrow. Of the body's granulocytic leukocytes, 90% are located here. They have the capability of performing an "oxidative burst" in which various lysosomal and peroxidative enzymes are released, as well as oxidants including H_2O_2, and transfered into the phagosomes and into the extracellular space. Myeloperoxidase belongs to these enzymes and makes up 5% of the dry matter in peripheral neutrophilic granulocytes. In the immature granulocytes of the bone marrow, the amount of the myeloperoxidase can be even higher; phenol, hydroquinone, and catechol seem to be potential substrates.

The "oxidative burst" of stimulated human leukocytes leads to a transformation of phenol into reaction products that covalently bind to cellular structures. Biphenols and 4,4′diphenoquinone were identified in

TABLE 1 Concentration of Benzene Measured in Blood and Tissues and Calculated Concentration of Benzene in the Fat of Blood and Tissues of Rats[a]

	Benzene content (μg/g fresh w, measured)	Fat content (mg/g tissue, measured)	Benzene content (μg/g fat, calculated)
Blood	11.5	35	329
Bone marrow	37.0	100	370
Adipose tissue	164.4	600	274

[a]See Fig. 1. The calculation results in approximately similar benzene levels in fat, and thereby enables an estimation of the total body burden on the basis of blood levels.

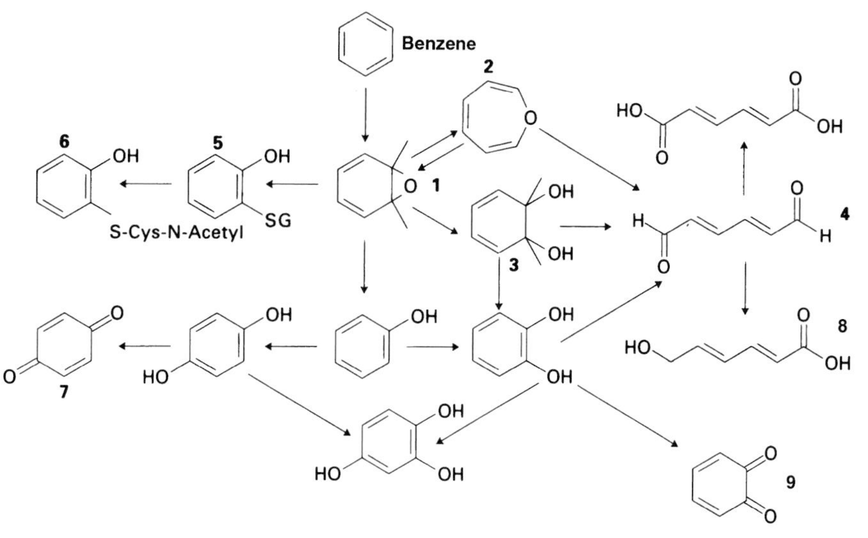

FIGURE 1 Proposed metabolism of benzene in the liver of mammals. Glucuronides and sulfates of the hydroxylated metabolites are not shown. Cytochrome P450 enzymes convert benzene to benzene oxide ("epoxide" 1), which is converted nonenzymatically to phenol and oxacycloheptane (2), or by an epoxide hydrase to benzene glycol (3). Metabolites 2, 3, and catechol undergo ring opening leading to *trans, trans*-muconaldehyde (4), which is oxidized to *trans, trans*-muconic acid and 6-hydroxy-2,4-*trans, trans*-hexadienoic acid (8), respectively. The epoxide becomes conjugated to glutathione via glutathione *S*-transferases, forming a glutathione conjugate (5), which is then converted to phenyl mercapturic acid (6). Stepwise oxidation of phenol to 1,4-hydroquinone leads to 1,4-benzoquinone (7) and via catechol to 1,2-benzoquinone (9). In mice, disproportionate amounts of hydroquinone conjugates and muconic acid are produced after inhalation of 16 mg benzene/m^3 and comparatively higher amounts of glutathione and phenyl sulfate conjugates at a exposure concentration of 1900 mg benzene/m^3. (Adapted from Cox, 1991.)

in vitro studies. Catalase and sodium azide inhibit the formation of such reaction products, presumably by detoxicating H_2O_2 by inhibition of the myeloperoxidase. The binding is further inhibited by GSH and ascorbic acid. Both factors have the property of an antioxidant through which, for instance, the phenoxy radical is reduced to phenol. In these tests the oxidative transformation of hydroquinone into 1,4-benzoquinone was observed. Phenol can stimulate myeloperoxidase-dependent hydroquinone oxidation. In addition, the hydroperoxidase component of the prostaglandin synthase plays a part in the hydroquinone activation. The impairment of the metabolic transformation of benzene in the liver via other substances, as well as a partial hepatectomy, decreases the extent of benzene-induced effects. Toluene antagonizes hematotoxic and genotoxic effects of benzene by competitive inhibition of microsomal biotransformation processes. Animal experiments show that the administration of both substances leads to larger neurotoxic effects, that is, an increase in concentration of biogenous amines in different regions of the central nervous system (CNS), than the separate application of both substances. This is probably due to a reduced biotransformation, resulting in a prolonged half-life and increasing concentration of both compounds in the central nervous system. The neurotoxicity observed is attributed to the parent compounds. A concurrent administration of benzene and lead or alcohol results in an impairment of the heme and protein synthesis in the precursors of the red blood cells.

The elimination kinetics of benzene are determined by the high biotransformation rate and by the high vapor pressure (118 mm Hg at 30°C). The elimination half-life of the unchanged substance in the tissue of rats varies between 0.4 and 0.8 h (in blood, bone marrow, liver, lung, kidney, spleen, and central nervous system) and 1.6 h (in adipose tissue). The elimination half-life of the major metabolite phenol in the blood is approximately 1 h. In contrast, the concentration of catechol and hydroquinone in the blood remains almost unchanged over a long period of time (9 h) after the end of exposure. The unchanged benzene (approximately 50%) is excreted mainly by exhalation. Ani-

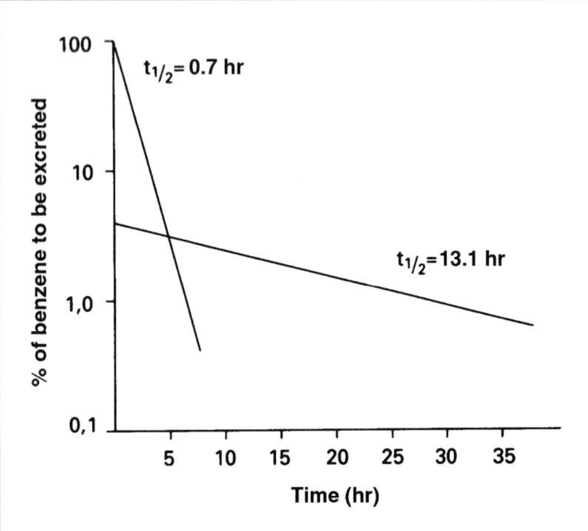

FIGURE 2 Percentage of benzene retained after cessation of a 6-h exposure of rats to 1.62 g benzene/m^3 air. The elimination curve is biphasic suggesting a two-compartment model. (Adapted from Rickert *et al.*, 1979.) From the first compartment, representing blood, bone marrow, liver, lung, kidneys, spleen, and brain, benzene is eliminated with a half-life of 0.7h. From the second compartment, representing adipose tissue and lipid fractions of other tissues, benzene is eliminated with a half-life of 13.1h.

TABLE 2 Symptoms after Acute Oral Benzene Exposure[a]

Mild intoxication	Severe intoxication
Dizziness	Staggering gait
Excitation	Visual disturbances
Euphoria	Shallow and rapid pulse
Vomiting	Breathlessness and constriction of the chest
Headache	Profound CNS depression
Fatigue	Loss of consciousness
Sleepiness	Collapse

[a]Adapted from Sandmeyer (1981).

mal experiments show various phases with an increasing half-life (Fig. 2). The half-life of the initial pulmonary elimination equals that of the benzene elimination in the blood. Later elimination phases have pronounced longer half-lives. The cause could be a not-yet-characterized deeper compartment. Via urine, mainly phenol and comparatively smaller amounts of hydroquinone, catechol, trihydroxyquinone, muconic acid (its conjugated form), and phenylmercapturic acid are excreted. Traces of retained benzene appear as CO_2 in the exhaled air and in metabolized form in the bile.

Acute and Chronic Toxicity

A concentration of approximately 2300 mg/m^3 air leads to unconsciousness after 30–60 min. A concentration of 65,000 mg/m^3 in air can have a lethal effect after 5 to 10 mins. Central depressory effects play the most important role. Mild forms of poisoning appear as subjective disorders (dizziness, numbness, headache, nausea, and feelings of drunkennes, as well ecstasy and euphoria). Severe forms of poisoning are mainly characterized by objectifiable symptoms (Table 2). Concentrations of 1–20 mg of benzene/liter blood can be reached. Microscopic changes of the blood cell count are not to be expected (for short exposures). Lesions of liver and kidney cannot be excluded after an intake of larger amounts of benzene.

TABLE 3 Hematopoietic Disorders following Chronic Benzene Inhalation

Erythropoietic system	Leukopoietic system	Thrombopoietic system
Anemia (aplastic)	Neutropenia	Thrombocytopenia
Erythroblastic myelosis	Leukopenia Leukocytosis	
Acute erythremia	Leukemia (acute myelogenous, acute myeloblastic, chronic myelogenous, chronic lymphatic) Lymphocytosis	
		Granulothrombopenia

The chronic exposure to benzene affects the hematopoietic system at three levels: erythropoiesis, leukopoiesis, and thrombopoiesis (Table 3). Casuistics from long-term occupational exposures prove the incidence of benzene-induced hemopathies with different severity and outcome. Signs of a severe benzene intoxication are panmyelophthisis, panmyelopathy, and pancytopenia, as well as isolated cytopenias of the three hematopoietic areas. The malfunction of one system (erythropoietic, leukopoietic, or thrombopoietic system) can co-occur with the hyperfunction of another of the systems. Benzene exposure can also induce a proliferation increase ("initial stimulation") in the erythropoietic and leukopoietic system as a first reaction, which is then followed by a malfunction. However, neither certain bone marrow lesions nor a certain sequence of them is regularly noted.

Myeloproliferative changes that might be preceded by a chronic pancytopenia can lead to a malignant illness, such as acute myelogenous leukemia. Due to its leukemogenic effect, benzene has been classified as a human carcinogen by numerous public health agencies, such as the International Agency for Research on Cancer (IARC) in 1982.

Neither the duration and dose of exposure nor the latency periods until the onset of hematotoxic effects can be clearly quantified. A depression of the blood-forming systems can be manifested within a few months when the benzene dose correlates with a concentration range of 6.5–81 mg/m^3 during a workshift. Leukoses (leukemias) appeared after an exposure period of 1.5–5 years and a latency period of up to 12 years after the end of exposure. The causal benzene concentrations ranged between an average of 513 and 5194 mg/m^3. In one case (chronic leukosis), a concentration level of 52 mg/m^3 was reported. Refined analyses of epidemiological data suggest that a critical benzene concentration is necessary for the development of leukemia.

At high benzene exposures, experimental animals (rats, mice) show a retardation of the cell cycle and changes of the mitotic index in the bone marrow, destruction of stem cells in specific stages of the cell cycle, inhibition of cellular functions, and lesions in the functional structure of the bone marrow in which stem-cell proliferation and stem-cell differentiation are disturbed. The suppressing effect of benzene metabolites on the cell division of promyelocytes, myelocytes, erythroblasts, and pronormoblasts leads to a reduction of the number of cells. This stimulates the stem cells to differentiate and it can lead to a reduction of the multipotent colony-forming unit stem cell (CFU-S). Bone marrow macrophages, which can induce stem-cell proliferation by producing hematopoietic growth factors (interleukin 1 and 6, erythropoietin), are seen as target cells of the myelotoxic effects of hydroquinone and other benzene metabolites.

In vitro studies with bone marrow cells of mice strains of different sensitivity toward benzene prove a high cytotoxic effect of benzoquinone and hydroquinone in precursor cells of erythrocytes [colony-forming unit erythroid (CFU-e)]. The cytotoxic effects take place especially during late DNA synthesis (S) or in the premitotic resting stage (G2) of the cell cycle.

Specific Toxicology

Reproductive Toxicity

The subcutaneous administration of 3 ml of benzene/kg on the 13th day of pregnancy in mice results in cleft palates and deformities of the jaw. Inhalative exposures to 950 and 6900 mg/m^3 for 6 h from the 6th to the 15th day of pregnancy lead to retarded ossification in rats in which the female fetus is affected to a greater extent than the male fetus. These effects were not observed after exposure to 320 mg/m^3. In the germ cell of male animals, benzene causes clastogenic changes after a single oral dose (1 ml/kg). In spite of teratogenic properties, there is no evidence that benzene influences the number of implantations and live births. Weight and length of the fetuses are strongly affected after exposure to 6900 mg/m^3 for 6 h daily from the 6th to 15th day of pregnancy but were not observed after exposure to 950 mg/m^3 or lower air concentrations. However, it cannot be excluded that these observed fetotoxic effects may be caused by reduced food intake by the dams.

Mutagenicity

Through a covalent binding of reactive benzene metabolites (hydroquinone, *p*-benzoquinone) with cell nucleus DNA (deoxyguanosine), biologically stable damages can be observed in somatic cells. Recently the participation of active oxygen species in benzene-metabolite-induced DNA damage has been suggested both from *in vivo* and *in vitro* studies. Furthermore, point mutations, as well as chromosomal deletions, inversions, and translocations, can appear after benzene exposure and be conducive to the development of tumors. Chromosomal changes in which DNA segments larger than a gene can activate proto-oncogenes or deactivate tumor-suppressor genes. Genotoxic damage not attributed to the development of cancer includes the induction of micronuclei in peripheral normo- and polychromatic erythrocytes and sister chromatid exchanges (SCE) in the peripheral lympho-

TABLE 4 Tumors in Organs of Rat and Mouse following Long-Term Intake of Benzene[a]

Ear, Zymbal gland	Ovary
Harderian gland	Preputial gland
Hematopoietic system	Skin
Mammary gland	Stomach
Nasal cavity	Vascular system
Oral cavity	

[a]The compilation is based on the Carcinogenic Potency Database, which includes results that were published in the general literature or in Technical Reports of the National Cancer Institute/National Toxicology Program.

cytes and in bone marrow cells. The appearance of micronuclei reflects chromosome fragmentation through a cumulative clastogenic effect. The extent of the cytotoxic and genotoxic effects is dependent on sex, age, and strain of mice. Male animals are more sensitive to clastogenic effects than females (including pregnant ones). Human peripheral lymphocytes respond *in vivo* and *in vitro* to sister chromatid exchange and other chromosomal aberrations to benzene exposure. In isolated peripheral human lymphocytes catechol, *p*-benzoquinone, hydroquinone, 1,2,4-benzenetriol, and phenol induce sister chromatid exchanges. This effect can be inhibited by adding glutathione.

Carcinogenicity

Medical surveys on humans revealed the first evidence of leukemogenic properties. Extensive studies of workers in the Turkish shoe industry proved the human carcinogenicity of benzene. Studies in experimental animals confirmed carcinogenicity in humans independent of species, sex, and mode of administration in different organs of the organism (Table 4). However, there is no adequate animal model to study benzene-induced leukemia. The correlation between the applied dose and tumor incidence is presumably nonlinear. In contrast, tumor formation seems to be linearly dependent on the number of the genotoxic changes (DNA adducts) in the target organ.

It is possible that benzene or a metabolite binds competitively to cell membrane receptors, resulting in a blockade of growth-regulating messenger substances. Furthermore, the transfer of intracellular messengers stimulated by benzene or its conversion products into the cell nucleus could be possible, inducing proliferation. In both cases benzene would be classified as a promoter. Protein kinase C is considered to be activated *in vitro* by benzene. A further epigenetic mechanism could be the inhibition of the gap-junction formation in target cells by phenyl, which has promoter qualities (Table 5).

Risk assessment based on dose-frequency relationships and dose–effect relationships is therefore connected with much uncertainty. A nonlinear dose-frequency relationship for the various tumor types is derived from the results of the American National Toxicology Program (NTP) study on rats and mice. According to these, the incidence of the Zymbal gland tumors increases by a factor of 3 to 5 when the daily dose is only doubled (from 25 to 50 mg/kg). An incidence of 28% was observed for uterus neoplasias at a daily intake of 100 mg/kg and of only 15% when the daily dose was 25 and 50 mg/kg. Epidemiological

TABLE 5 Effects and Sequels of Hypothetical Benzene-Induced Carcinogenesis and Leukemogenicity in the Benzene-Exposed Organism[a]

Effect	Sequel
DNA adduct formation	Initiation
Cytotoxic damage to partially differentiated bone marrow cells	Compensating stem cell proliferation
Cytotoxic damage to bone marrow stromal cells and stromal macrophages	Impairment of stem cell proliferation and differentiation (leukemia as a result of failure by the stroma to produce normal regulatory signals)
Immunotoxicity	Survival and proliferation of tumor cells
Chromosomal deletions, inversions, or translocation	Activation of protooncogenes or deactivation of tumor suppressor genes

[a]Adapted from Cox (1991).

surveys of occupationally exposed workers reveal that at exposure concentrations of 32.5–325 mg/m^3 for a life time during working time, an incidence of 140 and 170 cases of leukemia per 1000 workers was observed. With regard to environmental exposure of the general population, an additional life-time risk resulting from 1 μg/m^3 benzene has been calculated to be between 1 and 32 cases of leukemia per 1 million.

Immunotoxicity

Chronic exposure of humans to benzene has been associated with several immune alterations. Animal experiments show that benzene impairs the maturation and proliferation of the B-lymphocyte precursor cells and decreases the number of leukocytes, as well as of the B- and T-lymphocytes in bone marrow, spleen, and thymus. The reduction of the B-lymphocytes is dose-dependent and more dramatic than the reduction of the T-lymphocytes. Also a dose-dependent reduction of the relative weight of thymus and spleen is observed. Assumedly *p*-benzoquinone blocks the mitosis of the lymphocytes via its reaction with sulfhydryl groups of the tubulin. Furthermore, it inhibits the production of interleukin 2 and RNA synthesis. Hydroquinone, *p*-benzoquinone, and catechol inhibit the release of hydrogen peroxide from stimulated macrophages. *p*-Benzoquinone diminishes the phagocytic and cytolytic activity of macrophages towards tumor cells. The humoral immune response is affected by benzene, whereas the cell-mediated immune response remains unchanged or at higher exposures is stimulated by impairment of the suppressor T-cells.

Toluene

Coal and mineral oil are the essential original materials for the production of industrial toluene. Other accumulating alkylbenzenes and benzene are separated via distillation, washing with sulfuric acid, and redistillation. Highly purified toluene contains less than 0.01% benzene, whereas industrially used toluene can contain 10–20% benzene and other hydrocarbons. Toluene is the starting material for the synthesis of a number of organic compounds. The main sources of emissions are motor vehicles, paint and coatings (also indoor), affixed expanses of adhesives (also indoor), mineral-oil industry, industrial use of toluene, and wood fires.

Toluene has been of increasing importance during the last few years due to its function as a substitute solvent for benzene. Ambient concentrations in urban areas are about 8 μg/m^3, in traffic-influenced areas up to 60 μg/m^3, and in rural environments approximately 3 μg/m^3 or less. Indoor concentrations can reach levels up to 200 μg/m^3. For the general population, a daily intake of 0.2 mg per person is estimated (~60% originate from the air and ~40% from food). A larger intake in individual cases can result from the toluene contamination of fatty food, from the ambient indoor air, and from tobacco smoking. Keeping food and printed matters (newspapers and magazines) in the same room leads to an increase of the toluene amount in fatty food.

Absorption, Distribution, Metabolism, and Excretion

Humans absorb 40–60% of the inhaled toluene. The dermal absorption rate is 14–23 mg toluene/cm^2 skin per hour if toluene is administered in a lipophilic solvent but will be only 0.16–0.6 mg/cm^2 if the substance is administered in a saturated hydrous solution. The dermal uptake of toluene from the air reaches maximally 1% of the inhalative intake. After oral uptake, toluene is almost completely absorbed; however, it is lower than by inhalation.

The distribution of toluene in the organism is influenced by the lipid content of tissues and organs. The concentration ratio among blood, organs (liver, lung, kidney, CNS), and adipose tissue is 1:1–3:80. In the CNS of humans and rats, the distribution is not uniform. The toluene concentration is twice as high in the stem region (regulating cardiac activity, vasomotoricity, and respiration) than in the hippocampus (regulating endocrine and vegetative nervous functions) and the cerebral cortex. An increased blood circulation during exercise results in higher uptake in skeletal muscles, heart, CNS, and adipose tissue. Consequently, the toluene concentration in the liver, kidney, and gastrointestinal tract is comparatively low.

The metabolic transformation (Fig. 3) is performed mainly in the liver. Toluene interferes with the biotransformation of other related substances. For instance, it inhibits the metabolic transformation of benzene, styrene, xylene, and trichloroethane. Toluene—like *m*- and *p*-xylene—was shown to reduce the cytochrome-P450 content in rat lung and influence the benzo[*a*]pyrene metabolism by shifting the balance between intoxication and detoxication, which leads to an enhanced benzo[*a*]pyrene toxicity. Ethanol impairs the metabolic transformation of toluene, as surveys of printers show.

Approximately 20% of inhaled toluene is exhaled unchanged by humans and 80% is eliminated via the kidney after biotransformation. The elimination half-life of toluene from the subcutaneous adipose tissue of humans ranges between 0.5 and 2.7 days, and from blood between 6 and 8 h. In humans there is a corre-

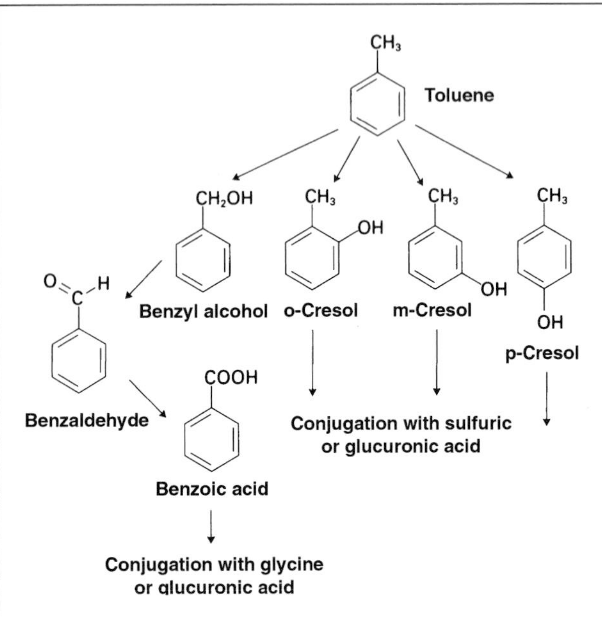

FIGURE 3 Metabolism of toluene in mammals. Oxidation of the methyl group and of the ring is catalyzed by microsomal cytochrome P450. Benzoic acid is formed gradually by the alcohol dehydrogenase and aldehyde dehydrogenase. Glucuronic acid conjugation (in some species but not in humans) takes place after saturation of the conjugation reaction with glycine to hippuric acid. About 80% of the absorbed toluene are conjugated with glycine after oxidation of the methyl group. About 1% of toluene is hydroxylated to cresol. 19% of the absorbed toluene is exhaled as parent compound. (Adapted from Dean, 1978.)

lation between the elimination half-life and the individual portion of the body fat in relation to the total body weight. This means that toluene is excreted more slowly with increasing amounts of body fat.

Acute and Chronic Toxicity

Toluene, as do many other solvents, evokes acute irritative and neurotoxic effects (Table 6). The latter can be classified into three clinical patterns.

1. Acute narcotic and subnarcotic states during several hours after exposure; at lower concentrations the impairment of vigilance results in lowered reliability of performance. Euphoria and irritation alternate with depressed mood; altered sleep quality leads to sleepiness and fatigue.
2. Pseudoneurasthenic syndrome in repeatedly exposed subjects, manifested as persistent mental and autonomic lability, sleep disturbances, and chronic fatigue, adversely affecting performance, quality of life, and adaptability to life stresses.
3. Psychoorganic syndrome in chronically exposed persons, including deeper and more stable changes in mental performance, sensorimotor coordination, and personality.

After long-term inhalative intake, functional disorders of liver and heart, as well as bone marrow lesions and changes in the blood count, can appear. However, the existing data do not allow us to quantify the influence of benzene, which may be present as an impurity in toluene. In a special context, toluene became known as drug for sniffers ("glue sniffing"). The resulting symptoms are motor weakness, intention tremor, ataxia, and, seldom, cerebral atrophy. Moreover, in workers occupationally exposed to toluene, otoneurological and audiological alterations were ascertained. With the exception of morphological damage, a recovery is mostly possible after a few months of withdrawal. To prevent chronic health effects, the WHO Air Quality Guideline (1997) proposes a value of 0.26 mg toluene/m^3 as a weekly average for the indoor and outdoor environments.

Specific Toxicology

Reproductive Toxicity

Cases in which children were born with CNS dysfunction, anomalies of the viscerocranium and the extremities, and growth retardations have been described. Their mothers had inhaled toluene during their pregnancies and in the preceding 4 to 5 years when using paint removers. However, no information about the toluene concentration in the air or about the intake of further solvents is known. Sniffing of toluene by pregnant women has been reported to cause intrauterine growth retardation among the infants. An elevated rate of spontaneous abortions was determined in a group (55 women with 105 pregnancies) of occupationally exposed (exposure range 190–570 mg/m^3) women.

In rats exposed to 6000 mg toluene/m^3 air daily from the 1st to 21st days of pregnancy, no signs of teratogenic properties of toluene were found. At a dose of 6000 mg toluene/m^3 daily during the entire pregnancy, about 1/6 of rat embryos died. In rabbits exposed to 1000 mg/m^3 air during the 6th to 20th days of pregnancy, spontaneous abortions were observed. When rats were exposed to 1000 mg toluene/m^3 air daily for 8 h from the 1st to 21st days of pregnancy, the fetal weights were reduced by 13%. This concentration was not toxic in the mother animals. Mice that had been given doses of 260–870 mg/kg body weight daily from the 6th to 15th days of pregnancy showed an increase in the embryonal lethality

TABLE 6 Dose–Response Relationship for the Acute Effects in Humans of Single Short-Term Exposures to Toluene Vapor[a]

Dose	Effect
1 mg/m^3	Odor threshold
140 mg/m^3	Probably perceptible to most human beings
188–375 mg/m^3	Subjective complaints (fatigue, drowsiness, or very mild headache), but probably no observable impairment of reaction time or coordination
750 mg/m^3	Mild throat and eye irritation; prolonged eye-to-hand reaction time; some impaired cognitive function; slight headache, dizziness, sensation of intoxication; aftereffects: fatigue, general confusion, moderate insomnia
1125 mg/m^3	Detectable signs of incoordination may be expected during exposure periods of up to 8 h
1500 mg/m^3	Irritation of the eyes and throat and lachrymation; skin paraesthesia, gross signs of incoordination, and mental confusion expected during exposure periods of up to 8 h
1875–2250 mg/m^3	Anorexia, staggering gait, nausea, nervousness (persisting to next day), momentary loss of memory, significant reduction in reaction time
3000 mg/m^3	Pronounced nausea (after 3-h exposure); confusion, lack of self-control; extreme nervousness, muscular fatigue, and insomnia lasting for several days
5625 mg/m^3	Probably not lethal for exposure periods of up to 8 h; incoordination likely, extreme weakness
15,000 mg/m^3	Probably cause rapid impairment of reaction time, and coordination exposures of 1 h or longer might lead to narcosis and possibly death
37,500–112,500 mg/m^3	Onset of narcosis within a few min; longer exposures may be lethal

[a]Adapted from WHO (1985).

for the whole dose range and a decrease in fetal weight for doses between 430 and 870 mg/kg body weight. Rabbits that had been exposed to a dose of 113–1875 mg toluene/m^3 air from the 6th to 18th days after insemination for 6 h daily exhibited no fetal changes (no soft tissue or skeleton changes). Therefore toluene has no embryotoxic, fetotoxic, or teratogenic properties in rabbits up to a concentration of 1875 mg toluene/m^3.

A simultaneous intake of toluene and aspirin leads to a dramatic increase in the extent of the maternal and embryotoxic effects. The reason seems to be the reduction of the glycine pool caused by both substances.

Mutagenicity and Carcinogenicity

Tests with various *Salmonella typhimurium* strains and with *Escherichia coli* showed no signs of genotoxic and mutagenic properties of toluene.

Occupational exposures to toluene and other solvents revealed no clear evidence for human carcinogenicity. A cohort mortality study in shoe-manufacturing factories found an elevated incidence of lung cancer among the men but not among the women. The possible contribution of smoking was suggested.

The carcinogenic properties of inhaled toluene were tested on rats up to a concentration of 1125 mg/m^3. No increase in neoplastic changes was observed, in males or in females. After an oral dose of 500 mg of toluene/kg body weight 4–5 days per week during a period of 2 y, rats showed no increased incidence of tumors. The results after administration to the skin of mice are equivocal.

Ethylbenzene

Like benzene, toluene, and xylene, ethyl benzene (BTEX) is contained in gasoline. It is used in styrene synthesis and as a solvent (as a benzene substitute). The main part of the exposure originates from motor vehicles and its use as a solvent. Through pyrolysis of ethyl benzene, benzene, toluene, phenantrene, styrene, biphenyl, and various other polycyclic aromatic hydrocarbons are formed. In the gas phase, ethyl benzene is converted into ethylphenols, benzaldehyde, acetophenone and *m*- and *p*-nitroethyl benzene when it reacts with OH radicals, developing by photolytic conversion of nitrogen oxides.

Inhalation is the major intake route for humans. Ambient air concentrations in urban areas range between 1 and 7 $\mu g/m^3$, with a traffic- or industrially influenced maxima of 40 $\mu g/m^3$. Indoor concentrations can reach up to 100 $\mu g/m^3$. A special source of contamination is tobacco smoke. It can be naturally contained in honey, jasmine, papaya, olive oil, and cheese.

Absorption, Distribution, Metabolism, and Excretion

The pulmonary and enteral absorption rates of humans have not yet been determined. Presumably they are comparable to those of other alkyl benzenes. The rat absorbs pulmonarily about 60%. Liquid ethyl benzene is absorbed dermally at a rate up to 22–33 mg/cm^2 per hour. The distribution pattern is not known. Only metabolites are excreted with urine. The metabolic conversion takes place predominantly at the side chain (Fig. 4). Ring oxidation is of only minor importance. The excretion of the ethyl benzene metabolites is slower than the excretion of *m*-xylene metabolites. Simultaneous intake of both compounds leads to a mutual metabolic inhibition, resulting in a delayed excretion of the metabolites.

Acute and Chronic Toxicity

The short-term exposure to 4400 mg/m^3 air leads to irritation of the eyes; however, tolerance is developed quickly. At 8800 mg/m^3, secretion of tears, irritation of the nasal mucosa, and dizziness occur. At 22,000 mg/m^3, irritation of the eyes and nose is no longer tolerable. This concentration is lethal in guinea pigs after 30–60 minutes and within few minutes at 44,000 mg/m^3 and higher. Signs of poisoning are pul-

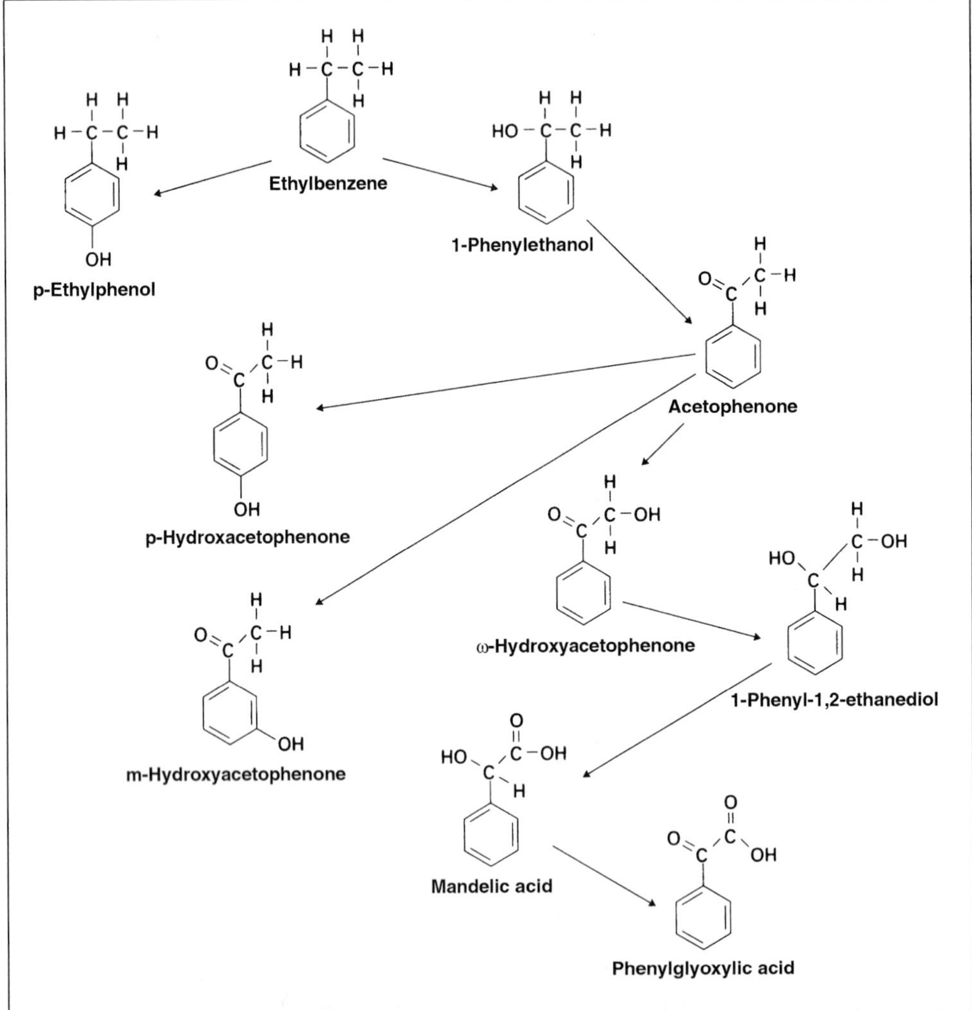

FIGURE 4 Metabolism of ethyl benzene in mammals. Conjugates of the metabolites are not shown. Urinary analyses suggest that 90% of the parent compound are converted to mandelic acid and phenylglyoxylic acid and only 4% are converted to ring-hydoxylated metabolites. Unknown glutathione conjugates and nonmetabolized ethylbenzene amount to about 6%. (Adapted from Fishbein, 1985c.)

monary edema and generalized visceral hyperaemia as a reaction to inflammation stimuli. Chronic intake of 1760–2640 mg/m^3 air results in a slight weight increase of the liver, kidneys, and testes of rats. There are no indications of hematotoxic effects.

Specific Toxicology

Reproductive Toxicity, Mutagenicity, and Carcinogenicity

No reproduction toxicity studies are available. Ames tests (for different *S. typhimurium* strains) with the metabolites mandelic acid, phenylglyoxyl acid, and hippuric acid yielded negative results.

Rats exposed to atmospheres containing 330–3300 mg/m^3(75–750 ppm) had increased incidences of kidney hyperplasia. Male mice exhibited higher incidences of lung tumors and female mice higher incidences of liver tumors. From these results, a clear evidence of carcinogenicity of ethyl benzene in male rats is concluded.

Xylene

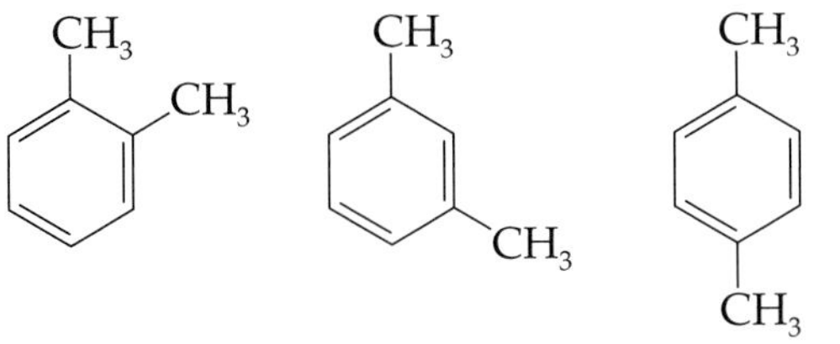

CH_3 CH_3 *ortho*-xylene; CH_3 CH_3 *meta*-xylene; CH_3 CH_3 *para*-xylene

Commercial products contain all three isomers of xylene, the portion of *m*-xylene being 60–70%. Furthermore, toluene, benzene, trimethylbenzene (pseudocumene), phenol, thiophene, pyridine, and aliphatic hydrocarbons can be present in xylene as impurities. The commercial product, mainly derived from mineral oil and coal, contains 10–20% *o*-xylene, 44–70% *m*-xylene, and 20% *p*-xylene, as well as about 10% ethylbenzene. This isomer mixture is contained in the BTX (benzene–toluene–xylene) components of gasoline. Furthermore, xylenes are used as solvents in paint and in the printing industry. The major sources of emission are refineries and cars. Indoor sources are mainly fresh coats of paint and adhesives. In the presence of NO_x and UV light, 80–90% of the xylenes in ambient air (and 30% of the benzene and 68% of toluene) are chemically converted within 6 h. Ambient air concentrations in urban areas range between 3 and 10 μg/m^3 for *o*-xylene and between 4 and 16 μg/m^3 for *m*- and *p*-xylene. Due to construction methods (hydrophobization of the outer walls), indoor air levels up to 300 μg/m^3 for *m*- and *p*-xylene and up to 40 μg/m^3 for *o*-xylene are found. The odor threshold of *m*- and *p*-xylene is about 800 μg/m^3 and for *o*-xylene approximately 3500 μg/m^3.

Absorption, Distribution, Metabolism, and Excretion

Inhalation is the major route of intake for humans. The pulmonary absorption rate for the three isomers ranges between 50 and 65%, depending on physical activity. The distribution ratio between blood and gas phase equals 29:1. Xylene is almost completely absorbed from the intestinal tract; dermal absorption is determined to be between 0.7 and 4.3 μg/cm^2 per minute. The organ and tissue distribution resembles those of other alkylbenzenes. Adrenal gland, bone marrow, CNS, spleen, and adipose tissue have comparatively high concentrations.

The main metabolic pathway for all three isomers in humans and animals is oxidation of one methyl group and subsequent conjugation with glycine (methyl hippuric acid). Ring hydroxylation and conjugation with glucuronic acid have a portion of approximately 2%. The occurrence of *o*-methyl benzylmercapturic acid in rats is an indicator for a conjugation reaction of *o*-xylene with glutathione (GSH). Unchanged xylene is eliminated by exhalation, whereas metabolites are excreted via urine. Xylene has a biphasic excretion pattern with an initial half-life of 1–2 h and a terminal half-life of about 20 h.

Acute and Chronic Toxicity

An acute exposure of 1–2 h at the most to a few hundred milligrams of xylene per cubic meter of air leads to sleepiness, numbness, headache, loss of concentration, and dizziness. After chronic exposure to a xylene concentration in the air of 1300 mg/m^3, signs of narcotic effects and functional disorders of liver, kidneys, and heart are observed. Among workers in the rubber industry using various aromatic solvents, an increased incidence of lymphocytic leukemia was observed. However, whether this effect is due to xylene or to a by-product is not known.

Specific Toxicology

Reproductive Toxicity

The exposure to 1500 mg/m^3 of *o*-xylene between days 7 and 14 of pregnancy resulted in reduced food intake in dams (in rats) followed by a retarded fetal development. Under the same conditions, at a concentration of 3000 mg/m^3, *m*- and *p*-xylene induce the appearance of supernumerary ribs and *o*-xylene fetal malossifications. In studies with mice, fetal malformation was observed after exposure to 500 mg/m^3 of *o*-, *m*-, and *p*-xylene. A significantly high portion of abnormal spermatozoa was noticed in rats after injection of 0.5 ml *o*-xylene/kg ip when they were kept in a heated room (30°C).

Mutagenicity and Carcinogenicity

Neither the bone marrow cell test nor the Ames test with various *S. typhimurium* strains (with or without metabolic activation) showed any signs of genotoxic effects. Studies with human lymphocytes revealed no evidence for xylene-induced chromosomal aberrations. Testing for possible clastogenic effect in rats exposed to 1320 mg/m^3 air for 18 weeks gave negative results.

Studies on the carcinogenicity are limited because only the isomer mixture was investigated and the chemical purity not sufficiently documented. In rats and mice the results were negative.

Styrene

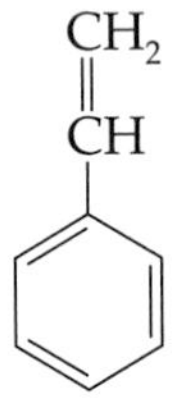

CH_2
||
CH

The compound, known also under the names cinnamene, phenethylene, phenylethene, styrolene, and vinyl benzene, is a colorless, highly volatile viscous liquid with a pungent odor. The odor perception threshold has been determined to be around 0.2 mg/m^3 for purified styrene. Styrene is an important monomer and is used mainly in the manufacturing of polymers and copolymers (polystyrene) and of reinforced fiber plastics. In 1992, the production of styrene in the United States was approximately 4 million tons. The highest human exposures to styrene occur in work-place air during polyester production. Peak concentrations as high as 800 mg/m^3 were determined in the personal breathing zone. Exposure to considerably lower levels can occur in ambient air. Concentrations in urban atmosphere range between 0.1 and 3 μg/m^3, automobile exhausts being the predominant source. Higher concentrations can be found in the vicinity of reinforced plastic processors. Indoor air may contain between 0.3 and 30 μg/m^3. Sources of contamination are styrene-containing polymers, tobacco smoking, and other combustion processes. To a minor extent, thermal degradation of polymers also releases styrene into the air. Polymerization of styrene and butadiene with latex is used for carpet backing. The smell of new carpets is mainly due to by-products, such as, 4-phenyl cyclohexene and 4-vinylcyclohexene, formed from styrene and butadiene in this process. Polystyrene and its copolymers are used as food-packaging materials, from which residual monomers may migrate into food.

Absorption, Distribution, Metabolism, and Excretion

Styrene is taken up by humans mainly via the lung, and 60–90% is absorbed; dermally only 2–5% is absorbed. The intestinal absorption in animal experiments is nearly complete. Due to its lipophilic properties, styrene is preferentially distributed in lipid-rich tissues; however, it does not accumulate there. The first important step in the metabolic pathway is the oxidation of styrene to the epoxide 7,8-styrene oxide by the microsomal cytochrome P450-dependent monooxygenase system (such as CYP2B6, CYP2E1, and CYP1A2). In the presence of the epoxide hydrase, glycol dehydrogenase and aldehyde dehydrogenase, mainly mandelic acid and phenylglyoxylic acid, are formed. Especially in animals, glutathione conjugation is a further side path of metabolism. The metabolism of styrene is competitively inhibited by the concurrent intake of ethanol. In humans, styrene metabolism is saturated at exposure concentrations of 430–860 m/m^3. Half-lives were measured in the blood of humans to be 2 and 41 min, and to be some hours in the lipid tissues. With a half-life of 4–6 h, styrene is excreted by humans at approximately 90% via urine as the metabolites mandelic acid and phenylglyoxylic acid. Further metabolites in the urine are 1- and 2-phenylethanol.

Acute and Chronic Toxicity

After acute exposure to 220–850 mg/m^3 for 1–3 hs, mucosa irritation of the eyes, nose, and lips can occur. Pulmonary effects (chronic bronchitis and obstructive pulmonary changes) were observed in chronically exposed workers. Acute exposures are associated with signs of CNS disorders, such as dizziness, headache, weariness, and lack of concentration. Abnormalities in the electroencephalographic recordings, the prolongation of the reaction time, and impairment of color vision have been noticed: The central and peripheral nervous systems are affected by styrene; for example, it slows down nerve conduction velocity. In experimental animals, sublethal concentrations of styrene evoked ataxia, tremor, convulsions, and unconsciousness.

Specific Toxicology

Reproductive Toxicity

Numerous studies were performed to study the potential risk of spontaneous abortions after occupational exposure to styrene. However, only one showed limited but equivocal results. After 60 days of oral uptake of 200 mg/kg, juvenile male rats showed degenerative changes of the testicular tubules and a decrease in the number of sperm. Inhalative exposures (200 or 1300 mg/m^3) 6 h per day on days 7–21 of gestation led to a reduction in body weight of the pup at delivery with no effect on the dams. Teratogenic properties are not known.

Mutagenicity

Genotoxic effects (chromosomal aberration, sister chromatid exchange, micronuclei) were observed in lymphocytes of workers who had been exposed from one-half year to one year or more to concentrations above 23 mg/m^3. This genotoxic effect is assumed to result from styrene 7,8-oxide, as in the Ames test without metabolic activation styrene is not mutagenic. In *in vitro* and *in vivo* cell systems of mammals, styrene and styrene-7,8-oxide cause DNA-strand breakage. After styrene exposure, protein and DNA adducts with styrene oxide are detected both in humans and experimental animals.

Carcinogenicity

Studies regarding carcinogenicity on workers in styrene production showed no increase in total cancer mortality. However, the largest study pointed out an increased incidence of lymphatic leukemias associated with latency time but not with exposure. Studies in rats showed an increase in mammary tumors after inhalative and oral exposures to styrene. However, these and further studies give no sufficient basis for assessing styrene's carcinogenic properties. In contrast to the unchanged substance, styrene 7,8-oxide induces tumors in the forestomach of rats and mice after oral intake at doses exceeding the metabolic capacity. The very low DNA-adduct formation after intake of styrene 7,8-oxide leads to the conclusion that its tumorigenic potency in the forestomach is the result of a tumor promotion process due to high-dose cytotoxicity and subsequent hyperplasia.

Polycyclic Aromatic Hydrocarbons

Polycyclic aromatic hydrocarbons, also referred to as polynuclear hydrocarbons, consist of two or more condensed rings. They are formed mainly during incomplete combustion processes of organic materials like wood, coal, mineral oil, and derived products. It is assumed that during pyrolysis, free carbon, hydrogen, and hydrocarbon radicals are produced and polymerize via agglomeration of acetylene molecules. Polycyclic aromatic hydrocarbons are contained in motor-vehicle exhausts both from gasoline and diesel engines. Pyrolysis of amino acids, fatty acids, and carbohydrates (in cooking) is another source of polycyclic aromatic hydrocarbon formation. They are also present in crude and refined oils; in commercial products, such as bitumen (asphalt), coal tars, and pitches; and as a major part in the pesticide creosote. Furthermore, they are contained in roasted coffee and can be found in dermatotherapeutic products. Of special toxicological importance is their presence in mainstream and sidestream tobacco smoke and in fried, grilled, and smoked food.

Mostly as a result of anthropogenic activities, polycyclic aromatic hydrocarbons are released into the environment and found in air, soil, water, and food. Some natural sources are known—forest fires, volcanic eruptions, and biosynthesis in plants (e.g., the phenanthrene derivative aristolochia acid) and microorganisms.

Polycyclic aromatic hydrocarbons are mainly distributed in the environment via air. Due to the low volatility of compounds with more than two rings, the majority is attached to particles (e.g., dust, soot, and pollen). The distribution of polycyclic aromatic hydrocarbons is further influenced by atmospheric factors (e.g., temperature and air humidity). During transport with increasing distance from the site of emission, the polycyclic aromatic hydrocarbons may shift from particle phase to gas phase.

Several hundred different polycyclic aromatic hydrocarbon congeners are known. Monitoring in the various environmental compartments usually detects only a few compounds (Fig. 5). Particularly in ambient air, benzo[*a*]pyrene serves as an indicator. Concentrations of benzo[*a*]pyrene in rural areas are less than 1 ng/m^3, in urban areas 1–10 ng/m^3, and in certain occupational settings more than 10 μg/m^3. The ambient air concentrations tend to be lower in North and South America than in Europe, and are higher during winter than during the summer. Both comparisons indicate the influence of heating and of fuel sources. In central Europe the ambient-air polycyclic aromatic hydrocarbon levels have been decreasing during the second half of the 20th century, at least partly because of the decreasing use of coal burning for heating. Indoor air concentrations above outdoor air levels are found in homes with special sources like

Substance	CAS Registry number	Chemical formula	EPA	Cancero-genicity	Substance	CAS Registry number	Chemical formula	EPA	Cancero-genicity
Naphthalene	91-20-3	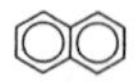	+		Benzo(k)fluoranthene	207-08-9	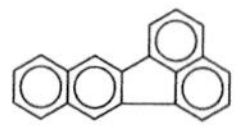	+	+
1-Methylnaphthalene	90-12-0	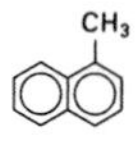			Benzo(e)pyrene	192-97-2	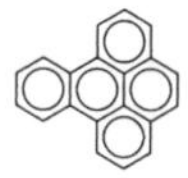		(+)
2-Methylnaphthalene	91-57-6	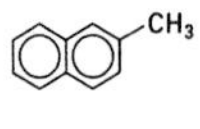			Benzo(a)pyrene	50-32-8	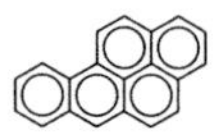	+	+
Acenaphthylene	208-96-8	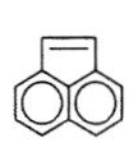	+		Indeno(1,2,3-cd)pyrene	193-39-5	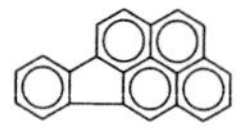	+	+
Acenaphthene	83-32-9	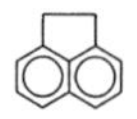	+		Dibenz(a,h)anthracene	53-70-3	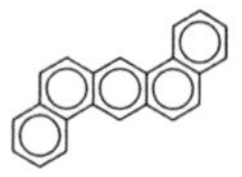	+	+
Fluorene	86-73-7	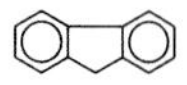	+		Benzo(g,h,i)perylene	191-24-2	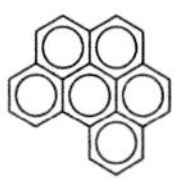	+	+
Phenanthrene	85-01-8	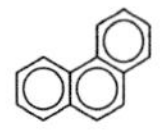	+		Benzo(j)fluoranthene	205-82-3	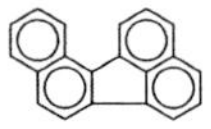		+
Anthracene	120-12-7	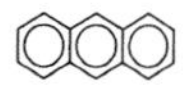	+	(+)	Dibenzo(a,e)pyrene	192-65-4	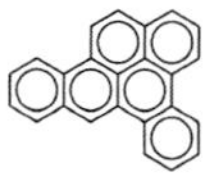		+
Fluoranthene	206-44-0	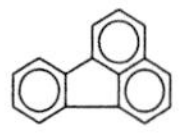	+		Dibenzo(a,h)pyrene	189-64-0	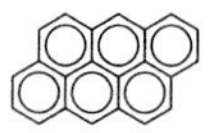		+
Pyrene	129-00-0	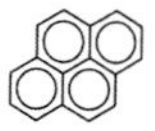	+		Dibenzo(a,i)pyrene	189-55-9	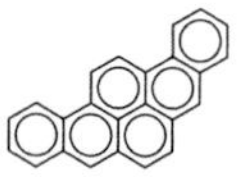		+
Benz(a)anthracene	56-55-3	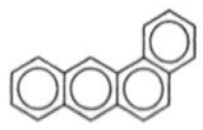	+	+	Dibenzo(a,l)pyrene	191-30-0	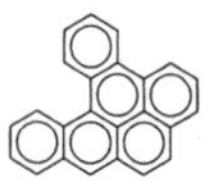		+
Chrysene	218-01-9	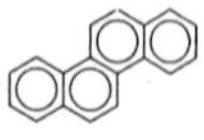	+	+	5-Methylchrysene	3697-24-3	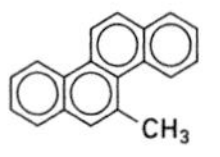		+
Benzo(b)fluoranthene	205-99-2	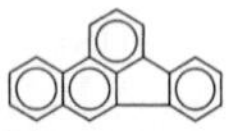	+	+	3-Methylcholanthrene	56-49-5	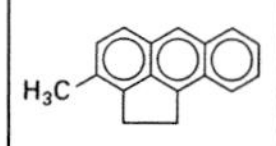		+

FIGURE 5 Polycyclic aromatic hydrocarbons with two to six condensed, mostly aromatic rings. For identification the CAS (chemical abstract system) number is listed. Further the compounds selected for environmental monitoring by the U.S. Environmental Protection Agency (EPA) are indicated as well as those compounds that are carcinogenic in animals.

unvented space heaters, coal-burning stoves, and food preparation.

The increasing traffic in cities has become the major source of polycyclic aromatic hydrocarbon air pollution. Monitoring a few selected polycyclic aromatic hydrocarbon congeners to obtain a polycyclic aromatic hydrocarbon profile reveals evidence for the identification of the source of polycyclic aromatic hydrocarbons. Some higher molecular weight particle-bound polycyclic aromatic hydrocarbons may be taken as markers for traffic sources. (Table 7).

The background level of polycyclic aromatic hydrocarbons in drinking water ranges form 4 to 24 ng/liter. In soil, benzo[a]pyrene concentrations between 0.8 and 4.3 μg/kg are found. Considerably higher levels can occur in the vicinity of hazardous-waste sites or where soils have been exposed to high atmospheric content of polycyclic aromatic hydrocarbons. This can lead directly or indirectly to the contamination of crops. The range of benzo[*a*]pyrene per net weight of food is between 0.004 and 1.2 μg/kg.

Excluding workplace exposures, the total uptake of polycyclic aromatic hydrocarbons can be dominated either by smoking or by the intake via food. Apart from smoked food, certain vegetables like lettuce, spinach, and cabbage can contain elevated amounts of polycyclic aromatic hydrocarbons, probably due to contamination via air. Differences in the total exposure within the general population have been estimated using various methods (including measuring DNA adducts). The monitoring of urinary metabolites (i.e., 1-hydroxyphenanthrene, 1-hydroxypyrene) has been employed as a biomarker of polycyclic aromatic hydrocarbon exposure and shown to detect environmentally higher exposed population subgroups.

Absorption, Distribution, Metabolism, and Excretion

Particles with adsorbed polycyclic aromatic hydrocarbons of three or more rings and a diameter more than 5 μm are retained in the upper respiratory tract (nasal pharynx area and main bronchi). Particles with a diameter of 1–5 μm are subject to sedimentation, mainly in the bronchial ramifications. Particles with a diameter less than 0.5 μm are deposited in the bronchioles according to the rules of diffusion. The retention time for particles in the respiratory tract depends on the site of deposition. A deposition in the upper respiratory tract leads to excretion via sputum and nasal discharge within from a few minutes to a few hours, or after uptake via the gastrointestinal tract with subsequent absorption and/or excretion. When deposited in the middle respiratory tract, the particles can be taken up by macrophages or they can be transported within several hours by mucociliary clearance into the pharynx area and enter the gastrointestinal tract. During transportation, polycyclic aromatic hydrocarbons that are adsorbed to particles can be solubilized and taken up by the tissue.

The particles in the upper respiratory tract contain few polycyclic aromatic hydrocarbons. Except for smokers, tumors in the nasal pharynx area are therefore rare. In the tracheobronchial respiratory system, presumably, a relatively dense deposition of particle takes place. It is not clear whether increased amounts of polycyclic aromatic hydrocarbons really do appear in the upper bronchial sections affecting epithelial cells. However, there seems to be a correlation between carcinoma frequency in the bronchi of the lung and the deposited amount of dust. In the terminal respiratory system, the portion of polycyclic aromatic hydrocarbons—after desorption is solubilized in surfactant—is presumably high.

After oral uptake, less than 50% of the polycyclic aromatic hydrocarbons are absorbed in the intestinal tract of animals, as calculated from the ratio between absorbed and excreted amount. Intestinal absorption of benzo[*a*]pyrene in humans is only about 10%. About 1 h after ingestion, smaller amounts of the dose appear in the lymph, biliary fluid, and in urine. Liver, kidney, and adipose tissue show higher concentra-

TABLE 7 Relative Composition[a] of Individual Polycyclic Aromatic Hydrocarbons in Traffic-Influenced Ambient Air[b]

Compound	Relative amount (%)	Compound	Relative amount (%)
Benzo[*b*]fluoranthene	87	Indeno[1,2,3-*cd*]pyrene	126
Benzo[*k*]fluoranthene	85	Dibenz[*a,h*]anthracene	73
Benzo[*e*]pyrene	150	Benzo[*b*]chrysene	64
Perylene	140	Benzo[*ghi*]perylene	77

[a]Benzo[*a*]pyrene set 100%.
[b]Adapted from Lee *et al.* (1995).

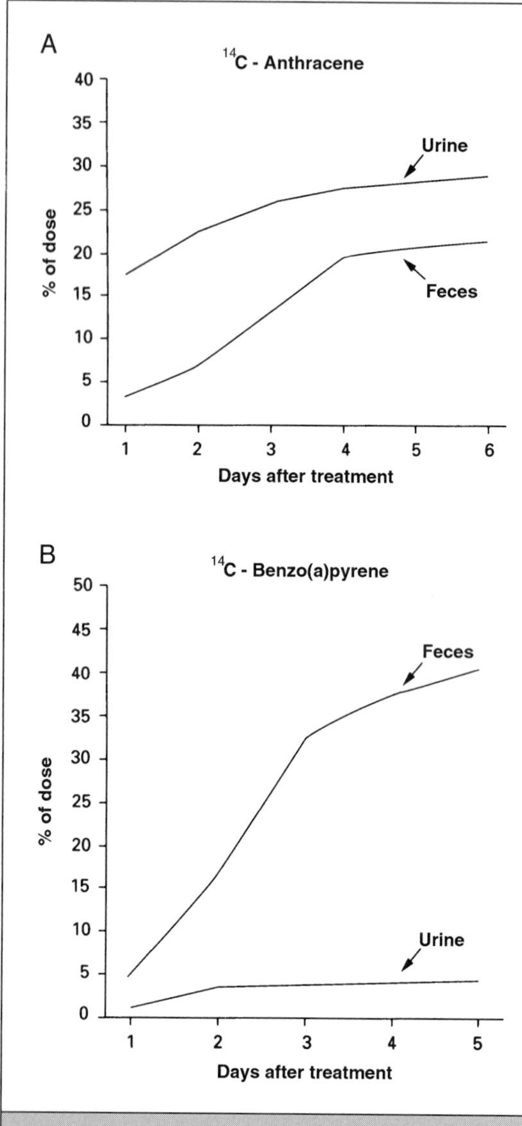

FIGURE 6 Excretion of radioactivity after administration of solved ^{14}C-anthracene (A) or benzo[*a*]pyrene (B) onto the skin of rats. The dose is 9.3 μg/m^2 skin surface. (Adapted form Yang *et al.*, 1986b.)

tions than blood, CNS, and muscular tissue. Within 3–4 days, a redistribution takes place into adipose tissue, adrenal glands, mesenteric lymph nodes, and ovaries, where the substances are detectable even months after administration. The milk of lactating rats contains polycyclic aromatic hydrocarbons even several days after oral intake. Comparable distribution pattern are observed after i.v. administration, however, without an accumulation in the mammary. Biliarily secreted conjugates (e.g., sulfates, glucuronides and GSH conjugates) can be deconjugated in the intestine and run through an enterohepatic circulation. After administration of a solution of anthracene or benzo[*a*]pyrene onto the skin, approximately one-half of the dose is absorbed and excreted relatively quickly via the kidney and intestine (Fig. 6). About 1% of the dose is found in the liver and kidney (anthracene) or in the intestinal wall and liver (benzo[*a*]pyrene). Animal experiments reveal that the placenta ("placenta barrier") and embryonic tissue apparently hinder the uptake of benzo[*a*]pyrene or its metabolites in the fetus.

In the 1930s dihydrodiols were described as conversion products of polycyclic aromatic hydrocarbons. In the 1960s the formation of *trans*-dihydrodiols from arene oxides (i.e., epoxides of originally aromatic double-bond structure) was shown. The enzyme involved, epoxide hydrase, was detected mainly in the microsomes. At the same time it was found that the oxygen necessary for the diol formation originates from water. Benzo[*a*]pyrene is transformed into different arene oxides, which are reactive intermediary products and precursors of phenols and dihydrodiols (Fig. 7).

Studies regarding carcinogenicity identified the 7,8-oxide and the 7,8-dihydrodiol as proximal carcinogens and the 7,8-diol-9,10-epoxide as strong mutagen and ultimate carcinogen. The last can appear in four isomers due to stereoselective properties of cytochrome P450 isoenzymes (Fig. 7).

In comparative studies with further polycyclic aromatic hydrocarbons, it became obvious that only those substances that have a bay region in the ring system and are epoxidized there have carcinogenic properties. The bay region theory deduced from these studies has been successfully applied to the prediction of the carcinogenic properties of various polycyclic aromatic hydrocarbons. An exception is phenanthrene (Fig. 5). The epoxidation of the ring system essential for the carcinogenic properties takes place where the character of the double bond is most distinct. This region was called "K region." However, the identification of DNA-binding metabolites revealed that mainly non-K-region metabolites—such as the bay region diolepoxides—enter into a covalent binding with the DNA. Benz[*a*]anthracene is moderately carcinogenic and is transformed step by step in the presence of *S*-adenosyl-*l*-methionine into the comparatively stronger carcinogen 7,12-dimethylbenz[*a*]-anthracene (Fig. 8). The same reaction probably leads to the conversion of benzo[*a*]pyrene into 6-methyl-benzo[*a*]pyrene.

Polycyclic aromatic hydrocarbons are bioactivated by metabolic conversion through cytochrome P450-dependent monooxygenases. An inactivation occurs through the epoxide hydrase by transformation of

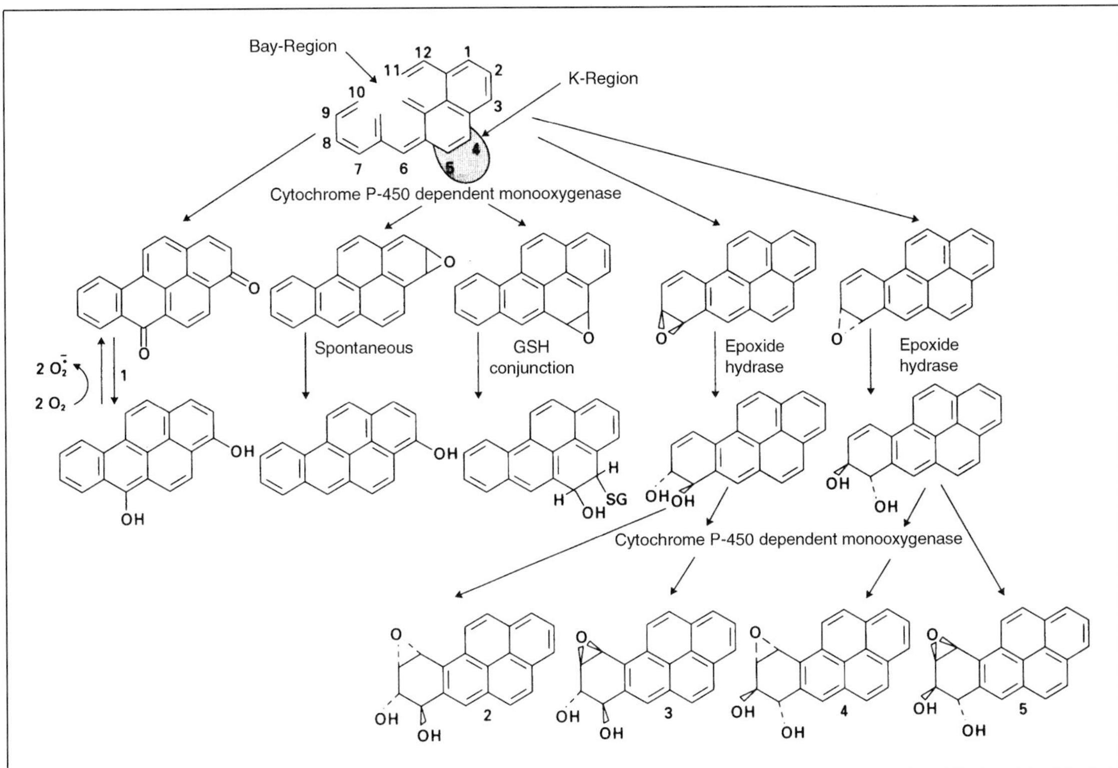

FIGURE 7 Selected steps of the metabolism of benzo [*a*] pyrene. Sulfate conjugation, glucuronidation of OH-groups and further GSH conjugates are not shown. 1, NADPH-dependent cytochrome P450 reductase, NAD(P)H quinone reductase, or DT-diaphorase; 2, *trans*-(+)-7β, 8α-dihydroxy-9α, 10α-epoxy-7, 8, 9, 10-tetrahydrobenzo [*a*] pyrene; 3, *cis*-(−)-7β, 8α-dihydroxy-9β, 10β-epoxy-7, 8, 9, 10-tetrahydrobenzo [*a*] pyrene; 4 = *cis*-(+)-7α, 8β-dihydroxy-9α, 10α-epoxy-7, 8, 9, 10-tetrahydrobenzo [*a*] pyrene; 5, *trans*-(−)-7α,8β-dihydroxy-9β, 10β-epoxy-7, 8, 9, 10-tetrahydrobenzo [*a*] pyrene. (Adapted from Conney, 1982.)

epoxides into less reactive vicinal diols. Via GSH *S*-transferases, sulfotransferases, and UDP-glucuronosyltransferases, the epoxides are conjugated with GSH and phenolic metabolites are transferred into sulfates and glucuronides (phase II reactions), reinforcing the elimination of nucleophilic and electrophilic metabolites.

Free oxygen radicals can also contribute to bioactivation. Epoxidation of the benzo[*a*]pyrene metabolites can result from lipid peroxidation, prostaglandin biosynthesis, and reduction of lipid peroxides. Furthermore, peroxi radicals can take part in the lipoxygenase-catalyzed epoxidation of 7,8-dihydroxy-7,8-dihydrobenzo[*a*]pyrene.

Benzo[*a*]pyrene stimulates its own metabolization. The benzo[*a*]pyrene hydroxylase or arylhydrocarbon hydroxylase located in the liver microsomes require NADPH and oxygen for catalytic activity. Benzo[*a*]pyrene metabolization is inhibited by ethionine; therefore, it was concluded that polycyclic aromatic hydrocarbons induce microsomal xenobiotic-metabolizing liver enzymes. Aryl hydrocarbon hydroxylase is a group of isoenzymes found in the liver, lung, kidney, gastrointestinal tract, placenta, lymphocytes, monocytes, and alveolar macrophages of various species. A comparatively high enzyme activity can be noted in the type II alveolar cells. In the mouse, benzo[*a*]pyrene leads to a prenatal induction of benzo[*a*]pyrene hydroxylase.

The activity of arylhydrocarbon hydroxylase and of epoxide hydrase is lower in the lung than in the liver of rats (Table 8). The bioactivation of polycyclic aromatic hydrocarbons is significant in lung carcinogenicity after inhalation. After administration of 3-methylcholanthrene and of other polycyclic aromatic hydrocarbons, cytochrome P450-dependent monoxygenases are strongly induced.

The polycyclic aromatic hydrocarbons contained in the main stream of cigarette smoke induce the aryl hydrocarbon hydroxylase in all tissues. Its activity in the placentas of female smokers can be 400 times higher than that in the placentas of female non-smok-

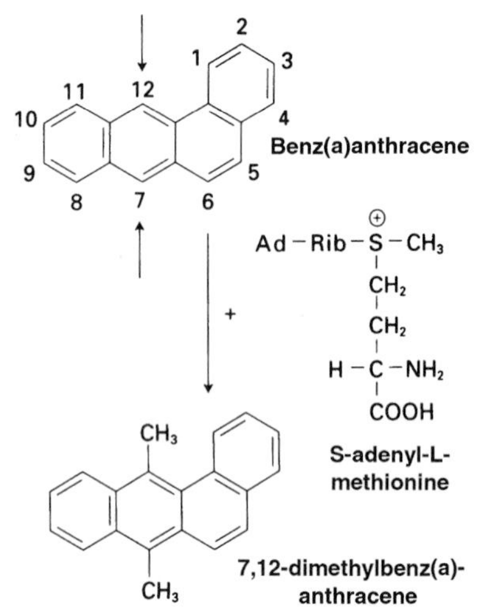

FIGURE 8 Alkylation of benz[*a*]anthracene (top) in the presence of cytosolic *S*-adenosyl-L-methionine into 7, 12-dimethylbenz[*a*]anthracene. The mesoanthracenic C-positions 7 and 12 are also referred to as L-region (arrows). (Adapted from Flesher *et al.*, 1984.)

ers. Also, vegetable (e.g., cabbage and Brussels sprouts) are capable of accelerating the metabolism of drugs (e.g., antipyrine) in humans. Indole-3-acetonitrile, indole-3-carbinol, and 3,3′-diindolylmethane are compounds with strong monooxygenase-inducing activity.

Acute and Chronic Toxicity

A single large dermal administration of 7,12-dimethylbenz[*a*]anthracene may lead to atrophy of the spleen and lymph nodes and, after oral intake, to growth retardation and leukopenia. In general a single high dose of polycyclic aromatic hydrocarbons impairs organs and tissues with a high mitotic activity (e.g., hematopoietic system, gonads, and intestinal mucosa). The mitochondria of the zona reticularis and fasciculata of the adrenal glands respond very sensitively, perhaps because of an inhibition of the DNA synthesis by metabolites. Benzo[*a*]pyrene and 3-methylcholanthrene given in solution into a rabbit's ear induce Ah-receptor-mediated acnegenic effects with hyperplasia and hyperkeratosis of the epidermal epithelium with a reduction of the sebaceous glands (Fig. 9).

Specific Toxicolgy

Reproductive Toxicity

Placental calcifications—associated with AHH induction—are more prevalent in the placenta of smokers. Effects of smoking on fertility seem to be attributed to polycyclic aromatic hydrocarbons in tobacco smoke, at least in part.

Benzo[*a*]pyrene, 3-methylcholanthrene, and 7,12-dimethylbenz[*a*]anthracene can cause the destruction of oocytes in rats and mice. In rats the administration of 7,12-dimethylbenz[*a*]anthracene during the initial phase of the estrus leads to necrosis in the corpora lutea, which may be correlated to the AHH activity in the rat ovary being elevated especially during the proestrus and estrus phases.

Mutagenicity

Despite the evident correlation between mutagenic and carcinogenic activity of the benzo[*a*]pyrene metabolites, which is supported by various studies of other polycyclic aromatic hydrocarbons, and the

TABLE 8 Comparison of the Activity of Arylhydrocarbon Hydroxylase (AHH) and of Epoxide Hydrase in the Liver and Lung of Rats[a]

Tissue and enzyme	Liver	Lung
Fresh weight (g)	6.9	1.37
Microsomes (mg protein/g fresh w)	23	1.62
AHH (nmol benzo[*a*]pyrene metabolized/min per mg microsomal protein)		
Control	0.5	0.09
Induced (3-methylcholanthrene)	4.0	0.6
AHH (total activity/g fresh w)		
Control	26	0.95
Induced (3-methylcholanthrene)	204	5.7
Epoxide hydrase (nmol styrene glycol formed/min per mg microsomal protein)	8	0.5
Epoxide hydrase (Total activity/g fresh weight)	408	4.75

[a]Adapted from De Pierre and Ernster (1978).

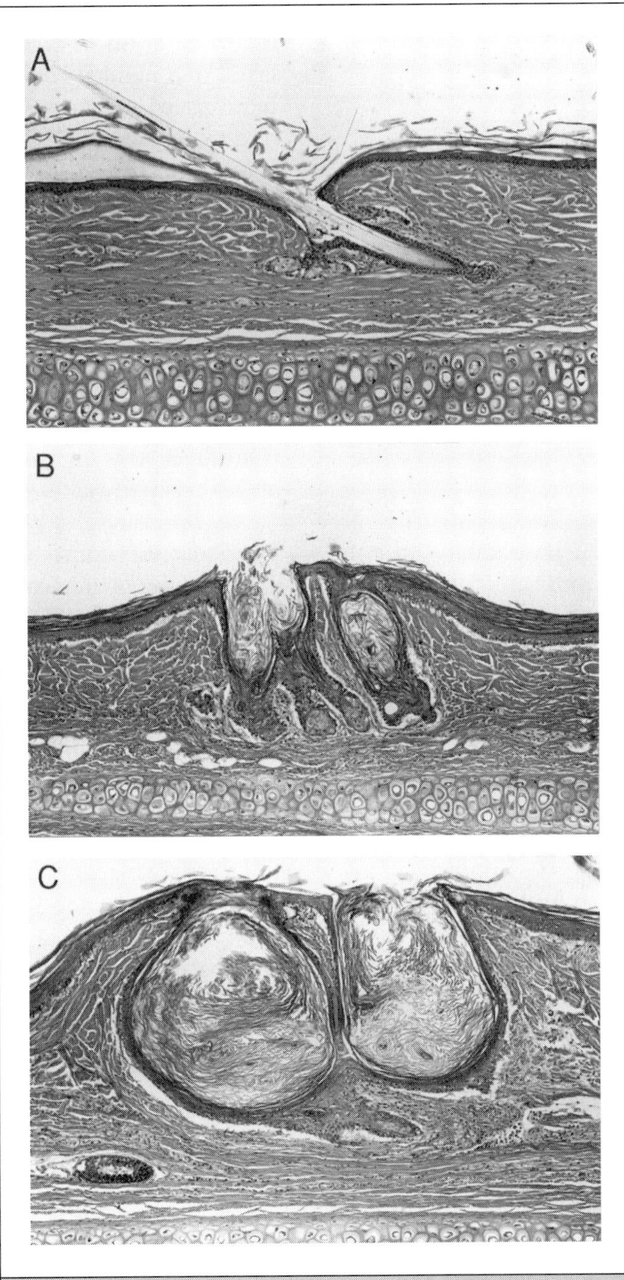

FIGURE 9 Histology of the inner ear surface (4 cm^2) of rabbits after four times administration of acetone: solvent control (A), 24 μg methylcholanthrene each (B), and 60 μg benzo[*a*]pyrene (C) each. H.E. × 80. (Adapted from Vos *et al.*, 1982.)

proven DNA adducts, the question concerning the target genes of the mutagenic and carcinogenic substances has not been answered. However, there are indications of preferred DNA regions and of the dependence of the oncogene transformation and mutation observed *in vitro* on the exposure time.

It is generally accepted that the chemically induced neoplastic transformation of a cell requires the alkylation of its DNA. The property of carrying out alkylation is especially distinct in the reactive electrophilic arene oxides. The demonstration of covalent binding (Fig. 10) is decisive. Animal studies reveal that low doses of polycyclic aromatic hydrocarbons show an almost linear correlation between the dose and the amount of DNA adducts. At present it is possible to measure one DNA adduct in the presence of 10^9–10^{10}

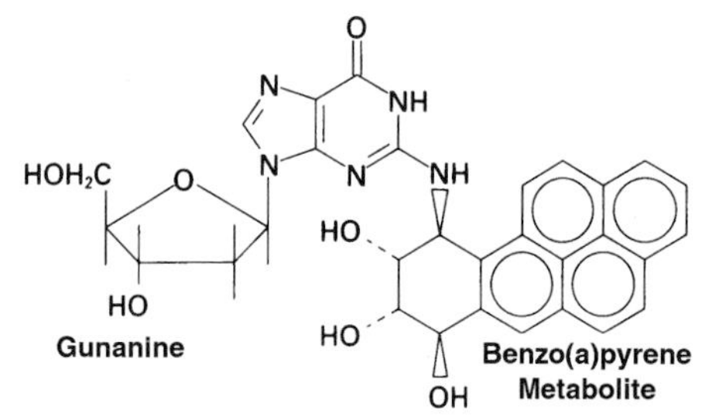

FIGURE 10 Isolated benzo[*a*]pyrene adduct of the benzo[*a*]pyrene metabolite and guanine of the DNA. (Adapted from Lawley, 1989.)

nucleotides. The detection limit is about one order of magnitude lower than the average adduct content. DNA adducts of different polycyclic aromatic hydrocarbons can be detected in practically all organs. The presence of DNA adducts in tissues is correlated with the distribution of the reactive metabolites (i.e., of epoxides) in the blood. The number of DNA adducts in skin and lung of mice correlates with the carcinogenic potency of the dibenzopyrenes after dermal administration. The amount decreases remarkably within 3 weeks in skin and lung. Traces can be detected after 3 months. Combinations of polycyclic aromatic hydrocarbons can result both in a decrease or an increase of adduct concentration. In humans, DNA adducts have been detected in the lymphocytes, lung, placenta, and fetal tissue (in the liver and lung). The number of DNA adducts in the lung tissue is different between smokers of filter-tipped and filterless cigarettes. In humans, DNA adducts of polycyclic aromatic hydrocarbons (in white blood cells) can be used as biomarkers of occupational and environmental exposure.

Carcinogenicity

In 1775 Percival Pott reported on the extraordinarily high incidence of scrotum cancer in London chimney sweeps, which he saw as having a causal connection with the exposure to soot and ashes. In 1892 the correlation to cancer of the skin and other organs in chimney sweeps, as well as in workers of the tar- and pitch-manufacturing industry, became accepted. The first experimental proof for the carcinogenic effect of compounds contained in soot and ashes was made in 1915 by Yamagiwa and Ichikawa, who applied undiluted coal tar to rabbits' ears and thereby induced sarcomas. Through identification of polycyclic aromatic hydrocarbons in tar, the cancer-inducing agent was determined. A self-experiment conducted by the German physician Klar a few years later confirmed that a solution of benzo[*a*]pyrene applied to the arm leads to a benign epithelioma. Several physical examinations of workers exposed to polycyclic aromatic hydrocarbons occupationally, as well as epidemiological studies on smokers, evidenced an increased risk of lung cancer after 10–15 years of exposure. A recent appraisal of epidemiological studies with mainly inhalative occupational exposure to polycyclic aromatic hydrocarbon mixtures revealed that the risks for lung and bladder cancer were dose dependent.

Human exposure to polycyclic aromatic hydrocarbons is always an exposure to complex mixtures; thus, the carcinogenic effect and potency of individual compounds in this mixture can only be investigated in animal experiments. In the mouse skin test—the "classical" model for carcinogenicity testing of compounds and compound mixtures—benzo[*a*]pyrene exhibits the same carcinogenic potency as dibenz[*a,h*]anthracene and a stronger effect than benz[*a*]anthracene. Tumors located in tissues distant from the place of administration develop after enteral and parenteral administration especially. Benzo[*a*]anthracene leads to tumors in liver and lung after oral intake. In rats 7,12-dimethylbenz[*a*]anthracene and 3-methylcholanthrene, like benzo[*a*]pyrene, induce mammary carcinomas after oral intake.

Dibenz[*a,h*]anthracene evokes carcinomas in lung and mammary gland, as well as papillomae and carcinomas of the forestomach in mice after oral intake. Newborn mice showed lung and skin cancer when their mothers had been given benzo[*a*]pyrene sc and ip on the 11th, 13th, and 15th days of pregnancy. The polycyclic aromatic hydrocarbons had been applied acutely and subacutely in relatively high doses. This way of inducing cancer clearly suggests that polycyclic aromatic hydrocarbons are solitary carcinogens. In two generations of mice, the transgeneration transmission of the carcinogenic action of 7,12-dimethylbenz[*a*]anthracene was studied. It was assumed that the carcinogenic effect of 7,12-dimethylbenz[*a*]anthracene can be transferred from parents to descendants via a germ-line mutation. In several inhalation studies in animals, benzo[*a*]pyrene, induced tumors in the respiratory tract, nasal cavity, pharynx, larynx, and trachea. Tumors were also observed in the esophagus and in the forestomach, but in hamsters no lung tumors occurred. Combined exposure with irritant gases, such as sulfur dioxide, enhanced the carcinogenicity of benzo[*a*]pyrene.

In the multistage model of the carcinogenisis, polycyclic aromatic hydrocarbons are initiators that lead to persistant changes (initiation) set off by genotoxic effects. A subsequent promotion through phenobarbital in the liver or through phorbolester on the skin then leads to the formation of tumors. The activity and substrate specificity of the cytochrome P450-dependent monooxygenase system of the different organs determines the carcinogenicity. The bay region theory allows an estimation of the carcinogenic potency; however, a quantitative statement regarding the biotransformation of the polycyclic aromatic hydrocarbons is not possible. Thus, for instance, benzo[*e*]pyrene and benz[*a*]anthracene are weak carcinogens not because of their Bay Region but because of their low affinity to the P450 system.

Immunotoxicity

Only animal experiments are available regarding the immunological effects of polycyclic aromatic hydrocarbons. Studies exist with selected compounds, with mixtures, and with different methods of administration (i.e., dermal, intraperitoneal, or subcutaneous). Polycyclic aromatic hydrocarbons have been shown to inhibit both the cell-mediated and the humoral immunity. 7,12-Dimethylbenz[*a,h*]anthracene affects the lymphoproliferative reaction towards the T-cell mitogens phytohemagglutinin and concanavalin A and the development of cytotoxic T cells, and it increases the death rate (apnea) after Listeria monocytogenes infection, observed up to 8 weeks after administration. A single dose inhibits the type IV hypersensitivity response (delayed type) toward 2,4,6-trinitro-1-chlorobenzene, as well as the activity of the helper T cells. Benzo[*a*]pyrene's lower effectiveness on these mentioned parameters is at least equivocal in some studies.

The immune response depends on the animal strain and the route of administration. Mice that respond with an increased activity of microsomal enzymes toward 3-methylcholanthrene (i.e., are AHH-inducible) also show a stronger impairment of the lymphoproliferation after phytohemagglutinin. 7,12-Dimethylbenz[*a,h*]anthracene evokes immunosuppression both in AHH-inducible and -noninducible strains following ip administration, the AHH-inducible strain being more susceptible. The AHH-noninducible strain showed a stronger response following oral administration. Addition of 3-methylcholanthrene to isolated peripheral human lymphocytes results in a decreased blastogenesis and cell-mediated cytotoxicity. Furthermore, interleukin-2 production and the lymphotoxin production are inhibited. The limited production of both mediators correlates with the reduced blastogenesis and cell activity. Complex mixtures of polycyclic aromatic hydrocarbons suppressed the splenic plaque-forming cell (PFC) response to T-cell-dependent and -independent antigens. Since the potency of the mixture was higher than expected based on the benzo[*a*]pyrene content, a possible synergistic interaction of different polycyclic aromatic hydrocarbons was suggested. Following dermal administration in mice, benzo[*a*]pyrene elicited a contact-allergic hypersensivity that was antigen specific. To a lesser extent, this effect was also observed in guinea pigs. Exposures to the noncarcinogen benzo[*e*]pyrene have practically no influence on the hypersensitivity response.

Carcinogenic polycyclic aromatic hydrocarbons (3-methylcholanthrene, dibenz[*a,h*]anthracene, and benz[*a*]anthracene) reduce the serum antibody titer against sheep erythrocytes in mice. However, polycyclic aromatic hydrocarbons without carcinogenic effect (phenanthrene) had no effect. In general the degree of immunosuppression correlates with the carcinogenic potency of the individual polycyclic aromatic hydrocarbon. Carcinogenic polycyclic hydrocarbons bind to the Ah receptor and a possible role of the Ah receptor in the polycyclic aromatic hydrocarbon-induced immunotoxicity has been suggested, but independent metabolic mechanisms must be considered as well.

Nitrated Polycyclic Aromatic Hydrocarbons (Nitro-PAH and Nitroarenes)

Nitrated polycyclic aromatic hydrocarbons show also mutagenic and carcinogenic potency. In general, nitrated polycyclic aromatic hydrocarbons can be expected anywhere that polycyclic aromatic hydrocarbons are found. They are formed by radical reactions in the gas phase and electrophilic reactions of particle-associated polycyclic aromatic hydrocarbons with NO_x. Furthermore, polycyclic aromatic hydrocarbons can react with sulfur oxides, molecular oxygen, ozone, free radicals, and aliphatic halogen compounds in the atmosphere. The toxicological relevance of the reaction products (e.g., oxa-, thia-, and azaarenes) is largely unclear.

The chemical stability of the nitrated polycyclic aromatic hydrocarbons varies. 1-Nitrobenzo[*a*]pyrene and 3-nitrobenzo[*a*]pyrene are photostable, whereas 6-nitrobenzo[*a*]pyrene and 9-nitroanthracene are subject to rapid light-induced degradation. Nitrated polycyclic aromatic hydrocarbons are emitted mainly by diesel engines; for example, 1-nitropyrene can reach concentrations as high as benzo[*a*]pyrene (10–30 $\mu g/g$ particle). The emission of nitropyrene in the toner of copying machines, observed in the past, has been largely reduced. Concentrations of nitrated polycyclic aromatic hydrocarbons in the air are generally

10 to 100 times lower than those of polycyclic aromatic hydrocarbons and urban air concentrations between 0.05 and 4.0 ng/m^3 have been reported.

Absorption, Distribution, Metabolism, and Excretion

After oral and intraperitoneal administration of 1-nitropyrene 50–70% is excreted with feces and a smaller percentage via the kidney. Inhalation of the substance as an aerosol results in mainly renal excretion. No data about distribution are available. However, studies on rats fed with [^{14}C]nitropyrene showed that DNA adducts could be detected in the liver, mammary gland, kidney, lung, and bladder. The adducts in the liver, mammary gland, and kidney have been identified as *N*-(deoxyguanosine-8-yl)-2-aminopyrene and *N*-(deoxyadenosine-8-yl)-2-aminopyrene.

Decisive for the formation of the DNA adducts is the biotransformation of nitrated polycyclic aromatic hydrocarbons (e.g., their bioactivation). The first step is the reduction of the nitro group, which possibly takes place mainly in the gastrointestinal tract. Nitroso and hydroxylamino compounds, as well as hydroxamic acid and aminopolycyclic aromatic hydrocarbons, can appear as metabolites. Important intermediary products are the nitreniumion, occurring spontaneously from nitroso compounds, and hydroxylamine. Both metabolites can covalently bind with DNA and other macromolecules. Furthermore, nitrated polycyclic aromatic hydrocarbons are subject to ring hydroxylation and subsequently to glucuronidation, epoxidation (1-nitropyrene), GSH conjugation, and acetylation of the amino group(s).

Specific Toxicology

Mutagenicity

In the Ames test without metabolic activation, 2-nitronaphthalene and 9-nitroanthracene (like benzo[*a*]-pyrene) are hardly mutagenic. However, 1-nitropyrene, 3-nitrofluoranthene, 2,7-dinitrofluorene, 2-nitrofluorene, and 8-nitrofluoranthene are remarkably stronger mutagenics than benzo[*a*]pyrene. Due to the catalytic activity of the nitroreductase, nitro aromatic compounds have a direct mutagenic effect. After metabolic activation, the mutagenicity of all the previously mentioned nitrated polycyclic aromatic hydrocarbons is shown. An inhibitory effect of benzo[*a*]pyrene and some other polycyclic aromatic hydrocarbons on the mutagenicity of 1-nitropyrene was attributed to the reduction of nitroreductase activity and to the modulatory effect on the formation of 1-nitropyrene DNA adduct. In mammalian cells, nitrated polycyclic aromatic hydrocarbons have been shown to induce DNA-strand breakage, sister chromatid exchange, unscheduled DNA synthesis, and cell transformation.

Carcinogenicity

Of the 15 nitrated polycyclic aromatic hydrocarbons investigated, only 6 have been shown to be carcinogenic (Fig. 11). The comparatively high mutagenic effect of 1-nitropyrene observed in the Ames test does not correlate with a high carcinogenic effect. Considering all tested nitrated polycyclic aromatic hydrocarbons, it can be shown that 1-nitropyrene is of only low effectiveness. Assuming an additive effect of the nitrated and nonnitrated polycyclic aromatic hydrocarbons, they contribute only to a minor part to the entire carcinogenic potency of diesel-engine emissions. The cancer risk from nitrated polycyclic aromatic hydrocarbons in humans is difficult to assess because no high risk group can be selected. From the detection of animal carcinogenic nitropyrenes and from data from patients with lung cancer, it has been suggested that nitrated polycyclic aromatic hydrocarbons participate in the induction of lung cancer in humans.

ALIPHATIC HYDROCARBONS

Alkanes

Methane, ethane, propane, and *n*-butane are volatile at room temperature; *n*-pentane to *n*-heptadecane are fluid and the higher homologous *n*-alkanes are solid. The isomers from butane on show different chemical and physical properties.

Higher alkanes are most commonly used (next to *n*-hexane) as solvents and paint diluents. In the Scandinavian countries the term "white spirits" is common for a commercially used solvent mixture that contains approximately 80% by weight octane, nonane, decane, dimethyloctane, undecane, and dodecane and about 20% by weight decaline, octene, tetraline, and alkylbenzenes. In the United States the regular grade of white spirits is called Stoddard solvent. It is a petroleum distillate characterized by a boiling range of 149–204°C and the absence of a rancid or objectionable odor. Test subjects who had been exposed to approximately 600 mg/m^3 of white spirits with an alkane portion of 99% by weight for 6 h daily for 5 days showed a significant increase in the creatine kinase and a significantly reduced amount of follicle-stimulating hormone (FSH) in the serum. The elimination half-life of the mixture was 46–48 h.

PAH	Name	Evidence
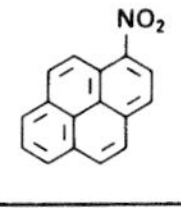	1-Nitropyrene	Sufficient
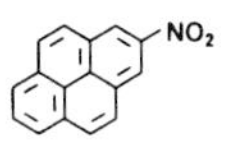	2-Nitropyrene	Inadequate
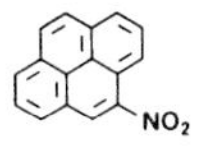	4-Nitropyrene	Sufficient
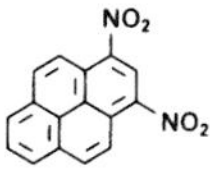	1,3-Nitropyrene	Limited
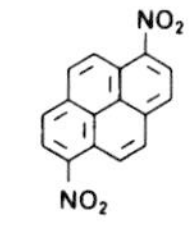	1,6-Nitropyrene	Sufficient
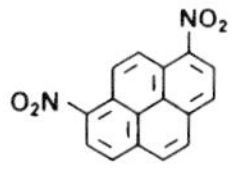	1,8-Nitropyrene	Sufficient
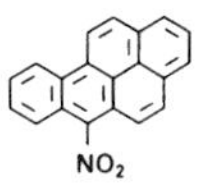	6-Nitro-benzo(a)pyrene	Limited
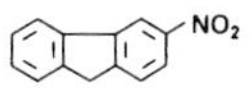	2-Nitrofluorene	Sufficient
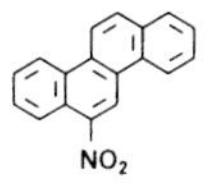	6-Nitrochrysene	Sufficient
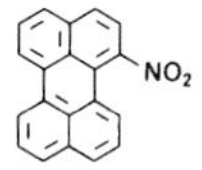	3-Nitroperylene	Inadequate
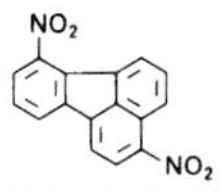	3,7-Dinitrofluor-anthene	Limited
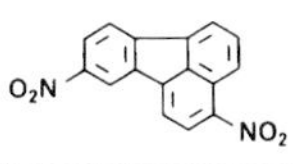	3,9-Dinitrofluor-anthene	Limited
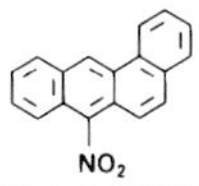	7-Nitrobenz(a) anthracene	Limited
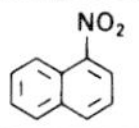	1-Nitro-naphthalene	Inadequate
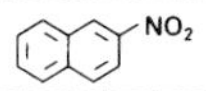	2-Nitro-naphthalene	Inadequate

FIGURE 11 Status of available data on the carcinogenicity of nitrated polycyclic aromatic hydrocarbons (adapted from Kouros and Dehnen, 1985; Rippe and Pott, 1988/89). Qualification of the criteria were performed according to the IARC (International Agency for Research on Cancer, Lyon) as sufficient, limited, or inadequate.

After several hours of exposure to pure *n*-decane (maximum, 5.82 mg/m^3 air) test subjects respond dose-dependently with increasing mucosa irritation, smell sensitivity toward *n*-butanol, a rising number of polymorphonuclear leukocytes in the tear fluid, and a decreasing stability of the fluid film on the cornea. The odor threshold is 0.5–5 mg/m^3. Long-term exposure to white spirits led to an increased incidence of complaints of memory impairment, impaired concentration, fatigue, irritability, dizziness, headache, anxiety, and apathy.

Hexane

Mineral oil and natural gas are the sources of *n*-hexane. It is used as solvent, extract medium (for the production of edible vegetable oil), detergent, and as original material for the production of pharmaceutical preparations. It is colorless, highly volatile, and inflammable. Technical hexane is a mixture of the isomers *n*-hexane, 2-methylpentane, 3-methylpentane, 2,3-dimethylbutane, cyclohexane, methylcyclopentane, pentane, heptane isomers, acetone, phthalate and adipate esters, and organophosphates (e.g., triphenyl phosphate). Occasionally it can contain traces (0.05%) of benzene. Purified *n*-hexane (95–99.5% *n*-hexane) contains different hexane isomers as impurities. In the environment, *n*-hexane is mainly distributed via air. In agglomeration areas, concentrations of more than 100 μg/m^3 can be measured. Indoor air concentrations of 8–100 μg/m^3 have been registered. The application in food production, as well as the transition via air onto food with a high-lipid content, can lead to a contamination with *n*-hexane.

Absorption, Distribution, Metabolism, and Excretion

In humans the pulmonary absorption rate ranges between 15 and 30%. Estimations reveal that workers absorb 112 mg *n*-hexane at a concentration of 180 mg/m^3 air within 8 h. The steady state of concentration in blood is linearly dose-dependent up to 704 mg/m^3. Both at low and at high physical activity, the blood concentration plateau is reached after only 15 min. After intake by inhalation *n*-hexane is found in various organs and tissues as well as in the bones of the rat. The content in fetal tissue equals that of the maternal blood. The same statement is valid for the metabolite 2,5-hexanedione. It is capable of producing pyrrol adducts of serum protein. Hexane has a biphasic kinetic with an intial half-life of 0.2 h and a terminal half-life of 1.5–2 h. The dermal absorption (in guinea pigs) of *n*-hexane is low. However, it is increased when other solvents are applied simultaneously. The biotransformation in humans correlates

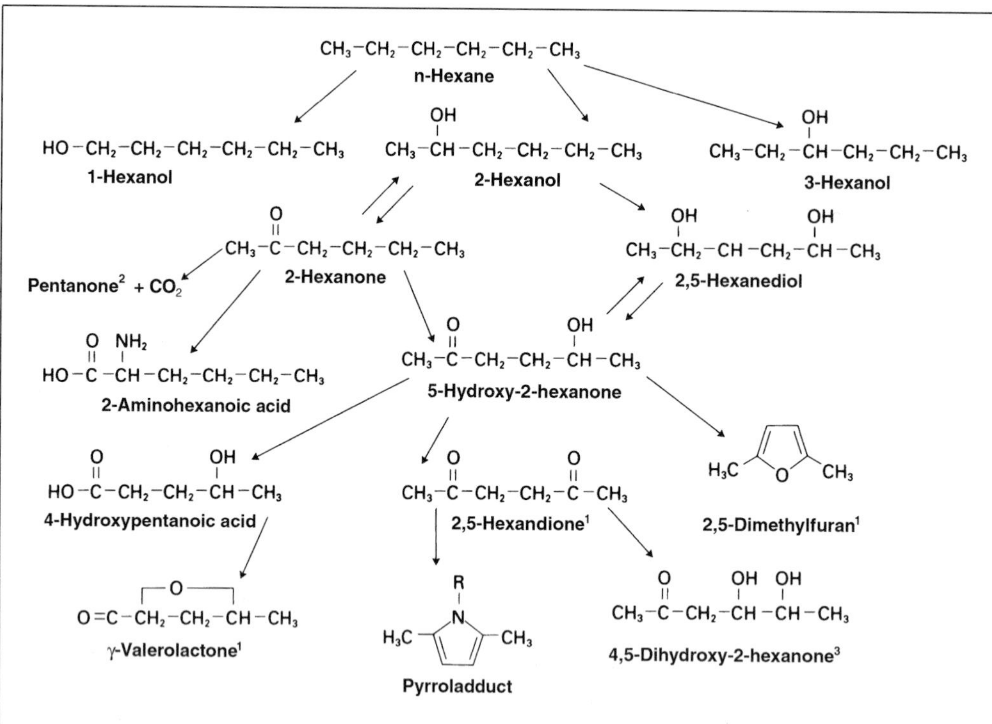

FIGURE 12 Metabolic pathways of *n*-hexane in animals. Oxidation is predominant. Following conversion to hexanoic acid, 1-hexanol is metabolized through β-oxidation. 5-Hydroxy-2-hexanone is presumably stepwise metabolized in 2,5-dimethylfuran via enolization, oxidation, and cyclization and in γ-valerolactone via α-oxidation, decarboxylation, and lactonization. (Adapted from WHO, 1991.) 1, Detected in human urine, major metabolite is 2,5-hexanedione; 2, isomeric structures are not characterized; 3, also know as methyl-*n*-butylketon.

qualitatively with that of the rat (Fig. 12). The excretion occurs mainly via the kidney. Rats eliminate *n*-hexane after inhalative absorption via the lung (17%), kidneys, and intestine. The major part of retained *n*-hexane is excreted within 24 h.

Acute and Chronic Toxicity

Intoxications were observed mainly in occupational settings (e.g., shoe production and the leather industry). Exposure was often not only to *n*-hexane but also to impurities in *n*-hexane and other solvents. Several reports support the hypothesis that the peripheral neuropathy that occurs with exposure to *n*-hexane is attributed to the appearance of 2,5-hexanedione. This metabolite can be used as parameter of *n*-hexane exposure because its concentration in the urine correlates with the concentration of the parent substance in the air. After a single short exposure (10 min) to 17,600 mg/m^3 *n*-hexane in the air, a feeling of dizziness was reported. After a 2-month exposure to about 8000 mg/m^3, neuropathies with paresthesia and weakness in the legs were observed. Preceding symptoms can be headache, anorexia, and dizziness. A decrease in conduction velocity in sensory and motoric nerves can occur. In the electromyography, abnormal changes can be observed. Larger axons show swelling in the area of the Ranvier's node, which is followed by a retraction of the myelin coat. Small and nonmyelinized fibers are less affected. Muscle biopsies show signs of myofibrillar atrophy. These poisonings were not only observed in workers but also in "sniffers." After the end of exposure, there is a recovery phase during which single signs of the neuropathy can persist for 3 to 4 years. With a lower concentration (243–475 mg/m^3 in the work place) an exposure- and dose-dependent decrease in conduction system's velocity of the motor nerves was observed. Records regarding functional disorders of other organs (e.g., the eye and kidney) are of only minor toxicological importance due to the simultaneous exposure to a variety of solvents. In mice it was observed that *n*-hexane and other *n*-alkanes activate the hypothalamic–pituitary–adrenal axis. The study concluded that this activation and the known behavioral impairment were closely associated.

An acute exposure in rats to 17,600 mg/m^3, *n*-hexane leads to reversible testicular changes; a 2-week exposure, however, results in irreversible testicular changes. The effect, occurring in the Sertoli cells as an increase in the tubulin synthesis, must be traced back to 2,5-hexanedione. Peripheral neuropathy appears after a 6-month inhalation of 17,600 mg/m^3 in rats. However, an exposure of the same duration to 440 mg/m^3 does not produce neuropathologic changes. Rabbits developed emphysema, pulmonary fibrosis, and Clara cell adenomas after inhalative intake of 10,000 mg/m^3 for 24 weeks. Impairments of liver function and kidney function of rats were noticed after inhalative and i.p. administration of *n*-hexane (as well as of *n*-heptane). Comparatively high oral doses of 2,5-hexanedione reduce liver growth and the weight of the spleen and thymus. Furthermore, they lead to impairments in the cell-mediated and humoral immune reaction in mice. Moreover, this metabolite induced testicular atrophy and defects in spermatogenesis in rat. Genotoxic effects of *n*-hexane have barely been investigated. It is certain that it induces chromatid breaks in the rat. Signs of a carcinogenic potential are not shown. Data on embryotoxicity and teratogenicity are equivocal.

Alcohols

Alcohols are used as organic solvents, detergents, and for chemical syntheses. Ethanol is also a luxury food. The substitution rate of the carbon atom, which contains the OH group, determines the classification into primary, secondary, and tertiary alcohols. Alcohol-induced effects can appear after inhalative, after oral, and, less distinctly, after dermal uptake. The neurotoxic effects that are the predominant effects of nearly 60 alcohols mainly originate from functional disorders of the membrane. The extent and velocity of the alcohol's distribution in membranes correlates with the dose for an induction of neurotoxic effects in animals. When sedation and ataxia are used as a measure, the effectiveness increases from methanol to 1-hexanol.

Methanol

Due to the high volatility of methanol (boiling point = 65°C), the use of methanol-containing lacquer, corrosives, extraction media, and solvent mixtures can cause poisoning symptoms. The odor threshold is 5.3 mg/m^3 air. In addition, methanol is emitted when used as and in gasoline. Several fatal cases of poisoning were described after drinking methanol that had been mistaken for ethanol or drinks containing high concentrations of methanol (distillates of fermented fruit) or to which methanol had been added. Tobacco smoke contains a small amount of methanol. During an acute intoxication, distinct ecstatic states (narcotic phase) appear about 1 day after intake of methanol, followed by a massive metabolic acidosis (blood pH value $\ll 7.0$). Depending on the severity of the intoxication, 5 to 6 days after methanol intake, visual disorders can occur that are irreversible. Women and children react more sensitively to methanol than men. Of great significance is the correlation between the amount of methanol in blood and the narcotic phase, as well as between the amount of formic acid and the appearance of visual disorders. Single doses between 100 and 250 ml are fatal, but even 30 ml can be life threatening. Respiratory paralysis, edemas of the CNS or the lung, circulatory collapse, and uremia are responsible for death.

Methanol is metabolized to formaldehyde via the alcohol dehydrogenase. This biotransformation rate is low. The subsequent oxidation of formaldehyde to formic acid by the aldehyde dehydrogenase is a rapid, whereas the oxidation of formic acid to CO_2 and H_2O is slow. Therefore 30–60% are exhaled as methanol and high concentrations of formic acid are accumulated in the blood. The half-life of both substances in the blood ranges between 1 and 2 days. In contrast, formaldehyde has a half-life of less than 1 min. Due to this metabolism of methanol, ethanol (0.1%) is used for therapy to inhibit the oxidation of methanol.

The chronic intake of smaller amounts of methanol (e.g., by inhalation of vapors) leads to mucosa irritation, numbness, dizziness, headache and body pains, cramps, functional disorders of the digestion and bladder, and visual disorders. Furthermore, ringing in the ear, loss of hearing, neuritis, and neuralgias can appear.

Ethanol (Ethyl Alcohol)

Alcohol (also known as anhydrol, ethyl hydroxide, ethyl hydrate, and grain alcohol) is a clear, colorless, flammable liquid with a vapor pressure of 44 mm Hg at 20°C. It is used as industrial solvent and as one of the alternative clean substitutes for gasoline. A gasoline blend with 10% ethanol is called "gasohol." Both uses contribute to exposure to ethanol in the work place and ambient air. Ethanol consumption is the most relevant toxicological means of exposure worldwide, and consumption and abuse of "alcohol" account for the greatest social–medical problems in civil communities.

Absorption, Distribution, Metabolism, and Excretion

When ingested, 20% of ethanol is absorbed via the stomach mucosa and the remaining part via the small intestine by passive diffusion. From an empty stomach, ethanol is absorbed within 1 to 2 h and from a full stomach within up to 6 h. Lipids and other components of the ingesta play an important role. Alcohol is absorbed more slowly from beer than from wine and more slowly from spirits. The odor threshold is 19 mg/m^3 air.

Ethanol is distributed to all organs, tissues, and body liquids. It crosses the blood–brain barrier and blood–liquor barrier, as well as the placenta. The ratio of distribution between alveolar air and blood is 1:2100. The ratio is determined by the diffusion velocity, vapor pressure, and alcohol concentration in the lung capillary blood and is important when measuring the blood-alcohol concentration from exhaled ethanol. The concentration of alcohol in the blood is determinated by the Widmark formula,

$$\text{blood-alcohol concentration (\%)} = \frac{\text{ml of ethanol intake} \times 0.8}{\text{body weight (g)} \times \text{dc}},$$

where the distribution coefficient (dc) 0.68 is for men and 0.55 for women; and 0.8 = specific weight of ethanol. Assuming that a man (75 kg) drinks 50 ml of ethanol on an empty stomach, the blood alcohol concentration (not considering elimination) will equal

$$\text{alcohol concentration} = \frac{50 \times 0.8}{75{,}000 \times 0.68} = 0.08\%.$$

When ingested, 90–98% of the alcohol is oxidized in the liver and 2–10% is excreted unchanged via lungs and kidneys. Biotransformation of ethanol in the kidneys and in the lungs is of no practical importance. The blood-alcohol concentration decreases by 0.01–0.02% per hour. Alcohol dehydrogenase and aldehyde dehydrogenase metabolize ethanol to acetic acid (Fig. 13). The alcohol dehydrogenase and aldehyde dehydrogenase in humans exhibit genetic polymorphisms. For instance, individuals lacking mitochondrial alcohol dehydrogenase are characterized by a low K_m value for acetaldehyde, and complain of facial flushing, vasodilation, and tachycardia after the intake of even minor amounts of alcohol.

Alcohol oxidation uses up to 80% of the disposable oxygen in the liver cells and is perhaps responsible for the development of liver cirrhosis. The decrease of the $NAD^+/NADH_2$ quotient leads to an inhibition of gluconeogenesis with resulting hypoglycemia, which can be critical in children, especially for those who repeatedly consume alcohol.

Interaction between Ethanol and Therapeutic Agents The simultaneous intake of ethanol and barbiturates, meprobamate, and oral anticoagulants can inhibit metabolism through substrate competition at the cytochrome P450 system, thereby increasing their half-lives. Chronic ethanol intake induces several xenobiotic- and drug-metabolizing enzymes, for example, cytochrome P450, and the biotransformation rates of doxycycline, meprobamate, phenytoin, tolbutamide, pentobarbital, propanolol, and rifampicin can be enhanced. The half-lives of these drugs are reduced by up to 50%. The consequence may be a suitable adaption of the therapeutic regimen. Metabolites of toxicological importance are formed from paracetamol and isoniazide. The same holds true for the metabolism of halothane and CCl_4. Disulfiram, originally used for the rubber vulcanization, is also used to treat alcohol addiction. However, it can lead to a critical drug concentration (e.g., of phenytoin) through the inhibition of the cytochrome P450 system. Due to the inhibition of acetaldehyde oxidation, disulfiram produces a hypersensitivity to ethanol. When disulfiram is administered together with ethanol, severe symptoms of alcohol intoxication may be provoked (e.g., antabus syndrome: circulatory-system collapse, cyanosis, dizziness, vomiting, reddening of the skin, and palpitation of the heart). These symptoms were also noticed in rural workers who drank an alcoholic beverage (e.g., beer) when handling calcium cyanamide, an inhibitor of aldehyde dehydrogenase activity.

The intended effect of all central-nervous-system effective drugs can be unpredictably reinforced, modified, or weakened through concomitant alcohol intake. Sedatives, narcotics, psychotherapeutic drugs, analgetics, remedies against motion sickness, antiepileptics, and antihistamines can belong to this group. Chronic ethanol intake can lead to the development of an unspecific tolerance by the CNS against alcohol itself, and also against barbiturates, inhalation anesthetics, and central-nervous-system depressants.

Acute and Chronic Toxicity

The effect of ethanol on the CNS is the same as that of a narcotic (e.g., diethyl ether). Smaller amounts of ethanol enhance motor and psychological reactions. Larger amounts induce symptoms of depression (Table 9).

Larger amounts of ethanol and its metabolic effects may cause tremor, exhaustion, vertigo, throbbing headaches, labile blood pressure, gastritis, dizziness, vomiting, acidosis, and dehydration with long-enduring thirst. Improvement can be achieved by taking liquids, aspirin, and sodium bicarbonate. However, an effective improvement may also be reached by taking a small amount of ethanol.

Chronic consumption of alcohol inhibits lipoprotein synthesis. The transportation and cell secretion of lipoproteins are almost completely inhibited. Furthermore, lipids are increasingly deposited because the

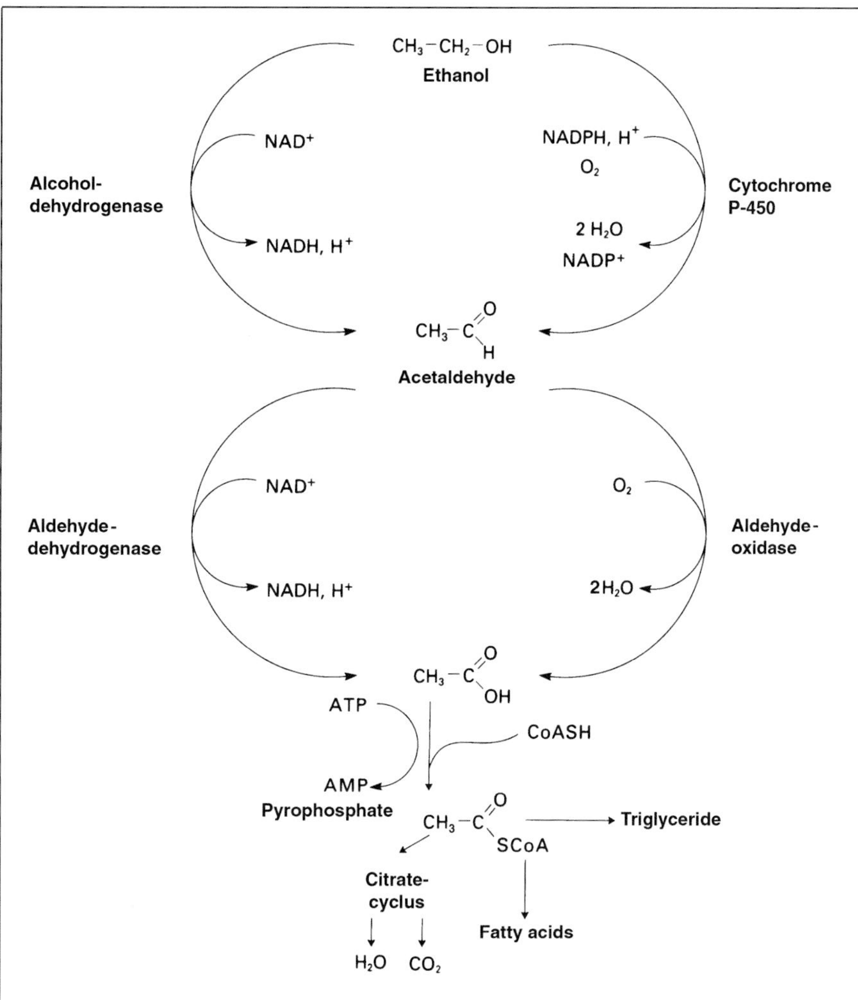

FIGURE 13 Metabolism of ethanol in liver cells. Following acute intake about 90% of ethanol is oxidized to acetaldehyde by the alcohol dehydrogenase and about 6% by the cytochrome P450-dependent enzyme system. Chronic ethanol intake causes induction of the cytochrome P450-dependent enzyme system, which leads to a conversion of only 80–90% ethanol to acetaldehyde. A major pathway to acetaldehyde is via acetaldehyde dehydrogenase. Aldehyde oxidase plays a minor role. About 10% of the ethanol is excreted unchanged or as glucuronic acid or sulfuric acid conjugates.

mitochondrial oxidation of fatty acids is disturbed and simultaneously fatty acid synthesis and esterification of the fatty acids to triglycerides ("alcohol fatty liver") are induced. A continuous supply of ethanol leads, via the reduction of the redox potentials, to an accumulation of acetaldehyde, which contributes to necrotic changes. Through its leukotactical properties, hyaline plays a role in the development of alcohol hepatitis. The toxic liver damage is, in contrast to alcohol fatty liver, not reversible and may lead to liver cirrhosis. Ethanol induces the microsomal cytochrome P450 system (CYP2E1) and in this way is conducive to its own metabolization. Animal experiments have further shown that free radicals (e.g., oxygen radicals and the 1-hydroxyethyl radical) are also produced; xanthinoxidase, nonbound iron, mitochondria, and peroxisomes contribute to this and are first expressed in the centrilobular hepatic lobule. Antioxidative factors, such as GSH, are reduced. Oxidative stress and lipid peroxidation cannot be excluded as further causes of toxic liver damage in alcohol abuse. Ethanol-induced radicals could play a role in the formation of extrahepatic effects (e.g., in the CNS, gastric mucosa, heart, testes, and uterus).

Vasodilation after alcohol consumption is explained as secondary effect (central depression is the

TABLE 9 Relationship between Blood Alcohol Concentration, Symptoms, Subjective Feeling, and Affected Brain Areas[a]

Blood alcohol concentration	Clinical description–symptoms	Affected brain area
0.05–0.10%	*Mild*	
	Decreased inhibitions; slight visual impairment; slowing of reaction time; increased confidence	Frontal lobe
0.15–0.30%	*Moderate*	
	Ataxia; slurred speech; decreased motor skills	Parietal lobe
	Decreased attention; diplopia	Occipital lobe
	Altered perception; altered equilibrium	Cerebellum
0.3–0.5%	*Severe*	
	Vision impariment	Occipital lobe
	Equilibrium	Cerebellum
	Stupor	Diencephalon
0.5%	Coma	
	Respiratory failure	Medulla

[a]Adapted from Gossel and Bricker (1984).

primary effect). The amounts of ethanol and acetaldehyde increase and decrease nearly simultaneously. A substance-related effect has not been observed. Both compounds have a strong vasodilating effect, resulting in a subjective feeling of heat. However, the loss of body temperature continues and cannot be regulated suitably; therefore, the risk of hypothermia, especially at low outdoor temperatures, must be taken into account. The primary sedative effect of ethanol can be accompanied by anxiolytical and euphoric effects. Gastric juice secretion is increased and the appetite is stimulated. In concentrated form, ethanol leads to irritation of the gastric mucosa and may be accompanied by hyperemia, prolonged evacuation time (pylorus spasm), reduced motility of the stomach, increased secretion of mucus, decreased secretion of acid, and, occasionally, vomiting and bleeding. Alcoholics can be affected by chronic atrophic gastritis. Through inhibition of the release of the antidiuretic hormone (ADH), ethanol leads dose-dependently to diuresis; however, chronic ethanol uptake can reduce this effect.

Chronic abuse of ethanol results in addiction. The psychological dependence on alcohol excludes somatic withdrawal symptoms; the physical dependence leads to somatic withdrawal symptoms (e.g., delirium tremens). The delirium can last in general for 2 days; in severe cases it can last up to 3–4 days. Hyperirritability, changes in hearing and eyesight, and hallucinations are typical ("toxic psychosis"). Fear, tremor, restlessness, agitation, sleeplessness, sweating, dizziness, vomiting, tachycardia, cramps, and self-deception and hallucinations can also appear. The mortality rate is high.

Specific Toxicology

Reproductive Toxicity The specific pattern of congenital changes after chronic alcohol consumption during pregnancy includes prenatal and postnatal growth retardation, microcephaly, and mental retardation (fetal alcohol syndrome). The incidence of fetal alcohol syndrome is estimated to be about 2–3 out of 1000 live births. Signs of the syndrome can be observed after a daily intake of 30 ml of ethanol during pregnancy.

Mutagenicity In experimental animals, ethanol induces dominant lethal mutations after oral uptake and, in fertilized egg cells of the mouse, sister chromatid exchange and aneuploidy. In the embryos of mice and rats, sister chromatid exchange has been noted when ethanol was given to the dams orally. The peripheral lymphocytes of alcoholics show an increased rate of sister chromatid exchange and aneuploidy.

The genotoxic effects (sister chromatid exchange, point mutation) shown *in vitro* with mammalian cells appear only after metabolic conversion of the ethanol; therefore, acetaldehyde is seen as the genotoxic agent.

Carcinogenicity In experimental animals the carcinogenicity of ethanol has not been sufficiently proven. The effects of ethanol (e.g., enzyme induction and tissue lesion) are understood as promotion leading to proliferation by initiation of changed cells.

For humans ethanol is seen as a weak risk factor. The daily consumption of four or more drinks is connected with an increased cancer risk (Fig. 14). Cancer located in the oral cavity and pharynx results from the consumption of spirits. Cigarette smoking increases the risk of alcohol-dependent cancer. Esophageal cancer is seen in connection with the consumption of alcohol as well. The increased incidence of cancer of the larynx in alcohol consumers is traced to the localized effects of hard drinks. The incidence of cancers of the liver, breast, large intestine, and rectum may be related to the chronic consumption of alcohol.

Propanol

1-Propanol

1-Propanol is used as solvent, for example, in textile manufacturing. Furthermore, it can be an additive in ink, cosmetics, detergents, polishes, and antiseptic preparations. The starting material is ethene. In nature, it can result from the microbial decomposition of organic material. It can also be a component in plants and mineral oil. 1-Propanol is often in alcoholic beverages with ethanol. In the environment, 1-propanol is dispersed mainly via air and less often via surface water. The main pathway of intake for 1-propanol in humans is through beverages and food.

After oral intake, absorption is almost complete. The absorption ratio after inhalative intake and dermal administration is not known. Proven data about mutagenicity and carcinogenicity are not available.

Volunteers who drank 2.53 mg/kg body weight (in addition to 650 mg of ethanol and 0.29 mg of 2-butanol/kg body weight) in a beverage in 15 min showed a blood concentration of 1 mg/liter after 3 h. In the liver, 1-propanol is oxidized to propionic acid. 1-Propanol is a better alcohol dehydrogenase substrate than ethanol and 2-propanol. It can therefore delay the metabolism of both alcohols. Furthermore, 1-propanol can be oxidized by cytochrome P450. The relative affinity of 1-propanol for the cytochrome P450 is three times higher than that of ethanol. The half-life of 1-propanol in the blood of rats and mice ranges between 45 and 57 min. The acute oral toxicity (LD_{50}) in various species lies between 1870 and 6800 mg/kg. Young rats are more susceptible (560–660 mg/kg). Signs of poisoning are hyperemia, vacuolization, and dilated sinusoids in the liver, as well as hyperemia. In addition, tubular swelling in and necrosis of the kidneys are described. An inhalation of 50 mg/liter for 2 h leads to a deep narcosis in mice.

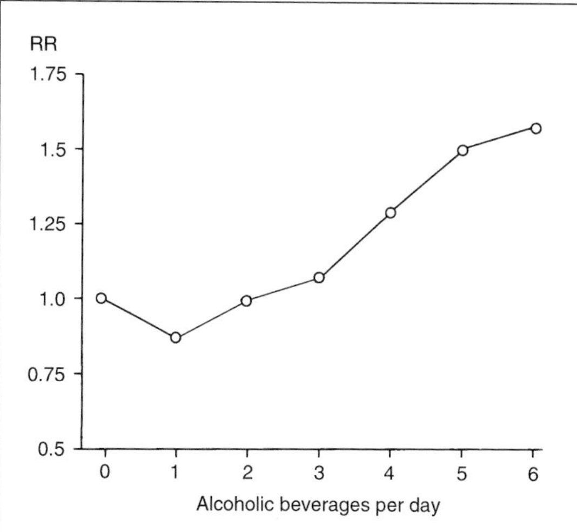

FIGURE 14 Relative risks (RR) of total cancer mortality according to number of alcoholic drinks (about 20 ml/drink) per day with a 60% smoking-adjusted excess risk in the heaviest alcohol consumption category. Data taken from a 12-year cohort followup of 276,000 American men. Remarkable is the known phenomenon of decreasing risks due to the daily intake of minor amounts of ethanol. (Adapted from Bofetta and Garfinkel, 1990.)

2-Propanol (Isopropyl Alcohol)

This alcohol is used as a solvent, heat-exchange medium, defroster (for car windows), and detergent, and in cosmetics and sprays of therapeutic agents and insecticides. It has antipyretic and antiseptic as well as skin-reddening properties. The smell equals that of a mixture of ethanol and acetone, its taste is slightly bitter, and the odor threshold is 7.5 mg/m^3 air. It is added to some luxury foods (e.g., tea and beer).

2-Propanol is mainly inhaled. Indoor air concentrations of 250 μg/m^3 can appear. The alcohol is quickly absorbed and distributed. Blood concentrations correlate with the dose. The main metabolite is acetone, which is exhaled or to a small extent excreted renally. The portion of exhaled acetone is inversely related to the dose of 2-propanol.

The biotransformation is catalyzed by the alcohol dehydrogenase. However, its activity for 2-propanol is about 90% lower than that for ethanol. The elimination half-life of 2-propanol in the blood of humans is 2.5–3 h in alcoholics and about 6.5 h in nonalcoholics. The half-life of the major metabolite acetone is 22 h. The acute oral toxicity (LD_{50}) in different species of animals ranges between 4475 and 7990 mg/kg. After inhalation for 8 h (19,680–64,206 mg/m^3), rats show severe irritation of the mucosa, as well as dose- and time-dependent CNS depression (e.g., ataxia, and narcosis).

In humans the oral uptake of 400 ml of 2-propanol can be lethal. However, it is reported that an uptake of 700 ml can be survived. The signs of poisoning are gastrointestinal complaints, hypothermia, drop in blood pressure, and shock. The causes of death are cardiac arrest and respiratory paralysis. Indications for genotoxic and carcinogenic effects in humans and animals do not exist. In studies in pregnant rats exposed to 2-propanol daily between the 1st and 19th day of pregnancy for 7 h per day, reduced food uptake and reduced weight were observed and the development of the fetuses decreased. The lowest observable effect level (LOEL) for maternal toxicity equaled 18,327 mg/m^3 and for fetal toxicity, 9001 mg/m^3. 2-Propanol induces the cytochrome P450 to a larger extent than 1-propanol but to a lesser extent than 1- and isobutanol. This could explain the over-additive effect of 2-propanol on the hepatotoxicity of carbon tetrachloride, 1,1,2-trichlorethane, chloroform, trichloroethene, and dimethylnitrosamine, on the metabolic activation of *n*-hexane. 2-Propanol is not genotoxic and is not an animal carcinogen.

Butanol (Butyl Alcohol)

Butanol exists in four isomer forms: 1-butanol, 2-butanol, tertiary butanol, and isobutanol. Through large-scale technical means, they are isolated from mineral oil. An exposure to higher concentrations mainly occurs at work places. Food can contain small amounts.

1-Butanol (n-Butanol)

1-Butanol is an odorous substance in food, beverages, and perfumes, with an odor threshold of 0.4 mg/m^3 air. It is the alcoholic component in solvents, detergents, textile manufacturing and brake-fluid additives and is used in the production of glass substitutes. Absorption via the skin, lung, and gastrointestinal tract is very rapid. C_{max} is reached 2 h after oral intake (in rats). Eight hours after uptake, only traces of the alcohol can be measured in urine. Within 24 h after oral uptake, 83.3% of the dose is excreted as CO_2, less than 1% is excreted unchanged via the intestine, and 4.4% is excreted in the urine (in rats), mainly as conjugates of sulfate and to a smaller extent as glucuronide. The LD_{50} (oral) in rats ranges between 0.8 and 2.0 g/kg. The inhalation of 24,624 mg/m^3 for 4 h has no lethal effect in animals.

Signs of acute poisoning are the same as those observed for ethanol. However, the toxic potency of 1-butanol is six times higher than that of ethanol. Fatal poisoning shows hyperemia of the liver and kidney, hemorrhage of the lung, and blood-count changes (i.e., reduction of erythrocytes and increase in lymphocytes). Irritation of the skin, eyes, and respiratory system can appear. Continuing exposure of rats to 1-butanol in the air shows no further effects at a concentration of 0.09 mg/m^3. However, the existing data are not sufficient to evaluate mutagenicity, carcinogenicity, and effects on reproduction. Humans respond to 1-butanol in the air with irritation of the eyes, tear flow and photophobia, headache, numbness, and narcosis. Healthy test subjects respond to a concentration of only 0.092 mg/m^3 with increased photosensitivity of dark-adapted eyes.

2-Butanol (Secondary Butyl Alcohol)

This isomer is used as a food additive because of its characteristic sweet smell and as a prestage of methyl ethyl ketone production. In rabbits, 2-butanol is transformed into methyl ethyl ketone, which is exhaled and excreted in the urine. The alcohol itself is glucuronidized. In the blood of rats, 2,3-butandiol and 3-hydroxy-2-butanone are the major metabolites. In rats the elimination half-life is 2.5 h; the LD_{50} (oral) is 6.5 g/kg. In rabbits butanol leads to irritation of the eyes but not of the skin. There are no data available from long-term studies of reproductive toxicity and carcinogenicity. In humans 2-butanol can lead to headache, numbness, and narcosis. Severe systemic effects are not known.

Tertiary Butanol

This alcohol (also called 2-methyl-2-propanol, butyl hydroxide, and trimethyl methanol) is mainly used as solvent and extraction medium and also as a prestage in the production of *tert*-butylchloride and of *tert*-butylphenol, as well as for the purification of polyolefins. It has a amphor-like odor. Two hours after oral uptake of *tert*-butanol (2 g/kg) C_{max} is reached in rats (1240 mg/liter). After another 6 h, the plasma concentration is only slightly decreased to 1100 mg/liter. The plasma half-life is 9.1 h. It is excreted unchanged and glucuronidized and after oxidation as acetone and CO_2. The metabolization is low because *tert*-butanol is not a substrate of the alcohol dehydrogenase. The LD_{50} after oral intake is 3.6 g/kg in rats. Signs of poisoning after inhalative intake are restlessness, mucosal irritation, ataxia, and narcosis. After exposure *in utero*, the alcohol leads to physical dependence and to postnatal effects (e.g., retardation of development).

In male rats *tert*-butanol increased renal tubular neoplasms. The underlying mechanism appears to be related to the known phenomenon of $\alpha 2\mu$-globulin accumulation in the renal tubule and the subsequent enhanced cell proliferation secondary to cytotoxicity and seems to be species and gender specific.

Isobutanol (2-Methylpropanol)

This alcohol is mainly used as solvent and in the production of esters, which are also used as solvents and as odorous additives in processed food and perfumes. Its odor threshold is 2.2 mg/m^3 air. Through natural methods, isobutanol is produced during fermentation of hydrocarbons. In some alcoholic beverages, it plays a role as impurity (e.g., in "rotgut"). Isobutanol can be absorbed via the lung or gastrointestinal tract. Even at higher doses (e.g., 2 ml/kg), the alcohol is no longer detectable in the blood of humans after 6 h. In the presence of alcohol dehydrogenase and of aldehyde dehydrogenase, isobutyric acid develops, which is channeled into the citric acid cycle. The oral LD_{50} in the rat varies between 2.5 and 3.1 g/kg.

The LC_{50} after inhalative intake ranges from 8 to 19.2 g/m^3. Signs of poisoning after oral uptake are numbness (narcosis) and after inhalation irritation of the respiratory system, decrease of the lymphocytes, reduction of the blood lactate value, retardation of bromphthalein elimination from the blood, and dystrophy of the hepatocytes and the olfactory neurons. The no observable effect level (NOEL) determined after long-term exposure is estimated at 0.1 mg/m^3. Two groups of rats that had been given alcohol twice a week orally in a lifetime study showed an increased number of carcinomas and sarcomas in the liver, of sarcomas in the spleen, and of carcinomas in the stomach, as well as leukemias. In summary, however, the data are insufficient and do not allow an evaluation of the carcinogenic potency in animals. There are no suitable data about mutagenicity and reproduction toxicity.

Glycol Ether

Diethylene Glycol

The compound ($HO{-}CH_2{-}CH_2{-}O{-}CH_2{-}CH_2{-}OH$) (also known as 2,2′-dihydroxydiethyl ether, bis-(2-hydroxyethyl)-ether, ethylene diglycol, 3-oxapentane-1,5-diol, and 2,2′-oxydiethanol) is slightly viscous, relatively nonvolatile, highly hygroscopic, and sweet-tasting. The odor threshold is about 4.4 mg/m^3. Diethylene glycol is used as a plasticizer and antifreeze formulation, as a component of cosmetics, in lubricants, and in the lacquer industry. In the mid-1980s it became known that some European wines and fruit juices contained diethylene glycol in concentrations up to 48 g/liter. Cases of intoxication, however, were not reported. Because it is water soluble and soluble in organic solvents, it was used in pharmaceutical products ("elixirs") and in this way led to dramatic poisonings worldwide (discussed later).

Absorption, Distribution, Metabolism, and Excretion

In rats, oral doses of 1.12 and 5.6 g/kg of a ^{14}C-labeled compound were rapidly and almost completely absorbed. Concentrations of radioactivity were found in the order kidneys > brain > spleen > liver > muscle > adipose tissue. Some of the treated animals showed a delay in the appearance of radioactivity in the blood and in distribution into the tissues. This phenomenon was traced back to diethylene glycol-induced CNS effects and cardiac depression. After about a half-hour, blood pressure returned to normal and consequently the velocity of invasion increased. Data for dermal and inhalative absorption are not available. In rats after a single dose, diethylene glycol is converted to 2-hydroxyethoxyacetic acid by liver alcohol dehydrogenase and aldehyde dehydrogenase, thereby increasing the ratio $NADH/NAD^+$. In long-term experiments, oxalic acid was identified as a further metabolite.

About 95% of labeled diethylene glycol and metabolites is excreted with the urine and the remainder is excreted with the feces. After an oral dose of 1.12 g/kg, radioactivity in rat blood decreased following a multicompartment model. The fast compartment has a half-life of 3.4 h.

Acute and Chronic Toxicity

After oral administration, the LD_{50} was 4.9 g/kg in rabbits, 13.2 g/kg in guinea pigs, 20.8 g/kg in rats, and 28.2 g/kg in mice. After iv injections in mice, the LD_{50} is 1.1–2.2 g/kg. As a cause of death, depression of the CNS (narcotic effect) was described. Lethally injured rats developed polyuria, and later oliguria with metabolic acidosis and even anuria. Tremors and spasms, with unpleasant body odor, cold limbs, ruffled coat, and turbid and pale-red lens are also described. Within 1–2 days the animals died in uremic coma. In the kidneys and liver, pathological alterations were diagnosed. In subacute studies on several animal species, nephrotoxic effects were predominant. Microscopic analyses revealed swelling and vacuolization of the tubulus epithelium, cell necroses, and increased connective tissue formation, including concurrent appearance of inflammation. Liver tissue samples showed fatty degeneration, centrilobular atrophy, and bile duct proliferations. The CNS was edematous. It showed hemorrhages and necrotic neurons with a compensatory growth of glia cells.

TABLE 10 Poisoning by Diethylene Glycol Used as Solvent in Formulations of Remedy Elixirs[a]

Year of poisoning	Country	Affected persons
1937	USA	34 children, 71 adults
1969	South Africa	7 children
1986	India	14 adults
1990	Nigeria	47 children
1990–1992	Bangladesh	339 children
1996	Haiti	86 children

[a]Adapted from Wax (1996).

In rats, chronic administration of diethylene glycol in the diet led to alterations similar to those observed after a subacute dosage. One outstanding finding was the occurrence of laminated mulberry bladder stones, which was accompanied by a marked chronic cystitis. Further analyses of the stones showed that the outer portion contained calcium oxalate and phosphate, while the inner portion consisted almost entirely of calcium oxalate.

The erroneous substitution of diethylene glycol for the less-toxic propylene glycol in medicinal elixirs used in the treatment of relatively minor ailments resulted in several dramatic poisonings and deaths. Poisonings also occurred in patients receiving glycerin that contained diethylene glycol as impurity (Table 10). In numerous cases, the patients suffered from renal failure. Postmortem examinations showed tubular nephrosis (vacuolar nephropathy) and centrilobular hepatic degeneration. Oxalate stones were not observed. It was estimated that a single or subchronic dose of about 1.12 g/kg diethylene glycol led to the symptoms observed in adults; children are expected to be more sensitive.

Specific Toxicology

Reproductive Toxicity In a two-generation study in rats, repeated administration of 11.2 g/kg body weight diethylene glycol in aqueous solution did not affect reproduction, and no embryotoxic effects were observed. In another two-generation study in mice, employing a continuous breeding protocol with diethylene glycol in water (> 6 g/kg body weight/d) for approximately 4 months, embryotoxicity, gross abnormalities, and decreased postnatal survival were observed. No adverse effects were observed on the outcome of pregnancy after exposure to 5% diethylene glycol in the diet (gestation days 0–20) or in mice after gavage of 11.2 g/kg (days 6–13). In rabbits dosed via gavage (1 g/kg; days 7–19), no compound-related effects on the dams or fetuses were observed.

TABLE 11 Glycol Ether and Their Acetates

Glycol ether	Formula
2-Methoxyethanol	$CH_3{-}O{-}CH_2{-}CH_2{-}OH$
2-Methoxyethyl acetate	$CH_3{-}O{-}CH_2{-}CH_2{-}O{-}CO{-}CH_3$
2-Ethoxyethanol	$CH_3{-}CH_2{-}O{-}CH_2{-}CH_2{-}OH$
2-Ethoxyethyl acetate	$CH_3{-}CH_2{-}O{-}CH_2{-}CH_2{-}O{-}CO{-}CH_3$

Mutagenicity and Carcinogenicity The Ames test, Chinese hamster ovary (CHO) gene mutation assay, sister chromatid exchange test, and chromosome aberration test with CHO cells revealed no genotoxic effects. In long-term experiments in which up to 2.5% diethylene glycol in drinking water was applied, no evidence was obtained for carcinogenic or promoting effects in rats.

2-Methoxy-, 2-Ethoxyethyl Ether and Their Acetates

The methyl ether and ethyl ether of the ethylene glycol, as well as the acetates of both glycol ethers (Table 11), are stable, colorless, and inflammable liquids with a slightly etheric smell. They can be mixed with water and organic solvents. They are components of paints and other coatings and are used as solvents in printer's ink, for dyes (e.g., in the manufacturing of textiles and leather goods), in synthetic resin, and as detergent, both domestically and commercially. Furthermore, they are used as antifreeze agents in the hydraulic oils and in fuels for airplanes. Humans are confronted with these substances mainly via inhalation.

Absorption, Distribution, Metabolism, and Excretion

Absorption via the lung, stomach, intestine, and skin is rapid and complete. The absorption rate via human skin is approximately 10 times higher than that of methanol, acetone, and methyl acetate. After oral intake of labeled 2-ethoxyethanol, the rat excretes within 96 h about 76–80% of the dose in urine. Distribution in pregnant mice after oral intake of labeled 2-methoxyethanol showed high amounts of radioactivity in the liver, blood, gastrointestinal tract, and placenta. The compound is metabolized rapidly in the liver. After a single ip application of 2-methoxyethanol, the rat excretes 50–60% of the dose as methoxyacetic acid and 18–25% as methoxyacetyl glycine within 48 h (Fig. 15). The intake of ethanol prior to 2-

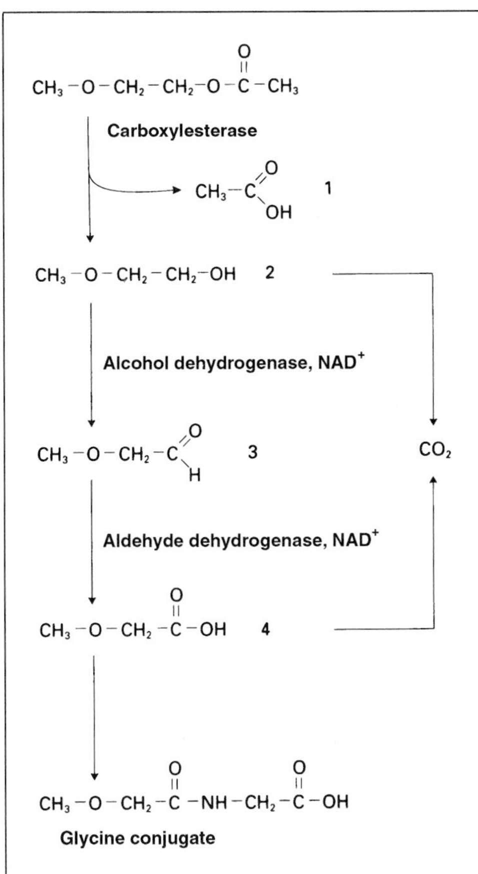

FIGURE 15 Major metabolic pathway of 2-methoxyethylacetate in rats. The ester is hydrolyzed to acetic acid (1) and methoxy ethanol (2), which is converted to methoxyacetaldehyde (3) and methoxyacetic acid (4). In a final step glycine conjugate is formed. (Adapted from WHO, 1990a.)

methoxyethanol and 2-ethoxyethanol leads to a longer retention of both glycol ethers in the blood of rats because of a competitive inhibition of alcohol dehydrogenase by ethanol. The elimination half-life of 2-methoxyacetic acid is 77 h in humans and of 2-ethoxyacetic acid 21–24 h. Women exposed to 2-ethoxyethanol and 2-ethoxyethyl acetate at their work places excreted 2-ethoxyacetic acid via urine even 12 days after the termination of exposure.

Acute and Chronic Toxicity

The intake of a mixture consisting of 400 ml of 2-methoxyethanol and ethanol (e.g., brandy) can have a lethal effect. Postmortem outcomes are acute hemorrhagic gastritis, fatty degeneration of liver, and black-colored kidney with remarkably degenerative changes of the tubuli. After intake of 44–100 ml of 2-methoxyethanol, agitation, confusion, nausea, cyanosis, hyperventilation, light tachycardia, metabolic acidosis, and kidney function disorders appear.

In animals, the acute toxicity of the four substances is low. After oral and dermal administration, the LD_{50} in rats, mice, and guinea pigs range between approximately 1000 and 5500 mg/kg. After inhalative administration of 2-methoxyethanol and 2-ethoxyethanol, the LC_{50} in mice are 4603 and 6698 mg/m^3, respectively. Signs of poisoning after a sublethal dose are dyspnea, somnolence, ataxia, and cachexia. In the kidney, degenerative and even necrotic changes can be observed. Rats showed testicular atrophy 24 h after an exposure for 4 h to 1866 mg of 2-methoxyethanol/m^3. After subchronic inhalative intake of 2-methoxyethanol, a decrease in the red and white blood cells counts, thrombocytes, hemoglobin, packed cell volume (PCV), and thymus weight was noticed in rats. After 22 days these changes had been reversed. Subchronic inhalation studies with 2-ethoxyethanol led to less distinct hematological parameters.

With respect to the blood parameters, 2-methoxyethanol seems to be more toxic than 2-ethoxyethanol. 2-Butoxyethanol, while inducing hemolytic anemia in rats, is presumably less toxic than 2-ethoxyethanol. The NOEL deduced from the inhalation studies are given at 93 mg/m^3 for 2-methoxyethanol and at 368 mg/m^3 for 2-ethoxyethanol. 2-Methoxyethanol inhibits antibody production and delays the rejection of skin grafts, which is not seen with 2-ethoxyethanol. Reversible changes in the liver (e.g., increased weight and decreased serum protein synthesis) were noted after subchronic exposure to 933 mg/m^3 of 2-methoxyethanol and 1104 mg/m^3 of 2-ethoxyethanol in various species. 2-Methoxyethanol induces irritation in the eyes. Nothing is known about the sensitization potential of either glycol ether.

Specific Toxicology

Reproductive Toxicity Both compounds have an influence on fertility. They induce a reduction of primary spermatocytes and also degenerative changes in secondary spermatocytes and in dividing spermatids; there are also changes in the sperms' motility, morphology, and concentration. The impairment of maturation of earlier primary spermatocytes is attributed to a reduction of the spermatid population, resulting from the fact that the tubuli contain only Sertoli cells, spermatogonia, and the early stages of primary spermatocytes. Many of these effects appeared after only 4 days of oral intake of 250 mg/m^3 of 2-methoxyethanol. Most of the effects were reversible within 8 weeks after 2-methoxyethanol administration. After an intake of 50 mg/kg, the effects were not noticed. These effects of 2-ethoxyethanol are observed after an oral dose of 500 or 1000 mg/kg for 11 days. After administration of 250 mg/kg, these changes were not noticed. A single oral treatment of 500 mg/kg 2-methoxyethanol in male rats leads to a dramatic reduction in the number of implantations after mating with nontreated female animals. This effect continues until the sixth week after the administration of 2-methoxyethanol. Signs of dominant-lethal mutations or abnormalities in the F_1 generation of rats have not been described.

After subchronic exposure of rabbits, rats, and mice to 2-methoxyethanol, degenerative changes of the testes were observed. Rabbits respond most sensitively. 2-Methoxyethanol orally administered to mice from day 7 to 14 of pregnancy induces a dose-dependent increase in the fetal death rate, encephalia, hernia umbilicalis, and skeleton anomalies, especially of the forepaws. It is remarkable that minimal skeleton changes appeared after a dose of only 31.25 mg/kg, which did not induce noticeable signs of poisoning in the dam. Cardiovascular defects and electrocardiogram changes were observed in pups if the dam had received 25 mg/kg of 2-methoxyethanol po from days 7 to 13 of pregnancy. 2-Ethoxyethanol provokes in rats a reduction of the fetal weight, skeleton anomalies, and cardiovascular changes, after inhalative as well as after dermal administration. Effects induced by inhaled 2-ethoxyethanol can be reduced by intake of ethanol in drinking water given together with glycol ether at the beginning of pregnancy. After dermal application of 2-ethoxyethanol or 2-ethoxyethyl acetate in rats from day 7 to 16 of pregnancy, fetotoxic effects also were observed.

Mutagenicity and Carcinogenicity Studies regarding carcinogenic properties of glycol ethers do not exist. Investigations of mutagenicity in bacteria and mammalian cells mostly showed negative results. With extremely high concentrations of 2-ethoxyethanol (3 to 7 mg/ml), chromosome aberrations and sister chromatid exchange on CHO cells were observed.

Formaldehyde

At room temperature, formaldehyde (also called methanal, methyl oxide, oxymethylene, and oxomethane) is a colorless gas with pungent odor. It is highly soluble in water, ethanol, and organic solvents. Formaldehyde available commercially as 30–50% (weight/weight) aqueous solution is called "formalin." In dilute aqueous solution, formaldehyde appears as monomeric hydrate (methylene glycol). The more concentrated the aqueous solution, the more polyoxymethylene glycol occurs as oligomers and polymers. To reduce the processes of polymerization, stabilizers, such as methanol (up to 15%) and amine-containing compounds, are added. In solid form, formaldehyde is marketed as its cyclic trimer (trioxane = CH_2O_3) or its polymer (paraformaldehyde) with 8–100 units of formaldehyde. Formaldehyde has natural and anthropogenic sources. Under atmospheric conditions in the presence of sunlight, formaldehyde is converted to CO_2. In the presence of NO_2, its half-life is 35 min; without NO_2, it is 50 min. Formaldehyde is still used as preservative and disinfectant in drugs and biological materials and also for disinfecting clothes and buildings (e.g., hospitals). Many cosmetic products contain formaldehyde because of its antimicrobial activity. Formaldehyde is widely used in the manufacture of resins with urea, phenol, melamine (cyanuric acid amide), and their derivatives, as well as in dyes, plastics, and other industrial chemical compounds. The release of formaldehyde into the atmosphere from industrial materials, consumer products, incomplete combustion of fossil fuels, and tobacco smoke contributes to the ubiquitous exposure to formaldehyde. In the United States, average outdoor levels of 0.005–0.01 mg/m^3 with peak concentrations of up to 0.1 mg/m^3 in urban air were determined. Mean levels in conventional homes are in the range of 0.025–0.06 mg/m^3. Modern office buildings contain concentrations of up to 0.45 mg/m^3. The highest exposures are encountered in occupational settings, as was shown for resin-production factories with 0.12–12mg/m^3.

Absorption, Distribution, Metabolism, and Excretion

After 2 h of exposure to 17.3 mg/m^3, the plasma of rats showed concentrations of 2.25 mg/liter; the controls showed 2.24 mg/liter. A blood concentration of 2.77 mg/liter was observed in persons exposed to 2.3 mg/m^3 for 40 minutes; before exposure the amount had equaled 2.61 mg/liter. Obviously a measurement of formaldehyde in plasma is no suitable method for biological monitoring. The same holds true for the metabolite formic acid in the blood and urine. Inhalation tests with labeled formaldehyde in animals revealed an almost complete absorption in the upper respiratory system. The absorption rate after oral intake has not been determined. Dermal administration of formaldehyde solutions to animals resulted in absorption rates up to 0.8%. In another study, where up to 0.9 μg/cm^2 was administered on the skin of monkeys, a percutaneous penetra-

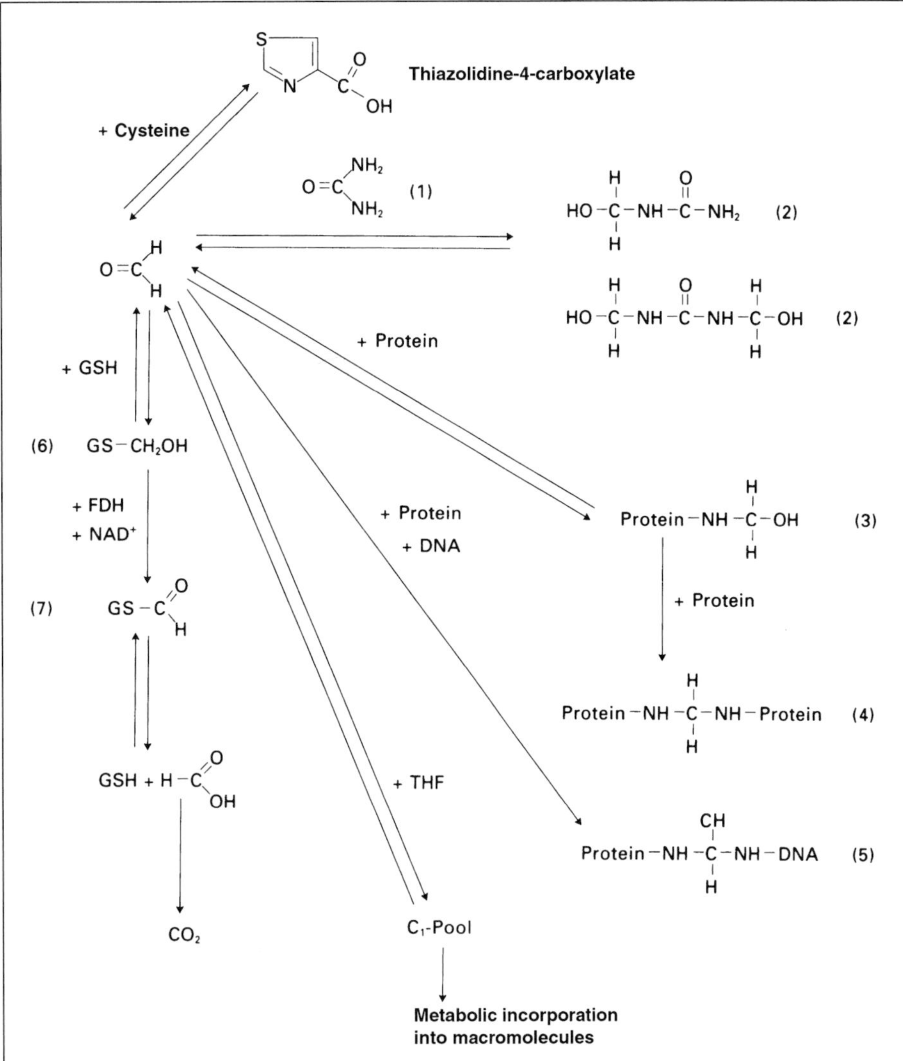

FIGURE 16 Biological reactions and metabolism of formaldehyde in rats. Formaldehyde undergoes reversible nonenzymatic reactions with cysteine, with urea (1) to hydroxymethyl adducts (2), with protein-to-protein adducts (3), and by repeated reaction with protein (not reversible) via a methylen bridge (cross-link) between two proteins (4) or with single-stranded DNA (not reversible) via a methylene bridge (cross-link) between protein and DNA (5). By the reversible formaldehyde dehydrogenase (FDH)-catalyzed addition of glutathione (GSH), *S*-hydroxymethylglutathione (6) is formed. The latter is metabolized to formylglutathione (7) in the presence of FDH and NAD$^+$. Formylglutathione dissociates to GSH and formic acid, which undergoes oxidation to water and carbon dioxide (Bolt, 1987.)

tion was observed, up to a maximum of 0.5% of the dose. Due to the relatively high formaldehyde concentration in the blood and tissues of humans and animals, definite data about the distribution of exogenous formaldehyde are only reliable from studies with labeled substance. After a 6-h inhalation of 18 mg/m^3 [^{14}C]formaldehyde, the highest amount of radioactivity was found in the esophagus and lower concentrations were found in the kidneys, liver, intestine, and lung of the rat. Autoradiographies show a major part of the radioactivity in the front part of the nasal cavity. After an intraperitoneal supply of labeled formaldehyde, 70–75% of the dose is excreted as CO_2 within 4 h (Fig. 16). The elimination half-life of formaldehyde registered in the plasma of various species is 1–1.5 mins. In contrast, the half-life of formic acid, which probands took in orally, equals 45 mins.

Acute and Chronic Toxicity

Its smell is perceived at 0.06 to 0.22 mg/m^3. This assumes that a longer exposure leads to a reinforced perception if the concentrations are lower. Thereby the simultaneous appearance of other contents of the air in the exterior (e.g., photochemical smog and motor-vehicle exhaust) as well as in the interior (e.g., building material, furniture and tobacco smoke) is normal or cannot be excluded. The known effects are irritation of the mucosa of the eye and the upper respiratory system. The effect threshold for irritation of the eye is 0.06 mg/m^3 and for the respiratory system 0.12 mg/m^3. Humans can respond to formaldehyde with discomfort of the respiratory system. Due to its sensitization, a subacute exposure at the work place and at home can lead to attacks similar to asthma, which can reappear after another exposure. Skin tests revealed that sensitized persons respond to a dose of only 0.05% formaldehyde in fluid solution, which can induce allergic contact dermatitis and contact urticaria. Data from several studies suggest that even at relatively high exposure levels, inhaled formaldehyde rarely induces a specific immune response. Children may show an increased tendency to develop specific antibodies after environmental exposure to formaldehyde. Their clinical significance, however, remains uncertain.

The acute oral LD_{50} is 800 mg/kg in rats and 260 mg/kg in guinea pigs. Injections sc and iv result in LD_{50} values of 420 and 87 mg/kg, respectively, for rats; inhalative intake for 4 h results in a LC_{50} of 984 mg/m^3. The signs of intoxication observed after more than 120 mg/m^3 were strong salivation, acute dyspnea, vomiting, and muscular spasms. Experiments with guinea pigs emphasize a dose-dependent sensitizing effect of formaldehyde solutions. A 5-day exposure of up to a maximum of 12 mg/m^3 led to irritation of the skin in guinea pigs.

Specific Toxicology

Mutagenicity and Carcinogenicity Chronic exposure to formaldehyde (up to 17 mg/m^3) in rats leads to cell degeneration, inflammation, necrosis, squamous metaplasia, and increasing cell proliferation of the epithelium of the nasal cavity. An increase in tumor incidence was observed after 6.7 mg/m^3; however, no increase in tumor incidence could be proven. During chronic exposure to 17.2 mg/m^3, mice developed tumors only in the nasal cavity; however, this result was not statistically significant.

The increase in the number of tumors in the nose and nasopharynx noted in workers is traced back to a direct inhalative contact with formaldehyde. This increase shows a direct dependence on the exposure. The suspicion that formaldehyde also induces leukemia and tumors of the CNS could not be confirmed. In contrast to animals, for which the carcinogenicity is classified with sufficient evidence, the carcinogenicity of formaldehyde for humans has only limited evidence.

Formaldehyde has been investigated as an initiator, promotor, and solitary carcinogen of the skin of mice, where phorbol esters were used as the promoter and benzo[*a*]pyrene and dimethylbenz(a)anthracene were used as initiators (i.e., a multistage model). According to this, formaldehyde has properties of neither an initiator nor a solitary carcinogen. With respect to its promoting properties, the results are negative or uncertain. In different test systems, gene mutations and chromosome mutations were proven when a high concentration of formaldehyde was used. After metabolic activation, genotoxicity was reduced. In mutagenicity tests with mammalian cells, the results were equivocal. Human lymphoblasts exposed to formaldehyde *in vitro* showed mutations and DNA–protein cross-links. The cross-links disappeared again after 24 h, probably due to repair mechanisms. Evidence that formaldehyde induces mutations *in vivo* does not exist. The cross-links measured *in vivo* appeared only in tissue where formaldehyde had been absorbed (stomach and upper small intestine) and at high doses (Fig. 16). Various species were examined regarding toxic effects in reproduction. The results gave no sign of a teratogenic potential when the substance was given orally and, dermally in amounts that exclude toxic effects in the dams.

However, after carefully considering the advantages of the use of formaldehyde in medicine and construction, we should take health-risk measures to keep the exposure to formaldehyde as low as possible for humans. The avoidance of formaldehyde is a part of these measures. Substitutes are preferred to formaldehyde only if they offer a lower health risk while having the same advantages. It is recommended in indoor environments that products that discharge formaldehyde into the air do not lead to a concentration exceeding 0.12 mg/m^3 (= 0.1 ppm).

Methyl tertiary-Butyl Ether (MTBE)

MTBE (also known as 2-methoxy-2-methylpropane and methyl-1,1-dimethylethyl ether) is a solvent with a boiling point of 55.3°C and a water solubility of 50 g/liter at 25°C. Its vapor pressure is 268 hPa at 20°C. In solution it is more stable than diethyl ether

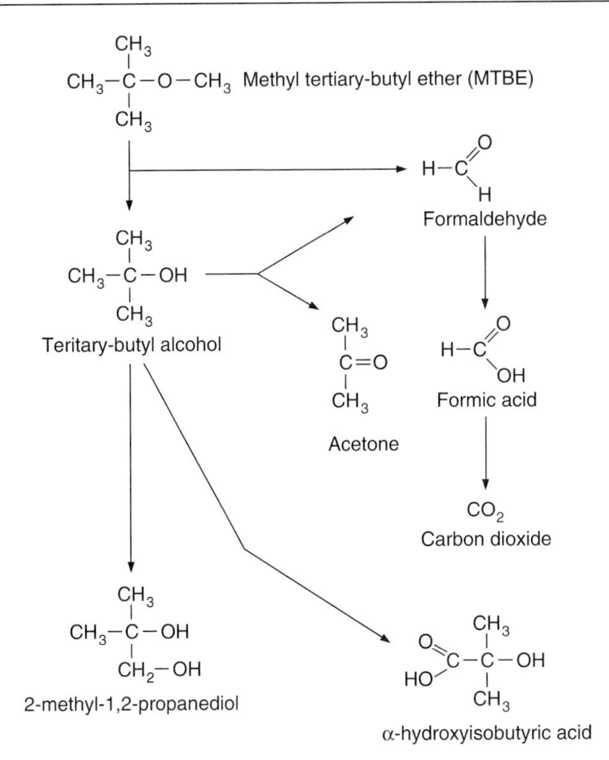

FIGURE 17 Metabolites of MTBE in rats. Biotransformation starts by demethylation, which is followed mainly by oxidative conversion reactions. Conjugation reactions (i.e., glucuronidation and glutathion conjugation) are omitted. The formation of acetone and carbon dioxide via formaldehyde is postulated on the basis of separate experiments with *tert*-butyl alcohol. (Adapted from Miller *et al.*, 1997, *J. Appl. Toxicol.* **17.** Copyright John Wiley & Sons Limited. Reproduced with permission.)

because it has a lower propensity to form peroxides. The conversion factor from parts per million volume to milligrams per cubic meter air is 3.6.

MTBE is currently used in two entirely different areas. First, it is approved by the Food and Drug Administration under investigational status for use in intraductal injection to dissolve cholesterol gallstones. This use has led to reports of toxicokinetics data and acute symptoms in humans and animals. Second, it is used as motor-vehicle-fuel additive. In 1993, 24,053 million pounds of MTBE were produced in the U.S. In the early 1970s, it was used as substitute for leaded octane enhancers, and more recently, because of its highly branched oxygenated structure, it has been added to gasoline to lower tailpipe carbon monoxide and other hydrocarbon emissions (resulting from incomplete combustion) so that communities can come into compliance with the standards set forth by the Clean Air Act. The Act's amendments stipulated that all regions that exceeded the national ambient air quality standard for carbon monoxide (referred to as "CO nonattainment areas") were required to use oxygenated fuels containing no less than 2.7% oxygen by weight or 15% by volume MTBE. In lower concentration, MTBE is used to enhance the octane rating in unleaded gasoline. With its increasing use, MTBE has tainted several drinking water supplies, leaking into groundwater from storage tanks and pipelines, or being spread from tailpipe emissions and leaching into the groundwater. The sources of exposure are manufacturing and transport, gasoline service stations, car repair garages, and car driving (as the emission of unburned fuel). Under the influence of reactive oxygen species in the atmosphere, MTBE undergoes oxidation to *tert*-butylformiate and via 2-methoxy-2-methylpropanol to formaldehyde and acetone. At 22°C, its atmospheric half-life is about 3.5 days.

Exposure to MBTE in air resulted in measurable concentrations in the blood. In gasoline-service-station attendants, values were in the range of 7.6–28.9 μg/liter. Blood levels in commuters ranged between < 0.05 and 2.60 μg/liter.

Absorption, Distribution, Metabolism, and Excretion

In humans, the absorption after respiratory uptake was estimated to be between 42 and 49%; it is almost complete after oral uptake and rather limited after dermal application. In rats, oral and intravenous administration of 40 mg/kg caused peak blood-MTBE values within 5–15 min. Maximum levels of the major metabolite *tert*-butyl alcohol were observed about 2 h after dosing. Following inhalative exposure to 1440 mg/m^3 for 6 h, blood levels of MTBE and *tert*-butyl alcohol reached peak values at the end of exposure and 30 min after exposure, respectively. Distribution into the tissues was studied after a single intraperitoneal administration of ^{14}C-labeled MTBE at a dose of 232 mg/kg. The highest concentrations of radioactivity 15 min after administration were detected in the adipose tissue, liver, kidneys, and CNS. It is remarkable that within the following 24 h, the concentrations of radioactivity in these tissues declined, while they increased in the lung and other tissues.

Metabolism of MTBE starts with demethylation yielding *tert*-butyl alcohol and a C_1 fragment. Both metabolites undergo further oxidative alterations (Fig. 17). The biotransformation rate can be deduced from elimination studies with ^{14}C-labeled MTBE in rats. After a 6-h inhalative exposure to 1440 mg/m^3, the males exhaled 17% and the females 22% of the radioactivity within 48 h. A single intravenous and oral administration of 40 mg/kg each resulted in an exhalation of 42 and 46% and of 46 and 54% in a 2-day period, respectively. Identification of the exhaled labeled compounds revealed that after inhalation, 65%, and after intravenous and oral administration, 26% and about 30%, of the radioactivity was represented by the *tert*-butyl alcohol. Regardless of the exposure route, about 1% of the radioactivity was contained in CO_2. The relative amount of the parent compound was in the range of one-third to more than two-thirds of the total exhaled compounds.

After inhalation, 65%, and after oral and intravenous dosing, 26–35%, of the administered radioactivity was detected in urine. The ^{14}C label was represented by *tert*-butyl alcohol, 2-methyl-1,2-propanediol, α-hydroxyisobutyric acid, and formic acid. Less than 1% of the administered doses was excreted via the feces. An additional route of excretion is milk.

Blood-elimination half-life values measured in rats were in the range of 0.5–0.6 h after inhalation and of 0.5–0.9 h after intravenous and oral administration, while *tert*-butyl alcohol has a half-life of 1.5–3.5 h, depending on the route of exposure and sex of the animals. In humans, after inhalation exposure the initial half-life of MTBE in the blood was approximately 10 min, that of *tert*-butyl alcohol about 7 h (Fig. 18).

Acute and Chronic Toxicity

In general, the acute toxicity of MTBE is low. The oral LD_{50} was determined to be about 3800 mg/kg for rats. Following sc administration, the LD_{50} is 4945 mg/kg for rats and 2646 mg/kg for mice. The intraperitoneal LD_{50} is 1249 mg/kg for rats and 1009 mg/kg for mice. Dermal LD_{50} values for rabbits exceed 10,000 mg/kg. Following a 4-h inhalation, the LC_{50} is 85–142,000 mg/m^3 for rats, and after 15 min inhalation the LC_{50} value is 141,000 mg/m^3 for mice.

A single iv injection of up to 14.8 mg/kg MBTE in rats and up to 37 mg/kg MBTE in rabbits was followed by a dose-dependent decrease in blood pressure and pulse. Cats given up to 74 mg/kg intravenously showed a more pronounced dose-dependent decrease in blood pressure and an increase in respiratory frequency and pulse. Single iv administration in mice led to reduced spontaneous activity and to a dose-dependent increase in pentobarbital-induced sleep time. Skin- and eye-irritation tests produced no or only mild alterations in rabbits. Rhesus monkeys of both sexes exposed to air concentrations between 12,400 and 341,000 mg/m^3 developed ataxia, emesis, prostration, unconsciousness, tremor, and bradypnoe. An 85-min inhalation of 341,000 mg/m^3 produced apnea.

Investigations in humans for the medical usage of MTBE have led to reports of symptoms such as nausea, vomiting, anorexia, hypotension, headaches, palpitations, angina, pain, and local tissue inflammation. Other effects were somnolence, sedation, coma, characteristic odor of MTBE on the breath, intravascular hemolysis, duodenitis, and, in one case, renal failure.

Repeated inhalative exposure of rats (13 weeks) to concentrations of up to 28,800 mg/m^3 resulted in an increase in the absolute and relative weight of the liver, kidneys, and adrenals. The highest dose group showed lymph-node hyperplasia, hemosiderosis in the spleen, and hyaline granula in the proximal kidney tubule. Signs of ataxia and hypoactivity occurred.

A 2-year oral administration of 250 and 1000 mg/kg MTBE did not lead to relevant differences in the mean body weights of male and female rats. There was a higher survival rate among male rats in the high-dose group 80 weeks after the start of the experiment, compared to the controls. In contrast, the survival of the females in both dosing groups decreased from week 16 of the treatment onward. MTBE-related behavioral changes were not observed.

Following a long-term inhalation exposure of mice (18 months) and rats (24 months) to 1480, 11,000, and 29,600 mg/m^3, high-dose-exposed mice showed MTBE-related reduced body-weight gain and early mortality, which—in the males—were traced back to uropathy or dysuria, symptoms occurring spontaneously in the mouse strain used. The brain and spleen weights were decreased, while, in the 11,000 and 29,600 mg/m^3 groups, the liver and kidney weights increased.

Both mice and rats of the high-dose groups developed reversible central nervous system depression for the first week of exposure, which continued in mice for the time of exposure. Male rats exposed to 11,000 and 29,600 mg/m^3 showed elevated mortality from a severe progressive nephrosis. Exposed females were comparable to controls. Hematological parameters were not influenced by MTBE. A decrease in corticosterone levels, however, was observed in the high-dose male rats. Liver and kidney weights were increased in the 11,000 and 29,600 mg/m^3 exposure groups.

Specific Toxicology

Reproductive Toxicity In a reproductive toxicity study, male and female rats were exposed to 1080, 4680, and 10,800 mg/m^3 for 6 h/day (for 2 and 3 weeks, respectively) before mating and subsequently during mating, gestation, lactation, and a second gestation period. In adult females and pups, dilated renal pelves were observed. In addition, a

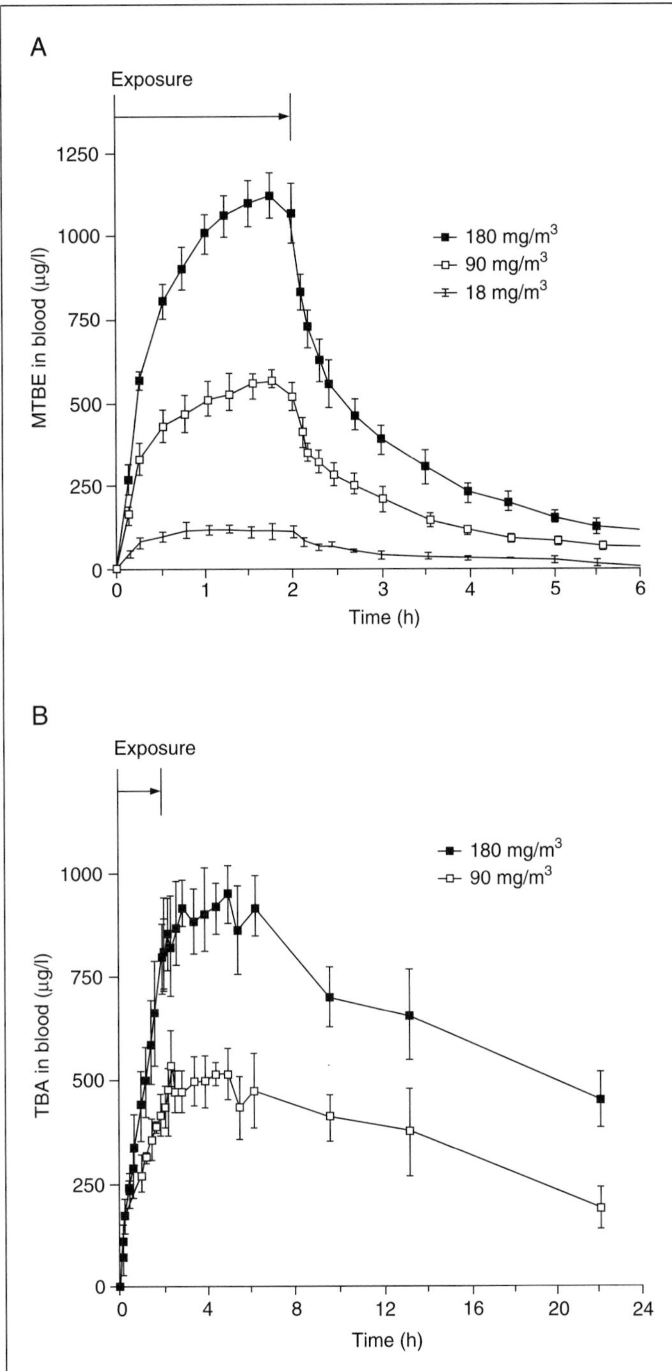

FIGURE 18 Concentration of MTBE (A) and *tert*-butyl alcohol (B) in capillary blood sampled from male volunteers during and after exposure to 18, 90, and 180 mg/m³ air for two hours in an exposure chamber. Vertical lines indicate mean values and 95% confidence intervals, $n = 10$. (Adapted from *Toxicol. Lett.* **82/83,** Johanson *et al.*, Toxicokinetics and acute effects of MTBE and ETBE in male volunteers, pp. 713–718, copyright 1995, with permission from Elsevier Science.)

Mechanism of the MTBE-Induced Kidney Tumors in Male Rats

Numerous chemicals (unleaded gasoline, 1,4-dichlorobenzene, α-limonene, isophorone, dimethyl methylphosphonate, hexachloroethane, and *tert*-butyl alcohol) that cause protein nephropathy in male rats have been shown to bind reversibly to α2μ-globulin, a low-molecular-weight protein. This globulin is sex-hormone related, and synthesized in the liver of the male rat, secreted into the blood, and filtered at the glomerulus, with approximately 50% being absorbed into kidney proximal tubule cells. Normally, α2μ-globulin is taken up by the lysosomes within the proximal tubule and digested by lysosomal enzymes to its constitutive peptides and amino acids. The hydrolysis of the globulin is slow compared to that of other proteins. Evidence suggests that chemical binding to α2μ-globulin makes the protein more resistant to hydrolysis, which accounts for its accumulation in the lysosome in the form of protein droplets.

The chemically induced accumulation of α2μ-globulin is thought to be responsible for cell necrosis, which, in turn, stimulates cell division as the kidney attempts to repair itself. With chronic chemical exposure, repeated cycles of cytolethality and reparative replication are proposed to be responsible for the cancer response in male rats.

As far as MTBE is concerned, three observations have emerged:

1. Accumulation of protein droplets related to MTBE exposure has been observed in the kidneys of male, but not female, rats after repeated inhalative and oral exposure.
2. By means of immuno-histochemical staining, MTBE-induced protein droplets were shown positive for α2μ-globulin. A dose-dependent linear increase in the intensity of the globulin, however, was not observed. Additionally, MTBE-exposed female rats did not show cell necrosis, protein accumulation, and positive staining for the α2μ-globulin in the kidneys.
3. After a short-term MTBE inhalation exposure, there was a concentration-dependent increase in kidney cell necrosis with minimal sloughing of epithelial cells in male rat kidney.

Moreover, another study confirmed that MTBE causes enhanced cell proliferation in male, but not in female, rat kidneys.

The first four compounds mentioned here that cause α2μ-globulin nephropathy bind reversibly to the globulin. Studies revealed that binding of MTBE to α2μ-globulin *in vitro* accounts for a high uptake of the ether into male rat kidney homogenate. In case of female rat kidney homogenate, the uptake of MTBE was comparatively low.

The uptake of MTBE in the male rat kidney cells is traced back to specific interactions between the chemical and protein. Interestingly, the addition of purified α2μ-globulin to a female rat kidney led to a four-fold increase in MTBE uptake into this tissue. Other proteins did not have the same effect.

With chronic MTBE exposure, there was an increase in the severity of chronic progressive nephropathy in male and female rats. Although the etiology of this pathological alteration is not known, it does not rule out the ability of α2μ-globulin nephropathy to mediate MTBE-induced male rat kidney cancer. In other words, chronic progressive nephropathy alone is not associated with increased incidence of kidney cancer.

A low or not identifiable risk for humans to develop chemically induced kidney cancer through the α2μ-globulin-mediated mechanism is indicated because the protein α2μ-globulin, or one similar to it, has not been detected in human kidneys.

slight decrease in pup viability and weight in the high-dose group were noticed. Male and female fertility indices were not affected.

In a two-generation study, rats of both sexes were exposed to concentrations up to 28,800 mg/m^3 for 10 weeks before breeding and for 7 days/week during mating, gestation, and the post-natal period. Fertility indices, live births and pup survival were not affected. In F_0 rats and F_1 litters, a decreased weight gain was observed. F_1 adults showed an increase in liver weight. In the F_2 generation, the perinatal deaths increased. Both F_0 and F_1 prebreed animals showed hypoactivity, lack of startle reflex, and ataxia. In pregnant rats exposed to concentrations up to 10,800 mg/m^3 during gestational days 6–15, no effects on maternal body and organ weights, uterine implantation, and fetal size were noticed.

Mice exposed to concentrations between 14,400 and 28,800 mg/m^3 during gestational days 6–15 exhibited a reduction in body weight, hypoactivity, ataxia, lacrimation, and labored respiration. The number of viable implants per litter and the fetal body weights were reduced. Exposure to 3600 mg/m^3 did not affect these parameters. At 14,400 and 28,800 mg/m^3, skeletal malformations occurred and at 28,800 mg/m^3 cleft palate occurred. Under similar conditions, mated rats and mice exposed by inhalation to concentrations up to 9000 mg/m^3 did not show adverse treatment-related effects. In the fetuses of mice only, the incidence of fused sternebrae was slightly increased. In pregnant rabbits exposed to concentrations of 3600–28,800 mg/m^3, a reduction of maternal weight gain and food consumption and an increased relative maternal liver weight were observed. Gestational parameters (corpora lutea, implantations, fetal body weight, and fetal malformation) were not significantly changed.

Mutagenicity and Carcinogenicity MTBE did not show mutagenic activity in tests with several *S. typhimurium* strains. In Chinese hamster ovary cells, no induction of sister chromatid exchanges or chromosomal aberrations occurred. The mouse lymphoma assay without microsomal activation likewise revealed negative results. In the presence of the microsomal fraction, however, there were positive results.

MTBE was proven to be carcinogenic in the experimental animal in 2-year cancer bioassays. In rats of both sexes given oral doses of 250 and 1000 mg/kg, MTBE caused an increase in Leydig interstitial cell tumors, and lymphomas, and leukemias in female rats. In another study in which male and female rats and mice were exposed via inhalation to high doses of MTBE (up to 28,800 mg/m^3), an increased incidence of renal tubular adenomas and carcinomas in male rats and liver cancer in female mice was observed.

The high-level exposure-related carcinogenic response may be traced back to nongenotoxic mechanisms (e.g., cytotoxicity, compensatory cell proliferation, and prolonged perturbations of hormones), which are of special relevance in cases of induced kidney cancer in male rats (see sidebar on previous page).

Bibliography

Agency for Toxic Substances and Disease Registry (1990) "Toxicological Profile for Polycyclic Aromatic Hydrocarbons." TP-90-20. U.S. Department of Health and Human Services, Washington, D.C.

Bevan, C., Tyl, R. W., Neeper-Bradley, T. L., Fisher, L. C., Pansson, R. D., Douglas, J. F., and Andrews, L. S. (1997). Development toxicity evaluation of methyl tertiary-butyl ether (MTBE) by inhalation in mice and rabbits. *J. Appl. Toxicol.* **17 (S1),** 21–29.

Bird, M. G., Burleigh-Flayer, H. D., Chun, J. S., Douglas, J. F., Kneiss, J. J., and Andrews, L. S. (1997). Oncogenicity studies of inhaled methyl tertiary-butyl ether (MTBE) in CD-1 mice and F-344 rats. *J. Appl. Toxicol.* **17,** S45–S55.

Boffetta, P., and Garfinkel, L. (1990). Alcohol drinking and mortality among men enrolled in an American Cancer Society prospective study. *Epidemiology,* **1,** 342–348.

Bolt, H. M. (1987). Experimental toxicology of formaldehyde. *Cancer Res. Clin. Oncol.* **113,** 305–309.

Borghoff, S. J., Prescott-Mathews, J. S., and Poet, T. S. (1996). The mechanism of male rat kidney tumors induced by methyl tert-butyl ether and its relevance in assessing human risk. *Chemical Industry Institute of Toxicology Activities* **16,** 1–6.

Cherng, S.-H., Lin, S. T., and Lee, H. (1996). Modulatory effects of polycyclic aromatic hydrocarbons on the mutagenicity of 1-nitropyrene: A structure-activity relationship study. *Mutat. Res.* **367,** 177–185.

Conney, A. H. (1982). Induction of microsomal enzymes by foreign chemicals and carcinogenesis by polycyclic aromatic hydrocarbons (G. H. A. Clowes Memorial Lecture). *Cancer Res.* **42,** 4875–4917.

Cox, L. A. (1991). Biological basis of chemical carcinogenesis: insights from benzene. *Risk Anal.* **11,** 453–464.

Dean, B. J. (1978). Genetic toxicology of benzene, toluene, xylenes and phenols. *Mutat. Res.* **47,** 75–97.

De Pierre, J. W., and Ernster, L. (1978). The metabolism of polycyclic hydrocarbons and its relationship to cancer. *Biochem. Biophys. Acta* **473,** 149–186.

Durant, J. L., Busby W. F., Jr., Lafleur, A. L., Penman, B. W., and Crespi, C. L. (1996). Human cell mutagenicity of oxygenated, nitrated and unsubstituted polycyclic aromatic hydrocarbons associated with urban aerosols. *Mutat. Res.* **371,** 123–157.

Farris, G. M., Robinson, S. N., Wong, B. A., Wong, V. A., Hahn, W. P., and Shah, R. (1997). Effects of benzene on splenic, thymic, and femoral lymphocytes in mice. *Toxicol* **118,** 137–148.

Fishbein, L. (1985a). An overview of environmental and toxicological aspects of aromatic hydrocarbons, II. Toluene. *Sci. Total Environ.* **42,** 267–288.

Fishbein, L. (1985b). An overview of environmental and toxicological aspects of aromatic hydrocarbons, III. Xylene. *Sci. Total Environ.* **43,** 165–183.

Fishbein, L. (1985c). An overview of environmental and toxicological aspects of aromatic hydrocarbons, IV. Ethylbenzene. *Sci. Total Environ.* **44,** 269–287.

Flesher, J. W., Myers, S. R., and Blake, J. W. (1994). Biosynthesis of the potent carcinogen 7,12-dimethyl-benz(a)anthracene. *Cancer Lett.* **24,** 335–343.

Gold, L. S., Slone, T. H., Manley, N. B., and Bernstein, L. (1991). Target organs in chronic bioassays of 522 chemical carcinogens. *Environ. Health Perspect.* **98,** 233–246.

Gossel, T. A., and Bricker, J. D. (1984). "Principles of Clinical Toxicology." Raven Press, New York.

Hard, G. C., Rodgers, I. S., Baetcke, K. P., Richards, W. C., McGaughy, R. E., and Valcovic, L. R. (1993). Hazard evaluation of chemicals that cause accumulation of $\alpha 2\mu$-globulin, hyaline droplet nephropathy, and tubule neoplasia in the kidneys of male rats. *Environ. Health Perspect.* **99,** 313–349.

Harper, N., Steinberg, M., and Safe, S. (1996). Immunotoxicity of a reconstituted polynuclear aromatic hydrocarbon mixture in B6C3F1 mice. *Toxicology* **109,** 31–38.

Heilmair, R., Lenk, W., and Löhr, D. (1993). Toxicokinetics of diethylene glycol (DEG) in the rat. *Arch. Toxicol.* **67,** 655–666.

Hellwig, J., Klimisch, H.-J., and Jäckh, R. (1995). Investigation of the prenatal toxicity of orally administered diethylene glycol in rabbits. *Fund. Appl. Toxicol.* **28,** 27–33.

Hiraku, Y., and Kawanishi, S. (1996). Oxidative DNA damage and apoptosis induced by benzene metabolites. *Cancer Res.* **56,** 5172–5178.

IARC (1988). "IARC Monographs on the Evaluation of Carcinogenic Risks to Humans, Vol. 44, Alcohol Drinking." International Agency for Research on Cancer, Lyon, France.

IARC (1994). "IARC Monographs on the Evaluation of Carcinogenic Risks to Humans, Vol. 60, Some Industrial Chemicals." International Agency for Research on Cancer, Lyon, France.

Johanson, G., Nihlén, A., and Löf, A. (1995). Toxicokinetics and acute effects of MTBE and ETBE in male volunteers. *Toxicol. Lett.* **82/83,** 713–718.

Klar, E. (1938). Über die Entstehung eines Epithelioms beim Menschen nach experimentellen Arbeiten mit Benzpyren. *Klin. Wochenschrift* **17,** 1279–1280.

Kouros, M., and Dehnen, W. (1985). Nitrierte polycyclische aromatische Kohlenwasserstoffe, mutagene und kanzerogene Wirkung—ein Überblick. *Funkt. Biol. Med.* **4,** 82–90.

Lawley, P. D. (1989). Mutagens as carcinogens—development of current concepts. *Mutat. Res.* **213,** 3–25.

Lee, W. J., Wang, Y. F., Lin, T. C., Chen, Y. Y., Lin, W. C., Ku, C. C., and Cheng, J. T. (1995). PAH characteristics in the ambient air of traffic source. *Sci. Total Environ.* **159,** 185–200.

Leuschner, U., Hellstein, A., Schmidt, K., Fischer, H., Güldütuna, S., Hübner, K., and Leuschner, M. (1991). Gallstone dissolution with methyl-tert-butyl ether in 120 patients—efficacy and safety. *Dig. Dis. Sci.* **36,** 193–199.

Lieber, C. S. (1997). Ethanol metabolism, cirrhosis and alcoholism. *Clin. Chim. Acta* **257,** 59–84.

Lioy, P. J., and Greenberg, A. (1990). Factors associated with human exposures to polycyclic aromatic hydrocarbons. *Toxicol. Ind. Health* **6,** 209–223.

Loktionov, A., Popovich, I., Zabezhinski, M., Martel, N., Yamasaki, H., and Tomatis, L. (1992). Transplacental and transgeneration carcinogenic effect of 7,12-dimethylbenz(a)anthracene: Relationship with *ras* oncogene activation. *Carcinogenesis* **13,** 19–24.

Mastrangelo, G., Fadda, E., and Mrzia, V. (1996). Polycyclic aromatic hydrocarbons and cancer in man. *Environ. Health Perspect.* **104,** 1166–1170.

Miller, M. J., Ferdinandi, E. S., Klan, M., Andrews, L. S. Douglas, F. J., and Kneiss, J. J. (1997). Pharmacokinetics and disposition of methyl t-butyl ether in Fischer-344 rats. *J. Appl. Toxicol.* **17(S1),** S3–S12.

Morris, H. J., Nelson, A. A., and Calvery, H. O. (1942). Observations on the chronic toxicities of propylene glycol, ethylene glycol, diethylene glycol, ethylene glycol mono-ethyl-ether, and diethylene glycol mono-ethel-ether. *J. Pharmacol.* **72,** 266–273.

National Toxicology Program (1997). Update, March 1997.

Nordmann, R., Ribiere, C., and Rouach, H. (1992). Implication of free radical mechanisms in ethanol-induced cellular injury. *Free Radical Biol. Med.* **12,** 219–240.

Ng, T. P., Foo, S. C., and Yoong, T. (1992). Risk of spontaneous abortion in workers exposed to toluene. *Br. J. Indust. Med.* **49,** 804–808.

Oesch, F. (1972). Mammalian epoxide hydrases: Inducible enzymes catalyzing the inactivation of carcinogenic and cytotoxic metabolites derived from aromatic and olefinic compounds *Xenobiotica* **3,** 305–340.

Pott, P. (1963). Chirurgical observations relative to the cancer of the scrotum, London, 1775. (Reprinted.) *Natl. Cancer Inst. Monograph* **10,** 7–13.

Rickert, D. E., Bakarrow, C. S., and Irons, R. D. (1979). Benzene disposition in the rat after exposure by inhalation. *Toxicol. Appl. Pharmacol.* **49,** 417–423.

Rippe, R. M., and Pott, F. (1988/1989). Kanzerogenitätsuntersuchungen von nitrierten PAK (Nitroarenen) im Hinblick auf ihre Bedeutung fur die krebserzeugende Wirkung von Dieselmotorabgas. (Umwelthygiene, Düsseldorf) *Jahresbericht.* **21,** 65–89.

Robinson, S. N., Shah, R., Wong, B. A., Wong, V. A., and Farris, G. M. (1997). Immunotoxicological effects of benzene inhalation in male Sprague-Dawley rats. *Toxicology* **119** 227–237.

Sandmeyer, E. E. (1981). Aromatic hydrocarbons. *In* "Patty's industrial Hygiene and Toxicology" (G. D. Clayton and F. E. Clayton eds.), 3rd rev. ed., Vol. 2, pp. 3253–3283. Interscience Publishers, New York.

Schnatter, A. R., Nicolich, M. J., and Bird, M. G. (1996). Determination of leukemogenic benzene exposure concentrations: refined analyses of the Pliofilm cohort. *Risk Anal.* **16,** 933–840.

Smedley, J. (1996). Is formaldehyde an important cause of allergic respiratory disease? *Clin. Exper. Allergy* **26,** 247–249.

Snyder, R., Witz, G., and Goldstein, B. D. (1993). The toxicology of benzene. *Environ. Health Perspect.* **100,** 293–306.

Tesseraux, I., Lommel, A., Ollroge, I., Kappos, A. D., and Koss, G. (1990). Human risk assessment of carcinogens from an administrative perspective. *Reg. Toxicol Pharmacol.* **11,** 63–67.

Tokiwa, H., Sera, N., Nakashima, A., Nakashima, K., Nakanishi, Y., and Shigematu, N. (1994). Mutagenic and carcinogenic significance and the possible induction of lung cancer by nitro aromatic hydrocarbons in particulate pollutants. *Environ. Health Perspect* **102(Suppl. 4)** 107–110.

Van Wijen, J. H., Slob, R., Jongmans-Liederkerken, G., Van de Weerdt, R. H. J., and Woudenberg, F. (1996). Exposure to polycyclic aromatic hydrocarbons among Dutch children. *Environ. Health Perspect.* **104,** 530–534.

Vos, J. G., Van Leeuwen; F. X. R., and De Jong, P. (1982). Acnegenic activity of 3-methylcholanthrene and benzo(a)pyrene, and a comparative study with 2,3,7,8-tetrachlorodibenzo-*p*-dioxin in the rabbit and hairless mouse. *Toxicology* **23,** 187–196.

Wax, P. M. (1996). It's happening again—another diethylene glycol mass poisoning. *Clin. Toxicol.* **34,** 517–520.

WHO (1985). "Toluene". Environmental Health Criteria 52. World Health Organization, Geneva.

WHO (1987). "Butanols—Four Isomers." Environmental Health Criteria 65. World Health Organization, Geneva.

WHO (1989). "Formaldehyde." Environmental Health Criteria 89. World Health Organization, Geneva.

WHO (1990a). "2-Methoxyethanol, 2-ethoxyethanol, and their acetates." Environmental Health. Criteria 115. World Health Organization, Geneva.

WHO (1990b). "1-Propanol." Environmental Health Criteria 102. World Health Organization, Geneva.

WHO (1990c). "2-Propanol." Environmental Health Criteria 103. World Health Organization, Geneva.

WHO (1991). "n-Hexane" Environmental Health. Criteria 122. World Health Organization, Geneva.

White, M. C., Johnson, C. A., Ashley, D. L., Buchta, T. M., and Pelletier, D. J. (1995). Exposure to methyl tertiary-butyl ether from oxygenated gasoline in Stamford, Connecticut. *Arch. Environ. Health* **50,** 183–189.

Yang, J. J., Roy, T. A., and Mackerer, C. R. (1986a). Percutaneous absorption of anthracene in the rat: Comparison of in vivo and in vitro results. *Toxicol. Indus. Health* **2,** 79–84.

Yang, J. J., Roy, T. A., and Mackerer, C. R. (1986b). Percutaneous absorption of benzo(a)pyrene in the rat: Comparison of in vivo and in vitro results. *Toxicol. Indus. Health* **2,** 409–416.

CHAPTER

26

Halogenated Hydrocarbons

HERMANN M. BOLT*, JÜRGEN T. BORLAK†

*Institute of Occupational Physiology, University of Dortmund, Dortmund, Germany

†Fraunhofer Institute, Hannover, Germany

INTRODUCTION

Because of their physicochemical properties, halogenated hydrocarbons are widely used. In general, they are highly lipophilic, are not flammable, and are often used as solvents for various applications such as in the dye and paint industry and to remove grease from metals or other materials that need to be cleaned. Most halogenated solvents have a high vapor pressure, and therefore the common route of exposure is via inhalation and to some extent via skin, although accidental ingestion has been reported. In the past large-scale production of halogenated solvents included chloroform and carbon tetrachloride; however, more recently dichloromethane, trichloroethene, tetrachloroethene, and 1,1,1-trichloroethane predominate.

Halogenated aliphatic and aromatic chemicals are anthropogenic compounds and do not normally occur in biological systems. Therefore, they need to be detoxified and the cytochrome P450-dependent monooxygenases play a key role in the oxidative metabolism. Metabolic activation leads frequently to reactive intermediates. It is of interest to note that halogenated hydrocarbons that are similar in chemical structure may develop different toxicological profiles upon metabolic activation. This can be demonstrated, for example, when the toxicities of 1,1,1-trichloroethane and 1,1,2-trichloroethane or those of chlorodifluoromethane and dichlorofluoromethane are compared.

The use of halogenated solvents becomes increasingly restricted in highly industrialized countries. In Germany, legislation that restricts the use of chloroaliphatics ("Chloroaliphatics Directive") has been enacted. This directive regulates the use of halogenated hydrocarbons such as carbon tetrachloride, 1,1,2,2- and 1,1,1,2-tetrachloroethane, and pentachloroethane, as well as of aliphatics containing fluorine, chlorine, and bromine.

Halogenated hydrocarbons tend to accumulate in lipid-rich tissues and organs, such as the brain, because of their high lipophilicity and may produce anesthesia at critical tissue levels. Below certain threshold concentrations, sedation is commonly observed and, for the purpose of human and environmental protection, legislation that defines maximum acceptable concentrations for human exposure is in place; these levels are based on the effects on behavior rather than the concentrations needed to produce anesthesia. Evidence suggesting that acute exposure to even small amounts of halogenated hydrocarbons may produce subtile but reversible behavioral changes has been obtained. Long-term exposure to high doses may result in irreversible damage to the central nervous system.

In the following, the toxicological properties of the most common halogenated solvents are described. As noted above, the toxicity of halogenated hydrocarbons is often brought about by metabolic activation. Therefore, biotransformation is a prerequisite to toxicity and the production of phase I metabolites is primarily catalyzed by CYP2E1, a specific isoenzyme of the cytochrome P450-dependent monooxygenases. Additional metabolism of halogenated hydrocarbons by glutathione *S*-transferases is of toxicological significance and the mechanisms of metabolic activation and its toxicological significance are given in detail.

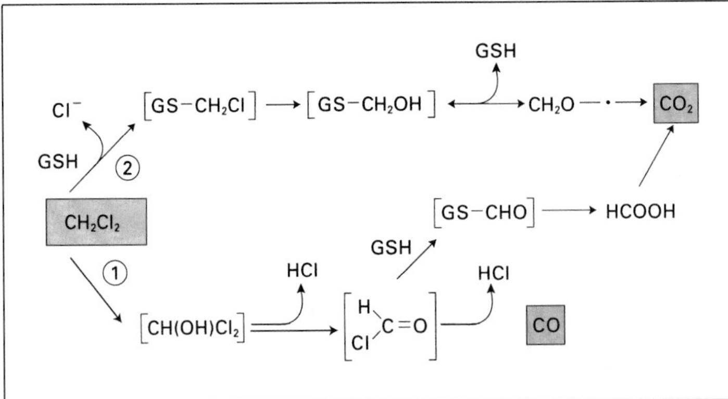

FIGURE 1 Metabolism of dichloromethane. Pathway 1: Oxidative metabolism by P450 monooxygenases (high-affinity reaction, but rapidly saturable) leading to the formation of carbon monoxide, a toxic metabolite. Pathway 2: Metabolism by glutathione *S*-transferases (low-affinity reaction, but less saturable).

DICHLOROMETHANE (METHYLENE CHLORIDE)

Dichloromethane is a weak cutaneous irritant and less potent than chloroform in its ability to depress the activities of the central nervous system (CNS). Nonetheless, in the past it was used as an anesthetic or to cause euphoria. Its inhalation provokes irritation, and occasionally pulmonary edema has been reported. In humans, concentrations of 1000 ppm and above can cause acute dizziness, and at concentrations of 10,000 ppm and higher anesthesia is noted.

Absorption, Distribution, Metabolism, and Excretion

Dichloromethane is rapidly absorbed from the lung and is metabolically converted to carbon monoxide by cytochrome P450-dependent monooxygenases and particularly via CYP2E1 (Fig. 1). This route of biotransformation can be saturated, as shown in rats and mice in which concentrations above 500 ppm caused saturation of the oxidative pathway. Dichloromethane can be metabolized by two routes. At high doses, the oxidative pathway becomes saturated and a shift in the biotransformation toward a gluthatione *S*-transferase-driven process becomes operational. At lower concentrations, conversion to carbon monoxide is the primary route of metabolic clearance and the formation of carbon monoxide is causally linked to the toxicity observed with dichloromethane. Alternatively, dichloromethane can be metabolized to carbon dioxide with formaldehyde as an intermediate. Dichloromethane is initially converted to chloromethylglutathione by glutathione *S*-transferases (Fig. 1). This intermediate is probably responsible for the genotoxic effects observed *in vitro*.

A linear relationship can be observed between time of exposure at various concentrations of CH_2Cl_2 (50–200 ppm) and the appearance of carbon monoxide (CO) bound to hemoglobin (Hb) in the blood of healthy human volunteers (Fig. 2). A 5% CO–Hb level is defined as the upper limit of acceptance and this level of CO–Hb can be reached at an exposure level of 100 ppm.

Acute and Chronic Toxicity

Rats exposed 8 h/day for 75 days, and then not exposed for 50 days, at 1300 ppm showed slight liver

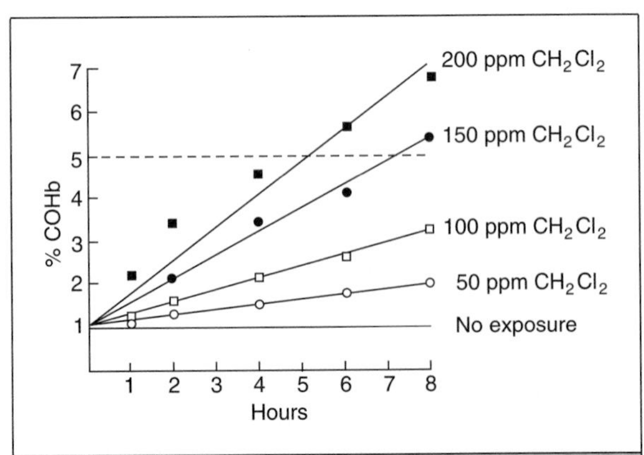

FIGURE 2 Metabolism of dichloromethane in healthy human volunteers at different exposure levels. 5% CO–Hb is considered to be the limit for exposure (dotted line).

changes. A mild hepatotoxic effect of dichloromethane was also found in other species (e.g., cats, dogs, and guinea pigs).

Specific Toxicity

The ability of dichloromethane to produce reproductive and developmental toxicity was studied in rats. No teratogenic effects were observed, but at very high doses (4500 ppm) prior to and during gestation, behavioral changes in the F_1 generation were noted. It is believed that the formation of CO–Hb is responsible for the change in the habitual behavior of rats and therefore dichloromethane might be potent in eliciting behavioral changes.

In the Ames test (*Salmonella typhimurium* TA 98, TA 100, TA 1535), dichloromethane was found to be mutagenic and it is thought that catalytic conversion via glutathione *S*-transferases leads to a genotoxic intermediate. In contrast, when dichloromethane was tested *in vivo* in mammalian species (micronucleus test, unscheduled DNA synthesis, and DNA binding), no evidence was obtained to suggest a mutagenic potential.

A total of seven carcinogenicity studies were carried out using rats, mice, and hamsters. The data are equivocal. No evidence was obtained in long-term bioassays to suggest dichloromethane to be a carcinogen for hamsters and rats, but there was a dose-dependent increase in lung and liver tumors in mice at inhalative doses of 2000 to 4000 ppm. This finding initiated further research into the species-dependent mechanism of carcinogenicity. As described above, it is reasonable to assume that the dose-dependent tumor formation in mice at high exposure levels of 2000–4000 ppm dichloromethane causes saturation of the oxidative pathway. Under these circumstances the glutathione *S*-transferase-driven pathway prevails, which leads to the formation of larger amounts of mutagenic intermediate(s) (i.e., chloromethylglutathione). Further evidence in pursue of a metabolically induced tumor formation comes from a species comparison, which shows that both *in vivo* and *in vitro* the species mentioned differed in their abilities to produce quantitatively metabolic breakdown products of the glutathione-dependent pathway in the order mice $>$ rats $>$ hamster. *In vitro* studies suggest that humans are less sensitive to a metabolically induced dichloromethane toxicity and particularly to the toxicity observed with intermediates of the glutathione *S*-transferase pathway. Therefore, the results obtained from mice need to be appraised with caution and may not be predictive for human risk assessment in view of the observed species differences.

The oxidative and CYP2E1-mediated metabolic pathway leads to the formation of carbon monoxide (Fig. 1). As carbon monoxide dissociates less rapidly than oxygen from hemoglobin iron, the capacity to transport oxygen declines with exposure time and level of exposure, resulting in a lowering of the oxygen available for tissues and organs. It is self-evident that a reduced oxygen availability results in a cascade of metabolic deregulations and dysfunctions. Further details of carbon monoxide poisoning are described elsewhere.

TRICHLOROETHENE (TRICHLOROETHYLENE)

Absorption, Distribution, Metabolism, and Excretion

Trichloroethene is primarily absorbed from the pulmonary system, although cutaneous absorption has been reported. It is extensively metabolized (Fig. 3). The oxidative pathway is the primary route of metabolic clearance. As depicted in metabolic pathway 1, the first intermediate, trichloroxirane, undergoes further biotransformation leading to several biotransformation products. Trichloroacetaldehyde is a stable intermediate that can readily be converted to trichloroethanol and trichloroacetic acid. The latter derivatives are important urinary metabolites. The ratio of trichloroethanol to trichloroacetic acid in urine differs remarkably among human individuals. Ratios ranging from 0.5:1 to 7:1 have been reported. It should be noted that trichloroethanol can partially be excreted as glucuronide, but the excretion of trichloroacetic acid is more common in humans than in other mammalian species, such as rabbit and rat.

When healthy human volunteers are uniformly exposed to trichloroethene, a steady-state concentration is reached in blood within 2 h (Fig. 4). The formation of trichloroethanol, however, increases linearly with time. The difference in the pharmacokinetic profiles of trichloroethene and trichloroethanol needs to be considered in detail when the toxicokinetic effects on the central nervous system are compared and exposure limits are to be determined.

The oxidative pathway involves the formation of an epoxide that is converted to dichloroacetic acid, oxal acid, and glyoxal acid, as well as the formation of the *N*-(hydroxyacetyl)-aminoethanol (Fig. 3). In addition, trichloroethene can be biotransformed via the glutathione *S*-transferase pathway leading to intermediates that become converted to mercapturic acid or are a substrate for β-lysase, which leads to toxicity

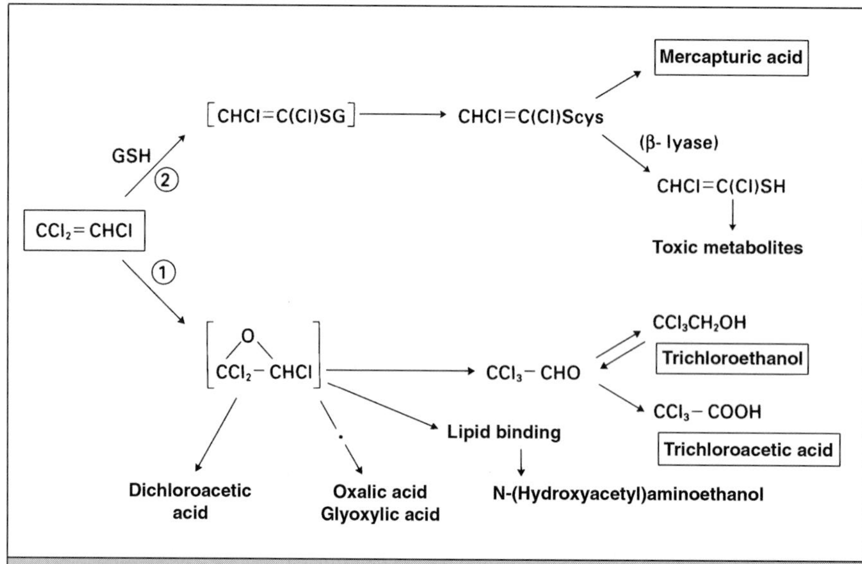

FIGURE 3 Metabolism of trichloroethene. Pathway 1: Oxidative metabolism (main route) leading to chloroethanol and trichloroacetic acid. Pathway 2: Metabolism by glutathione *S*-transferases (minor route).

in the parenchymal tissue of the kidney. Corroborative evidence for a metabolically induced toxicity comes from long-term studies in which laboratory animals developed kidney tumors when exposed to high levels of trichloroethene. The possible nephrocarcinogenic effects of trichloroethene after very high and long-term occupational exposures on humans are also discussed.

The formation of dichloroacetylene from trichloroethene needs to be considered further, as some specific neurotoxic effects have been observed with dichloroacetylene. Indeed, dichloroacetylene was found

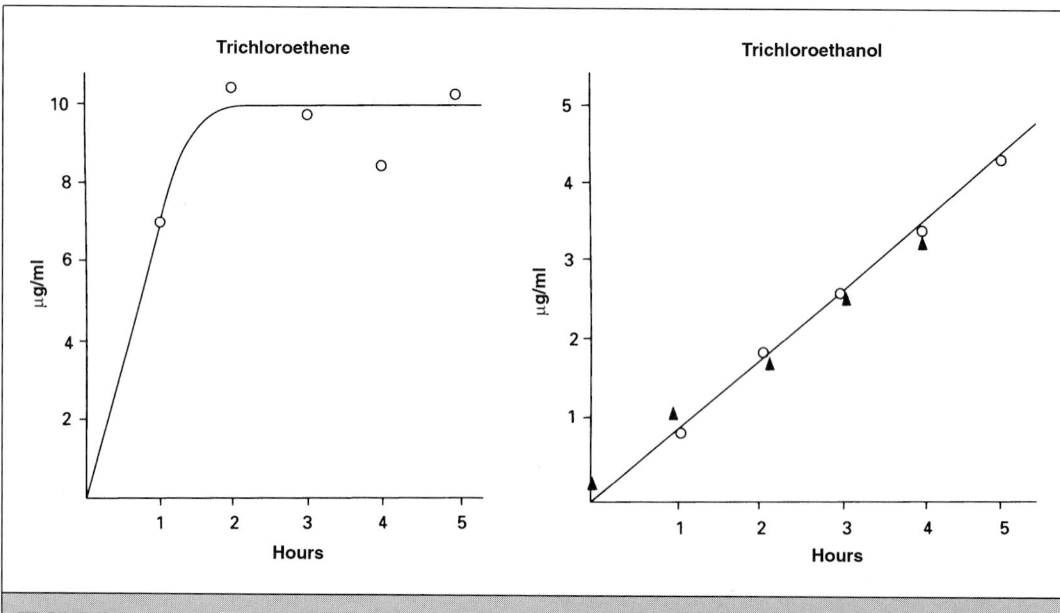

FIGURE 4 Plasma concentrations of (A) trichloroethene and (B) trichloroethanol in healthy human volunteers upon exposure to 100 ppm trichloroethene.

to be a specific toxin for the neuronal network of the brain. Corroborative evidence came from results with trichloroethene in closed exposure systems, where the exhaled carbon dioxide was absorbed onto soda lime, as well as from reports from accidents when trichloroethene was used as an anesthetic or as a solvent in submarines and spacecrafts where alkaline CO_2 absorbers are used.

In humans, trichloroethanol has a plasma half-life ($t_{1/2}$) of approximate 10 h, whereas the plasma half-life of trichloroacetic acid is approximately 100 h. The strong acidity of trichloroacetic acid and its high protein binding contribute to its rather slow plasma and urinary elimination. Trichloroacetic acid is also a peroxisome proliferator and this property might very well be linked to its ability to cause hepatocellular carcinoma after long-term administration of high doses of trichloroethene (300 ppm and higher). Similar results are obtained with tetrachloroethene.

Acute and Chronic Toxicity

As with other volatile chlorinated hydrocarbons, anaesthetic effects can be observed at 1000 ppm trichloroethene. Metabolism leads to the formation of trichloroethanol (Fig. 3). This metabolite has a pronounced depressive effect on the activities of the central nervous system, and indeed trichloroethanol is well known to be the active metabolite of the hypnotic drug chloralhydrate. These metabolites are responsible for most of the toxic effects of trichloroethene. After 4 h of inhalative exposure, the lethal concentration (LC_{50}) is 8000–12000 ppm for mice and rats. The oral LC_{50} was 3000 mg/kg body weight in mice and 5000 mg/kg body weight in rats and rabbits. Numerous studies have been carried out to assess the subchronic and chronic toxicity of trichloroethene in laboratory animals, and it can be concluded that exposure levels of above 400 ppm produce toxicity in liver and kidney as well as in the central nervous system.

Trichloroethene at high doses, or at lower doses with long-term exposure, causes damage to parenchymal tissues such as the liver and the kidney. Results obtained from animal studies and data from human exposure are in agreement and confirm liver and kidney to be targets for organ toxicity. Furthermore, trichloroethene can sensitize the myocardium toward catecholamines and causes potentially life-threatening arrhythmias due to its proarrhythmogenic potential. Again, studies with laboratory animals and results obtained from exposed humans provide corroborative evidence.

In the presence of alkaline materials, trichloroethene can readily be converted to dichloroacetaldehyde with the loss (removal) of HCl. As noted above, dichloroacetylene is severely neurotoxic and produces in its clinical manifestation a disorder similar to "polyneuritis cranialis." It is also a carcinogen and produces kidney tumors in laboratory animals. The interpretations of earlier studies are confounded, as impurities in the preparation of trichloroethene such as 1,1,2,2-tetrachloroethane, dichloroacetylene, or other ingredients cannot be excluded and these impurities could either contribute to or be even responsible for the observed toxicity.

Specific Toxicity

The ability of trichloroethene to produce reproductive and developmental toxicity was studied in rats and mice. Inhalative doses of 100 ppm produced a weak embryotoxic effect, but trichloroethene was not identified as a teratogen.

Numerous studies were carried out to assess its mutagenic and genotoxic potential. The results are equivocal, but evidence indicated that trichloroethene produced a positive result when liver homogenates from treated rats (Aroclor 1254-induced) were used. Similarly, an assessment of its mutagenic potential *in vivo* produced equivocal results. It is assumed that a reactive trichloroethene intermediate binds covalently to DNA, but studies with [^{14}C] trichloroethene could not confirm strong binding of radio-labeled material to DNA. Hitherto, the formation of stable DNA adducts still need to be confirmed.

The carcinogenic potential of trichloroethene was studied in rats and mice in several long-term bioassays after inhalative and oral doses. The target organs in mice are the lung and liver, whereas in rats toxic nephropathy and adenocarcinoma of the renal tubular cells are reported, leading to excessive mortality. On the one hand, it is of interest that lung tumors in mice are more frequent in the presence of stabilizing epoxide agents. On the other hand, lung and liver tumors are also observed in control animals in long-term bioassays and therefore trichloroethene might act as a tumor promoter rather than a tumor initiator.

Much attention has recently been focused on the development of renal cancer in humans, which has been linked to the glutathione-dependent pathway of trichloroethene (Fig. 5, pathway 2). Such tumors have been reported in workers occupationally exposed for years to high concentrations of trichloroethene (500 ppm and above), associated with frequent occurrence of prenarcotic symptoms. Because of these observations, a classification of trichloroethene as carcinogenic in humans is currently under review in different countries.

In several countries, such as the United States, Germany, France, and England, a concentration of 50 ppm trichloroethene has been defined as the upper limit for occupational exposure. This, in part, is due to the finding that an average exposure to 100 ppm trichloroethene produced effects on the central nervous system; the neurological effects have been described as a "psychoorganic syndrome" and include a number of neurological disorders, such as blurred vision. It is believed that the neurological effects are mainly the result of trichloroethanol acting directly on the central nervous system.

From a safety point of view, 5 mg trichloroethene/liter blood and 100 mg trichloroacetic acid/liter urine are considered to be the upper limits necessary to protect humans from potential intoxication. These recommendations do not take the carcinogenic potential of trichloroethene into account. In addition, a synergistic interaction between ethanol and trichloroethene has been reported, leading to an exaggerated pharmacodynamic and toxicokinetic response. Alcohol intolerance and skin reactions (flash) have also been reported when alcohol and trichloroethene are used simultaneously or consecutively. It is of importance that trichloroethene is an addictive agent and may be used by addicts as an inhalative drug or, in some cases, taken by ingestion.

TETRACHLOROETHENE (TETRACHLOROETHYLENE/ PERCHLOROETHYLENE)

Tetrachloroethene is an irritant to the mucous membranes at exposure levels > 100 ppm, whereas at concentrations between 500 and 1000 ppm, additional irritation of the respiratory tract is observed. Tetrachloroethene is more potent than chloroform as an anesthetic. It is absorbed through the skin, and, when applied as a liquid, a burning pain and erythema are observed. Similar to trichloroethene, it sensitizes the heart to the action of catecholamines and can cause extrasystoles. At prolonged exposures and at high concentrations, hepatotoxic effects in human beings have been reported.

Absorption, Distribution, Metabolism, and Excretion

As with other chlorinated hydrocarbons, tetrachloroethene is well absorbed upon inhalation. It is primarily exhaled as an unchanged substance. Nevertheless, some metabolic conversion to trichloroacetic acid occurs and the oxidative pathway is the common route of biotransformation (Fig. 5). Individuals differ in their abilities to metabolize tetrachloroethene and its metabolic conversion is dose-dependent.

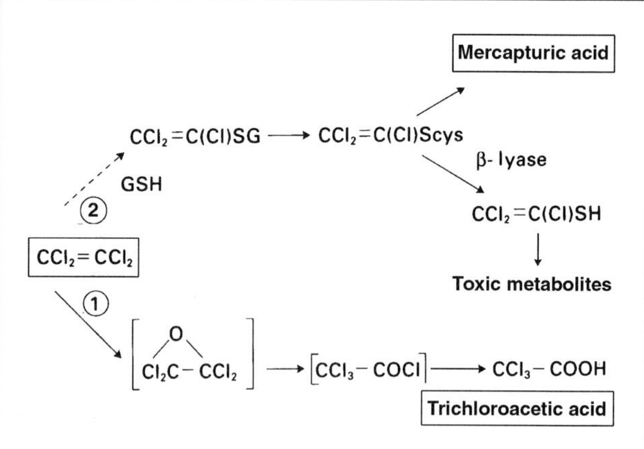

FIGURE 5 Metabolism of tetrachloroethene. Pathway 1: Oxidative metabolism (main route) leading to the formation of trichloroacetic acid. Pathway 2: Metabolism by glutathione *S*-transferases (minor route). Note: Most of the tetrachloroethene is exhaled as unchanged substance.

The glutathione *S*-transferase-mediated metabolism of tetrachloroethene leads to *S*-trichloroethenyl mercapturic acid, but this pathway represents only a minor route of biotransformation. β-Lyases are responsible for the further conversion of *S*-trichloroethenyl mercapturic acid (Fig. 5). This leads to a metabolically induced nephrotoxicity. In contrast, certain intermediate products from the oxidative pathway (e.g., tetrachloroxirane and trichloroacetyl chloride) are believed to be responsible for the hepatotoxic effects of tetrachloroethene.

Trichloroacetic acid is a major metabolite and, due to its high protein binding, a plasma half-life of about 100 h has been determined. This coincides with a rather protracted urinary excretion as at 70 h after dosing, only 1% of the dose is recovered as the urinary trichloroacetic acid metabolite.

Acute and Chronic Toxicity

In the course of acute intoxication (> 500 ppm) symptoms such as sickness, nausea, ebriety, and unconsciousness are often observed. Thereafter, hepato- and nephrotoxicity are common features of intoxication. During long-term exposure and at high doses, additional cerebral intoxication is noted, leading to

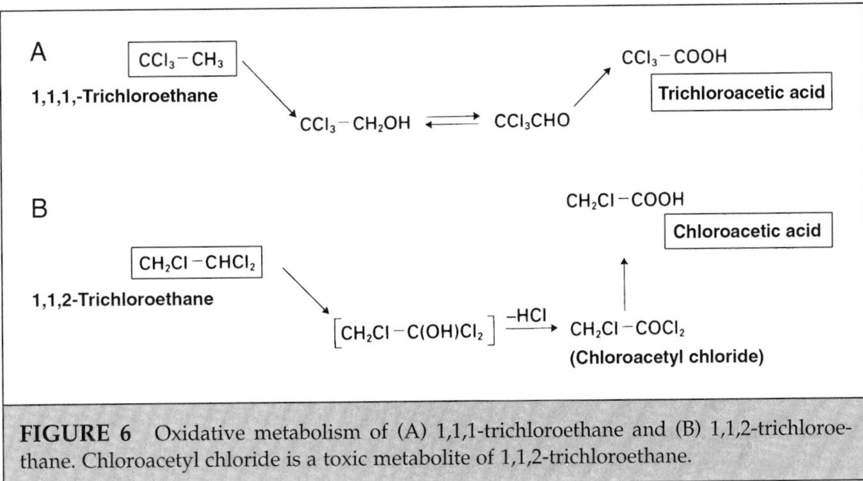

FIGURE 6 Oxidative metabolism of (A) 1,1,1-trichloroethane and (B) 1,1,2-trichloroethane. Chloroacetyl chloride is a toxic metabolite of 1,1,2-trichloroethane.

reduced functional capacity and changes in the behavior, including ataxia.

Specific Toxicity

The ability of tetrachloroethene to cause reproductive and developmental toxicity was studied in rats, mice, and rabbits. In general, no evidence was obtained to suggest that tetrachloroethene is teratogenic or mutagenic; however, not all the mutagenicity tests were negative. Therefore, no final appraisal is possible.

Long-term bioassays were carried out in several animals, including B6C3F1 mice and F344 rats. Studies reported by the National Toxicology Program (NTP) showed that in mice the most prominent findings were hepatocellular adenoma and hepatocellular carcinoma. In female rats, however, tubular kidney tumors, partly as adenoma or as adenocarcinoma, prevailed. The formation of the kidney tumors might be the result of high tissue concentrations of toxic metabolites, which are generated via the catalytic functions of β-lyase (Fig. 5). Based on the carcinogenicity finding, tetrachloroethene has been defined as a suspected carcinogen.

1,1,1-TRICHLOROETHANE (METHYL CHLOROFORM) AND 1,1,2-TRICHLOROETHANE

Similar to the halogenated solvents previously described, 1,1,1-trichloroethane has the potential to depress the activities of the central nervous system, but is not as effective as chloroform or trichloroethene. In humans, inhalative exposure to 500 ppm 1,1,1-trichloroethene for 3 h first causes signs of sedation; to achieve full anesthesia, exposure to 5000 ppm and higher is needed, as evidenced by cases of accidental intoxication.

1,1,1-Trichloroethene causes little irritation to the skin, but irritation of the respiratory tract is observed at higher concentrations (500 ppm and higher). Absorption through intact skin is rather limited and it is less potent in producing toxicity in parenchymal organs such as the liver and kidney than the previously described chlorinated solvents. Thus, the maximum occupational exposure level is higher and has been set at 200 ppm in the European Union. It is of considerable interest that the isomeric variant 1,1,2-trichloroethane is considerably more toxic (by a factor of approximately 20) than 1,1,1-trichloroethane and causes hepato- and nephrotoxicity. Its toxicological potential is comparable to that of chloroform. Occupational exposure levels have been set to 10 ppm in the United States (ACGH) and in Germany (MAK). Both isomers are metabolized via different routes and in the case of 1,1,2-trichloroethane, a reactive intermediate is formed (i.e., chloroacetyl chloride) (Fig. 6). This rather reactive metabolite is believed to be responsible for the hepato- and nephrotoxicity observed in animals and humans. Indeed, in the rat the LC_{50} for 1,1,1-trichloroethane is 20,000 ppm.

Absorption, Distribution, Metabolism, and Excretion

After inhalation, only 2% of 1,1,1-trichloroethane is metabolized in humans, whereas the remaining 98% is exhaled as the unchanged substance. Trichloroethanol and trichloroacetic acid are the predominant urinary metabolites. Inhalative doses between 150 and

1500 ppm caused saturation of plasma kinetics in rats. In contrast, 1,1,2-trichloroethane is extensively metabolized and 73 to 87% of a ^{14}C-labeled dose can be recovered from urine of mice as primarily chloroacetic acid, *S*-carboxymethylcysteine, and thiodiglycolic acid. The latter two metabolites are products of further metabolism of glutathione conjugates of chloroacetic acid. It is likely that the observed hepato- and nephrotoxicity of 1,1,2-trichloroethane can be attributed to the formation of chloroacetyl chloride, a toxic intermediate in the metabolism of 1,1,2-trichloroethane (Fig. 6). A similar toxic metabolite was not identified in the biotransformation of the isomeric variant 1,1,1-trichloroethane. Alcohol is less likely to potentiate the effects of 1,1,1-trichloroethane, in part due to its metabolic stability.

Acute and Chronic Toxicity of 1,1,1-Trichloroethane and 1,1,2-Trichloroethane

Exposures up to 450 ppm for 3 h did not result in adverse effects in human volunteers in various psychological and psychomotor tests, but at concentrations > 500 ppm (for 3 h) minor ocular irritation, partial headache, and drowsiness were noted. Only minor effects were seen in subchronic and chronic inhalation studies using rat, guinea pig, rabbit, dog, and monkey at concentrations below 1000 ppm. The most significant finding was fatty liver at anesthetic doses (> 1000 ppm). No evidence was obtained to suggest that 1,1,1-trichloroethane is a mutagen or a carcinogen, or produces reproductive and developmental toxicity.

1,1,2-Trichloroethane is a CNS depressant that is considered to be more potent than chloroform. Oral and intraperitoneal LD_{50} values in rats and mice vary between 400 and 900 mg/kg. It causes liver and kidney injury. Sixteen 7-h exposures at 30 ppm 1,1,2-trichloroethane resulted in hepatocellular damage (i.e., fatty changes) in the liver of female rats.

FURTHER EXAMPLES OF HALOGENATED SOLVENTS

In the past, chloroform (trichloromethane) and carbon tetrachloride (tetrachloromethane) were common halogenated solvents, but their use has now been restricted. From a toxicological point of view, chloroform and carbon tetrachloride are of considerable interest, as their mechanisms of action in causing liver- and nephrotoxicity are well understood (metabolically induced toxicity) and can be used as examples.

Chloroform (Trichloromethane)

Chloroform is a well-known anesthetic and analgetic substance and its use in medical practice dates back as early as 1847. The administration of chloroform is accompanied by side effects of respiratory changes, negative inotropism, and hepato- and nephrotoxicity. Its application in medicine has long been banned. Inhalative anesthesia with chloroform typically produced liver damage, including cellular necrosis and fatty degeneration in the centrilobular region of the liver. In accordance, liver transaminases and other target parameters of cellular damage were elevated with a maximum in enzyme activity around 3–4 days after exposure, but in most cases the liver function returned to normal thereafter. The observed liver damage in the centrilobular region, can, at least in part, be attributed to the distribution of cytochrome P450 monoxygenases, which are strongly expressed in this particular region of the liver.

Absorption, Distribution, Metabolism, and Excretion

Chloroform is well absorbed through the pulmonary system. It is readily metabolized in the liver (Fig. 7). During oxidation, removal of HCl results in the formation of carbonyl chloride (phosgene), a cell poison that reacts with functional groups to cause cellular damage.

Acute and Chronic Toxicity

Apart from its potential to produce liver damage, its ability to produce nephrotoxicity in male mice especially is well established. Because of the liver and kidney findings, a limit of exposure to 10 ppm has been set by the regulatory authorities in the European Union and the United States.

Specific Toxicity

The potential of chloroform to produce reproductive and developmental toxicity was studied in mice, rats, and rabbits, and the results depended on the route of application and the duration of exposure. After oral administration, only weak fetal and maternal toxicity was seen, but there was no evidence of chloroform being embryotoxic or teratogenic. In contrast, when chloroform was given to rats at inhalative doses of 30 ppm, embryo and fetal toxicity was noted and a teratogenic effect was seen at the 100-ppm exposure level. In mice, embryo and fetal toxicity and teratogenic effects were observed at 100 ppm.

Hepatocellular adenoma and hepatocellular carcinoma were the most significant findings in long-term bioassays with mice, whereas kidney tumors pre-

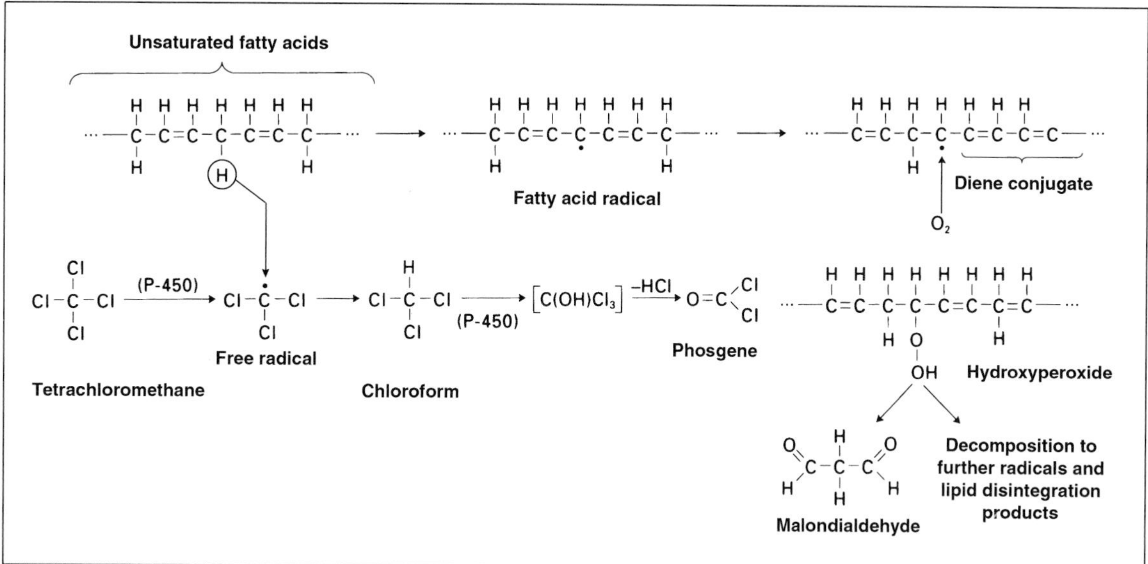

FIGURE 7 Metabolism of tetrachloromethane. Upon metabolic activation a CCl_3 radical is formed. This radical extracts protons from unsaturated fatty acids to form a free fatty-acid radical. This leads to diene conjugates. At the same time, O_2 forms a hydroperoxide with the C radical. Upon its decomposition, malondialdehyde and other disintegration products are formed. In contrast, the CCl_3 radical is converted to chloroform, which undergoes further oxidative metabolism.

vailed in rats upon oral administration. In view of these findings, chloroform is suspected to be a carcinogen. Its mechanism of action is viewed to be epigenetic because short-term genotoxicity tests are mostly negative.

Carbon Tetrachloride (Tetrachloromethane)

Carbon tetrachloride is used primarily in the production of chlorofluorocarbons.

Absorption, Distribution, Metabolism, and Excretion

Carbon tetrachloride is well absorbed across the respiratory system. Metabolic activation leads to the formation of a trichloromethyl radical, which is able to extract protons from normally esterifed desaturated fatty acids (Fig. 7). As a result, chloroform is formed *in vivo,* but lipid peroxidation also occurs. In consequence, esterifed fatty-acid radicals are formed and undergo diene conjugation; this reaction can be monitored *in vitro* at 233 nm. Furthermore, peroxides and hydroperoxides with the ability to cross-link or to undergo fragmentation are formed, leading to products such as malondialdehyde, ethane, and pentane. The chemical reactions described herein can be monitored spectrophotometrically (e.g., diene conjugation at 233 nm), and in the case of malondialdehyde formation a simple color reaction can be used (i.e., thiobarbituric acid assay). Ethane and pentane can be detected in exhaled air in *in vivo* studies. It is of interest that the chemically similar bromotrichloromethane is more effective in initiating lipid oxidation than carbon tetrachloride, as the removal of a bromide atom during dehalogenation is more readily obtained, which in turn leads to a more rapid generation of radicals (Fig. 7).

Carbon tetrachloride is a suicide substrate for cytochrome P450 and upon metabolic activation produces a trichloromethyl radical, which binds irreversibly to the monooxygenases and becomes the suicide substrate by this metabolic step. If an acute lethal dose is, however, given not as a bolus administration but is fractionized over a prolonged period of time, its toxicity becomes alleviated as the metabolic conversion to the trichlormethyl radical is reduced or even abolished; that is, the enzymes responsible for metabolic conversion are inhibited.

Acute and Chronic Toxicity

The LC_{50} (8 h) for mice is 10,000 ppm (inhalative dose), and in other laboratory animals oral LD_{50} values range from 3000–7000 mg/kg body weight. The cause of death is normally acute liver failure (necrosis). Characteristically, carbon tetrachloride poisoning produces centrilobular liver necrosis. Data obtained from occupational health studies suggest that prolonged and/or acute exposure to carbon tetrachloride is causally related to liver and kidney damage. Unfortunately, most of the older studies did not determine the exact concentrations of exposure, but it is generally accepted that subchronic and chronic inhalative doses of 10 to 100 ppm are deleterious. It is likely that the chronic liver damage observed in long-term animal studies (in mice) is a prerequisite for the onset of liver tumor formation. Corroborative evidence comes from occupational health studies in humans.

Specific Toxicity

Carbon tetrachloride is not teratogenic in rats, but it produces in fetal and maternal animals, concomitantly, toxicity (i.e., hepatotoxicity, nephrotoxicity, and death). A no-observable-effect level (NOEL) has not been determined as yet. Thus, further studies are needed to evaluate carbon tetrachloride's potential for causing fetotoxicity. In long-term bioassays, carbon tetrachloride produced liver tumors in rodents, probably as a result of chronic liver injury.

In view of its toxicological profile, an exposure limit of 10 ppm carbon tetrachloride has been set by the regulatory authorities in a number of countries. In biological monitoring, 0.07 mg carbon tetrachloride/liter blood is considered to be the upper limit of acceptance when the blood sample is taken at the end of an exposure.

CHLOROFLUOROCARBONS (CFC)

Since the convention in Montreal (in 1985), chlorofluorocarbons are less commonly used as solvents or degreasing agents, with the exception of 1,1,2-trichloro-1,2,2-trifluoroethane (chlorofluorocarbon 113). When compared with the previously discussed chlorinated solvents, most chlorofluorocarbons (mainly fluorinated and chlorinated methanes and ethanes) are less toxic. For instance, in the case of 1,1,2-trichloro-1,2,2-trifluoroethane, a maximum exposure limit of 1000 ppm has been set by both the ACGIH in the United States and by the European authorities because of its weak anesthetic properties and its metabolic stability. Indeed, due to its high vapor pressure, 1,1,2-trichloro-1,2,2-trifluoroethane is rapidly exhaled as an unchanged substance after exposure. Most chlorfluorocarbons are relatively nontoxic and thus higher occupational exposure concentrations are permitted. This is illustrated in the following comparison, which is taken from the German list of Occupational Exposure Levels (MAK values).

Compound	*MAK value*[a]
1,1,2,2-Tetrachloro-1,2-difluoroethane (chlorofluorocarbon 112)	200 ppm
Monchlorodifluoromethane (chlorofluorocarbon 22)	500 ppm
Chlorotrifluoromethane (chlorofluorocarbon 13)	1000 ppm
Trichlorofluoromethane (chlorofluorocarbon 11)	1000 ppm
1-Chloro-1,1-difluoroethane (chlorofluorocarbon 142b)	1000 ppm

[a]Maximum occupational exposure level for 8h/day or 40 h/week without adverse effect to humans.

In contrast, dichlorofluoromethane (chlorofluorocarbon 21, a fluorine analog of chloroform) is extensively metabolized and produces toxicological symptoms similar to chloroform. For this substance, a maximum exposure of 10 ppm is permitted by the European Union. It is of considerable interest that an isomeric variant of chlorofluorocarbon 21, chlorofluorocarbon 22, is practically inert. This exemplifies the importance of the relationship between substitution with halogen atoms and metabolically induced toxicity. 1,1,1-Trifluoroethane (chlorfluorocarbon 143a) was identified as a mutagen; however, chlorofluoromethane (chlorofluorocarbon 31) was more potent in the Ames test. The latter chlorofluorocarbon is also considered to be a carcinogen. The mutagenic and toxicological potential of chlorofluorocarbons can most certainly be attributed to a metabolically induced process. Corroborative evidence for this hypothesis can be obtained when the numerous chlorofluorocarbons are compared with respect to toxicity and metabolic stability. For instance, when chlorofluorocarbons with C_1 and C_2 substitution are compared, toxicity is rarely seen; this coincides with chemically and biologically inert behavior and also with their persistence in the environment. Much attention has focused on the use of chlorofluorocarbons because of their role in the ozone-depletion process. This property is described elsewhere.

MISCELLANEOUS HALOGENATED SUBSTANCES

A number of toxicologically important industrial chemicals are similar in structure and chemical properties to the previously described chlorinated solvents, for example, halogenated ethane and ethylene derivatives.

Halogenated Ethane and Propane

1,2-Dichloroethane (ethylene dichloride) and 1,2-dibromoethane (ethylene dibromide) are of considerable toxicological importance. These substances are used as scavengers in lead-containing fuel and as seed fumigants in agriculture. Ethylene dichloride and ethylene dibromide are metabolically activated via glutathione *S*-transferases to a reactive episulfonium ion, which is a strong alkylating agent. Ethylene dichloride and ethylene dibromide are mutagens and genotoxic carcinogens.

1,1,2,2-Tetrachloroethane is the most potent acute toxic substance among the halogenated ethanes. It also produces a more generalized toxicity in several organs and tissues. (e.g., CNS depression, hepatotoxicity, nephrotoxicity, cardiotoxicity, and pulmonary edema). Metabolic activation leads to dichloroacyl chloride, which is probably responsible for the observed toxicity. It is a suspected carcinogen and its toxicological profile is somewhat similar to that of 1,1,2-trichloroethane.

Halothane, a 2-bromo-2-chloro-1,1,1-trifluoroethane, is a well-known and commonly used inhalative anesthetic. Its mode of action and its toxicological profile are well described in pharmacology textbooks, to which the reader is referred. Halothane is only slowly metabolized, and the first step in its metabolic clearance involves the removal of the bromine atom. Further conversion leads to trifluoroacetic acid, which is excreted in urine. A limit of exposure has been set at 250 μg/dl blood and 10 mg/liter urine.

1,2-Dibromo-3-chloropropane has been used as a biozide (nematozide) as early as 1955. It has a low vapor pressure and is highly persistent in the soil. It can cause damage to the lung, intestinal mucosa, kidney, and testes in laboratory animals. Based on these findings, human occupational exposure levels were limited to 1 ppm as early as 1961. 1,2-Dibromo-3-chloropropane is an occupational health hazard and causes male sterility. When the exposed workers were examined in detail, different grades of oligospermia and even azoospermia were observed. Spermatogenesis returned to normal when minor oligospermia was diagnosed and no further exposure occurred, but this was not the case for workers suffering from azoospermia—these patients remained sterile. In animal studies, a dose-dependent toxic effect was seen with initial damage to the seminal epithelial cells and eventually total loss of spermatogenesis. Damage to the liver, kidney, and nasal tissue was also observed.

1,2-Dibromo-3-chloropropane is metabolically dehalogenated and the intermediate epoxide epichlorhydrine, a 1-chloro-2,3-epoxypropane is formed. This intermediate is a strong alkylating agent and a potent carcinogen. In long-term bioassays with rats and mice, 1,2-dibromo-3-chloropropane produced stomach cancer and upon inhalation nasal tumors. Its use is strictly regulated and it is a category 2 carcinogen according to European regulations (e.g., it is carcinogenic in experimental animals).

1,3-Dichloro-2-propanol is a genotoxic carcinogen. Carcinogenicity studies in rats demonstrated an increased tumor incidence for the tongue and mouth (for administration via drinking water), as well as the liver, kidney, and thyroid. Its metabolism and its mechanism of action are unknown.

Vinyl Chloride (Chloroethene)

The large-scale production of vinyl chloride dates back to the 1930s. It is the monomeric constituent of polyvinyl chloride (PVC). Its potential for causing liver damage was reported as early as 1949 in the USSR, but nonetheless it was considered safe for use as an anesthetic. Studies in dogs did, however, warrant concern about its use as an anesthetic, since vinyl chloride could produce arrhythmias in the canine heart.

The clinical signs of human vinyl chloride intoxication were initially reported in 1963. The symptoms described in this report were gastrointestinal and central nervous system disorders, Raynaud syndrome, sclerodermatoid changes of the skin, hepatosplenomegalia, and acroosteolysis of phalanx. Vinyl chloride's potential for causing cancer in animals and humans was discovered many years later. It typically produces hemangiosarcoma of the liver (hemangioendothelioma). Similar tumors were seen only in cases of arsenic and thorium dioxide poisoning. Hemangiosarcomas are rare tumors and thus epidemiological studies provide conclusive evidence for a causal relationship between vinyl chloride intoxication and the formation of hemangiosarcomata of the liver. Vinyl chloride is a potent carcinogen and is classified as a category-1 carcinogen (human carcinogen) according to European legislation. In the United States, it has been categorized as an A1 carcinogen by the ACGIH.

Vinyl chloride is metabolically activated via the CYP2E1 isoenzyme of the cytochrome P450-dependent monooxygenases (Fig. 8). After metabolic activation, a reactive and ultimately carcinogenic epoxide is formed (chloroxirane) and spontaneously rearranges to chloroacetaldehyde. Detoxification of the intermediates via glutathione conjugation leads to the formation of hydroxyethylmercapturic acid and thiodiglycolic acid, which are excreted into the urine. The latter metabolites are useful markers for monitoring vinyl chloride exposure.

The formation of the vinyl chloride epoxide occurs in the endoplasmic recticulum of hepatocytes. Chloroacetylaldehyde, as well as the epoxide, can react with adenosine to form a ethenoadenosine (Fig. 8), a known promutagen. These reactive intermediates also

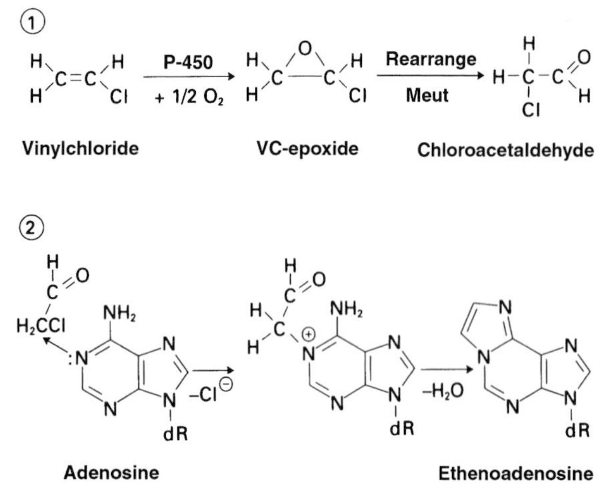

FIGURE 8 Metabolic activation of vinyl chloride (VC). Pathway 1: Cytochrome P450-catalyzed oxidation of vinyl chloride (VC) leads to the formation VC epoxide, which spontaneously rearranges to chloroacetaldehyde. Pathway 2: The aldehyde as well as the epoxide can react with nucleophilic DNA bases (e.g., adenosine), to form the promutagenic ethenoadenosine.

have the opportunity to damage the DNA of neighboring sinusoidal cells. The DNA damage in sinusoidal cells in conjunction with their more frequent cell division predestines the development of sinusoidal cell tumors (hemangiosarcoma of the liver) rather than tumors originating from the parenchymal cells, as hepatocytes divide less frequently. This agrees well with the finding that hepatocellular carcinoma are rarely observed in humans and in adult animals, compared to young animals, in which the growing liver is characterized by rapid cell proliferation. Therefore, the occurrence of hepatocellular carcinoma seems to be a logical consequence. As discussed above, vinyl chloride rapidly rearranges to form chloroacetaldehyde, which is further metabolized but may bind to proteins and nucleic acids.

Vinylidene Chloride (1,1-Dichloroethene)

1,1-Dichloroethene is a strong hepatotoxin and differs from vinyl chloride in its biological profile. A limit for human exposure of 2 ppm has been set because of its acute hepatotoxicity. Vinylidene chloride is metabolically activated to the epoxide 2,2-dichloroxirane, which is unstable and unlike the vinyl chloride epoxide is less potent in causing DNA damage. It is therefore not surprising that vinylidene chloride was either negative or only weakly positive in carcinogenicity trials. According to European legislation 1,1-dichloroethene is classified as a suspected carcinogen (category 3). In the United States, it has been classified as a A3 carcinogen by the ACGIH (i.e., as an animal carcinogen).

Bibliography

ACGIH (1996). Carbon tetrachloride. *In* "Documentation of Threshold Limit Values and Biological Exposure Indices," 6th ed., pp. 233–236, American Conference of Governmental Industrial Hygienists. Cincinnati, OH.

Benigni, R., Cotta-Ramusino, M., and Andreoli, C. (1991). Relationship between chlorofluorocarbon chemical structure and their Salmonella mutagenicity. *J. Toxicol. Environ. Health* **34,** 397–407.

Bornschein, R. L., Hastings, L., and Manson, J. M. (1980). Behavioural toxicity in the offspring of rats following maternal exposure to dichloromethane. *Toxicol. Appl. Pharmacol.* **52,** 29–37.

Clayton, J. W. (1967). Fluorocarbon toxicity and biological action. *Fluorine Chem. Rev.* **1,** 197–252.

Creech, J. S., and Johnson, M. N. (1974). Angiosarcoma of liver in the manufacture of polyvinyl chloride. *J. Occup. Med.* **16,** 150–151.

De Angelo, A. B., Daniel, F. B., McMillan, L., Wernsing, P., and Savage, R. E. (1989). Species and strain sensitivity to the induction of peroxisome proliferation by chloroacetic acid. *Toxicol. Appl. Pharmacol.* **101,** 285–298.

Di Vincenzo, G. D., and Kaplan, C. J. (1981). Uptake, metabolism and elimination of methylene chloride vapor by humans. *Toxicol. Appl. Pharmacol.* **59,** 130–140.

ECETOC (1987). The assessment of carcinogenic hazard for human beings exposed to methylene chloride. Technical Report No. 26. European Chemical Industry Ecology and Toxicology Centre, Brussels.

ECETOC (1988). Methylene chloride (dichloromethane): Human risk assessment using experimental animal data. Technical Report No. 32. European Chemical Industry Ecology and Toxicology Centre, Brussels.

ECETOC (1989). Methylene chloride (dichloromethane): An overview of experimental work investigating species, differences in carcinogenicity and their relevance to man. Technical Report No. 34. European Chemical Industry Ecology and Toxicology Centre, Brussels.

ECETOC (1990). Tetrachloroethylene: Assessment of human carcinogenic hazard. Technical Report No. 37. European Chemical Industry Ecology and Toxicology Centre, Brussels.

GDCH (Gesellschaft Deutscher Chemiker) (1992). "Beratungsgremium für umweltrelevante Altstoffe (BUA): Trichlorethen." VCH-Verlagsgesellschaft, Weinheim.

Gutacker, H. W., and Lelbach, W. K. (eds.) (1977). "Leberschäden durch Vinylchlorid: Vinylchlorid-Krankheit." Verlag Witzstrock, Baden-Baden.

Jongen, W. M. E., Harmsen, E. G. M., Alink, G. M., Koeman, J. H. (1982). The effect of glutathione conjugation and microsomal oxidation on the mutagenicity of dichloromethane in S. typhimurium. *Mutat. Res.* **95,** 183–189.

Longstaff, E., Robinson, M., Bradbook, C., Styles, J. A., and Purchase, I. F. H. (1984). Genotoxicity and carcinogenicity of fluorocarbons: Assessment by short-term in vitro tests and chronic exposure in rats. *Toxicol. Appl. Pharmacol.* **72,** 15–31.

Lorenz, H., Weber, E., Omlor, A., Walter, G., Haass, A., Steigerwald, F., and Buchter, A. (1990). Nachweis von Hirnschädigungen durch Tetrachlorethen. *Zbl. Arbeitsmed.* **40,** 355–364.

Maltoni, C., and Lefemine, G. (1974). Carcinogenicity bioassays of vinyl chloride. *Environ. Res.* **7,** 387–405.

Peter, H., Filser, J. G., v. Szentpály, L., and Wiegand, H. J. (1986). Different pharmacokinetics of dichlorofluoromethane (CFC 21) und chlorodifluoromethane (CFC 22). *Arch. Toxicol.* **58,** 282–283.

Snyder, R. (1987). "Ethel Browning's Toxicity and Metabolism of Industrial Solvents." 2nd ed. Elsevier, Amsterdam/New York.

Vamvakas, S., Dekant, W., Berthold, K., Schmidt, S., Wild, D., and Henschler, D. (1987). Enzymatic transformation of mercapturic acids derived from halogenated alkenes to reactive and mutagenic intermediates. *Biochem. Pharmacol.* **36,** 2741–2748.

WHO (1984). "Tetrachloroethylene." International Programme on Chemical Safety. Environmental Health Criteria, No. 31. World Health Organization, Geneva.

CHAPTER

27

Fluorocarbons

STEPHEN MAGDA

Solvay Pharmaceuticals, Hannover, Germany

INTRODUCTION

Fluorocarbons are chemical compounds that include chlorofluorocarbons (CFCs), hydrochlorofluorocarbons (HCFCs), and hydrofluorocarbons (HFCs). For many years, the fully halogenated chlorofluorocarbons (CFCs) performed an important role in society. They were used in a variety of applications, including refrigeration, air conditioning, insulation, and medical products. In 1974 they were cited as contributing to depletion of the Earth's protective ozone layer. In response to increasing concerns that certain chlorine-containing compounds, such as CFCs, may be catalyzing a decrease in stratospheric ozone levels, control measures and phase-out schedules were defined. Consequently, the search for potential substitutes was initiated.

OZONE DEPLETION AND CHLORINE

In the stratosphere, the ozone layer acts as a UV-B filter protecting from shortwave radiation. This radiation is biologically very active and causes cell changes in humans, animals, and plants. Reduction in ozone concentration can lead to increased rates of skin cancer (e.g., melanoma) and eye diseases (e.g., cataracts). Also, it can be damaging to living organisms (e.g., marine phytoplankton) and plants.

There are ozone-depleting processes, in particular resulting from the increasing emission of CFCs, which are the source of reactive chlorine in the stratosphere (Fig. 1). Because the rate of photolytic CFC decomposition is slower than the continuing emission rates, their atmospheric concentrations will steadily increase. Because chlorine-based substances are persistent, past emissions continue to cause the ozone damage. The emissions of today will be responsible for ozone depletion in the future. Model calculations show that if the emissions of these compounds are completely stopped, stratospheric chlorine concentrations are expected to peak in 2 to 4 years, and thereafter they will gradually decrease.

An international agreement, known as the Montreal Protocol on Substances That Deplete the Ozone Layer, was signed in 1987 and became effective in 1989. At subsequent meetings, the parties to the Montreal Protocol agreed to an accelerated phase-out schedule for controlled substances, including CFCs and HCFCs. Time-tables for developed countries are CFCs, 100% phase-out by the end of 1995; and HCFCs, 100% phase-out in 2030. A different schedule applies for developing countries (they have an additional ten years).

HCFCs and HFCs are considered environmentally superior to CFCs. Although the HCFCs, do contain chlorine, they are broken down mainly in the lower atmosphere and only a relatively small percentage of chlorine reaches the stratospheric ozone layer. HFCs contain no chlorine and thus do not contribute to ozone depletion.

An index called the Ozone Depletion Potential has been adopted under the Montreal Protocol. The Ozone Depletion Potential is an estimate of the total ozone depletion due to the release into the atmosphere of 1 kg of a compound divided by the total ozone depletion due to 1 kg of CFC-11. The Ozone Depletion Potentials of individual compounds are

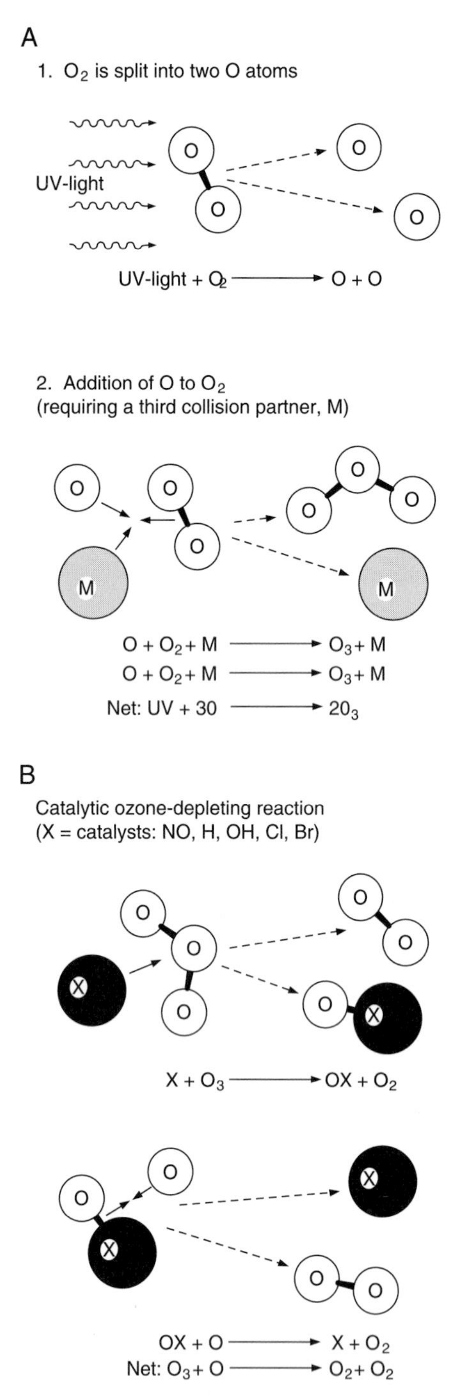

FIGURE 1 Schematic diagrams of (A) ozone formation and (B) catalytic destruction (X indicates catalysts NO, H, OH, Cl, Br). Adapted from Protecting the Earth's Atmosphere: An International Challenge; Interim Report of the Study Commission of the 11th German Bundestag "Preventive Measures to Protect the Earth's Atmosphere" (Publ. by the German Bundestag, Publ. Sect., Bonn, 1989).

shown in Fig. 2. These alternatives have been identified as promising substitutes for CFCs for a wide range of applications (e.g., refrigeration, foam blowing, cleaning, aerosols, fire fighting, and medicine).

To test the alternatives for health and safety characteristics, a cooperative research effort was organized by the leading CFC producers. The Programme for Alternative Fluorocarbon Toxicity Testing (PAFT) was designed to expedite the development of toxicology data for possible substitute fluorocarbons. Eight compounds—both HCFCs and HFCs—considered to be medium- or long-term replacements were evaluated. Only these new compounds will be discussed in this chapter.

PHYSICAL AND CHEMICAL PROPERTIES

The fluorocarbons described here are colorless liquids (HCFC 123, HCFC 141b, HCFC 225ca, HCFC 225cb) or gases (HCFC 124, HFC 125, HFC 134a, HFC 32) and with the exception of HFC 32 they are nonflammable.

ABSORPTION, DISTRIBUTION, METABOLISM, AND EXCRETION

Fluorocarbons are rapidly absorbed and equilibrated in tissues after inhalation and are eliminated from the blood by exhalation within few minutes. Metabolism studies in animals suggest that these compounds are oxidatively metabolized (i.e., there is a slight increase in urinary fluoride levels). For some compounds (HCFC 123, HCFC 134a, HCFC 124), trifluoroacetic acid (TFA) was also detected. The rate of metabolism appears to be low or very low.

ACUTE AND SUBCHRONIC–CHRONIC TOXICOLOGY

Fluorocarbons have a very low acute toxicity by inhalation (Table 1). In general, the symptoms are reversible effects on the central nervous system (CNS) (e.g., anesthetic-like affects such as lethargy and incoordination).

As with many other halocarbons and hydrocarbons, inhalation of these alternative fluorocarbons followed by intravenous injection of epinephrine, which simulates human stress reactions, results in a cardiac sensitization response in experimental screening studies with dogs. This response is observed at levels well above expected human exposures.

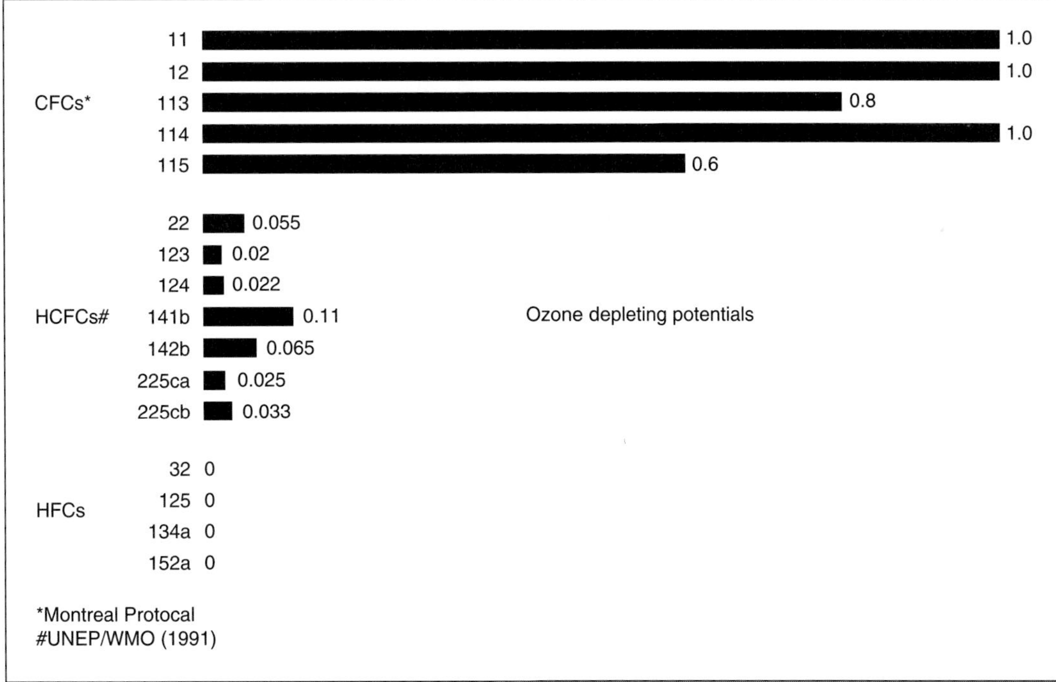

FIGURE 2 Comparison of ozone depletion potentials for Chlorofluorocarbons (CFCs) Montreal Protocol; hydrochlorofluorocarbons (HCFCs), UNEF/WMO (1991); and hydrofluorocarbons (HFCs). From Alternative Fluorocarbons Environmental Acceptability Study (AFEAS), September 1995.

TABLE 1 Acute and Subchronic–Chronic Toxicity of Fluorocarbons by Inhalation

	Acute studies			Subchronic–chronic studies			
Compound	Animal species	LC 50 (ppm)	NOEL (ppm)	Animal species	Duration (months)	Lowest toxic concentration (ppm)	NOEL (ppm)
HCFC 123 (1,1-dichloro-2,2,2-trifluoroethane)	Rat	32,000	5000	Rat	3 24	10,000–20,000 300	>5,000
HCFC 124 (1-chloro-1,2,2,2-tetrachloroethane)	Rat	>360,000		Rat	3 24	50,000[a]	15,000 >50,000
HCFC 141b (1,1-dichloro-1-fluoroethane)	Rat	62,000		Rat	3 24	20,000[a] 5,000	>8,000 1,500
HCFC 225ca (3,3-dichloro-1,1,1,2,2-pentafluoropropane)	Rat	37,000		Rat marmoset	1 1	5,000[a] 1,000	
HCFC 225cb (1,3-dichloro-1,1,2,2,3-pentafluoropropane)	Rat	37,000		Rat marmoset	1 1	5,000[a] 5,000[a]	1,000
HFC 134a (1,1,1,2-tetrafluoroethane)	Rat	>500,000		Rat	3 24	 50,000	>50,000 10,000
HFC 125 (pentafluoroethane)	Rat	>800,000		Rat	3		>50,000
HFC 32 (difluoromethane)	Rat	>760,000		Rat	3		>50,000

[a]Minimal effects.

The results of subchronic and chronic inhalation studies show a low toxicity for most of the compounds (Table 1).

In 2-year studies an increase of benign tumors was observed with HCFC 123 (in the liver, pancreas, and Leydig cells), with HCFC 141b (in the Leydig cells), and with 134a (in the Leydig cells). None of the benign tumors was life-threatening and all occurred near the end of the studies. In overall evidence obtained from genetic toxicity studies suggests that the increased incidence of benign tumors is not due to genotoxic effects.

DEVELOPMENTAL AND GENETIC TOXICOLOGY

The compounds were extensively tested *in vitro* and *in vivo*. Based on the weight of evidence from all these studies, the compounds are not developmental toxicants, they do not affect reproductive performance, and they are not genotoxic.

HUMAN EXPOSURE

There are no adverse health effects reported that can be ascribed to these compounds.

Bibliography

Anders, M. W. (1991). Metabolism and toxicity of hydrochlorofluorocarbons: Current knowledge and needs for the future. *Environ. Health Perspec.* **96,** 185–191.

Brock, W. J., Trochimowicz, H. J., Millischer, R.-J., Farr, C., Kawano, T., and Rusch, G. M. (1995). Acute and subchronic toxicity of 1,1-dichloro-1-fluoroethane (HCFC-141b). *Food and Chem. Toxicol.* **33(6),** 483–490.

Collins, M. A., Rusch, G. M., Sato, F., Hext, P. M., and Millischer, R.-J. (1995). 1,1,1,2-Tetrafluoroethane: Repeat exposure inhalation toxicity in the rat, developmental toxicity in the rabbit, and genotoxicity in vitro and in vivo. *Fund. Appl. Toxicol.* **25,** 271–280.

ECETOC (1990). "1-Chloro-1,2,2,2-tetrafluoroethane (HFA-124)." ECETOC Joint Assessment of Commodity Chemicals No. 12.

ECETOC (1994a). "1-Chloro-1,2,2,2-tetrafluoroethane (HCFC-124)." ECETOC Joint Assessment of Commodity Chemicals No. 25.

ECETOC (1994b). "Penta-fluoroethane (HFC-125)." ECETOC Joint Assessment of Commodity Chemicals No. 24.

ECETOC (1995a). "1,1-Dichloro-1-fluoroethane (HCFC-141b)." CAS No. 1717-00-6. ECETOC Joint Assessment of Commodity Chemicals No. 29.

ECETOC (1995b). "Difluoromethane (HFC-32)." CAS No. 75-10-5. ECETOC Joint Assessment of Commodity Chemicals No. 32.

ECETOC. (1995c). "1,1,1,2-Tetrafluoroethane (HFC-134a)." CAS No. 811-97-2. ECETOC Joint Assessement of Commodity Chemicals No. 31.

ECETOC (1996). "1,1-Dichloro-2,2,2-trifluoroethane." ECETOC Joint Assessment of Commodity Chemicals No. 33.

Kawano, T., Trochimowicz, H. J., Malinverno, G., and Rusch, G. M. (1995). Toxicological evaluation of 1,1,1,2,2-pentafluoroethane (HFC-125). *Fund. Appl. Toxicol.* **28,** 223–231.

Kurata, Y., Takechi, Toyotas, N., Tsuchitani, M., Katoh, M., Rusch, G. M., Trochimowicz, H. J., Shin-ya, S. (1997). Four week repeated inhalation study of HCFC 225ca and HCFC 225cb in the common marmoset. *Toxicol. Lett.* **92,** 209–219.

Malley, L. A., Carakostas, M., Hansen, J. F., Rusch, G. M., Kelley, D. P., and Trochimowicz, H. J. (1995). Two-year inhalation toxicity study in rats with hydrochlorofluorocarbon 123. *Fund. Appl. Toxicol.* **24,** 101–114.

Millischer, R.-J., de Rooij, C., Rusch, G. M., Farr, C. H., Hardy, C. J., Lewis, D., and Hodson-Walker, G. (1995). Evaluation of the genotoxicity potential and chronic inhalation toxicity of 1,1-dichloro-1-fluoroethane (HCFC 141b). *Food and Chem. Toxicol.* **33(6),** 491–500.

Molina, M. J., and Rowland, F. S. (1974). Stratospheric sink for chlorofluorocarbons, chlorine atom-catalyzed destruction of ozone. *Nature* **249,** 810–812.

Rusch, G. M., Millischer, R.-J., de Rooij, C., and Hughes, E. (1995). Inhalation teratology and 2-generation reproduction studies with 1,1-dichloro-1-fluoroethane. *Food and Chem. Toxicol.* **33(4),** 285–300.

Rusch, G. M., Trochimowicz, H. J., Malley, L. J., Kelly, D. P., Peckham, J., Hansen, J., and Charm, J. B. (1994). Subchronic inhalation toxicity studies with hydrochlorofluorocarbon 123. *Fund. Appl. Toxicol.* **23,** 169–178.

Study Commission of the 11th German Bundestag. (1989). Protecting the Earth's Atmosphere: An International Challenge. *In* "Preventive Measures to Protect the Earth's Atmosphere." Bundestag, Publ. Sect., Bonn, Germany.

Alternative Fluorocarbons Environmental Acceptability Study, September 1995.

CHAPTER

28

Pesticides

RANDY L. ROSE*, ERNEST HODGSON*, R. MICHAEL ROE[†]

*Department of Toxicology, North Carolina State University, Raleigh, North Carolina

[†]Department of Entomology, North Carolina State University, Raleigh, North Carolina

INTRODUCTION

Pesticides, as defined by the Federal Insecticide, Fungicide, and Rodenticide Act include "(1) any substance or mixture of substances intended for preventing, destroying, repelling or mitigating any pest [insect, rodent, nematode, fungus, weed, other forms of terrestrial or aquatic plant or animal life or viruses, bacteria or other organisms . . . which the Administrator declares to be a pest] and (2) any substance or mixture of substances intended for use as a plant regulator, defoliant or desiccant." The use of pesticides to control perceived pests has transformed our environment. Habitats previously uninhabitable due to vector-borne diseases are now habitable, crops are grown in large monocultures with minimal contamination by weeds and/or destruction by insects, and household pests can be easily eliminated.

Both food and fiber are affected by pests throughout all aspects of production, transport, and storage. Estimates of worldwide losses due to insects, weeds, and fungi have been estimated to be as high as 35%, with insects contributing 14%, fungi 11%, and weeds 10%. From another perspective, agricultural losses due to insect damage alone are approximately 10-fold greater than the amount spent by farmers for pesticides.

Pesticide use is validated by its many contributions to society; yet by their very nature, pesticides can also have deleterious effects. Insecticides and rodenticides are among the pesticides most likely to produce acute toxicity in humans and wildlife. Although many of the newer insecticide chemistries are more selective to insects and less persistent than older insecticides, they still are hazardous when used inappropriately. Incidents of acute human exposure by pesticides are relatively rare in developed countries, in part due to new chemicals with lower mammalian toxicity and also due to restrictions on the use of highly toxic chemicals. Indeed, most reported pesticide mortalities from acute poisoning have, in recent years, been suicidal or homicidal. Of greater concern, however, is the accumulation of data indicating that many pesticides can exert chronic effects.

The number of pesticides introduced over the years has seen an exponential increase, with cumulative totals of over 160 fungicides, 280 herbicides, and 295 insecticides introduced as of 1990. A more recent survey of pesticide use in the United States indicates that herbicides, fungicides, and insecticides (excluding oil) account for 454,000,000 lb/year, 129,000,000 lb/year, and 98,000,000 lb/year, respectively.

With the number of pesticide-active ingredients used in the U.S. alone exceeding 200, a comprehensive treatment of each pesticide is beyond the scope of this chapter. Pesticide classes discussed in this chapter were selected on the basis of frequency of use (Table 1) and/or known or suspected human health effects. Also, some of the newer insecticide chemistries have been included.

FUNDAMENTALS OF PESTICIDE TOXICITY

Acute toxicity is concerned, initially, with lethality through the estimation of the median lethal dose (LD_{50}) or the median lethal concentration (LC_{50}), but

TABLE 1 A Selection of Commonly Used Pesticidal Chemicals

Fungicides	Herbicides	Insecticides
Inorganics	Triazines	Chlorinated hydrocarbons
Sulfur	Atrazine	DDT
Copper sulfate	Cyanazine	Endosulfan
Substituted aromatics	Chloroacetamides	Organophosphates
Chlorothalonil	Alachlor	Parathion
PCNB	Metolachlor	Chlorpyrifos
Dithiocarbamates	Chlorophenoxy	Terbufos
Mancozeb	2,4-D	Phorate
Maneb	2,4,5-T	Malathion
Ziram	Nitroanilines	Acephate
Dicarboximides	Trifluralin	Carbamates
Captan	Pendimethalin	Carbofuran
Benzimidazoles	Phosphono amino acids	Carbaryl
Benomyl	Glyphosphate	Aldicarb
	Thiocarbamates	Pyrethroids
	EPTC	Permethrin
		Cypermethrin
		Cyhalothrin

other acute effects such as acute neurotoxicity, eye or skin irritation, and behavioral effects are also considered. The LD_{50} is the estimated dose that, when administered to the test organism, results in the mortality of 50% of the population. The LC_{50} is the estimated concentration in the environment to which animals are exposed that will kill 50% of the population.

While the use of the LD_{50} as a criterion for acute toxicity has been criticized, it is required as part of the data supporting pesticide registration. Data obtained from such testing is important in establishing the relative toxicities of pesticides, as well as in providing information on the cause of death, symptomatology, nonlethal acute effects, and reversibility. The tests not only act as a first approximation of hazard to workers but also form the basis for the design of subchronic tests, necessary for chronic study design.

For regulatory purposes, particularly the labeling of pesticide containers, the U.S. Environmental Protection Agency (EPA) has established four toxicity categories (I–IV). The criteria for these are listed in Table 2. Pesticides in category I have labels indicating "danger" and "poison" in conjunction with the skull-and-crossbones emblem. In addition, if the category I assignment was based on oral, inhalation, or dermal toxicity, the word "warning" must be prominently displayed. Pesticides belonging to categories II, III, and IV must carry the word "caution."

TABLE 2 Toxicity Categories

Category	Oral LD_{50}	Respiratory LD_{50}	Dermal LD_{50}	Ocular Effects	Dermal Effects
I	Up to 50 mg/kg	Up to 0.2 mg/liter	Up to 200 mg/kg	Corrosive; opacity of the cornea not reversible in 7 days	Corrosive
II	50–500 mg/kg	0.2–2.0 mg/liter	200–2000 mg/kg	Opacity of cornea reversible in 7 days; irritation persists for 7 days	Irritation severe at 72 h
III	500–5000 mg/kg	2.0–20.0 mg/liter	2000–20,000 mg/kg	No opacity of cornea; irritation reversible in 7 days	Irritation moderate at 72 h
IV	Over 5000 mg/kg	Over 20.0 mg/liter	Over 20,000 mg/kg	No irritation	Irritation mild at at 72 h

Toxic outbreaks or collective poisonings have resulted from the misuse of almost every type of pesticide: organochlorine insecticides such as DDT, lindane, and chlordecone; chlorinated camphenes such as toxaphene; the cyclodienes aldrin and dieldrin; organophosphates and carbamate cholinesterase inhibitors; organomercury fungicides; inorganics; and others. Other acute poisonings are usually occupational or are the result of suicide or homicide attempts.

The most common pesticide poisonings arise from exposure to organophosphates and carbamates. Exposure to these insecticides produces a broad spectrum of acute effects, all of which appear to be cholinergic in origin, although chronic effects are of increasing concern. They include nicotinic effects at the neuromuscular junction, such as muscular twitching and weakness, leading to paralysis. Although death is ultimately the result of respiratory failure, it is usually classified as neurotoxicity. Muscarinic effects on the autonomic nervous system lead to abdominal pain, diarrhea, and so on, and central nervous system effects include slurred speech, confusion, tremors, and, at high doses, convulsions.

In contrast to organophosphates and carbamates, pyrethroids are among the safest insecticides used worldwide. The safety of this insecticide class is probably the result of its rapid metabolism by most vertebrates, although fish can be adversely affected. The most common acute effect of pyrethroid use in agricultural workers is contact dermatitis.

Chronic toxicity is the result of continuous exposure to toxicants over a period of time at doses that do not generally produce noticeable toxic effects in the short term. Chronic effects of greatest concern include neurotoxicity, immunological effects, reproductive effects, developmental effects, and carcinogenicity. The extent to which pesticides are involved in chronic human health effects is largely unknown but constitutes a growing concern due to the effects that have been documented in other organisms. Similarly, the potential for chronic exposure and the mechanisms by which pesticides exert these effects are unexplored.

The best indications of human health effects, of course, are properly conducted epidemiological studies. While these can sometimes be conducted in the best case with groups that are occupationally exposed to specific chemicals, these studies are often complicated by exposure to multiple chemicals. Particularly in the case of agricultural workers, who appear to have a marginally increased risk of developing certain types of cancers such as leukemia, testicular cancer, myeloma, and Hodgkin's and non-Hodgkin's lymphomas, exposure to multiple pesticides and other agents makes it difficult to identify particular associations with certainty. Some epidemiological studies suggested that human exposure to phenoxy herbicides, such as 2,4,5-trichlorophenol (2,4,5-T), was likely to cause soft tissue carcinomas; however, other similarly conducted studies produced contradictory results, making clear causal relationships between pesticides and cancer difficult.

REPRODUCTIVE AND DEVELOPMENTAL EFFECTS

Evidence of adverse health effects associated with development and reproduction resulting from exposure to environmental chemicals continues to accumulate. Several pesticides have been demonstrated to directly affect the female reproductive system, including DDT, chlordecone, methoxychlor, and mirex. Many of these same pesticides also alter male reproductive parameters. An environmental example of these types of effects is found at Lake Apopka in Florida, where high concentrations of DDT and its metabolite DDE are probably the agents responsible for significant differences in sex-steroid concentrations, differences in the morphology and histology of gonads, and significant declines in the reproductive success of alligators.

More specific studies using laboratory animals have firmly demonstrated the estrogenic effects of several of these pesticides. Chlordecone induces defeminization in both rats and hamsters, resulting in persistent vaginal estrus in the former and persistent aberrant behavior in the latter. DDT exposure to prepubertal female rats resulted in precocious puberty, increased uterine weights, and persistent vaginal estrus. In male dogs, DDT exposure decreased reproductive capacity. Adverse effects on sperm development have been demonstrated for the pesticides chlordecone, dichlorvos, diquat, paraquat, dinoseb, and benomyl. Other pesticides such as dieldrin, chlordane, and 2,4,5-T have been shown to alter testosterone kinetics without causing any detectable effect on reproduction.

Human reproductive effects have also been observed in association with certain chemicals, including dibromochloropropane (DBCP), ethylene dibromide (EDB), chlordecone, carbaryl, and DDE. High levels of chlordecone exposure among factory workers at one site resulted in oligospermia and significant decreases in sperm count. Workers exposed to dioxins (by-products of pesticide manufacture) have been shown to have decreased serum testosterone and increased concentrations of leutinizing hormone.

CARCINOGENICITY

Cancer risks from occupational and environmental exposure to synthetic chemicals have been estimated to be about 10%. Although the overall risk of cancer due to these exposures may be small, some of these environmental agents may be highly carcinogenic. Because individuals exposed to high levels of pesticides may have a higher risk of developing cancer, it is extremely important that these chemicals be identified so that proper precautions can be observed.

The classification of pesticides as carcinogens relies primarily upon 2-year rodent carcinogenesis bioassays. Although these bioassays are complicated by species differences, use of high doses, sample size, and use of extrapolations from high doses to low doses for human risk assessment, they have remained the standard for human carcinogen classification.

The contribution of pesticides to overall cancer mortalities, though unknown, is perceived to be a major health risk by the population at large. In the United States and elsewhere, several pesticides have been banned or severely restricted because animal data indicated their oncogenic potential. In a positive epidemiological study, an association between occupational exposure to inorganic arsenic and lung cancer was demonstrated to be dose related. Studies of occupational exposure to organochlorine insecticides have indicated small increases of lung cancer (less than two fold). Increases in soft-tissue sarcoma, leukemia, and lymphoma among farmers and foresters exposed to various pesticides have also been noted. Many of the pesticides implicated in these studies have not been demonstrated to be carcinogenic in animal studies.

The majority of pesticides producing carcinogenic effects in animals are not genotoxic in assays such as the Ames test. A growing body of evidence indicates that chemicals may cause cancer as a result of a number of nongenotoxic processes, including promotion, peroxisome proliferation, hormone imbalances, and cytotoxicity leading to cellular compensation. Many of these effects are likely to be observed only at doses near the maximum tolerated dose, further complicating risk assessment of pesticides.

IMMUNOLOGICAL EFFECTS

Several pesticides have marked effects on the immune system. Among the more potent of these are TCDD, atrazine, captan, lead arsenate, and triphenyltin hydroxide. Rodents exposed to TCDD, a contaminant of 2,4,5-T production, demonstrated severe thymus atrophy accompanied by depressed antibody response and increased susceptibility to bacterial infections. Similar immunological responses have also been observed in humans exposed to TCDD. Surveys of immune responses elicited by insecticides, including organophosphates, organochlorines, and carbamates, suggest that some organochlorines and organophosphates are minimally immunosuppressive.

In contrast with immunosuppressive responses, exposure to some pesticides can result in increased immune responses, resulting in the development of allergies and autoimmune diseases. Contact dermatitis may develop as a result of repeated exposure to related pesticides. Symptoms include a red rash, swelling, itching, and possibly blisters. Often, symptoms manifest themselves after months or years of exposure. After sensitization, these symptoms appear within hours of contact with the sensitizing agent. Some pesticides known to cause allergic dermatitis include several pyrethroids, pentachlorobenzene, and chlorothalonil.

CLASSIFICATION OF PESTICIDES

Pesticides are classified in a number of different ways (e.g., by chemistry, mode of action, or type of application). Although pesticides of similar chemistry often share similar target sites, this is not always the case, as some pesticides with common structural features have varying toxicities to widely divergent organisms. For example, several insecticidal dithiocarbamates are not herbicidal and vice versa. However, structurally similar pesticides often impart similar toxicological actions on nontarget organisms.

Fungicides include a variety of chemicals ranging from the typically broad-spectrum metallic fungicides to pest-specific organic compounds. Classes of fungicides include copper- and sulfur-based fungicides, dithiocarbamates, aromatic hydrocarbons, benzimidazoles, phenylamides, and triazoles.

Herbicides are typically classified by chemistry as inorganic salts, halogenated alkanoic derivatives, (aryloxy)alkanoic acids, arylcarboxylic acids, esters of 2-[4-(aryloxy)phenoxy]alkanoic acids, nitriles, amides, anilides, phenols, diphenyl ethers, 2,6-dinitroanilines, carbamates, thiocarbamates, ureas, sulphonylureas, imidazolinones, pyrimidines, pyridazines, 1,3,5-triazines, bipyridinium compounds, miscellaneous heterocyclic compounds, oximes, organophosphates, organoarsenicals, and soil fumigants.

Insecticides have been traditionally classified into four major groups—chlorinated hydrocarbons, organophosphates, carbamates, and pyrethroids. Insect-growth regulators, such as methoprene, and bacterial endotoxins, such as that produced by *Bacillus thuringiensis,* were added to this list by the 1980s. Recently, several insecticides with novel modes of action have been identified (e.g., nicotinoids, fipronil, and the spinosids). Discussion of insecticide synergists is also included.

Fungicides

The relative importance of fungicides in the prevention of plant disease cannot be overestimated. In contrast with insect pests and weeds, fungal diseases are virtually impossible to control without chemical applications. Until the discovery of the Bordeaux mixture in 1882, farmers had little recourse against these diseases.

Among the several plant diseases that can be controlled by fungicides are storage rots, seedling diseases, root rots, gall diseases, leaf blights, rusts, smuts, mildews, and viral diseases. The majority of fungicides are surface or plant protectants. They are applied to the plant as dusts or sprays prior to potential infection by fungal spores. Other fungicides can be used therapeutically, that is, can be applied to diseased plants for control. Still others are used as systemic fungicides that are absorbed and distributed throughout the plant.

Although fungicidal activity of copper sulfate was first recognized as early as 1807, it was not until 1882 that its efficacy against grape downy mildew was first noticed. The mixture of copper sulfate and lime had been used on grapes to discourage pilfering along roadsides. Following experimentation, the use of this "Bordeaux mixture" to control potato late blight was suggested in 1885 and confirmed by 1888. Subsequent use of both copper and sulfur in several different combinations with other chemicals resulted in a wide variety of formulations effectively marketed as fungicides. Due to their low levels of toxicity, few if any levels of tolerance have been set for many of these compounds.

Several other inorganic fungicides were subsequently discovered and have found widespread use. These are based on metallic compounds, such as copper, zinc, sulfur, and mercury. These are generally broad spectrum in activity and often cause some plant toxicity. Inorganic and organic mercurial fungicides have been banned due to mammalian toxicity and environmental accumulation. It is interesting to note that many of the more recently discovered fungicides continue to have metals such as copper, zinc, and sulfur in their structures.

Sulfur-containing fungicides constitute more than 60% of the 130,000,000 lb of active fungicidal ingredients used in the U.S. each year. The first sulfur-containing fungicide was registered for use in the U.S. in 1920. Sulfur is currently registered for use as an insecticide, fungicide, and rodenticide on several hundred food and feed crops, ornamentals, turf, and residential sites, and it is an active ingredient in up to 300 registered pesticide products. As a fungicide, it is used to control brown rot in peaches; powdery mildew in apples, gooseberries, hops, ornamentals, grapes, peaches, strawberries, and sugar beets; apple scab; and mildew in roses. Sulfur can also be used as a fertilizer or as a soil amendment to reclaim alkaline soils.

Incorporation of sulfur into organic molecules resulted in the production of several new fungicides starting in 1931 with the discovery of thiram. Other organic sulfur-containing fungicides soon followed, including zineb (a dithiocarbamate) in 1943 and captan (a dicarboximide) in 1949. These newer organic fungicide classes presented several outstanding qualities over the inorganic compounds, because they were more efficient, longer lasting, and environmentally safer than the inorganic compounds. Many of these were also less phytotoxic and more readily degraded by soil microorganisms.

Representative chemical structures of several classes of fungicides, including the dithiocarbamates (thiram, mancozeb, maneb, and zineb), aromatic hydrocarbons (hexachlorobenzene, pentachloronitrobenzene, and chloroneb), benzimidazoles (benomyl and thiabendazole), phenylamides (metalaxyl and benalaxyl), and triazoles (propiconazole and hexaconazole), are shown in Fig. 1.

Several mechanisms of fungicide action have been elucidated, although many mechanisms remain unknown, particularly for several of the older fungicides. Newer fungicides tend to have modes of action that are site-specific, often resulting in the development of resistance; the older fungicides are nonsite-specific and have a broader spectrum of activity. Both fungicidal and fungistatic processes are mediated in fungi by the inhibition of respiration; metabolic pathways; and DNA, RNA, protein, and sterol biosynthesis.

The dithiocarbamates, including thiram, mancozeb, maneb, zineb, ferbam, and metamsodium, were developed in the 1930s and 1940s. This group of fungicides continues to be highly popular. Their toxicity has been attributed to the production of an isothiocyanate radical (−N=C=S), which inactivates the SH

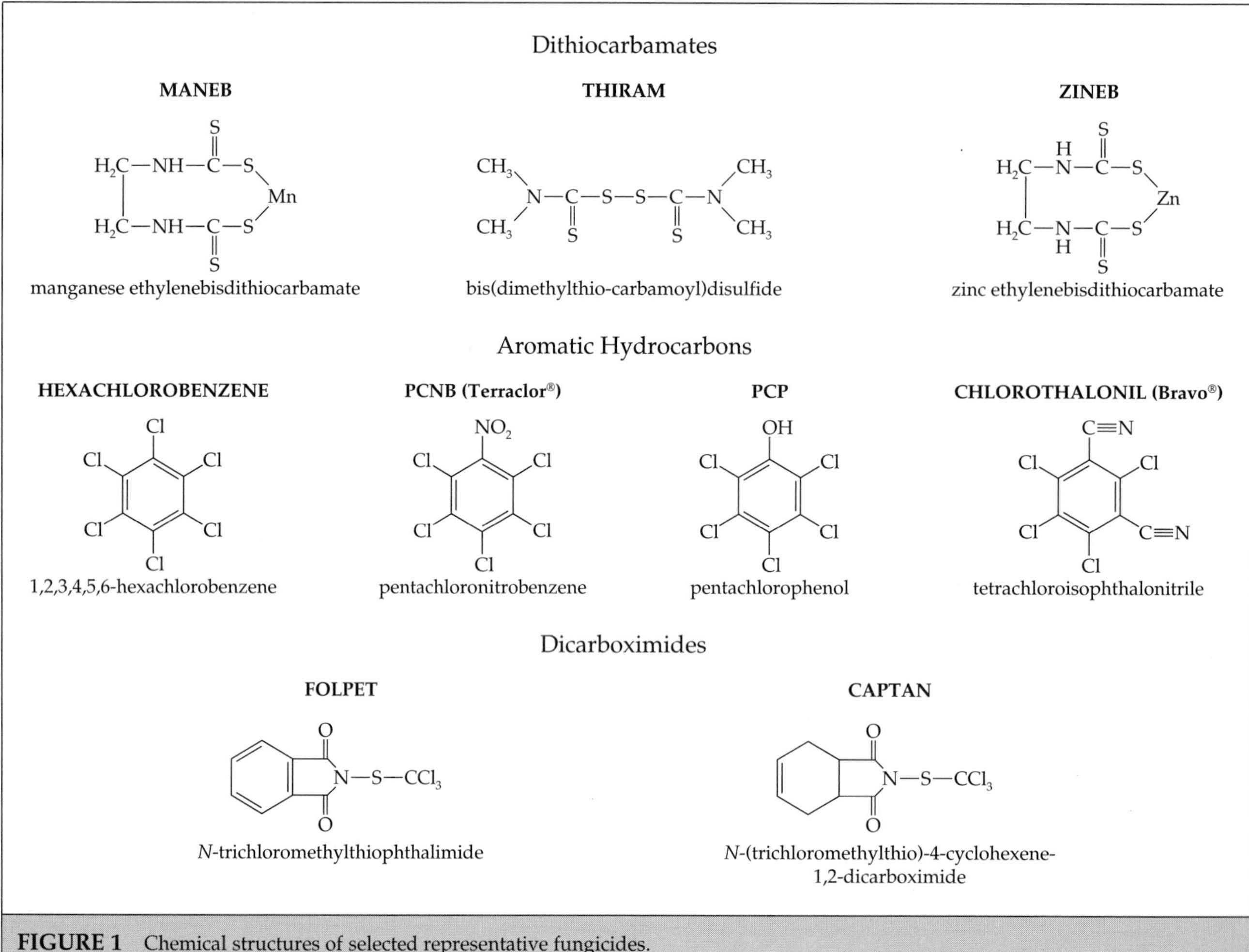

FIGURE 1 Chemical structures of selected representative fungicides.

groups in amino acids contained within individual pathogen cells. Aromatic hydrocarbon fungicides, such as pentachloronitrobenzene, reduce growth rates and sporulation of fungi by combining with NH_2 or SH groups of essential metabolic pathways. Dicarboximides such as captan and folpet are also thought to inhibit protein synthesis by interacting with the SH radical. Benzimidazoles, such as benomyl and imazalil, induce abnormalities in spore germination, cellular multiplication, and growth as a result of interference with DNA synthesis.

Two new groups of fungicides possessing systemic properties are the phenylamides and the triazoles. The phenylamides are active against soil-borne diseases caused by *Pythium* and *Phytophthora* as well as foliar diseases caused by *Phycomycetes*. These are used as foliar, soil, and seed treatments, and include metalaxyl, furalaxyl, and benalaxyl. The triazoles, which include triadimefon, propiconazole, and triadimenol, are effective against mildews and rusts. They are broad spectrum in action, causing toxicity by inhibition of sterol synthesis.

Fungicides as a group of pesticides have generally low mammalian toxicity when compared to many other pesticides (Table 3). Acute toxicity of many of these compounds is low with oral LD_{50}'s generally ranging from 1500 to > 10,000 mg/kg. Complaints of eye and skin irritation as well as respiratory effects are common among those using several fungicides. The majority of fungicides also have limited chronic effects, many of which are observed only at the highest doses that can be administered. However, the importance of chronic exposure to fungicides is easily illustrated by the fact that some of the most important epidemics of food poisoning were the result of fungicide treatments of grain that was subsequently used for human consumption.

Prior to 1970, several food-poisoning epidemics involved consumption of seed contaminated with fungicides. Most involved methyl mercury. The last and

Benzimidazoles

BENOMYL (Benlate®)

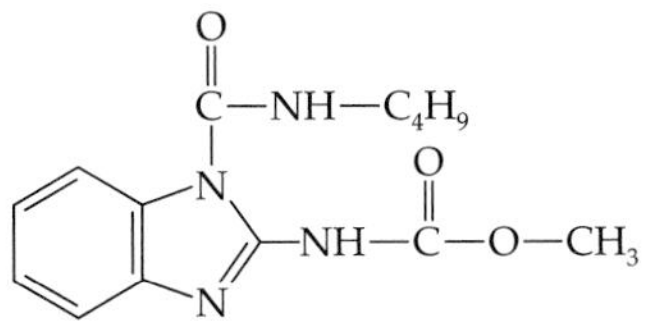

methyl 1-(butylcarbamoyl)-2-benzimidazolecarbamate

THIABENDAZOLE (TBZ)

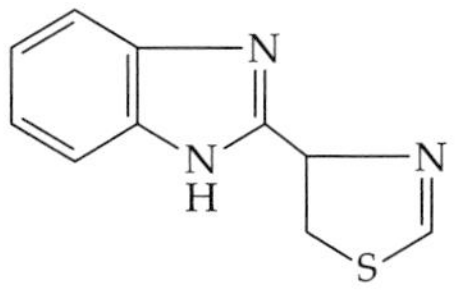

2-(4-thiazoyl) benzimidazole

Phenylamides

METALAXYL (Ridomil®, Dual®)

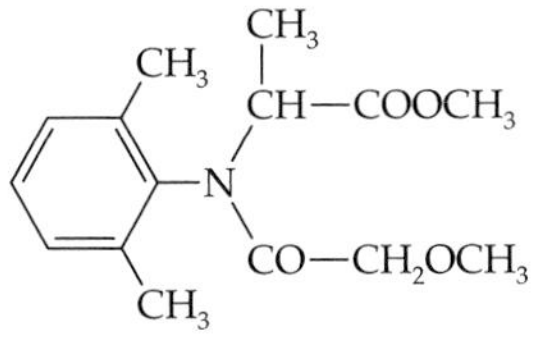

N-(2,6-dimethylphenyl)-*N*-(methoxy-acetyl)-alanine methyl ester

BENALAXYL (Galben®)

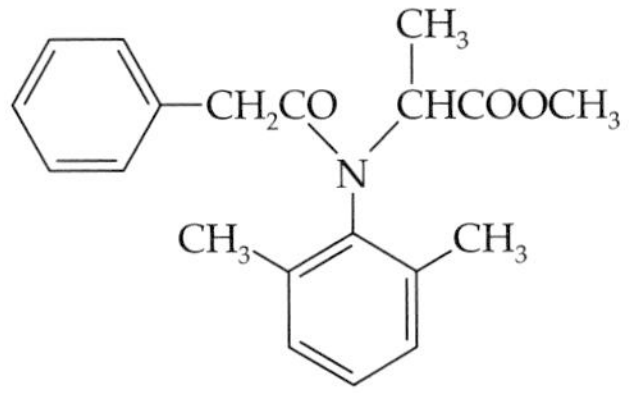

methyl-*N*-(2,6-dimethylphenyl)-*N*-(phenylacetyl)-DL-alaninate

FURALAXYL (Fongarid®)

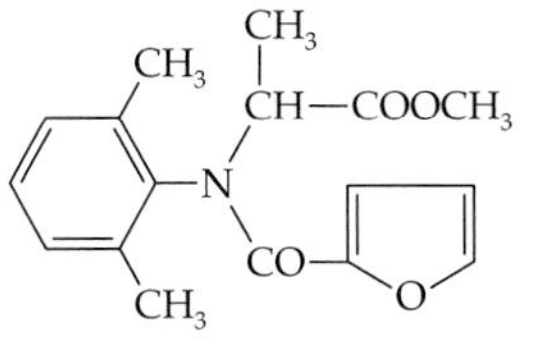

methyl-*N*-2,6-dimethylphenyl-*N*-furoyl-(2)-alaninate

Triazoles

TRIADIMEFON (Bayleton®)

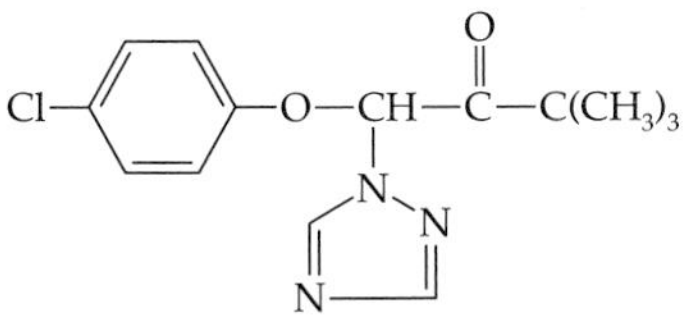

1-(4-chlorophenoxy)-3,3-dimethyl-1-(1H-1,2,4-triazol-1-yl)-2-butanone

PROPICONAZOLE (Tilt®)

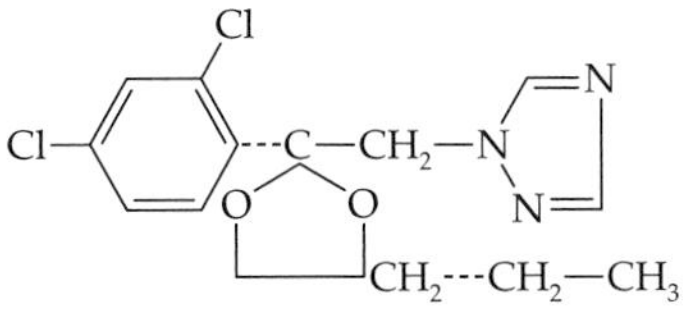

1-(2-(2,4-dichlorophenyl)4-propyl-1,3-dioxolan-2-ylmethyl)-1H-1,2,4-triazole

TRIADIMENOL (Baytan®)

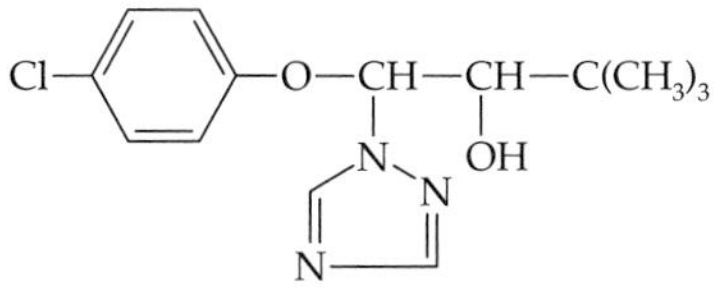

β-(4-chlorophenoxy)-α-(1,1-dimethyl-ethyl)-1H-1,2,4-triazole-1-ethanol

FIGURE 1 *(Continued)*

most serious episode occurred in Iraq in 1972, where 6530 people were admitted to hospitals and 459 deaths were attributed to this incident. Symptoms persisting among survivors included paresthesias, ataxia, paralysis, and blindness. Mortality was attributed to the direct failure of the central nervous system. Mercurial compounds are no longer in use as pesticides.

Another important epidemic associated with the consumption of seed intended for sowing occurred in three southeastern provinces of Turkey from 1955 to 1959. Hexachlorobenzene (not to be confused with the insecticide, lindane, γ-hexachlorocyclohexane) is a fungicide used as a seed treatment for wheat. It has a low acute toxicity but a high cumulative toxicity. The availability of seed treated with hexachlorobenzene after the planting season at a time of food shortage resulted in its consumption by humans. The resulting illness, called "black sore" or "monkey disease," was characterized by blistering and epidemolysis of the skin especially of the hands and face. Infant mortality was especially high.

One of the principal toxic effects of hexachlorobenzene, produced in all species, is porphyria. Other effects observed in rats include lethargy combined with hyper-responsiveness, weakness, and paralysis. Weight loss, constipation, and oligouria were also observed. Although many of the symptoms indicate neurological damage, there is no observable pathology of nervous system tissue. The most severe pathological changes were marked enlargement of the liver and liver cells following 5–9 weeks of exposure at

TABLE 3 Chronic Toxicity Profile of Selected Fungicides

Chemical group compound	Rat oral LD_{50} (mg/kg)	Chronic effects	Teratogenicity	Reproductive toxicity	Carcinogenicity
Sulfur-containing fungicides	>5,000	Miners experienced eye and respiratory effects	None	None	None
Aromatic hydrocarbons					
Pentachlorobenzene	>12,000 in water 1,500 in oil	Skin allergies	Possible defects in kidney formation (compromised by HCB)	None	Possible liver tumors at high doses (compromised by HCB)
Ethylenebisdithiocarbamates					
Maneb	5,000	Peripheral and central nervous system depression	Metabolite, ethylene-thiourea, a known teratogen	Adverse effects on fertility and development	Benign lung tumors; metabolite, ethylene-thiourea a known carcinogen
Benzamidazoles					
Benomyl	>10,000	Skin sensitization; liver cirrhosis at high doses	Limited evidence of birth defects	Decreased testicular function	Liver tumors in male and female mice; possible human carcinogen
Phenylamides					
Metalaxyl	669	Enlargement of liver noted in highest doses given	None	None	Parafollicular adenomas detected in thyroid
Substituted Aromatics					
Chlorothalonil	>10,000	Eye and skin irritation; at high doses, kidney toxicity	No effects	No effects	Tumors of kidney, ureter, bladder
Dicarboximides					
Captan	10,000	Decreased body weights at high doses	Limited evidence	No effects with oral dose. Inhalation produced fetal mortality.	Tumors of gastrointestinal tract and kidneys; probable human carcinogen

2000 ppm. Further treatment resulted in atrophy of the liver with focal necrosis. Other symptoms included hyperplasia of the adrenals, fibrosis, and inflammation of the lung.

Chloroalkyl thiofungicides (e.g., captan, captafol, and folpet) share structural similarities with the powerful teratogen thalidomide. Many studies were conducted in a variety of species, including rabbits and monkeys, both of which had been shown to respond to thalidomide in a manner similar to humans. In spite of the high rates that were often administered, there was no evidence of teratogenic effects with these fungicides.

Several dithiocarbamates, including thiram, ziram, maneb, zineb, and mancozeb, are widely used. The toxicity of these fungicides ranges from moderate to low toxicity, with a mean acute oral LD_{50} of 2500 mg/kg to rats. Although the mechanism of toxicity for these compounds is poorly understood, carbon disulfide is a common metabolite with many similar toxic effects. Areas of concern for these fungicides include interactions with alcohol, antithyroid effects, and teratogenic and carcinogenic potential. One dithiocarbamate, disulfiram (Antabuse), is used therapeutically to treat alcoholism by producing an intolerance to alcohol.

Animal studies indicate that several dithiocarbamates, including maneb, zineb, mancozeb, and disulfiram, are detrimental to the thyroid and cause cancer. Small doses administered to animals reduce the uptake of radioactive iodine and cause thyroid hypertrophy. The antithyroid effects of these compounds result in the suppressed synthesis of thyroxine, leading to hormonal imbalances. The carcinogenic responses observed with many of these compounds may be the result of these hormonal imbalances. Alternatively, the metabolite ethylenethiourea (a known teratogen and carcinogen) may be responsible. However, it is not known if sufficient ethylenethiourea would be formed from metabolism to cause these effects. Adverse reproductive effects observed with several of these compounds include infertility, early fetal deaths and abnormal development of the eye, ear, body wall, central nervous system, and the musculoskeletal system.

Occupational exposure to many dithiocarbamates can result in skin irritation, inflammation of the nose and throat, headache, fatigue, nausea, and, in extreme cases, convulsions and unconsciousness. Liver function, moderate anemia, and other blood changes have also been observed.

Herbicides

More than 200 herbicide active ingredients are used worldwide. In the United States, herbicide use makes up more than 54% of the total weight of active ingredients used for all pesticides. Although herbicides are generally less toxic than other pesticides, high use patterns combined with several health-related issues of concern make it important to understand all aspects of chronic health effects in relation to these important chemicals.

Herbicides can be classified by several methods, including selectivity, mode of action, method of use, and chemical structure. Nonselective herbicides are used to kill all vegetation (e.g., clearing of roadsides, in industrial areas, or before sowing a crop). Selective herbicides are those that are used to kill weeds without harming the crop. Selectivity may be obtained as a result of differences in metabolism, translocation, and mode of action. Although selectivity can also be obtained by timing and/or placement, true selectivity applies when the herbicide is active only against certain species of plants and not others. The recent development of herbicide-resistant crops through transgenic technology will allow once nonselective herbicides to be used as selective toxicants.

Herbicides may also be classified according to the manner in which they are applied to plants or soil. Contact herbicides are those that affect the portion of the plant that was treated. Translocated herbicides may be applied to the soil or above-ground parts of the plant, where they are absorbed by the plant and circulated to distant tissues. Soil-applied herbicides rely upon residual effects and translocation to the plant for effect.

Herbicides are often grouped together based upon their biochemical and physiological effects. Herbicide target sites include photosynthesis and respiration, regulation of growth characteristics, and inhibition of specific biochemical pathways such as those for amino acids, carotenoids, and lipids. Most recent advances in herbicide chemistry have targeted specific plant enzymes. These herbicides tend to be more selective, possessing high activity at low rates of application while also possessing low nontarget toxicity.

Although many herbicides are easily classified by chemical structure, such a classification scheme is difficult to use because a two-dimensional structural formula bears little relationship to the three-dimensional shape that determines biological behavior. Thus, two similar compounds with nearly identical structures may have very different effects. However, despite this difficulty, many herbicides with similarities in structure also possess similar mechanisms of action, both to the plants against which they are directed and to nontarget organisms including vertebrates. Common structural components shared among the herbicides reviewed in this chapter are chlorophenoxy, chloroacetamide, bipyridinium, and triazine herbicides. These structural families were selected based primarily on use patterns in the United States and evidence of some chronic toxicities present for these groups.

Chlorophenoxy Herbicides

The chlorophenoxy herbicides, which include 2,4-D, 2,4,5-T, MCPA, and silvex (Fig. 2), are plant growth regulators. These are characterized structurally by the presence of a simple acid, which is esterified onto a phenyl ring with one to three chlorine substitutions. These plant-growth regulators act as synthetic auxins or plant-growth hormones, altering plant metabolism and subsequent growth. Selectivity of these compounds is the result of inherent differences between the responses of enzyme systems of crops and those of weeds. Hormonal effects in mammalian systems have not been observed.

One of the most popular herbicides developed is 2,4-D. It was introduced in 1944 as the first of the "phenoxyacetic herbicides." Its effectiveness against broadleaf weeds, including lamb's quarters, pigweed, smartweed, and ragweed, provided the impetus for commercial searches for other organic herbicides. It was used in combination with 2,4,5-T as a component of Agent Orange during the Vietnam War. Currently it is often used in combination with other herbicides, particularly with linuron.

Toxicity of the chlorophenoxy herbicides is relatively low (LD_{50} ranges from 300 to 2000 mg/kg). Dogs are more sensitive to both 2,4-D and 2,4,5-T, with an LD_{50} to both compounds of approximately 100 mg/kg. The symptoms of poisoning for these compounds include myotonia, anorexia, excessive thirst, tremors, ataxia, rapid breathing, paralysis, and

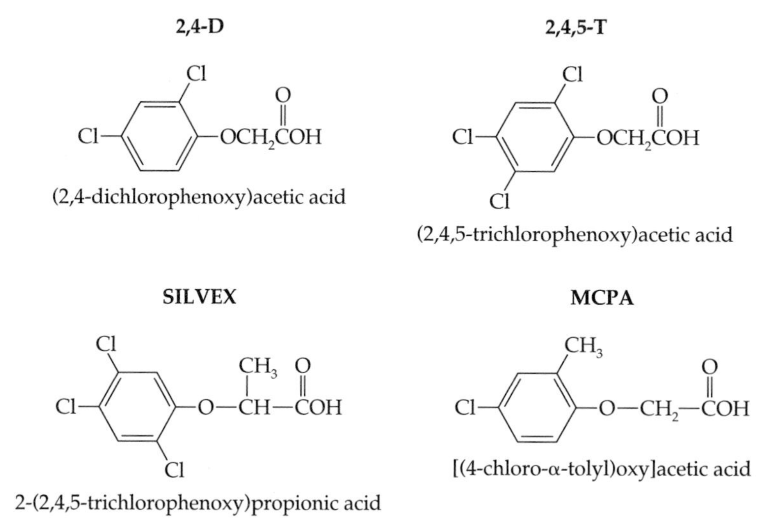

2,4-D

(2,4-dichlorophenoxy)acetic acid

2,4,5-T

(2,4,5-trichlorophenoxy)acetic acid

SILVEX

2-(2,4,5-trichlorophenoxy)propionic acid

MCPA

[(4-chloro-α-tolyl)oxy]acetic acid

FIGURE 2 Chemical structures of chlorophenoxy herbicides.

coma, with death resulting from ventricular fibrillation. These symptoms are accompanied by reduced body temperature and metabolic rate. Several cases of acute exposure in humans have resulted in severe poisoning and death. As with laboratory animals, most major organ systems are involved in human mortality, including the central and peripheral nervous systems, digestive system, respiratory system, skeletal muscles, liver, kidney, skin, and reproductive system.

Chronic human exposure to these herbicides, particularly for those involved in their manufacture, is characterized primarily by the presence of chloracne. This dermatological condition is known to have persisted for up to 20 years following the initial accidental exposure. Other signs of poisoning include several neurological disorders, including personality changes, sleep disturbances, loss of energy, impaired vision, and differences in taste and muscle coordination. These conditions are thought to be primarily due to the presence of the contaminant 2,3,7,8-tetrachlorodibenzo-*p*-dioxin (TCDD) (Fig. 3), which occurs during the production of 2,4,5-T. However, some cases of neurological disorders have also been reported among workers exposed to 2,4-D.

TCDD and a number of other closely related compounds, including 2,4,5-T, chloronaphthalenes, chlorobiphenyls, chlorodiphenyloxides, and chlorobenzenes, known collectively as dioxins, are contaminants in several manufacturing processes. Nearly all human exposures to these compounds involve highly complex mixtures of these and other chemicals.

Considerable efforts have been made to understand the toxicology of the chlorophenoxy herbicides and their contaminants as a result of the exposure of Vietnam War veterans and the Vietnamese people to Agent Orange. The chronic health effects of these chemicals are of particular interest in light of the many reproductive, teratogenic, and immunosuppressive effects of TCDD that have been observed experimentally. Signs of poisoning, other than chloracne, suggest that the liver is a major target organ. Several chronic neuropathies have also been reported among workers with industrial exposure. The symptoms include personality changes, sleep disturbances, loss of energy, impaired vision, and changes in taste and muscular coordination.

Several epidemiological studies of U.S. veterans and Vietnamese have failed to provide unequivocal evidence for increased risk of reproductive or teratogenic effects due to exposure to Agent Orange. Only one epidemiological study has demonstrated signifi-

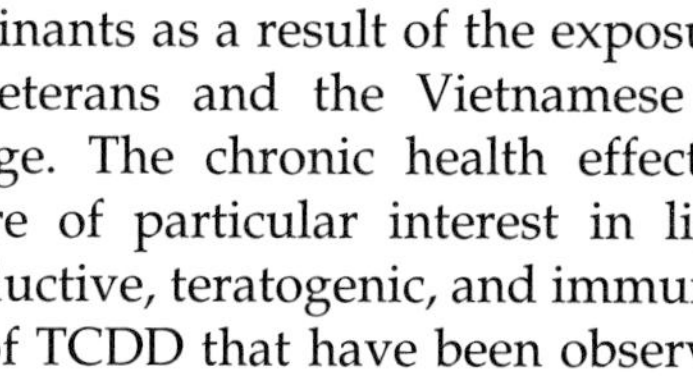

2, 3, 7, 8-Tetrachlorodibenzo-*p*-dioxin (TCDD)

FIGURE 3 Chemical structure of TCDD.

cant birth defects among offspring of Vietnam veterans. Observed defects included spina bifida, cleft lip, coloboma, and neoplasms in the first year of life. No studies of Vietnam veterans matched with an appropriate control group have demonstrated any association between the herbicide exposure and soft-tissue sarcomas. However, the latency period from the time of exposure to the time of development of a detectable tumor may have been insufficient for any increase in tumor incidence to have been noted among these individuals. In contrast, several small epidemiological studies have demonstrated an apparent association with increased incidence of soft tissue sarcoma and exposure to the chlorophenoxy herbicides. In one study, farmers who had been exposed to herbicides for more than 20 days per year had a sixfold increased risk of developing non-Hodgkins lymphomas compared to nonfarmers.

One of the initial studies of chronic health effects associated with 2,4,5-T exposure resulted in considerable concern for the safety of this chemical because of putative teratogenic and fetotoxic effects. It was later learned that the 2,4,5-T used in the study contained a high amount of TCDD (30 ppm), which compromised the results. Subsequent work using pure preparations demonstrated that in mice 2,4,5-T was indeed teratogenic, although evidence for this was lacking in rats and rabbits. 2,4-D has not been conclusively demonstrated to be teratogenic.

Investigations of the carcinogenic potential for 2,4-D and 2,4,5-T indicate that these herbicides are not carcinogenic in mice or rats. There was a published report that 2,4-D exposure in pet dogs resulted in increased malignant lymphomas, but this study has since been refuted based upon an absence of these effects in laboratory dogs and additional epidemiological evidence.

Immunological effects due to 2,4,5-T exposure are difficult to separate from exposure to TCDD. The initial investigations that identified TCDD as a toxic contaminant of 2,4,5-T production were the result of studies of chloracne in factory workers. Although chloracne is definitely a symptom of TCDD exposure, it is not clear that these effects are due to exposure to these herbicides. There is a report, however, in which a small group of women exposed to a mixture of 2,4,5-T and 2,4-D experienced contact eczema.

Chloroacetamide Herbicides

Chloroacetamide herbicides include alachlor, metolachlor, acetochlor, and propanil (Fig. 4). This class of herbicides is used principally in the selective preemergence control of annual grass, broadleaf weeds, and yellow nutsedge. The primary mode of action of these herbicides is not known. However, they are known to inhibit several metabolic processes including lipid biosynthesis and the syntheses of proteins,

ALACHLOR (Lasso®)

C_2H_5, CH_2OCH_3, N, $C.CH_2Cl$, C_2H_5, O

2-chloro-2′,6′-diethyl-*N*-(methoxymethyl) acetanilide

METOLACHLOR (Dual®)

CH_3, CH_3, $CH—CH_2O—CH_3$, N, O, $C—CH_2Cl$, C_2H_5

2-chloro-*N*-(2-ethyl-6-methylphenyl)-*N*-(2-methoxy-1-methylethyl)-acetamide

ACETOCHLOR (Harness®)

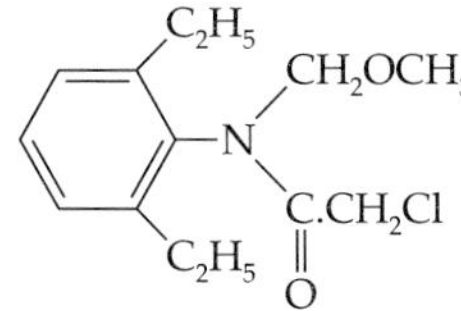

CH_3, $CH_2—O—CH_2—CH_3$, N, $C—CH_2—Cl$, $CH_2—CH_3$, O

2-chloro-*N*-(ethoxymethyl)-*N*-2-ethyl-6-methylphenyl) acetamide

PROPANIL (Stam®)

Cl, Cl, H, $N—C—C_2H_5$, O

N-(3,4-dichlorophenyl)-propanamide

FIGURE 4 Chemical structures of chloroacetamide herbicides.

gibberellins, and the products of the phenylpropanoid pathway. The herbicide pronamide inhibits mitosis by binding to tubulin and preventing the formation of microtubules. The mechanism contributing to selectivity is not known, although resistant plants are able to more rapidly metabolize these herbicides than susceptible plants. They are not generally persistent in the soil, most having a half-life of 1–3 months.

Alachlor was introduced in 1969 by Monsanto as a selective pre- and postemergent herbicide for annual broadleaf control. It became the largest selling herbicide in the United States, where it has been used successfully in several crops including beans, beets, cabbage, corn, cotton, ornamentals, peanuts, peas, potatoes, sorghum, soybeans, sugarcane, sunflowers, and tobacco. Due to reports of carcinogenic effects in rat nasal tissue, alachlor recently became a restricted-use pesticide and has largely been replaced in the U.S. marketplace by metolachlor.

The acute toxicity of the chloroacetamide herbicides is low, with LD_{50}'s ranging from 1400 to 2000 mg/kg. Chronic administration of alachlor in dogs resulted in hepatotoxicity at levels of 5 to 75 mg/kg over a 6-month period. In Long–Evans rats, a 2-year feeding study produced an ocular lesion (uveal degeneration syndrome) at all doses studied. An unusual dose-related increase in nasal turbinate adenomas was also observed in both sexes. In mice, broncheoalveolar tumors were observed only at the highest dose. Subsequent studies have suggested that alachlor is metabolized to a putative ultimate carcinogen 3,5-diethylbenzoquinone-4-imine (DEBQI). The preferential formation of DEBQI in rats (as compared to other animals, in which these adenomas have not been observed) was postulated to account for the formation of the nasal adenomas in these rodents. As a result of these studies, alachlor has been classified by the U.S. Environmental Protection Agency (EPA) as a probable human carcinogen (category B2).

Exposure of laboratory animals to these chloroacetanilide herbicides has not produced teratological or reproductive effects. Human exposures have been known to result in irritation of the skin, eyes, and mucus membranes. Ingestion causes nausea, vomiting, abdominal distress, and diarrhea. Skin sensitizations have also been reported.

Tests of the oncogenic potential of metolachlor were conducted in Sprague–Dawley rats, for which a weak response was noted only at the highest dose level (300 mg/kg/d). The benign hepatic tumors increased from 2% in the control to 15% in the 300 mg/kg/day group. This response was observed only in females. No tumors were observed at the highest doses tested in CD-1 mice. These results have led to the classification of metolachlor by the U.S. EPA as a possible human carcinogen (category C).

Bipyridinium Herbicides

The bipyridinium herbicides include paraquat, diquat, and difenzoquat (Fig. 5). These herbicides are the only herbicides containing quarternary nitrogen within two pyridyl rings. They are nonselective and are generally applied as postemergent contact pesticides. Plants treated with these herbicides quickly sustain a frostbitten appearance due to cell-membrane destruction. The result is rapid wilting and desiccation followed by leaf drop, making these materials desirable as preharvest desiccants for crops such as cotton, soybeans, potatoes, and sugarcane. In addition, diquat is used in aquatic weed control. Difenzoquat is used primarily for wild oat control in barley, wheat, flax, and rape.

The mechanism of paraquat and diquat toxicity involves the production of superoxides in response to cyclic oxidation–reduction of the compound in tissues. This mechanism of toxicity is similar in both plants and animals. In each, paraquat is reduced to a

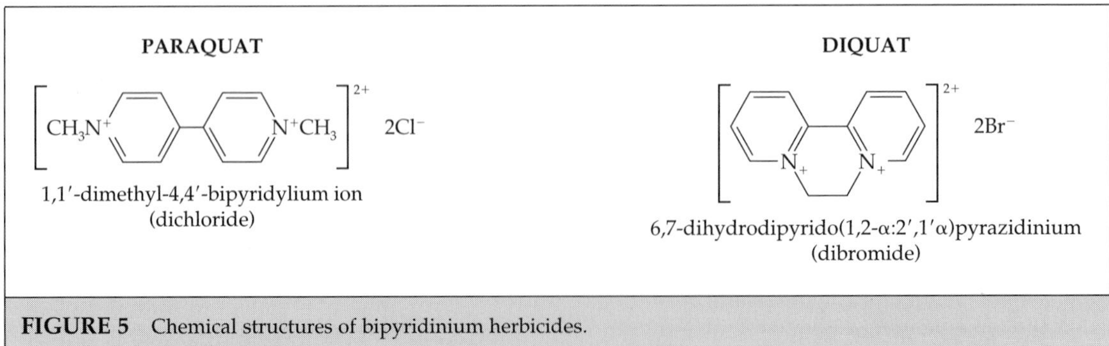

FIGURE 5 Chemical structures of bipyridinium herbicides.

radical anion due to electron flow from $NADP^+$. Subsequently, the free radical is reoxidized by molecular oxygen, resulting in the production of a superoxide radical. The superoxide radical then causes peroxidation of cellular membranes, resulting in the degradation of polyunsaturated fatty acids. These peroxidative reactions can be inhibited by superoxide dismutase and by a singlet oxygen-trapping agent, providing evidence that paraquat toxicity is mediated by superoxide free radicals. These findings also are consistent with the fact that oxygen enhances the toxicity of paraquat, which helps explain the preferential damage of lung tissue.

In comparison with many other herbicides, the mammalian toxicity of bipyridinium herbicides is quite high with oral LD_{50} values in rats of 100 mg/kg for paraquat. Similar levels of toxicity have also been observed when it is applied dermally. Paraquat toxicity is substantially increased by intraperitoneal administration, for which the rat LD_{50} is approximately 10 mg/kg. This difference in toxicity is probably the result of differences in absorption, although other aspects including alterations in tissue distribution or differences in metabolism may also be involved.

Following acute poisoning in rats and mice, there is a considerable variation in the time to mortality within the same species (2–12 days). Those individuals that die quickly demonstrate hyperexcitability, severe and varied ataxia, convulsions, or a combination of these symptoms. Animals in which death is delayed show increasing signs of respiratory difficulty and die of respiratory failure.

Many human deaths, mostly suicides, have been attributed to poisoning by paraquat. The symptoms of poisoning observed in humans are similar to those observed in laboratory animals. In cases of acute lethal poisoning (e.g., suicide attempts), deaths occurred within 48 h of ingestion as the result of direct toxicity to kidneys and liver or complications such as sepsis. Where moderate doses were involved (i.e., accidental poisoning), the interval between ingestion and death could be as long as 26–30 days, with a few cases extending much longer. In most cases, the initial toxic symptoms include gastrointestinal irritation followed by liver, kidney, and heart dysfunction. Irritation of the mouth, pharynx, esophagus, and stomach are common. These symptoms either fail to progress or actually regress with time and are replaced by a gradual onset of respiratory distress, eventually resulting in death. Patients who survive paraquat poisoning frequently show no symptoms of lung injury; however, there are a few exceptions in which some pulmonary dysfunction continues. The exceptions occur primarily in patients who either smoked or who had previous histories of respiratory disabilities.

It should be noted that although a fair number of deaths have been attributed to paraquat, the majority of these have been the result of intentional or accidental ingestion of concentrated solutions. Under normal conditions of use, few cases of symptomatic poisoning have been reported. In those rare cases, exposure was the result of either accidental spraying of the body or absorption through the lungs due to spraying under windy conditions. Fingernail injuries have also been reported as a result of exposure to concentrated material or to leakage of diluted material while spraying. Studies of skin absorption of paraquat in humans suggest that there is only slight absorption. However, workers exposed to fine mists have reported nosebleeds, skin irritation, inflammation of the mouth and upper respiratory system, cough, chest pain, asthmatic attacks, headache, and vomiting. Splashes to the eye have resulted in only a few initial symptoms but later progressed to near-blindness. In the few cases reported, however, the victims have all recovered fully within a few weeks.

Although diquat is structurally similar to paraquat, it is not quite as toxic, with a rat oral LD_{50} of 400 mg/kg. Administration of high concentrations of diquat, either orally or intraperitoneally, results in few symptoms of toxicity during the first 24 hs. Symptoms of acute diquat toxicity include lethargy, pupillary dilatation, respiratory distress, and weight loss, until death, which occurs between 2 and 14 days after exposure. Animals surviving 7 days or longer often have greatly distended abdomens, probably the result of increased fluid loss into the gastrointestinal tract.

Chronic studies of diquat conducted in rats at 1000 ppm (ca. 50 mg/kg/day) for 2 years demonstrated decreased food consumption and growth. At 500 ppm, food consumption, growth, and pathology are not affected, except in the eye, where cataracts are produced. Cataracts show a clear dose–response relationship, with higher doses producing the effects earlier and more frequently than lower doses. Similar results have also been observed in the dog.

Although the symptomologies of paraquat and diquat poisoning are markedly similar, particularly in cases of chronic toxicity, there are also significant differences. In particular, paraquat is more damaging to the lung tissue than diquat. In cases where death occurs rapidly, the lung is grossly congested, and hemorrhage and edema are indicated by a plum-like coloration. Where death is delayed significantly, signs of hemorrhaging and edema are no longer present. The tissue is scarred and consolidated, and in some cases honeycombing is evident. In contrast to paraquat, diquat produces little or no injury to the lung. The difference in the toxicities of these compounds is consistent with the fact that paraquat tends to accumulate in the lung, whereas diquat does not. It is not clear, however, whether the accumulation of paraquat is a consequence of injury or due to some other factor associated with absorption. Another difference in toxicity between these compounds involves the increased distribution of fluids to the gastrointestinal tract of diquat-poisoned animals. The role of this distribution of water in toxicity is not clear as tissue is dehydrated after a fatal oral dose but hydrated after a fatal subcutaneous dose.

Studies examining the mutagenic potential of paraquat and diquat using the Ames test, the mouse dominant lethal test, and recessive lethal mutation tests in *Drosophila* have all yielded negative data. However, paraquat increased chromosomal aberrations in the root cells of the spring onion, *Allium fistulosum,* and of spring barley, *Hordeum vulgare.* Similarly, positive effects of diquat have also been observed in assays of gene conversion in *Saccharomyces cerevisiae,* DNA repair in *Salmonella typhimurium,* and gene mutation in *Aspergillus nidulans.* These results suggest that these compounds are clastogens but not mutagens. Furthermore, there have been no reports of tumor formation, either in laboratory animals or in the human population. Reproductive and teratogenic effects were not significantly increased except at doses where toxicity in the dam was noted.

Triazines

The triazine herbicides consist of a six-member ring with three nitrogens arranged symetrically around the ring. In the 4 and 6 positions, amino substitutions are common, while in the 2 position chlorine, methoxyl, and methylthio substitutions occur. Triazoles are related to the triazines and consist of five-member rings with 2 carbons and 3 nitrogens.

The triazine and triazole products include herbicides, fungicides, and insecticides. Some of the more commonly used herbicides are atrazine, simazine, metribuzin, cyanazine, and propazine (Fig. 6). These products are strong inhibitors of photosynthesis and are used primarily as pre- and post-emergent herbicides. Some, including atrazine and simazine, can also be used selectively to control submerged pond weeds.

The triazine herbicides bind to the pigment protein of the photosystem II complex in the thylakoid membrane of chloroplasts, resulting in interference with electron transport necessary for photosynthesis. This is a mechanism similar to that of the urea herbicides, which include diuron and linuron. Crop selectivity is achieved by their rapid detoxication in tolerant crop plants and the judicious placement of the herbicide relative to the root zone of crop plants. They are readily absorbed by the roots and translocated to the leaves. Application to foliage does not result in translocation to other plant parts.

Acute oral toxicity of the triazine and triazole products in rats is low (LD_{50} 1000 to 5000 mg/kg). General symptoms of acute poisoning include excitation fol-

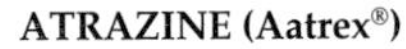
ATRAZINE (Aatrex®)
2-chloro-4(ethylamino)-6-(isopropylamino)-s-triazine
SIMAZINE (Princep®)
2-chloro-4,6-bis(ethylamino)-s-triazine
CYANAZINE (Bladex®)
2-[[4-chloro-6(ethylamino)-s-triazin-2-yl]amino]-2-methypropionitrile
PROPAZINE (Milogard®)
2-chloro-4,6-bis(isopropylamino)-s-triazine
METRIBUZIN (Lexone®, Sencor®)
4-amino-6-(1,1-dimethylethyl)-3-(methylthio)-1,2,4-triazin-5(4H)-one

FIGURE 6 Chemical structures of triazine herbicides.

lowed by depression, reduced respiratory rates, motor incoordination, spasms, and hyperthermia. In the case of amitrole, poisoning symptoms include increased intestinal peristalsis, pulmonary edema, and hemorrhages in various organs. Death generally results within 24 hours after oral administration.

Chronic toxicity testing of these herbicides indicates that generally there were few adverse effects. In one study of atrazine, however, 40% of rats fed oral doses of atrazine at 20 mg/kg/day for a period of 6 months suffered mortality following respiratory distress and limb paralysis. Morphological and biochemical changes in the brain, heart, liver, lungs, kidney, ovaries, and endocrine system were also observed. These results were contradictory to those of another 6-month study in which no pathology was observed at 25 mg/kg/day. Studies performed with amitrole, however, demonstrated adenomatous changes in the thyroid gland of rats fed high doses. These changes were reversable when feeding was discontinued.

Dietary levels of atrazine at 50 mg/kg/day were harmless to reproduction, although subcutaneous injections of 800 mg/kg/day on days 3, 6, and 9 of gestation resulted in death and resorption of some or all the pups in the litter. A similar study at 200 mg/kg/day did not affect the number of pups nor their weight at the time of weaning.

Numerous reproductive and mutagenic studies have been conducted on several of these herbicides, with particular focus upon atrazine. Tests for mutagenicity and carcinogenicity have largely been negative, with the exception that atrazine has produced mammary tumors in mice and in female Sprague–Dawley rats. Simazine also produced mammary tumors at the highest dose tested (100 ppm) in female Sprague–Dawley rats. Based on these results, atrazine has been classified by the EPA as a class 2B carcinogen.

Few human health effects have been observed with the triazine or triazole herbicides. Atrazine and related compounds have been known to result in dermatitis and to cause moderate-to-severe burning of the eyes.

Insecticides

One of the earliest records of the use of chemicals for insect control is Homer's mention (about 1000 BC) of the use of sulfur as a fumigant. Chinese records indicate the use of arsenic sulfides as early as 900 AD to control garden insects. In 1669 arsenic was mentioned as used in the Western Hemisphere as an ant bait, and tobacco smoke was used as a fumigant in the late 1700s. In the early 1800s, chrysanthemum flower heads were ground into powder and used as louse powder during the Napoleonic Wars. Up until the early 1940s, insecticide use was limited to several arsenicals, petroleum oils, nicotine, pyrethrum, rotenone, sulfur, hydrogen cyanide gas, and cryolite. It was not until the discovery of the insecticidal properties of DDT in 1939 that insecticides gained worldwide use.

Following the introduction of DDT, several organochlorinated compounds were introduced that revolutionized insect control. Some of the more important of these were benzene hexachloride and several cyclodienes, which were introduced between 1940 and 1958. Use of several of these compounds continued up until the mid 1960s, when insect resistance and problems of environmental persistance led to a curtailing of their use and their replacement by organophosphorus and carbamate insecticides.

The first organophosphorus insecticides were developed by Gerhard Schrader in the 1930s, although none was marketed until 1944. Shortly after the discovery of organophosphates, the carbamate class was also found. A period of intense research activity resulted, and structure–activity studies produced numerous organophosphorus and carbamate insecticides that dominated the insecticide market through the 1970s.

Use of pyrethrin extracts as insecticides was limited by production costs and their lack of stability. The first synthetic pyrethroid, allethrin, was introduced in 1949, however, it too lacked stability. During the 1970s important advances in pyrethroid synthesis allowed the exploitation of this chemical class of insecticides, resulting in the production of several different pyrethroids displaying not only high selectivity toward insects but also greater photostability.

Today, the discovery of novel insecticide classes remains problematic as the costs associated with discovery and development continue to escalate and new chemical leads are difficult to acquire. New areas of insect control have taken advantage of microbial agents such as *Bacillus thuringiensis* or insect-specific biological functions, such as the juvenile hormone as discussed in the following. Recently some novel insecticide chemistries have been discovered by routine screening of different chemistries (fipronil) and plant and soil samples (spinosyns), or by exploring derivatives of known natural products such as nicotine (chloronicotinyl insecticides).

Chlorinated Hydrocarbon Insecticides

Chlorinated hydrocarbon insecticides have been categorized into three groups, DDT-type compounds,

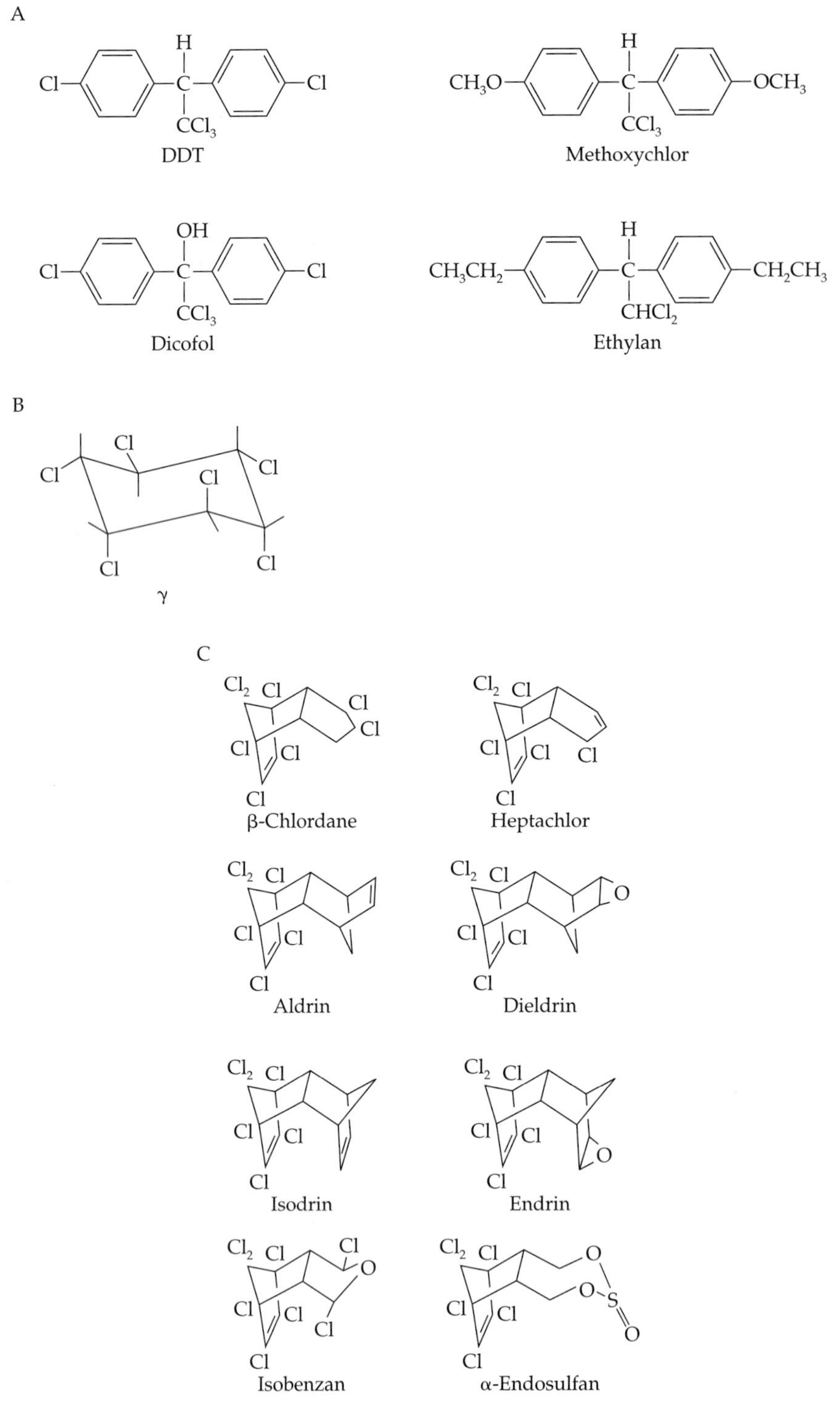

A

B

C

FIGURE 7 Chemical structures of chlorinated hydrocarbon insecticides. (A) DDT and DDT-like insecticides, (B) benzene hexachloride (lindane), (C) cyclodiene insecticides.

hexachlorocyclohexanes, and cyclodienes (Fig. 7). The DDT-type compounds include methoxychlor, dicofol, dimite and perthane (Fig. 7A). Hexachlorocyclohexanes (HCH) constitute a mixture of eight different isomers. The gamma isomer, lindane (Fig. 7B), is particularly toxic, and the toxicity of technical HCH is directly proportional to the percentage of lindane in the formulation. Cyclodienes are a group of highly chlorinated cyclic hydrocarbons that contain an endomethylene bridge. Important cyclodienes include chlordane, heptachlor, aldrin, dieldrin, endrin, and endosulfan (Fig. 7C).

Although chlorinated hydrocarbons have been studied for many years, the mode of action is still not complete. They are known to interfere with the axonal transmission of nerve impulses, resulting in the disruption of central nervous system function, which is discussed in more detail later. Typical symptoms of chlorinated hydrocarbon poisoning include salivation, nausea, tremors, convulsions, vomiting, and abdominal pain. Death is due to respiratory failure as a result of depression of the central nervous system.

The use of most organochlorine pesticides has been banned for several years in the United States. These insecticides typically are highly persistent and have a tendency to accumulate in the food chain. Some, such as methoxychlor, continue to have a limited use today in the United States while others, banned in the United States are still used in many developing countries.

DDT and DDT-like Insecticides

The first synthesis of DDT, 1,1,1-trichloro-2,2-bis(4-chlorophenyl)ethane, was by O. Zeidler in 1874. Following an independent synthesis of DDT, Paul Mueller discovered its potent insecticidal activity in 1939. During subsequent experiments using the blowfly, *Calliphora vomitoria,* the persistent nature of this chemical was discovered when carefully washed treatment cages proved to be toxic to the flies.

The efficacy of DDT was demonstrated as early as 1941 when DDT was used against the Colorado potato beetle to save the Swiss potato crop. This was at an especially critical time when the country was virtually isolated by World War II and food crops were of the utmost importance to the populace. Preliminary experiments conducted by Mueller and others at Geigy, as well as by R. Wiesmann, also demonstrated that DDT was effective against a wide range of agricultural pests. DDT was of even greater value to the field of medical entomology, due to its ability to control insects that transmit some of the world's most serious diseases, including typhus, malaria, and yellow fever.

In 1941, it was demonstrated that DDT could eliminate the human louse, *Pediculus humanus,* from infested individuals at a dose of 0.01%. In 1943, it was shown that DDT killed lice when applied directly and that garments treated with DDT remained louse-proof even after several washings. DDT did not kill eggs, but larvae exposed to treated garments died. The most spectacular use of DDT involved the control of louse-borne typhus in Naples, Italy, in 1943. During January 1944, 1,300,000 civilians were dusted with about a half-ounce of powder containing 5% active ingredient. No deleterious effects were observed among this large population, other than a few cases of skin irritation. Within weeks typhus disappeared from Naples. Several other campaigns to eliminate typhus were conducted with considerable success in Egypt, Mexico, Columbia, and Guatamala.

Other extraordinary successes of DDT were in the control of malaria and yellow fever. Due to the successful use of DDT to control malaria-carrying mosquitoes during the World War II, Professor A. Missiroli initiated a 5-year campaign to eliminate malaria from Italy in 1945. By 1949, mosquitoes had nearly disappeared altogether, and cases of malaria in Italy had dropped to near zero. Similar success stories can be told with respect to yellow fever and the eradication of its vector, *Aedes aegypti,* particularly in several South American countries.

Because of its unprecedented success, DDT gained extensive use throughout the world. In 1945 it became commercially available for use in agriculture, resulting in a steady increase in production until 1963 when restrictions were implemented to minimize food residues. This was especially a problem in the feed of animals used to produce milk and meat. Simultaneous with the concerns about DDT's persistence, several insect species developed resistance to DDT.

The acute oral toxicity of DDT to rats when formulated in oil is relatively low, with an LD_{50} of 250 mg/kg. Chronic toxicity studies with doses as high as 40 mg/kg/day produced no signs of illness for up to 18 months. At the end of the 18-month period, starvation mobilized DDT stored in fat reserves, resulting in marked tremors and other symptoms of DDT poisoning. These symptoms disappeared when food was again supplied.

Studies of human toxicity have been conducted with doses as high as 35 mg/person/day for up to 21.5 months. No symptoms associated with these doses were ever observed, even 5 years following treatment. Although there have been a few incidents of nervous symptoms, muscle tremors, and general malaise associated with DDT exposure, only four fatalities have been documented for this pesticide, each resulting from suicide attempts. All cases of individual poisoning involved ingestion, and mortalities may be attributed as much to the toxicity of the solvents as to DDT itself.

The toxicity of DDT is due to its ability to interfere with the sodium channel in the axonal membrane. The leakage of sodium ions results in an increase in the spontaneous firing of neurons, resulting in characteristic muscular twitching or the "jitters." This twitching increases with the dose until the onset of convulsions. DDT also is thought to inhibit the neuronal Na^+, K^+-ATPase pump that restores the potential across the axonal membrane following a signal transduction event. Other changes observed with DDT poisoning include increased brain concentrations of neurohormones, such as serotonin, glutamic acid, and γ-aminobutyric acid, and decreased levels of the neurotransmitter, acetylcholinesterase. Significant changes in brain–lipid metabolism have also been noted.

The reproductive effects of DDT have been very controversial. An early study in 1950 suggested that DDT produced estrogenic effects; high concentrations of DDT injected into cockerels resulted in an inhibition of testicular growth and produced secondary sexual characteristics. Prior to this time, DDT had been used extensively in chickens for the control of lice and mites without noticeable adverse effects. Several subsequent experiments were conducted in mice, rats, and dogs without definitive results. Two multigeneration studies conducted in dogs and ewes gave no evidence of reproductive or developmental effects. The results of one often-cited rat study suggesting that DDT significantly advanced puberty, induced persistent vaginal estrus, and caused other abnormalities was obtained by dosing 1-, 2-, and 3-day-old female rats with doses approximately 40-fold higher than are normally used in adult feeding trials. No teratogenic effects have been observed for this pesticide

Despite the controversial negative reproductive results, other evidence is accumulating that suggests that DDT and its metabolites, particularly DDE, may be estrogenic. One frequent contaminant of DDT, *o,p*-DDT, is a known estrogenic compound that can be metabolized to *o,p*-DDE. One of the most compelling studies involves changes in the reproductive status of alligators at Lake Apopka in central Florida, where an extensive pesticide spill released dicofol, DDT, and several of its metabolites. Female alligators from this lake had two fold increases in the level of plasma estradiol-17β and had abnormal ovarian morphology. Males demonstrated significantly depressed testosterone levels and had abnormal testes and phalli.

Several studies have been conducted in laboratory animals to investigate the potential of DDT as a carcinogen. Although DDT was hepatocarcinogenic in mice and rats, it was concluded that evidence for carcinogenicity in humans was inadequate. Several studies conducted in rats gave conflicting results, and studies in other animals including hamsters, dogs, and monkeys were also inconclusive. DDT appears to inhibit metabolic cooperation, resulting in a loss of control of cell proliferation. Since DDT has been demonstrated to be a tumor promoter in combination with 2-acetylaminofluorine and diethylnitrosamine, it is likely that the tumors observed in rats and mice were the result of tumor promotion rather than initiation. These results are bolstered by the fact that DDT was not found to be mutagenic in either the Ames test or the dominant lethal test in mice.

Several epidemiological studies of occupationally exposed men have provided no evidence to support a carcinogenic effect in humans. Similarly, reproductive and teratological effects in men, women, and children exposed to DDT have not been observed. The World Health Organization (WHO) made the following statement about DDT in 1979, "In practice, DDT has proved to be the safest pesticide used for residual spraying in vector control programs."

The concerns about DDT, however, are broader than those observed in studies relating to the health effects in humans or other mammalian species. Due to its high lipophilicity and its long half-life, DDT has the potential to bioaccumulate in other organisms. Although it is practically insoluble in water, DDT adsorbed onto minute particles of soil may act similarly to a solution, thereby exposing fish, insects, and crustaceans to its toxic effects. As a result of these characteristics, fish can biomagnify DDT concentrations to levels 3000-fold greater than the water concentration. When the fish are fed upon by birds of prey, this in turn, results in a further bioaccumulation of DDT through the food chain, eventually resulting in toxic effects. In many species of birds, but notably in the peregrine falcon, the result of DDT bioaccumulation is eggshell thinning, which dramatically reduced populations of these birds in many areas worldwide.

Methoxychlor is 1,1,1-trichloro-2,2-bis(4-methoxyphenyl)ethane, which is the *p,p'*-dimethoxy analog of *p,p'*-DDT. It is effective against a wide variety of insects, including pests of fruits, vegetables, forage crops, and livestock. In marked contrast to DDT, methoxychlor is not environmentally persistent, is readily metabolized, and does not accumulate in tissues.

These characteristics, combined with its low acute mammalian toxicity, are reflected in its wide use as an insecticide both in the U.S. and abroad.

The acute oral toxicity of methoxychlor is very low, with LD_{50}'s of 5000 and 1850 mg/kg in rats and mice, respectively. Rats dosed chronically at 10,000 ppm survived, but without weight gain, probably as a result of food refusal. Doses of 1600 ppm for 2 years resulted in a considerable weight reduction but did not affect longevity. No histological changes in tissues were observed. Dietary levels of 200 ppm (10 mg/kg/day) for 2 years were considered no-effect levels. Methoxychlor toxicity in dogs, swine, and chickens was also relatively low. In rabbits, doses of 200 mg/kg/d resulted in mortality within 15 days. In mice, methoxychlor is rapidly metabolized, and 98% is excreted within 24 hours. At dose levels of 25 ppm administered to rats, no methoxychlor was found in tissues. At higher doses of 100 and 500 ppm, storage in fat actually decreased after the ninth week although administration of the dose continued. Two weeks after dosing was discontinued, no methyoxychlor could be detected.

The symptoms of methoxychlor toxicity include depression of the central nervous system, tremors, diarrhea, and anorexia. Chronic administration at high doses results in severe reduction in growth, due to refusal to eat. No histological changes were observed at a dietary level of 1600 ppm for 2 years in rats, nor was a life-span reduction noted. Human volunteers fed 0.5 to 2 mg/kg/day for 8 weeks suffered no effects on health; clinical chemistry or morphology of blood, bone, marrow, small intestine, or testis.

Methoxychlor produces a multitude of effects on the reproductive systems of both male and female animals. Effects include histopathological changes in the reproductive organs and accessory glands, impaired pubertal development and reproductive function, and altered hormone levels. Early studies demonstrated that methoxychlor had estrogenic effects at high doses in swine. In rats, doses of 2500 and 5000 ppm resulted in a significant decrease in reproductive success. The reproductive success of rats fed doses of 1000 ppm prior to mating and through lactation was not affected; however, female pups had early vaginal opening and reduced reproduction when mature. Male pups displayed abnormal reproductive behavior. At dietary levels of 10,000 ppm or greater, testicular atrophy was noted in rats. Male rats fed at 100–200 mg/kg/day for 70 days showed inhibition of spermatogenesis and folliculogenesis. Degenerative changes were also noted in the Sertoli cells, spermatogonia, and spermatocytes. Females treated in the same manner also experienced atresia of the ovarian follicles. Accumulations of lipid in ovarian cells suggested that the cells have retained their ability to synthesize lipids but have lost the ability to convert these to steroid hormones. If this is true, the resulting loss of hormone balance might explain many of the changes observed in the female reproductive system. No teratogenic responses have been observed with methoxychlor.

Several lines of evidence suggest that methoxychlor has carcinogenic potential. Methoxychlor is metabolized to active intermediates, which can potentially form DNA adducts and mutations. Several mutagenicity studies have also indicated that metabolically activated methoxychlor increases mutation frequency at the thymidine kinase locus. Metabolites of methoxychlor are estrogenic, and estrogen has been linked to the etiology of cancers of endocrine-sensitive tissues such as the gonads, adrenals, prostrate, and breast. In spite of these effects, the results of many bioassays conducted on laboratory animals have been mostly negative, as listed later. One epidemiological study indicated that leukemia risk was slightly increased in farmers exposed to methoxychlor.

Evidence for the carcinogenic effects of methoxychlor in both rats and mice is inconclusive. In one study, rats fed 1600 ppm for 2 years had the identical number and type of tumors as the controls. Another 2-year study found that the occurrence of neoplasms increased somewhat with dose; however, carcinomas were found only at the highest dose of 2000 ppm. In a 2-year mice study, only one of two strains showed an increase in carcinomas of the testes at a dose of 750 ppm. No tumors were found in a study of dogs fed 10,000 ppm. These results led the National Cancer Institute to conclude that methooxychlor is not an animal carcinogen.

Benzene Hexachloride (Lindane)

Lindane is the γ isomer of benzene hexachloride (BHC, 1,2,3,4,5,6-hexachlorocyclohexane) (Fig. 7B). BHC is composed of eight separable steric isomers, one of which exists in two enantiomorphic forms. Six of these are relatively stable and are found in the technical product. The discovery that the γ form, lindane, is responsible for insecticidal activity has led to its widespread use in agriculture.

Lindane and BHC have been used against a variety of insect pests including those on agricultural food products, as well as for seed protection, treatment of poultry and livestock, and treatment of humans for lice and mites. Since BHC tended to produce an "off-flavor" in certain food items, its use on a number of crops was impractical. Due to environmental concerns over persistence as well as toxicity, lindane is classified as a restricted-use chemical, and its manufacture in the United States has been discontinued.

Lindane is very toxic, with oral LD_{50}'s in mice and rats ranging from 100 to 200 mg/kg. The lowest estimated oral dose for child mortality is 180 mg/kg. Lotions administered for the treatment of scabies have resulted in severe intoxication in some children and infants. The symptoms of poisoning occur rapidly and include central nervous system excitation, clonic and tonic convulsions, respiratory failure, pulmonary edema, and dermatitis. Acute exposure in humans can also include mental and motor retardation.

Lindane has a greater inhibitory effect on Na^+,K^+-ATPase than on Mg^{2+}-ATPase, in contrast with DDT and chlordane. It is possible that some of the subtle differences observed in the actions of these chlorinated hydrocarbon insecticides are due to different inhibitory activities, as cation transport across the nerve membrane is mediated by these enzymatic processes. Significant increases in serotonin metabolism are also known to occur with the first few doses of lindane but this returns to normal levels with further exposure. Recent findings suggest that lindane and dieldrin bind to the picrotoxin binding site of the GABA-receptor–ionophore complex. It has been suggested that the degree of binding for the picrotoxin site for lindane, other BHC isomers, dieldrin, and other chlorinated insecticides correlates with the acute toxicities of these compounds.

The different isomers of BHC have different toxicogical actions. Lindane is stimulatory, while the α, β, and δ isomers are depressants of the nervous system. These differences are so significant that equivalent or slightly greater doses of the α, β, and δ isomers can counteract the effects of lindane. Since approximately 70% of technical BHC is composed of the alpha isomer, symptoms of BHC poisoning are typical of the predominant form.

Surveys of workers exposed to lindane or BHC indicated that there have been cases of mild acute intoxication. Abnormal EEG patterns have been observed in some workers exposed to BHC, but in a group of 60 workers with exposures ranging from 1 to 30 years, no significant neurophysiological, neuromuscular, or other poor health effects were detected. Some mortalities have resulted from the use of lindane and/or BHC in vaporizing devices used in homes. These devices were later restricted.

Lindane treatments in female rats at doses of 0.5 mg/kg for 4 months resulted in disturbances in the reproductive cycle and reduced fertility. Lindane is slightly estrogenic to female rats and caused atrophy of the seminiferous tubules of male rats at doses of 8 mg/kg/day over a 10-day exposure period. No teratological effects have been observed in dogs or rats, although lindane can pass through the placenta.

Significant liver lesions have been observed in rats at low doses, while in mice no effects were observed. Tumor studies have produced conflicting results. In one study, mice given 20 mg/kg/day produced tumors, while in another study no sign of tumors was observed at 100 to 500 mg/kg/day. Rats fed over a life time at doses ranging from 5 to 1600 mg/kg also had no increase in tumor incidence. Based on these results, lindane has been judged to be carcinogenic, though there is insufficient evidence to establish carcinogenicity of the other isomers. Animal studies involving low doses of lindane (1.5 to 25 mg/kg) fed to rabbits and rats resulted in immune system suppression, which adversely affected their ability to fight disease.

Cyclodiene and Related Insecticides

The cyclodiene insecticides include aldrin, dieldrin, isodrin, endrin, isobenzan, endosulfan, chlordane, and heptachlor (Fig. 7C). Two pairs of stereoisomers are included among these insecticides: (1) aldrin and isodrin and (2) dieldrin and endrin. Aldrin is rapidly metabolized to its epoxide isomer dieldrin, while isodrin is similarly metabolized to endrin. In both cases, metabolism results in a greater toxicity in the organism.

As with DDT, cyclodiene pesticides generally have a tendency to bioaccumulate in animal adipose tissue as well as in the environment. Although the storage of these chemicals is partly accounted for by their lipophilicity, other factors such as their ability to be metabolized and excreted are also important. For example, dieldrin is readily stored in adipose tissue, while its isomer, endrin, is rapidly metabolized and excreted.

Cyclodienes are highly toxic in comparison with DDT, with the majority of cyclodienes having acute oral LD_{50}'s in rats of approximately 50 to 100 mg/kg. The symptoms of poisoning by the various cyclodienes are similar, first appearing as convulsions. This symptom contrasts with poisoning by the DDT analogs, in that tremors resulting from DDT exposure generally progress in severity until the point of convulsions.

Although the symptoms of cyclodiene poisoning are similar to those of DDT, they appear to act at the synapse rather than at the nerve membrane, as in the case of DDT. Cyclodiene toxicity tends to increase in temperature in contrast to DDT. Cyclodienes bind to the picrotoxin binding site of the GABA-receptor–ionophore complex. The degree of binding is positively correlated with acute toxicity and convulsions. The GABA receptor is inhibitory and when activated, reduces chloride-ion uptake into neurons. Cyclodienes antagonize the GABA receptor, preventing chloride-ion uptake and thereby stimulating the mammalian central nervous system. Cyclodienes have also been demonstrated to alter brain concentrations of amines such as epinephrine, norepinephrine, and serotonin.

Studies of reproductive effects of dieldrin and chlordane indicate that testosterone kinetics are altered, but the influence on reproduction itself is unknown. In contrast, chlordecone and, to a lesser extent mirex significantly impair reproductive function in mice and rats. In humans, although chlordecone has been shown to cause oligospermia and decreased sperm motility, there have been no reports of infertility. These effects are probably due to the ability of chlordecone and mirex to mimic estrogen. Multigenerational studies with hepatochlor in rats indicated that male fertility is significantly reduced when they are fed diets of 0.25 mg/kg/day, particularly in the second generation. At this dose level, however, survival of the F_1 progeny of treated rats was significantly reduced.

As with DDT and methoxychlor, studies of carcinogenicity have been conducted with the cyclodiene pesticides with equivocal results. Many of the cyclodienes tested produce tumors in mice, but the results in rats are less conclusive. Similarly, these chlorinated hydrocarbons are negative in mutagenicity tests. There is ample evidence, however, that many of these compounds are effective tumor promoters. The changes in liver morphology are similar to those observed with phenobarbital, which results in dramatic increases in smooth endoplasmic reticulum with significant enlargement of most cells. Other changes in liver cell morphology include increases in fat droplets or "lipospheres" and the displacement of cytoplasmic granules to the periphery of the cell.

Several epidemiological studies have been performed. No human epidemiological studies have shown increases in tumors that have had a positive association with chlorinated hydrocarbon exposure. In one case, occupational exposure of a single group of workers to chlordecone resulted in significant nervous-system toxicity, which was manifested by tremors, visual difficulties, muscle weakness, gait ataxia, incoordination, headache, and increased cerebrospinal fluid pressure.

Organophosphate Insecticides

The toxic properties of organophosphates were first recognized in 1932, when Lang and Krueger observed poisoning in rats. Subsequent work with organophosphates during World War II by Saunders in his search for potential nerve gases resulted in the discovery of diisopropyl fluorophosphate (DFP). Schrader was the first to discover the insecticidal properties of these compounds and developed some of the first organophosphate insecticides, including schradan and tetraethylpyrophosphate (TEPP), the first marketed organophosphate insecticide.

Organophosphates are a large and well-defined class of pesticides with a characteristic basic structure as follows.

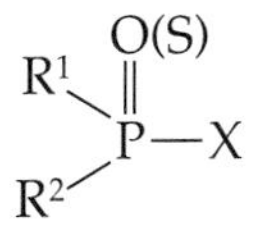

$$(R^1)(R^2)P(=O(S))\text{—}X$$

R^1 and R^2 are usually simple alkyl- or aryl- groups, both of which may be bonded directly to the phosphorus atom or linked by an –O- or an –S- bridge. The characteristics of the leaving group, X, result in the placement of most organophosphates into one of four major categories: (1) X contains quarternary nitrogen, (2) X = F, (3) X = CN, OCN, SCN or a halogen other than F, and (4) X = other moieties such as alkyl, alkoxy or alkylthio, aryl, or heterocyclic. Of these categories, most pesticides are in category 4, which can be subdivided into as many as eight subcategories based on structure, as discussed in detail by Gallo and Lawryk (1991). Many common organophosphate insecticides are depicted in Fig. 8.

Organophosphates can range from acutely toxic to relatively nontoxic. The toxicity is the result of excessive stimulation of cholinergic nerves and is dependent upon the ability to inhibit acetylcholinesterase. The function of the enzyme is to rapidly hydrolyze acetylcholine at the postganglionic membrane of the synapse. Hydrolysis terminates the stimulatory activity at the nerve membrane and normally occurs almost instantaneously (Fig. 9). Organophosphates, however, bind more tightly to the enzyme's active site at the serine hydroxyl group than does acetylcholine, resulting in significant inhibition of the phosphorylated enzyme. Spontaneous breaking of the phosphorous enzyme bond requires hours to weeks, depending on the strength of the bond (the turnover number for dimethyl phosphates is 0.008 molecule/min/acetylcholinesterase compared to 300,000 for acetylcholine). Inhibition results in the accumulation of acetyl-

ETHYL PARATHION

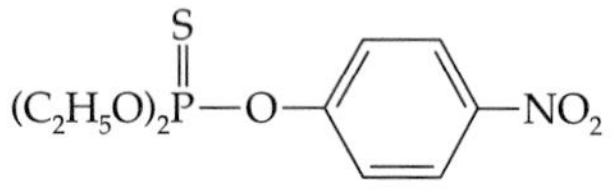

O,O-diethyl O-p-nitrophenyl phosphorothioate

CHLORPYRIFOS

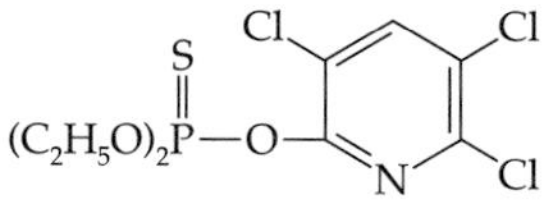

O,O-diethyl O-(3,5,6-trichloro-2-pyridyl) phosphorothioate

AZINPHOSMETHYL

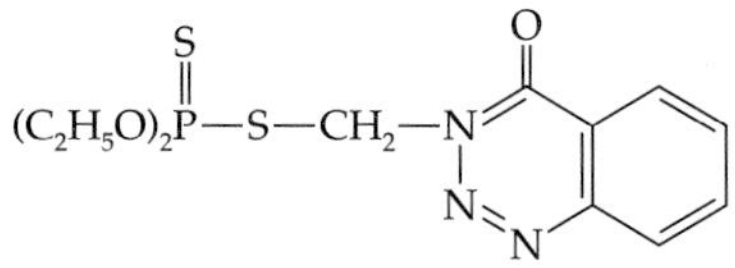

O,O-dimethyl S-(4-oxo-1,2,3-benzotriazin-3(4H)-ylmethyl) phosphorodithioate

ACEPHATE

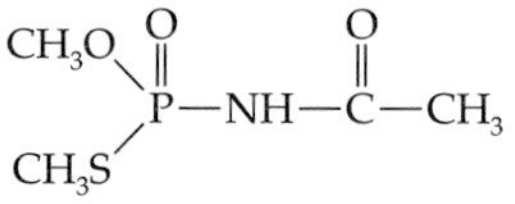

O,S-dimethyl acetylphosphoramidothioate

DIAZINON

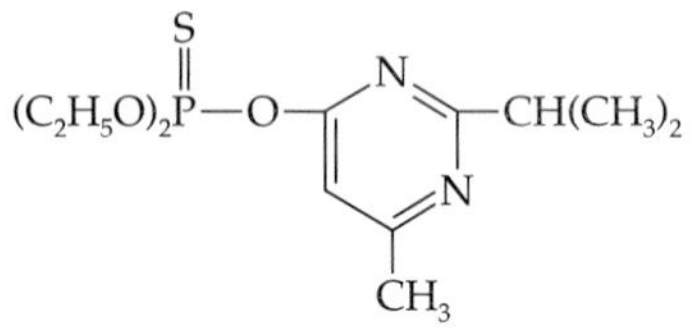

O,O-diethyl O-(2-isopropyl-4-methyl-6-pyrimidinyl) phosphorothioate

FONOFOS

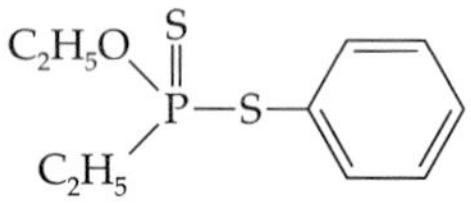

O-ethyl S-phenyl ethylphosphonodithioate

MALATHION

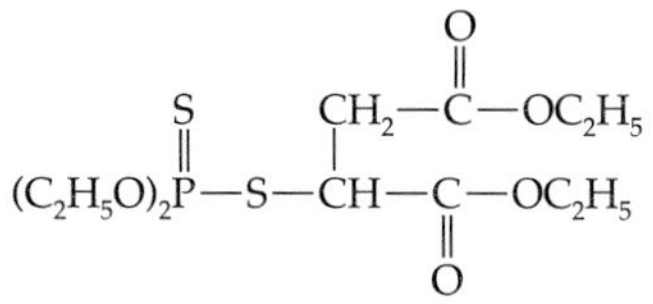

O,O-dimethyl-S-1,2-di(carboxyethoxy) ethyl phosphorodithioate

PROFENOFOS

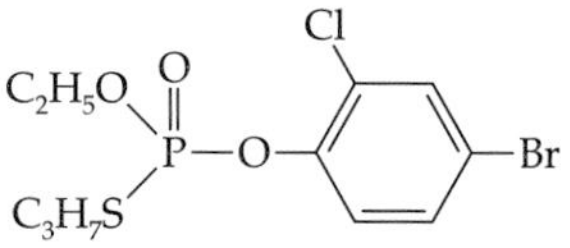

O-(4-bromo-2-chlorophenyl)-O-ethyl-S-propyl phosphorothioate

FIGURE 8 Chemical structures of selected organophosphates.

choline at the receptor, initially resulting in an excess stimulation in the postsynaptic neuron. Continued stimulation eventually results in the opposite effect, producing profound weakness followed by paralysis.

The symptoms of toxicity are a direct result of cholinesterase inhibition. They include headache, giddiness, nervousness, blurred vision, weakness, nausea, cramps, diarrhea, and discomfort in the chest. Signs include sweating, miosis, tearing, salivation, excess respiratory tract secretions, vomiting, cyanosis, and uncontrollable muscle twitches followed by muscular weakness, convulsions, coma, loss of reflexes, and loss of sphincter control. Cardiac arrhythmia, various degrees of heart block, and cardiac arrest may also occur. Generally death is the result of respiratory failure.

In cases of organophosphate poisoning as the result of suicide or murder, death has occurred within 5 min following ingestion. In cases of occupational or accidental exposure to nonlethal concentrations, symptoms can appear anywhere from 1 to 12 h after exposure. In these cases, initial giddiness, blurred vision, and headaches may precede the more serious effects of nausea, cramps, muscular twitching, and discomfort in the chest. Miosis could be a diagnostic symp-

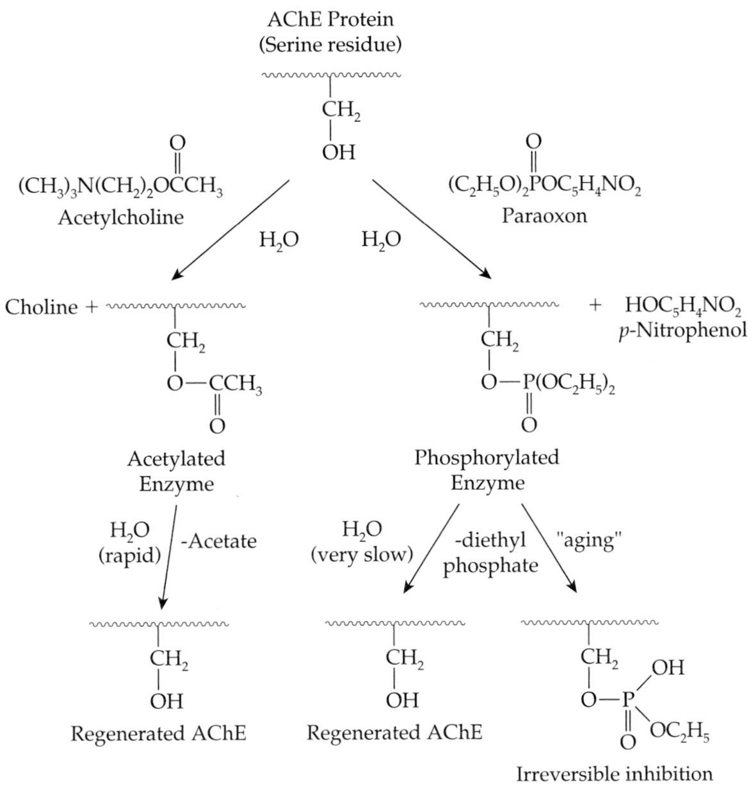

FIGURE 9 Schematic illustrating hydrolysis of ACh and parathion by the enzyme AChE.

tom of organophosphate poisoning; however, it may not appear until late in the progression of poisoning. For this reason, treatment following exposure should not be delayed because of the absence of miosis.

Multiple and/or severe acute exposures may lead to behavioral changes, including increased irritability, memory deficits, and lethargy. Lapses of attention have also been observed. Other symptoms observed in some cases include delirium, combativeness, hallucinations, depression, and psychosis. These may be the result either of impurities in the pesticide preparations or due to side effects of the atropine used in treatment.

Treatment of organophosphate poisoning involves the use of artificial respiration in combination with the administration of atropine and *N*-methylpyridinium 2-aldoxime (2-PAM). Atropine is a cholinergic-blocking agent that effectively competes with acetylcholine at the binding site, alleviating many poison symptoms, the most important being respiratory tract secretions. Use of oxime derivatives such as 2-PAM prior to "aging" results in the reactivation of the inhibited cholinesterase enzyme.

"Aging" is the phenomenon in which dealkylation of the phosphorylated-enzyme complex effectively eliminates acetylcholinesterase reactivation. After aging, regeneration of cholinesterase activity relies entirely upon resynthesis of the enzyme. Therefore, it is important to administer the oxime as early as possible to achieve a maximum effect; phosphorylation of aged enzyme cannot be reversed by oximes. Reactivation of the cholinesterase enzyme is not indicated in carbamate poisoning, since the carbamylated enzyme does not age. In fact, its use in carbamate poisoning is contraindicated, since the oxime derivatives also act as acetylcholinesterase inhibitors.

Certain organophosphates have been known to produce a delayed neuropathy. This condition arises following an apparent recovery from the acute symptoms of organophosphate poisoning for certain but not all organophosphates. The symptoms of this condition begin in the distal portions of the lower limbs of both humans and other susceptible animals. Some patients experience symptoms ranging from numbness and tingling in their extremeties to permanent partial paralysis. These symptoms are the result of a delayed distal axonapathy, known as organophosphorus-induced delayed neuropathy (OPIDN). The initial symptoms of this condition do not occur until 7 to 10 days following acute exposure. In cases of prolonged chronic exposure, the symptoms may take several months to appear. Organophosphates known to cause this condition include triorthocresyl phosphate (TOCP), diisopropyl fluorophosphate, mipafox, leptophos, and EPN. Most of these compounds are not in use due to this problem.

The first outbreak of delayed neuropathy occurred in the 1930s during Prohibition in the United States. As many as 20,000 people suffered "Ginger Jake" paralysis as a result of drinking Jamaica ginger, which had been fortified with TOCP. Although many of the victims of paralysis recovered promptly, some were affected for life. Several other serious episodes of poisoning as a result of unintentional food contamination with TOCP have occurred since.

Delayed neuoropathy is characterized morphopathologically by the degeneration of peripheral axons with subsequent degeneration of the myelin sheath. The nerves that are affected primarily include the sciatic, peroneal, and tibial nerves. The long ascending and descending tracts of the spinal cord are also affected, but not the brain. The mechanism is thought to be the result of disturbed metabolism of the nerve-cell body in spinal tracts such that the synthesis and transport of nutrients essential to the maintenance of the long axons of major nerves are not supported.

Certain species appear to be more vulnerable; humans, cats, and adult chickens are particularly vulnerable. Young animals, with the exception of chick embryos, are less susceptible. Some studies indicate that phosphorylation of 80% or more of neurotoxic esterase is highly correlated with the neuropathology.

Attempts to examine the chronic effects of organophosphates on reproduction, teratogenicity, and carcinogenicity have been difficult due to the fact that these pesticides are acutely toxic, making long-term studies difficult. Reproductive and teratogenic studies conducted with organophosphates at doses producing a marked inhibition of plasma and red blood cell cholinesterase levels failed to cause harmful effects in offspring other than those caused by cholinesterase inhibition.

Because dichlorvos is a chemical alkylating agent, several long-term studies were conducted to examine its mutagenic and carcinogenic potential. In these studies, increases in mutations were observed in some bacterial strains but not others. Long-term feeding studies conducted with dichlorvos in mice, rats, and dogs failed to increase tumor incidence even at doses high enough to cause weight reduction. Dimethoate has been shown to induce benign and malignant neoplasms in ovaries of the rat.

Carbamate Insecticides

Carbamates are derivatives of carbamic acid, RO-C-N(CH_3)R′, where R can be an alcohol, an oxime, or a phenol. R′ is often hydrogen or a methyl group (Fig. 10). In some cases, R′ can be one of several N- or S-substituted moieties that result in the formation of a proinsecticide that requires metabolism to become insecticidal.

Carbamate insecticides, like organophosphates, are acetylcholinesterase inhibitors. The signs and symptoms of poisoning are similar to those for organophosphates. The first signs, occurring within 15 to 30 min after oral administration, include excessive salivation and increased and irregular respiration. Other symptoms include lacrimation, urination, defecation, and muscular fasciculations and tremors. Mortality occurs in cases of severe poisoning as a result of respiratory failure accompanied by excessive bronchial constriction, excessive respiratory secretions, and paralysis of the respiratory muscles.

Although the symptoms of poisoning are nearly identical for organophosphates and carbamates, there are also some significant differences. For example, in contrast to the organophosphates, carbamate doses resulting in the first toxic symptoms are widely separated from doses resulting in mortality. This is the result of differences between the binding properties of organophosphates and carbamates to acetylcholinesterase. Also, in comparison to the organophosphates, recovery from carbamate poisoning is rapid, due to the significantly more facile rate of reactivation of acetylcholinesterase (the turnover number for methyl carbamates is 0.04 molecule/min/molecule of enzyme). Therefore, the use of oximes as an organophosphate antidote is contraindicated, as the rate of spontaneous reactivation of the carbamylated cholinesterase is similar to that of 2-PAM reactivation.

The mammalian acute toxicity of insecticidal carbamates varies from the highly toxic aldicarb (LD_{50} of 0.5 to 1.2 mg/kg) to the moderately toxic and widely used carbaryl (LD_{50} of 233 to 850 mg/kg). Monkeys have been shown to tolerate carbaryl at doses of 600 mg/kg/day for up to 6 months. In cases of accidental or intentional human exposures to carbamates, recov-

CARBARYL

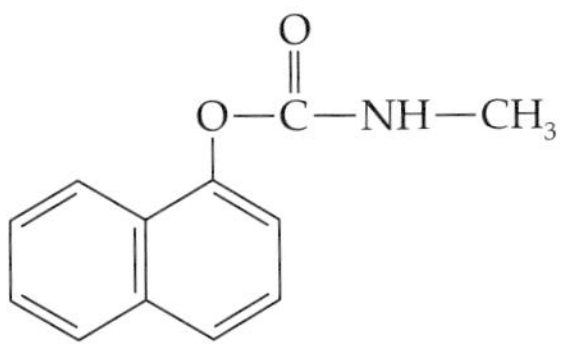

1-naphthyl methyl carbamate

CARBOFURAN

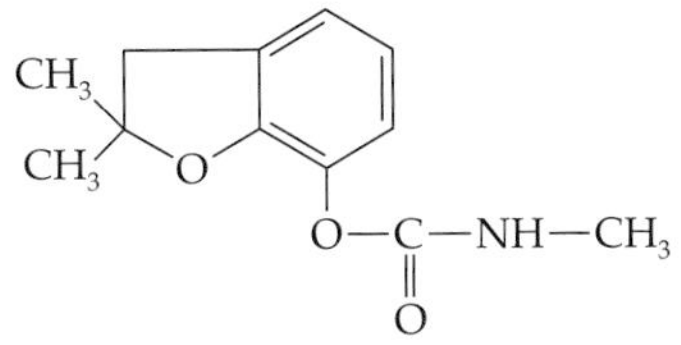

2,3 dihydro-2,2-dimethyl-7-benzofuranyl methylcarbamate

METHOMYL

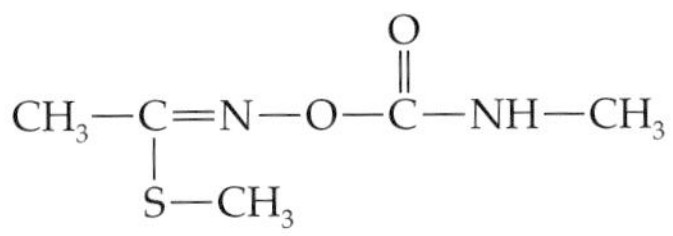

$CH_3-C(-S-CH_3)=N-O-C(=O)-NH-CH_3$

methyl N-[(methylcarbamoyl)oxy] thioacetimidate

ALDICARB

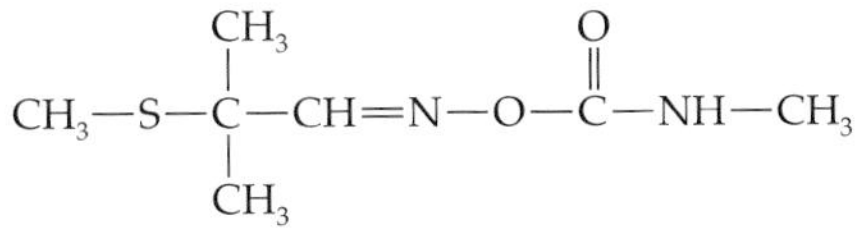

$CH_3-S-C(CH_3)_2-CH=N-O-C(=O)-NH-CH_3$

2-methyl-2-(methylthio)propionaldehyde,*O*-(methylcarbamoyl) oxime

FIGURE 10 Chemical structures of selected carbamates.

ery is rapid and complete, often within 24 hours of exposure. Although recovery from carbamate poisoning is often spantaneous, the use of atropine as an antidote is important in cases of severe poisoning.

Numerous tests for reproductive and teratogenic potential show little evidence for significant effects, other than embryotoxicity occurring at doses that are also maternally toxic. Several reports from the former USSR indicated reproductive effects for carbaryl. These studies reported functional and focal histological changes in the testes, changes in sperm function, inhibition of oogenesis, and increased hypophyseal secretion of gonadotropic hormones. Increased estrous cycle duration has also been reported. Western studies examining similar parameters following carbaryl application produced conflicting results. Depending in part on the mode of application, some studies indicated sperm abnormalities in the absence of degenerative changes in the testes, while others produced no effects on testes weight, sperm count, or frequency of sperm abnormalities.

The mutagenicity of carbamates has been thoroughly explored using a variety of assays. In general, the evidence suggests that carbamates are not mutagenic. There are some studies in which carbamates have been demonstrated to be weakly mutagenic. For example, weak mutagenicity was demonstrated in *Salmonella typhimurium* for aminocarb, carbaryl, carbofuran, and ethiofencarb. Similarly, weak mutagenicity was reported in cultured rodent cells for aminocarb, carbaryl, carbofuran, formetanate HCl, and mecarbam. Primary DNA damage has also been reported for aldicarb in *S. typhimurium,* for thiodicarb in *Saccharomyces cerevisiae,* and for carbaryl in human fibroblasts *in vitro.* In spite of these studies, feeding of carbaryl, carbofuran, ethiiofencarb, formetanate HCl, and propoxur to mice did not cause chromosomal aberrations in bone marrow erythrocytes.

Although several noninsecticidal carbamates are carcinogenic, most insecticidal carbamates are not. In the case of insecticides such as carbaryl, administration of maximum tolerated doses to mice and rats for 18 months and 2 years, respectively, did not affect tumor incidence. There is no evidence suggesting that methyl and dimethyl carbamates are carcinogenic.

Pyrethroids

The discovery in the early 1800s that pyrethrum flowers (genus *Chrysanthemum*) ground to a fine powder had insecticidal activity ultimately led to the commercialization of "insect powder." The ground dried flowerheads were used originally to control body lice during the Napoleonic wars. By 1851, the use of pyrethrum powders for insect control was worldwide. However, in comparison with DDT, they were costly to produce and highly unstable until the advent of synthetic pyrethroids.

Naturally occurring pyrethrum, when isolated from extracts, consists of six active ingredients collectively known as the pyrethrins. These six insecticidally active pyrethrins are composed of esters of two acids and three alcohols. A wide range of acute oral toxicities in rats have been reported (LD_{50}'s of 200 to 1870 mg/kg). However, in contrast to their toxicity to mammals, the pyrethrins are highly toxic to houseflies as well as a variety of other insect pests. For these reasons, there are more uses for pyrethrum approved by the EPA than for any other insecticide.

Using the basic chemistry of pyrethrum, a variety of synthetic pyrethroids have been successfully introduced over several years (Fig. 11). The first synthetic pyrethroid, available in 1949, was allethrin. Allethrin is a synthetic duplicate of one of the four insecticidal components of pyrethrum, with a slightly more stable side chain requiring as many as 22 synthetic steps to produce the final product. A second generation of pyrethroids, including tetramethin, resmethrin, bioresmethrin, and phenothrin, became available during the 1960s. These lacked photostability; therefore, they have been confined mostly to indoor use against flying and crawling insects. In the 1970s, a third generation, including fenvalerate and permethrin, was synthesized. These were the first pyrethroids to gain wide agricultural use due to their exceptional insecticidal activity and photostability. They can remain as stable residues on foliage for up to 7 days. A fourth generation of pyrethroids containing an α-cyano group had even greater stability and insecticidal activity. The addition of the cyano group made these compounds less susceptible to metabolic degradation, resulting in 10-fold increases in toxicity compared to the third-generation pyrethroids. Included among these compounds are cyhalothrin, cypermethrin, bifenthrin, cyfluthrin, deltamethrin, esfenvalerate, fenpropathrin, fluvalinate, and tralomethrin. Although the stability of these compounds has increased substantially compared to the first-generation pyrethroids, they retain their ability to be nonpersistent in the environment. This, combined with their high degree of selectivity towards insects, has made them the standard against which new chemical insecticides are compared.

Pyrethroids have a high degree of selective toxicity to insects since most vertebrates rapidly hydrolyze the pyrethroids to their nontoxic acid and alcohol components. The ability of insects to metabolize pyrethroids is often counteracted by the addition of synergists to the formulated material to inhibit oxidative metabolism.

Pyrethroids exert their toxic effects primarily as a result of their ability to interact with the sodium channel of the nervous system. Their affinity for the sodium channel is high, with dissociation constants on the order of 4×10^{-8} M. Toxicity results largely from neuronal hyperexcitability. Other less important effects noted with pyrethroids include their ability to antagonize GABA-mediated inhibition, modulate nicotinic cholinergic transmission, and enhance noradrenalin release or actions on calcium ions.

Pyrethroids mainly interact at the sodium channel by inhibiting the inactivation of the sodium current following membrane depolarization. Although pyrethroids have a high affinity for open sodium channels, they possess little or no effect on closed or inactive channels, nor do they affect the activation of the sodium current by membrane depolarization. Thus, the amplitude and duration of action potentials are not affected. Instead the pyrethroids inhibit the regeneration of the current to normal levels. The result is that at low concentrations the tail current continues to act as a stimulus to the nerve membrane. At high concentrations (such as those that may never occur *in vivo*), the effect is to block the nerve entirely.

The symptoms of pyrethroid toxicity fall into two general classes, which are defined by differences in the inhibition of the sodium channel. Type I pyrethroids include most of the traditional pyrethroids that lack the α cyano substituent. They, like DDT, produce

ALLETHRIN

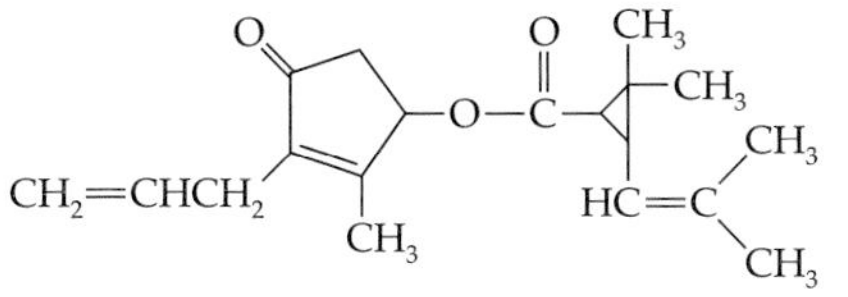

2-methyl-4-oxo-3-(2-propenyl)-2-cyclopenten-1yl 2,2 dimethyl-3-(2-methyl-1 -propenyl)cyclopropanecarboxylate

RESMETHRIN

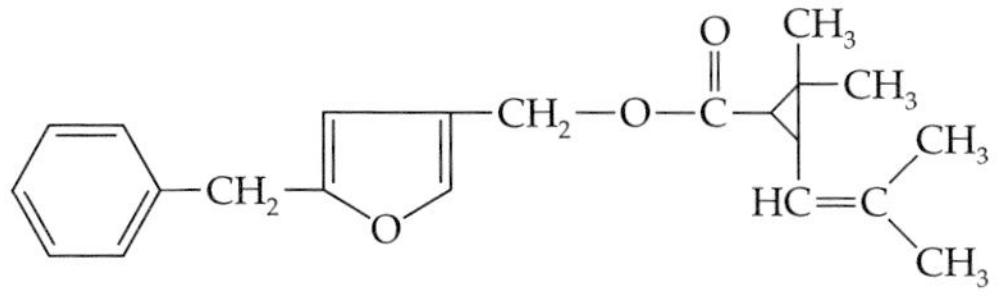

(5-phenylmethyl-3-furanyl)methyl 2,2-dimethyl-3-(2-methyl-1-propenyl) cyclopropanecarboxylate

PHENOTHRIN

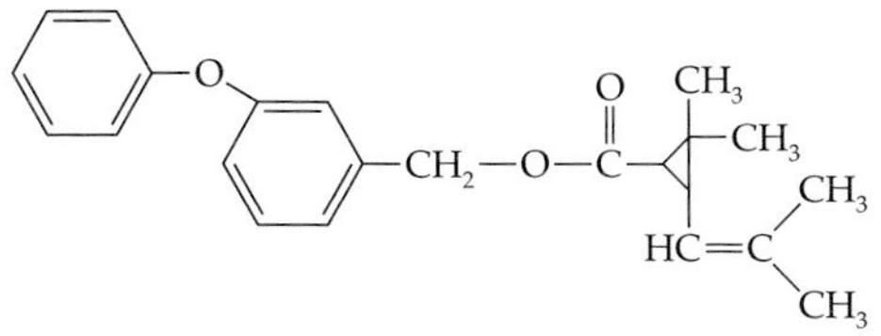

(3-phenoxyphenyl)methyl 2,2-dimethyl-3-(2-methyl-1-propenyl)-cyclopropanecarboxylate

PERMETHRIN

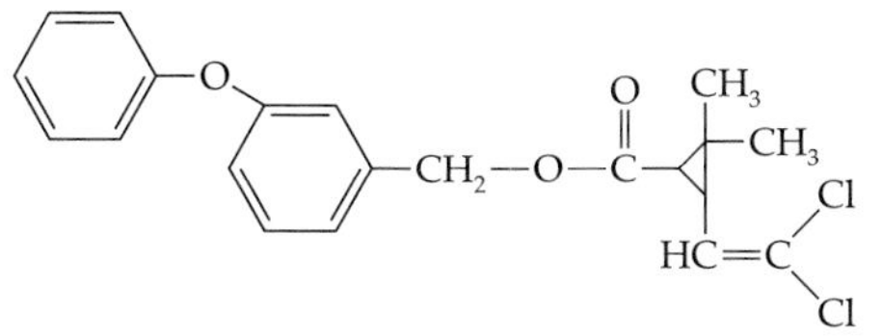

m-phenoxybenzyl (±)-cis, trans-3-(2,2-dichlorovinyl-2,2-dimethyl) cyclopropanecarboxylate

CYPERMETHRIN

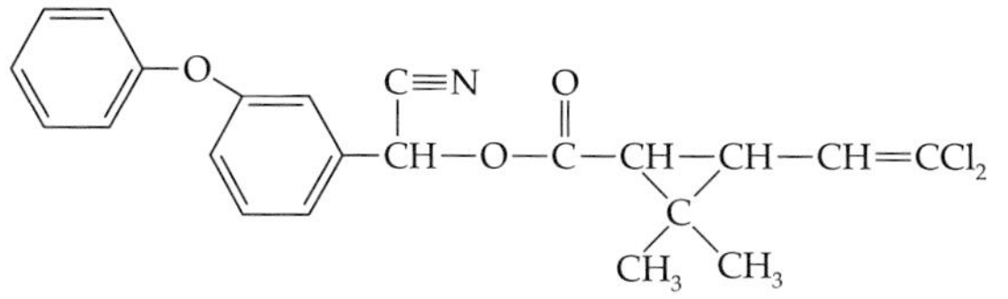

(±)-a-cyano (-phenoxyphenyl)-methyl (±)cis, trans 3-(2,3-dichloroethenyl)-2,2 dimethyl cyclopropanecarboxylate

FENVALERATE

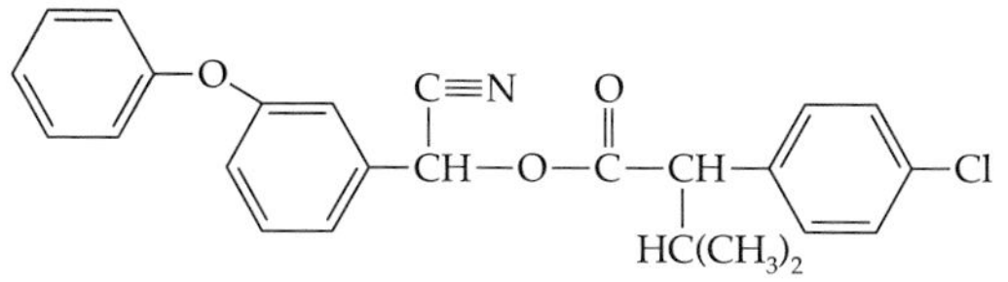

cyano (3-phenoxyphenyl)-methyl 4-chloro-a-(1-methyl-ethyl)-benzeneacetate

DELTAMETHRIN

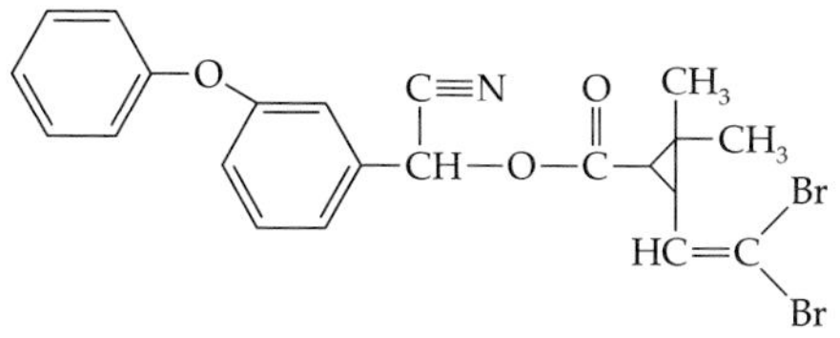

(1R(1(S),3))-cyano (3-phenoxyphenyl)-methyl 3-(2,2-dibromoethenyl)-2,2-dimethyl cyclopropanecarboxylate

TRALOMETHRIN

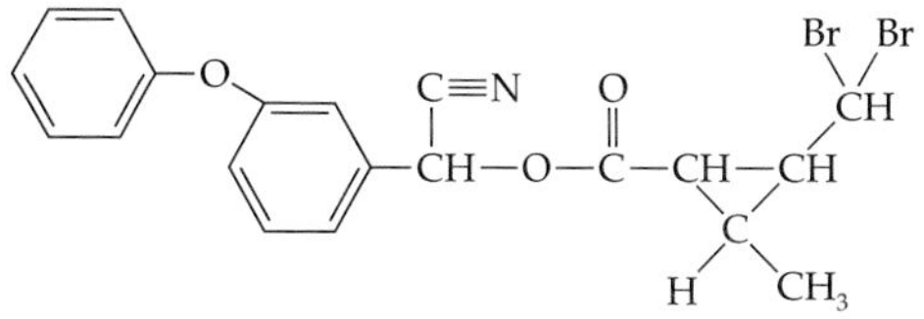

cyano (3-phenoxyphenyl)-methyl 2,2-dimethyl-3-(1,2,2,2-tetrabromomethyl) cyclopropanecarboxylate

FIGURE 11 Chemical structures of selected pyrethroids.

sodium tail currents with relatively short time constants. Poisoning involves a progressive development of fine whole-body tremor, exaggerated startle response, incoordinated twitching of dorsal muscles, hyperexcitability, and death. The tremors produced by pyrethroid poisoning result in large increases in the metabolism leading to hyperthermia, metabolic exhaustion, and death.

In contrast, type II pyrethroids, characterized structurally by the presence of the α-cyano group (in most cases), produce longer delays in sodium channel inactivation than those observed for type I. A greater variety of symptoms are expressed, including intense salivation, increased extensor tone in the hind limbs, incoordination, and the development of whole-body tremors, leading to tonic seizures, apnea, and death. Unlike with type I pyrethroids, animals treated with type II compounds generally have a decreased startle response to sound, although this is a complex response with high innate variability. Type II pyrethroids also do not produce the repetitive activity in the sensory nerves observed with type I pyrethroids.

Mammalian toxicity to pyrethroids is low. Only one human mortality has been attributed to pyrethroid poisoning, a 2-year-old child who consumed 14,000 mg of pyrethrum powder. Most injuries to humans have been due to the allergenic properties of the material. Because of the low toxicity to humans, pyrethroids are used in applications to control head lice.

Chronic studies of pyrethroid toxicity indicate that they cause liver enlargement, accompanied by bile duct proliferation and focal necrosis of liver cells. Pyrethroids have not been implicated as teratogens or mutagens. As a rule they do not cause cancer, although permethrin has been demonstrated to be carcinogenic in rats and mice. Allergenic responses have mostly been associated with pyrethroid powders or extracts, suggesting that they are not reactions to the chemicals themselves.

Novel Insecticide Chemistries

Modern insecticides must be highly active against the most economically important insects in order to be commercially viable and at the same time must demonstrate a high margin of safety for the environment, people, and animals. New chemistries often must represent novel modes of action, demonstrate minimal risk for the development of insect resistance or cross-resistance to other insecticides, be inexpensive to produce, and be commercially competitive in a changing market that includes approaches such as transgenic plant technologies. A surprisingly large number of new insecticide chemistries have recently been commercialized, some of which will be discussed here. Others not included here are avermectins, formamidines and pyrroles, and the insect growth regulators, discussed elsewhere.

Spinosyns

Recently, a new family of macrolides possessing insecticidal activity was produced by an actinomycete, *Saccharopolyspora spinosa*, discovered in soil samples collected in the Caribbean in 1982. These compounds are referred to as the spinosyns, the predominant forms being spinosyns A and D (Fig. 12). The compound contains a tetracyclic core consisting of a 12-member macrocyclic lactone fused to a 5,6,5-*cis-anti-trans*-tricyclic ring system. Also attached to the core is the amino sugar forosamine and a neutral sugar, 2,3,4-tri-*O*-methylrhamnose. This structure has been confirmed both by X-ray diffraction and chemical synthesis. Interestingly, spinosyns A and D differ only by the addition of a C_6 methyl group. A mixture of spinosyns A and D is currently registered for insect control in cotton and in vegetables.

The spinosyns truly represent a novel insecticide class in terms of both structure and mode of action. The symptoms of insect poisoning include lack of coordination, prostration, tremors, and involuntary muscle contraction, leading to paralysis and death. These characteristics suggest that the spinosyns are acting as nerve poisons. Electrophysiological studies support this hypothesis. Spinosyn A activates the nicotinic receptor via a novel mechanism and alters the function of the GABA-gated chloride channels. The exact mechanism is unknown but is different from that of the chloronicotinyl insecticides.

The spinosyns are highly active against economically important Lepidoptera (moths) with additional activity demonstrated against Coleoptera, Diptera, Hymenoptera, Isoptera, Orthoptera, Siphonaptera, Arachnida, and Thysanoptera. Using third instar tobacco budworm, *Heliothis virescens*, as an example, spinosyn A has an LD_{50} of 1.28 mg/kg, which compares favorably with that for the pyrethroid insecticide cypermethrin at 0.52 mg/kg. The level of insecticidal activity of spinosyn is similar to a variety of pyrethroids and is significantly higher than that of the organophosphorus and carbamate insecticides. The spinosyns act slightly slower than the pyrethroids but are rapid relative to *Bacillus thuringiensis* and act both by contact and ingestion. It also appears that they are

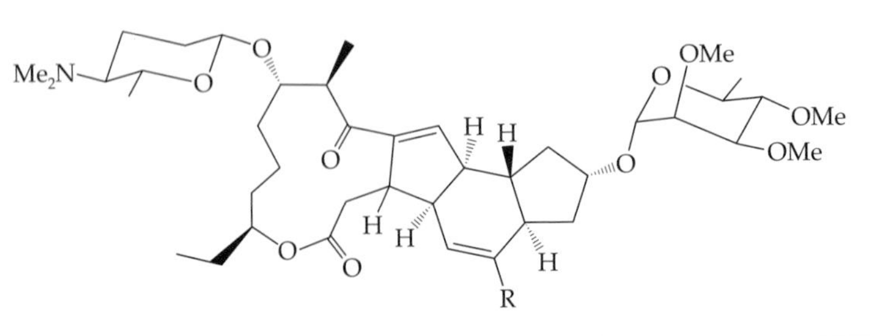

FIGURE 12 Chemical structure of spinosyn.

poorly metabolized by insect systems. Almost no metabolism was noted in the tobacco budworm after 24 hours, and piperonyl butoxide (an inhibitor of monooxygenase activity) increased permethrin toxicity but not the insecticidal activity of spinosyn A.

Spinosyn is nontoxic to many beneficial insects, including Neuroptera, Hemiptera, and Coleoptera and, although some toxicity was noted for honeybees and whitefly parasitoids, the activity was 10-fold less than that for cypermethrin. The spinosyns also demonstrate minimal toxicity in mammals, fish, and birds. In rats the oral LD_{50} for spinosyn A ranges from 3800 to 5000 mg/kg, compared to 9 mg/kg for the organophosphate methyl parathion, 307 for the carbamate carbaryl, and 247 for the pyrethroid cypermethrin. Spinosyn has no reproductive effects and is nonmutagenic, nonteratogenic, noncarcinogenic, and nonneurotoxic in mammals. It is classified by the U.S. EPA in the reduced risk category.

Chloronicotinyl Insecticides

Another natural product with insecticidal activity is nicotine (Fig. 13), extracted from the tobacco plant, *Nicotiana tabacum.* Although its insecticidal properties have been known for decades, the commercial development of this compound was minor because of its high mammalian toxicity and relatively low insecticidal activity.

In 1979 nithiazine, a nitromethylenyl heterocyclic compound (Fig. 13), was discovered. Interestingly, nithiazine resembled, in part, the structure of nicotine and also acted at the same receptor but, unlike nicotine, was highly active against insects while possessing minimal mammalian toxicity. As a result of this discovery, a new insecticide class was born, the chloronicotinyl insecticides, which emphasize essential structural similarities and the same mode of action as nicotine. In 1992, imidacloprid (Fig. 13) was introduced as a new insecticide. Later the open-ringed nitenpyram and the cyanoimine acetamiprid (Fig. 13) were introduced. Imidacloprid and nitenpyram are most active against sucking insects, while acetamiprid is especially toxic to the economically important lepidopterous pests. These insecticides are noteworthy because of their unique plant-systemic and translaminar properties. This allows their use as seed and seedling treatments, which is important in accurate plant dosing and in minimizing field treatments.

Imidacloprid poisoning in the American cockroach, *Periplaneta americana,* is characterized in sequence by a loss of leg strength, leg tremors followed by body shaking, and death. The symptoms are similar to those of the housefly poisoned with nicotine and suggest the involvement of the nervous system in intoxication. Neurophysiological studies have confirmed that imidacloprid is an agonist at the postsynaptic nicotinic acetylcholine receptor (nAChR). It appears that the nitro group in imidacloprid and nitenpyram and the cyano group in acetamiprid along with the tandem amine (Fig. 13) are the essential moieties for chloronicotinyl binding with nAChR. The pyridyl portions of imidacloprid, nitenpyram, and acetamiprid are, in comparison, subsidiary in receptor bonding. The selectivity of the chloronicotinyl compounds for insects as opposed to mammals can be partly explained by the differences in the ionization of the pyrrolidine nitrogen from that found in nicotine. Imidacloprid is poorly ionized in neutral media, in contrast to nicotine, and thus passes easily through insect lipophilic barriers. This difference in ionization and the

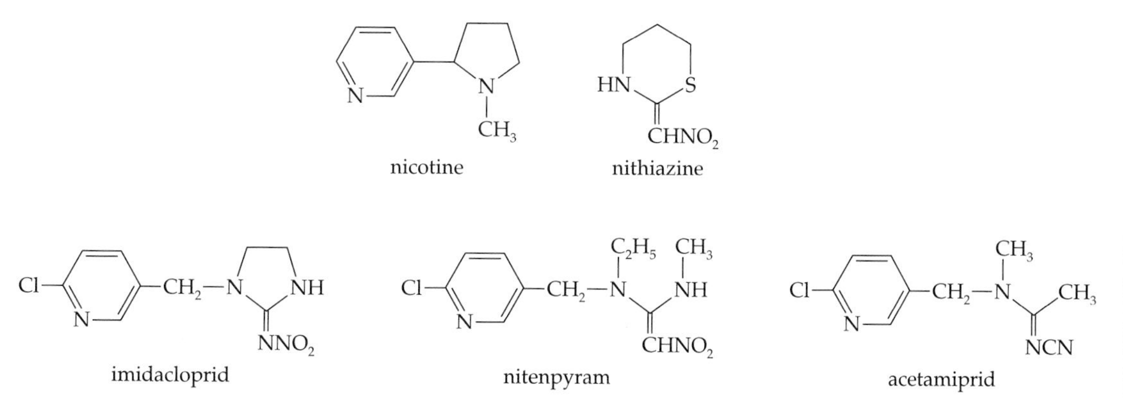

FIGURE 13 Chemical structures of nicotine, nithiazine, and commercial chloronicotinyl insecticides.

expected differences in the nAChR receptor between insects and vertebrates are most likely responsible for the lower mammalian toxicity of imidacloprid.

The chloronicotinyl insecticides have limited mammalian toxicity. The imidacloprid acute oral LD_{50}'s in mouse and rat are approximately 100 and 435 mg/kg, respectively. These values were similar to those for acetamiprid (190 and 180 mg/kg, respectively) and lower than the acute toxicity for nitenpyram (1070 and 1630 mg/kg, respectively). Acute dermal toxicity is > 2000 mg/kg for all these compounds. Chronic studies failed to detect significant problems.

Imidacloprid is toxic to birds with an LD_{50} ranging from 25 to 50 mg/kg, although it appears to also be a repellent. The insecticide can essentially be excluded as a hazard to algae, water fleas, and fish. Soil microbial activity, respiration, and nitrogen mineralization were unaffected by imidacloprid.

Fipronil

A common target for insecticide research and development in the past has been the insect nervous system and this has resulted in numerous insecticide classes. Fipronil is the first commercial insecticide developed from phenyl pyrazole chemistry (Fig. 14) and is another example, along with the nicotinoids, of the importance of target-based research in insecticide discovery and development.

Fipronil was discovered in 1987 and commercialized in 1993 for pest control in agriculture, animal health, and public health. Its major strengths include broad-spectrum activity, lack of cross-resistance with existing commercial products, good soil and foliar persistence, effectiveness at low dosages, excellent crop tolerance, selectivity against pest species, bird repellency, limited soil mobility, some plant systematic activity, plant growth enhancement, and fungicidal activity. It is also used as a systemic pesticide for tick and flea control on dogs and cats.

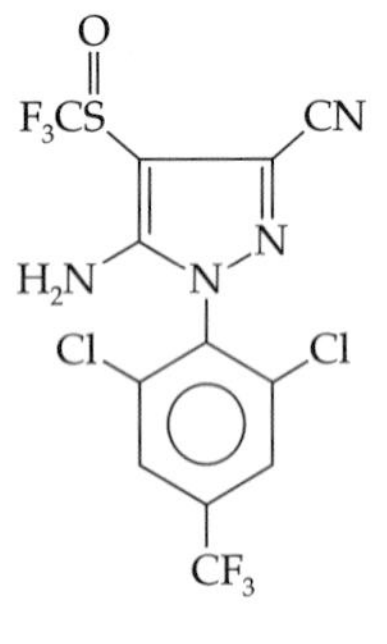

$F_3CS(O)$, CN, N, H_2N, N, Cl, Cl, CF_3

FIGURE 14
Chemical structure of fipronil.

The site of action of fipronil is the GABA-gated chloride channel in the insect nervous system. Fipronil acts as an antagonist to alter chloride ion movement, resulting in disruption of central nervous system activity and death. Insect specificity relative to mammals is the result of differences in the binding affinity of fipronil to chloride channel membranes. This is a unique mode of action from other insecticides.

Fipronil is a reversible GABA-receptor inhibitor with moderate mammalian toxicity. The acute oral LD_{50}'s for rat and mouse are 97 and 95 mg/kg, respectively, while the acute dermal LD_{50}'s in rat and rabbit are > 2000 and 354 mg/kg, respectively. The acute inhalation LC_{50} in rat is 0.682 mg/l. Fipronil produced no skin or eye irritation in rabbit, is not mutagenic, is not teratogenic, and has no effects on reproduction. Based on life-time feeding studies in rodents, the insecticide is not a human carcinogen. Fipronil is considered toxic to birds in the family Galliformes and nontoxic to other species. However, because of the high aversion of birds to fipronil-treated seeds, the risk to avian species is greatly reduced. There is no effect on bird reproduction. Fipronil is highly toxic to some aquatic fish. The acute 96-h LC_{50}'s for bluegill sunfish, rainbow trout, and European carp are 85 (NOEC = 43), 248 (33.8), and 430 (73) $\mu g/l$, respectively. However, because of the high insecticidal activity and low field rates needed for fipronil, its low water solubility, and its high binding coefficient to soil, its bioavailability to fish is greatly minimized and its toxicity should not limit its use even in rice paddies. Fipronil is considered nontoxic to aquatic plants, earthworms, and soil microflora. The insecticide is degraded in the environment by sulfoxide reduction, oxidation to the sulfone, degradation of the CN moiety to an amide, and photolytic elimination of the sulfoxide. Fipronil is absorbed passively across the mammalian digestive system and becomes widely distributed, with the highest concentration in the fatty tissues. The major route of elimination is the feces.

Juvenile Hormone Analogs

Most insecticides target the insect nervous system and achieve their specificity based on receptor and/or pharmacokinetic differences that exist between economically important insect pests and other organisms. An alternative approach is to identify biological functions that are exclusive to insects. Good examples of this are the insect juvenile hormones, methyl esters of farnesoic acid C10,11 epoxide (JH III) (Fig. 15) and their related homologs. The juvenile hormone regulates many aspects of insect life, including insect embryogenesis, larval growth and development, metamorphosis, reproduction, diapause, and migration. Because the juvenile hormone for the most part is not found outside of Insecta, its analogs are selective and safe insecticides.

Some common juvenile hormone analogs registered as insecticides include methoprene for the control of mosquitoes and fleas and hydroprene for the control of cockroaches (Fig. 15). Because these compounds are sensitive to photodegradation, their application has been somewhat limited to indoor uses. Fenoxycarb is effective both for household insects and agricultural pests like the leafroller and Codling moth. Pyriproxyfen (Fig. 15) is the most recent juvenile hormone analog. It has been registered for use both indoors and in the field against urban and medically important pests, such as fleas, mosquitoes, and roaches, and against agricultural pests, including thrips, aphids, and scales. Because these compounds are highly active against insects and considered to be very safe for animals and humans, they can be used in and around the home and in aquatic environments. The IC_{50} of pyriproxyfen in water for control of the mosquito, *Aedes aeqypti,* is as low as 0.0039 ppb, and the topical dose in houseflies, *Musca domestica,* to inhibit 50% emergence from the pupa is 0.00033 μg/prepupa.

Juvenile hormone analogs such as methoprene, hydroprene, fenoxycarb, and pyriproxyfen mimic the structure and function of the natural insect hormone and presumably bind to the insect juvenile hormone receptor. Critical structural features for juvenile hormone biological activity include the 12-carbon juvenile hormone backbone (JH III), the C10,11 epoxide, and the methyl ester. Precisely controlled changes in juvenile hormone esterase and juvenile hormone epoxide-hydrolase activity correlated with changes in the rate of juvenile hormone biosynthesis are responsible for the regulation of the titer and insect development. The insecticidal analogs contain functional mimics of the epoxide and ester moieties of the juvenile hormone that are poorly metabolized or not metabolized at all by juvenile hormone metabolic enzymes.

The stages most sensitive to control by insecticidal juvenoids are early embryogenesis, late larval development, metamorphosis, and adult reproduction. The timing of the applications to these stages is critical to insecticidal activity. Since young larvae are not susceptible, larval pests are not usually the target for juvenile hormone mimics. However, the development and commercialization of juvenile hormone insecticidal mimics were important breakthroughs, demonstrating that basic knowledge of insect function could

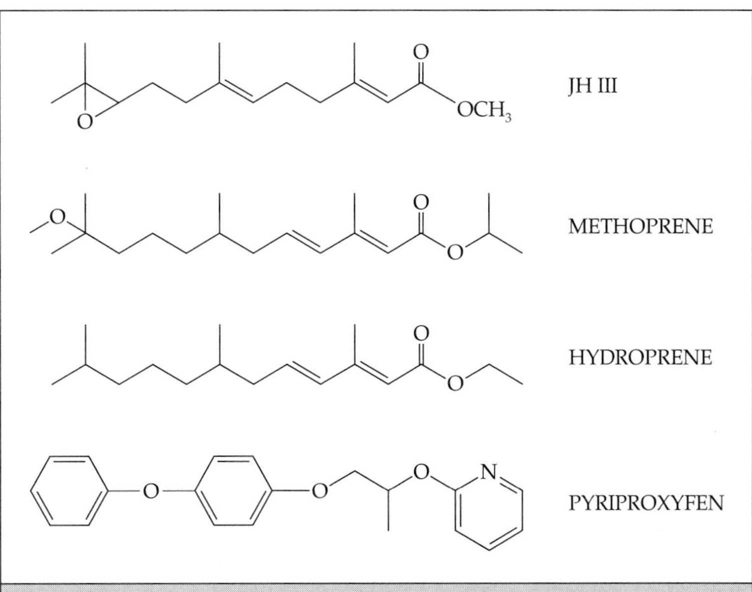

FIGURE 15 Chemical structures of juvenile hormone III and the insecticidal juvenoids: methoprene, hydroprene, fenoxycarb, and pyriproxyfen.

be used a priori to direct insecticide structure–activity studies and the development of new insecticide chemistry.

Bacillus thuringiensis (Bt) and Bt Recombinant Plant Technology

The sporangium of the bacteria *Bacillus thuringiensis* produces a parasporal, proteinaceous crystalline inclusion with widespread application as a biological control agent. Several varieties of *Bt* have been described on the basis of antigenic activity and varying selective toxicities against numerous insect species. Much of the *Bt* research has concentrated on *Bt* var. *kurstaki* because of its larvicidal activity against agricultural pests in the insect order Lepidoptera. However, there has also been considerable interest in *Bt tenebrionis* because of its activity against agriculturally important beetles and *Bt israelensis* because of its activity against medically important flies and mosquitoes. Today, the *Bt* genes are classified based on their structures and biological activities. The *cry*I, *cry*II, *cry*III, and *cry*IV genes are toxic to Lepidoptera, Diptera and Lepidoptera, Coleoptera, and Diptera, respectively. *Bt* poisoning results from insect ingestion of the toxin. *Bt* toxin proteins bind to the gut brush border, disrupting the normal function of the insect ventriculus.

Bt recombinant plant technologies have revolutionized our current thinking about insect pest management. *Bt* genes are expressed in a wide variety of commercial crop plants, the most noteworthy being cotton and corn. In the summer of 1996, over 1.8 million acres of farmland in the southern United States was planted in genetically engineered cotton expressing one of the *Bt* genes toxic to moths. The future expansion of this technology is expected to have important environmental benefits due to a reduction of the use of broad-spectrum insecticides. The *Bt* toxins are different from many of the conventional chemical insecticides in having high specificity for a small number of target pests with no toxicity to beneficial insects, wildlife, or humans. Because the recombinant insecticide is synthesized by the plant, the pest species are only exposed to the toxin at the time of feeding. The primary concern regarding the use of *Bt* genes in transgenic crops is the risk of insect pest populations evolving a genetically based resistance to the toxin. Although there was at one time some skepticism about the potential of insects to evolve resistance to *Bt*, there is now a significant set of laboratory and field data suggesting that many insect pest species are capable of evolving high levels of resistance to a number of commonly used *Bt* toxins.

The commercially available *Bt* toxins (especially those used in transgenic crops) demonstrate no toxic activity outside of Insecta and have limited activity even among insects. This is partly due to the selectivity of the *Bt* toxin for receptors in the insect digestive system. In addition, the alkaline insect gut along with protease activity dissolves the protein crystal form of the toxin produced by the bacteria and activates its insecticidal activity. In contrast, the vertebrate stomach is highly acidic and the toxin is rapidly hydrolyzed to amino acids. However, the solubilized parasporal crystalline protein of *Bt israelensis* is highly toxic to vertebrates when injected into the peritoneal cavity. For example, the LD_{50}'s for mouse and Japanese quail are 1.3 and 22.7 mg/kg, respectively. The toxin is not lethal when introduced by intratracheal, intranasal, intravenous, subcutaneous, and oral administration, demonstrating even in this unique case the safety of this insecticide. The toxic activity in mice was attributed to a low-molecular-weight protein component of the natural protein crystal different from the mosquito protein toxin.

Synergists

Synergists are chemicals that, when co-administered, increase the toxicity of other toxicants. As used in the agrochemical field, synergism describes those cases where the synergist is relatively nontoxic when administered alone. The word "potentiation" is used to describe those cases where both chemicals are toxic but where the toxicity upon co-administration is significantly more than additive.

The best-known insecticide synergists are methylenedioxyphenyl (benzodioxole) compounds, particularly piperonyl butoxide but also including sesamex, sulfoxide, and propyl isome (Fig. 16), all of which function by the inhibition of cytochrome P450. MGK 264, a substituted dicarboximide, also functions by inhibition of cytochrome P450 (Fig. 16).

The mode of action of the methylenedioxyphenyl insecticide synergists involves the formation of a stable metabolite-inhibitory complex with cytochrome P450. This results from the interaction of a carbene with the heme iron of the cytochrome. This carbene is formed by the elimination of water from the hydroxylated product formed by cytochrome P450 attack on the methylene carbon. Thus, insecticide synergists such as piperonyl butoxide are suicide substrates for cytochrome P450. Although MGK 264 is also known to be an inhibitor of cytochrome P450, a stable inhibitory complex has not been demonstrated. Herbicide synergists, of which tridiphane is an excellent exam-

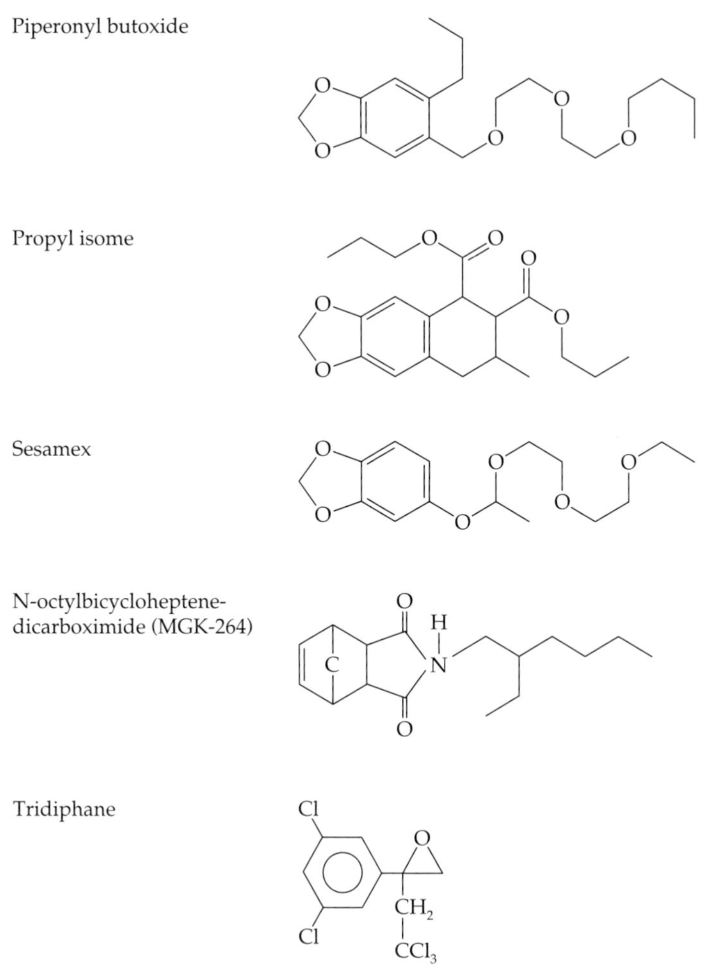

FIGURE 16 Chemical structures of several synergists.

ple, function by the inhibition of the plant glutathione *S*-transferases involved in herbicide detoxication.

The acute toxicity of commercial synergists to mammals is uniformly low. For example the LD_{50}'s in rats are MGK 264, 2800 mg/kg; piperonyl butoxide, >7500 mg/kg; propyl isome, 1500 mg/kg; sesamex, 2000 to 2270 mg/kg; and tridiphane, 1743 mg/kg. When dealing with chemicals whose mode of action is the inhibition of xenobiotic-metabolizing enzymes, the possibility of interactions with other chemicals, for example prescription drugs, should always be considered a potential hazard.

In mammals, methylenedioxyphenyl synergists act as both inhibitors and inducers of cytochrome P450. Because the time course for cytochrome P450 inhibition is considerably more rapid than that for induction, the overall time course for enzyme activity affected by a methylenedioxyphenyl compound is typically biphasic. Following an acute dose, first inhibition is apparent, followed by a return to the control levels and, subsequently, an increase in activity above the control levels. As indicated previously, the inhibition in both insects and mammals is due to the formation of a stable complex with the heme iron of the cytochrome. Induction is more complex and recently has been related to specific isoforms. Insecticide synergists such as piperonyl butoxide can, in the mouse, induce Cyp 1A1, 1B2, and 2B10. Cyp 1A1 is induced only at the highest doses by an Ah-receptor-dependent mechanism. Cyp 1A2, on the other hand, is induced by both Ah-receptor-dependent and Ah-receptor-independent mechanisms. The latter mechanism was recently confirmed by the use of Ah-receptor-knock-out mice.

Although tridiphane is known to function in plants as an inhibitor of glutathione S-transferase, in mammals it is both an inhibitor and an inducer of cytochrome P450. Tridiphane is a peroxisome proliferator in rodents and, like other peroxisome proliferators, induces CYP4A1 and epoxide hydrolase. The CYP4A enzymes are constitutive proteins involved in the hydroxylation of fatty acids. The importance of peroxisome proliferation in human health has not yet been clearly defined because many aspects appear to be rodent specific. Tridiphane is also a cytochrome P450 inhibitor in mammals, although the isoform specificity is quite different from that for induction, with the effect being selective for CYP2B10. It is not known whether the observed ability of tridiphane to function as an insecticide synergist in houseflies is due to its ability to inhibit glutathione S-transferase, cytochrome P450, or both.

Some methylenedioxyphenyl compounds, particularly the natural products, safrole and isosafrole, have been known to be carcinogenic. Various members of this chemical class have also been shown to be cocarcinogens, to induce fatty livers, and to affect drug metabolism and clearance. It is only recently, however, with the demonstration that very high doses of piperonyl butoxide cause tumors in rodents, that any of the commercial synergists have been shown to have carcinogenic properties.

FUTURE DIRECTIONS

As we look into the future, pesticides will become an increasingly more important factor in the production of food and fiber. This will be driven by population increases, reductions in farmland as a result of urbanization, and simple agroeconomics, which are driven by increasing fuel and labor costs as well as global competition. The need for safe pesticides will also become more intense due to increased pesticide use in the urban environment and because of increased demands by the general public for land and water resources free of contaminants.

There is no question that the older-generation pesticides like the organophosphates and organochlorines will have a diminishing role in pest control due to their relatively high mammalian toxicity and demonstrated carcinogenicity. This is especially true compared to the newer pesticides such as the spinosyns, *Bt*, and others. Future pesticides are more likely to be highly selective, possessing minimal vertebrate toxicity, which will allow their use at ultralow levels for control. Pesticide toxicology will focus less on acute toxicity and more on long-term chronic effects. The discovery of protein toxins like *Bt* with no practical vertebrate toxicity, as well as applications in transgenic–recombinant technologies, has produced a new standard of pesticide safety that is not likely to be exceeded soon. However, the economic success of genetic engineering in crop protection and pest control is still not certain and threatens this approach.

One inescapable reality, which will continue as long as pesticides are used, is the evolution of biological resistance to these control measures. Resistance can be delayed by better technologies in resistance detection and improved management strategies in pesticide use. However, until we fully understand resistance mechanisms and develop methods to reverse resistance, this problem will continue to require us to develop new pesticides with novel modes of action. The possible targets for new pesticide research and development is finite, limited by the physiology of the target organism. We will need to continue to be innovative in pesticide discovery, management, and toxicology to maintain our current edge in pest control.

Bibliography

Bauer, L. S. (1995). Resistance: a threat to the insecticidal crystal proteins of *Bacillus thuringiensis*. *Fla. Ent.* **78,** 4 414–443.

Berg, D., and Plempel, M. (eds.) (1988). "Sterol Biosynthesis Inhibitors." Ellis Horwood Ltd., Chichester, England.

Birnbaum, L. S. (1994). Endocrine effects of prenatal exposure to PCBs, dioxins, and other xenobiotics: Implications for policy and future research. *Environ. Health Perspect.* **102,** 676–679.

Colburn, T., Dumanoski, D., and Myers, J. P. (1996). "Our Stolen Future. Are We Threatening Our Fertility, Intelligence, and Survival? A Scientific Detective Story." Dutton, New York.

Cole, L. M., Nicholson, R. A., and Casida, J. E. (1993). Action of phenyl pyrazole insecticides at the GABA-gated chloride channel. *Pestic. Biochem. Physiol.* **46,** 47–54.

DeAmicis, C. V., Dripps, J. E., Hatton, C. J., and Karr, L. L. (1997). Physical and biological properties of the spinosyns: Novel macrolide pest control agents from fermentation. *In* "Phytochemicals for Pest Control" (P. A. Hedin *et al.* eds.), pp. 144–154. American Chemical Society, Washington D.C.

Fischhoff, D. A. (1996). Insect-resistant crop plants. *In* "Biotechnology and Integrated Pest Management" (G. J. Persley, ed.), pp. 214–227. CAB International, Cambridge, UK.

Gallo, M. A., and Lawryk, N. J. (1991). Organic phosphorus pesticides. *In* "Handbook of Pesticide Toxicology, Vol 2" (W. J. Hayes, Jr. and E. R. Laws, Jr., eds.), pp. 917–1123. Academic Press, San Diego, CA.

Gant, D. B., Bloomquist, J. R., Ayad, H. M., and Chalmers, A. E. (1990). A comparison of mammalian and insect GABA receptor chloride channels. *Pestic. Sci.* **30,** 355–357.

Gasser, C. S., and Fraley, R. T. (1989). Genetically engineering plants for crop improvement. *Science* **244,** 1293–1299.

Gill, S. S., Cowles, E. A., and Pietrantonio, P. V. (1992). The mode of action of *Bacillus thuringiensis* endotoxins. *Annu. Rev. Entomol.* **37,** 615–663.

Gould, F., Anderson, A., Jones, A., Sumerford, D., Heckel, D. G., Lopez, J., Micinski, S., Leonard, R., and Laster, M. (1997). Initial frequency of alleles for resistance to *Bacillus thuringiensis* toxins in field populations of *Heliothis virescens. Proc. Nat. Acad. Sci.* USA **94,** 3519–3523.

Guillette, L. J., Jr., Gross, T. S., Masson, G. R., Matter, J. M., Percival, H. F., and Woodward, A. R. (1994). Developmental abnormalities of the gonad and abnormal sex hormone concentrations in juvenile alligators from contaminated and control lakes in Florida. *Environ. Health Perspect.* **102,** 680–688.

Hance, R. J., and Holly, K. (1990). The properties of herbicides. *In* "Weed Control Handbook: Principles" (R. J. Hance and K. Holly, eds.), pp. 75–125. Blackwell Scientific Publications, Oxford.

Harrison, S. K., and Loux, M. M. (1995). Chemical weed management *In* "Handbook of Weed Management Systems" (A. E. Smith, ed.), pp. 101–153. Marcel Dekker, New York.

Hayes, W. J., Jr., and Laws, E. R., Jr. (eds.) (1991). "Handbook of Pesticide Toxicology." Academic Press, San Diego, CA.

Hodgson, E., and Levi, P. E. (1996). Pesticides: An important but underused model for the environmental health sciences. *Environ. Health Perspect.* **104,** 97–106.

Hodgson, E., Ryu, D-Y., Adams, N., and Levi, P. E. (1995) Biphasic responses in synergistic reactions. *Toxicology* **105,** 211–216.

Höfte, H., and Whiteley, H. R. (1989). Insecticidal crystal proteins of *Bacillus thuringiensis. Microbiol. Rev.* **53,** 242–255.

Institute of Medicine (1994). "Veterans and Agent Orange: Health Effects of Herbicides Used in Vietnam." National Academy Press, Washington, D.C.

Kavlock, R. J., Daston, G. P., DeRosa, C., Fenner-Crisp, P., Gray, L. E., Kaattari, S., Lucier, G., Luster, M., Mac, M. J., Maczka, C., Miller, R., Moore, J., Rolland, R., Scott, G., Sheehan, D. M., Sinks, T., and Tilson, H. A. (1996). Research needs for the risk assessment of health and environmental effects of endocrine disruptors: A report of the U.S. EPA-sponsored workshop. *Environ. Health Perspect.* **104,** 715–740.

Kirst, H. A., Michel, K. H., Mynderse, J. S., Chio, E. H., Yao, R. C., Nakatsukasa, W. M., Boeck, L. D., Occlowitz, J., Paschal, J. W., Deeter, J. B., and Thompson, G. D. (1992). Discovery, isolation and structure elucidation of a family of structurally unique, fermentation derived tetracyclic macrolides. *In* "Synthesis and Chemistry of Agrochemicals III" (D. R. Baker *et al.*, eds.), pp. 214–225. ACS Symposium Series No. 504. American Chemical Society, Washington D.C.

Kuhr, R. J., and Dorough, H. W. (1976). "Carbamate Insecticides: Chemistry, Biochemistry and Toxicology." CRC Press, Boca Raton, FL.

Mellanby, K. (1992). "The DDT Story." The British Crop Protection Council, Farnham, UK.

Mertz, F. P., and Yao, R. C. (1990). *Saccharopolyspora spinosa sp. nov.* isolated from soil collected in a sugar mill rum still. *Int. J. Syst. Bacteriol.* **40,** 34–39.

Minamida, I., Iwanaga, K., Tabuchi, T., Uneme, H., Dantsuji, H., and Okauchi, T. (1993). Synthesis and insecticidal activity of acyclic nitroethene compounds containing a 3-pyridylmethylamino group. *J. Pestic. Sci.* **18,** 31–40.

Nene, Y. L., and Thapliyal, P. N. (1993). "Fungicides in Plant Disease Control." International Science Publisher, New York.

Pfluger, W., and Schmuck, R. (1991). Ecotoxicological profile of imidacloprid. *Pflanzenschutz Nachr. Bayer.* **44,** 145–158.

Roe, R. M., Burton, J. D., and Kuhr, R. J. (1997). "Herbicide Activity: Toxicology, Biochemistry and Molecular Biology," Ios Press, Amsterdam.

Roe, R. M., Kallapur, V. L., Dauterman, W. C., Edens, F. W., Mayes, M. E., Held, G. A., Kawanishi, C. Y., Alford, A. R., and Clifford, C. W. (1991). Vertebrate toxicology of the solubilized parasporal crystalline proteins of *Bacillus thuringiensis* subsp. *israelensis. In* "Pesticides and the Future: Toxicological Studies of Risks and Benefits" (E. Hodgson *et al.*, eds.), pp. 119–130. North Carolina State University, Raleigh, NC.

Roe, R. M., and Venkatesh, K. (1990). Metabolism of juvenile hormones: Degradation and titer regulation. *In* "Morphogenetic Hormones of Arthropods" (A. P. Gupta, ed.), Vol. 1, pp. 126–179. Rutgers University Press, New Brunswick, NJ.

Rosenstock, L., Kiefer, M., Daniell, W. E., McConnell, R., and Claypoole, K. (1991). Chronic central system effects of acute organophosphate pesticide intoxication. *Lancet* **338,** 223–227.

Schoonover, J. R., and Larson, L. L. (1995). Laboratory activity of spinosad on non-target beneficial arthropods, 1994. *Arthropod Management Tests* **20,** 357.

Schroeder, M. E., and Flattum, R. F. (1984). The mode of action and neurotoxic properties of the nitromethylene heterocycle insecticides. *Pestic. Biochem. Physiol.* **22,** 148–160.

Soloway, S. B., Henry, A. C., Kollmeyer, W. D., Padgent, W. M., Powell, J. E., Roman, S. A., Tieman, C. H., Corey, R. A., and Horne, C. A. (1979). Nitromethylene insecticides. *In* "Advances in Pesticide Science, Part 2" (H. Geissbuhler *et al.*, eds.), pp. 206–227. Pergamon, Oxford.

Sone, S., Nagata K., Tsuboi, S., and Shono, T. (1994). Toxic symptoms and neural effect of a new class of insecticide, imidacloprid, on the American cockroach, *Periplaneta americana* (L.). *J. Pestic. Sci.* **19,** 69–72.

Sparks, T. C. (1996). Toxicology of insecticides and acaricides. *In* "Cotton Insects and Mites: Characterization and Management," (E. G. King *et al.*, eds.), pp. 283–322. The Cotton Foundation Publisher, Memphis, TN.

Sparks, T. C., Thompson, G. D., Larson, L. L., Kirst, H. A., Jantz, O. K., Worden, T. V., Hertlein, M. B., and Busacca, J. D. (1995). Biological characteristics of the spinosyns: A new class of naturally derived insect control agents. *In* "Proceedings of the 1995 Beltwide Cotton Production Conference," pp. 903–907. National Cotton Council, Memphis, TN.

Tabashnik, B. E. (1994). Evolution of resistance to *Bacillus thuringiensis. Annu. Rev. Entomol.* **39,** 47–79.

Yamamoto, I. (1965). Nicotinoids as insecticides. *In* "Advances in Pest Control Research" (R. L. Metcalf, ed.), pp. 231–260. Interscience Publishers, New York.

Ware, G. W. (1989). "The Pesticide Book." Thomson Publications, Fresno, CA.

CHAPTER

29

Dioxin and Dioxin-like Polychlorinated Hydrocarbons and Biphenyls

GÜNTER KOSS*,†, DETLEF WÖLFLE†,‡

*Department of Labor, Health and Social Affairs, Hamburg, Germany

†Department of Toxicology University of Hamburg Medical School Hamburg, Germany

‡Federal Institute for Health Protection of Consumers and Veterinary Medicine, Berlin, Germany

INTRODUCTION

Prominent members of the class of polychlorinated hydrocarbons are characterized by the molecular structure of dibenzo-*p*-dioxin, dibenzofuran, and biphenyl, with different chlorine substitution patterns at the aromatic rings (Fig. 1). The physical and chemical stability of the higher chlorinated compounds along with their lipophilicity contributes to their ubiquitous occurrence and to efficient bioaccumulation via the aquatic and terrestrial food chains. Other related products, such as the polychlorinated naphthalenes, quarterphenyls, and azoxybenzenes, are of minor relevance because of their limited use.

Of more regional interest are the polybrominated biphenyls, brominated analogs of chlorinated biphenyls. From a chemical and analytical point of view, brominated and mixed halogenated hydrocarbons should be mentioned as well. The group of mixed brominated and chlorinated dibenzo-*p*-dioxins and dibenzofurans are combustion products. Preliminary data suggest that there are minor differences in their toxic potencies compared to the chlorinated analogs. Although the release of polychlorinated hydrocarbons into the environment was substantially decreased during the last decade, their global occurrence has not ceased.

POLYCHLORINATED DIBENZO-*p*-DIOXINS AND DIBENZOFURANS

2,3,7,8-Tetrachlorodibenzo-*p*-dioxin (TCDD) has been described as the most toxic human-made chemical in sensitive rodent species such as guinea pig. Worldwide attention has been focused on the toxicity of TCDD especially since the 1976 accident at a chemical plant in Seveso, Italy, where thousands of residents in the area were heavily exposed to TCDD. Only a few other chemicals are discussed as equivocally as the ubiquitous dioxin-like compounds. The different approaches of national and intergovernmental organizations to risk assessment are a major challenge in appraising very low environmental concentrations and body burdens. More than two decades of intensive research brought a basic understanding of the molecular mechanism of action of TCDD via high-affinity binding to a cellular receptor protein; however, the complex interactions of factors leading to the

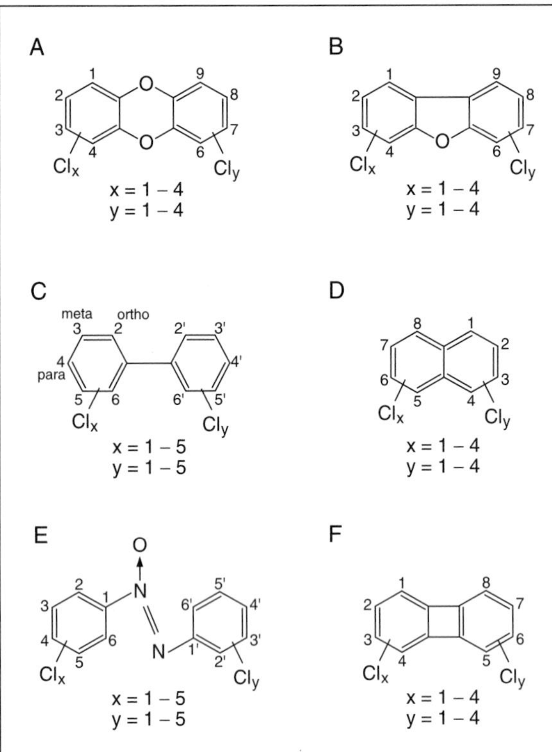

FIGURE 1 General molecular structure and numbering of polychlorinated dibenzo-*p*-dioxins (A), dibenzofurans (B), biphenyls (C), naphthalenes (D), azoxybenzenes (E), and biphenylenes (F). Numbers identify the position of carbon bound chlorine. x and y indicate the number of chlorine atoms per ring. Ring positions of biphenyl structure are also characterized by the terms ortho, meta, and para, as shown for the numbers 2, 3, and 4, respectively.

highly cell-specific effects of dioxin-like compounds are yet unknown.

TCDD serves as the prototype congener for a large series of halogenated aromatic hydrocarbons, including chlorinated and brominated dioxins (PCDDs and PBDD), furans (PCDFs and PBDFs), and biphenyls (Fig. 1). These compounds are approximate isosteromers and produce a characteristic pattern of biochemical and toxic responses in animals of the same species, strain, sex, and age as does TCDD. TCDD is one of 75 possible chlorinated dibenzo-*p*-dioxin congeners. The toxic potency of these congeners is due to the number and position of chlorine substitutions on the dibenzo-*p*-dioxin molecule. Dioxins and furans with decreased lateral (2,3,7,8) or increased nonlateral chlorine and bromine substituents are less potent than TCDD. A relative ranking scheme for the toxic potencies of congeners has led to the toxic equivalency factor (TEF) approach based on the congeners potency compared to TCDD.

Dioxins have no industrial or commercial use and have been produced as inadvertent trace contaminants in the synthesis of chlorophenol-based pesticides, chlorine bleaching, and other industrial (e.g., metallurgical) processes. Furans are also formed as inadvertent by-products in the production and use of PCBs. High-temperature pyrolysis, combustion of organic compounds (e.g., in municipal, hazardous-and medical-waste incinerators, and sintering processes) are the major sources of emission of dioxins and furans. The contribution of accidental fires, cable burning, wood combustion, coal-fired utilities and diesel engines to dioxin emissions is less reliably established. In the 1990s dioxin sources were substantially reduced or eliminated due to changes in the paper industry, technological improvements in waste incineration, the ban imposed to the use of pentachlorophenol in wood preservatives, and the decreasing use of leaded gasoline with halogenated scavengers. These decisions may be responsible for decreasing dioxin body burdens in people in industrialized countries.

Atmospheric chlorinated aromatic hydrocarbons emitted from all sources are deposited in the environment as highly complex mixtures of isomers and congeners on soil, grass, vegetation, and surface water. Subsequent uptake via various food chains results in the preferential bioaccumulation of the 2,3,7,8-substituted dioxins and furans (as compared to congeners lacking chlorines in the lateral positions) in fish, reptiles, birds, and mammals. Tetra- to octachlorinated dioxins are resistant to metabolism and are extremely persistent in both environmental and biological systems.

The major route of human exposure to dioxins and furans is through food consumption ($> 90\%$), for example, from milk, dairy products, fish, meat, and eggs. Current background exposure to dioxins and furans results in a daily intake of approximately 1–3 pg TEQ (toxicity equivalents) /kg body weight. The total PCDD–PCDF levels in blood and fat in the normal population in industrialized countries increase during an individual's life time and range between 10 and 110 pg TEQ/g blood lipid.

For breast-fed infants, the average daily intake of PCDDs and PCDFs (110 pg TEQ/kg body weight at age 2 months) is about 50-fold higher than that for formula-fed babies and adults. Considering the relative short time period of breast-feeding and the increasing body weight of the children, the infant's body burden was calculated to be only 2- to 4-fold higher than that of the mothers. Moreover, the infant's shorter half-life of TCDD (about 4 months in newborns compared to 5–9 years in adults) contributes to

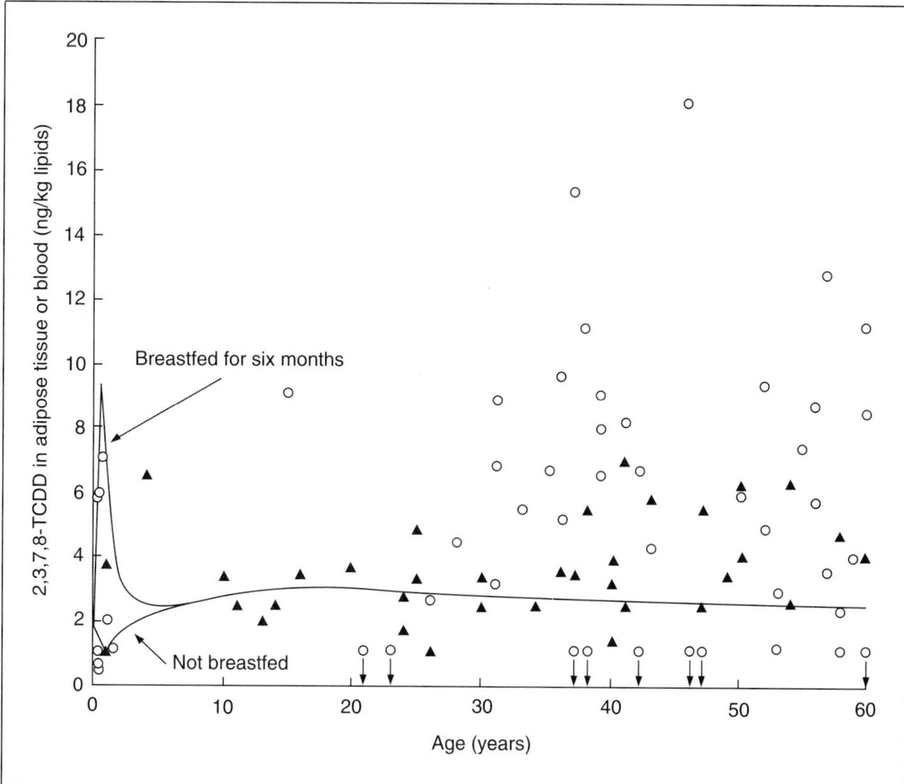

FIGURE 2 Predicted and measured TCDD concentration for a time span of 60 years. TCDD concentrations were determined in lipids of adipose tissue (○) or blood (Δ) (↓ represent values ≤ 1.0 pg/g lipid). TCDD concentrations predicted from a toxicokinetic model for male subjects with or without breastfeeding for 6 months are represented by the curves (Kreuzer *et al.*, 1997, *Arch. Toxicol.* **71**, 383–400, copyright notice of Springer-Verlag.).

the relatively rapid decline of the dioxin body burden to average background concentrations during 5 years after breast-feeding. Subsequently, the average background concentration of TCDD remains at about 3 pg/g fat (Fig. 2).

Toxicokinetics of Polyhalogenated Dioxins and Furans

The toxicokinetics of PCDDs and PCDFs are congener-, dose-, and species-specific, with urinary and biliary excretion dependent on the exposure routes and the metabolism of these compounds; for example, TCDF is excreted more rapidly than TCDD (this may partly explain the lower toxic potency of TCDF). Pulmonary, oral, and dermal exposure of male rats to a single low TCDD dose results in an absorption of about 95, 90, and 40%, respectively. A similar oral absorption was found in humans. While tetra- and pentachlorinated congeners are well absorbed from the gastrointestinal tract, the molecular size of PCDDs and PCDFs becomes a limiting factor for the absorption of hepta- and octachlorinated congeners. Following environmental exposure, absorption is determined by the dioxin-binding matrices (e.g., PCDDs and PCDFs are very poorly absorbed from fly ash and soil particles).

Upon absorption, 2,3,7,8-substituted PCDDs and PCDFs are bound to chylomicrons, lipoproteins, and other serum proteins, followed by vascular transport. In addition to passive diffusion, cellular uptake may partly be facilitated through the cell membrane low-density lipoprotein receptor, the hepatic receptor for albumin and/or other systems. The partitioning of ingested dioxins in various tissues is mainly a function of their lipophilicity and tissue affinity; major tissue depots include liver and fat. Tissue levels are also dependent on the halogenation grade of the congeners, the administered doses, and the exposure routes. For most of the penta- to octachlorinated congeners, the relative liver retention tended to be higher than that observed for TCDD and TCDF. In laboratory animals (rodents, marmosets), low TCDD and TCDF doses are distributed to equal or higher extents into the liver compared to the fat. The high concentrations found in the liver may be related to CYP1A2 levels, which represent a primary hepatic binding site for these chemicals in rodents. The liver–fat concentration ratio declines time-dependently (e.g., for TBDD, 1 nmol/kg in rats, from around 30 to 0.15 over a 56-day period). Discrepancies between liver–fat-concentration ratios in rodents and humans may be related in part to dose-dependent dispositional differences between relatively high experimentally administered doses and much lower environmental exposures. Intra- and interspecies variations in the induction of hepatic-binding proteins, hepatic lipid content, and whole-body adipose tissue content may also contribute to the differences in the disposition of dioxins. Following environmental exposure, most of the dioxin-like chemicals are sequestered in human adipose tissue (concentrations in the fat are about 10 times higher than those in the liver).

Although TCDD is highly resistant to biotransformation, small amounts of metabolites have been identified in rats and dogs. The hydroxylated or conjugated metabolites are rapidly eliminated through bile and feces. The mechanism of elimination of PCDDs and PCDFs in humans is still unknown; first-order kinetics via bile and feces are assumed. After chronic exposure to TCDD, much higher concentrations are accumulated under steady-state conditions in humans than in rats. The elimination half-life of TCDD in humans is approximately 7–9 years, while in rats the half-lives for TCDD range between 17 and 31 days. The long half-lives of dioxin-like compounds depend on the lateral position of the halogen substituents and increase with a higher degree of halogen substitution of the molecules. For the hexa- to octachlorinated congeners, half-lives between 75 days and 7 years have been calculated for the rat and between 15 and 50 years have been estimated for humans. Nonlateral substituted congeners are metabolized and excreted more rapidly than TCDD.

Mechanism of Action

The unusual high potency of TCDD to induce cytochrome P450-dependent enzymes (e.g., ary hydrocarbon hydroxylase (AHH) activity (CYP1A1 and CYP1A2)) and the excellent structure–induction relationships for a series of halogenated aromatics led to the hypothesis that the actions of these compounds are mediated via an "induction receptor." Studies of AHH induction with different inbred mice strains indicated that the high (C57BL/6 strain) and the low (DBA/2 strain) responsiveness to *a*romatic *h*ydrocarbons is regulated by a distinct genetic locus, the Ah locus. Using [^{3}H]TCDD as a radioligand in binding assays with liver fractions of C57BL/6 mice, the cytosolic binding *a*ryl *h*ydrocarbon (Ah) receptor was identified in 1976. TCDDs reversibly binds to the Ah receptor with a high affinity ($K_D < 1$ nM). Various coplanar ligands of different chemical classes competitively bind to the Ah receptor, including halogenated (PCDDs, PCDFs, and PCBs) and nonhalogenated (benzo[*a*]pyrene and methyl cholanthrene) aromatic hydrocarbons, as well as heterocyclic aromatic compounds (indole-3-carbinol, flavones, and benzocoumarins). The Ah receptor is expressed in multiple tissues of humans (at high concentrations in the placenta, lung, liver, pancreas, and heart) and in diverse animal species, such as rodents, fish, and birds. Inter- and intraspecies differences exist in the molecular properties of the Ah receptor (e.g., in the apparent molecular mass and binding affinity). In both human and mouse, two forms of Ah receptor have been identified which show a 5- to 10-fold difference in binding affinity.

The current model of Ah-receptor-mediated signal transduction hypothesizes that the latent form of the Ah receptor exists in association with the heat-shock protein hsp90 and other proteins, possibly including the protein kinase c-Src in a multiprotein complex primarily within the cytoplasmic compartment of cells. Upon ligand binding, the Ah receptor is dissociated from these proteins, translocated into the nucleus, and dimerized with a structurally related protein, the Ah-receptor nuclear translocator protein (ARNT). The heterodimeric Ah-receptor–ARNT complex functions as a transcriptional enhancer by binding to specific DNA sequences that is, the *d*ioxin or *x*enobiotic *r*esponsive *e*lements (DREs or XREs) present in one or several copies in the promoter region of dioxin-inducible genes (Fig. 3). The prototypical member of the genes is the *CYP1A1* gene. Analysis of the 5′-flanking region of various TCDD-inducible genes identified DREs, which contain a core 5′-GCGTG-3′ sequence that binds the Ah-receptor complex and are essential for Ah-receptor-mediated transcriptional activation. Ah-receptor-complex binding causes changes in the chromatin structure, increasing the accessibility of the promoter to the transcriptional machinery required for gene expression. However, no relationship between the strength of DNA binding and Ah-receptor-mediated inducibitity has been observed, indicating that binding is not sufficient to cause induction of a target gene, as shown for the murine Ah gene battery, coordinately regulated genes encoding drug-metabolizing enzymes (Table 1).

It has also been suggested that the Ah-receptor-complex binding to a nonfunctional response element

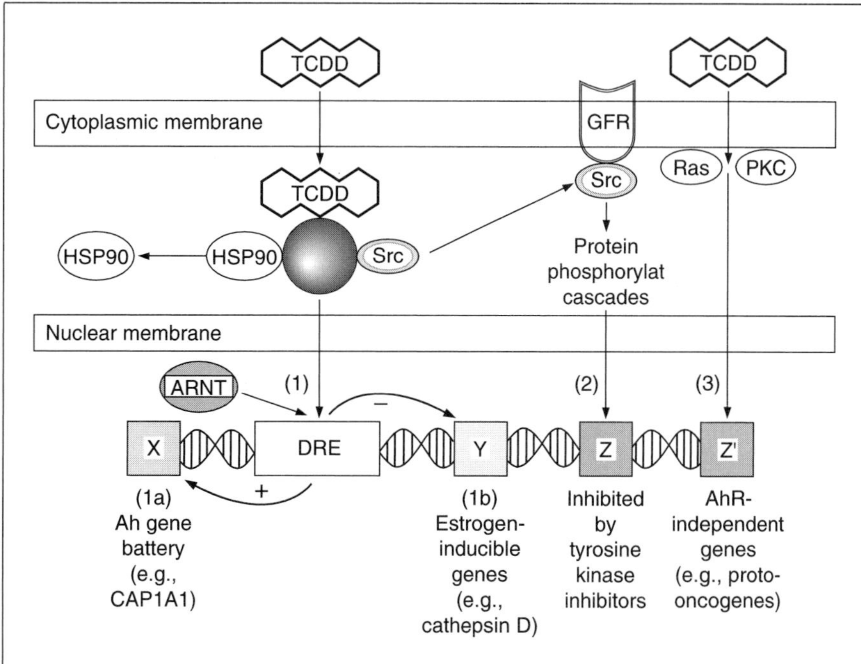

FIGURE 3 Hypothetical scheme of TCDD-mediated signal transfer pathways. Upon TCDD binding to the Ah receptor (AhR), the heat-shock protein(hsp)90 and the tyrosine protein kinase Src are released from the receptor complex. The liganded Ah receptor heterodimerizes with the ARNT protein and triggers gene expression via binding to dioxin-responsive elements (DREs) in the promoter or 3′ region of TCDD-responsive genes (1). TCDD repression of gene transcription can be mediated by interference of negative DREs with the induction process by other factors such as estrogens (1b). Moreover, gene transcription can be modified by TCDD-enhanced protein phosphorylation (2), (i.e., via tyrosine phosphorylation cascades) and via growth-factor-receptor (GFR)-induced signal transfer pathways, possibly resulting in the phosphorylation of nuclear transcription factors (e.g., AP-1). Ah-receptor-independent pathways including activation of Ras proteins, protein kinase C (PKC), may lead to enhanced proto-oncogene expression (e.g., *c-fos* and *junB*). (Adapted from Safe, 1995; Matsumara *et al.*, 1997.)

causes the disruption of the gene transcriptional machinery, resulting in transcriptional repression. Moreover, transcriptional regulation may also be mediated by protein–protein interactions (e.g., the Ah receptor can modulate cathepsin D gene transcription by interfering with the DNA-binding ability of an estrogen-receptor complex); the exact mechanism of these interactions has not been fully elucidated. Interestingly, similar inhibitory effects of estradiol on TCDD-induced mRNA accumulation are known, demonstrating a mutual cross-talk between the signal transfer pathways triggered by estrogens and Ah-receptor ligands.

The genes for Ah receptor and ARNT have been cloned and sequenced. Both proteins contain a basic region helix–loop–helix (bHLH) domain, which is required for recognition of specific DNA sequences and for protein–protein dimerization. Another domain designated as PAS (*P*ER, *A*h receptor or *A*RNT, *S*IM) domain is involved in dimerization and also contains

TABLE 1 Proteins Attributed to the Murine Ah Gene Battery

Cytochrome P450 1A1 (CYP1A1)	Aldehyde-3-dehydrogenase
Cytochrome P450 1A2 (CYP1A2)	UDP-glucuronosyltransferase (UGT1 06)
NAD(P)H:menadione oxidoreductase	Glutathione *S*-transferase Ya (GST 1a1, Ya)

the ligand-binding site interacting with hsp90. Deletion analysis has defined glutamine-rich regions in the carboxyl terminus of the Ah receptor as important in transactivation of responsive genes.

The expression of dioxin-regulated genes (e.g., CYP1A1 and CYP1A2) is reduced by a number of other factors, such as hormones (insulin), growth factors (epidermal growth factor, EGF), and cytokines (interleukin 1β). Moreover, various TCDD-induced pathological responses including the alteration of growth regulation and the enhancement of malignant cell transformation are, at least *in vitro,* inhibited by antioxidants and inhibitors of arachidonic acid metabolism. Thus, modulations of the highly cell-specific actions of TCDD may occur at different levels of the signal transduction pathway: (1) phosphorylation (protein kinase C and/or other protein kinases) and dephosphorylation of the Ah receptor and ARNT regulate the heterodimerization and binding to DRE; (2) different bHLH proteins may compete with the Ah receptor for recruitment of ARNT (e.g., the hypoxia-inducible factor 1α exhibiting a very high affinity for ARNT); (3) binding of the Ah-receptor–ARNT complex to the DNA recognition sequence is reduced by cystein methylation of CpG dinucleotides in that sequence, often in a tissue-specific fashion; (4) the activity of DREs may be further modulated by tissue-specific repressors, cooperative protein–protein interactions (C/EBPα, a positive DRE regulator), and cross-talk with other response elements; and (5) TCDD-induced transcription may be inhibited by serine–threonine-specific protein phosphatases.

TCDD can also inhibit gene expression by a direct interaction of the nuclear Ah-receptor complex with inhibitory DREs; such DRE sequences have been identified in the promoter or 3′ region of several estrogen-inducible genes, possibly resulting in an anti-estrogenic effect of TCDD (Fig. 3).

In addition to the Ah-receptor–DRE signaling pathway, further mechanisms may contribute to the dioxin-mediated regulation of proteins involved in inflammation and the regulation of growth and differentiation (Table 2). Phosphorylation via tyrosine kinases, possibly by a Src kinase released from the Ah receptor subsequent to ligand binding, may be an alternative signaling pathway for TCDD-mediated effects. Further evidence for the important role of a phosphorylation pathway is supported by studies with c-*src*-deficient mice (c-$src^{-/+}$), in which some toxic effects of TCDD are not fully expressed (e.g., lethality at a high TCDD dose, loss of weight in the adipose tissue, thymus, and body). The possibilitiy that TCDD may affect multiple pathways, some of which are Ah-receptor independent is raised by *in vitro* studies on biochemical effects of TCDD, including activation of protein kinases, phospholipase C, and increases in the immediate-early proto-oncogenes *c-fos* and *junB.*

Ah-receptor-deficient transgenic mice are resistant to thymic and hepatic toxicities. However, high doses of TCDD induce—apparently via Ah-receptor-independent mechanisms—vasculitis and cell necrosis in the lungs and livers of these mice. It is remarkable that livers of Ah-receptor-deficient mice exhibit a threefold increase in retinoids, which inhibits the toxic effects of TCDD.

Acute and Long-Term Toxicity

Animal and cell culture studies are essential for the elucidation of biochemical pathways and types of biological events of dioxin-like compounds. However, the species, strain, sex, and cell specifities of these effects complicate attempts to assess TCDD's potential hazard to human health.

Since the 1970s, many epidemiological studies have been published on populations with potential exposure to PCDDs, including phenoxy herbicide production workers and users, workers in paper and pulp production, Vietnam War veterans, and members of the general population (e.g., after the Seveso accident). High exposures to PCDFs have occurred in Japan (e.g., Yusho poisoning) and Taiwan (e.g., Yu Cheng poisoning), involving contamination of rice oil with PCDFs and PCBs (see the section on "Polychlorinated Biphenyls (PCB)") and in accidents involving electrical equipment containing PCBs.

After the Seveso accident, in which effluent containing TCDD was released from a chemical plant, TCDD effects were examined by "zones" of exposure and TCDD levels in the serum of many residents were determined. A major problem in environmental studies is that the body burden of individuals resulting from a similar dioxin exposure (e.g., residents of the same area) are very different. TCDD concentrations in the plasma of highly contaminated children from Seveso were up to four orders of magnitude greater than those in the general unexposed population. However, statistical evaluation of the epidemiological data is difficult because of the relatively small number of highly exposed individuals.

The largest known TCDD contamination occurred between 1962 and 1970, when 12 million gallons of Agent Orange, a defoliant mixture contaminated with TCDD (average concentration, 3 mg/kg), were sprayed during the Vietnam War. Studies of Agent Orange plus TCDD have focused mainly on American veterans. The U.S. military personnel who applied

TABLE 2 TCDD-Mediated Modulation of Factors Related to Growth and Differentiation

TCDD-induced effects	Species, tissues, and cells
Endogenous factors/hormones and receptors	
Increased EGF receptor phosphorylation and decreased EGF receptor binding	Human keratinocytes, mouse, rat, guinea pig, and fish liver
Stabilization of TGFα mRNA	Human keratinocytes
Decrease in insulin receptor binding	Rat hepatocytes
Decrease in glucocorticoid receptor binding	Rat and mouse liver
Transcriptional downregulation of TGFβ_2	Human keratinocytes and hepatoma cells
Decrease in vitamin A levels	Rat liver
Downregulation of estrogen receptors	Rat liver, murine hepatoma and human breast cancer cells
Inhibition of prolactin receptor expression	Human breast cancer cells
Decrease in testosterone levels	Rat
Modulation of thyroid hormones	Rat
Members of signal transfer pathways	
Enhancement of activities of protein kinases	Rat and mouse liver
Increase in the expression and tyrosyl phosphorylation of $p34^{cdc2}$ kinase	Murine hepatocytes
Transient increase in Ca^{2+} influx	Murine hepatoma cells
Elevated levels of $p21^{ras}$ protein	Rat liver
Increased expression and phosphorylation of p53	Mouse liver
Induction of $p21^{WAF1}$ CDK inhibitory protein	Mouse liver
Induction of immediate early genes: *c-fos* and *junB*	Murine hepatoma cells
Increased expression of c-ErbA	Mouse liver
Decrease in connexin 32 gap junction mRNA	Rat hepatocytes
Proteins associated with inflammatory processes	
Enhanced expression of cyclooxygenase-2	Canine kidney cells
Induction of plasminogen activator inhibitor type 2	Human keratinocytes, hepatocytes, monocytic cells
Increased expression of interleukin 1β mRNA	Human keratinocytes, mouse liver, lung, thymus
Stimulated secretion of tumor necrosis factor α (TNFα), increase in TNFα mRNA	Murine macrophages, human breast cancer cells

Agent Orange in Vietnam (Ranch Handers) had higher TCDD body burdens than the general population or the ground troops who served in Vietnam. The potential health effects of Agent Orange are of particular concern to the people of the contaminated areas of Southern Vietnam, where the highest TCDD concentration reported in human milk (>1800 pg/g lipid) has been found in nursing women in 1970. In adipose tissues collected in the 1980s in this area, TCDD concentrations up to 103 pg/g were detected and pooled blood collected in 1991–1992 also showed elevated TCDD concentrations up to 33 pg/g (compared to 2.9 pg/g in tissues from Northern Vietnam).

Many epidemiological studies have focused on workers in chemical production or processing or sprayers exposed to chlorinated phenoxy herbicides and/or chlorophenols contaminated with TCDD or higher-chlorinated dioxins; extrapolated TCDD serum concentrations for the time of employment were up to 32,000 pg/g (assuming a TCDD half-life of 7.1 years). The largest study in U.S. production workers—5000 men probably exposed to TCDD in chemical manufacturing—was conducted by the United States National Institute for Occupational Safety and Health. In 1997 another international-cohort study examined the cancer mortality among 21,863 workers from 12 countries. Exposure was re-evaluated using job records, company exposure questionnaires, and serum and adipose tissue dioxin concentrations, which were considerably higher in the production workers than in the general population. The evaluation of these data is complicated by the possible interaction of TCDD with other components of the chemical mixtures to which the workers and sprayers had been exposed.

Dioxin-like compounds are known to cause qualitatively different symptoms, and their toxicities vary widely among species. The skin and liver are the major targets of TCDD toxicity in humans and animals. The most prominent effect of high exposure to dioxin-like compounds in humans, monkeys, hairless mice, and rabbits is chloracne, a persistent acneiform skin disease characterizied by comedones and cysts of the skin, which has been suggested to be a disturbance of the normal differentiation process of keratinocytes. In severe cases inflammatory pustules, hyperpigmentation, abscesses, and large cysts may occur and persist for months or even years after exposure. Data from chloracne cases among exposed chemical workers or Seveso residents show no strict correlation between serum–adipose tissue concentrations of PCDDs and the development of chloracne. Serum-lipid concentrations of TCDD in Seveso residents with chloracne—except children < 11 years of age—ranged from 820 to 56,000 pg/g, while other individuals without chloracne—>30 years—had TCDD concentrations ranging from 1770 to 10,400 pg/g. Children in Seveso may have been more heavily exposed to TCDD by skin contact than adults. In chloracne patients that were chemical workers, adipose concentrations of >200 pg/g lipid TCDD and >2000 pg/g lipid hexachlorinated dibenzo-*p*-dioxin were estimated. It should be taken into consideration that the exposure route (dermal or oral) may play an important role in the development of skin lesions, in addition to the individual susceptibility to chloracne. Other dermal disorders reported among workers exposed to TCDD were hyperpigmentation and hypertrichosis (abnormal distribution of hair).

A consistent marker of liver toxicity induced by TCDD-like compounds in animals is hepatomegaly due to hypertrophy and hyperplasia of parenchymal cells. Liver enlargement in humans has been reported in only a few cases, including some trichlorophenol production workers and in Seveso residents with severe chloracne.

Other signs of liver toxicity that vary among species are necrosis (in rabbit), centrilobular lesions (in mouse), lipid accumulation, pigment deposition, infiltration of inflammatory cells, and fibrous proliferation in necrotic areas (in rat). Liver damage by TCDD in female rats is associated with increased serum activities of γ-glutamyl transferase (GGT), alkaline phosphatase, and glutamic–pyruvic transaminase. Elevated concentrations of GGT were also reported among Seveso children with chloracne. A long-lasting elevation of the GGT concentrations is observed in trichlorophenol workers with above-average alcohol consumption.

In rats and mice, TCDD induces alterations in the porphyrin biosynthesis, including a decrease in uroporphyrinogen decarboxylase activity and an increase in δ-aminolevulinic acid synthetase (the rate-limiting step in heme synthesis). Urinary excretion of coproporphyrin and possibly uroporphyrin is increased in female rats by long-term treatment with TCDD (100 ng/kg). Porphyrin excretion is unspecific for TCDD exposure and is also induced by other aromatic chlorinated hydrocarbons like hexachlorobenzene.

The evidence for a TCDD-mediated effect on serum cholesterol and triglycerid levels is conflicting. An increase in high-density lipoprotein cholesterol concentrations has been observed in highly TCDD-exposed chemical workers. However, neither adults nor children from Seveso showed elevated lipid concentrations. An association between TCDD exposure and adverse effects on the cardiovascular system is not yet proven. An increased mortality attributed to cardiovascular diseases was observed among a small number of residents of the most contaminated region in Seveso.

Various toxic effects of TCDD, including elevated cholesterol concentrations, might be related to alterations of the thyroid function. Administration of a single nonlethal dose of TCDD reduces the serum concentrations of thyroxine (T_4), indicating hypothyroidism. TCDD-induced T_4 glucuronidation by UDP-glucuronosyltransferase-1 and an enhanced biliary excretion of the glucuronide may decrease T_4 concentrations and reduce the negative feedback inhibition on the pituitary, resulting in an increased secretion of thyroid-stimulating hormone (TSH). Continuous elevation of TSH concentrations following chronic TCDD treatment in rodents results in hypertrophy and hyperplasia of thyroid follicular cells and ultimately leads to thyroid adenomas and carcinomas, very sensitive endpoints of the action of TCDD in rodent carcinogenicity bioassays. However, in human studies the results of TCDD-mediated alterations of the thyroid function are equivocal. Conflicting data from human and animal studies have also been ob-

TABLE 3 Acute Oral LD_{50} of TCDD in Different Animal Species

Species	Dose (μg/kg)
Guinea pig	0.6–2.5
Mink	4
Sprague–Dawley rat (male)	22
Rhesus monkey	<70
C57BL/6 mouse (male)	114–280
Dog	>300
Syrian hamster (female, male)	1150–5000

Factors Contributing to the Cell Type Specificity of TCDD Effects

Induction of cell proliferation by TCDD is associated with receptor down-regulation in hepatocytes, unchanged EGF receptor concentrations in mouse skin, and increased EGF receptor levels in the developing ureteric epithelium. Thus, proliferation, apoptosis, and differentiation are regulated in a cell-type-specific manner controlled by a variety of growth factors and hormones. EGF, estrogen, insulin, and glucocorticoids modulate the proliferative responses to TCDD. The stimulation of hepatocyte growth by TCDD involves the interaction with endogenous hormones (e.g., of estrogens for TCDD-stimulated hepatocyte proliferation in normal female rats but not in ovariectomized ones). That TCDD enhances the growth of periportal hepatocytes but not of centrilobular cells may be due to gradients of the hormones in the liver acinus. The dependence of TCDD-induced stimulation of DNA synthesis on insulin and glucocorticoids was shown in the primary rat hepatocyte. In contrast, CYP1A1 induction, reduced by insulin and growth factors, is more pronounced in the centrilobular region, suggesting different control mechanisms in the expression of the genes involved in drug metabolism and those associated with growth regulation.

tained for serum-glucose concentrations and diabetes after TCDD exposure. While human studies suggest a slightly greater risk of diabetes for highly TCDD-exposed individuals and elevated fasting glucose concentrations, animal studies generally show a decrease after short-term and high-dose exposure to TCDD. The animal data might be explained by the TCDD-mediated inhibition of glucagon-induced phosphoenolpyruvate carboxykinase, the key enzyme of gluconeogenesis, in the liver of rats. However, this effect is partially counterbalanced by an increased renal phosphoenolpyruvate carboxykinase activity after TCDD treatment in rats. Changes in the carbohydrate and lipid metabolisms are very prominent symptoms of high doses of TCDD-like chemicals in animals, resulting mostly in the loss of fat and muscle. The severe forms of body-weight loss are described as "wasting syndrome." The loss of body weight (up to 50%) is not entirely attributable to the lack of food intake. A drastic TCDD-mediated decline in the adipose lipoprotein lipase activities is considered to induce lipolysis in the adipose cells and an increase in serum lipids. This phenomenon is apparently not associated with changes in the plasma concentrations of triiodothyronine or epinephrine. The wasting syndrome is lethal and develops over a period of a few weeks (e.g., in guinea pig, 1–2 weeks; in rat, 2–3 weeks; in monkey, 6–8 weeks). The lethality of TCDD is not correlated to the wasting syndrome because parenterally fed, TCDD-treated rats die despite a body weight gain. The acute lethality of TCDD is characterized by exceptionally wide inter- and intraspecies differences in susceptibility (Table 3). The hamster, regarded as the most resistant species, tolerates an oral dose 5000-fold higher than the lethal dose for the guinea pig, the most sensitive species. In rats, the LD_{50} values range from 10 μg/kg with Long–Evans (TCDD-sensitive) to >7200 μg/kg with Han–Wistar (TCDD-resistant) substrains. Studies with TCDD-sensitive and TCDD-resistant rat substrains do not demonstrate a correlation between lethality and typical Ah-receptor-mediated TCDD effects, such as CYP1A1 induction. Thus, the hypothesis that all the toxic and biochemical effects of TCDD are mediated by the Ah receptor does not readily explain the large differences in TCDD sensitivity.

A difference in the biochemical effects of TCDD-sensitive and TCDD-resistant rat strains has been reported for the binding of the epidermal growth factor (EGF) to liver membranes after TCDD treatment. Down-regulation of growth factor receptors and a decreased binding of EGF and the transforming growth factor α (TGFα; Table 2) are consistent TCDD effects in hepatocytes and keratinocytes. The proposed mechanism of EGF-receptor down-regulation in keratinocytes is overexpression of TGFα. Enhanced TGFα concentrations in keratinocyte cells and increased receptor phosphorylation in the liver membranes of TCDD-treated species are followed by the internalization and degradation of the EGF receptor. Down-regulation by TCDD is also known for insulin and glucocorticoid receptors. These phenomena are associated with alterations in the regulation of growth and differention by dioxin-like compounds.

TCDD causes various anti-estrogenic effects, including down-regulation of estrogen receptors and a reduction of estrogen-induced increases in uterine wet weights in rats and mice. In human breast cancer cell lines, TCDD results in the decreased secretion of the tissue plasminogen activator and of estrogen-induced proteins, such as cathepsin D. TCDD also blocks the estradiol-dependent proliferation response and the occurrence of multicellular foci in postconfluent cultures of human breast cancer cells. The structure–activity relationship for anti-estrogenic responses of dioxin-like compounds correlates with their potencies for cytochrome P450-dependent enzyme induction. No anti-estrogenic responses of TCDD are found in Ah-receptor-defective, ARNT-deficient, or mutant cells. Studies analyzing the interference of TCDD with the promoter or 3′ regions of estrogen-inducible genes suggest that these regions contain core DRE sequences that may bind the Ah receptor complex and thus may decrease the estrogen-induced expression of these genes.

The disruption of the normal homeostasis of growth- and differentiation-related processes by dioxin-like compounds is reflected by hyper-, hypo-, meta-, and dysplastic responses in different tissues. Hyperplasia is induced by TCDD in the gastric mucosa and bile duct of monkeys, in the urinary bladder of guinea pigs, and in liver and skin of various species. TCDD-induced hypoplasia is observed in lymphoid tissues. Squamous metaplasia occurs in the meibomian gland of the eyelid, resulting in blepharitis and in the ceruminous glands of the ears, leading to waxy exudates. Ectodermal dysplasia with alterations in teeth and nails occurs in humans and primates following high dioxin exposure. Ectodermal effects on skin, nails, meibomian glands, and accelerated tooth eruption were hallmarks of fetal and neonatal toxicity in children of mothers exposed to rice oil contaminated with PCBs and PCDF (in the Yusho and Yu Cheng episodes).

Reproductive Toxicity

Several PCDDs and PCDFs are developmental and reproductive toxicants in experimental animals. Major structural malformations, such as cleft palate and hydronephrosis, are observed as species-specific effects in mice following prenatal exposure to TCDD-like compounds at maternally nontoxic doses. The apparent absence of cleft palate in nonmurine species is in accord with a much lower responsiveness of cultured palatal shelves from rats and humans. In both mouse and human palates, TCDD exposure was associated with inappropriate epithelial cell differentiation and proliferation and altered expression of EGF, TGFα, TGFβs, and the EGF receptor. Evidence from studies with TCDD-sensitive and -insensitive mouse strains suggest that the TCDD-induced cleft palate is dependent on the presence of the Ah receptor. The hydronephrosis response of TCDD is caused by hyperplasia of the ureteric lumenal epithelium, resulting in ureteric obstruction. Excessive proliferation of ureteric cells is associated with increased expression of EGF receptors.

The common fetotoxic effects of TCDD in most laboratory animals are thymic and splenic atrophy, subcutaneous edema, decreased fetal growth, and prenatal mortality. Gastrointestinal hemorrhage occurs in rats and guinea pigs and embryonic-blood hemorrhage into the maternal circulation has been observed in mice following prenatal exposure to TCDD and 2,3,4,7,8-pentaCDF. In general the embryo or the fetus is more sensitive to TCDD than the adult, and dose levels associated with fetotoxicity are similar across species. The maternal doses of TCDD that cause prenatal mortality in hamsters, Sprague–Dawley rats, and rhesus monkeys are 1 to 2 orders of magnitude lower than the LD_{50} of TCDD in the adult animals. The prenatal mortality is mostly associated with maternal TCDD toxicity indicated by decreased maternal weight gain and/or marked subcutaneous edema of the dam.

TCDD decreases female fertility and litter size. Several studies indicate that the anti-estrogenic action of TCDD is related to the menstrual–estrus cycle and to reduced uterine weights. In female rats and hamsters prenatally exposed to TCDD, a delayed vaginal opening and structural abnormalities of the external genitalia are observed. Antiandrogenic effects (e.g., decreased testis weights and spermatogenesis) and reduced fertility are associated with decreased testosterone concentrations after high doses of TCDD in male rats. However, the male rodent reproductive system is very sensitive to *in utero* and lactational TCDD exposure. Prenatal exposure of rats to low doses of TCDD (64 ng/kg) reduces the ventral prostate weight and decreases sperm production and numbers.

In contrast to the species-specific reproductive effects in animals, epidemiologic studies fail to show associations between exposure to dioxin-like compounds and birth defects or perinatal mortality, with the exception of a few studies, including the investigation of the Yusho and Yu Cheng incidents. Occupational studies have focused on paternally mediated reproductive effects. In accord with animal studies, alterations in the male sex-hormone concentrations (low testosterone and high gonadotropin levels) have been reported following occupational exposure. Given the high percentage of pregnancy loss (30–

50%) in all conceptions and the high exposure misclassification (40–50%) mainly based on self-reported dioxin exposure, which correlates poorly with serum TCDD levels, the impact of dioxin exposure on early pregnancy loss remains unknown. Epidemiological studies are generally hampered by a selection bias (the population at risk is often defined by the proximity of the residence to a contaminated site) and volunteer bias (subjects responding to publicized requests). Studies of the Seveso accident have not reported any significant indication of teratogenic or embryotoxic effects. A significant effect was an excess of daughters born to heavily exposed parents (high serum TCDD concentrations) as observed nine months after the Seveso accident. This observation and the changes mentioned here in the male sex-hormone concentration after dioxin exposure support the hypothesis that the sex ratio of newborns is changed by the altered hormone concentrations of contaminated males.

Mutagenicity

TCDD is not mutagenic in most short-term mutagenicity assays *in vitro* and *in vivo.* No consistent evidence exists for increased frequencies of chromosomal aberrations in human populations exposed to TCDD, either accidentally or occupationally. Using radioactive-labeling methods for the detection of very low levels of carcinogen adducts with DNA, no adduct formation is detected with DNA from dioxin-treated rats. Thus, TCDD does not damage DNA directly. However, TCDD enhances the oxidative DNA damage by endogenous compounds (e.g., TCDD-induced cytochrome P450-dependent enzymes metabolize endogenous estrogens to catechols; subsequently, enhanced catechol formation may increase oxidative DNA damage). Furthermore, very high doses of TCDD (50–100 μg/kg) induce single-strand breaks in Sprague–Dawley rats, presumably as a result of increased lipid peroxidation.

Carcinogenicity

TCDD is an animal carcinogen in the rat, mouse, hamster, and fish. It causes tumors at multiple sites in both sexes at doses well below the maximum tolerated dose. In chronic feeding experiments, a daily TCDD intake (0.1 μg/kg) for two years resulted in an increased number of hepatocellular carcinomas and squamous cell carcinomas of the lung, hard palate, and nasal turbinate in female Sprague–Dawley rats. Tumor data exhibit a positive dose-dependent incidence of liver tumors (adenomas and carcinomas) of nearly 50%. The evaluation of data from multistage carcinogenicity bioassays in rats suggests that TCDD is an extraordinarily potent tumor promoter and a weak or noninitiator. The promoting activity is in accordance with a nongenotoxicity of TCDD and is thought to result from an Ah-receptor-mediated pleiotropic response leading to alterations of growth and differentiation. Therefore, treatment with TCDD is associated with an enhanced hepatocellular growth and a suppression of apoptosis in liver foci. TCDD-mediated growth and tumor-promoting effects have been found only in the livers of intact female rats but not in ovariectomized rats. Hence, the induction of estrogen-mediated DNA damage by TCDD is related to TCDD-mediated carcinogenicity in rats. In contrast to its action in the liver, ovariectomy sensitizes rats to the promoting action of TCDD in the lung. As an early indication of TCDD's anti-estrogenic action, long-term treatment with TCDD caused a dose-dependent reduction of spontaneous mammary and uterine tumors in female rats. In the livers of mice, tumor promotion by TCDD is observed in both sexes but there was no tumor-promoting activity in Ah-nonresponsive mice. In the skin of hairless mice, TCDD promotes tumor formation at 1% of the dose of the skin-tumor-promoter 12-*O*-tetradecanoylphorbol 13-acetate. Further targets for its carcinogenic potential in the mouse are the thyroid gland, lung, and lymphopoietic system. In hamsters TCDD produces squamous-cell carcinomas of the facial skin. Tumor-promoting effects in female rat liver were also observed with 1,2,3,7,8-pentachlorodibenzo-*p*-dioxin, 1,2,3,4,6,7,8-heptachlorodibenzo-*p*-dioxin, and a defined mixture of 49 PCDDs. Surprisingly, at extremely low doses (0.0001–0.001 μg/kg/day) TCDD is an apparent "anti tumor promoter" that is, it inhibits formation and growth of preneoplastic lesions in rat liver. In summary, the extrapolations of the effects observed after high exposure (e.g., cancer in rats) to low environmental exposure in humans are complicated by species- and tissue-specific effects and an unknown mechanism of action of TCDD after low doses.

There is still controversy about the potential carcinogenic effect of dioxins in humans. Epidemiological studies have shown an increase in overall cancer mortality after high exposure to dioxins and after a long latency. Dose–response relationships for dioxin-like chemicals are hampered by the frequent lack of individual exposure data. Significantly increased incidence of cancers is reported for various organs (e.g., the liver, respiratory tract, hematopoietic system, and connective and other soft tissues), but no consistent site specificity for TCDD in humans can be derived

TABLE 4 Biochemical and Immunomodulatory Effects of TCDD at Different Doses

Dose (μg/kg body weight)	Effect	Species
0.001	Induction of CYP1A1 mRNA	Rat
0.0015	Induction of CYP1A1, CYP1A2 enzymatic activities	Mouse
0.01	Increased mortality to influenza virus	Mouse
0.01	Changes in the pattern of lymphocyte subpopulations	Marmoset
0.3	Suppression of primary antibody response	Mouse
1	Induction of thymus involution	Mouse
1	Induction of interleukin 1β mRNA	Rat
3	Induction of thymus involution	Rat
3	Suppression of influenza virus; augmented natural killer activitiy	Rat

from epidemiological studies. Evidence for a slightly increased risk of lung cancer has been provided by cohort follow-up studies among highly TCDD-exposed chemical workers; however, tobacco smoking and occupational carcinogens cannot be excluded as confounding factors. Data from an international retrospective cohort study (including phenoxy herbicide production workers) indicate that exposure to herbicides contaminated with dioxins are associated with a slight increase in overall cancer risk and an increase in specific cancers. Exposure to phenoxyacetic acids and chlorophenols contaminated with dioxins and dibenzofurans are apparently a risk-factor for soft-tissue sarcoma, based on a small number of deaths; however, the risk of soft-tissue carcinoma may also be increased by TCDD-free phenoxy herbicides and/or chlorophenols themselves. The Seveso studies showed an excess for cancers of the gastrointestinal sites and of the lymphatic and hematopoietic tissue. The anti-estrogenic effect of TCDD and a TCDD-mediated reduction of estrogen-dependent malignancies in rats may reflect human cancer data from Seveso, indicating a decreased incidence of breast and uterus cancer. According to the overall evaluation of the International Agency for Research on Cancer, TCDD is "carcinogenic to humans (Group 1)" while other PCDDs and PCDFs are "not classifiable as to their carcinogenicity to humans (Group 3)."

Immunotoxicity

An impairment of immunological functions may result in an increased susceptibiltiy to infectious and neoplastic diseases. Numerous studies using animal-host resistance models indicate that TCDD enhances susceptibility to bacterial (*Salmonella*), viral (*Herpes*), parasitic (*Plasmodium*), and neoplastic (tumor cells) challenges. One of the most sensitive adverse effects of TCDD is an enhanced mortality to influenza virus in mice at a single dose of 10 ng/kg body weight (Table 4). The mechanism of this TCDD effect remains to be elucidated. TCDD has immunomodulatory effects in rodents and is capable of interfering with B-cell maturation and with humoral antibody production, increasing the activity of natural killer cells, altering T-cell differentiation, and inducing thymic atrophy. TCDD decreases the expression of surface proteins on splenic B-cells and macrophages in response to a tumor-cell challenge and inhibits B-cell proliferation triggered by surface immunoglobulin cross-linking. TCDD also suppresses cytotoxic T-lymphocyte activity following an alloantigen challenge as in a toxic dose range in which thymus involution is also induced (Table 4). Treatment with low doses of TCDD changes the number of B-cell, natural-killer-cell, and T-cell subpopulations in the venous blood of marmosets. The $CD4^+$ subset most affected by TCDD is the $CDw29^+$ "helper-inducer" or "memory" subset, with significant effects observed after a TCDD dose of 10 ng/kg. In contrast, after a very low TCDD dose (0.3 ng/kg per week for 24 weeks) the opposite effect on the $CD4^+$-$CDw29^+$ subset was observed, a significant increase in this population. Thus, the extrapolation of the dose-response curves to very low levels of TCDD is again difficult or even impossible. In *in vitro* studies mouse, monkey, and human lymphocytes are responsive to very low TCDD concentrations.

The information on immunomodulatory effects of TCDD in humans is sparse and no consistent pattern of effects can be derived from the different studies. In volunteers with slightly enhanced TCDD body burdens, significant increases in globulins, IgG, and $CD8^+$ cells were observed compared to a reference group, but no evidence of clinical immunosuppression was found. The same holds for accidentally exposed individuals, such as children from the area of highest contamination in Seveso (partially with chloracne). Moreover, no relationship between pre- and post-na-

TABLE 5 Examples of Tradenames and Country of Origin of Technical PCB Mixtures

Trade name	Country of origin
Aroclor, Pyranol, Pyroclor	U.S./U.K.
Clophen, Elaol	Germany
Phenochlor, Pyralene	France
Fenchlor, Apirolio	Italy
Delor	(former) Czechoslovakia
Sovcol	(former) Soviet Union
Kanechlor, Santotherm	Japan

tal PCDD–PCB exposure and respiratory-tract symptoms or humoral antibody production were detected in environmentally exposed (breast-fed) children in the Netherlands; a transiently decreased number of monocytes and granulocytes was associated with higher TCDD exposure in these children. A decreased T-helper-cell function was observed in 11 workers after 20 years of exposure to TCDD in trichlorophenol production.

Neurotoxicity

Case reports and epidemiological studies demonstrate that TCDD exposure is associated with symptoms consistent with mood disorders, including fatigue, nervousness, anxiety, and decreased libido. The neurologic effects occur shortly following TCDD exposure and, in some cases, last many years. However, the results suggest that the effects observed in adults are transient even after exposure to high levels of TCDD. No significant effect on mental development and neurological status was observed in infants exposed to PCDD and PCBs through breastfeeding.

POLYCHLORINATED BIPHENYLS (PCBs)

PCBs are a group of compounds derived from biphenyl by the replacement of 1 to 10 atoms of hydrogen by chlorine. They are also called chlorinated biphenyls, chlorobiphenyls, or polychlorobiphenyls. The following terms are used in connection with PCB. *Homologs* differ from one another in the numbers of chlorine atoms; there are 10 PCB homologs. *Isomers* differ from one another in the substitution pattern of the chlorine atoms. Each homolog has a particular number of isomers, for example, monochlorobiphenyl, 3; di, 12; tri, 24; tetra, 42; penta, 46; hexa, 42; hepta, 24; octa, 12; nona, 3; and decachlorobiphenyl, 1. *Congener* denotes each individual polychlorinated biphenyl, in other words, any isomer of any homolog. There are 209 different PCB congeners. Each congeners has been designated with a number from 1 to 209 in accordance with the rules of the International Union of Pure and Applied Chemistry (IUPAC).

PCBs were first synthesized in 1881 and commercially produced in 1929 in the United States and later they were produced throughout the world. The estimated domestic production of PCBs in North America between 1930 and 1975 was 570,000 tonnes, and an additional 1400 tonnes were imported. Further manufacturing in the U.S. was banned in 1979. In 1984 the total cumulative world's production was estimated to 1,200,000 tonnes.

The tradename (Table 5) is usually followed by a number that indicates an average degree of chlorination of the product. For example, Aroclor is followed by a four-digit number, the first two (12) indicating the type of compound (biphenyl) and the other two the average percentage of chlorine. The only exception is Aroclor 1016, which contains about 40% chlorine and is similar to Aroclor 1242. Delors are designated with a three-digit number, the first two (10) indicating the type of the molecule and the third the average number of chlorine atoms in the molecule. PCBs have extensive applications because of their physicochemical properties (e.g., stability or inflammability) (Table 6).

Commercial products of PCBs are mixtures of a large number of congeners. During the manufacture of PCBs by the reaction of gaseous chlorine with molten biphenyl under specified conditions, the chlorination is thermodynamically controlled. As a result, certain substitution patterns are favored and others are more abundant.

The congener compositions of samples from different areas of the environment and biological materials are influenced by the physicochemical properties (e.g., water solubility), as well as by their environmental and biological kinetic behavior (e.g., absorption, distribution, metabolism, and excretion). Furthermore, contamination may originate from more than one source. It has been shown that a number of PCB congeners are produced, for example, during the combustion of chloride-containing wastes in incinerators or during the syntheses of azo dyes, phthalocyanine pigments, chlorinated paraffins, and phenolic resins. The determination of a few analytically selected congeners enables an accurate monitoring of total PCBs in humans and environmental samples. For regulatory purposes, several laboratories only use the six standard congeners 28, 52, 101, 138, 153, and 180.

TABLE 6 Examples of Applications of PCB

PCB in open systems (dissipative uses)	PCB in closed systems
Formulation of lubricating and cutting oils	Dielectric in transformer and capacitors
Additives in dyes	Heat transfer and hydraulic systems
Additives in formulations of pesticides	
Plasticizer in paints, copying paper	
Adhesives, sealants and plastics	
Additives in antifouling formulations	
Oil immersion for microscopy	

PCBs have been used for almost 70 years, but their presence in the environment was not apparent until the electron-capture detector was extensively applied in gas chromatography. In 1966 PCBs were first identified as pollutants and subsequently as ubiquitous compounds. Concentrations are given usually in pg/m^3 in the atmosphere, ng/kg in surface waters, μg/kg in sediments and soils, and mg/kg in eggs of aquatic birds, fat of fishes, and adipose tissue, and milk fat of humans. For a 70-kg person, an average dietary intake of PCB was estimated to amount to a maximum of approximately 0.2 μg/kg body weight. The U.S. Food and Drug Administration analysis of data for the dose–response assessment for PCBs based on animal experiments and of epidemiological results derived from the Yusho incident (see following) led to an estimated tolerable daily intake (TDI) of 1 μg PCB/kg body weight/day for a 70-kg person. For breast-fed infants, the daily intake is about 1–2 orders of magnitude higher. Compared with a lifetime intake, a 6-month breastfeeding period contributes less than 5% of the total body burden from lifetime exposure. The amount of PCBs in the global environment has been estimated to be about 3.7×10^8 kg, and a further 7.8×10^8 kg were estimated to be still available for use or deposition in different ways.

Structurally related to PCBs are polybrominated biphenyls (PBB), theoretically also comprising 209 different congeners. PBB are primarily used as flame retardants in polymeric materials. In North America, FireMaster BP-6, consisting mainly of 2,2′,4,4′,5,5′-hexabromobiphenyl, was the principal product. As a commercial fire retardant it contained 2% calcium trisilicate and was sold under the name FireMaster FF-1. Highly brominated biphenyls were also produced in Germany (Bromkal 80–90) and France (Adine 0102). Inadvertent substitution of FF-1 for a mineral feed supplement added to dairy cattle feed in Michigan 1973 resulted in PBB exposure in farmers and in consumers through contaminated meat and other agricultural products. Contaminated cows had a dramatic reduction in feed consumption and milk production, along with other toxic signs.

It was estimated that the most highly exposed people consumed 5–15 g PBB over a 230-day period through milk. Some additional exposure may have occurred through meat. Most studies that were carried out suffered from major design weaknesses and the use of confounders that made it difficult, or impossible, to draw conclusions about the potential health effects of PBB. The follow-up time has not been long enough to evaluate possible carcinogenic effects.

The possible impact of the PBB exposure on human health is a major concern due to their presumed long half-life ($t_{1/2}$ = 12 years; range: 4–97 years) in highly exposed PBB individuals of both sexes in the Michigan study.

Structure–activity studies using individual PCB congeners have been performed to elucidate the mechanisms of PCB-induced toxicity. The data obtained show that toxic equivalency factors (TEFs) as calculated and used to evaluate the toxicity of PCDD–PCDF mixtures could be developed to assess the potential toxicity of PCB mixtures for certain specific target-organ effects (e.g., the liver, and immune system) but would be inappropriate for other effects (e.g., thyroid function and neurochemical effects). For risk evaluation in humans, it should be considered that the PCB mixtures responsible for human exposure and determined to be in human tissues, milk, and excreta predominantly consist of congeners not covered by TEFs for PCBs.

Absorption, Distribution, Metabolism, and Excretion

Of the polychlorinated biphenyls contained in the human tissue, 90–95% are absorbed from food rich in lipids, such as milk and milk products, meat, and fish. The lipophilic properties of the polychlorinated bi-

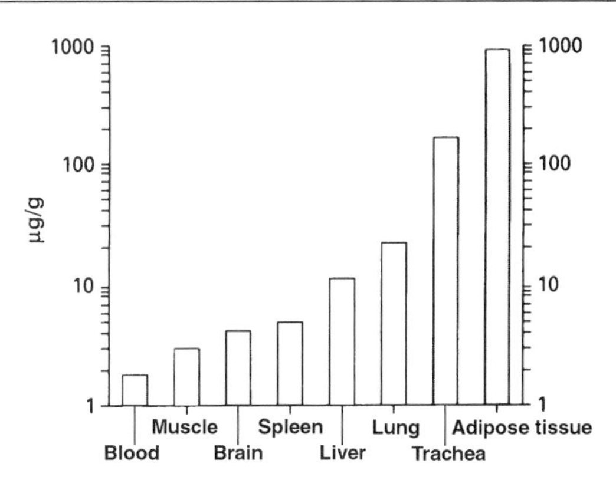

FIGURE 4 Content of 2,2′,3′,4,4′,5,5′-heptachlorobiphenyl (PCB 180) in blood and tissues of female rats after oral administration of 7 mg/kg body weight every other day for 3 months. One day after cessation of treatment, groups of five animals were investigated. The substance was dissolved in olive oil. The relatively high concentration in the trachea can be seen in a causative connection with structural particularities in its tissue. (Adapted from Koss *et al.*, 1993).

phenyls enable an almost complete distribution of the substances from the gastrointestinal tract into the mucosa cells. Active intake mechanisms seem not to play an important role. After oral administration of mono- up to hexachlorobiphenyl, rats absorbed more than 90% from the intestine, depending on the dose or the grade of chlorination. The absorption rate of the various congeners for humans is higher than 90%, but for higher chlorinated congeners it is likely to be lower. For example, 75% of octachlorobiphenyls are absorbed from the intestine by rats. The pulmonary absorption rate of the polychlorinated biphenyls is unknown. The dermal absorption depends on exposure time by the polychlorinated biphenyl and the matrix by which the polychlorinated biphenyls are applied. Rhesus monkeys absorb 2.4% of a technical compound (Aroclor 1242) via skin within 24 hours if the dose equals 4.1 $\mu g/cm^2$ applied in a mineral-oil solution. Rats treated dermally with 573 μg of 2,2′,4,4′,5,5′-hexachlorobiphenyl (PCB 153) in an acetone solution (5.6 cm^2 of back skin) absorbed 11% of the dose within 24 h and 43% within 5 days.

The polychlorinated biphenyls are distributed into all tissues by means of the blood circulation and the lymph—especially that inside the intestinal wall. However, the portion distributed by the lymph was estimated to be much lower than that distributed by blood.

In the blood, polychlorinated biphenyls are mainly associated with the lipoprotein and plasma proteins. In the liver tissue, central nervous system (CNS), and adipose tissue, tetrachlorobiphenyls are found mainly in the lipid fraction. In contrast, hexachlorobiphenyls in the liver tissues and CNS are mainly found in the lipid fraction (90%) but also partly in the protein fraction (10%). The distribution from the blood into the tissues is chiefly determined by the lipophilic properties of the congeners and the lipophilicity of the tissues. As expected the concentrations are much higher in adipose tissue than in the blood and muscle tissue (Fig. 4). The distribution of the polychlorinated biphenyls seems to be independent on the route of intake, dose, and duration of administration. A distinctive feature of all lipophilic xenobiotics is their accumulation in the tissues with a high percentage of lipid. The relative concentrations of PCBs in tissues depend on the physicochemical properties of the polychlorinated biphenyls and in addition on the position of the chlorine atoms in the molecule. A study on humans (in Japan in 1989) showed that the number of polychlorinated biphenyls in adipose tissue increases the higher the number of chlorine substitutes is in ortho-position.

Studies in human adipose tissue showed the following:

1. The average PCB content increases linearly with time.
2. The tissue content of PCB congeners is dominated by compounds with a 2,4-chlorine-substitution pattern.
3. The concentration of hexa- and heptachlorine congeners is mainly explained by the continuous intake of persistent polychlorinated biphenyls via the food chain.
4. The concentrations of tri- and tetrachlorine congeners, in general, are due to a short-termed exposure to PCB compounds with 20–42% weight portion of chlorine.
5. An accumulation of 2,4,4′-trichlorobiphenyl and 2,4,4′,5-tetrachlorobiphenyl (PCB 28, PCB 74) is dependent on a long-term exposure only, for example, in the work place.
6. If the content of polychlorinated biphenyls in human serum and adipose tissue (normal exposure) on the basis of the six indicator PCBs is measured, 25–28% of the total polychlorinated biphenyls can be recorded. If, additionally, the congeners PCB 18, 33, 66, 74, 99, 118, 146, 156, 187, 183, and 170 are analytically determined, 88% (77% in serum) of all polychlorinated biphenyls can be monitored.

Human (Fig. 5) and animal studies show that polychlorinated biphenyls cross through the placenta. Mice without experimental exposure to polychlorinated biphenyls during pregnancy had an average PCB

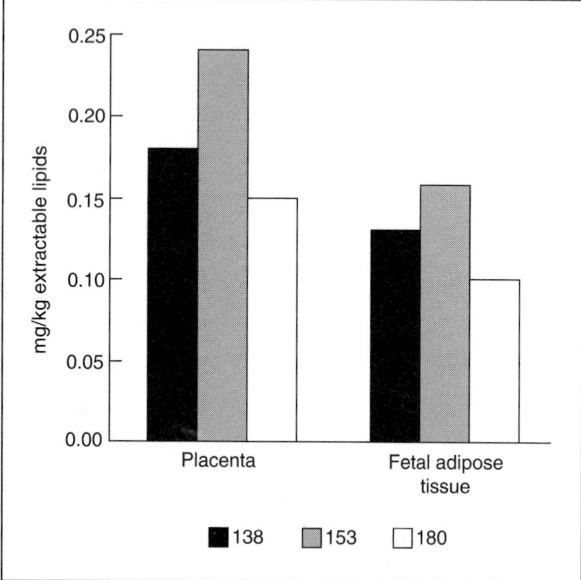

FIGURE 5 Concentration of higher chlorinated congeners (PCB 138, PCB 153, PCB 180) in human placenta (n = 9) and fetal subcutaneous adipose tissue (n = 9). Tissue samples were obtained after miscarriage between the 13th and 40th weeks of pregnancy. Results are based on extractable lipids. (Adapted from Bosse *et al.*, 1996.)

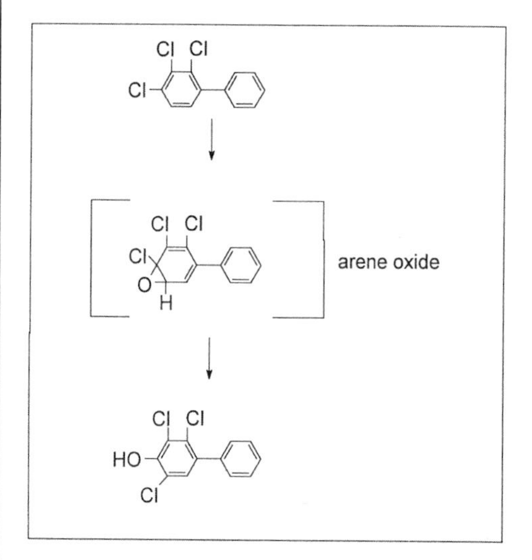

FIGURE 6 Hydroxylated PCB metabolite representative for congeners with a 3,4-dichloro- or 2,3,4-trichloro-substituted phenyl ring after an arene oxide formation in 4,5- position and subsequent shift (NIH-shift) of the chlorine atom at 4- position to 5-position. (Adapted from Kuroki *et al.*, 1996.)

concentration that was between six times higher (2,4,4′-trichlorobiphenyl, PCB 28) and 20 times higher (2,2′,4,4′,5,5′-hexachlorobiphenyl, PCB 153) than the concentration in fetus tissues. An administration of polychlorinated biphenyls during pregnancy resulted in an accumulation in the dams 40–50 times higher than in the fetuses due to the higher content of lipids of the mothers' tissues. Surveys in humans show that the PCB concentration in the maternal blood is significantly higher than that in the umbilical cord blood. The liver proves to have the highest enzymatic capacity for a metabolic conversion of the polychlorinated biphenyls, followed by the lungs, kidney, and intestinal wall. Metabolism shows the following characteristics.

- Biotransformation is inversely related to the number of chlorine atoms in the molecule. The biotransformation rate of 4-chlorobiphenyl (PCB 3) = 96–97%; the biotransformation rate of 2,2′,3,4,4′,5,5′-heptachlorobiphenyl (PCB 180) = 5%; octachlorobiphenyls and decachlorobiphenyls are practically not metabolized.
- Hydroxylation predominates over the production of sulfur-containing metabolites and reductive dechlorination. It primarily occurs in the meta- and para-positions, provided that no chlorine is bound.
- Metabolism of some polychlorinated biphenyls presumably procedes via an arene oxide (epoxide). By means of the exchange of the substitutes' positions, metabolites can develop from the arene oxide, whose chlorine atoms have a different position than in the parent substance (Fig. 6).
- Sulfur-containing metabolites (thioether) are products due to transformation of di- to heptachlorobiphenyls. The main part results from a conjugation reaction with glutathione. In further reactions during the enterohepatic circulation they can be transferred into sulfoxides and sulfones (Fig. 7).
- Polychlorinated biphenyls are mainly metabolized by cytochrome P450-dependent monooxygenases and glutathione *S*-transferases.

In humans, the metabolism of polychlorinated biphenyls leads to hydroxylation and sulfur-containing compounds. The extent of the hydroxylation and thioether formation is not clear. On the one hand, the biotransformation leads to a detoxification of the polychlorinated biphenyls. The water solubility is increased by introducing phenolic OH-groups and conjugation reactions with glucuronic acid, sulfuric acid, and glutathione. As a rule, the free metabolites, as well as the conjugates, are excreted more quickly via the kidney and intestine than are the parent compounds. Lactation is an additional way of excretion—

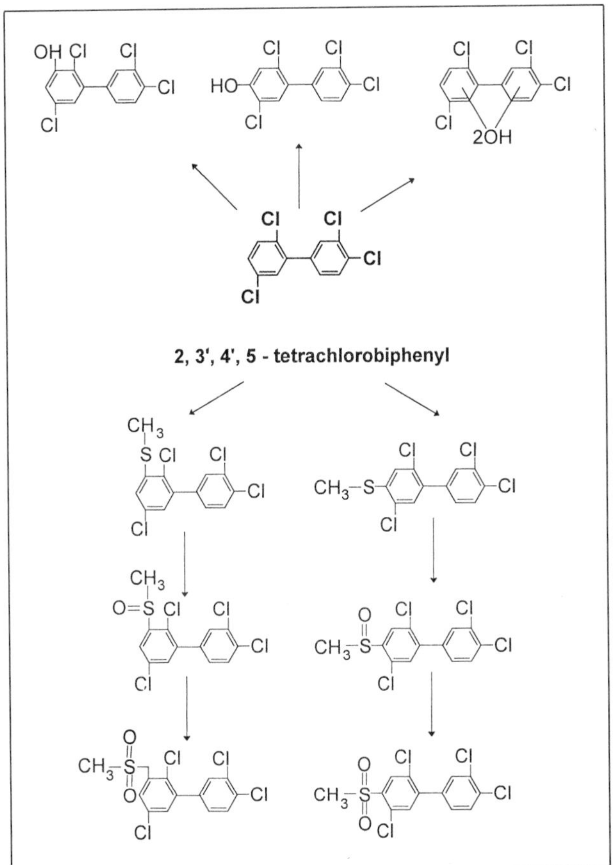

2, 3′, 4′, 5 - tetrachlorobiphenyl

FIGURE 7 Hydroxylated and sulphur-containing metabolites in the feces of male Wistar rats three days after oral administration of 50 mg/kg body weight of 2, 3′,4′,5-tetrachlorobiphenyl (PCB 70). Arrows indicate postulated pathways, in case of the sulphur-containing metabolites the stepwise oxydation of the methylthio via the methyl sulphoxide to the methyl sulfonyl compounds. (Adapted from Kuroki *et al.*, 1996.)

especially for the lipophilic methylsulfone metabolites.

However, biotransformation also must be considered as a possibility in toxification. The postulated arene oxides possess distinct electrophilic features. They are able to form adducts with proteins, RNA, and DNA. A remarkably high concentration of the metabolites 4-OH-3,3′,4′,5-tetrachlorobiphenyl and 4-OH-2,3,3′,4′,5-pentachlorobiphenyl could be demonstrated in mouse plasma after giving 3,3′,4,4′-tetrachlorobiphenyl (PCB 77) and 2,3,3′,4,4′-pentachlorobiphenyl (PCB 105), respectively. The cause of this high concentration seems to be the binding of metabolites with transthyretin, which has a higher affinity than thyroxine. The exposure of pregnant mice to PCB 77 resulted in an accumulation of 4-OH-3,3′,4′,5-tetrachlorobiphenyl in fetal mouse plasma, where it binds to transthyretin, accompanied by a decrease in fetal plasma thyroxine levels.

There is growing interest in the proof of the selective concentration of various methylsulfone metabolites in the bronchial mucosa, pulmonary parenchyma, kidney, intestine, and liquid of the tracheobronchial lavage in experimental animals (Fig. 8). Methylsulfone metabolites were detected in the bronchioalveolar lavage in humans poisoned by Kanechlor and in unexposed individuals. Up to 60 different methylsulfone metabolites are found in the liver, lung, and adipose tissue of poisoned persons.

The extent of the renal excretion is limited by the water solubility, which is inversely related to the increasing number of chlorine substitutes (Table 7). After an iv injection of 4,4′-dichloro[^{14}C]biphenyl, dogs excrete 7% of the radioactivity via the kidneys and 43% via the intestine within 24 h. Three days after injection of 2,2′,4,4′,5,5′-hexachloro[^{14}C]biphenyl (PCB 153), 3% of the radioactivity is excreted via the urine and 63% is excreted via the feces. These results demonstrate that the major part of the parent compound and metabolites is excreted via the bile into the intestine.

The direct distribution from the blood into the intestinal lumen plays only a minor role. Many of the metabolites reaching the intestine via bile enter an enterohepatic circulation. In the intestine they are deconjugated, are re-absorbed, and reach the liver metabolism once again. This could explain the existence of dithioethers, which—originating from glutathione conjugates—additionally have a methylthio- or methylsulfone group. The excretion velocity is determined by the elimination of polychlorinated biphenyls from the adipose tissue and by the extent of their metabolism. The metabolism depends especially on the positions of the chlorine substitutes. In rats PCB 136 is excreted with a half-life of 5.5 days and PCB 133 with a half-life of 69 days (Fig. 9).

Chronic animal experiments proved that the elimination of polychlorinated biphenyls does not follow biphasic kinetics but rather triphasic, especially if the concentrations in the adipose tissue are low. In this case the terminal half-life in the adipose tissue of rats is 465 days for 2,2′,4,4′,5,5′-hexachlorobiphenyl (PCB 153) and about a half-year for 2,2′,3,4,4′,5,5′-heptachlorobiphenyl (PCB 180). Workers exposed to Aroclor 1242 and 1254 showed a half-life of 2.6 and 4.8 years (median value) according to the analysis of serum. On the basis of measurements in the serum lipids between 1982 and 1990, a half-life of 10.4 years for 3,3′,4,4′,5,5′-hexachlorobiphenyl (PCB 169) was determined for a Yusho-affected person. The determination

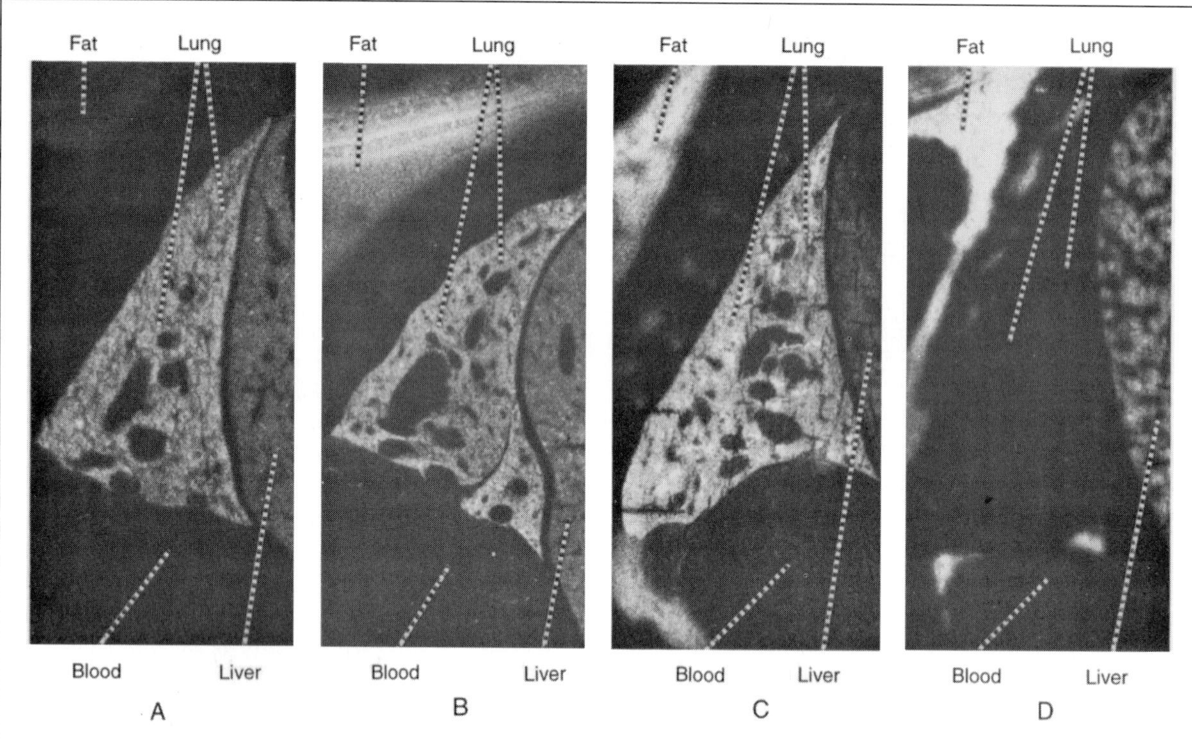

FIGURE 8 Details of autoradiograms of mice 4 days after i.v. injection of ^{14}C-labeled 2,2′,3,3′,6-pentachlorobiphenyl (PCB 84, A), 2,3,3′,4′,6-pentachlorobiphenyl (PCB 110, B), 2,2′,3,5′,6-pentachlorobiphenyl (PCB 95, C) and 2,3′,4,5,5′-pentachlorobiphenyl (PCB 120, D). Light areas represent tissues with high concentration of radioactivity. The autoradiograms show a highly selective uptake and retention of the three 2,3,6-substituted ^{14}C-pentachlorobiphenyls in the lung parenchyma of mice. In (D) there is an accumulation in the adipose tissue only. The doses per animal were: PCB 84 = 0.22 μmol, 2.6 μCi, PCB 110 = 0.20 μmol, 2.4 μCi, PCB 95 = 0.21 μmol, 2.4 μCi, and PCB 120 = 0.15 μmol, 4.0 μCi. (Adapted from Brandt *et al.*, 1981, *Toxicology* **21,** 317–322, with kind permission from Elsevier Science Ireland Ltd., Bay 15K, Shannon Industrial Estate, Co. Clare, Ireland.)

TABLE 7 Water Solubility of PCB Congeners[a]

Congener	Water solubility at room temperature (μg/liter)	Congener	Water solubility at room temperature (μg/liter)
2-Monochlorobiphenyl (PCB 1)	6000	2,2′,4,5,5′-Pentachlorobiphenyl (PCB 101)	10
2,2′-Dichlorobiphenyl (PCB 4)	1100	3,3′,4,4′,5-Pentachlorobiphenyl (PCB 126)	1
4,4′-Dichlorobiphenyl (PCB 15)	56	2,2′,3,4,4′,5′-Hexachlorobiphenyl (PCB 138)	1.8
2,2′,5-Trichlorobiphenyl (PCB 18)	410	2,2′,4,4′,5,5′-Hexachlorobiphenyl (PCB 153)	0.9
2,2′,5,5′-Tetrachlorobiphenyl (PCB 52)	29	2,2′3,4,4′,5,5′-Heptachlorobiphenyl (PCB 180)	0.63
3,3′,4,4′-Tetrachlorobiphenyl (PCB 77)	9.2	2,2′,3,3′,4,4′,5,5′,6,6′-Decachlorobiphenyl (PCB 209)	0.0013

[a]Adapted from Abramowitz and Yalkowsky (1990) *Chemosphere* **21,** 1221–1229, with kind permission from Elsevier Science Ltd, The Boulevard, Langford Lane, Kidlington OX5 1GB, UK.

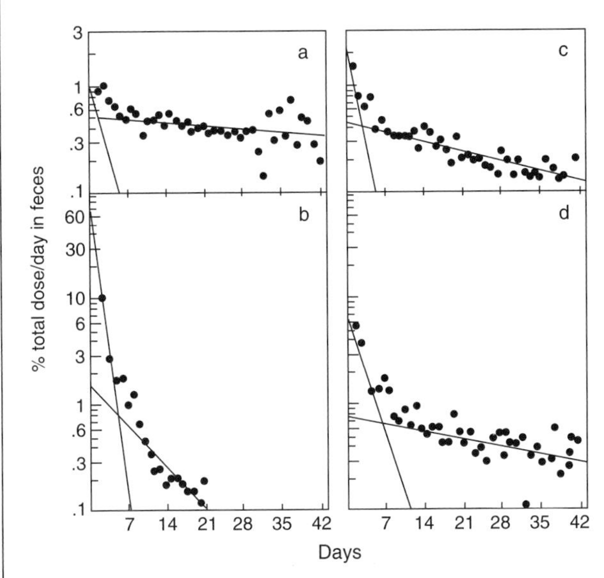

FIGURE 9 Daily excretion of total hexachlorobiphenyl derived radioactivity versus time after an i.v. dose of 0.6 mg/kg (2 mCi/mmol). The lines represent the components of the biexponential excretion rate curve for each congener. (a) 2,2′,3,3′,5,′-hexachlorobiphenyl (PCB 133), (b) 2,2′,3,3′,6,6′ -hexachlorobiphenyl (PCB 136), (c) 2,2,4,4′,5,5′ -hexachlorobiphenyl (PCB 153), (d) 2,2′,4,4′,6,6′-hexachlorobiphenyl (PCB 155). (From Matthews and Tuey, 1980.)

of the various PCB congeners in the blood of Yu Cheng-affected people showed a half-life of 1.1–5.7 years (Table 8). There is evidence that the concentrations of polychlorinated biphenyls in the blood of humans linearly correspond to those in the adipose tissue, as can be noted for 2,3,7,8-TCDD.

In females, lactation is another route of elimination. At the beginning of lactation, the lipophilic xenobiotics, such as polychlorinated biphenyls and their methylsulfone-containing metabolites, continuously disperse in the milk. The volume of the milk and lipid concentrations are decisive. The conveyed polychlorinated biphenyls that are transferred via the milk to the newborn lead to concentrations that are one or two orders of magnitude higher than those in an infant immediately after delivery (Fig. 10).

Investigations of women's milk (1990–1991) revealed that the three highly chlorinated indicator PCBs, 138, 153, and 180, in milk fat showed concentrations between 0.2 and 0.3 mg/kg. These values equal the concentrations in the adipose tissue of the approximately 30-year-old population. Apart from the three indicator PCBs mentioned, which represent about 30% of the total amount of PCBs in women's milk according to a current estimation, 24 other congeners were recorded, altogether about 60–70%. It is remarkable that the PCB concentration in milk fat is reduced by approximately 30% during the first two weeks of breastfeeding by reaching a steady state. As shown for several countries, the concentration of the total polychlorinated biphenyls in breast milk decreased by 50% between 1980 and 1990.

Acute Toxicity

Generally the acute oral toxicity (LD_{50}) of technical PCB mixtures is low (e.g., in rats 11.3 g/kg for Aroclor

TABLE 8 Elimination of Seven PCB Congeners from the Blood of Three Yu Cheng Individuals on a Whole Weight Basis[a,b]

Congener	Elimination half-life (years)
2,3′,4,4′-Tetrachlorobiphenyl (PCB 66)	2.0–2.6
2,3′,4,4′,5-Pentachlorobiphenyl (PCB 118)	1.1–1.3
2,2′,4.4′,5.5′-Hexachlorobiphenyl (PCB 153)	3.6–5.4
2,2′,3,4,4′,5′-Hexachlorobiphenyl (PCB 138)	3.3–4.9
2,3,3′,4,4′,5′-Hexachlorobiphenyl (PCB 156)	3.3–5.4
2,2′,3,4,4′,5,5′-Heptachlorobiphenyl (PCB 180)	3.7–5.7
2,2′,3,3′,4,4′,5-Heptachlorobiphenyl (PCB 170)	3.4–5.0

[a]Determination was performed from 1980 to 1989. The results stem from the individual with the lowest and highest value, respectively. Total PCB concentration in 1980 amounted to 156–398 μg/kg and in 1989 to 29.8–36.4 μg/kg.

[b]Adapted from Ryan *et al.* (1993).

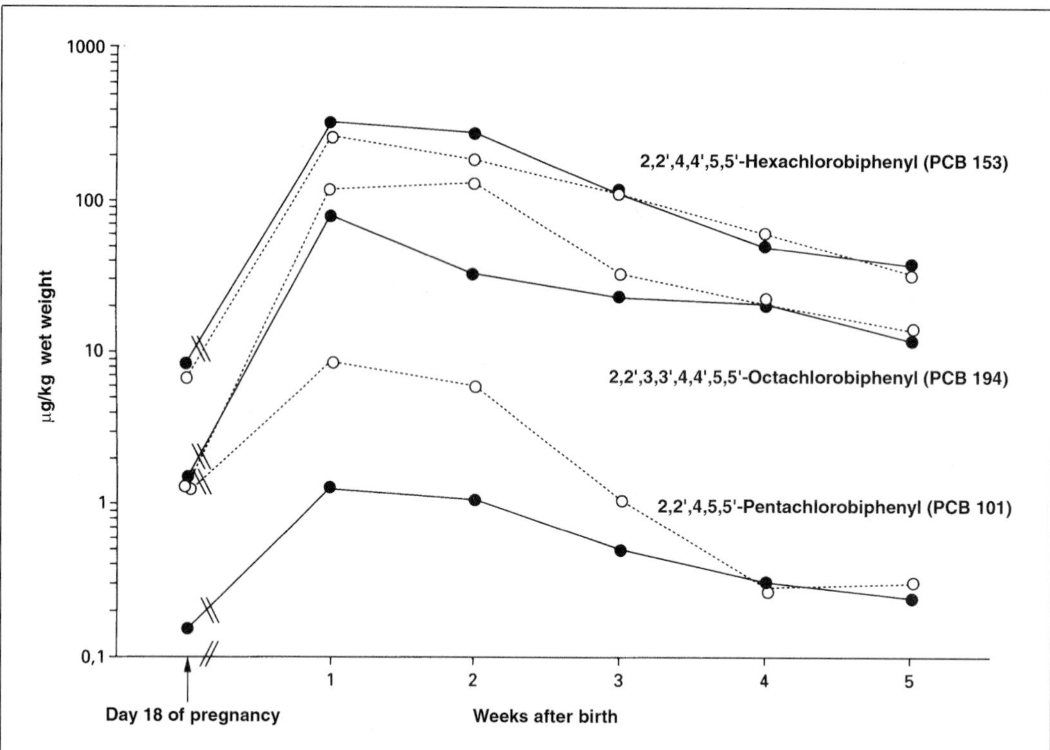

FIGURE 10 Concentrations of PCB in fetuses and offspring of mice after oral administration of congeners for 18 days before (○) or during (●) pregnancy. The PCB were administered in a diet with concentrations of 0.44 mg/kg PCB 153, 0.23 mg/kg PCB 194 and 0.42 mg/kg PCB 101. It is shown that the amount of each compound transferred through milk is larger than the amount transplacentally transferred. (Adapted from Masuda *et al.*, 1979.)

1254 and 1262). The LD_{50} for Aroclor 1221, which has a lower chlorination level, is 4.25 g/kg. The signs of poisoning were ulcerations in the small intestine and glandular stomach. A single oral intake of 50 mg/kg Aroclor 1254 caused growth of the liver and an induction of hepatic microsomal enzymes within 12 hours.

After applying Aroclor 1221, 1242, 1248, and 1260 to the skin of rabbits, LD_{50} values of 0.79 to 3.17 g/kg were noted. After i.v. injection of Aroclor 1254, the average lethal dose for rats was 0.4 g/kg, and for mice after i.p. injection between 0.9 and 1.2 g/kg.

There are no toxicity data after inhalation. Studies regarding the average lethal dose of individual congeners were made with guinea pigs, among others. Here the LD_{50} after oral intake of 3,3′,4,4′,5,5′-hexachlorobiphenyl (PCB 169) is 0.5 mg/kg and of 2,2′,4,4′,5,5′-hexachlorobiphenyl (PCB 153) 10 mg/kg. Rats, which are much more insensitive to polychlorinated biphenyls, respond to a single i.p. injection of 1 mg/kg of 3,3′,4,4′,5-pentachlorobiphenyl or to a single oral intake of 50 mg/kg of 3,3′,4,4′,5,5′-hexachlorobiphenyl with an increase in liver weight and deposit of neutral fat in liver cells, with thymus atrophy, and with reduction of the relative weight of the spleen. Similar reactions with reference to hexa- and heptachlorobiphenyls were not noted with diorthochlorine substitutes.

Chronic Toxicity

Symptoms of chronic poisoning in humans became known after the consumption of highly contaminated food. Toxic symptoms were also noticed after contact with polychlorinated biphenyls in the work place.

Yusho

In 1968, an accumulated appearance of chloracne was noticed in Japan. Investigations revealed that the patients had eaten rice oil (Yusho means rice oil illness) that had been put on the market five months previously. It was highly contaminated with Kanech-

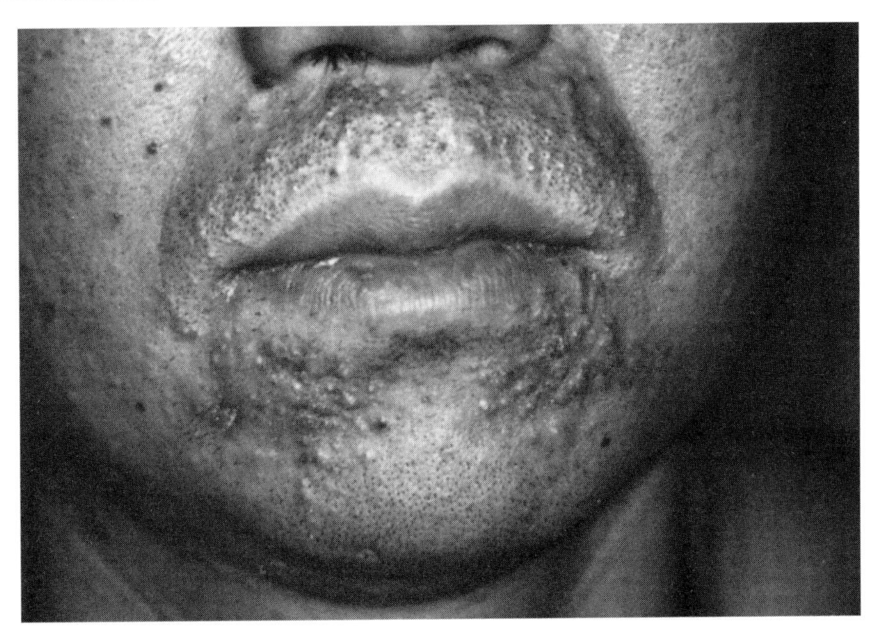

FIGURE 11 The clinical appearance of acneiform in eruptions in Yusho patients. (Adapted from Nakayama *et al.*, 1996.)

lor 400. The rice oil contained not only polychlorinated biphenyls but also chlorinated dibenzofurans and quarterphenyls, which can develop from the dimerization of polychlorinated biphenyls at high temperatures. Theoretically more than 100,000 chlorinated quarterphenyls are possible. The estimated average intake was 157 μg polychlorinated biphenyls, 148 μg chlorinated quarterphenyls, and 0.9 μg PCDF/kg body weight per day. The duration of intake is not known. Later it was assumed that the clinically remarked signs of poisoning appeared 20 to 190 days after consumption of the rice oil. Estimates revealed that 14000–15000 people had eaten the rice oil. By 1982 there were 1788 clinically registered patients.

Besides the eye-catching chloracne (Fig. 11), the first signs of poisoning were enlargement and strong excretion of the meibomian gland at the eyelid, swelling of the eyelids, beginning of pigmentation of nails and mucosas, and extraordinary exhaustion, dizzines, and vomiting. Secondary symptoms were hyperkeratosis and strong pigmentation due to the accumulation of melanin in the basal cells of the epidermis; enlargement of the hair follicles; and acne-similar eruptions partly with secondary staphylococcal infection, mainly in the area of neck and chest, and occasionally also throughout the whole body. Some patients showed edemas on the arms and legs and increased values of serum transaminases, serum triglycerides, and alkaline phosphatase.

Many patients suffered from continuous disorders of the respiratory system, showing symptoms such as chronic bronchitis. The liver tissue of one of the patients showed a growth of the smooth endoplasmatic reticulum. Serum bilirubin was obviously reduced. Tests of sputum proved that polychlorinated biphenyls can accumulate in the bronchial mucosa depending on dose and molecular structure. Difficulties in breathing were due to disorders of the small respiratory systems (inflammatory changes), whereas certain cells (Clara cells) were especially affected.

In the early stages of the poisoning the values of serum IgA and serum IgM were reduced, the latter especially in patients with chloracne. Furthermore, a strongly restricted cell-mediated immunocompetence could be noted.

Women affected by Yusho during pregnancy endured stillbirths. Live births showed hyperpigmentation of the skin and mouth mucosa, hyperplastic changes of the gums, abnormal calcification of the skull bones, early teething, and low birth weight. These disorders, described as "fetal PCB syndrome," were explained by impairments of the sex-hormone and calcium balance caused by the polychlorinated biphenyls. A deformation of the foot known as "rocker bottom heel" with an upright heel was noticed in some children. Discomfort resulting from central nervous disorders is not mentioned. However, complaints about numbness in the arms and legs were made and decreased peripheral-nerve-conduction velocities were observed.

By 1983, 120 Yusho patients had died; 41 of these had had cancer. The liver, stomach, and lungs were primarily affected. A statistically significant high percentage of cancer mortality was noticed only in men. An evaluation of the cause is under preparation. Measurements of the organohalogens in the blood after the end of the exposure had not been made. After 11 years, the average blood concentrations of 6 μg polychlorinated biphenyls/liter and 2 μg quarterphenyls/liter were measured.

Yu Cheng

In 1979, a remarkably large number of changes of the skin similar to acne were noticed in Taiwan. As in Japan, the rice oil highly contaminated with polychlorinated biphenyls (in Chinese, Yu Cheng means rice oil illness) was found to be the cause. The technical mixtures of Kanechlor 400 and 500 used in a heat exchanger in rice-oil production had penetrated through a leak and contaminated the rice oil. It was estimated that about 700–1840 mg polychlorinated biphenyls, 586 mg polychlorinated quarterphenyls, and 3.8 mg polychlorinated dibenzofurans were taken up. The contaminated rice oil was consumed for up to one month. After cessation of exposure, values of 3–1156 μg/liter organohalogens were measured in the blood. Six months later, the concentrations had decreased to 12–50 μg/liter polychlorinated biphenyls, 1.7–11 μg/liter polychlorinated quarterphenyls, and 0.062–0.24 μg/liter of PCDF. The first appearance of toxic signs was observed after 3 to 4 months in about 2000 people.

Frequent symptoms were eruptions similar to acne involving the hair follicles, strong pigmentation of the skin and nails, swelling of the eyelids with suppuration, headache, nausea, and numbness of the extremities. The number of erythrocytes, as well as the concentrations of hemoglobin and IgA and IgM, were reduced; the number of leukocytes; the concentrations of the triglycerides, serum glutamate oxalacetate transaminase, and serum glutamate pyruvate transaminase, and the activity of the alkaline phosphatases, were increased. Furthermore, a high excretion of δ-aminolevulinic acid and uroporphyrine was noticed in urine. In the placenta a remarkable increase in the activity of arylhydrocarbon hydroxylase and a diminished autophosphorylation of the epidermal-growth-factor receptor were recorded, correlating with the reduction of birth weight.

Babies showed a higher excretion of total porphyrins and a hyperpigmentation of the skin. By 1985 12 cases of severe liver damage, including hepatoma, were recorded. The symptoms of Yusho and Yu Cheng were very similar. However, the extent of the skin changes was higher in Japan than in Taiwan.

Exposure in the Workplace

Symptoms noted in Yusho and Yu Cheng poisoning were also observed after occupational exposure. However, the intake of the polychlorinated biphenyls in the work place occurred via the skin, and presumably via the air as a smaller percentage. A high prevalence of comedos and acne was noticed, and there were also irritations of the skin and erythemas in workers exposed to Kanechlor 300 and 500 for 1 to 24 years. The polychlorinated biphenyl concentration in the plasma ranged between 21 and 117 μg/liter; the extent of the skin changes correlated with the amount of PCB. Exposure to Aroclor for 5 to 25 years produced irritation of the mucosas of the upper respiratory systems, as well as gastrointestinal, neurological, and dermatological symptoms. In addition, hepatomegaly and increased activity of plasma enzymes were observed.

After exposure to Aroclor 1016, 1242, and/or 1254 with plasma concentrations of 363 μg/liter (low-chlorinated PCBs) and 30 μg/liter (higher-chlorinated PCBs), diminished bilirubin values and an increase of γ-glutamyl transpeptidase activity and lymphocytes were observed. There was evidence for an increased excretion of porphyrins in workers who had been exposed to Pyralone and Apirolio. Some work place surveys recorded a correlation between PCB contents in the blood and changes of liver-enzyme activity, hepatomegaly, and changes in the skin. In contrast, other studies did not show these correlations.

Studies in Animals

Technical Mixtures

Long-term studies were first performed mainly with technical mixtures. These studies were a major factor in finding a tolerable PCB dose for humans. A toxicological evaluation of polychlorinated biphenyls relevant to humans' daily uptake is only possible when toxicological data about the effects of the congeners in question and the mechanisms of action of these compounds are available. Rats fed Aroclor 1254 and 1260 in different concentrations ranging between 20 and 1000 mg/kg (corresponding to 1.5–72 mg/kg body weight) showed a dose-dependent increase of the relative liver weight, enlarged hepatocytes with increased lipid amount, and adenofibrosis and cholangiofibrosis. The last is due to the proliferation and adenomatosis of the bile duct, as well as fibroadenoma.

Female rats of a sensitive strain were given a diet containing 10, 30, and 100 mg of Aroclor 1254/kg (0.5, 1.5, and 5 mg/kg body weight) for 20 weeks. The higher doses led to body-weight reduction. All doses were associated with loss of hair, reddening and thickening of the skin with hyperkeratosis, subcutaneous edema, and infiltration of polymorphonuclear leucocytes in the skin. The highest dose showed changes mainly in the areas of the nose, tail, and extremities.

A wider spectrum of PCB-induced changes was noted in rhesus monkeys. The intake of about 1 mg/kg body weight of Aroclor 1248 for 2 months produced weight reduction, loss of hair, subcutaneous edema, swollen eyelids, erythema, and acneiform changes involving especially those skin areas affected by the loss of hair. Furthermore, anemia, hyperproteinemia, hemorrhages, ulcerations of the gastric mucosa, and bone-marrow hypoplasia were noticed. Animals that received 0.1 and 0.2 mg/kg body weight in their food for 1.5 years showed necrotic areas in the liver, enlarged hepatocytes, and signs of a changed lipid metabolism. After oral intake of 0.28 mg/kg body weight for more than 2 years, rhesus monkeys showed profound changes in the spleen and lymph nodes, erosion and ulceration of gums, hypertrophic gastropathies with cystic dilatation of certain glands, enlarged and necrotic liver cells, hypertrophy of the bile duct and gall bladder epithelium, hyperplasia of the bile duct, and a not yet-clearly-proven increase in the number of the lysosomes in the thyroid's follicular epithelial cells.

Congeners

The hepatic cytochrome P450-dependent monooxygenase system is induced after a single administration of polychlorinated biphenyls and more pronounced after a long-term administration. This holds true in all species of experimental animals and in humans, which can be demonstrated with the reduced half-life of antipyrine in workers who had been exposed to Aroclor 1016. Furthermore, experimental animals show an increased activity of the monooxygenase in the kidneys, adrenal glands, lungs, intestinal wall, skin, and testis. This effect is also caused by the transfer of polychlorinated biphenyls via the placenta and milk in a fetus or a suckling pup. Animal experiments have proven that the activity of the monooxygenase is correlated with the degree of chlorination of the compounds. Comparative congener-specific studies revealed a "structure–activity relationship" (SAR) for enzyme induction; congeners that have chlorine substitutes in both para-positions and at least two chlorine substitutes in the meta-positions induce the same microsomal-monooxygenase system (cytochrome P450-dependent enzyme activities, e.g., CYP1A1 and CYP1A2) as 2,3,7,8-TCDD and 3-methylcholanthrene. These congeners have a co-planar arrangement in phenyl rings (Fig. 12): 3,3′,4,4′,5-pentachlorobiphenyl (PCB 126), 3,3′,4,4′,5,5′-hexachlorobiphenyl (PCB 169), and 3,3′,4,4′-tetrachlorobiphenyl (PCB 77).

Congeners like 2,2′,4,4′,5,5′-hexachlorobiphenyl (PCB 153), which are chlorinated in at least two *ortho*-positions, induce the same monooxygenase system as phenobarbital (cytochrome CYP2B1 and CYP2B2). Congeners like 2,3′,4,4′,5-pentachlorobiphenyl (PCB 118), which are not substituted symmetrically on both rings, having only one chlorine atom in ortho-position and more chlorine atoms on both neighboring rings in the meta-position and para-position, induce CYP1A as well as CYB2B (mixed-type inducer). *In vitro* and *in vivo* studies have shown that the extent of the induction of arylhydrocarbon hydroxylase and of ethoxyresorufin-*O*-deethylase, as well as of the body-weight loss ("wasting syndrome"), thymus atrophy, immunologic toxicity, and teratogenicity, correlates with planarity of the congeners. Furthermore, there was a positive correlation between the enzyme induction (CYP1A1) and the toxic effects. A receptor for polychlorinated biphenyls of the phenobarbital type which induces, for example, aminopyrine *N*-demethylase and aldrin epoxidase, is not known. Some of these congeners have a neurotoxic potential because they inhibit the activity of tyrosine hydroxylase, which is the rate-limiting enzyme of the dopamine synthesis.

Co-planar and nonplanar congeners—analogous to the polychlorinated dioxins and hexachlorobenzene—produce massive hepatic disorders of the heme biosynthesis (hepatic porphyria), affecting the uroporphyrinogen decarboxylase with subsequently increased concentrations of uro- and heptacarboxyporphyrin in the liver. The inhibition of enzyme activity could be induced by the direct interaction of the congeners with the active center or the sulfhydryl groups of the enzyme, resulting in an accumulation of highly carboxylated porphyrins, which can also occur many months after the cessation of treatment with polychlorinated biphenyls (and also of polybrominated biphenyls). The reason for this delayed onset of porphyria seems to be the associated complex changes of aging tissue (e.g., lacking detoxification of free rad-

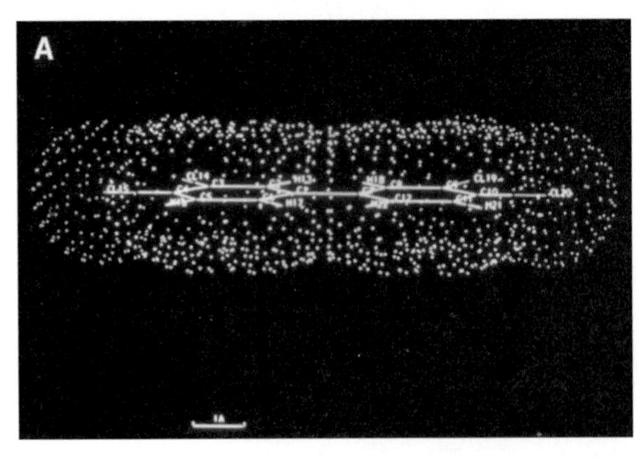

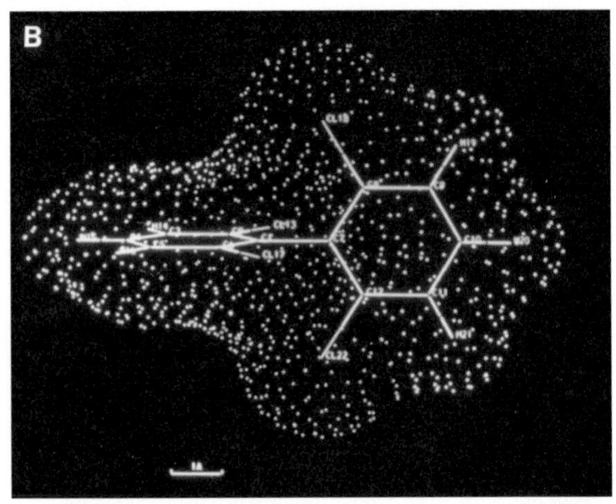

FIGURE 12 Computer-generated three-dimensional structure of (*A*) 3,3′,4,4′,-tetrachlorobiphenyl (dihedral angle = 0°) and (*B*) 2,2′,6,6′-tetrachlorobiphenyl (dihedral angle = 90°) . Each dot represents the van der Waals surface and the dot density is equal to five dots/0.01 nm^2. The total dimensions of 3,3′,4,4′-tetrachlorobiphenyl are 0.34 nm × 1 nm × 0.34 nm. (Adapted from Sassa *et al.*, 1986.)

icals) with the concurrent presence of the accumulated congener (e.g., 2,2′,3′,4,4′,5′,5-heptachlorobiphenyl, PCB 180). Co-planar as well as nonplanar congeners lead to a reduction of the serum content of the thyroide hormone and vitamin A in experimental animals. Hydroxylated PCB metabolites impede hepatic thyroxine-5′-deiodinase activity and impair mitochondrial oxidative phosphorylation. The nonplanar 2,2′,4,4′,5,5′-hexachlorobiphenyl adversely affects vitamin-K-dependent blood coagulation, which could play a role in PCB-induced hemorrhage. Various congeners that have three or four chlorine atoms in the ortho-position have axial enantiomerism and therefore appear as racemate. The enantiomers show different properties, which, however, are not elucidated. For instance, the (+)-enantiomer (in comparison with the (−)-enantiomers) of the 2,2′,3,4,4′,6-hexachlorobiphenyl induces high uroprophyrin accumulation and high ethoxyresorufin-*O*-deethylase activity after the addition of δ-aminolevulinic acid to liver-cell cultures of chicken embryos. Under the same conditions, (−)-2,2′,3,4,6-pentachlorobiphenyl induces a higher uroporphyrin accumulation and benzphetamine *N*-demethylase activity without changing the activity of the ethoxyresorufin-*O*-deethylase.

Specific Toxicology

Reproduction Toxicity

Kanechlor 500 administered to mice for 5 days during pregnancy led to cleft palates in the fetuses. In this experiment maternal toxic effects were also noted. In further experiments, lower doses were given to exclude maternal effects. Afterward, teratogenic effects were no longer observed. Aroclor 1254 can antagonize the effect of 2,3,7,8-TCDD in mice. In contrast to the technical mixtures, teratogenic effects occurred after administration of single PCB congeners without maternal toxicity. If the dams were treated with 2 mg/kg per day of 3,3′,4,4′,5,5′-hexachlorobiphenyl (PCB 169), fetuses showed an increased number of cleft palates. After doubling the dose, an increased number of hydronephrosis was observed. An intake of 1 mg/kg per day did not lead to this effect. 3,3′,4,4′-Tetrachlorobiphenyl induced cleft palates and hydronephrosis after an intake of 4 mg/kg per day but not after 1 and 2 mg/kg. However, 3,3′,5,5′-tetrachlorobiphenyl had no effect on the fetuses up to 64 mg/kg per day.

After a 10-week intake of Clophen A 60 at a daily dose of 0.8 mg/kg body weight, mice showed prolonged estrus cycles. The same effect was noted in rats that received 10 mg/kg per day Aroclor 1254 over a period of 6 weeks. The cycles were not influenced after the intake of Aroclor 1242 at 3.7 and 7.5 mg/kg per day for 36 weeks. In spite of the unchanged length of the cycles, the animals showed a reduced progesterone content in the plasma and histological changes in the stroma of the ovaries. Female rhesus monkeys treated orally with 0.08 mg/kg body weight of Aroclor 1254 daily showed no change in the cycle length nor in the estrogen and progesterone concentrations in the plasma. Male rhesus monkeys that received

Aroclor 1248 for more than 12 months showed reduced spermatogenesis and libido.

In the area affected by Yusho poisoning, a total of 851 births were registered between 1968 and 1972. Of these, 34 of the children (3.9%) suffered from fetal-PCB syndrome. All children had an dark-brown-skin pigmentation ("cola babies"), which also affected the mucosas. Biopsy material disclosed signs of hyperkeratosis and a high concentration of melanin. After the ages of 2 to 5 months, this pigmentation disappeared. The faces of the children were edematous. Three children suffered from exophthalmus. Frontal and occipital fontanels showed comparatively larger openings. The sagittal suture (between right and left parietal bones) stayed further apart than normal. Abnormal bone calcification was proven via X-ray in the parietaloccipital skull area. Immediately after birth, some children already had teeth. Hepatomegaly was observed in one child, the liver function test, however, was to be normal. No child showed any signs of neurological or cardiovascular abnormalities. In a few cases, increased SGOT values, enlarged hepatocytes, minimal fibrosification, and pigmentation in the histological liver preparation were observed; in one case anemia and in another case retarded bony growth were observed. The percentage of children who were under-weight was 17.4%.

As in Yusho, Yu Cheng also showed a complex spectrum of toxicity. Additionally, 16 out of 125 newborn developed a noticeable acne. The children who were examined in 1985 at the ages of 5 to 6 years still suffered from hyperpigmentation and deformations of their nails. Several children suffered from bronchitis. It is assumed that prenatal exposure to polychlorinated biphenyls and also to other organohalogens led to neurological deficits, as well as to deficits in behavior. Prenatal exposure to high doses of the polychlorinated compounds apparently has a much greater toxic effect on a child's development than post-natal exposure via breast milk.

Neurotoxicity

The high exposures to PCBs in Japan and Taiwan have had significant effects on the behavioral and cognitive development of the children who were exposed *in utero* and during breastfeeding. More recent epidemiological studies on exposure to low doses reported effects on psychomotor development and cognitive function of PCB-exposed children. Animal research concerning the developmental neurotoxicity of PCB mixtures and single congeners is generally consistent with findings in humans.

Following the exposure of rat dams to 20 or 100 mg/kg Kanechlor 500 during gestational days 8–14 or 15–21, the offspring made errors in a water-maze task, which is interpreted as an alteration in learning ability. Exposure of rats to Fenclor 42 (2–10 mg/kg) before and during gestation and lactation affected cliff-avoidance behavior (lactation), decreased swimming performance, increased circling behavior (for any of the three periods of exposure), and depressed active avoidance learning (second trimester or lactation) in the offspring. Pregnant female rhesus monkeys were exposed to either Aroclor 1016 or Aroclor 1248 in their diet during gestation. The offspring showed changes in locomotor activity and deficits in spatial, shape, and color discrimination reversal tasks. Specific distribution and neurochemical studies with technical mixtures and congeners elucidated the mechanisms of the PCB-induced neurotoxic action. Orthochlorine-substituted congeners accumulated in the brains of rat groups by a factor of 100, as compared to the concentration of PCB mixtures to which the dams were exposed. 3,3′,4,4′-Tetrachlorobiphenyl (PCB 77) was not detected in the brains of rats; however, it was in mice, as shown by a ^{14}C-labeled congener. Mice perinatally exposed to PCB 77 exhibited decreased hind-limb strength, hyperactivity, and uncoordinated circling. Decreases in the striatal concentrations of dopamine and decreased concentrations of dopamine-receptor-binding sites were noted and it was concluded that this congener also affects the muscarinic acetylcholine receptors.

Studies of adult nonhuman primates (*Macaca nemestrina*) revealed that relatively low doses of Aroclor 1260 (30 mg/kg diet) result in neurochemical changes largely restricted to dopamine. However, not all brain regions containing dopamine were affected. The congeners present in the brain are *ortho*-chlorine substituted (responsible for decrease of dopamine). The effects of PCB exposure persist beyond the period of exposure. There is evidence, however, that some effects related to PCB exposure may dissipate with age.

Mutagenicity

Aroclor 1242, 1254, and 1268, Clophen A 30, 50, and 60, and Kanechlor 500 were tested with the Ames test (*Salmonella typhimurium* with and without metabolic activation), on hamster ovary cells, with the mouse-micronucleus test, in human lymphocytes (chromosome aberration), in the bone marrow cells and spermatogoniums of rats, in *Drosophila melanogaster*, and in rats in the dominant–lethal test with reference to a genotoxic potential. All the results were negative. Tests using 2,2′,5,5′-tetrachlorobiphenyl in the Ames test with and without metabolic activation did not show any effects as well. 3,3′,4,4′-Tetrachlorobiphenyl induced dose-dependent chromosomal breakages in human lymphocytes. 2,2′,5,5′-Tetrachlorobiphenyl showed no effect. When both congeners were combined, the effect was synergistic compared to an application of the co-planar congener alone. The same combination induced a clear increase in polyploidy and in the percentage of cells with chromosome aberrations in the bone marrow cells of rats that received both congeners at concentrations of 0.1 and 10 mg/kg per day, respectively, for more than a year.

Carcinogenicity

Chronic administration of Kanechlor 300, 400, or 500 and of Aroclor 1254 in mice leads to hepatocellular carcinoma, nodular hyperplasia, and hypertrophy of the liver. In rats, hepatic nodular hyperplasias were recorded after intake of Kanechlor 400 and 500. These changes were not observed after intake of Kanechlor 300. Aroclor 1242, 1254, and 1260 induce carcinomas and nodular hyperplasia in the liver of rats. In a study of rats that received Clophen A30 or A60 at a dose of 100 mg/kg diet each for 800 days, a possible influence of the technical mixtures' chlorination grade was investigated. Polychlorinated dibenzofurans were not contained in both mixtures; however, information regarding the detection limits were missing. After 700 days, the first tumors were seen. At the end of the study, 61% of the animals had hepatocellular carcinomas after the administration of Clophen A60, 3% of the animals after Clophen A30, and 2% of the control animals. The frequency of developing neoplastic nodes and carcinomas increased with time. It was remarked that the incidence of thymomas and inflammatory changes of the urogenital tract decreased and the mortality due to the Clophen supply was reduced. These results led to the assumption that the PCB mixtures involved not only have tumorigenic effects but can also lead to a certain protection of the immune system.

In animal experiments, PCB mixtures and certain congeners were surveyed with respect to their tumor-promoting potential. In order to initiate the formation of lung and liver tumors 4-day-old mice received an ip dose of 5 mg/kg of dimethyl nitrosamine and four days later, a single dose of 500 mg/kg Aroclor 1254. The incidence of alveologenic adenomas 16 weeks later was twice as high as when dimethyl nitrosamine alone was given. Aroclor alone did not induce lung adenomas. In the liver, an additional dose of Aroclor led to tumors and focal hepatocellular proliferative lesions, which were fewer in quantity but much larger than those noted after only nitrosamine had been given.

Several studies in rats showed a promoting effect of PCB mixtures and of 3,3′,4,4′,5-pentachlorobiphenyl, 2,3,3′,4,4′-pentachlorobiphenyl and 2,2′,4,4′,5,5′-hexachlorobiphenyl. Inhibition of neoplasms in the liver was recorded after a simultaneous administration of PCB mixtures and substances with initiating properties or when the mixtures were given before the initiator. This "antitumor effect" is caused by the induction of the cytochrome P450-dependent monooxygenases, resulting in an extensive biotransformation of the initiating substances.

One week after oral administration of diethyl nitrosamine, rats received 2,2′,4,4′- or 2,2′,5,5′-tetrachlorobiphenyl (100 mg/kg each) for 28 weeks. Both polychlorinated biphenyls had a promoting effect with regard to the development of enzyme-altered foci in the liver. Rats first given diethyl nitrosamine and then treated with a mixture of 2,2′,5,5′- and 3,3′,4,4′-tetrachlorobiphenyl for one year showed an eight- to ninefold higher number of preneoplastic foci per liver than after treatment with each individual substance. The number of foci was only four times higher when the individual polychlorinated biphenyls were administered after diethyl nitrosamine. The larger number of neoplastic nodes and the aneuploidy in many hepatocytes is seen as an indicator for the induction of the transition from a benign to a malignant tumor (progression).

The co-planar 3,3′,4,4′,5-pentachlorobiphenyl (PCB 126) and 3,3′,4,4′-tetrachlorobiphenyl (PCB 77) have approximately 10% and 0.1% of TCDD's tumor-promoting potency, respectively. Additive promoting effects have been shown for 3,3′,4,4′,5-pentachlorobiphenyl (PCB 126) and TCDD. However, a more complex mixture of dioxin-like compounds (TCDD, pentachlorodibenzo-*p*-dioxin, 3,3′,4,4′,5-pentachlorobiphenyl (PCB 126), 2,3′,4,4′,5-pentachlorobiphenyl (PCB 118), and 2,3,3′,4,4′,5-hexachlorobiphenyl (PCB 156)) that is relevant for human exposure had a significantly lower tumor-promoting effect in rat liver as compared to a TCDD dose that was nearly equivalent based on Toxic Equivalency Factor values. Moreover, the diortho-substituted 2,2′,4,4′,5,5′-hexachlorobiphenyl (PCB 153), a phenobarbital-like cytochrome P450 inducer, has also been found to have tumor-promoting activity. Tumor-promotion studies with mixtures of PCB 153 and co-planar PCB have given equivocal results. PCB 153 in combination with PCB 126 caused a more than additive effect on the formation of hepatic foci. However, a significant decrease in the number of hepatic foci per volume was observed after treatment with PCB 153 and PCB 77, as compared a treatment with PCB 77 alone. This antagonistic effect is in accord with the inhibition of TCDD-mediated teratogenic and immunosuppressive effects by PCB 153.

No strong evidence exists for a causal relationship between the intake of polychlorinated biphenyls and cancer or morbidity in humans. This assessment is based first on studies of Yusho-affected individuals and then on other cohorts who were exposed to technical PCB mixtures in their work place for a longer period of time. One must assume that polychlorinated biphenyls may promote the formation of neoplasias in humans. The conclusions are equivocal. It is said that human carcinogenicity of PCB is not fully evidenced (WHO) and it is also said that the carcinogenicity studies on animals are sufficient evidence.

Immunotoxicity

PCB mixtures produce changes in the primary lymphatic organs (e.g., thymic atrophy and bone marrow depression) and in the secondary lymphatic organs (e.g., hypoplasia and atrophy of the spleen and loss of the germinal center of lymph nodes). They must be regarded as immune-depressive effects and are more distinct the higher the concentration of polychlorinated dibenzofurans in the technical mixture. In these

TABLE 9 PCB-Mixture-Caused Immunologic Alterations in Experimental Animals[a]

Technical mixture	Animal species	Immunologic alteration
Aroclor 1016 Aroclor 1242	Mouse	Increased mortality to microbiological infection
Aroclor 1242	Mouse	Decreased formation of splenic plaque-forming cells in response to sheep red blood cells
Aroclor 1016, 1232, 1242, 1248, 1254, 1260	Mouse	Reduction in antibody production to sheep red blood cells
Kanechlor 500	Mouse	Modulation of T-cell function
Aroclor 1016	Mouse	Altered graft vs. most response
Aroclor 1254	Rabbit	Splenic and thymic gamma globulin reduction
Aroclor 1260, Clophen A 60	Guinea pig	Reduction in tetanus antitoxin producing cells
Aroclor 1260	Guinea pig	Reduction in gamma globulin producing cells
Aroclor 1254, Kanechlor 400	Monkey	Reduction in antibody production to sheep red blood cells
Aroclor 1254	Monkey	Modulation of several nonspecific and specific immune parameters
Aroclor 1254	Rat	Reduced natural killer cell activity

[a]Adapted with permission from Safe (1994) *Crit. Rev. Toxicol.* **24,** 87–149, Copyright CRC Press, Boca Raton, Florida.

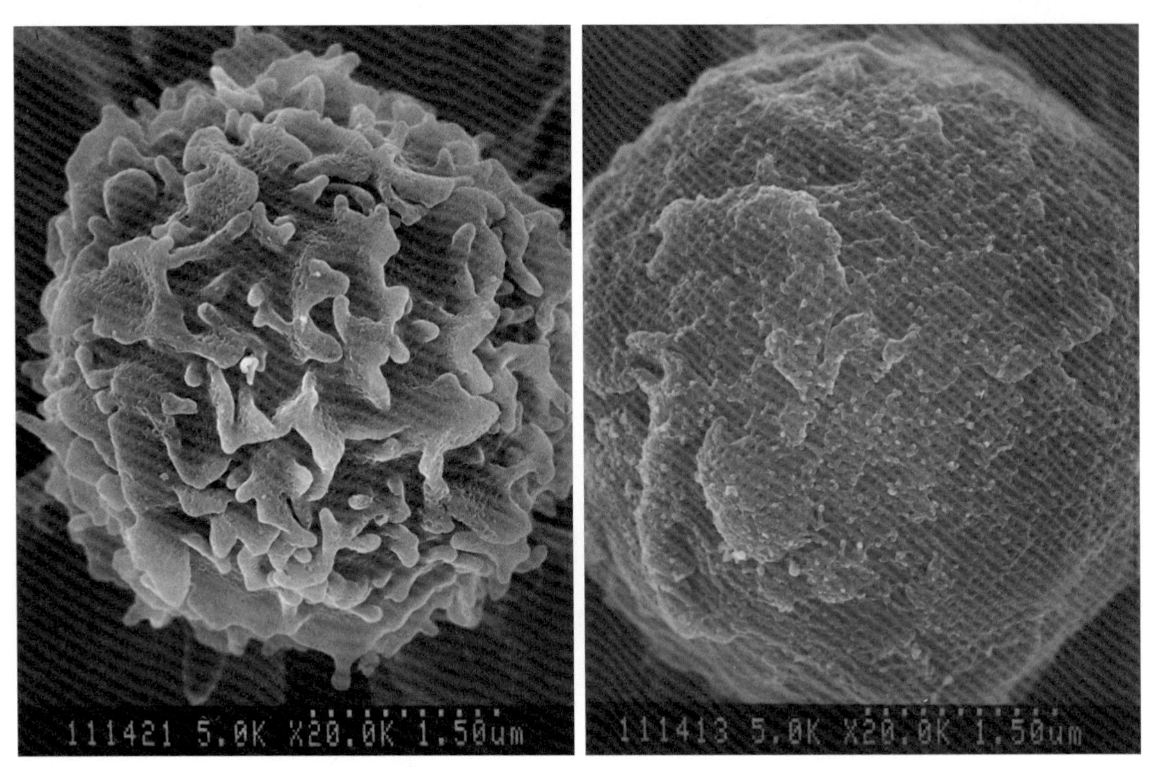

FIGURE 13 Scanning electron micrograph of a normal T-helper cell (left) and an abnormal T-helper cell (right) isolated from the peripheral blood of a rat fed a diet containing 0.1 mg/kg 3,3′,4,4′-tetrachlorobiphenyl and 10 mg/kg 2,2′,5,5′-tetrachlorobiphenyl for one year (× 5000). (Adapted from Sargent *et al.*, 1991, *Carcinogenesis* **12**, 793–800, by permission of Oxford University Press.)

studies, rhesus monkeys and rabbits were the most sensitive species. The results of animal studies largely support the observations in humans, suggesting a complex interaction of the immunomodulatory and immunotoxic effects of PCB (Table 9). Higher-chlorinated PCB mixtures are apparently more immunotoxic than the lower-chlorinated Aroclors.

Congener-specific studies reveal that co-planar polychlorinated biphenyls are much more toxic to lymphocytes than are nonplanar polychlorinated biphenyls. The number of B lymphocytes in the blood of rats was reduced after treatment with 3,3′,4,4′-tetrachlorobiphenyl (PCB 77); however, it was not reduced after treatment with 2,2′,5,5′-tetrachlorobiphenyl (PCB 52). In the same study, an influence of both congeners on the number of circulating T-helper, suppressor, and cytotoxic cells was not registered. However, the surface structure of a large number of T-helper cells was changed (Fig. 13).

The distinct immunotoxic effect of the co-planar congeners is apparently mediated by the binding to the Ah receptor in the lymphatic organs and immunocompetent cells. The hereby other synthesized proteins with enzymatic activity, and presumably other functional and morphological properties, could have a regulating influence on the immune response. Congeners that have the inductive property of 3-methylcholanthrene and phenobarbital (e.g., 2,3,3′,4,4′,5-hexachlorobiphenyl) probably have an immunosuppressive effect on the formation of antibodies against sheep erythrocytes due to their interaction with the Ah receptor. However, no effect has been observed on the thymus. This observation allows the conclusion that the thymus is not a target organ of this congener and that there are different Ah-receptor-mediated mechanisms in the organs. This conclusion is supported by the fact that β-naphthoflavone induced growth of the spleen and that 2,3,3′,4,4′,5′-hexachlorobiphenyl (PCB 156), also a ligand of the Ah receptor, causes spleen atrophy.

Bibliography

Abbott, B. D., Birnbaum, L. S., and Diliberto, J. J. (1996). Rapid distribution of 2,3,7,8-tetrachlorodibenzo-*p*-dioxin (TCDD) to embryonic tissues in C57BL/6N mice and correlation with palatal uptake *in vitro*. *Toxicol. Appl. Pharmacol.* **141,** 256–263.

Abramowitz, R., and Yalkowsky, S. H. (1990). Estimation of aqueous solubility and melting points of PCB congeners. *Chemosphere* **21,** 1221–1229.

Bertazzi, P. A., Zocchetti, C., Guercilena, S., Consonni, D., Tironi, A., Landi, M. T., and Pesatori, A. C. (1997). Dioxin exposure and cancer risk: A 15-year mortality study after the "Seveso accident." *Epidemiology* **8,** 646–652.

Borlakoglu, J. T., and Wilkins, J. P. G. (1993). Metabolism of di-, tri-, tetra-, penta- and hexachlorobiphenyls by hepatic microsomes isolated from control animals and animals treated with Aroclor 1254, a commercial mixture of polychlorinated biphenyls (PCBs). *Comp. Biochem. Physiol.* **105, C1,** 95–125.

Bosse, U., Bannert, N., Niessen, K. H., Teufel, M., and Röse, I. (1996). Fetal organ and tissue content of organohalogens and polychlorinated biphenyl. *Zbl. Hyg.* **198(4),** 331–339.

Boyer, I. J., Kokoski, C. J., and Bolger, P. M. (1991). Role of FDA in establishing tolerable levels for dioxin and PCBs in aquatic organisms. *J. Toxicol. Environ. Health* **33,** 93–101.

Brandt, I., Mohammed, A., and Slanina, P. (1981). Persistence of 2,3,6-substituted pentachlorobiphenyls in the lung parenchyma: A new structure-dependent tissue localization of polychlorinated biphenyls in mice. *Toxicology* **21,** 317–322.

Burleson, G. R., Lebrec, H., Yang, Y. G., Ibanes, J. D., Pennington, K. N., and Birnbaum, L. S. (1996). Effect of 2,3,7,8-tetrachlorodibenzo-*p*-dioxin (TCDD) on influenza virus host resistance in mice. *Fund. Appl. Toxicol.* **29,** 40–47.

Darnerud, P. O., Morse, D., Klasson-Wehler, E., and Brouwer, A. (1996). Binding of a 3,3′,4,4′-tetrachlorobiphenyl (CB 77) metabolite to fetal transthyretin and effects on fetal thyroid hormone levels in mice. *Toxicology* **106,** 105–114.

Hankinson, O. (1995). The aryl hydrocarbon receptor complex. *Ann. Rev. Pharmacol. Toxicol.* **35,** 307–340.

Hofer, A., Chang, C.-Y., and Puga, A. (1996). Dioxin induces transcription of *fos* and *jun* genes by *Ah* receptor-dependent and -independent pathways. *Toxicol. Appl. Pharmacol.* **141,** 238–247.

Huff, J., Lucier, G., and Tritscher, A. (1994). Carcinogenicity of TCDD: Experimental, mechanistic, and epidemiologic evidence. *Ann. Rev. Pharmacol. Toxicol.* **34,** 343–372.

IARC (1997). "Polychlorinated Dibenzo-*para*-dioxins and Polychlorinated Dibenzofurans." IARC Monographs on the evaluation of carcinogenic risks to humans. Vol. 69. Lyon, France.

Jacobsen, J. L., and Jacobson, S. W. (1996). Intellectual impairment in children exposed to polychlorinated biphenyls in utero. *New Eng. J. Med.* **335,** 783–789.

Kimbrough, R., and Jensen, A. A. (eds.) (1989). "Halogenated Biphenyls, Terphenyls, Naphthalenes, Dibenzodioxins and Related Products." 2nd ed. Elsevier Science Publishers, Amsterdam.

Kogevinas, M., Becher, H., Benn, T., Bertazzi, P. A., Boffetta, P., Buenode Mesquita, H. B., Coggon, D., Colin, D., Flesch-Janys, D., Fingerhut, M., Green, L., Kauppinen, T., Littorin, M., Lynge, E., Mathews, J. D., Neuberger, M., Pearce, N., and Saracci, R. (1997). Cancer mortalitiy in workers exposed to phenoxy herbicides, chlorophenols, and dioxins: An expanded and updated international cohort study. *Am. J. Epidemiol.* **145,** 1061–1075.

Koss, G., Meyer-Rogge, D., Seubert, S., Seubert, A., and Losekam, M. (1993). 2,2′,3′,4,4′,5,5′-heptachlorobiphenyl (PCB 180)—on its toxicokinetics, biotransformation and porphyrinogenic action in female rats. *Arch. Toxicol.* **67,** 651–654.

Kreuzer, P. E., Csanády, Gy. A., Baur, C., Kessler, W., Päpke, O., Greim, H., and Filser, J. G. (1997). 2,3,7,8-Tetrachlorodibenzo-*p*-dioxin (TCDD) and congeners in infants. A toxicokinetic model of human lifetime body burden by TCDD with special emphasis on its uptake by nutrition. *Arch. Toxicol.* **71,** 383–400.

Kuroki, H., Ishimura, N., Fuzino, K., Masuda, Y., Koga, N., Yoshimura, H. (1996). Formation and distribution of hydroxylated and methylsulfonyl metabolites of 2,3′,4′,5-tetrachlorobiphenyls in rats. *In* "Organohalogen Compounds," Vol. 29, pp. 481–484 16th Symposium Chlorinated Dioxins and Related Compounds, Amsterdam; Conference Office University of Amsterdam, The Netherlands.

Lambert, G. H., Schoeller, D. A., Humphrey, H. E. B., Kotake, A. N., Lietz, H., Campbell, M., Kalow, W., Spielberg, P., and Budd, M. (1990). The caffeine breath test and caffeine urinary metabolic ratios in the Michigan cohort exposed to plybrominated biphenyls: A preliminary study. *Environ. Health Perspect.* **89,** 175–181.

Lang, V. (1992). Polychlorinated biphenyls in the environment. *J. Chromatogr.* **595,** 1–43.

Luotamo, M., Järvisalo, J., and Aitio, A. (1991). Assessment of exposure to polychlorinated biphenyls: Analysis of selected isomers in blood and adipose tissue. *Environ. Res.* **54,** 121–134.

Masuda, Y., Kagawa, R., Kuroko, H., Tokudome, S., and Kuratsune, M. (1979). Transfer of various polychlorinated biphenyls to the foetuses and offspring of mice. *Fd Cosmet. Toxicol.* **17,** 623–627.

Matsumura, F., Enan, E., Dunlap, D. Y., Pinkerton, K. E., and Peake, J. (1997). Altered *in vivo* toxicity of 2,3,7,8-tetrachlorodibenzo-*p*-dioxin (TCDD) in c-src deficient mice. *Biochem. Pharmacol.* **48,** 215–224.

Matthews, H. B., and Tuey, D. B. (1980). The effect of chlorine position on the distribution and excretion of four hexachlorobiphenyl isomers. *Toxicol. Appl. Pharmacol.* **53,** 377–388.

Mocarelli, P., Brambilla, P., Gerthoux, P. M., Patterson, D. J., Jr, and Needham, L. L. (1996). Change in sex ratio with exposure to dioxin. *Lancet* **348,** 409.

Nakayama, J., Urabe, A., and Hori, Y. (1996). The clinical course of dermatological symptoms in Yusho patients over the past 25 years. *In* "Yusho—A Human Disaster Caused by PCBs and Related Compounds" (M. Kuratsune *et al.* eds.), pp. 182–196. Kyushu University Press, Fukuoka, Japan.

Nebert, D. W., Puga, A., and Vasiliou, V. (1993). Role of the Ah receptor and the dioxin-inducible [Ah] gene battery in toxicity, cancer, and signal transduction. *Ann. NY Acad. Sci.* **685,** 624–640.

Neubert, R., Stahlmann, R., Korte, M., Van Loveren, H., Vos, J. G., Golor, G., Webb, J. R., Helge, H., and Neubert, D. (1993). Effects of small doses of dioxins on the immune system of marmosets and rats. *Ann. NY Acad. Sci.* **685,** 662–686.

Pesatori, A. C., Zocchetti, C., Guercilena, S., Consonni, D., Turrini, D., and Bertazzi, P. A. (1998). Dioxin exposure and non-malignant health effects: a mortality sutdy. *Occup. Environ. Med.* **55,** 126–131.

Peterson, R. E., Theobald H. M., and Kimmel G. L. (1993). Developmental and reproductive toxicity of dioxins and related compounds: Cross-species comparisons. *CRC Crit. Rev. Toxicol.* **23,** 283–335.

Poland, A. and Knutson, J. C. (1982). 2,3,7,8-Tetrachlorodibenzo-*p*-dioxin and related halogenated aromatic hydrocarbons: Examination of the mechanism of toxicity. *Annu. Rev. Pharmacol. Toxicol.* **22,** 517–554.

Ryan, J. J., Levesque, D., Panopio, L. G., Sun, W. F., Masuda, Y., and Kuroki, H. (1993). Elimination of polychlorinated dibenzofurans (PCDFs) and polychlorinated biphenyls from human blood in the Yusho and Yu Cheng rice oil poisonings. *Arch. Environ. Contam. Toxicol.* **24,** 504–512.

Safe, S. H. (1990). Polychlorinated biphenyls (PCBs), dibenzo-p-dioxins (PCDDs), dibenzofurans (PCDFs), and related compounds: environmental and mechanistic considerations which support the development of toxic equivalency factors (TEFs). *Crit. Rev. Tox.* **21,** 51–88.

Safe, S. H. (1994). Polychlorinated biphenyls (PCBs): Environmental impact, biochemical and toxic responses, and implications for risk assessment. *Crit. Rev. Toxicol.* **24,** 87–149.

Safe, S. H. (1995). Modulation of gene expression and endocrine response pathways by 2,3,7,8-tetrachlorodibenzo-*p*-dioxin and related compounds. *Pharmac. Ther.* **67,** 247–281.

Sargent, L., Dragan, Y. P., Erickson, C., Laufer, C. J., and Pitot, H. C. (1991). Study of the separate and combined effects of the non-planar 2,5,2′,5′-and the planar 3,4,3′,4′-tetrachlorobiphenyl in liver and lymphocytes in vivo. *Carcinogenesis* **12,** 793–800.

Sassa, S., Sugita, O., Ohnuma, N., Imajo, S., Okumura, T., Noguchi, T., and Kappas, A. (1986). Studies of the influence of chloro-substituent sites and conformational energy in polychlorinated biphenyls on uroporphyrin formation in chickembryo liver cell cultures. *Biochem. J.* **235,** 291–296.

Schecter, A., Le, C. D., Le, T. B. T., Hoang, T. Q., Dinh, Q. M., Hoang, D.C., Constable, J. D., Baughman, R., Päpke, O., Ryan, J. J., Fürst, P., and Räisänen, S. (1995). Agent Orange and the Vietnamese: The persistence of elevated dioxin levels in human tissues. *Am. J. Public Health* **85,** 516–522.

Schrenk, D., Buchmann, A., Dietz, K., Lipp, H.-P., Brunner, H., Sirma, H., Münzel, P., Hagenmaier, H., Gebhardt, R., and Bock, K. W. (1994) Promotion of preneoplastic foci in rat liver with 2,3,7,8-tetrachlorodibenzo-*p*-dioxin, 1,2,3,4,6,7,8-heptachlorodibenzo-*p*-dioxin and a defined mixture of 49 polychlorinated dibenzo-*p*-dioxins. *Carcinogenesis* **15,** 509–515.

Seegal, R. F., and Shain, W. (1992). Neurotoxicity of polychlorinated biphenyls. *In* "The Vulnerable Brain and Environmental Risks, Vol. 2, Toxins in Food" (R. L. Isaacson, and K. F. Jensen, eds.), pp. 169–193. Plenum Press, New York.

Sewall, C. H., and Lucier, G. W. (1995). Receptor-mediated events and the evaluation of the Environmental Protection Agency (EPA) of dioxin risks. *Mutat. Res.* **333,** 111–122.

Sundström, G., Hutzinger, O., and Safe, S. (1976). The metabolism of chlorobiphenyls. A review. *Chemosphere* **5,** 267–298.

Tilson, H. A., and Harry, G. J. (1994). Developmental neurotoxicology of polychlorinated biphenyls and related compounds. *In* "The Vulnerable Brain and Environmental Risks, Vol. 3, Toxins in Air and Water" (R. L. Isaacson, and K. F. Jensen, eds.), pp. 267–279. Plenum Press, New York.

U.S. Dept. of Health and Human Services (1992). "Toxicological Profile for Polychlorinated Biphenyls (Draft)." Agency for Toxic Substances and Disease Registry, Atlanta, GA.

Van den Berg, M., De Jong, J., Poiger, H., and Olson J. R. (1994). The toxicokinetics and metabolism of polychlorinated dibenzo-*p*-dioxins (PCDDs) and dibenzofurans (PCDFs) and their relevance for toxicity. *Crit. Rev. Toxicol.* **24,** 1–74.

Weber, L. W. D. (1997). The toxicity of brominated and mixed-halogenated dibenzo-p-dioxins and dibenzofurans: An overview. *J. Toxicol. Environ. Health* **50,** 195–215.

Whitlock, J. P., Jr. (1993). The regulation of gene expression by 2,3,7,8-tetrachlorodibenzo-*p*-dioxin. *Pharmacol. Rev.* **39,** 147–161.

WHO (1993). "Polychlorinated Biphenyls and Terphenyls." 2nd ed. Environmental Health Criteria 140. World Health Organization, Geneva.

WHO (1994). "Polybrominated Biphenyls." Environmental Health Criteria 152. World Health Organization, Geneva.

Wölfle, D., and Marquardt, H. (1996). Antioxidants inhibit the enhancement of malignant cell transformation induced by 2,3,7,8-tetrachlorodibenzo-*p*-dioxin. *Carcinogenesis* **17,** 1273–1278.

CHAPTER

30

Aromatic Amines, Nitroarenes, and Heterocyclic Aromatic Amines

G. SABBIONI, E. RICHTER

Walther Straub Institute of Pharmacology and Toxicology Ludwig Maximillians University, Munich, Germany

AROMATIC AMINES

Aromatic amines are important intermediates for the production of polymers, pesticides, rubber chemicals, dyes, pigments, and pharmaceuticals. Since the discovery of aniline in 1826, the number of arylamines has risen exponentially. The toxicity of the aromatic amines has been recognized since the early industrial use of aniline, when the clinical picture of "anilism" was first seen. Hematuria, methemoglobinemia, cystitis, and dermatitis were the main manifestations of this toxicity. Such symptoms and signs could be reduced by improved manufacturing practices. In 1895, Rehn reported four cases of bladder tumors in workers involved in the production of fuchsin for periods up to 20 years. These cancers were labeled aniline cancer because Rehn suggested that aniline was the carcinogenic agent. In 1898, Leichtenstern implied that naphthylamines could cause bladder cancer. Rehn reported 38 further cases of bladder tumors and indicated the involvement of naphthylamine and benzidine. In the following years, more cases of bladder tumors were found among industrial workers. In a landmark epidemiological study, it was demonstrated that 2-naphthylamine and benzidine are the main causes of bladder tumors in dye workers. Aniline was not found to be carcinogenic. The following compounds have been classified as carcinogens in humans: 4-aminobiphenyl, benzidine, 4-chloro-2-methylaniline, and 2-naphthylamine.

Chemical and Physical Properties, Major Uses, and Importance

Aromatic amines or arylamines are aromatic hydrocarbons in which one or more hydrogen atoms are replaced by amino groups. Aromatic amines are either liquids or solids at room temperature. The ones without other functional groups are colorless and have a characteristic odor. Most compounds oxidize on exposure to air and darken. They are usually soluble in organic solvents, such as alcohol, benzene, and ether; but are slightly soluble in water. In contrast to the aliphatic amines, the aromatic amines are only weakly basic. Aromatic amines are used as dye intermediates for azo dyes and as intermediates for pharmaceuticals and agricultural chemicals; in polyurethanes; and as antioxidants in polymers. The oldest use of aromatic amines is as intermediates for dyes. Today, the largest share of aniline consumption is by the manufacture of isocyanates, primarily for 4,4′-methylenediphenyldiisocyanate (MDI). Analgesics and sulfonamides are examples of important pharmaceuticals synthesized from aromatic amines. Arylamines are directly used in inks for pens, in shoe cream, and in dyes for ink pads. 4-Methoxy-*m*-phenylenediamine and *o*- or *p*-phenylenediamines are used in hair dyes. The bicyclic diamino compounds, such as benzidine, 3,3′-dimethylbenzidine, 3,3′-dimethoxybenzidine, and 3,3′-dichlorobenzidine, have been used for the production of azo dyes. Because benzidine can be metabolically released from azo dyes, all dyes with a benzidine base have been banned. Urine metabolites and hemoglobin adducts of carcinogenic arylamines have been found in workers, exposed for example, to benzidine, 4,4′-methylenebis(2-chloroaniline), 4,4′-methylenedianiline, and 2-methylaniline. The main exposures of the general population to aromatic amines is through cigarette smoke or products that contain products synthesized from aromatic amines. Among other compounds, arylamines as 2-, 3-, and 4-methylaniline; 4-aminobiphenyl; and 3-aminobiphenyl are present in the cigarette smoke. Significantly higher amounts of 4-aminobiphenyl, 3-aminobiphenyl, and 2-naphthylamine have been found as hemoglobin adducts in smokers. Other arylamines, such as 2-, 3-, 4-methylaniline; the dimethylanilines; and the ethylanilines, did not correlate with the smoking. Therefore, other sources of exposure to arylamines in the environment must be present. In animal experiments, it has been shown that arylamines can be metabolically released from a large array of structurally different compounds. Hemoglobin adducts of the parent arylamine were found after giving lidocaine, propham, monuron, monolinuron, chlorpropham, chlordimeform, diuron, metolachlor, metalaxyl, acetoacetanilide, *N*-ethylaniline, *N,N*-dimethylaniline, *N*-methylaniline, and the azo dye direct red 28.

Absorption, Distribution, Metabolism, and Excretion

Arylamines are absorbed by the gastrointestinal tract, by the respiratory system, and through the skin. Usually the amines are excreted after metabolism. The monocyclic arylamines are excreted mainly through the kidney and the bicyclic amines excreted more via feces than with urine. Most arylamines are excreted in 2–3 days. The half-life times are between 3 and 4 hours. Some substituted monocyclic arylamines, such as, *p*-phenylenediamine and especially the benzidine congeners, are much more persistent, with half-lifes between 2 and 4 days. The metabolism of arylamines has been studied intensively. Ring oxidation, N-glucuronidation, N-acetylation, and N-oxidation are the major metabolic pathways of arylamines in mammals. N-Oxidation is a crucial step in the metabolism of arylamines and aromatic amides to toxic products. Three classes of enzymes are mainly responsible for the N-oxidation: cytochrome P450 (CYP), flavine adenine dinucleotide-containing monooxygenases (FMO), and prostaglandin H synthase (PHS). In humans, N-oxidation of nearly planar arylamines (e.g., 4-aminobiphenyl, 2-naphthylamine, and 2-aminofluorene) is preferentially catalyzed by CYP1A2. For nonplanar arylamines such as, 4,4′-methylenebis(2-chloroaniline) and dapsone, it could be shown that CYP3A4 is the main enzyme that catalyzes the N-oxidation. The two other enzyme systems (FMO and PHS) play only a minor role in the toxicity and the metabolism in the liver. Only in organs such as the bladder, where little CYP is present, is PHS important for the formation of toxic and genotoxic intermediates. FMO can catalyze the formation of *N*-hydroxy-arylamines from secondary arylamines, such as, *N*-methylbenzidine and *N*-methyl-4-aminobiphenyl.

Arylamines are metabolized in the liver by monooxygenases to yield highly reactive *N*-hydroxyarylamines (Fig. 1). *N*-Hydroxyarylamines can be further metabolized to *N*-sulfonyloxyarylamines, *N*-acetoxyarylamines, or *N*-hydroxyarylamine *N*-glucuronide. These highly reactive intermediates are responsible for the genotoxic and cytotoxic effects of this class of compounds. The O-activated hydroxyarylamines react with DNA and proteins. Typically arylamines react with the C-8 of guanine. DNA adducts of arylamines have been located in different organs of animals and humans. DNA adducts of 4,4′-methylenebis(2-chloroaniline), benzidine, and 4-aminobiphenyl have been identified in the exfoliated urothelial bladder cells in human urine. DNA adducts of 4-aminobiphenyl have been retrieved from human lung tissue. The formation of hemoglobin adducts and glutathione adducts in erythrocytes is a complicated process. In brief, *N*-hydroxyarylamines are oxidized in the erythrocytes to the nitrosoarenes, which react with the thiol group of cysteine to semimercaptals. The elimination of water from the nitrenium ion and subsequent reaction of sulfur with water yields the sulfinamide. Hemoglobin adducts are stable, but glutathione adducts are reduced by glutathione reductases back to the parent compounds. Arylamines react with cysteine 93 of the β-chain of human hemoglobin. Only the adduct of 4-aminobiphenyl with albumin has been characterized. In experiments with radioactively labeled arylamines, it could be shown that the hemoglobin binding correlates with DNA binding. This has been demonstrated, for example, for 2-aminofluorene, benzidine, and 4,4′-methylenebis(2-chloroaniline). The release of the arylamines from the hemoglobin adducts upon mild base hydrolysis indicates the presence of sulfinamide-type adducts. This implies the biological availability of the *N*-hydroxyarylamine in the erythrocyte and in the tissue. The detoxification pathway of arylamines is strongly dependent on the *N*-acetyltransferase 2 (NAT2), for which two phenotypes are known, fast and slow acetylators. Fast acetylators have a lower risk of bladder

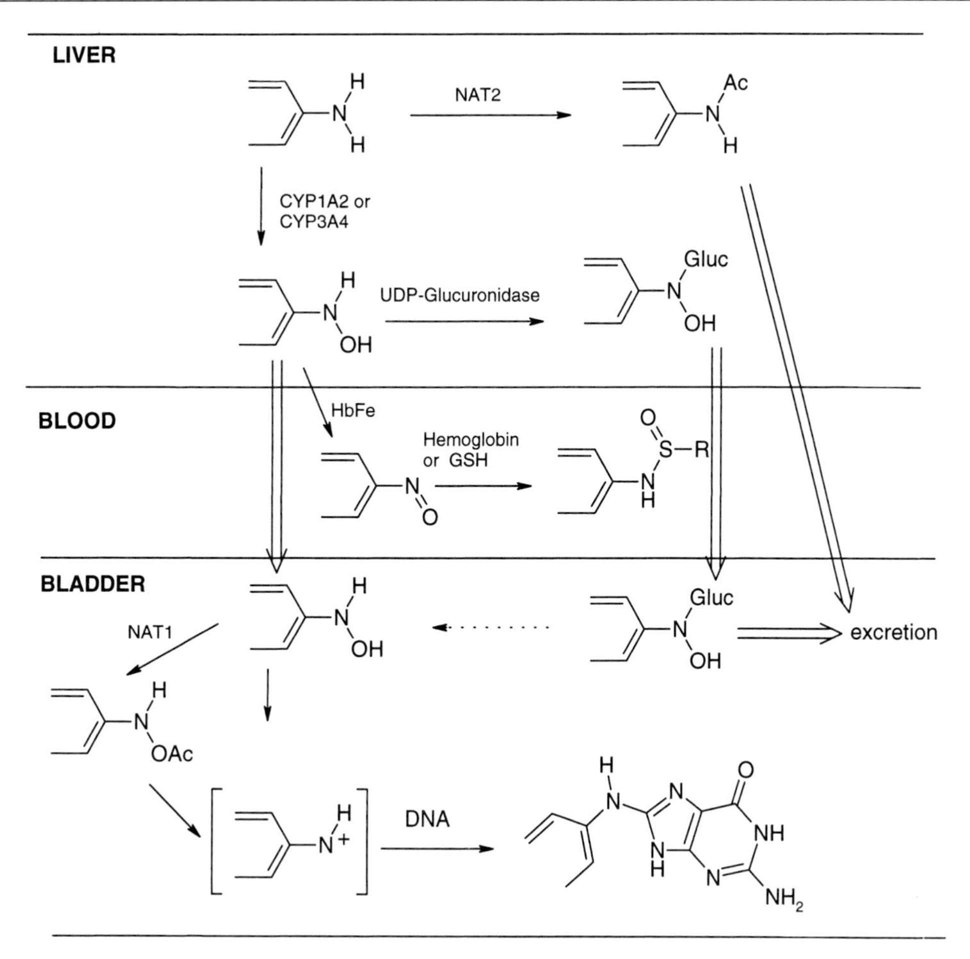

FIGURE 1 Postulated mechanism for the generation of the ultimate carcinogen leading to DNA-adducts in the bladder urothelial cells. Arylamines are detoxified by polymorphic *N*-acetyltransferase 2 (NAT2) and excreted in the urine. The arylamines are oxidized to the potentially genotoxic *N*-hydroxy-arylamines by CYP1A2 for planar arylamines and by CYP3A4 for bulky arylamines. The arylamines or the *N*-hydroxyarylamines can be glucuronidated. The *N*-hydroxyarylamines and the *N*-glucuronide are transported through the blood into the bladder. The acidic pH of the bladder catalyzes the formation of the nitrenium ion, which gives a DNA-adduct with guanine. Alternatively, *N*-hydroxyarylamines can be activated by *O*-acetylation with *N*-acetyltransferase 1(NAT1) in the urothelium. In the blood, the *N*-hydroxyarylamines are taken up by the erythrocytes and oxidized to the nitrosoarenes under the formation of methemoglobin; this process is known as the Kiese redox cycle. The nitroso arenes react to sulfinamides with glutathione and/or hemoglobin (Hb).

cancer and are less susceptible to methemoglobin formation. However, not only N-oxidation products can lead to toxic reactions. For example, the formation of quinoneimine intermediates after the oxidation of arylamines in *para*-position can yield cytotoxic reactions. The toxic effects might result from the reaction of quinoneimine with thiols of glutathione or protein or from the formation of superoxide anion radicals in a redox cycle with oxygen. The possible reactions evolving from benzoquinoneimine intermediates have been shown by many research groups in studies on acetaminophen.

In humans there are toxicologically important, individual polymorphisms of the slow *N*-acetyltransferase 2 (NAT2) and of the CYP that are important for the individual susceptibilities that lead to diseases. Slow acetylators have a larger bladder cancer risk but a lower colon cancer risk than fast acetylators. For the urinary bladder, putative arylamine DNA adducts are predominant and are significantly elevated in active smokers. Rapid CYP1A2 and slow NAT2 phenotypes have been previously implicated in the activation (N-oxidation) and detoxification (N-acetylation) of arylamines for human bladder carcinogenesis. New data now indicate that NAT1, which is expressed in the human urothelium and catalyzes the O-acetylation of *N*-hydroxyarylamines, is significantly correlated with DNA-adduct levels and is bimodally distributed in this tissue.

The glucuronidation and sulfation of the amino or hydroxy group are further important pathways for toxification and detoxification. *N*-Glucuronides are excreted through the bile with the feces, depending from the size of the amine. *N*-Sulfate is excreted in urine. The sulfotransferases (SULT) and the UDP-glucuronosyltransferases (UGT) are probably present in polymorphic forms. The characterization of these forms is researched by several laboratories. UGT catalyzes the N-glucuronidation of *N*-hydroxyarylamines and is probably responsible for their transport to the colon. UGT, SULT, and NAT2 can form more toxic products with the *N*-hydroxyarylamines by introducing a glucuronide, sulfate, or acetylgroup into the hydroxy function. The leaving-group properties of the hydroxy group are increased and the ultimate carcinogen can be obtained at a physiological pH. It has been shown in dogs that about 70% of the *N*-hydroxy-4-aminobiphenyl reaches the bladder in unconjugated form, while the remaining 30% is in the form of the *N*-glucuronide. The glucuronides of 4-aminobiphenyl and *N*-hydroxy-4-aminobiphenyl are acid labile at pH 5.5, but this is not true of the glucuronide of *N*-hydroxy-*N*-acetyl-4-aminobiphenyl. The glucuronide of 4-aminobiphenyl was the most acid labile conjugate examined. A large portion of the *N*-hydroxy-4-aminobiphenyl will be oxidized in erythrocytes to nitrosobiphenyl, which then forms a sulfinamide with the cysteine of hemoglobin or glutathione. In animals and in humans it could be shown that *N*-hydroxy-4-aminobiphenyl reacts with urethelial bladder DNA and with hemoglobin (Fig. 1).

Acute and Chronic Toxicity

Arylamines are moderately to extremely toxic. The main hazards associated with arylamine exposure are methemoglobinemia and carcinogenesis. Both of these effects are attributed to the products resulting from N-oxidation. The chloroanilines and nitroanilines are the strongest methemoglobin inducers among the arylamines. Many aromatic amines cause irritant contact dermatitis because of their alkaline properties. One of the best examples are dyes, rubber products, and other formulations containing *p*-phenylenediamine. This causes a delayed hypersensitivity reaction (type IV allergy), which can be detected by a skin patch test. However, there is a cross-reaction between *p*-phenylenediamine and other anilines and benzidines. *m*-Phenylenediamine, used as a curing agent for epoxy resins, also induces irritant and allergic contact dermatitis. 4,4′-Methylenedianiline causes jaundice. In Epping (Essex, UK) 84 individuals who ate bread made from flour contaminated with 4,4′-methylenedianiline developed cholestatic jaundice. The jaundice was reversible on recovery.

In the past years, numerous cases of severe intoxication manifested by methemoglobinemia have occurred after skin contact with commercial products said to contain aniline dyes. Indelible marking ink (laundry ink) has been a source of exposure. These were often dissolved in aniline or nitrobenzene for their application; thus, it appears likely that the major signs of poisoning produced by the inks were due to the vehicles rather to than the colorants. Infant deaths have been caused by the absorption of aniline from diapers stenciled with cloth-marking ink containing aniline as the vehicle for the dye. Pathologic findings in acute fatalities from aniline and nitrobenzene derivatives include chocolate color of the blood; injury to the kidney, liver, and spleen; and hemolysis. Bladder-wall ulceration and necrosis will also occur.

Chronic poisoning with aniline leads to general weakness, tiredness, lack of appetite, abominal pain, dizziness, light depressions, low-levels cyanosis, anemia with Heinz-inclusion-body formation, and uremia.

Genetic Toxicology

The majority of the arylamines are mutagenic and carcinogenic (Table 1). Many amines are mutagenic in *Salmonella* tester strains TA98 and TA100, but metabolic activation with the S9 microsomal preparation mix is required for activity for most of the active ones. 2,4-Diaminotoluene, 2,4-diaminoethylbenzene, and a few amines containing a nitro-group are direct mutagens. In general, the mutagenic potency increases with oxidizability and with the lipophilicity of the arylamines.

In humans, benzidine, 2-naphthylamine, 4-chloro-2-methylaniline, and 4-aminobiphenyl have been classified as clearly carcinogenic for the human bladder. The carcinogenicity of arylamines has been tested in mice and rats (Table 1). Arylamines induce tumors in different sites in the different species. Ashby compared the mutagenicity and carcinogenicity of the compounds from the National Toxicology Program (NTP) studies with his predictive model. Most carci-

TABLE 1 Toxicological Properties of Arylamines

			Carcinogenicity			
		Mutagenicity[b]		Classification for humans[d]		
	LD_{50}[a]	TA98/TA100	Target organs in animals[c]	DFG	IARC	ACGIH
Monocyclic arylamines						
Aniline	440	−/−	Sp	IIIB	3	A3
N,N-Dimethylaniline	1300	−/−	Sp	IIIB	3	A4
2-Chloroaniline	1104	+/+		n.l.	n.l.	n.l.
4-Chloroaniline	300	+/+	Sp	IIIA2	2B	n.l.
2-Methylaniline	635	nt/−	Bl, Va	IIIA2	2B	A3
4-Methylaniline	656	−/−	Bl, Va	IIIB	—	A3
2,4-Dimethylaniline	467	+/+		IIIB	3	A3[e]
2,6-Dimethylaniline		nt/−		n.c.	2B	A3[e]
2,4,5-Trimethylaniline	1585	+/+		IIIA2	3	n.l.
4-Chloro-2-methylaniline	1058	−/+	H	IIIA1	2A	n.l.
5-Chloro-2-methylaniline	464	nt	H	IIIB	—	n.l.
2-Methoxyaniline	2000	−/−		IIIA2	2B	A3
4-Methoxyaniline	1400	−/−		n.c.	3	A4
2-Methoxy-5-methylaniline	1450	+/+	Bl, Lu, No	IIIA2	2B	n.l.
o-Phenylenediamine	973	+/+	Lu	IIIB	3	A3
m-Phenylenediamine	650	+/+	Sk	IIIB	3	A4
p-Phenylenediamine	80	+/−	Sk	IIIB	3	A4
4-Methoxy-*m*-phenylenediamine	460	+/+	Th	IIIA2	2B	n.l.
2,4-Toluenediamine	230	+/+	Lu, Bl	IIIA2	2B	n.l.
2-Methyl-5-nitroaniline	574	−/nt	Lu	IIIA2	3	n.l.
Bicyclic arylamines						
4-Aminobiphenyl	500	+/+	Bl, Li	IIIA1	1	A1
Benzidine	309	+/+	Bl, Li	IIIA1	1	A1
3,3′-Dichlorobenzidine		+/+	Va	IIIA2	2B	A3
3,3′-Dimethylbenzidine	404	+/−	Zy, Va	IIIA2	2B	A3
3,3′-Dimethoxybenzidine	30–100	+/+	Va	IIIA2	2B	n.l.
4,4′-Methylenedianiline	547	+/+	Th, Li	IIIA2	2B	A3
4,4′-Methylenebis(2-chloroaniline)		−/+	Li, Lu	IIIA2	2A	A2
4,4′-Methylenebis(2-methylaniline)		+/+		IIIA2	2B	n.l.
4,4′-Methylenebis(*N,N*-dimethylaniline)	3160 (mice)	+/+	Th, Li	IIIA2	3	n.l.
2-Naphthylamine	727	+/+	Bl	IIIA1	1	A1
4,4′-Oxydianiline	725	+/+	Th, Li	IIIA2	2B	n.l.
4,4′-Thiodianiline	1100	+/+	Th, Li	IIIA2	2B	n.l.

[a]The LD_{50} refers to single-oral-dose rat experiments.
[b]nt = not tested.
[c]The main location of the tumors listed: Bl (bladder), H (hemangiosarcoma), Sk (skin), Li (liver), Lu (lung), No (nose), Th (thyroid), Sp (spleen), Va (various), Zy (Zymbal gland).
[d]Classification according to the DFG (German Research Foundation): IIIA1 = carcinogenic in humans, IIIA2 = carcinogenic in animal experiments with comparable conditions to occupational exposure, IIIB = compound with carcinogenic potential. Classification according to IARC (International Agency of Research on Cancer): 1 = carcinogenic, 2A = probably carcinogenic; 2B = possibly carcinogenic; 3 = not classifiable as carcinogenic. Classification according to ACGIH (American Conference of Governmental Industrial Hygienists): A1 = confirmed human carcinogen; A2 = suspected human carcinogen, A3 = animal carcinogen; A4 = not classifiable as a human carcinogen; A5 = not suspected as a human carcinogen; n.l. = not listed; n.c. = not classified as a carcinogen.
[e]The values are given for the mixture of all isomers.

nogenic arylamines are mutagenic, except for two compounds. However, in a few cases, compounds were mutagenic but not carcinogenic. Aniline, 4-chloroaniline, and *N,N*-dimethylaniline cause tumors of the spleen. In rats 2,4-diaminoanisole, 4,4′-thiodianiline, 3,3′-dimethoxybenzidine, and 5-nitro-2-methoxyaniline induce tumors of the Zymbal gland in rats. 3,3′-Dimethylbenzidine, 5-nitro-2-methoxyaniline, and

2,4,5-trimethylaniline induce lung tumors in rats; 4,4′-methylenedianiline and 1,5-naphthyldiamine induce lung tumors in mice. In mice, the most important site for tumors are the liver, vascular system, bladder, stomach, hematopoietic system, and thyroid. In rats more organs are affected; the target organs are the mammary, liver, Zymbal gland, kidney, small intestine, and lung (data include the nitroarenes).

NITROARENES

Chemical Properties, Major Uses, and Importance

Nitroarenes are much more lipophilic than the corresponding arylamines. Monocyclic nitroarenes have a sour to almond odor and taste, which are very prominent for nitrobenzene. Nitroarenes play an extremely important role in the chemical industry. In 1980, 5% of the total benzene–toluene–xylene production was used to produce nitroaromatic compounds. Two consumer end-use classes of nitroaromatics are distinguished, those used directly, which still contain a nitro group, and those in which the ultimate consumer product is a nitro-group derivative. Four percent of the total benzene–toluene–xylene–nitro production is direct consumer good. These are pharmaceuticals (e.g., chloramphenicol), pesticides (e.g., parathion, trifluralin, and pendimethalin), explosives (e.g., 2,4,6-trinitrotoluene or TNT), and cosmetics (e.g., musk xylene, musk ambrette, musk ketone, and musk tibetene).

Dinitrotoluenes are very important intermediates for the production of 2,4- and 2,6-diaminotoluene, which are used in the production of toluenediisocyanates. TNT was the most important explosive used during the Second World War. Soil, rivers, and lakes close to ammunition plants have been found to be highly contaminated with several derivatives and byproducts of TNT (over 500 of these sites in Germany). Nitrobenzene, nitrotoluene isomers, and chloronitrobenzenes have repeatedly been observed in samples from the river Rhine (in Germany). Other significant pollutants are the nitroaromatic fragrances and perfumes, which are now ubiquitous in the environment. Musk xylene (2,4,6-trinitro-1,3-dimethyl-5-*tert*-butylbenzene), a synthetic musk often used in fragrances and soaps as a substitute for natural musk, has been found in human breast milk, blood, and adipose tissue. Nitroarenes found in the air can result, for example, from combustion of fuel (especially diesel), atmospheric nitration of aromatic compounds, and kerosene-heater emissions. The following compounds have been found in the vapor phase or particle phase of the air: 1-nitropyrene, 9-nitroanthracene, 2-nitrofluorene, 1-nitronaphthalene, 3-nitrobiphenyl, 4-nitrobiphenyl, 2-nitrobiphenyl, 3-nitrotoluene, 2-nitrofluoranthene, dinitropyrenes, and several nitrophenols.

Absorption, Distribution, Metabolism, and Excretion

Nitroarenes are absorbed by the gastrointestinal and respiratory tracts and through the skin. The first metabolic step for nitroarenes is the reduction of the nitro group or the oxidation in the aromatic ring. After nitro reduction, the same metabolites are found as after arylamine exposure. Nitroarenes are reduced by the microflora in the gut and by several enzymes in the liver to nitro radical anions, nitrosoarenes *N*-hydroxyarylamines, and/or the amine. Several studies have been done to establish which is the more important organ for the reduction of nitroarenes. In male Fischer 344 rats, the urinary metabolites after an oral dose of nitrobenzene, *p*-hydroxyacetanilide, *p*-nitrophenol, and *m*-nitrophenol, are excreted as sulfate ester conjugates. The metabolism and excretion of 2-nitrotoluene, 3-nitrotoluene, and 4-nitrotoluene were studied in male Fischer 344 rats (Fig. 2). The major metabolites excreted 72 hours after administration were the corresponding benzoic acids, acetamidobenzoic acids, and nitrohippuric acids. However, the percentage of these metabolites varied within the isomers. In humans exposed to TNT, 2-amino-4,6-dinitrotoluene (2A46DNT) and 4-amino-2,6-dinitrotoluene (4A26DNT) were found in the urine and as hydrolyzable covalent hemoglobin adducts.

Acute and Chronic Toxicity

In general, the same acute toxic effects (Table 2) are seen after nitroarene exposure as after arylamine exposure, as the same reactive intermediates, *N*-hydroxyarylamine and nitrosoarene, are biologically available. Inhalation of nitrobenzene caused methemoglobinemia, splenomegaly, and increased fetal malformations in rats. In humans, nitrobenzene and other nitroarenes generate methemoglobin more slowly than aniline, dinitrobenzene, or nitroaniline, but cyanosis is more persistent. The symptoms from inhaling nitrobenzene are headache, vertigo, nausea, vomiting, depressed respiration, disturbed vision, coma, and death from respiratory failure. The skin is bluish gray or intensively cyanotic. Repeated exposure may be

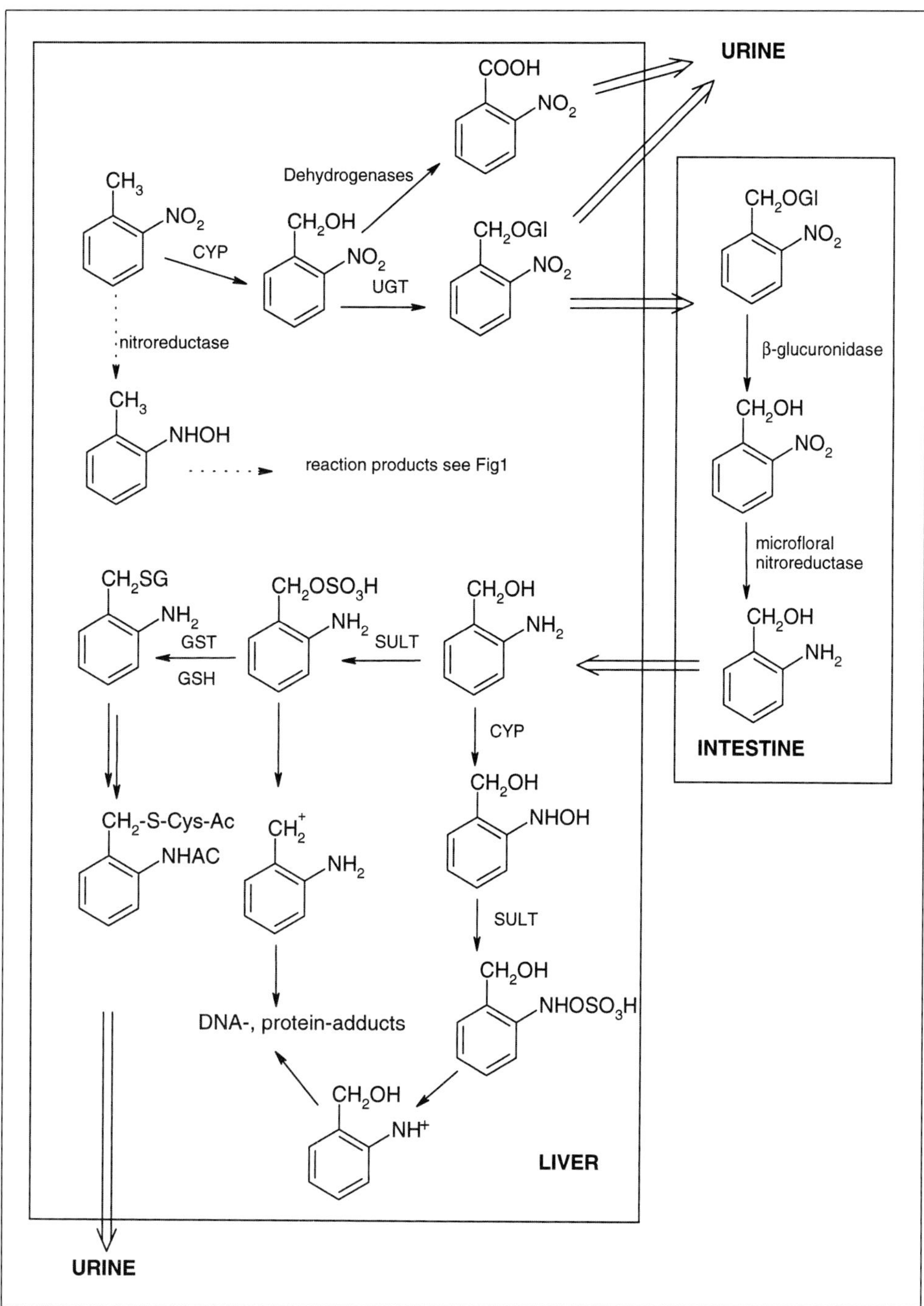

FIGURE 2 Putative route of disposition of 2-nitrotoluene. The minor metabolic pathways have been expressed with a dashed arrow line.

followed by liver impairment up to yellow atrophy, hemolytic icterus, and anemia at various degrees with presence of Heinz inclusion bodies in the red cells. Nitrotoluenes are toxic by inhalation, ingestion, and dermal absorption.

In TNT-exposed humans, the notable toxic manifestations have included aplastic anemia, toxic hepatitis, and cataracts. Similar conditions have been observed in animals. High doses are needed to observe acute toxic effects in rodents. The toxic properties of

TABLE 2 Toxicological Properties of Nitroarenes						
			Carcinogenicity			
		Mutagenicity[a]		Classification for humans[a]		
	LD_{50}	TA98/TA100	Target organs in animals[a]	DFG	IARC	ACGIH
Nitrobenzene	640	−/−			2B	A3
4-Chloro-nitrobenzene	420	−/+	(Lu, Sp)[b]	IIIB	3	A3
2-Chloro-nitrobenzene	270	+/+	(Va)	IIIB	3	n.l.
2-Nitrotoluene	890–2546	nt/+	(Sk)	IIIA2	3	n.l.
3-Nitrotoluene	1072	nt/+		n.c.	3	n.l.
4-Nitrotoluene	1960–4700	nt/+		n.c.	3	n.l.
2-Methoxy-nitrobenzene	874	+/+	Bl, Va	IIIA2	2B	n.l.
Dinitrobenzene (all isomers)	ca. 100	+/+		IIIB		n.l.
2,4-Dichlornitrobenzene	640–1070	nt/+				
Dinitrotoluene (6 isomers)	177–1122	+/+	Li, Va	IIIA2	2B[c]	A2
2,4,6-Trinitrotoluene	820	nt/+		IIIB	3	—
4-Nitrobiphenyl	2230	+/nt	(Bl)	IIIA2	3	A2
l-Nitronaphthalene	120	+/+	(Bl)	IIIB	3	n.l.
2-Nitronaphthalene	4400	+/+	(Bl)	IIIA2	3	n.l.
Musk ambrette	4800	−/+		n.l.	3	n.l.
Musk ketone	>10000	−		n.l.		n.l.
Musk xylene	>10000	−		n.l.	3	n.l.

[a]The abbreviations are given in the legend of Table 1.
[b]Tumor experiments requiring confirmation
[c]Classification for 2,4-dinitrotoluene and 2,6-dinitrotoluene

the major metabolites of TNT, 4A26DNT and 2A46DNT, remain largely unknown.

Genetic Toxicology

Most nitroarenes are mutagenic in the *Salmonella* TA100 and TA98 tests. Including the nitroheteroaromatic compounds, only 30 of 162 nitroarenes tested were not mutagenic. The cytotoxicity of nitroarenes is related to their ease of reduction to nitro radical anions and nitrosobenzenes. The most cytotoxic compounds have the strongest electron-withdrawing substitutent (e.g., 1,4-dinitrobenzene).

4-Nitrobiphenyl, 2-nitronaphthalene, 2-nitrotoluene, 2-methoxy-nitrobenzene, and six isomers of dinitrotoluenes taken as group have been classified by the German MAK commission as carcinogenic in animal experiments that were performed under conditions comparable to occupational exposure. The IARC classified 2,6-dinitrotoluene, 2,4-dinitrotoluene, nitrobenzene, and 2-methoxy-nitrobenzene as possible carcinogens in humans. All other monocyclic and bicyclic nitroarenes were unclassifiable as to carcinogenicity to humans. Only 3,7-dinitro- and 3,9-dinitrofluoranthene, 1,6- and 1,8-dinitropyrene, 6-nitrochrysene, 2-nitrofluorene, 1-nitropyrene, and 4-nitropyrene were classified as possibly carcinogenic to humans.

HETEROCYCLIC AROMATIC AMINES

The finding that extracts of cooked meats produce a potent response in the Ames test led to the isolation and identification of a number of heterocyclic aromatic amines. These potent mutagens have been shown to be carcinogenic in laboratory animals, and their importance in the etiology of diet-related human cancer is of growing interest.

Chemistry and Sources

The cooked food mutagens all have a characteristic heterocyclic structure and an exocyclic amino group (Fig. 3). Chemically they can be subdivided into two major classes, aminoimidazoazaarenes and carbolines. The main precursors of the heterocyclic aromatic amines found in meat and fish are creatine or creatinine, free amino acids, and sugars. The formation of the mutagenic agents increases with the temperature

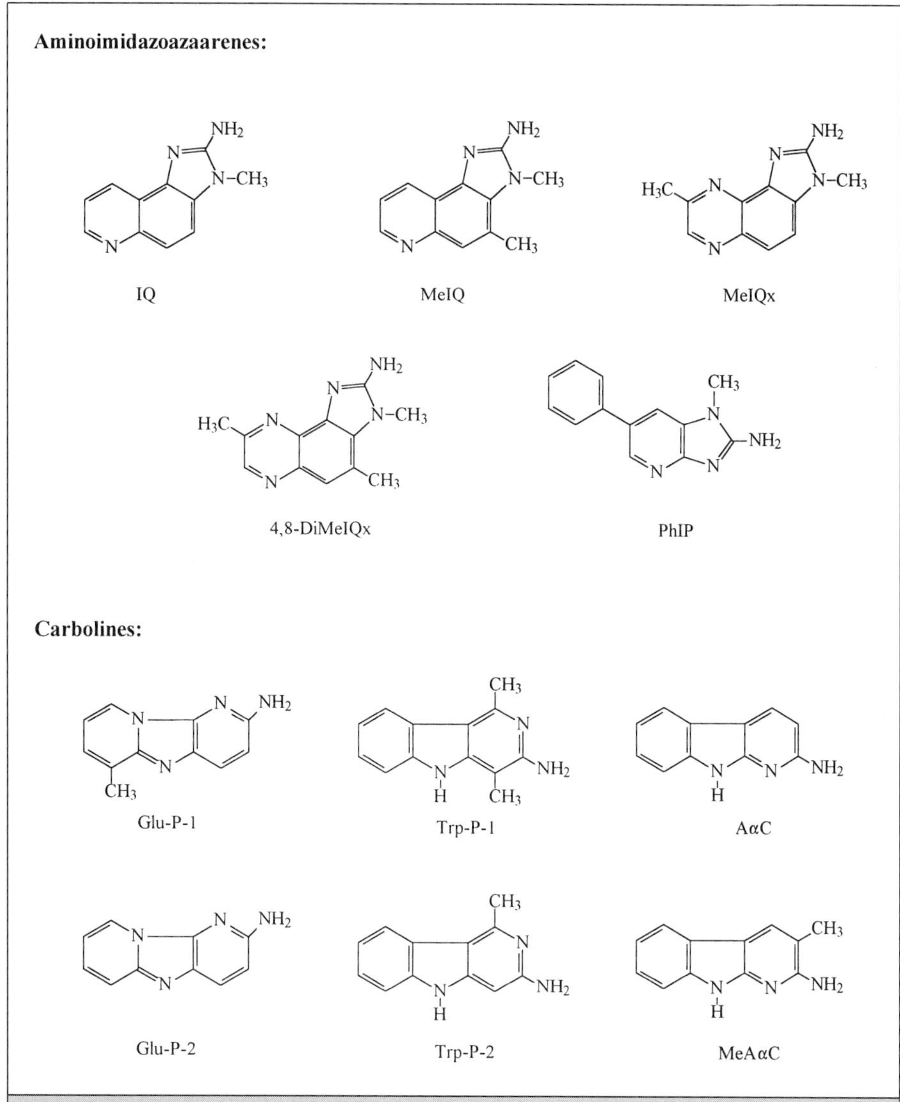

FIGURE 3 Structures of some important heterocyclic amines. For chemical names, see Tables 3 and 4.

and cooking time. The Western diet contain the highest levels of heterocyclic aromatic amines due to the abundance of meat in the diet cooked at temperatures above 200°C. No measurable quantities of heterocyclic aromatic amines are formed by cooking at temperatures around 100°C or using microwave ovens. Gravy is also an important source of exposure in countries where gravy and brown sauce are prepared from the pan residue after the meat has been fried (Table 3). Because of the many factors influencing the formation of heterocyclic aromatic amines, these values should be regarded only as a measure of the order of magnitude of possible contamination. In most reports, PhIP is the most abundant among the food mutagens, followed by MeIQx and 4,8-DiMeIQx. Although present in processed food in the same order of magnitude, concentrations of AαC, MeAαC, Trp-P-1, and Trp-P-2 have been determined in a few reports only. These four heterocyclic aromatic amines have also been detected in cigarette-smoke condensate (up to 260 ng/cigarette) and various components of the environment, such as airborne particles, rainwater, cigarette-smoke-polluted indoor air, and diesel-exhaust particles. PhIP was detected in cigarette-smoke condensate (11–26 ng/cigarette), wine (12–66 ng/liter), and beer (8–25 ng/liter).

TABLE 3 Heterocyclic Aromatic Amines in Cooked Meat and Fish (ng/g cooked product)[a]

Heterocyclic aromatic amines	Beef	Chicken	Lamb	Pork	Fish
2-Amino-9-*H*-pyrido[2,3-*b*]indole (AαC)	651	180	2.5		109
2-Amino-3-methyl-9-*H*-pyrido[2,3-*b*]indole (MeAαC)	63		0.2		
2-Amino-3-methylimidazo[4,5-*f*]quinoline (IQ)	8			0.04	20
2-Amino-3,4-dimethylimidazo[4,5-*f*]quinoline (MeIQ)	0.1			0.02	17
2-Amino-3,8-dimethylimidazo[4,5-*f*]quinoxaline (MeIQx)	42	9	1.0	27	6.4
2-Amino-3,4,8-trimethylimidazo[4,5-*f*]quinoxaline (4,8-DiMeIQx)	28	4	0.67	9.3	5.4
2-Amino-1-methyl-6-phenylimidazo[4,5-*b*]pyridine (PhIP)	68	480	43	36	73
3-Amino-1,4-dimethyl-5*H*-pyrido[4,3-*b*]indole (Trp-P-1)	53				13
3-Amino-1-methyl-5*H*-pyrido[4,3-*b*]indole (Trp-P-2)	14		0.15		13

[a]Maximal concentrations reported by Layton *et al.* (1995), Galceran *et al.* (1996), Knize *et al.* (1997), and Sinha *et al.* (1995).

Absorption, Distribution, Metabolism, and Excretion

After oral administration, heterocyclic aromatic amines are taken up efficiently and are subject to extensive metabolism prior to excretion with the urine and feces. In rat experiments, a high proportion of unchanged PhIP is excreted via the bile and feces, thereby reaching the colon, one of its major target organs. No data on biliary excretion in humans are available. However, heterocyclic aromatic amines can be detected consistently in the urine of healthy people but not in patients receiving parenteral alimentation. Normal human volunteers excreted about 2% the ingested MeIQx and about 1% PhIP in the urine. After hydrolysis of acid-labile conjugates, about 11% and 1.4% MeIQx and PhIP, respectively, ingested with well-done cooked beef patties were recovered in the urine after 24 h. In animal experiments, heterocyclic aromatic amines are distributed throughout the body without any significant enrichment in fatty tissues. At later times after administration, enrichment in certain tissues occurs, which is due to covalent binding to DNA and proteins. For PhIP the highest binding occurs in the colon and rectum mucosa, but high levels are also measured in nontarget organs such as the liver, pancreas, and small intestinal mucosa. The inhibition of biliary excretion of PhIP and/or its metabolites did not affect the extent of DNA binding in the colon mucosa. This is in contrast to the hypothesis that the enterohepatic circulation of heterocyclic aromatic amines is important for tumor induction in the large intestine. Hemoglobin adducts of Trp-P-1 have been detected in humans. In rat experiments, hemoglobin adducts of Trp-P-1 correlated highly with liver DNA adducts Although 0.2% of the PhIP dose was bound to hemoglobin in the rat, hemoglobin adducts of PhIP have not yet been reported in humans. Some of the other heterocyclic aromatic amines are bound to a higher extent to the serum albumin. Prior to covalent tissue binding, heterocyclic aromatic amines require metabolic activation, as described previously for aromatic amines (Fig. 1). Hydroxylation of the exocyclic nitrogen by CYP1A2 followed by O-acetylation by NAT2 are thought to be the major activation pathways. Recently, it has been suggested that CYP1B1 and NAT1 play a significant role in the target-organ-specific metabolism of PhIP (Fig. 4). This is consistent with the observation of only a 70% inhibition of PhIP metabolic clearance in humans pretreated with a dose of furafylline sufficient to inhibit >99% of CYP1A2 activity *in vivo*. In contrast, metabolic clearance of MeIQx was inhibited >90% *in vivo*, whereas N-hydroxylation of PhIP was inhibited even more effectively than that of MeIQx, 98.5 versus 91.5%, respectively. Detoxification pathways, such as 4′-hydroxylation of PhIP, seem to be of minor importance in humans.

Genetic Toxicology

Heterocyclic aromatic amines have been discovered as the major mutagens in cooked meat and fish. They require metabolic activation in the Ames test. All of these food mutagens tested so far have shown strong carcinogenic properties (Table 4). AαC was the only compound that tested negative in rats. It was, however, positive in mice. The carcinogenic potencies were ranked in the order IQ > 4,8-DiMeIQx > MeIQx > PhIP > AαC, which is almost the reverse order of the dietary intake. No carcinogenicity data are available for an additional heterocyclic aromatic amine of potential dietary significance, 4,8-DiMeIQx. From its

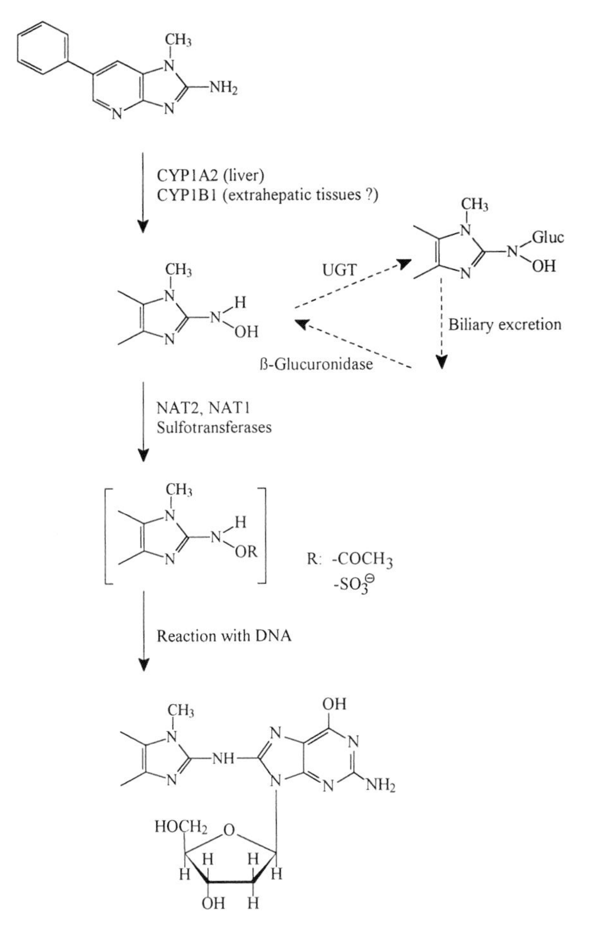

FIGURE 4 Major activation pathways of 2-amino-1-methyl-6-phenylimidazo[4,5-*b*]pyridine (PhIP).

high mutagenic potency it was estimated to be one of the strongest carcinogens in this class of compounds. Heterocyclic aromatic amines produce a broad spectrum of tumors, with the liver and colon as the two major sites. Even more important, the spectrum includes other major tumors sites such as the breast, pancreas, and lung, for which, as for the colon tumors, a significant contribution of dietary factors is evident from epidemiological studies. For these tumor sites, synergistical effects have been observed in rats when consuming several heterocyclic aromatic amines together. In a comparative study on mammary tumorigenesis in rats, the carcinogenic potency of PhIP was equal to benzo[*a*]pyrene. A possible contribution of heterocyclic aromatic amines to human cancer is further supported by the observation that in human tissues *in vitro* the same DNA adducts are produced as in animal experiments. Using highly sensitive detection by accelerator mass spectrometry, MeIQx DNA binding to rat liver followed a linear dose–response relationship down to the concentrations in the ng/g range that are expected to occur in humans. However, the extent and tissue distribution of DNA binding from heterocyclic aromatic amines in animal tissues does not always correlate with the major sites of tumor formation in the same animals. In Fischer F344 rats treated with PhIP, extraordinarily high DNA-adduct levels were induced in the pancreas, a nontarget organ of PhIP in this species. Heterocyclic aromatic amines leave a mutational fingerprint in rat experiments that is specific for each compound. *APC* gene mutations in PhIP-induced rat colon tumors have characteristics in common with human cancers. In experiments with nonhuman primates, IQ but not MeIQx has been shown to be a potent hepatocarcinogen. The different potency of these two heterocyclic aromatic amines could be correlated with *in vivo* metabolic activation that is high for IQ and very poor for MeIQx. Studies with PhIP indicate that PhIP is metabolically activated in monkeys and is a likely carcinogen in this species.

Recent work in rats and monkeys has shown that some cooked-food mutagens preferentially produce damage in heart cells. This cardiac toxicity was correlated with dose- and time-dependent adduct formation in the mitochondrial DNA. It is speculated that heterocyclic aromatic amines may contribute to diet-dependent cardiomyopathies and congestive heart disease.

Relevance for Human Carcinogenicity

The heterocyclic aromatic amines MeIQ, MeIQx, and PhIP were classified by the IARC as possible human carcinogens, and IQ as a probable carcinogen. Based on extrapolation from animal experiments, the incremental risk for the average consumption of heterocyclic aromatic amines by the U.S. population was estimated to be between 1×10^{-5} and 3.8×10^{-4}. However, for risk assessment, it is essential to know the individual consumption of heterocyclic aromatic amines. Therefore, it is practically impossible to appreciate the potential risk because of the diversity of human diets and age-related changes in dietary habits. In a recent study combining information on food consumption and the chemical analysis of 22 standard dishes, the total mean daily intake of heterocyclic aromatic amines in an elderly Swedish population from 50 to 75 years of age was determined to be < 200 ng, with an individual range of 0–865 ng/day for PhIP, 0–1388 ng/day for MeIQx, and 0–171 ng/day for 4,8-

TABLE 4 Mutagenicity and Carcinogenicity of Heterocyclic Aromatic Amines[a]

	Mutagenicity, log MP[b]	TD_{50}[c]		Carcinogenicity, target organs[d]
		Rat	Mouse	
AαC	2.08	—	50	Liver, vascular
MeAαC	1.11	8.7	22	Liver, vascular, skin, bladder, pancreas, salivary glands
Glu-P-1	4.07	4.7	5.4	Liver, large and small intestine, Zymbal gland, clitoral gland, lung, vascular, lymphoma, skin
Glu-P-2	2.64	42	16	Liver, large and small intestine, Zymbal gland, clitoral gland, lung, vascular, lymphoma
IQ	4.50	1.9	20	Liver, lung, forestomach, large and small intestine, breast, pancreas, Zymbal gland, clitoral gland, skin, bladder
MeIQ	5.30	0.54	12	Liver, lung, forestomach, large and small intestine, breast, Zymbal gland, oral cavity, skin, bladder
MeIQx	4.33	2.0	24	Liver, lung, forestomach, small intestine, Zymbal gland, clitoral gland, skin, lymphoma
PhIP	2.80	4.3	29	Large intestine, breast, lymphoma, prostate, lung
Trp-P-1	4.03	0.58	41	Liver, lymphoma, bladder, skin
Trp-P-2	4.21	6.7	13	Liver, vascular, bladder, clitoral gland

[a]Full chemical names: 2-amino-6-methyldipyrido[1,2-*a*:3′,2′-*d*]imidazole (Glu-P-1); 2-aminiodipyrido[1,2-*a*:3′,2′-*d*]imidazole (Glu-P-2); for others, see Table 3.

[b]MP, mutagenic potency, was determined from the slope of the linear part of the dose–response curves (number of revertants/nmol) in a standardized Ames test using *Salmonella* strains TA98 and TA1538 in the presence of liver S9 mix from PCB-induced rats or hamsters (Hatch *et al.*, 1992).

[c]TD_{50}, daily dose in mg/kg body weight given with the food, which induces tumors in 50% of animals (Gold *et al.*, 1994).

[d]Target organs taken from Eisenbrand and Tang (1993), Bogen (1994), Hasegawa *et al.* (1994), and Tamano *et al.* (1994).

DiMeIQx. This is much lower than earlier estimates for the daily intake of total heterocyclic aromatic amines in Germany (800–8400 ng) and Japan (400–16,000 ng). Based on concentrations in the urine, a daily uptake of 200–2600 ng MeIQx/day was estimated in Japan. Several methods for the determination of biomarkers of the internal dose, such as protein and DNA-adducts, have been developed. Epidemiological studies using these new tools may show a relationship of exposure to heterocyclic aromatic amine with colon cancer and other diet-related cancers. From the present data it can be concluded that high-temperature heating of meat and fish is an avoidable risk with regard to heterocyclic aromatic-amine eposure.

Bibliography

Ashby, J., and Paton, D. (1993). The influence of chemical structure on the extent and sites of carcinogenesis for 522 rodent carcinogens and 55 different human carcinogen exposures. *Mutat. Res.* **286,** 3–74.

Augustsson, K., Skog, K., Jägerstad, M., and Steineck, G. (1997). Assessment of the human exposure to heterocyclic amines. *Carcinogenesis* **18,** 1931–1935.

Babu, S. R., Lakshmi, V. M., Huang, G. P., Zenser, T. V., and Davis, B. B. (1996). Glucuronide conjugates of 4-aminobiphenyl and its N-hydroxy metabolites. pH stability and synthesis by human and dog liver. *Biochem. Pharmacol.* **51,** 1679–1685.

Badawi, A. F., Stern, S. J., Lang, N. P., and Kadlubar, F. F. (1996). Cytochrome P-450 and acetyltransferase expression as biomarkers of carcinogen-DNA adduct levels and human cancer susceptibility. *Prog. Clin. Biol. Res.* **395,** 109–140.

Benigni, R., Andreoli, C., and Giuliani, A. (1994). QSAR models for both mutagenic potency and activity: Application to nitroarenes and aromatic amines. *Environ. Mol. Mutagen.* **24,** 208–219.

Bogen, K. T. (1994). Cancer potencies of heterocyclic amines found in cooked foods. *Food Chem. Toxicol.* **32,** 505–515.

Case, R. A. M., Hosker, M. E., and McDonald, D. B. (1954). Tumors of urinary bladder in workmen engaged in the manufacture and use of certain dyestuff intermediates in British chemical industry. Part 1. The role of aniline, benzidine, alpha-naphthylamin and beta-naphthylamine. *Br. J. Ind. Med.* **11,** 75–104.

Culp, S. J., Roberts, D. W., Talaska, G., Lang, N. P., Fu, P. P., Lay, J. O., Jr., Teitel, C. H., Snawder, J. E., Von Tungeln, L. S., and Kadlubar, F. F. (1997). Immunochemical, ^{32}P-postlabeling, and GC/MS detection of 4-aminobiphenyl-DNA addducts in human peripheral lung in relation to metabolic activation pathways involving pulmonary *N*-oxidation, conjugation, and peroxidation. *Mutat. Res.* **378,** 97–112.

Debnath, A. K., Debnath, G., Shusterman, A. J., and Hansch, C. (1992). A QSAR investigation of the role of hydrophobicity in regulating mutagenicity in the Ames test: 1. Mutagenicity of aromatic and heteroaromatic amines in Salmonella typhimurium TA98 and TA 100. *Environ. Mol. Mutagen.* **19,** 37–52.

Eisenbrand, G., and Tang, W. (1993). Food-borne heterocyclic amines. Chemistry, formation, occurrence and biological activities. A literature review. *Toxicology* **84,** 1–82.

Eyer, P., and Gallemann, D. (1996). Reactions of nitrosoarenes with SH groups. *In* "The Chemistry of Amino, Nitroso, Nitro and Related Groups" (S. Patai, ed.), Supplement F2, pp. 999–1039. John Wiley & Sons, New York.

Galceran, M. T., Pais, P., and Puignou, L. (1996). Isolation by solid-phase extraction and liquid chromatographic determination of mutagenic amines in beef extracts. *J. Chromatogr. A* **719,** 203–212.

Garner, R. C., Martin, C. N., and Clayson, D. B. (1984). Carcinogenic aromatic amines and related compounds. *In* "Chemical Carcinogens" (C. E. Searle, ed.) pp. 175–276. ACS Monograph 182. American Chemical Society, Washington, D.C.

Glatt, H. R. (1997). Bioactivation of mutagens via sulfation. *FASEB J.* **11,** 314–321.

Gold, L. S., Slone, T. H., Manley, N. B., and Ames, B. N. (1994). Heterocyclic amines formed by cooking food: Comparison of bioassay results with other chemicals in the carcinogenic potency database. *Cancer Lett.* **83,** 21–29.

Gold, L. S., and Zeiger, E. (1997). "Handbook of Carcinogenic Potency and Genotoxicity Databases." CRC Press, Boca Raton, FL.

Hartter, D. R. (1985). The use and importance of nitroaromatic compounds in the chemical industry. *In* "Toxicity of Nitroaromatic Compounds" (D. E. Rickert, ed.), pp. 1–13. Hemisphere Publishing, Washington, D.C.

Hasegawa, R., Tanaka, H., Tamano, S., Shirai, T., Nagao, M., Sugimura, T., and Ito, N. (1994). Synergistic enhancement of small and large intestinal carcinogenesis by combined treatment of rats with five heterocyclic amines in a medium-term multi-organ bioassay. *Carcinogenesis* **15,** 2567–2573.

Hatch, F. T., Knize, M. G., Moore, D. H., and Felton, J. S. (1992). Quantitative correlation of mutagenic and carcinogenic potencies for heterocyclic amines from cooked foods and additional aromatic amines. *Mutat. Res.* **271,** 269–287.

Henschler, D., and Greim, H., eds. (1996). Toxikologisch-arbeitsmedizinische Begründung von MAK-Werten, 23.Lieferung, Wiley-VCH-Verlag, Weinheim.

Ippen, H. (1994). Nitromoschus, *Bundesgesundheitsblatt* **37,** 255–260, 291–294.

Kadlubar, F. F. (1994). DNA adducts of carcinogenic aromatic amines. *In* "DNA Adducts: Identification and Biological Significance" (K. Hemminki *et al.,* eds.), pp. 196–216. International Agency for Research on Cancer, Lyon, France.

Knize, M. G., Salmon, C. P., Hopmans, E. C., and Felton, J. S. (1997). Analysis of foods for heterocyclic aromatic amine carcinogens by solid-phase extraction and high-performance liquid chromatography. *J. Chromatogr. A* **763,** 179–185.

Lawrence, F. R., and Marshall, W. J. (1985). Aniline. *In* "Ullmann's Encyclopedia of Industrial Chemistry," 5th ed., Vol. A2 (W. Gerhartz *et al.,* eds.), pp. 303–312. Wiley-VCH, Weinheim.

Layton, D. W., Bogen, K. T., Knize, M. G., Hatch, F. T., Johnson, V. M., and Felton, J. S. (1995). Cancer risk of heterocyclic amines in cooked foods: An analysis and implications for research. *Carcinogenesis* **16,** 39–52.

Miller, J. A. (1994). Research in chemical carcinogenesis with Elizabeth Miller—a trail of discovery with our associates *Drug Metab. Rev.* **26,** 1–36.

Neumann, H.-G. (1984). Dosimetry and dose response relationships. *In* A. Berlin, M. Draper, K. Hemminki and H. Vainio, eds. "Monitoring Human Exposure to Carcinogenic and Mutagenic Agents" (A. Berlin *et al.,* eds.), pp. 115–126. IARC Scientific Publications No. 59. International Agency for Research on Cancer, Lyon, France.

O'Brien, P. J., Wong, W. C., Silva, J., and Khan, S. (1990). Toxicity of nitrobenzene compounds towards isolated hepatocytes: Dependence on reduction potential. *Xenobiotica* **20,** 945–955.

Rickert, D. E. (1987). Metabolism of nitroaromatic compounds. *Drug Metab. Rev.* **18,** 23–53.

Sabbioni, G., and Sepai, O. (1995). Comparison of hemoglobin binding, mutagenicity and carcinogenicity of arylamines and nitroarenes. *Chimia* **49,** 374–380.

Sabbioni, G., Wei, J., and Liu, Y.-Y. (1996). Determination of hemoglobin adducts in workers exposed to 2,4,6-trinitrotoluene. *J. Chromatogr. B.* **682,** 243–248.

Sinha, R., Rothman, N., Brown, E. D., Salmon, C. P., Knize, M. G., Swanson, C. A., Rossi, S. C., Mark, S. D., Levander, O. A., and Felton, J. S. (1995). High concentrations of the carcinogen 2-amino-1-methyl-6-phenylimidazo-[4,5-*b*]pyridine (PhIP) occur in chicken but are dependent on the cooking method. *Cancer Res.* **55,** 4516–4519.

Skipper, P. L., and Tannenbaum, S. R. (1994). Molecular dosimetry of aromatic amines in human populations. *Environ. Health Perspect. Suppl.* **102,** 17–21.

Sugimura, T. (1997). Overview of carcinogenic heterocyclic amines. *Mutation Res.* **376,** 211–219.

Tamano, S., Hasegawa, R., Hagiwara, A., Nagao, M., Sugimura, T., and Ito, N. (1994). Carcinogenicity of a mutagenic compound from food, 2-amino-3-methyl-9*H*-pyrido[2,3-*b*]indole (MeAαC), in male F344 rats. *Carcinogenesis* **15,** 2009–2015.

Vogt, P. F., and Gerulius, J. J. (1985). Amines, aromatic. *In* "Ullmann's Encyclopedia of Industrial Chemistry," 5th ed., Vol A2 (W. Gerhartz *et al.,* eds.), pp. 37–53. Wiley-VCH, Weinheim.

Wakabayashi, K., Ushiyama, H., Takahashi, M., Nukaya, H., Kim, S.-B., Hirose, M., Ochiai, M., Sugimura, T., and Nagao, M. (1993). Exposure to heterocyclic amines. *Environ. Health Perspect.* **99,** 129–133.

Ward, E. M., Sabbioni, G., DeBord, D. G., Teass, A. W., Brown, K., Talaska, G., Roberts, D., Ruder, A., and Streicher, R. P. (1996). Biological monitoring of aromatic amine exposures at a chemical plant with a known bladder excess. *J. Natl. Cancer Inst.* **88,** 1040–1052.

Weisburger, J. H. (1988). Past, present and future role of carcinogenic and mutagenic N-substituted arylcompounds in human cancer causation. *In* "Carcinogenic and Mutagenic Responses to Aromatic Amines and Nitroarenes" (C. M. King *et al.,* eds.), pp. 3–19. Elsevier, New York.

CHAPTER

31

N-Nitroso Compounds

WERNER KOEHL*, GERHARD EISENBRAND†

*Department of Toxicology, Henkel KGaA, Duesseldorf, Germany

†Department of Food Chemistry and Environmental Toxicology, University of Kaiserslautern University, Kaiserslautern, Germany

N-Nitroso compounds are important environmental carcinogens. They are chemically relatively simple substances that are classified into two groups according to their chemical structure, reactivity and effects, *N*-nitrosamines and *N*-nitrosamides (Fig. 1).

OCCURRENCE, CHEMISTRY, AND EXPOSURE

Nitrosamines originate from the nitrosation of amine precursors by nitrosating agents like nitrite or nitric oxides. In acidic aqueous solutions, the active nitrosating agent is nitrous acid (Fig. 2). Other potent nitrosating agents are N_2O_3 and nitrosyl halogenides. The pK_a of the amine and the pH value of the solution are important factors for the nitrosation rate. The reaction is second order with respect to nitrite and first order with respect to amine. At a given pH value, weakly basic amines in general react faster than stronger basic amines. In most cases the nitrosation rate is significantly lower for tertiary than for secondary amines. The nitrosation of primary amines leads to unstable alkylating agents that react with compounds of the reaction mixture to produce a variety of products, especially alcohols.

The two main sources of human exposure are exogenous and endogenous exposure to *N*-nitroso compounds (Fig. 3). *Endogenous burden* results from the formation of nitrosamines by nitrosation processes inside the body; nitrosatable precursors, such as, amines, amides, or amino acids, can react with agents like nitrite or nitric oxides. Nitrite can be formed in the gastric system (are oral cavity, stomach, intestine, and infected bladder) by the reduction of nitrate, which is found in food in considerable amounts (Fig. 4). The relevance of endogenous formation of carcinogenic *N*-nitroso compounds as risk factors for certain types of human cancer is still a matter of debate. The results of various epidemiological studies are not conclusive. The potential for endogenous formation of *N*-nitroso compounds from amino acids, such as proline in the gastrointestinal tract, can be easily assessed by monitoring the excretion in the urine of *N*-nitrosoproline, which is non-carcinogenic and quantitatively excreted with the urine.

In addition to chemical nitrosation in an acidic medium (e.g., the stomach), endogenous nitrosation is also mediated by bacteria and stimulated macrophages. Bacteria of the gastrointestinal tract, such as *Escherischia coli* or *Proteus,* can catalyze the formation of nitrosamines from nitrate, specifically nitrite and amine, respectively. In these reactions there is a participation of bacterial molybdenum-containing enzymes. These processes are considered potential risk factors for stomach cancer in patients suffering from achlorhydria and for bladder cancer in patients with chronical infection of the urinary system (e.g., bilharzia), as well as in paraplegic patients.

Whether nitrogen monoxide (NO), known as a transmitter for biological signaling and also formed

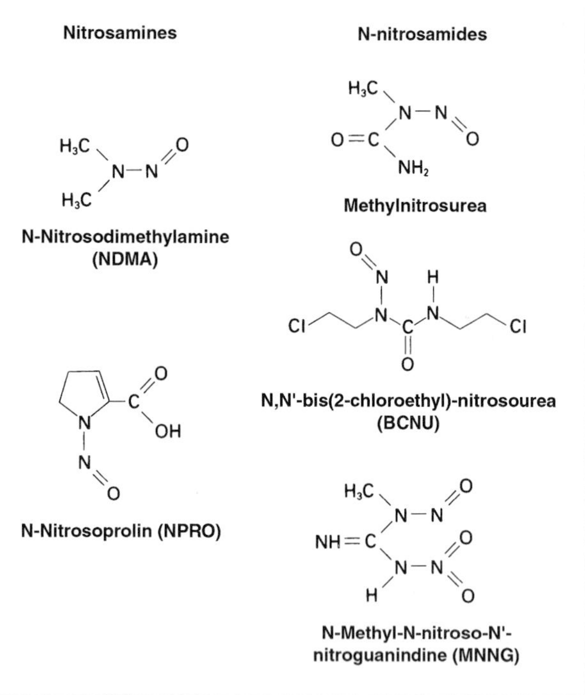

Nitrosamines

N-Nitrosodimethylamine (NDMA)

N-Nitrosoprolin (NPRO)

N-nitrosamides

Methylnitrosurea

N,N'-bis(2-chloroethyl)-nitrosourea (BCNU)

N-Methyl-N-nitroso-N'-nitroguanindine (MNNG)

FIGURE 1 Structure of *N*-nitroso compounds.

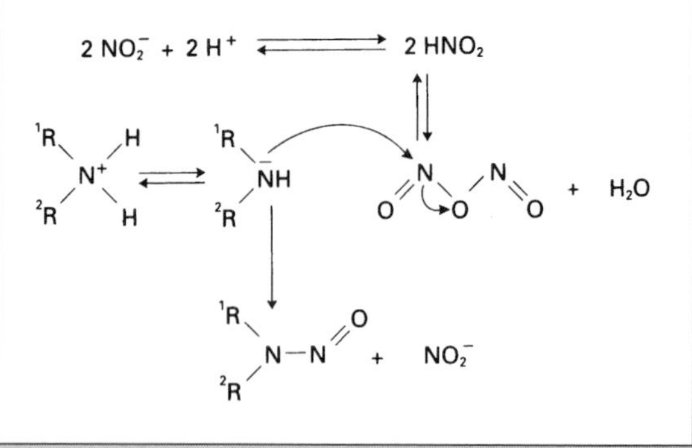

$2\,NO_2^- + 2\,H^+ \rightleftharpoons 2\,HNO_2$

FIGURE 2 Mechanism of the nitrosation of secondary amines. Nitrosating agent is N_2O_3. Only the free amine (unprotonated form) is undergoing nitrosation. For strong basic amines, the fastest nitrosation reaction is observed at pH levels of 3–4.

during inflammation from the amino acid arginine by activated macrophages, contributes significantly to endogenous nitrosation is a matter of debate. A reliable assessment of exposure to endogenous *N*-nitroso compounds is not possible, as a multitude of parameters are individually influential. However, the sensitive tools available for the detection of promutagenic lesions, as well as mutations in certain maker genes, are promising with regard to the further elucidatation of the role of endogenous nitrosation in human cancer risk, especially in connection with high exposure to either amine precursors or nitrate uptake.

For drugs containing nitrosatable groups, toxicological testing at the preclinical stage includes a nitrosatability test. The drug aminophenazone was taken from the market in most countries because of the high risk of its being nitrosatated and generating the potent carcinogen *N*-nitrosodimethylamine.

The *exogenous burden* might result from consumption-related exposure (i.e., lifestyle) via food, tobacco, cosmetics and household commodities, and occupa-

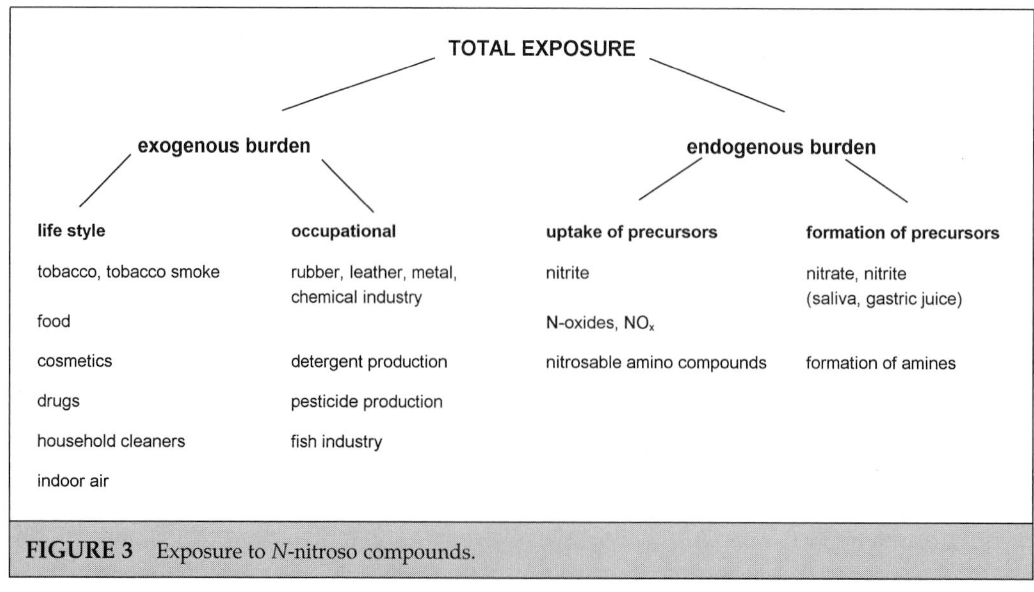

FIGURE 3 Exposure to *N*-nitroso compounds.

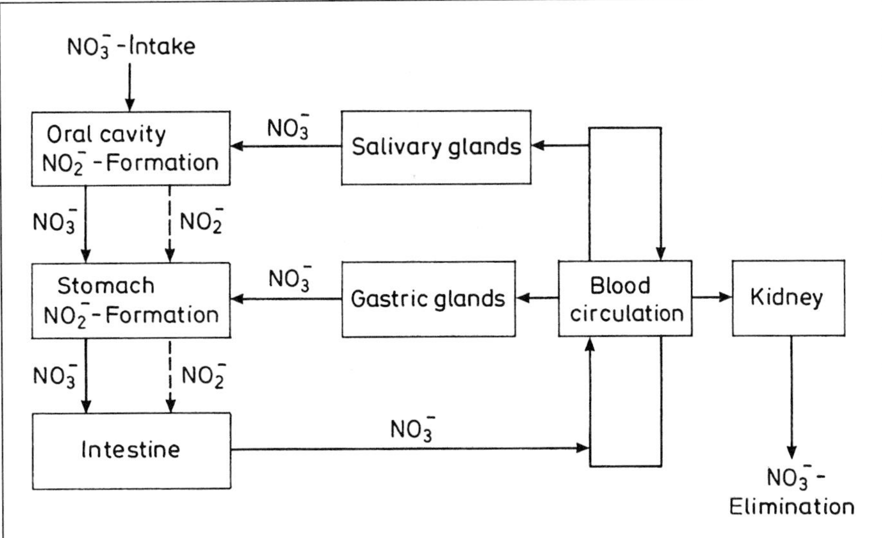

FIGURE 4 Flow diagram of gastrointestinal nitrate circulation. Ingested nitrate is absorbed in the small intestine, circulated in the blood, excreted by elimination in to the urine (65–70%) and feces (3–10%), and partially secreted into the oral cavity by the salivary glands. There, up to 7% of nitrate is converted by microorganisms (bacterial nitrate reductase) to nitrite within 24 h. Under the acid conditions in the stomach, nitrite can react with amines to form nitrosamines (endogenous nitrosation).

tional exposure. In western Europe, the intake of volatile *N*-nitroso compounds (especially *N*-nitrosodimethylamine) from food today is less than 0.5 μg/day. In contrast, the consumption of cigarettes or smokeless tobacco (e.g., snuff and chewing tobacco) leads to substantial exposure. With 20 cigarettes per day, the total intake of nitrosamines increases to 17–85 μg. In specific cases, the intake of tobacco-specific nitrosamines (TSNA) via sniffing has reached up to 400 μg/day. TSNA are formed from nicotine and homologous alkaloids during processing and fermentation of tobacco.

N-Nitrosonornicotine (NNK), 4-(methylnitrosamino)-1-(3-pyridyl)-1-butanone, and 4-(methylnitrosamino)-1-(3-pyridyl)-1-butanol, which is a reducted form of 4-(methylnitrosamino)-1-(3-pyridyl)-1-butanone, are potent carcinogens in laboratory animals, leading to tumors of the upper respiratory tract, lung, and/or pancreas in several rodents. These substances are found in mainstream smoke, as well as in sidestream smoke. They are therefore considered risk factors for passive smoking. For passive smokers after one hour in a tobacco-smoke-saturated room, an uptake of 0.6 μg nitrosamine (total) was determined.

Comparing the total doses of 4-(methylnitrosamino)-1-(3-pyridyl)-1-butanone and NNK, which clearly induce tumors in laboratory animals, with the total life-time exposure of a smoker or snuff-user shows that the tobacco-related uptake is within the dose range that is carcinogenic in laboratory animals. 4-(Methylnitrosamino)-1-(3-pyridyl)-1-butanone is considered a major risk factor causally related to tumor induction in the lung, esophagus, oral cavity, and pancreas of smokers.

With respect to occupational exposure, specific work, places in the metal, rubber, leather, and fish industries, as well as in the pesticide and detergent industries, are of special importance. In addition to volatile nitrosamines, such as *N*-nitrosodimethylamine (NDMA), *N*-nitrosomorpholine (NMOR), and *N*-nitrosodibutylamine (NDBA), the nonvolatile *N*-nitrosodiethanolamine (NDELA) is important. This last is frequently found as contamination in cutting fluids used in the metal industry. *N*-Nitrosodiethanolamine penetrates the skin, leading to systemic exposure. In the urine samples of workers in the metal industry, levels up to 40 μg *N*-nitrosodiethanolamine/day were found.

The uptake of volatile nitrosamines in the metal industry was in the range of 40 μg/day and in the rubber industry up to 150 μg/day. In Germany, the technical guidelines for dangerous substances recommend a maximum level of 1 $\mu g/m^3$ total nitrosamine in the air, with the exception of certain working areas in rubber industry, where a maximum level of 2.5 $\mu g/m^3$ is allowed. Because these guidelines still allow daily uptakes by inhalation as high as 0.1 μg/kg body wt, these values need to be reduced further.

N-Nitrosamides do not appear to play a role as environmental carcinogens. Bisfunctional alkylating chloroethylnitrosoureas, especially *N,N'*-bis(2-chloroethyl)-nitrosourea (BCNU), are of a some clinical importance as antineoplastic agents.

ABSORPTION, DISTRIBUTION, METABOLISM, AND EXCRETION

The absorption of nitrosamines can occur via the lung (volatile nitrosamines, such as *N*-nitrosodimethylamine or aerosol-bound tobacco-specific nitrosamines), via the gastrointestinal tract, and via the skin (e.g., *N*-nitrosodiethanolamine).

Orally administered *N*-nitrosodimethylamine is absorbed from the stomach only to a small extent. In rats, the absorption takes place mainly in the upper small intestine ($t_{1/2} < 5$ min) and to a smaller extent in the jejunum and the cecum. Most of the nitrosamines are metabolized very efficiently by the liver (first-pass effect). Smaller doses of up to 40 μg/kg body wt of *N*-nitrosodimethylamine are totally metabolized during first pass in the liver. At higher doses, the metabolic capacity of the liver is saturated and *N*-nitrosodimethylamine is systematically distributed. This effect is considered responsible for the induction of kidney tumors after higher oral doses.

The systemic blood clearance for short-chain. *N*-dialkylnitrosamines is very high (40 ml/min/kg *N*-nitrosodimethylamine in rats) due to their efficient metabolism. Plasma binding has not been reported for these compounds.

Up to about 60% of the short-chain *N*-nitrosodialkylamines are degraded to CO_2 and exhaled, a small amount is excreted via the urine, and a negligible part via the feces. After an ip application of 30 mg/kg body wt *N*-[^{14}C]nitrosodimethylamine to rats, complete biotransformation was observed within 6 hours, as measured by $^{14}CO_2$ exhalation.

Well-water-soluble *N*-nitrosohydroxyalkylamines are preferentially excreted via the urine. After oral or intravenous administration to rats, unmodified *N*-nitrosodiethanolamine is excreted in the urine up to more than 60% of the applied dose.

Sex-specific differences in the liver clearance of rats were observed for *N*-nitroso-*N*-methylhydroxyethylamine. The higher rate of metabolism in the liver of female rats correlated with a higher incidence of liver tumors, whereas in males more tumors in the mucosa of the nose were found.

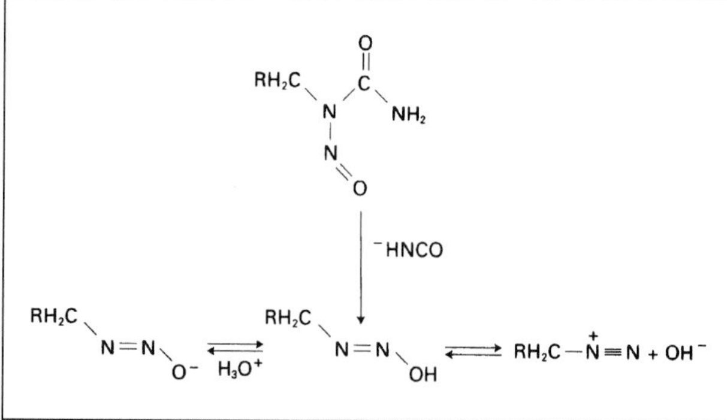

FIGURE 5 Spontaneous decomposition of *N*-nitrosurea to alkylating intermediates.

In the case of the bladder carcinogen *N*-nitrosodibutylamine, in addition to biotransformation in the liver, first-pass metabolism in the small intestine was found to be especially important for the formation of *N*-nitroso-*N*-butyl-(3-carboxypropyl-)amine (BCPN) in rats, the crucial metabolite for the induction of bladder tumors. Differential isoenzyme distribution appears to be responsible for this effect.

Ethanol can influence the metabolism and pharmacokinetics of nitrosamines. The sequence of application of ethanol and nitrosamine is important for the observed biological effects. Simultaneous application of ethanol and *N*-nitrosodimethylamine in rats leads to a delayed clearance of the nitrosamine and a shift in the target organ, as observed for *N*-nitrosodiethylamine in rats and mice.

Nitrosamines can also appear in milk. In goats after a dose of 30 mg/kg body wt, a *N*-nitrosodimethylamine concentration of 11.4 mg/kg was found in milk and 11.9 mg/kg in the blood after 1 h.

METABOLISM AND MECHANISMS OF TOXICITY

DNA damage is considered to be the main cause of the carcinogenic effect of *N*-nitroso compounds. The relevant reactive intermediates are electrophilic diazohydroxides, diazonium, and carbenium ions that result from the spontaneous decomposition of nitrosoureas in aqueous solution (Fig. 5) or from the metabolic activation of nitrosamines (Fig. 6).

NITROSAMIDES

The spontaneous decomposition of *N*-nitrosoureas leads to electrophiles that alkylate nucleophilic cen-

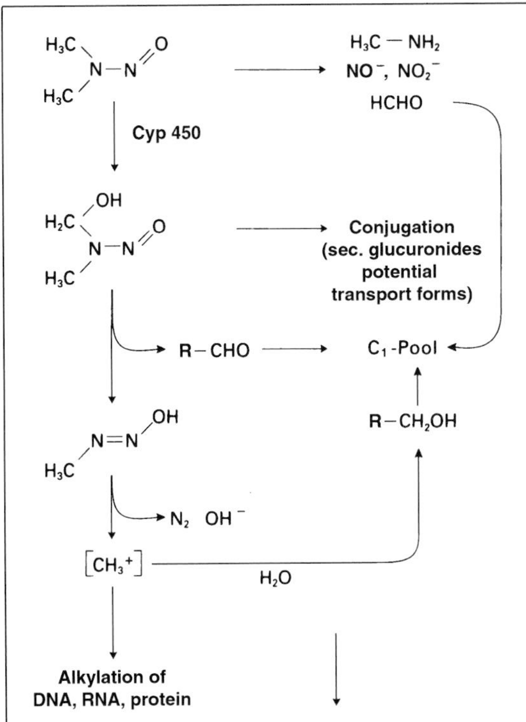

FIGURE 6 Biotransformation of *N*-nitrosodimethylamine. The key step in the activation is the cytochrome P450-mediated α-C-hydroxylation. The generated unstable α-hydroxyalkylnitrosamine decomposes spontaneously via the elimination of formaldehyde to the ultimate carcinogen, the methyldiazohydroxide (diazonium or carbenium intermediate). The latter is able to alkylate cellular macromolecules like DNA, RNA, and proteins.

ters of cellular macromolecules. DNA alkylation results in various DNA base adducts (N-1, N-3, and N-7 of adenine; N-3, O^6, and N-7 of guanine; O^2, N-3, and O^4 of thymidine; and O^2 and N-3 of cytosine), as well as alkyl-adducts of the sugar–phosphate backbone. The resulting methyl- and ethylphosphotriesters are highly stable. In contrast, 2-hydroxyethyl phosphotriesters are unstable and lead to high rates of DNA single-strand breaks. The formation of DNA–DNA cross-linked adducts has been demonstrated for bifunctionally alkylating *N*-nitrosoureas, such as *N,N'*-bis(2-chloroethyl)-nitrosourea.

Certain regions in cellular oncogenes (for example, in c-H-*ras*, c-*mos* or c-*myc*) and in viral promotor sequences (for example from Epstein–Barr and SV 40) are rich in guanine–cytosine (G-C)-containing sequences. It is assumed that the high antineoplastic efficacy of some alkylating agents can be attributed at least partly to the preferential alkylation of G-C-rich regions in cellular or viral DNA.

For the *N*-methylnitrosourea-induced mammary tumors in rats, an activation of the *H-ras* gene through G ⇒ A transition in codon 12 was observed. The same transition leads to an activation of the K-*ras* gene in *N*-methylnitrosourea-induced kidney tumors. For *N*-methylnitrosourea-induced colon tumors in rats, point mutations in the K-*ras* gene (G ⇒ A transition in codon 12 and 13) have been detected. *N*-Methylnitrosourea-induced carcinomas or papillomas of the esophagus and *N*-ethylnitrosurea-induced nephroblastomas showed high incidences of G ⇒ A transitions in the p53, suppressor gene, predominantly at the first base in codon 204 (GAG ⇒ AAG) and the second base of codon 213 (CGG ⇒ CAG).

NITROSAMINES

In contrast to *N*-nitrosoureas, nitrosamines are precarcinogens (see the section on carcinogenesis) that need metabolic activation. This metabolic activation of the ultimate carcinogen occurs via cytochrome-P450 monooxygenase (CYP)-mediated α-C-hydroxylation. Various cytochrome P450 isoenzymes have been shown to differ in their metabolic activity towards individual *N*-nitrosamines. For the metabolism of various *N*-nitrosamines, often at least one high-affinity isoenzyme has been described in addition to several isoenzymes with low affinity. Metabolic activation of *N*-nitrosodimethylamine in humans is essentially mediated by the isoenzymes CYP2E1 and CYP2A3, for activation of 4-(methylnitrosamino)-1-(3-pyridyl)-1-butanone CYP1A2, CYP2E1, and CYP2D6 are relevant.

There are significant variations in the metabolism of nitrosamines among different species. For instance, some *N*-nitrosamines are not measurably activated by liver microsomes from rats but are substantially activated by liver microsomes from hamsters. Depending on the localization of the corresponding isoenzymes in different tissues, metabolic activation can also take place in extrahepatic tissues like the esophaus, small intestine, or lung. The activation sequence for cytochrome P450-mediated α-C-hydroxylation is shown for *N*-nitrosodimethylamine (Fig. 6).

The *N*-nitroso-*N*-alkyl-α-hydroxyalkylamine generated via α-C-hydroxylation represents an unstable proximal carcinogen that spontaneously eliminates an aldehyde. The ultimate alkylating species alkyldiazohydroxide, alkyl diazotate, or the corresponding diazonium ion can react with biopolymers (DNA, RNA, or protein) in the cell, and equivalently with carbenium ions. Deuterium labeling at the α-C-atom reduces the metabolic activation and diminishes the muta-

TABLE 1 Carcinogenic Potency and Main Target Organ in the Rat of Selected N-Alkylnitrosamines

Nitrosamine	Carcinogenic activity[a]	Mode of administration	Main target organ
N-Nitrosodimethylamine	+++	Oral	Liver
N-Nitrosodiethylamine	+++	Oral	Liver
N-Nitrosodi-*n*-propylamine	+++	Oral	Liver
N-Nitroso-iso-propylamine	+	Oral	Liver
N-Nitrosodibutylamine	++	Oral, subcutaneous	Liver (bladder)
N-Nitrosomethylpentylamine	+++	Oral, subcutaneous	Esophagus
N-Nitrosomethylbenzylamine	+++	Oral	Esophagus
N-Nitrosomorpholine	+++	Oral, intravenous	Liver
N-Nitrosopiperazine	+++	Oral, intravenous	Esophagus

[a]Activity levels: + low; ++ medium; +++ high.

genic and carcinogenic potency of *N*-nitrosomorpholine or *N*-nitrosodimethylamine, due to the more stable C–D bond (i.e., deuterium-isotope effect). The role of α-C-hydroxylation as the key event for metabolic activation and for the resulting carcinogenic effect also becomes evident when considering the biological efficacy of nitrosamines with a sterically hindered α-position. Methyl substitution at the α-C-position leads to decreased carcinogenic efficacy, as demonstrated by comparing the potency of *N*-nitroso-di-*n*-propylamine with that of *N*-nitroso-diisopropylamine (Table 1). The presence of a *tert*-butyl group at the α-C-position totally abrogates carcinogenicity, as shown for the noncarcinogenic *N*-nitroso-*N*-methyl-*tert*-butylamine. In contrast, *N*-nitroso-α-acetoxyalkylamines (Fig. 7) are stabilized α-C-hydroxylated nitrosamines and potent carcinogens, which generate the corresponding alkylating agents by hydrolysis or via esterase-mediated cleavage.

The cytochrome P450-mediated oxidative denitrosation represents a main detoxification pathway of nitrosamines, generating a primary amine, the corresponding aldehyde, and NO or nitrite. In special cases, a reductive denitrosation to a secondary amine might also take place, as seen with *N*-nitrosodibenzylamine. In addition, glucuronide conjugation of *N*-nitroso-*N*-alkyl-1-hydroxyalkylamine is also relevant. However, only the formation of primary glucuronides is considered to represent a detoxification reaction. Secondary glucuronides are discussed as potential transport forms for *N*-nitroso-*N*-alkyl-1-hydroxyalkylamines that might liberate alkylating species in target tissues by glucuronidase-mediated cleavage. In the urine of smokers, in addition to 4-(methylnitrosamino)-1-(3-pyridyl)-1-butanol, the corresponding glucuronide was also detected; this was not found in nonsmokers.

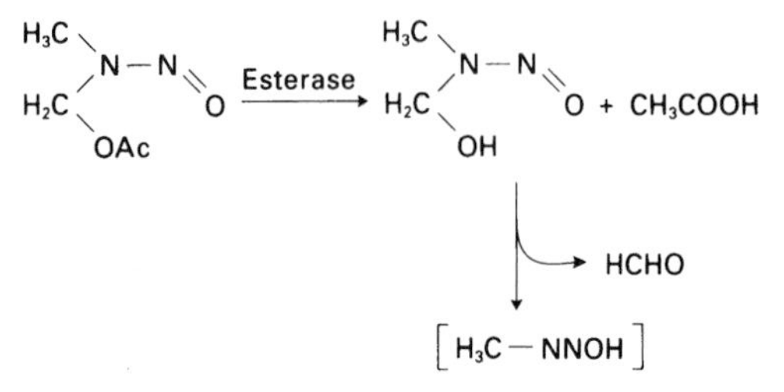

$$H_3C(H_2C(OAc))N{-}N{=}O \xrightarrow{\text{Esterase}} H_3C(H_2C(OH))N{-}N{=}O + CH_3COOH$$

$$\downarrow -HCHO$$

$$[H_3C{-}NNOH]$$

FIGURE 7 Activation of *N*-nitroso-α-acetoxydimethylnitrosamine by esterase.

FORMATION OF ADDUCTS

N-Nitrosodialkylamines can alkylate DNA bases *in vivo*. *N*-Nitrosodimethylamine methylates DNA in rat liver at the positions N-7, O^6, and N-3 of guanine; and N-1, N-3, and N-7 of adenine. The main adduct is *N*-7-methylguanine. *N*-Nitrosodiethylamine ethylates DNA bases at positions N-7 and O^6 of guanine; N-3 of adenine; and O^2 of thymine. The last shows a substantially longer persistence because of the low rate of repair. In general, the alkylation rate decreases with increasing chain length. Promutagenic lesions such as O^6-guanine-alkyl-adducts appear to be useful as markers for molecular epidemiology.

Methyl adducts and pyridyloxobutyl adducts from 4-(methylnitrosamino)-1-(3-pyridyl)-1-butanone found in the lung tissue of mice lead to mutations of the *K-ras* gene. This tobacco-specific nitrosamine also inhibits the repair enzyme O^6-alkylguanine DNA-alkyltransferase, leading to delayed repair of a promutagenic lesion.

Alkylation was also demonstrated for proteins, as evidenced by formation of 5-methyl cysteine in hemoglobin after the application of *N*-nitrosodimethylamine in animals. The extent of 5-methylcysteine formation in hemoglobin and the urinary excretion of *N*-7-methylguanine or *N*-3-methyladenine can be used to determine human exposure.

In smokers, hemoglobin adducts derived from tobacco-specific nitrosamines, as well as DNA-adducts in lung tissue, have been detected. *In vivo* studies in rats have shown that about 20–40% of the radioactivity from 4-[5-^{3}H] (methylnitrosamino)-1-(3-pyridyl)-1-butanone is covalently bound to hemoglobin. The metabolic pathways relevant for the formation of DNA and hemoglobin adducts are summarized in Fig. 8.

4-Hydroxy-1-(3-pyridyl)-1-butanone (HPB) can be quantified after hydrolysis (alkaline conditions) of the corresponding hemoglobin adduct. About 22% of the investigated smokers showed a significantly elevated

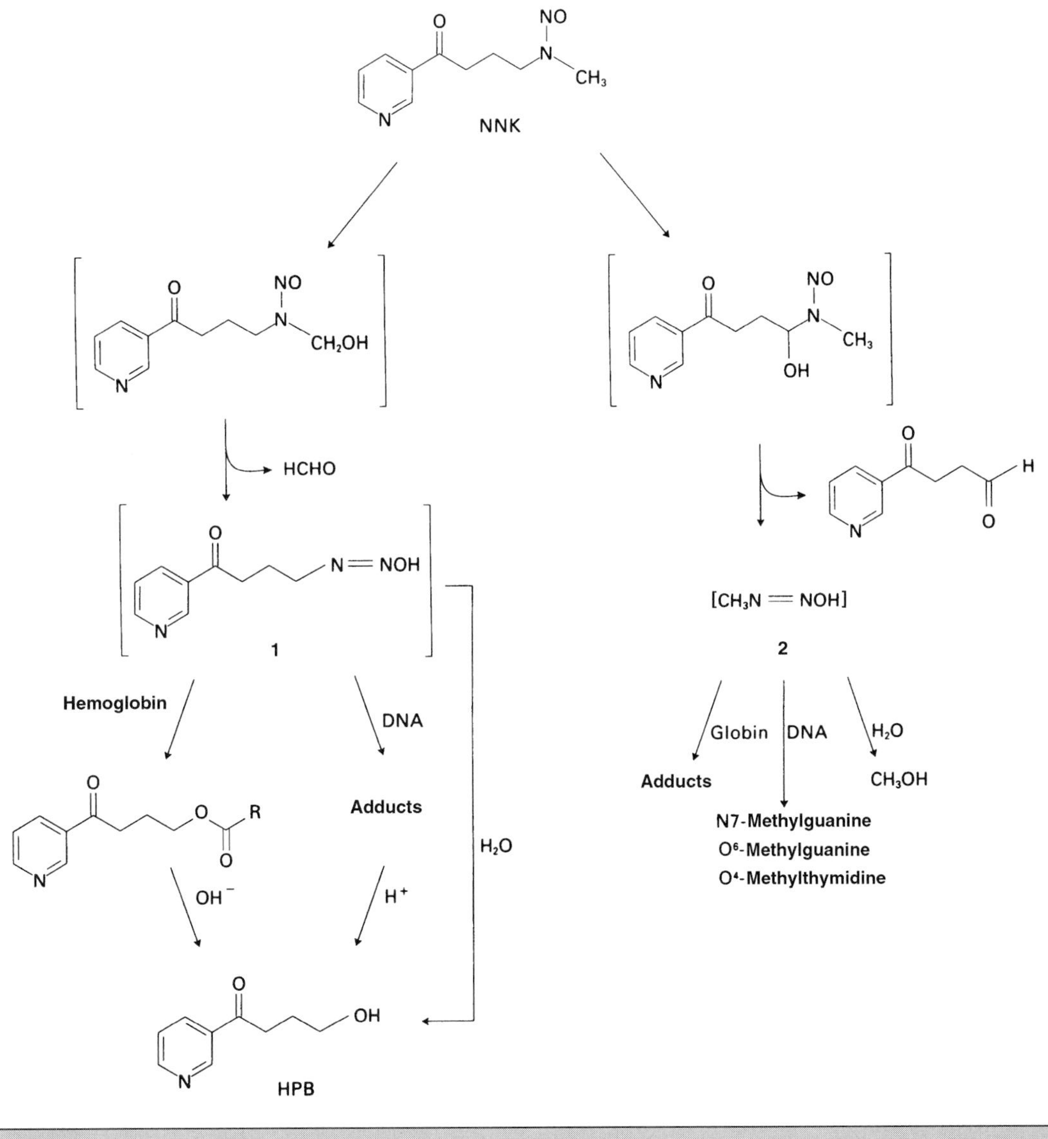

FIGURE 8 Generation of alkylating and pyridyloxobutylating intermediates after cytochrome P450-mediated α-C-hydroxylation of NNK. The reactive intermediates are able to alkylate biopolymers like DNA or proteins (hemoglobin). These adducts can be determined directly or after hydrolytic cleavage of hemoglobulin-adducts, for example, 4-hydroxy-1(pyridyl)-1-butanone (HPB).

level of HPB (200–1600 fmol/g hemoglobin); for nonsmokers the HBP-levels were usually below the detection limit.

In smokers, the average DNA adduct levels from 4-oxo-4-(3-pyridyl)-1-butyldiazohydroxide (Fig. 8) were 11 and 16 fmol/mg DNA for lung and bronchial tissue, respectively, with highest values reaching 50 fmol/mg DNA. These adducts were not detectable in nonsmokers. In bronchial tissue samples of smokers about 17 *N*-7-methylguanine adducts per 10^7 nucleotides (for nonsmokers about 5) were detected. In lymphocytes, the corresponding value was 12 *N*-7-methylguanine adducts per 10^7 nucleotides (for nonsmokers).

For the organ specificity of *N*-alkylnitrosamine-induced carcinogenesis, locally different activation or detoxification and repair ratios appear to be relevant. As an example, the potent esophageal carcinogen *N*-nitrosobenzylamine is metabolized differently in the esophagus and liver. The main metabolic pathway (>80%) in the esophagus is the hydroxylation of the methylene group at the benzyl side chain, resulting in the formation of benzaldehyde and the reactive methyldiazohydroxide, whereas in the liver only 50% is metabolized via this route. This correlates well with the formation of O^6-methylguanine, which is six-fold higher in the esophagus than in the lung and nine-fold higher in the esophagus in the liver. In addition, the ratio of *N*-7 to O^6-methylguanine-adducts in the esophagus points to a lower repair capacity of O^6-alkylguanine DNA-alkyltransferase, leading to a further accumulation of the promutagenic lesion. Moreover, detoxification by glucuronide conjugation of *N*-nitroso-*N*-alkyl-1-hydroxyalkylamines apparently does not take place. The marked organ specificity of the carcinogenic effect therefore appears to result from stronger metabolic activation, as well as a reduced rate of DNA repair in the target organ.

Similar results were obtained in studies with *N*-nitroso-*N*-methylalkylnitrosamines (alkyl chains of C1 to C12) with respect to their ability to form O^6-methylguanine in the DNA of the target organs, the liver and esophagus. The DNA-alkylation levels in the target organs were found to correlate well with the organ specificity of the compounds. Whereas *N*-nitrosodimethylamine, a strong liver carcinogen, induces high adduct rates in the liver and practically no DNA adducts in the esophagus, the strong esophageal carcinogens *N*-nitroso-*N*-propylmethyl nitrosamine and *N*-nitroso-*N*-pentylmethylamine induce only few adducts in the liver but high rates of O^6-methylguanine in the esophagus.

Besides α-hydroxylation there are, however, other biotransformation pathways important for the organ-specific activation of certain nitrosamines. One example is the activation of *N*-nitrosodibutylamine, which has been founder in certain work places in the rubber industry as a work-place carcinogen. *N*-Nitrosodibutylamine leads to liver and bladder tumors. When applied subcutaneously in low doses, bladder tumors are induced exclusively. The organ-specific effect of *N*-nitrosodibutylamine in the bladder is most probably due to a specific biotransformation pathway; as a

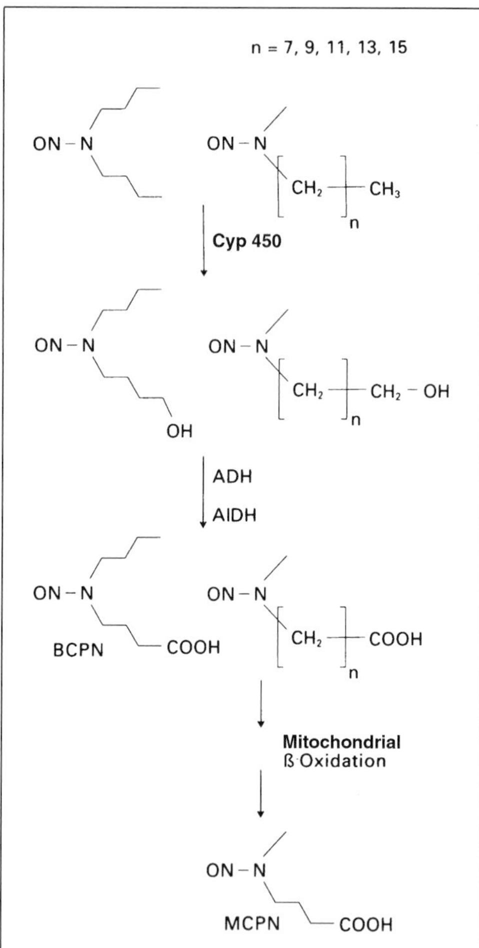

FIGURE 9 Biotransformation of nitrosamines that are almost exclusively carcinogenic to the bladder. Important for the generation of an ω-carboxypropyl side chain after ω-oxidation is the following β-oxidation taking place in the mitochondria, similar to the fatty-acid catabolism. *N*-Nitrosodibutylamine is converted to *N*-nitroso-*N*-butylcarboxy-propylamine (BCPN). *N*-Nitroso-*N*-methylalkylamines with an even-number C chain (C8–C12) are converted first to the corresponding acid and further activated to *N*-nitroso-*N*-methylcarboxypropylamine (MCPN) via β-oxidation.

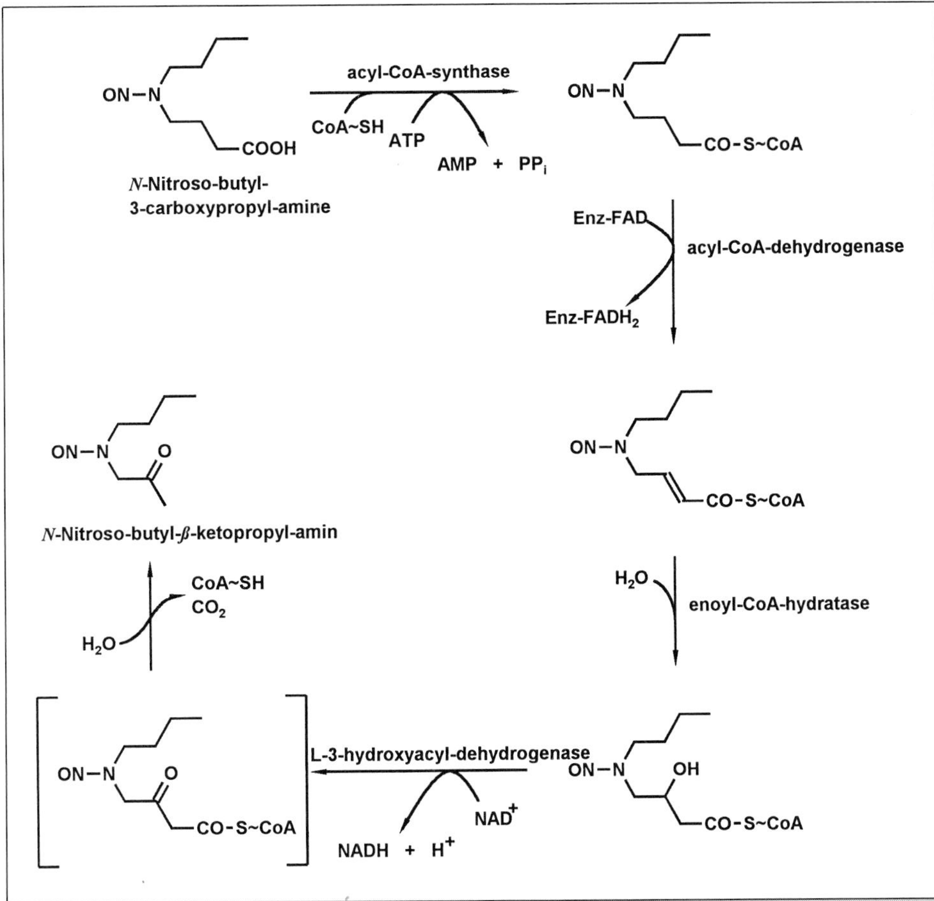

FIGURE 10 Biotransformation of ω-carboxypropyl metabolites via enzymes of the fatty-acid catabolism in mitochondria. The polar *N*-nitroso-*N*-butyl-3-carboxylpropylamine (BCPN) is converted via decarboxylation and β-oxidation to the lipophilic *N*-nitroso-*N*-butyl-oxopropylamine (BOPN), which can be further activated by cytochrome P450.

result of ω-hydroxylation *N*-nitrosobutyl-4-hydroxybutylamine is formed, which is further oxidized rapidly to *N*-nitroso-*N*-butyl-(3-carboxypropyl-)amine (BCPN) (Fig. 9) by alcohol dehydrogenase (ADH) and aldehyde dehydrogenase (AIDH). *N*-Nitroso-*N*-butyl-(3-carboxypropyl-)amine is excreted at high concentrations in the urine. *N*-Nitroso-*N*-butyl-4-hydroxybutylamine and *N*-nitroso-*N*-butyl-(3-carboxypropyl-)amine are potent carcinogens for the urinary bladder. *N*-Nitroso-*N*-butyl-(3-carboxypropyl-)amine is assumed to be the key metabolite for the bladder carcinogenicity of *N*-nitrosodibutylamine. It induces bladder tumors after direct instillation into the bladder. Detailed investigations have shown that nitrosamines causing carcinogenic effects in the bladder in general give rise to a 3-carboxypropyl intermediate. Such an intermediate, is also for instance, formed by sequential metabolic ω-oxidation and chain-shortening β-oxidation of *N*-nitroso-*N*-methylalkyl-nitrosamines with even-number carbon chains from C12 to C18.

N-Nitroso-*N*-alkyl-3-carboxypropylamines can further be biotransformed by mitochondrial β-oxidation and decarboxylation to generate the corresponding β-ketopropyl compounds. In contrast to the highly water-soluble transport-metabolites (*N*-nitroso-*N*-alkyl-3-carboxypropylamines) the latter are highly lipophilic and represent good substrates for cytochrome P450 (Fig. 10). By cytochrome P450-mediated α-C-hydroxylation of *N*-nitroso-β-ketopropylalkylamines methylating agents are generated. (Fig. 11). The corresponding (butyl- and methyl-) adducts were detected in the bladder after the application of *N*-nitroso-*N*-butyl-4-hydroxybutylamine.

The key reaction relevant for bladder carcinogenicity, though, is the ω-oxidation. Blocking of this reaction, for example by the exchange of the terminal CH_3 groups of *N*-nitrosodibutylamine by CF_3 groups,

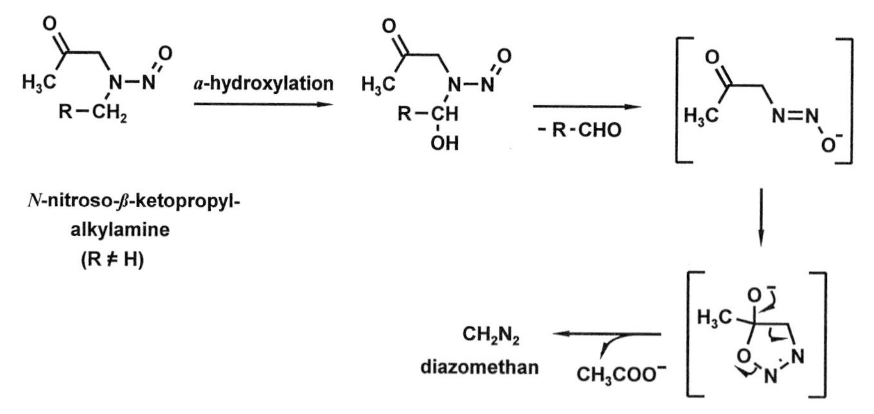

FIGURE 11 Mechanism of cytochrome P450-mediated generation of alkylating agents (diazomethan) from *N*-nitroso-*N*-alkyl-*β*-ketopropylamine.

which are resistant to oxidative metabolism, prevents the induction of bladder tumors.

ACUTE AND CHRONIC TOXICITY

The acute toxicity of *N*-nitroso compounds is highly variable and does not correlate with their carcinogenic potency. The most toxic nitrosamine, *N*-nitroso-*N*-methylbenzylamine, has an acute LD_{50} of 0.12 nmol (18 ng) per kg body wt in the rat. On the other hand, the potent liver carcinogen *N*-nitrosodiethanolamine, with an LD_{50} value of > 7500 mg/kg body wt, does not show acute toxicity.

The spectrum of organ toxicity displayed by various nitrosamines is quite similar, with few exceptions. Lethal doses of dialkylnitrosamines induce a slowly progressing kachexia, often accompanied by an icterus. Depending on the dose, death usually is observed between day 3 and day 7 after administration. The section normally shows strong damage to the liver parenchyma with centrilobular necroses and fatty degeneration, as well as hemorrhagic lung edema. After accidental intoxication or poisoning, a comparable pattern of lesions was observed in humans. For nitrosamides, damage of rapidly proliferating tissues like the bone marrow and the lymphatic tissue are characteristic. After few days, a strong lymphopenia occurs and the animals die. The section shows massive hemorrhages and ulcerations in the gastrointestinal tract. A marked delayed bone marrow toxicity caused by damage of the stem cell compartment is also the most critical and dose-limiting side effect of clinically applied *N*-nitrosureas in cancer therapy.

In principle, the chronic toxicity of nitrosamines displays intoxication patterns similar to those for acute toxicity. Liver damage and liver failure are the prevailing causes of death in most cases. The total dosage causing death, however, is generally much higher than the acute LD_{50} values. In many cases, tumors develop after chronic application before other lethal effects are seen.

REPRODUCTIVE TOXICOLOGY

Certain *N*-nitrosoureas are not only highly potent transplacental carcinogens but also teratogens. A single dose of *N*-ethylnitrosourea applied on day 15 postcoitum, thus, induced deformations of the paws in the offspring. Practically all animals of the F_1 generation died later with neurogenic tumors, even at a dosage as low as 5 mg/kg (2% of the LD_{50}), which did not induce tumors in the dams. Obviously, the fetus is much more sensitive toward these carcinogens than adult animals.

Nitrosamines, such as *N*-nitrosodiethylamine and *N*-nitrosodimethylamine, are not considered to pose a teratogenic risk but are reported as acting as transplacental carcinogens when given to pregnant animals at high doses just before birth. The application of 50–200 mg/kg body wt *N*-nitrosodiethylamine to pregnant mice and hamsters leads to an increased rate of stillbirths. Moreover, animals of the F_1 generation displayed an increased rate of lung adenomas and kidney tumors.

MUTAGENICITY

Various nitrosamines are mutagenic in bacteria, yeast, and mammalian cells. When activated either with liver S9 mix or microsomes, *N*-nitrosodimethylamine and *N*-nitrosodiethylamine show a moderate mutagenicity in bacterial assays using *Salmonella typhimurium* (TA 100 and TA 1530), *Escherischia coli*, and yeast cells (*Saccharomyces cerevisiae*). They also induce recessive lethal mutations in the fruit fly *Drosophila melanogaster*.

Chromosomal aberrations and sister chromatide exchanges (SCE) were detectable in a range of 8–135 mM in Chinese hamster ovarian cells (CHO). DNA damage in human fibroblasts was detectable after treatment with *N*-nitrosodimethylamine by measurement of [^{3}H]thymidin incorporation into the DNA (i.e., unscheduled DNA synthesis, UDS). Epithelial rat liver cells in culture are transformed by *N*-nitrosodimethylamine. Such transformed cells are capable of inducing local tumors in neonatal rats at the injection site when applied subcutaneously.

CARCINOGENICITY

The first report by Magee and Barnes (1956) of *N*-nitrosodimethylamine being a liver carcinogen in rats induced intensive research activities. More than 300 compounds have been tested for carcinogenicity, among them more than 200 *N*-nitrosodialkylamines. About 90% of all substances tested were carcinogenic and no species has been found to be resistant. Because pharmacokinetics and biotransformation in the animal species studied appear to be very similar to those in humans, it can be assumed that these compounds also can induce malignant tumors in humans. Moreover, after acute intoxication with *N*-nitrosodimethylamine, the same DNA-adducts were found in human tissue as in laboratory animals.

Epidemiological data corroborate the indications of the carcenogenic activity of nitrosamines in humans. Studies of the use of a specific type of chewing tobacco ("snuff-dipping") in the southern United States showed that the frequency of snuff dipping was correlated to an increased incidence of oral cavity cancer. The only carcinogens this tobacco product contains in relevant amounts are *N*-nitrosonornicotine (up to 64 ppm) and 4-(methylnitrosamino)-1-(3-pyridyl)-1-butanone (up to 3.4 ppm).

Another unique characteristic of this class of substances is the striking organ specificity regarding tumor induction, which made nitrosamines attractive as model compounds for cancer research. Typical target sites for tumors induced by these compounds in animal studies are the brain and nervous system, oral cavity, esophagus, stomach, gastrointestinal tract, liver, kidney, urinary bladder, pancreas, hematopoetic system, heart, and skin. The organ specificity is influenced by various factors, such as animal species, mode of application, dose, and length of exposure. The most important factor, however, is the chemical structure of the nitrosamine itself. For symmetrically substituted nitrosamines (both alkyl chains are identical) the main target organ is the liver. In general, the route of administration is of minor importance with regard to the target organ (Table 1).

In contrast, unsymmetrical nitrosamines induce preferentially esophageal tumors in the rat, also after parenteral administration. Unlike these groups, cyclic nitrosamines do not show such uniform organ specificity but induce instead a broad spectrum of tumors in different tissues. Individually, however, each compound does shows charateristic organotropism. *N*-Nitroso amino acids, such as *N*-nitrosoprolin and *N*-nitrosohydroxyprolin, are considered not to be carcinogenic. They are excreted unmodified and quantitatively in the urine.

Nitrosamides induce tumors at the administration site and systemically. Epidermal or subcutaneous application (i.e., skin and subcutaneous tissue) almost invariably leads to local tumor formation.

Alkylnitrosoureas often induce tumors in the forestomach after oral application, whereas after i.v. application, leukemias and neurogenic tumors are induced, especially in the central nervous system. *N*-Nitroso-*N*-methyl-*N*′-nitroguanidine (MNNG) is used as a standard carcinogen for the induction of stomach and gut tumors in various animal species.

DOSAGE IN LONG-TERM EXPOSURE

The doses of *N*-nitroso compounds needed to induce tumors are low to very low. At 2 μg/kg body wt/day of *N*-nitrosodimethylamine, hyperplastic nodules are induced in the livers of male rats. The lowest tumoregenic total dose has been determined to be 7.2 mg/kg body wt.

In an extensive study with more than 5000 rodents, *N*-nitrosodiethylamine was found to be a stronger carcinogen than *N*-nitrosodimethylamine after oral administration (about factor 3). An oral dose of 1 μg/kg body wt/day of *N*-nitrosodiethylamine increased the probability of a tumor as cause of death by 0.06% in male and by 0.1% in female Colworth rats. At the same dosage, the tumor incidence is increased with earlier onset of administration. In inhalation experiments with a total dose as low as 2 mg/kg body wt of *N*-nitrosodimethylamine, mucoepidermal tumors in the nasal cavity were induced in more than a third of the treated rats (36%). Total doses of the tobacco-specific nitrosamine 4-(methylnitrosamino)-1-(3-pyridyl)-1-butanone, which in long-term studies induces lung tumors in rats, are in a similar range. These data clearly demonstrate that nitrosamines without doubt belong to the most potent carcinogenic substances humans can be exposed to.

Bibliography

Bartsch, H., O'Neill, I. K., and Schulte-Hermann, R. (eds.) (1987). "The Relevance of N-nitroso Compounds to Human Cancer: Exposure and Mechanisms." IARC Scientific Publications No. 84. International Agency for Research on Cancer, Lyon, France.

Eisenbrand, G., Bozler, G., and v. Nicolai, H. (eds.) (1990)."The Significance of N-Nitrosation of Drugs" Gustav Fischer Verlag, Stuttgart.

Eisenbrand, G., Fuchs, A., and Koehl, W. (1996). N-nitroso compounds in cosmetics and cutting fluids. *Eur. J. Cancer Prev.* **5**(Suppl. 1), 41–46.

Gangolli, S. D. *et. al.* (1994). Nitritate, nitrite and N-nitroso compounds. *Eur. J. Pharmacol.* **292,** 1–38.

Hill, M. J. (ed.) (1988). "Nitrosamines: Toxicology and Microbiology." VCH Verlagsgesellschaft, Weinheim.

Hotchkiss, J. H. (1989). Preformed N-nitroso compounds in foods and beverages. *Cancer Surv.* **8,** 295–321.

Lijinsky, W. (1992). "Chemistry and Biology of N-Nitroso Compounds." Cambridge University Press, Cambridge, UK.

Loeppky, R. N., and Michejda, C. J. (1994). "Nitrosamines and Related N-Nitroso Compounds: Chemistry and Biochemistry." ACS Symposium Series 553. ACS, Washington, DC.

Magee, P. N., and Barnes, J. M. (1956). The production of malignant hepatic tumours in the rat by feeding dimethylnitrosamine. *Brit. J. Cancer* **10,** 114.

National Academy of Sciences (1981). "The Health Effects of Nitrate, Nitrite and N-Nitroso Compounds." National Academic Press, Washington, DC.

C H A P T E R

32

Metals

SIEGFRIED G. SCHÄFER*, R. L. F. DAWES†, BERND ELSENHANS‡, WOLFGANG FORTH‡, KLAUS SCHÜMANN‡

*Solvay Pharmaceuticals, Hannover, Germany, and Department of Toxicology, University of Hamburg, Hamburg, Germany

†Solvay Pharmaceuticals, Weesp, The Netherlands

‡Walter Straub Institute of Pharmacology and Toxicology, Ludwig Maximilians University, Munich, Germany

INTRODUCTION

About 80% of the elements described in the periodic system are metals or metalloids. Some of them are biologically essential, for example, sodium, potassium, calcium, iron, cobalt, zinc, and copper. Others are known toxic elements, such as cadmium, arsenic, lead, mercury, and thallium. The importance of metal toxicity has changed over the centuries. Between the 14th and 18th centuries lead acetate was used to sweeten wine (sopa), while arsenic played a major role in homocides until specific analytical methods permitted the diagnosis of such poisonings. Thallium changed its role from a therapeutic to a toxic agent during the course of the 19th century. It was discovered in 1861 by Sir William Crookes and was at first used to treat nightsweats in tubercular patients. Later thallium was used for depilation in children instead of X-ray treatments to support therapy of infectious diseases of the scalp. The use in cosmetics for depilation was stopped during the 1930s when some casualities were observed. Organotin compounds were used in France to treat furuncles and the arsenic-containing drug Salvarsan® was the first chemotherapeutic. Other heavy metals, such as cadmium (causing Itai-Itai disease), mercury (causing Minamata disease), and lead (causing deficits of intellectual development), are well-known environmental and occupational hazards. Their growing industrial use and the resulting occupational exposure has increased the public and scientific interest in these metals.

For metal toxicity in animals and humans, the behavior of metals in biological fluids is more important than their pure physicochemical properties (Table 1). Metals form ionic (e.g., NaCl, $HgCl_2$) or organic (e.g., $CH_3{-}Hg{-}CH_3$; $(CH_3)_4Pb$) bonds. Organic metal compounds, such as, alkylated mercury, and organic germanium, tin, and lead, are at least of the same toxicological relevance as the numerous inorganic metal compounds. The future will show to what extent the substitutes for tetraethyl lead in gasoline, such as cyclopentadienyl-mangan-tricarbonyl $((C_X{}^5{-}C_2H_5)Mn(CO)_3)$, have toxicological potentials.

PRINCIPLES OF METAL KINETICS

Metals cannot be destroyed metabolically. However, toxic metals may bind to organic molecules or compete with physiological metals, which may result in a metal-specific toxic effect, for example, the lead effect on δ-aminolevulinic acid. Toxic metals have specific target organs (e.g., cadmium on the kidneys). Because of such changes, a metal can be detoxified or become more toxic. The methylation of mercury by microorganisms in contaminated sediments is a case in point. A threshold value in metals that provokes toxic effects is common.

Principles of Therapy of Metal Intoxication

Removal of toxic metal ions from the organism by chelation is the principal therapeutic action in metal intoxication because metals cannot be catabolized, in contrast to organic compounds. Chelating agents decrease the body burden of toxic metals by the formation of nontoxic complexes, which are excreted rapidly via urine or feces. Metal chelation is supposed to work in a simple way. The chelating agent (H—C) is administered orally or intravenously to a patient contaminated by a toxic dose of a known heavy metal (M—X).

$$H{-}C + M{-}X \longrightarrow C{-}M + H^{+} + X^{-}$$

The chelated metal (C—M) is excreted and then the body burden is reduced continuously. For some metals, effective chelating agents for human use are available (Table 2). The therapeutic use of chelating agents in the treatment of metal intoxication, however, is not without risks because of the adverse effects of the chelating agents, as well as the potential redistribution of metal ions to sensitive organs. The chelation of metal ions is highly sensitive to changes in pH (e.g., in plasma and urine). For example, thallous ions are redistributed from the plasma compartment to the central nervous system (CNS) if dithiocarb is used as chelating agent. Chelation of cadmium or mercury can be reduced substantially in acidic urine, resulting in an increased concentration of free metal ions, which may lead to impaired kidney function. In addition, chelating agents may increase excretion of essential metals, such as zinc, copper, and electrolytes. Therefore, chelating agents should be used intermittently to reduce treatment-attributed side effects.

TABLE 1 Comparison of Physicochemical Properties and Behavior of Metals in Biological Fluids

Physicochemical properties	Properties in biological fluids
Metallic sheen resulting from a high reflectivity	Formation of cations by release of one or more electrons; this reaction is observed in biological fluids (pH ~ 7.0) in the presence of electrolytes.
Good thermic conductance	
Good electrical conductance	
Stability and plasticity	

TABLE 2 Examples of Chelating Agents Used Therapeutically in Intoxications by Toxic Metals or after Contamination with Radioactive Actinides

Metal	Chelating agent[a]	Therapeutically used
Aluminum	Deferoxamine	Yes
Arsenic	BAL, DMSA, DMPS	Yes
Cadmium	BAL, DDTC	Not fully evaluated
Copper	D-Penicillamine, TRIEN	Yes
Lead	DMSA, EDTA (after low exposure)	Yes
Mercury	DMSA, DMPS	Yes
Nickel ($Ni(CO)_4$)	DDTC	Yes
Plutonium, Americum	DTPA	Yes
Thallium	Prussian Blue	Yes

[a]Abbreviations used: BAL, British Anti-Lewisite (2,3-dimercapto-1-propanol); DDTC, Na-diethyldithiocarbamate; DMPS, Na-2,3-dimercaptopropane-1-sulfonate; DMSA, meso-2,3-dimercaptosuccinate; DTPA, diethylentriaminepentaacetic acid; Prussian Blue, ferro(II)hexacyanoferrate.

ALUMINUM

Aluminum in its compounds makes up 8.1% of the mass of Earth's crust, thus representing the third most abundant element and the most abundant metal. The metal was first isolated in 1827 by Woehler by reduction of aluminum chloride with metallic potassium. The discovery of a feasible mass production by electrode deposition soon made the metal available for industrial applications. Owing to its physicochemical properties, the metal has multiple uses in aircraft, packaging, and other industries.

Chemical Properties, Occurrence, and Use

Aluminum (Al, atomic weight 27.0) belongs to the light metals. Its density is about one-third that of iron. Essentially, only inorganic compounds are of toxicological interest; all of these contain aluminum as Al^{3+} ion. The oxide Al_2O_3, depending on the degree of hydratization, is of limited solubility, particularly in water. Aluminum salts are soluble in acids, in strong alkali hydroxide solutions, and in water, although they hydrolize at neutral pH, forming less soluble hydroxides. More theoretically oriented studies employing pure aqueous systems lead to the assumption that soluble aluminum in the physiological range (pH 6 to 8) is mainly present in form of $Al(OH)_2^{1+}$, dissolved $Al(OH)_3$, and $Al(OH)_4^{1-}$, although the data about the quantitative composition, dependent on pH and concentration, of such mixtures vary a lot.

The metal is produced from bauxite or kaolin (also called "china clay"), which are essentially iron oxide-containing mixtures of various forms of aluminum oxides and hydroxides. Potash alum (*"Terra aluminis"*) has been known since ancient times (since approximately 500 A.C.). The most important deposits are found in the United States, G.U.S. Canada, Japan, and Norway.

Cooking food in aluminum dishes and storing it in aluminum foil are harmless, the increase in the aluminum content of human nutrition being estimated as being in the range of 5–30 mg/kg of dry matter. Exceptions are possible when particularly acidic food items (e.g., fruit juice) are stored in aluminum dishes. Vegetables typically contain between 100 and 120 mg Al/kg (ww). In root vegetables, such as comfrey and carrots, aluminum levels are even higher and reach 200–400 mg/kg (ww). Data about the exposure to aluminum via nutrition vary extensively, as they are influenced by different food habits. A range from 2 to 160 mg Al/day is generally accepted; an average supply of about 5 to 20 mg Al/day appears to be likely.

Gels of aluminum hydroxide play an important role in medicine for the therapeutic treatment of gastritis (i.e., antacids); they are also used as phosphate binders for dialysis fluids. Administration is normally not under medical supervision. Previous intake was between 6 and 8 g/day; more recent maximum daily doses amount to 3–4 g.

Al^{3+} ions are released from polymeric $Al(OH)_3$ gels. Aluminum ions are formed in the stomach by reaction with hydrochloric acid and absorbed in the gastrointestinal tract. Based on this reaction, antacids are phosphate binders that were used previously to reduce the frequency of dialysis in renal-insufficiency patients.

Neutralization

$$Al(OH)_3 + 3\,HCl \longrightarrow AlCl_3 + 3\,H_2O \longrightarrow Al(OH)Cl_2 + HCl + 2\,H_2O$$

Phosphate binding

$$Na_2HPO_4 + NaH_2PO_4 + 2\,AlCl_3 \longrightarrow 2\,AlPO_4 + 3\,NaCl + 3\,HCl$$

For this indication, the use of phosphate-binding calcium carbonate is steadily increasing, as the risk of dialysis encephalopathy as a result of an excessive intake of aluminum can thus be reduced.

Aluminum has an important role in self-medication (e.g., as acetate of aluminum). Alum ($KAl(SO_4)_2$) or basic aluminum chloride ($Al(OH)_2Cl$) is used as a local deodorant and in hyperhydrosis; these compounds possess astringent and, at higher concentrations, protein-denaturating properties.

Absorption, Distribution, and Excretion

The dermal uptake of aluminum is negligible. Uptake by inhalation is only of interest in occupational medicine. Larger uptakes of aluminum, particularly of Al_2O_3 dust, only occur in work places. Increased aluminum concentrations have been detected in the urine of industrially exposed persons, but because they were not appropriate for determining uptake and excretion rates, no data are available from pulmonary absorption for kinetic evaluations. Investigations of the toxicokinetics of aluminum are generally hampered by the lack of an appropriate radioactive isotope.

The gastrointestinal absorption of Al^{3+} ions follows the kinetics of other metal ions. The absorption rate is not determined exactly. Data about dietary exposure to aluminum differ greatly, as they are influenced by different food habits. A range of 2 to 160 mg Al/day is generally accepted; an average supply of about 5 to 20 mg Al/day seems to be likely. Aluminum is absorbed by the gastrointestinal tract only in small amounts. If 2 to 40 mgAl/day is consumed with food, 20 to 30 μg Al is excreted with urine, which leads to an estimated absorption rate of 0.05–3.0%; in the case of aluminum-containing antacids, when larger quantities are consumed (several grams) the absorption rate can drop to about 0.01%. When 5 to 125 mg Al/day is consumed, healthy male test subjects show a negative or an even aluminum balance, with no accumulation of aluminum in the organism. Only when amounts of 1 to 3 g Al/day are ingested over an extended period are positive balances observed, so that increasing retention is expected.

After gastrointestinal or inhalative uptake, aluminum is distributed via blood, where transferrin exhibits transport functions for Al^{3+} ions. In addition to transferrin, other plasma proteins can probably bind aluminum, but it is not yet clear whether aluminum species of low molecular weight can be found in the plasma only when the binding capacity of these proteins is saturated. Al^{3+} ions not associated with proteins are mainly bound to physiological ligands of low molecular weight; of these, citric acid seems to be the most important one. Recent investigations stating that

89% of Al^{3+} ions in plasma are bound to transferrin and 11% to citrate demonstrate that there are no free Al^{3+} ions but an ultrafiltrable fraction, which is directly available for renal excretion or uptake into the tissue.

Distribution occurs into the soft tissues and bone. Because aluminum forms insoluble phosphates, it is considered a "bone-seeking" element. In all studies of organ levels of nonexposed persons, the lung tissue consistently shows high aluminum levels (5–100 mg/kg dry matter), which is certainly due to the inhalation of hydrated aluminum oxides and silicates, which are frequent components of various soils. Bone and muscle also show comparably high levels of aluminum (>10 mg/kg). In the CNS, aluminum levels increase with age; hence, patients with renal insufficiency accumulate significantly more aluminum than healthy persons (approximately 2- to 100-fold; Table 3).

Absorbed aluminum is excreted via the kidneys, which play a predominant role in the elimination of Al^{3+} ions; in the absence of renal function, aluminum is not eliminated. Biliary excretion is probably negligible. The half-life of the major fraction of Al^{3+} in plasma is 4–12 hours. About one-third of the Al^{3+} quantity applied parenterally is excreted via the urine after approximately 2 h; others have found half-lives of about 8 h.

Healthy individuals readily eliminate rather high oral aluminum loads (1.0–3.8 g/day), whereby renal excretion of the normal 20 to 60 μg Al/day can increase up to values of 300 to 500 μg Al/day. In steady-state absorption tests with healthy persons, the amount of aluminum excreted with the urine increased from 39 to 129 μg Al/day if the chronic oral intake was increased up to 125 mg Al/day. As no positive aluminum balance was observed in this study, it can be assumed that an amount of about 130 μg Al/day absorbed chronically does not cause any side effects in persons with healthy kidneys. This applies also for higher exposures due to the intake of antacids. A risk may emerge, however, from a sustained ingestion of large doses in cases of renal insufficiency.

Aluminum Concentrations in the Plasma and Urine

Aluminum determinations in the plasma exhibit a remarkable tendency; between the years 1962 and 1982, the average plasma concentrations decreased from 800 μg Al/liter to <10 μg Al/liter, which is considered normal. This "normalization" was certainly due to an increasing awareness of the problems associated with aluminum analyses. The most widely used method of quantitative analysis available for the relevant concentration range, electrothermic atomic absorption spectrometry, is difficult and requires exceptional experience in sampling, processing, and measuring. As ubiquitous element, aluminum can very easily lead to contamination and, thus, its determination requires a level of extreme care in sampling that often cannot be fulfilled in the routine of a clinic. In general, a urinary excretion between 0.4 and 23 μg Al/g creatinine is considered normal. Based on a threshold limit value of 6 mg/m^3 in the work place, a renal aluminum excretion of 170 μg/liter urine is regarded as a maximum tolerable measure at the end of an 8-h shift.

Acute and Chronic Toxicity

The concentration of aluminum in the plasma is considered a primary parameter for toxicological evaluations. The actual normal value is up to 10 μg/liter. Values up to 60 μg/liter indicate an increased aluminum absorption, the reasons for which should be elucidated. A plasma concentration between 60 and 100 μg/liter is critical and should be controlled. Values higher than 200 μg/liter can result in CNS symptoms. It is generally accepted that the normal concentration of aluminum in plasma can be considerably exceeded without the typical clinical

TABLE 3 Aluminum Concentrations in Brain Tissue of Dialysis Patients[a]

	White and grey matter	White matter	Grey matter
Controls	1.3 ± 0.7 (6)	2.0 ± 0.6 (5)	2.2 ± 0.7 (5)
Hemodialysis patients without symptoms	7.6 ± 4.6 (6)	3.8 ± 1.8 (7)	6.5 ± 2.9 (7)
Hemodialysis patients with clinical symptoms of encephalopathy	8.9 ± 4.3 (12)	5.6 ± 1.9 (7)	25.0 ± 9.1 (6)

[a]Values in mg Al/kg dry matter; M ± SEM; (*n*) indicates number of determinations (according to Alfrey *et al.*, 1976).

symptoms of aluminum intoxication. There are findings of aluminum concentrations up to 180 μg/liter in dialysis patients without any sign of dementia and of concentrations higher than 170 μg/liter in patients with manifest dementia. Plasma concentrations of up to 190 μg Al/liter probably do not lead to pathological symptoms in storage organs. Thus, concentrations of 170 to 180 μg/liter would be critical, especially if aluminum exposure continues for an extended period (i.e., for weeks and months). In cases of occupational aluminum exposure in the work place, even over an extended period no neurotoxic symptoms occur when plasma levels do not exceed 150 μg Al/liter.

The systemic effects of aluminum are usually not found in persons with a normal renal function. The local effects of aluminum are seen in the lungs of workers in aluminum smelters and other aluminum-processing plants. Formerly, this lung fibrosis, also called Shaver's disease, was quite frequently seen in workers of industries where exposure to aluminum dust was common. Since bauxite also contains silicates, it is not clear to what extent aluminum contributes to this disease, as its symptoms largely resemble those of lung silicosis.

It is plausible that toxic effects of aluminum are observed mainly in renal insufficiency. Furthermore, infants, particularly preterm infants, are at risk because of their not yet fully developed renal functions. The three most important toxic effects of aluminum are anemia, osteopathy, and encephalopathy.

Anemia

Observations of the development of a microcytic hypochromic anemia in uremic patients who later developed an aluminum-derived osteomalacia and encephalopathy are considered to be due to a toxic effect of Al^{3+} ions on erythropoiesis. For physicians, anemia itself or its exacerbation normally represents the first indication of aluminum overload. It is remarkable that this anemia can occur in aluminum-loaded uremic patients in the presence of normal iron stores (i.e., normal or only slightly reduced serum ferritin levels) and does not react to iron supplementation, but is reversible by reducing the aluminum overload. The most common anemia in dialysis patients, however, is a normocytic and normochromic anemia, which can be treated with iron preparations. The findings show that a continuously high, chronic aluminum overload can affect the iron metabolism as well as the hemoglobin synthesis. The exact nature of this effect of aluminum is not clear, however. In cases of sustained and chronic intake of antacids, a reduced bioavailability of iron is suggested as being responsible.

Osteopathy

This disease was initially interpreted as a consequence of hyperparathyroidism caused by renal insufficiency. Under the influence of parathyroid hormone (parathormone, PTH) osteoclasts as well as osteoblasts are activated; on total balance, however, a deossification of the bone tissue predominates. Animal studies show that parenteral administration of aluminum may cause osteomalacia. Several methods clearly demonstrate the correlations between uremic osteomalacia and Al^{3+} deposits at the interface of osteoid and mineralized bone matrix. However, the underlying pathogenesis is still unclear. Histologically, the mineralization defects show an excessive reproduction of the osteoid. In dialysis patients with predominant osteomalacia, Al^{3+} ions can be detected at the mineralization front (i.e., at the border of the mineralized and nonmineralized matrices), which has led to the assumption that Al^{3+} ions, at least partially, impede mineralization directly. This interpretation, however, is controversial. The deposit of Al^{3+} ions at the interface of osteoid and mineralized bone matrix could as well be merely secondary, and the impairment of mineralization could actually have other causes.

Furthermore, the parathyroids, in the secretory granules in which Al^{3+} ions can accumulate, appears to be sensitive to Al^{3+} ions, as their presence impairs secretion of PTH. In addition, the secretion of PTH by the parathyroids after hypocalcemic stimuli is distinctly reduced in aluminum-loaded patients. In fact, these patients do not suffer from those with hyperparathyroidism but, on the contrary, from hypoparathyroidism and therefore a parathyroidectomy may worsen the osteopathic symptoms.

Dialysis Encephalopathy

The signs of dialysis encephalopathy are related to aluminum levels in brain tissue (Table 3). In the 1970s, progressive dementia was observed in dialysis patients. These symptoms have been positively correlated with the aluminum concentrations in the water in England, Chicago, and Denver by the end of that decade. In this respect, one must consider that the blood of dialysis patients is exchanged for 18,000–36,000 liters of dialysis fluid yearly. It appears to be fully established that the formerly high aluminum concentrations in dialysis fluids were responsible for the incidence of encephalopathy. With the application of electroosmosis, dialysis fluids are produced with drastically reduced aluminum concentrations, which, in general, amount to 10 μg/liter; European regulations require concentrations of less than 30 μg Al/liter.

The symptoms of progressive dialysis encephalopathy are listed in Table 4. In approximately 60% of the patients, convulsions were noticed, which are likely to have been triggered by Al^{3+} ions. In animal experiments, aluminum ions can produce Jackson epilepsy when administered to the cerebral cortex directly. In animal studies, electrophysiologically recordable disturbances can be expected when the aluminum concentration in brain tissue exceeds levels of 5 μg/g dry weight.

To lower the plasma aluminum concentrations in dialysis patients, aluminum can be removed with deferoxamine by means of peritoneal dialysis, a procedure successfully carried out to relieve aluminum-overload symptoms. Deferoxamine is also employed in mobilization tests for differential diagnosis of osteopathy in dialysis patients.

Aluminum and Alzheimer's Disease

Alzheimer's disease is considered to be a genetically determined disease, in the course of which amyloid beta protein (plaques) is formed, causing the degeneration of the affected cells. The appearance of detectable denaturated parts of cytoplasmatic fibers (tangles) is regarded as merely a consequential event. All investigations attempting to connect the disease with an excessive or chronic exposure to aluminum failed to produce conclusive results. In animal studies, amyloid beta protein plaques were not produced by exposure to aluminum nor were tangles found that might be considered characteristic of Alzheimer's disease. Furthermore, observations in humans exposed to excessive amounts of aluminum lack findings on amyloid beta protein plaques, although tangles have been observed.

TABLE 4 Frequency of Symptoms in 42 Patients with Progressive Dialysis Encephalopathy[a]

Symptom	*n*	Percent
Dementia	41	98
Speech disorder	40	95
Myoclonia	34	81
Convulsions	24	57
Psychotic symptoms	22	52

[a] According to Ledermann and Henry (1978).

ARSENIC

Inorganic arsenicals and their toxic effects have been well known since ancient times. In particular, minerals such as realgar (As_4S_4) and auripigment (As_2S_3) were used in ancient Greece and Rome as depilatories and cosmetics. Aristotle was aware of the toxic effects of realgar, which are due to its transformation into auripigment and arsenic trioxide (As_2O_3) by exposure to the weather. In the Middle Ages and Renaissance, arsenicals, essentially arsenic trioxide, were the preferred murder poisons in France and Italy. The discovery of a sensitive detection test for arsenic by Marsh (in 1836) certainly reduced the attraction of that use. In biological systems (e.g., bacteria, mammals), inorganic arsenicals can be methylated, which is considered to represent detoxification. Therefore, metabolism of inorganic arsenic always has to be considered in humans.

Chemical Properties, Occurrence, and Use

Arsenic (As, atomic weight, 74.92) is a metalloid occurring in various oxidation states (−3, 0, +3, and +5). In air it burns, forming arsenic trioxide, the most important arsenic compound; this is also formed when arsenic-containing ores are roasted or arsenic-containing coal is burned. It is poorly soluble in pure water but readily dissolved in alkaline solutions, forming arsenites. Oxidation forms arsenates, the alkali salts of which are also readily soluble. In addition to naturally occurring methylated arsenic compounds, other organic arsenicals can be synthezised preferentially from arsenic trichloride. Phenyl arsenic compounds and derivatives are characterized by a rather stable As–C bond. Owing to its special toxicity, arsine (AsH_3) is of particular significance. This extremely toxic gas can be formed from arsenides or by the reduction of inorganic arsenicals under acidic conditions.

Elemental arsenic is rarely found in nature. Inorganic arsenic mainly occurs in sulfidic copper-, zinc- or lead-containing ores, from which it is obtained as a by-product during mining, roasting, and melting. Owing to biological methylation, organic arsenicals are widespread and found in many organisms. Monomethylarsonic and dimethylarsinic acid are the the main organic arsenic compunds found in most mammals. Various methylarsines are produced by microbial reduction and methylation. Fish and other sea organisms are rich in methylated arsenic compounds, such as arsenobetaine and arsenocholine.

Metallic or elemental arsenic plays a substantial role as a component of some special lead and copper

TABLE 5 Arsenic (As_2O_3) Consumption per Year in 1979[a]

	United States		Federal Republic of Germany	
	t/year	Percentage	*t*/year	Percentage
Agriculture and forestry	13,000	70	0	0
Industrial chemicals	4000	20	290	37
Glass industry	960	5	300	38
Alloys and electronics	600	3	171	22
Others (pharmaceuticals, catalysts, feed additives)	360	2	30	4
Total	19,420		791	

[a]From Hanusch *et al.* (1988).

alloys. Some important uses of arsenicals are in glass industries and for purifying electrolyte solutions in the electrolytic production of zinc (Table 5). Zinc, chromium, and copper arsenates are used as wood preservatives, which can cause some problems when such materials are burned. In agriculture and forestry, inorganic and organic arsenicals are used as pesticides and herbicides; however, this application is declining worldwide and in some countries this use is becoming more and more restricted. Arsanilic acid is used as feed additive, but the use of other arsenicals in animal breeding and veterinary medicine is negligible. High-purity arsenic, in the form of gallium or indium arsenide, is increasingly used in the electronics industry.

Absorption, Distribution, Metabolism, and Excretion

Inhalative Uptake

Inhalative uptake of inorganic arsenic is mainly from the work-place environment or tobacco smoking. In comparably unpolluted areas, the arsenic concentration in air is around 1 ng/m^3 or less. In more urbanized regions without any particular arsenic pollution, concentrations in air range between 1 and 20 ng/m^3. In heavily urbanized areas with intensive coal burning, concentrations can rise to between 0.07 and 0.5 μg/m^3. Much higher concentrations can be found in industrialized regions where, especially in the vicinity of copper- and lead-processing plants, concentrations are up to 0.5–5 μg/m^3. Arsenic in tobacco smoke is mainly due to the use of arsenic-containing pesticides.

Quantitative data on the absorption rate after inhalative uptake of arsenic are rare. In studies employing cancer patients in the final stage, arsenic retention after inhalative uptake via tobacco smoke was about 20% after 4 days, as determined using a radioactive arsenic isotope. In general, a substantial absorption of arsenic can be assumed, as there was a good correlation between the arsenic concentration in the air and the urinary excretion of arsenic in workers at a copper smelter (Fig. 1). There are no quantitative data on the extent and rate of arsenic absorption after inhalative uptake of organic arsenicals.

Intestinal Absorption

For all inorganic arsenicals that are soluble in water, essentially the arsenites and arsenates of alkali metals, absorption after oral uptake is high. Studies of patients who received a dose of 9.5 mg arsenic as a solution of arsenite (Fowler's solution) showed a rather small fecal excretion of arsenic, which amounted to about 3.5% after a period of 10 days, demonstrating a high oral absorption. Similar results were obtained from administering arsenate orally. The oral uptake of relatively insoluble compounds, such as the trisulfide (As_2S_3) or triselenide (As_2Se_3), does not increase the urinary excretion of arsenic. These compounds have little toxicity. As the decomposition or reduction can lead to toxic reaction products (As_2O_3 or AsH_3), the handling of these compounds always requires some precautions; this also applies to indium and gallium arsenide.

Intestinal absorption of organic arsenicals is difficult to assess, as there are only limited data available. A few studies have demonstrated that ingested amounts of "natural" arsenic ingested with fish (a single dose of 0.5–2.2 mg As/person) are rapidly exreted with the urine (83% of the dose within 2 days). In another study, after oral administration of a single dose of arsanilic acid (1.3–3.0 mg As/person), 74% of the dose was excreted with the feces within 6

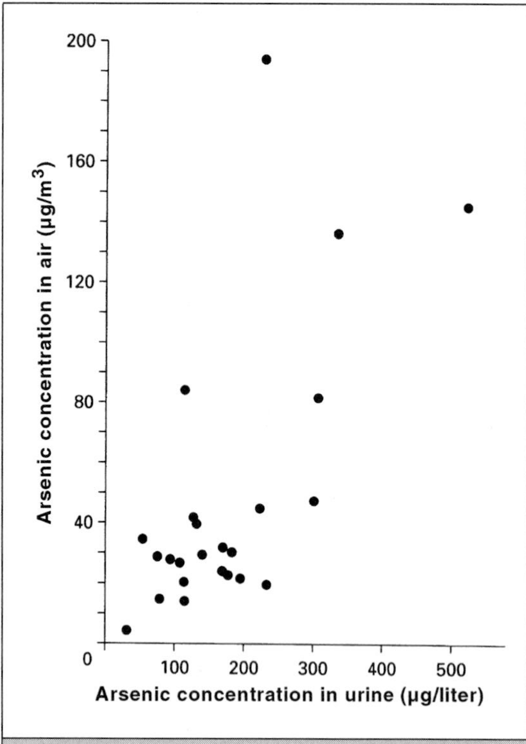

FIGURE 1 Correlation between concentration of arsenic in urine of workers of a smelter and air in the work place. (Adapted from Pinto *et al.*, 1977.)

days. This demonstrates that "natural" organic arsenicals in food, particularly in fish, are absorbed quite well, while phenyl arsenic compounds show lower absorption rates.

Dermal Absorption

There have been no investigations of dermal absorption of arsenicals in humans. However, systemic intoxication was observed in workers who accidentally came into contact with arsenic acid and arsenic trichloride. The signs of systemic intoxication were also seen after treatments with arsenic-containing ointments. These findings certainly indicate that dermal absorption of arsenic is possible. Data on the dermal uptake rates of organic arsenicals are not available.

Distribution

Arsenic from inhaled and ingested inorganic arsenicals initially appears in the blood. Animal studies demonstrate that arsenic concentrations in the blood decline rather quickly after single doses of arsenites and arsenates. In mice, guinea pigs, rabbits, and primates, less than 1% of a single dose is found after 1–2 days. An exception is the rat; in this species arsenic is efficiently taken up by the erythrocytes and exhibits a half-life of about 70 days.

The elimination of arsenic from blood is rapid after intravenous administration; this is also the case in humans. Elimination is best described using a model employing three phases. The half-life of the first phase is quite short (< 1 h) (i.e., the main fraction of the iv-administered dose is eliminated quickly), after 24 h, less than 0.1% of the dose per liter was found. The second phase has a half-life of 30 h. The last phase shows a half-life of approximately 200 h and is responsible for the elimination of less than 0.02% of the dose.

In humans as well as in most mammals, radioactively labeled arsenite is rapidly distributed all over the body. Within the initial phase, most of the arsenic is taken up by liver and kidneys. In addition, the spleen, lungs, and small intestine exhibit high arsenic tissue concentrations, as is known from animal studies. The accumulation of arsenic in the small intestine was also observed after intravenous administration, which indicates biliary excretion of arsenic, a pathway experimentally established in animals. Since little arsenic is excreted with the feces, reabsorption by the small intestines can be assumed. Whether such an enterohepatic circulation operates in humans, too, is not proven but is very likely. The elimination of arsenic is rather rapid from the these organs. However, subsequently, a more persistent accumulation can be observed in the skin, hair, epididymis, thyroid gland, lens, and skeleton (i.e., in the organs and tissues exhibiting the highest arsenic levels after chronic exposure and from which arsenic is rather slowly eliminated). Animal studies reveal a similar distribution after arsenite and arsenate administration, although slightly higher tissue levels in kidneys and bone were found after administration of arsenite.

No human data are available for the distribution of organic arsenicals. The results of animal studies suggest a higher hepatic and renal retention of monophenylic arsenicals than of methylated compounds, which are readily excreted with the urine. Retention and distribution appear to depend on the substitution at the phenyl group and the oxidation state of arsenic; thus, the retention of phenylarsonic acid (As-V) is lower than that of phenylarsenic oxide (As-III). Systematic investigations on that subject are lacking, however.

Metabolism and Excretion

Inorganic arsenic is predominantly excreted via the kidneys, whatever the route of uptake. Results obtained in male volunteers administered a single oral dose of radioactively labeled arsenate yielded a urinary excretion of 22% within the first 24 h. Total urinary excretion amounted to 58% after 5 days; unfortunately the fecal excretion was not determined in this study. Analyses of whole-body measurements describing total arsenic elimination fit into a three-compartment model. About 66% of a dose is eliminated with a half-life of 2.1, 30% with a half-life of 9.4, and the other 4% with a half-life of 38.4 days. When arsenic trioxide was administered daily (in solution, 0.8 mg As/day), the urinary arsenic excretion reached a steady state after 5 days, with a daily excretion of 70% of the dose.

The excretion of arsenic after the uptake of organic arsenicals has hardly been investigated. Arsenic from methylated arsenicals occurring in fish and other sea organisms is rapidly excreted with the urine. After the uptake of such "natural" organic arsenicals with a meal of fish (total dose, 0.5–5 mg As), between 50 and 70% was renally excreted within the first 24 h. Phenyl arsenic compounds are less well absorbed, so more arsenic is excreted with the feces than with the urine; for example, after the oral uptake of arsanilic acid, 64–74% of the dose was excreted fecally.

Dimethylarsinic acid represents the main arsenic metabolite in the urine after the administration of inorganic arsenic to humans and most other mammals. Analyses of the urinary metabolites of arsenic in four volunteers yielded 66% dimethylarsinic acid, 8% monoarsonic acid, 17% arsenate, and 8% arsenite. In another study administering radioactively labeled arsenate (mentioned previously), 51% of the urinary metabolites was found to be dimethylarsinic acid, 21% monomethylarsonic acid, and 27% inorganic arsenic.

These results demonstrate the effective methylating mechanism in humans, as in most other mammalian species. Prior to methylation, the reduction of arsenate to arsenite is required. Whether reduction is exclusively enzymatic or whether a chemical process is also involved is not clear. For the transfer of methyl groups, physiological compounds such as *S*-adenosylmethionine and related intermediate metabolites and precursors are of importance. Animal experiments indicate that high doses of inorganic arsenic impair the formation of methylated metabolites, which is consistent with the enzymatic nature of this process. Because the investigation of the quantitative distribution of the various metabolites in human organs is hardly possible and in animals is extremely difficult, corresponding findings are based on analyses of the blood and urine. How far these metabolite patterns in the blood and urine are representative of the patterns in tissue and organs is not known yet. Compared to most other laboratory animals, in humans monomethylarsonic acid represents a larger fraction of the urinary arsenic.

The human metabolism of organic arsenicals is less clear. Arsenobetaine is excreted unmetabolized. From animal studies, it can be concluded that dimethylarsinic acid orally administered is not further metabolized; the same applies to arsanilic acid. Substituted phenylarsonic acids are metabolically transfomed into more or less toxic organic arsenicals, but not into inorganic arsenic.

Mechanism of Toxicity

The toxic symptoms after acute or chronic exposure to inorganic arsenicals are quite similar, although dependent on the dose and availability of the substance. In general, the trivalent compounds are slightly more toxic than the pentavalent ones. In contrast, the toxicity of organic arsenical depends much more on the chemical form. While "natural" methylated arsenicals (e.g., monomethylarsonic acid, dimethylarsinic acid, arsenobetaine, and arsenocholine) are of low toxicity, some phenyl arsenic compounds are fairly toxic.

The toxic mechanisms of inorganic and most organic arsenicals, in particular of the derivatives of the trivalent form, are based on their reaction with SH groups in enzymes, intermediate metabolites, and other proteinaceous structures. From the results of animal studies, it can be assumed that the inhibition of glycogenolysis and gluconeogenesis substantially contributes to the lethal effect of inorganic arsenic. In addition, disturbances of electrolyte and water balance, probably by impairing membrane processes, play an important role.

Acute and Chronic Toxicity

Acute Toxicity

Inhalative Toxicity

Arsine (AsH_3) poisoning differs from intoxication by most inorganic or organic arsenicals. The lethal dose of arsine gas in air for humans is 250 mg/m^3 for a 30-min exposure (Table 6). After exposure to concentrations of 3–10 mg/m^3, toxic symptoms occur after a few hours. Depending on the dose inhaled, the initial symptoms usually occur between 2 and 24 h, with typical signs including paresthesia in the lower extremities, nausea, vomiting, abdominal pain, hematuria, and jaundice. The most important clinical symptom is severe hemolysis, which can lead to nephrosis and renal failure.

TABLE 6 Toxicity Data of Selected Arsenicals

Compound	Species		Toxicity parameter[a]
Arsenite	Mouse	LD_{50}	25–45 mg/kg, po
	Rat	LD_{50}	15–110 mg/kg, po
	Rabbit	LD_{Lo}	4 mg/kg, iv
	Human	LD_{Lo}	0.6–3 mg/kg, po
Arsenate	Mouse	LD_{50}	55 mg/kg, po
	Rat	LD_{50}	110 mg/kg, po
Arsenic trichloride	Cat	LC_{Lo}	100 mg/m^3, inhal.
Arsine	Human	LC_{Lo}	250 mg/m^3, inhal.
Monomethylarsonic acid	Mouse	LD_{50}	970 mg/kg, po
Dimethylarsinic acid	Mouse	LD_{50}	650 mg/kg, po
	Rat	LC_{50}	2100 mg/m^3, inhal.
Roxarsone	Rat	LD_{50}	23 mg/kg, po
	Mouse	LD_{50}	70 mg/kg, po
	Hund	LD_{50}	15 mg/kg, po
Phenoxarsinoxide	Rat	LD_{50}	7–12 mg/kg, po
Phenarsazinoxide	Rat	LD_{50}	25 mg/kg, po

[a]All data related to mg As; inhal, inhalative uptake.

There are no reports of deaths due to the inhalation of inorganic arsenicals (except for arsine), not even at concentrations of 1–100 mg As/m^3, concentrations that were occasionally reached at extremely exposed work places in former times. However, the systemic symptoms of poisoning are well documented; these are mainly respiratory, often gastrointestinal, and to a lesser degree hematological and dermal symptoms. Workers occupationally exposed to airborne inorganic arsenic (i.e., essentially As_2O_3 in the form of dust) often suffer from acute damage to the mucous membranes of the respiratory tract. The subsequent symptoms are irritation of the nasal mucosa, larynx, bronchia, conjunctiva, and occasionally skin. The inhalative uptake of arsenic can lead to a perforation of the nasal septum within 2 weeks. There are not sufficient data available to estimate the threshold concentration for respiratory effects; however, it is generally assumed that below concentrations of 0.1–1 mg As/m^3, acute effects are negligible or lacking (Table 7).

The inhalative and dermal toxicity of organic arsenic compounds is difficult to assess because of the lack of quantitative investigations. Since the LC_{50} values of dimethylarsinic acid range between 2000 and 4000 mg As/m^3 for laboratory animals, the inhalative toxicity in humans can be assumed to be low.

Oral Toxicity

Depending on the solubility, the oral LD_{50} of inorganic arsenic (i.e., of arsenic trioxide, arsenic pentoxide, and their corresponding acids and alkali salts) range between 20 and 300 mg As/kg body weight for rats and between 10 and 150 mg As/kg body weight for other laboratory animals. For humans, the minimal lethal dose of arsenic trioxide can be estimated to 70–180 mg (~1–3 mg As/kg body weight). The most critical signs of acute arsenic poisoning are gastrointestinal, cardiovascular, neurological, and hematological effects. Among the gastrointestinal symptoms, nausea, abdominal pain vomiting, and diarrhea are the dominant ones. For doses below 0.01 mg As/kg body weight/day, acute intoxications probably do not occur. The cardiovascular effects are mainly represented by myocardial depolarization and arrhythmia with typical changes in the electrocardiogram. The neurological effects of large doses of inorganic arsenic (1 mg As/kg body weight/day) often cause encephalopathy accompanied by headache, signs of irritation, hallucinations, and seizures leading into coma. An impairment of the peripheral nervous system mostly affecting sensory nerves is often seen in acute arsenic poisoning. In addition, in acute poisoning hematological alterations, such as anemia and leukopenia, can be seen. The acute toxicity of organic arsenicals cannot easily be assessed for humans because not enough data are available. Animal studies indicate that some phenyl arsenic compounds are of toxicological significance but that "natural" methyl derivatives is certainly of minor importance (Table 6).

Chronic Toxicity

Inhalative Toxicity

The primary symptoms of chronic toxicity after inhalative exposure to inorganic arsenicals are damage to the mucous membranes of the respiratory airway and respiratory distress. In addition, neurological

TABLE 7 Selection of Regulations and Guidelines for Arsenicals

Time-weighted average concentration (TWA; ACGIH, 1991; U.S.)	
As and soluble compounds	0.20 mg/m^3
Arsine	0.16 mg/m^3
Guideline value for drinking water WHO, 1984	0.05 mg As/liter
Germany, BMFFJG, 1990	0.01 mg As/liter
Tolerable daily intake (ADI, WHO)	2 μg inorg. As/kg/day

symptoms and skin damage and irritation can be observed. In some cases, an impairment of hepatic and cardiovascular functions were reported. Differences between trivalent and pentavalent arsenic are not significant.

Regarding the respiratory effects in humans, two types of symptoms can be distinguished—first, symptoms of the upper respiratory airway with perforation of the septum, rhinitis, pharyngitis, and laryngitis; and second, symptoms such as bronchitis and signs of pulmonary insufficiency, often due to emphysemic alterations. While the first mentioned symptoms were characteristic of the exposure to pure arsenicals, other symptoms were observed in workers concomitantly exposed to sulfur dioxide during the roasting and converting processes, so these symptoms may not exclusively due to arsenic exposure. The neurological effects are mainly characterized as functional and morphological disturbances of the peripheral nerves. Reversibility is likely but a lengthy regeneration is typical. Hyperkeratosis and melanosis are the main skin alterations described.

The inhalative toxicity of organic arsenicals cannot easily be assessed for humans. Investigations of workers exposed to arsanilic acid (average concentration, 0.13 mg As/m^3) for 1–2 years did not show an increased incidence for gastrointestinal, hematologic, or dermal alterations.

Oral Toxicity

Except for the effects in the respiratory tract, all the other symptoms are also observed in chronic intoxication after enteral exposure. Some of the signs, particularly the dermal ones, however, might be more pronounced. This suggests higher doses after enteral than after inhalative exposure. Based on epidemiologic studies, the highest dose not leading to any noticeable neurologic, hematologic, cardiovascular, or gastrointestinal alterations (the NOAEL, no observed adverse effect level) can be established at 0.001 mg As/kg/day; the corresponding value for dermal effects only is 0.0005 mg As/kg/day. Because, in these studies, dietary exposure to arsenic was not taken into account, a NOAEL of 0.001 mg As/kg/day for all effects represents a realistic estimate.

Limited information is available on the chronic toxicity of organic arsenicals in humans. Essentially most of this is based on the observations of side effects after the administration of therapeutic arsenicals; thus, encephalopathy was diagnosed in 1.5% of 1000 patients treated with tryparsamide ([4-[(2-amino-2-oxoethyl)-amino]-phenyl]-arsonic acid). Another side effect was atrophy of the optic nerve, which led to visual impairment in 3–4% of these patients. Rarer symptoms were dermatitis, and hepatic and hematologic disturbances. The chronic uptake of "natural" methylated arsenicals in the diet (e.g., marine fish contains approximately 0.1–5 mg As/kg wet wt, other species and shellfish 10-fold that and more) appears to be harmless for normal eating habits.

Special Toxicity

Reproduction Toxicity

There are observations of teratogenic effects in animals after the administration of inorganic arsenic, but the rather high doses needed do not suggest any relevance for humans. An epidemiologic study of the progenies of female workers in a copper smelter with high arsenic concentrations suggest an increased incidence of malformations and spontaneous abortions; the findings, however, are not conclusive.

Mutagenicity

Mutagenic effects of inorganic arsenicals were found in various systems, both *in vitro* and *in vivo*. However, not all of these results correspond to each other. Thus, positive mutagenic effects were found in DNA recombination tests with *Bacillus subtilis*, while negative results were obtained with the Ames test. Other investigations employing bacteria and isolated mammalian cells indicate that there is an effect of arsenicals on repair mechanisms. In this connection, an interaction of arsenic with the SH groups of DNA polymerases or other chromosomal proteins appears conceivable.

Chromosome aberrations in lymphocytes were more frequently found in patients exposed to arsenic than in the unexposed controls; the correlation between the number of chromosome aberrations found and the estimated exposure level was rather weak, however. Whether the inorganic arsenicals produce these aberrations directly or inhibit repair steps is not clear. The mutagenic effects of organic arsenicals in humans are not known. Methylated compounds are not found to be mutagenic in animal experiments.

Carcinogenicity

Epidemiologic studies point to the carcinogenic effects of inorganic arsenicals in humans. For this assessment, studies in which workers were exposed to relatively pure arsenicals and not to complex mixtures of various substances are of particular importance. But most data are derived from workers employed in

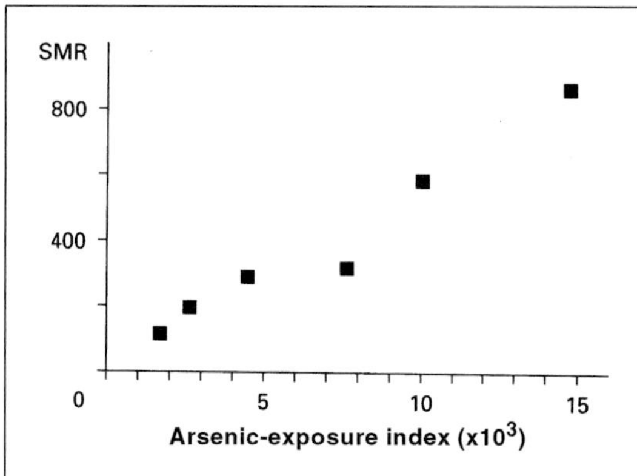

FIGURE 2 Standardized mortality rate (SMR) for deaths by cancer of the respiratory system and dependence on the arsenic exposure index of 527 retired male workers in a U.S. copper smelter. The normal standardized mortality rate is 100 and the arsenic exposure index for a normal urine concentration (50 μl As/liter) and 25 years of employment amounts to 1250 (adapted from Pinto *et al.*, 1977).

mining and smelters. Based on standardized mortality rates (SMR), a significantly increased incidence was observed for mortality from cancer of the trachea, bronchus, and lung in men, (Fig. 2). Differences in the carcinogenic potential of trivalent and pentavalent inorganic arsenicals could not be established. The oral uptake of arsenic with drinking water (i.e., most likely inorganic arsenic) is primarily related to cancer of the skin; how far this correlates with cancer of other organs is unknown. Inorganic arsenicals are therefore considered carcinogens for humans (group A, EPA; group 1, WHO). In the main, animal studies employing various species (e.g., rat, mouse, hamster, and dog) did not confirm a carcinogenic effect for arsenite or arsenate, however. Therefore, it is suggested that inorganic arsenic represents a progressor but not an initiator in carcinogenesis. At present, no findings indicate a carcinogenic potential for organic arsenicals.

Therapeutic Measures

Urinary arsenic concentrations are good indicators for the evaluation of acute arsenic poisoning. Levels above 200 μg/liter indicate severe exposure. In addition to conventional measures, such as gastric lavage, the use of cathartics, and the instillation of activated charcoal, chelation therapy should be administered. BAL (British Anti-Lewisite, Dimercaprol) is one of the agents used for this purpose. BAL is dissolved in oil and administered intramuscularly and repeatedly in single doses of 3 mg/kg until the symptoms clear or urinary arsenic levels fall below 50 μg/24 h. Penicillamine might be administered orally as adjunct treatment after the ingestion of arsenic. Newer chelating agents such as *meso*-2,3-dimercaptosuccinic acid (DMSA, Succimer, Chemet) or the even less toxic 2,3-dimercaptopropanesulfonate (DMPS, Unithiol, Dimaval) are now recommended for oral therapy. DMPS has also been administered parenterally in animals.

CADMIUM

Cadmium was discovered in 1817 by the German chemist and physician Friedrich Strohmeyer. Its toxic potential became obvious with its increasing industrial use at the beginning of the 20th century. Because of its extraordinarily long biological half-life, cadmium tends to accumulate in the body. Exposure to cadmium fumes resulted in the first occupational cadmium intoxications. Occupational exposure, however, has decreased continously since the 1950s because of improved safety precautions. In the 1950s, Itai-Itai disease was observed in Japan, the result of eating Cd-contaminated rice. This epidemic intoxication drew public attention to the relevance of cadmium as a dangerous environmental contaminant.

Chemical Properties, Occurrence, and Use

Cadmium (Cd, molecular weight 112.4; oxidation status +2) forms a number of inorganic compounds, such as CdS, CdO, $CdSO_4$, $CdCl_2$, and $Cd(CH_3-COO)_2$. Some of the salts are soluble. The oxide and sulfide, however, are nearly insoluble in water. Geologically, cadmium is widely distributed and is often associated with lead, zinc, and phophates. Worldwide production is about 12,000 to 15,000 tons/year. Fifty to sixty percent of the production is used in alloys or for galvanization (i.e., as protection against corrosion). Roughly 10% is used in pigments. Furthermore, cadmium is used as a stabilizer in plastics and is used in radiation screens and batteries.

Absorption, Distribution, Metabolism, and Excretion

The kinetics of cadmium is characterized by a very long biological half-life (10–30 years). Humans are exposed to cadmium mainly via contaminated food (Table 8). Cadmium air concentrations (1 to 5 ng/m^3; in a few highly industrialized towns, up to 40 ng/m^3) do not contribute substantially to the total body bur-

TABLE 8 Estimated Uptake of Cadmium per Week from Normal Food[a]

Food	Consumption (kg/week)	Concentration (μg/kg w.w)	Uptake (μg/week)
Wheat	1.58	56 ± 51	89
Potatoe	1.23	48 ± 51	59
Beer	6.99	3.9 ± 7.9	27
Drinking water	4.45	2.0	9.1
Vegetable	0.11	72 ± 194	27
Egg	0.36	12 ± 14	4.3
Coffee	0.18	17 ± 12	3.0
Wine	0.61	5	3.0
Pork	0.39	12 ± 20	3.9
Kidney (pork)	0.004	692 ± 849	2.8
Carrot	0.08	245 ± 430	19
Milk	1.25	2.9 ± 3.9	3.6

[a]Values were calculated from average consumption and mean cadmium concentration in normal food in Germany. Data show that consumption behavior determines body burden more than absolute Cd concentration. From Diehl and Boppel (1985).

den in most areas. A remarkable inhalative uptake may be observed during occupational exposure to cadmium dust or aerosols. Cadmium-containing particles may be retained in the alveoli. Animal experiments suggest that 50% or more of inhaled cadmium is absorbed from respiratory tract. Corresponding human data are not available. However, a comparison of cadmium concentrations in the inhaled air and in the blood of smokers and nonsmokers supports the assumption that in humans between 40 and 50% of inhaled cadmium is absorbed. Therefore, smoking about 20 cigarettes a day is assumed to result in an additional uptake of about 1 to 2 μg Cd/day, which is more than the average daily uptake with food. The absorption rate for cadmium from the respiratory tract into the plasma is determined by the particle size and water solubility of the inhaled particles. The mechanism of absorption is not known.

The absorption of cadmium from the gastrointestinal tract is as low as 2 to 8%. It is influenced by the composition of intestinal contents. In rats, cadmium absorption is increased by the presence of meat, bread, milk, and calcium. From interaction studies, it is suggested that cadmium ions probably bind to the calcium-binding protein (CBP); in the intestinal mucosa, a low Ca concentration in food enhances Cd absorption. Furthermore, Cd absorption is increased four- to fivefold in animals and humans with iron deficiency. Investigations of transfer kinetics showed that the Michaelis–Menten constant (K_m) is increased without changing of the maximal transport velocity (V_{max}). Therefore, it is assumed that cadmium may share the intestinal transport mechanism for iron. The intestinal aborption of cadmium ions has two steps.

1. Cd^{2+} ions are bound to the apical membrane of the mucosal cells of the small intestine. This process is fast, saturable, and can be inhibited by Ca^{2+} ions.
2. In the mucosal cells, cadmium is bound in part to metallothionein and, thus, in part is excreted with feces after cell desquamation. The absorption from the mucosal cells into the plasma determines the rate of the cadmium absorption. The transport mechanism of cadmium across the basolateral membrane is unknown.

Cadmium does not cross the placenta. Therefore, neonates are essentially cadmium free. The cadmium body burden increases continuously with age and reaches its maximum at about 50 years (Fig. 3). The highest Cd concentration is measured in the kidneys. In unexposed nonsmokers, the renal Cd concentration varies between 9 and 30 mg/kg. In Cd-contaminated areas in Japan, up to 60 mg/kg may be reached in the kidneys, which corresponds to about one-third of the total body burden, while the liver stores about 20%. In smokers the tissue concentrations can become more than twice this value. Cadmium concentrations in blood of unexposed nonsmokers will vary between 0.2 and 1.1 μg/liter and in smokers between 0.7 and 3.9 μg/liter. Cd^{2+} is bound to anionic sites, mainly to sulfhydryl groups of intra- and extracellular proteins, such as metallothionein and albumin. After absorption from the lung or gastrointestinal tract in a first stage, cadmium is mainly bound to the albumin and

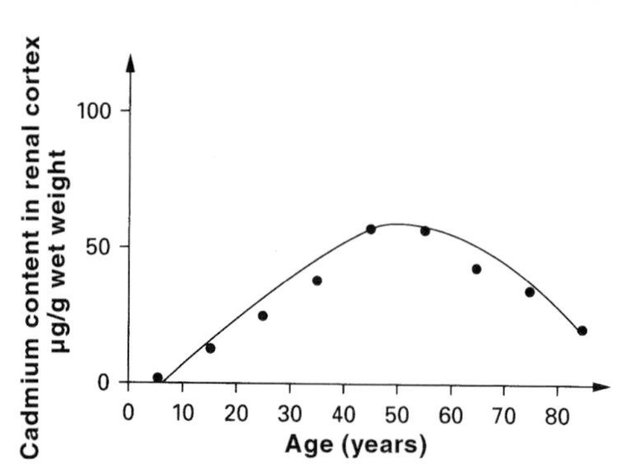

FIGURE 3 Age-dependent cadmium concentration in renal cortex of humans in South Bavaria (Germany). The data are based on biopsies from 263 dead people without occupational exposure. The age was symmetrically matched. It is to be emphasized that smokers were overrepresented, showing always higher cadmium concentrations in renal cortex than nonsmokers. A differentiation between nonsmoker [NS], smokers (< 20 cigarettes)[S], heavy smokers [HS], and pipe smokers [PS] between 44 and 55 years was made. The subgroups showed the following Cd concentrations in the renal cortex (μg/gww): NS = 24; S = 42; HS = 73; PS = 53. From Schäfer (1990).

other plasma proteins with a molecular weight >70,000. The protein-bound cadmium is taken up by the liver cells, is bound to metallothionein, and may be excreted again into the blood (Fig. 4). In hepatocytes as well as in variety of other cells, the synthesis of metallothionein is induced by cadmium. Metallothionein (molecular weight, ~6000 to 7000) has a high capacity for storing and transporting zinc. In the plasma, cadmium is almost completely bound to metallothionein and albumin. The largest concentration of cadmium is found in the erythrocytes.

In the kidney Cd-metallothionein passes the glomerulae and is reabsorbed in tubular cells by pinocytosis. Within the renal tubular epithelium the metal–protein complexes are metabolized. The unbound cadmium induces a further synthesis of metallothionein. Thus, the equilibrium between bound and unbound cadmium ions is shifted nearly completely to bound metal. It is suggested that free cadmium ions represent the toxic species that causes kidney damage if a total critical Cd concentration exceeds 200 μg/g. All renal cadmium concentrations measured in humans were not higher than 15 to 30% of this critical limit. Only 0.01 to 0.02% of the body burden is excreted with feces per day.

The intestinal absorption is small; therefore about 95% of the ingested cadmium is directly excreted with feces. In contrast, renal Cd elimination is related to the body burden and, in addition, increases with age. The individual variation is high. An increase of renal Cd excretion is observed during cadmium-associated kidney damage. The biological half-life ($t_{1/2}$) for the renal cortex, liver, and muscles is estimated to be between 10 and 30 years, reflecting 15 to 40% of the human life expectancy. Cd excretion in unexposed nonsmokers is <2 μg/liter, while the urine of smokers contains significantly higher Cd concentrations. Biliary and intestinal excretions of Cd are of minor importance. WHO has recommended (in 1972) that food for human use should contain less than 0.1 ppm Cd (0.1 mg/kg). These values correspond to a provisional tolerable weekly intake (PTWI) of 400—500 μg Both values were calculated to prevent a critical Cd concentration in the kidney, even after life-long exposure. The recommendation is based on a mathematical model that assumes an absorption rate of 5%. The average cadmium uptake from food is probably much lower.

Mechanism of Toxicity

Many effects related to cadmium have been described; however, a definite explanation of the mechanism of toxicity for acute and chronic effects is not available. Chronic oral exposure to cadmium results in iron-deficient anemia, osteomalacia, kidney damage, and other symptoms, as mentioned previously. Animal experiments suggest that chronic-inhalation Cd intake bears a carcinogenic risk. The mechanisms of these effects are obviously different. Iron-deficient anemia is caused by the competition between iron and cadmium during intestinal absorption. Osteomalacia may be due to the inhibited hydroxylation of 25-OH-D_3 to 1,25-$(OH)_2$-D_3, resulting in bone mineralization disturbances (Fig. 5). The renal cortex is the primary target organ for cadmium toxicity. The tubular cells seem to have only a limited capacity to sequester cadmium ions in metallothionein. If the capacity is exceeded, the free concentration of cadmium ions will increase and interfere directly the metabolic functions (e.g., the adenylate cyclase), which may cause cell death in the renal cortex.

Acute and Chronic Toxicity

Acute and chronic intoxication can be associated with cadmium exposure. However, based on its toxicokinetic properties, cadmium is a typical cumulative poison. After occupational exposure and once following the consumption of highly Cd-contaminated food

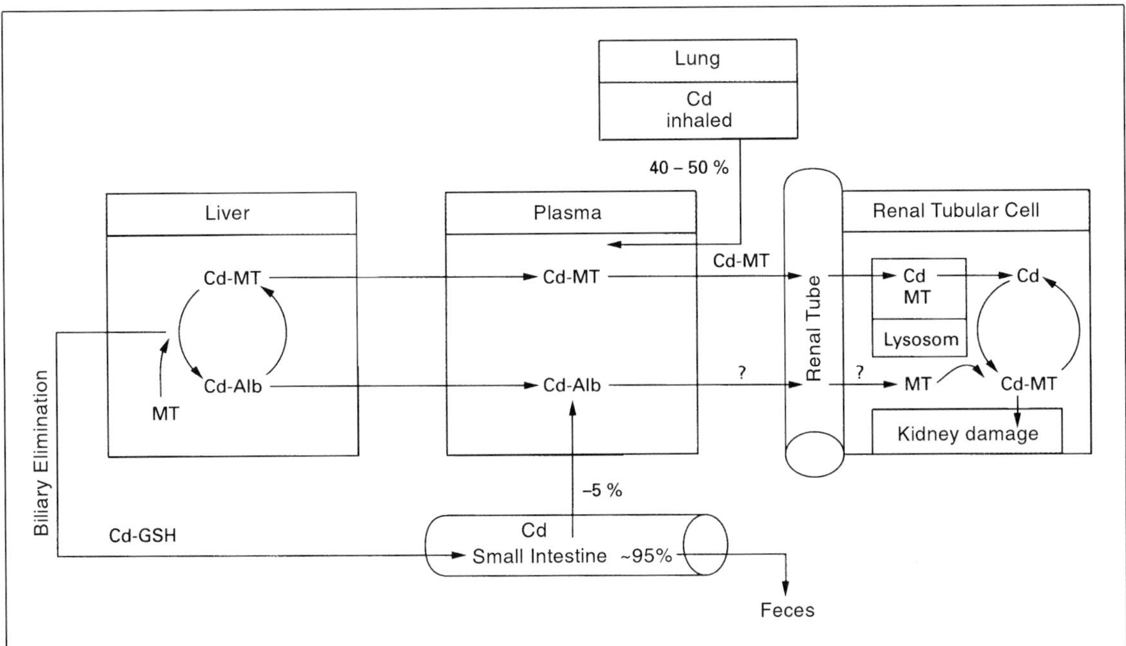

FIGURE 4 Absorption, distribution, metabolism, and excretion of cadmium. After absorption from the small intestine (~5%) or lung (40–50%) Cd is bound to albumin (Alb) and taken up into hepatocytes. Within hepatocytes, cadmium stimulates the synthesis of metallothionein that binds cadmium. Biliary excretion of glutathion-bound cadmium is of minor importance. Cd-metallothionein is released from hepatocytes into plasma. From plasma Cd-metallothionein is transported to renal tubules via glomerular filtration. A small fraction is excreted with urine. The major part is reabsorbed by the tubular cells. In lysosomes Cd-metallothionein is metabolized. Cd is released and induces metallothionein synthesis again. When a critical Cd concentration is exceeded (>200 mg/kg) in the renal cortex, kidney damage cannot be excluded. Modified from Friberg *et al.* (1986).

in Japan, chronic cadmium diseases have been observed.

Cd ions may contribute to the denaturation of proteins and cause damage to the capillary structures and barrier functions of membranes (e.g., in the lungs and mucosal epithelia of the gastrointestinal tract). The inhalation of highly contaminated air can result in lethal lung edema or pneumonitis (Table 9). The mechanism of toxicity in the respiratory tract is probably due to the damage of specific alveolar cells (Type I).

Acute Toxicity

Acute intoxication is a rare event and is restricted to occupationally exposed workers in nickel–cadmium refineries, in galvanizing industries, or during cadmium roasting. The initial symptoms are dry mucous membranes in the nose and throat, cough, headache, dizziness, fever, and/or retrosternal pain. Lung edema may develop 24 h after exposure. Therefore, after exposure medical care is needed for at least 2 to 3 days. As a late consequence, bronchiolitides cannot be excluded, which may result in delayed mortality. Animal experiments show that acute exposure to Cd dust, aerosols, or smoke may provoke persistant morphological changes in the lung tissue and even edemas. The sensitivity to Cd-induced damage is species dependent and is worse after CdO inhalation than after $CdCl_2$ uptake (Table 10). The lethal concentration of cadmium in the air for humans is estimated to be ~5–6 mg/m^3 over 8 h. An exposure to as low as 1 mg/m^3 for 8 h must be considered dangerous.

Years ago, acute oral Cd intoxication was occasionally observed when fruit juice or ice cream was stored in cadmium-plated containers. A considerable amount of cadmium ions was released into the food and induced vomiting, diarrhea, and colic-like pain. The slow absorption rate and the emetic effect of cadmium, however, frequently prevented severe intoxication. Cd concentrations above 15 mg/liter provoke vomiting.

Chronic Toxicicty

Leaving aside the epidemiological intoxication in Japan (Itai-Itai), which was attributed to Cd-contaminated food, oral cadmium exposure plays a minor role

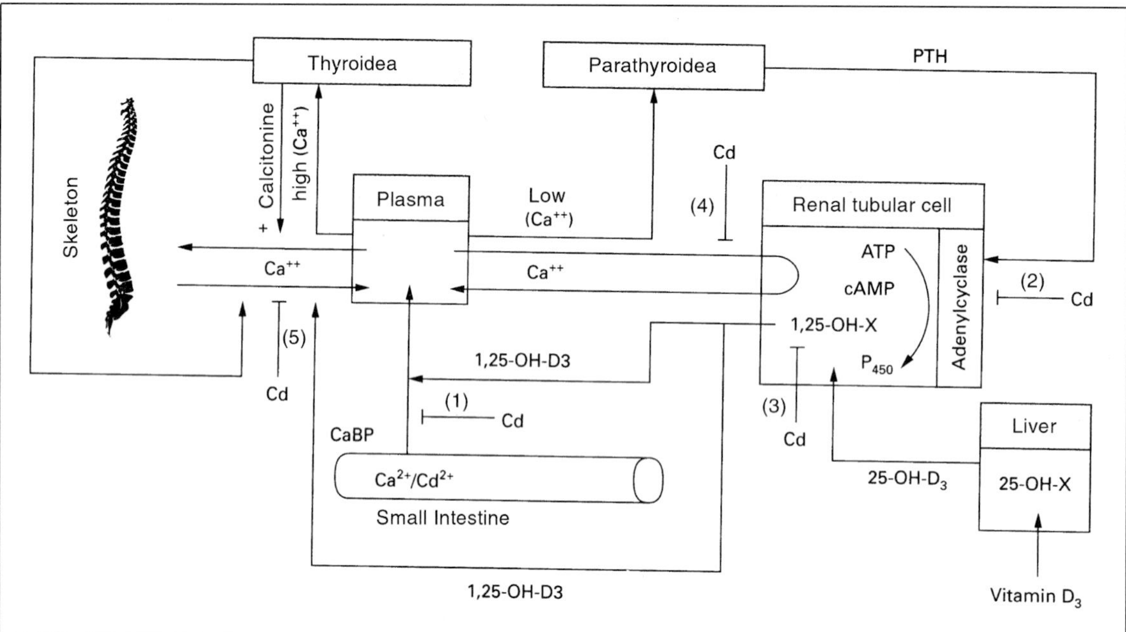

FIGURE 5 Potential mechanism of Cd-attributed osteomalacia. Vitamin D_3 is metabolized to 1,25-dihydroxy-D_3 (1,25-$(OH)_2$-cholecalciferol) in renal tubular cells. This metabolite of the vitamin is engaged in the regulation of Ca absorption from the small intestine and the release of Ca from skeleton and mineralization of bone matrix. Ca^{2+} absorption in the small intestine is mediated by calcium-binding protein (CBP). This protein may be the first interaction site between Cd and Ca (1). Depending on the Ca concentration in plasma either more calcitonin (high concentration) or more parathyroid hormone is excreted by stimulation of the thyroid. Calcitonin increases the uptake of Ca into the bone. Parathyroid hormone stimulates the release of Ca from bone as well as the adenylate cyclase in renal tubular cells; this effect can be inhibited by Cd (2). In the liver cells vitamin D_3 is hydroxlated to 25-OH-D_3. The renal tubular cells metabolize it to 1,25-$(OH)_2$-D_3. This hydroxylation can be inhibited by cadmium (3). In addition, uptake of Ca into the tubular cells is inhibited by Cd (4). It is also supposed that Cd may affect bone mineralization directly. Modified from Friberg *et al.* (1986).

in chronic toxicity compared to occupational inhalative intake. The kidney is the target organ after both oral and inhalation exposure. After occupational exposure for many years, specific symptoms can develop. In some cases, the inflammation of the nasal mucous membrane and the throat was described. The teeth at the gingival margin may show yellow rings, attributed to cadmium sulfide deposits. Besides the typical cadmium rhinitis, progressive degenerative changes of the olfactoric epithelia may lead to hyposmia and anosmia. Severe obstructive diseases of the respiratopry tract have been observed. Dose-dependent lung lesions were described for all inhaled cadmium compounds. Cd smoke, however, seems to be the most dangerous. The lowest concentration to provoke the first symptoms is 70 $\mu g/m^3$. These results, however, were not confirmed by later investigations. A dose–response relationship for the pulmonary effects is not

TABLE 9 Cadmium Concentrations that Provoked an Increase of Lung Weight in Animals after Acute Inhalative Exposure to CdO or $CdCl_2$[a]

Species	Compound	Cd concentration (mg/m³)	Exposure time (min)	Dose (mg × min/m³)
Rat	$CdCl_2$	6.5	120	780
	CdO	10	15	150
	CdO	6.5	60	390
Rabbit	CdO	<22	15	330

[a]From Elinder (1986).

TABLE 10 Inhalative LD_{50} of Cd Smoke Compared to the Lethal Dose in Humans[a]

Species	LD_{50} (mg × min/m³)	Lethal dose in humans (mg × min/m³)
Rat	500[b]	
Mouse	500[b]	
Guinea pig	2,500[b]	
Dog	4,000[b]	
Monkey	15,000[b]	
Human		2500–2900

[a]From Friedberg *et al.* (1986).
[b]Values were estimated.

described for humans. Therefore, a maximal tolerable dose cannot be given for human respiratory tract.

An excessive uptake of cadmium with food has been observed only in Japan, resulting in Itai-Itai disease, with kidney damage, severe osteomalacia and osteoporosis, iron-deficient anemia, and disturbances of intestinal absorption and liver metabolism. Osteomalacia was observed in Itai-Itai patients and in a few cadmium workers (i.e., Franconi syndrome) and may be an indirect effect of a Cd-related kidney damage. Due to Cd-induced kidney dysfunction, calcium and phosphate are excreted to a larger extent than physiologically appropriate. At the same time, the hydroxylation of vitamin D_3 metabolites in the renal tubular cells is possibly inhibited by cadmium in the renal tubular cells (Fig. 5). Chronic oral exposure to very high cadmium concentrations in the food (>1 mg/kg) causes microcytic iron-deficient anemia in animals and humans, which can be corrected by appropriate therapeutic iron doses. In contrast, in non-cadmium-induced iron deficiency, cadmium absorption is increased by factor 4 to 5.

Although the kidney and liver mainly accumulate cadmium, there is no unequivocal evidence that cadmium exposure and liver damage are linked. A relationship between cadmium exposure and hypertension has been discussed for a long time, but could not be confirmed in four studies of Cd workers between 1950 and 1980, as well as of an unexposed population in 1984. Osteoporosis is likely to be enhanced in high Cd exposure, due to an interference between the cadmium and calcium metabolisms. Whether the development of an osteoporosis-like status is typical of severe Cd exposure is not known. Even in heavily exposed Cd workers, it was rarely diagnosed.

Cd-attributed kidney damage results in proteinuria and an increased excretion of albumins, globulins, and β_2-microglobulins, and increased serum creatinine. In addition, glucosuria, phosphaturia, and/or urinary amino acid excretion may occur. In general, the urinary concentrations of calcium and phosphate are increased. Cd-induced kidney damage is progressive even after the cessation of exposure. The role of metallothionein has not been definitively clarified.

Itai-Itai Disease

Itai-Itai disease was observed for the first time in 1946 in the prefecture of Toyama (Japan). It affected mainly postmenopausal multiparial women between 40 and 70 years of age. Dr. Hagino called this illness "Itai-Itai" (which means ouch-ouch), because patients suffered from extreme pain in the back and legs. Massive osteoporosis, leading to severe deformations and up to a 30-cm shrinking of the skeleton, was reported. Minor traumas resulted in multiple bone fractures. In addition, the patients suffered from enteropathia and pancreatic diarrhea. Treatment with high doses of vitamin D alleviated the symptoms. The pathogenetic mechanisms are not fully understood. The osteomalazia and osteoporosis may result from a disturbance of the renal calcium, phosphate, and vitamin D metabolisms. On the one hand, epidemiological studies emphasize that these symptoms are linked to cadmium exposure; on the other hand, malnutrition from diets low in proteins, calcium, and vitamin D may have contributed to and enhanced the severity of the Itai-Itai symptoms.

Specific Toxicity

Reproduction Toxicity

Animal experiments suggest that cadmium is teratogenic and mutagenic at high doses. There are no data in support of teratogenic effects in humans. An investigation of heavily exposed Russian women in 1970 showed no teratogenic potential. However, the newborn babies frequently had birth weights below the average. In addition, a few cases of rachitis were observed in these children.

A single injection of a high cadmium dose (3 mg/kg) showed teratogenic effects in hamsters and rats. In mice, chronic Cd administration with the drinking water (10 mg Cd/liter) caused teratogenic effects.

Mutagenicity and Carcinogenicity

Some *in vitro* studies using high Cd doses show remarkable effects on the DNA. In spite of numerous studies on Cd mutagenicity, it is not clear whether cadmium is mutagenic in humans.

Carcinogenicity was described in animal experiments only after subcutaneous and intramuscular injections and chronic inhalation. After chronic oral up-

TABLE 11 Selection of Epidemiological Studies on Carcinogenicity in Cd Workers[a]

Organ	Incidence observed	Incidence expected	Year of investigation
Lung	12	5.1[b]	1976
	7	3.9	1980
	3	2.5	1983
	89	70.2[b]	1983
	199	185.6	1983
	20	11.43[b]	1985
Prostata	4	0.58[b]	1967
	3	1.6	1973
	4	0.88[b]	1976
	4	2.69	1979
	2	1.2	1979
	8	6.6	1983
	23	23.3	1983
	4	2.6	1985

[a]The results are from studies that investigated the carcinogenic potential of Cd after inhalative exposure (>1 mg Cd/m^3) in workers of Cd-processing plants. The simultaneous exposure to other heavy metals (Ni, As) has to be taken into consideration. From Elinder (1986).

[b]Statistically significant; $p < 0.05$.

take, no carcinogenic effect was observed. Therefore, inhalation may be the only important route for humans with regard to Cd-attributed carcinogenicity. Rats treated continuously for 18 months with aerosols containing 0, 12.5, 25, and 50 μg Cd/m^3 as cadmium chloride aerosol developed primary lung tumors in a dose-dependent manner. This study is of extraordinary importance as it is the only study and because the highest dose reflects the maximal acceptable concentration of cadmium allowed in the work place in Germany. Animal data suggest that cadmium has an affinity for prostate tissue and that cadmium may induce prostate neoplasms. Data from epidemiological studies, however, are equivocal (Table 11). A questionable increased incidence of prostate and lung tumors was observed after long-term occupational exposure to high concentrations that are not relevant for the general population. Cadmium concentrations in the environment probably do not contribute to increases in lung cancer. Cadmium uptake via food and drinking water bears no remarkable carcinogenic risk.

Therapeutic Measures

The therapy for a severe acute oral or inhalative Cd intoxication is restricted to life-saving activities (e.g., keeping airways open, assisting respiration, and stabilizing the circulation). Based on animal experiments, BAL (British Anti-Lewisite) may be helpful in acute inhalative Cd intoxication. It must be considered that treatment with complexing agents can cause a redistribution of Cd from other tissues to the kidneys. Thus, the therapeutic measures may cause renal damage. For long-term treatment, complexing agents are not suitable and should only be administered intermittently.

COPPER

Bronze, an alloy of tin and copper, gave its name to an entire age (about 3500 B.C.) Quantitatively, copper is the most important essential biological metal after iron and zinc. The body store contains between 80 and 150 mg copper. Copper functions in the catalytic center of many metalloenzymes (Table 12). Copper metabolism is based on a sensitive balance between absorption and excretion. About 2% of the total body store has to be replaced each day. A copper deficit, as well as an overload, shows typical clinical

TABLE 12 Selected Copper-Containing Metalloenzymes with Locations and Functions or Effects[a]

Enzyme	Location	Function or effect
Ferrooxidase I (ceruloplasmin)	Plasma	Oxidation Fe^{2+} Fe^{3+} Deficit: microcytic anemia
Ferrooxidase II (lipoprotein)	Plasma	Oxidation Fe^{2+} Fe^{3+} Deficit: microcytic anemia
Aminooxidase	Mitochondria	Oxidation from primary amines to aldehydes $R\text{-}CH_2\text{-}NH_2$ to R-CHO
Zn-Cu-superoxiddismutase	Cytosol	Metabolism of $2\ O_2^{-} + 2H^+ \xrightarrow{SOD} H_2O_2 + O_2$
Cytochrome C oxidase	Mitochondria	Respiratory chain
Lysyl oxidase	Bones	Metabolism of elsatin and collagens
Tyrosinase	Bones	Tyrosine hydroxylation; biosynthesis of melanine and other polyphenolic compounds

[a]From Schäfer and Schümann (1991).

symptoms, which are well known from congenital copper metabolism disorders. Menke (1962) first described the X-chromosomal recessive genodermatosis ("Kinky Hair disease") attributed to copper deficiency resulting from malabsorption. "Wilson disease," in contrast, is characterized by a hepatic copper overload, resulting probably from a decreased biliary copper excretion causing hepatolenticular degenerations. Both congenital diseases are rare; they occur with a frequency of about 1 in 100,000 births. From the viewpoint of toxicology, copper is of minor importance, with the rare exception of occupational exposure and a disease referred to as "Indian–German Childhood Cirrhosis," which is attributed to massive copper overloading in infants.

Chemical Properties, Occurrence, and Use

Copper (Cu, molecular weight 63.54) is soluble only in nonoxidizing acids in the presence of oxygen (e.g., amonium or potassium cyanide solutions). In water, copper goes through a disproportioning reaction from Cu^0 to CU^{2+} ($2\ Cu(I) \rightleftharpoons Cu(O) + Cu(II)$). Copper is found ubiquitously. Large deposits exist in the United States, Canada, Chile, Russia, Zimbabwe, Zambia, and Zaire. More than 50% of the world's copper production is used for cables and electrical equipment. Other uses are in heating pipes and in alloys like bronze. Wine growers spray copper sulfate ($CuSO_4$) with slaked lime as a pesticide ("Bordeaux mixture").

Absorption, Distribution, Metabolism, and Excretion

About 10 to 15% of the total body stores (80–150 mg) are found in the liver. The daily requirement is estimated by WHO to be about 2 mg. The steady state is balanced via gastrointestinal absorption and biliary excretion. A temporary deficiency can be counter-balanced by endogenous stores, while an overload would be compensated for mainly by enhanced biliary excretion, which matures in infants during the first years of life.

Ten to fifteen percent of copper is absorbed through the stomach. In healthy adults, the absorption rate from the gastrointestinal tract (GIT) is estimated to be between 30 and 50%. It is substantially influenced by the composition of the GIT contents. Copper absorption is increased by proteins, amino acids, citrate, and oxalate; but decreased by phytates, high concentrations of calcium and phosphates, and fibers. A metal–metal interaction is observed between zinc and copper.

Copper is almost quantitatively bound to plasma albumin. It is taken up mainly by hepatocytes (first pass), where it is bound to metallothionein and finally to ceruloplasmin. Ceruloplasmin is excreted from the liver cells back into the plasma and distributed to various tissues (Fig. 6). Ceruloplasmin is a single-strand glycoprotein (molecular weight, 132,000) containing six copper atoms per molecule.

Copper is excreted mainly by the bile when it is associated with amino acids, glutathione, and unknown high-molecular-weight compounds. The active biliary excretion mechanisms have not been characterized. However, they play an important role in the maintenance of a steady state for copper. Copper elimination by perspiration is of minor importance; renal excretion is small (<1% in 72 h vs. 9% with feces). Biliary excretion plays a major role and seems to be reduced in Wilson disease. The biological half-life ($t_{1/2}$) of copper in a healthy human is estimated to be about 2 weeks.

Mechanism of Toxicity

The mechanism of copper toxicity is not fully understood. In addition to gastrointestinal irritation, the target organ for copper is the liver, as observed in the congenital Wilson disease or the anthropogenic copper overload in childhood cirrhosis. Copper is transported from the plasma to the liver cells by albumin. In the liver cells, copper ions are transfered to metallothionein and to ceruloplasmin (Fig. 6), a process of limited capacity. At the same time, copper ions are secreted with the bile. In cases of a reduced elimination capacity (Wilson disease, childhood cirrhosis) and an exhaustion of intracellular binding proteins, free copper ions are likely to become available. The cytotoxicity of free copper ions is well known. It may result in hepatic cirrhosis, as is observed in copper-overload diseases.

Acute and Chronic Toxicity

Acute and chronic copper intoxications are extremely rare. Anecdotal reports are published about contaminated drinking water resulting in intoxication. The toxic effects are attributed to ionized metal compounds. An occupational exposure is reported in copper refineries or in vineyards if "Bordeaux mixture" (1–2% $CuSO_4$ neutralized by slaked lime) is widely used.

Acute Toxicity

The acute inhalation of copper-containing fumes or dusts may cause irritation of the upper respiratory tract. Airway disorders resulting from copper inhalation are not reported. The acute toxic effects of copper

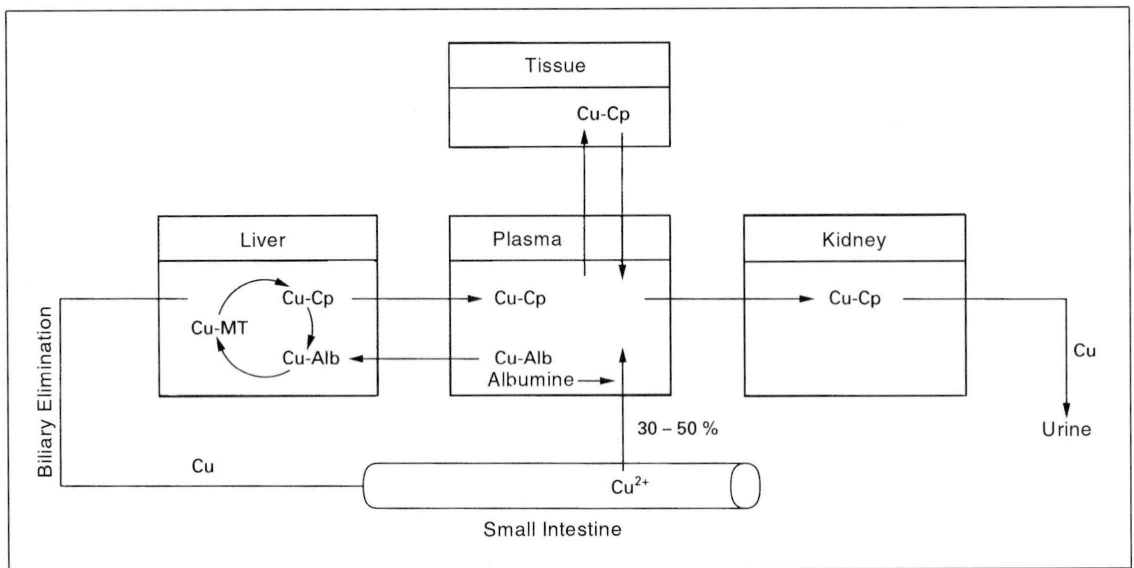

FIGURE 6 Absorption, distribution, metabolism, and excretion of copper. About 2–3 mg Cu^{2+} are ingested daily with the food and between 30 and 50% are absorbed. In plasma copper is bound quantitatively to albumin (Alb) and transported into hepatocytes. Cu-Alb is metabolized and copper is temporary bound to metallothionein (MT) and finally to ceruloplasmin (CP). Cu-CP is released back to plasma. On the one hand, this protein has a transport function for Cu into the tissue; on the other hand, it has an enzymatic function. Biliary elimination is the most relevant excretion pathway (1–2 mg/day). It has not matured during the first 2 years of age and is insufficient in Wilson disease. There is no substantial enterohepatic circulation. Renal excretion is of minor importance (Schäfer *et al.*, 1994).

sulfate result from GIT irritation. This effect was the reason that copper was used as emetic in Europe. Nausea, vomiting, and irritation of the GIT and possibly hemorrhagic gastroenteritis may result from ingestion of copper salts. After an intake of a large quantity (>10 g), severe liver and kidney injuries are observed because copper is absorbed well compared to most of the other heavy metals. Contact allergies are rare (~1%). The acute toxicity of the various copper compounds is low (Table 13) compared to other metals or metaloids, such as thallium or arsenic. *In vitro* investigations show that copper(II) ions are cytotoxic (~ 10^{-6} molar).

A unique case of lethal copper intoxication was described in a 58-year-old woman in New Jersey (U.S.) in 1987, who suffered from nausea, vomiting, lethargy, and icterus. She died in the clinic briefly after transportation. The women had swallowed a total of 275 coins, mostly copper coins. The copper concentration in the liver tissue was increased by several orders of magnitude to 1.16 mg/g (normal concentration in adults, 0.007 mg/g).

TABLE 13 Acute Toxicity of Selected Organic Copper Compounds after Oral Administration to Rats

Compound	LD_{50} (mg/kg body weight)
Copper(II) carbonate ($CuCO_3 \times 2\ H_2O$)	159
Copper chloride ($CuCl_2$)	140
Copper nitrate ($Cu[NO_3]_2 \times 3\ H_2O$)	940
Copper(I) oxide (Cu_2O)	470
Copper oxychloride ($(CuCOCl)_2$)	700
Copper sulfate ($CuSO_4$)	300

[a]From MAK list (1977).

Chronic Toxicity

Chronic copper intoxication attributed to Cu-contaminated food is not described. However, the chronic intake via drinking water can be considerable. An extensive copper uptake via contaminated water induced chronic copper intoxication in a family in Vermont (U.S.). They drank water containing between 2.8 and 7.8 mg copper per liter for a long period of time (Environmental Protection Agency (EPA) recommendation, < 1 mg/liter; Europe, 0.1 mg/liter). Gastrointestinal irritation developed. Their hair and nails contained extremely high copper concentrations, whereas all other metal concentrations were in the

TABLE 14 Copper Concentrations of Selected Organs in Healthy Adults and Infants[a]

Organ	Adults (A)	Infants (I)	Ratio (I/A)
Brain	6.3 (5.1–8.3)	3.7 (1.5–9.1)	0.59
Heart	3.0 (1.5–3.8)	2.6 (1.3–4.0)	0.87
Liver	5.1 (3.0–9.5)	19.0 (2.9–56.5)	3.73
Spleen	0.8 (0.2–1.1)	2.6 (0.8–4.7)	3.25
Kidney	2.0 (1.2–3.1)	3.1 (0.9–8.6)	1.25
Plasma (mg/100 ml)	0.08–0.15	—	—

[a]In μg/g wet weight; brackets show the measured range (Schäfer and Schümann, 1991).

normal range. The symptoms disappeared after the consumption of the contaminated water was stopped.

Indian–German Childhood Cirrhosis

The name of the disease reflects the fact that it has been observed only in India and Germany. Only children younger than 4 years of age were affected. In India, the food for infants was prepared and stored in copper containers, resulting in a high copper contamination. The copper concentrations in fresh milk stored overnight in copper containers rose, for example, from 40 μg/100 ml to between 2500 and 3500 μg/100 ml. The consumption of such milk resulted in a dangerous increase in the copper concentration in the liver because the infants had not yet developed the mechanism for biliary copper excretion. Consequently, cirrhotic degeneration of the hepatic tissue developed. The prognosis for these infants is poor. A relationship between the development of the Indian childhood cirrhosis and massive copper intake is generally accepted (Table 14).

In the few cases of German childhood cirrhosis, breastfeeding was stopped early. Powdered milk was resuspended in water from a private well, which had a relative low pH (6.2, vs. 7.6 normal value). Therefore, Cu^{2+} ions accumulated in the drinking water overnight. Drinking water from a public supply avoids such a contamination, mainly because of the higher pH. Between 1979 and 1991, 13 babies died in two small villages in Germany due to a massive copper overload in the infants' liver tissue. The tissue copper concentration was increased dramatically (1.27–1.87 mg/g dry weight exposed vs. 0.022–0.041 mg/g unexposed). At the same time, the iron concentration in liver tissue decreased remarkably (0.072–0.167 mg/g exposed vs. 1.5–2.73 mg/g unexposed). In addition, a long-lasting disturbance of the immune system was observed, reflected by a pathological ratio of lymphocyte–monocyte functions.

Specific Toxicity

There is no evidence for a teratogenic, mutagenic, or cancerogenic effect of copper. The increased incidence of lung cancer in workers from copper refineries is likely due to contamination from metalloids, such as arsenic, that are deposited in the lungs via respiration.

Therapeutic Measures

The therapeutic measures in cases of copper overload derive mostly from the therapy for Wilson disease. The elimination of copper ions can be increased by the oral administration of D-penicillamine (dimethylcysteine). Renal elimination mainly is enhanced. In case of D-penicillamine intolerance (incidence <5%), TRIEN (triethylentetramine hydrochloride) could be used. During long-term treatment, the side effects have to be considered.

LEAD

The first reports of lead intoxication (saturnism) date back to the Roman Empire where 80,000 t of lead were produced per year as a by-product of silver mining. The worldwide consumption of lead in modern times is estimated to be 5.3 million tons. For comparison, the lead content of 5000-year-old human bones from the Sudan was as low as to 0.6 μg Pb/g compared to values between 6.5 and 9.0 μg/g in Germany in the 1980s. Thus, the anthropogenic contribution to the human lead load is substantial. In the past decades, however, industrial lead pollution has decreased in western Europe. Thus, the Rhine at the Dutch–German border carried 2000 t Pb/year in 1971 and only 500 t Pb/year in 1984.

Chemical Characteristics, Sources, and Uses

Lead (chemical symbol, Pb, atomic weight 207.2; specific density 11.3 g/cm^3, melting point 327.5°C) is a silvery-gray soft metal. Lead occurs in the oxidation states Pb^0, Pb^{2+}, and Pb^{4+}. In most of its salts, such as lead oxide and lead sulfide, lead is bivalent and poorly water soluble. Lead acetate, lead chlorate, and to a certain extent lead hydroxide are exceptions to this. The physiologic behavior of Pb^{2+} is similar to that of Ca^{2+}. Most salts of Pb are poorly water soluble.

Lead is mined in the United States, Australia, Russia, and Germany. The United States, Europe, and Japan consume 80% of the world's lead production; about 40% of lead is used in batteries, 7% in color pigments, and smaller amounts in chemical agents, cable mantels and pipes, radiation protection screens, printing characters, and ballast weights. In highly industrialized countries, more than 40% of the lead consumed is recycled.

Absorption, Distribution, Metabolism, and Excretion

The current provisional tolerable weekly intake (PTWE) is 25 μg Pb/kg body weight. These values are reached or exceeded, for example, in Cuba, India, and Thailand. The intakes reported for Italy, Germany, and New Zealand were half or more of the PTWI; lower intakes were found in Sweden, Denmark, and in the United States.

Even in cities, air lead concentrations rarely exceed 1 μg/m^3. In lead smelters and refineries, however, lead air concentrations between 80 and 4000 μg/m^3 may be found. Depending on their diameter (0.01–5 μm), 10–60% of inhaled lead particles are deposited in the alveolar regions of the lung. The major part of the retained fraction is absorbed; some, however, is removed by tracheobronchial clearance. In consequence, there is no substantial lead accumulation in the lung after inhalation. Cigarette smoke leads to an additional lead accumulation in the body.

The worldwide daily oral lead intake is estimated to be 200–300 μg/liter; in western Europe and in the United States, it is estimated to be below 100 μg/liter. Food and water usually contain less than 1 mg Pb/kg and 50 μg Pb/liter, respectively, although the food lead content may exceed 6 mg/kg in extreme cases, which may be caused by contamination during production, processing, or storage in lead-soldered tin cans. In houses with lead water pipes, the concentration in the drinking water may be as high as 3000 μg Pb/liter. Mother's milk and cow's milk may contain 5 to 12 μg Pb/liter and 40 μg Pb/liter, respectively. The average lead concentration in selected French and Italian wines was 65 μg/liter, which may triple when the wines are kept in crystal glass decanters for some hours. Intestinal absorption depends on the interaction of lead with food components. On an empty stomach, 60% of lead doses between 4 and 400 μg are absorbed. In adults, these high absorption rates decrease to 4–21% when lead is taken with food that has a normal calcium and phosphate content. A high phytate and zinc content in the food will inhibit lead bioavailability, while lactose and milk intake will increase it. When there are calcium, vitamin D, and iron deficiencies, lead absorption increase. The absorption of lead salts via the skin can be neglected (Table 15).

Children between 2 months and 6 years absorb between 42 and 50% of oral lead doses, which is five times that of adults. The mechanisms of increased lead absorption in children are incompletely understood. High milk consumption and the high frequency of deficiency states for iron, calcium, and phosphate during growth, as well as the increased overall absorption capacity of the intestine in early childhood (e.g., for macromolecular substances), may serve as an explanation.

In the blood, lead is transferred from the plasma to erythrocytes within a few minutes, where it is bound to the cell membranes and to hemoglobin. Lead shows a 16-fold enrichment in erythrocytes compared to plasma, where it mainly binds to albumin. The uptake into erythrocytes seems to be saturable. Blood-lead concentrations are frequently lower in women, prob-

TABLE 15 Estimated Daily Lead Intake and Absorbtion

	Lead intake		Lead absorption
Pb intake with food	200–300 μg/day	10% absorption	20–30 μg/day
Pb contents of drinking water	>20 μg/liter	10% absorption, 2 liter/day	>4 μg/day
Pb contents of air	1 μg/m^3	30% absorption, 20 m^3/day	6 μg/day
Total absorption in adults			30–40 μg/day

ably because of their often lower average hemoglobin concentration. From the blood, lead distributes into the soft tissues, such as the liver (about 1 mg Pb/kg), the kidney (about 0.8 mg Pb/kg), and the brain (about 0.1 mg Pb/kg). In the cells, lead mainly binds to the membranes and mitochondria. In soft tissues, lead has a half-life of approximately 20 days. The lead content of bones (9–34 mg/kg) increases with age and makes up approximately 70% and 90% of total body load in children and adults, respectively. Its half-life in the skeleton is 5–20 years. Therefore, the bone-lead content is an index of chronic lead exposure; it can be measured by X-ray fluorescence spectrometry in the tibia or finger bones.

Glomerular filtration makes up 76% of total lead excretion; 16% is eliminated with the feces via the bile or via pancreatic and intestinal secretion. Less than 8% is eliminated through hairs, nails, and perspiration.

Acute and Chronic Toxicity

Acute Toxicity of Inorganic Lead

The risk of occupational exposure to inorganic lead was substantially reduced by automation and protective measures. Cases of acute lead intoxication are rare in modern industrial facilities, such as battery manufacturing, lead smelters, and spray painting; however, they may still occur. After past exposure, substantial amounts of lead can be mobilized from the skeleton during pregnancy or after bone fractures. Mobilized lead quantities can induce symptoms of acute lead intoxication (lead crisis).

Intestinal colics frequently are the first symptom of acute lead intoxication, with loss of appetite, nausea, constipation, diarrhea, and diffuse abdominal pain. In acute lead intoxication, patients are often pale due to capillary spasms of the dermal capillaries. The pulse rate may be low and the blood pressure increased. These symptoms are caused by vagal irritation and contraction of smooth muscles. Acute lead encephalopathy is observed at blood-lead concentrations between 80 and 300 μg Pb/100 ml, with disorientation, insomnia, vomiting, apathy, stupor, ataxia, hyperkinesis, and aggressiveness. Motor and sensory disturbances, seizures, parkinsonism, and cortical atrophies (Table 16) are among the neurological sequels of encephalopathy after acute lead exposure; and, in extreme cases, this also include debility and hydrocephalus. Papillary edema is a common complication; coma and deaths from cardiac failure are a possible outcome. Children are more sensitive than adults; the first symptoms in children may be cramps or delirium.

Chronic Toxicity of Inorganic Lead

Chronic exposure to toxic amounts of lead affects the hematopoietic system, the gastrointestinal tract, the central and peripheral nervous systems and the kidneys. Other toxic effects occur at very high concentrations or are controversial. At lead-exposure levels found in the environment, children run a higher risk than adults because of their higher intestinal-absorption rate and their higher calorie demand as related to body weight. In addition, children ingest up to 5.6 g of dirt/day (average approximately 0.5 g/day), a phenomenon that is called "pica." Children living in the vicinity of lead smelters show blood-lead levels of about 40 μg/100 ml compared to approximately 9 μg Pb/100 ml in children that live 40 km away from such facilities. The ingestion of lead-containing paint flakes or particles can lead to severe chronic intoxication. The use of leaded fuel and lead pigments is restricted in western Europe and the U.S. In addition to reduced industrial lead emissions, these measures explain the decrease in human lead exposure.

Hematopoietic system

Chronic occupational lead exposure may lead to micro- to normocytic anemia as the lead interferes with hemoglobin synthesis and the life span of erythrocytes, which is reduced at concentrations over 40 μg Pb/100 ml blood. The permeability of the

TABLE 16 Correlation between Blood Lead Concentrations and Effects

Blood lead concentration (μg/100 ml)	Effect
>15	Inhibition of δ-aminolevulinic acid dehydratase
10–20	Impaired intellectual and cognitive development in children
20–60	Increased erythrocyte protoporphyrin concentrations
>40	Increased urinary coproporphyrin and δ-ALA concentration
50–60	Chronic encephalopathy in children
>80	Chronic encephalopathy in adults
60–80	Peripheral neuropathy
70–100	Impaired renal function
80–300	Acute lead encephalopathy

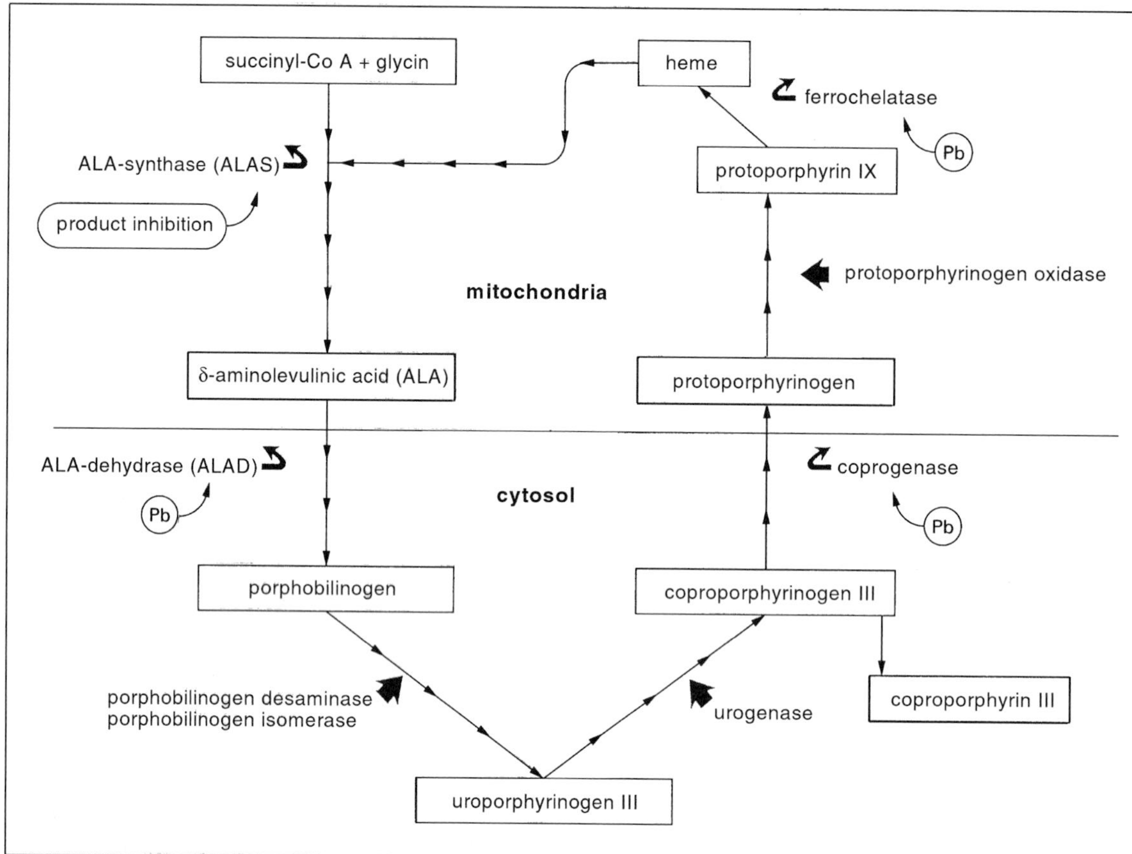

FIGURE 7 Interference of lead with hemebiosynthesis. Lead inhibits of δ-aminolevulinic acid dehydratase; high heme concentrations inhibit the synthesis of δ-aminolevulinic acid synthetase. Both effects lead to an accumulation of δ-aminolevulinic acid in plasma and urine. In addition, lead inhibits ferrochelatase and coprogenase, leading to increased concentrations of coproporphyrin III contents in urine and to an elevated protoporphyrine content in erythrocytes.

erythrocyte membrane is 10 times higher for lead than for calcium. Thus, lead accumulates in erythrocytes and interacts with different stages of hemoglobin synthesis. In consequence, some intermediates of heme synthesis accumulate in the serum, which is quantitatively related to the degree of exposure and has prognostic value.

The activity of δ-aminolevulinic acid synthetase (ALAS) is rate limiting in heme biosynthesis. The activity of this enzyme is inhibited by high concentrations of its terminal product, the heme (i.e., negative feedback). Lead inhibits the activity of δ-aminolevulinic acid dehydratase (ALAD), probably by interacting with the Zn ion in the enzyme (Fig. 7). ALAD inhibition reduces heme concentration, which, in turn, increases ALAS activity and thus the concentration of δ-aminolevulinic acid. This enzyme is used as a diagnostic parameter in the blood and urine. In addition, ALA is neurotoxic. An increased concentration may mediate lead neurotoxicity.

The ALAD activity is inhibited at 15 μg Pb/100 ml blood; the ALA concentration, however, does not increase at urine concentrations below 40 μg Pb/100 ml. It is used to diagnose occupational lead exposure. In contrast, ALAD activity in erythrocytes is very sensitive and is inhibited at low blood-lead concentrations (Fig. 8).

In addition, lead inhibits ferrochelatase activity. This enzyme catalyzes the incorporation of iron into the porphyrin ring to form heme. Its inhibition contributes to the development of anemia and leads to increased protoporphyrin IX concentrations in the erythrocyte, which correlate almost linearly with blood-lead levels in the critical lead concentration range between 20 and 60 μg Pb/100 ml. The inhibition of pyrimidine 5-nucleotidase causes basophilic strippling of erythrocytes in lead-exposed patients. The reduced survival time of erythrocytes is caused by the inhibition of Na^+,K^+-ATPase in the cells and contributes to anemia.

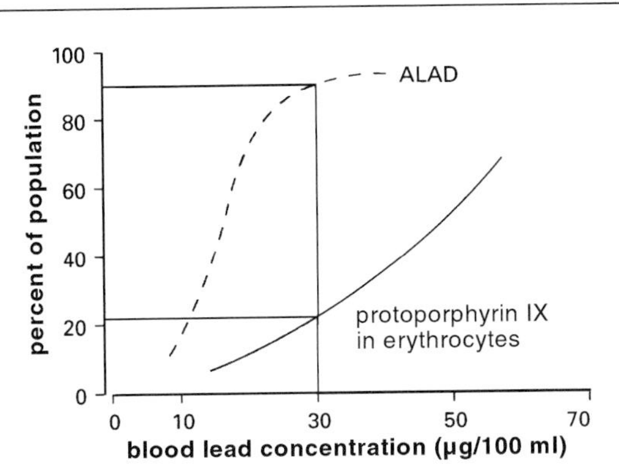

FIGURE 8 Dose–effect curve for the inhibition of δ-aminolevulinic acid dehydratase (δ-ALAD) by lead and the concentration of erythrocyte protoporphyrine IX (EP). The dashed line shows the percentage of a population that shows a 40% inhibition of δ-ALAD activity in erythrocytes at increasing blood-lead concentrations. The full line shows the percentage of a population with increased erythrocyte porphyrin concentrations. At concentrations below 30 μg Pb/100 ml inhibition of erythrocytic δ-ALAD is a very sensitive parameter. Above 30 μg Pb/100 ml blood erythrocyte protoporphyrin is the better parameter for diagnosing the extent of a lead intoxication (reprinted with permission from the Committee on Lead in the Human Environment. Copyright 1980 by the National Academy of Sciences. Courtesy of the National Academy Press, Washington, DC).

Nervous system

In workers, exposure to inorganic lead has resulted in impaired memory, concentration, and psychomotor performance, while the parameters of intelligence remained unaltered. In children, chronic encephalopathy occurs at lower blood levels than in adults (50–60 μg Pb/100 ml blood vs. > 80 μg Pb/100 ml blood). The symptoms of chronic lead intoxication include hallucinations, excitation states, and mental disorders. The accumulation of neurotoxic ALA concentrations, which may interact with the γ-aminobutyric acid (GABA) system, as well as interference of lead with catecholamines and the cholinoceptor system, has been proposed as pathophysiological mechanism. There are unequivocal results as to the extent that the interactions between lead and calcium play a role in the neurological effects of lead. A disturbed energy metabolism may impair the blood–brain barrier and the tryptophane metabolism.

Low lead concentrations (20 and 30 μg Pb/100 ml) are assumed to have a negative impact on intelligence, learning ability, and behavior in children. Early epidemiological studies of the problem were unequivocal and did not sufficiently control for sociological stratification. Marginal increases in blood-lead concentrations may be regarded as markers of an unfavorable social environment, which, in turn, may impair the development of intelligence and learning behavior. Large studies in the United States and Australia strongly support the assumption of a causal relationship between blood-lead concentrations as low as 10 to 20 μg Pb/100 ml during pregnancy and childhood and an impaired mental development. A negative correlation between blood-lead concentrations and the results of psychomotoric intelligence and visual–motor integration tests was also found in eight cross-sectional studies in European children. However, the variance explained by low-level lead exposure was as low as 1%. Social and hereditary influences on a child's mental development must, indeed, be included in these considerations.

Peripheral lead neuropathy has become rare. It occurs at high lead concentrations (60–80 μg Pb/100 ml) and mainly affects the extensor muscle groups (e.g., wrist and ankle drops). Sensory nerves are rarely affected. These symptoms may be due to axonal degeneration and segmental demyelinization of the peripheral nerves. Impairment of peripheral-nerve function, such as reduced conduction rate, have been observed at blood lead levels between 30 and 45 μg Pb/100 ml. Such changes may be a consequence of an impaired energy metabolism in the mitochondria due to the effects of lead on cytochrome C-oxidase. These functional disturbances are reversible, at least in part. However, they may also be regarded as the early stages of the morphological damage discussed previously.

Gastrointestinal and Hepatic Effects of Lead

Chronic lead exposure leads to loss of appetite, abdominal pain, constipation, and diarrhea. However, the gastrointestinal symptoms show no strict dose–effect relationship. Lead sulfate precipitation in the gingiva due to a high oral lead exposure (lead lines or Burtonian lines) has become extremely rare.

No serious functional and morphological liver damage due to high lead exposure has been described. However, increased lead concentrations were correlated with increased concentrations of serum glutamic oxalacetic transaminase (SGOT); the ratio between albumin and globulin in the plasma was increased.

Renal Lead Effects

Nephropathy following lead exposure is rare. Increased plasma urea and plasma creatinine concentrations are more frequent in lead-exposed workers than in an unexposed population. However, no correlation was found between the severity of these symptoms and blood-lead concentrations. In adults, tubular damage has been observed after chronic lead exposure (e.g., due to the consumption of lead-contaminated whisky). Eosinophilic inclusion bodies consisting of a lead–protein complex were found in the renal tubuli after lead damage, as well as in other organs (e.g., in the liver and brain). Functional impairment after lead exposure is characterized by increased renal excretion of amino acids, glucosuria, hyperphosphaturia, hyperphosphatemia, and leakage of enzymes from the tubular tissue into the urine (e.g., *N*-acetyl-β-D-glucosaminidase). Blood-lead concentrations in excess of 70 μg Pb/100 ml over extended periods of time may lead to interstitial fibrosis and tubular atrophy, as well as arterosclerotic kidney changes resulting in azotemia and eventually in hyperuricemia. In one study, 13% of hemodialyzed patients showed elevated blood-lead concentrations (< 30 μg/dl), which is significantly more frequent than in healthy controls. Lead exposure during childhood does not seem to increase the risk of nephropathy in later life.

Cardiovascular Lead Effects

Reports of a causal relationship between lead exposure and hypertension date back to 1886. Since then, increased cardiovascular risks have been observed in animal experiments and seem probable after substantial occupational lead exposure. Doubling the blood-lead concentration seems to increase blood pressure by 1–2 mm Hg; the effect levels off at high blood-lead concentrations. However, a causal relationship has not been established because confounding factors, such as sex, age, and alcohol and cigarette consumption, were not adequately considered. Hypertension after chronic lead exposure may be secondary to kidney damage; kidney damage, in turn, could also lead to reduced lead excretion and cause elevated blood-lead levels.

Organic Lead Compounds

Tetraethyl and tetramethyl lead have been used extensively as antiknock agents to improve the octane rating in gasoline. It is distributed on a global scale and was detected in Greenland shelf ice corresponding to 1940 and later. Both compounds are colorless, liquid, and volatile. They decompose at temperatures between 100 and 200°C. The addition of ethyldihalides (Cl, Br), which are used to clean motors of lead, turns lead residues into Pb, Br, and Cl, which consequently appear in the exhaust after gasoline combustion. Leaded gasoline contains less than 0.1% lead as tetraethyl lead. Because of high gasoline consumption, more than 90% of the lead emissions in cities was derived from this source before the lead content of fuels was reduced. At gasoline stations, substantial concentrations of tetraethyl lead could be found, which represented a risk for people working at the gasoline stations. Another cause of intoxication from organic lead compounds is gasoline sniffing, which was reported to have induced high mortality rates in Australian aborigines. It is controversial, however, to what extent this is due to hydrocarbon toxicity.

Tetraethyl lead is a lipophilic compound that is absorbed quickly and to a great extent after inhalation, via the skin, and via the gastrointestinal tract. The highest concentrations are found in the liver, followed by the kidney, pancreas, brain, and heart. In most tissues, tetraethyl lead is quickly decomposed to triethyl lead, showing a half-life in the organism of more than 20 days and being excreted via the kidneys, partly as inorganic lead.

The early symptoms of tetraethyl lead intoxication are nausea, vomiting, diarrhea, fearfulness, and headache. Later the patients may suffer from cramps, delirium, and coma. Animal experiments suggest that lead trialkyl impairs the polymerization of tubulin dimers to microtubuli, causing these symptoms. However, the pathophysiological sequence of events is not completely understood. There is no specific therapy for intoxication from organic lead compounds. Chelating agents cannot influence the cause of the disease. If the intoxication is survived, the symptoms vanish within 2 to 3 months without sequels. The frequency of organic lead intoxication has decreased markedly since unleaded fuels were introduced.

Special Toxicity

Reproduction

Lead reduces spermatogenesis, sperm motility, and may cause testicular atrophy. Pb^{2+} passes the blood–placenta barrier. Bone deformations after lead exposure *in utero* were observed in hamsters. However, there is no convincing evidence for genotoxic lead effects in humans. In rats, implantation failure, reduced birth weights, and reduced survival rates of the offspring were observed after lead exposure *in utero.* In Roman days, lead compounds were used to induce abortion. Paul reported in 1860 that severely lead-poisoned women are more likely to abort or to deliver stillborn babies. These early findings were confirmed by increased stillbirth rates and preterm deliveries in women living in the vicinity of a lead smelter more than 120 years later.

Carcinogenicity

High lead exposure can induce renal neoplasia in mice and rats. However, the carcinogenicity of lead could not be demonstrated in epidemiological investigations in humans, though the single case of a 48-year-old worker describes a renal carcinoma with a lead-tissue content of 2.49 μg Pb/g. Therefore, IARC has classified lead as group 2B (i.e., chemicals that are possibly carcinogenic for humans). Organic lead compounds are classified as group 3 (i. e., chemicals for which carcinogenity is not classified for humans).

Therapeutic Measures

The determination of blood-lead concentrations and of zinc protoporphyrin IX in the erythrocyte are suitable methods of assessing the severity of lead intoxication at all exposure levels. The delta-aminolevulinic acid dehydratase activity increases at low lead-exposure levels. In severe cases, the hemoglobin concentration is reduced and erythrocytes may show a basophilic stippling.

As about 90% of the life-long cumulative lead body burden accumulates in the skeleton and can be measured by X-ray fluorescence spectrometry, blood-lead concentrations return to normal when the exposure is terminated and the lead has been distributed into the bones. In this case, the lead load can be estimated by the use of the EDTA provocation test. The cumulative lead load of the patient is too high if the urinary lead excretion during 24 h exceeds 1 mg. The renal lead excretion in an unexposed control population is below 600 μg Pb/4 days.

Acute and chronic lead intoxications are both treated with chelating agents. Thus, D-penicillamine can be given orally for lead intoxication. However, serious adverse effects have been noted (e.g., bleeding, leucopenia, neutropenia, and penicillin allergy). For several decades the recommendation was to treat children with blood-lead concentrations above 70 μg/100 ml with a parenteral combination of British Anti-Lewisite (BAL) plus $CaNa_2$–EDTA and with $CaNa_2$–EDTA alone in less severe cases (1000 mg/m^2/day, in three divided doses). The intramuscular administration of BAL is associated with nausea and vomiting in the majority of children. The administration of $CaNa_2$–EDTA goes along with the excretion of essential metals, particularly of zinc. Adverse reactions may be lacrimation, dry nasal mucosa, sneezing, muscle pain, and hypotension. Renal toxic effects were observed in particular in patients who were not adequately hydrated. In chronic renal failure with restricted renal clearance, the application of $CaNa_2$–EDTA is contraindicated. Since 1991 the U.S. EPA has approved the oral administration of *meso*–2,3-dimercaptosuccinic acid (DMSA = Succimer) for the treatment of children with blood-lead concentrations of 45 μg/dl and above.

Anemia and gastrointestinal and neurological symptoms can improve if diagnosed and treated in time. Lead encephalopathy in childhood will often lead to residual symptoms, as mentioned previously. Tubular damage in the kidney is mostly reversible in early stages, as long as it has not induced morphological damage.

MERCURY

Mercury is one of the metals known since antiquity. Acute intoxication from mercury and its compounds results mostly from their uses in agriculture and industry accidents, and improper or careless handling. Mass intoxications of epidemic extent occurred through ingestion of mercury-contaminated food, such as grain (Iraq) and fish (Minamata, Japan). Microbial methylation of mercury in the biosphere is an important process in the accumulation of mercury in the food chain.

Chemical Properties, Occurrence, and Use

At room temperature, mercury (Hg; atomic weight 200.59; oxidation states; 0, + 1, and + 2) is a liquid and volatile metal with a high vapor pressure (saturation at 20°C, 14 mg Hg/m^3); it is soluble in water to some extent (at 25°C, 0.06 mg/liter; at 90°C, 1.1 mg/liter). In addition to salts in the oxidation states +1 and +2, mercury forms organic compounds of the type RHgX or R_2Hg (where R are alkyl- or aryl-groups). Salts of mercury(I) are almost insoluble in water, exept for the nitrate and perchlorate, which are more readily soluble. In general, the salts of mercury(II) are soluble in water and because of their lipophilic nature are often also soluble in ethanol or ether. Compounds of the type RHgX are crystalline, the properties of which largely depend on the anionic rest X; with halogenides highly lipophilic compounds are formed, whereas oxygen-containing anions render the compounds more saline. Compounds of the type R_2Hg are partly volatile and highly lipophilic; most of these organic mercury compounds are chemically stable but thermally labile and light sensitive.

Mercury occurs in nature mainly as sulfidic ores, from which it is separated by roasting. A ubiquitous exposure to mercury comes from natural emissions as mercury degases from Earth's crust and the oceans (~120,000 t/year). Production is in the range of 8000 to 12,000 t/year. Large amounts of the metal are used in the production of chlorine and sodium hydroxide (chloralkali industries). The largest portion of the metal is used in electrical and electronic equipment, instruments, and apparatus. Compounds of mercury are employed as catalysts, pigments, and fungicides. In medicine, the metal is still used in dental amalgam and in a few compounds as antiseptic agents.

Absorption, Distribution, Metabolism, and Excretion

Absorption

Elemental mercury vapor is taken up from the atmosphere via the respiratory tract. A concentration of around 2 ng/m^3 is typical for entirely unpolluted areas in the Northern Hemisphere. In more polluted regions, the concentrations increase to about 3–4 and in heavily urbanized and industrialized regions concentrations of up to 20 ng/m^3 have been measured. Of mercury vapor that is inhaled, about 80% is retained in the lungs. Of this amount, 80% is taken up by the blood and the rest is retained in the lung tissue. There are no quantitative data available on the inhalative uptake of the inorganic compounds of mercury. Volatile organic mercury compounds (e.g., dimethylmercury ($CH_3 \cdot Hg \cdot CH_3$)) are absorbed by the lungs to a considerable extent (> 80%).

After ingestion, the metal is absorbed from the gastrointestinal tract. However, the absorption rate is generally rather slow (< 0.01%). Since metallic mercury is covered by a sulfidic layer within the lumen of the gastrointestinal tract, solubilization and thus absorption are markedly decreased. It is certain that the absorption rates depend also on gastrointestinal residence times and on the surface area of the metal.

No data are available for estimating the intestinal absorption rates of mercury(I) salts; however, it must be assumed that little absorption takes place. There are findings about the accumulation of mercury in the kidneys (> 0.5 mg Hg/g wet tissue) after several years of intake of mercury(I) chloride as laxative. In humans, the absorption rate of mercury(II) chloride is between 2 and 15% of the dose. As young unweaned animals can absorb up to 50% of a dose, one assumes that there is markedly higher absorption in babies and infants than in adults.

For the general population, the uptake of organic mercury compounds, particularly methylmercury ($CH_3 \cdot Hg^+$), through nutrition represents the major exposure pathway. Freshwater and marine fish, as well as other sea organisms showing concentrations of 0.2 mg Hg/kg (ww) on an average, are foods with the highest mercury levels. Freshwater herbivores are the least contaminated species (~0.02 mg/kg ww), whereas carnivores may accumulate a considerable amount, up to 20 mg/kg (ww) depending on the degree of water pollution. The intestinal absorption of methylmercury is of 90–95% in humans, independent of the form of oral administration (e.g., with or without food).

It is suggested that the dermal uptake of elemental mercury is rather low and that inhalative uptake plays a much larger role after contact of the skin or clothes with mercury; however, this is difficult to judge as quantitative data are not available. From results of animal experiments, it is known that lipophilic mercury compounds can be dermally absorbed (e.g., in guinea pigs, 8% of a dose of $HgCl_2$ within 5 h). Therefore, one should assume a certain dermal absorption of mercury compounds, although human studies are lacking.

Distribution and Metabolism

The distribution of mercury depends on the chemical form, exposure pathway, and dose. Accordingly, the distribution of mercury is different after the intake of elemental mercury vapor, mercury(II) salts, or methylmercury. These differences are predominantly seen after acute or subacute short-term exposure to these compounds, due to their different physicochemical properties. The nonpolar compounds, like mercury vapor and methylmercury chloride can cross the various blood–tissue barriers more easily than the polar ones, like mercury(II) chloride. This is of particular significance for transport across the blood–brain barrier and explains the different effects of the various compounds on the CNS.

Mercury and its compounds are metabolized in the mammalian organism. Dissolved, elemental mercury (Hg^0) is oxidized to Hg^{2+} intracellularly. In the erythrocytes, the liver, and the brain, oxidation is mainly, if not exclusively, a matter of catalase activity. After uptake as elemental vapor, it is this enzymatic oxidation that causes mercury to accumulate in the brain, as the Hg^{2+} formed does not readily diffuse back across the blood–brain barrier. This mechanism is responsible for the high risks of long-term exposure to even small concentrations of mercury vapor. Within the organism, mercury(I) salts disproportionate into Hg^0 and Hg^{2+}. Furthermore, Hg^{2+} can be reduced to Hg^0, as small amounts of elemental mercury are exhaled after the uptake of mercury(II) salts. It can be assumed from these reactions that chronic ingestion of inorganic mercury compounds facilitates mercury accumulation by the CNS.

Methylmercury and other alkylmercury compounds are slowly metabolized into Hg^{2+}. Particularly after chronic exposure, through the consumption of contaminated diets, inner organs contain mainly inorganic mercury. After high oral loads of methylmercury in humans, the following amounts of Hg^{2+} could be found: in total blood 7, in plasma 22, in milk 39, in liver 16–40, and in urine 73%. Demethylation of $MeHg^{+}$ to Hg^{2+} is predominantly performed by the intestinal flora. Owing to the marked enterohepatic circulation of methylmercury, this step results in a partial reabsorption of Hg^{2+}. This is certainly not the only source of Hg^{2+} after exposure to methylmercury, as macrophages in the spleen contribute to this demethylation. The mechanisms of the cleavage of the Hg–C bond is not clear, but it has been suggested that selenium compounds are involved. Phenyl and other arylmercury compounds appear to be more readily transformed into Hg^{2+} than alkyl derivatives.

Elemental mercury is rapidly distributed in the body within 24 h after a single exposure to mercury vapor. The appearance in the blood is relatively rapid (about 2% of the dose/liter). Uptake by erythrocytes is complete within 10 min, whereas maximal concentrations in plasma are reached after 5 to 10 h. Distribution into the brain region (after short-term exposure, about 7%) appears to be slower, as the maximum is obtained after 2–3 days. Animal studies show that mercury taken up as elemental vapor is predominantly bound to ecto- and endodermal epithelia and, therefore, in addition to its accumulation in the brain cortex, kidneys, liver, pancreas, and testes, it accumulates in the intestinal mucosa, salivary and sweat glands, the squamous epithelium of the skin, and hair.

After the uptake of mercury(II) salts, almost equal amounts of mercury are transported by the blood plasma and erythrocytes. After a single dose, most of the mercury is accumulated by the kidneys; the results of animal studies show that after 3 days, one-third and after 14 days, up to 90% is found in the kidneys. Mercury preferentially accumulates in the renal cortex where it is bound to tubular metallothionein. In addition to renal uptake, the accumulation in the liver, intestinal mucosa, skin, and testes is most important. The blood–brain barrier is not very permeable for inorganic mercury(II). In subchronic experiments with rats, the renal uptake amounted to 3% of the dose, while uptake into the brain was only 0.01%.

Methylmercury, as well as other short-chain alkyl derivatives, is distributed throughout the entire organism, yielding remarkably uniform tissue levels of mercury compared to those after the administration of other mercury compounds. This mobility results from the lipophilic properties and a fast and general exchange between SH ligands. Therefore, the blood–brain and placental barriers are crossed readily. Thus, the concentration ratio between blood and brain is about 5–10 and that between the blood of a newborn and the blood of its mother approximately 1–2. Certainly, these ratios depend on the dose and time of exposure. Particularly after chronic exposure, methylmercury accumulates in the CNS owing to its gradual transformation into Hg^{2+}.

Excretion

After the inhalative uptake of mercury vapor, the elimination of mercury occurs mainly through renal and fecal excretion of Hg^{2+}. Elemental mercury, however, can also be exhaled. Particularly after short-term exposure, exhalative elimination predominates over renal. Within the first week after a 20-min exposure to 0.1 mg Hg/m^3, 50% of the dose is excreted with the feces, 37% with the expired air, and only 13% with the urine. After several years chronic exposure to 0.05–0.2 mg Hg/m^3, the daily excretion of mercury was more equally divided between the urine (58%) and feces (42%). Therefore, it is conceivable that a high rate of exhalation immediately after short-term exposure results from a high portion of unmetabolized Hg^0. The organ half-lives vary considerably. The highest values are obtained for the CNS, the testes, and the kidneys, organs in which mercury accumulates predominantly after chronic exposure to Hg^0 (e.g., in humans, half-lives are 19 days for the brain and 64 days for the kidneys). Since renal accumulation is the most substantial one, the biological half-life of Hg^0 (about 58 days) is mainly determined by the kidneys.

The elimination of mercury after the intake of Hg^{2+} compounds is mainly by the excretion of equal amounts through the urine and feces. Small amounts can be excreted by saliva, sweat, and exhalation. Animal studies show that three phases can be distiguished in the elimination kinetics, a fast, ($t_{1/2}$ ~5 days), a medium ($t_{1/2}$ ~30 days), and a slow ($t_{1/2}$ ~90 days) phase. A similar process can be assumed for humans, for which the elimination half-life was determined to 42 days for 80% of the excreted amount.

The elimination of methylmercury appears to depend on the rate of the transformation of $MeHg^{+}$ into Hg^{2+}. Approximately 90% of a single dose of methylmercury is excreted by the feces. This is the result of the predominant biliary excretion of $MeHg^{pl}$ together with Hg^{2+}, probably mainly in form of glutathione complexes. While the reabsorption of methylmercury is high, that of Hg^{2+} is low. Part of the biliary-excreted methylmercury is demethylated by intestinal bacteria and about 10% of that is reabsorbed. This explains the fecal output of mainly Hg^{2+} and the partial accumulation of inorganic mercury after methylmercury uptake. The elimination half-life of mercury after methylmercury uptake is about 70 days and, thus, slightly higher than that after uptake of inorganic mercury. An explanation could be the accumulation of alkylmercury compounds in the erythrocytes.

Mechanisms of Toxicity

There is no doubt that the toxic effects of mercury and its compounds are based upon their reactivity with amino and sulfhydryl groups in proteins, enzymes, and other physiological components and structures. This inevitably leads to changes in the rates of enzymatic synthesis and carrier-mediated transport, in particular, when optimal functions depend on the presence of free SH groups. In these interactions, inorganic mercury(II) compounds (Hg^{2+} ions) can react with two SH-groups, whereas monoalkymercury compounds ($MeHg^+$) react only with one. By means of this feature, one explains the higher mobility and the lesser tissue accumulation of monoalkymercury compounds compared to those of mercury(II) salts. In addition, metal–mercury interactions, in particular the displacement of essential zinc ions, can play a role in mercury toxicity. These findings, however, are not specific enough to describe the mechanisms of the toxicity of mercury for the various organs and mercury compounds in detail. Since the complex interactions between kinetic and metabolic processes are not elucidated to a great extent for the various mercury compounds, subsequent alterations in cellular events are not be correlated.

Acute and Chronic Toxicity

Acute Toxicity

Acute intoxication by the inhalation of mercury vapor is rare but extremely critical. In particular, the lung is the most critical organ. Patients suffer from respiratory insufficiency and eventually become cyanotic, which are severe signs of bronchitis and bronchiolitis with interstitial pneumonia and pulmonary emphysema. Such intoxications can be observed after several hours of exposure to mercury vapor at levels around 1—3 mg Hg/m³ or above. Besides respiratory distress, fever and headache are the most frequent symptoms within the first few hours. Complications may emerge by the air insufflation of the mediastinal connective tissue (pneumomediastinum) and the development of a pneumothorax. Acute symptoms are unlikely to occur below concentrations of 0.1 mg Hg/m³ (Table 17). The inhalation toxicity of inorganic and organic mercury compounds cannot be evaluated due to the lack of corresponding findings.

When taken orally, metallic mercury is normally not very harmful. In a single case of ingestion of 204 g of metallic mercury, no signs of intoxication were observed. Occasional intoxications through enteral uptake of metallic mercury cannot be excluded, however. Altered gastrointestinal residence times due to the presence of diverticula or abscesses and the degree of dispersion of the mercury ingested may affect absorption.

The oral uptake of mercury(II) salts can lead to erosive damages of the oral and nasal cavities and the esophagus, which often are accompanied by nausea and vomiting (also hemorrhagic). Edema of the glottis may cause further complications. When after oral intake larger amounts of mercury(II) salts reach the stomach and small intestine, gastroenteritis develops together with losses of protein and electrolytes. The circulatory collapse and shock can be fatal; if not, renal damage is observed, mostly polyuria, subsequently oligouria or anuria accompanied with uremia; and finally acute kidney failure. In laboratory animals, the LD_{50} of mercury(II) salts averages

TABLE 17 Regulations, Limits, and Threshold Values for Mercury

Threshold limit values in the work environment[a]	
Alkylmercury	0.01 mg Hg/m³
Arylmercury	0.10 mg Hg/m³
Mercury (metallic)	0.05 mg Hg/m³
Inorganic mercury	0.10 mg Hg/m³
Drinking water standard[b]	3 μg Hg/liter
Guideline concentrations in food (examples)[c]	
Fresh water fish	1.00 mg Hg/kg ww
Pork	0.03 mg Hg/kg ww
Potatoes	0.02 mg Hg/kg ww
Vegetables	0.05 mg Hg/kg ww
Eggs	0.03 mg Hg/kg ww
Tolerable weekly intake[d]	<0.30 mg Hg/person

[a] ACGIH, 1988.
[b] US EPA, 1985.
[c] Guidelines, German Health Department (BVV), 1986.
[d] WHO, 1989 (provisional tolerable weekly intake).

TABLE 18 Toxicological Data for Selected Mercury Compounds

Compound	Species		Toxic dose
Mercury(II) chloride	Mouse	LD_{50}	5–7 mg Hg/kg, ip
	Rat	LD_{50}	30–50 mg Hg/kg, po
	Human	LD_{Lo}	3–15 mg Hg/kg, po
Mercury(I) chloride	Human	LD_{Lo}	30–40 mg Hg/kg, po
Methylmercury chloride	Mouse	LD_{50}	14 mg Hg/kg, ip
	Rat	LD_{50}	10 mg Hg/kg, po
	Human	LD_{Lo}	5 mg Hg/kg, po
Ethylmercury chloride	Rat	LD_{50}	14 mg Hg/kg, ip
	Rat	LD_{50}	50 mg Hg/kg, po
Phenylmercury acetate	Mouse	LD_{50}	8 mg Hg/kg, ip
	Mouse	LD_{50}	16 mg Hg/kg, iv
	Mouse	LD_{50}	26 mg Hg/kg, po
	Rat	LD_{50}	60 mg Hg/kg, po
	Human	LD_{Lo}	5 mg Hg/kg, po

5 mg Hg/kg body weight after parenteral and is about 10-fold higher after oral administration. In humans the minimal lethal oral dose is in the range of 3–5 mg Hg/kg body weight (Table 18).

In contrast to the toxicity of phenyl and alkoxymercury compounds, which resembles that of the inorganic mercury salts, the toxicity of methyl- and other short-chain alkyl mercury compounds is primarily characterized by CNS effects. Initially unspecific symptoms like nausea and paresthesia occur, followed by the loss of sensation in the extremities, incoordination (ataxia), difficulty in speaking (dysarthria) and hearing (dysaudia), and constriction of the visual fields. Most severe intoxications lead to coma and death. After uptake of high doses of methylmercury, as happened in the Iraq epidemic, an impairment of the peripheral nervous system (damage to the neuromuscular endplate) can be observed, in addition. Methylmercury poisoning is characterized by an extended latent period (Fig. 9), which appears to be dose dependent. Thus, in the Iraq epidemic ($MeHg^+$ intake, 5–15 mg Hg/day) a mean latency of 16–38 days was recorded, whereas after ingestion of mercury-contaminated fish ($MeHg^+$ intake, 1.5–4 mg Hg/day) in a Japanese epidemic (Minamata), latent periods of several years were observed.

Chronic Toxicity

Chronic intoxication by the inhalation of elemental mercury vapor mainly occurs in the work place (e.g., via spillage of metallic mercury). Akrodynia and nephrotic syndrome are the dominant signs. Inflammations of the gingiva and the oral cavity as well as tremor (tremor mercurialis) and a morbid excitability (erethism) are among the most characteristic symptoms. Furthermore, polyneuropathy frequently develops.

Mercury concentrations in the urine, blood, and hair are used to diagnose chronic mercury intoxication and to evaluate its degree of severity. Legal requirements and threshold values for industrial safety and hygiene purposes certainly differ among countries. However, the values adopted by most industrialized countries in the Western Hemisphere mostly fall in a narrow range. In Germany the BAT value describes concentration limits in the blood and urine of persons working with mercury that can be tolerated without medical intervention (Table 17). Tremor and other psychomotoric changes are very likely to occur above urinary concentrations of 500 ng Hg/ml. However, they may develop at urinary concentrations of 100 ng Hg/ml, above which an increase in unspecific signs such as loss of appetite and insomnia can also be observed. Symptoms of early nephrosis (proteinuria) have been noticed in workers exposed to mercury vapor at concentration of up to 0.1 mg Hg/m^3; in these workers urinary excretion amounted to 53 μg Hg/24 h. Chronic intoxication by inorganic mercury is rare; for occupational intoxication generally a simultaneous inhalation of mercury vapor can be assumed.

The symptoms of chronic intoxication by methylmercury correspond with those of acute intoxication. Accordingly, with increases in dose, a gradual transition to more severe symptoms is generally observed. Data obtained from the Iraqi epidemic intoxication by methylmercury indicate a risk for paresthesia of approximately 0.3% after an oral uptake of 50 μg Hg/day and of 8% when uptake increases to 200 μg Hg/day (Fig. 9). This is in agreement with

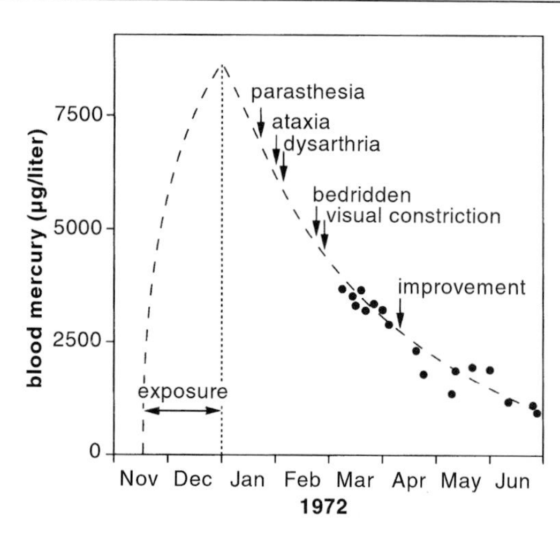

FIGURE 9 The sequence of appearance of signs and symptoms of methyl mercury poisoning in a patient exposed to methyl mercury in homemade bread in the Iraq outbreak. The patient was admitted to hospital in March 1972, when measurements of mercury in blood (open circles) were started. The dashed line prior to March is a recapitulation of blood levels based on patient's history of exposure, bread intake, and the biological half-time in blood. Paresthesia, usually the first symptom of methylmercury poisoning, did not appear until approximately 3 weeks after the peak blood level. More serious signs of brain damage appeared later and the full syndrome took approximately 2 months to develop completely. Later, some functional improvement was observed, and the patient was no longer bedridden. (From Clarkson, 1983).

data indicating a 5% prevalence of initial symptoms after long-term methylmercury uptake of daily 3–7 μg Hg/kg body weight which leads to 200–500 ng Hg/ml in the blood and 50–125 μg Hg/g in the hair. In a Japanese epidemic (Minamata), however, the symptoms of a chronic methylmercury intoxication were observed at hair concentrations of 10 μg Hg/g (30 ng Hg/ml blood), indicating that the threshold values might be lower in cases of extremely extended exposure times.

Amalgam fillings contribute to the mercury exposure of humans. A continuous and mobilizable (e.g., through tooth brushing) release of mercury vapor can be detected; in exhaled air, concentrations between 0.1 and 62 μg Hg/m^3 have been measured. Mercury can also be released in form of mercury(II) ions and metallic particles. The significance of this release for the overall exposure to mercury and its impact on the chronic toxicity of mercury is, however, highly controversial. On average, amalgam tooth fillings add 0.5–30 μg Hg/day to a dietary and environmental uptake of 1–6 (without fish) or 2–25 (with fish) μg Hg/day. Although there is an increase in mercury concentrations in the urine and blood depending on the number of amalgam fillings, for the majority of these concentrations, levels fall within a range considered normal and tolerable in most industrialized countries. In about 90% of the population not occupationally exposed to mercury, the blood and urine levels are below 20 and 10 ng Hg/ml, respectively. Occasionally, levels are observed above these figures, with a subsequent normalization after the removal of the amalgam fillings, these are arguments for a more critical evaluation of the use of dental amalgam.

Special Toxicity

Reproduction Toxicity

Teratogenic effects of mercury(II) salts are known only from animal studies. It is unclear whether this applies also to humans. The epidemics of Iraq and Japan demonstrate that methylmercury excerts toxic effects on fetal growth and development. Methylmercury permeates the placenta and accumulates in the fetal blood, in a concentration that is about twice that of the maternal blood. In newborns of heavily exposed Iraqi mothers, blood levels between 40–4000 ng Hg/ml were found. As these levels were not measured directly after delivery, but at various later times, one has to assume there were higher levels at birth. These children exhibited the following symptoms: prolonged persistance of primitive reflexes, mental impairment, retarded growth and development, disturbance in mastication and swallowing, disturbance in motility and impairment of coordination (ataxia), and constriction of the visual fields. All of these toxic symptoms may not necessarily be observed at early stages, probably depending on the prenatal dose; some may develop later in childhood, such as hyperreflexia and disturbances in motor activity and speech. Maternal blood-mercury concentrations of 700–2000 ng Hg/ml were associated with the most severe symptoms in the newborns, several of which died either in early infancy or childhood. On the basis of the risk assessments, after exposure to methyl mercury, maternal blood levels of 50 ng Hg/ml are considered as a threshold value for the onset of neurological symptoms in the fetus.

Mutagenicity and Carcinogenicity

The results from animal studies suggest the induction of chromosome aberrations by mercury. However, the small number of studies of chromosome aberrations in humans by inorganic and organic mercury compounds are contradictory, so that this issue is not settled. There are a few statistical suggestions concerning an increased frequency of aneuploidy in dental personnel exposed to amalgam. However, *in vitro* investigations with mercury(II) chloride in mammalian cells did not indicate chromosome aberrations and studies employing human lymphocytes could not detect sister chromatid exchanges.

Single findings hint of some carcinogenic potential of mercury. In rats, injections of metallic mercury can produce sarcoma and after the administration of methylmercury, renal carcinomas were observed; in addition, methylmercury may enhance the carcinogenic potency of sodium nitrite and methyl nitrosourea. The significance of these findings for humans is rather low because there is no evidence of any carcinogenic effect of mercury in humans.

Therapeutic Measures

The intestinal absorption of mercury(II) salts can be interrupted by the administration of activated charcoal. A complex-forming agent that is recommended as an antidote for inorganic mercury poisoning is Dimercaprol (BAL, British Anti-Lewisite); it can also be administered after intoxication from aryl mercury compounds, as these are readily metabolized to mercury(II). Dimercaprol is, however, not indicated in cases of intoxication by mono- or dialkymercury compounds because it results in an enhanced accumulation of mercury in the CNS; also in case of elemental mercury poisoning, its use is rather questionable.

Instead of Dimercaprol, more water-soluble antidotes have been recommended for enhancing mercury elimination after inorganic mercury poisoning. Dimercaptosuccinic acid (DMSA) and the less toxic 2,3-dimercaptopropane-1-sulfonate (DMPS) are used to increase the urinary excretion of mercury. DMPS decreased the elimination half-lives from 33.1 days to 11.2 days in workers exposed to excessive concentrations of mercury vapor. DMPS might even be useful in the treatment of methylmercury poisoning, as it reduced the elimination half-life in blood from about 65 to 10 days. In addition, D-penicillamine and its derivatives appear to be appropriate antidotes for the treatment of elemental and inorganic mercury poisoning.

Complex-forming agents increasing urinary excretion of mercury should only be administered if no renal insufficiency has been developed. In cases of anuria, hemodialysis together with infusions of cysteine might remove enough mercury to allow a regeneration of damaged tubuli.

NICKEL

Functional roles for nickel have been defined for bacteria, fungi, plants, and invertebrates, where it serves essential functions in ureases and in Ni,Fe-hydrogenases. For humans no defined essential function is reported. However, nickel has a wide variety of technical uses. Its yearly production is 750,000 t and it is part of more than 3000 alloys.

Chemical Characteristics, Sources, and Uses

Nickel (atomic weight 58.7, specific density 8.9 g/cm^3, melting point 1453°C) is a silvery-white tractable metal occurring mostly in the oxidation states Ni^0 and Ni^{2+}, but also Ni^{1+}, Ni^{3+}, and Ni^{4+}. Nickel oxide and nickel subsulfide (insoluble in water), as well as the water-soluble nickel sulfate and nickel chloride, are of toxicological interest. Nickel carbonyl ($Ni(CO)_4$) is a volatile fluid with a boiling point of 43°C, which decomposes at temperatures over 50°C. It is used in nickel purification, as a catalyst in the petroleum and plastics industries and in nickel-vapor plating. It is highly toxic. More than 90% of nickel for technical purposes is extracted from nickel sulfide ore (pentlandide, $(FeNi)_9S_8$). Nickel ores are mined mainly in Canada, New Caledonia, and Russia. Forty percent of yearly nickel production is used in the production of stainless steel and 20% is used for galvanization. Dry batteries, for example, contain nickel together with cadmium.

Absorption, Distribution, Metabolism, and Excretion

The kinetics and toxicity of nickel depend on whether it is taken up in a metallic, soluble, or non-soluble form or as organic compound. In Germany the maximum permissible concentration in the air for different nickel compounds is set between 0.05 and 0.5 mg/m^3; in Sweden these values are set 5 times lower.

The average daily nickel intake in the United States is in the range of 0.3 to 0.5 mg per capita. Air nickel concentrations in rural areas are as low as 6–25 ng/m^3, in New York city approximately 150 ng Ni/m^3 have been determined. As coal and oil contain up to 20 and 400 mg Ni/kg, respectively, these differences are explained by much higher energy consumption in the cities. In the vicinity of nickel refineries, nickel concentrations may rise to 1.2 $\mu g/m^3$. In consequence, an urban population inhales between 2 and 14 μg Ni/day. For comparison, a cigarette contains about 2.3 ng nickel. The nickel content in food varies between 0.1 and 6.5 $\mu g/g$, and nickel intake varies between 150 and 700 μg/day. A diet with a nickel content above 250 μg Ni/g induced toxic symptoms in rats, mice, dogs, cows, pigs, and monkeys.

About 1% of nickel is absorbed when it is administered with food compared to about 30% after the administration of nickel dissolved in water on an empty stomach. Intestinal nickel absorption is mediated partly by energy-consuming active-transfer processes in the small intestine and partly by simple diffusion. Insoluble Ni salts are phagocytized. Nickel is absorbed by the skin, mainly via the sweat ducts and hair follicles. Significant nickel quantities are bound by the epidermis. Surgical implants may release substantial nickel amounts which, however, rarely leads to allergic manifestations.

In human plasma, nickel is mainly bound to albumin. Smaller fractions bind to nickeloplasmin or they form nickel–histidine or nickel–histidine–albumin complexes. The average serum nickel concentration is in the range of 0.1–0.6 μg/liter; older studies found values between 1.5 and 5.0 μg/liter. The serum nickel concentration may rise above 7.5 μg/liter after high nickel exposure which, besides increased urinary nickel concentrations, is regarded as a reliable sign of excess nickel intake. In the urine the nickel content ranges between 0.4 and 3.1 μg/liter.

The adult organism contains about 10 mg nickel. After intravenous application of soluble nickel salts to rats, the highest nickel concentrations were found in the kidney. The liver and lungs may also contain a substantial amount of nickel, but only the pulmonary nickel content increases with age. Insoluble nickel salts are phagocytized by the reticuloendothelial system and subsequently deposited in the lymph nodes, liver, and kidneys. Crystalline nickel subsulfide is phagocytized to a greater extent than amorphous nickel subsulfide. Nickel passes through the placenta.

After absorption, nickel carbonyl is decomposed to nickel and carbon monoxide. The CO moiety binds to hemoglobin and represents no toxic risk. Up to 50% of the released nickel circulates with the blood and accumulates in parenchymal organs. Up to 30% is found in muscles and fat and approximately 15% in bones and connective tissue. Nickel carbonyl is excreted via the lung during the first hour after intravenous application. After metabolic decomposition to CO and Ni, the nickel moiety is excreted via the kidney.

After parenteral application, about 90% of nickel is excreted via the kidney with a biological half-life >7 days. Only a small fraction is excreted via the bile. Enterohepatic circulation has not been described. To a small extent, nickel is excreted via salivation and perspiration. After inhalation, insoluble nickel species are retained in the lung while soluble nickel salts, such as nickel sulfate and nickel chloride, are cleared more rapidly. The half-life for the clearance of soluble nickel compounds from the plasma is 14–40 hours.

Acute and Chronic Nickel Toxicity

Acute Toxicity

Nickel salts show little acute toxicity. After high quantities are ingested, nickel may induce nausea and vomiting. Nickel tetracarbonyl is the most toxic nickel compound. It is generated during the refining process according to Mond. Because of its high lipid solubility nickel carbonyl is absorbed well in the lung and passes through the blood–brain barrier. The LD_{50} of nickel carbonyl was 67 and 240 mg/m^3 after inhalative exposure in mice and rats, respectively. Severe alveolar damage was observed in mice and rats 4 to 6 days after a short nickel carbonyl exposure (30 minutes). In humans the first symptoms after the inhalation of nickel carbonyl are nausea, vomiting, headache, dyspnea, fatigue, vertigo, insomnia, and chest pain, which appear with the characteristic odor of nickel cabonyl in the exhaled breath. After an asymptomatic interval that may last between 12 h and 5 days, pneumonia may develop with dyspnea, coughing, substernal pain, tachycardia, and muscular weakness. Death may result from respiratory failure as well as from cerebral edema and hemorrhage. The liver, kidneys, and adrenal glands may be damaged. Surviving patients recover slowly. The threat of a nickel carbonyl intoxication correlates with the nickel concentration in the urine. Concentrations above 500 μg Ni/liter characterize a serious situation. Diethyldithiocarbamate is generally accepted as the most suitable antidote in nickel carbonyl toxicity, although its effectiveness has not been proven by clinical trials.

Chronic Toxicity

In inhalation trials with poorly soluble nickel compounds, rats showed sinusitis and ulcerations of the nasal mucosa. Adenoid cell transformations in the lung as well as metaplasia and abscesses were observed in mice. Nickel accumulates in the nasal mucosa. The removal half-life of nickel from the nasal mucosa in retired nickel workers is about 3.5 years. Exposure to nickel aerosols caused damage of the nasal mucosa in workers in galvanic plants. Epithelial dysplasia of the nasal mucosa is more frequent in nickel workers than in a matched control population. Its extent depends on the kind and duration of nickel exposure, as well as on smoking habits.

Nickel also accumulates in the alveolar septa, where it may cause damage leading to emphysema and pneumoconiosis. The soluble nickel salts, such as nickel chloride, inhibit mucociliary clearance and increased the incidence of viral pneumonia in mice in some studies. In addition, inhalation of Ni^{2+} salt containing dusts may cause asthma and pneumoconiosis in humans in rare cases. A mixed exposure to nickel and additional hazardous substances in dust has not been excluded in the pathogenesis of occupational pneumoconiosis.

A concentration of more than 250 μg Ni/g in the diet was required to produce toxic nickel symptoms in rats, dogs, and monkeys. Accidental oral ingestion of an estimated amount of 0.5–2.5 g of soluble Ni^{2+} salts leads to nausea and abdominal cramps, diarrhea, vertigo, and lassitude. The symptoms last from a few hours to a few days; at oral doses up to 18 μg Ni/kg body weight, no adverse effects were observed in humans. The intravenous application of nickel doses above 1 mg/kg to animals damaged the kidneys and inhibited glucose metabolism. Such systemic effects have not been observed in humans.

Allergic Manifestations

Nickel dermatitis is the prototype of a delayed-type hypersensitivity. After occupational exposure, nickel dermatitis usually starts as a papular or maculopapular efflorescences in the hands. Chronic nickel dermatitis tends to lichenification. The prevalence of nickel dermatitis is between 7 and 10% in women and 1 and 2% in men in industrialized countries. Up to 20% of females reacted positively to clinical patch testing with nickel. Nickel dermatitis is regarded as the most widespread allergy among women, as nickel alloys are contained in jewelry, coins, and cooking pots. Work-related nickel dermatitis is common among skin diseases as a cause of permanent disability. After oral ingestion of large doses of nickel (>7 μg Ni/kg/day) nickel eczema tends to be exacerbated. The average dietary nickel intake is approximately 2–3 μg Ni/kg/day. Accordingly, in clinical studies the ingestion of 2.5 mg nickel sulfide worsened chronic nickel eczema in 17 of 28 cases; a diet with low nickel content improved the clinical symptoms in 9 of 17 patients.

Special Toxicology

Nickel has a low nephrotoxicity; in humans cardiovascular risk is not related to nickel exposure.

Reproductive Toxicity

The application of 5 mg Ni/liter in the drinking water over three generations increased the mortality of rat pups and caused stunted growth. The parenteral application of nickel acetate i.v. on the eighth day of pregnancy caused malformation in hamsters; application of nickel chloride caused abortions and stillbirths in mice and rats. Nickel carbonyl showed teratogenic effects in hamsters and rats after inhalation. In humans no malformations have been reported after nickel exposure.

Carcinogenity

Carcinogenic effects after occupational nickel exposure have been known for more than 60 years; they are well documented. Accordingly, the IARC classifies nickel salts, such as nickel carbonate, nickel hydroxide, nickel subsulfide, nickel sulfate, and nickel tetracarbonyl as group 1 (known carcinogenic agent in humans). In contrast, metallic nickel is classified as group 2 B (i.e., possibly carcinogenic in humans). After inhalation, nickel workers tend to develop neoplasia in the nasal and paranasal mucosa after shorter latency periods than in the lung. The nickel content of the nasal mucosa is increased after occupational exposure, showing a half-life of 3.5 years in these tissues. Nasal carcinoma after nickel exposure are squamous in 48% and adenocarcinomas in 6% of the cases. Anaplastic carcinomas or anaplastic areas were found in 49%.

Inhalation of nickel concentrations over 1 mg/m^3 is recognized prerequisite for the carcinogenic effect of nickel. Since the 1930s the cancer risk for nickel-exposed workers has been markedly reduced by suitable protective measures. Still, the risk of developing a nasal carcinoma is 40 times higher than in a matched control population. Oral and dermal nickel exposures are not related to an increased risk for cancerous diseases. Nickel carbonyl has been shown to be carcinogenic in animal but not so in humans.

Mechanisms of Carcinogenic Effects

The carcinogenic potential of nickel compounds is correlated to their cellular uptake and access to nuclear chromatin. Potent nickel carcinogens such as crystalline Ni subsulfides and crystalline Ni sulfides lead to a high incidence of cancer at exposure sites, such as nasal and lung cancer after inhalation in occupational settings. In animal experiments, tumors in the muscle, kidneys, and testes can be produced by the local injection of such nickel compounds. Water-insoluble nickel compounds, as with the strong nickel carcinogens mentioned are readily phagocytized, while the less carcinogenic amorphous nickel sulfide is not. Water-soluble nickel salts cannot enter cells as readily. In consequence, these compounds were carcinogenic only after intraperitoneal injection in rats and mice.

Nickel has a very low binding constant for DNA. High intracellular levels of Mg and Mn were shown to inhibit nickel carcinogenesis, which is thought to be due to competitive interaction for binding sites at nuclear proteins. However, because of homeostatic regulation, intracellular Mg and Mn concentrations are difficult to elevate *in vivo*. When bound to chromatin, nickel may generate oxidative DNA damage, which may lead to DNA–DNA and DNA–protein cross-linking and to deletion of DNA sequences. As nickel binds preferentially to heterochromatin, such deletions will mainly occur in highly concentrated DNA–protein structures (i.e., in transcriptonally inactive areas of the DNA). In addition, as in chemical carcinogenesis, nickel carcinogenesis involves mediation via onocogenes and tumor-suppressor genes such as the *ras* gene on chromosome 12, the suppressor gene p53 on chromosome 17, or deletion of senescence genes.

Therapeutic Measures

Nickel excretion can be increased by lipid-soluble chelating agents, such as triethylentetramine (TETA) and cyclan. Hydrophilic chelating agents, such as EDTA, are less effective, probably because they do not reach nickel in intracellular compartments. Sodium diethyldithiocarbamate is the chelator of choice in nickel carbonyl intoxication. Other chelating agents are less effective and may even worsen the symptoms in some cases.

PLATINUM METALS

Compared to other heavy metals, platinum metals did not receive much toxicological interest in the past. Use of noble elements as metals in alloys or by themselves was not considered problematic for the public in general. Industrial progress and the increasing use of platinum metal as catalysts and in complex compounds in medicine, however, have contributed to an increase in the toxicological significance of these metals and their compounds in recent years.

Chemical Properties, Occurrence, and Use

Platinum metals (Table 19) are transition metals and belong to Group VIII of the periodic table. The majority of their compounds are anionic and cationic complexes, particularly in aqueous systems. Based on the electronic structure of the elements and their ions, one can assume in biological systems the formation of stable compounds with a coordination number of six and an octahedral configuration. Exceptions to this scheme are likely to occur with palladium and osmium. A stable square planar configuration can be proposed only for palladium(II) and platinum(II); for the other elements this configuration is too labile to be of biological relevance.

In principle, all platinum metals occur in mixtures. Besides elemental occurence in iron and nickel ores, platinum metals are found in various minerals as sulfides and arsenides. Although most well-known as a precious metal in jewelry, platinum metals and their compounds have found numerous applications (e.g., in the chemical industry as catalysts for synthesizing organic chemicals). Owing to their resistance to corrosion, the metals are applied in the electrical, electronic, glass, and textile industries. In the 1990s, platinum metals have gained the most widespread use as automobile exhaust catalysts. Probably the most special application is found in the medical use of planar

TABLE 19 Platinum Metals

Element	Symbol	Atomic number	Atomic weight	Prefered oxidation state in compounds
Ruthenium	Ru	44	101.1	+2, +3, +4, +6, +8
Rhodium	Rh	45	102.9	+1, +3
Palladium	Pd	46	106.4	+2, +4
Osmium	Os	76	190.2	+2, +3, +4, +6, +8
Iridium	Ir	77	192.2	+1, +3, +4
Platinum	Pt	78	195.1	+2, +4

cis-platinum complexes (e.g., diamminodichloro platinum(II), cisplatin) in chemotherapy for cancer.

Absorption, Distribution, Metabolism, and Excretion

All these processes depend on the chemical form of the metal compounds, and thus on their solubility, reactivity, and stability in aqueous media. Limited information is available on the inhalative absorption of platinum metals and their compounds. In the case of ruthenium and platinum and their compounds, the inhalative uptake may be more substantial than the gastrointestinal. About half the amount inhaled is retained by the lungs; subsequent redistribution from the lung tissue is rather slow. In this respect, the compounds of rhodium behave in a similar manner. In contrast, the inhalative absorption of palladium is low but retention in the lung tissue high. Osmium is readily inhaled as osmium(VIII) oxide (osmium tetroxide, OsO_4), which represents a very volatile substance (boiling point 131.2°C) released from aqueous solutions into the air at room temperature. Although more labile, ruthenium(VIII) oxide exhibits similar features. No information is available concerning the inhalative absorption of iridium.

Quantitative investigations of the enteral absorption and distribution of platinum metal compounds in humans are rare. Animal studies demonstrate gastrointestinal absorption rates for platinum metal salts that are lower than for iron salts (<5–10%). Owing to the low absorption rate, platinum metal compounds enterally administered are predominantly excreted with the feces.

Animal studies indicate that more unstable compounds, such as the oxides of the highest oxidation state, which are strongly oxidative and therefore reduced to the elemental metal within the organism (e.g., OsO_4), are deposited at the site of administration. From these deposits, platinum metals are distributed and subsequently excreted at an extremely low rate. More stable compounds (e.g., chloropalladinates, hexachloroiridates, and chloroplatinates) are distributed to the inner organs, particularly to the kidneys, and excreted relatively quickly; thus, between 20 and 50% can be excreted renally 24 h after administration. For most stable complexes (e.g. tris-1, 10-phenanthroline ruthenium perchloride) renal excretion reaches 90% in the first 24 h, followed by a phase of slower excretion. There are findings of the sustained retention of ruthenium in bone. As chloroplatinates are excreted fecally after parenteral administration, biliary excretion is suggested.

Mechanism of Toxicity

Beyond a description of the chemical reactivity to hydroxy, amino, and sulfhydryl groups and suggestions on subsequent interactions, a more detailed explanation of the mechanisms by which platinum metal compounds cause toxic symptoms cannot be provided. Nothing is known about how the metallic dust of these metals affects the organism. The oxidative potential of compounds of the highest oxidation state certainly results in local damage to tissues in contact with these compounds, but to state more is speculative. Similarily unknown are the mechanisms of induction as well as of inhibition of tumor growth. In case of the action of *cis*-platinum complexes, complex formation with heterocyclic bases of the DNA is thought to be responsible.

Acute and Chronic Toxicity

There is little quantitative data on the acute toxicity of platinum metals and their compounds in humans. Except for the dusts, the metals themselves are not considered to be very toxic. The human intradermal lowest toxic dose (TD_{Lo}) is about 40 mg/kg for potassium hexachloroplatinate and platinum tetrachloride, and the i.v. TD_{Lo} for *cis*-diamminodichloro platinum is around 2.5 mg/kg. Animal studies provide more data on the toxicity of particular compounds (Table 20). In these studies renal damage is the most common toxic sign from palladium, osmium, and platinum compounds either after i.v. or i.p. administration. Among planar platinum complexes, cis complexes are more toxic than the corresponding trans isomers, one reason for the limited use of *cis*-platinum complexes in chemotherapy of cancer. Besides gastrointestinal disturbances, such as nausea and vomiting, sensitization reactions such as eczema and dermatitis, are observed after the administration of *cis*-platinum complexes. More serious are the ototoxic, neurotoxic, and particularly nephrotoxic symptoms, however. In addition to their renal toxicity, rhodium compounds may also cause toxic symptoms in the CNS. The readily volatile osmium tetroxide is highly toxic to the mucous membranes. At concentration levels of around 0.1 mg OsO_4/m^3 conjunctivitis, headache, and respiratory insufficiency are observed. The acute effects of iridium compounds are unknown.

A platinum allergy (platinosis) set off by contact to soluble platinum compounds, essentially chloroplatinates, represents one of the most predominant chronic effect of platinum metals. Conjunctivitis, acute rhinitis, irritation and inflammation of the oral cavity

TABLE 20 Toxicity of Selected Compounds of Platinum Metals

Compound	Species	Toxic doses (mg metal/kg body weight)	
Ruthenium trichloride	Rat	LD_{50}	360 ip
Ruthenium dioxide	Rat	LD_{50}	4850 po
Rhodium trichloride	Rat	LD_{50}	140 ip
	Rat	LD_{50}	200 iv
	Rabbit	LD_{50}	215 iv
Palladium dichloride	Mouse	LD_{50}	60 ip
	Rat	LD_{50}	200 po
	Rabbit	LD_{Lo}	11 iv
Platinum dichloride	Rabbit	LD_{Lo}	17 iv
Platinum tetrachloride	Rat	LD_{50}	15 iv
Diamminodichloro platinum	Rat	LD_{50}	8 ip

and the upper respiratory tract, and bronchial asthma belong to the characteristic symptoms of this type-I allergy, which is assumed not to be caused by finely dispersed metallic platinum. Similar allergenic properties are described for soluble palladium salts. Whether other platinum metals and their compounds possess an allergenic potential is largely unknown. Chronic inhalation of small amounts of osmium tetroxide leads to lower counts of erythrocytes and leukocytes in guinea pigs, which is thought to reflect an impairment of reticulocytosis. The chronic toxicity of rhodium and iridium compounds is essentially unknown. In occupational health, similar threshold-limit values restricting exposure in the work place are established in most industrialized countries (Table 21).

Owing to the use of platinum metals in automobile exhaust catalysts, platinum, rhodium, and palladium are emitted into the atmosphere; 90% of this is in the elemental form. There is some controversy as to the ecotoxicological significance of these emissions. At present, the concentrations in air do not exceed values between 10 and 100 ng/m^3; the hazardous potential is certainly much lower than that of nitrogen oxides, hydrocarbons, and carbon monoxide emitted without the application of these catalysts.

TABLE 21 Threshold Limit Values for Platinum Metals and Compounds in the Work Environment[a]

Substance	Concentration
Rhodium (metallic dust)	1.0 mg/m^3
Rhodium compounds (insoluble)	1.0 mg Rh/m^3
Rhodium compounds (soluble)	0.01 mg Rh/m^3
Osmium tetroxide	0.002 mg Os/m^3
Platinum (metallic dust)	1.0 mg/m^3
Platinum compounds (soluble)	0.002 mg Pt/m^3

[a]TLV, ACGIH (1988).

Special Toxicity

Reproduction Toxicology

The teratogenic potential of platinum metals and their compounds in humans is unknown. Studies in chick embryos demonstrate teratogenic properties of rhodium trichloride as signs of micromelia (reduction of limb size) and an inhibition in the feather growth have been noticed; palladium dichloride was without effect in these studies.

Mutagenicity

Similarily incomplete are data on the mutagenic properties of platinum metal compounds. Complexes of ruthenium and platinum exhibit positive reactions in the Ames test.

Carcinogenicity

Single findings indicate carcinogenic properties of some platinum metal compounds. The administration of rhodium trichloride (5 mg/liter) produced lymphoma–leukemia tumors in mice. Based on studies in mice leading to the induction of lung adenomas, cisplatin can be classified as a moderately active carcinogen; skin papillomata have also been observed.

PLUTONIUM

Substantial amounts of plutonium were released into the environment by the explosion of two nuclear bombs, in Hiroshima and Nagasaki, in 1945. The actinide present in the fall-out from nuclear-weapon explosions in the atmosphere is mainly plutonium. Traces of americum, curium, and neptunium can be measured. The most frequent plutonium isotope is ^{239}Pu. During atmospheric testing of nuclear weapons (1954–1962) about 6 metric tons of plutonium (^{239}Pu) were distributed into the stratosphere (Fig. 10). The fall-out mainly precipitated over the Northern Hemisphere. Plutonium is used mainly in nuclear power plants (reprocessing) and for the production of nuclear weapons.

Chemical Properties, Occurrence, and Use

Plutonium (Pu; molecular weight 240) is a silver-white metal. Between room temperature and melting point, there are six temperatures at which plutonium shows different heat coefficients of expansion. Because of this property, its low melting point (640°C), and its tendency to form alloys with a large number of metals, pure plutonium is not suitable as nuclear material.

The transuranic metal oxidizes easily, especially in the presence of water. The reactivity of the metal is increased by a self-heating process resulting from alpha decay. The chemistry of plutonium in solution is complex because of hydrolysis, formation of polynuclear ions, complexing with anions (exceptional perchlorates), and disproportioning reactions at some oxidation states. Chelating agents form stable complexes mainly with Pu(IV) and Pu(VI). The most important oxide is PuO_2. There are 15 isotopes of plutonium (Table 22). They are formed by multiple neutron capture from ^{238}U. During reprocessing, these isotopes can be isolated. Since ^{244}Pu was found in the mineral bastnesite plutonium is considered to be a naturally occuring element; however, more than 99.9% of the plutonium measured in the environment is anthropogenic.

Absorption, Distribution, Metabolism, and Excretion

In occupational exposure, inhalative and percutaneous absorption plays a major role (e.g., in aerosols and solutions). Oral uptake from contaminated drinking water or food is the most important pathway for the general population. Plutonium-containing aerosols are the main source for inhalative plutonium uptake. The particle size is of particular importance for its deposition in the respiratory tract, as well as for its bioavailability. Presently it is assumed that 25 to 50% of an aerosol will be retained in the lungs if the average particle size is about 1 μm. The remaining 50 to 75% are eliminated rapidly from the respiratory to gastrointestinal tract by ciliary clearance. The total lung clearance of inhaled plutonium shows a rapid intial half-life ($t_{1/2} \sim 1$ day) and slows down considerably in a second phase ($t_{1/2} \sim 500$–700 days). The absorption of plutonium from the respiratory tract to the blood is slow.

The intestinal absorption of plutonium is very small compared to other heavy metals (~0.01% compared to 5–50% for Fe and Cu). Plutonium has an extraordinarily long biological half-life in target organs, as well as a long half-life for its radioactive decay. Therefore, even small quantities of plutonium, due to alpha-particle emission, can be of toxicological importance (Table 22). Limited animal data suggest that plutonium shows nonlinear absorption kinetics. The absorption rate of plutonium seems to increase at

TABLE 22 Selection of the Most Important Plutonium Isotopes and Their Radioactive Characteristics[a]

Isotope	Half-life (y)	Type of radiation	Radiation energy (MeV)
^{238}Pu	86	α	5.50
^{239}Pu	2.4×10^4	α	5.15
^{240}Pu	6.6×10^3	α	5.16
^{241}Pu	13	β	0.021
^{242}Pu	3.8×10^3	α	4.90
^{244}Pu	7.6×10^7	α	—

[a]Schäfer *et al.* (1994).

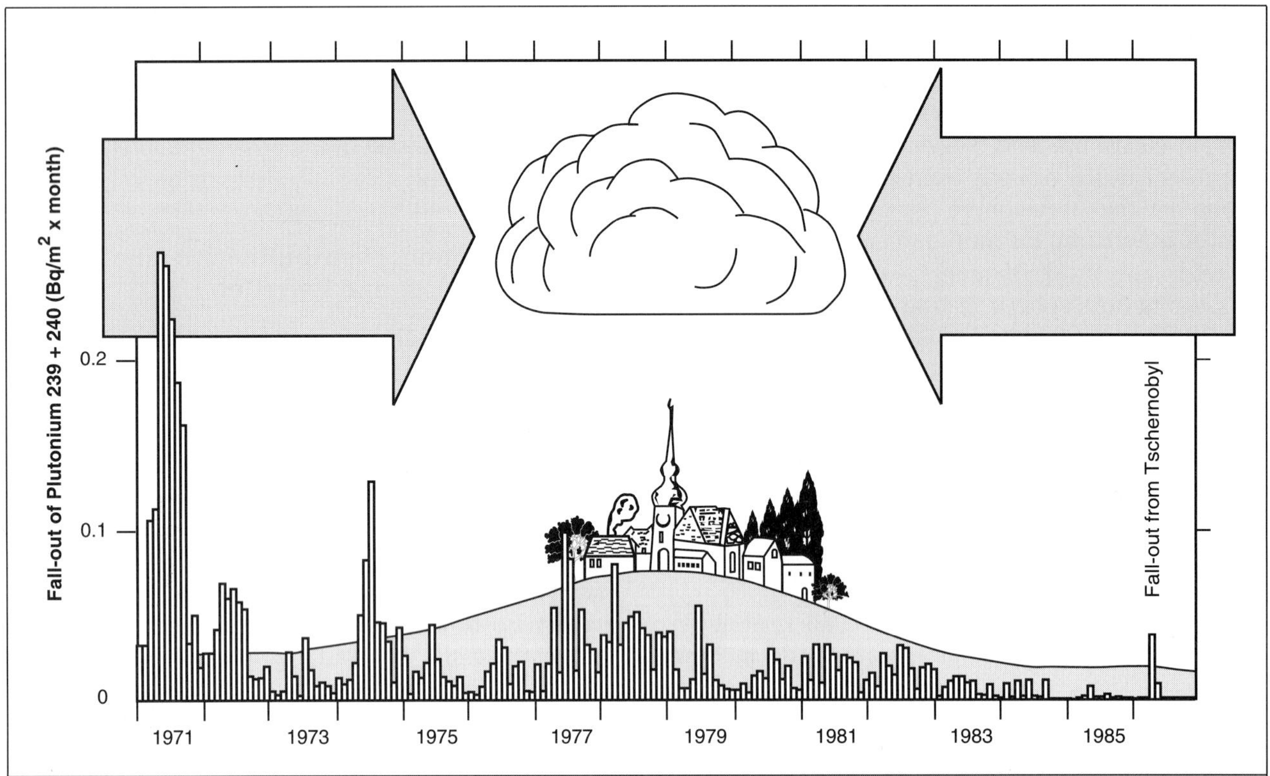

FIGURE 10 Plutonium-239 + 240 fall-out at Munich (Southern Germany) between 1971 and 1986. The data represent the average monthly monitoring values as measured by the GSF (Society for Radiation and Environmental Research) in Neuherberg (north of Munich). The increase in Plutonium-239 + 240 fall-out in the summer 1971 reflects the Chinese atmospheric nuclear weapon tests in 1969 and 1970. Tests performed in 1973 and 1976 resulted in a retarded fall-out in 1974 and 1977. Test of small Chinese nuclear weapons between 1978 and 1980 did not contribute substantial amounts of Pu-239 + 240 to the total fall-out. After 1980 the plutonium fall-out decreased continuously. The nuclear-power-plant accident in Tschnernobyl in 1986 did not contribute significant amounts of Pu-239 + 240 to the total fall-out, which increased to the average values of the 1980s. Caesium-137 fall-out, however, was about five times the values measured before the accident. (Anonymous (1989), Plutonium, GSF, Neuherberg, p16.)

higher doses and shows substantial species differences. Therefore, it is difficult to extrapolate animal data to humans.

As in the case of other heavy metals, intestinal absorption of plutonium is affected by the physiological situation of the organism. For example, intestinal absorption seems to be increased by a factor of 100 in infants (<1 year) compared to adults. In iron-deficient or fasting humans, bioavailability is also increased. High iron or calcium concentrations reduce plutonium absorption. Absorption is observed mainly in the upper small intestine; the mechanism is unknown.

There are no reliable data for humans regarding the bioavailability of plutonium. The ICRP (International Committee on Radiological Protection) assumes that about 0.01% of Pu hydroxides and oxides and 0.1% of other soluble compounds are absorbed in adults. In infants (<1 year), the absorption rate is estimated to be about 1%. The largest fraction of ingested plutonium (>99.9%) is excreted immediately with the feces or after desquamation of intestinal epithelial cells.

Cutaneous absorption occurs very slowly and to a lesser extent. One hour after contamination, about 0.01% has penetrated the upper skin layers. Diffusion of plutonium follows Fick's law of diffusion along hair follicles and sebaceous glands. In cases of injuries and cutaneous erosions, uptake can be substantially increased.

The distribution in the organism is very slow. From animal experiments it is shown that plutonium binds to plasma transferrin, a plasma protein that binds iron and transports it to liver and erythropoetic tissue. These organs are the most important target organs for plutonium. About 10% of absorbed plutonium is excreted with the urine, whereas the remaining 90% is distributed in the organism. About 50% is accumulated in the bones, about 30% in the liver tissue, and another 10% in the rest of the body. This distribution pattern was confirmed in humans.

Studies in human bones showed that the largest amount of plutonium was deposited in the bone trabeculae. These bone structures are close to the hematopoetic cells of the bone marrow. Therefore, this specific accumulation of radioactive plutonium is regarded as an explanation for the typical plutonium-related osteosarcomas and leukemias. Plutonium passes through the human placenta and accumulates in the fetus. Once plutonium is bound to the tissue, its excretion via the urine and bile is extremely slow. The biological half-life for plutonium retention in the organism is estimated to be between 40 and 100 years.

Currently the average plutonium body burden in the population—as referred to alpha radiation—lies between 2 and 20 μSv/year. For comparison, the radiation from natural sources is estimated to be between 1000 and 10,000 μSv/year. The recommendation of the ICRP for the maximal tolerable dose was for ^{239}Pu = 300 Bq (Bequerel), corresponding to 130 ng Pu.

Specific Toxicity

For plutonium, the acute and chronic toxicity data, as usually studied for other heavy metals, are not relevant because chronic radiation effects play the major toxicological role. Long-term radiation exposure of distinct cells to alpha particles affects mainly DNA. Therefore, the mutagenicity and carcinogenicity are to be appraised.

An appraisal of the toxic potential has to differentiate among the isotopes ^{237}Pu, ^{238}Pu, ^{239}Pu, ^{240}Pu, and ^{241}Pu. The rate of alpha radiation differs extensively among these isotopes. As result of nuclear reactions, these isotopes are produced in very variable amounts. From a toxicological point of view, plutonium plays an exceptional role among the radioactive elements, because of its long decay half-life ($t_{1/2} \sim 2.4 \pm 10^4$ years), as well as because of its very long biological half-life ($t_{1/2} \sim$ 40–100 years). These properties, coupled with its intensive alpha emissions, explain its classification as carcinogenic metal.

Reproduction Toxicity, Mutagenicity, and Carcinogenicity

Plutonium causes chromosomal abberations, sister chromatide exchanges and/or carcinogenic transformations by alpha irradiation of cellular DNA, as do other radioactive metals (e.g., radium or uranium). In addition, anomalies of the germ cells and effects on spermatogenesis were observed after high exposure.

Carcinogenicity of plutonium has also been confirmed for humans. In animal erxperiments, plutonium caused liver tumors and osteosarcomas. It is assumed that both types of neoplasms are related to the long biological half-life in the target organs and to the long lasting "punctual alpha radiation," especially in bones (osteosarcomas, leukemia).

The cells of the hematopoetic system and the proliferating cells of the bones are most sensitive to alpha irradiation. These cells have a diameter of about 10 μm, which can be reached by alpha particles from plutonium deposited in trabeculae, because alpha irradiation reaches across a distance of 30 to 35 μm. This explains the development of neoplasms of the hematopoetic system. Animal data show that an intrauterinal contamination leads to an increased risk of myeloic leukemia in the next generation. Retrospectively, cancers of the lymphopoetic system, leukemias, thyroid tumors, or neoplasms of the prostate, stomach, or colon all were shown to be increased after high exposure (<100 mrem).

Therapeutic Measures

Plutonium should be decorporated as soon as possible. This is not easy because in the organism Pu(IV) behaves in a way similar to Fe(III). Pu(IV) binds tightly to transferrin, the transport protein for iron. Zn–DTPA (zinc diethylenetriaminepentaacetic acid) (Table 2) enters the cells only in very limited amounts. Therefore, only plutonium circulating in the plasma can be chelated. Redistribution between tissues and plasma is slow, and an intermittent therapy with Zn–DTPA over several years could become necessary.

A new group of compounds, the LICAM family (Fig. 11), did not prove to be more effective. Siderophores, such as hydroxypyridinone derivatives (3,4,3-LIHOPO), may be more effective. However, clinical experience is still scarce. A therapy with complexing agents must take into consideration the specific adverse events. For example, in animal experiments de-

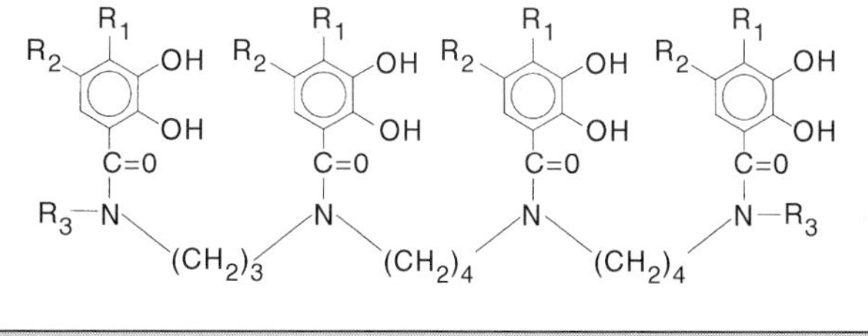

FIGURE 11 Principal structure of LICAM-complexing agents. (1) 3,4,3-LICAM, $R_1 = R_2 = R_3$ = H; (2) 3,4,3-LICAM(C), $R_1 = CO_2Na$, $R_2 = R_3$ = H; (3) 3,4,3-LICAM(S), $R_1 = R_3$ = H, $R_2 = SO_3Na$. (With permission from Jones, 1991.)

generative changes in the liver tissue and in the renal proximal tubules were observed after the administration of 3,4,3-LIHOPO (30 μmol/kg).

THALLIUM

Thallium was discovered in 1861 by Crookes. One year later it was isolated from lead sludge by Lamy. Its name derives from the green color that it produces in a flame. Until the 1930s, it was used as a depilatory agent. Thallium is not an environmental pollutant; its concentrations in drinking water, air, and in the soil are very low. Occupational exposure is rare. Intoxication is mostly due to accidental, suicidal, or homocidal ingestion of thallium-containing compounds.

Chemical Characteristics, Sources, and Uses

Thallium (Tl, atomic weight 204.4; density 11.9 g/cm^3, melting point 449°C) occurs in two oxidation states: Tl^{1+} (thallous ions) and Tl^{3+} (thallic ions). Thallous sulfate, thallous nitrate, thallous iodide, thallous phosphate, and thallous acetate dissolve freely in water; in contrast, thallium sulfide is almost insoluble. Thallium is purified from lorandite and crookesite ores, which are mined mainly in the United States and in Brazil.

The technical uses of thallium are limited. Seventy percent of worldwide production is used in the electrics industry to produce semiconductors and scintillation counters. In the chemical and optical industries, thallium is used as a catalyst and to increase the refraction index of glass. Due to its low melting point, thallium alloys are used in thermometers for very low temperatures. In addition, thallium alloys are extremely stable against corrosion. The isotope Tl^{201} is used in medicine for scintigraphy of the heart.

Absorption, Distribution, Metabolism, and Excretion

Thallous ions are almost completely absorbed from the respiratory system and the gastrointestinal tract; 81.4 and 64.4% were absorbed within 2 h from ligated jejunal and ileal loops, respectively, in rats after the administration of 10 nmol Tl_2SO_4. Thallium is also absorbed via the skin. Once absorbed, the thallous ions are rapidly cleared from the circulation and distributed into the tissue by mediation of Na^+,K^+-ATPase. The interaction between Tl^+ and K^+ ions with Na^+,K^+-ATPase was investigated in erythrocytes.

After parenteral administration to mice, radioactively labeled thallium accumulated preferentially in epithelial structures, such as renal tubuli and colonic mucosa, which are active in electrolyte transport. Persistently high concentrations of radioactive thallium were found in the epididymis, in the periosteum of long bones, and in hyaline cartilages. After a subject eats thallium-contaminated food ($\leq$0.5 mg Tl/day) for several months, the liver and kidney may accumulate 1.0 mg Tl/kg.

In humans thallous ions have a biological half-life of about 30 days. The main excretional pathways are via the intestine, where thallium is reabsorbed extensively (entero–enteral circulation), and via the kidney. The excretion of thallous ions via the skin and with milk and bile is of minor importance. The small intestine and the colon of the rat can actively transport Tl^+ ions from the blood into the intestinal lumen (Fig. 12). There is an electronegative charge at the luminal surface and an electropositive charge at the serosal surface. The potential difference between both sides was determined to be 10–15 mV in the colon, and 4–6 mV in the jejunum. The analysis of Tl^+ ion movements in the rat colon showed that excretion of Tl^+ ions against an electrochemical gradient depends on metabolic energy. The absorption of Tl^+ ions in the opposite direction follows an electrochemical gradient.

Mechanisms of Toxicity

The physicochemical similarity between thallium and potassium (ionic radius Tl^+/K^+ = 133/144) explains the high intracellular accumulation of thallium ions; both ions use the same transport systems (Na^+, K^+-ATPase, Na^+–K^+–Cl_2 cotransporter). However, the intracellular accumulation of Tl^+ does not seem to explain the toxic thallium effects, as shown by the following examples.

1. Tl^+ ions can substitute for K^+ ions in all cells, as well as in isolated enzyme systems such as the Na^+, K^+-ATPase. Thallous ions substitute for K^+ ions at low and intermediate concentrations and can maintain particular cell functions. At high concentrations, Tl^+ ions may induce the same toxic effects in the heart as high K^+ concentrations. This explains the cardiac symptoms that may be fatal at the height of thallium intoxication. The renal symptoms of thallium intoxication do not seem to depend on the thallium tissue content; they cannot be observed before long periods of exposure.
2. The toxic symptoms after thallium exposure de-

velop very slowly. Thallium concentrations in the cerebrospinal fluid, in peripheral nerves, and in different parts of the CNS are lower than in the heart, kidney, and intestinal tissue. The highest accumulations in the CNS are found in the thalamus, nucleus caudatus, frontal lobe, and in the cerebellum. Vital organs, such as the CNS, peripheral nerves, liver, and kidney, show mitochondrial damage in thallium intoxication. There may be an increased formation of mitochondrial cristae or complete vacuolization, which presages a complete destruction of mitochondria. In the Golgi apparatus, electron microscopy shows "dense bodies." It is frequently wrapped in multiple layers, resembling an onion bulb. The determination of enzyme activities in the damaged parts of the CNS did not help in the understanding of the mechanisms of toxic thallium effects.

3. There are doubts as to whether Tl^{+} is the toxic species. An interesting hypothesis assumes a slow generation of Tl^{3+} ions in the cell, which may be responsible for mitochondrial destruction. Depending on intracellular pH, Tl^{3+} can oxidize glutathione to GSSG (pH 7.0–7.2) or sulphen and sulphine acids (pH 7.4–7.8). The latter reaction is likely to take place in the mitochondrial compartment and is likely to cause mitochondrial damage. This hypothesis needs further clarification. The oxidation of Tl^{+} to Tl^{3+} has been demonstrated in mitochondrial cristae of yeast cells.

Acute and Chronic Toxicity

Accidental intoxications were caused by the ingestion of thallium-containing rodenticides, especially in children. Environmental thallium contamination from cement plants was discussed. There are marked dif-

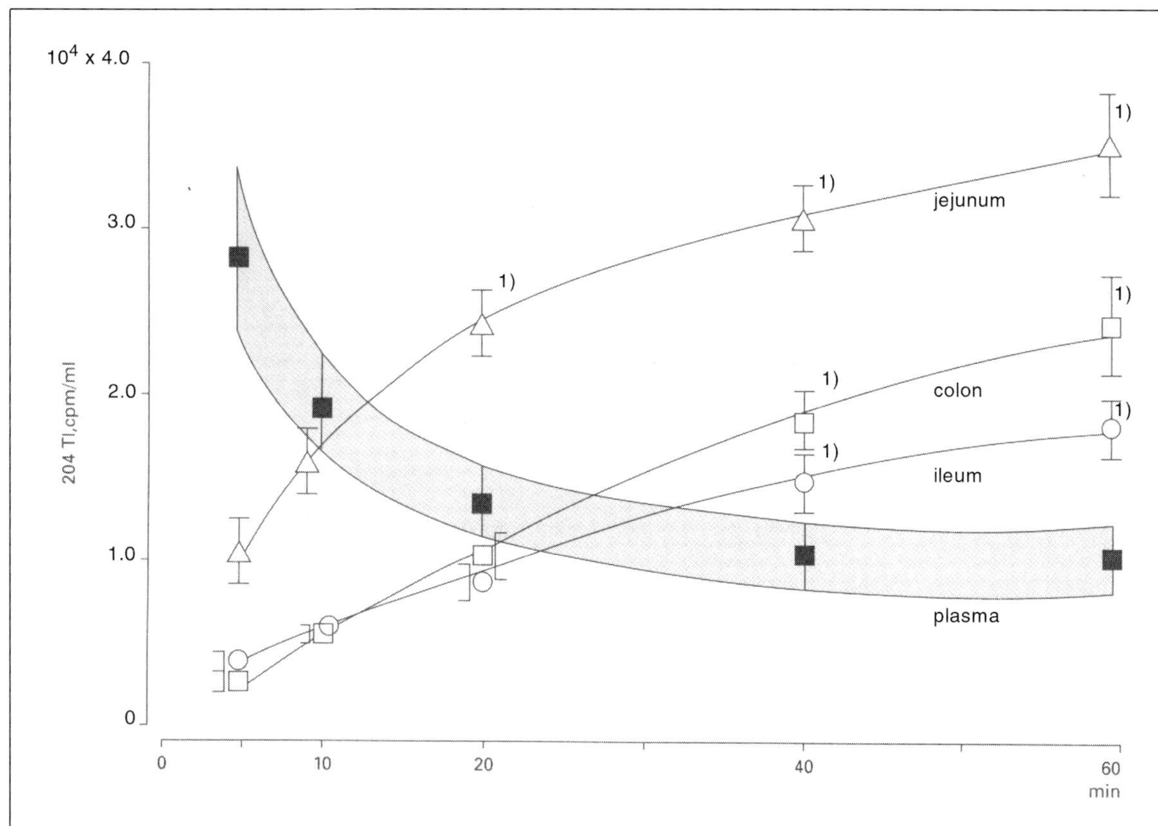

FIGURE 12 Secretion of Tl^{+} ions into intestinal lumen. Pendular perfusion of intestinal segments in the rat. Points represent the means of 5–36 determinations. Changes in the ^{204}Tl concentration show that the intraluminal ^{204}Tl concentration in the jejunum exceeds the corresponding plasma concentration after 20 minutes, that in ileum and colon after 40 minutes. Thus, Tl^{+} ions are secreted from plasma into the lumen against a concentration gradient (1) indicates a statistically significant difference between the Tl^{+} concentration in the plasma and in the intestinal lumen ($p < 0.05$). (Forth and Henning, 1982, *Arch. Toxicol.* **49,** 149–158, Fig. 2, copyright notice of Springer Verlag, with permission).

ferences in the thallium load of different plant species; cabbage species and parsley are specially prone to the accumulation of thallium, which in some plants seems to inhibit the synthesis of chlorophyll.

The thallium load in food is low. Vegetables and fruits contain between 0.005 and 0.08 mg Tl/kg. In areas that are contaminated by the thallium emission, e.g., from cement plants, these values were 10 to 20 times higher. Thallium is also accumulated in mushrooms that may contain between 0.05 and 1.22 mg Tl/kg. Food of animals origin contains 0.02 to 0.1 mg Tl/kg.

In adults 0.8–1 g thallium is fatal. Lower doses may cause severe intoxication but with partial recovery. The initial phase of acute thallium intoxication lasts up to 4 days. There are few, unspecific symptoms, such as gastrointestinal disturbances with diarrhea followed by constipation (Fig. 13). At this stage, thallium may cause blackish discoloration (thallium sulphide) at the hair roots, which can be analyzed by microscopy (Widy's syndrome). In the early phase of intoxication (between the 7th and the 10th day after thallium ingestion) unspecific symptoms, such as insomnia and psychological alterations appear. Polyneuritis leads to hypersensitivity of the legs and pretibial pains that cause the slighest touch to be unbearable. The soles of the feet are also involved.

The intoxication reaches its summit between day 10 and day 20. At approximately day 13 the patients lose their hair (alopecia); this does not involve all parts of the body to the same extent. On the head, alopecia areata is frequent and may be accompanied by alopecia of the axial and pubic hairs. Although alopecia is characteristic of thallium intoxication, it is not a specific symptom. In the eyebrows the medial parts are frequently spared. These hairs seem to be more resist-

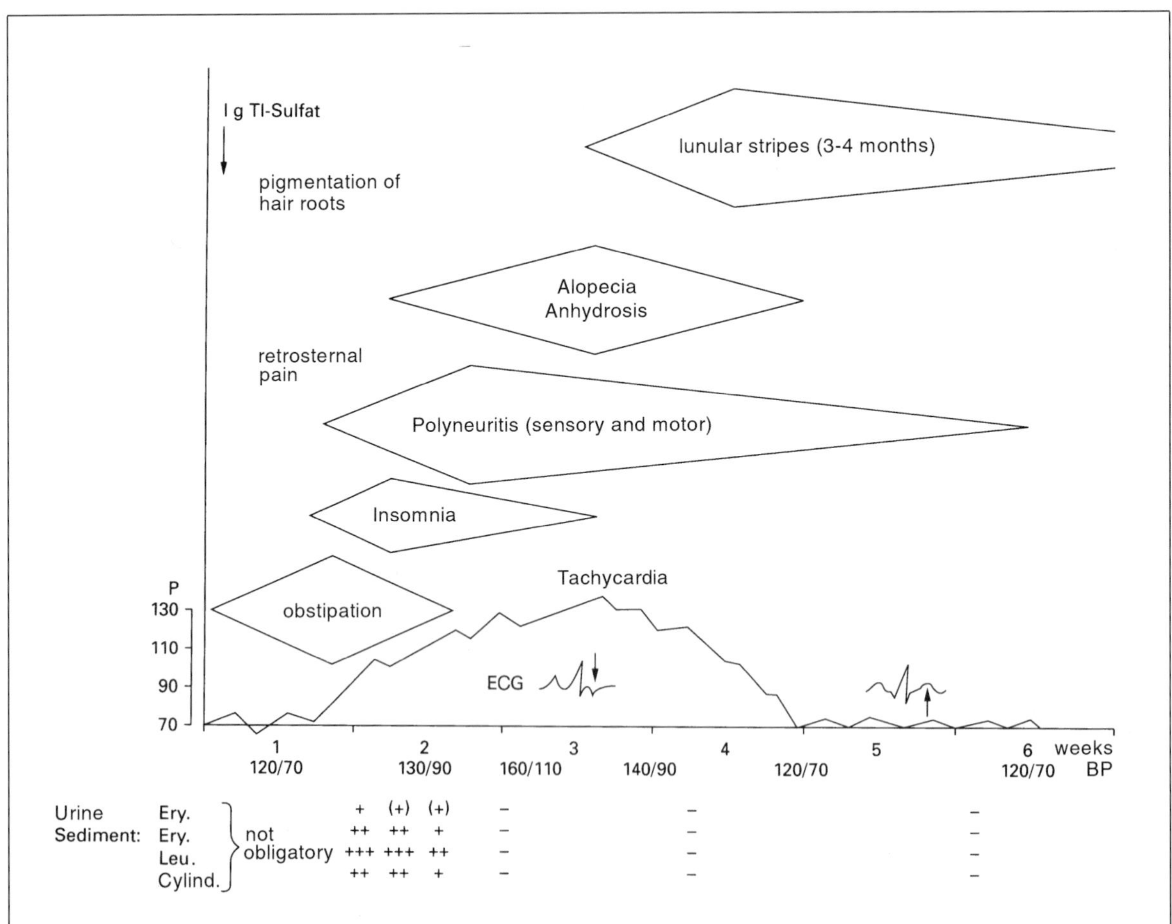

FIGURE 13 Time course of symptom development in thallium intoxication. Ordinate gives the pulse rate and relates to the curve marked "tachycardia." BP is the blood pressure in mm Hg. Renal damage shows in the urine sediment findings at the beginning of the intoxication. (Modified from Moeschlin, 1980, with permission.)

ant to thallium intoxication, similar to the sensory pili of animals. As was shown in animal experiments, mitotic dysfunction at the hair follicles may be associated with a disturbed energy supply.

As intoxication proceeds, the symptoms of toxic polyneuritis worsen. The skin becomes extremely sensitive to the touch. Sometimes partial or irreversible lesions of the optic nerve with impaired vision are observed. Cranial nerves may be paralyzed, leading to ptosis and impaired eye muscle coordination. Impaired hearing is in part reversible. Respiratory insufficiency and tachycardia are frequently observed. The ECG shows signs of a myopathy with impaired stimulus production and conduction. Pseudobulbar paralysis or cardiac arrhythmia with disturbed artroventricular conductance are the most frequent causes of death.

Recovery requires between 3 months and 1 year and may be incomplete. The legs may become athrophic, showing residual paresis and pathological reflexes. The nerve conduction is impaired. After 1–2 months, the hair has regrown, sometimes more densely than before. The nails may show Mees' stripes, which are caused by disturbed growth during the intoxication. The residues may lead to an impaired CNS performance in some cases. Another possible residual effect is renal impairment, which may go along with an increased albumin concentration in the urine. After thallium intoxications, the libido frequently remains impaired. Erection may be difficult and painful; menstruation may cease.

Chronic thallium intoxication is a rare event that is distinguished from acute intoxication by the severity of the symptoms. The patients are not confined to bed as early. Because the symptoms are unspecific, chronic thallium intoxication is frequently misdiagnosed in its early stages. Surveillance of occupational exposure is simple. Normal urinary thallium excretion is 0.05 to 1.5 μg/liter; 300 μg/liter urine is the upper limit after short-term exposure in thallium-processing plants.

Special Toxicology

Thallium passes through the placenta and is fetotoxic. Data on thallium mutagenicity are equivocal. No data are available on carcinogenic effects of thallium compounds, either from animal experiments or from epidemiological investigations.

Therapeutic Measures

The renal excretion of thallium ions can be increased by forced diuresis and by potassium infusion. The latter method makes use of the competition between Tl^+ and K^+ ions in tubular reabsorption. Mineral corticoids increased Tl^+ excretion in animal experiments. The thallous ion (Tl^+) is difficult to chelate by common chelators. The application of dithiocarb may even lead to increased thallium concentrations in the CNS. Colloidal Prussian Blue, however, increases thallium excretion via the intestine. It is a suitable therapy in thallium intoxication. This therapy was inaugurated by A. Catsch in the 1950s; he showed that the excretion of radioactively labeled cesium can be increased by oral administration of Prussian blue. He recognized that all ions with an ionic radius similar to that of K^+ can be chelated by Prussian blue (Fig. 14); in addition to rubidium, this includes thallium. At first it was assumed that the oral application of nonabsorbable Prussian blue prevents the intestinal absorption of orally administered thallium. However, Prussian blue will also bind Tl^+ ions after intestinal secretion. A continuous oral supply of Prussian blue can scavenge the excreted Tl^+ ions in the intestinal

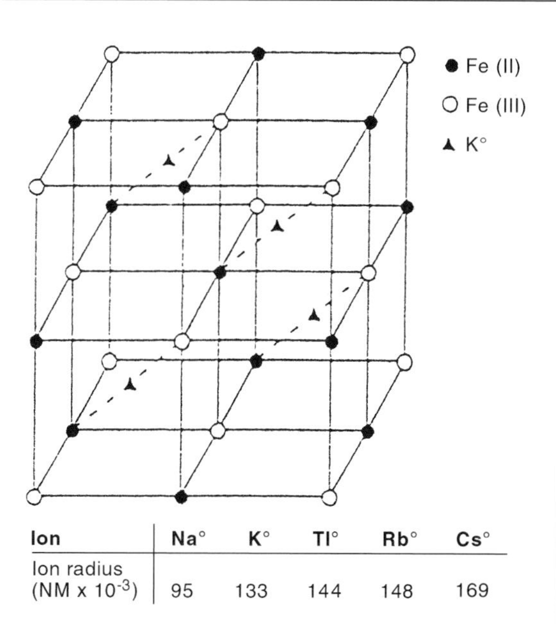

Ion	Na°	K°	Tl°	Rb°	Cs°
Ion radius (NM x 10^{-3})	95	133	144	148	169

FIGURE 14 Structural frame work of Prussian Blue (ferrohexacyanoferrat(II). Metal salts form mixed hexacyanoferrates(II). These complexes contain protons or sodium or potassium ions in varying ratios. Thus, Prussian Blue can act as cation exchangers. The stability of the complex increases in proportion to the ionic radius. The structure of Prussian Blue was analyzed by Keggen and Miles (1936) by use of X-ray structure analysis. The CN^- groups are arranged at the corners of the cube. To maintain electroneutrality, every Fe^{3+} ion must be accompanied by a K^+ ion.

lumen so that they are excreted fecally; eight oral doses of 20–24 g of Prussian blue per day together with a laxative, such as mannitol, have been shown to be effective for this purpose. Even at high doses, Prussian blue releases only minor amounts of cyanide, which do not exceed the detoxifying capacity of endogenous rhodanase. The Prussian blue therapy has been most effectively applied in the Netherlands; no casualties due to thallium intoxication have been reported there since. Treatment of thallium intoxication uses forced diuresis and administration of Prussian blue together. In severe intoxication, renal excretion is supported by dialysis.

TIN

Tin has been used by humans for more than 5000 years. The most prominent tin alloy is bronze, which gave its name to an entire epoch. The processing of bronze was developed about 3500 B.C. Until the 17th century bronze was of extraordinary importance in weapon and gun production. Therefore, humans have been exposed "occupationally" to tin for a very long time. Nicolas Appert proposed in 1810 to use closed tinned cans to cook and store food for Napoleon's army. Afterwards, this became popular and a larger part of the population is still exposed orally to tin.

From a toxicological point of view, inorganic and organic tin compounds have to be discussed separately. The toxicity of inorganic compounds is relative low. In contrast, some organotin compounds like trimethyl or triethyl tin are extremely toxic. However, toxicity decreases with the increasing length of the organic side-chain.

Chemical Properties, Occurrence, and Use

Tin (Sn; molecular weight: 118.7; oxidation states +2 and +4) can form either SnX_2 or SnX_4 compounds. The bivalent tin is found in ionic compounds fourvalent tin forms covalent compounds. The most important inorganic tin compounds are oxides, chlorides, and fluorides or otherwise halogenated compounds. There are mono-, di-, tri- or tetraorganotin compounds. Methyl, ethyl and butyl tin deserve the highest toxicological interest, as are the important triphenyl and tricyclohexyl tins (Table 23).

The most important deposits are found in Bolivia, China, Great Britain, Russia, Indonesia, Malaysia, and Thailand. More than 50% of the world's tin production is used for processing tinned iron and a variety of other tin alloys. Organotin compounds are used as stabilizer for PVC production, to process silicon, or as a catalytic agent for polyurethane production. In some cases organotin compounds are used as molluscicides; fungicides, or insecticides.

Absorption, Distribution, Metabolism, and Excretion

Absorption from respiratory tract has not been investigated either for inorganic or for organic tin compounds.

Inorganic Compounds

Only few toxicokinetic studies were performed with inorganic tin. Controlled studies in humans are not available. The absorption of Sn(II) is poor. It depends on the dose administered, as well as on the composition of the ingesta. Investigations in rodents showed that up to 50% of the dose was absorbed after the administration of very small amounts. In contrast, only 3% is absorbed at high concentrations. Citric acid (i.e., fruit juice) increases tin bioavailability in rats 4- to 5-fold. The same may also hold true for humans.

Data about the distribution and metabolism of inorganic tin are available from animal experiments only and from single-case reports about acute intoxications in humans observed after the consumption of fruit juice stored overnight in tin containers. After i.v injection in rats, about 46% of tin was found in the bones, 5.3% in the kidneys, and only 0.2% in the liver. Uptake into the bones is particularly high. Therefore, the bones seem to be the target organ for tin, without provoking remarkable toxic effects. The metabolism of inorganic tin has scarcely been investigated.

Again, data about the excretion of Sn(II) are available from animal experiments only and show substantial species differences. While dogs excrete about 60% within 3 days via the kidneys, mice eliminate only 20% via the urine in the same period. Fecal excretion is low in all species (5 to 10%); therefore, a remarkable species difference has to be expected with regard to the biological half-life.

The biological half-lives of tin in human beings indicate distinct compartments (C): C_1 (~20%), $t_{1/2}$ ~ 4 days; C_2 (~20%), $t_{1/2}$ ~ 25 days; C_3 (~60%), $t_{1/2}$ ~ 400 days. The compartment with the longest elimination half-life is probably represented by the skeleton.

Organotin Compounds

In contrast to inorganic, tin organotin compounds are absorbed dermally. After transdermal absorption, triphenyl, trimethyl, and tributyl tin can provoke severe intoxication. Dermal absorption rates are unknown.

TABLE 23 Physicochemical and Toxic Properties of Selected Organotin Compounds

Compound	Formula	Molecular weight	Water solubility	Toxic effects
Trimethyl-Sn	$Sn(CH_3)_4$: $H_3C-Sn(CH_3)_2-CH_3$	199.26	No data	Damage of neurones
Triethyl-Sn	$H_3C-H_2C-Sn(CH_2CH_3)_2-Br$	285.81	No data	Edema in CNS
Bis(tributyl)-tin oxide	$(CH_2-CH_2-CH_2-CH_2)_3-Sn-O-Sn-(CH_2-CH_2-CH_2-CH_2)_3$	596.16	Low solubility	Damage of neurones and edema in CNS
Triphenyl-Sn	$(C_6H_5)_3Sn-Cl$	385.47	Not soluble	Liver injuries
Dibutyl-Sn	$H_3C-H_2C-H_2C-H_2C-Sn(CH_3)_2-CH_2-CH_2-CH_2-CH_3$	308.85	Soluble in hot water	Degeneration of the ductus choledochus

The absorption from the gastrointestinal tract varies between 2% (tricyclohexyl tin) and nearly 100% (triethyl tin), depending on the chemical structure (Table 24). Confirmed data in humans are not available. In 1954 an epidemic intoxication was observed in France after the administration of the drug Stalinon®, which was used in the treatment of osteomyelitis, anthrax, and acne. The toxic agent was triethyl tin. The oral toxic dose was estimated retrospectively to be about 70 mg.

After a single, as well as chronic, exposure to trimethyl or triethyl tin, the relative distribution can be measured among the organs, ranked in order is blood > liver > kidney > brain; the actual percentages can vary extensively.

The uptake of organotin compounds into the neuronal structures is extremely hazardous because they are neurotoxins. Organotin compounds accumulate in the brains of experimental animals to the relative extents triethyl > trimethyl > tripropyl > tributyl > triphenyl > tricyclohexyl tin. The distribution among the blood, liver, and kidney differs depending on the compound used (e.g., for trimethyl tin, the ratio of the concentrations between erythrocytes and plasma is ~120; in comparison, for triethyl tin it is only 20). To estimate exposure and uptake, the organotin concentration in whole blood samples must be determined.

Organotin compounds are dealkylated in liver microsomes by a cytochrome P450-dependent monoox-

TABLE 24 Absorption Rates of Various Organotin Compounds from the Gastrointestinal Tract of Different Species

Sn(IV) compounds	Absorption rate (%)	Species
Tricyclohexyl	2	Rat
Monoethyl	8	Rat
Triphenyl	10	Cow
Triethyl	~100	Rat
Tributyl	No data	—
Dibutyl	No data	—

[a]Magos (1986).

igenase. *In vivo* dealkylation from tetraethyl to triethyl tin and from diethyl to monoethyl tin is a rapid reaction. In contrast, from triethyl to diethyl tin, it is very slow. The presence of radicals results in a further decreased metabolic rate. Triphenyl tin is not metabolized by the monoxygenase system; the metabolic mechanism is not known for this compound.

The excretion of the various organotin compounds with the urine and feces differs substantially. Monoethyl tin is mainly excreted with the urine. In contrast, diethyl or dibutyl tin are excreted to a large extent by the bile and, thus, via the feces. An enterohepatic circulation cannot be excluded. The biological half-life ($t_{1/2}$) in the various organs shows a large variation. The toxicokinetic data for humans are not available.

Mechanisms of Toxicity

The mechanisms of toxicity of organotin compounds are not described in detail. The chemical structures are similar to the organic lead compounds. Therefore it is assumed that organotin compounds inhibit the mitochondrial enzyme systems (respiratory chain) and the cellular ATP metabolism. Triethyl tin accumulates in the mitochondria of the CNS and inhibits oxidative phosphorylation, glucose oxidation, and the utilization of phosphates in phospholipids of the CNS.

Acute and Chronic Toxicity

Intoxication from inorganic tin compounds is extremely rare and is limited in general to acute intoxication. Chronic intoxication is unknown.

Inorganic Compounds

The uptake of relatively large amounts of tin may result in a temporary inhibition of some enzymes (e.g., succinate dehydrogenase or acid phophatase). However, toxic symptoms were observed only after the uptake of highly contaminated food (>1400 ppm). For example, an acute intoxication was observed in participants of a celebration where orange juice was served that has been stored overnight in tin containers. The juice contained about 2000 ppm Sn(II). No lethal intoxication or severe long-lasting toxic effects have been reported for inorganic tin compounds. This holds true also for chronic inhalative exposure to tin-containing dust, which resulted in benign pneumoconiosis in the worst case.

Organotin Compounds

The most toxic organotin compounds are di- and trialkylated compounds. Tetraalkylated compounds are metabolized to trialkylated compounds, which increases the toxicity. Monoethyl tin is about 20-fold less toxic than triethyl tin.

The toxicity of organotin compounds differs with regard to the toxic dose and the toxic effects. Trimethyl, triethyl, dibutyl and triphenyl tin intoxications show characteristic symptoms, whereas all other organotin compounds cause a less characteristic pattern of symptoms or are even nontoxic, for example, octyl tin. However, all organotin compounds—independent of the chain length—provoke a decrease of the thymus weight coupled with a reduction of the number of thymus cells.

Occupational exposure is occasionally observed. Brief dermal exposure, as observed in cases of cloth contamination, can result in skin irritation or diffuse dermatosis.

Trimethyl and triethyl tin intoxications provoke typical neurotoxic effects. Trimethyl tin can destroy the neurons in the CNS, leading to agressiveness, tremor, dizziness, or hyperactivity in rats. Only a few cases of intoxication by trimethyl tin in humans are known. The initial symptoms are hyperactivity, sleeplessness, and loss of appetite. A continued exposure results in confusion and generalized convulsions. The patients recovered completely. Triethyl tin provokes edemas in the brain and the spinal cord in humans and other species. An epidemic intoxication resulted from the use of the antiseptic drug Stalinon® in France (in 1954). More than 100 patients died from an intoxication attributed to triethyl tin, which was a by-product of dibutyl tin, used as a cream to treat furuncles. Dibutyl tin causes degeneration of the bile duct (ductus choledochus) in some species, as well as liver and pancreas damage. Triphenyl tin seems to be responsible for liver damage after oral uptake. Unspecific symptoms, such as headache, dizziness and hepatomegalias, were observed as well.

Special Toxicity

There are no indications of reproduction toxicology, mutagenicity, or carcinogenic effects of inorganic or organic tin compounds from any animal experiments or from epidemiological observations. The data, however, are limited and do not allow a definite appraisal. More recent data show that organotin compounds like dibutyltin, tributyltin, bis(tributyl)-tin oxide, dimethyl tin, and trimethyl tin may be genotoxic.

Bibliography

Alfrey, A. C., Legendre, G. R., and Kaehny, W. D. (1976). The dialysis encephalopathy syndrome. *New Engl. J. Med.* **294**, 184–188.

Anonymous (1989). Plutonium aus dem weltweiden Fallout. Mensch and Umvelt, Plutonium, GSF, Neuherberg.

Berlin, M. (1986). Mercury. *In* "Handbook on the Toxicology of Metals" (L. Friberg *et al.*, eds.), 2nd ed., pp. 387–445. Elsevier, New York.

Bowden, C. A., and Krenzelok, E. P. (1997). Clinical applications of commonly used contemporary antidotes. *Drug Safety* **16,** 9–47.

Burkinshaw, L. *et al.* (1987). Plutonium content of tissues of members of the general public. *J. Soc. Radiol.* **7,** 27–32.

Carson, B. L., Ellis, H. V., III, and McCann, J. L., (1987). "Toxicology and Biological Monitoring of Metals in Humans." Lewis Publishers, Chelsea.

Chadwick, D. J., and Whelan J. (1992). "Aluminium in Biology and Medicine." Ciba Foundation Symposium 169. John Wiley & Sons, Chichester, U.K.

Clarkson, T. W. (1983). Methylmercury toxicity to the mature and developing nervous system: Possible mechanisms. In "Biological Aspects of Metals and Metal-Related Diseases" (B. Sarkar, ed.), pp. 183–197. Raven Press, New York.

Clarkson, T. W., Hursh, J. B., Sager, P. R., and Syversen, T. L. M. (1988). Mercury. *In* "Biological Monitoring of Toxic Metals" (T. W. Clarkson *et al.*, eds.), pp. 199–246. Plenum Press, New York.

Cohen, M., Latta, D., Coogan, T., and Costa, M. (1990). Mechanisms of metal carcinogenesis: The reactions of metals with nucleic acids. *In* "Biological Effects of Heavy Metals" (E. C. Foulkes, ed.), Vol. 2, pp. 19–75. CRC Press, Boca Raton, FL.

Committee on Lead in the Human Environment (1980). "Lead in the human environment." National Academy Press, Washington, D.C.

Crapper, D. R., and De Boni, U. (1980). Aluminium. *In* "Experimental and Clinical Neurotoxicology" (P. S. Spencer and H. H. Schaumburg, eds.), pp. 326–335. Williams and Wilkins, Baltimore, MD.

Diehl, J. F., and Boppel, B. (1985). Dietary cadmium: A re-evaluation. *Trace Elements Med.* **2,** 167–174.

Durbin, P. W. (1989). Chelation of ^{238}PU(IV) in vivo by 3,4,3-LI-CAM(C): Effects of ligand methylation and pH. *Health Physics* **56,** 839–855.

Ellenhorn, M. J., and Barceloux, D. G. (1988). "Medical Toxicology." Elsevier, New York.

Elinder, C. G. (1985). Respiratory effects. *In* "Cadmium and Health: A Toxicological Appraisal" (L. Friberg *et al.*, eds.), Vol. 2, pp. 1–20. CRC Press, Boca Raton, FL.

Elinder, C. G. *et al.* (1985). Cancer mortality of cadmium workers. *Brit. J. Indus. Med.* **42,** 655–657.

Elinder, C.-G., and Sjögren, B. (1986) Aluminium. *In* "Handbook on the Toxicology of Metals" (L. Friberg *et al.*, eds.), Vol. II, pp. 1–25. Elsevier/North-Holland Biomedical Press, Amsterdam.

Ewers, U., and Schlipköter, H. W. (1991). Lead. *In* "Metals and Their Compounds in the Environment" (E. Merian, ed.), pp. 971–1014. VCH Verlagsgesellschaft, Weinheim.

Forth, W. (1989). Zur Toxizität von Platin und Platinmetallen. *Dtsch. Z. Onkol.* **21,** 110–114.

Forth, W., and Henning, H. (1982). The excretion of thallium(I)-ions into the gastrointestinal tract in situ of rats. *Arch. Toxicol.* **49,** 149–158.

Friberg, L. *et al.* (1986). Cadmium. *In* "Handbook on the Toxicology of Metals" (L. Friberg *et al.*, eds.), Vol. II, pp. 130–184. Elsevier/North-Holland, Biomedical Press, Amsterdam.

Friberg, L. and Vostal, J. (eds.) (1992). "Mercury in the Environment." CRC Press, Cleveland, CH.

Goyer, R. A. (1992). Toxic effects of metals. *In* "Casarett and Doull's Toxicology" (M O Amdur *et al.*, eds.), 4th ed., pp. 623–680. Pergamon Press, New York.

Hanusch, K., Grossmann, H., Herbst, K.-A., Rose, G., and Wolf, H. U. (1988). Arsenic and arsenic compounds. *In* "Ullmann's Encyclopedia of Industrial Chemistry" (W. Gerhartz *et al.*, eds.) 5th Ed., Vol. A3, pp. 113–141. Verlag Chemie, Weinheim.

Harrison, J. D. (1991). The gastrointestinal absorption of the actinide elements. *Sci. Total Environ.* **100,** 43–60.

Henning, H. V. (1989). Die Toxizität des Aluminiums. *Klin. Wochenschr.* **67,** 1221–1228.

Inskip, M. J., and Piotrowski, J. K. (1985). Review of the health effects of methylmercury. *J. Appl. Toxicol.* **5,** 113–133.

Ishinishi, N., Tsuchiya, K., Vahter, M., and B. A. Fowler (1986). Arsenic. *In* "Handbook on the Toxicology of Metals" (L. Friberg *et al.*, eds.), 2nd ed., pp. 43–83. Elsevier, New York.

Jones, M. M. (1991). New development in therapeutic chelating agents and antidotes for metal poisoning. *Critical Rev. Toxicol.* **21,** 209–233.

Kemper, F. H., and Bertram, H. P. (1991). Thallium. *In* "Metals and Their Compounds in the Environment" (E. Merian, ed.), pp. 1101–1126. VCH Verlagsgesellschaft, Weinheim.

Kurtzman, N. A. (1986). Toxicity from aluminum and iron: Recognition, treatment and prevention. *Sem. Nephrol.* **4 (Suppl. 1).**

Lataillade, G., M. *et al.* (1989). Gastrointestinal absorption of large amounts of plutonium. Effect of valency state on transfer. *Rad. Protec. Dosimetry* **26,** 307–311.

Lederman, R. J., and Henry, C. E. (1978). Progressive dialysis encephalopathy. *Ann. Neurol.* **4,** 199–204.

Léonard, A. (1991). Arsenic. *In* "Metals and Their Compounds in the Environment" (E. Merian, ed.), pp. 751–774. Verlag Chemie, Weinheim.

Magos, L. (1986). Tin. *In* "Handbook on the Toxicology of Metals" (L. Friberg, *et al.*, eds.), Vol. II, pp. 568–593. Elsevier/North-Holland, Biomedical Press, Amsterdam.

Merian, E. (1991). "Metals and Their Compounds in the Environment." Verlag Chemie, Weinheim.

Moeschlin, S. (1980). Klinik und Therapie der Vergiftungen, 6th ed. Georg Thiewe, Stuttgart.

Mushak, P. *et al.* (1989). Prenatal and postnatal effects of low-level lead exposure: Integrated summary of a report to the U.S. Congress on childhood lead poisoning. *Environ. Res.* **50,** 11–36.

Nieboer, E., and Nriagu, J. U. (eds.) (1992). "Nickel and Human Health." John Wiley & Sons, New York.

Norseth, T. (1986). Nickel. *In* "Handbook on the Toxicology of Metals" (L. Friberg *et al.*, eds.), 2nd ed., Vol. 2, pp. 462–481. Elsevier, Amsterdam.

Pinto, S. S., Enterline, P. E., Henderson, V., and Varner, M. O. (1977). Mortality experience in relation to a measured arsenic trioxide exposure. *Environ. Health Perspect.* **19,** 127–130.

Renner, H. (1992). Platinum group metals and compounds. *In* "Ullmann's Encyclopedia of Industrial Chemistry" (B. Elvers *et al.*, eds.), 5th Ed., Vol. A21, pp. 75–126. Verlag Chemie, Weinheim.

Rosner, G. (1989). Plutonium aus dem weltweiten Fall-out. *In* "Plutonium" (G.S.F München, ed.), Vol. 6, pp. 15–18.

Schäfer, S. G. (1990). Cadmium—ein aktuelles Risiko? *Hamburger Ärzteblatt* **43,** 74–80.

Schäfer, S. G., Elsenhans, B., and Forth, W. (1988). Iron and cadmium: What is known about the interaction of these metals in the organism? *In* "Environmental Toxin, Series 2" (M. Stoeppler and M. Piscator, eds.), pp. 27–31. Springer Verlag, Berlin.

Schäfer, S. G., Elsenhans, B., Forth, W., and Schümann, K. (1994). Metalle. In "Lehrbuch der Toxikologie" Marguardt, H., and Schäfer, S. G., eds.), Spektrum Akademischer Verlag, Heidelberg, Berlin.

Schäfer, S. G., and Femfert, U. (1984). Tin.—A toxic heavy metal? A review of the literature. *Reg Toxicol. Pharmacol.* **4,** 57–69.

Schäfer, S. G., and Forth, W. (1985). The interaction between cadmium and iron: A review of the literature. *Trace Elements Med.* **2,** 158–162.

Schäfer, S. G., and Forth, W. (1987). Thallium(I) secretion across the isolated mucosa of rat descending colon. *Arch. Toxicol.* **59,** 413–420.

Schäfer, S. G., and Schümann, K. (1991). Zur Toxikologie des Kupfers. *Bundesgesundheitsblatt* **34,** 323–327.

Schaller K. H. (1988). Aluminiumkonzentrationen im biologischen Material—Analytische Aspekte und Grenzwerte. *In* "Aluminium in der Therapie—Nützlich oder Schädlich?" (W. Rösch und C. Kori-Lindner, eds.), pp. 31–47. L. Brunner Nürnberg.

Schümann, K., Elsenhans, B., Schäfer, S., Kolb, K., and Forth, W. (1990). Cadmium absorption and its interaction with essential transition metals. *Toxicol. Environ. Chem.* **27,** 81–90.

Sharma, J. *et al.* (1986). Hazards and analysis of thallium—A review. *Tox. Environ. Chem.* **11,** 93–116.

Sigel, H. (ed.) (1986). "Metal Ions in Biological Systems," Vol. 20. Marcel-Dekker, New York.

Simon, M., Jönk, P., Wühl-Couturier, G., and Daunderer, M. (1988). Mercury, mercury alloys, and mercury compounds. *In* "Ullmann's Encyclopedia of Industrial Chemistry" B. Elvers *et al.*, eds.), 5th Ed., Vol. A16, pp. 269–298. Verlag Chemie, Weinheim.

Smith, J. M., Miller, S. C., and Jee, W. S. S. (1984). The relationship of bone marrow type and microvasculature to the microdistribution and local dosimetry of plutonium in the adult skeleton. *Radiation Res.* **99,** 324–335.

Solomons, N. W. (1984). Biomedical, metaboloic, and clinical role of copper in human nutrition. *J. Am. Coll. Nutr.* **4,** 83–105.

Sorensen, J. R. J., Campbell, I. R., Tepper, L. B., and Lingg, R. D. (1974). Aluminium in the environment and human health. *Environ. Health. Perspect.* **8,** 3–95.

Sunderman, F., W., and Oskarsson, A. (1991). Nickel. *In* "Metals and Their Compounds in the Environment" (E. Merian ed.), pp. 1101–1126. VCH Verlagsgesellschaft, Weinheim.

Takenaka, S. *et al.* (1983). Carcinogenicity of cadmium chloride aerosols in W rats. *J. Natl. Cancer Inst.* **70,** 367–373.

Thorne, M. C. (1991). "The Metabolism of Plutonium and Related Elements." Annals of the ICRP 48. Pergamon Press, Oxford.

Tsuchiya, K. (1969a). Causation of ouch-ouch disease (Itai-Itai Byo)—An introductory review, Part I. Nature of the disease. *Keio J. Med.* **18,** 181–194.

Tsuchiya, K. (1969b). Causation of ouch-ouch disease (Itai-Itai Byo)—An introductory review, Part II. Epidemiology and evaluation. *Keio J. Med.* **18,** 195–211.

Tsuchiya, K. (1986). Lead. *In* "Handbook on the Toxicology of Metals" (L. Friedberg *et al.*, eds.), 2nd ed., Vol. 2, pp. 198–343. Elsevier, Amsterdam.

Umweltbundesamt (1983). "Umwelt- und Gesundheitsrisiken fur Arsen." Berichte 4/83. Erich Schmidt Verlag, Berlin.

Vahter, M. (1988). Arsenic. *In* "Biological Monitoring of Toxic Metals" (T. W. Clarkson *et al.*, eds.), pp. 303–321. Plenum Press, New York.

Venugopal, B., and Luckey T. D. (1978). "Metal Toxicity in Mammals," Vol. 2. Plenum Press, New York.

Webb, W. (1979). "The chemistry, Biochemistry and Biology of Cadmium." Elsevier/North-Holland, Biomedical Press, Amsterdam.

Weiner, J. A., Nylander, M., and Berglund, F. (1990). Does mercury from amalgam restorations constitute a health hazard? *Sci. Total Environ.* **99,** 1–22.

Wilkinson, G. S. *et al.* (1987). Mortality among plutonium and other radiation workers at a plutonium weapon facility. *Am. J. Epidem.* **125,** 231–249.

Winge, D. R. (1984). Normal physiology of copper metabolism. *Seminars in Liver Disease* **4,** 239–251.

CHAPTER

33

Gases

PETER EYER

Walther Straub Institute of Pharmacology and Toxicology, Ludwig Maximilians University, Munich, Germany

INTRODUCTION

Toxic gases are airborne poisons that normally occur in the gaseous state and gain entrance to the body mainly by inhalation. Exposure to airborne poisons is unavoidable unless special devices are used to remove toxic contaminants before they enter the respiratory tract. As an adult inhales a mass of some 15 kg of air per day and simultaneously exposes the largest surface area of his or her body to xenobiotics, acute toxic effects may develop very rapidly, either systemically (e.g., with hydrocyanic acid and hydrogen sulfide) or locally in the respiratory tract (e.g., with chlorine or sulfur dioxide). On the other hand, chronic exposure to sulfur dioxide, nitrogen dioxide, and ozone, even at the very low levels found in urban environments, can affect lung function. While low concentrations of airborne toxicants often present little more than a nuisance, high concentrations as found in chemical disasters due to fires, explosions, or blasts may quickly cause death or injury to so many people that normal health and emergency services are overburdened. Hence, different disciplines, such as disaster and military medicine, industrial hygiene, and toxicology, are equally concerned with airborne poisons.

From this it is obvious that various aspects of toxic gases are dealt with in more than one chapter of this book. This chapter encompasses the classical systemically acting asphyxiants, carbon monoxide, carbon dioxide, and hydrocyanic acid. In view of the similarity of their toxic actions, hydrogen sulfide and hydrazoic acid are also included. The methemoglobin-forming gases NO and NO_2 form a bridge between systemic and pulmonary toxicants. Similar actions and mutual chemical reactions suggest also placing ozone among this group of gases, although it is admitted that such an arrangement may be somewhat arbitrary.

Most of the toxic effects of airborne poisons do not obey Haber's law, which states that the product of the concentration of a gas and the duration of exposure required to produce a specific effect is equal to a constant, that is, $C \times t = k$. This is true for carbon monoxide and carbon dioxide, which are metabolically inert, and for hydrocyanic acid, and probably also for hydrogen sulfide and ozone, which are quickly biotransformed, thus allowing nontoxic thresholds. The situation is less clear with the nitrogen oxides and with hydrazoic acid because of their inherent mutagenic potentials. Hence, the establishment of a maximum safe concentration is difficult and may change with the enlargement of our knowledge.

Exposure to toxicants from industrial or urban environments has become a subject of considerable public interest and regulatory action. The "Workplace Exposure Guidelines" have been taken from the American Conference of Governmental Industrial Hygienists (ACGIH, 1996). They are mostly presented as TWA, that is, the time-weighted average exposure concentration for a conventional 8-h workday and a 40-h work week. They may include short-term exposure limits of no more than 15 min (STELs). Other occupational exposure values have been published by the National Institute of Occupational Safety and Health (NIOSH, 1994) as recommended exposure limits (RELs) and by the Occupational Safety and Health Administration (OSHA, 1993) as permissible exposure limits (PELs). These limits and the German MAK values (Maximum Concentrations in the Workplace; DFG 1996) are comparable to the TWA values. Their concentrations are given in ppm (ml/m^3) or in mg/m^3, the latter referring to 20°C and a barometric pressure of 1013 hPa.

CARBON MONOXIDE

Worldwide, some 600 million tons of carbon monoxide (CO) are released into the atmosphere each year, mainly by the combustion of hydrocarbons. A similar amount originates from the tropospheric oxidation of methane emanating from swamps and manure. Another major amount results from the catabolism of porphyrin-containing material, mainly of chlorophyll from algae and leaves. CO also arises from heme oxygenase-catalyzed degradation of hemoglobin at the α-methene bridge, which is the most important endogenous source of CO in humans. In recent years, evidence has been accumulating that CO generated by the two iso-forms of heme oxygenase also has neuromessenger functions in the brain and in the periphery, in analogy to NO.

Despite this huge CO challenge, the global ecosystem is hardly affected because CO is continuously eliminated from the higher atmosphere by oxidation to CO_2 via hydroxyl radicals. CO is also degraded by soil bacteria. Hence, the atmospheric half-life of CO is rather short and amounts to less than half a year. The mean atmospheric concentration is approximately 0.1 ppm. Thus, CO is not a global threat but rather a regional one. In the United States, CO is the main cause of deaths due to poisoning, accounting for some 4,000 annual fatalities, roughly two-thirds of these occurring in fire victims.

Properties, Sources, and Exposure Potential

Carbon monoxide (CO, molecular weight 28.01, 1 ppm = 1.16 mg/m^3) is a nonirritating, colorless and odorless gas with a relative specific gravity of 0.97 (air = 1); it therefore tends to rise in the air and to seep unperceived through cracked conduits, ceilings, and walls. In humid air, CO burns with a blue flame and produces CO_2 exothermically. Its property of combining with oxygen at high temperatures is exploited to reduce metal oxides, such as in iron smelting. Palladium salts are reduced by CO at ambient temperatures; this can be used as a sensitive CO test. Mixtures of CO (12.5 to 74%) with air are explosive. At higher temperatures, CO disproportionates to carbon and CO_2, the equilibrium (Boudouard equilibrium) approaching unity at 700°C.

In the 19th century, synthetic cracked-coal gas containing 6 to 40% CO was introduced for lighting, cooking, and heating. It caused many accidental fatalities from leaking fixtures and became the favorite means of committing suicide by "taking the gas pipe." Nowadays, the households are usually provided with natural gas that does not contain CO.

In conflagrations and mine explosions in confined spaces, atmospheres containing 0.5 to 8% CO prevail. Under these conditions, most fire victims die from CO poisoning rather than from burns. This also happened in 1906, when some 1,100 miners died from a mine explosion in Northern France. Most CO accidents occur due to incomplete combustion of carbonaceous fuel. Automobile exhaust may contain up to 10% CO, and car engines being warmed up in garages located under the living rooms of single-family dwellings have been a source of CO poisoning. Catalytic converters substantially reduce the CO level to below 1%, which is still enough to cause intoxication. Hence, all garage doors and windows should remain open as long as a car engine is running, and prolonged operation of an automobile engine in a garage should be avoided. In 68 cases of accidental CO poisoning, 20 cases concerned children riding in the back of pickup trucks, most of them under a rigid, closed canopy. In all these cases, the truck exhaust system had a known leak or a tailpipe with an outlet at the rear rather than at the side of the pickup truck. Another source of repeated accidents are ice-resurfacing machines with internal combustion engines in closed rinks. Skaters in particular may be at risk for CO poisoning, as physical exercise is attended with increased respiration. CO levels on expressway may approach 25 to 100 ppm. A 90-min Los Angeles freeway exposure produced ECG abnormalities in 40% of patients with preexisting cardiovascular disease.

About one-third of fatal CO accidents are caused by faulty heating equipment, such as improperly vented gas water heaters and kerosene space heaters. Intoxication occurred in inappropriately ventilated rooms in which charcoal grills or ceramic kilns were used.

Tobacco smokers have chronically elevated HbCO levels. The consumption of two to three packs per day results in 7 to 9% HbCO. Nonsmokers may passively

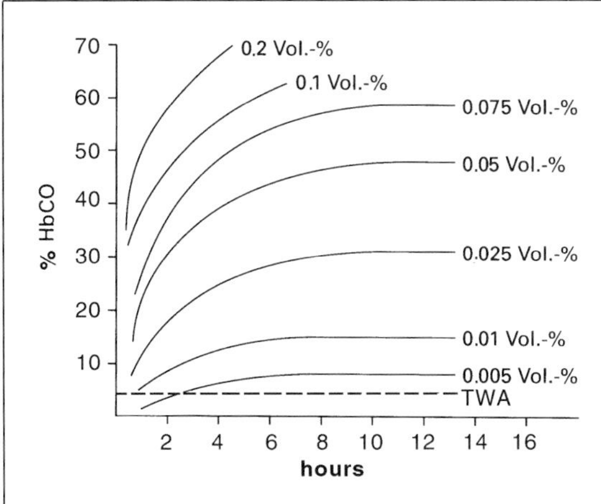

FIGURE 1 Formation of HbCO upon inhalation of various CO concentrations at a respiratory minute volume of 10 liters/min (resting conditions). 100 ppm (0.01%) CO results in 12% HbCO at normal oxygen concentration. The dashed line indicates the TWA (25 ppm).

inhale the CO equivalents of five cigarettes in a smoky room over an 8-hour period. Tobacco smoke contains between 1.5 and 4.5% CO.

CO is formed as a metabolite of dichloromethane that is used as a paint and varnish remover. In poorly ventilated spaces, the use of such a paint remover may cause myocardial infarction in predisposed patients. An unexpected source of CO exposure may be found during anesthesia. Anecdotal reports suggest that CO_2 absorbents can produce CO from inhaled anesthetics containing a CF_2H moiety. Peak CO concentrations of 10,000 and 4000 ppm were detected over 1 min when 4% desflurane and 1.2% enflurane, respectively, passed through a completely dry absorbent (20% $Ba(OH)_2$, 80% $Ca(OH)_2$) at a flow rate of 12.5 ml/min. The associated chemical reactions have not been fully elucidated. At any rate, the CO generation could be greatly reduced by using absorbents containing some percentage of water. Although no reports indicate that injury has resulted from CO due to the degradation of an anesthetic, this issue is of considerable concern during prolonged closed-circuit anesthesia in patients who are at an increased risk from CO.

Absorption, Distribution, Metabolism, Excretion, and Mechanisms of Toxicity

The lungs rapidly absorb carbon monoxide, which avidly combines with hemoglobin to impair the transport and delivery of oxygen to the cells. The competition of oxygen and carbon monoxide for the same ferrous heme binding sites on hemoglobin is described by the Haldane equation:

$$[Hb(CO)_4]/[Hb(O_2)_4] = M\, pCO/pO_2.$$

The value of the constant M is approximately 250 at pH 7.4 for human blood.

Therefore, if $pCO = 1/250\ pO_2$, the hemoglobin will be half-saturated with CO. Hence, 0.1% of CO in inspired air results in more than 50% HbCO (Fig. 1). The high affinity of CO is caused by the very low dissociation-rate constant (2500 times lower than that of oxygen), while the rate of CO association is 10 times lower than that of oxygen.

The rate at which the arterial blood approaches equilibrium with the inspired gas depends on the diffusion capacity of the lungs and the alveolar ventilation; both are related to the level of exercise (Fig. 2). Several other factors govern the toxicity of CO (e.g., duration of exposure, cardiac output, oxygen demand of the tissues, and blood hemoglobin concentration). Therefore, anemic persons are more susceptible to CO than individuals with normal amounts of hemoglobin.

An increased metabolic rate enhances the severity of the symptoms of CO poisoning, so that children will succcumb earlier than adults if exposed to a given concentration of the gas. For this reason, small animals such as canaries have been used for the detection of toxic CO concentrations in mines.

CO reduces the oxygen delivery to the tissue by an additional important mechanism. The affinity of oxygen for the tetrameric hemoglobin decreases with

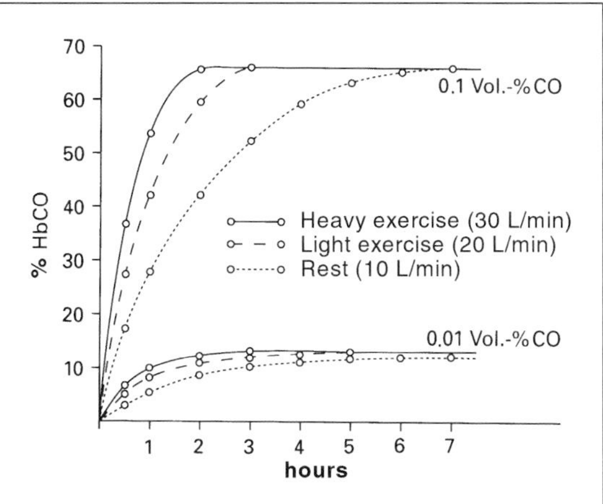

FIGURE 2 Influence of the respiratory minute volume on the rate of HbCO formation. Heavy exercise shortens the time to reach equilibrium.

gradual deoxygenation, as the conformation of deoxyhemoglobin has a smaller affinity for ligands than does hemoglobin in the tetrameric R-state (fully liganded). This phenomenon causes the sigmoidal shape of the oxyhemoglobin dissociation curve. The affinity of oxygen for $Hb(O_2)_2$ is smaller by a factor of 10 than it is for $Hb(O_2)_3$, and is even smaller for $Hb(O_2)_1$ and $Hb(O_2)_0$. Hence, at the oxygen partial pressure of the tissue most hemoglobin species are in the form of $Hb(O_2)_4$ and deoxyhemoglobin with only small percentages of the partially saturated intermediates. Correspondingly, the hemoglobin hybrid $Hb(CO)(O_2)_3$ has a much higher oxygen affinity than $Hb(O_2)_3$, resulting in a distortion and less sigmoidal shape of the oxyhemoglobin dissociation curve (Fig. 3). Although no method has been devised to test the existence of hybrid species in which both oxygen and carbon monoxide are found on the same tetramer, the demonstration of hybrid species with similar properties in the case of methemoglobin lends credence to the hybrid hypothesis for carboxyhemoglobin. For this reason, the oxygen delivery from the hemoglobin hybrids will be much smaller than expected from the reduced oxygen-binding capacity of the blood. However, an anemic patient with a similarly low binding capacity will not suffer from hypoxia to the same extent as in the case of CO intoxication.

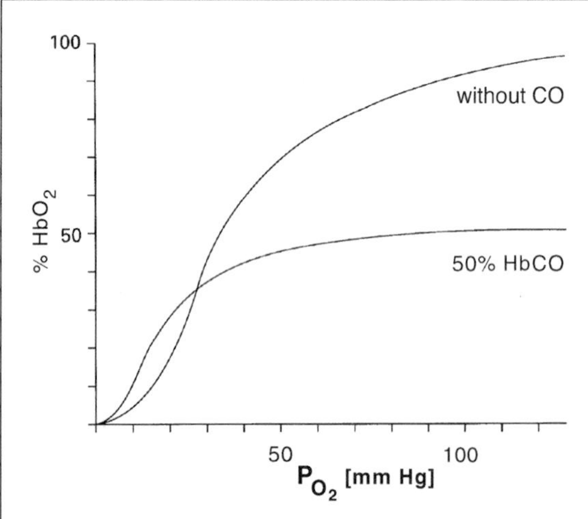

FIGURE 3 Dissociation curves of normal oxyhemoglobin and hemoglobin hybrids containing 50% HbCO. Normal hemoglobin shows oxygen half-saturation at an oxygen partial pressure of 27 mm Hg, while hybrids containing 50% HbCO give this figure at 15 mm Hg. At 27 mm Hg, 50% oxygen will be released from normal oxyhemoglobin, but only 15% from hemoglobin hybrids containing 50% HbCO.

This effect is not observed with the monomeric myoglobin. Therefore, the oxygen delivery from myoglobin (particularly in the heart muscle) to the mitochondrial respiratory chain may be expected to be less affected, the more so because the affinity of CO for myoglobin is only 40 times that of oxygen. However, the percentage of carboxymyoglobin is higher than that of carboxyhemoglobin because the concentration of competing oxygen is much lower in the heart muscle cell than in the venous blood.

Apart from its influence on the oxygen affinity, CO also reduces the oxygen dissociation rate, which further impairs the oxygen supply to the tissues. Another function of hemoglobin is altered by CO; the affinity of CO_2 for the N-terminal amino groups of hemoglobin (reversible carbamate formation) is diminished in HbCO when compared to deoxyhemoglobin.

Other heme proteins that form an intermediate ferrous iron (e.g., cytochrome P450, cytochrome *c*, and cytochrome oxidase) are significantly inhibited by exogenous CO only at supralethal concentrations that cause severe tissue hypoxia. However, if CO arises during biotransformation of halogenated hydrocarbons by means of cytochrome P450 2E1, it may have easy access to the neighboring mitochondria, resulting in inhibition of cytochrome oxidase.

Recently, CO has been discussed as activating guanylate cyclase, in analogy to NO, leading to vasodilatation. In fact, CO has been shown to dilate coronary arteries in the isolated heart, and studies *in vivo* have demonstrated a significant decrease in the blood pressure of rats exposed to 500 ppm CO for 31 days. Moreover, CO exposure increased the release of NO from platelets several hundred-fold, possibly by binding to the nitric oxide synthase. NO and NO-derived oxidants such as peroxynitrite have a high affinity for sulfur–iron proteins. They are able to inactivate mitochondrial enzymes, to impair electron transport and to accelerate the production of reactive oxygen species.

The CO-induced delayed neurologic sequelae cannot be explained by tissue hypoxia alone. Neuroimaging studies suggest that perivascular damage and secondary hemorrhagic necroses give rise to the focal pathology that is typical of CO poisoning. The individual molecular events are not clear, but it appears that systemic hypotension due to decreased cardiac output, together with vasodilation, compromises the cerebral blood flow. These changes have been linked to oxidative injury in the brain. In addition, excitatory amino acids may also play a role in CO neuropathology, effects that can be prevented by glutamate-receptor-blocking agents, such as dizolcipine. At any rate, CO toxicity should not be regarded as an exclusive hemoglobinotoxicity.

Acute and Chronic Toxicity

Acute Toxicity

Acute poisoning with CO is a rare event and requires concentrations of >2000 ppm (Fig. 1). The clinical signs and symptoms of intoxication do not correlate with the concentration of CO in the inspired air but with the degree of carboxyhemoglobinemia. The symptoms can be described as follows:

[HbCO] <20%: Shortness of breath and impaired motor skill comparable to the effects seen at high altitudes; impairment of decision making, visual threshold, and visual discrimination. Such effects suggest alcoholic inebriation and may contribute to industrial and car accidents. CO decreases light sensitivity and dark adaptation of the eyes.

[HbCO] 20–30%: Fatigue, headache, dizziness, dimness of vision, confusion, and impaired judgment. The patient may be unable to make clear decisions for escape despite the physical ability to do so.

[HbCO] 30–50%: Decided headache, fainting on exertion, collapse, and confusion.

[HbCO] >50%: Usually, unconsciousness, intermittent convulsions, and respiratory failure ensue; and unless treatment is instituted, collapse, cardiac standstill, and death are likely to follow. The color of HbCO in the dilated skin capillaries can often be seen as a cherry-red blush.

Subacute Toxicity

Most of the severe accidents with CO show a subacute development. Toxic signs and symptoms proceed within several hours at CO levels between 500 and 2000 ppm (Fig. 2). This type of intoxication is characterized by severe lactacidosis, which is considered a more reliable parameter than the CO content of blood for grading the severity of intoxication. The cherry-red hue of the skin is seldom observed on admission to the hospital because the patients have been treated with oxygen during transport and the circulatory shock may have caused centralization. If hypoxia and acidosis have lasted for longer periods, the patients become deeply unconscious, exhibiting signs of cerebral edema, muscle spasm, hyperreflexia, and convulsions. Cheyne–Stokes respiration may indicate precipitating respiratory arrest. Patients with cardiovascular disease are particularly sensitive to CO and may show disturbances in ECG conduction, atrial fibrillation, premature ventricular contractions, and signs of myocardial infarction.

The cardiotoxic effects of CO have been confirmed in animal experiments. The exposure of rats to 2300 ppm of CO for 10 min with HbCO levels of 45% was associated with an increase in the heart-specific plasma creatine phosphokinase activity. The number of ectopic beats in response to norepinephrine stress increased and microscopic focal lesions appeared in the myocardium.

Chronic Toxicity

Chronic toxicity of CO is uncommon because it does not accumulate in the body. However, repeated exposure to toxic concentrations, which individually do not precipitate any gross symptoms, may cause accumulated damage. It should be considered that CO toxicity is increased by several factors, including decreased barometric pressure (e.g., at higher altitude), lowered oxygen content (e.g., in fires within confined spaces), and high metabolic rate (e.g., in pregnant women or hyperthyroidism). The fetus is particularly vulnerable to CO poisoning because of the lower fetal pO_2 levels (20–30 mm Hg) compared to 100 mm Hg in adults. Furthermore, the fetal hemoglobin dissociation curve is shifted to the left compared to the curve for adults, resulting in more pronounced tissue hypoxia.

The teratogenic risk of CO has not received special attention in the past. However, a review of 60 case reports of acute CO poisoning involving pregnant women shows a striking correlation between CO exposure and fetal death or toxic effects, including anatomical malformations and functional alterations. The high teratogenic risk of CO is also supported by animal data. The neonatal mortality in the children of intensively smoking mothers was elevated and their weight at birth was decreased. Neonates are more susceptible towards CO due to residual fetal hemoglobin and to the increased hemoglobin degradation *post partum.*

Anemia, particularly hemolytic anemia with enhanced endogenous CO production due to hemoglobin degradation, reduces the threshold for exogenous CO. The same holds true for heavy smokers with basal HbCO values between 5 and 15%. Patients suffering from reduced vascular perfusion (e.g., because of a cardiovascular, peripheral, or cerebral vascular disease) are at increased risk.

Therapeutic Measures

Immediate removal from the contaminated area, control of the airway, and support of breathing with artificial ventilation are the priorities. It should be emphasized that first-aid personnel must be aware of the dangerous atmosphere. It has happened more than once that, when a victim was treated in the odorless contaminated atmosphere, the treating physician was overcome. Care has to be taken to avoid switching on electric lights or other equipment because an explosive atmospheric mixture of CO and oxygen may be present. Of course, the same applies to open flames.

The elimination of CO should be initiated immediately by vigorous ventilation with 100% oxygen (half-life of HbCO is 60 to 80 min at normobaric O_2). Placing victims in a pressure chamber containing oxygen at 2.5–3 atm immediately results in a sufficient oxygen supply to the tissue by the oxygen physically dissolved in plasma and, moreover, in a rapid clearance of blood from CO. The HbCO half-life has been estimated at 10–20 min under hyperbaric conditions. This measure, however, requires the proximate availability of such a facility and the presence of trained personnel. Hyperbaric oxygen therapy is not without risk in view of the possibility of decompression sickness as a result of intravascular and intracellular distension, mainly by dissolved nitrogen.

In parallel to the vigorous ventilation, the institution of intravenous lines and the correction of acidosis are mandatory. After that, the addition of 5% CO_2 to the oxygen can powerfully stimulate respiration, as is illustrated by the effect of carbogen ventilation on the decrease of HbCO in a poisoned dog (Fig. 4).

Especially in the cases of fire victims, other toxic gases (e.g., hydrogen cyanide and nitric oxides) have to be considered and identified before initiating any further specific treatment.

The possible development of cerebral edema has to be monitored by serial neurological examinations (e.g., fundoscopy and CAT scans). Corticosteroids have been administered, but their value has not been definitively proven. To reduce the intracranial pressure, mannitol infusion (20% solution; 0.5 g/kg within 30 min) has been recommended.

The early therapy of acute poisoning is particularly successful and has a good prognosis. Due to its poor water solubility, physically dissolved CO is rapidly removed from the plasma by exhalation. In contrast, severe subacute intoxication is often associated with permanent neurological sequels. Patients may develop neurological symptoms, such as temporospatial disorientation, amnesia, apathy, dysphasia, memory loss, urinary incontinence, gait disturbance, and franc psychosis, 2 to 3 weeks after the initial recovery. Rarely, Parkinson's disease develops. The degree of recovery varies, with up to 75% resolving after 1 year, but memory deficits and gait disturbances may remain.

It has been stressed repeatedly that the outcomes poorly correlate with the HbCO levels found on admission to the hospital. On this basis, survivors cannot be distinguished from nonsurvivors.

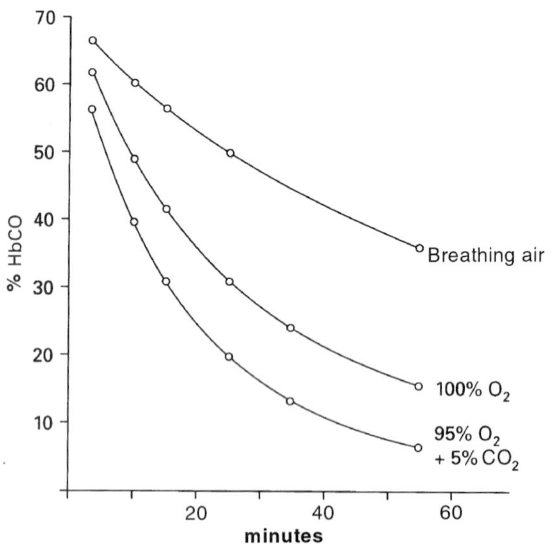

FIGURE 4 Time course of the decrease of HbCO in dogs breathing air, pure oxygen, or a mixture of 95% oxygen and 5% carbon dioxide. The half-life of CO elimination is reduced from 60 min (air) to 20 min (pure oxygen) and 12 min (carbogen), respectively.

Work-Place Exposure Guidelines

The TWA values are 25 and 30 ppm (ACGIH and MAK, respectively), at which maximum HbCO levels of 5% are expected during an 8-hour period on the assumption of normal physical activity. OSHA recommends a TWA of 50 ppm and NIOSH 35 ppm with a STEL of 200 ppm. These concentrations hold for normal altitudes; at heights between 5000 and 8000 ft (1500–2400 m) only half of the above value is accepted. Currently, the recommended values are felt to be too high; if persons at increased risk, such as pregnant women, are considered, HbCO concentrations should not exceed 2.7%.

Analysis

HbCO in freshly drawn blood is easily detected spectroscopically after deoxygenation of oxyhemoglobin with sodium dithionite. Small percentages of HbCO can be detected by GC or infrared spectroscopy. Draeger tubes are available with a sensitivity ranging from 5 to 70,000 ppm. The catalytic reduction by CO of iodine pentoxide liberates iodine, which is detectable by its color.

CARBON DIOXIDE

The atmosphere contains about 0.03% carbon dioxide, a value that was constant in previous centuries. Increased emissions from the combustion of fossil fuels, however, has led to a global increase of carbon dioxide from 0.028% at the beginning of the 19th century to approximately 0.035% in the late 20th century. Humans produce carbon dioxide via the oxidative metabolism of carbohydrates, fatty acids, and amino acids at a rate of 20 l/h under resting conditions. Thus, enhanced concentrations of carbon dioxide are formed in crowded halls, such as in a university auditorium where 0.09% was found at the end of a lecture. Concentrations below 1% are usually well tolerated and without immediate health effects. Of more concern, however, are the physical properties of carbon dioxide in the troposphere. Carbon dioxide is transparent to the incoming short-wave radiation, but it absorbs the long-wave radiation emitted from Earth's surface. Carbon dioxide is estimated to contribute by some 50% to the Greenhouse Effect.

Properties, Sources, and Exposure Potential

Carbon dioxide (CO_2, molecular weight 44.01, 1 ppm = 1.83 mg/m^3) is a nonirritating, colorless, odorless, nonflammable gas with a slightly sour taste. It has a relative specific gravity of 1.5 (air = 1), therefore tending to spread along the ground. CO_2 does not exist as a liquid at atmospheric pressure; it sublimes from the solid state (i.e., from dry ice, at −78.5°C). At 20°C, CO_2 can be liquefied at 55 atmospheres; in this form it is usually distributed in steel cylinders.

CO_2 is expelled into the atmosphere from Earth via springs, wells, and volcanoes. Various other sources include the respiration of plants and animals, decay of organic material, and industrial processes, such as lime-burning and the production of hydrogen and ammonia. CO_2 is removed from the air by photosynthesis, the weathering of rocks, and the metabolism of certain bacteria. All these processes give rise to a dynamic equilibrium of global CO_2.

About half of all the technical CO_2 recovered is used at the point of production to make further chemicals, such as urea and methanol. CO_2 is used as an inert gas; it is particularly suitable for use in fire extinguishers (a candle is extinguished by 8 to 10% CO_2), as shielding gas in arc welding, and for the handling and transportation of materials and foodstuffs sensitive to autoxidation. CO_2 is an excellent medium for heat transfer in (nuclear) power stations and is used as a refrigerant.

When solid CO_2 is handled, there is a risk of skin burns, similar to severe frostbite. Of more toxicological concern, however, is gaseous CO_2 at higher percentages. Fatalities have occurred in mines, well pits, and confined spaces during the fermentation of carbonaceous material, such as in breweries, wineries, farm silos, and ship cargo holds loaded with grain, soja, potatoes, and fruit. CO_2 emanating from dry ice during the cooling of sensitive material has caused intoxication on cargo airplanes.

Absorption, Distribution, Metabolism, Excretion, and Mechanisms of Toxicity

When inhaled, CO_2 freely penetrates the cellular membranes. The diffusion rate of CO_2 through the alveolar membrane into the blood is about 20 times that of O_2. Catalyzed by carbonic anhydrase of erythrocytes, 90% of the CO_2 in the blood reacts with water to form carbonic acid, which in turn is ionized to bicarbonate. About 5% of the CO_2 in the blood is physically dissolved in the water of plasma and cells. The remaining 5% of CO_2 is bound to hemoglobin in the carbamino form. The normal partial pressure of CO_2 in the plasma of mixed venous blood is about 46 mm Hg.

Most of the CO_2 is eliminated from the body via exhalation, amounting to 220 and 1700 ml/min in healthy humans at rest and during moderate exercise, respectively. Normally, CO_2 is exhaled at the same rate at which it is produced, leaving a partial pressure of about 40 mm Hg in the alveoli and in the arterial blood. The CO_2–bicarbonate couple functions as the major buffering system in the blood. When CO_2 is inhaled or when alveolar ventilation is decreased, the pCO_2 in the arterial blood rises and pH falls, which is referred to as respiratory acidosis. CO_2 is a potent stimulus to ventilation, particularly under hypoxic conditions. Under normoxic conditions very little respiratory stimulation occurs until the inspired CO_2 concentration exceeds about 2%. Upon increasing CO_2 to 10%, the respiratory minute volume increases up to 75 liters/min. Respiratory stimulation involving both rate and tidal volume begins within seconds, and the maximal effect is usually attained within less than 5 min. The mechanism by which CO_2 acts on the peripheral arterial and the medullary chemoreceptors probably involves a decrease in pH. Moreover, elevated pCO_2 causes bronchodilation and widespread activation of the sympathetic nervous system. As a result, cardiac contractility, heart rate, and cardiac output increase. Sympathetic effects on the blood vessels are counteracted by the local effects of CO_2, leading to a decrease in peripheral resistance. Cerebral blood vessels, which are devoid of functionally important innervation, undergo dilatation when CO_2 is inhaled.

Elevated levels of CO_2 in the blood depress the excitability of the CNS and raise the threshold for pain stimuli and the onset of seizures. Pre-existing CNS depression can be accentuated by CO_2. However, inhalation of CO_2 at concentrations above 25% can activate the cortical regions and elicit seizures.

Acute and Chronic Toxicity

Acute Toxicity

Dyspnea is usually observed at CO_2 concentrations above 3% during 30 min of exposure. While normal subjects can tolerate a fivefold increase in breathing for a short time period, increased ventilation for longer periods becomes unpleasant and distressing. In addition to dyspnea, acute exposure to CO_2 usually causes a headache that is more intense during exercise. It has been supposed that headache is caused by CO_2-induced vasodilation of meningeal vessels. However, headache does usually not appear immediately upon CO_2 exposure but rather at the end of the trials. Hence, CO_2-induced acidosis may be another cause for headache. The plasma pH has been found to drop from 7.40 to 7.30 during a 1-h exposure to 7% CO_2. At this concentration, a deterioration of mental competence rapidly becomes evident. In addition, hearing and vision may be impaired within several minutes of exposure to 6% CO_2.

At 15 to 20% CO_2 in the inspired air, respiratory distress is abrupt and violent in onset, accompanied by a rapid loss of consciousness and spasmodic muscular twitching. With 20 to 30% inspired CO_2 (with oxygen for safety), convulsions occur within 1 to 3 min after the beginning of the exposure. Death may ensue, probably due to severe acidosis.

Chronic Toxicity

Chronically elevated pCO_2 is found in submarines, in diving, and in similar work. The problem of increased concentrations of CO_2 is of more concern at higher ambient pressure than during spacecraft activities, where the ambient pressure is considerably reduced. Hence, 5% CO_2 may be detrimental at a pressure of 5 atmospheres, but of no concern at 0.2 atmospheres. In addition to the acute symptoms already described, pCO_2 when increased over longer periods may influence the levels of calcium, magnesium, and inorganic phosphate. The results, however, found in submarine crews exposed to about 1% CO_2 for several weeks are equivocal. At any rate, it appears that the specific influences of CO_2 exposure are completely reversible.

Therapeutic Measures

Acutely intoxicated patients usually recover rapidly in fresh air. Rescuers should be aware that oxygen may be lacking on the ground of confined spaces. Hence they should only enter with a self-contained breathing apparatus (SCBA). If hypoxia prevails, artificial ventilation with oxygen and correction of the acidosis are mandatory. Pulmonary edema may ensue from longer-lasting hypoxic states.

Work-Place Exposure Guidelines

The TWA value is 5000 ppm with a STEL of 30,000 ppm (ACGIH, OSHA, NIOSH, MAK).

Analysis

On passing a solution of freshly filtered barium hydroxide, CO_2 forms poorly soluble barium carbonate. Draeger tubes are available, covering a range between 0.01 and 60% CO_2. Carbamate formation with hydrazine, used to keep crystal violet in the reduced state, is exploited to detect CO_2 by violet discoloration.

CYANIDES

Hydrogen cyanide (hydrocyanic acid) is one of the fastest acting poisons; it is well known to most lay persons because of its use in spectacular murders (e.g., the Marcov poison umbrella), suicides, and judicial executions. The homicidal misuse of hydrogen cyanide is associated with the incomprehensible genocides during the Nazi regime and the collective suicide in Jonestown, Guyana, when 900 adults and children followed a sect leader into death. Insidious assassinations made the headlines in 1982 when seven persons in the metropolitan Chicago area were fatally poisoned with potassium-cyanide-laced capsules. The role of hydrogen cyanide and its derivatives in prebiotic evolution of our planet's atmosphere is probably less known. Curiously, the deadly hydrogen cyanide was the prerequisite for the prebiotic formation of the majority of biochemical compounds necessary for life (i.e., purines, pyrimidines, and amino acids).

Munitioning of hydrogen cyanide as a potential chemical-warfare agent is a principle that Mother Nature has made use of for eons. Thus, hydrogen cyanide is liberated from various seeds and fruits to discourage predators, but animals and humans have learned to cope with small amounts of cyanide by metabolic inactivation.

Properties, Sources, and Exposure Potential

Hydrogen cyanide (HCN, molecular weight 27.03, 1 ppm = 1.12 mg/m^3) is a colorless liquid (density 0.687; mp −14°C; bp 26°C). Anhydrous HCN dimerizes in the liquid state. Due to its relative density of 0.94 (air = 1) HCN vapor rises in the air. HCN is completely miscible with water and ethanol. It is a weak acid (pK_a = 9.2), and aqueous solutions of its alkali salts are strong alkaline caustics. HCN vapor has a characteristic smell reminiscent of bitter almonds, which is recognized by some people at very low concentrations. The limit of detection, however, varies widely (0.2 to 5 ppm), and a considerable proportion of the population has an inborn deficiency for smelling HCN. Another warning sign of HCN vapor is a burning sensation in the throat.

HCN is a prototypical fumigant that has been formerly widely used in the elimination of insects and rodents from orchards, buildings, greenhouses, ships, and stored merchandise and foodstuffs. Sodium and potassium cyanide are hygroscopic salts, from which atmospheric carbon dioxide can liberate the less acidic HCN with formation of the corresponding hydrogen carbonates. HCN and the alkali cyanides are used for the extraction of gold and silver from their ores. This process, cyanidation, involves the leaching of stable soluble cyanide complexes that can be directly used for electroplating.

Cyanides are used in case-hardening procedures and iron-cyanide blue pigments (Chinese, Prussian, and Milori blues) in photography, blueprints, carbon paper, and pigment manufacture. Thiocyanates (rhodanides), derivatives of HCN, are used in photography and film processing.

Calcium cyanamide is an important source of fixed nitrogen and therefore extensively exploited as plant fertilizer. It is also used as an herbicide, a defoliant for cotton and tomatoes and as a pesticide. Cyanogen chloride is used in the synthesis of triazine herbicides, cyanogen bromide as a pesticidal fumigant. Of the nitriles, nitrilotriacetic acid is used for calcium complexation (e.g., in washing powders). Acetonitrile and acrylonitrile are important components for the synthesis of rubbers and plastics.

Naturally occurring nitriles (Fig. 5) include amygdalin and prunasin, which are found in bitter almonds and the pits of fruits such as cherry, peach, and apricot. During absorption from the gut, amygdalin is hydrolyzed in the mucosal cell first-pass metabolism, liberating a glucose molecule and the monosaccharide prunasin. By the reaction with another β-glucosidase, benzaldehyde cyanohydrin (mandelonitrile) is formed, which easily releases HCN. Hence, these precursors are termed cyanogenic. It has been suggested that cyanogenesis may have a protective function in plants. In fact, a correlation was found between the concentration of HCN released from dhurrin when the grain sorghum is bitten by the African grasshopper (*Locusta migratoria*) and the unpalatability of individual sorghum plants to the locust. Similarly, the grasshopper is normally deterred from eating cassava (*Manhiot esculenta*) by the production of relatively large amounts of HCN liberated from linamarin. The contents of cyanide found in various plants and foodstuffs are shown in Table 1. Even arthropods use cyanide for their defense. The millipede *Haraphe haydeniana,* for example, synthesizes mandelonitrile from phenylalanine. The cyanogen can be stored and mixed in a reaction chamber with an α-hydroxynitrile lyase that enables the quick release of HCN. By this device, potential predators such as birds or lizards may be quickly deterred from feeding by this cyanogenic secretion.

Cyanide intoxication from cyanogenic glycosides repeatedly occurs in tropical regions and has been associated with motoneuron diseases such as "konzo" and "mantekassa." An epidemic outbreak occurred in Mozambique in 1981. It followed a severe drought and the failure of the harvest of maize and sorghum. Even the production of cassava was severely reduced. The short-cut method of fermentation did not allow

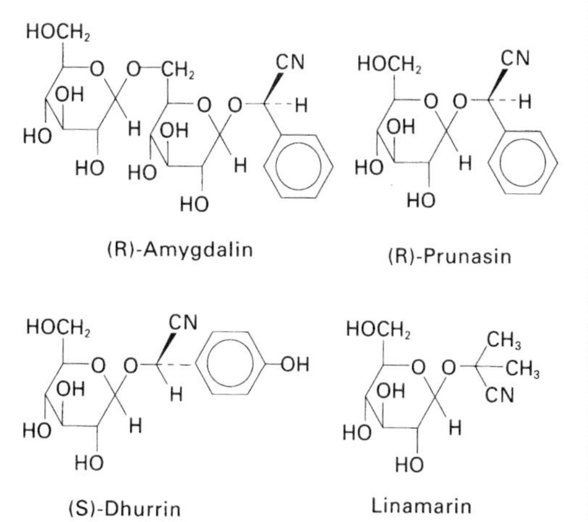

(R)-Amygdalin

(R)-Prunasin

(S)-Dhurrin

Linamarin

FIGURE 5 Cyanogenic glycosides found in various foodstuffs.

TABLE 1 Cyanogen Content of Foodstuffs

Cyanogenic glycoside	Content (g HCN/kg)	Source
Amygdalin	2.5–5	Seeds of bitter almonds, peach, and apricot
	<1	Seeds of plum, pear, and apple
Prunasin	1.0–1.5	Cherry laurel
Linamarin	0.3–2.5	Cassava tubers
	up to 8	Bamboo sprouts
	up to 3	Lima beans
	up to 0.5	Linseeds
Dhurrin	0.1–0.3	Sorghum

the elimination of the cyanhydrin and, together with a low protein intake (i.e., shortage in sulfur uptake, see the following), led to the neurological disease.

There have been a number of fatalities from acute cyanide poisoning following the ingestion of cyanogenic compounds by paramedic intention. Amygdalin has been promoted commercially, mostly in the United States, for the treatment of a number of diseases, including cancer. This controversial preparation can give rise to high levels of cyanide, especially if ingested together with foods containing β-glucosidases that degrade amygdalin into mandelonitrile. The seeds of apples and pears are especially rich in these enzymes. Hence, the combination of amygdalin with fruit may have produced a particularly dangerous cocktail. Another potential source of cyanide intoxication is sodium nitroprusside, which is used in malignant hypertension and may require concomitant administration of sodium thiosulfate. The thermostabile HCN is also produced during the combustion of nitrogenous material, thus being a significant factor in mortality from fires. The increased use of plastics and synthetic materials for buildings and furnishings has been associated with the increase in morbidity and mortality from the inhalation of smoke. In comparison with natural materials, such as wool and silk, nitrogenous synthetic materials (e.g., polyacrylonitrile, nylon, polyurethane, and melamine) tend to be easily ignited and, when burning, produce intense fires with thermal decomposition.

Absorption, Distribution, Metabolism, and Excretion

HCN is very rapidly absorbed from the lungs, and good absorption occurs across both mucous membranes (e.g., in the oral cavity and stomach) and intact skin. The cyanide salts are less permeable. In dogs, following administration of 24 mg KCN/kg by gavage, 31% of the dose was still present in the stomach 2 h later (pH 9.5). When 0.5 equivalents of hydrochloric acid were co-administered, only 4% of the dose remained in the stomach (pH 8.5).

Small amounts of cyanide are sequestered in the red blood cells by binding to endogenous methemoglobin (0.5 to 1%). The apparent dissociation constant is 2×10^{-6} M at pH 7.4. Cyanide is reversibly bound to plasma proteins (approximately 60%). Hence, the proportion of free cyanide in plasma water is much smaller than expected from the total cyanide content in blood, particularly at low cyanide load. Therefore, the apparent volume of distribution largely depends on cyanide concentration and methemoglobin content. The very widely varying compartmentation of cyanide also has an impact on its elimination half-life. In the dog 15 to 50 min have been reported; upon artificial methemoglobinemia (30%), the value increased to 80 min. A half-life of 1.2 h was found in patients with cyanide inhalation during fires.

Small, though detectable (by smell), amounts of cyanide are exhaled; the excretion of unchanged cyanide by urine is insignificant. The various metabolic routes depend on the cyanide load. Quantitatively most important is thiocyanate (rhodanide) formation. This reaction is catalyzed by the enzyme rhodanese (thiosulfate: cyanide sulfotransferase [EC 2.8.1.1]), using sulfane sulfur (RSO_xS) as a donor and a thiophile such as cyanide or sulfite as an acceptor. In the first step, the sulfur atom is transferred to the enzyme, followed by sulfuration of the acceptor. In the reaction of cyanide with thiosulfate, thiocyanate and sulfite are formed.

The enzyme is mainly located in the mitochondria of the liver and skeletal muscles. According to calculation for dogs, the total amount of rhodanese should be able to detoxify 5 g of cyanide within 15 min. In fact, detoxication is by two orders of magnitude slower because the diffusion of thiosulfate across the mitochondrial membranes is rate limiting.

Sulfane sulfur is also metabolically produced from 3-mercaptopyruvate by catalysis of a 3-mercaptopyruvate sulfur transferase (EC 2.8.1.2).

3-Mercaptopyruvate is formed by transamination of cysteine and transfers its sulfur atom to a sulfide or sulfite to yield persulfides and thiosulfate, respectively. Alternatively, the enzyme-catalyzed sulfur transfer to cyanide results in thiocyanate and pyruvate formation also within the mitochondria (Fig. 6). If sulfur donors are sufficiently available, most cya-

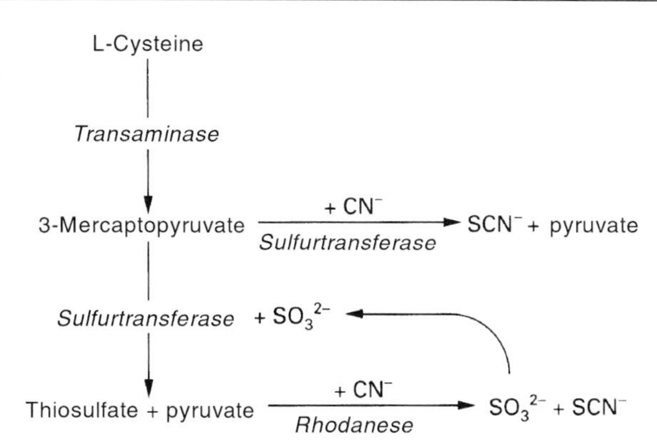

FIGURE 6 Routes of thiocyanate formation from cyanide and cysteine in mammals. 3-Mercaptopyruvate sulfurtransferase cleaves the carbon-sulfur bond of 3-mercaptopyruvate that is formed by transamination of cysteine. Cyanide accepts the sulfane sulfur with formation of thiocyanate. Alternatively, the enzyme catalyzes the sulfur transfer from 3-mercaptopyruvate to sulfite under formation of thiosulfate, from which rhodanese transfers the sulfur to cyanide, generating the sulfite ion needed in the preceding reaction. The final products are pyruvate and thiocyanate, irrespective of the metabolic route. (Adapted from Ballantyne and Marrs, 1987, with permission.)

nide is excreted by the kidneys as thiocyanate (80% in dogs). Small amounts of cyanide enter the C_1 pool of the body and are ultimately excreted as carbon dioxide, thus explaining the delayed elimination of radioactive compounds following the administration of ^{14}CN. The incorporation of the ^{14}C label most probably occurs via cyanate and formic acid.

Mechanisms of Toxicity

As revealed by O. Warburg in the 1920s, cyanide exerts its toxic actions mainly by binding to the heme iron in the cytochrome oxidase complex (cytochrome a–a_3), thereby inhibiting the final step of oxidative phosphorylation in the respiratory chain. As a result, the most effective ATP regeneration and the removal of catabolically formed hydrogen are impeded. The mechanism of cytochrome oxidase inhibition by cyanide is intricate because the enzyme complex contains 2 heme iron and 2 copper atoms and each of them is capable of binding cyanide. The binding rate to the reduced enzyme ($Fe^{2+}Cu^{+}$) is higher than that to the oxidized one, while the binding affinity to the oxidized form ($Fe^{3+}Cu^{2+}$; $K_{Dox} \sim 10^{-6}$ M; $K_{Dred} \sim 10^{-4}$ M) is higher.

Besides cytochrome oxidase, other metalloenzymes are also inhibited by cyanide (e.g., catalase (Fe^{3+}) and peroxidases (Fe^{3+}); succinate dehydrogenase by the interaction of cyanide with the iron–sulfur complex, superoxide dismutase (Cu, Zn), carbonic anhydrase (Zn), alkaline phosphatases (Zn), alcohol dehydrogenase (Zn); molybdenum-containing enzymes such as xanthine oxidase, xanthine dehydrogenase, aldehyde oxidases, sulfite oxidases, and selenium-containing glutathione peroxidase).

Besides ligation with metals, cyanide reacts under cyanohydrin formation with various enzymes containing a carbonyl function in the active center (e.g., pyridoxal-phosphate-dependent enzymes). Thus, the inhibition of glutamate decarboxylase, leading to the depletion of the inhibitory transmitter GABA, may predispose one to the development of convulsions. Cyanide causes slow but virtually irreversible inactivation of some enzymes by the scission of essential disulfide linkages, and it destroys xanthine oxidase activity by the elimination of sulfur as thiocyanate from the protein. Hydroxyproline degradation is impaired because 2-keto-4-hydroxyglutarate aldolase is irreversibly inhibited by cyanide.

A huge body of evidence indicate that the brain is the primary functional target in acute cyanide poisoning because the maintenance of sufficiently high levels of ATP and creatine phosphate is of principal importance for neuronal activity. In experimental acute lethal cyanide poisoning, cyanide concentrations are consistently high in the brain, irrespective of the species or the route of exposure. Biochemical measurements of cytochrome oxidase activity in the brain of killed animals indicate a mean reduction by 50% with concomitant permanent EEG silence. The comparably small degree of inhibition is somewhat surprising because, if oxygen is available in quantity, the electron flow through the respiratory chain is primarily regulated via the ATP/ADP quotient and the cytochrome oxidase activity is not rate limiting. Hence one may ask whether the post-mortem enzyme activity indeed reflects the situation during the impairment of brain function.

The inhibition of oxidative phosphorylation with a decrease in ATP and an increase in ADP and P_i stimulates glycolysis by de-inhibition of phosphofructokinase. NADH as produced in the glyceraldehydephosphate dehydrogenase reaction cannot be oxidized in the respiratory chain and shifts the lactate dehydrogenase equilibrium towards lactate. The ensuing lactacidosis coincides with a decreased bicarbonate reserve because CO_2 production in the tricarboxylic acid cycle is impaired. Finally, also anerobic glycolysis stops because phosphofructokinase is inhibited by acidosis. There is no way out of this metabolic vicious circle. Respiration stops and the circulation collapses due to cardiac arrhythmia and failure.

Acute and Chronic Toxicity

Acute Toxicity

The onset of symptoms depends on dose, route, and duration of exposure. Inhalation of small amounts of HCN induces hyperventilation, resulting from direct stimulation of chemoreceptors in the carotid and aortic bodies. Reflexive hyperventilation is also observed when pure nitrogen is inhaled for a short period. It appears that the signal transduction of the oxygen sensor has cyanide-sensitive structures such as cytochrome oxidase. The tachypnoic response can be suppressed if pure oxygen has been inhaled in advance. This phenomenon has been exploited in a clinical pulmonary function test, as oxygen abolishes the inspiratory gasp in normal individuals, whereas those who have impaired gaseous diffusion continue to exhibit this gasp. Cyanide also stimulates the nociceptors, which is characterized by a brief sensation of dryness and burning in the nose and throat, retrosternal pain, and itching of the conjunctivae. Frontal headache, palpitations, air hunger, and nausea are frequently seen, while vomiting is rarely reported. These events are short-lived and may disappear rapidly by sequestration or metabolic elimination if small amounts of cyanide have been inhaled. On exposure to high doses, the first breath is immediately followed by hyperpnea, sometimes associated with a brief outcry; apnea, a few gasps, collapse, and convulsions occur in less than a minute, often together with cardiovascular failure. The heart may continue to beat, though with various irregularities and blocks, for as long as 3 to 4 min after the last gasp. Death ensues with maximally dilated pupils. The skin acquires a rose-colored hue because the venous blood contains high proportions of oxyhemoglobin because oxygen cannot be consumed due to a blockade of cytochrome oxidase. Rose-colored skin or bright-red blood are not consistently found in fatal cases of acute cyanide poisoning due to oxygen-consuming processes that are not inhibited by cyanide (cyanide-insensitive autoxidation reactions).

Upon oral ingestion of cyanide salts, rapid intoxication is observed as long as gastric acid is available for protonation of cyanide to HCN. There are some cases in which even patients with rapid loss of consciousness, late arrival at the hospital, and ingestion of several lethal doses of potassium cyanide survived. Analysis of the gastric juice showed an alkaline reaction with copious unabsorbed cyanide. Hence it appears that the energy-dependent proton pump in the gastric mucosa is also quickly inhibited by cyanide.

Mild intoxications are usually survived without any remaining ailment. Recovery from more severe intoxication, however, may not be complete due to hypoxic brain damage similar to that seen after carbon monoxide poisoning. Even prolonged exposure to 20–40 ppm is usually tolerated; exposure to 100 ppm is life-threatening and exposure to 200–300 ppm is lethal in a few minutes. The lethal dose for adults taken as a bolus either by inhalation or by ingestion is approximately 1 mg HCN/kg, corresponding to 0.2 g of KCN or to 50 bitter almonds.

Chronic Toxicity

Chronic exposure to cyanide occurs under conditions of low-temperature combustion of vegetable matter (e.g., tobacco smoke, which contains 100 to 1600 ppm of HCN). Other sources are found in the diet, as already mentioned. Chronic exposure due to industrially produced HCN is quite uncommon. The degree of chronic cyanide intoxication largely depends on cyanide detoxication, which may be inadequate due to inborn metabolic errors or to a dietary deficiency. Thus, low protein and vitamin B_{12} intake are important nutritional factors, often associated with large intake of cyanogenic food. Typical diseases are tobacco amblyopia, tropical ataxic neuropathy (konzo, mantekassa, West Indian neuropathy, lathyrism) and tropical goiter. Low birth weight and sterility have been associated with the cyanide intake of heavy smokers. Leber's hereditary optic atrophy results from an inborn error of thiocyanate formation. One of the common pathophysiological endpoints of increased cyanide load is a shift of hydroxocobalamine to cyanocobalamine, which is more readily lost via the kidneys than the former. In fact, hydroxocobalamine infusion ameliorates most sequelae due to chronic cyanide intoxication. Reducing cyanide intake (discontinue smoking!) and increasing proteinaceous food uptake are rational therapeutic precepts, which, however, may remain utopian in countries with notorious undernourishment.

Therapeutic Measures

The therapy of acute cyanide intoxication pursues three strategies:

1. Detoxication of cyanide via the formation of thiocyanate, which is by two orders of magnitude less toxic.
2. Complexation of cyanide outside of cyanide-sensitive cells.

3. Symptomatic measures that should be instituted as early as possible.

Detoxication of Cyanide

Thiocyanate formation is drastically increased upon the administration of a sulfane sulfur donor, mostly thiosulfate. Thus, the biotransformation of cyanide increased 13-fold and respiration recovered spontaneously in a cyanide-poisoned dog following the administration of sodium thiosulfate, 500 mg/kg iv (Fig. 7). Nonetheless, the plasma cyanide concentration decreased only slowly because it was distributed into the central compartment from body stores such as erythrocytes (containing approx. 0.15 mM methemoglobin) and metmyoglobin in muscles (Fig. 8). Pretreatment with thiosulfate increases the LD_{50} of cyanide several-fold. Toxic effects of sodium thiosulfate are observed at doses of $>$1g/kg due to the high sodium load. The therapeutically recommended dose in humans is 0.25 g/kg iv. Sodium thiosulfate is rapidly eliminated by the kidneys with an apparent half-life of 15 to 20 min.

Complexation of Cyanide

Cobalt(II) salts, for example, dicobalt ethylenediamine tetraacetic acid (dicobalt edetate in Kelocyanor) form stable cyanide complexes that are excreted with the urine. Unfortunately, cobalt compounds are quite toxic by themselves. In animals, the toxicity has mainly been associated with circulatory depression and decreased cerebral blood flow. Moreover, cobalt edetate produces hyperventilation, metabolic acidosis, and increases in plasma lactate. There is a mutual antagonism in the toxicity of cobalt edetate and cyanide. Hence, the use of dicobalt edetate should only be used, if at all, in unequivocally cyanide-poisoned patients.

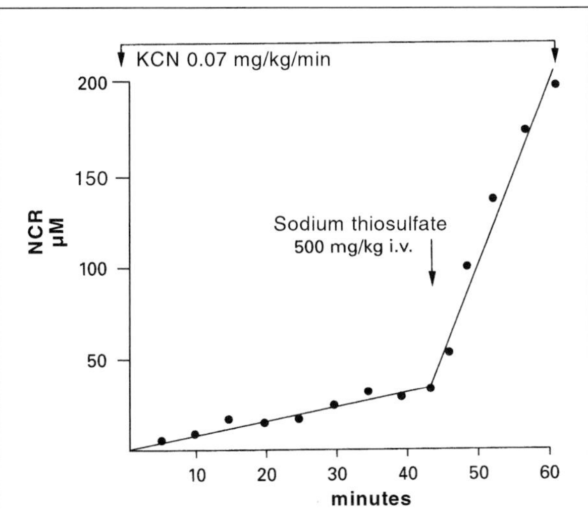

FIGURE 7 Effect of thiosulfate on the rate of metabolite formation from cyanide. Upon intravenous infusion of ^{14}C-labeled KCN in a dog (16.5 kg; 0.07 mg KCN/kg/min) metabolites in plasma increased slowly (NCR indicates non-cyanide radioactive compounds). Injection of sodium thiosulfate (500 mg/kg iv) increased the metabolic rate 13-fold. (From Christel *et al.*, 1977, *Arch. Toxicol.* **38,** 181–183, © Springer-Verlag, with permission.)

Hydroxocobalamine is a less toxic cobalt compound that has been shown to be highly effective in human cyanide poisoning. It is able to penetrate into cyanide-loaded cells and to complex cyanide to the nontoxic cyanocobalamine, which is easily excreted by the kidneys. A certain disadvantage of this elegant therapeutic concept is the high molecular weight of the antidote (molecular weight 1388), which can only bind one mole of cyanide (molecular weight 26). To detoxify one lethal dose of cyanide, that is, 1 mg/kg, some 50 mg/kg of hydroxocobalamine are needed. Moreover, the possibility of an anaphylactic reaction should be taken into consideration. From a practical point of view, these features indicate that hydroxocobalamine may be suitable in intoxications from moderate doses of cyanide that can be antagonized by small volumes of the hydroxocobalamine solution.

Another, possibly more versatile method to complex cyanide makes use of limited methemoglobin formation by 20 to 30%. Methemoglobin binds cyanide with an affinity similar to cytochrome oxidase. Because of the much larger pool of methemoglobin, cyanide is rapidly sequestered into the red blood cells. An amount of 30% methemoglobin (about 13 mmol in adults) binds maximally 350 mg HCN (i.e., approximately five lethal doses). Sufficiently low plasma cyanide concentrations are obtained only if free methemoglobin is in excess. The apparent dissociation constant for the reaction between methemoglobin and cyanide is approximately 2×10^{-6} M at pH 7.4 and 37°C. Figure 9 illustrates the influence of methemoglobin formation on cyanide distribution in a dog. 4-Dimethylaminophenol was used as the methemoglobin-forming agent. This compound has been successfully administered in human cyanide poisoning. The recommended regimen is intravenous administration of 3.5 mg of 4-dimethylaminophenol hydrochloride/kg body weight immediately followed by sodium thiosulfate, 0.1 to 0.25 g/kg iv. While 4-dimethylaminophenol leads to rapid sequestration but not to detoxication of cyanide, sodium thiosulfate induces thiocyanate formation with definite detoxication (see previous discussion). The particular advantages of 4-dimethylaminophenol over other methemoglobin-

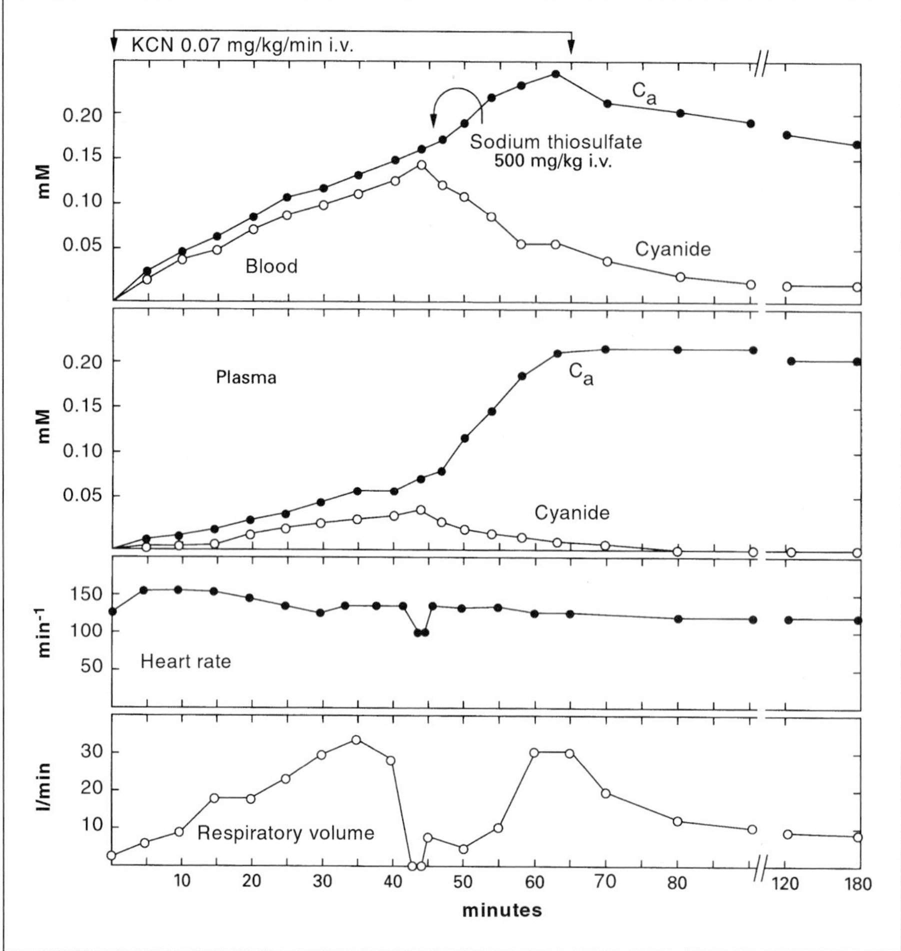

FIGURE 8 Influence of cyanide and sodium thiosulfate on heart rate and respiration. Upon intravenous infusion of ^{14}C-labeled KCN in a dog (16.5 kg; 0.07 mg KCN/kg/min) most of the cyanide was found within erythrocytes. While heart rate was hardly affected, respiratory minute volume steadily increased until the plasma cyanide concentration approached 0.04 mM; thereafter respiration stopped. Infusion of sodium thiosulfate reduced total and plasma cyanide and restored respiration. (From Christel *et al.*, 1977, *Arch. Toxicol.* **38,** 181–183, © Springer-Verlag, with permission.)

forming agents are its fast onset of action (15% methemoglobin within 1 min), the quick termination of methemoglobin formation (30 to 35%, T_{max} 15 min), and the lack of influence on respiration, blood pressure, and heart rate.

In contrast, methemoglobin formation by sodium nitrite, which is the standard in the United States, proceeds much more slowly. Thus, 6% methemoglobin is formed within 30 min after 4 mg/kg iv. This dose lowers the blood pressure by 20%, resulting in orthostatic dysregulation. The usually recommended dose of 6 to 10 mg sodium nitrite/kg forms 20% methemoglobin in 60 min and is associated with a remarkable decrease in blood pressure. Nevertheless, sodium nitrite in conjunction with sodium thiosulfate is effective in cyanide poisoning. It is unclear whether the vasodilating effects of nitrites are of value during cyanide intoxication. It has been suggested that NO liberated from nitrite or amyl nitrite, another cyanide antidote, which is practically inefficient in producing ferrihemoglobin, may be responsible for the antidotal activity. Experiments with mice have shown that a longer-acting NO derivative is indeed able to reduce cyanide toxicity. Because this compound also produced methemoglobin, it cannot be decided whether the antidotal action is based on vasodilatation or simply on methemoglobin formation.

At present, intravenous administration of 4-dimethylaminophenol and sodium thiosulfate is probably the fastest-acting measure to safely detoxify cyanide. It has the major advantage of not being harmful to unpoisoned people, as compared to cobalt edetate.

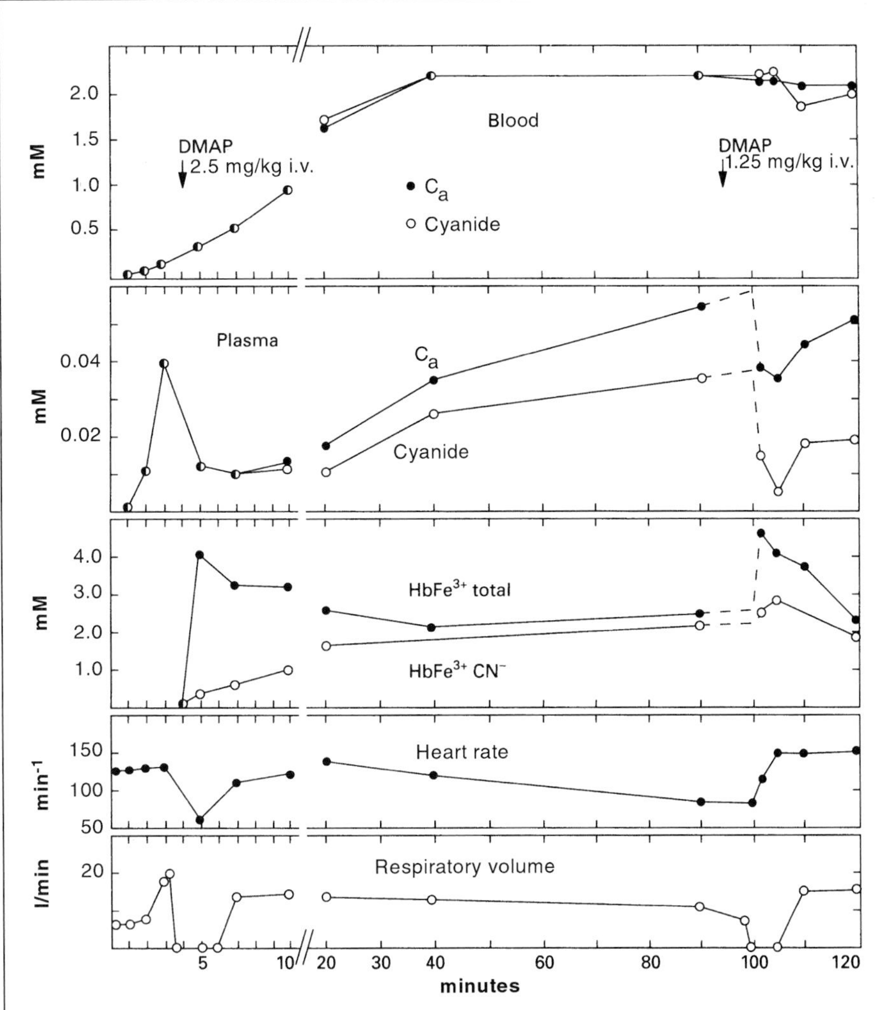

FIGURE 9 Influence of therapeutic methemoglobinemia on cyanide distribution, heart rate, and respiratory minute volume. A dog (10.5 kg) received 24 mg/kg KCN (approximately 7 LD) through a gastric tube. The plasma cyanide concentration rose quickly and, after a short period of tachypnea, caused respiratory arrest. The iv injection of 4-dimethylaminophenol (DMAP) produced some 40% methemoglobin within 1.5 min, leading to a rapid fall in plasma cyanide and restoring respiration. Further absorption of cyanide along with the spontaneous reduction of methemoglobin diminished the cyanide-binding capacity and allowed an increase in plasma cyanide, whereupon respiration stopped again. A second DMAP injection (half of the initial dose) induced spontaneous respiration. (*Ca* indicates the sum of all radioactive compounds) (From Christel *et al.*, 1977, *Arch. Toxicol.* **38,** 181–183, © Springer-Verlag, with permission.)

The adverse effects of 4-dimethylaminophenol are insignificant hemolysis and sometimes pain at the site of injection. Overdosing may produce dangerous methemoglobinemia and nephrotoxic effects, as observed in rats after 100 mg/kg iv. 4-Dimethylaminophenol has been shown to be mutagenic in the V79 HPRT test but not in the Ames test. The significance of these results needs to be assessed, but it may be felt that the mutagenicity of a drug unlikely to be used on more than one occasion does not necessarily represent an unacceptable risk in lethal cyanide intoxication.

In mixed intoxications with carbon monoxide and HCN, such as in fires, any methemoglobin formation further reduces the oxygen-carrying capacity of the blood. Here, hydroxocobalamine may be the antidote of choice, provided the cyanide ingested does not require too large a volume of infusions.

Symptomatic Therapeutic Measures

The presence and intensity of lactacidosis indicate the severity of acute cyanide poisoning and can be taken as a prognostic indicator of the ultimate outcome. Infusion of sodium bicarbonate is essential if the blood pH has fallen below 7.2. Concomitantly, oxygen should be administered. At first glance, this recommendation appears strange because oxygen consumption is reduced and venous blood is oxygenated above normal. Many experiments, however, have shown that the toxicity of cyanide is reduced when the animals are allowed to breathe pure oxygen; moreover, thiosulfate appears to be more effective in the presence of high oxygen partial pressure. Some possible explanations have been offered.

- The whole potential of oxidative phosphorylation is only partially (60%) exploited at pO_2 40 mm Hg and can be improved by higher oxygen pressure.
- The cyanide-insensitive respiration (autoxidation of the ubiquinone pool) is increased by higher oxygen concentrations, thus leading to NAD^+ regeneration, which is necessary for other metabolic reactions and particularly important in the glyceraldehyde-phosphate dehydrogenase and/or phosphoglycerate kinase reaction to restore ATP.
- Oxygen may activate rhodanese for thiocyanate formation.

While no single explanation is satisfying, clinical experience is in favor of normobaric oxygen therapy. Particularly after smoke inhalation, when mixed intoxication with CO/HCN may prevail, artificial respiration with pure oxygen may be life-saving.

Prophylactic Measures

Prophylactic measures are mandatory if high doses of sodium nitroprusside are infused. In addition, any expected attack with cyanide in chemical warfare requires an effective prophylaxis and therapy. While sodium thiosulfate infusion is suitable during nitroprusside therapy, it is less effective at high lethal concentrations of the airborne toxicant, which require a very rapid antidotal action. Among the orally effective methemoglobin-forming agents, 4-dimethylaminophenol is less suitable because it underlies an extensive first-pass metabolism in the liver. On the other hand, a short-acting drug does not produce long-lasting methemoglobin levels because of the efficient reduction of methemoglobin by methemoglobin reductases (5–7%/h). From a theoretical point of view, *p*-aminopropiophenone and *p*-aminooctanoylphenone may appear to be more appropriate for prophylaxis. These compounds are slowly N-oxygenated in the liver, yielding hydroxylamino derivatives, which are potent methemoglobin-forming intermediates. They are able to produce methemoglobin levels of some 15% for 10 h. It must be argued, however, that these derivatives may have a carcinogenic potential (via O-esterified *N*-hydroxyarylamines). More recently, 8-aminoquinolines with antileishmanial and antimalarial activity have attracted major interest because of the induction of long-lasting methemoglobinemia after oral administration.

Work-Place Exposure Guidelines

The TWA value is 10 ppm (OSHA, MAK), while ACGIH and NIOSH recommend a STEL value of 4.7 ppm only.

Analysis

HCN vapor is most easily detected by a Draeger HCN detector (2–30 and 10–150 ppm). The method makes use of the complexation of $HgCl_2$ with HCN with release of hydrochloric acid that is detected by a methyl red indicator. For quick analysis of cyanide in the blood, it has been suggested that 1 ml of blood be taken and shaken with acid (e.g., 10% sulfuric acid) and the escaping HCN be picked up by the Draeger tube.

Quantitative determination includes microdiffusion of HCN into an alkali trap and oxidation of cyanide to cyanogen chloride with chloramine-T, followed by the Zinke-König reaction. Glutaconaldehyde, which is formed from cyanogen chloride and pyridines, reacts with pyrazolinones or barbiturates to give an intense blue condensation product (detection limit 10 ng/ml).

HYDROGEN SULFIDE

Although hydrogen sulfide is one of the leading causes of sudden death in the work place, detailed knowledge is scarce with regard to its toxic mechanisms, toxicokinetics in humans, and appropriate treatment. The nasty smell of hydrogen sulfide may have deterred scientists from performing more detailed investigations. The excellent olfactory warning properties of this gas may have prevented its use in suicides and homicides, despite the fact that it resembles hydrocyanic acid in its toxicity.

Properties, Sources, and Exposure Potential

Hydrogen sulfide (H_2S, molecular weight 34.08; 1 ppm = 1.41 mg/m^3) is a colorless, irritating, and highly toxic gas with a relative specific gravity of 1.19

(air = 1). H_2S has a characteristic odor resembling rotten eggs, which is recognized at 0.025 to 1 ppm. H_2S is a weak acid with pK_a values for the first and second dissociation step of 7.04 and 11.96, respectively. Hence, about 70% of H_2S exists as the hydrosulfide anion, HS^-, at physiological pH. H_2S is relatively lipophilic, and its solubility in diethylether is five times higher than in water. Though H_2S easily penetrates biological membranes, its absorption through the skin appears to be minimal in humans.

H_2S is produced from numerous environmental sources including bacterial decomposition of vegetable and animal proteinaceous material. In addition, H_2S is found in crude petroleum, natural gas, volcanic gases, and sulfur springs. It is released into the environment from petroleum refineries, natural gas plants, sulfur production, coke-oven plants, iron smelters, paper mills, viscose rayon manufacture, tanneries upon depilation with CaS, food-processing plants, dairies, and wool-scrubbing plants. In some areas natural gas may contain as much as 50% H_2S, indicating the anerobic decomposition of fossils.

Owing to its intense smell, H_2S is usually recognized before toxic concentrations are reached. Its warning properties, however, are rapidly lost at high concentrations (>500 ppm), leading to insidious exposures and serious intoxications. Fatalities have occurred in poorly ventilated spaces after the agitation of underground manure tanks, upon the addition of sulfuric acid to a drain and of hydrochloric acid to a well, and upon the cleaning of propane tanks. Workers as well as rescuers were affected in many cases when entering sewers or ship holds loaded with fish meal. Thus, it is highly important that rescuers be fully protected and use a self-contained breathing apparatus (SCBA). The latter is preferable to gas masks because oxygen may be lacking, too.

Absorption, Distribution, Metabolism, Excretion, and Mechanisms of Toxicity

H_2S is primarily a respiratory poison; cutaneous absorption is negligible. The toxicokinetics of H_2S have apparently not been studied in humans. In animals, elimination by the lungs is minimal while rapid metabolic transformation to sulfate is the predominant route. The mechanism of the oxidative H_2S metabolism has not been completely elucidated. Two other metabolic pathways include methylation of H_2S to the less toxic methanethiol and dimethylsulfide. Reactions with metalloenzymes, such as cytochrome oxidase, are likely to contribute to the toxicity of H_2S, but the reduction of disulfide bridges in proteins may be of additional importance. H_2S is oxidized by hemoproteins, including oxyhemoglobin, without the formation of sulfhemoglobin. Similar to CN^-, HS^- binds to methemoglobin with formation of sulfmethemoglobin (not sulfhemoglobin). The affinity of HS^- is by two to three orders of magnitude lower than that of CN^-. This difference, however, is much smaller at pH 7.4 if one considers the different dissociation constants (pK_a HCN = 9.2, H_2S = 7.04).

As many organs are susceptible to the effects of H_2S, this toxic gas has often been regarded as a broad-spectrum toxicant. The most sensitive tissues are those with exposed mucous membranes and high oxygen demand, pointing to impaired oxidative phosphorylation by blocking the cytochrome oxidase. Newer results have revealed elevated neurotransmitter contents in the brains of exposed animals. H_2S increases the levels of GABA, serotonin, dopamine, and norepinephrine in the brain stem, probably due to the inhibition of monoamine oxidase (MAO). Because the reversal of MAO inhibition was achieved by the removal of bound sulfide with dithiothreitol, reaction of H_2S with enzyme disulfide bonds has been suggested. Moreover, H_2S causes K^+-channel-mediated hyperpolarization of neurons and potentiates other inhibitory mechanisms.

Acute and Chronic Toxicity

Acute Toxicity

The direct action of H_2S on mucous membranes is usually first manifested as an eye irritation with local inflammation of the conjunctiva and cornea. These symptoms occur between 10 and 50 ppm of H_2S. The latter concentration also causes inflammation and dryness of the respiratory tract with rhinitis, pharyngitis, laryngitis, bronchitis, and pneumonia. Similar to CN^-, H_2S may also increase the respiratory rate by the stimulation of peripheral chemoceptors. In acute intoxications with high concentrations of H_2S (>500 ppm), rapid olfactory paralysis occurs and death may ensue from respiratory failure with consequent asphyxia and cardiac failure. It should be pointed out that in those cases where death has been instantaneous, autopsy has not revealed any characteristic finding. The clinical picture only may consist of a nonspecific hemorrhagic pulmonary edema, visceral congestion, and scattered petechial hemorrhages in the pleura.

Subacute Toxicity

The most prevalent respiratory symptoms upon accidental exposure to H_2S are dyspnea, sore throat, cough, and chest pain. Other respiratory signs and symptoms, such as pulmonary edema, cyanosis, and hemoptysis, are less frequently seen. One of the complications ensuing from H_2S exposure is the development of pneumonia, which may be related to the inhibitory effect of H_2S on alveolar macrophages and their ability to inactivate bacteria. Cardiac symptoms include arrhythmias, myocardial depression, conduction defects, and abnormal ventricular repolarization. The inhibition of oxidative phosphorylation may result in a switch to anerobic glycolysis with lactacidosis.

Chronic Toxicity

The existence of a chronic intoxication with H_2S in terms of a distinct clinical entity has been questioned. It is possible that the symptoms of chronic intoxication represent sequelae to acute or subacute toxicity rather than to chronic toxicity. Fatigue, headache, dizziness, and irritability may be interpreted as neurasthenic symptoms. Asthmatics appear to be more susceptible to H_2S, and even 2 ppm for 30 min caused symptoms of increased airway resistance. There has been very little research concerning carcinogenic, mutagenic, teratogenic, or developmental effects of H_2S in humans and nonrodents. Here, some studies provide evidence that chronic exposure to low concentrations of H_2S may affect the central nervous system (CNS) development and contribute to long-term abnormalities in motor function and behavior. However, no systematic studies are available.

Therapeutic Measures

Immediate supportive care at the scene is the most important measure to take. Rescuers must very cautiously enter areas that may contain H_2S. Thus, closed spaces such as manure pits or storage tanks require self-contained breathing apparatus, safety harness, and outside observation. Despite unconsciousness, most victims appear to recover spontaneously by breathing fresh air, most probably due to rapid elimination of H_2S. Maximum oxygen flow has been recommended, and several anecdotal case studies suggest that hyperbaric oxygen therapy may be useful.

Antidotal therapy consists of scavenging sulfide with methemoglobin either formed with nitrites or by *p*-aminopropiophenone. In fact, these approaches did prophylactically protect against subsequent poisoning in animals, but there are few cases in which treatment after exposure affected the outcome. It has been suggested that nitrites may be of value only if given within minutes after H_2S exposure. The same probably holds true if methemoglobin is formed by 4-dimethylaminophenol (see the section on cyanide). Interventions that actively remove sulfide from the sites where it causes enzyme inhibition, such as the administration of dithiothreitol, may have the advantage of preventing some of the long-lasting sequelae. Nonetheless, the value of all these antidotal measures is not yet proven and their clinical efficacy remains to be determined.

Work-Place Exposure Guidelines

The TWA and STEL values are 10 and 15 ppm, respectively (ACGIH, MAK). The threshold limit value is intended to prevent injury to the eye. Interestingly, odor thresholds are much lower. OSHA permissible exposure limits are 20 ppm with a ceiling value of 50 ppm (10 main peak; once per 8-h shift), while NIOSH recommends a STEL of 10 ppm (10 min).

Analysis

A specific ion electrode in combination with a microdiffusion cell has been developed to detect elevated sulfide ion in blood. Sulfide-ion levels must be measured as soon as possible, because of the endogenous destruction of the sulfide ion on storage. Concentrations measured immediately after H_2S-induced death ranged from 1.7 to 3.75 mg/liter. For air analysis, several Draeger tubes are available, covering a range between 1 and 70,000 ppm. H_2S is detected by its reaction with lead acetate under the formation of black lead sulfide.

HYDRAZOIC ACID (HYDROGEN AZIDE)

Hydrazoic acid and its salts are easily decomposable compounds that disintegrate with a minor energy supply from outside (e.g., pressure, blow, warming) with the liberation of nitrogen. Explosions also occur in the absence of oxygen.

Properties, Sources, and Exposure Potential

Hydrazoic acid (HN_3, molecular weight 43.03; 1 ppm = 1.79 mg/m^3) is a colorless explosive liquid with a boiling point of 37°C and a rotten, garlic-like odor. The p*K* of the acid is comparable to that of acetic acid, thus giving an alkaline reaction with alkali salts. The relative specific gravity of vaporous HN_3 (1.49) exceeds that of air (=1).

Sodium and potassium azide are employed as biocides and preservatives for technical liquids containing water in order to inhibit the growth of microbials and algae. Heavy metal azides (e.g., $Cu(N_3)_2$, $Pb(N_3)_2$, and $Hg(N_3)_2$ (mercuric fulminate)) are used as primary explosives. Air bags installed in automobiles for protection from accidental impacts are a novel source of azide intoxication because sodium azide (several hundred grams) is employed together with copper and iron oxides to initiate the gas generation.

Absorption, Distribution, Metabolism, Excretion, and Mechanisms of Toxicity

Like cyanide the azide ion binds to trivalent porphyrin-bound iron. The cytochrome oxidase is extensively inhibited at azide concentrations of $>10^{-3}$ M only. Catalase and peroxidases are more sensitive to inhibition. The affinity of azide for ferrihemoglobin is markedly less than that of cyanide or hydrogen sulfide. In contrast to earlier assumptions, the affinity of the azide anion for trivalent iron is likely to be of minor toxicological importance. The toxic effects are, rather, produced by the NO arising metabolically. They consist of a drastic fall in blood pressure and in convulsions, which may be accounted for by an NO-mediated increase in the synthesis of excitatory amino acids. Unlike NO, which avidly binds to ferrohemoglobin upon systemic administration, sufficient azide remains available to pass the blood–brain barrier for subsequent NO production in the CNS. Azide is completely metabolized in the body, yielding 1 mol of nitrogen per mole of azide.

Mutagenic actions of sodium azide have been found in plants and bacteria. Mutagenicity of azide has also been shown in cell cultures from Chinese hamsters and in mouse lymphoma cells. The mutagenic action is assumed to come about by base substitution.

Acute and Chronic Toxicity

In laboratory workers with acute exposure to hydrazoic acid, strong stimulation and swelling of nasal mucosa, a balloon sensation in the head, headache, flaming red in the face, tachypnea, and tachycardia occurred. The decrease in blood pressure may be massive, resembling that seen with nitroprusside sodium. These symptoms can be adequately explained by NO formation. Tachypnea is likely to come about by the stimulation of the carotid body, much like the action of cyanide at this site. High doses can elicit central convulsions and respiratory-center paralysis. Irritation of the mucous membranes, headache, and general weakness may occur at >0.5 ppm. Heavy intoxication symptoms were observed following 150 mg sodium azide taken orally.

Chronic exposure to hydrazoic acid with occasional episodes of headache, flush, and decrease in blood pressure was not followed by obvious pathological changes.

Therapeutic Measures

There is no specific therapy for azide intoxication. Therapeutic attempts with methemoglobin production were disappointing. Upon massive inhalative absorption prophylaxis of pulmonary edema with a glucocorticoid aerosol may be useful.

Work-Place Exposure Guidelines

The MAK value is 0.1 ppm. Presently, the azides are reexamined with respect to carcinogenic effects. No data are available from the United States.

Analysis

Azide forms a deep-red $Fe(N_3)_3$ complex with $FeCl_3$.

NITROGEN OXIDES

Nitrogen can occur in seven different oxidation states, thus allowing the formation of several nitrogen oxides in the ambient air: N_2O, NO, N_2O_3, NO_2, N_2O_4, NO_3, and N_2O_5. NO, NO_2 and NO_3 are free radicals; NO and NO_2 can be present indoors and outdoors at toxicologically significant concentrations. The mixture of NO and NO_2 is usually called NO_x. N_2O, being a product of mainly biological processes, is of minor immediate health concern, but is considered an important Greenhouse gas. NO is the main primary nitrogen oxide (85 to 95%) formed during combustion at elevated temperatures. NO_2 gradually decomposes completely to NO and 1/2 O_2 between 150 and 620°C.

The most important sources of NO_x are automobile and aircraft exhausts, which contribute to half of the total emissions, followed by emissions from power plants, domestic burning, and industrial activities such as welding. In the atmosphere, NO_x is subject to various photochemical reactions in the upper troposphere (up to approximately 15 km). NO_2 efficiently absorbs longer-wavelength UV light, resulting in the formation of atomic oxygen that combines with O_2 to form O_3. This process is cyclic, because NO_2 is regenerated by a reaction between NO and O_3. In the absence of hydrocarbons, this series of reactions would approach a steady state.

$$NO_2 \xrightarrow{h \times \nu} NO + (O)$$

$$(O) + O_2 \longrightarrow O_3$$

$$NO + O_3 \longrightarrow NO_2 + O_2$$

In the presence of hydrocarbons, particularly olefins and substituted aromatics, atomic oxygen is consumed, resulting in oxidized compounds and free radicals reacting with NO to produce more NO_2. Hydrocarbons emanate from anthropogenic and natural sources for example, from swamps (methane) or woods (isoprene, ethylene, α-pinene). All these photochemical reactions are very complex and involve the formation of unstable intermediate radicals that undergo a series of additional reactions, for example, the formation of aldehydes or peroxyacetyl nitrate (PAN). Depending on the season and the intensity of the sun, the mean residence time of $(NO)_x$ is 24 to 36 h in the lower troposphere.

In the 1980s, NO was still considered to be a potentially toxic agent of tobacco smoke and automobile exhaust polluting our environment and destroying the ozone layer in the upper troposphere. Now, NO has been identified as the endothelium-derived relaxing factor (EDRF). There has been an explosion of publications establishing a central role of NO in mammalian physiology. It is formed in many different cell types through a common biochemical pathway with oxidation of guanidino nitrogen of L-arginine by nitric oxide synthase (NOS). Several NOSs (EC 1.14.23) include both constitutive and inducible forms, all of which belong to the cytochrome P450 enzyme superfamily. NO is involved in cardiovascular physiology, neuron signaling, endotoxic shock, host defense, platelet aggregation, and sexual function. It now appears that organic nitrates (e.g., nitroglycerin and nitroprusside), which have been used in medicine for years as antispasmodic, antianginal and antihypertensive agents, act by elevating NO levels in smooth muscle cells. Apart from its ability to mediate signal transduction via stimulation of guanylate cyclase-controlled cGMP synthesis, NO is also capable of modulating reactions and pathological processes long associated with the excess production and the biological effects of reactive oxygen species.

In addition, NO and its descendants also have prooxidant effects and may lead to DNA damage and cell death in the cells producing them or in their adjacent cells. This dichotomy of physiologic and toxic reactions appears to depend critically on the balance of various competing reactions. Currently, we are realizing that NO reacts with the superoxide anion to generate peroxonitrite, which has a reactivity comparable to that of the hydroxyl radical. Peroxonitrite reacts with CO_2 to form a putative nitrosoperoxycarbonate, which may constitute a further novel oxidant.

Dinitrogen Oxide (Nitrous Oxide)

Properties, Sources, and Exposure Potential

N_2O (molecular weight 44.01; 1 ppm = 1.83 mg/m^3) is a nonirritating colorless gas with a slightly sweetish odor and a relative specific gravity of 1.53 (air = 1). Although N_2O is not flammable, it supports combustion like oxygen when present in proper concentration with flammable gases. Besides xenon, N_2O is the only inorganic gas that is used as an analgesic in dentistry and minor surgery. In the presence of 70% N_2O in oxygen, the concentration of potent halogenated anesthetics can be reduced by a factor of approximately 2.5, resulting in less respiratory and circulatory depression and a more rapid recovery from general anesthesia. N_2O is also used in whipped cream preparations.

Absorption, Distribution, Metabolism, Excretion, and Mechanisms of Toxicity, as Well as Toxicity

The uptake and distribution of N_2O are influenced in a relatively unique way by its physical properties. When breathing 70% N_2O, approximately 10 liters of N_2O will be absorbed in an adult within 15 min. If air is abruptly substituted upon the discontinuation of N_2O breathing, the rediffusion of N_2O from tissue and blood to alveolar gas produces a substantial decrease in the alveolar oxygen tension, with subsequent diffusional hypoxia. This complication can be avoided by the administration of pure oxygen during the early period of N_2O discontinuation. Because the blood:gas partition coefficient for N_2O is 34 times that for N_2, pockets of gas trapped in the body will expand when nitrogen is replaced by N_2O. Such pockets may be found in an occluded middle ear, pneumothorax, intestinal loops, lung, or renal cysts.

N_2O has been shown to oxidize Co^+ in vitamin B_{12} with the inhibition of methionine synthetase and subsequent decreases in hepatic *S*-adenosyl-L-methionine and tetrahydrofolate concentrations, formate oxidation, and thymidine synthesis. Because hematopoiesis in humans strongly depends on the methylcobalamin coenzyme, inactivation by prolonged exposure to N_2O may cause megaloblastic changes of the bone marrow, similar to those observed in cobalamin deficiency. Moreover, neurologic disorders, which are well known in cobalamin deficiency, may occur after repeated exposure to N_2O. In severely ill patients and folate- or cobalamin-deficient subjects these effects may be provoked by N_2O within a few hours. It appears that the complete recovery of methionine synthase activity requires several days, even after a short exposure to N_2O.

There has been increasing concern that inhalation anesthetics may have teratogenic effects and reduce fertility among women exposed to these agents in operating rooms or in dentistry. In most of the epidemiological studies, "working in operation theaters" rather than actual exposure to a single anesthetic agent has been investigated. Confounding factors may be more easily excluded from studies on dentists and their staff, due to the fact that the dentists can readily be divided into two groups differing only in the use of N_2O for analgesia. While no significant increase in tumor rates was observed in N_2O-exposed male dentists and female assistants, N_2O-exposed U.S. women had twice the rate of spontaneous abortion and a 1.5-fold increase in congenital abnormalities compared to unexposed women. In contrast, in Swedish and Finnish studies no association of spontaneous abortion and congenital abnormalities could be shown between exposed and unexposed pregnant women working in operating theaters.

A more recent study examined the fertility of American female dental assistants exposed to N_2O by assessing the time elapsed between the start of unprotected intercourse and conception. Although the design of the study may be criticized, there was a dose-dependent delay in conception in N_2O-exposed women. Therefore, it appears to be advisable to administer N_2O by techniques that guarantee minimum contamination of the room air.

Work-Place Exposure Guidelines

The TWA values are 50 and 25 ppm (ACGIH and NIOSH, respectively). The MAK is 100 ppm.

Analysis

Due to its specific infrared absorption (4.5 μm), N_2O is most easily quantified spectroscopically in gas cuvettes. Continuous and discontinuous measurements are possible, ranging between 1 and 1000 ppm.

Nitrogen Monoxide (Nitric Oxide)

Properties, Sources, and Exposure Potential

NO (molecular weight 30.01; 1 ppm = 1.25 mg/m^3) is a colorless gas with a relative specific gravity of 1.04 (air = 1). Industrial publications suggest that the odor threshold is 0.3 to 1 ppm and that it has a sharp, sweet smell. Pure NO without higher oxides of nitrogen appears to have no irritant properties. Neutral NO (better depicted as $NO^{\bullet}$) has a single electron in its 2p-π antibonding orbital. The removal of this electron forms NO^+; conversely, the addition of an electron results in NO^- (pK_a ~ 4.5). NO reacts with various redox forms of (di)oxygen and with transition metals. The reaction of NO with O_2 under formation of NO_2 in the gas phase and in aqueous solution is a complicated process that is second order in [NO]. The velocity can be described using $k \times [NO]^2 \times [O_2]$, k being $1.4 \times 10^4\ M^{-2}\ s^{-1}$ at 27°C. This means that 5 ppm NO_2 are produced in 60 min at 20 ppm NO, but in 2.4 min only at 100 ppm NO.

In aqueous solution NO_2 reacts with the educt NO to yield N_2O_3, which comproportionates into nitrite:

$$NO_2 + NO \rightleftharpoons N_2O_3$$

$$2\ N_2O_3 + 2\ H_2O \rightleftharpoons 4\ NO_2^- + 4\ H^+.$$

$NO^{\bullet}$ also reacts extremely rapidly (close to diffusion limit) with $O_2^{\bullet -}$ in aqueous solution ($k \sim 10^9\ M^{-1}\ s^{-1}$), yielding peroxynitrite ($ONOO^-$) and its corresponding acid (ONOOH; pK_a ~ 6.8). This compound reacts with moderate velocity with a variety of biological compounds including thiols, thioethers, amino acids bearing aromatic moieties, lipids, carbohydrates, and ascorbic acid. It has been suggested that peroxynitrite generated by the reaction between $NO^{\bullet}$ and $O_2^{\bullet -}$ has a *cis* configuration that contributes to the relatively low reactivity. The energy barrier to form the *trans* configuration is quite high, but it may be lowered in peroxynitrous acid. The *trans* peroxynitrite may be similarly reactive to the $OH^{\bullet}$ radical. Thus, *cis* peroxynitrite may diffuse from the site of production and exert its deleterious effects after conversion into the *trans* form.

Biologically most significant, however, may be the reaction of peroxynitrite with bicarbonate-CO_2 that is abundant at ~25 mM, the second-order rate constant being $3 \times 10^4\ M^{-1}\ s^{-1}$ at pH 7.4 and 37°C. The biological and toxicological roles for the reaction of CO_2 and peroxynitrite with the formation of $ONO_2CO_2^-$ are unclear, but a matter of much investigation. In the presence of transition metals, peroxynitrite also yields a species with a reactivity similar to the nitronium ion, NO_2^+, that easily nitrates phenolic groups, including tyrosine residues.

Dealing with the toxicity and reactivity of NO is a difficult task, and it would be premature to attribute toxic effects to a single toxic species. It must be remembered that the NO formed in our body has dichotomic properties, and we are faced with the problem that an endogenous, probably very important, biomolecule and its reactive descendants are able to produce DNA deamination, DNA oxidation, DNA-strand breaks and DNA cross-links, while inhibiting several repair mechanisms.

Exogenous NO, originating from farm silos due to plant decomposition, fires, domestic heaters (indoor), or even activated air bags, is usually contaminated with NO_2, depending on the NO concentration and reaction time. Hence, the toxicological effects of exogenous NO can be evaluated only when purified NO is carefully insufflated, such as during therapeutic administration.

Absorption, Distribution, Metabolism, Excretion, and Mechanisms of Toxicity

Due to its low water solubility, NO descends to the alveoli and enters the bloodstream. Some 80 to 90% of inhaled NO is absorbed, depending on the depth of respiration. In the blood, NO readily penetrates the red-cell membrane and reacts with hemoglobin. With oxyhemoglobin NO forms methemoglobin and nitrate, the reaction being complete within 0.1 s. No nitrite is formed, and the concentration of HbNO is low. With deoxyhemoglobin NO forms a very tight complex because the rate of dissociation is about 3×10^{-5} times that of oxygen. Nevertheless, this complex is very unstable if oxygen is present, as it is in the bloodstream. Ultimately, methemoglobin and nitrite or nitrate are formed. Studies in rats with ^{15}NO have shown that some 60% of the label is found in urinary nitrate and urea. It has been suggested that nitrite may be reduced by bacteria in the gut with the liberation of ammonia. Upon reabsorption, the labeled ammonia may be transferred into urea or incorporated into biomolecules, such as amino acids and purines, thus explaining the incomplete balance.

Acute Toxicity

The acute toxicity of pure NO is due to methemoglobinemia and to a lesser extent to impaired oxygen liberation from HbNO-HbO_2 hybrids. Mice exposed to 3500 and 400 ppm NO died within 5 and 30 min, respectively, and exhibited deep cyanosis. Rats developed 20% methemoglobin when exposed to 200 ppm for 60 min. While a linear relationship could be observed between the concentrations of NO and HbNO formation, an exponential increase in methemoglobin was observed when NO was increased.

Some hundred patients with pulmonary hypertension received 80 ppm NO for various time intervals. No patient coughed or objected to breathing. In 23 subjects receiving prolonged NO therapy for an average of 40 h, methemoglobin amounted to $2.5 \pm 0.4\%$ (range of 0 to 14%). Methemoglobinemia in a native American rose from 0.9 to 9.6% within 6 h of administration of 80 ppm NO. This was attributed to a deficiency in methemoglobin reductase that is more common in this population. In a neonate, the concentration increased to 14% after 18 h of treatment and decreased to about 7.5% in response to the administration of vitamin C (500 mg) and blood transfusion. Again, immature methemoglobin reductase was assumed to be responsible for this effect.

Mutagenicity and Carcinogenicity

When discussing the genotoxicity of NO one has to consider the effects of the various descendants of NO during the interaction, particularly of dioxygen species. Thus, it is difficult to assign genotoxic actions to a single nitrogen oxide species. Although there is some ambiguity about the mutagenic activity of NO, the majority of the studies have shown that NO is a mutagen both in bacteria and in mammalian cell systems, although less active than NO_2. Studies of the carcinogenicity of pure NO are not available. Of course, such a task may be difficult due to the ease of autoxidation of NO. From a practical standpoint it is probably more important to study the effects of nitrogen oxides as airborne toxicants in the environment.

Nitrogen Dioxide

Properties, Sources, and Exposure Potential

NO_2 (molecular weight 46.01, 1 ppm = 1.91 mg/m^3) is a reddish-brown, poorly water-soluble, irritant gas with a relative specific gravity of 1.58 (air = 1) and a boiling point at 21.2°C. It has an odor reminiscent of chlorine with a rapidly increasing threshold of detection, beginning at approximately 0.1 ppm. Depending on its concentration, NO_2 is in a dynamic equilibrium with its colorless dimer, N_2O_4. In aqueous solutions and humid air NO_2 decomposes into nitric acid and N_2O_3 that, in turn, disproportionates into NO and NO_2. Thus, a variety of nitrogen oxides are in a rapid dynamic equilibrium. NO_2 does not burn but supports the combustion of oxidizable materials.

Besides the occurrence in ambient air, NO_2 is a chemical intermediate of fertilizer and nitric acid production. Occupational exposure may occur during gas welding, in agriculture (silo fillers), in nitration processes (e.g., production of nitrocellulose, explosives, and rocket fuels), in mining when using dynamite, and during exposure to fire fumes and exhausts from combustion engines in confined areas. Fire victims and firemen are at particular risk. A curious outbreak of nitrogen dioxide-induced respiratory illness was observed among 116 ice-hockey players, cheerleaders, and band members attending a hockey game in an indoor ice arena. The ice resurfacer was found to be malfunctioning. If these engines, powered by an internal combustion engine using propane fuel, are not properly tuned and the fuel mixture in the carburetor receives too much oxygen, elevated levels of NO_2 may occur. Conversely, elevated concentrations of CO may come about due to an oxygen shortage.

Absorption, Distribution, Metabolism, Excretion, and Mechanisms of Toxicity

Inhalation studies with healthy volunteers exposed to NO_2 (0.3 up to 7.2 ppm) showed that between 75% and 90% were absorbed during normal and maximal ventilation, respectively. Similar values were found in asthmatic subjects. The mechanisms by which NO_2 is removed from the inspired air are not fully understood. Once deposited, NO_2 dissolves in the epithelial lining fluid, and various chemical reactions may occur, giving rise to products found in the blood and other body fluids. In experimental animal models some 70% of absorbed $^{15}NO_2$ appeared in the lung effluent as nitrite in addition to some nitrate, and the remainder was found in the lung tissue. Ultimately, most of the NO_2 absorbed was excreted as nitrate in the urine. In conclusion, NO_2 reacts with tissue components and the epithelial lining fluid with conversion to nitrite. This may enter the bloodstream and react with oxyhemoglobin with the formation of nitrate, which is eventually eliminated by the kidneys.

Due to its radical character, NO_2 rapidly reacts with polyunsaturated fatty acids, causing lipid peroxidation, as well as with certain amino acids in proteins, thus affecting enzyme activities and structural proteins in the lung. NO_2 exerts an oxidative stress on antioxidant defense systems with the depletion of ascorbic acid, glutathione, and vitamin E. NO_2 affects the ciliated epithelial cells, apparently without impairing the mucociliary transport. It has been suggested that the airway epithelium has an overcapacity in mucus transport. The host defense systems are also affected by NO_2, and a decreased function of alveolar macrophages has been observed upon subchronic exposure. In addition, NO_2 induces an increased susceptibility to bacterial and viral infections. The relevance of these *in vitro* studies and animal experiments for humans is not clear.

Acute and Chronic Toxicity

Acute Toxicity

At concentrations between 100 and 150 ppm, toxic symptoms occur within 30 to 60 min, and at 200 to 700 ppm fatalities result after short exposure. The clinical symptoms depend on duration and intensity of exposure. Typically, there is a triphasic pattern. Initially, mild irritation of the upper respiratory tract predominates with cough, sore throat, conjunctivitis, dyspnea, headache, vertigo, nausea, and, less commonly, loss of consciousness and chest tightness. Methemoglobinemia and hypotension may accompany the NO_2 exposure. The severity of the initial symptoms does not correlate well with the extent of the pulmonary damage. After a lag period of 3 to 30 h, pulmonary edema may develop, resulting in acute respiratory failure. About half of the patients surviving the pulmonary edema show bronchiolitis obliterans within 2 to 3 (up to 6) weeks.

The symptoms of the silo-filler's disease (fermentation of silage produces up to 4000 ppm of NO_2) resemble influenza with fever, chills, cough, chest pain, and dyspnea. While most patients fully recover, some may develop the adult respiratory distress syndrome and bronchiolitis obliterans. Three American astronauts who were exposed to about 250 ppm of NO_2 for 4–5 min, owing to the inadvertent firing of the reaction control system in the Apollo–Soyuz spacecraft, had radiological evidence of pulmonary edema the day after splashdown. Controlled exposure studies at low NO_2 concentrations have shown bronchoconstriction at levels above 2.5 ppm. Below 1 ppm, no significant effect on lung function has been reported. For asthmatics, however, some studies indicate slight but statistically significant effects on spirometry and airway resistance at NO_2 concentrations above 0.25 ppm. Asthmatics appear to respond more readily to carbachol in the presence of 0.1 ppm NO_2. Because people with asthma make up a considerable proportion of the population (about 5%) it has been proposed that NO_2 concentrations of 0.1 ppm be judged as the lowest observable adverse effect level (LOAEL).

Chronic Toxicity

Several animal studies on rats continuously exposed to 0.4 ppm for up to 2 years indicate morphological (proliferation of type II alveolar epithelium and edematous extension of interstitial tissue) and biochemical changes (e.g., increased lipid peroxidation with elevated ethane and pentane exhalation). Despite a large body of human data on NO_2 exposure, the assessment of occupational exposure is confounded by other pulmonary reactive substances such as SO_2 and particulates. Epidemiological data showing some correlation between the exposure of indoor NO_2 from heating and cooking facilities are likewise confounded (e.g., by household allergens, cigarette smoke, climate, and indoor vs. outdoor activities). Thus, it is difficult to obtain a valid LOAEL.

Mutagenicity and Carcinogenicity

NO_2 is mutagenic in bacteria and clastogenic in mammalian cells *in vitro*. The few *in vivo* studies gave mostly negative results. According to the available studies, there is no clear evidence for a carcinogenic potential of NO_2, but the few relevant studies do not allow a proper evaluation of this risk. Nitrite and nitrosamines arising from NO_2 are suspected of being carcinogens. However, the contribution of inhaled NO_2 is probably small when compared with the descendants ingested.

Therapeutic Measures

Acutely exposed, symptomatic persons should be observed for at least 24 h (rescuers should be cautious and wear protective gear if the ambient concentrations are critical, e.g., >5 ppm NO_2). Early use of corticosteroids has been suggested for the prevention of pulmonary edema. In fact, rats exposed to 105 ppm of NO_2 for 30 min were effectively protected from the development of pulmonary edema by previous inhalation of an aqueous aerosol of dexamethason-21-isonicotinate. In another study, guinea pigs pretreated with methylprednisolone (i.p.) exhibited a four-fold reduction in the mortality from NO_2 exposure as compared to unprotected controls. However, methylprednisolone administration after NO_2 exposure for 76 to 130 min was without beneficial effect. In the case of a pulmonary edema, which responds poorly to diuretics, corticosteroids and mechanical ventilation with positive end-expiratory pressure (PEEP) offer the best chance of reducing mortality, which may be as high as 40% in severe cases. Prolonged administration of corticosteroids for at least 2 months has been reported to prevent bronchiolitis obliterans. It should be noted, however, that no controlled human study exists conclusively demonstrating the beneficial effect of corticosteroids after the inhalation of toxic gases. Thus, the effectiveness of post-exposure corticosteroids remains a matter of debate.

Work-Place Exposure Guidelines

The TWA values are 25 ppm for NO (ACGIH, OSHA, NIOSH) and 3 ppm for NO_2 with a STEL of 5 ppm NO_2 (ACGIH). OSHA gives a STEL value of 5 ppm, while NIOSH recommends 1 ppm NO_2. The MAK value is 5 ppm NO_2, a value currently under discussion.

Analysis

NO is oxidized by Mn^{IV} or Cr^{VI} to NO_2. NO_2 can be detected after diazotation of sulfanilic acid followed by coupling with N-naphthyl-1-ethylenediammonium chloride. The detection limit is 0.07 ppm NO_2. Alternatively, NO_2 is converted to NO, which reacts with O_3 with the formation of NO_2 and concomitant light emission that is monitored by a chemiluminescence analyzer. The detection limit is 0.003 ppm. Draeger tubes are available, covering a range between 0.5 and 5000 ppm $(NO)_x$.

OZONE

Ozone is the primary oxidant of concern in photochemical smog due to its inherent bioreactivity. It differs from other volatile poisons because a great proportion of the population is exposed to concentrations that are not in compliance with ambient air quality standards. It has been estimated that, depending on the meteorologic pattern of a given year, 60 to 135 million Americans live in areas with ozone exceeding the 1-h National Ambient Air Quality Standard (NAAQS) of 0.12 ppm. In Los Angeles, for example, ozone concentrations exceeded this value for 141 days in 1985. Due to human activities the former background level of some 0.02 ppm has reached a level of 0.04 ppm worldwide, and current mitigation strategies with the significant reduction of automobile emissions have been offset by population growth.

Properties, Sources, and Exposure Potential

Ozone (O_3, molecular weight 48.00; 1 ppm = 2.0 mg/m^3) is a bluish, explosive, irritating, and highly toxic gas with a relative specific gravity of 1.65 (air = 1). Pure O_3 has a characteristic odor resembling hay that is recognized at 0.01 to 0.05 ppm. Owing to its polarized state, O_3 is about 14 times more water soluble than oxygen.

O_3 is a powerful oxidizing agent with a standard redox potential of 2.07 V and is capable of participating in many chemical reactions with inorganic and organic substances. O_3 strongly absorbs ultraviolet light and is subject to photolysis, yielding atomic oxygen, which, in the presence of H_2O vapor, produces highly reactive OH radicals.

In the stratosphere, there is sufficient short-wave ultraviolet light (<242 nm) to directly split molecular O_2 into atomic oxygen, which combines with O_2 to form O_3. Build-up and photolytic decomposition upon irradiation are in a dynamic equilibrium, leading to stratospheric O_3 concentrations that approach

10 ppm O_3 at an altitude of 20 to 25 km. Due to its efficient absorption of UV light (<310 nm) in the stratosphere, O_3 gradually decreases at lower altitudes, while protecting the surface of the Earth from hazardous irradiation. In the upper troposphere with O_3 concentrations around 1 ppm, NO_2 efficiently absorbs longer-wavelength UV light (<400 nm) to decompose to NO and atomic oxygen, thereby feeding O_3 formation in a cyclic process.

O_3 in ambient air is attributable to several sources. One is the stratosphere, from which O_3 enters especially during the springtime when the stratospheric–tropospheric air exchange is most pronounced. The other sources are driven by complex photochemical reaction sequences requiring inputs of organic vapors, nitrogen oxides (NO_x), and solar radiation. Interestingly, local O_3 concentrations are reduced in the vicinity of heavy vehicular traffic due to scavenging by NO. On the other hand, less-trafficked areas downwind may have higher O_3 concentrations due to the enrichment of the air mass with motor vehicle exhaust chemicals (NO_2 and volatile organic compounds) and more intensive radiation. Thus, rural settings surrounding metropolitan areas usually have higher O_3 peaks in the afternoon and less pronounced troughs at night than the centers of the emissions, and summer peaks (due to prolonged solar radiation) of O_3 are usually particularly high.

Indoor concentrations of O_3 are almost always substantially lower than those outdoors due to efficient scavenging by indoor surfaces. Higher indoor concentrations may be measured when copying machines, electrostatic air cleaners, or sun lamps are operating. A mean half-life of 7 min has been estimated for O_3 in the ambient air. Because most people spend more than 80% of their time indoors, their exposure is much lower than estimates based on outdoor concentrations.

Commercially, O_3 is generated from atmospheric oxygen in a corona discharge on a demand basis and at its point of use. Modern water treatment plants use O_3 as an oxidant for disinfection and facilitation of the filtration process. The main advantages of O_3 over chlorine are disinfection from bacteria, viruses, and waterborne parasites, and removing odors and discoloration from water without the formation of residues of toxicological relevance. In fact, public concern about the quality of municipal water supply has risen sharply since the early 1970s when naturally occurring organic compounds were found to be converted to chloroorganics, principally trichloromethane, in chlorinated drinking water. Similarly, O_3-treated wastewater is safe for the receiving body of water and carries the maximum dissolved oxygen concentration. O_3 is currently used by the beverage industry to remove organic compounds in feed water, which could contribute to taste and odor problems. Furthermore, O_3 is replacing chlorine in wood-pulp bleaching. Occupational exposure involves electric arc welding, mercury vapor lamps, office photocopy machines, X-ray generators, and high-voltage electrical equipment.

Absorption, Distribution, Metabolism, Excretion, and Mechanisms of Toxicity

Because of its poor water solubility, a substantial portion of O_3 penetrates deeply into the lung although some 40% is scrubbed by the nasopharynx of humans. The region of the lung that is predicted to have the largest O_3 deposition is the bronchoalveolar duct junction. Exercise increases the dose to the target area because O_3 penetration increases with increased tidal volume and flow rate. By means of $^{18}O_3$, it has been shown that the dose penetrating to the distal lung and the degree of damage to the lung in exercising humans (0.4 ppm for 2 h) are similar to those found in resting rats exposed to 2 ppm for 2 h. In mice, ^{18}O accumulated in the lung and decreased with a half-life of approximately 6 h.

One of the biological actions of O_3 is the reaction with unsaturated fatty acids. The strongly electrophilic nature of O_3 enables it to attack carbon double bonds (ozonolysis). The mechanism proceeds through electrophilic addition with the formation of an intermediate carbonium ion, which further reacts to form a cyclic ozonide (Criggee-ozonide). In the presence of water, the ozonide undergoes hydrolysis with the formation of a carbonyl species and an intermediate zwitterion that ultimately decomposes into another carbonyl compound along with hydrogen peroxide. Each carbonyl group is located at the site of one of the parent olefinic carbon atoms. The ozonization of these fatty acids is essentially equivalent to lipid peroxidation and occurs primarily on biomembranes.

Sulfhydryl compounds may scavenge O_3 with the formation of disulfides and sulfonic acids. During the reactions of O_3 with oxidizable compounds, reactive oxygen species are produced, such as singlet oxygen, OH radicals, and hydrogen peroxide. These secondary reactive compounds may be responsible for subsequent reactions with amino acids and DNA. In fact, a variety of oxygenated DNA bases have been detected upon the incubation of DNA with O_3. Thus, O_3 poses an intense oxidative stress by various pathways. Its toxic effects may be mitigated by antioxidants. Following subtoxic O_3 exposure, a variety of adaptive mechanisms have been observed to counteract the oxidative stress, including enzyme induction of superoxide dismutase, catalase, glutathione peroxidase, and glutathione reductase.

Acute and Chronic Toxicity

Acute Toxicity

Acute intoxications with high doses exceeding 1 ppm O_3 are rare events. The inhalation causes irritation of the respiratory tract, cough, frontal headache, and, in some persons, nausea and retching. O_3 inhalation may be followed by rhinitis and anosmia. At concentrations of 0.25 to 0.75 ppm it causes shallow rapid breathing, a decrease in pulmonary compliance, and subjective symptoms, such as cough, tightness in the chest, and dryness of the throat. Owing to its poor water solubility, pure O_3 hardly provokes lacrimating, in contrast to other compounds of photochemical smog.

Healthy subjects exposed to 0.4 ppm for 2 h with concurrent heavy intermittent exercise showed decreases in forced vital capacity and forced expiratory volume in 1 s and increases in specific airway resistance. Interestingly, these parameters had coefficients of variation ranging from 80 to 100%. The observed scattering was attributed to interindividual differences, probably due to differences in the delivered dose of O_3, as determined primarily by the minute volume. Such dose-dependent decrements in pulmonary function have been observed at concentrations above 0.08 ppm. Reduced respiratory functions are reflected in reduced athletic performance.

The mechanism by which O_3 impairs the pulmonary functions is not well understood. In contrast to sulfated pollutants, functional impairment by O_3 does not correlate with enhanced sensitivity towards a bronchoconstrictor challenge and is not enhanced in asthmatics. Cholinergic and β-adrenergic mechanisms are apparently not important. More attention has been paid to the role of inflammatory effects, which have been observed in nose and lung as early as 1 h after exposure. Following a 2-h exposure to 0.4 ppm O_3, the bronchoalveolar lavage fluid showed an increase in polymorphonuclear leukocytes together with arachidonic acid descendants, such as the prostaglandins, PGE_2 and PGF_α. Pretreatment with nonsteroidal antiphlogistics decreased the pulmonary function deficit and PGE_2 production. Other lavage compounds indicative of inflammation include thromboxane B_2, interleukin 6, lactate dehydrogenase, albumin, and fibronectin. Inflammatory mediators in the bronchoalveolar lavage fluid and decrements in lung function have also been found in humans exposed to about ambient air O_3 concentrations for 6.6 h.

In addition to its effects on respiratory function and inflammation, O_3 adversely affects the immune response that protects the lung from infectious diseases. In animal models and humans, O_3 impairs the phagocytic capacity of alveolar macrophages. In fact, O_3 increased the susceptibility of rodents to several pathogenic bacteria, possibly by impairing the ability of the macrophage to produce bactericidal superoxide radicals during the oxidative burst.

Systemic effects caused by O_3 itself are quite unlikely due to its high reactivity, which excludes its intact transfer to sensitive targets via the blood. Accordingly, O_3 was not found to be teratogenic in animal experiments.

Chronic Toxicity

Animal experiments with various species have revealed pulmonary function deficits at threshold concentrations as low as 0.1 ppm. Histomorphological changes included hyperplasia of type I and type II pneumocytes and changes in cilial and Clara cells. High concentrations (0.5 ppm) resulted in irreversible lung fibrosis. It should be pointed out that continuous exposure was less deleterious than an intermittent one, even at half the continuous dose.

An important aspect in the long-term toxicity of O_3 is its ability to induce tolerance. This adaptive phenomenon begins after single exposure, is complete after some days, and has been observed in animal experiments and humans with regard to lung function tests and inflammatory phenomena.

Mutagenicity and Carcinogenicity

O_3 has been shown to be mutagenic in almost all *in vitro* systems. Genotoxic effects on the lung macrophages of rats following O_3 inhalation have been reported. A recent National Toxicology Program (NTP) study indicates "some evidence" of carcinogenicity (bronchoalveolar adenomas and carcinomas) in female mice (B6C3F1) exposed to 1 ppm of O_3 for 2 years (6 h/day, 5 days/week), while "equivocal evidence" was found in male mice. However, metaplasia of the epiglottis, nose, and lung occurred in male mice and rats. These effects were not observed at 0.12 ppm of O_3. In addition, O_3 may have promoting effects due to its inflammatory activity.

Conceivably, adaptive mechanisms coping with the oxidative stress and reducing reactive oxygen species that are thought to be responsible for DNA effects may cause a threshold phenomenon, similar to that applicable to formaldehyde.

Therapeutic Measures

Acutely exposed, symptomatic persons should be observed for at least 24 h. The early use of corticosteroid aerosols has been suggested for the prevention of pulmonary edema. Otherwise, treatment is supportive.

Work-Place Exposure Guidelines

The TWA values are 0.1 ppm, 0.16 ppm, and 0.2 ppm for heavy, moderate, and light work, respectively. There is a notice of intended changes to halve these values (ACGIH). OSHA recommends a TWA of 0.1 ppm, NIOSH a STEL of 0.1 ppm. The MAK value was 0.1 ppm O_3 until 1994. This figure was suspended in 1995 because O_3 was classified as a substance suspected of having carcinogenic potential.

Analysis

The methods mostly employed to analyze gaseous samples are the direct ultraviolet-absorbance method and the O_3-dependent chemiluminescence of ethylene. Draeger tubes are available with a sensitivity ranging from 0.05 to 300 ppm (bleaching of indigosulfonate). Ozone in liquid samples can be analyzed by using a iodometric procedure or following the bleaching of indigosulfonate.

Bibliography

ACGIH (1996). "Guide to Occupational Exposure Values—1996." ACGIH, Cincinnati, OH.

Allred, E. N., Bleecker, E. R., Chaitman, B. R., Dahms, T. E., Gottlieb, S. O., Hackney, J. D., Pagano, M., Selvester, R. H., Walden, S. M., and Warren, J. (1989). Short-term effects of carbon monoxide exposure on the exercise performance of subjects with coronary heart disease. *N. Engl. J. Med.* **321,** 1426–1432.

Anders, J. C., Chung, H., and Theoharides, A. D. (1988). Methemoglobin formation resulting from administration of candidate 8-aminoquinoline antiparasitic drugs in the dog. *Fund. Appl. Toxicol.* **10,** 270–275.

Astier, A., and Baud, F. J. (1996). Complexation of intracellular cyanide by hydoxocobalamin using a human cellular model. *Hum. Exp. Toxicol.* **15,** 19–25.

Ayres, S. M., Evans, R., and Licht, D. (1973). Health effects of exposure to high concentrations of automotive emissions. *Arch. Environ. Health* **27,** 168–177.

Ballantyne, B., and Marrs, T. C. (1987). "Toxicology of Cyanides." Wright, Bristol, U.K.

Baskin, S. I., Neally, E. W., and Lempka, J. C. (1996). Cyanide toxicity in mice pretreated with diethylamine nitric oxide complex. *Hum. Exp. Toxicol.* **15,** 13–18.

Baumeister, R. G. H., Schievelbein, H., and Zickgraf-Rüdel, G. (1975). Toxicological and clinical aspects of cyanide metabolism. *Arzneim. Forsch./Drug Res.* **25,** 1056–1064.

Beauchamp, R. O., Jr., Bus, J. S., Popp, J. A., Boreiko, C. J., and Andjelkovich, D. A. (1984). A critical review of the literature on hydrogen sulfide toxicity. *Crit. Rev. Toxicol.* **13,** 25–97.

Benignus, V. A., Hazucha, M. J., Smith, M. V., and Bromberg, P. A. (1993). Prediction of carboxyhemoglobin formation due to transient exposure to carbon monoxide. *J. Appl. Physiol.* **76,** 1739–1745.

Boström, C.-E. (1993). Nitrogen oxides in ambient air—properties, sources and concentrations. *Scand. J. Environ. Health* **19, Suppl. 2,** 9–20.

Bunn, H. F., and Forget, B. G. (1986). Carboxyhemoglobin and Carboxyhemoglobinemia. *In* "Hemoglobin: Molecular, Genetic and Clinical Aspects" (??, ed.), pp. 663–675. W.B. Saunders, Philadelphia.

Bylin, G. (1993). Health risk evaluation of nitrogen oxides. Controlled studies on humans. *Scand. J. Work Environ. Health* **19 Suppl. 2,** 37–43.

Casarett L. J., Klaassen, C. D., Amdur, M. O., and Doull, J. (1996). "Casarett and Doull's Toxicology: The Basic Science of Poisons," 5th ed. McGraw-Hill, New York.

Christel, D., Eyer, P., Hegemann, M., Kiese, M., Lörcher, W., and Weger, N. (1977). Pharmacokinetics of cyanide in poisoning of dogs, and the effect of 4-dimethylaminophenol or thiosulfate. *Arch. Toxicol.* **38,** 177–189.

Culotta, E., and Koshland, D. E. (1992). NO news is good news. A startling simple molecule unites neuroscience, physiology, and immunology and revises scientists' understanding how cells communicate and defend themselves. *Science* **258,** 1862–1865.

Dale, O., and Husum, B. (1994). Nitrous oxide: A threat to personnel and global environment? *Acta Anaesthesiol. Scand.* **38,** 777–779.

Devlin, R. B., McDonnell, W. F., Becker, S., Madden, M. C., McGee, M. P., Perez, R., Hatch, G., House, D. E., and Koren, H. S. (1996). Time-dependent changes of inflammatory mediators in the lungs of humans exposed to 0.4 ppm ozone for 2 h: A comparison of mediators found in bronchoalveolar lavage fluid 1 and 18 h after exposure. *Toxicol. Appl. Pharmacol.* **138,** 176–185.

DFG (1996a). "Gesundheitsschädliche Arbeitsstoffe. Toxikologisch-arbeitsmedizinische Begründungen von MAK-Werten." VCH, Weinheim.

DFG (1996b). "List of MAK and BAT Values 1996." VCH, Weinheim.

Ellenhorn, M. J., Schonwald, S., Ordog, G., and Wasserberger J. (1996). "Ellenhorn's Medical Toxicology: Diagnosis and Treatment of Human Poisoning," 2nd ed. Williams & Wilkins, Baltimore.

Elstner, E. F. (1996). "Ozon in der Troposphäre: Bildung, Eigenschaften, Wirkungen." Akademie für Technikfolgenabschätzung in Baden-Württemberg, Stuttgart.

Engelhardt, G. (1987). Effect of corticosteroids on the toxic pulmonary oedema induced by nitrogen dioxide inhalation in the rat. *Arzneim.-Forsch./Drug Res.* **37,** 519–523.

Ermens, A. A. M., Refsum, H., Rupreht, J., Spijkers, L. J. M., Guttormsen, A. B., Lindemans, J., Ueland, P. M., and Abels, J. (1991). Monitoring cobalamin inactivation during nitrous oxide anesthesia by determination of homocysteine and folate in plasma and urine. *Clin. Pharmacol. Ther.* **49,** 385–393.

Eyer, P. (1994). Gasförmige Verbindungen. *In* "Lehrbuch der Toxikologie" (H. Marquardt and S. G. Schäfer, eds.), pp. 550–570. BI-Wissenschaftsverlag, Mannheim.

Fang, Z. X., Eger, E. I., Laster, M. J., Chortkoff, B. S., Kandel, L., and Ionescu, P. (1995). Carbon monoxide production from degradation of desflurane, enflurane, isoflurane, halothane, and sevoflurane by soda lime and baralyme®. *Anesth. Analg.* **80,** 1187–1193.

Feelisch, M. (1993). Biotransformation to nitric oxide of organic nitrates in comparison to other nitrovasodilators. *Eur. Heart J.* **14,** 123–132.

Forbes, W. H., Sargent, F., and Roughton, F. J. W. (1945). The rate of carbon monoxide uptake by normal men. *Am. J. Physiol.* **143,** 594–608.

Gerrity, T. R., McDonnell, W. F., and House, D. E. (1994). The relationship between delivered ozone dose and functional responses in humans. *Toxicol. Appl. Pharmacol.* **124,** 275–283.

Goldsmith, J. R., and Landaw, S. A. (1968). Carbon monoxide and human health. *Science* **162,** 1352–1359.

Hardman, J. G., Limbird, L. E., Molinoff, P. B., Ruddon, R. W., and Goodman Gilman, A. (1996). "Goodman & Gilman's The Pharmacological Basis of Therapeutics," 9th ed. McGraw-Hill, New York.

Hardy, K. R., and Thom, S. R. (1994). Pathophysiology and treatment of carbon monoxide poisoning. *Clin. Toxicol.* **32,** 613–629.

Ignarro, L., and Murad, F. (1995). "Nitric Oxide: Biochemistry, Molecular Biology, and Therapeutic Implications." Academic Press, San Diego, CA.

Kaplita, P. V., Borison, H. L., McCarthy, L. E., and Smith, R. P. (1984). Peripheral and central actions of sodium azide on circulatory and respiratory homeostasis in anesthetized cats. *J. Pharmacol. Exp. Toxicol.* **231,** 189–196.

Kiese, M., and Weger, N. (1969). Formation of ferrihaemoglobin with aminophenols in the human for the treatment of cyanide poisoning. *Eur. J. Pharmacol.* **7,** 97–105.

Kirschner, M. J., (ed.) (1991). Ozone. *In* "Ullmann's Encyclopedia of Industrial Chemistry" (W. Gerhartz, ed., 5th ed., Vol. A18, pp. 343–357 VCH, Weinheim.

Klimmek, R., Fladerer, H., and Weger, N. (1979). Circulation, respiration, and blood homeostasis in cyanide-poisoned dogs after treatment with 4-dimethylaminophenol or cobalt compounds. *Arch. Toxicol.* **43,** 121–133.

Klimmek, R., Krettek, C., Szinicz, L., Eyer, P., and Weger, N. (1983). Effects and biotransformation of 4-dimethylaminophenol in man and dog. *Arch. Toxicol.* **53,** 275–288.

Lambertsen, C. J. (1980). Effects of excessive pressure of oxygen, nitrogen, helium, carbon dioxide, and carbon monoxide. *In* "Medical Physiology" (V. B. Mountcastle, ed.), pp. 1901–1944. Mosby, St. Louis, MO.

Lane, G. A., Nahrwold, M. L., Tait, A. R., Taylor-Busch, M., Cohen, P. J., and Beaudoin, A. R. (1980). Anesthetics as teratogens: Nitrous oxide is fetotoxic, xenon is not. *Science* **210,** 899–901.

Lippmann, M. (1989). Health effects of ozone: A critical review. *J. Air Pollution Control. Ass.* **39,** 672–695.

Meredith, T. J., Jacobsen, D., Haines, J. A., Berger, J.-C., and van Heijst, A. N. P. (1993). "Antidotes for Poisoning by Cyanide." Cambridge University Press, Cambridge, U.K.

Moldéus, P. (1993). Health risk evaluation of nitrogen oxides. Toxicity induced by nitrogen dioxide in experimental animals and isolated cell systems. *Scand. J. Work Environ. Health* **19 Suppl 2,** 28–36.

Nunn, J. F. (1993). Carbon dioxide. *In* "Nunn's Applied Respiratory Physiology" (J. F. Nunn, ed.), 4th ed., pp. 219–246. Butterworths, London.

Reiffenstein, R. J., Hulbert, W. C., and Roth, S. H. (1992). Toxicology of hydrogen sulfide. *Ann. Rev. Pharmacol. Toxicol.* **32,** 109–134.

Rowland, A. S., Baird, D. D., Weinberg, C. R., Shore, D. L., Shy, C. M., and Wilcox, A. J. (1992). Reduced fertility among women employed as dental assistants exposed to high levels of nitrous oxide. *New Eng. J. Med.* **327,** 993–997.

Smith, R. P., and Gosselin, R. E. (1964). The influence of methemoglobinemia on the lethality of some toxic anions. II. Sulfide. *Toxicol. Appl. Pharmacol.* **6,** 584–592.

Smith, R. P., Lousi, C. A., Kruszyna, R., and Kruszyna, H. (1991). Acute neurotoxicity of sodium azide and nitric oxide. *Fund. Appl. Toxicol.* **17,** 120–127.

Stamler, J. S., Singel, D. J., and Loscalzo, J. (1992). Biochemistry of nitric oxide and its redox-activated forms. *Science* **258,** 1898–1902.

Stewart, R. D. (1975). The effect of carbon monoxide on humans. *Ann. Rev. Pharmacol.* **15,** 409–423.

Topham, S. (1986). Carbon dioxide. *In* "Ullmann's Encyclopedia of Industrial Chemistry": (W. Gerhartz, ed.), Vol. A5, pp. 165–183. VCH, Weinheim.

Vennesland, B., Conn, E. E., Knowles, C. J., Westly, J., and Wissing, F. (1981). "Cyanide in Biology." Academic Press, London.

Verma, A., Hirsch, D. J., Glatt, C. E., Ronnett, G. V., and Snyder, S. H. (1993). Carbon monoxide: A putative neural messenger. *Science* **259,** 381–384.

Victorin, K. (1993). Health risk evaluation of nitrogen oxides. Genotoxicity. *Scand. J. Work Environ. Health* **19 Suppl. 2,** 50–56.

Wagner, M. (1993). Ozon—somatische und psychische Auswirkungen. *München. med. Wschr.* **135,** 367–470.

Way, J. L. (1984). Cyanide intoxication and its mechanism of antagonism. *Ann. Rev. Pharmacol. Toxicol.* **24,** 451–481.

Wong, K. L. (1992). "Carbon Dioxide." Internal report, Johnson Space Center, National Aeronautics and Space Administration, Houston, TX.

CHAPTER

34

Fibers

DAVID B. WARHEIT,* GEORGIA A. HART†, THOMAS W. HESTERBERG†

*Haskell Laboratory, E. I., du Pont de Nemours and Company, Newark, Delaware 19714

†Health Safety and Environmental Department, Johns Manville Corp., Denver, Colorado 80162

INTRODUCTION

Numerous types of synthetic inorganic and organic fibers are used for a vast array of purposes. As with any occupational exposure, the safety of workers handling fibrous materials should be evaluated. Because inhalation exposure to asbestos fibers is associated with fibrotic lung disease and cancer, the safety of fibrous dusts are of particular concern. Safety evaluations of fibers are generally more complex than those of nonfibrous dusts, because fiber toxicity is not only affected by chemical composition but also by the aspect ratio (length/diameter). For determining workplace exposure levels of airborne fibers, the World Health Organization (WHO) has defined a respirable fiber (one that can be inhaled into the lower lung) as a particle with an aspect ratio of at least 3:1, a length greater than 5 μm, and a diameter less than 3 μm. Fiber dimensions determine the lung dose (i.e., the quantity of fibers that are inhaled and deposited in the lower lung) and greatly impact both the lung biopersistence (length of time that fibers persist in the lung) and biological reactivity. The long–thin geometry of fibers permits the inhalation and lower lung deposition of fibers as long as 100–200 μm. However, this long–thin geometry is problematic for lung clearance, which depends to a large extent on translocation by mobile phagocytic cells to the upper airways. Thus, long fibers ($>$20 μm in length) of very durable compositions can remain in the lung indefinitely. Longer fibers are also more biologically reactive than short fibers. When cells attempt to ingest (phagocytize) long fibers, the fibers may disrupt cell division, alter genetic material, and/or trigger the release of inflammatory agents, all of which can eventually lead to lung disease.

In addition to the respiratory route, humans can be exposed to fibers by two other routes, oral and dermal. Oral ingestion of fibers has not resulted in toxic effects in rodents and is probably of no concern for humans. Skin irritation can be caused by a mechanical reaction to the sharp ends of thicker vitreous fibers and is generally not persistent. Inhalation is the route of exposure that poses the greatest potential for harm to humans and will be the subject of this chapter. The next section of this chapter outlines the major types of fibers and describes some of the biophysical aspects of fibers that influence lung responses following inhalation. The remaining sections review the critical inhalation toxicity studies of the major inorganic and organic fibers, with the primary focus on synthetic fibers.

CONCEPTS IN FIBER TOXICOLOGY

Types of Fibers

Fibrous materials are used for a vast array of commercial, industrial, and even medical functions. Some major uses of fibers are for thermal and acoustical insulation, filtration, and reinforcements. Thus, fibrous products aid in energy conservation (thermal insulation) and the abatement of pollution (filtration). Medical uses of fibers include blood filtration and implant reinforcements.

Fibers can be classified as naturally occurring or synthetic. The best-known family of natural inorganic fibers is asbestos (e.g., crocidolite, chrysotile, and amosite) (Fig. 1). Inhalation exposure to asbestos is associated with lung fibrosis (asbestosis, a permanent untreatable debilitating lung scarring) and thoracic cancers (lung cancer and mesothelioma of the lung pleura). Asbestos was widely used several decades ago but is now avoided or prohibited in most technologically developed nations. Numerous synthetic fibers have been developed to serve as substitutes for asbestos, as well as for a host of newer functions.

Three additional types of natural inorganic fibers are erionite, wollastonite, and attapulgite. Erionite and other natural zeolites are crystalline minerals that contain alkaline metal and alkaline earth elements in a hydrated aluminum silicate structure. Small, highly respirable erionite fibers (diameters of 0.1 μm) have been reported from natural outcroppings in Turkey and have been associated with the development of mesotheliomas in exposed humans and in laboratory animals. Wollastonite is an acicular or fibrous monocalcium silicate, which is mined in the United States, Mexico, and Finland and is mainly used in ceramics. Wollastonite fiber diameters range from 1 to 10 μm, with an average of 3.5 μm. Wollastonite is highly soluble. Attapulgite is composed of magnesium and aluminum silicate and is used as an absorbent and a thickening agent. The morphology varies according to its source; fibers mined in the United States are relatively short (0.1 to 2.5 μm) in comparison to the longer and thicker fiber from Spanish mines.

Synthetic fibers include numerous types of inorganic and organic fibers. Most of the important commercial inorganic fibers belong to the family of synthetic vitreous fibers (SVF), which are made from clay, rock, slag, and other inorganic materials and have an amorphous (glassy) composition. The three major classes of SVFs are fiberglass, mineral wool (slag wool and rock or stone wool), and refractory ceramic fiber. Numerous types of organic fibers are made from various synthetic and semisynthetic polymers, such as polyolefin, polyvinyls, polyamides, and derivatives of cellulose.

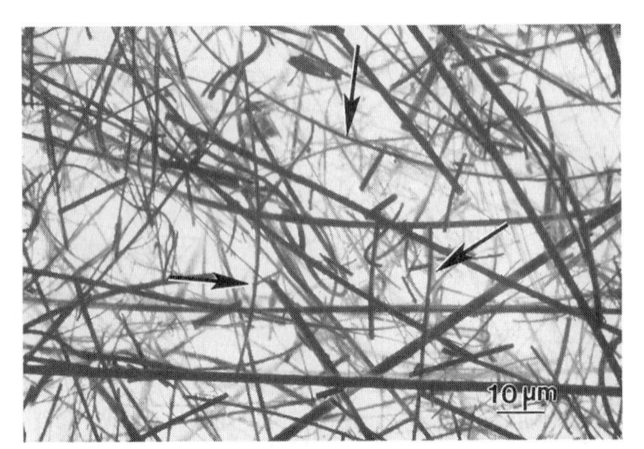

FIGURE 1 Backscatter scanning electron microscopy (SEM) image of crocidolite asbestos fibers (arrows).

Fiber Dimensions

Fiber dimensions and the aspect ratio (length/diameter) play important roles in the pathogenesis of fiber-associated lung disease. These are the primary critera that differentiate the effects of fibers from the effects of nonfibrous particulates. In general, the longer the fiber, the greater the potential for causing pulmonary effects. In a study reported in 1986, rats were exposed for 1 year by inhalation to aerosols of amosite asbestos that had been processed to be either "short" (<5 μm in length) or long (>20 μm). No significant histopathological pulmonary effects were observed in rats exposed to short fibers, but one-third of the rats exposed to similar mass concentrations of long fibers developed lung tumors and pulmonary fibrosis (permanent lung scarring). In other studies, similar fiber-length-related effects were observed in rats exposed by inhalation for 1 year to long or short chrysotile asbestos fibers. The influence of fiber dimension is not exclusively associated with asbestos fibers. In earlier studies, intratracheal instillation (injection of fibers into the trachea) of long glass fibers produced considerable pulmonary fibrosis, while instillation of shorter samples of these fibers caused no significant effects. (Instillation and injection studies inject quantities of fiber into the lung, thoracic cavity, or abdominal cavity of animals. These studies can provide useful mechanistic data but are not valid for hazard assessment of fibers because these routes of exposure bypass the normal defense and clearance mechanisms and expose animals to quantities and sizes of fibers that could not reach the lung by the normal route of exposure, i.e., inhalation.)

Deposition of Inhaled Fibers

The deposition of inhaled fibers in the distal portions of the lung is the initial event that can lead to the development of fiber-related lung disease (Fig. 2A). Size, shape, and density determine whether or not a fiber is respirable and where in the lung it will deposit. "Aerodynamic diameter" is a term that combines all three of these characteristics. The aerodynamic diameter of a fiber is equivalent to the diameter of a sphere with a specific gravity of 1 that settles in

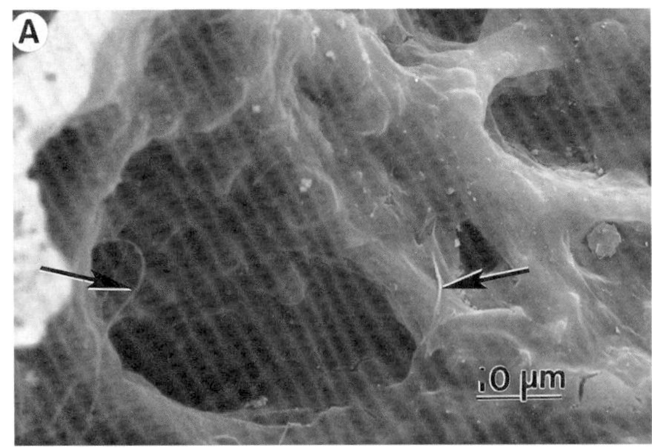

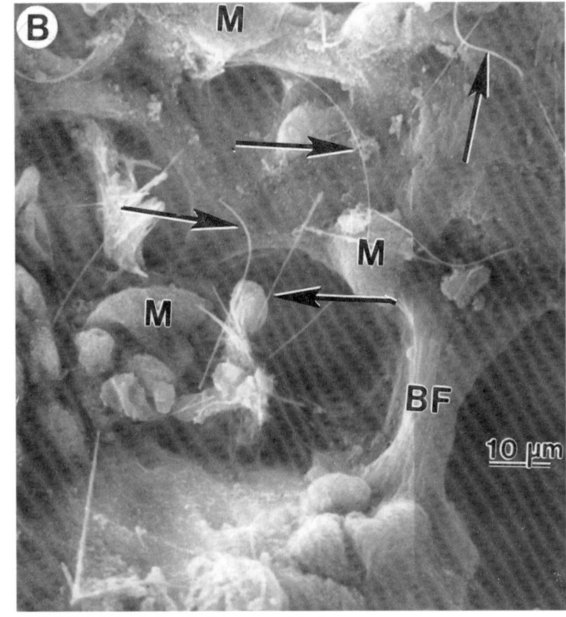

FIGURE 2 (A) Scanning electron micrograph demonstrating deposition of inhaled chrysotile asbestos fibers (arrows) in the distal lung of a rat. (B) Scanning electron micrograph demonstrating deposition of inhaled crocidolite asbestos fibers (arrows) on an alveolar duct bifurcation (BF) of a rat after a 6-h exposure. Alveolar macrophages (M) have migrated to sites of fiber deposition.

air at the same rate as the fiber and is determined by the formula $D_A = 1.3p^{1/2}\ d^{5/6}L^{1/6}$ (D_A = aerodynamic diameter; p = density; d = diameter; L = length). From this formula, it can be seen that fiber diameter is more important than length in determining the aerodynamic diameter of a fiber and, hence, the lung depth to which it will penetrate. Fibers having an aerodynamic diameter greater than 12 μm for humans and 6 μm for rodents are generally considered to be nonrespirable, that is, not likely to reach the gas-exchange regions of the lung (bronchioles and alveoli). Fibers with actual diameters less than or equal to 3 μm are respirable in humans, even with lengths as great as 100–200 μm.

The primary mechanisms of fiber deposition in the lung are impaction, sedimentation, and interception. Impaction increases under conditions of high flow velocity and occurs in the larger airways. Sedimentation is favored under conditions of low flow velocity, long residence time, and small airway size. The likelihood of interception increases directly with fiber length. The early pulmonary effects associated with fiber-induced lung diseases are probably governed to a large extent by the initial patterns of fiber deposition in the lung. In humans, the larger bronchial airway bifurcations are the preferred sites of particle deposition, as well as of bronchial cancer. Little is known about the deposition sites at the respiratory bronchiolar or alveolar levels in humans. However, studies using rodents have demonstrated that inhaled fibers and particulates small enough to pass through the rodent airways deposit primarily on the epithelial surfaces of alveolar duct bifurcations and at the junctions of terminal bronchioles and alveolar ducts, perhaps as a consequence of air-flow characteristics (Fig. 2A). In these studies, alveolar deposition decreased with increasing fiber length and increasing aerodynamic diameter, while tracheobronchial deposition increased with increasing fiber length.

Fiber Migration and Lung Clearance

Intact fibers can migrate from the initial site of deposition to foci at the bronchiole-alveolar junction, up the ciliated epithelium of the airways (Fig. 2B), and into and through the lung epithelium. Fibers with diameters greater than 3 μm deposit in the upper airways and are quickly cleared to the throat by the ciliated epithelium, and are thus probably not important in lung pathology. Some fiber migration is mediated by mobile lung cells (macrophages), which can ingest (phagocytize) and translocate shorter fibers (with lengths less than 15 μm). Alveolar macrophages clear shorter fibers from the lower lung by carrying them up to the ciliated epithelium of the upper airways where they are transported up to the throat. Other pathways and processes of fiber migration are not clearly understood. Inhaled fibers that are not cleared from the lung (due to greater length and chemical persistence) may be taken up by phagocytic cells in the lung wall and translocated through the epithelium, into interstitial storage sites in the lung parenchyma, along lymphatic drainage pathways, or to the pleura and/or other sites distant from the lung.

Fiber Biopersistence

Biopersistence can be defined in its broadest sense as the ability of inhaled fibers to resist changes in number, dimension, surface chemistry, chemical composition, surface area, and other characteristics. Any or all of these parameters can be altered during a fiber's residence in the lung, and such alterations affect the lung's long-term response to the fiber. Fiber biopersistence in the lung is determined by macrophage-mediated clearance, the fiber's dissolution rate, and the tendency of the fiber to undergo transverse fragmentation. For fibers that are too long to be cleared out of the lung by alveolar macrophages, the principal alternative clearance mechanisms are translocation to other thoracic compartments, dissolution, and/or transverse breakage into shorter segments. *In vitro* fiber dissolution experiments demonstrate a broad range of dissolution rate constants (k_{dis} = ng/cm^2/h, or ng of fiber dissolved per cm^2 fiber surface area per hour in physiological saline solution) for the various synthetic vitreous fibers, from 3 for refractory ceramic fiber (RCF) to $>$400 for slag wool and $>$600 ng/cm^2/hr for X607 (a developmental fiber). *In vitro* fiber-degradation experiments demonstrate a direct relationship between the fiber's rate of leaching (some components dissolve more rapidly than others, leaving a depleted silica matrix) and its tendency to undergo transverse fragmentation. While synthetic vitreous fibers tend to break transversely, asbestos fibers tend to split longitudinally. This is significant for pathogenesis because over time in the lung the number of long asbestos fibers can actually increase due to splitting while the number of long SVFs decreases due to transverse fragmentation. In an intratracheal injection experiment, SVFs were instilled into the lungs of rats; lung clearance by macrophages and the mucociliary escalator was more efficient for short segments than for longer fibers. Thus fibers that have a rapid rate of leaching and fragmentation in the lung are likely to be nonbiopersistent, even though they may not completely dissolve.

Fiber biopersistence was studied in rats for 1 year following short-term inhalation exposure to either chrysotile or crocidolite asbestos. Fibers in the lungs of crocidolite-exposed rats underwent a progressive increase in mean length but no significant change in mean diameter over time. In the chrysotile-exposed rats, mean fiber length also underwent a progressive increase, but, in this case, mean diameter underwent a significant reduction. The researchers concluded that long fibers were selectively retained in the lungs of both chrysotile- and crocidolite-exposed rats; however, longitudinal splitting with a corresponding decrease in mean fiber diameters occurred only with the chrysotile asbestos fibers. These findings were confirmed in a 2-year study of fiber clearance following intratracheal instillation. In rats instilled with crocidolite, the number of short fibers per lung declined slowly, but the number of fibers longer than 5 μm did not change significantly during 1 year of observation. In contrast, the number of chrysotile fibers per lung longer than 5 μm increased continuously over a 2-year period, which was probably a result of longitudinal splitting of fibers.

Surface Chemistry

Despite the fact that the toxicity of asbestos is now well established, little attention has been given to its surface chemistry and to its early biochemical interactions with tissues and body fluids, which could set the stage for subsequent biological responses in the lung. With nonfibrous dusts, a chemical origin of toxicity is quite obvious. With fibers, however, the physical characteristics (length and diameter) dominate the mechanisms of toxicity, and thus the roles of chemical composition are difficult to determine. It is interesting to note that more surface chemistry studies have been performed on isometric dusts, such as silica or carbons, than on fibers such as asbestos.

Several investigators have postulated a chemical origin of fiber toxicity that is based on the generation of reactive oxygen species and other free radicals when some fiber compositions come into contact with biological fluids. Strong oxidants are destructive to living tissues and can trigger a host of inflammatory reactions. Erionite is a fibrous zeolite and is one of the most potent carcinogenic minerals known. In one study, nearly 100% of rodents exposed by inhalation to erionite developed mesothelioma, a rare form of cancer of the pleura. Like other zeolites, erionite has a very large internal surface area and exchanges ions with surrounding media. It is postulated that the surface characteristics of erionite contribute to its carcinogenic potential in humans and experimental animals.

STUDIES OF SYNTHETIC VITREOUS FIBERS

Rodent Inhalation Studies

The only valid laboratory method for evaluating the respiratory toxicity of a fibrous dust has been the animal inhalation model. In the 1970s and 1980s, a number of rodent inhalation studies evaluated the toxicity of different types of SVFs and reported mostly negative results. However, questions still remained as to the safety of SVFs for workers, who may be exposed for extended periods. In 1988 a new generation of rodent inhalation studies was initiated to thoroughly test the biological effects and lung biopersistence of representatives of each class of SVF. Seven long-term and a number of short-term studies have been completed, several studies are currently in progress, and more are in the planning stages.

The newer studies incorporate the following important features that distinguish them from most of the earlier studies.

1. The test fibers are uniform in length and diameter and have approximate arithmetic mean dimensions of 20 μm $\times$ 1 μm. These dimensions are representative of airborne fibers in occupational exposures and are rat respirable. Earlier test fibers often had broad ranges of fiber dimensions and smaller average lengths.
2. The aerosolization system creates uniformly high concentrations of airborne fibers without destroying the biologically important long–thin fibers.
3. A nose-only inhalation exposure system is used in which each individual animal inhales fresh fiber aerosol that has not been affected by the exhalation of other animals. Earlier studies often used whole-body exposure, which may not deliver uniform and high doses to the lungs.
4. To simulate occupational exposure, animals inhale fibers for 6 hours per day, 5 days per week for a life time or for shorter periods, depending on the objectives of the study.
5. Aerosol and lung fibers are evaluated (counted, measured, and chemically and morphologically analyzed) at regular intervals using scanning electron microscopy. For both the aerosols and lung burdens, concentrations of fibers longer than 5 μm and longer than 20 μm ($F > 20$ μm) are reported. The World Health Organization has identified fibers >5 μm as biologically relevant. However, fibers >20 μm may be more significant for lung pathology by virtue of their inability to be cleared from the lung by macrophages and their greater biological activity.
6. Pathology is evaluated at regular intervals by veterinary pathologists.

These new rodent inhalation studies include three main protocols. Chronic inhalation studies evaluate thoracic fibrogenesis and tumorigenesis during lifetime exposure. Biopersistence studies expose rodents for 5 days and then evaluate lung fiber burdens during a period of post-exposure recovery up to 1 year. Subchronic studies evaluate early signs of toxicity and are used to predict the maximum tolerated lung-dose (MTD) of SVF for rodents and to aid in the selection of doses for a chronic study. A variety of other subchronic inhalation protocols are also being investigated for their possible utility as fiber-screening assays that could predict long-term pathogenesis. Most of these studies have been conducted in rats; however, hamsters have also been used. The new generation of studies include constant monitoring and numerous measurements to ensure the uniformity of animal handling, exposure aerosols, and analytical procedures.

Three types of asbestos (chrysotile, crocidolite, and amosite) have been evaluated in one or more of the newer studies as positive control fibers and to validate the test system with fibers that are known human carcinogens. Life-time exposure to 10 mg/m^3 crocidolite asbestos induced early pulmonary fibrosis and tumors in rats, thus demonstrating a response in the rat experimental model that is similar to that observed in occupationally exposed humans. The studies also included negative control animals that were exposed to filtered air.

In these post-1988 studies, test SVFs representing a variety of compositions but having similar fiber dimensions and administered to laboratory rodents at similar aerosol concentrations induced a broad range of different biological effects. Some SVF compositions induced only minimal transient lung irritation, while others induced severe pulmonary inflammation and fibrosis, and three were associated with increased incidences of thoracic cancers. These more recent studies demonstrate a relationship between lung biopersistence and pathogenicity. The next several subsections deal with specific results and possible interpretations.

Chronic Inhalation Studies

Fiberglass

In the 1980s, seven rodent inhalation studies found no tumorigenesis as a result of exposure to several types of fiberglass. In a recent chronic inhalation study, rats were exposed to two fiberglass insulation wools, coded MMVF10 and MMVF11, for 2 years at a maximum dose of 30 mg/m^3 (250 fibers/cc longer than 5 μm). In agreement with the earlier studies, these fiberglasses induced only transient lung inflammation that resolved after brief recovery periods. In contrast, crocidolite asbestos induced pulmonary fibrosis and tumors.

A more recent hamster chronic inhalation study compared the biological effects of amosite asbestos and two forms of fiberglass, MMVF10a and MMVF33.

MMVF33 is composed of 475 glass, a special application glass that is relatively durable. Exposures to each of the three fiber types were similar in average dimensions (approximate mean dimensions 1 μm diameter $\times$ 20 μm length) and concentrations (250–320 fibers/cc > 5 μm, 100 fibers/cc > 20 μm). As in the previous study with rats, MMVF10 insulation fiberglass induced no permanent lung changes in hamsters during the 18-month exposure period or the subsequent 2–3-month recovery period (Table 1). However, hamsters exposed to 475 fiber glass developed minimal lung fibrosis and one mesothelioma in 125 hamsters exposed. Hamsters exposed to a comparable concentration of amosite asbestos also developed fibrosis, but earlier and more severe than that in the animals exposed to 475 glass, and 19.5% mesotheliomas.

This more recent hamster study is significant because it provides the first known published report of permanent lung damage in a laboratory animal following inhalation of a fiber glass composition. In the preliminary results of another study, researchers observed fibrosis and pulmonary tumors in rats exposed by inhalation to high concentrations of microfibers composed of another relatively durable special application glass, E glass (in the United States and Europe, E glass is produced as a continuous filament that is too thick to be respirable but is no longer produced as a microfiber). However, in contrast to the hamster study, rats exposed to 475 glass fibers exhibited no more lung problems than rats exposed to air (Table 1).

In the hamster chronic inhalation study, toxicity paralleled the biopersistence of fibers in the lung. After 12 months of exposure, the fibers/lung ratio for fibers longer than 20 μm was 7–8 times greater for high-dose amosite than for 475 glass (MMVF33) and 3–4 times greater for 475 glass than for insulation glass (MMVF10a). However, initial lung depositions after 5 days of exposure were equivalent for these three fibers. Thus, the greater lung accumulation of long fibers of amosite compared with the fiberglasses, and of 475 glass compared with insulation glass, demonstrates that the glass fibers, insulation glass in particular, are clearing from the lung more rapidly than amosite. In agreement with previous rat studies, the hamster data link fiber length and biopersistence to pathogenicity.

Mineral Wool

Three pre-1990 rodent inhalation studies reported no fibrosis or tumors with chronic exposure to mineral wool. A more recent study exposed rats by nose-only inhalation to two compositions of mineral wool—rock wool (MMVF21) and slag wool (MMVF22)—in 3 concentrations, the maximum of which was 30 mg/m^3 (approximately 250 fibers/cc > 5 μm), for 6 hours/day, 5 days/week, for 2 years. Test fibers were size-selected to have average dimensions of approximately 1 μm $\times$ 20 μm. In agreement with the earlier studies, neither of the mineral wools was tumorigenic. However, in the more recent study, the rats exposed to rock wool (MMVF21) developed minimal lung fibrosis late in the inhalation period.

Refractory Ceramic Fibers

Earlier rodent inhalation studies of the chronic toxicity of refractory ceramic fiber (RCF1) reported conflicting results. In the more recent studies, rodents were exposed to four types of RCF (RCF1–4) for 6 hours/day, 5 days/week, at a maximum dose of 30 mg/m^3 (200–250 fibers/cc longer than 5 μm). Again, test fibers were size-selected to have average dimensions as close to 1 μm $\times$ 20 μm as possible. In rats, RCF1 induced lung fibrosis, 13% lung tumors, and 1.6% pleural mesothelioma. In hamsters, RCF1 induced lung fibrosis, no lung tumors, and 38% mesotheliomas. These studies present a striking difference between rat and hamster responses to the same test fiber, which opens questions of species-related differences and which species, if either, is representative of humans. As noted above, species-related differences in response were also reported for 475 fiberglass.

Inhalation Studies of Fiber Biopersistence

Because chronic inhalation studies have suggested that the pathogenicity of a fiber is linked to its ability to persist in the lung, fiber researchers have recently turned their attention to developing ways to study and measure fiber biopersistence. Lung biopersistence is here defined as the ability of a fiber to persist, chemically and physically, in the lung after it has been inhaled.

To study fiber biopersistence in the lung, rats were exposed by nose-only inhalation to 8 SVFs and two asbestos types (Table 2) for 6 hours per day for 5 days and then held without further exposure for 1 year. Lung fiber burdens were evaluated at 8–9 time points during the post-exposure year. Each of the 10 fibers had also been tested for pathogenicity in previous rodent chronic inhalation studies. All of the SVFs had similar dimensions. The amosite asbestos fiber dimensions were similar to those of the SVFs, but the crocid-

TABLE 1 MMVF-Induced Lung Pathology, Rodent Inhalation Studies, 1988–1997

Fiber	F diameter GMD ± SD (μm)	Aerosol: F > 5 μm/cc	Aerosol: F > 20 μm /cc	Fibers–Lung, 12-mo. inhalation: F > 5 μm × 10^6	Fibers–Lung, 12-mo. inhalation: F > 20 μm × 10^6	Fibers–Lung, 24-io. inhalation: F > 5 μm × 10^6	Fibers–Lung, 24-io. inhalation: F > 20 μm × 10^6	Thoracic tumors: Lung fibrosis[a]	Thoracic tumors: Lung tumors[d]	Thoracic tumors: Meso-theliomas
Rats—RCC[b]										
Air Control		0	0					—	1–3%	0
Crocidolite (LF)	0.28 (1.54)	1610 ± 989	236 ± 145	1000	46			+ (3)	15 (14%)	1 (0.9%)
Chrysotile	0.07 (1.73)	10600 ± 11400	0	1020 ± 450	0	1600 ± 1150	0	+ (3)	13 (18.5%)	1 (1.4%)
RCF1	0.86 (1.96)	187 ± 53	101 ± 15	119 ± 46	20 ± 6	143 ± 23	25 ± 7	+ (6)	15 (12.4%)	2 (1.7%)
RCF2	0.88 (1.92)	220 ± 52	87 ± 37	148 ± 72	24 ± 8	304 ± 97	42 ± 25	+ (9)	9 (7.4%)	3 (2.5%)
RCF3	0.85 (1.99)	182 ± 66	102 ± 14	100 ± 59	16 ± 9	106 ± 38	18 ± 8	+ (6)	19 (15.7%)	2 (1.7%)
RCF4	1.22 (1.68)	153 ± 49	34 ± 28	51 ± 21	1 ± 1	148 ± 18	2 ± 1	+ (12)	4 (3.4%)	1 (0.8%)
MMVF10	1.13 (1.77)	232 ± 56	73 ± 19	42 ± 9	3 ± 1	82 ± 11	5 ± 2	—	7 (5.8%)	0
MMVF11	0.76 (1.92)	246 ± 76	92 ± 25	69 ± 8	7 ± 1	182 ± 65	6 ± 3	—	3 (2.6%)	0
MMVF21	0.98 (1.74)	243 ± 67	114 ± 32	94 ± 13	16 ± 5	88 ± 25	14 ± 5	+ (12)	5 (4.4%)	0
MMVF22	0.87 (1.75)	213 ± 62	99 ± 31	58 ± 13	1 ± 0.6	62 ± 9	4 ± 2	—	3 (2.6%)	0
MMVF34a[a]		264	82					—	?	0
X607		170 ± 74	47 ± 23	62 ± 16	0.5 ± 0.5	58 ± 14	1 ± 1	—	0	0
Rats—IOM[c]										
Air Controls									2 (6%)	0
Amosite-D (LF)		981	91		123 ± 44			+ (?)	16 (38%)	2 (5%)
'MMVF32-D'		1022	109		not done			+ (?)	10 (23%)	2 (5%)
'MMVF33-D'		1119	137		11 ± 27			+/—(?)	4 (11%)	0
Hamsters—RCC[b]										
Air Control		0	0	0	0			—	0	0
Chrysotile	0.08 (1.71)	10600 ± 11400	0 ± 0	460 ± 20	0			+ (3)	0	0
Amosite (LF), lo				37 ± 2	7 ± 0.4			+ (3)		3 (2.7%)
Amosite (LF), hi	0.59 (0.24)	255 ± 89	67 ± 27	260 ± 11[f]	36 ± 7.0[f]			+ (3)	0	17 (14.9%)
MMVF10a	0.95 (0.46)	323 ± 57	151 ± 22	32 ± 5	1 ± 0.4			—	0	0
MMVF33	0.91 (0.75)	283 ± 42	106 ± 20	49 ± 7	6 ± 1.6			+ (6)	0	1 (0.9%)
RCF1	0.78 (1.93)	215 ± 56		40 ± 1	13 ± 3.0			+ (6)	0	42 (41%)

[a]In parentheses, inhalation month when fibrosis first observed (i.e., when avg. Wagner score was >3).

[b]For RCC studies, inhalation exposure was 2 years for rats (except crocidolite, 10 months) and 18 months for hamsters. Inhalation was by nose only.

[c]IOM (Institute of Occupational Medicine, Edinburgh, Scotland) studies inhalation exposure was 1 year and was followed by 1 year recovery. Test fibers were similar to those used in RCC studies but compositions and dimensions may have had minor differences. IOM studies were whole-body inhalation exposure. Davis *et al.* (1995) and unpublished data by personal communication. Amosite LF = long fiber amosite. MMVF32-D and 33-D were similar to MMVF32 and 33 of the RCC Studies.

[d]Incidence of carcinomas + ademonas.

[e]Study conducted at RCC, sponsored by Rockwool International.

[f]Chrysotile was carcinogenic in rats (18.5% lung tumor incidence) but had no detectable fibers longer than 20 μm and was not carcinogenic in hamsters. Hamster exposure to crocidolite was terminated after 44 weeks due to high mortality in this exposure group.

LF = Long fiber (i.e., fibers selected for increased average length).

TABLE 2 Fiber Biopersistence, *In Vitro* Dissolution Rate and Pathogenicity, Listed in Order of Pathogenicity

Fiber	Type	Biopersistence T-90[a]	*In vitro* dissolution k_{dis} at pH 7.4[b]	Pathogenicity: Fibrosis	Pathogenicity: Tumors
Crocidolite	Asbestos	2715	<1	+	+
Amosite	Asbestos	2095	<1	+	+
MMVF32	E glass	371	9	+	+
RCF	Refractory ceramic	226	3	+	+
MMVF33	475 glass	240	12	+/−[c]	+/−[c]
MMVF21	Rock Wool	264	20	+	−
MMVF10	Fiberglass	123	300	−	−
MMVF11	Fiberglass	38	100	−	−
MMVF22	Slag wool	37	400	−	−
MMVF34	HT stone wool	19	59	−	−

[a]T-90 = 90% clearance time, days.

[b]k_{dis} = ng/cm² h; *in vitro* flow-through system; Eastes *et al.* 1996); and O. Kamstrup (personal communication).

[c]+/−; in inhalation studies, exposed hamsters developed fibrosis and 1 mesothelioma (<1% incidence), but exposed rats did not differ from negative controls.

olite asbestos fibers were considerably thinner and shorter.

The data for fibers/lung longer than 20 μm were modeled by using the two pool first-order kinetic equation given below. The 90% clearance time (T-90) of long fibers (i.e., longer than 20 μm) was calculated from the mathematical model of each fiber type and used as an index of biopersistence.

$$y = ae^{-bx}$$

or

$$y = a_1e^{-b_1x} + a_2e^{-b_2x}$$

where x = recovery times (days); y = fibers/lung; a_1 and a_2 = fibers/lung in the faster and slower pools, respectively, when time (x) = 0; and b_1 and b_2 are the rate constants for the fast and slow pools, respectively.

The weighted clearance half-life ($WT_{1/2}$) of long fibers is another measure of biopersistence. The $WT_{1/2}$ is an attempt to provide one index that reflects the clearance rates of both pools in a two-pool model by "weighting" the clearance half-life ($T_{1/2}$) of the faster and slower pools according to their respective proportions of the total lung fiber population. The $T_{1/2}$ of each pool is calculated from the equation provided above. The $WT_{1/2}$ is then calculated from the equation

$$WT_{1/2} = p \cdot T1/2_1 + (1 - p) \cdot T1/2_2$$

where $T1/2_1$ and $T1/2_2$ = 50% clearance half-lives of the faster and slower pools, and p = the proportion of the lung fibers in the faster pool at time 0.

The T-90 has several advantages over the $WT_{1/2}$. The $WT_{1/2}$ is strongly influenced by the presence of a very small stagnant pool of lung fibers (i.e., a very small proportion of lung fibers that clear very slowly or not at all). That such a pool could have an equivalent impact on the actual lung toxicity is not supported by the data available. The T-90, on the other hand, is not strongly influenced by a very small stagnant pool. The T-90 also reflects a later phase of clearance than half-life clearance ($T_{1/2}$ or $WT_{1/2}$), and therefore the T-90 may be mechanistically more related to pathogenesis. Additionally, the T-90 is a simpler calculation and is not dependent upon the type of mathematical modeling (i.e., one-or two-pool model). Unlike the $WT_{1/2}$, the T-90 is easily determined and easily defined.

The 90% clearance times (T-90s) of long (>20 μm) fibers fell into three groups: 19–123 days (MMVF10, 11, 22, and 34), 260–370 days (RCF1, MMVF32, 33, and 21), and more than 2000 days (amosite and crocidolite asbestos) (Table 2). Each of the two asbestos fibers underwent very slow or stagnant clearance during the last three-quarters of the postexposure year.

The four less biopersistent SVFs (MMVF10, 11, 22, and 34) showed chemical and morphological changes over time in the lung, but the more biopersistent fibers did not. For example, after 6 months in the rat lung, the relatively nonbiopersistent MMVF22 (slag

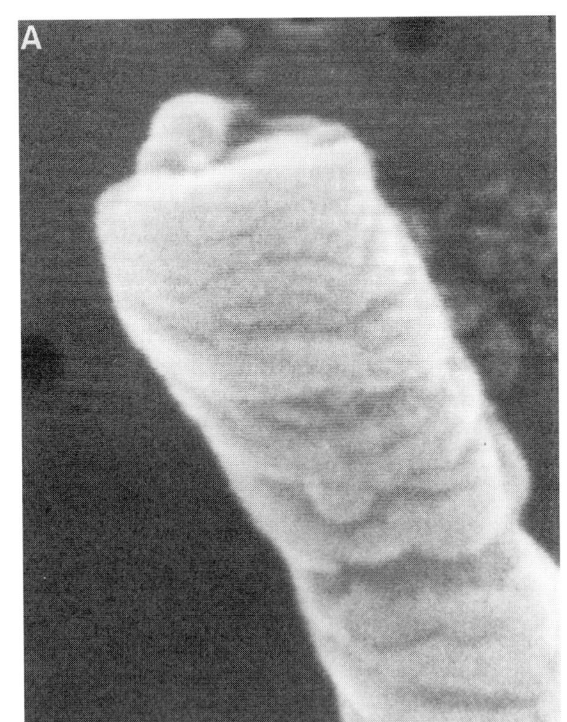

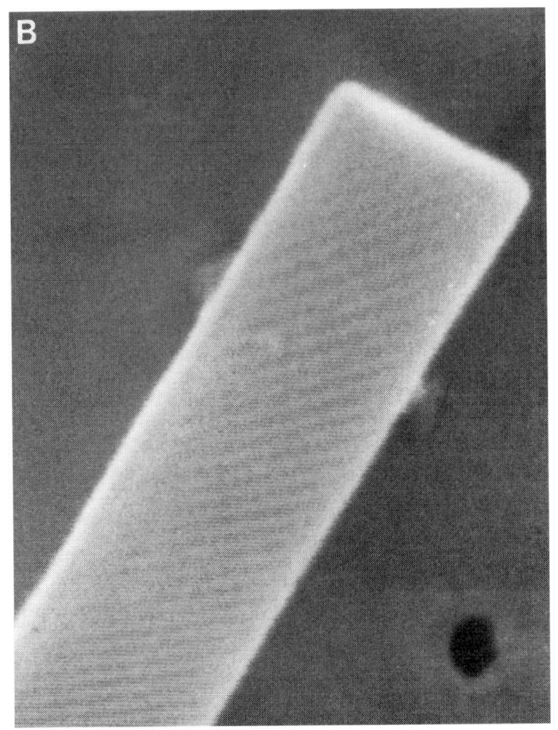

FIGURE 3 Fibers after 6 months in the rat lung. (A) MMVF22 (slag wool), showing major surface degradation; (B) (MMVF21) rock wool, showing no surface degradation.

wool), showed deep furrowing of the surface, but MMVF21 (rock wool) and the other persistent fibers retained smooth surfaces and sharp ends (Figs. 3A and B). Also, in lung burdens of the four less biopersistent fibers, the numbers of long fibers/lung declined more rapidly than the numbers of shorter fibers/lung. This was especially true for MMVF34, which cleared the most rapidly of all the fibers (Fig. 4A). After 30 days of post-exposure recovery, the percentage of MMVF34 fibers retained in the lung was 3% for long fibers but 42% for short fibers. In contrast,

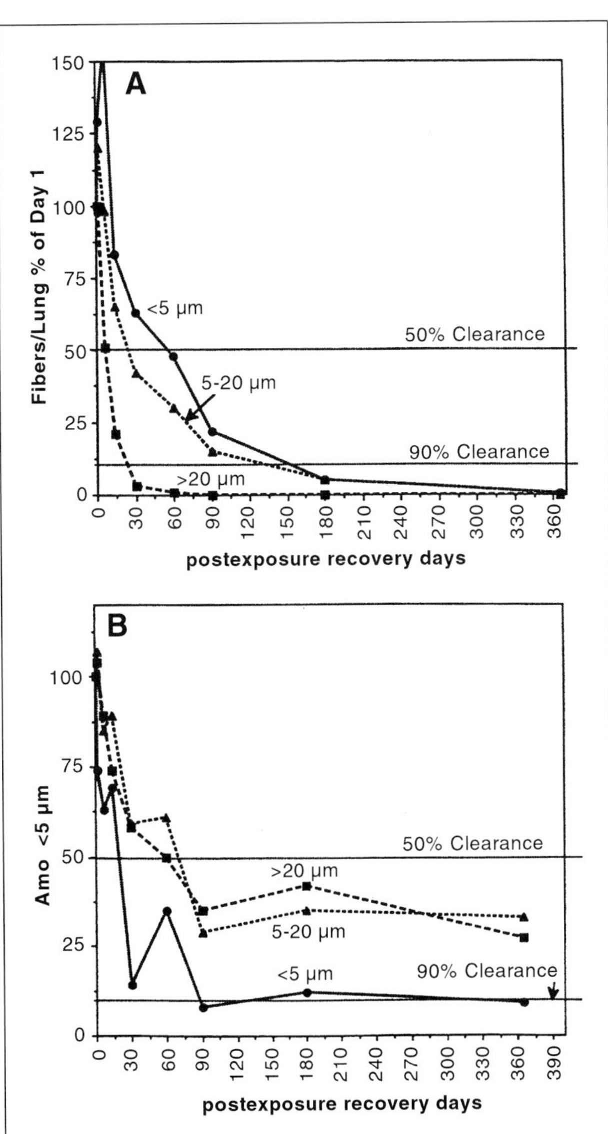

FIGURE 4 Lung clearance of fibers from the rat lung. (A) MMVF34 (HT stone wool), a nonbiopersistent fiber, showing more rapid clearance of long fibers than of short fibers; (B) amosite asbestos, a very biopersistent fiber, showing more rapid clearance of short fibers.

in lung burdens of the more durable fibers, short fibers cleared as rapidly or more rapidly than long fibers, which would be expected if clearance were primarily or solely by macrophage-mediated translocation and fiber dissolution. The more rapid clearance of long fibers observed in the less biopersistent compositions is probably a result of transverse fragmentation of long fibers into shorter segments; the short segments add to the subpopulation of short fibers, but the short fibers are, at the same time, being removed by macrophages. Thus the dynamics would result in a shrinking long-fiber population and a short-fiber population that grows initially and then also declines. Thus, transverse fragmentation may be as important as dissolution in the lung clearance of fibers.

Biopersistence and Pathogenicity

Biopersistence as represented by the T-90 values for long fibers agrees quite well with toxicity; compositions with long-fiber T-90s greater than 200 days were all fibrogenic, and all but MMVF21 were associated with tumorgenesis (Table 2). The relationship between fiber biopersistence and lung injury could be explained as follows. Fibers that are too thick to be inhaled into the lower lung or are short enough to be transported by alveolar macrophages are quickly cleared from the respiratory tract and will probably cause nothing more than transient pulmonary inflammation. Long fibers with a diameter less than 3 μm are able to penetrate into the lower lung; however, these fibers will also be innocuous if they dissolve rapidly or break transversely into small segments that can be cleared by alveolar macrophages and the ciliated epithelium. However, long thin fibers that reach the lower lung in sufficient doses will be pathogenic if they do not dissolve or fragment.

This scenario does not take into account fiber surface chemistry, which apparently plays a role in the toxicity of at least some fibers, such as erionite. In recent rat inhalation studies, E glass fibers were very pathogenic but 475 glass fibers were relatively innocuous; but both fiber types appeared to clear from the rat lungs at about the same rate. However, during a year of post-exposure recovery, 475 glass fibers underwent significant changes in chemistry due to leaching. Thus, the concept of biopersistence must be broader than the simple visible retention of fibers in the lung; in addition to fiber numbers and dimensions, changes in fiber surfaces due to leaching and other processes could impact bioreactivity.

In Vitro Studies of Inorganic Fiber Degradation

Rodent inhalation studies demonstrate a broad range of lung biopersistences for the different SVFs and suggest that dissolution, leaching, and fragmentation determine the lung residence time of inhaled fibers. At the same time, *in vitro* studies have begun to reveal some of the molecular mechanisms of fiber degradation in simulated body fluids. For these studies, fiber samples are sandwiched between two filters and placed in a cartridge, which is then placed in either a flow-through system or a high-volume static system, both of which contain a physiological saline solution. The saline solution is typically set at pH 7.4 to mimic extracellular fluid. However, fiber dissolution studies are also conducted with saline at pH 4.5, which mimics the pH of the phagolysosomes of macrophages; the reasoning here is that fibers are subjected to this pH in the lung when they are ingested by macrophages. Fluid from the test system is analyzed at intervals for dissolved fiber components, and the dissolution rate constant, k_{dis}, is determined (ng/cm^2/h, or mass loss per unit surface area over time). Fibers are also removed from the system at intervals and examined for chemical and physical changes.

In vitro dissolution studies demonstrate a broad range of dissolution rates for the different compositions of inorganic fibers. Some examples of some *in vitro* k_{dis} values at near-neutral pH (expressed as ng/cm^2/h) are less than 1 for crocidolite or amosite asbestos, 8 for RCF1, and 140–260 for fiberglass insulation. HT stone wool insulation fiber (MMVF34) has a modest k_{dis} of 59 at pH 7.4 but a very rapid dissolution rate at pH 4.5 of more than 700 ng/cm^2/h. The *in vitro* dissolution rates of fibers at near-neutral pH tend to parallel their lung biopersistence and their pathogenicities, with the exception of MMVF34 (Table 2). Apparently the lung biopersistence of MMVF34 is determined by factors other than just simple dissolution, such as macrophage action and/or transverse fragmentation.

In one study, fibers were placed in saline solution at pH 7.4 for 500 hours, and then removed and cut transversely. The different compositions showed varying zones of leaching in the outer perimeter. The relatively nonbiopersistent fibers (insulation glass MMVF10 and slag wool MMVF22) had broad leached zones, while the relatively persistent and moderately toxic rock wool (MMVF21) had no leached zone (Fig. 5). In a similar study, insulation fiberglass (MMVF10) showed an average of 20 transverse breaks per fiber after approximately 500 hours in simulated *in vitro* in saline solution (Fig. 6).

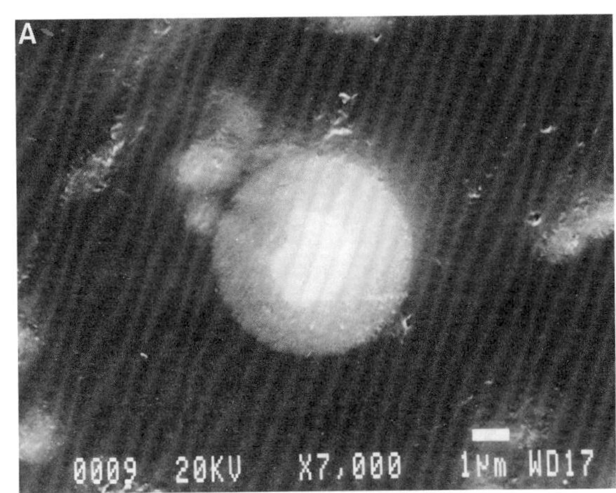

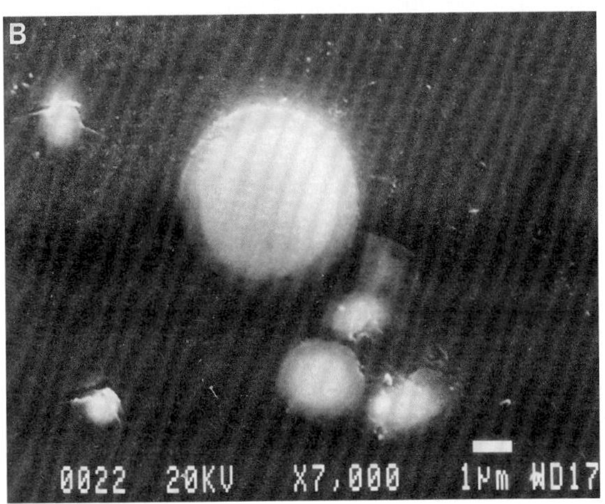

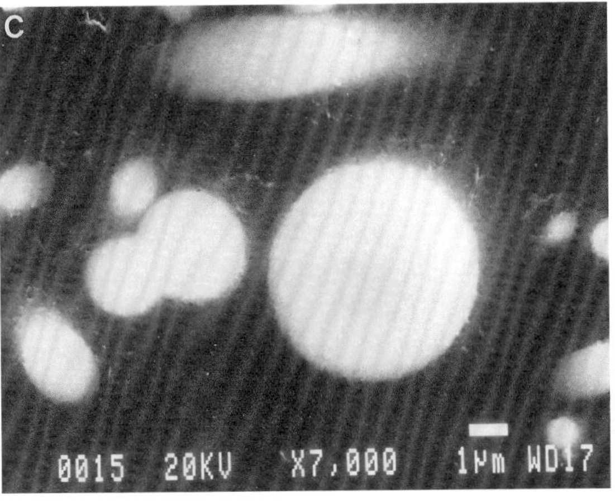

FIGURE 5 Cross sections of fibers after 500 hours in simulated extracellular fluid (*in vitro*). (A) MMVF10 (insulation fiberglass), showing a broad zone of peripheral leaching; (B) MMVF22 (slag wool), showing an intermediate zone of peripheral leaching; (C) MMVF21 (rock wool, a relatively biopersistent fiber), showing no zone of surface leaching.

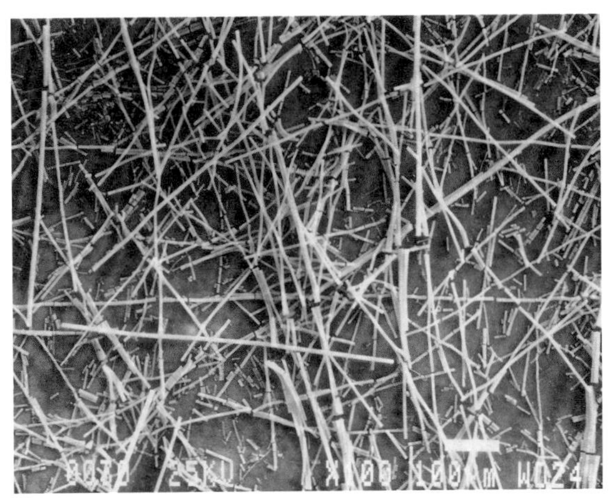

FIGURE 6 Transverse breakage of insulation fiberglass (MMVF10) after 500 hours in simulated extracellular fluid (*in vitro*). An average of 20 transverse fractures/fiber was observed.

Cell Culture Studies

In vitro cell culture studies have shown fairly consistently that fiber toxicity to cells in culture is directly related to fiber length and perhaps indirectly related to fiber diameter. *In vitro* studies are less conclusive about whether there is a relationship between chemical composition and toxicity, whether fibers can induce cancer-like neoplastic changes in cultured cells, and whether fibers can induce gene mutation or chromosomal damage. Fiber toxicologists have long sought, but without success, a battery of short-term cell culture tests that could be used to screen fibers for their toxicological potential. Such a battery could save millions of dollars and months and years of time that are required for long-term animal studies. After nearly two decades of research such a battery has not been found.

However, *in vitro* studies have contributed to a better understanding of the molecular mechanisms of fiber-induced lung injury. Recently, a number of studies have focused on the role of inflammatory mediators in particle-induced lung injury. In their critical role in lung defense, macrophages and other leukocytes inactivate and clear foreign agents and recruit additional inflammatory cells to the site of invasion in the lung. During this process, activated inflammatory cells release biodestructive factors, such as active oxygen species and proteolytic enzymes, that not only destroy microbes but also can injure lung tissues. Recruitment of other cells and the release of biodestructive agents are at least in part mediated by cytokines

TABLE 3 Examples of Organic Fibers

Natural plant fiber	
Cellulose	
Semi-synthetic fibers (derived from natural cellulose)	
Regenerated cellulose	
Viscose rayon	
Cuporcellulose	
Cellulose acetate	
Cellulose triacetate	
Synthetic polymeric fibers	**Polymer Monomer**
Polyolefins	
Polyethylene	$-CH_2-CH_2-$
Polypropylene	$-CH(CH_3)-CH_2-$
Polyvinyls	
Polyacrylonitrile	$-CH(CN)-CH_2-$
Polyvinylchloride	$-CH(CL)-CH_2-$
Polyamides	
Aliphatic (nylon)	$-NH-CO-(CH_2)_4-CO-NH-(CH_2)_5-$
Aromatic (para-aramid)	-NH-**R**-NH-CO-**R**-CO-
Polyester	-O-CO-**R**-CO-O$(CH_2)_n$-
Others	
Polyimide	
Polyurethane	
Elastomer	
	R =

and arachadonic acid metabolites that are released by the first wave of phagocytic cells that come into contact with the foreign agent.

Recently, researchers have determined some of the cytokines that are involved in particle-induced lung responses and what they do. Soon after an irritant particle is deposited in the lung, a cytokine called TNF-α (tumor necrosis factor alpha) appears in the lung fluid and is followed by a large influx of inflammatory cells into the lung fluid. TNF-α is released *in vitro* by macrophages that were cultured from the lungs of animals that had been exposed to crocidolite asbestos. TNF-α stimulates other cultured lung cells to release chemoattractant cytokines called MIPs (macrophage inflammatory proteins). MIPs induce macrophages and other inflammatory cells to migrate *in vitro* along the MIP concentration gradient (*in vivo,* this could induce migration toward the source of the irritant).

Thus, a mechanistic model of fiber-induced lung damage at the cellular level could be as follows: Fibers and other inflammatory particles (e.g., crystalline silica) stimulate macrophages to release TNF-α, which stimulates macrophages and other lung cells to release MIPs, which recruit more inflammatory cells to the irritant in the lung. The activated inflammatory cells release biodestructive agents, which would destroy microbial invaders, and have of little or no effect on nonliving particles but would injure lung tissue. Tissue repair and cell proliferation take place in response to the injury. If the initiating fibers are biopersistent and in high concentrations, the cell recruitment–injury–repair cycle continues and expands and could eventually result in permanent lung damage, such as fibrosis and even tumorogenesis.

The mechanisms whereby fibers activate inflammatory cells and induce them to release bio-active agents may be both mechanical and chemical. Long fibers that are phagocytized by cells may perturb their cell membranes to the extent that the cells release their internal contents into the extracellular space, thereby initiating a cascade of inflammatory effects. The surface chemistry of some fibers could also contribute to cell membrane destruction; some *in vitro* studies have suggested a greater free radical activity for pathogenic fibers than for nonpathogenic fibers. Free radical formation on the surface of certain fiber compositions (amosite and RCF1) could be mediated by the release of iron from the fiber.

ORGANIC FIBERS

Composition and Structure

Numerous synthetic and semisynthetic polymers have been used to produce organic fibers. Table 3 lists some examples of organic fiber-forming materials. A generic term such as "nylon" or "acrylic" indicates a group of polymeric materials that have a common type of chemical link between monomers. However, it is important to note that different members of a group like "nylon" may have very different physical and chemical properties. Semisynthetic fibers based on cellulose differ from natural cellulose fibers in structure, molecular weight of the (reconstituted) cellulose polymer, and in functional endgroups attached to the cellulose molecules.

Synthetic organic molecules are often referred to as microfibrils. Microfibrils have diameters of 0.1–1.0 nm and lengths of several μm. Microfibrils are composed of flexible macromolecules in the oriented state with alternating amorphous layers and crystalline regions. The amorphous layers are more vulnerable to chemical breakdown and enzymatic digestion than the crystalline regions, and are thus important in determining lung biopersistence. In microfibrils of *para*-aramid and other polymers with more rigid rod-like macromolecules, a radially oriented "pleated sheet" structure is microscopically visible, and these regions may be vulnerable to physicochemical attack in the lung. The term RFP (respirable-sized, fiber-shaped particulate) is used to distinguish respirable-sized organic fibers from nonrespirable fibers.

Animal Studies of *p*-Aramid

Para-aramid (*p*-aramid) is one of the very few synthetic organic fibers that have been evaluated in inhalation studies, and it has been investigated extensively. The studies outlined below evaluate the toxicity and biopersistence of RFPs of Kevlar, a representative *p*-aramid fibril (Fig. 7). Recently, the terms *p*-aramid RFP and *p*-aramid fibrils have become interchangeable. The results of many of the studies with *p*-aramid RFP are summarized in a recent IARC monograph.

Biopersistence Studies of p-*Aramid*

In an earlier study, rats were exposed to *p*-aramid RFP for two weeks, then maintained for a period of post-exposure recovery. Rats exposed to lower levels (up to 26 fibers/cc) showed only a macrophage response, and those exposed to higher levels (≥280 f/cc) developed granulomatous lesions at the alveolar duct bifurcations with fibrotic thickening. By 6 months post-exposure, the granulomatous lesions were nearly recovered and the fibrotic lesions were much reduced. During lung residence, the fibers fragmented and decreased in size at a rapid rate.

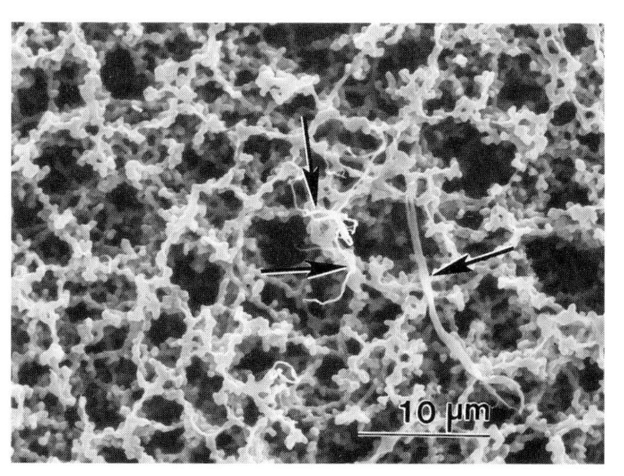

FIGURE 7 Scanning electron micrograph demonstrating aerosolized *para*-aramid fibrils (arrows) caught on a filter during an inhalation exposure.

In a more recent study, rats were exposed for 5 days to aerosols of *p*-aramid fibrils (900–1344 f/cc, 9–11 mg/m^3) or wollastonite fibers (800 f/cc; 115 mg/m3). The wollastonite fibers cleared from the lung rapidly, with a clearance half-life of less than 1 week. During 1 month in the lung, wollastonite mean fiber length progressively decreased from 11 to 6 μm. The number of *p*-aramid fibrils/lung showed a transient increase at 1 week post-exposure and then a rapid decrease thereafter; lung clearance half-life was approximately 30 days. During the 6 months in the lung, the *p*-aramid fibril mean length progressively decreased from 12.5 μm to 7.5 μm. The study demonstrated that both inhaled *p*-aramid and wollastonite fibers have low biopersistence in the rat lung.

In another study, the lung deposition and clearance of *p*-aramid fibrils were investigated in rats exposed by inhalation for as long as 2 years. The initial mean dimensions of the inhaled *p*-aramid fibrils were 12 μm length and <0.3 μm diameter. After a 2-year exposure at 2.5, 25, and 100 fibrils/cc, or a 1-year exposure plus a 1-year recovery at 400 fibrils/cc, mean lengths of lung-retained fibrils approached 4 μm. The time required for the fibrils to be reduced to <5 μm in the lung was markedly less at lower exposure concentrations. These data suggest that *p*-aramid fibrils are less biopersistent in the lungs of rats than would be expected from the known chemical resistance of *p*-aramid commercial yarn.

Searl (1997) conducted a study to evaluate the relative biopersistence of inhaled *para*-aramid fibrils, chrysotile asbestos, and code 100/475 glass fibers in the lungs of rats following 2 weeks of exposure to similar aerosol concentrations (700 fibers/cc). All three fiber types underwent large reductions in number and volume of retained fibers during the 16-month post-exposure period. The data from the *p*-aramid-exposed rats demonstrated rapid clearance of the longest fibrils during the first month following exposure, concomitant with an initial increase in the numbers of shorter fibrils. This is consistent with a mechanism of transverse breakage of *p*-aramid fibrils into shorter fragments that could be more readily cleared by macrophages. The 475 glass fibers also underwent rapid clearance of the longest fibers with a concomitant increase in the numbers of very short fibers consistent with the removal of long fibers through transverse fragmentation. In contrast, the chrysotile data showed a preferential clearance of

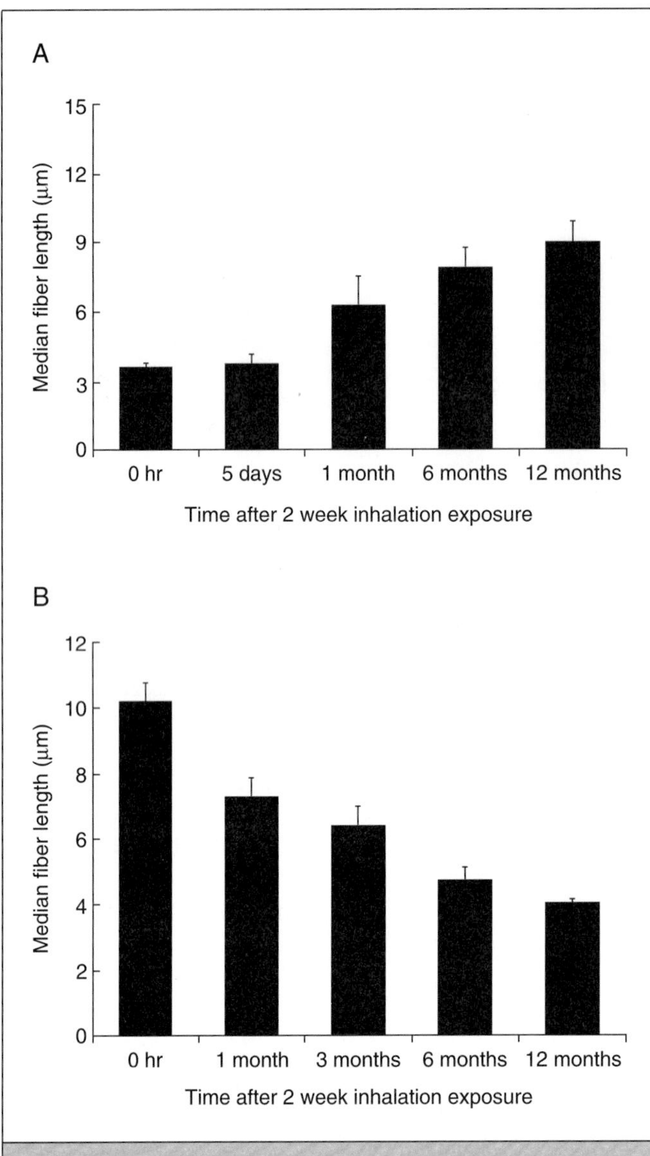

FIGURE 8 (A) Chrysotile asbestos fiber dimensions in lung tissue of rats following a 2-week inhalation exposure. Note the progressive increase in median fiber lengths with increased residence time in the lung, indicating that the short fibers are cleared over time while the longer fibers are retained. This indicates that inhaled chrysotile asbestos fibers are biopersistent in the lungs of exposed rats. (B) *p*-Aramid fibril dimensions in lung tissue of rats following a 2-week inhalation exposure. Note the progressive decrease in median fiber lengths with increased residence time in the lung, indicating that inhaled *p*-aramid fibrils are biodegradable in the lungs of exposed rats.

short fibers and minimal transverse breakage of fibers. The biopersistence of long (>15 um) chrysotile fibers was very much greater than that of long fibers of the 475 glass or *p*-aramid.

In yet another study, rats were exposed for 2 weeks to size-separated *p*-aramid fibrils or chrysotile asbestos at target concentrations of 400 and 750 fibers/cc. Because the vast majority of chrysotile fibers are very short compared to the synthetic test fibers, chrysotile was size-selected to eliminate the shorter fibers and thereby increase the proportion of longer fibers. Following exposure, the lung burdens were evaluated at six time points up to 1 year post-exposure. Median lengths of lung fibers were 8.6 μm for *p*-aramid but only 3.5 μm for chrysotile. Lung clearance of long chrysotile fibers was negligible. In contrast, *p*-aramid fibrils cleared rapidly. Median lengths of chrysotile lung fibers increased over time, while median lengths of *p*-aramid fibrils decreased over time (Figs. 8A and B).

A study was conducted in hamsters to determine whether the *p*-aramid fibrils would behave in the lungs of hamsters as they did in the lungs of similarly exposed rats. Hamsters were exposed whole-body to aerosols of size-separated *p*-aramid fibrils for 2 weeks at target fiber concentrations of 350 and 700 fibers/cc. Lung burdens were evaluated at several intervals during a post-exposure period of 3 months. Mean lengths of *p*-aramid fibrils recovered from hamster lungs were 10.4 μm at time 0 (immediately after the 2-week exposure), 6.3 μm at 1 month, and 6.1 μm at 3 months. Thus, the biodegradability of inhaled *p*-aramid fibrils observed in hamsters was similar to that observed in rats, in that, for both species, the mean and median lengths of lung fibrils were progressively reduced during their residence time in the lungs.

Chronic Inhalation Studies of p-Aramid

In a chronic inhalation study, groups of 100 male and female rats were exposed to ultrafine *p*-aramid fibrils at concentrations of 0, 2.5, 25, and 100 fibrils/cc (0, 0.8, 0.31, and 0.63 mg/m^3) for 5 days/week for 2 years. An additional group of 100 animals was exposed during the same period to 400 fibrils/cc. The 400 fibril/cc exposure was terminated at 12 months due to toxicity, and the animals were followed for an additional year. For this study, fibrils were separated from the *p*-aramid pulp matrix by high-pressure air impingement. Lungs exposed at 2.5 fibrils/cc exhibited normal alveolar architecture and a few dust-laden macrophages in the alveolar air spaces—this constituted a NOAEL (no observable adverse effect level). In rats exposed to 25 and 100 fibrils/cc, the following were observed: a dose-related increase in lung weight, a dust cell response, slight type II pneumocyte hyperplasia, alveolar bronchiolarization, and a negligible amount of collagenized fibrosis in the alveolar duct region. In addition, 6% of the female rats (but none of the males) exposed to 100 fibrils/cc developed foci that were termed "cystic keratinizing squamous cell carcinomas (CKSCC)," which were later reevaluated and termed "proliferative keratin cysts (PKCs)" by an expert panel of pathologists. Female rats also had more prominent foamy alveolar macrophages, cholesterol granulomas, and alveolar bronchiolization. In the group exposed to 400 fibrils/cc for up to 1 year, 29 males and 14 females died due to obliterative bronchiolitis resulting from dense accumulation of inhaled *p*-aramid fibrils in the ridges of alveolar duct bifurcations. Rats in this exposure group that survived for 1 year post-exposure had markedly reduced lung dust content, average fiber lengths, and the pulmonary lesions. However, these rats exhibited slight centriacinar emphysema and minimal fibrosis in the alveolar duct region; one male rat (1/36; 3%) developed a carcinoma and six female rats (6/56; 11%) developed PKCs.

Since the publication of these studies, considerable discussion has occurred regarding the nature of the CKSCC and PKC. A panel of pathologists agreed that these cystic lesions found in the *para*-aramid exposed rats should be referred to as "proliferative keratin cysts." These lesions were lined by well-differentiated stratified epithelium with a central keratin mass and were not considered by the majority of the panel to be neoplastic in nature or to be relevant for carcinoma development. In 1995, a pathology workshop on keratinizing lesions in the rat lung, organized by the Deutsche Forschungsgemeinschaft, reached an agreement on the criteria for the classification of cystic lesions. The cystic keratinizing lung lesions produced following exposure to *p*-aramid and many other dusts appear to be unique to the rat, and further investigation is necessary to better understand their biological nature. The general opinion is that these lesions are probably not relevant for human risk assessment of pulmonary cancer.

Para-aramid fibrils (RFP) were evaluated in 1997 by the International Agency for Research on Cancer (IARC) and were judged to be a category 3 material (i.e., inadequate evidence for carcinogenicity). This decision was based primarily on the lack of carcinogenic effects in rats following long-term inhalation exposures and after intraperitoneal injection, and on strong evidence of the biodegradability of inhaled *p*-aramid fibrils in the lungs of exposed rats and hamsters.

Polyolefins

Groups of rats were exposed nose-only 6 h/day, 5 days/week for 90 days to 12, 20, or 46 polypropylene fibers/cc (15, 30, or 60 mg/m^3) that had been size-selected to have an average diameter of 1.6 μm and an average length of 20 μm. Rats were evaluated during the exposure period and at one post-exposure time point. The rats developed dose- and duration-dependent lung changes characterized by increased cellularity and early bronchiolitis but no fibrosis. These cellular changes are considered to be reversible.

Carbon Fibers

Groups of male rats were exposed nose-only to aerosols of respirable-sized pitch-based carbon fibers or nonrespirable polyacrylonitrile-(PAN-) based carbon fibers (7 μm diameter) at target concentrations of 50 or 100 mg/m^3 (47 or 62 fibers/cc) for 1 to 5 days (6 h/day) and evaluated at several post-exposure time points. After 5 days exposure, respirable-sized, pitch-based carbon fibers produced dose-dependent transient inflammatory and cell proliferative responses in the lungs. Pigment-laden alveolar macrophages, as well as minimal type II epithelial cell hyperplasia were observed primarily at the junctions of the terminal bronchioles and alveolar ducts. After 10 days of post-exposure recovery, the lungs had returned to a normal appearance. The nonrespirable PAN-based carbon fibers produced no significant pulmonary effects, and few fibers were observed in the lungs of exposed animals, indicating that the 7 μm diameter fibers did not deposit in the distal lungs of exposed rats.

Other Organic Fibers

In a 1975 study, 28 guinea pigs were exposed to manually pulverized nylon and 10 guinea pigs were exposed to acrylonitrile dust for nearly 1 year. Eighteen nylon-exposed and 10 acrylonitrile-exposed animals were histologically examined either at terminal sacrifice or after interim deaths (six animals). Intraseptal granulomas were found in 14 of the 18 nylon-exposed animals and in all 10 of the acrylonitrile-exposed animals. The lesions contained microscopically visible birefringent material. Unfortunately, no respirable dust concentrations or particle dimensions were reported in this study.

SUMMARY

Safety evaluations associated with inhalation exposure to fibers require toxicological evaluations that are more complex than those required for study of nonfibrous particulate materials in general. Fiber toxicology has different biophysical elements, which must be understood as a first step in the understanding of the mechanisms related to fiber-induced lung disease. First, fibers are particulate materials that are defined by length/diameter aspect ratios. Second, it is generally considered that physical dimensions, biopersistence in the lung, and surface characteristics, play important roles in producing fiber-induced toxic effects in the lungs of exposed animals and humans.

Some of the important concepts of fiber toxicity have been outlined in the first part of this chapter. These describe the biophysical aspects of fibers that influence the response of the lung following deposition in the respiratory tract. In the remaining sections of this chapter, some of the important studies related to synthetic vitreous fibers (SVF) have been described. In addition, although the database for synthetic organic fiber types is limited, some of the critical inhalation toxicity studies have been briefly reviewed. It is important to recognize that there exists a wide range of potencies for various fiber types and many of these effects are related to their physical and surface properties.

Bibliography

Bellmann, B., Muhle, H., Pott, F., Konig, H., Kloppel, H., and Spurny, K. (1987). Persistence of man-made mineral fibers (MMF) and asbestos in rat lungs. *Ann. Occup. Hyg.* **31,** 693–709.

Bernstein, D. M., Morscheidt, C., Grimm, H. G., Thevenaz, P., and Teichert, U. (1996). Evaluation of soluble fibers using the inhalation biopersistence model, a nine-fiber comparison. *Inhal. Tox.,* **8,** 345–385.

Bernstein, D. M., Thevenaz, P., Fleissner, H., Anderson, R., Hesterberg, T., and Mast, R. (1995) Evaluation of the oncogenic potential of man-made vitreous fibers: The inhalation model. *Ann. Occupat. Hygiene* **39(5),** 661–672.

Boorman, G. A., Brockmann, M., Carlton, W. W., Davis, J. M. G., Dungworth, D. L., Hahn, F. F., Mohr, U., Reichhelm, R., Turusov, V. S., and Wagner, B. M. (1996). Classification of cystic keratinizing squamous lesions of the rat lung: Report of a workshop. *Toxicol. Pathol.* **24,** 564–572.

Brown, D. M., Fisher, C., and Donaldson, K. (1997) Free radical activity of manmade fibers: Iron chelation inhibits hydroxyl radical generation by refractory ceramic fiber. *J. Tox. Environ. Health* (in press).

Carlton, W. W. (1994). "Proliferative keratin cyst," a lesion in the lungs of rats following chronic exposure to para-aramid fibrils. *Fundam. Appl. Toxicol.* **23,** 304–307.

Davis, J. M. G. (1986). A review of experimental evidence for the carcinogenicity of man-made vitreous fibers. *Scand. J. Work Environ. Health* **12(1),** 12–17.

Davis, J. M. G., Addison, J., Bolton R. E., Donaldson, K. *et al.* (1986). The pathogenicity of long versus short fiber samples of amosite asbestos administered to rats by inhalation or intraperitoneal injection. *Br. J. Exp. Pathol.* **67,** 415–430.

Davis, J. M. G., Brown, D. M., Cullen, R. T. Donaldson, K., Jones A. D. Miller, B. G., McIntosh, C. and Searl, A. (1996). A comparison of methods of determining and predicting the pathogenicity of mineral fibers. *Inhal. Tox.* **8,** 747–770.

Davis, J. M. G., and Jones, A. D. (1988). Comparison of the pathogenicity of long and short fibers of chrysotile asbestos in rats. *Br. J. Exp. Pathol.* **69,** 717–737.

Driscoll, K. E. (1994). Macrophage inflammatory proteins: Biology and role in pulmonary inflammation. *Exper Lung Res.* **20,** 473–490.

Driscoll, K. E. (1995). The toxicology of crystalline silica studied in vitro. *Appl Occupat Environ Hygiene* **10(12),** 1118–1124.

Driscoll, K. E., Hassenbein, D. G., Carter, J. M. Kunkel, S. L. Quinlan, T. R. and Mossman, B. T. (1995). TNF alpha and increased chemokine expression in rat lung after particle exposure. *Toxicol. Lett.* **82–83,** 483–489.

ECETOC (1996). "Toxicology of Man-Made Organic Fibers (MMOF)." "Technical Report No. 69. European Centre for Ecotoxicology and Toxicology of Chemicals, Brussels.

Frame, S. R., Brockmann, M. Hahn, F. F., Slone, T. W., and Warheit, D. B. (1997). Microscopic review of para-aramid -induced cystic keratinizing squamous lesions in the lungs of rats. *Inhal. Toxicol.* **9,** 189–198.

Hart, G. A., Kathman, L. M., and Hesterberg, T. W. (1994). In vitro cytotoxicity of asbestos and man-made vitreous fibers: Roles of fiber length, diameter and composition. *Carcinogenesis* **15,** 971–977.

Hart, G. A., Newman, M. Bunn, W. B., and Hesterberg, T. W. (1992). Cytotoxicity of refractory ceramic fibers to Chinese hamster ovary cells in culture. *Toxicology In Vitro* **6(4),** 317–325.

Hesterberg, T. W., Axten, C., Hadley, J. Oberdörster, G. McConnell, E. E. Everitt, J. Miiller, W. Chevalier, H. J. Chase, G. and Thevenaz, P. (1997). Chronic inhalation study of fiber glass and amosite asbestos in hamsters: Twelve month results. *Environ. Health Perspect.* (in press).

Hesterberg, T. W., and Barrett, J. C. (1984). Dependence of asbestos- and mineral dust-induced transformation of mammalian cells in culture on fiber dimension. *Cancer Res.* **44,** 2170–2180.

Hesterberg, T. W. Chase, G. Axten, C., Miiller, W. C. Musselman, R. P. Kamstrup, O. Hadley, J. Morscheidt, C. Bernstein, D. and Thevenaz, P. (1998) Biopersistence of synthetic vitreous fibers and amosite asbestos in the rat lung following inhalation, a joint study of NAIMA and EURIMA. *Inhal. Toxicol.* (in preparation).

Hesterberg, T. W., Hart, G. A., and Bunn, W. B. (1993). In vitro toxicology of fibers: Mechanistic studies and possible use for screening assays. *In* "Fiber Toxicology" (D. Warheit ed.), pp. 139–170. Academic Press, San Diego, CA.

Hesterberg, T. W., Miiller, W. C., Hart, G. A., Bauer, J., and Hamilton, R. D. (1996). Physical and chemical transformation of synthetic vitreous fibers in the lung and in vitro. *J. Occup Health Safety, Aust. NZ* **12(3),** 345–355.

Hesterberg, T. W., Miiller, W. C., Musselman, R. P., Kamstrup, O., Hamilton, R. D., and Thevenaz, P. (1996) Biopersistence of man-made vitreous fibers and crocidolite in rat lung following inhalation. *Fund. Appl. Toxicol.* **29,** 267–279.

Hesterberg, T. W., Miiller, W. C., McConnell, E. E., Chevalier, J., Hadley, J., Bernstein, D. M., Thevenaz, P., and Anderson, R. (1993). Chronic inhalation toxicity of size-separated glass fibers in Fischer 344 rats. *Fund. Appl. Toxicol.* **20,** 464–476.

Hesterberg, T. W., McConnell, E. E., Miiller, W. C., Chevalier, J., Everitt, J., Thevenaz, H., Fleissner, H., and Oberdorster, G. (1996). Use of lung toxicity and lung particle clearance to estimate the maximum tolerated dose (MTD) for a fiber glass chronic inhalation study in the rat. *Fund. Appl. Toxicol.* **32,** 31–44.

IARC (1997). "IARC Monographs on the Evaluation of Carcinogenic Risk to Humans, Vol. 68, Silica, Some Silicates, Coal Dust and Para-Aramid Fibrils." IARC, Lyon, France.

Kelly, D. P., Merriman, E. A., Kennedy, G. L. Jr., and Lee, K. P. (1993). Deposition, clearance and shortening of Kevlar para-aramid fibrils in acute, subchronic and chronic inhalation studies in rats. *Fund. Appl. Toxicol.* **21,** 345–354.

LeBouffant, L., Daniel, H., Henin, J. P., Martin, J. C., Normand, C., Thichoux, G., and Trolard, F. (1987). Experimental study on long-term effects of inhaled SVF on the lung of rats. *Ann. Occup. Hyg.* **31,** 765–790.

Lee, K. P., Barras, C. E., Griffith, E. D., Waritz, R. S. and Lapin, C. A. (1981). Comparative pulmonary responses to inhaled inorganic fibers with asbestos and fiberglass. *Environ. Res.* **24,** 167–191.

Lee, K. P. Kelly, D. P., O'Neal, F. O., Stadler, J. C., and Kennedy G. L., Jr. (1988). Lung response to ultrafine Kevlar aramid synthetic fibrils following 2-year inhalation exposure in rats. *Fund. Appl. Toxicol.* **11,** 1–20.

Levy, L. S. (1994). Squamous cell lesions associated with chronic exposure by inhalation of rats to p-aramid fibrils (fine fiber dust) and to titanium dioxide: Finding of a pathology workshop. *In* "Toxic and Carcinogenic Effects of Solid Particles in the Respiratory Tract" (U. Mohr *et al.*, pp. 253–266. ILSI Press, Washington, D.C.

Lippmann, M. (1993). Biophysical factors affecting fiber toxicity. *In Fiber Toxicology,* (D. B. Warheit, ed) Academic Press, San Diego, CA.

Mast, R. W., McConnell, E. E., Anderson, R., Chevalier, J., Kotin, P., Bernstein, D. M., Thevenaz, P., Glass, L. R., Miiller, W. C., and Hesterberg, T. W. (1995). Studies on the chronic toxicity (inhalation) of refractory ceramic fiber in male Fischer 344 rats. *Inhal. Toxicol.* **7,** 425–467.

Mast, R. W., McConnell, E. E., Hesterberg, T. W., Chevalier, J., Kotin, P., Thevenaz, P., Bernstein, D. M., Glass, L. R., Miiller, W. C., and Anderson, R. (1995) A multiple dose chronic inhalation study of size-separated kaolin refractory ceramic fiber in male Fisher 344 rats. *Inhal. Toxicol.* **7,** 469–502.

McConnell, E. E., Kamstrup, O., Musselman, R., Hesterberg, T. W., Chevalier, J., Miiller, W. C., and Thevenaz, P. (1994). Chronic inhalation study of size-separated rock and slag wool insulation fibers in Fischer 344/N rats. *Inhal. Toxicol.* **6(6),** 571–614.

McConnell, E. E., Mast, R. W., Hesterberg, T. W., Chevalier, J., Kotin, P., Bernstein, D. M., Thevenaz, P., Glass, L. R., and Anderson, R. (1995). Chronic inhalation toxicity of a kaolin based refractory ceramic fiber (RCF) in Syrian golden hamsters. *Inhal. Toxicol.* **7,** 503–532.

McConnell, E. E., Wagner, J. C., Skidmore, J. W., and Moore J. A. (1984). A comparative study of the fibrogenic and carcinogenic effects of UICC Canadian chrysotile B asbestos and glass microfiber (JM 100). *In* "Biological effects of man-made mineral fibers," Vol. 2, pp. 234–252. World Health Organization, Copenhagen.

Morgan, A. and Holmes, A. (1984). The deposition of MMMF in the respiratory tract of the rat, their subsequent clearance, solubility in vivo and protein coating. *In* "Biological Effects of Man-Made Fibers," Vol. 2, pp. 1–7. World Health Organization, Copenhagen.

Mossman, B. T., Jimenez, L. A., BeruBe, K., Quinlan, T., and Janssen, Y. M. W. (1995). Possible mechanisms of crystalline silica-induced lung disease. *Appl. Occup. Environ. Hyg.* **10(2),** 1115–1117.

Mossman, B. T., and Sesko, A. M. (1990). In vitro assays to predict the pathogenicity of mineral fibers. *Toxicology* **60(1–2),** 53–61.

Mossman, B. T., Surinrut, P., Brinton, B. T., Marsh, J. P., Heintz, N. H. Lindau-Shepard, B., and Shaffer, J. B. (1996). Transfection of a manganese-containing superoxide dismutase gene into hamster tracheal epithelial cells ameliorates asbestos-mediated cytotoxicity. *Free Radical Biol. Med.* **21,** 125–131.

Muhle, H. Bellmann, B., and Pott, F. (1991). Durability of various mineral fibers in rat lungs. *In* "Mechanisms in Fiber Carcinogenesis" (R. Brown *et al.*, eds.), Vol. 223, pp. 181–187. NATO ASI Series A: Life Sciences. Plenum Press, New York.

Oshimura, M., Hesterberg, T. W., Tsutsui, T., and Barrett, C. J. (1984). Correlation of asbestos-induced cytogenetic effects with cell transformation of Syrian hamster embryo cells in culture. *Cancer Res.* **44,** 5017–5022.

Poole, A., Brown, R. C., and Rood, A. P. The in vitro activities of a highly carcinogenic mineral fiber–potassium octatitanate. *Br. J. Exp. Pathol.* **67,** 289–296.

Roggli, V. L., and Brody, A. R. (1984). Changes in numbers and dimensions of chrysotile asbestos fibers in the lungs of rats following short-term exposure. *Exp. Lung Res.* **7,** 133–147.

Roggli, V. L., George, M. H., and Brody, A. R. (1987). Clearance and dimensional changes of crocidolite asbestos fibers isolated from lungs of rats following short-term exposure. *Environ. Res.* **42,** 94–105.

Searl, A. (1997). A comparative study of the clearance of respirable para-aramid, chrysotile and glass fibers from rat lungs. *Ann. Occup. Hyg.* **41,** 217–233.

Seilikoff, I. J., Churg, J. and Hammond, E. C. (1965). The occurrence of asbestosis among insulation workers in the United States. *Ann. NY Acad. Sci.* **132,** 139.

Sincock, A., and Seabright, M. (1925). Induction of chromosome changes in Chinese hamster cells by exposure to asbestos fibers. *Nature* **257,** 56–58.

Tilkes, F., and Beck, B. G. (1980). Comparison of length-dependent cytotoxicity of inhalable asbestos and man-made mineral fibers. *In* "Biological Effects of Mineral Fibers" (J. C. Wagner, ed.), pp. 475–483. IARC Scientific Publications No. 30. IARC, Lyon, France.

Wagner, J. C., Berry, G. B., Hill, R. J., Munday, D. E., Skidmore, J. W. (1984). Animal experiments with MMM(V)F effects of inhalation and intrapleural inoculation in rats. *In* "Biological Effects of Manmade Mineral Fibers," Vol. 2, pp. 209–233. World Health Organization, Copenhagen.

Warheit, D. B. (1995). A review of inhalation toxicology studies with *para*-aramid fibrils. *Ann. Occup. Hyg.* **39,** 691–697.

Warheit, D. B., and Hartsky, M. A. (1990). Species comparisons of alveolar deposition patterns of inhaled particles. *Exp. Lung Res.* **16,** 83–99.

Warheit, D. B., Hartsky, M. A., Butterick, C. J., and Frame, S. R. (1995). Pulmonary toxicity studies with man-made organic fibers: Preparation and comparisons of size-separated para-aramid with chrysotile asbestos fibers. *In* "Toxicology of Industrial Compounds" (H. Thomas, ed.) pp. 119–130. Taylor and Francis, London.

Warheit, D. B., Hartsky, M. A., and Frame S. R. (1996). Pulmonary effects in rats inhaling size-separated chrysotile asbestos fibers or p-aramid fibrils: Differences in cellular proliferative responses. *Toxicol. Lett.* **88,** 287–292.

Warheit, D. B., Hartsky, M. A., McHugh, T. A., and Kellar, K. A. (1994). Biopersistence of inhaled organic and inorganic fibers in the lungs of rats. *Environ. Health Perspec.* **102(Suppl 5),** 151–157.

Warheit, D. B., and Johnson, N. F. (1990). Symposium on health effects of inhaled fibrous materials. *Fund. Appl. Toxicol.* **15,** 633–640.

Warheit, D. B., Kellar, K. A., and Hartsky, M. A. (1992). Pulmonary cellular effects in rats following aerosol exposures to ultrafine Kevlar aramid fibrils: Evidence for biodegradability of inhaled fibrils. *Toxicol. Appl. Pharmacol.* **116,** 225–239.

Warheit, D. B., Snajdr S. I., Hartsky, M. A., and Frame, S. R. (1997). Pulmonary responses to inhaled para-aramid fibrils in hamsters: Evidence of biodegradability in the lungs of a second rodent species. *Inhal. Toxicol.* **9,** 181–187.

Wright, G., and Kuschner, M. (1977). The influence of varying lengths of glass and asbestos fibers on tissue responses in guinea pigs. *In* "Inhaled Particles IV, Part 2" (W. H. Walton, ed.), pp. 455–474. Pergamon Press, Oxford.

Zoitos, B., Rouyer-Archer, E., De Meringo, A., Thelohan, S. Bauer, J. Law, B., Boymel, P., Olson, J., Christensen, V. Guldberg, M. Koenig, A. and Perander, M. (1997). In vitro measurement of fiber dissolution rate. *Inhal. Toxicol.* **9,** 525–540.

CHAPTER

35

Chemical and Biological Agents

LADISLAUS SZINICZ*, STEVEN I. BASKIN†

*Institute for Pharmacology and Toxicology, Akademie des Sanitäts der Bundeswehr, Garching-Hochbrück, Germany

†Medical Research Institute of Chemical Defense, U.S. Army, Aberdeen Proving Ground, Maryland

CHEMICAL AGENTS

Introduction

The use of poisons as weapons and efforts to ban them dates from ancient times. Despite the Hague Convention (1899/1907) and Geneva Protocol (1925), chemical warfare agents were used in World War I, World War II, and various other conflicts, and remained a serious threat for civilians and military personnel, (e.g, during the Gulf War I (GWI) between Iraq and Iran (1980–1988) and Gulf War (GWII) between Iraq and the allied forces (1991).

Based on the recent protocol (Paris 1993) signed by 160 nations and ratified by the 65th signatory nation (Hungary) in November 1996, the Chemical Weapons Convention (CWC) came into force on April 29, 1997. The ban of the production, stockpiling, use, and spread of chemical weapons will be controlled by the Organization for the Prohibition of Chemical Weapons in The Hague, Netherlands. Nevertheless, several countries did not sign the protocol, and the destruction of the present stocks of weapons will take some time. The attacks using chemical agents in Japan in Matsumoto 1994 (sarin) and Tokyo 1995 (sarin and cyanide) show that terroristic organizations may also produce highly toxic chemicals in sufficient amounts to cause mass poisoning.

The state-of-the-art knowledge of the risks of chemical agents, protection against them, and treatment of poisoning seem to be important not only from a military point of view but also to be imperative for protection against terroristic attacks and for effective disarmament and its control.

History

The use of poison for the acquisition of food or protection of living territory belongs to the evolution of life on Earth. The use and misuse of poisons by humans go back to prehistoric times. In ancient Greek and Roman history, reports can be found of the use of poisons in wars. The tempestuous development of chemical science and technology (and also by grievous accidents) during the 19th and 20th centuries brought the knowledge of new highly toxic chemicals and their large-scale production. The German chlorine gas attack on April 22, 1915, in Flanders during WWI is considered to be the "birthday" of "modern" chemical warfare, although other synthetic chemicals (irritants) were used before this and also by other parties (e.g., France). Sulfur mustard was used in WWI. The G series of nerve agents (Table 1) were developed between 1937 and 1943 and the V agents during the 1950s.

During WWII, chemical weapons were not used in Europe in the military, but the use of toxic chemicals in concentration camps of the Third Reich should be mentioned here. GWI and the actions of Iraq against the Kurdish population (in 1988) are more recent uses of chemical weapons. GWII (in 1991) was the latest conflict with a high chemical-agent threat, leading to

TABLE 1 Classification of Chemical Agents Relative to the Target Organ

Group and chemical name	Common name	Symbol[a]
Nerve Agents		
Ethyl-*N*,*N*-dimethyl phosphoramidocyanidate	Tabun	GA
Isopropyl methyl phosphonofluoridate	Sarin	GB
Cyclohexyl methyl phosphonofluoridate	Cyclosarin	GF
Pinacolyl methyl phosphonofluoridate	Soman	GD
O-Ethyl-*S*-(2-diisopropylamino-ethyl)-methyl phosphonothiolate	—	VX
Vesicant Agents		
Bis(2-chloroethyl)sulfide	Sulfur Mustard, Yperite, S-Lost	H, HD
Tris(2-chloroethyl)amine	Nitrogen Mustard	HN-3
2-Chlorovinyl dichloroarsine	Lewisite	L
Hydrogen cyanide	—	AC
Cyanogen chloride	—	CK
Arsine	—	SA
Lung-damaging Agents		
Carbonyl chloride	Phosgene	CG
Trichloromethyl chloroformate	Diphosgene	DP
Incapacitating Psychochemicals		
3-Quinuclidinyl benzilate	—	BZ
Lacrimators		
2-Chloroacetophenone	—	CN
2-Chlorobenzalmalononitrile	—	CS
Vomiting Agents		
Diphenylchloroarsine	Clark I	DA
Diphenylcyanoarsine	Clark II	DC
10-Chloro-5,10-dihydrophenarsazine	Adamsite	DM

[a]U.S. Department of Defense symbols.

extensive protective measures including pyridostigmine pretreatment by the allied forces. Large stocks of sarin, cyclosarin (also as binary products) and sulfur mustard were found during UN inspections after the war in Iraq.

Terminology

Chemical agents are synthetic chemicals produced to be used in wars. Chemical weapons are agents that are ready to use, in ammunition, bombs, rockets, and other delivery systems. From the medical–toxicological point of view, the most common classification of chemical agents relates to the organ or tissue that is mainly involved (Table 1). Inconsistencies are included; for example, cyanide is classified as blood agent, although there is no specific effect on the blood or blood constituents.

Several countries use their own symbols for classification. The U.S. Department of Defense codes are commonly used also in other Western countries and are given in Table 1. During WWI, color codes on ammunition were used in Germany—a white cross for eye irritants, blue cross for sternutators, green cross for choking agents, and yellow cross for corrosives (i.e., vesicants).

The use of precursors, which are mixed to produce the parent agent in the casing only during delivery, allows a safer handling of chemical agents for the user. Binary (two-precursor) delivery systems were described for the nerve agents sarin and VX. Precursor systems may simplify unstable agent use and complicate disarmament controls.

The agents presented here were chosen with respect to the military threat, demilitarization and disarmament control, destruction of improperly disposed of old agents, and hazards as peace-time irritant use for self-defence and riot control.

During the U.S. Chemical Disarmament Program, great efforts were made to increase the knowledge of chemical agent toxicology in order to establish safety standards for their destruction (Table 2).

Cyanides are broadly used industrial chemicals. Their very rapid action and very short persistence, making incapacitating protective gear unnecessary for

TABLE 2 Control Limits (mg/m^3) for Chemical Agents

Agent	General population	Workers	Maximum allowable stack concentration
GA, GB	0.000003	0.0001	0.0003
VX	0.000003	0.00001	0.0003
H, HD, HT	0.0001	0.003	0.03
L	0.003	0.003	0.03
Averaging time	72 hours	8 hours	—

the assailant, make them of interest for an aggressor. The usual aerosol-charcoal filters are not effective against cyanides; a special impregnation is necessary. However, the toxicity of cyanides is much lower compared to nerve agents after inhalation, decreasing their military importance. The toxicology, mechanism of action, and treatment of poisoning are described elsewhere (Gases). Prophylactics and/or drugs for immediate treatment would be most useful against cyanide in the field because of the fast onset of toxic effects. Prophylactics based on methemoglobin-forming antimalarials are under investigation, but they are not available; antidotes for self-administration or use on others are also not available.

Phosgene and analogs were responsible for about 80% of chemical-agent-caused deaths during WWI. Phosgene and analogs are common industrial chemicals that cause lung edema by alveolar damage, similar to other respiratory irritants. Similarly acting compounds have been discussed because of the increased penetration of activated charcoal filter by the combustion of polyfluorinated hydrocarbons (i.e., perfluoroisobutene and analogs).

In 1996 the use of psychotropic agents was reported in Bosnia. The intended effects are central nervous system (CNS) incapacitation, leading to impairment of memory, concentration ability, and performance. The most important representatives of these agents are the central anticholinergic 3-quinuclidinylbenzilate (BZ) and the sympathomimetic and 5-HT_2 agonist lysergic acid diethylamide (LSD).

Other chemicals, such as herbicides, were also used in wars. Compounds as 2,4-dichlorophenoxyacetic acid (2,4-D), 2,4,5-trichlorophenoxyacetic acid (2,4,5-T), picloram, and cacodylic acid are common herbicides with broad nonmilitary uses. A special toxicological problem appeared in Vietnam because of the contamination of phenoxyacetic acid herbicides with dioxins during production.

Physicochemical Properties

The important chemical agents are mostly liquids. The highest toxicity is reached by vapor or aerosol inhalation, but being highly lipophilic, they may penetrate the skin very well, where metabolism influences penetration.

The persistence of chemical agents in the target area varies from hours to days, depending on their physicochemical properties and the climatic and environmental conditions (Table 3). Contaminated living and nonliving matter may become a source of secondary contamination. Main parameters influencing persistence are evaporation and hydrolysis.

Buried or sunken chemical agents are much less prone to evaporation or hydrolysis and may remain active for decades. Skin damage was reported in fishermen who caught rotten sulfur-mustard casings from WWII with their nets in prohibited areas in the Baltic Sea.

Principles of Protection

Prevention of exposure, immediate decontamination, prophylactic medical measures, and the timely use of antidotes, with basic and advanced life support, are the mainstays of protection and therapy.

Physical Protection

A protective mask with an appropriate filter, an impermeable rubber, plastic, or semipermeable charcoal-impregnated overgarment with impermeable boots and gloves protect from exposure for a limited time. Collective protection using a filtered air supply is necessary for longer periods.

Decontamination

For exposure of limited skin areas, dry decontaminants containing only adsorbents (e.g., fuller's earth) or including hypochlorite (e.g., Dutch powder con-

TABLE 3 Persistence of Chemical Agents

Agent	Environmental conditions		
	Sunny, light breeze, 15°C	Wind and rain, 10°C	Calm, snow on the ground, −10°C
HD	2–7 days	0.5–2 days	2–8 weeks
GA	1–4 days	0.5–6 hours	1–14 days
GB	0.25–4 hours	0.25–1 hours	1–2 days
GD	2.5–5 days	3–36 hours	1–6 weeks
VX	3–21 days	1–12 hours	1–16 weeks

taining magnesium oxide and calcium hypochlorite) are very useful. The application of household flour followed by wiping with wet tissue paper also showed good decontamination properties.

Adsorbents are not to be used on the mucous membranes (e.g., eyes) or wounds, as they will not be absorbed and may cause granulomas. Concentrated hypochlorite is a strong irritant and may cause damage to the mucous membranes and eyes. Contaminated clothing should be removed. For decontamination of the eyes, tap water or low-strength alkaline solutions (2–5% $NaHCO_3$) can be used. Wounds and other mucous surfaces can be irrigated with low-strength calcium hypochlorite (1–2%) solution. It must not be used in the cavities (cranial, thoracic, abdominal); there isotonic neutral solutions such as sterile 0.9% NaCl are more appropriate.

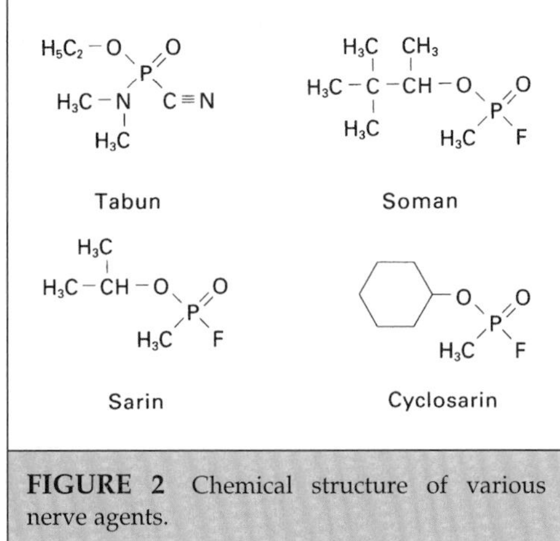

FIGURE 2 Chemical structure of various nerve agents.

Organophosphorus Compounds

The general formula for organic phosphorous anticholinesterases was first given by G. Schrader (in 1952) (Fig. 1). Tabun, sarin, cyclosarin, soman, and VX are the most significant agents of military interest (Table 1, Figs. 2–3).

As technical products, they may have a (weak) distinct odor, which becomes negligible at high purity. The agents are liquids of increasing viscosity, from that of gasoline to that of heavy diesel oil (Table 4).

Several other highly toxic anticholinesterases were classified as possible nerve agents (i.e., 2-dialkylaminoalkyl-(dialkylamido)-fluoro-phosphates (G-compounds) and bis quaternary carbamates). The development of new V-type agents with the code name "novichok" (newcomer) in Russia has been discussed in public domain; however, chemical structures have not been published. None of these agents is known to have been used as a weapon.

Toxicity, Toxicokinetics, and Metabolism

Nerve agents, being very lipophilic, can enter the circulation very rapidly by inhalation, ingestion, and percutaneous absorption, showing a rapid penetration into the CNS.

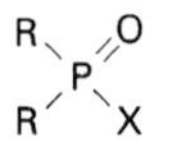

R = Alkyl-, Alkoxy-, Dialkylamidogroup

X = Halogen, Cyanide, Thiocyanate, Alkyl/Aryl-Oxy, Alkyl-/Aryl-Thio, Pyrophosphates, Quaternary Ammonium Compounds

FIGURE 1 General formula of organophosphorus anticholinesterases, according to Schrader (1952).

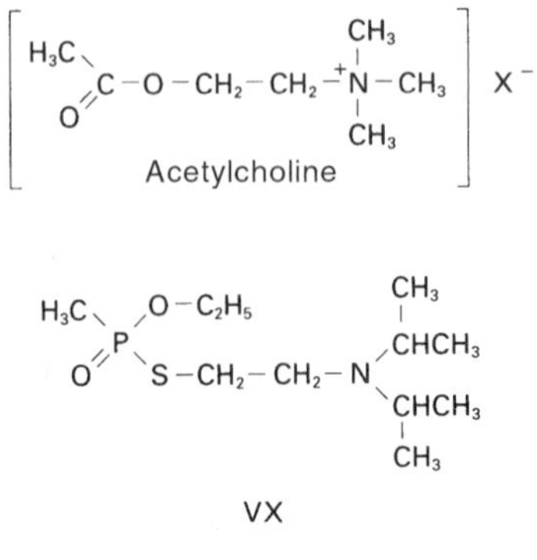

Organic phosphorus compounds hydrolyze spontaneously in plasma and other aqueous solutions. Enzymatic hydrolysis occurs via α-esterases and phosphoryl phosphatases. Binding to β-esterases as carboxylesterases and cholinesterases, the latter being also the target of toxicity, contributes also to its elimination. Structural asymmetries are common in organophosphorus compounds. The isomers may exhibit different biological activities, degradation velocities and patterns, and responses to antidote treatment. Experiments with anesthetized atropinized rats and guinea pigs show a very rapid degradation of P(+) sarin or soman isomers after iv injection, mostly due to enzymatic hydrolysis. The much more toxic P(−) isomers were relatively stable and could be measured in the circulation for at least 1 hour. The elimination

Acetylcholine

VX

FIGURE 3 Chemical structure of acetylcholine and VX.

TABLE 4 Physicochemical Properties of Several Chemical Agents

Physicochemical property	GA	GB	GF	GD	VX	HD	HT	HN-3	L	DA	DC	DM	CN	CS
Molecular weight	162.3	140.1	180.1	182.2	267.4	159.1	263.2	204.5	207.35	264.5	255	277.57	154.6	188.5
Specific gravity (g/cm^3; 25°C)	1.073	1.089	1.133 (20°C)	1.022	1.008	1.27 (20°C)	1.23 (20°C)	1.23 (20°C)	1.89 (20°C)	1.42 (20°C)	1.45 (20°C)	1.65 (20°C)	1.32 (20°C)	—
Boiling point (°C; 760 mm Hg)	246	147.3	—	167	298	228.8	174 (2 mm Hg)	230–235	190	307	290	410	245	310–315
Melting point (°C)	−48	−56	−12	−80	−39	14.4	32	−4	−14.4	44	30	19.5	59	94
Vapor pressure (mm Hg; 25°C)	0.073	2.9	0.068	0.3	0.0007	0.07 (20°C)	—	0.011	0.394	1.6×10^{-5} (20°C)	4.7×10^{-5} (20°C)	2×10^{-15} (20°C)	5.4×10^{-5} (20°C)	3.4×10^{-5} (20°C)
Volatility (mg/liter; 20°C)	0.6	11.3	0.66	3–10	0.01	0.625	0.002	0.07	2.3	7.2 (mg/m^3)	2.79 (mg/m^3)	0.02 (mg/m^3)	105	0.31–0.7
Water solubility (g/liter, 20°C)	72	Not limited	—	15 (25°C)	30 (25°C)	0.8	Not soluble	0.2–0.5	0.5	0.2%	0.2%	Not soluble	0.1–0.5	Almost insoluble
Hydrolysis ($t_{1/2}$; 20°C; h)	8.5 (pH 7)	46 (pH 7.5)	—	Slower than GB	428 (pH 7.5)	8.5 (25°C)	—	Very slow	Very rapid	Rapid	Slow	Rapid	Almost none	12 min (25°C)

of the P(−) isomers was mostly related to covalent binding to β-esterases.

Although experiments with ^{3}H sarin and soman in mice and rabbits show relatively a high accumulation of radioactivity in the lung, only 3% were found in exhaled air. Free ^{3}H-isopropylmethylphosphonic acid or ^{3}H-pinacolylmethylphosphonic acid were identified as the main metabolites in the urine of mice treated with ^{3}H-labeled sarin or soman, respectively. In contrast to sarin, very little degradation of VX occurs in the skin. Data on toxicity of various nerve agents are given in Table 5.

Mechanism of Action

Nerve agents inhibit acetylcholinesterase (AChE), causing acetylcholine (ACh) accumulation with uncontrolled stimulation and functional impairment of cholinergically innervated tissues and organs, and death of the organism (Table 6).

Hypothermia, decrease in motor performance, and dopamine increase in the brain were observed at sublethal soman doses in mice. The reversal by atropine, methylatropine, or the oximes HI 6 or HLö-7 indicates a cholinergic origin for the effect. Seizures with subsequent morphological brain damage may be ameliorated by antimuscarinics, GABA, and NMDA antagonists, also indicating a primary cholinergic (muscarinic) involvement, with consequent loss of inhibitory control and subsequent recruitment of other excitatory transmitter systems, sustaining convulsions and producing brain damage. Cardiac toxicity and necroses of the skeletal muscles by organophosphorus compounds are presumably also due to AChE inhibition.

Neuropathy target esterase (NTE) -inhibition may lead to organophosphate-induced delayed polyneuropathy (OPIDN), but more than 10 times the lethal dose is necessary for the inhibition of the enzyme by nerve agents. The interference of anticholinesterases in the formation or degradation of biologically active peptides is described, but the contribution to the toxicity is unclear.

Signs of Poisoning

In general, the effects of nerve agents and the related pesticides are similar. Contact with a nerve agent first causes local effects, but soon signs of systemic toxicity follow. At very low concentrations or amounts, local effects (i.e., eyes, lung, skin, or gut) can predominate. The clinical symptoms are mainly governed by signs of peripheral muscarinic hyperstimulation. Death occurs mostly by asphyxiation, central respiratory depression, inhibited neuromuscular transmission with the impairment of respiratory muscles, or bronchorrhea and bronchoconstriction (Table 6). Cardiocirculatory parameters remain

TABLE 5 Toxicity of Nerve Agents

Parameter	GA	GB	GD	VX
LD_{50} iv (mg/kg)	0.31	0.1	0.064	0.014
Mouse				
Rat	0.07	0.045	0.05	0.008
LD_{50} oral (mg/kg)				
Rat	3.7	1.06	0.4	0.1
Human (estimate)	5	0.14	0.14	0.07
LD_{50} percutaneous (mg/kg)				
Rat	12.6	2.5	14.3	0.1
Human (estimate)	14–21	24	15	0.04
LCt_{50} inhalative (mg × min/m^3)[a]				
Mouse	—	240	—	40
Rat	450	220	—	—
Human (estimate)	200–400	100	70	36
Minimal effective concentrations (mg × min/m^3), human				
Miosis (vapor)	0.9	2–4	0.5	0.5
Tremor	—	4	—	1.6
No effect	—	0.5	0.3	0.02

[a] LCt_{50} indicates concentration time product causing 50% lethality.

TABLE 6 Pathophysiology and Clinical Appearance of Nerve Agent Poisoning

Target receptor, organ, tissue	Signs and symptoms
Central nervous system	
Respiration	Decreased respiratory frequency and tidal volume, cyanosis, dyspnea, central respiratory paralysis
Circulation	Transient initial hypertension, hypotension
Activity	Restlessness, tremor, ataxia, weakness, tonic–clonic convulsions
Behavior	Anxiety, giddiness, emotional lability, nightmares, insomnia, failure to concentrate, confusion
Perpipheral nervous system	
Muscarinic	
Eye	
+ Smooth muscle	
Iris	Miosis, impaired vision at twilight
Ciliary muscle	Failure of accommodation, frontal headache
+ Exocrine glands	Lacrimation (severe exposure)
Respiratory tract	
+ Smooth muscles	Bronchoconstriction, chest tightness, dyspnea
+ Exocrine glands	Rhinorrhea, salivation, bronchorrhea, dyspnea
Gastrointestinal tract	
+ Smooth muscles/exocrine glands	Nausea, vomiting, abdominal cramps, diarrhea, involuntary defecation
Urinary tract	
+ Smooth muscle	Increased micturition frequency, involuntary micturition
Heart	Bradycardia
Skin	
+ Exocrine glands	Sweating
Nicotinic	
Skeletal muscles	Weakness, fasciculation, weakness of respiratory muscles, dyspnea, cyanosis, peripheral respiratory paralysis
Autonomic ganglia	Pallor, initial transient hypertension and tachycardia

mostly stable up to the terminal state with severe hypoxia, but at lower doses and a protracted course of poisoning, circulatory depression may complicate the respiratory impairment.

Laboratory Findings

Acetylcholinesterase (AChE; erythrocyte cholinesterase) or butyrylcholinesterase (BuChE; plasma cholinesterase) activity can be used for diagnostic purposes. AChE activity is thought to reflect the central and peripheral synaptic enzyme more accurately. The therapeutic effect of atropine and adaptive receptor changes will not be reflected by these enzymes. The recovery of AChE is very slow, 1% per day by *de novo* synthesis. BuChE synthesis in the liver is much faster, the recovery of plasma activity being complete after 1 to 3 weeks. An increase in BuChE activity indicates the absence of toxicologically relevant concentrations of the agent in the blood.

A 15–20% increase in BuChE activity during 3–5 days indicates past exposure. It should be confirmed by regular measurements of the enzyme to assess baseline values. Employees with less than 75% of the baseline activity should not be allowed to work with anticholinesterases.

Late Effects

Severe organophosphorus anticholinesterase poisoning may cause long-term neuropsychopathological changes: impaired vigilance, reduced concentration, reduced information processing and psychomotor speed, memory deficit, speech disorders, depression, anxiety, and irritability. In contrast, the available data do not indicate that asymptomatic (low-dose) exposure is connected with an increased risk of delayed or permanent neuropsychopathological changes. Some very subtle EEG changes observed in monkeys 1 year after asymptomatic sarin exposure were without any clinical correlate.

A muscular weakness and paralysis syndrome affecting the neck and respiratory muscles (intermediate syndrome) was described, which may lead to respira-

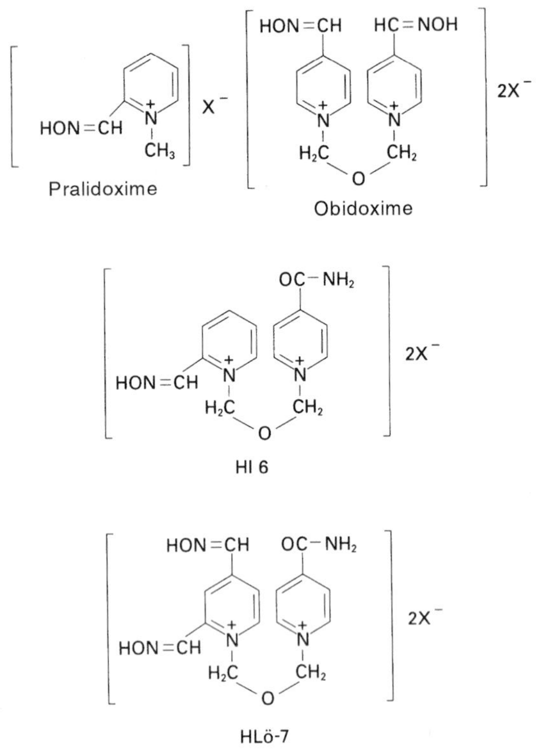

Pralidoxime

Obidoxime

HI 6

HLö-7

FIGURE 4 Chemical structure of various oximes.

tory muscle paralysis. It is probably due to protracted AChE inhibition, which may lead to muscular necrosis due to inadequate treatment of the acute phase of poisoning (e.g., inadequate amounts and times of administration of the oxime and inadequately assisted ventilation). In dogs (beagles), a syndrome similar to the intermediate syndrome, with weakness of the neck muscles so that the dogs were unable to lift their heads, but without the respiratory paralysis, was reported after soman poisoning (5 LD_{50}).

Special Toxicology

There is no evidence for the mutagenicity of sarin, soman, and VX *in vitro* and *in vivo.* Weak mutagenicity was reported for tabun. No evidence was found for teratogenicity or carcinogenicity of nerve agents, including tabun.

Therapeutic Measures

Atropine

Atropine is a competitive antagonist of acetylcholine at the muscarinic receptors. Central respiratory depression, hypersecretion, increased activity of smooth muscles, bradycardia, and other muscarinic signs will be ameliorated. Nicotinic signs, such as fasciculations of the striated muscles and neuromuscular block, will not respond. Seizures will initially respond, but later the addition of GABA agonists become necessary.

Repeated doses of 2 mg iv, or in cases with marked respiratory depression 4–6 mg iv (children 0.015–0.05 mg/kg), with tight control of muscarinic signs are necessary (*in vivo* titration of the effect, mainly secretions). Miosis may not reflect the degree of muscarinic stimulation in the body because of local absorption of the agent into the eye. Pulse frequency should not exceed 90–100 bpm to prevent arrhythmia. Overatropinization may cause heat stress, constipation, bladder dysfunction, ileus, and worsen the outcome, as observed in severe insecticide poisoning.

Massive atropine doses, as have been reported to be necessary in "mega-dose" oral suicidal insecticide poisoning, are presumably not realistic for the scenario of a nerve agent in the field. A cumulative dose of 10–20 mg over the first 2–3 hours was proposed to be sufficient.

Oximes

Several pralidoxime salts and obidoxime are approved for the treatment of organophosphorus compound poisoning in most countries. HI 6 and HLö 7 are the most effective newer oximes developed by I. Hagedorn ("H"-oximes) to improve soman-poisoning treatment (Fig. 4).

Oximes act by binding to the phosphyl moiety of the agent at the enzyme. The bimolecular reaction results in the formation of a phosphyl–enzyme–oxime complex, similar to the Michaelis complex. The second step is the splitting of the complex to give free enzyme and phosphyloxime (i.e., the reactivation process) (Fig. 5). It follows first-order kinetics and can be quantified using the half-life.

The optimal "therapeutic" oxime concentration, frequently and uncritically adopted from Sundwall (1961) as 4 μg/ml, irrespective of oxime, agent type, and species, should be dismissed, as it varies due to these parameters. In general, obidoxime is a fast and effective reactivator in concentrations of 10–30 μmol/liter for AChE inhibited by most pesticides, sarin, and cyclosarin, and more effective than HI 6 and pralidoxime for the reactivation of tabun-inhibited AChE. HI 6, 30 μmol/liter, shows a higher efficacy for sarin-, soman-, cyclosarin-, and VX-inhibited enzyme, compared to obidoxime and pralidoxime, although obidoxime was also rather effective with VX. In all cases, pralidoxime showed a low efficacy, indicating that high doses are necessary to achieve an effect.

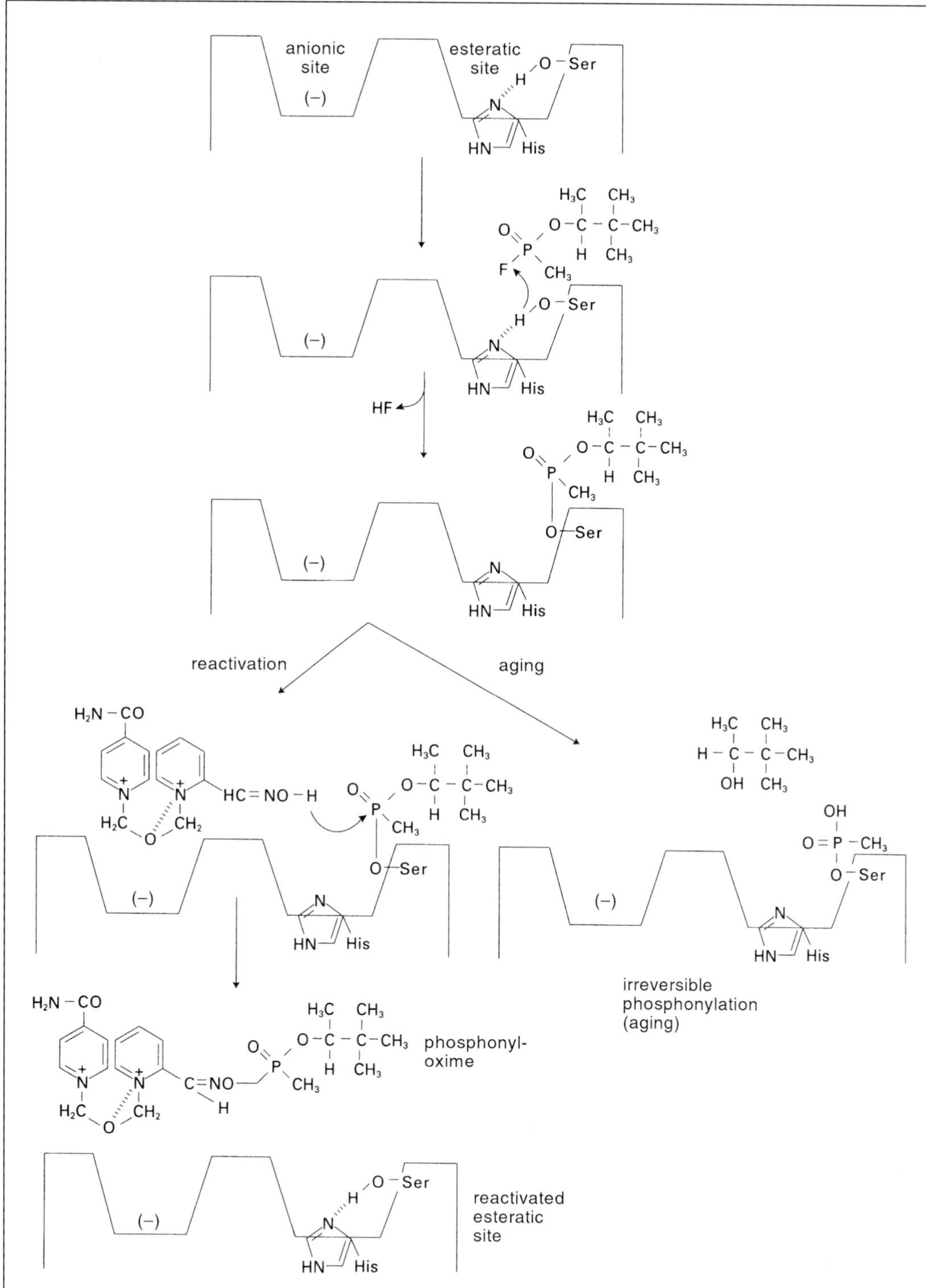

FIGURE 5 Steps of acetylcholinesterase (AChE) inhibition by soman, reactivation of the enzyme by HI 6, and aging of the enzyme-soman complex. Soman binds to the OH group of serine at the esteratic site of AChE, as other organophosphorus and carbamate anticholinesterases. The soman-AChE complex "ages" rapidly in human tissues (half-life 2 min), by losing the alkyl moiety of the agent (right branch). The inhibition becomes completely irreversible, and can not be split by oximes as HI 6. In the unaged complex, the phosphorus of the agent is prone to the nucleophilic attack by an oxime (HI 6). A phosphonyloxime is formed and split off, leaving the regenerated enzyme (left branch).

Oxime efficacy may be limited by the aging of the AChE-agent complex and reinhibition of AChE by a persisting agent, and by phosphyloximes. The half-life is 2 min for soman in human AChE, 5 hours for sarin, 48 hours for VX and 13 hours for tabun. Phosphylated 4-pyridinium aldoximes are much more stable and thereby more relevant inhibitors compared to the 2-oxime analogs.

Oximes, being polar quaternary ammonium compounds, act mainly peripherally by the improvement of respiratory muscle function due to the improvement of neuromuscular transmission. Although barely effective themselves in organophosphorus-compound poisoning, they may markedly potentiate the therapeutic effect of atropine.

Other Measures

Artificial respiration is necessary in severe cases. Diazepam im or iv is used to prevent neurotoxicity and to control seizures, although the improvement of survival is doubtful. For full efficacy it has to be used early.

Pretreatment

Pyridostigmine, a carbamate, inhibits AChE reversibly and prevents phosphylation by nerve agents. After the agent and pyridostigmine are eliminated, the carbamylated enzyme will become free for its physiologic function by spontaneous decarbamylation. The half-life of pyridostigmine in human plasma *in vivo* after oral intake is about 4 hours and the half-life of the spontaneous reactivation of human erythrocyte dimethylcarbamyl-AChE is about 30 min. Initially, the two anti-ChE compounds would increase AChE inhibition concurrently, and aggravate or precipitate symptoms. The charged pyridostigmine molecule acts mainly peripherally to improve neuromuscular transmission. Pretreated nerve-agent poisoning always needs atropine and oxime treatment. Pyridostigmine pretreatment is recommended only in the case of soman threat, as no improvement of the therapeutic effect of atropine and oxime treatment by the carbamate could be shown in sarin and VX poisoning in several animal experiments. Decarbamylation rates will be slightly decreased by pralidoxime, increased by HI 6, and remain unchanged by obidoxime. The direct effects of pyridostigmine and physostigmine at the striated muscle nicotinic receptor were also shown, but not after usual pretreatment doses.

The administration of 30 mg pyridostigmine every 8 hours orally is recommended to maintain AChE activity at 60–80% of control. No serious acute impairment is to be expected at this dose, only a slight peripheral cholinergic stimulation. No late or chronic effects of pyridostigmine are known, although it is used in the long term in much higher doses for the treatment of myasthenia gravis.

Physostigmine, a centrally acting carbamate anticholinesterase, was shown to be more effective than pyridostigmine in preventing incapacitation and mortality by the nerve agents soman and sarin. It is mostly used in combination with an anticholinergic drug such as scopolamine or aprophen to prevent carbamate side effects. Scavaging enzymes also belong to the experimental prophylactic measures against nerve agents.

Alkylating Agents

Of the highest military significance is bis(2-chloroethyl)sulfide (Fig. 6), with the symbol H for the compound synthesized by the Levinstein process and HD for the *d*istilled product. It is also called mustard gas for the odor of the first technical product, yperite (in France and Russia) for the place of the first military use in WWI (in Ypres, Belgium, July 11, 1917), and lost (in Germany) for the chemists who investigated the use of the compound, *Lo*mmel and *St*einkopf. A nitrogen analog, tris(2-chloroethyl)amine (HN-3) was stockpiled by the German army during WWII.

Mixtures of HD with the similarly acting bis(2-chloroethyl-thioethyl)ether (HT) (Fig. 6) and with the organoarsenic compound Lewisite are known. The odor of sulfur mustard resembles mustard, garlic, rotten cabbage, and/or sulfur compounds.

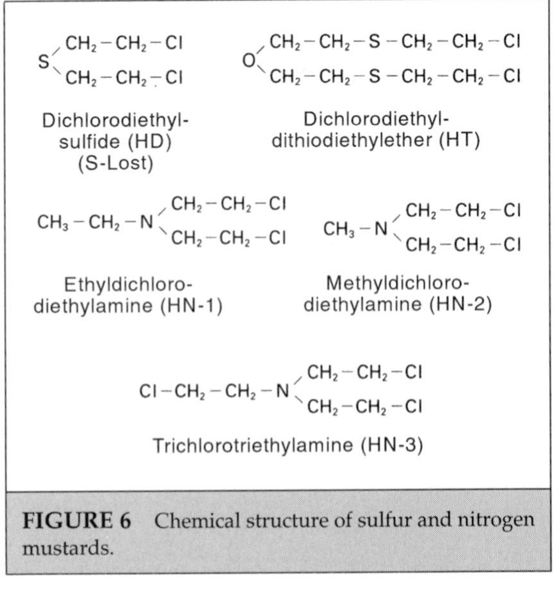

$S(CH_2-CH_2-Cl)_2$
Dichlorodiethylsulfide (HD) (S-Lost)

$O(CH_2-CH_2-S-CH_2-CH_2-Cl)_2$
Dichlorodiethyldithiodiethylether (HT)

$CH_3-CH_2-N(CH_2-CH_2-Cl)_2$
Ethyldichlorodiethylamine (HN-1)

$CH_3-N(CH_2-CH_2-Cl)_2$
Methyldichlorodiethylamine (HN-2)

$Cl-CH_2-CH_2-N(CH_2-CH_2-Cl)_2$
Trichlorotriethylamine (HN-3)

FIGURE 6 Chemical structure of sulfur and nitrogen mustards.

Nitrogen mustards may have a fishy odor. The physicochemical properties of the relevant agents are given in Table 4.

Toxicity, Toxicokinetics, and Metabolism

Mustards are very lipophilic and reactive agents with a pronounced local damaging capacity and high systemic toxicity. The data are summarized in Table 7.

Nitrogen or sulfur mustard will disappear within few minutes from the circulation. In aqueous solutions, sulfur mustard is rapidly hydrolyzed to semimustard and thiodiglycol. Somewhat in contrast, sulfur mustard was found in several tissues of an Iranian patient who died several days after exposure, with highest concentrations in the brain and fat tissue. About 70% of the radioactivity from ^{35}S-labeled sulfur mustard injected iv in mice and rats was excreted in the urine within 12 hours (about 80% at 24 hours). In contrast, only 17% was excreted in humans in the same period (22% at 24 hours) and the major portion was retained for very long time in the body. Essentially, the metabolites found in the urine of rodents and humans imply a similar metabolism, that is, the formation of glutathione and cysteine conjugates and their decomposition products. No radioactivity was found in exhaled air or the feces.

After administration, 80% of a liquid sulfur mustard drop will evaporate, 2% will be fixed in the skin for a long period, and the remaining 18% will reach the circulation. In rabbits 80% of inhaled sulfur mustard and 90% of nitrogen mustard will be removed by the nasal mucosa.

Mechanism of Action

In aqueous solutions the 2-chloroethyl side chains of mechlorethamine undergo a first-order (S_N1) molecular cyclization to form the highly reactive ethyleneiminium intermediate under the liberation of chlorine. The intermediate can react avidly through formation of a carbonium ion, or a transition complex intermediate, with a broad variety of organic radicals or inorganic ions with phosphate, amino, sulfhydryl, hydroxyl, carboxyl, and imidazole groups, by reactions resembling a second-order (S_N2) nucleophilic substitution. Most favored are reactions with the nucleic acids in DNA, mainly the 7 nitrogen in guanine. Both chloroethyl groups may react, causing cross-linking of the nucleic acids to other nucleophiles. The sensitivity towards mustards increases with the proliferation fidelity of the cell type, where the efficiency of the cell DNA-repair system appears to be decisive. Sulfur mustard reacts in analogy, forming a cyclic ethylenesulfonium ion intermediate (Fig. 7). The reaction with nucleophiles appears to be faster, compared

TABLE 7 Toxicity of Alkylating Agents

Parameter	HD	HT	HN-3
LD_{50} iv (mg/kg)			
Mouse	3.3	—	0.7
LD_{50} oral (mg/kg)			
Rat	17	—	—
Human (estimate)	—	—	2
LD_{50} percutaneous (mg/kg)			
Rat	9–18	—	4.9
Human (estimate)	40–60	—	15
LCt_{50} inhalative (mg × min/m^3)[a]			
Mouse	860–1320	820–1100	—
Rat	800–1512	—	—
Human (estimate)	1500	—	400
Minimal effective doses, human			
Erythema (mg/cm^2)	0.01	—	0.001
Blistering (mg/cm^2)	0.1–0.15	—	0.1
Conjunctivitis (mg/l)	0.0012 (30 min)	—	0.0007 (15 min)
No effect (mg × min/m^3)	2	—	—

[a]LCt_{50} indicates concentration time product causing 50% lethality.

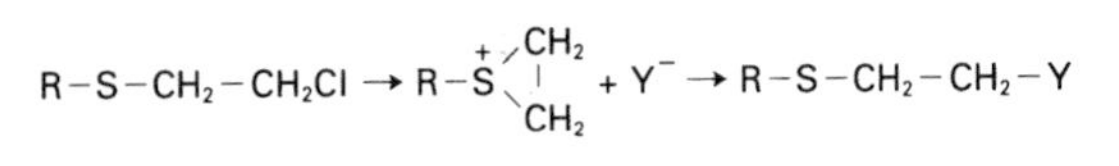

$$R-S-CH_2-CH_2Cl \rightarrow R-\overset{+}{S}\langle^{CH_2}_{CH_2} + Y^- \rightarrow R-S-CH_2-CH_2-Y$$

FIGURE 7 Alkylation of nucleophilic groups (Y) by sulfur mustard.

to the nitrogen mustards. Mechlorethamine may actively enter cells using the choline uptake system.

Extensive research on the mechanism of vesication led to the "Papirmeister Hypothesis" of cell damage by mustards. The repair of DNA activates the chromosomal enzyme poly(adenosine diphosphate ribose)polymerase, causing the depletion of its substrate nicotinamide adenine dinucleotide (NAD), which results in glycolysis inhibition, energy metabolism impairment, hexose monophosphate shunt activation, protease release, and finally cell death.

Also, glutathione depletion by mustard and subsequent alkylation of critical sulfhydryl groups in Ca^{2+} adenosine triphosphatase may prevent Ca^{2+} extrusion from the cell. Intracellular Ca^{2+} accumulation, causing membrane damage, could result. Some effects of mustards are attributed to central nervous cholinergic stimulation, such as nausea and vomiting.

Signs of Poisoning

The course and signs of poisoning by sulfur mustard and the nitrogen analogs are very similar. In contrast to earlier reports (from WWI), the Iranian victims from GWI reported at exposure, in addition to the garlic odor, a pungent sensation, and burning and pain in the eyes and throat, which may be explained by the short distance to the target area and dust formation due to the explosion. It is unclear whether synthesis by-products may have contributed to this. Although the "biochemical lesion" occurs within minutes, hours or even days may elapse before the first symptoms develop. In general, the symptoms develop slowly with little initial sequelae and need several days to reach the maximum. Immunosuppression with increased susceptibility to infection and delayed healing are also characteristic features.

Skin

Hours after exposure itching, erythema and, subsequently blisters with initially little pain develop. Open blisters and uncovered necrotic areas become very painful. Erythematous areas become dark livid-brownish after about two weeks and finally a dark-brown pigmentation remains in the area for years. Deeper ulceration leaves mostly unpigmented flat scars. The coincidence of unpigmented, tanned, and unaffected skin may give a "geographic map" appearance to the affected area. The classification of the injury as erythematous, superficial bullous, deep bullous, and ulcerative remains only a local description, as all these stages can coincide, one next to the other. Late vesication is a typical feature and can appear several weeks after mustard exposure. The fluid of early and late blisters is free of the active agent.

The sensitivity of the skin increases with the density of the sweat and sebaceous glands, as well as the thickness and moisture content of the skin's horny layer. Increased friction by movement and free room for vapor accumulation from contaminated clothing may further aggravate the damage, as in the arm pits and genital area. Early tanning, especially pronounced in stronger pigmented people such as the Iranian victims, with superficial epidermolysis can also occur.

Eyes

The mucous membranes are much more prone to damage by mustard compared to the skin. Without protection, the eyes are almost always involved. In general, one to several hours after vapor exposure, grittiness, photophobia, erythema, lacrimation, and blepharospasm develop. After more severe exposure, conjunctivitis, initially serous and later suppurative, corneal opacity, and ulceration occur. Visual impairment by blepharospasm and corneal opacity are generally reversible. Liquid exposure may cause symptoms within minutes, with extensive tissue damage and irreversible loss of vision.

Respiratory System

Following a sign-free period, early symptoms include sneezing, painful coughing, discharge of mucus from nose and throat with increasing irritation, and loss of sense of smell and taste. More severe exposure results in pharyngitis, laryngitis, aphonia, dysphagia, difficulty in swallowing, and bronchitis.

A pseudomembrane from secretions and debris can appear in the larynx and the bronchi, with loosening of casts after days and acute obstruction of the airways, leading to a lethal outcome. Severe exposure causes ulceration in the pharynx and larynx and bronchial necroses, leading to secondary bronchopneumonia. Lung edema is not a characteristic feature of mustard poisoning.

Gastrointestinal Tract

During the first hours after exposure, nausea, vomiting, and epigastric distress develop. After 1 to 3 days diarrhea with water, electrolyte, and occasionally blood loss can occur.

Systemic Poisoning

Symptoms known from cancer patients receiving irradiation or chemotherapy are caused by nitrogen and sulfur mustards (radiomimetic effects). Anorexia, recurrent nausea, vomiting, epigastric distress, lassitude, and depression are typical for low doses. Higher doses may cause, in addition, general malaise, diarrhea, hemoconcentration, fever, headache, cachexia, bone marrow depression with progressive leucopenia, hyperexcitability, convulsions, and death.

Laboratory Findings

Thiodiglycol, cysteine, and glutathione adducts may be found in the urine. The common early leukocytosis and fever should not be uncritically misdiagnosed as a sign of infection. Later, related to the turnover rate of the respective cell types, leukopenia, thrombopenia, and finally also reduced red cell count can be observed.

Late Effects

Superficial skin damage needs weeks and deep lesions several months to heal. About 100,000 chemical casualties were reported in Iran during GWI, where 10% died soon after exposure. From 30,000 surveyed cases 55% showed some degree of disability. Of all symptomatic individuals, 78% suffer from respiratory symptoms, that is, asthmatic bronchitis (9.5%), chronic suppurative bronchitis with bronchiectasis (80.8%), major airway obstruction due to granulation formation (4.8%), and nonpulmonary respiratory impairment (5%). Of GWI victims surveyed by Balali, 70% suffered from complications of the airways (mostly chronic asthmoid bronchitis), 41% of the skin (mostly abnormal pigmentation in affected skin areas), 36% of the eyes (mostly chronic conjunctivitis), and 45% suffered from neurotic disturbances such as depression and personality changes. Essentially, these late complications resembled the findings from WWI. Chronic gastritis and late neurotic disturbances may occur. Some cases with recurrent conjunctivitis and ulceration of the cornea or persistant ulceration of the skin over more than 10 years were also reported. Hypersensitivity to sulfur mustard is also known.

Special Toxicology

Sulfur mustard is considered by the U.S. Department of Health to be a mutagen and human carcinogen, although less potent than tobacco, radon, and chromates. Interestingly, the proof for sulfur mustard as animal carcinogen could not be settled.

In British veterans from WWI exposed to sulfur mustard, a similar frequency of bronchial cancer was observed in the exposure and nonexposure chronic bronchitis group, which was twice as high as the amputee group (no exposure, no chronic bronchitis). A similar conclusion was drawn in a study on American veterans from WWI.

More stringent evidence for human carcinogenicity comes from tracing the workers in factories producing sulfur mustard. An increased frequency of laryngeal carcinoma in a British factory (7 observed/0.75 expected), bronchial carcinoma in a German factory (11/5), and in a Japanese factory (Okunojima)(33/0.9) was reported. The occurrence of Bowens disease, intraepidermal squamous cell carcinoma, and basalioma was also reported in workers from Okunojima factory and in workers exposed during the closure of a former poison gas plant in Germany (Heeresmunitionsanstalt St. Georgen).

An increased leukemia frequency by adjuvant chemotherapy with nitrogen mustards was shown. An increased frequency of squamous cell carcinoma and basalioma of the skin after local treatment of mycosis fungoides and T-cell lymphoma is known.

With nitrogen mustards, teratogenicity, embryotoxicity, and fetotoxicity were observed after doses not toxic to the mothers. In contrast, several studies in mice, rats, and rabbits with sulfur mustard showed teratogenicity only at doses toxic to the mothers. No abnormal findings were reported in the descendants of the Okunojima chemical-agent factory. In contrast, more female births were reported in the former workers of a German chemical-agent plant, where also abnormal spermiogenesis and damaged sperm were found, attributed to sex-linked fetal mutations with a higher mortality in male fetuses. It should be noted that in this factory sulfur and nitrogen mustard (HN-3) were produced.

Therapeutic Approach

Antidotes

Sodium thiosulfate binds active mustard mainly in the extracellular space. A high dose iv is necessary (500 mg/kg), its efficacy being limited to the very short period of mustard persistence in the blood. The charged molecule penetrates the membranes only poorly and thereby iv administration will not influence local lesions. Local use of dimercaprol (BAL) (e.g., for the prevention of mustard-Lewisite damage) may be effective if applied early, but increases the sensitization against BAL.

Other Measures

Cooling bland lotions (e.g., calamine) can relieve itching. Antihistamines and analgesics should be given systemically. Damaged skin areas should be irrigated and dressed under sterile conditions, using sterile Vaseline gauze to prevent sticking. Sulfasalazine cream was used when there was evidence of infection. Eyes should also be irrigated and sterile Vaseline used to prevent the eyelids from sticking. Mydriatics containing eye drops (e.g., homatropine) can be used to prevent the sticking of the iris to the lens and to relieve iris spasm. The local use of antimicrobial eye drops becomes necessary. Dark glasses alleviate photophobia. Cough suppression using codeine is necessary. Inhaled air should be moistened. Regular inspection of the airways and bronchial lavage help to prevent obstruction by pseudomembrane casts. Diarrhea may generate the need for electrolyte and water substitution.

Organic Arsenicals

Chemical agents include only trivalent arsenicals, which may have one or two reactive groups, mostly substituted with a halogen (Figs. 8 and 14). Both types react with thiol. The bireactive arsenicals are mainly attracted by vicinal sulfhydryl groups to form stable ring structures, causing more instant inhibition of enzymes and cytotoxicity. The monoreactive arsenicals are primarily reversible irritants of the upper respiratory tract.

Skin-Damaging Arsenicals

In WWI methyldichloroarsine (MD) and ethyldichloroarsine (ED) were first used by German forces. Lewisite synthesis is attributed to W. L. Lewis (Fig. 9). It was not used in WWI, but was used by Japan forces in China during WWII. The large stockpiles of the former Soviet Union, including a mixture with sulfur mustard to decrease its melting point, await destruction. Technical Lewisite is a violet-black or green volatile liquid with geranium-like odor. The pure compound is colorless and almost odorless and tasteless (Table 4).

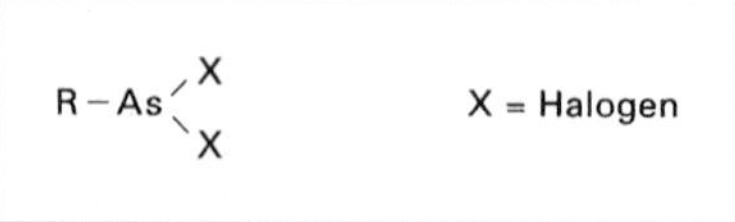

R – As(X)(X)   X = Halogen

FIGURE 8 General formula of bireactive skin-damaging arsenicals.

Toxicokinetics

Lewisite will penetrate and damage tissues it contacts to rapidly reach the systemic circulation and cause systemic poisoning, either by inhalation, percutaneous, or oral route. Lewisite hydrolyzes rapidly in aqueous solutions to the dihydroxyde and thereafter to the more lipophilic and still toxic oxide (Fig. 10).

The persistence of a drop of Lewisite on human forearm skin *in vivo* is 3–5 min, compared to 20–30 min for sulfur mustard. The disappearance by evaporation (<10%) is much lower compared to sulfur mustard (80%; see previous section). In human skin ^{74}As from labeled Lewisite was fixed mainly in the epidermis, with only small amounts in the dermis. It was mostly distributed in the hair and hair follicles. Nails, with their high keratin content, exhibit high arsenical deposition.

A subcutaneous injection of Lewisite in rabbits produced peak arsenic concentrations in the lung, liver, and kidney after about 4 hours. The concentrations were five- to seven-fold higher than in the blood, brain, spinal cord, testes, and skin. In organs with a blood–organ barrier, as the CNS and testes, maximum arsenic concentrations occurred much later (i.e., 12–24 hours after injection). The clearance of Lewisite arsenic in this study was 112 ml/min/kg after the injection of 2.4 mg/kg (LD_{10}) and 129 ml/min/kg after 3.5 mg/kg (LD_{40}); the volume of distribution was 7.7 and 12.7 l/kg; and the terminal half-life 54.7 and 75 hours, respectively.

Toxicity and Mechanism of Action

The basic data on Lewisite toxicity are given in Table 8. In contrast to sulfur mustard, the risk of lethal poisoning is prominent with Lewisite, even after percutaneous exposure. Lewisite and inorganic trivalent arsenicals form a stable six-member ring with reduced lipoic acid (Fig. 11), essential for the activity of two

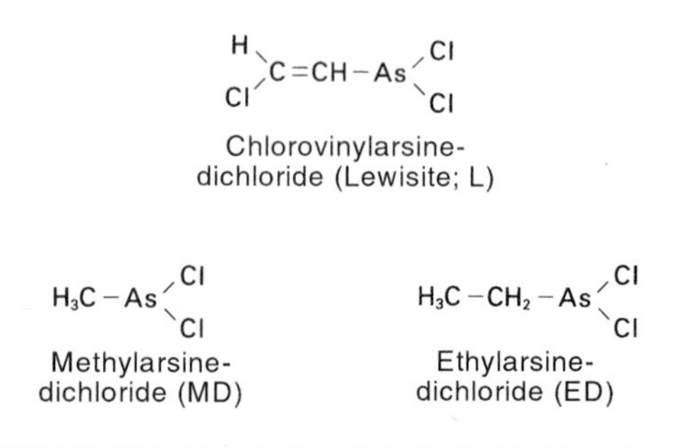

H(Cl)C=CH–As(Cl)(Cl)
Chlorovinylarsine-dichloride (Lewisite; L)

H_3C–As(Cl)(Cl)
Methylarsine-dichloride (MD)

H_3C–CH_2–As(Cl)(Cl)
Ethylarsine-dichloride (ED)

FIGURE 9 Chemical structure of several skin-damaging arsenicals.

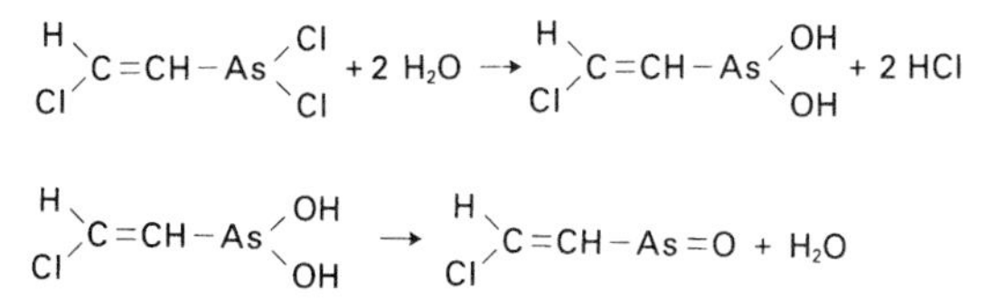

$$\mathrm{ClHC{=}CH{-}AsCl_2 + 2\,H_2O \rightarrow ClHC{=}CH{-}As(OH)_2 + 2\,HCl}$$

$$\mathrm{ClHC{=}CH{-}As(OH)_2 \rightarrow ClHC{=}CH{-}As{=}O + H_2O}$$

FIGURE 10 Hydrolysis of Lewisite in aqueous media.

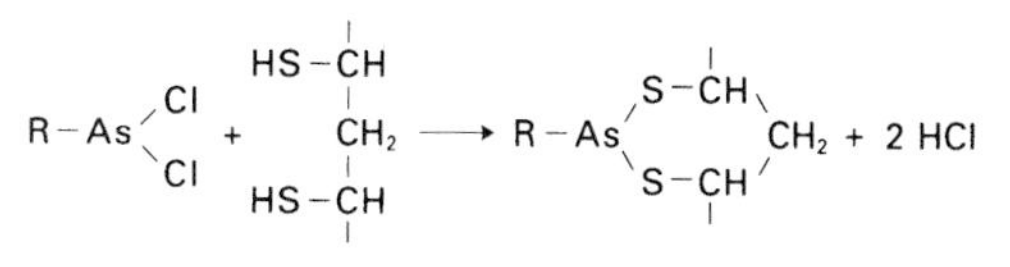

$$\mathrm{R{-}AsCl_2 + HS{-}CH{-}CH_2{-}CH{-}SH \rightarrow R{-}As(S{-}CH{-}CH_2{-}CH{-}S) + 2\,HCl}$$

FIGURE 11 Reaction of Lewisite with sulfhydryl compounds.

key enzymes of oxidative metabolism, the pyruvate and *a*-ketoglutarate dehydrogenase complex (PDH, KGDH). The entry of carbohydrates in the citric acid cycle becomes inhibited, with increased blood pyruvate content *in vivo,* decreased formation of reduced pyridine nucleotides (NAD(P)H) and adenosine triphosphate (ATP), and inhibition of gluconeogenesis. Lewisite is a capillary poison causing endothelial damage with edema, extravasation of fluid and proteins, hemoconcentration, hypotonia, and finally "Lewisite shock."

Signs of Poisoning

Skin

In contrast to sulfur mustard, a substantial drop of Lewisite on the skin immediately causes burning, extensive erythema within 15–30 min and vesication within 12 hours. A further increase in erythema, edema, discomfort, and blister size occurs up to the fourth day, remaining unchanged for the next 3 days.

TABLE 8 Toxicity of Lewisite

Parameter	Lewisite
LD_{50} iv (mg/kg)	
Rabbit	0.5–2
LD_{50} oral (mg/kg)	
Rat	50
LD_{50} percutaneous (mg/kg)	
Rat	15–24
Human (estimate)	38–54
LCt_{50} inhalative (mg × min/m^3)[a]	
Mouse	1500
Rat	1400–1600
Human (estimate)	1200–1500
Minimal effective doses, human	
Erythema (mg/cm^2)	0.05–0.1
Blistering (mg/cm^2)	0.2
Conjunctivitis (mg/l)	0.01 (15 min)
Minimal lethal dose (inhalative; mg/m^3; 30 min)	48

[a] LCt_{50} indicates concentration time product causing 50% lethality.

Steady improvement follows, with complete healing after 4 weeks. Most blisters rupture 1 to 3 days after exposure. The contents are a light, clear, yellow liquid containing arsenic. In contrast to sulfur mustard, abnormal pigmentation is not observed.

Eyes

Lewisite exposure results in the immediate irritation of the eyes without a symptom-free interval. Consequently immediate first aid efforts lead to less pronounced damage than with mustard. Although the course of damage and the healing are faster, the pathology is very similar to the damage by mustard.

Respiratory Tract

Immediate irritation with sneezing, coughing, headache, nausea, and vomiting develop on inhalation. Weakness for days with retrosternal pain may follow. Necroses of the bronchial epithelium with pseudomembrane formation and later bronchopneumonia follow severe exposure. Involvement of the capillary endothelia in the lung is common in more severe poisoning, accompanied by lung edema.

Systemic Poisoning

Animal experiments indicate that hypotension, shock, depressed cardiac activity, gastrointestinal impairment, nausea, vomiting, diarrhea, and liver and kidney disorder may occur. Bronchial involvement and pulmonary edema were also observed in animals with systemic Lewisite poisoning.

Restlessness, confusion, paresthesias, memory loss, ataxia, unconsciousness, and finally stupor and coma were reported from methyldichloroarsine poisoning. A case of percutaneous human phenyldichloroarsine poisoning was reported in 1996, with blistering at the exposed right hand a few hours after exposure, and severe vomiting and diarrhea with slight jaundice occurring after two days. The vomiting lasted for about 1 week, diarrhea for 2 weeks, and jaundice for 3 weeks. The skin damage healed after 10 days. In this case of percutaneous phenyldichloroarsine poisoning, the patient suffered recurrent diarrhea over a period of 3 years.

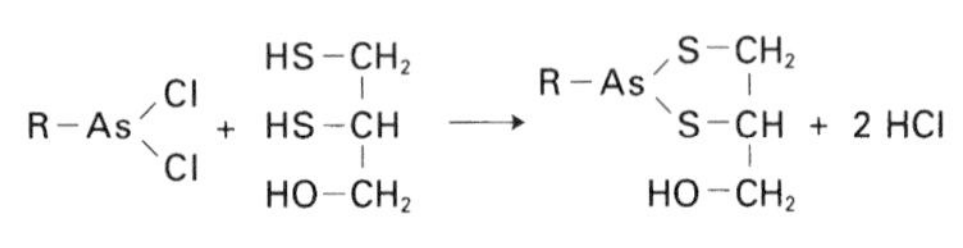

$$R{-}As{<}^{Cl}_{Cl} + \begin{matrix} HS{-}CH_2 \\ HS{-}CH \\ HO{-}CH_2 \end{matrix} \longrightarrow R{-}As{<}\begin{matrix} S{-}CH_2 \\ S{-}CH \\ HO{-}CH_2 \end{matrix} + 2\,HCl$$

FIGURE 12 Reaction of Lewisite with dimercaptopropanol (BAL).

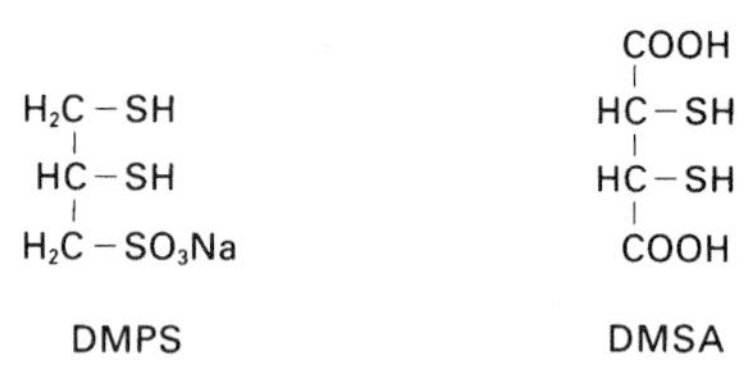

About 2 ml of Lewisite percutaneously is reported to cause lethal systemic poisoning.

Special Toxicology

Various mutagenicity, teratogenicity and carcinogenicity studies gave negative results. In contrast, inorganic arsenicals are considered human carcinogens (intraepidermal squamous-cell and superficial basal-cell carcinoma of the skin and lung, and suspected liver cancer). As the employees of the Okunojima plant, which produced Lewisite among other agents, later showed excessive mortality from respiratory and digestive tract cancer and the occurrence of skin neoplasias, the U.S. Department of Health (in 1988) considered that "some evidence suggests that Lewisite might also be a carcinogen."

Therapeutic Measures

Pharmacotherapy

2,3-Dimercaptopropanol (dimercaprol; BAL) forms a five-member ring with bireactive arsenicals. This is more stable than the six-member ring with lipoic acid. Mobilization of the toxicant, increased elimination, and reversal of enzyme inhibition are the results (Fig. 12). In severe poisoning, up to 3 mg/kg BAL im every 4 hours until relief of the abdominal symptoms should be given, continued on days two and three with 200–400 mg/day, and on days 4–12 with 100–200 mg/day. Ointments to alleviate eye (3–5%) and skin (5–10%) damage were used.

The lack of iv and oral preparations, relatively high toxicity, and increased arsenic content in the brain during treatment, led to the search for alternatives to BAL. The more water-soluble and, by a factor of 10–20, less toxic analogs 2,3-dimercaptopropane sulfonate (DMPS) and 2,3-dimercaptosuccinic acid (DMSA) are the most prominent successors (Fig. 13). Both allow iv and oral administration; both compounds were effective in animal Lewisite poisoning, without accumulation of arsenic in the brain. Systemic application of the dithiols, including BAL, is ineffective against local damage by Lewisite (e.g., on the skin). The efficacy of local treatment seems to increase with the lipophilicity of the dithiol, BAL being most effective.

DMPS	DMSA
	COOH
$H_2C{-}SH$	$HC{-}SH$
$HC{-}SH$	$HC{-}SH$
$H_2C{-}SO_3Na$	COOH

FIGURE 13 Chemical structure of dimercaptopropane sulfonate (DMPS) and dimercaptosuccinic acid (DMSA).

Other Measures

The opinion on irritant-caused pulmonary edema treatment by glucocorticoids is equivocal. Glucocorticoid therapy can only be effective if high-dose treatment, no matter how, is started immediately after exposure. Treatment by inhalation at free airways and systemic injections were used after exposure to respiratory irritants. Physical stress should be avoided. Positive end-expiratory pressure respiration with 60% oxygen improves tissue oxygenation. Intensive bronchial toilet is necessary. Codeine can be used for cough control.

Arsenical Irritants

Diphenylchloroarsine (DA; Clark I) (1917) and diphenylcyanoarsine (DC; Clark II) (1918) were first used by German forces (Fig. 14). Set free by heating, the vapors condensed to a very fine aerosol that penetrated the gas masks of the time. The name Clark

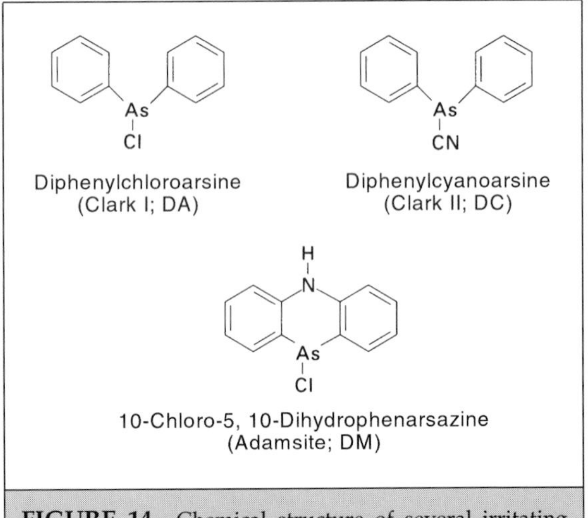

FIGURE 14 Chemical structure of several irritating arsenicals.

TABLE 9 Toxicity of Several Irritating Arsenicals

Parameter	DA	DC	DM
LCt_{50} (mg × min/m^3)[a]	15000	10000	15000
ICt_{50} (mg/m^3)	12 (15 min)	20 (5 min) 30 (0.5 min)	8 (60 min) 22 (1 min)
Maximal tolerable dose (mg/m^3)	1.0	0.25	0.4
Minimal irritating dose (mg/m^3)	0.1	0.005	0.1

[a]LCt_{50} indicates concentration time product causing 50% lethality.
[b]ICt_{50} indicates concentration time product causing 50% incapacitation.

comes from Ch*l*or-*A*rsen-*K*ampfstoff or chlorine-arsenic agent. Diphenylamine chloroarsine (DM), also called Adamsite (Fig. 14), named for the chemist in charge of its development, was synthesized in the U.S. but did not come into use in WWI.

Depending on purity, DA is a white to brown, DC a white to pink, and DM a yellow to green powder. The odor of DC resembles bitter almonds and garlic; the other two are odorless (Table 4).

Toxicokinetics

The agents are rapidly taken up by the skin and mucous membranes. The symptoms appear after seconds to few minutes. No data on the distribution and metabolism are available.

Toxicity, Mechanism of Action, and Signs of Poisoning

The agents are used as aerosols to cause irritation. Tissue damage or lethality occur at about 500 times the concentration causing irritation (Table 9), and are rare in open spaces. The mechanism of action is unknown. A reaction with the thiol groups of the cell constituents is suspected. In the older literature, the stimulation of pain receptors also was proposed.

Exposure causes, within seconds to minutes, violent sneezing; burning in the nose and pharynx; severe headache caused by mucous membrane congestion in paranasal cavities; pain in the teeth, jaws, and ears; nausea; and vomiting. The eyes are less sensitive. After the termination of exposure, the symptoms persist for about 30 min to several hours. The inhalation of high concentrations may cause, in addition, tightness in the chest, anxiety, retrosternal pain radiating to the back and arms, and pulmonary edema. Systemic poisoning is characterized by general weakness, weight loss, malaise, hypotension, severe limb pain, ataxia, paresthesias, paralysis, unconsciousness, and kidney damage. Skin exposure to concentrated agents rapidly exhibits local erythema, edema, blistering, and pain. Severe skin lesions can exacerbate after months. Enhanced sensitivity may persist. Chronic conjunctivitis was reported.

Therapeutic Measures

The irritation, nausea, and vomiting are reversible. No specific antidote is known. Dithiols are ineffective. For pulmonary edema management, see Lewisite-poisoning treatment.

Lacrimators

Chloroacetophenone (CN), was developed in the U.S. but was not used in WWI. In 1928 Corson and Stockton synthesized 2-chlorobenzalmalononitrile (CS) and described its properties. Its introduction is a result of British efforts to replace CN in the 1950s (Fig. 15). Hand-held spray devices with CN (chemical mace) or CS are marketed in various countries for individual protection. CS was used in the Vietnam War on a large scale by U.S. forces.

Toxicokinetics

CN and CS are white powders with an apple-blossom and pepper-like stinging odor, respectively (Table 4). The predominant route of exposure is by inha-

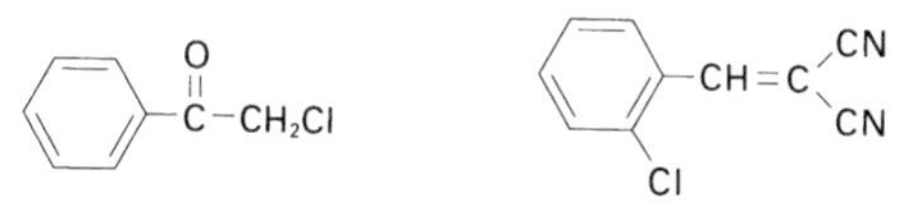

FIGURE 15 Chemical structure of 2-chloroacetophenone (CN) and 2-chlorobenzalmalononitrile (CS).

lation, although some material may be swallowed with mucous secretions. CN is very lipophilic and prone to hydrolysis.

Immediately after exposure, no unchanged agent could be found in the blood of guinea pigs. The main metabolites of CS are *ortho*-chlorobenzyl malononitrile (CBM), and *ortho*-chlorobenzaldehyde (CBA), the later being excreted in the urine as *ortho*-chlorohippuric acid. The blood half-lives of CS, CBA, and CBM are shorter than 1 minute. After administration, 75% of CS is hydrolyzed to CBA and 15% reduced to CBM, the metabolism being largely confined to the liver.

The hydrolysis product malononitrile is degraded further to CO_2 and cyanide. After inhalation of CS, cyanide concentrations remain irrelevant, but after parenteral injection cyanide contribution to systemic toxicity in rabbits was reported.

Toxicity and Mechanism of Action

In general, the ratio of the irritating dose to the toxic dose is much higher for CS than for CN (Table 10). CN and CS are S_N2 type alkylating agents. Most reactive cell constituents are thiols and amines. CS may cause bradykinin release and thereby cause irritation and pain. Lacrimators were assumed to exert their irritating effect by being reduced in the cell, thereby oxidizing NADH. Extensive NADH oxidation would disturb the action of cellular oxidoreductases and thereby energy metabolism. CS reacts very avidly with glutathione, cysteine, and dithiothreitol, and even faster with lipoic acid.

Clinical Signs

Sensory irritation of the eyes and upper respiratory tract appear 10–30 seconds after exposure. Increasing doses cause burning and stinging pain in eyes, nose, and mouth; conjunctivitis; blepharospasm with impairment of the vision; lacrimation; sneezing; and rhinorrhea. Coughing, increased tracheobronchial secretion, nausea, vomiting, headache, and chest tightness may develop. Unexperienced persons may react with agitation and panic. Most symptoms persist only for minutes after termination of the exposure. The eye symptoms may persist for 30 min.

The development of short-lived human tolerance (45 min) to CS was reported.

A burning sensation of the skin and stinging pain at already-injured areas may develop. Higher concentrations may cause erythema and blistering, intensified in a humid and warm environment. Inhalation of extreme concentrations may result in lung edema.

Short-distance spraying and shots from cartridges containing CN or CS into the eye can cause corneal ulcers, severe eye injuries, and permanent blindness; this is more prominent with CN. Both agents may cause sensitization with allergic reactions and contact dermatitis on repeated exposure.

TABLE 10 Toxicity of Several Lacrimators

Parameter	CN	CS
LD_{50} iv (mg/kg)		
Rat	35–41	28
LD_{50} oral (mg/kg)		
Rat	127	1248 (male) 1366 (female)
LD_{50} i.p. (mg/kg)		
Rat	36–56	48
LCt_{50} inhalative (mg × min/m^3)[a]		
Mouse	18,200–73,500	36,000–76,000
Rat	3700–23,330	26,000–88,848
Effective concentrations, human		
Minimal irritative (mg/m^3)	0.15–0.4	0.004
Maximal tolerable (mg/m^3)	1–4.5	1–5
ICt_{50} (mg × min/m^3)[b]	80	10–20
LCt_{50} (mg × min/m^3)(estimate)	600	3800
LCt_{50} (mg × min/m^3)(estimate)[a]	4000–11,000	25,000

[a] LCt_{50} indicates concentration time product causing 50% lethality.
[b] ICt_{50} indicates concentration time product causing 50% incapacitation.

Special Toxicology

No evidence for the mutagenicity or genotoxicity of CN and CS was found in the Ames test and in Chinese hamster ovary cells, except at cytotoxic doses. No evidence for carcinogenicity of CN was found in mice and rats. A significant increase in mammary gland adenomas was observed, but the rate in the control group was unusually low compared to other animals of the same strain. Promotion of epidermal papilloma formation by dimethylbenzanthracene was found in mice treated locally with CN. Incubation of chick embryos with CN (0.3–3 mmol/liter) caused disturbances in brain development.

No evidence of binding to DNA of CS, and no impairment of repair was found but evidence for mutagenicity was found in V79 Chinese hamster cells, Chinese hamster ovary cells, and mouse lymphoma cells at high doses. Binding to the spindle apparatus of the cell was discussed.

No evidence for carcinogenicity after inhalation of CS was found in mice, rats, and guinea pigs. No teratogenicity was reported in rats and rabbits. No evidence of increased frequency of abortions, still births, or malformations were observed in a population frequently exposed to CS.

Therapeutic Measures

Irritation disappears rapidly after termination of exposure (by aeration). Irrigation of the eyes may become necessary after heavy exposure. Visible agent should be decontaminated using copious amounts of water. Hypochlorite may worsen the symptoms. Full body washing may increase the uptake of the agent by the skin, and cause a severe itching and burning sensation. Lung edema should be treated as described in section on Lewisite-poisoning treatment.

BIOLOGICAL AGENTS

General Toxicology

The earliest nonconventional weapons for hunting and war were probably of biological origin. Their use goes back to prehistoric times. In 1972, many countries signed the Convention on the Prohibition of Development, Production and Stockpiling of Bacteriological and Toxin Weapons and on Their Destruction, commonly called the Biological Weapons Convention (BWC). This treaty prohibits the stockpiling of biological agents for offensive military purposes and also forbids research into such offensive employment of biological agents. However, despite this historic agreement, biological warfare research continued to flourish in many countries. The accidental release of anthrax at Sverdlovsk 1979 and Iraq's offensive biologic program, made available to the United Nations in 1995, are prominent examples from countries that signed the convention. Moreover, after the attacks with sarin and cyanide in Tokyo it became known that biological agents were also produced by the Aum Shinrikyo. This shows that knowledge of the effects of biological agents and state-of-the-art protective, prophylactic, diagnostic, and therapeutic measures are necessary for control and disarmament in this area.

History

The earliest reports mention the use of rye ergot for the poisoning of wells by the Assyrians and Solon's use of the purgative herb hellebore during the siege of Krissa in sixth century BC. In 1346 the Tartar army was reported to have hurled the bodies of those who had died of plaque over the city walls during the the siege of Kaffa (at Feodosiya in the Crimea). The plague epidemic that followed forced the defenders to surrender. Some infected people who left Kaffa may have started the Black Death pandemic that spread throughout Europe. Sir Jeffery Amherst provided Native Americans loyal to the French with smallpox-laden blankets during the French and Indian War of 1754 to 1767. Native Americans defending Fort Carillon sustained epidemic casualties, which directly contributed to the loss of the fort to the English.

In 1940, a plague epidemic in China and Manchuria followed reposed overflights by Japanese planes dropping plague-infected fleas. By 1945, the Japanese program had stockpiled 400 kilograms of anthrax to be used in a specially designed fragmentation bomb.

In 1943, the U.S. began research into the offensive use of biological agents. The program was stopped by President Nixon in 1969 and the stocks, including spores of *Bacillus anthracis*, botulinum toxin, *Francisella tularensis*, *Coxiella burnetii*, Venezuelan equine encephalitis virus, *Brucella suis*, and Staphylococcal enterotoxin B were destroyed in 1971–1972.

Through the United Nations inspections of 1991–1995 it became known that, all in all, Iraq produced 19,000 liters of concentrated botulinum toxin (nearly 10,000 liters in munitions), 8500 liters of concentrated anthrax (6500 liters in munitions) and 2200 liters of aflatoxin (1580 liters munitions).

Terminology

Many bacteria, fungi, viruses, rickettsial agents, and toxins have been mentioned in the literature as possible biological warfare agents. Those mentioned most often include *Bacillus anthracis* spores (anthrax), botulinum toxin (botulism), *Yersinia pestis* (plague), ricin, Staphylococcal enterotoxin B (SEB), and Venezuelan equine encephalitis virus (VEE) (Table 11 and 12).

Properties

Despite the very different characteristics of these organisms, viruses, and toxins, biological agents used as weapons share some common characteristics. They can be dispersed in aerosols of particle size 1 to 5 micrometers (microns), which may remain suspended (in certain weather conditions) for hours and if inhaled will penetrate into the distal bronchioles and terminal alveoli of the victims (particles larger than 5 microns would tend to be filtered out in the upper airway). Thereby, the main path for uptake is by inhalation, although oral uptake is also possible via contaminated food or water. In the case of trichothecene mycotoxins percutaneous uptake and skin damage is also possible.

The presently known biological agents in the open literature are natural products, causing known diseases. Nevertheless, by changing the path of uptake (e.g., inhalation), unexpected symptoms and courses of the disease can appear compared to the natural disease. Although not known at present, genetic manipulations and microencapsulation may also lead to changed properties of the microorganisms and their effects.

Person-to-person spread, resulting in epidemics, could be important for some agents, such as smallpox and pneumonic plague, and local disease cycles might occur if a competent vector for a bacterium or virus is present in the environment (such as fleas and rats for *Y. pestis* and certain mosquitoes for an arboviral encephalitis such as the Venezuelan equine encephalitis virus).

Principles of Protection

A major problem of protection is early detection and warning, as microorganisms exhibit a delayed onset of action. A protective mask with an aerosol filter prevents agent inhalation. Protective garments are necessary against trichothecene mycotoxins. The skin can be decontaminated by using soap and copious amounts of water. Against microorganisms, this should be followed by disinfection with 0.5% sodium hypochlorite solution. A solution of 0.5% sodium hy-

TABLE 11 Comparative Lethality of Selected Toxins in Laboratory Mice

Agent	LD_{50} (μg/kg ip)	Molecular weight	Source
Botulinum toxin	0.001	150,000	Bacterium
Shiga toxin	0.002	55,000	Bacterium
Tetanus toxin	0.002	150,000	Bacterium
Abrin	0.04	65,000	Plant (rosary pea)
Diphteria toxin	0.1	52,000	Bacterium
Maitotoxin	0.1	3400	Marine dinoflagellate
Palytoxin	0.15	2700	Marine soft coral
Ciguatoxin	0.4	1000	Marine dinoflagellate
Textilotoxin	0.6	80,000	Elapid snake
C. Perfringens toxin	0.1–0.5	35,000–40,000	Bacterium
Batrachotoxin	2.0	539	Poison-arrow frog
Ricin	3.0	64,000	Plant (castor bean)
ω-Conotoxin	5.0	1500	Cone snail
Taipoxin	5.0	46,000	Elapid snake
Tetrodotoxin	8.0	319	Pufferfish
α-Tityustoxin	9.0	8000	Scorpion
Saxitoxin	10.0 (inhalation 2.0)	299	Marine dinoflagellate
Staphylococcus enterotoxin G (rhesus/aerosol)	27.0 (ED_{50} pg range)	28,494	Bacterium
Anatoxin-A(s)	50.0	500	Blue-green algae
Microcystin	50.0	994	Blue-green algae
Aconitine	100.0	647	Plant (monkshood)
T-2 toxin	1210.0	466	Fungal mycotoxin

TABLE 12 Properties of Various Biological Agents

Agent/desease	Likely method of dissimination	Transmissible human to human	Infective dose	Incubation period	Duration of illness	Lethality	Persistence	Vaccine efficacy (aerosol exposure)
Bacillus anthracis/ inhalation anthrax	Spores in aerosol	No (except cutaneous)	8–10,000 spores	1–5 days	3–5 days	High	Very stable (spores remain viable for years in soil)	2 doses of vaccine protect against 200–500 LD_{50} in monkeys
Vibrio cholerae/ cholera	Sabotage (food and water); aerosol	Rare	$>10^6$ organisms	12 hours–6 days	≥1 week	Low	Unstable in aerosols and freshwater; stable in saltwater	No data on aerosol
Yersinia pestis/ pneumonic plague	Aerosol	High	<100 organisms	1–3 days	1–6 days	High unless treated within 12–24 hours	For up to 1 year in soil; 270 days in bodies	3 doses not protective against 118 LD_{50} in monkeys
Francisella tularensis/ tularemia	Aerosol	No	1–50 organisms	1–10 days	≥2 weeks	Moderate if untreated	For months in moist soil or other media	80% protection against 1–10 ID_{50}
Coxiella burnetii/ Q fever	Aerosol; sabotage (food and water)	Rare	10 organisms (aerosol)	14–26 days	Weeks	Very low	For months on wood and sand	94% protection against 1–3500 ID_{50} in guinea pigs
Ebola virus/Ebola fever	Direct contact (endemic); aerosol (BW)	Moderate	1–10 plaque forming units for primates	4–16 days	Death between 7–16 days	High for Zaire strain, moderate for Sudan	Relatively unstable	No vaccine
Variola virus/ smallpox	Aerosol	High	Assumed low	10–12 days	4 weeks	High to moderate	Very stable	Vaccine protects against large doses in primates
Venezuelan equine encephalitis virus/VEE	Aerosol; infected vectors	Low	Assumed very low	1–6 days	Days to weeks	Low	Relatively unstable	TC 83 protects against 30–500 LD_{50} in hamsters
Botulinum toxin/ botulism	Aerosol; sabotage (food and water)	No	Human LD_{50} p.o. 1 ng/kg	Hours to days	Death in 24–72 h; lasts months if not lethal	High without respiratory support	Weeks in food and nonmoving water	3 doses efficacy of 100% against 22–250 LD_{50} in primates
T-2 mykotoxins	Aerosol; sabotage	No	Moderate	2–4 hours	Days to months	Moderate	Years at room temperature	No vaccine
Ricin	Aerosol; sabotage (food and water)	No	LD_{50} 3–5 $\mu g/kg$	Hours to days	Days, death 10–12 days after ingestion	High	Stable	No vaccine
Staphylococcal enterotoxin B	Aerosol; sabotage (food and water)	No	Clinical illness from picogram range	1–6 hours	Hours	<1%	Resistant to freezing	No vaccine

pochlorite can also be used for wound irrigation, but it must not be used in body cavities. Materials can be decontaminated by using a 5% sodium hypochlorite solution, dry heat (4 hours, 160°C) or steam 121°C at 1 atmosphere over pressure for 20 min (autoclaving).

In general, vaccine prophylaxis and treatment is possible for B agents. Against most bacterial agents, treatment with certain chemotherapeutics is also known (Table 13). Andidotes are in development for botulinum toxin but have not been introduced.

Toxins

Numerous toxins are known; however, only the most relevant can be treated in more detail in this chapter. Several others are mentioned in Tables 11–13.

Botulinum Toxin

The botulinum toxins are among the most toxic compounds known to humans (Table 11). They are a group of seven related neurotoxins produced by the bacillus *Clostridium botulinum*. These toxins, types A through G, can be delivered by aerosol. When inhaled, these toxins produce clinical signs very similar to foodborne intoxication, although the time to onset of paralytic symptoms may actually be longer than for foodborne cases and may vary by type and dose of toxin. The clinical symptoms produced by one or more of these toxins is known as "botulism." Botulinum toxins act by binding to and entering the presynaptic nerve terminal at the neuromuscular junction and at cholinergic autonomic sites. These toxins then act to prevent the release of acetylcholine presynaptically and thus to block neurotransmission. This interruption of neurotransmission causes both bulbar palsies and the skeletal muscle weakness seen in clinical botulism.

The onset of symptoms of inhalation botulism may vary from 24 to 36 hours to several days following exposure. Bulbar palsies are prominent early, with eye symptoms such as blurred vision due to mydriasis, diplopia, ptosis, and photophobia, in addition to other bulbar signs such as dysarthria, dysphonia, and dysphagia. Skeletal muscle paralysis follows, with a symmetrical, descending, and progressive weakness, which may culminate abruptly in respiratory failure. Progression from the onset of symptoms to respiratory failure has occurred in as little as 24 hours in cases of foodborne botulism.

Respiratory failure secondary to the paralysis of the respiratory muscles is the most serious complication and, generally, the cause of death. Reported cases of botulism prior to 1950 had a mortality of 60%. With tracheostomy or endotracheal intubation and ventilatory assistance, fatalities should be less than 5%. Intensive and prolonged nursing care may be required for recovery, which may take several weeks or even months. A prophylactic vaccine and a heptavalent antitoxin for specific therapy are available as investigational new drugs (IND) (Table 13).

Ricin

Ricin is a potent protein toxin derived from the beans of the castor plant (*Ricinus communis*) (Table 11). It is actually made up of two hemagglutinins and two toxins. The toxins, RCL III and RCL IV, are dimers of about 66,000 daltons molecular weight. The toxins are made up of two polypeptide chains, an A and a B chain, which are joined by a disulfide bond. Castor beans are ubiquitous worldwide, and the toxin is fairly easily produced from them. Ricin is therefore a potentially widely available toxin.

Ricin is very toxic to cells. The B chain binds to cell surface receptors and the toxin–receptor complex is taken into the cell; the A chain has endonuclease activity and extremely low concentrations will inhibit protein synthesis. When inhaled as a small particle aerosol, this toxin may produce pathologic changes within 8 hours and severe respiratory symptoms followed by acute hypoxic respiratory failure in 36–72 hours. When ingested, ricin causes severe gastrointestinal symptoms followed by vascular collapse and death. This toxin may also cause disseminated intravascular coagulation, microcirculatory failure, and multiple organ failure if given intravenously in laboratory animals.

There are little toxicity data in humans. Accidental sublethal aerosol exposures that occurred in humans in the 1940s were characterized by the onset of the following symptoms in 4 to 8 hours: fever, chest tightness, cough, dyspnea, nausea, and arthralgias. The onset of profuse sweating some hours later was commonly the sign of termination of most of the symptoms. In rodents, the histopathology of aerosol exposure is characterized by necrotizing airway lesions causing tracheitis, bronchitis, bronchiolitis, and interstitial pneumonia with perivascular and alveolar edema. Intravascular injection can cause pulmonary perivascular edema due to vascular endothelial injury. Ingestion causes gastrointestinal hemorrhage with hepatic, splenic, and renal necrosis. Intramuscular administration causes severe local necrosis of muscle and regional lymph nodes with moderate visceral organ involvement.

Specific treatment is not available. A candidate vaccine is under development. The treatment is primarily supportive, depending on the route of exposure (Table 13).

Trichothecene Mycotoxins

The trichothecene mycotoxins are low molecular weight (250–500 daltons) nonvolatile compounds produced by filamentous fungi (molds) of the genera *Fusarium, Myrotecium, Trichoderma, Stachybotrys,* and others (Table 11). The structures of approximately 150 trichothecene derivatives have been described in the literature. These substances are relatively insoluble in water but are highly soluble in ethanol, methanol, and propylene glycol. The trichothecenes are extremely stable to hypochlorite, heat, and ultraviolet light inactivation, while brief exposure to NaOH destroys toxic activity. These toxins are very toxic to cells by the inhibition of protein synthesis. Skin exposure results in erythema and ulceration. The potential for use as a BW toxin was demonstrated shortly after World War II when flour contaminated with species of *Fusarium* was baked into bread that was ingested by civilians (Siberia). Some developed a protracted lethal illness called alimentary toxic aleukia (ATA), characterized by initial symptoms of abdominal pain, diarrhea, vomiting, prostration, and, within days, fever, chills, myalgias, and bone marrow depression with granulocytopenia and secondary sepsis. Survival beyond this point allowed the development of painful pharyngeal–laryngeal ulceration and diffuse bleeding into the skin (petechiae and ecchymoses), melena, bloody diarrhea, hematuria, hematemesis, epistaxis, and vaginal bleeding. Pancytopenia and gastrointestinal ulceration and erosion were secondary to the ability of these toxins to profoundly arrest bone marrow and mucosal protein synthesis and cell cycle progression through DNA replication. No specific treatment is known. Early use of dexamethasone was effective in animals (Tables 12 and 13).

Microbial Agents

Many microorganisms can be misused as biological agents. Only some details for anthrax are given in this chapter. Several others are mentioned in Tables 12 and 13.

Anthrax

Bacillus anthracis is a rod-shaped, gram-positive, sporulating organism, the spores constituting the usual infective form. Anthrax is a zoonotic disease, with cattle, sheep, and horses being the chief domesticated animal hosts, but other animals may be infected. The disease may be contracted by the handling of contaminated hair, wool, hides, flesh, blood, and excreta of infected animals and from manufactured products such as bone meal, as well as by purposeful dissemination of spores. Transmission is made through scratches or abrasions in the skin, wounds, inhalation of spores, eating infected meat that is insufficiently cooked or by flies. All human populations are susceptible. Recovery from an exposure to the disease may be followed by immunity. The spores are very stable and may remain viable for many years in soil and water. They will resist sunlight for varying periods.

Anthrax may appear in three forms in humans: cutaneous, inhalational, and gastrointestinal. The cutaneous form, or skin form (also referred to as malignant pustule), occurs most frequently on the hands and forearms of persons working with infected livestock. It is characterized by carbuncles and swelling at the site of infection. The scab that typically forms over the lesion is black as coal, hence the term anthrax (Greek for "coal"). Sometimes this local infection will develop into a systemic infection. The inhalational form, known also as woolsorters' disease, is an infection of the lungs contracted by the inhalation of the spores; this form occurs mainly among workers handling infected hides, wool, and furs. The intestinal form, which is rare in humans, is contracted by the ingestion of insufficiently cooked meat from infected animals. In humans, the mortality from untreated cutaneous anthrax ranges up to 25%; in inhalational and intestinal cases, the case fatality rate is almost 100%.

After an incubation period varying from 1–6 days, presumably dependent on the dose of inhaled organisms, onset is gradual and nonspecific. Initially fever, malaise, and fatigue may be present, sometimes in association with a nonproductive cough and mild chest discomfort. These initial symptoms are often followed by a short period of improvement (from hours to 2–3 days), followed by the abrupt development of severe respiratory distress with dyspnea, diaphoresis, stridor, and cyanosis. Shock and death usually follow within 24–36 hours after respiratory distress onset. Physical findings are usually nonspecific. A chest X-ray may sometimes reveal a widened mediastinum with pleural effusions but typically is without infiltrates. *Bacillus anthracis* will be detectable by gram stain of the blood and by blood culture with routine media, but often not until late in the course of the illness. Studies of inhalation anthrax in nonhuman primates (rhesus monkey) showed that the bacilli and toxin appear in the blood late on day 2 or early on day 3 post-exposure. The toxin parallels the appear-

TABLE 13 Protective and Therapeutic Measures Against Various Biological Agents

Agent	Vaccine prophylaxis	Drug/therapeutic	Chemotherapeutic regime or supportive therapy	Chemoprophylactic regime	Comments
Anthrax	Michigan Department of Public Health Vaccine 0.5 ml at 0, 2, 4 weeks and 6, 12, 18 months then annual boosters	Ciprofloxacin[a]	400 mg iv every 8–12 h	500 mg po bid × 4 wks, also 2 doses of vaccine 2 weeks apart if unvaccinated	Alternated are ciprofloxacin[a], clindamycin, erthromycin, and chloramphenicol
		Doxycycline[a]	200 mg, then 100 mg every 12 h	100 mg po bid × 4 wks, plus vaccination	
		Penicillin	2 million units iv every 2 h		For penicillin sensitive organisms
Cholera (toxin)	Wyeth–Ayerst Vaccine (50% efficacy, short-term) 0.5 ml im at 0 and 4 weeks, then boosters every 6 months	Oral rehydration therapy: 3.5 g NaCl, 2.5 g $NaHCO_3$, 1.5 g KCl, and 20 g glucose per liter of water (WHO)	During period of high fluid loss		Vaccine not recommended for routine protection in endemic areas; Swedish SBL oral vaccine effective but not available in the United States
		Tetracycline[b]	500 mg every 6 h × 3 days		Pediatric treatment includes tetracycline[b], erthromycin, trimethoprim-sulfamethoxazole, and furazolidone
		Ciprofloxacin[a]	500 mg every 12 h × 3 days	For tetra-/doxycycline resistant strains	
		Norfloxacin	400 mg every 12 h × 3 days		
Q fever	IND 610, inactivated whole-cell vaccine given as single 0.5 ml sc injection	Tetracycline[b]	500 mg oral every 6 h × 5–7 days	Useful for prophylaxis; start 8–12 days post-exposure × 5 days.	Currently testing vaccine to determine the necessity of skin testing prior to use
	Qvax (CSL Ltd, Parkvill, VIC, Australia)	Doxycycline[b]	100 mg oral every 12 h × 5–7 days	Useful for prophylaxis; same regimen	Licensed vaccine in Australia
Plague	Greer Laboratory vaccine 1.0 ml im, then 0.2 ml im at 1–3 and 3–6 months, and boosters at 6, 12, 18 months, and 1–2 years	Streptomycin	30 mg/kg/day im in divided dose × 10 days	Plague vaccine not protective against aerosol challenge in animal studies	
		Doxycycline[b]	200 mg iv then 100 mg every 12 h × 10–14 days	100 mg every 12 h × 7 or more days	Alternates: trimetoprim-sulfa, methoxazole, or ciprofloxacin
		Chloramphenicol	1 g iv every 6 h		For plague meningitis

Tularemia	LVS, live attenuated vaccine (IND), one dose by scarification	Streptomycin	1 g im every 12 h for 10–14 days		
		Gentamicin	3–5 mg/kg/day for 10–14 days		
		Doxycycline[b]		100 mg po every 12 h for 14 days	Can also use tetracycline[b]
Venezuelan equine encephalitis	TC-83 live attenuated vaccine (IND) 0.5 ml sc (1 dose) C-84 (formalin inactivation of TC-83 [IND]) 0.5 ml sc for up to 3 doses every 2 weeks	No specific anti-viral	Supportive therapy, analgesics, anticonvulsants		Reactogenic in 20%; no seroconversion in 20% Vaccine used for nonresponders to TC-83
Marburg/Ebola virus	No vaccine available	No specific anti-viral	Supportive therapy, shock, hypotension, and DIC management		Isolation and barrier nursing required
Smallpox virus	Wyeth Vaccine: 1 dose by scarification, booster every 3 years for V. major	Vaccinia Immune Globulin (VIG)		0.6 ml/kg im (within 3 days of exposure, best within 24 hours)	Pre- and post-exposure vaccination recommended if >3 years since last vaccine
Botulinum toxin	IND pentavalent toxoid (A–E) sc at 0, 2, and 12 weeks, then yearly boosters	IND heptavalent anti-toxin (A–F) (equine despeciated)	1 vial (10 cc) iv every 20 min until no further improvement		Need to skin test before uses of anti-toxin.
		Trivalent equine anti-toxin (A, B, and E)			Licensed CDC products; need to skin test.
Staphylococcus enterotoxin B	No vaccine available	No specific anti-toxin	Ventilatory support for inhalation exposure		
Ricin toxin	No vaccine available	No specific antitoxin	Inhalation: supportive therapy for acute lung injury and pulmonary edema Oral: gastric lavage, superactivated charcoal, cathartics		
T-2 mycotoxins	No vaccine available	No specific antitoxin		Decontamination of clothing and skin	

[a]Ciprofloxacin has been shown to impair cartilage growth in beagles and, therefore, is not recommended for use in children and during pregnancy. However, no serious adverse consequences have been reported in children who have used ciprofloxacin, and it would be recommended for use in a life-threatening situation.

[b]Staining of teeth in fetuses and children <8 years old with use of tetra- or doxycycline has been documented only after >6 cycles of treatment of at least 6 days each. In pregnant women and children, doxycycline should be used only if disease is life threatening.

ance of the bacilli in the blood and tests are available to rapidly detect the toxin. Vaccines and chemotherapeutics are known for protection and treatment (Table 13).

Bibliography

Aldrige, W. N., and Reiner, E. (1972). "Enzyme Inhibitors as Substrates. Interactions of Esterases with Esters of Organophosphorus Compounds and Carbamic Acids." North Holland, Amsterdam.

Aposhian, V. H., Carter, D. E., Hoover, T. D., Hsu, C.-A., Maiorino, R. M., and Stine, E. (1984). DMSA, DMPS, and DMPA—as arsenic antidotes. *Fund. Appl. Toxicol.* **4,** S58–S70.

Ballantyne, B. and Marrs, T. C. (1992). "Clinical and Experimental Toxicology of Organophosphates and Carbamates." Butterworth-Heinemann, Oxford.

Barbieri, L., Balteil, M., and Stirpe, F. (1993). Ribosomes-inactivating proteins from plants. *Biochem. Biophys. Acta.* **1154,** 237–282.

Beebe, G. (1960). Lung cancer in World War I veterans: Possible relation to mustard gas injury and 1918 influenza epidemic. *J. Natl. Cancer. Inst.* **25,** 1231–1252.

Benschop, H. P., de Jong, L. P. A., and Langenberg, J. P. (1995). Inhalation toxicokinetics of C(±)P(±)-soman and (±)-sarin in the guinea-pig. *In* "Enzymes of the Cholinesterase Family" (D. M. Quinn, *et al.*, eds.), pp. 361–368, Plenum Press, New York.

Büscher, H. (1937). "Giftgas! Und Wir?" Barth Verlag, Leipzig, Germany.

Butler, T. (1983). "Plague and Other Yersina Infections." Plenum Press, New York.

Calabresi, P., and Chabner, B. A. (1990). Antineoplastic agents. *In* "Goodmans and Gilman's the Pharmacological Basis of Therapeutics" (A. Goodman Gilman *et al.*, eds.), pp. 1209–1263. Pergamon Press, New York.

Dacre, J. C., and Goldman, M. (1996). Toxicology and pharmacology of the chemical warfare agent sulfur mustard. *Pharmacol. Rev.* **48,** 289–326.

Davison, C., Rozman, R. S., and Smith, P. K. (1961). Metabolism of bis-β-chloroethyl sulfide (sulfur mustard gas). *Biochem. Pharmacol.* **7,** 65–74.

Dawson, R. M. (1994). Review of oximes available for treatment of nerve agent poisoning. *J. Appl. Toxicol.* **14,** 317–331.

Duffy, F. H., and Burchfiel, J. L. (1980). Long term effects of the organophosphate sarin on EEG's in monkeys and humans. *Neurotoxicology* **1,** 667–689.

Dunn, M. A., and Sidell, F. R. (1989). Progress in medical defense against nerve agents. *JAMA* **262,** 649–652.

Eyer, P. (1995). Neuropsychopathological changes by organophosphorus compounds—a review. *Hum. Exp. Toxicol.* **14,** 857–864.

Evans, M. E., and McGee, Z. A. (1983). Tularemia. *In* "Current Therapy in Infectious Diseases" (E. H. Kass and R. Platt, eds.), pp. 18–19. B.C. Decker, Philadelphia, PA.

Gear, J. H. S. (1989). Clinical aspects of African viral hemorrhagic fevers. *Rev. Infect. Dis.* (May–June) S777–S782.

Geissler, E., ed. (1986). "Biological and Toxin Weapons Today." Oxford University Press, Stockholm International Peace Institute, Oxford.

Goldman, M., and Dacre, J. C. (1989). Lewisite: Its chemistry, toxicology, and biological effects. *Rev. Environ. Contam. Toxicol.* **110,** 75–115.

Graham, A. F., Levy, G. A., and Chance, A. C. (1947). The fate of arsenical vesicants in the skin and the effect of BAL. *Biochem. J.* **41,** 352–357.

Grob, D. (1963). Anticholinesterase intoxication in man and its treatment. In "Handbuch der experimentellen Pharmakologie Vol. 15, Choliesterases and Anticholinesterase Agents" (G. B. Koelle, ed.), pp. 989–1027, Springer Verlag, Berlin.

Hanslian, R. (1937). "Der chemische Krieg." Mittler und Sohn, Berlin.

Harris, R., and Paxman, J. (1984). "A Higher Form of Killing," Hill and Wang, New York.

Henderson, D. A. (1986). The eradication of smallpox. *In* "Maxcy-Rousenau Public Health and Preventive Medicine" (L. M. Last, ed.) 12th ed., pp. 129–138. Appeton-Century-Crofts, Norwalk, CT.

Himsworth, R. H., and Snowden, L. (1971). "Report on the inquiry into the medical and toxicological aspects of CS." Her Majesty's Stationery Office, London.

Holmstedt, B. (1959). Pharmacology of organophosphorus cholinesterase inhibitors. *Pharmacol. Rev.* **11,** 567–688.

Huxoll, D. L., Parrott, C. D., and Patrick, W. C., III (1989). Medicine in defense against biological warfare. *JAMA* **265,** 677–679.

Jones, G. R. N. (1972). CS and its chemical relatives. *Nature* **235,** 257–261.

Keeler, J. R., Hurst, C. G., and Dunn, M. A. (1991). Pyridostigmine used as a nerve agent pretreatment under wartime conditions. *JAMA* **266,** 693–695.

Klehr, N. W. (1984). Spätmanifestationen bei ehemaligen Kampfgasarbeitern unter besonderer Berücksichtigung der cutanen Befunde. *Z. Hautkr.* **59,** 1167–1170.

Leadbeater, L. (1973). The absorption of o-chlorobenzylidene malononitrile by the respiratory tract. *Toxicol. Appl. Pharmacol.* **25,** 101–110.

Lohs, K. (1975). Delayed toxic effects of chemical warfare agents. Stockholm International Peace Research Institute (SIPRI), Almquist and Wiksell International, Stockholm, Sweden.

Marrs, T. C., Colgrave, H. F., Cross, N. L., Gazzard, M. F., and Brown, R. F. (1983). A repeated dose study of the toxicity of inhaled 2-chlorobenzylidene malononitrile (CS) aerosol in three species of laboratory animal. *Arch. Toxicol.* **52,** 183–198.

Marrs, T. C., Edginton, J. A. Price, P. N., and Upshall, D. G. (1986). Acute toxicity of T2 mycotoxin to the guinea-pig by inhalation and subcutaneous routes. *B. J. Exp. Path.* **67,** 259–268.

Marrs, T. C., Maynard, R. L., and Sidell, F. R. (1996). "Chemical Warfare Agents, Toxicology and Treatment." John Wiley and Sons, Chichester, UK.

Montecucco, C. (1995). "Clostridial Neurotoxins. The Molecular Pathogenesis of Tetanus and Botulism." Springer, Berlin.

Morris, C. D. (1988). Eastern equine enchephalitis. *In* "The Arboviruses: Epidemiology and Ecology" (I. P. Monath, eds.), Vol. 3. pp. 203–231. CRC Press, Boca Raton, FL.

National Research Council, Division of Biological Sciences, Committee on the Effects of Herbicides in Vietnam (1974). "The Effects of Herbicides in South Vietnam." National Academy of Sciences, Washington D.C.

Norman, J. (1975). Lung cancer mortality in World War I veterans with mustard gas injury. 1919–1965. *J. Natl. Cancer. Inst.* **54,** 311–317.

O'Neill, J. J. (1981). Non-cholinesterase effects of anticholinesterases. *Fund. Appl. Toxicol.* **1,** 154–160.

Papirmeister, B., Feister, A. J., Robinson, S. I., and Ford, R. D. (1991). "Medical Defense Against Mustard Gas; Toxic Mechanisms and Pharmacological Implications." CRC Press, Boston, MA.

Pechura, M. C., and Rall, D. P. (eds.) (1993). "Veterans at Risk, the Health Effects of Mustard Gas and Lewisite." U.S. Institute of Medicine, Commitee to Survey the Health Effects of Mustard Gas and Lewisite, Division of Health Promotion and Disease Prevention, National Academy Press, Washington, D.C.

Peters, R. A. (1955). Biochemistry of some toxic agents. I. Present state of knowledge of biochemical lesions induced by trivalent arsenical poisoning. *Bull. John Hopkins Hosp.* **97,** 1–20.

Rauber, A., and Heard, J. (1985). Castor bean toxicity re-examined: A new perspective. *Vet. Hum. Toxicol.* **27,** 498–502.

Reisen, W. K., and Monath, T. P. (1988). Western equine enchephalitis. *In* "The Arboviruses: Epidemiology and Ecology" (T. P. Monath, ed.), Vol. 5 pp. 203–231. CRC Press, Boca Raton, FL.

Robinson, J. P., and Leitenberg, M. (1971). The rise of CB weapons. *In* "The Problem of Chemical and Biological Warfare," Vol. 1. Stockholm International Peace Research Institute (SIPRI), Almquist and Wiksell, Stockholm, Sweden.

Salas, R., De Manzione, N., Tesh, R. B. *et al.* (1991). Venezuelan haemorrhagic fever. *Lancet* **338,** 1033–1066.

Schrader, G. (1952). "Die Entwicklung neuer Insktizide auf Grundlage von organischen Fluor und Phosphorverbindungen." Monographie Nr. 62, 2. Aufl. Verlag Chemie, Weinheim, Germany.

Seeley, S. D., Nowicke, J. W., Meselson, M., Guillemin, J., and Akratanakul, P. (1985). Yellow rain. *Sci. Am.* **253,** 128–137.

Senanayake, N., and Karalliedde, L. (1987) Neurotoxic effects of organophosphorus insecticides. An intermediate syndrome. *N. Engl. J. Med.* **306,** 761–763.

Shih, T.-M., Koviak, T. A., and Capacio, B. R. (1991). Anticonvulsants for poisoning by the organophosphorus compound soman: Pharmacological mechanisms. *Neurosci. Biobehav. Rev.* **15,** 349–362.

Sidell, F. R., Takafuji, E. T., Franz, D. R. (1997). "Textbook of Military Medicine, Part 1, Medical Aspects of Chemical and Biological Warfare" U.S. Department of the Army, Office of the Surgeon General, and Borden Institute, Washington, D.C.

Somani, S. M. (1992). "Chemical Warfare Agents." Academic Press, San Diego, CA.

Sohrabpour, H. (1995). The current status of mustard gas victims in Iran. *ASA Newsletter* **47(2),** 1, 14–15.

Stade, K. (1964). "Pharmakologie und Klinik synthetischer Gifte." Deutscher Militärverlag, Berlin.

Stephen, J. (1986). Anthrax toxin. *In* "Pharmacology of Bacterial Toxins" (F. Dorner and J. Drews eds.), pp. 381–395. Pergamon Press, Oxford.

Strauss, J. H., and Strauss, E. G. (1994). The alphaviruses: gene expression, replication, and evolution. *Microbiol. Rev.* **58,** 491–562.

Sundwall, A. (1961). Minimum concentration of N-methylpyridinium-2-aldoxime methane sulphonate (P2S) which reverse neuromuscular block. *Biochem. Pharmacol.* **8,** 413–417.

Szinicz, L., Mückter, H., and Kreppel, H. (1992). Effect of dithiol compounds on lewisite and mustard toxicity. *In* Proceedings 4th International Symposium Prot. Chemical Warfare Agents," pp. 299–304. FOA Report A 40067-4.6,4.7, National Defence Research Establishment, Department of NBC Defense, Umea, Sweden.

Tacket, C. O., and Rogawski, M. A. (1989). Botulism. *In* Simpson, L. L., ed. "Botulinum Neurotoxin and Tetanus Toxin" (L. L. Simpson, ed.), pp. 351–378. Academic Press, New York.

Tu, A. T. (1996). Basic information on nerve gas and the use of sarin by Aum Shinrikyo. *J. Mass. Spectrom. Soc. Japan* **44,** 293–320.

Ueno, Y. (1989). Trichothecene mycotoxins: Mycology, chemistry, and toxicology. *Adv. Nutr. Res.* **3,** 301–353.

Ulrich, R. G., Bavari, S., and Olson, M. (1995). Bacterial superantigens in human diseases: Structure, function and diversity. *Trends Microbiol.* **3,** 463–468.

U.S. Department of the Army (1988). "Chemical Stockpile Disposal Program; Final Programmatic Environmental Impact Statement, Appendix B." Program Executive Officer - Program Manager for Chemical Demillitarization. Aberdeen Proving Ground, MD.

U.S. Department of Health and Human Services (HHS), Centers of Disease Control (CDC) (1988). Final recommendations for protecting the health and safety against potential adverse effects of long-term exposure to low doses of agents: GA, GB, VX, mustard agent (H,HD,T), and lewisite (L). *Fed. Reg.* **53,** 8504–8507.

U.S. Department of Health and Human Services (HHS), National Toxicology Program (1990a). "Toxicology and Carcinogenesis Studies of 2-Chloroacetophenone in F344/N Rats and B6C3F1 Mice (Inhalation Studies)." Technical Report Series No. 379, Pub. No. 90-2834. National Institute of Health, Washington D.C.

U.S. Department of Health and Human Services (HHS), National Toxicology Program (1990b). "Toxicology and Carcinogenesis Studies of CS (94% o-Chlorobenzalmalononitrile) in F344/N Rats and B6C3F1 Mice." Technical Report Series No. 377, Pub. No. 90-2832. National Institute of Health, Washington D.C.

Von Däniken, A. (1983). "Literaturübersicht über die Toxikologie der Tränengase." Giftabteilung des Bundesamtes für Gesundheitswesen, Bern, Switzerland.

Wallenfels, K., Ertel, W., Hockendorf, K., Rieser, J., and Überschar, K. H. (1975) Tränenreizstoffe als Akzeptoren für Dihydropyridinwasserstoff. *Naturwissenschaften* **62,** 459–467.

Willems, J. L. (1989). Clinical management of mustard gas casualties. *Ann. Med. Milit. Belg.* **3,** 1–61.

Williams, J. C. (1991). Infectivity, virulence, and pathogenicity of Coxiella burnetii for various hosts. *In* "Q fever: The Biology of Coxiella burnetii" (J. C. Williams and H. A. Thompson, eds.). CRC Press, Boca Raton, FL.

Worek, F., Bäcker, M., Thiermann, H., Szinicz, L., Mast, U., Klimmek, R., and Eyer, P. (1997). Reappraisal of indications and limitations of oxime therapy in organophosphate poisoning. *Hum. Exp. Toxicol.* **16,** 466–472.

C H A P T E R

36

Active and Passive Smoking

DIETRICH HOFFMANN, ERNST L. WYNDER

Naylor Dana Institute for Disease Prevention, American Health Foundation, Valhalla, New York, 10595

INTRODUCTION

Early indications of the use of tobacco are related to us through the artifacts of the Mayas of the Yucatan region of Mexico, where the people were smoking string-tied cigars (Fig. 1). Five hundred years later, the vessel *Santa Maria* brought Christopher Columbus to San Salvador in the Bahamas where he was presented with dried tobacco leaves by the House of Arawaks. Columbus and his crew thus were the first Europeans who became acquainted with tobacco smoking and the *Santa Maria* brought it to Portugal on its return voyage. The first person known to have grown tobacco in Europe was Jean Nicot, the French ambassador to Portugal. In 1570, the French botanist Jean Liebault gave the tobacco plant the name *herba nicotiana* in honor of Jean Nicot. In 1828, the chemists Reimann and Posselt in Heidelberg isolated and characterized nicotine as the major pharmacoactive ingredient in tobacco. In 1885, A. Pinner confirmed the chemical structure of nicotine through the total synthesis of 3-(1-methyl-2-pyrrolidinyl) pyridine. Today, the tobacco alkaloid nicotine is recognized as the major inducer of tobacco dependence among tobacco chewers, snuff dippers, and smokers.

The first clinical report about the cancer-inducing potential of tobacco smoke was recorded in 1795 by the surgeon Sömmering in Frankfurt on Main, Germany, who had observed the frequent occurrence of carcinoma of the lower lip of pipe smokers. In 1859, M. Bouisson of the University of Montpellier, France, reported that cigar smokers frequently developed cancer of the lip and of the mouth. Clinical observations of lung cancer among cigarette smokers were published in 1939 by F. M. Müller in Cologne, and in 1943 by Schairer and Schön in Jena, Germany.

In 1950, publications by E. L. Wynder and E. A. Graham in the United States, and by R. Doll and A. B. Hill in the United Kingdom, reported the results of the first major epidemiologic studies on cigarette smoking and lung cancer. The American investigators had found that among the 684 proven cases of lung cancer in men, 649 were cigarette smokers while 21 of the smokers had used cigars. In the following decades more than 200 epidemiologic studies in more than 15 countries confirmed that the smoking of cigars and pipes and especially the inhalation of cigarette smoke were causally associated with cancer of the lung. Many large cohort and case control studies have documented a dose–response relationship between the duration of exposure and lung cancer death rates in cigarette smokers (i.e., higher rates for smokers who began the habit when they were between 15 and 19 years of age than for those who began at age 20 years or older). After an initial 3- to 5-year increase, the lung cancer risk for ex-smokers declines progressively with the number of years since smoking ceased. The smoking of cigarettes, cigars, and pipes is also causally associated with cancer of the upper aerodigestive system and with cancer of the urinary bladder. In addition, cigarette smoking is causally linked to cancer of the pancreas and of the renal pelvis, and it is associated with cancer of the nasal cavity, the liver, and the uterine cervix, and with myeloid leukemia Table 1 presents the estimates of the contribution of

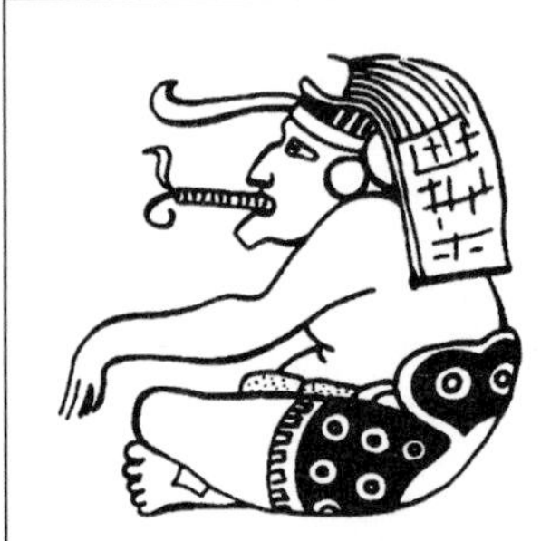

FIGURE 1 Maya smoking a cigar (10th century). (Courtesy of the General Research Division, The New York Public Library, Astor, Lenox and Tilden Foundations.)

cigarette smoking to the numbers of deaths from cancer at various sites in men and women in the United States in 1991. At that time, 38.8% of the 272,000 cancer deaths among men, and 21.4% of 242,000 cancer deaths among women were attributed to cigarette smoking.

In addition to cancer, cigarette smokers also face higher mortality rates from chronic obstructive lung disease and coronary heart disease. Prospective studies have shown that chronic bronchitis and emphysema occur far more frequently among smokers than among nonsmokers. The risk of heavy smokers for these chronic respiratory illnesses is actually 20- to 30-fold greater than that of nonsmokers. By far the highest numbers of tobacco-related deaths are attributable to myocardial infarction. Even though smoking is an independent risk factor, synergistic effects, such as those from hypercholesterolemia and hypertension, have a significant role in heart disease and coronary heart disease.

The smoker's tobacco dependence and how he or she smokes are largely determined by his or her need for nicotine. Nicotine from the inhaled smoke is absorbed in the lung and then transported to the central and peripheral nervous systems and also to the heart, liver and other organs with endogenous secretion. The nicotine levels in the blood reflect the intensity of smoke uptake, which is governed by the degree of each smoker's nicotine addiction.

TABLE 1 U.S. Cancer Deaths Caused by Cigarette Smoking, 1991[a]

International classification of diseases, revision 9 category	Cancer site	Cancer deaths expected 1991[b]	Smoking-attributable risk (%)[c]	Estimated deaths due to smoking[d]
		Males		
140–149	Oral	5275	91.5	4827
150	Esophagus	7300	78.2	5709
157	Pancreas	12,000	28.6	3460
161	Larynx	2900	81.2	2355
162	Lung	92,000	90.3	83,076
188	Bladder	6400	46.5	2976
189	Kidney	6300	47.6	2999
Total		272,000		105,402
		Females		
140–149	Oral	2875	61.2	1760
150	Esophagus	2500	74.3	1858
157	Pancreas	13,200	33.3	4396
161	Larynx	750	86.7	650
162	Lung	51,000	78.5	40,035
180	Cervix	4500	32.4	1458
188	Bladder	3100	36.7	1138
189	Kidney	4300	12.3	529
Total		242,000		51,824

[a]Shopland *et al.* (1991).
[b]Total male and female cancer deaths expected in 1991 = 514,000.
[c]Percent attributed to cigarette smoking, males and females combined = 30.6.
[d]Total excess deaths due to cigarette smoking = 157,226.

Nicotine crosses the blood–brain barrier and is enriched in the brain where it binds to specific cholinergic receptors. Although the mechanisms of the effects of nicotine on the central nervous system are not yet fully understood, experiments with laboratory animals have documented that the binding of nicotine to specific receptors in the brain leads to dependence, as well as to stimulation, depression and mood changes.

CONSUMPTION OF CIGARETTES

After World War II, most developed countries experienced a major increase in cigarette consumption, at first, among men, and since the 1970s, also among women. Table 2 reveals that in countries with intense antismoking campaigns, a modest, and in some cases a major decrease in lung cancer mortality began to show among men. These countries were Australia, England, and Wales. In other countries where cigarette consumption decreased between 1970–1972 and 1990–1992, the decline of lung cancer mortality rates slowed down. In countries with a major increase in cigarette consumption between 1970–1972 and 1990–1992 there were also drastic increases in lung cancer mortality. These included Poland, Hungary, Japan, and France. In developing countries where major increases in cigarette consumption have occured, there is also a prediction of significant increases of lung cancer in future years.

PHYSICOCHEMISTRY OF TOBACCO SMOKE

The results of epidemiologic investigations as well as the experimental induction of tumors in laboratory animals have raised the question, "Why does tobacco smoke elicit such a variety of diseases?" Some answers to this question can be derived from our knowledge about the physicochemical composition of tobacco smoke. The burning of tobacco yields combustion products that can be designated as mainstream and sidestream smoke. While mainstream smoke is a combustion product that is inhaled by the smoker immediately upon its generation, sidestream smoke is produced during the smoldering of the tobacco product and is the major contributor to environmental tobacco smoke. Table 3 presents some key data regarding the physicochemical parameters of mainstream and sidestream smoke of a nonfilter cigarette. Aerosol particles in urban air are usually found at a concentration of 10^5 per ml with particle diameters between 0.1 and $> 10.0 \mu m$; the mainstream smoke of cigarettes when inhaled contains 5×10^9 particles per ml with a mean diameter of 0.2 μm in a range of 0.1–1.0 μm. Thus, all of the particles in the smoke aerosol are within the size range of lung-damaging particles, known to be between 0.1 and 3.0 μm. Moreover, the mainstream smoke contains $>10^{10}$ highly reactive radicals. Overall, the mass of the mainstream smoke of a nonfilter cigarette weighs about 500 mg, of which 20–30 mg are particulate phase (tar). To

TABLE 2 Estimated Per Capita Consumption of Cigarettes Per Adult (≥15 Years), Percent Adult Men and Women Who are Smokers, and Age-adjusted Lung Cancer Death Rates Per 100,000[a]

Country	Per capita consumption per year		Smokers (%)		Lung cancer death rates (per 100,000) 1970–1971		1990–1993	
	1970–1972	1990–1992	Males	Females	Men	Women	Men	Women
Poland	3,010	3,620	51.0	29.0	36.42	4.89	71.3	10.2
Hungary	2,940	3,260	40.0	27.0	40.76	7.62	81.6	16.6
Japan	2,950	3,240	59.0	14.8	16.12	5.13	30.6	8.1
Switzerland	3,700	2,910	36.0	26.0	20.51	3.55	43.6	8.3
Australia	3,400	2,710	29.0	21.0	42.54	6.52	40.4	13.0
U.S.	3,700	2,670	28.1	23.5	46.77	9.44	57.1	25.6
Canada	3,910	2,540	31.0	29.0	40.46	6.39	55.1	21.8
Germany (West)	2,430	2,360	36.8	21.5	44.17	4.77	47.0	8.4
England and Wales	3,250	2,210	28.0	26.0	72.42	12.41	55.9	21.0
France	1,860	2,120	40.0	27.0	30.12	3.31	47.0	5.2
Sweden	1,700	1,550	22.0	24.0	20.51	8.71	23.7	10.6

[a]Source: World Health Organization.

TABLE 3 Mainstream and Sidestream Smoke of One Cigarette without Filter Tip

	Mainstream smoke	Sidestream smoke[a]
Temperature in the burning cone	860–900°C	500–650°C
Temperature of the smoke	20–50°C[b]	20–60°C[c]
pH[d]	5.8–6.2	6.8–7.5
Particles/ml	5×10^9	10^5–10^6
Size of the particles (μm)	0.2 (0.1–1.0)	0.5 (0.1–1.5)
Radicals/ml	2–3×10^{10}	N/A
Total weight (mg)	500	N/A
Weight of the particle phase (mg)	20–30	25–40

[a]N/A-indicates not available.
[b]First puff 20°C, last puff 50°C.
[c]8 mm distance from the smoldering cone.
[d]Bright tobacco or tobacco blend; pH of the mainstream smoke of the barley cigarettes 6.6–7.1; pH of sidestream smoke 7.5–8.7.

date, about 400–600 chemical compounds have been identified as gas-phase constituents and more than 4,000 of the particulate-phase constituents have been characterized.

The gas phase of cigarette mainstream smoke consists mainly of nitrogen, oxygen, carbon dioxide, and carbon monoxide. These major constituents make up 85–95 % of the total weight of the mainstream smoke (Table 4). The most important compounds in terms of toxic and/or tumorigenic potential of the gas phase are carbon monoxide, ammonia, nitrogen oxides, hydrogen cyanide, formaldehyde, acetaldehyde, benzene pyridine, and volatile *N*-nitrosamines.

The major components of the particulate phase include the *Nicotiana* alkaloids, nicotine itself being the most important one (Table 5). Significant constituents of the cuticular layer of the tobacco leaves are specific terpenes, fatty acid esters, and long-chain hydrocarbons (paraffins). Hentriacontane ($C_{31}H_{64}$) is the main representative of the long-chain hydrocarbons. A substantial portion of the naphthalenes and practically all of the polynuclear aromatic hydrocarbons in mainstream and sidestream smoke are formed by pyrolysis during the burning of tobacco. Among 60 polynuclear aromatic hydrocarbons identified in tobacco smoke are 11 compounds with carcinogenic activity in bioassays with laboratory animals.

Another important group of carcinogens in tobacco and tobacco smoke are the tobacco-specific *N*-nitrosamines. These are formed by *N*-nitrosation of the alkaloids during the curing and aging of tobacco and also during smoking (Fig. 2). Bioassays have documented that phenolic compounds in the particulate phase of smoke are promoters of epithelial tumors, while catechols are considered to be cocarcinogens in epithelial tissue.

Tobacco tar also contains traces of aromatic amines. These are known bladder carcinogens. In addition, N and O heterocyclic hydrocarbons, fatty acids, fatty-acid esters, phytosterols, and polyphenols are found in tar. The term "tar" was chosen for didactic reasons; the authors acknowledge that its use in connection with tobacco smoking is not correct in terms of chemical definition because tobacco smoke particulates are not formed in an oxygen-free atmosphere.

The quantitative data presented in Tables 4 and 5 are based on standardized smoking conditions and on standardized analytic techniques. Since about 1960, machine-smoking of cigarettes for analytical purposes used a 35-ml puff of 2 seconds duration, drawn once per minute. These conditions no longer reflect "average" smoking parameters of men and women who use contemporary filter-tipped cigarettes. It has been observed that such smokers may choose to draw 2 to 4 puffs per minute and puff volumes can be as large as 55 ml, depending on nicotine yield in the mainstream smoke.

Tobacco contains up to 30 metals as oxides or salts, mostly as trace elements. Thus, one finds in the smoke of one cigarette the salts, or oxides, of 38 mg potassium, 22 mg calcium, and 5.5 mg magnesium. Because <1% of these compounds in tobacco transfer into the mainstream smoke during the burning of a cigarette, they are not specifically mentioned as important smoke constituents in Table 4. Similarly, data on insecticides, pesticides and other agricultural chemicals used in the cultivation of tobacco are not listed because of their high degrees of variation among countries and from season to season. Yet, it is important to mention that some countries or provinces produce tobacco that may contain high ppm levels of DDD, DDT, or maleic hydrazide and that 20% of such residual amounts may transfer into the mainstream smoke.

The smoke of low-yield filter cigarettes lacks flavor. The rising demand for low-yield cigarettes has therefore led to the practice of adding flavor compounds or plant extracts to the tobaccos. Menthol (0–10 mg/cigarette) is probably the most well known of these additives; others are usually patented or formulated in a way that preserves their status as trade secrets. Their composition is thus known only to manufacturers. In adherence to strict laws in many developed countries that prohibit use of additives, the cancerogenic coumarin is rarely used nowadays.

TABLE 4 Major Constituents of the Vapor Phase of the Mainstream Smoke of Nonfilter Cigarettes

Compound	Concentration/cigarette (% of total effluent)
Nitrogen	280–320 mg (56–64%)
Oxygen	50–70 mg (11–14%)
Carbon dioxide	45–65 mg (9–13%)
Carbon monoxide	14–23 mg (2.8–4.6%)
Water	7–12 mg (1.4–2.4%)
Argon	5 mg (1.0%)
Hydrogen	0.5–1.0 mg
Ammonia	10–130 μg
Nitrogen oxides (NO_x)	100–600 μg
Hydrogen cyanide	400–500 μg
Hydrogen sulfide	20–90 μg
Methane	1.0–2.0 mg
Other volatile alkanes [20][a]	1.0–1.6 mg[b]
Volatile alkenes [16]	0.4–0.5 mg
Isoprene	0.2–0.4 mg
Butadiene	25–40 μg
Acetylene	20–35 μg
Benzene	6–70 μg
Toluene	5–90 μg
Styrene	10 μg
Other volatile aromatic hydrocarbons [29]	15–30 μg
Formic acid	200–600 μg
Acetic acid	300–1700 μg
Propionic acid	100–300 μg
Methyl formate	20–30 μg
Other volatile acids [6]	5–10 μg[b]
Formaldehyde	20–100 μg
Acetaldehyde	400–1400 μg
Acrolein	60–140 μg
Other volatile aldehydes [6]	80–140 μg
Acetone	100–650 μg
Other volatile ketones [3]	50–100 μg
Methanol	80–180 μg
Other volatile alcohols [7]	10–30 μg[b]
Acetonitrile	100–150 μg
Other volatile nitriles [10]	50–80 μg[b]
Furan	20–40 μg
Other volatile furans [4]	45–125 μg[b]
Pyridine	20–200 μg
Picolines [3]	15–80 μg
3-Vinylpyridine	7–30 μg
Other volatile pyridines [25]	20–50 μg[b]
Pyrrole	0.1–10 μg
Pyrrolidine	10–18 μg
N-Methylpyrrolidine	2.0–3.0 μg
Volatile pyrazines [18]	3.0–8.0 μg
Methylamine	4–10 μg
Other aliphatic amines [32]	3–10 μg

[a]Brackets enclose the number of individual compounds identified in a given group.
[b]Estimated amounts.

TABLE 5 Major Constituents of Particulate Matter of the Mainstream Smoke of Nonfilter Cigarettes

Compound	Concentration (μg/cigarette)[a]
Nicotine	100–3,000
Nornicotine	5–150
Anatabine	5–15
Anabasine	5–12
Other tobacco alkaloids [17][b]	n.a.
Bipyridyls [4]	10–30
n-Hentriacotane [*n*-$C_{31}H_{64}$]	100
Total nonvolatile hydrocarbons [45][a]	300–400[c]
Naphthalene	2–4
Naphthalenes [23]	3–6[c]
Phenanthrenes [7]	0.2–0.4[c]
Anthracenes [5]	0.05–0.1[c]
Fluorenes [7]	0.6–1.0[c]
Pyrenes [6]	0.3–0.5[c]
Fluoranthenes [5]	0.3–0.45[c]
Carcinogenic polynuclear aromatic hydrocarbons [11][d]	0.1–0.25
Phenol	80–160
Other phenols [45][c]	60–180[c]
Catechol	200–400
Other catechols [4]	100–200[c]
Other dihydroxybenzenes [10]	200–400[c]
Scopoletin	15–30
Other polyphenols [8][c]	n.a.
Cyclotenes [10][c]	40–70[c]
Quinones [7]	0.5
Solanesol	600–1,000
Neophytadienes [4]	200–350
Limonene	30–60
Other terpenes [200–250][c]	n.a.
Palmitic acid	100–150
Stearic acid	50–75
Oleic acid	40–110
Linoleic acid	150–250
Linolenic acid	150–250
Lactic acid	60–80
Indole	10–15
Skatole	12–16
Other indoles [13]	n.a.
Quinolines [7]	2–4
Other aza-arenes [55]	n.a.
Benzofurans [4]	200–300
Other *O*-heterocyclic compounds [42]	n.a.
Stigmasterol	40–70
Sitosterol	30–40
Campesterol	20–30
Cholesterol	10–20
Aniline	0.36
Toluidines	0.23
Other aromatic amines [12]	0.25
Tobacco-specific *N*-nitrosamines [6][d]	0.34–2.7
Glycerol	120

[a]n.a. indicates not available.
[b]Brackets enclose the number of individual compounds identified.
[c]Estimate.
[d]For details, see Fig. 2 and Table 6.

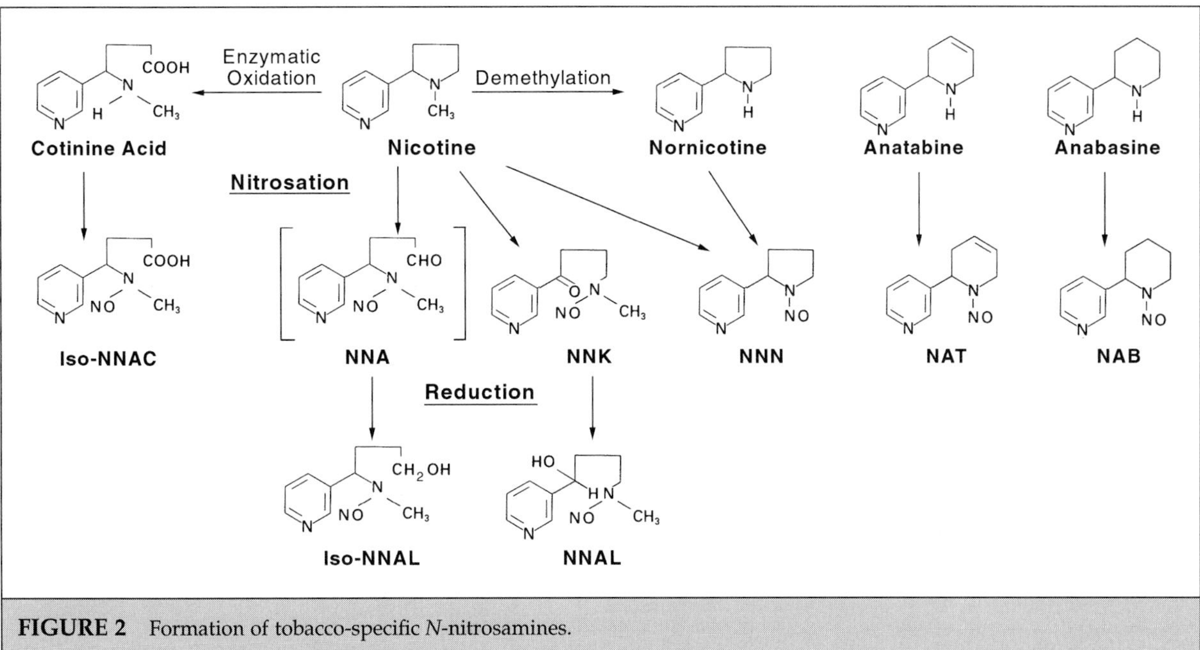

FIGURE 2 Formation of tobacco-specific *N*-nitrosamines.

Cigarette additivies that are used in the United States can be gleaned from a list of 599 ingredients that is published by the industry.

The Changing Cigarette

The dose–response relationship of tobacco smoking and lung cancer has also been substantiated by means of smoke-inhalation bioassays with Syrian golden hamsters. A reduction of the dose appeared to be first step toward a reduction of the cancer risk. Consequently, cigarette production has undergone many changes that were designed a priori to lower the smoke yields of cigarettes. Thus, the sales-weighted average smoke condensate and nicotine emissions of cigarettes in Germany declined from 22 mg and 1.5 mg in 1960 to 13.7 mg and 0.85 mg in 1987. Similar trends were observed in England, in the United States, in Canada, and in many western European countries (Fig. 3). The technology that has contributed to these developments is foremost that of the development of filter tips from cellulose acetate (more than 90% of all cigarettes sold in developed nations are filter-tipped brands). Also, the use of reconstituted tobaccos and of expanded tobacco leaf and ribs in the blends, and tobacco selection have aided these developments. The use of perforated filter tips since about 1975 has been especially effective in lowering smoke yields by enabling air dilution of the mainstream smoke (Fig. 4).

Legislative regulation in western Europe mandated for 1993 that only cigarettes with tar yields ≤ 15 mg could be sold. By 1998, regulation prescribed adherence to ≤ 12 mg tar as the highest permissible smoke yield. However, nicotine yields were not regulated. Accordingly, they are expected to remain in the range of 0.8–1.2 mg. The pharmacological effect of nicotine is regarded as the motivating reason for smoking tobacco. The number of cigarettes smoked each day is therefore determined foremost by the nicotine dependence of the user and only secondarily by other smoke constituents. The reduction of tar in the mainstream smoke by filtration has the added advantage that certain compounds, like phenols and volatile nitrosamines are selectively removed. Perforated filter tips also serve to reduce the amounts of carbon monoxide, hydrogen cyanide, phenols, and volatile aldehydes.

As previously discussed, the smoker reacts to lower nicotine emissions in the smoke by smoking more cigarettes per day, drawing puffs more frequently and more intensely, and by inhaling the smoke more deeply into the lung. Until the late 1960s and early 1970s, the smoker of filter-tipped cigarettes had a 20–40% lower risk for cancer of the lung, larynx, oral cavity, and esophagus than the smoker of nonfilter cigarettes. However, today, the smoker of filtered cigarettes with low nicotine delivery (1.2 mg/cigarette according to standard laboratory machine smoking) inhales deeply, takes up to 4 puffs per minute, and inhales smoke volumes up to 50 ml. The result is that adenocarcinoma of the lung has drastically increased, and smokers of filtered cigarettes today have

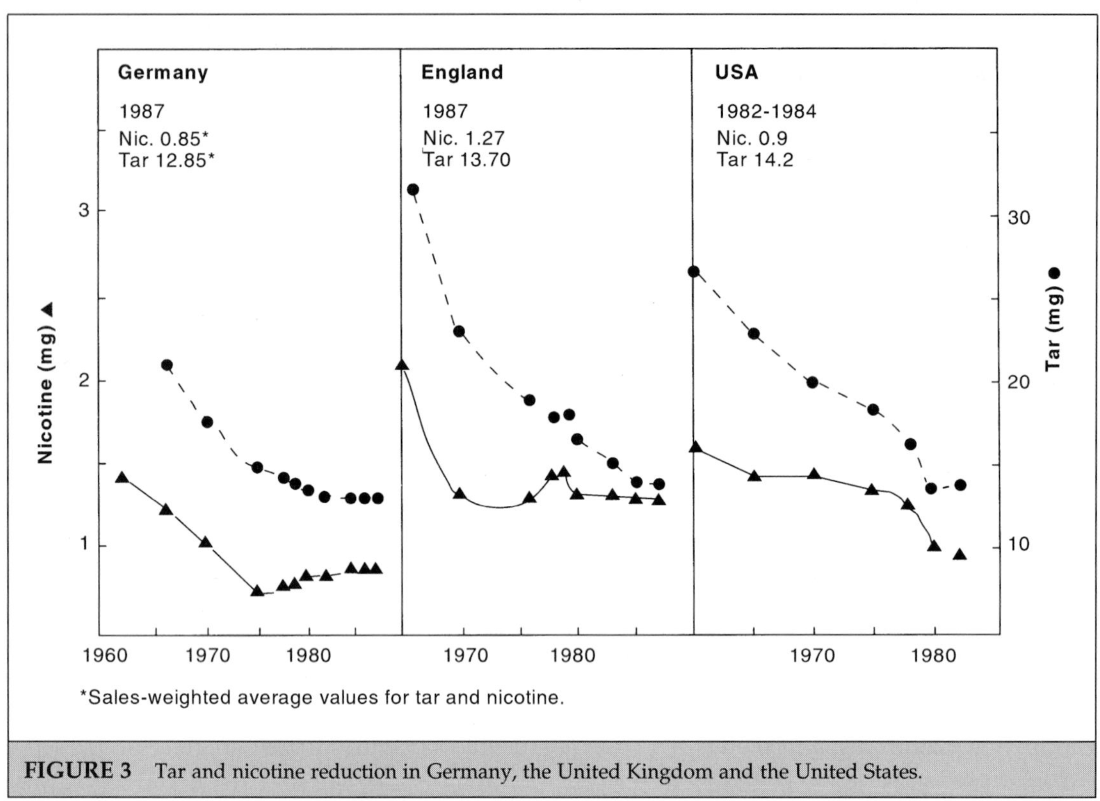

FIGURE 3 Tar and nicotine reduction in Germany, the United Kingdom and the United States.

the same risk of lung cancer as smokers of nonfilter cigarettes.

Toxic Smoke Constituents

Like acetylcholine, nicotine liberates noradrenaline in the adrenal gland and in the hypothalamus. This liberation of catecholamines by nicotine raises their blood levels and thus impacts the arterial walls and coagulating factors. This in turn leads to elevated blood pressure and a higher pulse rate. Therefore, smokers who have hypertension or hyperchosterolemia have an increased risk for angina pectoris.

Carbon monoxide, inhaled as a smoke constituent, has 200-fold greater affinity for hemoglobin than does oxygen. Consequently, oxygen in circulating blood and its diffusion (distribution) into the tissues and cells is strongly reduced upon smoke inhalation. Carbon monoxide is also known to form adducts with myoglobin in the muscle tissues, and this could lead to oxygen deficiency in the mitochondria of the heart muscles. The elevated COHb concentration in smokers is therefore also regarded as the reason why healing processes after accidents or after surgery are slowed down in smokers. Patients with heart disease who smoke are especially vulnerable to the toxic effects of nicotine, carbon monoxide, hydrogen cyanide, nitrogen oxides, CS_2, and cadmium.

Smoke inhalation assays with laboratory animals and pathologic findings in humans have clearly demonstrated that the inhalation of cigarette smoke causes temporary paralysis of the ciliated epithelium in the respiratory tract. In chronic cigarette smokers, the ciliated epithelium degenerates, resulting in bronchial mucus stagnation so that the self-cleansing mechanism of the respiratory defenses is impaired. A symptom indicating this condition is the 'smokers cough', which most often occurs in the morning. Smoke constituents with high cilia toxicity are hydrogen cyanide, acrolein, acetaldehyde, ammonia, and nitrogen dioxide. The inhibition of ciliary clearance mechanisms in the bronchi and trachea by tobacco smoke increases the toxic and carcinogenic potential of smoke constituents and thus elevates the risk for chronic bronchitis, emphysema, and precancerous changes in lung tissues.

Carcinogens in Tobacco Smoke

Smoke inhalation bioassays with Syrian golden hamsters have elicited benign and malignant tumors in the respiratory airways, predominantly in the larynx. Exposure of hamsters to the gas phase of ciga-

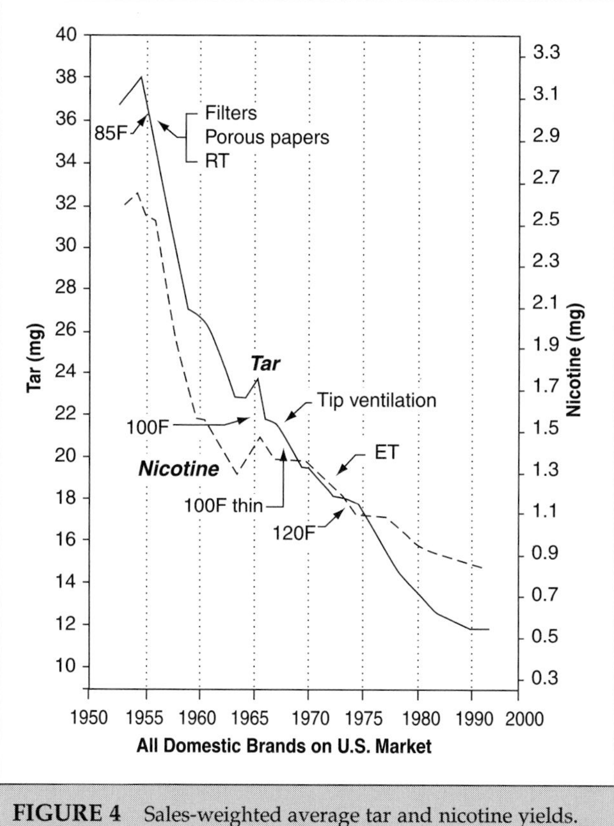

FIGURE 4 Sales-weighted average tar and nicotine yields.

rette smoke did not lead to tumor development. This indicates that most of the tumorigenic potential of the smoke resides in the particulate matter (tar). Applications of solutions of tar from cigarettes, cigars, and pipes have produced skin tumors in mice and rats and tumors in the ear of rabbits and in the subcutaneous tissues of rats. Fractioning cigarette tars and bioassays of all fractions have led to the identification of the neutral portion and its subfractions B and B 1 as the most active tumorigenic materials (Fig. 5). These fractions contain polynuclear aromatic hydrocarbons as major known carcinogens; yet by themselves these compounds cannot account for the observed carcinogenic potential of tobacco tars. When these polynuclear aromatic hydrocarbons are assayed in tumor-promotion experiments with the fraction containing noncarcinogenic phenolic compounds of the tar (9.3% of whole tar) about 75–90% of the tumor activity of whole tar on mouse skin is explained. The phenolic fraction contains phenol and other tumor promoters as well as the cocarcinogenic catechols. In addition, in tobacco smoke we also find organ-specific carcinogens, such as the aromatic amines, which are known human bladder carcinogens, and the tobacco-specific *N*-nitrosamines. The latter have structurally related organ-specific carcinogenic activity.

Polynuclear Aromatic Hydrocarbons (PAH)

The neutral fraction B1 is the only truly carcinogenic portion of tobacco tar (Fig. 5). The PAH that are concentrated in this subfraction comprise 10 cancerogenic compounds. The most prevalent carcinogenic PAH is benzo[*a*]pyrene (BaP) (Fig. 6 and Table 6). Most induce tumors of the skin and other sites they come in contact with, such as subcutaneous tissue, esophagus, and lung. They are called contact carcinogens because their metabolic activation proceeds via enzymes in the host tissues. Inhaling PAH from aerosols in inhalation carcinogenesis assays leads to tumors of the larynx and of the lung in hamsters. The doses of PAH inhaled as tobacco smoke carcinogens are in line with the importance of PAH as factors that induce lung cancer. Benzo[*a*]pyrene, a major representative of the compounds in this class of chemicals, leads to a high incidence of skin tumors in mice when solutions containing 5 μg of the carcinogen are applied on mouse skin three times weekly for 60 weeks at a total dose of 36 mg/kg. A single instillation of 5 mg benzo[*a*]pyrene on an iron oxide carrier into the trachea of hamsters (50 mg/kg) leads to tumors in the upper-respiratory airways of the animals. A smoker who consumes 40 cigarettes per day over a 40-year period will have inhaled about 28 mg benzo[*a*]-pyrene (0.4 mg/kg). The carcinogenic activity of benzo[*a*]pyrene and other PAH in the smoke is potentiated through the presence of promoters like phenol and cocarcinogens like catechol. Therefore benzo[*a*]pyrene and the other carcinogenic PAH play a major role in the pathogenesis of epithelial lung cancer in smokers.

N-Nitrosamines

N′-Nitrosonornicotine (NNN) and 4-(methylnitrosamino)-1-(3-pyridyl)-l-butanone (NNK) are the most significant *N*-nitrosamines identified in tobacco smoke (Fig. 2). In rats, NNK elicits benign and malignant tumors in the lung, in the nasal mucosa, in the pancreas, and in the liver. In hamsters, NNK induces tumors in the lung, the trachea, and the nasal mucosa; and in mice it elicits adenocarcinoma of the lung. *N*′-Nitrosonornicotine is a lung carcinogen in mice, an esophageal carcinogen and inducer of nasal mucosal tumors in rats, and a laryngeal and nasal mucosal

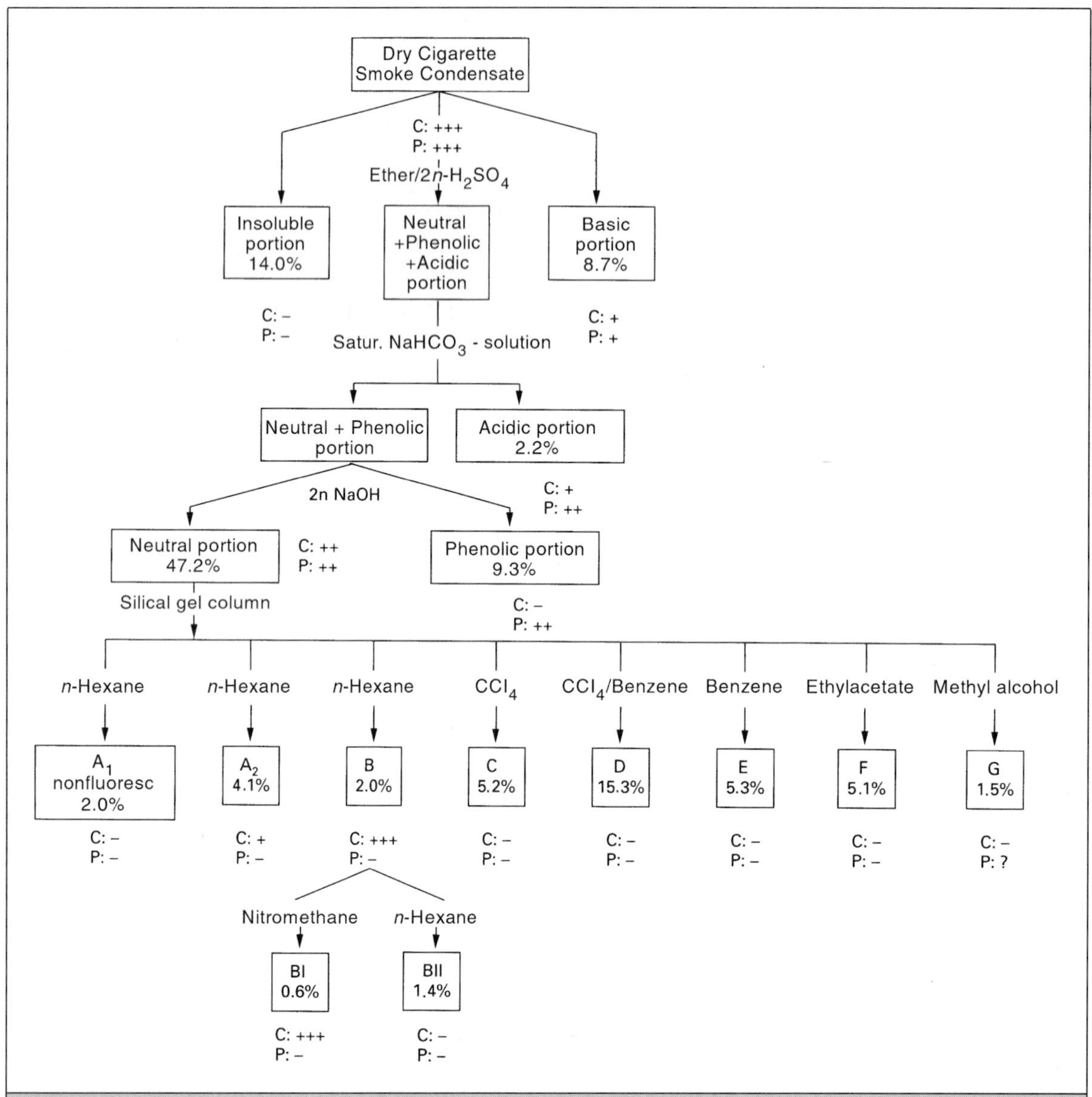

FIGURE 5 Fractionation of cigarette-smoke condensate. Abbreviations: C, carcinogenic activity; P, tumor-promoting activity.

carcinogen in hamsters. In mink, NNN also elicits tumors of the nasal mucosa.

Of special interest are the organ-specific effects of these nitrosamines. These compounds have systemic effects, independent of their oral, subcutaneous, intraperitoneal, or intramuscular administration. Each animal species reflects the organ-specificity of the compounds in its own way. 4-(Methylnitrosamino)-1-(3-pyridyl)-1-butanone induces primarily lung tumors in rats, mice, and hamsters, even in cases of transplacental exposure. A single subcutaneous application of 0.6 mg 4-(methylnitrosamino)-1-(3-pyridyl)-1-butanone (9 μmol/kg) leads to adenocarcinoma of the lung in rats. Administration of 6.9 mg 4-(methylnitrosamino)-1-(3-pyridyl)-1-butanone (73 μmol/kg) in the drinking water elicits also tumors of the exocrine pancreas in rats. An estimate of the exposure of a smoker of 40 cigarettes per day over a 40-year period leads to a total dose of 100 mg 4-(methylnitrosamino)-1-(3-pyridyl)-1-butanone (7 μmol/kg). Even though it is not possible to compare exposures in bioassays with laboratory animals with calculated human exposures to these tobacco carcinogens, it is apparent that 4-(methylnitrosamino)-1-(3-pyridyl)-1-butanone is of signifi-

Polynuclear Aromatic Hydrocarbons

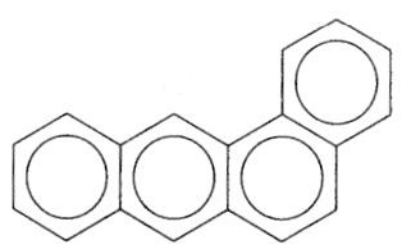

Benz(*a*)anthracene

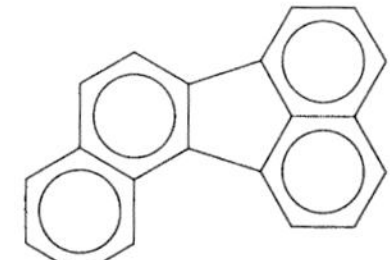

Benzo(*j*)fluoranthene

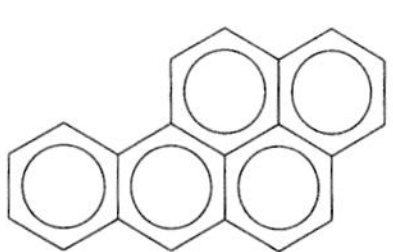

Benzo(*a*)pyrene

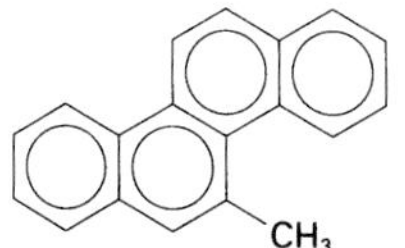

5-Methylchrysene

Aza-Arenes

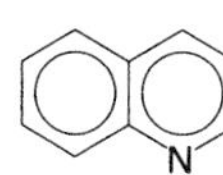

Quinoline

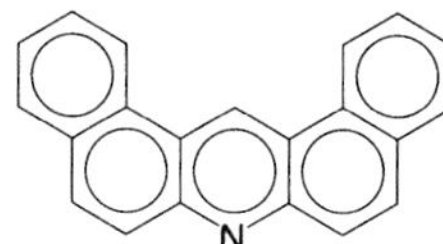

Dibenz(*a,j*)acridine

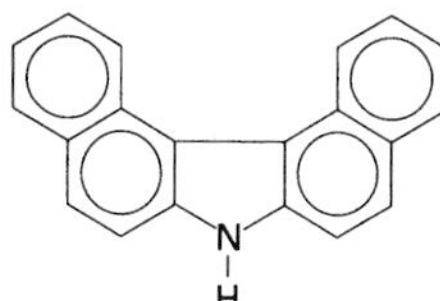

7H-Dibenzo(*c,g*)carbazole

***N*-Nitrosamines**

$(CH_3)_2N{-}N{=}O$

N-Nitrosodimethylamine

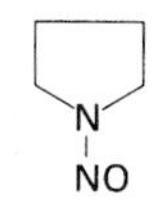

N-Nitrosopyrrolidine

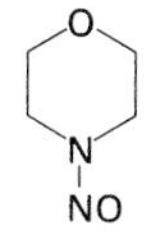

N-Nitrosomorpholine

$(HO{-}CH_2{-}CH_2)_2N{-}NO$

N'-Nitrosodiethanolamine

Tobacco-specific *N*-Nitrosamines

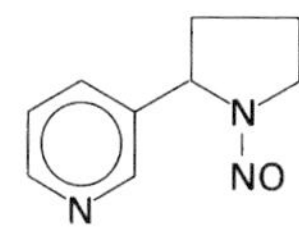

N'-Nitrosonornicotine (NNN)

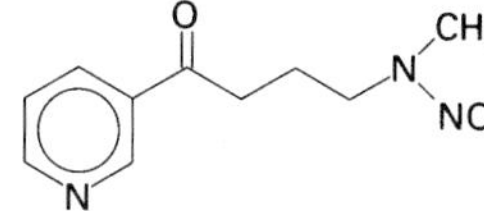

4-(Methylnitrosamino)-1-(3-pyridyl)-1-butanone (NNK)

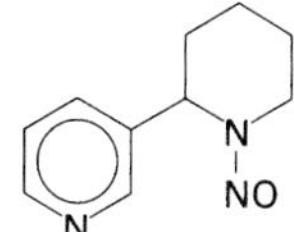

N'-Nitrosoanabasine

Aromatic Amines

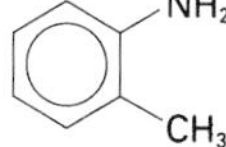

2-Toluidine

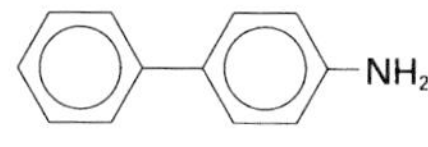

4-Aminobiphenyl

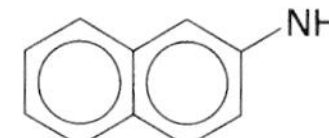

2-Naphthylamine

Various Organic Compounds

$CH_2{=}CH{-}CN$	$CH_3{-}CH{=}CH{-}CHO$	$CH_3{-}CH(NO_2){-}CH_3$	$CH_2{=}CH{-}Cl$
Acrylonitrile	Crotonaldehyde	2-Nitropropane	Vinyl Chloride

$(CH_3)_2N{-}NH_2$

1,1-Dimethylhydrazine

$O{-}C(OC_2H_5)(NH_2)$

Ethylcarbamate (Urethan)

HCHO

Formaldehyde

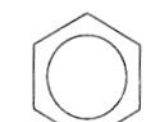

Benzene

Inorganic Carcinogens

$H_2N{-}NH_2$

Hydrazine

^{210}Po

Polonium-210

FIGURE 6 Chemical structures of tumorigenic agents in tobacco smoke.

TABLE 6 Probable Causative Agents for Cigarette-Smoke-Related Disorders

Disorder	Contributing agents[a]	Possible enhancing or associated agents
Tobacco dependence	Major: nicotine Minor: secondary *Nicotiana* alkaloids, flavor components	Acetaldehyde (?)
Cardiovascular disease	Major: carbon monoxide, nitrogen oxides, hydrogen cyanide, "tar" Minor: cadmium, zinc, carbon disulfide	Nicotine Alkylating species
Chronic obstructive lung disease	Hydrogen cyanide, volatile aldehydes, nitrogen oxides, carbon monoxide, "tar"	
Lung and larynx cancer	Major: PAH, NNK Minor: ^{210}polonium, formaldehyde, acetaldehyde, butadiene, metals (Cr, Cd, Ni)	Catechol, tumor promoters Acetaldehydes Diet Alkylating species
Oral cavity cancer	Major: NNN, NNK Minor: PAH	Herpes simplex, irritation Ethanol, diet
Esophageal cancer	NNN	Ethanol, diet
Urinary bladder	4-Aminobiphenyl, 2-naphthylamine, other aromatic amines	Urinary infection
Pancreas cancer	NNK, NNAL	Diet

[a]Abbreviations: PAH, polynuclear aromatic hydrocarbons; NNK, 4-(methylnitrosamine)-1-(3-pyridyl)-1-butanone; NNN, *N*′-nitrosonornicotine; NNAL, 4-(methylnitrosamino)-1-(3-pyridyl)-1-butanol.

cance to the smoker's risk of pancreas cancer. *N*′-Nitrosonornicotine may also be responsible in large measure for the increased rate of esophageal cancer among tobacco smokers. In rats, a total dose of 630 mg *N*′-nitrosonornicotine (10 mmol/kg) led to tumors of the esophagus. Within a 40-year period, a smoker of 40 cigarettes per day inhales a total of 290 mg of *N*′-nitrosonornicotine (0.025 μmol/kg).

Aromatic Amines

In this class of chemicals, 4-aminobiphenyl, 2-naphthylamine, and 2-toluidine have been identified among tobacco-smoke constituents. Both 4-aminobiphenyl and 2-naphthylamine are bladder carcinogens in humans. 2-Toluidine may also be an aromatic amine with potential bladder carcinogenic activity. Concentrations of aromatic amines in tobacco smoke are relatively low so that it is not clear whether they are indeed responsible for an elevated bladder cancer risk among smokers. Epidemiologists imply a role for these chemicals as smoke constituents that are involved in bladder carcinogenesis because of comparisons of bladder cancer incidences among smokers and persons with occupational exposure (gas-oven workers). It is also remarkable that the smoke of cigarettes made with 'black' tobacco contains higher concentrations of aromatic amines than the smoke of Virginia tobaccos or blended tobaccos. This is reflected in 4-aminobiphenyl hemoglobin adducts in the blood of smokers. Smokers of dark (black) tobaccos have a higher incidence of bladder cancer than the smokers of Virginia tobaccos or blends. In summary, these observations strengthen the hypothesis that aromatic amines are of significance as bladder carcinogens in smokers.

Aldehydes

Long-term inhalation assays with formaldehyde (14 ppm) and acetaldehyde (1000–3000 ppm) have indicated unambiguously that exposure to these aldehydes leads to tumors in the nasal mucosa. Because rats are obligatory nose breathers, this means that the aldehydes are contact carcinogens. For smokers who inhale tobacco smoke deeply into their lungs, this indicates that the aldehydes inhaled as smoke constituents are most likely also toxic to lung tissues. The experiments with rats do not indicate the dose levels of the aldehydes that were directly in contact with the nasal mucosa; thus, it is difficult to compare bioassays in animals with the inhalation of smoke by tobacco smokers. After all, the concentrations of aldehydes in smoke (i.e., 100 μg formaldehyde and 1,000 μg acetaldehyde per cigarette) are remarkably high. For the smoker of 40 cigarettes/day this translates into a total dose of 58 g formaldehyde (26 mmol/kg) and 580 g acetaldehyde (177 mmol/kg) over a 40-year period. These doses lie 1000- to 10,000-fold above those of polynuclear aromatic hydrocarbons and nitrosamines.

Benzene

Compared to the nonsmoker, the cigarette smoker's risk of myelocytic leukemia is two- to threefold higher. At this time, it is impossible to document a causal association of this elevated cancer risk with specific smoke constituents. However, it is important to consider that each cigarette smoker inhales 54–73 μg (47–67 ppm) of benzene with the mainstream smoke of cigarettes. Smokers exhaled 22–29 $\mu g/m^3$ benzene, while nonsmokers had 5–8 μg benzene/m^3 in their breath. The MAK list (maximum allowable concentrations list) of the Deutsche Forschungsgemeinschaft (German Research Association) describes benzene as an industrial (occupational) carcinogen that induces myelocytic leukemia. The urine of nonsmokers contains two to three times as much *t,t*-muconic acid, a metabolite of benzene, than the urine of nonsmokers.

Trans, trans-muconic acid can be employed as an indicator of benzene exposure because its concentration in urine is correlated with the degree of exposure. This observation supports the hypothesis that benzene may be responsible for the increased risk of leukemia among smokers.

Other Organic Compounds

The levels of an adduct formed from hemoglobin in blood with ethylene oxide are significantly higher in smokers than in nonsmokers. A group of investigators in Sweden calculated that up to 15% of the lung cancer rate in smokers may be attributed to endogenous formation of ethylene oxide from inhaled ethylene (176–250 μg/cigarette). The International Agency for Research on Cancer regards ethylene oxide as a human carcinogen. Cigarette smoke contains 7 μg ethylene oxide/cigarette.

Among the aza-arenes present in tobacco smoke are dibenz[*a,j*]acridine, dibenz[*a,h*]acridine, and 7*H*-dibenzo[*c,g*]carbazole. All three compounds are animal carcinogens, however, their concentrations in tobacco smoke are relatively low (Table 5). Quinoline, a liver carcinogen in rats and in newborn mice, is found in cigarette smoke at 1–2 μg, per cigarette. Acrylonitrile (3–15 μg/cigarette) is carcinogenic in bioassays, but it has not been possible to evaluate its significance and contribution to tobacco carcinogenesis.

Whether vinyl chloride is formed in tobacco smoke depends on the Cl concentration in tobacco (0.2–1%). Even though the presence of this occupational carcinogen in cigarette smoke has been established (1–16 ng/cigarette), its concentration is too low to warrant attributing major significance to this compound in tobacco carcinogenesis. 2-Nitropropane (1.0 μg/cigarette) and ethyl carbamate (urethane 0.03 μg/cigarette) may also play merely a minor role in this context.

In recent years, nanogram amounts of nine N-heterocyclic amines have been identified in cigarette smoke (e.g., PhlP-11–23 ng/cigarette). All of these compounds are carcinogenic in laboratory animals, and PhlP is also regarded as a possible human carcinogen. However, on the basis of current knowledge, it is not possible to assign a role in tobacco carcinogenesis to any of these N-heterocyclics.

Inorganic Compounds

Cigarette smoke contains traces of arsenic, nickel, chromium, cadmium, and lead (Table 5). It is not possible at this time to assign or to dismiss a role in tobacco carcinogenesis to any of these elements. In the case of nickel, of which 10–20% may transfer into the smoke, there may be some significance if sufficient nickel tetracarbon $Ni(CO)_4$, were formed. This compound is readily volatilized (bp 42°C) and was proven to be a lung carcinogen in bioassays with laboratory animals. There is no evidence, however, to document the type of nickel compound that occurs in the mainstream smoke of tobacco. Inhalation experiments with cadmium chloride (12.5, 25, and 50 $\mu g/m^3$) have shown that this compound is capable of inducing lung tumors in rats. In humans, cadmium is regarded as carcinogenic. It is present in tobacco mainstream smoke (47–350 ng/cigarette). Traces of hydrazine (24–43 ng/cigarette) were shown to occur in cigarette smoke. Hydrazine, given orally to mice and rats, induced tumors in the liver and in the lung; in inhalation assays with rats it elicited tumors in the nasal mucosa. Because of only trace amounts of hydrazine in tobacco smoke, a significant role in tobacco carcinogenesis can probably be ruled out. Polonium-210 is present in tobacco (0.2–1.2 pCi/g) and also in the smoke of cigarettes (0.03–1.0 pCi/cigarette). Because this element emits α-radiation, it is a strong lung carcinogen in humans, rats, and hamsters. Among smokers, deposition of ^{210}Po in the lungs has been three times greater than among nonsmokers. The U.S. Commission for Radiation Protection and Measurement estimated that in men about 1% of lung cancer risk for cigarette smokers after 50 years of smoking is due to ^{210}Po in the cigarette smoke. Table 6 presents a list of those compounds that contribute to the cancerogenic activity of tobacco smoke.

THE BIOCHEMISTRY OF TOBACCO CARCINOGENESIS

The biochemistry and molecular biology of tobacco cancerogenesis contribute not only to an understanding of mechanisms of carcinogenesis with respect to the various fractions of tar and individual smoke constituents, but also point to concepts for preventive strategies among smokers and nonsmokers. The delineation of the processes of metabolic activation and detoxification of smoke carcinogens and the quantification of specific adducts formed with them in humans is essential to such approaches. The analytical assessment of the dosimetry of uptake of carbon monoxide, thiocyanate, and nicotine by measuring these themselves, or by measuring their metabolites or adducts, can lead to objective evaluations. Mutagenicity tests of smokers' urine and the determination of chromosomal aberrations in the lymphocytes in peripheral blood can indicate the carcinogenic potential of cigarette smoke. However, such assessments are unspecific in view of the individuality of host responses to environmental carcinogens among smokers. One of the best approaches to determining specific host reactions is the quantitative assessment of adducts formed by the metabolites of xenobiotics with cellular macromolecules in individual smokers. This type of dosimetry of uptake and effect is based on the metabolic activation of procarcinogens. Most of the carcinogenic substances in tobacco smoke are procarcinogens that require metabolic activation by enzymes, and primarily by P450 isozymes.

Polynuclear Aromatic Hydrocarbons (PAH)

Biochemical studies have shown that procarcinogenic PAH are enzymatically converted into diolepoxides. These metabolites are the biologically active forms of PAH when a carbon atom is attached to an epoxy ring in the bay region of the structure. For benzo[*a*]pyrene, the biologically most active form is (+)7α, 8β-dihydroxy-9β,10β-epoxy-7,8,9,10-tetrahydro-benzo[*a*]pyrene [(+)-anti BPDE]. Activation of methylated PAH may lead to similar metabolites with even higher biological activity. The tobacco carcinogen 5-methylchrysene is converted into 1,2-dihydroxy-3,4-epoxy-1,2,3,4-tetrahydro-5-methylchrysene (Fig. 7). In 5-methylchrysene and in all of the other

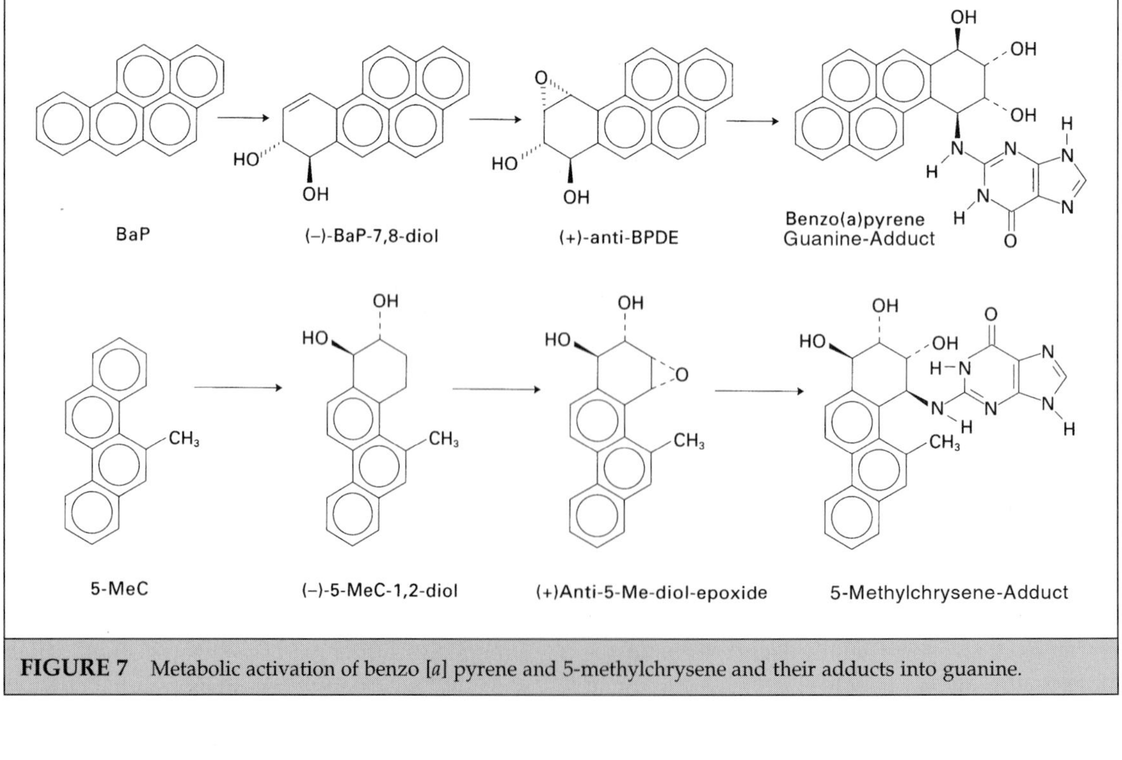

BaP → (−)-BaP-7,8-diol → (+)-anti-BPDE → Benzo(a)pyrene Guanine-Adduct

5-MeC → (−)-5-MeC-1,2-diol → (+)Anti-5-Me-diol-epoxide → 5-Methylchrysene-Adduct

FIGURE 7 Metabolic activation of benzo [*a*] pyrene and 5-methylchrysene and their adducts into guanine.

carcinogenic methyl-PAH, the methyl group and epoxide group are in the same bay region. The significance of the carcinogenic PAH and methyl PAH in tobacco carcinogenesis lies primarily in their role as initiators of tumorigenesis because their presence in the smoke is at a relatively low concentration. Their effects are potentiated by the tumor-promoting and carcinogenic properties of other tobacco-smoke constituents and become evident only because of this potentiation. The sum of all polynuclear aromatic hydrocarbons in the neutral subfraction B1 of tobacco tar can explain only a minor proportion of the total carcinogenic activity of the tars. However, when subfraction B1 is applied to mouse skin or rabbit ear together with solutions of the weakly acidic fraction of the tar, tumor yields reach 75–90% of the effects observed with whole tar. The weakly acidic fraction, as such, does not induce tumors; it contains phenols that function as tumor promoters and catechols with cocarcinogenic potential. The metabolically activated forms of carcinogenic PAH form adducts with DNA, RNA, and proteins. Tests with the ^{32}P-post-labeling method have shown that tissues excised from the lungs of smokers during surgery contain multiple DNA adducts. Such DNA adducts occur at different levels and in various forms in the tissues of the lung and of the respiratory airways. They have also been found in the lungs of nonsmokers. The frequency of their occurrence in smokers can be correlated with cigarette consumption and with the intensity of smoke uptake.

An HPLC fluorimetric analysis has shown that hydrolysis of DNA adducts in tumor-free tissues harvested from lung cancer patients liberates 7,8,9,10-tetrahydroxy,7,8,9,10-tetrahydrobenzo[*a*]pyrene. This benzo[*a*]pyrene metabolite was also identified upon hydrolysis of DNA adducts in the lung tissues from a majority of smokers. The correlation between concentration of benzo[*a*]pyrene-DNA adducts and aryl hydrocarbon hydroxylase activity in lung tissues appears to be significant. These studies strengthen the hypothesis that smokers have different sensitivities to tobacco carcinogens due to individual capacities for metabolic activation of procarcinogens and DNA adduct formation.

Tobacco-Specific *N*-Nitrosamines

Among seven tobacco-specific *N*-nitrosamines identified in tobacco smoke (Fig. 2), *N*-nitrosonornicotine and 4-(methylnitrosamino)-1-(3-pyridyl)-l-butanone are especially potent animal carcinogens. They are converted enzymatically to labile hydroxynitrosamines, which then decompose into diazohydroxides, aldehydes, and ketones (Fig. 8). *In vitro* studies with tissues from animals and humans, and also *in vivo* research with laboratory animals, have shown that DNA adducts with 4-(methylnitrosamino)-1-(3-pyridyl)-1-butanone are formed via methylation and pyridylbutyl oxidation pathways. Thus, *N*-7-methylguanine, O^6-methylguanine, and O^4-methylthymidine have been found in DNA isolated from lung tissues of smokers. O^6-methylguanine is a promutagenic base that is enriched in the DNA of lung tissues of animals treated with 4-(methyl-nitrosamino)-1-(3-pyridyl)-1-butanone because 4-(methylnitrosamino)-1-(3-pyridyl)-1-butanone inhibits methyl transferase activity and thus DNA repair. Besides the fact that 4-(methylnitrosamino)-1-(3-pyridyl)-1-butanone forms O^6-methylguanine in DNA of lung tissues, which leads to changes in the genetic code, it is remarkable that adenocarcinoma formed from such lesions were found to contain activated K-*ras* oncogenes. The latter have also been identified in lung adenocarcinoma of 41 (29%) among 141 cigarette smokers; among nonsmokers, activated K-*ras* oncogene was found only in 2 (5%) of 40 patients. Activation of K-*ras* oncogene on codon 12 appears to be a significant event in the pathogenesis of lung adenocarcinoma. A study published in 1990 found that a group of cancer patients with activated K-*ras* oncogene in their lung adenocarcinoma has especially poor prognoses. In summary, it can be stated that nicotine leads to the formation of 4-(methylnitrosamino)-1-(3-pyridyl)-l-butanone during post-harvest processing of tobacco and during smoking. Upon inhalation, the DNA adduct O^6-methylguanine is formed in the lung tissues of smokers and it activates the K-*ras* oncogene. This is a basic step towards lung cancer development.

The metabolic activation of 4-(methylnitrosamino)-1-(3-pyridyl)-1-butanone leads not only to methylhydroxide formation (Fig. 8) but also to 4-(methylnitrosamino)-l-(3-pyridyl)-4-oxobutyldiazohydroxide. This same compound is also formed by α-hydroxylation of *N'*-nitrosonornicotine. *In vivo* this intermediate reacts with DNA and proteins. Hydrolysis of such protein adducts yields a keto alcohol that is also obtained upon hydrolysis of hemoglobin adducts from animals treated with *N'*-nitrosonornicotine or with 4-(methylnitrosamino)-1-(3-pyridyl)-l-butanone. Thus, the determination of this keto alcohol via hemoglobin-adduct analysis can serve to assess the dosimetry of uptake in smokers. Among 40 smokers examined for the presence of hemoglobin adducts with the metabolites of tobacco-specific *N*-nitrosamines, seven showed increased levels of such adducts. This is prob-

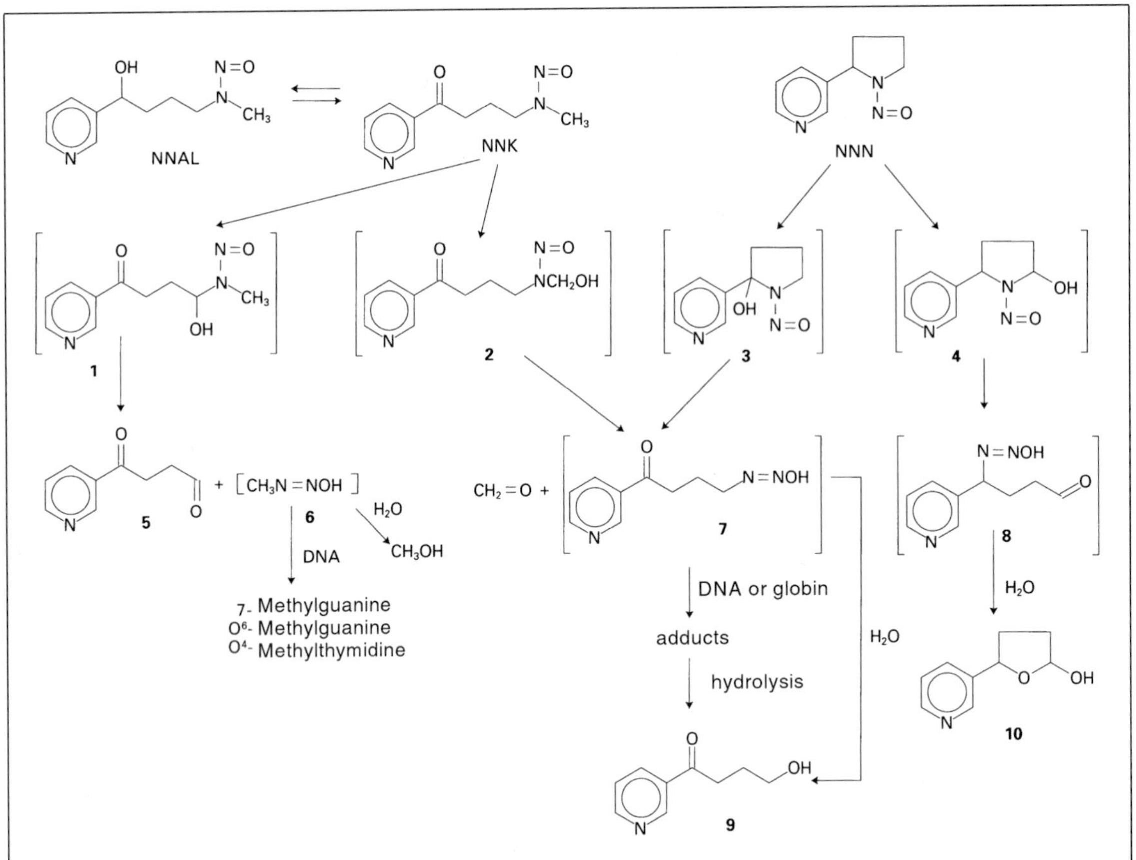

FIGURE 8 Metabolic activation of 4-(methylnitrosamino)-1-(3-pyridyl)-1-butanone (NNK) and of *N′*-nitrosonornicotine (NNN).

ably related to their individual capacity for metabolic activation of tobacco-specific nitrosamines.

AROMATIC AMINES

On the basis of epidemiologic and experimental studies, 4-aminobiphenyl and 2-naphthylamine are regarded as bladder carcinogens that are probably responsible for the elevated bladder cancer risk among smokers. It is known that activation of these compounds proceeds via N-acetylation and N-hydroxylation and that in the epithelium of the bladder DNA adducts are formed with metabolites of these aromatic amines. Also protein adducts are formed. In the case of 4-aminobiphenyl, a sulfonic acid amine is bound to β-cysteine. When hemoglobin from smokers is treated with mild acid, traces of aminobiphenyl can be obtained. A newly developed, highly sensitive gas chromatography-mass spectrometry (GC/MS) method enables the determination of 4-aminobiphenyl adducts with hemoglobin. Comparative studies among men smoking different types of cigarettes documented that significantly higher adduct formation takes place among smokers of black-tobacco cigarettes. These smokers are known to have a higher risk for cancer of the bladder than smokers of bright or blended cigarettes. It is also fact that the smoke of these types of cigarettes contains more of the aromatic amines than does smoke from cigarettes made of blond tobaccos.

PASSIVE SMOKING

The respiratory burden of tobacco-smoke-derived indoor air pollutants causes an increased susceptibility of infants to bronchitis and lung infections. Whether such burden also leads to lung cancer among nonsmokers has been examined in epidemiologic studies since about 1980. The International Agency for Research on Cancer (IARC) in Lyon, France, concluded a review of literature on this topic in 1985 with the following statement, "The observations on nonsmokers that have been made so far are compatible with either an increased risk from 'passive' smoking or an absence of risk." Retrospective and prospective epidemiologic investigations that have dealt with the question have determined risk factors below 2.0. On closer examination of the data, there is still a lack of fulfillment of the criteria for causality of a relationship between (passive) exposure to environmental tobacco smoke and lung cancer. These criteria include magnitude of the association, consistency of findings, logical agreement of temporal factors of exposure and effect, and biological plausibility. When risk factors lie below 3.0, one needs to consider whether the data collection and interpretation may suffer from bias, confounding, or an incorrect selection of the population that was examined. With regard to consistency of the data, the histologic confirmation of lung tumors is important. Among smokers, Kreyberg type I lung cancer (squamous cell cancer) predominated for many years over Kreyberg type II (glandular) lung cancer. Among nonsmokers with lung cancer, it was primarily Kreyberg type II, mostly in the form of adenoma and adenocarcinoma, that is most frequently seen. However, the ratios of Kreyberg type I and type II lung cancers among smokers have heavily shifted in recent decades towards an increasing preponderance of type II. Whether there is truly a causal relationship between lung cancer and exposure to environmental tobacco smoke and what the significance of the histological type of tumor is in this relationship remains to be examined through further research.

It is not easy to determine the relationship between passive-smoke exposure and the appearance of lung cancer through epidemiologic assessment because the recollection of facts regarding past exposure during childhood can be blurred by ignorance or by the bias of those questioned. To elucidate the biological plausibility of a causal relationship of passive smoking with lung cancer, it is helpful to rely on knowledge of the composition of mainstream and sidestream smoke and data about dosimetry, uptake, and metabolism of key constituents of tobacco smoke. The IARC deduces from this knowledge and from evidence on dose and effect relationships in chemical carcinogenesis that passive smoking may cause "some risk of cancer." A more detailed evaluation of this question is based on examining the physicochemical and chemical–biological properties of tobacco-smoke-polluted environments. A major source for such air pollutants is the sidestream smoke that is formed when cigarettes, cigars, and pipes smolder during puff intervals. In addition, the smoke emitted from the mouthpiece of the tobacco product and from the exhaled breath of smokers after smoke uptake by inhalation make minor contributions to this type of air pollution.

Table 7 presents a quantitative comparison of some select constituents of sidestream smoke and mainstream smoke. Generally, the levels of compounds in the sidestream smoke exceed those in the mainstream smoke by 30–100%. Lesser amounts in sidestream smoke are found only for hydrogen cyanide, catechol, hydroquinone, and benzoic acid. Chemical compounds that are formed during smoldering are, of course, especially prevalent in sidestream smoke. Among these are primarily the volatile *N*-nitrosamines, such as nitrosodimethylamine and the aromatic amines, 4-aminobiphenyl, and 2-naphthylamine. In evaluating health risks from passive smoking, one needs to be mindful of the fact that sidestream smoke becomes substantially diluted with air before the environmented tobacco-smoke pollutants are inhaled. Table 8 is a list of measurements of pollution levels in various indoor atmospheres. None of the measurements in these examples exceeds the maximal permissible concentrations of pollutants in occupational environments that were established by the American Conference of Governmental Industrial Hygienists and by the German Research Association (Deutsche Forschungsgemeinschaft), except for those tobacco-smoke constituents in indoor air that are carcinogenic but should not normally be present in occupational environments. These include 4-aminobiphenyl, 2-naphthylamine, benzene, volatile nitrosamines, and polynuclear aromatic hydrocarbons that result from pyrolysis of organic matter.

SUMMARY

Epidemiologic studies have clearly documented that cigarette smoking causes cancer of the lung, trachea, larynx, oral cavity, esophagus, kidneys, and bladder. Smokers of cigars and pipes also face an increased risk for these cancers, although except for cancer of the oral cavity, larynx, and esophagus, this risk is lower than that for the cigarette smoker. Smokers also are more prone to develop chronic bronchitis and emphysema than are nonsmokers. By far the greatest number of tobacco-related deaths is attributable to myocardial infarction. Inhalation experiments with cigarette smoke lead to benign and malignant tumors of the respiratory airways and especially in the larynx in the Syrian golden hamster. Because the gas phase of cigarette smoke does not induce tumors in this animal model, most of

TABLE 7 Distribution of Constituents in Fresh Undiluted Mainstream Smoke (MS) and Diluted Sidestream Smoke (SS) from Nonfilter Cigarettes[a]

Constituent	Amount in MS	Range in SS/MS
Vapor phase		
Carbon monoxide	10–23 mg	2.5–4.7
Carbon dioxide	20–40 mg	8–11
Carbonyl sulfide	18–42 μg	0.03–0.13
Benzene	12–48 μg	5–10
Toluene	100–200 μg	5.6–8.3
Formaldehyde	70–100 μg	0.1–≃50
Acrolein	60–100 μg	8–15
Acetone	100–250 μg	2–5
Pyridine	16–40 μg	6.5–20
3-Methylpyridine	12–36 μg	3–13
3-Vinylpyridine	11–30 μg	20–40
Hydrogen cyanide	400–500 μg	0.1–0.25
Hydrazine	32 ng	3
Ammonia	50–130 μg	40–170
Methylamine	11.5–28.7 μg	4.2–6.4
Dimethylamine	7.8–10 μg	3.7–5.1
Nitrogen oxides	100–600 μg	4–10
N-Nitrosodimethylamine	10–40 ng	20–100
N-Nitrosodiethylamine	ND–25 ng	<40
N-Nitrosopyrrolidine	6–30 ng	6–30
Formic acid	210–490 μg	1.4–1.6
Acetic acid	330–810 μg	1.9–3.6
Methyl chloride	150–600 μg	1.7–3.3
Particulate phase		
Particulate matter	15–40 mg	1.3–1.9
Nicotine	1–2.5 mg	2.6–3.3
Anatabine	2–20 μg	<0.1–0.5
Phenol	60–140 μg	1.6–3.0
Catechol	100–360 μg	0.6–0.9
Hydroquinone	110–300 μg	0.7–0.9
Aniline	360 ng	30
2-Toluidine	160 ng	19
2-Naphthylamine	1.7 ng	30
4-Aminobiphenyl	4.6 ng	31
Benz[*a*]anthracene	20–70 ng	2–4
Benzo[*a*]pyrene	20–40 ng	2.5–3.5
Cholesterol	22 μg	0.9
γ-Butyrolactone	10–22 μg	3.6–5.0
Quinoline	0.5–2 μg	8–11
Harman	1.7–3.1 μg	0.7–1.7
N′-Nitrosonornicotine	200–3,000 ng	0.5–3
NNK	100–1,000 ng	1–4
N-Nitrosodiethanolamine	20–70 ng	1.2
Cadmium	100 ng	7.2
Nickel	20–80 ng	13–30
Zinc	60 ng	6.7
Polonium-210	0.04–0.1 pCi	1.0–4.0
Benzoic acid	14–28 μg	0.67–0.95
Lactic acid	63–174 μg	0.5–0.7
Glycolic acid	37–126 μg	0.6–0.95
Succinic acid	110–140 μg	0.43–0.62

[a]National Research Council (1986).

TABLE 8 Some Toxic and Tumorigenic Agents in Indoor Environments Polluted by Tobacco Smoke

Pollutant	Location	Concentration (m^3)
Nitric oxide	Workrooms	50–440 μg
	Restaurants	17–240 μg
	Bar	80–520 μg
	Cafeteria	2.5–48 μg
Nitrogen dioxide	Workrooms	68–410 μg
	Restaurants	40–190 μg
	Bar	2–116 μg
	Cafeteria	67–200 μg
Hydrogen cyanide	Living room	8–122 μg
Benzene	Public places	20–317 μg
Formaldehyde	Living room	23–50 μg
Acrolein	Public places	30–120 μg
Acetone	Public places	360–5800 μg
Phenols (volatile)	Coffee houses	7.4–11.5 ng
N-Nitrosodimethylamine	Restaurants, public places	0–240 ng
N-Nitrosodiethylamine	Restaurants, public places	0–200 ng
Nicotine	Public places	1–6 μg
	Restaurants	3–10 μg
	Workrooms	1–13.8 μg
Benzo[*a*]pyrene	Restaurants, public places	3.3–144 ng
N′-Nitrosonornicotine	Bar, restaurant, car	4–32 ng
4-(Methylnitrosamino)-1-(3-pyridyl)-1-butanone	Bar, restaurant, car	1–120 ng

the carcinogenic potential of tobacco smoke is attributed to its particulate phase, the tar. Biochemical studies have delineated that most of the tobacco carcinogens, (i.e., the polynuclear aromatic hydrocarbons, the tobacco-specific nitrosamines, and the aromatic amines) are procarcinogens. As such, they are metabolically activated through enzymatic action to become biologically reactive. Active metabolites of the procarcinogens react *in vitro* and *in vivo* to form adducts with cellular macromolecules like DNA, RNA, and proteins. Certain DNA adducts, primarily O^6-methylguanine and O^4-methylthymidine are promutagenic bases that are regarded as the first step in the induction of neoplasms. The quantitative assessment of DNA adducts and hemoglobin adducts formed with metabolites of benzo[a]pyrene and of tobacco-specific *N*-nitrosamines and/or aromatic amines are used as markers of dosimetry and uptake and of individual patterns of enzyme activities (phenotypic propensity for carcinogen activation).

The possibility that nonsmokers face a substantial cancer risk from passive tobacco smoke exposure continues to be criticially examined. Some qualitative similarities of carcinogens in mainstream tobacco smoke and in smoke-polluted indoor environments indicate that the passive smoker inhales carcinogens, albeit at a far lower dosage than the smoker of cigarettes. To verify whether the burden of environmental tobacco-smoke exposure poses a risk for nonsmokers remains a challenge for translational epidemiology, researchers in the natural sciences, and public health agencies.

Bibliography

Hoffmann, D., and Hecht, S. S. (1989). Advances in tobacco carcinogenesis. *In* "Springer Handbook of Experimental Pharmacology—Chemical Carcinogenesis and Mutagenesis" (C. S. Cooper and P. L. Grover, eds.) pp. 63–102. Springer Verlag, Berlin.

International Agency for Research on Cancer (1986). "Tobacco Smoking." IARC Monographs on the Evaluation of the Carcinogenic Risk of Chemicals to Humans 38. IARC, Lyon, France.

Landis, S. H., Murray, T., Bolden, S., and Wingo, P. A. (1999). Cancer Statistics. *CA-A Cancer J. Clinicians* **49,** 8–31.

Parkin, D. M., Pisani, P., and Ferlay, J. (1999). Global Cancer Statistics. *CA-A Cancer J. Clinicians* **49,** 33–64.

Royal College of Physicians (1962). "Smoking and Health." Pittman, London.

Shopland, D. R., Eyre, H. J., and Pechacek, T. F. (1991). Smoking-attributable cancer mortality in 1991. *J. Nat. Cancer Inst.* **83,** 1142–1148.

U.S. Surgeon General (1964). "Smoking and Health" Publication No. 1103. U.S. Public Health Service, Rockville, MD.

U.S. Surgeon General (1986). "The Health Consequences of Involuntary Smoking." DHHS (CDC) 87-8398. Washington D.C.

U.S. Surgeon General (1989). "The Health Consequences of Smoking: 25 Years of Progress." DHHS Public No. (CDC) 89-8411. Washington D.C.

Wynder, E. L. (1998). The past, present, and future of lung cancer. *Cancer Epidemiol. Biomarkers Prev.* **7,** 735–748.

Wynder, E. L., and Hoffmann, D. (eds.) (1967). "Tobacco and Tobacco Smoke: Studies in Experimental Carcinogenesis." Academic Press, New York.

CHAPTER

37

Cosmetic Toxicology

JOHN F. CORBETT, RAJ K. SHARMA, WILLIAM E. DRESSLER

Bristol-Myers Squibb Worldwide Beauty Care, Stamford, Connecticut

INTRODUCTION

Decorative cosmetics and fragrances have been part of almost every culture for many thousands of years but a formal approach to the toxicological evaluation of cosmetic products has only evolved during the 20th century. Initially; the evaluation involved only dermal, ocular, and, in some cases, mucous membrane irritation toxicity and allergenicity via the Draize eye and skin tests in rabbits and guinea pigs. This was sometimes followed by clinical studies in humans.

The recognition that the skin was not an impermeable barrier to topically applied materials required that systemic toxicity, including both acute and chronic effects, also be taken into account. For the most part, and for obvious reasons, ingredients used in products subject to incidental ingestion, such as lipstick, have received particular attention, followed by those used in the eye area and products applied to and left on the skin, while rinse-off products, except for hair dyes, have been of least concern.

This chapter will consider the scope of testing that is generally accepted as desirable for cosmetic products, together with the chemical nature of the active ingredients used in selected specialized hair products such as dyes, bleaches, permanent waves, and straighteners. For other varied types of cosmetic products, use experience and some general principles regarding safety evaluation and risk assessment will be discussed. In addition, reference will be made to the particular requirements for and methods of reviews of safety data in the European Union, the United States and Japan.

COSMETIC SAFETY REGULATION

The United States

In the U.S., the Food, Drug and Cosmetic Act designates the Food and Drug Administration as the agency responsible for cosmetic safety.

For this purpose, the FDA has defined cosmetics as "articles to be rubbed, poured, sprinkled, or sprayed on or introduced into, or otherwise applied to the human body or any part thereof for cleansing, beautifying, promoting attractiveness, or altering the appearance, and articles intended for use as a component of any such articles; except that such term shall not include soap." The exemption for soap applies only to a composition consisting of an alkali metal salt of a fatty acid that is intended only for cleansing.

Certain cosmetic products that are "intended for use in the diagnosis, cure, mitigation, treatment or prevention of disease" are classified by FDA as drugs. This category includes sunscreen products, anticavity toothpastes, antiperspirants (as opposed to deodorants, which are "cosmetics"), antidandruff preparations, "medicated" skin lotions and liquids, skin protectants, and hair restorers.

Under the regulations, the active ingredients in cosmetic drug products must be safe and effective according to the appropriate monograph covering the claimed indication.

The only category of cosmetic ingredient subject to FDA approval is colors used for purposes other than dyeing the hair. There are only 36 "certified colors" and 23 "permitted" colors available for general use in cosmetics, and a further 7 that are permitted only for specific uses. In addition, a number of lakes of the soluble certified colors are available.

For all other cosmetic ingredients, the safety evaluation is the responsibility of the manufacturer. In order to assist its members in this, the Cosmetic, Toiletry, and Fragrance Association (CTFA) established in 1976 the Cosmetic Ingredient Review (CIR) to review all the available data on an ingredient and to decide whether the ingredient is safe under the conditions of use. The CIR expert panel comprises six independent scientists as voting members and a nonvoting member representing each of the CTFA, the FDA, and the consumer. By 1996, the CIR had reviewed over 600 ingredients, finding 64% to be safe as used, 27% to be safe for use under defined conditions, 8% to have insufficient data, and five ingredients to be unsafe.

The CIR expert panel currently requests the following as a minimum data requirement for reviewing the safety of the cosmetic ingredients that are on its priority list:

1. Current concentration of use data.
2. Chemistry data, including method of manufacture and impurities.
3. UV-absorption data; if absorption occurs in the UVA or UVB range, photosensitization data are needed.
4. Skin-irritation and -sensitization data at concentrations of use in humans.
5. Dermal-absorption data; if significant dermal absorption occurs, 28-day dermal-toxicity and development-toxicity data are needed.
6. Two genotoxicity studies, one using a mammalian system; if positive, a 2-year dermal carcinogenicity assay performed using NTP methods is needed.

Additional studies may be requested based on the nature and use of the ingredient.

The European Union

In the European Union, cosmetics are regulated under the Cosmetics Directive (76/768/EEC) of 1976 and amendments thereto. For the purpose of regulation, cosmetics are more broadly defined than in the United States, viz. "any substance or preparation intended to be placed in contact with various external parts of the human body (epidermis, hair system, nails, lips and external genitalia) and with the teeth or mucous membranes of the oral cavity with a view exclusively or mainly to cleaning them, perfuming them, changing their appearance and/or correcting body odors and/or protecting them or keeping them in good condition." This definition covers many of the product categories that are considered to be over-the-counter drugs in the U.S.

In common with the United States, cosmetics do not require premarket clearance in Europe. However, certain ingredients, notably colorants (other than hair dyes), preservatives, and sunscreens, do require approval before they can be used in cosmetic products. The list of permitted colorants (Annex IV) is broader than the U.S. list, comprising 157 materials.

The approval process involves the submission of data via COLIPA, the European trade association, to the European Commission. The data is evaluated by a group of independent experts who make up the Scientific Committee for Cosmetology and Non-Food Products (SCCNFP) and who decide whether the ingredient can be accepted for listing in the appropriate Annex. Data requirements are similar to those listed above for the CIR.

The General Toxicological Requirements for Cosmetic Ingredients (1996 revision) state:

> When requested, the manufacturer shall provide the Commission with the information set out below:
>
> 1. Acute toxicity
> 2. Dermal absorption
> 3. Dermal irritation
> 4. Mucous membrane irritation
> 5. Skin sensitization
> 6. Sub-chronic toxicity
> 7. Mutagenicity
> 8. Phototoxicity and Photomutagenciny (in case of UV-light absorbing substances)
> 9. Human data (if available)
>
> When considerable oral intake can be expected or when the data or dermal absorption do indicate a considerable penetration of the ingredients through the skin, taking into account the toxicological profile of the substance and its chemical structure, the following further information may be necessary:
>
> 10. Toxicokinetics
> 11. Teratogenicity, Reproduction toxicity, Carcinogenicity, and additional Genotoxicity.

Additionally, there is now a legal requirement, formalized in Article 7a of the sixth amendment to the Cosmetics Directive, that cosmetic companies hold a technical dossier of information on each of their products. This requirement applies to every cosmetic product, both retail and professional, including imported products.

This dossier must include information or product composition, specifications, and method of manufacture, as well as an assessment of product safety carried out by an appropriately qualified expert. The assessment must take account of the general toxicological profile of the ingredients, their chemical structures, and the potential levels of exposure.

The SCC is also responsible for recommending the listing of substances prohibited for use in cosmetics (Annex II) and substances that can be used with certain limitations with regard to product category, concentration, and/or special labeling requirements (Annex III).

In addition to these requirements, the EU regulation for the Notification of New Substances must be followed by companies introducing new chemicals. These regulations state that "a material is considered to be a new substahce within the EU if it is not listed in EINECS (European Inventory of Existing Chemical Substances)." EINECS is a closed list (closed in 1981), that is, no new substances can now be added.

Substances not in EINECS must be notified according to Council Directive 92/32/EEC (seventh amendment to the EC Dangerous Substances Directive) prior to marketing in the EU. Notified substances are issued in ELINCS (European List of New Chemical Substances). ELINCS is an open list, that is, new substances may be added once notified according to the Directive.

The precise contents of a notification depend on the quantity of the substance to be placed or already placed on the market. The notification system is banded, the information required increasing as the quantity of a substance placed on the market increases.

Japan

The Japanese regulation of cosmetics is the most restrictive. While the definition of a cosmetic is similar to that in the U.S., the number of product types considered to be "quasi-drugs" (analogous to cosmetic drugs or O.T.C. products) is much greater. Thus, in addition to the U.S. categories, products to combat bad breath, bath preparations, hair dyes, permanent waves, talcum powder, depilatories, shaving lotions, and skin packs are considered "quasi-drugs."

In Japan, all cosmetic products are subject to premarket approval by the Ministry of Health and Welfare and can contain only those ingredients included in the Comprehensive Licensing Standards of Cosmetics by Category (CLS) and these must conform to certain defined specifications. New ingredients can be added to the list on the basis of the submission of appropriate toxicological data.

For quasi-drugs, there are lists of permitted active ingredients for use in hair dyes, permanent waves, and medicated toothpastes. Lists for other categories are being developed.

For countries other than those discussed here, ingredients acceptable in the United States and/or Europe would usually be acceptable.

HAIR COSMETICS

Permanent Waves

The conformational integrity of the hair fiber is maintained by various interactions between protein chains making up the cortex. These comprise polar (electrostatic) and nonpolar interactions between the side chains of the amino acids, hydrogen bonding, and covalent bonding—in particular the interchain disulfide bonds of the amino acid cystine.

A temporary set can be imparted to hair simply by wetting the hair, restraining it in the desired new conformation, and drying it while still constrained. On the release of the constraint, the hair will retain the new conformation until it is again exposed to water or even to high humidity.

If a more permanent effect is desired, it is necessary to break and reform covalent bonds, as is done in the process of permanent waving. For this purpose, thiols (compounds containing the -SH group) have been found to be the most effective at reducing the disulfide bond.

Essentially the permanent wave process involves about six or seven steps:

1. Rolling, in which a section of hair is wound onto a perm rod. In this step the hair may be first dampened with water or with the waving lotion.
2. The application of waving lotion, if the hair was dry-rolled or water-rolled, to the hair on the rods in such a way as to saturate each hair mass.
3. The creep step, in which the reduced hair is left on the rods for about 20 minutes to allow movement of segments within the individual cortex.
4. Water rinsing, which is then carried out with the hair still on the rods.
5. Neutralization, in which the disulfide bonds are rebuilt. This step can be performed on or off the rods depending on the desired end result.
6. Rinsing to remove the excess neutralizer and other chemicals, which is performed after removal of the rods.
7. Styling and drying.

Because of the complexity of the process and the skill required to obtain satisfactory results, the market for home perms is small compared to that for salon products. As a consequence, professional hairdressers have greater exposure to perm chemicals than do the general public.

Although literally thousands of thiol compounds have been investigated as reducing agents for the keratin disulfide bonds, only derivatives of thioglycolic acid, cysteine and, to a lesser extent, ammonium bisulfite and ammonium thiolacetate have achieved commercial importance.

The thiols work best at pH levels slightly below the pK_a of the thiol group. Most "cold wave" or "alkaline" perms are based on ammonium thioglycolate at a pH of about 9.2 (the pK_a of thioglycolic acid is 10.4), while the "acid waves" employ glyceryl monothioglycolate (GMT), which has a pK_a of 7.8 and is applied in a composition having a pH of about 6.8, the reduction step generally being performed under a heating device such as a hair dryer of infrared lamp.

The reduction step can be represented as

$$\text{K-S-S-K} + \text{RS}^- \rightarrow \text{K-S-S-R} + \text{KS}^-$$

$$\text{K-S-S-R} + \text{RS}^- \rightarrow \text{K-S}^- + \text{R-S-S-R}$$

where K represents a keratin protein chain and RS^- is the thiolate perming agent.

The rebuilding step, which usually employs hydrogen peroxide, although the previously widely used potassium bromate neutralizer is still occasionally used, can be represented as

$$2\text{K-S-H} + H_2O_2 \rightarrow \text{K-S-S-K} + 2H_20$$

In the case of bisulfite perms, which give much weaker results, the reduction step is performed at pH 6 and involves the formation of a Bunte salt.

$$\text{K-S-S-K} + HSO_3^- \rightarrow \text{K-S-H} + \text{K-S-}SO_3^-$$

Neutralization is performed by reversing the above reaction by treatment with a solution buffered at pH 8 and containing a little hydrogen peroxide, which serves to oxidize the liberated sulfite to sulfate.

Apart from occasional cases of skin irritation, dermal problems among recipients of permanent waves are rare. More common are problems with dryness and brittleness of the hair due to overprocessing in the form of too strong a lotion for the particular hair type, too long a residence time of the waving lotion, or inadequate rinsing or neutralization.

The use of ammonium thioglycolate in the cold wave process has the advantage that evaporation of the ammonia results in lowering of the pH and, with that, the possibility of over-reduction of the disulfide bonds. The use of alkanolamines in place of ammonia has the advantage of better odor but carries with it the possibility of over-reduction.

There have been few examples of sensitization from exposure to the alkaline thioglycolate waves, even among hairdressers. On the other hand, glyceryl monothioglycolate has been shown to be a sensitizer and allergies to it are reported to be common among hairdressers in some countries, notably Germany and Holland.

Adverse reactions can be minimized by the adherence to certain guidelines.

1. Commercial use of single-dose rather than bulk GMT to avoid contamination of work surfaces and measuring equipment.
2. Water rolling rather than lotion rolling of the hair.
3. The use of suitable disposable gloves while handling the hair and rinsing of the gloves before disposal.
4. General good work practices to avoid contamination of work surfaces and equipment.

Hair Straighteners

Conventional thioglycolate and sulfite permanent waving products are relatively ineffective when used to straighten African hair because the hair tends to revert to the curly state within a short time.

Treatment with highly alkaline compositions (pH ~ 13), known in the trade as relaxers, is the most effective way to achieve a long-lasting result. The most widely used products contain 2–4% sodium hydroxide in an emulsion system containing petrolatum, fatty alcohols, mineral oil, and 40–50% water.

Products promoted as "no lye relaxers" employ either guanidinium hydroxide or lithium hydroxide as the alkali.

Under these highly alkaline conditions it is believed that a C–S bond in cystine is broken to give an aminoacrylic residue that reacts with the disulfide to give lanthiomine or with an aminoalkyl side chain to give lysinoalanine. These new interchain linkages are unreactive to chemicals used in hair products, including alkaline and reducing agents, thus creating a permanent conformational change.

Due to their high alkalinity, great care must be exercised in the use of relaxers. Every effort must be made to avoid contact with the scalp, which would result in a chemical burn. Sometimes a base coat of petrolatum is applied to the scalp and around the hair line, although this is very difficult given the density of the hair.

In use, the thick composition is applied to the hair, section by section, and pulled through with a comb vertically away from the scalp. If the hair is combed parallel to the scalp, a right angle will be set into the hair where it emerges from the follicle and, after about two weeks of new hair growth this will become a point of breakage when the hair is combed. Contact time for these products is about 15 minutes and should not exceed 20 minutes.

Hair Dyes

There are a wide variety of products marketed for changing the color of human hair and they can conveniently be divided into three groups according to the type of coloring materials.

The most important of these groups, representing about 80% of the market in the U.S., is the oxidation dyes, which employ colorless precursors and an oxidizing agent (usually hydrogen peroxide) that together are capable of producing colored molecules inside the hair. This class is often referred to as "permanent" because the dyes formed do not readily diffuse out of the hair during subsequent shampooing. A unique feature of this class of product is the ability to formulate them to simultaneously lighten the hair's natural color and deposit the synthetic color. This is because hydrogen peroxide is a good bleaching agent for the melanin, which constitutes the natural hair pigment. Thus, oxidation dyes can be used to change the color of hair to darker or lighter shades that may have warm red, gold, neutral, or cool ash nuances, as well as to cover grey without necessarily producing a darker shade than that of the individual's naturally pigmented hair.

The second group in commercial importance is the direct or preformed dyes. This group can be further subdivided into semipermanent dyes, which withstand six to twelve shampoos, and temporary dyes, which wash out in one shampoo.

A smaller segment of the market is the group based on natural dyes extracted from plants, which have lasting properties similar to those of the semipermanent dyes.

Finally, there is the group for products based on metal salts. In Europe and the United States, these usually contain a solution of lead acetate and are known as progressive dyes, which are mainly used by men for grey coverage. In Asia, there are also products that employ polyhydric phenols, particularly pyrogallol, and ferrous salts. These are used by both men and women exclusively for covering grey hair.

Oxidation Dyes

The oxidation dyes have been in use for over 100 years and were based on the discovery that a mixture of *p*-phenylenediamine and an oxidizing agent could produce color on hair. This color was shown to be due to the formation of Bandrowski's base.

Modern oxidation dyes contain four essential classes of ingredients in a suitably thickened detersive base.

p-Phenylenediamine and other para diamines, and *o*- and *p*-aminophenols, referred to as the primary intermediates, are materials that individually are capable of being oxidized to give colored reaction products.

The second class contains the couplers, which are aromatic compounds that do not themselves produce colored products on oxidation but, when present during the oxidation of the primary intermediates, result in the production of colored species.

The couplers are generally meta di-functional benzene derivatives such as *m*-phenylenediamines, *m*-aminophenols, and resorcinols. Additionally, certain monohydric phenols, such as 1-naphthols and thymol, are useful as couplers.

The color-forming reactions have been shown to involve the initial oxidation of the primary intermediate to form a *p*-benzoquinonediimine from *p*-diamines, or monoamine from *p*-aminophenols. These imines are highly reactive toward the nucleophilic couplers and react to form diphenylamine leuco-dyes, which are rapidly oxidized to indo-dyes, (Fig. 1).

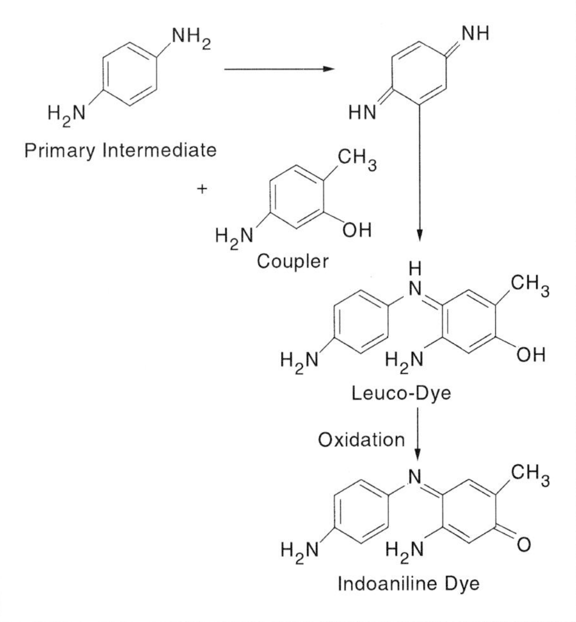

FIGURE 1 Dye formation in oxidative dyeing of human hair.

TABLE 1 Primary Intermediates Used in Oxidation Dyeing

p-Phenylenediamine
2,5-Diaminotoluene
N-Phenyl-*p*-phenylenediamine
N,N'-bis(2-Hydroxyethyl)-phenylenediamine
2-β-Hydroxyethyl-phenylenediamine
N,N'-bis-(β-Hydroxyethyl)*N,N'*-bis-(4'-aminophenyl)-1,3-diamino-2-hydroxypropane
p-Aminophenol
3-Methyl-4-aminophenol
N-Methyl-*p*-aminophenol
o-Aminophenol

The oxidant of choice is hydrogen peroxide (generally 3% in the applied mixture), although some products employ solid oxidants, such as urea peroxide, sodium percarbonate, or perborate. These latter are efficient in initiating the color-forming reactions but have little bleaching power for melanin.

The chemistry involved in the color formation and in melanin bleaching occurs optimally at a pH of 9.0–9.5 and the preferred alkalizing agent is ammonia. Monoethanolamine can also be used and has a better odor but at the cost of some bleaching efficiency. If no bleaching is required, as in the "no-lift," "demipermanent," "tone on tone," or "deposit only" colorants, then a higher alkanolamine such as aminomethylpropanol can be used. Secondary alkanolamines, such as diethanolamine, are now avoided because of the possibility of nitrosamine formation.

The *m*-difunctional benzene couplers, such as resorcinol and *m*-aminophenol, having no substituent para to either of the functional groups, react beyond the initial indo-dye stage to produce trinuclear or even polymeric dyes that are drabber in color than the binuclear indo-dyes formed with couplers having a blocking group para to one of the functional groups and serve to provide a background brownish or blackish coloration. In contrast, the blocked couplers produce intense bright colors.

Using the ingredients listed in Tables 1 and 2, it is possible to formulate a full line of natural-looking shades and many "fashion" shades. Occasionally certain red and yellow direct dyes of the nitroaminophenol or nitrophenylenediamine type are added when a particularly bright shade is desired.

Direct Dyes for Hair

The temporary hair dyes include a variety of acid and/or basic dyes mainly chosen from among those used in textile dyeing. In the truly temporary dyes, which are removed by a single shampoo treatment, acid dyes are precipitated by the addition of a cationic surfactant to give a fine dispersion of colored particles, which is applied to the hair and left on to dry without rinsing, thus leaving a colored surface coating on the hair.

Semipermanent colorants, which withstand 6 to 12 shampoos, employ low-molecular-weight dyes that were specifically designed for use in hair dyes (Fig. 2). These are generally nitro phenylenediamines or nitroaminophenols and their *N*-substituted derivatives, which cover the color range of yellow to violet, together with a small number of azo or anthraquinone dyes, which provide violet to blue tones. These dyes are small enough to diffuse into the hair under ambient conditions and, consequently, will also diffuse out slowly during subsequent washings of the hair.

Typical dyes used in semipermanent colorants are shown in Table 3. The dyes are presented in a low-foaming surfactant base and are applied to the hair

TABLE 2 Couplers Used and Colors Produced in Oxidation Dyeing

Coupler	Color produced with *p*-Diamine	*p*-Aminophenol
Resorcinol	greenish brown	beige
2-Methylresorcinol	yellowish brown	beige
m-Aminophenol	warm brown	pinkish beige
m-Phenylenediamine	blue-black	reddish beige
2,4-Diaminophenoxyethanol	blue-violet	orange-red
1-Methoxy-2-amino-4-β-hydroxyethylaminobenzene	blue-violet	orange-red
1,3-Bis-(2,4-diaminophenoxy-propane)	blue-violet	orange-red
5-Amino-2-methylphenol	magenta	red-orange
5-β-Hydroxyethylamino-2-methylphenol	magenta	red-orange
1-Naphthol	blue-violet	red

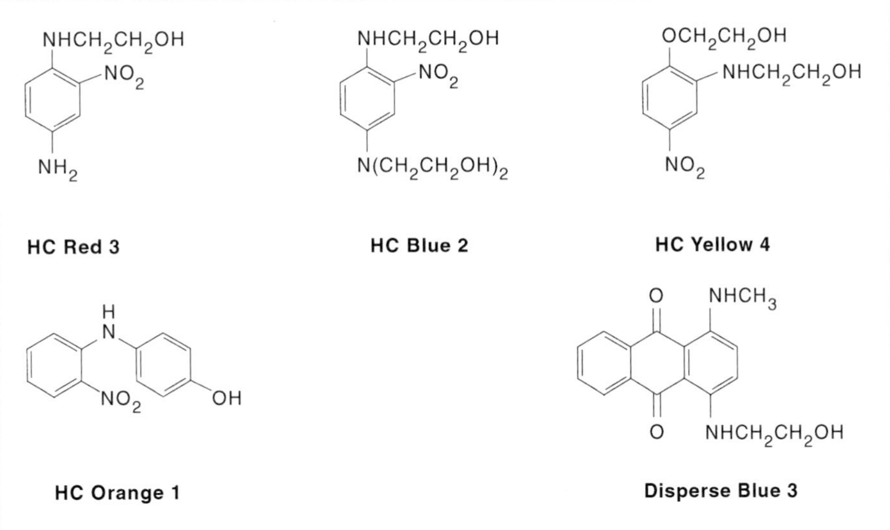

HC Red 3

HC Blue 2

HC Yellow 4

HC Orange 1

Disperse Blue 3

FIGURE 2 Typical dyes used in semipermanent hair colorants.

and left for 10 to 30 minutes before the composition is rinsed from the hair.

Natural Dyes for Hair

The practice of using plant extracts to dye the hair goes back over 2500 years when henna was employed for this purpose by the Egyptian nobility.

Henna is made from the dried macerated leaves of shrubs of the Lawsonia family. The major coloring agent is lawsone (2-hydroxy-1,4-naphthoquinone) together with a smaller amount of luteolin, 2-(3′,4′-dihydroxyphenyl)-5,6-dihydroxyflavone, which is extracted when leaves are mixed with hot water. The resulting paste is applied to the hair and left on for up to 1 hour, imparting an orange-red color that is quite resistant to shampooing.

In order to extend the range of shades, henna is sometimes mixed with other plant materials, such as indigo, logwood, chamomile, and hematin.

Natural dyes have a particular advantage in being essentially nonsensitizing. However, the coloring results and, in particular the grey coverage do not encourage their widespread use.

In some parts of the world, henna is mixed with powdered *p*-phenylenediamine and used to dye both the hair and the skin. Such a practice should certainly be discouraged on toxicological grounds.

Metallic Dyes for Hair

The use of lead acetate solutions containing sulfur to develop a gradual darkening of the hair derives from the ancient practice of dipping lead combs in vineger and combing the hair.

The modern products command less than 1% of the market and are mainly used by men for masking grey hair. The product is applied to the hair on a daily basis and, by interaction with the air and hydrogen sulfide, possibly produced by bacterial action on the sulfur, produces a deposit of lead oxide and lead sulfide on the surface of the hair. With repeat application, a significant brown coloration develops. Studies have shown that use of these products does not increase the body burden of lead, provided that the scalp is intact.

The other metallic dyes are used mainly in Asia and have one of two component systems, one containing a ferrous salt and the other containing pyrogallol.

Hair-Dye Toxicology

Sensitization

Because a number of the oxidative dye intermediates are known to be sensitizers, it is an almost universal requirement that these products carry a cautionary notice saying that the product may cause a reaction in some individuals. Additionally, instructions for carrying out a preliminary skin-patch test must be included. In the U.S., the mandatory warning reads, "This product contains ingredients which may cause skin irritation on certain individuals and a preliminary test according to accompanying directions should first be made. This product must not be used for dyeing the eyelashes or eyebrows: to do so may

TABLE 3 Dyes Currently Used in Semipermanent Hair Colorants

N-(2-Hydroxyethyl)-*o*-nitroaniline (HC Yellow 2)
4-Nitro-*o*-phenylenediamine
N^1-(2-Hydroxyethyl)-4-nitro-*o*-phenylenediamine (HC Yellow 5)
2-Amino-3-nitrophenol
O,N-Bis(2-hydroxyethyl)-2-amino-5-nitrophenol (HC Yellow 4)
N-(2-Hydroxyethyl)-2-amino-5-nitrophenol
4-Amino-3-nitrophenol
N-2-Hydroxyethyl)-2-amino-3-nitrophenol
N-2-(Hydroxyethyl)-4-amino-3-nitroanisole
1-(3-Methylamino-4-nitrophenoxy)propane-2,3 diol
3-Methylamino-4-nitrophenoxyethanol
2-Nitro-*p*-phenylenediamine
N^1-(2-Hydroxyethyl)-2-nitro-*p*-phenylenediamine (HC Red 3)
N^4-(2-Hydroxyethyl)-2-nitro-*p*-phenylenediamine (HC Red 7)
N^1-Methyl-2-nitro-*p*-phenylenediamine
N^1,N^4,N^4-Tris(2-hydroxyethyl)-2-nitro-*p*-phenylenediamine (HC Blue 2)
N^4-(2-Hydroxyethyl)-N^1,N^4-dimethyl-2-nitro-*p*-phenylenediamine
4-Nitro-*m*-phenylenediamine
Picramic acid
N-Methyl-iso-picramic acid
4-Amino-2-nitrodiphenylenediamine (HC Red)
2-Hydroxy-2′-nitrodiphenylenediamine (HC Orange)
4-(*p*-Aminophenylazo)-*N*,*N*-bis(2-hydroxyethyl)aniline
4-(*p*-Aminophenylazo)-3-methyl-*N*,*N*-bis(2-hydroxyethyl) aniline (Disperse Red 17)
1,4,5,8-Tetraminoanthraquinone (Disperse Blue 1)
1,4-Diaminoanthraquinone
1-Amino-4-methylaminoanthraquinone
1-(2-Hydroxyethylamino)-4-methyaminoanthraquinone (Disperse Blue 3)

cause blindness". There is no evidence to suggest that the use around the eye would cause blindness. In fact most of the ingredients have been subjected to *in vivo* animal tests and the incidence of accidental instillation of the product during use is not insignificant; yet no evidence of permanent injury has been documented. In Europe the warning states, "Can cause allergic reactions. Contains phenylenediamines. Do not use to dye eyelashes or eyebrows," and, on products for professional use, "wear suitable gloves."

Clinical tests have shown some of the nitro and anthraquinine dyes to be weak allergens and that there is some cross-sensitivity with *p*-phenylenediamine.

Mutagenicity

Much attention has been focused on the mutagenicity of hair dyes since the initial report by Ames of a study conducted as part of a biochemistry class experiment that showed positive responses for a number of dyes in *Salmonella tymphimurium*. While positive activity has also been reported for a number of dye materials in cultured mammalian cells, there have been only infrequent reports of positive results using *in vivo* test systems. Accumulated experience has shown that Ames mutagenicity is not a reliable predictor of rodent carcinogenic potential, particularly for aromatic amines. Such compounds were among the 33/301 NTP-tested chemicals, and invariably showed Ames-positive results for both transpecies, as well as for noncarcinogens. Batteries of short-term mutagenicity tests, despite some initial promise of facilitating the detection of rodent carcinogens, do not appear to improve substantially on the overall performance of the *Salmonella* assay for chemicals in general, and for hair dyes specifically. As an example, a highly purified sample of HC Blue 1, which was negative in a battery of short-term tests, produced hepatocellular carcinomas in mice, as did an unpurified mutagenic commercial material. However, other investigators subsequently found very small amounts of mutagenic impurities in ethanol-recrystallized HC Blue 1 using an Ames-directed HPLC fractionation assay. They speculated that these impurities may have been present in insufficient quantities to express an effect at a 5 mg maximum dose in the Ames test.

The consideration of the chemistry of the oxidative hair color process and *in vitro* assay conditions also have implications for the interpretation of hair dye mutagenicity data. For example, it was found that aqueous and freshly prepared DMSO solutions of *p*-phenylenediamine were nonmutagenic in Ames tests (TA98 and TA1538), while DMSO solutions allowed to stand at room temperature for 4 hours were active. The mutagenicity of *p*-phenylenediamine in the Ames test, the mouse lymphoma assay, and in human lymphocytes *in vitro* has been attributed to the formation of Bandrowski's base, a trimer of *p*-phenylenediamine. The addition of adequate amounts of couplers and restricted incubation times prevented the mutagenic activity in these assays. This is especially relevant because Bandrowski's base is not formed under conditions of actual hair dyeing in formulations that contain materials that preferentially couple with *p*-phenylenediamine to produce the desired colored dye polymer.

In view of these observations and complexities, the interpretation of the *in vitro* or *in vivo* mutagenic effects of individual hair dye materials and the possible relevance of such findings to the carcinogenic or mutagenic potential of dye materials under actual conditions of use needs to be carefully considered in a risk-assessment process.

Carcinogenicity

A substantial number of hair-dye ingredients have been subjected to subchronic toxicity, chronic toxicity, and life-time or multigeneration carcinogenicity studies, as well as to evaluations of teratologic and mutagenic potential. A number of these studies have involved composite oxidative and semipermanent (direct) hair-dye formulations given by topical application, dietary administration, or oral gavage (Table 4). These composite formulations reflected complete palettes of individual dyes used to produce various hair color shades.

Other than local irritant-type effects at the sites of topical application, none of these formulation studies have found any evidence of tumorigenicity of skin or internal organs, or clear evidence of other systemic nontumor pathology.

In addition to carcinogenicity tests involving topical application of composite hair dye formulations, the U.S. National Toxicology Program (NTP) has evaluated a number of individual dye materials by feeding or gavage routes using maximally tolerated doses (MTDs) determined from preliminary 14- and 90-day subchronic studies.

The results from these studies are summarized in Table 5 (direct dyes) and Table 6 (oxidative dyes). A few of these dyes, none of which remain in use, have elicited positive responses or "clear evidence" of carcinogenicity in one or more species or sex (e.g., 2,4-diaminoanisole, 2,4-toluenediamine, and HC Blue 1). Other materials have produced lesser degrees of evidence ("some" or "equivocal" responses) or "clear evidence" isolated to an individual sex or species. A number of dyes have been prohibited in Europe on the basis of such oral studies or because of a close structural relationship to the tested dyes (Table 7).

TABLE 4 Hair Dye Formulation Studies

Type of study—species	Number of formulations		Reference
	Permanent	Semipermanent	
Subchronic			
13 wk topical application—rabbits	9	3	Burnett *et al.* (1976)
Chronic			
2 year dietary administration—dogs		1	Wernick *et al.* (1975)
Carcinogenicity			
18 month topical application—mice	3	—	Burnett *et al.* (1975)
Life-time topical application—mice	6	3	Burnett *et al.* (1980)
Life-time topical application—mice	2	12	Jacobs *et al.* (1984)
Multigeneration topical application—rats	7	3	Burnett *et al.* (1988)
Teratology			
Oral gavage—rabbits	—	1	Wernick *et al.* (1975)
Dietary administration—rats	—	1	Wernick *et al.* (1975)
Topical application—rats	9	3	Burnett *et al.* (1976)
Mutagenicity			
Heritable translocation, topical—rats	1	1	Burnett *et al.* (1981)

TABLE 5 Semipermanent (Direct) Hair Dyes Evaluated in Two-Year NTP Bioassays[a,b]

Dye	Route	Overall call	F344/N rats		B6C3F1 mice		Source
			Male	Female	Male	Female	NTP TR, year
HC Blue 2	Gav	NEG	NE	NE	NE	NE	293, 1985
HC Yellow 4	Feed	NEG	EE-PIT AD	NE	NE	NE	419, 1992
HC Red 3	Gav	NEG	NE	NE	EE-LIV AD/CA	IS	281, 1986
Acid Orange 3	Gav	POS	NE	CE-KID TC CA	NE	NE	335, 1988
Disperse Blue 1	Feed	POS	CE-UBLAD CA	CE-UBLAD CA	EE-LIV AD/CA	NE	299, 1986
HC Blue 1[c]	Gav	POS	EE-LIV CA	CE-LUNG CA	CE-LIV/THY CA/AD	CE-LIV CA	271, 1985

[a]Summary data can be found in compendium of abstracts from long-term cancer studies reported by The National Toxicology Program from 1976 to 1992 (*Environ. Health Perspectives* **101** (Supplement 1), April 1993). Overall calls were given in 1993 correspondence from NTP Position paper on "Hair dyes, NTP research findings" (January 22, 1993).

[b]Abbreviations: AD = ademoma; CA = carcinoma; CE = clear evidence; EE = equivocal evidence; IS = inadequate study; IT = pituitary gland; KID = kidney; LIV = liver; NEG = negative; NE = no evidence; POS = positive; SE = some evidence; TC = transitional cell; THY = thyroid gland; UBLAD = urinary bladder.

[c]Not in current use.

However, in some instances the positive findings in such oral studies are of unlikely relevance to human health, in view of mechanistic and exposure considerations, as well as in light of potential confounding influences that may have affected the study outcomes.

For example, urinary bladder tumors produced in rats by Disperse Blue 1 (squamous- and transitional-cell tumors, and leiomyosarcomas) were highly associated with urinary bladder calculi and were not found at the low dose in the three-dose level NTP bioassay. This was suggestive of a secondary mechanism for tumor induction. Quantitative risk assessments, assuming a threshold effect, indicated the safe level was 20-fold higher than the maximum average daily-applied dose associated with product use.

For HC Red No. 3, the NTP concluded that there was "equivocal evidence of carcinogenicity" in male B6C3F$_1$ mice due to an increased incidence (35/50 mice) of combined liver tumors (adenomas and carcinomas) in the high-dose group (250 mg/kg/day) as compared to the control group (25/50 mice). However, there was also a significant reduction in these tumors in the low-dose group (15/50 mice at 125 mg/kg/day). The possible importance of these findings is reduced by the known variability of hepatic cell neoplasms in this strain. Moreover, a perfect dose–response (15/50; 25/50; 35/50) association was found between cage shelf heights and tumor incidence on reanalysis of these data (and other NTP bioassay results) for "systematic" effects unrelated to chemical treatment.

For 2-amino-5-nitrophenol, the NTP call of "some evidence of carcinogenicity" for male rats was based on an increased incidence of acinar cell adenomas of the pancreas. The dye was administered by gavage in corn oil. Subsequently, NTP found increases in the incidence of pancreatic exocrine hyperplasia and adenoma with either corn oil, safflower oil, tricapyrilin alone, and with dichloromethane given in corn oil. NTP concluded that the use of corn oil as a gavage vehicle may have a confounding effect on the interpretation of chemical-induced proliferative lesions of the exocrine pancreas (as well as on mononuclear cell leukemias) in male F344/N rats.

Exposure is an important consideration with respect to risk assessment for hair dyes, which may display a carcinogenic hazard in rodent studies but are used on an infrequent basis and display a relatively low potential for percutaneous penetration. For 2,4-diaminoanisole, an oxidative hair dye that induced thyroid tumors in mice and rats, as well as tumors of the integumentary system in rats, exposures based on percutaneous penetration data obtained *in vivo* in rhesus monkeys (about 0.032% of the applied dose) and risks estimated by conservative mathematical approaches (Mantel–Bryan and linear models) yielded cancer risks in the range of 6.1×10^{-8} to 2.8×10^{-11} for dark shades and 4.1×10^{-11} to 4.9×10^{-19} for light shades of hair color containing this material. Subsequent human data on 2,4-diaminoanisole obtained under actual-use conditions showed a lower absorption of about 0.02% of the applied dose. Such risks are clearly in the range of being *de minimus*. *In vivo* human studies with other dye materials have shown percutaneous absorption values to generally less than 1% of the applied dose. For representative oxidative and direct hair dyes, this translated to exposures in the range of about 2 to 7 mg per applica-

TABLE 6 Permanent (Oxidative) Hair Dyes Evaluated in Two-Year NTP Bioassays[a,b]

Dye	Route	Overall call	F344/N rats		B6C3F1 mice		Source
			Male	Female	Male	Female	NTP TR, year
2,5-Toluenediamine	Feed	N	N	N	N	N	126, 1978
p-Phenylenediamine	Feed	N	N	N	N	N	174, 1979
4-Nitro-*o*-phenylenediamine[c]	Feed	N	N	N	N	N	180, 1979
N-Phenyl-*p*-phenylenediamine	Feed	N	N	N	N	N	82, 1978
2-Chloro-*p*-phenylenediamine	Feed	N	N	N	N	N	113, 1978
Resorcinol	Gav	N	NE	NE	NE	NE	403, 1992
2,4-Diaminophenol	Gav	N	NE	NE	SE-KID; tubular AD	NE	401, 1992
2-Amino-4-nitrophenol	Gav	N	SE-KID cortical AD	NE	NE	NE	339, 1988
2-Amino-5-nitrophenol	Gav	N	SE-pancreas acinar AD	NE	NE	NE	334, 1988
Hydroquinone	Gav	(N)	SE-KID; cortical AD	SE-MLCLEUC leukemia	NE	SE-LIV AD	366, 1989
2-Nitro-*p*-phenylenediamine[c]	Feed	P	N	N	N	P-LIV AD	169, 1979
4-Amino-2-nitrophenol[d]	Feed	P	P-UBLAD TC CA	EE-UBLAD TC CA	N	N	94, 1978
2,4-Toluenediamine[d]	Feed	P	P-LIV CA	P-LIV CA; MAMGL CA/AD	N	P-LIV CA	162, 1979
2,4-Diaminoanisole[d]	Feed	P	P-skin & assoc glands, AD/CA	P-skin & assoc glands, AD/CA	P-THY FC AD	P-THY FC AD/CA	84, 1978

[a]Summary data can be found in compendium of abstracts from long-term cancer studies reported by the NATIONAL TOXICOLOGY PROGRAM from 1976 to 1992 (*Environ. Health Perspectives* **101** (Supplement 1), April 1993). Overall calls were given in 1993 correspondence from NTP position paper on "Hair dyes, NTP research findings" (JANUARY 22, 1993). Calls noted in ( ) applied similar criteria.

[b]Abbreviations: AD = ademoma; CA = carcinoma; CE = clear evidence; EE = equivocal evidence; FC = follicular cell; IS = inadequate study; KID = kidney; LIV = liver; MAMGL = mammary gland; MLCLEUL = mononuclear cell leukemia; NE = no evidence; N = negative; P = positive; PIT = pituitary gland; SE = some evidence; TC = transitional cell; THY = thyroid gland; UBLAD = urinary bladder.

[c]Direct dye used as toner in oxidative hair color.

[d]Not in current use.

TABLE 7 Ingredients Not Permitted in Hair Dye Products in the European Union

o-Phenylenediamine[a]
2,4-Diaminotoluene[a]
2,4-Diaminoanisole[a]
2,4-Diaminophenetole[b]
2,4-Diaminophenylethanol[b]
2,5-Diaminoanisole[b]
2-Amino-4-nitrophenol[a]
2-Amino-5-nitrophenol[a]
4-Amino-2-nitrophenol[a]
Catechol[c]
Pyrogallol[c]

[a]Positive bioassay data.
[b]Structural similarity to 2,4-diaminoanisole.
[c]Suspected as benzene metabolites.

tion for relatively dark shades or about 1–4 μg/kg/day, taking into account a 4-week use frequency.

Relevant to the extrapolation of risks to low-level human exposures from high-dose rodent tumorgenicity studies is an observation based on an evaluation of 139 NTP studies. It was found that the MTD/740,000 provides an esimate of the 10^{-6} life-time risk, which was generally within a factor of 10 of that dose estimated by applying linear multistage models to the 2-year bioassay data. Thus, for materials exhibiting MTDs in the range of 1 gm/kg/day (10^6 μg/kg/day) in 2-year rodent bioassays, life-time average daily exposures of about 1.4 μg/kg/day (i.e., $10^6/(0.74 \times 10^6)$ would generally be expected not to pose significant carcinogenic risk. Extended use of hair dyes containing the materials would pose a risk of considerably less than the *de minimus* one in a million.

Hair Bleaches

Lightening of the natural hair color requires destruction of the brown–black eumelanin and/or the yellow to red phaeomelanin pigments that occur as granules in the cortex of the hair.

Hydrogen peroxide, particularly under alkaline conditions, is effective in disintegrating the eumelanin granules and in bleaching some of the dispersed pigment. However, the end result is a reddish brown that requires modulating with oxidation dyes if a natural shade is desired.

Complete decolorization of the natural pigment requires the use of "boosters" with the hydrogen peroxide. Ammonium and potassium persulfates are very effective in this role. While the persulfates alone have no effect on the pigment granules, when used in admixture with ammonium hydroxide and hydrogen peroxide in the form of a paste, they are very effective in completely destroying the natural pigments. Application time varies from 20 minutes to more than 1 hour, depending on the original color of the hair.

Unfortunately, the strong oxidizing mixture also results in the oxidation of the hair keratin, particularly at the cystine moiety. Injudicious use of bleaches can thus result in brittle hair that requires careful handling and the extensive use of conditioners. This phenomenon is often referred to as "drying," which is a misnomer resulting from the feel of hair with a roughened cuticle. Indeed, damaged hair has a higher water content than virgin hair under the same ambient conditions.

The persulfates have been reported to be sensitizers, but such reactions appear to be rare.

OTHER COSMETIC PRODUCT CATEGORIES

It is beyond the scope of this chapter to detail the toxicological profiles and issues associated with individual cosmetic ingredients used in the wide variety of available product types. However, it is relevant to put the associated risks into an appropriate perspective based on actual-use history and experience.

Accidental and Emergency-Related Human Exposures

In 1995, cosmetic and other personal-care products accounted for 8.5% (n = 171,426) of the human exposures reported to poison control centers in the United States, ranking third, below cleaning substances and analgesics. It is important to acknowledge that materials with a high frequency of involvement may not necessarily be the most toxic but may be merely the most accessible, particularly to children. Indeed, it is reassuring that only a small proportion (9.5%) of such exposures involved treatment in a health-care facility, while that the majority resulted in no significant outcome (33.2%) or a minor outcome (21.4%) associated with minimally bothersome and generally resolvable signs and symptoms. Major effects were relatively infrequent (n = 69) and largely associated with alcohol-containing mouthwashes. Deaths were associated with exceptional circumstances, such as intentional abuse of a hair spray (n = 1) or suicides involving mixed chemical exposures (n = 2).

Other Adverse Reactions

U.S. FDA Reports

Industry Data

Until recently, the U.S. cosmetic industry reported to the FDA the incidence of adverse reactions received via toll-free 800 telephone numbers or other correspondence, together with the numbers of units distributed as part of the Voluntary Cosmetic Registration Program. In turn, the FDA would calculate the number of such cosmetic experience reports (CERs) per million units sold, fit the data to a linear regression model and report back to the individual manufacturers which of their products had reaction rates that were more than one standard deviation above the calculated mean rate. It was then the responsibility of the manufacturer to determine the relevance, if any, of the reported observations and take any appropriate action. Representative rates (CERs per 10^6 units sold) for various product types are shown for the years 1989–1992 in Table 8.

While such data provide a general idea of the propensity of various cosmetic product types to produce undesired reactions in consumers, the lack of detailed information and standardized medical follow-up limits more meaningful analysis of the causative ingredient(s) and the relative severity or importance of the reported adverse experiences.

TABLE 8 Cosmetic Experience Reports (CER) to the U.S. FDA (1989–1992): Voluntary Reports by Industry

CER (10^6 units)	Product types	
20–30	Baby shampoo	Bath soaps and detergents
	Other baby products	Skin cleansers
	Permanent waves	Skin moisturizers
	Hair rinses	Night creams
		Indoor-tanning preparations
10–19	Noncoloring shampoos	Hair sprays
	Deodorants	Hair straighteners
	Other skin-care preparations	Hair dyes and colors
	Other suntan preparations	Hair lighteners
		Hair bleaches
		Foundations
5–9	Baby lotions, oils	Skin fresheners
	Bath oils, tablets	Suntan gels, creams
	Eyeliners	
	Eye shadows	
	Eye-makeup removers	
	Powders	
<5	All other categories	

TABLE 9 Cosmetic Injury Reports to the FDA by Consumers (July 1987–1995)

Number of reactions[a]	Product types
262	Skin moisturizers, cleansers, night creams, and other skin care
111	Hair dyes
70–89	Shampoos; Nail products
50–69	Permanent waves; eye products; hair conditioners/sprays
30–49	Suntan products; facial foundations; hair straighteners[b]; deodorants; depilatories
20–29	Fragrances; toothpastes and oral-hygiene products; lipsticks; hair tonics
10–19	Bath soaps and detergents; bath products; baby products
≤10	Hair bleaches and lighteners; other hair colors; shaving products

[a] $n = 1305$.

[b] Excludes 157 injury reports that were related to one particular product.

Consumer Complaints Reported Directly to the FDA

The FDA continues to report cosmetics injuries reported directly to them organized by the same product categories as the industry data. Reports provide details of the brand name, injury complaints (e.g., dermatitis, pain, tissue damage, and respiratory effects), and affected body part or area. An analysis of the incidence of the complaints by cosmetic product type for the period July 1987 through 1995 is shown in Table 9. Skin-care products (e.g., moisturizers, cleansers, and night creams), hair dyes, shampoos, nail products, permanent waves, eye products, and hair sprays and conditioners showed the highest incidence of adverse reactions. A high incidence of reports associated with hair straighteners for this period was primarily attributable to a single product and, while not representative of the product category in general, points to ability of the system to detect (and react to) problematical materials.

The availability of such data through Freedom of Information Act requests to the FDA affords individual manufacturers the opportunity of examining the type and frequency of adverse reactions associated with their material compared to those for related or competitive products. It is likely that there is overlap in these databases, in that those consumers reporting adverse reactions directly to the FDA would also inform the manufacturer, particularly if medical costs were incurred.

Swedish MPA Reports

Adverse reactions to cosmetics and toiletries are reported to the Swedish Medical Products Agency (MPA) in a voluntary system introduced in 1989. In the period from 1989–1994, 191 cases involving 253 products were evaluated and causality was established by dermatologists using World Health Organization (WHO) criteria for suspected adverse drug reactions. The large majority of adverse reactions (90%) involved moisturizers, followed by hair-care and nail products, sunscreens and tanning products, eye makeup, and perfume. Most of the effects were limited to the skin and eczematous reactions were often (7%) classified as contact allergic in nature, as confirmed by patch-test reactions to the product or its individual components. The most frequent components implicated were fragrances (22/79), toluene sulfonamide-formaldehyde resin (19/79), various preservatives (19/79), and glyceryl monothioglycolate (7/79).

Dermatological Reactions

U.S. Experience

In a 5-year prospective study of cosmetic reactions conducted by the North American Contact Dermatitis Group, 713 cosmetic-related cases of contact dermatitis were identified among 13,216 of their patients. Of these, 89% of the cosmetic reactions were confirmed by patch testing, with the remainder based on case history and medical examination. The majority of the reactions were related to skin-care products (28%), hair preparations including hair color (24%), and facial makeup (11%), with lesser contributions associated with other product types. Fragrance (usually unspecified) accounted for the majority of reactions, followed by preservatives, (Quaternium 15, imidazolidinyl urea, parabens, 2-bromo-2-nitropropane-1,3 diol, formaldehyde); *p*-phenylenediamine; lanolin and its derivatives; glyceryl monothioglycolate; propylene glycol; toluene sufonamide-formaldehyde resin; sunscreens and other UV absorbers; and acrylate or methacrylate. The group acknowledged that their data might not have been representative of the country at large because of the specialized interest of the dermatologists involved.

Belgium Experience

The European experience with respect to dermatological reactions appears to be quite consistent. Among 3970 patients evaluated in a contact allergy unit from 1985–1990, 11.9% (462) represented cosmetic contact dermatitis. The majority of the reactions were associated with face- and body-care products (29%), followed by perfumes and toilet waters (22%), sun products (7%), and a variety of other cosmetic products with lower reaction incidences (1–5%). In patients who had positive patch tests, the most frequent allergens among ingredient types were fragrance mix, oak moss, balsam of Peru, preservatives (e.g., [chloro] methylisothiazoline, formaldehyde, and parabens), vehicles and emulsifiers (e.g., wood alcohol, cocamidopropylbetaine, and propylene glycol), active ingredients and hair dyes (e.g., *p*-toluene sulfonamide formaldehyde resin, glyceryl, or ammonium thioglycolate, and paraphenylenediamine), and sunscreens (e.g., benzophenone-3, Eusolex 8021, and *p*-aminobenzoic acid).

COSMETIC INGREDIENTS

Fragrances

Fragrances are used widely in cosmetic products, either to provide a direct end benefit as in the case of perfumes, toilet waters, and deodorants, or to increase the acceptability of other cosmetic product types by masking undesired odors or imparting a pleasant scent to enhance the consumer's product-use experience.

The potential for fragrance materials to elicit allergic contact dermatitis and, in some cases, contact urticaria of immunologic or nonimmunologic origin is well recognized and extensively studied (see the review by Scheinman, 1996). Self-regulatory initiatives by the Research Institute for Fragrance Materials (RIFM) and the International Fragrance Research Association (IFRA) has led to the systematic review of fragrance components for toxicological, ecotoxicological, and sensitization potential. As a result, certain components have been prohibited for use or have had limits imposed based on their concentrations.

North American, European, and Japanese dermatologists have routinely included either fragrance mixtures or a screening series of selected individual fragrance components in their diagnosis and surveillance of cosmetic allergic reactions. The use concentration and use circumstances (i.e., leave on or rinse off), extent and location of product application, use frequency, integrity of the skin barrier, and underlying skin disease can all impact the propensity of potential sensitizers to elicit dermatological reactions. Therefore, after exclusion of known strong sensitizers, the routine safety evaluation for finished cosmetic products invariably incorporates a human prophetic patch test to ascertain the potential of the material to induce an allergic response under exaggerated (e.g., occlusive patches) conditions.

Based on the chemical analysis of fragrance components from 17 common cosmetic products (8 leave-on and 9 wash-off types) in Denmark, from one to five constituents of the European fragrance mix materials were present in each of the products. However, patch testing performed in 500 consecutive eczema patients revealed that not all cases of perfume allergy were detected by the mix, as reflected by positive concordance values of 52.4% and 81.3% for wash-off and leave-on products, respectively. Conversely, 70% of the subjects that were fragrance-mix positive did not react to the product perfumes. This emphasizes the importance of establishing the clinical relevance of observed patch-test reactions based on actual product testing.

In a worldwide multicenter investigation of fragrance contact dermatitis involving the diagnostic patch testing of 67 subjects at seven centers, atopic individuals were over-represented as compared to the general population. The face and hands were the most common sites of eczematous dermatitis. Racial differences included a higher likelihood of reactions to fragrance mix in white persons and a higher prevalence of reactions to benzyl salicylate among Asians.

In addition to the clinically related issues associated with fragrance materials, the chemical reactivity of certain fragrances may predispose them to more toxicologically significant findings in animal studies, such as reproductive and carcinogenic effects. These are discussed with regards to an important class of fragrance materials, the nitromusks and the polycyclic musks.

Nitromusks

The terms "musk" and "nitromusk" are nonchemical classifications that are used in the perfume industry to describe substances that have a typical "musky" odor. There are currently four nitroaromatic compounds of interest to the fragrance industry, musk xylene, musk ketone, musk tibetine, and moskene. Musk xylene and musk ketone are the most important of these, while musk tibetine and moskene are used in much smaller amounts. These compounds have had a safe history of use as perfume ingredients for over 100 years and there are no reports of adverse effects in humans. A fifth nitromusk, musk ambrette, was found to cause neurotoxicity and testicular atrophy in rats via both oral and topical routes. In addition, musk ambrette was also found to be phototoxic in a few individuals. As a result, musk ambrette is banned from all fragrances and was placed on Annex II of the European Cosmetics Directive in 1995. The RIFM has evaluated the other nitromusks and concluded that they did not produce the same toxicity as musk ambrette.

In studies for potential mutagenicity and carcinogenicity, musk xylene was found to produce hepatocellular carcinomas and adenomas when fed to mice for 2 years. Musk xylene was subsequently categorized as a nongenotoxic carcinogen causing hepatic tumors in mice by mechanisms similar to those observed for the barbiturate phenobarbital, and thus it is not considered to represent a carcinogenic risk for humans. Through mechanistic studies, musk ketone and musk tibetine were shown to be metabolized differently and hence unlikely to show the same toxicity as musk xylene. As a result of the musk xylene observations, the RIFM proceeded to evaluate more extensively the genotoxic potential of the nitromusks. Musk xylene was tested in the mouse lymphoma assay, in an *in vitro* cytogenetics assay in Chinese hamster ovary (CHO) cells, in an *in vitro* UDS assay, and in an *in vivo* unscheduled DNA synthesis (UDS) assay. When these were combined with the negative Ames assay performed earlier, the RIFM concluded that musk xylene showed no evidence of genotoxic potential.

The RIFM also evaluated the genotoxicity of musk ketone in a battery of short-term tests and found no evidence of genotoxic potential based on results from the mouse lymphoma, *in vitro* cytogenetics, and *in vitro* UDS assays. In addition, musk ketone was found to be negative in an *in vivo* mouse micronucleus assay.

Recent studies indicate that trace amounts of nitromusks have been detected in mother's milk and in environmental samples. Although nitromusks have been the subject of an extensive testing program examining both human health and environmental safety, due to these relatively recent findings the SCCNFP has requested specific toxicological data from the industry on these compounds in order to evaluate their significance for human health. Because these four ingredients are, in fact, four different chemical substances with different toxicological profiles, each substance is being evaluated separately by the SCCNFP.

The RIFM has undertaken research to provide additional data to help in the risk assessment. Studies have been conducted to determine the effects of musk ketone and musk xylene on developmental toxicity. These studies demonstrated that developmental toxicity was not a biologically significant factor in the risk assessment for musk ketone or musk xylene when assessed in relation to expected human exposure through the use of cosmetics.

Using dermal-absorption figures obtained from rat studies and NOELs (no observed effect levels) determined from subchronic dermal studies also in rats, large safety factors can be calculated for musk xylene and musk ketone, 2000 and 3000 respectively, under simulated conditions of human use. Large safety factors have also been demonstrated for indirect human exposure through the environment.

The SCCNFP is currently evaluating the toxicological data submitted by industry on musk ketone and musk xylene. For the other two nitromusks, musk tibetine and moskene, the SCCNFP considered the available data to be insufficient to enable a safety evaluation and classified these as 2b and not to be used in cosmetic products. The SCCNFP has indicated that there are no adverse findings or identified health hazards on musk tibetine and moskene and is prepared to reassess its opinion subject to additional data submissions.

Polycyclic Musks

These ingredients have been widely used in fragrance formulations for a wide variety of consumer products, including perfumes, soaps, shampoos, and detergents, for over 40 years. Extensive safety dossiers have also been submitted to the SCCNFP for both HHCB (1,3,4,6,7,8-hexahydro-4,6,6,7,8,8,-hexamethylcyclopenta-γ-2-benzopyran) and AHTN (6-acetyl-1,1,2,4,4,7-hexamethyltetraline). As in the case of the nitromusks the SCCNFP will review an extensive battery of mutagenicity assays, subchronic studies, skin absorption, and teratology and developmental toxicity studies investigating exposure via maternal milk.

As part of the environmental risk assessment for AHTN, a chronic fish study was conducted on fathead minnows. An absent tail fin was observed in the majority of fish at the lowest observed-effect concentration level of 67 μg. All fish at the no-observed-effect concentration level of 35 μg/liter and below had normal tail fins. This finding was reported to the U.S. EPA (Environmental Protection Agency); however, it is not considered to be of environmental concern or to be relevant to human health. The SCCNFP is yet to complete its evaluation of HHCB and AHTN.

Preservatives

As with fragrances, cosmetic use experience has demonstrated a relatively high propensity for allergic reactions to this widely used ingredient category. Examples of potential contact sensitizers used in cosmetics have included formaldehyde, paraben esters, sorbic acid, isothiazoles, and organic mercurial compounds. Skin irritation is also a potential limiting factor with preservatives, and cosmetic-formulation goals strive to achieve adequate microbial preservation using the lowest feasible preservative levels. Human repeat-insult patch tests and cumulative irritation studies on prototype or finished cosmetic products can usefully serve in identifying such potential issues prior to marketing.

In a study among 19,546 unselected dermatitis patients in Italy, positive patch-test incidences of 1.9% with parabens and 0.3% with formaldehyde were reported. In subsets of this population, comprising from 980 to 14,897 patients, incidences ranged between 0.1% (Quaternium 15) to 1.6% (chloromethylisothiazolone and methylisothiazolone). Except for sodium metabisulfite and chloracetamide, with incidences of 1.4% and 1.0%, respectively, all of the other preservatives tested (triclosan, butylated hydroxyanisole, imidazolidinyl urea, bronopol, and butylated hydroxytoluene) showed reaction rates of less than 0.3%. Temporal analysis showed that the incidence of contact allergy to parabens declined from about 2.5–2.7% in the period between 1968 and 1982 to about 1.0–1.3% in the period between 1983 and 1991. Paraben allergy appeared to be associated more with local remedies applied to diseased or compromised skin than with cosmetic products *per se.* For parabens, the hands and face were considered to be moderate and low risk areas, respectively, while for chloromethylisothiazolone and methylisothiazolone, the hands and face were the predominant cutaneous sites of contact allergy.

As is the case for fragrances, the presence of positive patch-test results for preservatives may not be indicative of intolerance to the material under use conditions. For example, 24/27 subjects with positive patch-test reactions to 100 ppm chloromethylisothiazolone and methylisothiazolone tolerated a 2-week use period with a shampoo formulated at 15 ppm. The authors emphasize that it still may be prudent to suggest alternative products to patients with known sensitivities. They also point to the paucity of controlled clinical trials evaluating positive patch-test allergens under use conditions.

In the European Union, cosmetic preservatives are systematically reviewed and the maximum authorized concentrations and other limitations and requirements are listed in Annex VI, Part 1 (allowed) and Part 2 (provisionally allowed).

Surfactants

Surfactants are another broadly used cosmetic ingredient class employed at varied concentrations in diverse product types, such as shampoos, body washes, and other types of skin cleansing products, and at relatively lower concentrations as emulsifiers and wetting agents in many other product categories. The toxicology of surfactants used in cosmetics has been reviewed recently by Sterzel (1997). Their biochemical properties include interactions with membranes involving adsorption to surfaces and alterations in membrane permeability and, at higher concentrations, cell lysis and solubilization of integral membrane proteins. Cationic and anionic surfactants also interact with proteins, with consequent swelling of the stratum corneum, and may also inactivate enzymes due to conformational changes or binding to active enzyme sites.

The skin compatibility of anionic surfactants appears to vary by chain length and, for sodium soaps, alkyl sulfates, and alkylbenzene or α-olefin sulfonates, compounds with a saturated side chain of 10–12 carbon atoms are usually the least compatible. It is generally acknowledged that for mucous membranes, the rank order of surfactant compatibility is nonionic > anionic > cationic. While surfactants as a class have a concentration-dependent potential of inducing skin and mucous membrane irritation, they are not generally regarded as having a significant sensitization liability because of their inability to act as haptens by forming strong bonds to endogenous proteins.

Because of their relatively low potential for percutaneous absorption under normal cosmetic use conditions, the likelihood of systemic adverse effects from surfactants are low, and feeding or drinking water toxicology studies with these materials have generally shown substantial safety margins.

Other Ingredients

In addition to the fragrances, preservatives, and surfactants that are used widely in a variety of cosmetic products, there is a diversity of other product and ingredient categories with more specialized toxicological issues, which presents a significant challenge to summarize adequately. Some examples include UV absorbers with potential for photoxicity, photosensitization and, possibly, photomutagenicity; hair sprays; nail-polish solvents; powdered materials with inhalation potential; lipstick components for which oral exposure may be an expected exposure route; and nail-polish resins with sensitization issues. Nater and DeGroot (1988) have compiled comprehensive lists of representative cosmetic formulations, their ingredients, and their reported side effects, including contact allergy, urticaria, irritant dermatitis, and systemic effects such as respiratory symptoms associated with an immediate-type allergy. Included are recommended skin patch-test concentrations and vehicles for diagnostic patch testing. The reader is referred to this text for detailed information.

EXPOSURE AND RISK ASSESSMENT CONSIDERATIONS FOR COSMETIC PRODUCTS AND INGREDIENTS

The toxicological evaluation of cosmetic ingredients serves usefully to identify potential hazards, which then need to be put into appropriate perspective via a risk assessment that incorporates an estimation of exposure and a calculation of the margin of safety by relating the human exposure dose to the no-observed-adverse-effect level obtained from animal tests. Key exposure parameters include the amount of product and the concentration of ingredient applied, the route and site of application, and the frequency and duration (e.g., rinse off or leave on) of application. Although, there are no good quantitative data that adequately reflect the variations in consumer habits and practices, particularly for several of the newer cosmetic types and forms, some conventions that are used for cosmetic exposure assessment are given in Table 10. Because demographics and cultural differences would be expected to have a significant influence, particularly on use frequency or on amounts, there may be considerable variations in the actual exposures, which often may be remarkably overestimated using conservative exposure assumptions.

While the intended route of exposure for most cosmetic products, by definition, is topical, inadvertent exposure may also occur via the mucous membranes, orally, or via inhalation for aerosol or powdered cosmetic forms. Inhalation may also be a potential exposure route for ingredients, including contaminants, that may be volatilized under use conditions. In some cases, such as for hair cosmetics, skin (scalp) exposure is an inadvertent but unavoidable consequence of product use. While it is important to consider the relative contribution of various exposure routes to an ingredient on a case-by-case basis, oral and inhalation exposures would generally be considered to potentially engender higher risks than would topical application.

TABLE 10 Typical Use Amounts and Use Frequencies for Various Cosmetic Product Types[a]

Exposure type	Use frequency	Amount (gm/application)	Product types
Rinse off	3–6/day	0.8	Soap bar
	1/day	2.0	Shave cream
	1–7/week	12.0	Shampoo
	1–4/week	10.0	Shower gel
	1–3/week	14.0	Hair conditioner
	1–2/week	17.0	Foam bath (undiluted)
	8–18/year	30.0	Semipermanent hair dye
	8–12/year	50.0	Permanent hair dye (ready-to-use)
Leave on	2/day	0.80	Face cream
	1–5/day	0.75	Toilet water
	1–3/day	3.0	Antiperspirant/deodorant (spray)
	1–3/day	0.5	Antiperspirant/deodorant (others)
	1–2/day	1 (mg/cm^2)	General-purpose cream
	1–2/day	1.2	After shave
	1–2/day	2.5	Make-up remover
	1–2/day	2.5	Talcum powder
	1–2/day	7.5	Body lotion
	1–2/day	10.0	Hair spray
	2–3/week	0.25	Nail product
	1–2/week	12.0	Setting product
	1–2/week	12.0	Temporary hair dye
	2–3 day for 2 wk/year	8.0	Sun cream
Mucous membrane contact	1–6/day	0.01	Lipstick
	1–3/day	12.0	Mouthwash (ready-to-use)
	1–3/day	0.01	Eye make-up: powder
	1–2/day	0.5	Eye make-up remover (wipe-off)
	1–2/day	1.5	Toothpaste
	1/day	0.025	Eye make-up: mascara
	1/day	0.005	Eye make-up: liner

[a]Adapted from ECETOC (1993).

INGREDIENT, TOXICOLOGY AND PRODUCT SAFETY

While the toxicologic potential of cosmetic ingredients, some of which have a broader use in other consumer, industrial, and pharmaceutical products or in food applications, has traditionally been characterized in conventional animal studies such as those listed earlier in this chapter, the European Union sixth amendment to the Cosmetics Directive has brought increased emphasis on the use of nonanimal study alternatives for both ingredients and finished products. The use of selected individual *in vitro* tests or test batteries shows good promise for cosmetic materials in certain areas, such as skin irritation, percutaneous absorption, and photoirritation or photosensitization. While considerable progress has been made in understanding their utility and limitations, there is less of a consensus on alternative methods for testing eye irritation and, particularly, skin sensitization. It is generally acknowledged that for the evaluation of systemic effects, such as studies of chronic toxicity, reproductive toxicity, and immunotoxic potential as currently required or requested by international cosmetic regulations and guidelines, there appear to be no near-term alternatives to animal testing.

In many circumstances, finished product testing may be accomplished without or with minimal use of animals by a stepwise approach involving the thorough evaluation of the available toxicological data on the ingredients and consideration of prior experience with related ingredients and formulations ("paper" toxicology); the conservative application of controlled clinical studies with appropriate ethical considerations and close medical supervision; and the use of *in vitro* methods that have been validated for a specific purpose with the appropriate known "benchmark" materials. This scheme, incorporating the option of conducting limited animal tests under selected circumstances to resolve outstanding issues or, alterna-

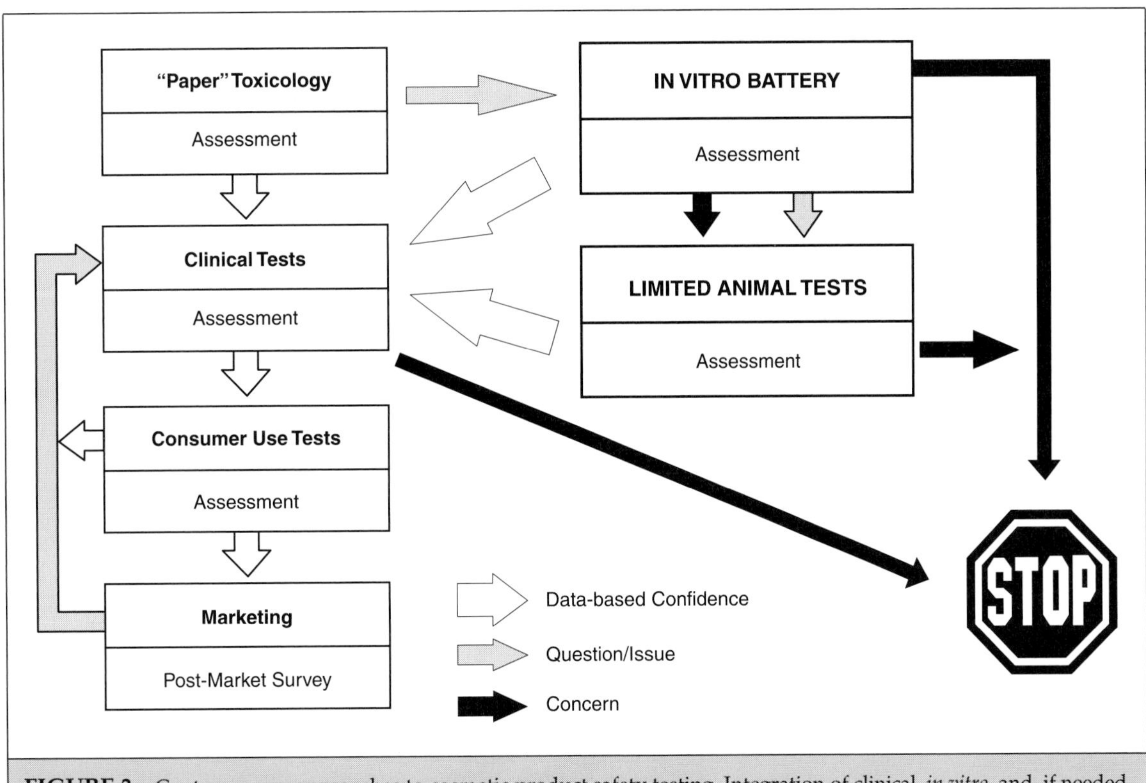

FIGURE 3 Contemporary approaches to cosmetic product safety testing. Integration of clinical, *in vitro*, and, if needed, animal tests.

tively, to suspend development, is shown in Fig. 3. An important element in such a process is the inclusion of feedback loops to address issues that may develop during the various stages of product development, including the exposure of a broader numbers of individuals under less controlled circumstances, such as consumer-use tests or test marketing. Post-market surveillance is an important element of cosmetic product safety in that low-frequency events may only be ascertained after broad consumer use.

The viability of maintaining the option to include animal tests of finished products, even on a selected basis, remains to be determined by future international regulatory activities and by the policy and practices of individual cosmetic companies.

Bibliography

Abu-Shakra, A., Johnson, L., Earlley, K., Jamson, C. W., Kari, F. W., Gupta, R., and Langenbach, R. (1991). Isolation of the mutagenic and DNA adduct-inducing components from a commercial preparation of HC blue 1 using *Salmonella* (TA98) bioassay-directed HPLC fractionation. *Mutat. Res.* **260,** 377–385.

Adams, R. M., and Maibach, H. I. (1985). A five-year study of cosmetic reactions. *J. American Academy of Dermatology* **13(6),** 1062–1069.

Ames, B., Kammen, H. O., and Yamasaki, E. (1975). Hair dyes are mutagenic: Identification of a variety of mutagenic ingredients. *Proc. Nat. Acad. Sci. USA* **6,** 2423–2427.

Angelini, G., Vena, G. A., Foti, C., and Grandolfo, M. (1997) Contact allergy to preservatives and perfumed compounds used in skin care products. *J. Appl. Cosmetol.* **15,** 49–57.

Anonymous (1993). Compendium of abstracts from long term cancer studies reported by the National Toxicology Program from 1967 to 1997. *Environ. Health Perspectives* **101,** Supplement 1.

Api, A. M., Ford, R. A., and San, R. H. C. (1995). An evaluation of musk xylene in a battery of genotoxicity tests. *Food Chem. Toxicol.* **33 (12),** 1039–1045.

Api, A. M., Pfitzer, E. A., and San, R. H. C. (1996). An evaluation of genotoxicity tests and musk ketone. *Food Chem. Toxicol.* **34,** 633–638.

Ashby, J., and Tennant, R. W. (1991). Definitive relationships among chemical structure, carcinogenicity and mutagenicity for 301 chemicals tested by the U.S. NTP. *Mutat. Res.* **257(3),** 229–306.

Berne B., Boström, A., Grahnén, A. F., and Tammela, M. (1996). Adverse effects of cosmetics and toiletries reported to the Swedish Medical Products Agency 1989–1994. *Contact Dermatitis* **34,** 359–362.

Bracher, M., Faller, C., Grötsch, W., Marshall, R, and Spengler, J. (1990). Studies on the potential mutagenicity of *p*-phenylenediamine in oxidative hair dye mixtures. *Mutat. Res.* **241,** 313–323.

Burnett, C. M. and Corbett, J. F. (1987). Failure of short-term *in vitro* mutagenicity tests to predict the animal carcinogenicity of hair dyes. *Food Chem. Toxicol.* **25(9),** 703–707.

Burnett, C., and Goldenthal, I. E. (1988). Multigeneration reproduction and carcinogenicity studies in Sprague-Dawley rats exposed topically to oxidative hair colouring formulations containing *p*-phenylenediamine and other aromatic amines. *Food Chem. Toxicol.* **26(5),** 467–474.

Burnett, C., Fuchs, C., Corbett, J., and Menkart, J. (1982). The effect of dimethylsulfoxide on the mutagenicity of the hair dye *p*-phenylenediamine. *Mutat. Res.* **103,** 1–4.

Burnett, C., Goldenthal, I. E., Harris, S. B., Wazeter, F. X., Strausburg, J., Kapp, R., and Voelker, R. (1976). Teratology and percutaneous toxicity studies on hair dyes. *J. Toxicol. Environ. Health* **1,** 1027–1040.

Burnett, C., Jacobs, M. M., Seppala, A., and Shubik, P. (1980). Evaluation of the toxicity and carcinogenicity of hair dyes. *J. Toxicol. Environ. Health* **6,** 247–257.

Burnett, C., Lanman, B., Giovacchini, R., Wolcott, G., and Scala, R. (1975). Long-term toxicity studies on oxidation hair dyes. *Food Chem. Toxicol.* **13,** 353–357.

Burnett, C., Loehr, R., and Corbett, J. (1981). Heritable translocation study on two hair dye formulations. *Fund. Appl. Toxicol.* **1,** 325–328.

Cronin, E. (1984). Photosensitivity to musk ambrette. *Contact Dermatitis* **11,** 88–92.

De Groot, A. C., and Frosch, P. J. (1997). Adverse reactions to fragrances: A clinical review. *Contact Dermatitis* **36,** 57–86.

Dooms-Goossens, A., Kerre, S., Drieghe, J., Bossuyt, L., and Degreef, H. (1992). Cosmetic products and their allergens. *Eur. J. Dermatol.* **2,** 465–468.

Dressler, W. E. (1998). Percutaneous absorption of hair dyes. *In* "Dermal Absorption and Toxicity Assessment" (M. Roberts and K. A. Walters eds.) Vol. 21. Marcel Dekker, New York (in press).

ECETOC (1993) "Percutaneous Absorption." Monograph No. 20. European Centre for Ecotoxicology and Toxicology of Chemicals. Brussels, Belgium.

FDA. (1994). "Cosmetic Injury Reports from Consumers as Reported to Office of Cosmetics & Colors Division of Programs and Enforcement Policy Cosmetic Programs and Regulations Branch, Food and Drug Administration, Washington, D.C. 20204, July 1987 through 1995." U.S. Food and Drug Administration, Washington, D.C.

FDA. (1996) "Regression Line and Other Pertinent Statistical Data Based on Cosmetic Product Experience Information Reported Voluntarily by Some Cosmetic Firms under 21 CFR 730 for the Years 1989–1992" U.S. Food and Drug Administration, Washington, D.C.

Ford, R. A., Api, A. M., and Newberne, P. M. (1990). 90-Day dermal toxicity study and neurotoxicity evaluation of nitromusks in the albino rat. *Food Chem. Toxicol.* **28(1),** 55–61.

Frosch, P. J., Lahti, A., Hannuksela, M., Andersen, K. E., Wilkinson, J. D., Shaw, S., and Lachapelle, J. M. (1995). Chloromethylisothiazolone/methylisothiazolone (DMI/MI) use test with a shampoo on patch-test-positive subjects—Results of a multicentre double-blind crossover trial. *Contact Dermatitis* **32,** 210–217.

Gaylor, D. W., and Gold, L. S. (1995). Quick estimate of the regulatory virtually safe dose based on the maximum tolerated dose for rodent bioassays. *Regulatory Toxicol. Pharmacol.* **22,** 57–63.

Haws, L. C., Jackson, B. A., Turnbull, D., and Dressler, W. (1994). Two approaches for assessing human safety of Disperse Blue 1. *Regulatory Toxicol. Pharmacol.* **19,** 80–96.

Jacobs, M. M., Burnett, C. M., Penicnak, A. J., Herrera, J. A., Morris, W. E., Shubik, P., Apaja, M., and Granroth, G. (1984). Evaluation of the toxicity and carcinogenicity of hair dyes in Swiss mice. *Drug Chem. Toxicol.* **1,** 573–586.

Johansen, J. D., Rastogi, S. C., Andersen, K. E., and Menné, T. (1997). Content and reactivity to product perfumes in fragrance mix positive and negative eczema patients—A study of perfumes used in toiletries and skin-care products. *Contact Dermatitis* **36,** 291–296.

Larsen, W., Nakayama, H., Lindberg, M., Fisher, T., Elsner, P., Burrows, D., Jordan, W., Shaw, S., Wilkinson, J., Marks, J., Jr., Sugawara, M., and Nethercott, J. (1996). Fragrance contact dermatitis: A worldwide multicenter investigation (part I). *Amer. J. Contact Dermatitis* **7(2),** 77–83.

Litovitz T. L., Felberg, L., White S., and Klein-Schwartz, W. (1996). 1995 annual report of the american association of poison control centers toxic exposure surveillance system. *Amer. J. Emergency Med.* **14(5),** 487–537.

Maekawa, A., Matsushima, Y., Onodera, H., Shitutani, M., Ogasawara, H., Kodame, Y., Kurokawa, Y., and Hayashi, Y. (1990) Long-term toxicity/carcinogenicity of musk xlol in B6C3F1 mice. *Food Chem. Toxicol.* **28(8),** 581–586.

Nater, J. P., and de Groot, A. C. (1985). "Unwanted Effects of Cosmetics and Drugs Used in Dermatology" Elsevier, New York.

National Toxicology Program (1993). Hair dyes NTP research findings (personal communication).

National Toxicology Program (1994). "Comparative Toxicology Studies of Corn Oil, Safflower Oil, and Tricaprylin (CAS Nos. 8001-30-7, 8001-23-8, and 538-23-8) in Male F344/N Rats as Vehicles for Gavage." NTP Technical Report, Series No. 426. NIH Publication No. 94-3157. NIH, Bethesda, Maryland.

The Nutrition Foundation (1983). "The Relevance of Mouse Liver Hepatoma to Human Carcinogenic risk." Report of the International Expert Advisory Committee to the Nutrition Foundation.

Scheinman, P. L. (1996). Allergic contact dermatitis to fragrance: A review. *Amer. J. Contact Dermatitis* **7(2),** 65–76.

Sterzel, W. (1997). Toxicology of surfactants used in cosmetics. *In* "Surfactants in Cosmetics" 2nd ed.; pp. 557–571. Marcel Dekker, New York.

Stuard, S. B., Johnson, D. R. Caudill, D., and Lehman-McKeeman, L. D. (1996). Structure-activity relationsuips for induction and inactivation of cytochrome P-450 2B enzymes (Cyp2b) by synthetic nitro musks. *Fund. Appl. Toxicol.* (supplement) **30(1),** 274–275.

Tennant, R. W., Margolin, B. H., Shelby, M. D., Zeiger, E., Haseman, J. K., Spalding, J., Caspary, W., Resnick, M., Stasiewicz, S., Anderson, B., and Minor, R. (1987). Prediction of chemical carcinogenicity in rodents from *in vitro* genetic toxicity assays. *Science* **236,** 933–941.

Wernick, T., Lanman, B., Fraux. J. L. (1975). Chronic toxicity, teratologic and reproduction studies with hair dyes. *J. Toxicol. Appl. Pharmacol.* **32,** 450–460.

Yoshikawa, K. (1996). Anomalous nonidentity between *Salmonella* genotoxicants and rodent carcinogens: Nongenotoxic carcinogens and genotoxic noncarcinogens. *Environ. Health Perspect.*: **104,** 40–46.

Young, S. S. (1989). Are there location/cage/systematic nontreatment effects in long-term rodent studies? A question revisited. *Fund. Appl. Toxicol.* **13(2),** 183–188.

CHAPTER

38

Polymers

ECKHARD LÖSER, GISELA STROPP

Institute of Industrial Toxicology, Bayer-AG, Wuppertal, Germany

INTRODUCTION

Polymers are high-molecular-weight substances produced from a variety of identical or similar low molecular units. The characteristics and specific physical and chemical properties of polymers are a function of the type of polymers from which they are produced. The typical properties of the various polymers, however, are a function of the monomers and the additives used to modify the plastics materials. Additives are, for example, stabilizers, plasticizers, lubricants, and catalysts. Polymers are differentiated according to their production methods into polymerisates (e.g., polyethylene, polyvinylchloride, and polystyrene), polycondensates (e.g. phenol resins, silicones, polyester, polycarbonates, and polyamides), and polyadducts (e.g., epoxy resins, and cross-linked polyurethanes). Polymers are differentiated according to their properties into thermoplasts, duroplasts, and elastomeres. Natural polymers for technical use are wood, cotton, and wool; the natural polymers are not discussed further in this chapter.

Important polymer materials and their respective monomers are listed in Table 1.

MONOMERS

Monomers are normally low-molecular-weight units from which the polymers are formed. Monomers are predominantly reactive substances produced extensively using fossil raw material, such as oil. The basic requirement for the reactivity of the monomers are unsaturated bindings or easily reacting moieties. Unsaturated bindings allow polymerization, whereas easily reacting moieties allow polyaddition or polycondensation.

Technically important monomers are alkenes (e.g., ethylene, propylene, and butadiene), aromatic-substituted alkenes (e.g., styrene), nitrogen-substituted alkenes (e.g., acrylonitrile), acrylic acid compounds (e.g., acrylates and methacrylates), chloro- and fluoro-substituted alkenes (e.g., vinyl chloride, vinylidene chloride, vinyl fluoride, vinylidene fluoride, 2-chloroprene, and tetrafluoroethylene), diisocyanates, amino compounds (e.g., hexamethylenediamine, caprolactam, and melamine), dicarbonic acids (e.g., adipic acid and terephthalic acid), anhydrides (e.g., phthalic acid anhydride), aldehydes (e.g., formaldehyde), phenol compounds (e.g., phenol and bisphenol A), alcohols (e.g., ethylene glycol, propylene glycol, butanediol, and the ethoxylated and propoxylated derivates of butanediol), carbonylic compounds (e.g., phosgene), epoxide compounds (e.g., ethylene oxide, propylene-oxide, and epichlorohydrine), and silanes (e.g., methylchlorosilane).

Unsaturated Monomers

Alkenes

Ethylene (C_2H_4, CAS No. 74-85-1) is mainly used in the production of polyethylene. Ethylene in liquid form may produce skin and eye irritation in humans and freezing effects.

Ethylene, under normal pressure, is a gas with narcotic properties in animals and humans. Prolonged exposure to high concentrations of the gas is associated with the disturbance of vision in humans. Ethyl-

TABLE 1 Polymers and Monomers

Polymer (abbreviation)	Monomers
Thermoplastics	
Polyethylene (PE)	Ethylene
Polypropylene (PP)	Propylene
Polyvinyl chloride (PVC)	Vinyl chloride
Polyvinyl fluoride (PVF)	Vinyl fluoride
Polyvinyl acetate (PVA)	Vinyl acetate
Polystyrene (PS)	Styrene
Polyamides (PA)	Diamine (e.g., hexamethylenediamine), dicarbonic acids (e.g., adipinic acid) Lactamderivates
Polyethyleneterephthalate (PET)	Dimethylterephthalic acid, Ethylene glycol
Acrylonitrile-butadiene-styrene (ABS)	Acrylonitrile, styrene, butadiene
Polycarbonate (PC)	Bisphenol A and diphenyl carbonate
Polytetrafluoroethylene (PTFE)	Tetrafluoroethylene
Celluloseacetate (CA)	Cellulose
Duroplasts	
Phenolic resins (PF)	Phenols and formaldehyde
Unsaturated polyester (UP)	Hydroxy- or dicarbonic acids and alcohols (e.g., ethylene glycol)
Polyurethane (PUR)	Isocyanate, dicarbonic acids, and low-molar-mass hydroxy compounds polyols)
Epoxy resins (EP)	Bisphenol A and epichlorohydrine, BADGE
Melamine-formaldehyde resins (MF)	Melamine and formaldehyde
Elastomeres	
Polyisoprene (IR)	Isoprene
Polybutadiene (BR)	Butadiene
Styrene-butadiene co-polymer (SB)	Styrene, butadiene
Styrene-acrylonitrile co-polymer (SAN)	Styrene, acrylonitrile
Polychloroprene (CR)	Chloroprene
Silicone resins (SI)	Methylchlorosilane
Natural rubber (NR)	Isoprene, proteine, fat, carbohydrates
Polyvinyl acetate resins (PVAC)	Vinyl acetate

ene is a low-level by-product of physiological processes in human. The inhalative uptake is very rapid. In the mammalian metabolism, it is partly oxidized to the carcinogen ethyleneoxide. The Ames mutagenicity assay was negative. The inhalation of ethylene leads to DNA adducts in different species. In a long-term inhalation study in rats and in a liver foci test, however, there was no evidence of carcinogenic effects of ethylene. For example, an exposure to 50 ppm leads to an internal ethylene oxide burden comparable to an exposure to 1 ppm ethylene oxide. A study in volunteers showed that 2% of inhaled ethylene was metabolized, whereas 98% was exhaled unchanged.

Propylene (C_3H_6, CAS No. 115-07-1) is a gas used as a starting material in the production of polypropylene plastics and various other chemical materials (e.g., propyl alcohol, propylene oxide, and allyl chloride). No irritant effects were observed with propylene in high concentrations in gaseous form, but, when compressed to a liquid, freezing effects on tissue may occur in humans. High concentrations of propylene are analgesic and narcotic. At very high concentrations, propylene may cause asphyxia by displacement of oxygen. The target organs of toxicity after repeated inhalation of propylene are the liver, kidney, and respiratory tract. The genotoxicity data are inconclusive.

Similar to ethylene, propylene also induced no tumor formation in long-term inhalation studies, although the corresponding epoxide (propylene oxide) is mutagenic and carcinogenic in animal experiments. With propylene there is evidence of a saturable metabolism with a maximal body burden of propylene oxide. Similar to ethylene and ethylene oxide, propylene oxide is also not produced in amounts capable of inducing tumors.

1,3-Butadiene (divinyl, C_4H_6, CAS No. 106-99-0) is a colorless gas used mainly for the synthesis of copolymers, for example, ABS (the polymer from acrylonitrile-butadiene-styrene), but it is also a chemical intermediate. As a liquid, it leads to frostbite after skin contact. In humans, very high concentrations in the air led to irritation and to a central-nervous-system depression and/or narcosis. The acute oral toxicity in the rat is low and the LC_{50} is 285,000 mg/m^3 after a 4-hour inhalation exposure. At very high concentrations 1,3-butadiene may cause asphyxia by displacement of oxygen.

The repeated-dose toxicity gave evidence of species differences of the toxic effects, the mouse being particularly susceptible. In rats up to concentrations of 18,000 mg/m^3, no specific symptoms were recorded, whereas in mice there was an increase of mortality at this concentration. Butadiene is a well-defined multisite carcinogen (the most sensitive response is in the lung) in the mouse, whereas it has a low or no carcinogenic potency in rats. This difference of sensitivity is due to more effective biotransformation to mono- and diepoxides of butadiene in mice. The mono- and diepoxides are metabolic intermediates that have been identified as the ultimate agents for the carcinogenic and mutagenic potential of butadiene (see Fig. 1 for the metabolism of butadiene). Genotoxicity tests *in vitro* were positive only in the presence of a metabolic system. *In vivo* studies indicate that butadiene is mutagenic in the mouse but not in the rat or the hamster. In mice, positive results in dominant lethal studies indicate that butadiene is also a germ cell mutagen. The genotoxic potential of butadiene in humans has been evaluated in a number of studies in exposed workers. From these studies there is some evidence that butadiene causes genetic damage in humans. Butadiene is not teratogenic, as shown in animal experiments. Extensive epidemiologic studies have been conducted in workers from butadiene-monomer production plants and polymerizing plants. In workers from polymerizing plants, only increased incidences of lymphohematopoetic malignancies of different types have been reported. Combined styrene and benzene exposures is a confounding factor in this studies.

Isoprene (2-methyl-1,3-butadiene, CAS No. 78-79-5) occurs naturally and is widely present. It is emitted from plants and produced endogenously by humans and rodents. Isoprene is a precursor of polycyclic aromatics and a constituent of natural rubber. Industrially, isoprene is used for the synthesis of various types of elastomers; *cis*-1,4-polyisoprene is the most important. Isoprene is of low toxicity following single oral, dermal, or inhalative exposure. In humans, isoprene causes irriation to skin, eyes, and respiratory tract. After repeated skin contact, the human skin becomes dry and flaky.

In animals, the elimination of isoprene and metabolites occurs mainly via the urine. The principal reactive metabolites *in vitro* are mono- and diepoxides. *In*

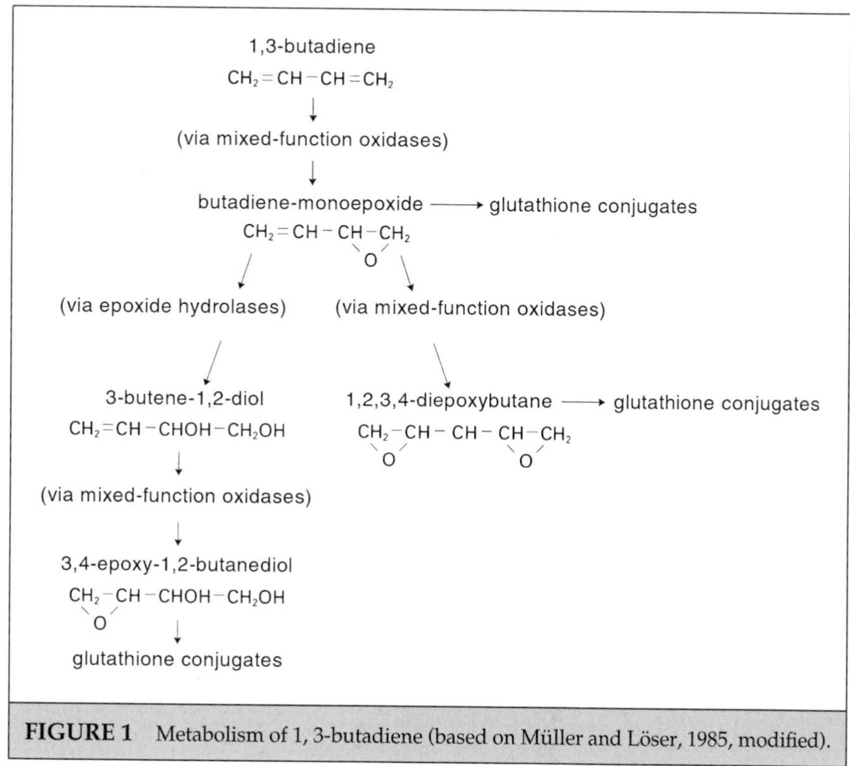

FIGURE 1 Metabolism of 1, 3-butadiene (based on Müller and Löser, 1985, modified).

vivo a saturation of isoprene metabolism was observed at exposure concentrations between 266 and 1480 ppm after a 6-hour exposure. Repeated exposure in experimental animals showed reduction in red blood cell count, olfactory epithelial degeneration, testicular atrophy, and forestomach epithelial hyperplasia. Isoprene is nonmutagenic in *in vitro* tests. It induces micronuclei in the bone marrow and peripheral blood and sister chromatid exchanges (SCE) in the bone marrow in mice. There is lack of mutagenic response of the monoepoxides of isoprene, but the diepoxide is positive in a bacterial mutagenesis assay. Inhalation carcinogenicity studies showed multiorgan tumor induction (e.g., in the liver, forestomach, lungs, and Harderian gland) in mice but not in rats. This tumor pattern is similar to the pattern seen in butadiene-exposed mice. T-cell lymphomas, however, were not seen in the isoprene experiment. The carcinogenic potency of isoprene is lower than that of butadiene. Isoprene was not embryotoxic or teratogenic after oral administration in rats.

Aromatic Substituted Alkenes

Styrene (vinylbenzene, C_8H_8, CAS No. 100-42-5) is a liquid widely used in the production of plastics, synthetic rubber, and polyester resins. It irritates the eye and the respiratory tract. Chronic local contact leads to defattening of the skin in humans. After exposure to high concentrations via inhalation (up to 800 ppm), fatigue, increased reaction times, and changes in the electroencephalogram (EEG) were recorded. Styrene is well absorbed after inhalation in humans, whereas dermal absorption is low. Styrene is of low toxicity following repeated exposure in different species. The mouse is the most susceptible species. Styrene is metabolized through 7,8-styreneoxide (Fig. 2). Elimination takes places as mandelic acid (60–80%) or phenylglyoxylic acid (approximately 30%) via the urine. The metabolite 7,8-styreneoxide is a mutagen and carcinogen, whereas similar studies with styrene gave no evidence of a carcinogenic potential. This is due to a rapid detoxification of styrene and the short half-life of the epoxides during metabolism. Additional long-term studies are ongoing. Animal and human data indicate that styrene is not genotoxic *in vivo*.

Nitrogen-Substituted Alkenes

Acrylonitrile (vinyl cyanide, propenenitrile, C_3H_3N, CAS No. 107-13-1) is a colorless, highly flammable, and volatile liquid. It is widely used as monomer for acrylic fibers and in co-polymers with styrene and butadiene. Acrylonitrile is well absorbed from the respiratory tract, the gastrointestinal tract, and the skin.

Biotransformation occurs via two major pathways, direct glutathione (GSH) conjugation and cytochrome P450-mediated oxidation to the epoxide 2-cyanoethylene oxide (glycidonitrile) (Fig. 3). The elimination is mainly via the urine. Symptoms in humans after exposure to toxic concentrations are icterus, anemia, cyanosis, nausea, vomiting, and headache and resemble those of intoxication with hydrogene cyanide (HCN). In liquid form and as a vapor, acrylonitrile is an irritant to the skin and mucous membranes and has sensitization properties. Long-term experiments with oral (via drinking water) or inhalation exposure showed increased tumor incidences (e.g., mammary tumors, brain tumors, forestomach tumors, and Zymbal gland tumors). *In vitro* genotoxicity studies revealed positive results, whereas *in vivo* studies in mammals were mostly negative. Acrylnitrie–DNA binding has been shown in the rat liver. Acrylonitrile is teratogenic at maternally toxic exposure doses.

Epidemiological studies of workers with potential exposure to acrylonitrile revealed inconsistent results. The carcinogenicity of acrylonitrile in humans is unresolved.

Acrylic Acid Compounds

Acrylic compounds of technical importance are acrylates (e.g., *n*-butyl acrylate, ethyl acrylate, and methyl acrylate) and methacrylates (e.g., methylmethacrylate, ethylmethacrylate and *n*-butylmethacrylate).

Acrylates and methacrylates are liquids used in the synthesis of plastics and resins. The toxicity of the compounds decrease with an increase of the chain length. Acrylates show higher acute toxicity than methacrylates with LD_{50} values of 500 to 5000 mg/kg body weight for the acrylates. The irritation potential of methacrylates is higher than that of acrylates. The acute toxicity of the methacrylates is low with LD_{50} values of more than 5000 mg/kg body weight. Acrylates and methacrylates show skin-sensitization properties to different degrees. Cross-reactivity is also described. The repeated-dose toxicity is dominated by the local irritation caused by the compounds. Acrylates and methacrylates are hydrolyzed to their respective alcohols.

In vitro genotoxicity studies were partly positive at cytotoxic test concentrations. Carcinogenicity studies with acrylates showed that tumorigenic response after oral and dermal exposure can be attributed to the local reactivity of these compounds. Long-term studies with methylmethacrylate showed no increase of

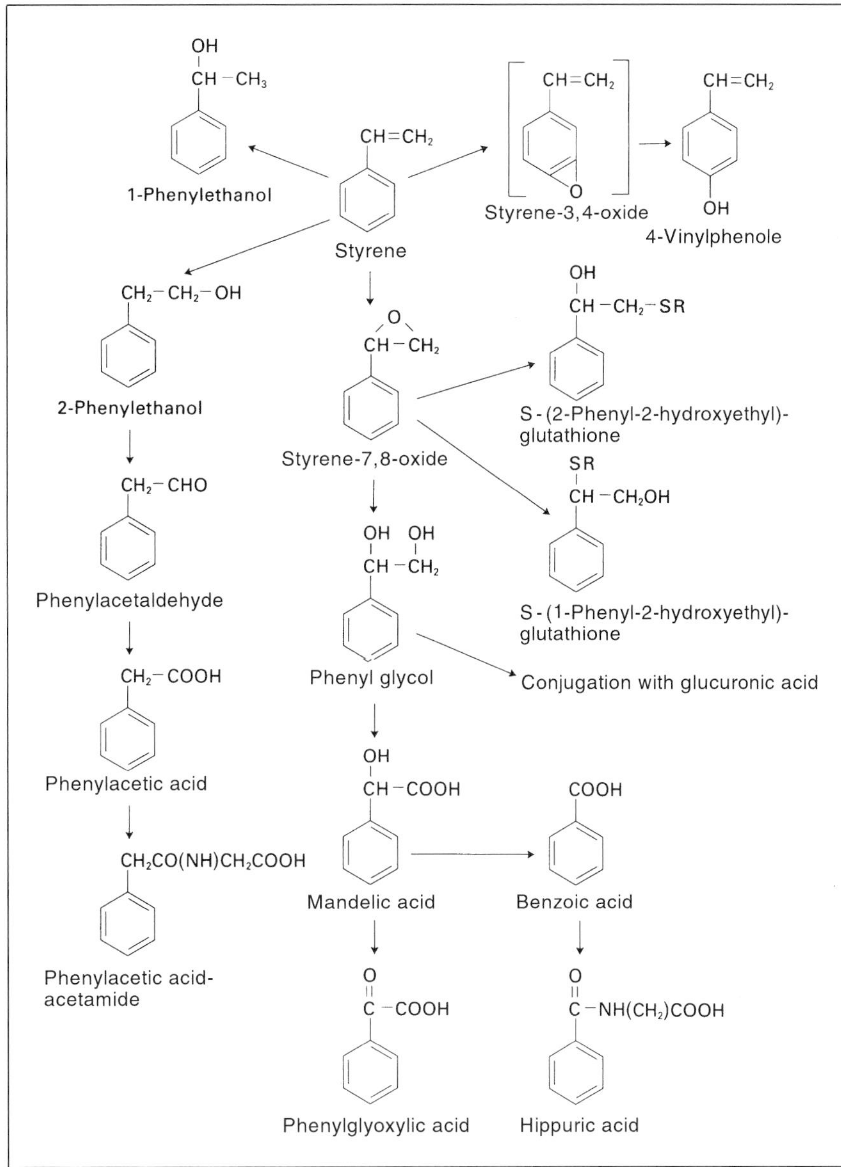

FIGURE 2 Metabolism of styrene (according GDCh) The quantitatively most important path of metabolism is the oxidation of the lateral chain to styrene-7, 8-oxide with following metabolism to phenyl glycol, catalyzed by epoxide hydrolase.

tumor incidence after oral and inhalation exposure. Acrylates showed teratogenic effects at maternal toxic doses in mice but not in rats.

Acrylamide (C_3H_5NO; CAS No. 79-06-1) is a water-soluble solid primarily used in the production of polymers and co-polymers, but also for other industrial uses. Rapid absorption leads to a rapid onset of toxic effects. Acrylamide shows neurotoxic properties in humans (e.g., hallucination, confusion, and peripheral neuropathy) and in animals (e.g., peripheral axonopathy and axonal swelling in the medulla oblongata and spinal cord) after repeated intake. The neurotoxicity was reversible in most cases.

After skin contact in humans, acrylamide led to irritations of the skin, mucous epithelium, and eyes. Animal experiments showed binding of acrylamide to DNA, RNA, and protein and can be detected in erythrocytes. In *in vivo* and *in vitro* genotoxicity studies, acrylamide showed mostly clastogenic activity. Carcinogenicity studies led to tumors in a number of tissues and organs in rats and mice. Acrylamide was not teratogenic in animal experiments, but transport

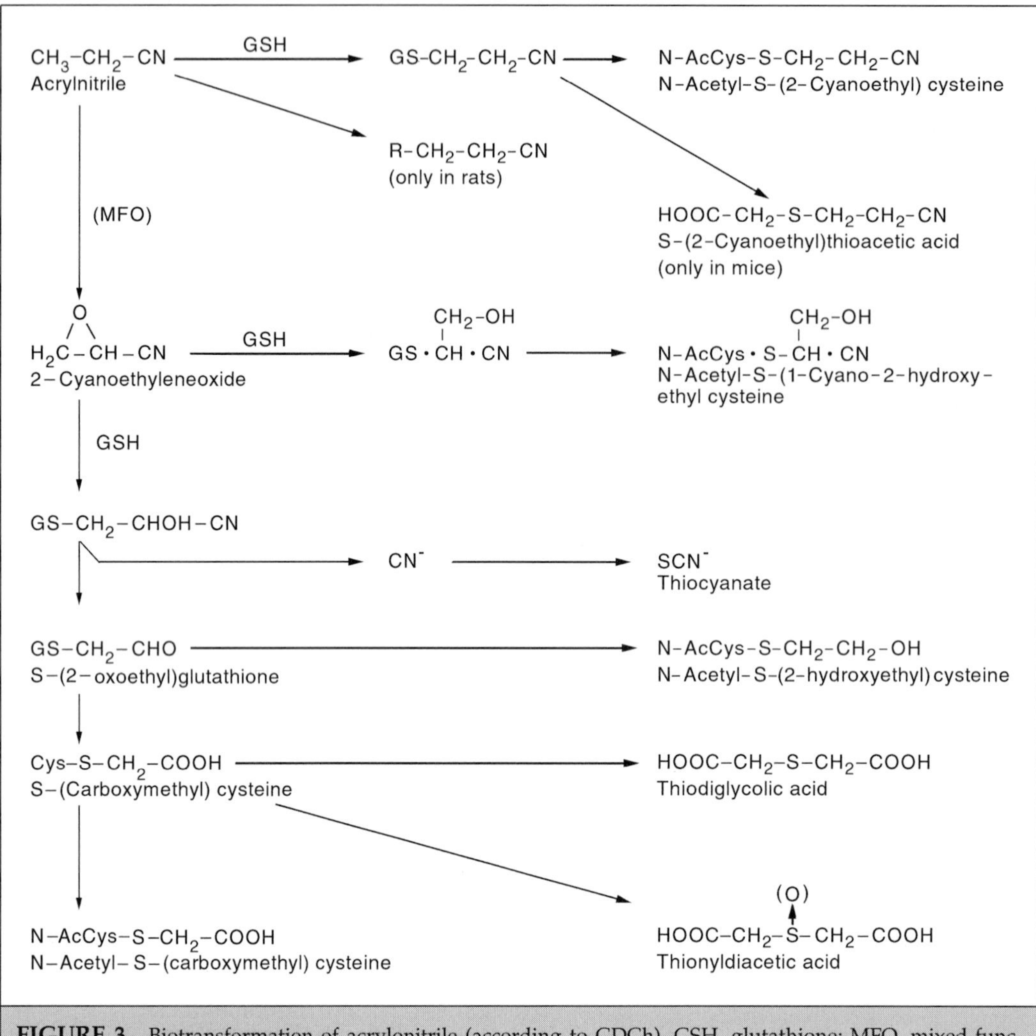

FIGURE 3 Biotransformation of acrylonitrile (according to GDCh). GSH, glutathione; MFO, mixed functional oxidases.

through the placental barrier and exposure during pregnancy may lead to neurotoxic effects in the offspring. Reduced fertility in male rodents has also been demonstrated.

Chloroalkenes

Vinyl chloride (chloroethene, C_2H_3Cl, CAS No. 75-01-4) is a colorless, explosive gas of low acute toxicity in humans and experimental animals. It is used in the production of vinyl chloride homopolymer and mixed-polymer resins. Inhalation of high concentrations (e.g., 7% in the air) led to narcosis. In contact with the skin, liquid vinyl chloride freezes tissue (frostbite). Animal data indicate a rapid absorption of vinyl chloride after inhalation or oral administration. The metabolism of vinyl chloride is dose dependent and saturable. Chloroacetaldehyde and chloroethylene oxide are the major metabolites. The relevant pathways appear to be oxidation to 2-chloroethanol, to 2-chloroacetalaldehyde, and finally to 2-chloroacetic acid by alcohol dehydrogenase or the oxidation by mixed-function oxidases to 2-chloroethylene oxide, with rearrangement to chloralaldehyde or the oxidation by catalase to 2-chloroethylhydroperoxide, followed by dehydration to form 2-chloroacetalaldehyde.

Glutathione conjugation with further rearrangements leads to thiodiglycolic acid and hydroxyethylmercapturic acid, the main urinary metabolites (Fig. 4).

Due to the low acute toxicity, workers were exposed in the past to very high concentrations of vinyl chloride vapor. This resulted in a syndrome characterized as "vinyl chloride disease." The clinical effects are liver fibrosis leading to portal hypertension and

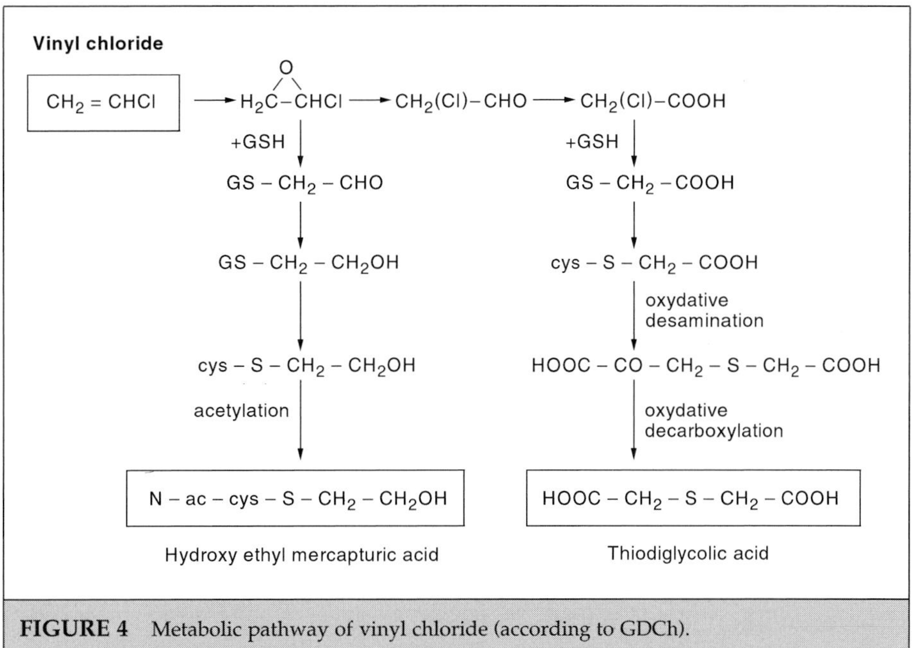

FIGURE 4 Metabolic pathway of vinyl chloride (according to GDCh).

esophagus varices, increased spleen weight with thrombocytopenia and a Raynaud-like condition with reversible arteriole constriction causing cyanosis of the fingers and osteolysis of the terminal phalanges of the fingers as a late effect. The vinyl chloride disease was no longer observed when the exposures were drastically reduced. Hemangiosarcoma in the liver and other tumors (mainly lung tumors and mammary carcinomas) are associated with occupational vinyl chloride exposure at levels of 100 ppm and higher. Inhalation and ingestion of vinyl chloride in experimental animals confirmed the carcinogenic potential of vinyl chloride (mammary gland tumors, liver tumors, lung tumors, and hemangiosarcoma in different organs) seen in humans. Vinyl chloride is mutagenic in *in vitro* and *in vivo* mutagenicity assays. The mutagenicity data implicate 2-chloroethylene oxide and 2-chloroacetalaldehyde as being the mutagenic agents. 2-Chloroethylene oxide has DNA-alkylating properties and is therefore considered to be the ultimate agent for the carcinogenicity.

Vinylidene chloride (1,1-dichloroethene, VDC, $C_2H_2Cl_2$, CAS No. 75-35-4) is a volatile, colorless liquid that polymerizes rapidly and is used as a copolymer in the production of vinyl chloride co-polymers and of fibers largely based on acrylonitrile with small amounts of vinylidene chloride and other monomers. Exposure to high concentrations results in CNS depression and narcosis. Mice are more sensitive than rats to acute or long-term exposure to vinylidene chloride. Males are generally more sensitive than females. The liver and kidneys are the target organs of toxicity. The more pronounced sensitivity of mice is due to a saturation of metabolism at lower exposure concentrations compared to rats. The oxidation of vinylidene chloride to the corresponding epoxide occurs in both species, but in rats the epoxide is rapidly detoxified by the formation of the intermediate monochloroacetic acid and conjugation reactions (glutathione, cysteine), whereas in mice the conjugated epoxide is eliminated with the urine.

No teratogenic effects were observed in rats or rabbits. Several long-term studies have been conducted. In one inhalation study with mice, vinylidene chloride nephrotoxicity and kidney tumors occur, particularly in the males. Genotoxicity was shown in *E. coli* and *S. typhimurium,* but not in mammalian cells or *in vivo.* Therefore, a nongenotoxic mechanism as a result of the nephrotoxicity, especially in male mice, is suggested as the cause of carcinogenicity. In a small cohort study (n = 138), no adverse health effects attributable to vinylidene chloride were found.

2-Chloroprene (2-chlor-1,3-butadiene, C_4H_5Cl, CAS No. 126-99-8) is a flammable, colorless liquid used mainly in the production of polychloroprene elastomers. Acute intoxication is characterized by a depression of the central nervous system and in high concentrations by liver and lung damage. 2-Chloroprene is an irritant to the skin and the eyes. Epidemiological studies provide no firm evidence for a carcinogenic potential. In earlier long-term studies on rats and hamsters, 2-chloroprene showed no carcinogenic effect. A recent study using a different quality of test materials and different exposure system, however, showed a multiorgan carcinogenic effect in mice and rats. Chloroprene is mostly not mutagenic in *in vitro* and *in vivo* tests. Maternal toxic air concentrations of pure chloroprene caused fetal toxicity but no teratogenic effects. A two-generation study did not give evidence of reproductive impairment.

As are other unsaturated hydrocarbons, chloroprene is assumed to be metabolized via epoxide formation and conjugation with glutathione and eliminated as thioether. The elimination of glutathione conjugate may lead to a depletion of glutathione after saturation at high-concentration exposures.

Fluoroalkenes

Vinyl fluoride (Fluoroethylene, C_2H_3F, CAS No. 75-02-5) is a colorless gas used in the production of polyvinyl fluoride and other fluoropolymers. It is of low toxicity after single or repeated inhalation. Rapid equilibrium occurs in tissues following inhalation. Vinyl fluoride is transformed to the reactive metabolites, the epoxide intermediate. The fluoride ion appears in the urine of exposed animals. The metabolism of vinyl fluoride is saturable at concentrations higher than 75 ppm. The metabolic rate is lower in comparison with vinyl chloride or vinyl bromide.

Vinyl fluoride is mutagenic in several test systems. Rats exposed to vinyl fluoride developed ATPase-deficient (preneoplastic) hepatic foci, but the extent was lower than was seen after a similar exposure to vinyl chloride and vinyl bromide. Long-term studies revealed hepatic tumors and Zymbal gland carcinoma related to fluoride exposure in rats and hepatic tumors, bronchoalveolar tumors, mammary gland tumors, and Harderian gland tumors in mice. This spectrum of lesions is similar to vinyl chloride, but vinyl chloride induces, in addition, tumors at other sites (e.g., hemangiosarcoma).

Vinylidene fluoride (1,1-difluoroethene, $C_2H_2F_2$, CAS No. 75-38-7) is a colorless gas used in the production of polyvinylidene fluoride. It is of low acute toxicity with a lethal dose of 128,000 ppm after 4 hours exposure. No specific target organ of toxicity is described. Narcosis is the predominant symptom of acute intoxication. Vinylidene fluoride is slowly metabolized and the metabolic elimination is saturatable. Rats exposed to vinylidene fluoride developed ATPase-deficient (preneoplastic) hepatic foci, but the extent was much lower than after a comparable exposure to vinyl chloride. A limited carcinogenicity study showed some but no clear evidence of carcinogenicity (increase of lipoma) in the rat. The *Salmonella* mutagenicity assay revealed a marginal positive response.

Tetrafluoroethylene (C_2F_4, CAS No. 116-14-3) is a colorless gas used mainly in the synthesis of polytetrafluoroethylene (PTFE). Tetrafluoroethylene is of low acute toxicity with lethal doses ranging from 25,000 to 45,000 ppm. At high concentrations, the gas is an irritant to the respiratory tract. The primary pathological effects of acute high exposure and repeated inhalation toxicity are kidney changes. Rats appear to be more sensitive to the kidney-damaging effect than hamsters. There is evidence that tetrafluoroethylene undergoes conjugation with glutathione followed by degradation of the *S*-conjugate resulting in cytotoxicity in the kidney. The urinary fluoride content increases dose-dependently after repeated exposure in experimental animals. *In vitro* and *in vivo* mutagenicity studies gave no evidence of a genotoxic potential of tetrafluoroethylene.

Monomers with Easily Reacting Moieties

Diisocyanates

Industrially important diisocyanates are diphenylmethane 4,4′-diisocyanate (MDI), toluene diisocyanate (TDI), and hexamethylene diisocyanate (HDI). TDI and MDI have a melting point of approximately 22 and 40°C and are mostly solid materials. HDI, with a melting point of −67°C, is a liquid. Diisocyanates are used in the production of polyurethane, which are the the basic materials for flexible or rigid foam, coatings, and elastomers.

The toxicity of the diisocyanates is to a great extent influenced by the reactivity of the isocyanate (−N=C=O) moiety. The acute oral toxicity in general is low, whereas the inhalation toxicity, especially of the aerosols, is high. Inhalation leads to a concentration-dependent irritation at the respiratory tract. The acute skin- and eye-irritation properties of the diisocyanates vary. Animal experiments show respiratory hypersensitivity. The skin-sensitization potential of the diisocyanates is of less importance. Long-term and high-concentration occupational exposure to diisocyanates led to irritation and impairment of the lung function in humans. Asthmatic symptoms (isocyanate asthma) are based on a bronchial hyperreagibility, which is correlated with specific antibodies, as observed in some of the persons affected.

The 2,4- and 2,6-toluene diisocyanate mixture (80 : 20) gave no evidence of reprotoxicity in the animal experiment.

Mutagenicity test results differ due to the different vehicles used in the experiments. Chronic inhalation of toluene diisocyanate and hexamethylene diisocyanate gave no evidence of carcinogenicity in animal experiments, whereas an aerosol of diphenylmethane 4,4′-diisocyanate-prepolymer (containing approximately 50% monomer diphenylmethane 4,4′-diisocyanate) led to lung adenoma. The lung adenoma are most probably the result of the chronic irritation effect to the lung tissue. Chronic oral administration of 2,4- and 2,6-toluene diisocyanate in corn oil via gavage led to an increased incidence of subcutanous fibroma and fibrosarcoma, as well as mamma tumors, pancreas adenoma, and pancreas islet adenoma in rats and hemangioma, hemangiosarcoma, and liver adenoma in female mice. This tumor spectrum is very similar to that in studies of the carcinogen 2,4-diaminotoluene. It was shown that in the long-term oral study with 2,4-/2,6-toluene diisocyanate, the test material was partly decomposed in the vehicle used (corn oil). Further formation of the amine is expected as a reaction product under the acidic conditions in the stomach. Another shortcoming for using corn oil as vehicle is its well-established contribution to the production of pancreas adenoma in rats.

Aliphatic Amines

1,6-Hexanediamine ($C_6H_{16}N_2$, CAS No. 124-09-4) is a solid with high solubility in water. 1,6-Hexanediamine is widely used as a corrosion inhibitor in lubricants and as an intermediate in the synthesis of resins, especially polyamide resins. The acute toxicity is moderate; due to the alkaline reaction corrosion of the skin and eyes may occur after local contact. Vapor and dust led to irritation of the upper respiratory tract in animal experiments. The principal route of excretion is via the urine. 1,6-Hexanediamine causes retardation of fetal development in rats and mice, but no teratogenic effects have been found. 1,6-Hexanediamine was not genotoxic.

Caprolactam (6-aminohexanoic acid cyclic lactam, $C_6H_{11}NO$, CAS No. 105-60-2) is a white solid with high solubility in water. It is used primarily as a monomer for synthetic fibers and plastics and as a cross-linker for polyurethanes. Caprolactam stimulates the central nervous system, and is shown to be a convulsant in animals and humans. Caprolactam vapor or dust irritates the skin and the respiratory tract. Some isolated cases of contact dermatitis cannot be considered to be evidence for caprolactam as a skin sensitizer. Experimental data suggest that caprolactam at high doses depresses circulatory functions and leads to respiratory stimulation. The chronic exposure of rats and mice via the diet did not increase the tumor incidences. No genotoxic effects of caprolactam have been seen. In rats and rabbits, caprolactam is not a teratogen. A three-generation reproduction study in the rat showed no effects on the reproductive performance.

Melamine (2,4,6-triamino-1,3,5-triazine, $C_3H_6N_6$, CAS No. 108-78-1) is a solid of low acute toxicity used for the synthesis of resins, predominantly formaldehyde-melamine resin. Melamine shows no irritation effects to the skin and the eyes and is no skin sensitizer in the animal experiment. Comprehensive studies on genotoxicity *in vivo* and *in vitro* showed no genotoxic potential. Melamine causes diuresis and is eliminated up to 90% via the urine within 1 day after oral intake. After uptake of high doses, crystalization in the urinary tract may occur and may lead to the formation of urinary calculi. Urinary calculi formation in long-term animal experiments with high doses of melamine produced chronic irritation effects in the urinary tract, which resulted in the formation of tumors of the urinary bladder epithelium (transitional-cell carcinoma) in male rats.

Dicarbonic Acids

Terephthalic acid ($C_8H_6O_4$, CAS No. 110-21-0) is a solid used for the synthesis of polyethyleneterephthalate. The acute toxicity is low. Terephthalic acid is not an irritant to skin and mucous epithelium. The available animal tests showed no signs of intoxications. Repeated dose toxicity after oral dosing in rats resulted in urinary calculi formation resulting in urinary bladder calculi and hyperplasia of the urinary bladder epithelium. Consequently, bladder carcinoma were observed at low incidences. Terephthalic acid is not genotoxic. In high maternal toxic doses of 1000 mg/kg body weight and higher doses, fetal loss was observed in rats.

Adipic acid ($C_6H_{10}O_4$, CAS No. 124-04-9) is a solid used for the production of polyesters and polyester-urethanes and polyamides. It is of low toxicity after single and repeated oral or inhalative exposure in animal experiments. Irritative effects to the eye were more pronounced than to the skin. Adipic acid shows no genotoxic potential in various *in vivo* or *in vitro* genotoxicity tests. No carcinogenic or teratogenic potential was demonstrated in animal experiments. Adipic acid is readily absorbed after oral administration. Excretion of the unmetabolized adipic acid via urine or as CO_2 via the airways are the main paths of elimination.

Alcohols

Important alcohols for the production of polyesters are ethylene glycol and propylene glycol.

Ethylene glycol ($C_2H_6O_2$; CAS No. 107-21-1) is a colorless liquid that is used in the production of polyester films and fibers, polyethylene terephthalate

(PET) solid-state resins, elastomers, and other products. Another use is as antifreeze in coolants. It is well absorbed following administration by various routes. Metabolism is via glycol aldehyde to glyoxalate and oxalate to CO_2. Oxalate may crystalize and form bladder stones. CO_2 in the exhaled air and glycolate and unchanged ethylene glycol are the major excretory end product. Ethylene glycol is of low acute toxicity. Irritation effects on the skin, eyes, and respiratory system have been described. The kidneys are the target organs of repeated-dose toxicity. Ethylene glycol is not genotoxic in various test systems. Long-term studies showed no evidence of carcinogenic activity in rats and mice. In reproductive toxicity studies after very high oral doses, embryotoxic and teratogenic effects have been shown.

Propylene glycol ($C_3H_8O_2$; CAS No. 57-55-6) is a liquid used as an intermediate in the production of polyester resins and polyurethanes. Other uses are as an antifreezing agent or flame retardant. It is of low acute toxicity and is absorbed after oral exposure, dermal contact, or inhalation. It is metabolized via lactic aldehyde and methoxy glyoxal to lactate or pyruvate. Propylene glycol has no skin-sensitizing properties in experimental animals; however, some cases of positive patch-test reactions in humans are documented. Propylene glycol is not genotoxic in various test systems or carcinogenic in experimental animals and shows no reproductive toxicity.

Aldehydes

Formaldehyde (CH_2O, CAS No. 50-00-0) is an irritant gas that is used in the production of phenolic resins and as a chemical intermediate. It is easily recognized by the stinging and prickling smell. Symptoms of toxicity are dominated by the irritant action to the mucous membranes of eyes and respiratory tract (e.g., lacrimation, catarrh, and laryngospasmus). Skin sensitization after skin contact was described after contact with an aqueous solution of formaldehyde but not after contact with the gas. The positive results of *in vitro* genotoxicity tests could not be confirmed by most of the *in vivo* experiments. Chronic inhalation in the rat, and to a lesser extent in the mouse, induced local tumors at the mucous membranes in the nose and the sinuses. However, despite the extensive use of formaldehyde in various applications, formaldehyde did not reveal any evidence of tumor formation in the respiratory tract in humans, even at very high exposures. A causal relationship with the irritation is suggested for the effects in animals.

Anhydride

Phthalic anhydride ($C_8H_4O_3$; CAS No. 85-44-9) occurs as white crystalline needles with a mild odor and is used as an industrial chemical and for the manufacture of resins and polyesters. It is a potent irritant to the skin and mucous membranes (e.g., eye and respiratory tract) but, in comparison to other industrial acid anhydrides such as maleic acid anhydride, the irritation is of lower degree.

Sensitization, particularly at the respiratory tract (anhydride asthma), is a well-known disease in humans. The anhydride is hydrolyzed to phthalic acid, which is eliminated rapidly in unconjugated form via the urine. Phthalic anhydride shows no genotoxic or carcinogenic properties.

Phenol Compounds

Phenol (hydroxybenzene; C_6H_5OH; CAS No. 108-95-2) is a crystalline solid with a distinctive odor that is used as the starting product for a variety of industrial chemicals, for example, in the manufacture of synthetic resins and plastics. Phenol penetrates the skin rapidly, irrespective of whether it is solid, liquid, or gaseous. By hydroxylation of phenol, isomeric dihydroxybenzenes (e.g., hydroquinone, catechol, benzoquinone, and 1,2,4-trihydroxybenzene) are formed to a limited degree. The elimination occurs rapidly, mainly via the urine as the main metabolites, phenylsulfate and phenylglucuronide. Dermal contact is the main route of incorporation. Lethal accidents due to dermal resorption are described. Rapid decontamination after dermal contact is therefore essential. The main symptoms of acute lethal intoxication are local effects, central nervous symptoms, and congestion. After long-term exposure, the effects on the nervous system and dermatitis predominate, whereas long-term studies revealed no effect on tumor formation. Malformations or variations were not seen in fetuses from phenol-treated dams. The only effect seen in developmental studies was an decrease of the fetal body weight.

Bisphenol A ($C_{15}H_{16}O_2$; CAS No. 80-05-7) is a white solid with a mild phenolic odor that is used for the production of epoxy resins, phenol resins, and polycarbonate. It is of low toxicity. The skin irritation potency is minimal; however, it is more pronounced at the mucous membranes of nose and throat after exposure to bisphenol A dust. The repeated oral administration led to minor damage in the liver and urinary bladder. After long-term inhalation exposure, inflammatory reactions of the mucous membranes in the nose appeared as a result of the irritation properties. The wide range of genotoxicity tests, as well as the carcinogenicity data, in rats and mice gave no evidence of a genotoxic or carcinogenic potential. Animal experiments found no teratogenic effect. Embryotoxic effects were seen in maternally toxic doses with increased maternal mortality. The effect on fertility at doses causing systemic toxic effects in various tissues can be regarded as secondary to general intoxication. The guinea pig maximization-sensitization test with bisphenol A did not induce skin sensitization. Cross-reactivity was described in humans with expoxy resin exposure. Persistent light-responsive dermatitis was described in animal experiments and in bisphenol A-exposed workers. Some short-term assays indicate a very low estrogenic potential of bisphenol A; long-term and reproductive toxicity studies, however, gave no indication of an estrogenic effect or hormonal imbalance in mammals.

Carbonyl Compounds

Phosgene (carbonyl chloride, $COCl_2$, CAS No. 75-44-5) is an intermediate in the production of many industrial chemicals, such as isocyanates, carbamates, and related resins. It is an easily liquified, nonflammable gas of high primary irritancy. The inhalation of very low concentrations of phosgene may damage the alveolar membrane in the lung and may lead to toxic lung edema with a long latency period of up to 24 hours. After exposure to higher concentrations, the local irritation of the respiratory tract predominates and lethality may occur without induction of lung edema. Lethality was observed in animal experiments with concentrations of 10 ppm or higher. Recent animal data suggest effects in the lung at the current occupational exposure limit of 0.1 ppm. Due to the rapid hydrolysis, a systemic or cumulative damage to organs other than the lung is not likely.

Epoxy Compounds

Ethylene oxide (C_2H_4O, CAS No. 75-21-8) is an intermediate in the chemical industry, a monomer in the production of polymers and widely used in the health-care sector, for example, for the vapor sterilization of medical supplies. At room temperature it is a reactive gas with an ether-like odor. The acute toxicity in humans is dominated by the irriation properties to skin and respiratory tract and by central nervous effects (headache, nausea, vomiting, narcosis, and unconsciousness). Ethylene oxide is well absorbed. The elimination takes place rapidly and mainly via the urine.

Ethylene oxide alkylates haemoglobin and DNA and is genotoxic in various test systems *in vivo* and *in vitro*. Ethylene oxide tested by intragastric intubation in rats produced local tumors in the forestomach. Long-term inhalation resulted in tumors, mainly in the lung. Ethylene oxide produced slight developmental toxicity after inhalation (depression of fetal body weight and delays in ossification), but was non-teratogenic in animal experiments. Hemoglobin alkylation allows the biomonitoring of ethylene oxide exposure at the work place.

Propylene oxide (epoxypropane, C_3H_6O, CAS No. 75-56-9) is a liquid used as an intermediate in the manufacture of polyols, propylene glycol, and a variety of other chemicals. Propylene oxide is a primary irritant and a depressant of central nervous system. The acute oral toxicity is moderate. Propylene oxide, like other epoxides, has alkylating properties and therefore is genotoxic. Teratogenicity could not be shown, even in maternally toxic doses in animal experiments. As in the case of ethylene oxide, propylene oxide has a carcinogenic potential shown in animal experiments (mammary gland tumors, thyroid adenoma, and hemangiosarcoma).

1-Chloro-2,3-epoxy propane (epichlorohydrine; C_3H_5ClO; CAS No. 106-89-8) is a liquid used in the production of epoxy resins. It is of high acute toxicity and a primary irritant to the skin, eye and respiratory tract. Skin sensitization occurs. The target organs of toxicity are the central nervous system, the respiratory tract, and the kidneys. 1-Chloro-2,3-epoxy propane *is* a potent alkylating agent reacting with macromolecules, such as DNA. Consequently a genotoxic and carcinogenic potential was demonstrated. After maternally toxic doses, retardation of fetal development and resorptions have been shown. Biotransformation in mammals occurs via hydrolysis to 3-chloro-1,2-propanediole and oxidation to chloroacetic acid and oxalic acid or epoxidation to 2,3-epoxypropane-1-ole, with further hydrolysis to glycerin.

Bisphenol-A-diglycidylether (BADGE, $C_{21}H_{24}O_4$; CAS No. 1675-54-3) is a liquid that is used as a curing agent in combination with polyamines and acidic anhydrides in the production of epoxy resins. It is of low acute toxicity. Skin sensitization was described in exposed persons. The positive results of some *in vitro* genotoxicity test could not be confirmed by a variety of *in vivo* studies. BADGE is not carcinogenic in mice and rabbits after dermal application. Teratogenicity or reproductive toxicity could not be shown in animal experiments.

Silanes

Methylchlorosilanes (e.g., dimethyldichlorosilane, methylhydrogendichlorosilane, methyltrichlorosilane, and trichlorophenylsilane) are important starting materials for the production of polydimethylsiloxanes, the most important silicone polymers.

Silanes are highly reactive, liquid compounds that hydrolyze very rapidly. After skin contact, burns may occur. Inhalation exposure leads to the irritation of the upper respiratory tract. The acute oral toxicity is less than inhalation toxicity. *In vitro* and *in vivo* methylchlorosilanes were not genotoxic.

POLYMERS

Polymers are long-chain molecules composed of small simple repeating units (monomers). Linear and branched chains are typical for the thermoplasts, whereas elastomers are weakly cross-linked and duroplasts are strongly cross-linked polymers. Due to the high molecular weight and the inability to penetrate membranes, solid polymers are in general considered to be biologically and physiologically inert. The toxicity of the polymers is determined mainly by the content of the residual monomers and additives. The local tumorigenic potential after implantation of different polymers, mostly subcutaneously and intraperitoneal, however, depends on the physical form of the implant and not on the chemical identity. Local factors at the implantation site (e.g., a disruption of exchange of oxygen, electrolytes, or nutritients) are the cause of the tumor formation ("solid-state carcinogenesis").

Polystyrol (PS) and polyethylene (PE), when implanted subcutaneously or intraperitoneal, produced variable tumor incidences depending on the form and size of the polymer implant. Polystyrol discs und polyethylene film induced local tumors after sc implantation in rats, whereas perforated polystyrene discs and small polystyerene particles (rods, sphers, and fibers) produced tumors less frequently. Polystyrene and polyethylene powder, however, did not lead to tumors after sc implantation.

Similar data are available for most of the following polymeric materials. Polypropylene (PP) is used mainly for injection moulding, as well as for the production of fibers and films.

Polymethyl methacrylate is the major constituent of thermoplastic acrylic resins. Polytetrafluorethylene (PTFE) is the thermoplastic polyester produced from tetrafluoroethylene.

Polyvinyl chloride (PVC) is one of the most often used plastic material produced from the monomer vinyl chloride. Based on the carcinogenicity of the monomer vinyl chloride, the monomer content in the polymer is critical for the safety evaluation of the polymer. Earlier PVC technology resulted in a high monomer content in the polymer. The use of effective stripping decreased the monomer content. Food-grade materials contain less than 1 ppm monomer. PVC dust is neither acutely toxic nor locally irritating. Long-term occupational exposure to the dust may lead to pneumoconiosis. Epidemiological studies and animal testing revealed no carcinogenic potential of PVC dust.

Polyurethanes are produced from diisocyanates und dihydroxy compounds (polyols) by polyaddition. Polyurethane foams are produced as flexible or rigid foam. Solid-state carcinogensis was also shown when implanting polyurethanes. No association could be made between the lung-tumor rate in rats and inhalative, intratracheal, or intrabronchial application of polyurethane dust.

Epoxy resins are oligomeric compounds with epoxide groups. Most of the epoxy resins are produced from bisphenol A and epichlorohydrine. The oligomeric reaction products of bisphenol A and epichlorohydrine are strong skin sensitizers in animal experiments. Bisphenol A diglycidylether (BADGE) may be detected as a migrant after contact with epoxy resins.

Amino resins are condensation products of formaldehyde with amino-group-containing chemicals such as melamine. A long-term feeding study in rats with concentrations of ≤10% melamin-formaldehyde resin produced no specific toxicity. A two-generation study in rats showed no evidence of reproductive toxicity. There are case reports with sensitization to melamin-formaldehyde resin.

Polyamide are used in the production of fibers or resins. Polyamide is produced by polycondensation of dicarbonic acids and diamines or lactames.

Polyvinyl acetate (PVAc) is the homopolymer of vinyl acetate. It is manufactured using vinyl acetate, peroxide catalysts, or other initiators. It is a white to pale solid used in cosmetics as a latex emulsion or emulsion stabilizer. PVAc at a concentration of 50% showed no irritation reaction or allergic contact sensitization in human.

Silicone polymers, materials of high diversity, are built using a wide range of monomers (e.g., monochlorosilanes, see previous discussion) with silicon atoms bearing organic rests linked together via oxygen. Silicone oils, silicone resins, and silicone rubber are in use. The typical products, *polydimethylsiloxanes* (PDMS), are a group of silicone fluids with a wide range of molecular weights and viscosities. Polydimethylsiloxanes are not skin irritants or sensitizers in humans and experimental animals. The acute toxicity of PDMS is low after oral, dermal, or inhalation exposure. Repeated-dose toxicity studies did not identify any target organ. Animal studies have provided no evidence of teratogenicity, genotoxicity, or carcinogenicity. The accidental intravenous or intraarterial injection may lead to embolism of silicon droplets with the occlusion of blood vessels and damaging of the supplied organs. Foreign-body reactions also may occur. PDMS is also used orally for the treatment of flatulence or as antifoaming agent after intoxication with foaming substances, in medical devices and as implant material (see the section on "Special Aspects").

ADDITIVES AND MODIFIERS

Additives are of importance for the polymerization of monomers (e.g., initiators and cross linkers), whereas modifiers (e.g., stabilizers, plasticizers, lubricants, and flame retardants) modify the properties of the plastics. Additives may migrate from the polymer, so that exposure of the consumer may occur.

Stabilizers

Antioxidants, thermostabilizers, and light absorbers belong to the group of stabilizers.

Common antioxidants are phenols (e.g., butylhydroxytoluene, BHT, and other derivatives with high molecular weight), secondary aromatic amines (e.g., phenylenediamine compounds, such as stabilizers for rubber materials), phosphites (e.g., tris (nonylphenyl)-phosphite), phosphonite, and thio compounds (e.g., dilaurylthiodipropionate). Heavy metals (e.g., organotin compounds and metal stearate) are used as thermostabilizers. Stabilizers against UV radiation are, for instance, hydroxybenzophenone and hydoxyphenylbenzotriazole, hindered aliphatic amines, and nickel-chelate compounds.

Butylhydroxytoluene (BHT, $C_{15}H_{24}O$; CAS No. 128-37-0) is a solid used as an antioxidants in polymers. It is of low acute toxicity and leads to slight irritation of the skin and eye.

Metabolism is via oxidation of the methyl group at the benzene ring, the tertiary butyl moiety, or the aromatic ring. BHT is an enzyme inducer, which leads to an increase of activity of monooxygenase, epoxide hydrolase, und glutathione transferase. The elimination takes place mainly as glucuronide via the urine. The repeated administration of high doses of BHT in experimental animals leads to tissue damage in the liver, lung, and kidneys. Due to the vitamin-K-antagonistic action of BHT, hemorrhagic diathese may occur. The wide variety of genotoxicity assays performed with BHT gave no reasonable evidence of a mutagenic potential. Most long-term studies gave no evidence of carcinogenicity in rats and mice. Limited cases of increased tumor rates are assumed to be initiated due to a promoting action of BHT. An antitumor effect and a protecting effect against chemical carcinogens were also reported. In nonmaternally toxic doses, there is no evidence of teratogenicity. Breeding studies showed no reproductive effects of BHT. Relative high maternally toxic doses may result in the growth retardation of offspring.

Metal salts of fatty acids are called metal soaps. These compounds are of great technical importance. As stabilizers for polyvinyl chloride, metal soaps of cadmium (cadmium stearate) or of barium, lead, calcium, and zinc are used. *Stearic acid, cadmium salt* ($C_{36}H_{72}O_4Cd$, CAS No. 2223-93-0) is poisonous by inhalation and moderately toxic by ingestion. Heating leads to the emission of toxic fumes. Cadmium oxide may lead to toxic lung edema after a latent period. The primary target organ for chronic intoxication is the kidney. Chronic intake results in the accumulation of cadmium in the kidneys, which may lead to kidney damage after exceeding a threshold concentration. Metal fumes may lead to pulmonary emphysema, yellow discoloration of the teeth, and anosmia. Cadmium-containing compounds that contain bioavailable cadmium are carcinogenic in animal experiments after inhalation. There is also a debate on the carcinogenicity in humans after inhalation of Cd aerosols. After oral intake, cadmium is not regarded as carcinogen.

Organotin compounds typically used as stabilizers are organotin mercaptide and organotin carboxylate. Organic tin compounds are in general of high toxicity and are local irritants. *Tributyl tin oxide,* for example, is of high acute toxicity and a strong irritant but is not sensitizing, mutagenic, or teratogenic. A carcinogenicity study showed benign tumors in the endocrine organs. These tumors are probably due to an immunosuppressive effect and endocrine disregulation.

Plasticizers

Plasticisers are added to polymers to confer different degrees of flexibility to the plastic.

The following substances are used as plasticizers.

- Phthalates (e.g., di-2-ethylhexylphthalate and dibutyl phthalate).
- Phosphates (tricresyl phosphate [see also flame retardants]), diphenyl cresyl phosphate, and tributyl phosphate).
- Adipates (diethylhexyladipate)
- High-molecular polyester, mainly of the adipic acid.

Di-2-ethylhexylphthalate (DEHP; $C_{24}H_{38}O_4$; CAS No. 117-81-7) is a colorless to yellow oily liquid and is used as plasticizer in PVC, cellulose ester plastics, and synthetic elastomers. The DEHP-plasiticized materials are used for medical devices (e.g., for plastic blood bags). It is highly lipophilic. Acute inhalation toxicity and acute oral toxicity are low. The liver is the target organ. DEHP is a peroxisome proliferator. The liver carcinogenicity of DEHP in laboratory animals is most probably the result of a species-specific peroxisome proliferation. Peroxisome proliferators normally are not mutagenic. Tumor formation is due to stimulation of growth and of oxidative stress leading to DNA damage. Whereas peroxisome proliferation is a well-known phenomenon in rats and mice, this effect is only minor in primates and humans. The effects shown in rodents therefore are considered to be of no relevance for humans. A number of studies in experimental animals have demonstrated that DEHP induces testicular effects with changes in the seminiferous tubules at high doses, as well as teratogenic effects in rats and mice. No teratogenic effects have been found in chickens and rabbits.

Dibutyl phthalate ($C_{16}H_{22}O_4$, CAS No. 84-74-2) is a colorless oily liquid of low acute toxicity and does not have skin or eye irritation properties, or a skin-sensitization potential. Repeated-dose administration leads to mild peroxisome proliferation in rodents. In addition, there is evidence of testicular damage. The available data on genotoxicity give no evidence of a mutagenic potential. In mice oral administration of maternally toxic doses led to teratogenic effects.

Diphenyl cresyl phosphate ($C_{19}H_{17}O_4P$, CAS No. 26444-49-5) and tricresyl phosphate (a flame retardant and plasticizer) in technical grade forms are liquid mixtures of positionally isomeric cresyl derivatives. The content of esterized *o*-cresol depends on the production process. There is little experimental data on the toxicokinetics and metabolism of diphenyl cresyl phosphate. It is assumed that the *o*-cresyl isomer is metabolized by animals to phenylsaligenin phosphate, a neurotoxic compound. Technical grades therefore may show neurotoxic properties dependent on the content of *o*-cresyl in the mixture. Technical-grade diphenyl cresyl phosphate is of low acute toxicity and is not irritating to slightly irritating to the skin and eyes. There is no evidence of skin-sensitization effects based on the limited animal data. Genotoxicity was not shown in Ames tests.

Tributyl phosphate ($C_{12}H_{27}O_4P$; CAS No. 126-73-8) is of low acute toxicity. Local irritation or skin sensitization was not shown in laboratory animals. Repeated intake in mammals led to damages in the liver, urinary bladder, and kidneys. Extensive studies showed that tributyl phosphate is nongenotoxic in a number of *in vitro* and *in vivo* tests. In addition, there is no evidence of reproductive toxicity in experimental animals. Actual studies could not show a neurotoxic potential in mammals and chickens. Tributyl phosphate is rapidly absorbed and eliminated mainly in the urine. The metabolism is via dibutyl phosphate. To some extend the butyl groups are oxidized up to the acid. Long-term oral administration of tributyl phosphate leads to benign liver tumors in mice and to urothelial damage and tumors in the urinary bladder in rats. Hyperplasia of the urinary epithelium correlates with necrosis and ulcerations in the epithelium and is reversible within 10 weeks after cessation of the exposure.

Di-(2-ethylhexyl) adipate (DEHA; $C_{22}H_{42}O_4$; CAS No. 103-23-1) is a liquid of low acute toxicity in laboratory animals by oral and dermal routes of administration. In repeated-oral-administration studies DEHA has effects on the liver and induces peroxisome proliferation. An increase in liver tumor incidence was seen in mice but not in rats. Most of the genotoxicity assays have failed to demonstrate a genotoxic potential. DEHA is not an irritant and there is no evidence of a sensitization potential. Specific effects on reproduction could not be demonstrated in experimental animals. In mammalian metabolism, DEHA is rapidly hydrolyzed to the mono-ester. Subsequent conversion to more oxidized forms (2-ethylhexanol and 2-ethylhexanoic acid) depends on the examined species and correlates to the amount of peroxisome proliferation.

Lubricants

Lubricants are auxiliaries used during the production process of thermoplastic materials. Mineral oil, waxes, alcohols (e.g., cetyl alcohol), stearate (e.g., butyl, calcium, magnesium, or zinc stearate), and other fatty acid esters and long-chain alcohols are used.

Paraffin (CAS No. 8002-74-2) is a mixture of saturated aliphatic hydrocarbons of various molecular weights. The toxicity is very much dependent on the molecular weight.

Cetyl alcohol (CAS No. 36653-82-4) is a long-chain aliphatic alcohol (solid and crystals) of low acute toxicity. Cetyl alcohol is considered to be slightly irritating. In human volunteers, cetyl alcohol produced no skin-sensitization reactions.

Flame Retardants

The flame retardants can be differentiated into the following groups.

1. Anorganic compounds (e.g., aluminum oxidehydrate, antimon oxide, magnesium hydroxide, metal borate, and elemental phosphor).
2. Halogenated organic compounds (e.g., chloroparaffin, tetrabromobisphenol A and derivatives, polybrominated diphenylether, and tetrabromophthalic acid derivatives).
3. Organic phosphorous compounds (triaryl phos-

phate as, for example, tricresyl phosphate, tris[2-ethylhexyl]-phosphate, and triphenyl phosphate).

4. Halogenated organic phosphor compounds (e.g., tri (2,3-dichloropropyl)-phosphate and tris (2,3-dichloroethyl)-phosphate).
5. Nitrogen-containing compounds (e.g., melamine).

Aluminum, aluminum oxide hydrate (AlH_3O_3; CAS No. 21645-51-2), and other aluminium oxide compounds may as respirable particles induce lung fibrosis (e.g., aluminum lung and aluminosis). The "aluminum lung" could also be induced in rabbits and guinea pigs but not in hamsters and rats. Carcinogenic, genotoxic, or skin-sensitizing properties were not recorded after inhalation of aluminum dust or aluminum oxides. The clinical relevance of an aluminum enrichment in patients with chronic dialysis is currently under discussion.

Antimontrioxide (O_3Sb_2, CAS No. 1327-33-9) is a white solid of low acute oral toxicity and shows irritation effects of the eyes and skin. In humans, inhalation of the dust leads to irritation in the respiratory tract. Repeated inhalation in rats revealed a fibrogenic and tumorigenic activity. Epidemiologic data did not show a clear correlation between occupational exposure to antimontrioxide and tumor incidence.

The chlorinated paraffins are a group of complex mixtures with different lengths of carbon atom chains and different amounts of chlorination. The short- and medium-chain chlorinated paraffins are oily liquid materials, whereas long-chain chlorinated paraffins are solid and waxy. The acute toxicity of the chlorinated paraffins is low and independent of the structure. The skin-irritation potential is mild and decreases with the length of the chain. Animal experiments identified the liver and kidneys as the target organs; short-chain chlorinated paraffins, in addition, affect the thyroid gland. There is no evidence of teratogenic or genotoxic activity. Carcinogenicity studies with long-chain chlorinated paraffins showed equivocal evidence of a tumorigenic activity, but short-chain paraffin caused an increase of tumor incidences in the liver, kidneys, and thyroid gland after high doses.

Tetrabromobisphenol A (TBBPA; $C_{15}H_{12}Br_4O_2$; CAS No. 79-94-7) is a solid used mainly as an additive or reactive flame retardant. TBBPA is of low acute toxicity. Absorption via the gastrointestinal tract is limited and elimination occurs via the feces. The local-irritation potential is mild. An animal experiment showed no skin sensitization potential. No systemic toxicity was seen after repeated exposure, but there was evidence of irritation of the respiratory tract. Genotoxicity and teratogenicity could not be shown.

Other brominated flame retardants, in particular polybrominated diphenyl ether, generate brominated furanes, and to a lesser extent also dioxines, under pyrolytic conditions. These compounds are no longer is use.

Tri (2-ethylhexyl-phosphate) (TEHP; $C_{24}H_{51}O_4P$; CAS No. 78-42-2) is used in plastics as a flame retardant and plasticizer. The compound is moderately irritating to the skin and eyes but is not sensitizing to guinea pig skin. Repeated oral administration or inhalative exposure did not produce systemic toxicity, but the analogous di (2-ethylhexylphosphate) induces peroxisome proliferation. TEHP was not genotoxic in a variety of *in vitro* tests. A long-term oral study in rats and mice showed a higher liver tumor incidence in female mice only. Because TEHP is expected to hydrolyze to DEHP, peroxisome proliferation is also expected after TEHP application. No delayed neuropathy occured in chickens after oral or intramuscular administration of TEHP.

Tricresyl phosphate ($C_{21}H_{21}O_4P$, CAS No. 1330-78-5) is produced and used as a mixture of isomers. Depending on the production process, differences in the distribution pattern and occurrence of the isomers are known. The material is used as flame retardant and lubricant. Esterized *o*-cresol is capable of inducing polyneuropathy ("organophosphate induced delayed neuropathy"). The neurotoxicity is caused by the metabolite cyclic saligenin-*o*-tolylphosphate. Main metabolites, however, are di- and monocresyl phosphate. An epidemic intoxication in humans with tri-*o*-cresylphosphate occurred 1930 in the U.S. due to an alcoholic ginger extract containing tri-*o*-cresylphosphate as an impurity ("Jamaica ginger paralysis"); later, contaminated salad oil or wheat led to epidemic intoxications in Morocco. Tri-*o*-cresylphosphate causes impairment of fertility.

The esterized *o*-cresol content of technical-grade tricresyl phosphate amounts less than 0.1%. Tricresyl phosphate is of low acute toxicity and irritation. The material is not teratogenic in rats and not mutagenic. Uncharacterized material also showed impairment of fertility and limited evidence of neurotoxicity.

Triphenyl phosphate ($C_{18}H_{15}O_4P$; CAS No. 115-86-6) is a solid used as a plasticizer and fireproofing agent. The acute toxicity and irritation potential is low. Triphenyl phosphate is not considered to be a skin sensitizer. Actual studies on neurotoxicity did not produce effects. Triphenyl phosphate is neither fetotoxic nor teratogenic in animals. Limited evidence of the induction of micronuclei was seen in an *in vitro* genotoxicity assay, but in the Ames test no activity has been demonstrated.

Tris-(1, 3-dichloro-2-propyl)phosphate ($C_9H_{15}Cl_6O_4P$; CAS No. 13674-87-8), another flame retardant, is well absorbed via oral or dermal route. Decomposition occurs via hydrolyzation to the main metabolite di-(1,3-dichloro-2-propyl) phosphate. Elimination is mostly completed within 1 day. Oxidative dealkylation could also be a route of decomposition. The acute toxicity is low, as well as the local-irritation potency. Genotoxicity assays *in vitro* produced evidence of a mutagenic activity, whereas *in vivo* no effects were observed. A carcinogenicity study in rats showed an increase of tumors in the liver, kidneys and testes.

Other Additives

Examples of fillers are talc, quartz, glass fibers, metals, and metal oxides. Important colorants are titanium and zinc oxide as white pigments and carbon black and ferrous oxide as black pigments. Colored pigments are ferrous-, manganese-, chromium-, zinc-, and molybdenum-containing pigments, as well as organic pigments. Because these compounds are fixed in the polymer matrix, consumer exposure due to migration or leaching may not occur.

As curing agents, organic peroxides are used. As blowing agents, for example, azo compounds (e.g., azodicarbonamide) and hydrazine derivates are in use. The use of azodicarbonamide may lead to respiratory sensitization. Some of the peroxides are known to be carcinogens. Corrosive and sensitizating effects are caused by peroxides.

SPECIAL ASPECTS

Plastics Used for Food-Contact Materials or for Medical Devices

Plastic material is widely used for the production of articles for daily use, such as packaging materials, kitchen utensils, dishes, and other objects that may come in contact with food, toilet requisites, or toys.

Concern about the safety of the use of polymers in food-contact material may arise from the possible toxicity of the monomers, additives, and modifiers. Food laws are established in various countries to regulate polymers in food-contact material.

Medical devices, such as transfusion packs, blood storage bags, syringes, catheters, and implants, are regulated mostly under the drug regulations. The polymers are evaluated with respect to the extraction or leaching of components of the polymer and their biocompatibility.

Polymers Used as Implants in Human Medicine

Polymers have found widespread use in medical applications. They are the most important materials for medical implants, following metals and ceramics. Commonly used polymers are silicones, fluoropolymers, polyalkenes, and polymethacrylates. In general the biocompatibility of the polymers used for medical implants has been demonstrated. Reports of side effects are mostly due to the underlying morbidity of the patients.

Polymethylmethacrylate is used for artificial eye lenses. Polyethylene forms the basis for the artificial lubricant for hip prostheses. Artificial heart valves are produced using polytetrafluoroethylene or polypropylene.

Polytetrafluoroethylene is also used in artificial blood vessels, such as hemodialysis shunts, and in bone replacement. Another use of polypropylene is in joint replacements. Intrauterine contraceptive devices and penile implants were produced using polyethylene. Polyvinyl pyrrolidones are plasma expanders.

Methylmethacrylate and other methacrylates are used in dentistry. Silicones are used in intraocular tamponade in retina detachment, plastic surgery, and joint replacement for rheumatic diseases. In plastic surgery, silicone oil is injected or silicone-filled prostheses are implanted.

Foreign-body reactions are the most common adverse effects and may aggravate up to granulomas and fibrotic encapsulation of the implants. Auto-immune diseases due to implants and the association of breast implants and mammary tumors are under debate.

Recycling

The recycling of plastics is desirable to limit waste and save ressources. The recycling of single-grade wastes (primary recycling) is easily possible with thermoplastic waste (e.g., polyethylene, polypropylene, PVC, and ABS) after separation and cleaning.

Recycling of mixed plastic wastes can only be achieved by degradation to small fragments by hydrolysis, alcoholysis, aminolysis, hydrogenation, or pyrolysis. The ultimate recycling may be to use the energy of the plastics (energy recycling). However, some plastics, such as PVC, release hazardous substances during combustion. Therefore, extensive flue-gas washing and thermic control are essential.

Degradation of Polymers and Plastics

The degradation of plastics, limiting their durability, is caused by heat, UV radiation (photochemical reactions), and mechanical treatment. This degradation is probably of no toxicological relevance, whereas the flue-gas toxicity from plastics incineration requires attention. The combustion of plastics may lead to exposure to asphyxiants, such as carbon monoxide or cyanides; halogenated dibenzodioxines and -furanes; and mixtures of benzene, aromatic carbohydrates, heavy metals, and acids, depending of the polymer material.

Acute inhalation toxicity tests examine the fire effluents of plastics and natural polymers, such as wood and wool, under standardized conditions. This test system allows the comparison of the toxicity of the plastics combustion products to that of natural polymers, such as wood or wool.

Biodegradable polymers have been developed to optimize waste management. Degradable polymers are, for example, cellulose derivatives, aliphatic polyesters, polyesteramide, and thermoplastics based on poly(hydroxycarboxylic acids) and polylactones from glycolic acid, lactic acid, or β-hydroxybutyric acid.

Bibliography

Agency for Toxic Substances and Disease Registry (1990). "Toxicological Profile for Acrylonitrile." ATSDR, Atlanta, Georgia, USA.

American Conference of Governmental Industrial Hygienists Inc. (1996, 1995). "Documentation of the threshold limit values and biological exposure indices." Fifth Edition (1986), Sixth Edition, Supplement on Sixth Edition (1996), ACGIH, Cincinnati, Ohio, USA.

Anonymous (1994). "Toxicology update vinyl chloride." *J. Appl. Toxicol.* **14,** 301–307.

Anonymous (1996). Amended final safety assessment of polyvinyl acetate. *J. Amer. College Toxicol.* **15,** 166–176.

Anonymous (1996). Final report on the safety assessment of melamin/formaldehyd resin. *J. Amer. College Toxicol.* **14,** 373–385.

Anonymous (1996). Special issue: Evaluation of butadiene and isoprene health risks. *Toxicology* **113.**

Arbete Och Hälsa vetenskaplig skriftserie (1995). "The Nordisk Expert Group for Criteria Documentation of Health Risks from Chemicals. 117. Propene." Arbets Miljö Institutet, Solna, Sweden.

Bischoff, F. (1972). Organic polymer biocompatibility and toxicology. *Clin. Chem.* **18,** 869–894.

Bogdanffy, M., Makovec, G. T., and Frame, S. R. (1995). Inhalation oncogenicity bioassay in rats and mice with vinyl fluoride. *Fundam. Appl. Toxicol.* **26,** 223–238.

Clayton, G. D., and F. E. Clayton (eds.). "Patty's Industrial Hygiene and Toxicology." 3rd/4th ed.

Dearfield, K. L., Abernathy, C. O. *et al.* (1988). Acrylamide: its metabolism, developmental and reproductive effects, genotoxicity and carcinogenicitiy. *Mutat. Res.* **195,** 45–77.

Greim, H. (ed.) (current editor) (1998). "Occupational toxicants, critical data evaluation for MAK values and classification of carcinogens. Volume 1–10. Wiley-VCH Weinheim, New York, Chichester, Brisbane, Singapore, Toronto.

Eckard, R. E. and Hindin, R. (1973). The health hazards of plastics. *J. Occup. Med.* **15,** 808–819.

ECETOC (1983). "Joint Assessment of Commodity Chemicals No 1: Melamine." European Chemical Industry Ecology & Toxicology Centre, Brussels, Belgium.

ECETOC (1986). "Joint Assessment of Commodity Chemicals No. 5: Vinylidene chloride." European Chemical Industry Ecology & Toxicology Centre, Brussels, Belgium.

ECETOC (1992). "Hepatic Peroxisome and Proliferation." Monograph 17. European Chemical Industry Ecology & Toxicology Centre, Brussels, Belgium.

ECETOC (1992). "Joint Assessment of Commodity Chemicals No. 20: Tris-/Bis-/Mono-(2-ethylhexyl) phosphate." European Chemical Industry Ecology & Toxicology Centre, Brussels, Belgium.

ECETOC (1994). "Joint Assessment of Commodity Chemicals No. 26: Linear Polydimethylsiloxanes (viscosity 10–100,000 centistoes)." European Chemical Industry Ecology & Toxicology Centre, Brussels, Belgium.

ECETOC (1995). "Joint Assessment of Commodity Chemicals No. 30: Methyl Methacrylate." European Chemical Industry Ecology & Toxicology Centre, Brussels, Belgium.

GDCh Advisory Committee on Existing Chemicals of Environmental Relevance (BUA) (1990). "BUA Report 48 on Styol." VCH-Verlag. Weinheim, New York, Basel, Cambridge.

GDCh Advisory Committee on Existing Chemicals of Environmental Relevance (BUA) (1994). "BUA Report 142 on Acrylnitril." S. Hirzel Wissenschaftliche Verlagsgesellschaft, Stuttgart.

Illing, H. P. A., and Shillaker, R. O. (1985). "Toxicity Review II, 1,3-Butadiene and Related Compounds." Health and Safety Executive. H. M. Stationery Office, London.

International Agency for Research on Cancer [IARC] (1986). "1,3-Butadiene." IARC Monographs on the Evaluation of the Carcinogenic Risk of Chemicals to Humans. World Health Organization, Geneva, Switzerland. IARC Press, Lyon, France.

International Agency for Research on Cancer [IARC] (1979). "Chloroprene." IARC Monographs on the Evaluation of the Carcinogenic Risk of Chemicals to Humans. World Health Organization, Geneva, Switzerland. IARC Press, Lyon, France.

International Agency for Research on Cancer [IARC] (1979). "Some monomers, plastics and synthetic elastomers, and acrolein." IARC Monographs on the Evaluation of the Carcinogenic Risk of Chemicals to Humans. Volume 19. World Health Organization, Geneva, Switzerland. IARC Press, Lyon, France.

International Programme on Chemical Safety [IPCS] (1983). "Styrene," Volume 26. Environmental Health Criteria Series, World Health Organization, Geneva, Switzerland.

International Programme on Chemical Safety [IPCS] (1984). "Epichlorohydrin," Volume 33. Environmental Health Criteria Series, World Health Organization, Geneva, Switzerland.

International Programme on Chemical Safety [IPCS] (1985). "Ethylene oxide," Volume 55. Environmental Health Criteria Series, World Health Organization, Geneva, Switzerland.

International Programme on Chemical Safety [IPCS] (1990). "Vinylidene chloride," Volume 100. Environmental Health Criteria Series, World Health Organization, Geneva, Switzerland.

International Programme on Chemical Safety [IPCS] (1990). "Tricresyl phosphate," Volume 110. Environmental Health Criteria Series, World Health Organization, Geneva, Switzerland.

International Programme on Chemical Safety [IPCS] (1991). "Triphenyl phosphate," Volume 111. Environmental Health Criteria Series, World Health Organization, Geneva, Switzerland.

International Programme on Chemical Safety [IPCS] (1990). "Tributyltin compounds," Volume 116. Environmental Health Criteria Series, World Health Organization, Geneva, Switzerland.

International Programme on Chemical Safety [IPCS] (1995). "Tetrabromobisphenol A and derivatives," Volume 172. Environmental Health Criteria Series, World Health Organization, Geneva, Switzerland.

International Programme on Chemical Safety [IPCS] (1992). "Di[2-ethylhexyl] phthalate," Volume 131. Environmental Health Criteria Series, World Health Organization, Geneva, Switzerland.

International Programme on Chemical Safety [IPCS] (1984). "Toxicological Evaluation of Certain Food Additives and Food Contaminants." World Health Organization, Geneva, Switzerland.

Kennedy, G. L. (1990). "Toxicology of fluorine-containing monomers." *Crit. Rev. Toxicol.* **21,** 149–170.

Lickly, T. D., Lehr, K. M., and Welsh, G. C. (1995). "Migration of styrene from polystyrene foam food-contact articles." *F. Chem. Toxic.* **33,** 475–481.

Müller, H. J., and Löser, E. (1985). "Butadiene." "Ullmann's Encyclopedia of Industrial Chemistry." W. Gerhartz (ed). Volume A4, pp. 431–446. VCH Verlagsgesellschaft mbH, D-6940 Weinheim.

National Toxicology Program (1993). "Technical Report 24 on 1, 6-Hexanediamine Dihydrochloride," National Toxicology Program, P.O. Box 12233, Research Triangle Park, NC 27709, U.S. Department of Health and Human Services. Public Health Services.

National Toxicology Program (1979). "Technical Report No. 170 on Styrene," National Toxicology Program, P.O. Box 12233, Research Triangle Park, NC 27709, U.S. Department of Health and Human Services. Public Health Services.

National Toxicology Program (1983). "Technical Report 245 on Melamine," National Toxicology Program, P.O. Box 12233, Research Triangle Park, NC 27709, U.S. Department of Health and Human Services. Public Health Services.

National Toxicology Program (1985). "Technical Report 272 on Propylene." National Toxicology Program, P.O. Box 12233, Research Triangle Park, NC 27709, U.S. Department of Health and Human Services. Public Health Services.

Serrone, D. M., Birtley, R. D. N., Weigand, W. and Millischer, R. (1987). Toxicology of chlorinated paraffins. *Fd. Chem. Toxicol.* **25,** 553–562.

CHAPTER

39

Radiation

R. J. MICHAEL FRY*, ULRICH F. W. HAGEN†
JOHANN KUMMERMEHR†, R. JULIAN PRESTON‡

*Life Sciences Division, Oak Ridge National Laboratory, Oak Ridge, Tennessee
†Institute for Radiobiology, National Center for Environment and Health, Neuherberg, Germany
‡Chemical Industry Institute of Toxicology, Research Triangle Park, North Carolina

INTRODUCTION

Only a few textbooks on toxicology describe the biological effects of radiation. This may be due to the opinion that radiation effects have to be described by physical analysis, whereas toxicology deals mostly with the biological effects of chemicals. In the following chapter it will be shown that radiation also should be considered as an agent that damages biological organisms and we have to protect humans and nature against the harmful effects of radiation. Radiation research has become a leading field in understanding the mechanisms of harmful agents, and in the area of risk assessment, radiation research developed convincing concepts useful also for the analysis of the harmful effects of chemicals.

The main topic of this chapter is the effects of ionizing radiation, such as gamma rays and X-rays, particle radiations (electron, protons, and neutrons), and the effect of "nonionizing radiation", such as UV light, radar, radiowaves, microwaves, laser, and electromagnetic fields.

To understand the biological effects of radiation, the events following the absorption of the radiation energy and the damaging of biomolecules by radical reactions need to be analyzed. The final outcome depends on the ability of the cell to repair the initial damage, otherwise this will lead, by incomplete or inaccurate repair, to mutation or to cell death (genotoxic and cytotoxic effects of radiation). The cellular radiation effect is also responsible for complex syndromes in animals and in humans, resulting in acute and late diseases. The genotoxic effects may cause late effects, such as cancer or inheritable diseases, in future generations.

Biological effects of radiation have to be analyzed by a whole dose–effect response. Cellular radiation effects follow the laws of probability. Such stochastic effects are defined as those events for which the probability of occurrence increases as a function of dose, but not of the severity, in the absence of a threshold. In contrast, the probability and the severity of deterministic effects (acute and late radiation syndromes) are observed only above a threshold dose ("nonstochastic" effects).

IONIZING RADIATION

Types of Radiation and Primary Events after Absorption and Dosimetry

Electromagnetic waves and particles of high energy lead after absorption in matter to ionized molecules. If the energy of X-rays or gamma rays is less than 10 keV, the photon will transfer its energy to the orbital electrons and liberate them from the atom (photoabsorption). If the energy is higher than 10 keV, only a part of the energy of the photon is absorbed directly; the photon with lower energy continues on its way with deflected direction until the whole energy is used up (Compton effect). By these events, the energy of electromagnetic waves is transferred (up to 99%) to the energy of free electrons (secondary electrons). Charged particles, such as protons, alpha particles, or heavy ions, produce ionization after absorption into the tissue by interacting with the orbital electrons in the atom. Neutrons, not charged, interact with the nuclei of the atoms, liberating (setting in motion) fast-recoil protons, alpha particles, and heavier nuclear fragments.

The fundamental dosimetric quantity is the absorbed dose (energy dose), in units of joules per kilogram or gray (Gy). Different radiations produce different densities of ionization in matter. This density is expressed as the energy per unit length of the radiation track with the dimension keV/μm (linear energy transfer, LET). Co-gamma radiation produces LET values of 0.3 keV/μm, X-rays of around 3 keV/μm, and fission neutrons of about 45 keV/μm. The biological effectiveness depends on the LET; thus the energy dose is multiplied with a special radiation weighting factor (w_R), resulting in the equivalent dose (H_T) in the unit sievert (Sv); (Gy $\times$ w_R = Sv). The equivalent dose in a tissue T is given by the equation

$$H_T = \Sigma w_R \times D_{T,R}$$

where $D_{T,R}$ is the absorbed dose averaged over the organ or tissue T due to radiation. The w_R values are recommended 1991 by the International Commission for Radiation Protection (ICRP) (Table 1). In biological experiments, however, the term "relative biological effect" (RBE) is used to describe the biological effect of different types of radiations under special experimental conditions.

TABLE 1 Radiation Weighting Factors (w_R)[a]

Type and energy range	w_R
Photons, all energies	1
Electrons and muons, all energies	1
Neutrons, energy <10keV	5
10–100 keV	10
>100 keV–2 MeV	20
>2MeV–20 MeV	10
>20 MeV	5
Protons, no recoil protons >2MeV	5
Alpha particles,	20
Fission fragments, heavy ions	20

[a]The factors have been selected based on values for relative biological effectiveness (RBE) for relevant endpoints.

TABLE 2 Examples of Tissue Weighting Factors (w_T)

Tissue/organ	w_T	Tissue/organ	w_T
Skin	0.01	Bone surface	0.01
Bladder	0.05	Breast	0.05
Liver	0.05	Esophagus	0.05
Thyroid	0.05	Remainder	0.05
Bone marrow	0.12	Lung	0.12
Colon	0.12	Stomach	0.12
Gonads	0.20	Total	1.00

The various organs of mammals and humans have different radiation sensitivities with regard to acute and late effects. To judge a given exposure in an organ for the total biological radiation effect, the equivalent dose has to be multiplied by the "tissue weighting factors" (w_T) resulting in the "effective dose" (E), expressed also in sievert. For radiation protection purposes, tissue weighting factors make it possible to ensure that an effective dose would produce a comparable degree of detriment (Table 2). These values are independent of the type of radiation. From a radiobiological viewpoint, w_T and the radiation weighting factors w_R are approximations and should be updated as soon as more precise data are available.

For the dosimetry of incorporated radionuclides specific dose factors have to be evaluated and used between the incorporated radioactivity (in bequerel (Bq) = disintegrations per second) and the resulting absorbed dose (in Sv). These factors, expressed in Sv/Bq, which depend on the radionuclide, the range of its radiation in tissue, and the physical and biological half-lives, are found in tables for radiation protection. For example, after the uptake of 1000 Bq of Cs-137 by adults (e.g., in milk), the dose factor is 1.4×10^{-8}, which means that in the following 50 years 14 μSv are absorbed.

Human Radiation Exposure

All human beings are exposed to radiation from natural as well as from human-made sources. Natural exposure is received from the sky (cosmic), soil (terrestic), and incorporated radionuclides (Table 3). The intensity of the cosmic irradiation depends on the height above sea level; at 10,000 feet it is about 1 mSv/year, compared to 0.3 at sea level. Flying from New York to Europe, a passenger receives about 0.03–0.05 mSv. The terrestial doses depend on the soil; for example, in the Colorado plateau area (U.S.) the dose is around 0.9 mSv/year whereas on the east and the Caribbean coasts (U.S.) it is about 0.23 mSv/year. In addition, the exposure from radon varies con-

TABLE 3 Annual Natural and Anthropogenic Radiation Exposure in Germany

Radiation source	Effective equivalent dose (mSv ± S.E.)
External	
Cosmic radiation (gamma rays, neutrons)	0.30
Terrestic radiation (K-40, U-238 series)	0.42 ± 0.15
Internal (ingestion, inhalation)	
K-40	0.18
C-14	0.01
Rb-87	0.005
Radon and decay products (lung exposition only)	1.0 ± 0.5
Medical diagnostics	1.0 ± 0.05
Medical genetic significant dose	0.1–0.2
Total dose, whole body	2.0–2.5
Lung dose by radon, in addition	1.0
Total genetic significant dose	1.2–1.5

siderably depending on the soil and the specific surrounding in houses or in mines.

Among anthropogenic radiation sources, the exposure by medical diagnostics is predominant. The annual patient dose from diagnostic radiology depends on the standard for a particular health organisation. In less-developed countries, lower human-made doses are evaluated than in those with a high-standard health organisation. However, more modern technology allows a reduction of the dose. On average, about 1.0 ± 0.5 mSv/person/year for medical diagnostics can be assumed, but it should be considered that there is a wide individual range. Some patients are exposed only occasionally; others with severe illnesses are exposed repeatedly with higher doses (e.g., CT of abdomen 20 mSv and chest 0.3 mSv). Thus an average value is not useful in evaluating the individual risk of exposure by medical diagnosis. In addition, the gonadal dose has to be taken into consideration. For example, a lung examination leads to a bone marrow dose of 0.05 mGy; the corresponding gonadal doses are 0.002 mGy for females and 0.0005 mGy for males.

Molecular Radiation Biology

Basic Radiation Chemistry

To understand the biological effects of radiation, the primary physicochemical events have to be analyzed, that is, the radiation chemistry, which is actually a chemistry of radicals (Fig. 1). Eqs. (1–3), describe the radiation chemistry of water, and Eq. (4) the influence of oxygen on water radicals. There are several types of reactions of biomolecules with water radicals producing electrons, H atoms, and OH radicals. Electrons and H atoms are liberated from organic molecules (Eq. (7)). H·, OH·, and organic radicals may recombine leading to a stable dimer molecule (Eqs. (5), (6), and (9)) or to two different stable molecules (i.e., disproportion, Eq. (10)). The OH· radical is able to abstract hydrogen from an organic molecule or to add on an organic double bond as shown in Eq. (11).

Equations (1), (2), and (7) are reversible. In the presence of oxygen, however, peroxy radicals are formed (Eq. (8)). This latter reaction is irreversible; thus the radical concentration is higher than in the absence of oxygen. This is the basis for explaining the oxygen effect in radiation biology. Understanding the radiation chemistry of biological macromolecules (e.g., nucleic acids, protein, or membranes) is important. The irradiation of proteins leads to changes of conformation and to subsequent denaturation, to cross-links between different molecules or with DNA by radical–radical interaction and to loss of enzymatic activity. In or at membranes, radiation produces mostly peroxides.

DNA Damage In Vitro and In Vivo

Radiation-induced damage of the DNA can be considered to be responsible for most of the biological radiation effects. The radiation chemistry of DNA has been studied *in vitro* with DNA solutions as well as in irradiated cells. According to the radical reactions shown in Fig. 2, there is a splitting of the

$$H_2O \rightleftharpoons H^\bullet + OH^\bullet \quad (1)$$

$$H_2O \rightleftharpoons H_2O^+ + e^-_{aq} \quad (2)$$

$$H_2O^+ \longrightarrow H^+ + OH^\bullet \quad (3)$$

$$e^-_{aq} + O_2 \longrightarrow O_2^{-\bullet} \quad (4)$$

$$2\,OH^\bullet \longrightarrow H_2O_2 \quad (5)$$

$$2\,H^\bullet \longrightarrow H_2 \quad (6)$$

$$RH \rightleftharpoons R^\bullet + H^\bullet \quad (7)$$

$$R^\bullet + O_2 \longrightarrow ROO^\bullet \text{ (Peroxyradical)} \quad (8)$$

$$2\,R_3C^\bullet \longrightarrow R_3C{-}CR_3 \quad (9)$$

(10)

(11)

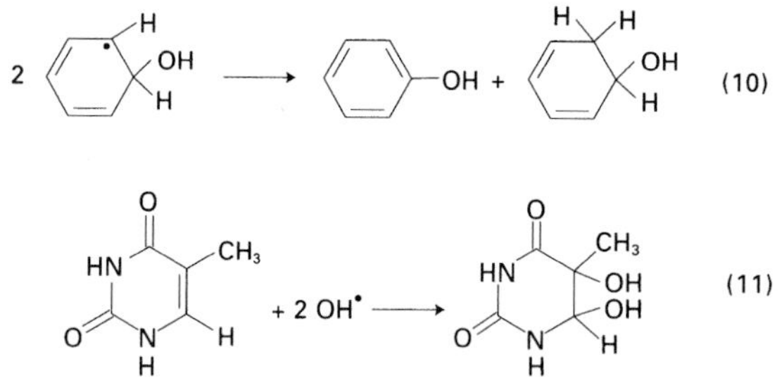

FIGURE 1 Important radiation-induced radical reactions in water. Presence of oxygen, recombinations of radicals, H abstraction, and addition of OH radicals on double bonds.

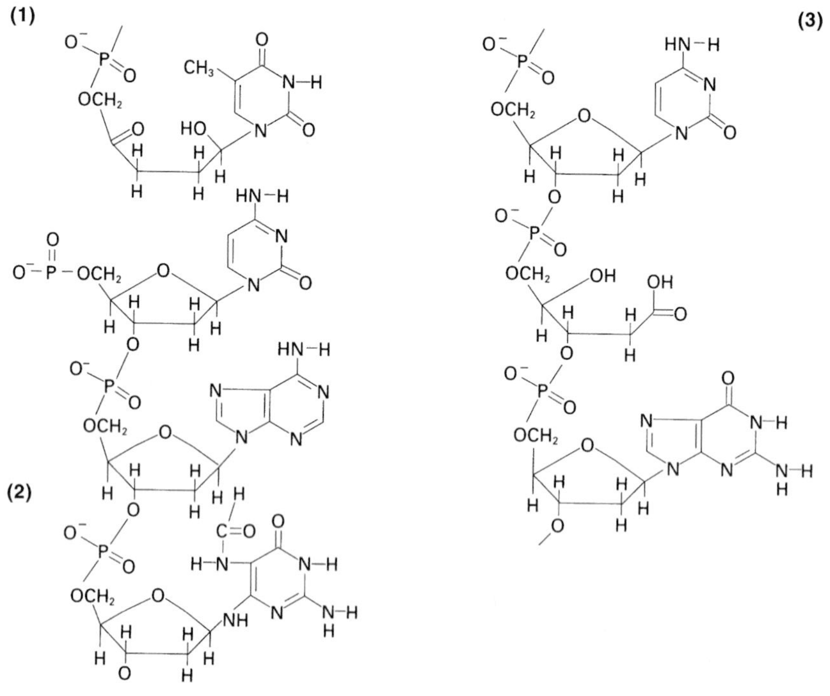

(1)

(2)

(3)

FIGURE 2 Radiation-induced damage in DNA. Changes in the structure of DNA moieties after irradiation of aqueous DNA solution: (1) single-strand breaks with oxidized sugar; (2) base damage—formation of an aminoformamido pyrimidine; (3) loss of a base, leading to an alkali-labile lesion.

phosphodiester bond by sugar oxidation (Fig. 2) leading to single-strand breaks, which are also formed by a loss of a whole nucleotide with phosphoester end groups at both sides. DNA double-strand breaks are formed in irradiated DNA solutions but only by coincidence of two single-strand breaks that are opposite each other (within about 7 base pairs).

A number of base damages have been identified after irradiation; predominant are the additions of $H^{\cdot}$ or $OH^{\cdot}$ on the double bond of pyrimidines (e.g., thymine-glycol; Eq. (11) in Fig. 1), as well as a splitting of the heterocycle of purines leading to aminoformamido pyrimidines (Fig. 2). Another type of radiation damage in DNA is the loss of a base leading to the oxidation of the sugar and the formation of an "abasic site" in the DNA.

Base and sugar damage will also be observed in DNA of irradiated cells. In addition DNA damage is also due to a direct hit in DNA in the cell, where the energy is deposited unevenly forming a number of radicals close together. Such an event leads to double-strand breaks and also to a cluster with about 2–5 primary ionizations without a break, called "locally multiply damaged sites" and DNA–protein cross-links. These events are induced in cellular DNA linearly with the dose. In mammalian cells irradiated in air with 1 Gy, about 1000 single-strand breaks, 1000 base damages, 40 double-strand breaks, 40 local multiply damaged sites, and 100 DNA–protein cross-links are formed. This is the dose producing, on average, one lethal hit per cell, where 37% of the cells survive. From these data it follows that in this dose range most of the DNA damage must be repaired in the cell within a short time.

DNA Repair

The molecular aspects of DNA repair include a very complete understanding of the nucleotide excision repair pathway for UV-induced DNA damage, the base excision repair pathway, and DNA mismatch repair. More recently the mechanism of the repair of ionizing radiation-induced double-strand breaks has been partially unraveled. What is apparent is that for ionizing and nonionizing radiation the repair pathways are complex and involve multiple enzymes. This is a consequence of damage recognition and repair pathways being exquisitely accurate.

Nucleotide Excision Repair

The nucleotide excision repair process removes DNA damage by incising the damaged DNA strand on either side of the lesion. The types of damage that are recognized by this process are UV-induced pyrimidine dimers and 6-4 photoproducts, and bulky lesions, such as those induced by benz[*a*]pyrene. Following the incision and release of the DNA fragment containing the damage, repair synthesis fills the gap using the undamaged DNA strand as a template by a DNA polymerase (repair synthesis) with ligation completing the process. The excised fragments are about 12–30 nucleotides in length. The complexity of the enzymatic process differs between prokaryotes and eukaryotes. In humans, 16 polypeptides are required for the production of the two incisions; seven are xeroderma pigmentosum (XP) proteins, trimeric replication protein A, single-stranded DNA-binding protein, and the multisubunit general transcription factor TFIIH. The latter provides a link between transcription and nucleotide excision repair. In fact, a transcription–repair coupling factor allows for the preferential repair of DNA damage in the transcribed strand.

Base Excision Repair

A number of endogenous cellular processes can give rise to DNA damage that can be repaired by base excision repair. These include hydrolytic events, such as deamination or base loss, oxygen free-radical attack, and methylation of ring nitrogens. In general the modified base is excised in free form by hydrolysis of the N-glycosyl bond that links the base to sugar of the DNA chain. This base-release process is catalyzed by the class of enzymes known as DNA glycosylases.

There is a DNA glycosylase with a specificity for each set of DNA lesions. An apurinic or a apyrimidinic site remains at the position of the released base, and this site is cleaved by a specific endonuclease. The process of base excision repair is completed by the removal of the 5′ terminal deoxyribose-phosphate residue generated by the apurinic–apyrimidinic endonuclease, and the subsequent repair synthesis and ligation. The size of the repair patch is variable, from as small as a single nucleotide to several nucleotides.

Mismatch Repair

Mismatched bases can arise from DNA replication (including repair synthesis), from recombination between divergent DNA sequences, and from modification of bases via chemical and radiation exposures or by cytosine deamination. The mismatch repair system has been highly conserved during evolution; homologs of bacterial MutS and MutL have been characterized from yeast and mammalian cells. This process of damage recognition and repair are functionally related to the base excision and nucleotide excision repair processes in that segments of DNA incorporating the base are involved in the mismatch. In prokaryotes, the choice of the base that is excised allows for a return to the normal DNA sequence, and the selection is controlled by the adenine methylation pattern in d(GATC) sequences. Corresponding processes may occur also in eukaryotes.

Double-Strand Break Repair

There is some evidence that radiation-induced double-strand breaks can be repaired by a ligation process, following modification of the broken ends. However, the more frequent mode of repair of radiation-induced double-strand breaks is via a recombination process. Recent studies have demonstrated that this recombination process is the same as the one used to produce the diversity of maturing immunoglobulin genes by V(D)J rejoining.

The DNA-dependent protein kinase (DNA-PK) is required for nomal DSB rejoining in mammalian cells and also for correct V(D)J rejoining. DNA-PK consists of a 465-kD catalytic subunit (DNA-PK_{CS}) and an associated binding component, the Ku complex, consisting of two subunits (Ku 70 and Ku 80). The DNA-PK holoenzyme is activated by binding to DNA ends via the Ku component. Upon activation, it is able to phosphorylate a number of protein substrates *in vitro* in particular transcription factors. A range of other proteins have a role in the repair of DSB, including the p53 tumor-suppressor gene, a complex of Rad51 (a yeast gene that has homology to *E. coli* Rec A, a gene involved in recombination), and two tumor-suppressor genes BRCA1 and BRCA2 associated with early onset of breast cancer.

Human Disorders Associated with a DNA-Repair Deficiency

A large number of examples of a cellular radiosensitivity that is proposed to be associated with human genetic disorders have been presented. However, many of these are rather tenuous. Table 4 provides a list of 13 human disorders that affect DNA repair and the maintenance of genomic integrity for which there is more reliable evidence for an increased sensitivity at the cellular level to ionizing and/or nonionizing radiations.

Defective nucleotide excision repair in humans is associated with three diseases, xeroderma pigmentosum (XP), Cockayne's syndrome (CS), and trichothiodystrophy (TTD). XP is a consequence of an absence or greatly reduced level of excision repair and results almost exclusively in skin cancer. CS appears to be more of a transcription-defect disease than a repair-deficiency disease, although some CS mutants cause an uncoupling of transcription with repair, and others affect transcription factor TFIIH activity that has also an involvement in DNA repair. The disease manifestations are cathetic dwarfism, mental retardation, and progressive neurological symptoms. TTD also involves alterations in transcription control that reduce nucleotide excision repair capacity. The affected individuals have sulfur-deficient brittle hair and suffer from dental caries, ichthyosis, skeletal abnormalities, and progressive mental retardation.

Individuals with hereditary nonpolyposis colorectal cancer (HNPCC) contain frequent mutations in simple DNA sequence repeat units that are typically tumor-specific. This instability has been shown to be the result of a mutation in one of four genes responsible for DNA mismatch repair (MSH2, MLH1, PMS1, and PMS2). Individuals with ataxia telangiectasia (AT) are hypersensitive to X-rays and gamma irradiation, and the syndrome is characterized by cerebellar ataxia as a consequence of progressive neurodegeneration. The recent cloning of the ATM (mutated in AT) gene and subsequent characterization have shown that it is broadly involved in DNA-damage recognition, DNA rearrangement, and cell-cycle arrest. While a direct role in DNA repair has not been demonstrated, the increased radiosensitivity, mutagenicity, and clastogenicity are all strongly indicative of such a role. For other disorders (Table 4), there is currently insufficient evidence to define a link between the syndrome, a DNA-repair defect, and a cellular sensitivity to ionizing and/or nonionizing radiations.

Chromosomal Aberrations

There is general agreement that unrepaired or misrepaired double-strand breaks lead to cell death. These repair errors become visible at metaphase as distortions and breaks of the chromosomal structure. Chromosome breaks have the ability to rejoin with other breaks (Fig. 3). This recombination either occurs between the original strands (no changes of chromosomes) or between fragments of another chromosome, resulting in deletions, rings, acentrics, dicentrics, translocations, and inversions in metaphase.

Exchanges of the broken ends between two chromosomes can occur symmetrically (symmetrical exchange or reciprocal translocation) or asymmetrically, leading to a chromosome with two centromeres (dicentric) and an acentric fragment. Whereas dicentrics are easily analyzed by light microscopy, symmetrical translocations are difficult to detect. Recently "painting" specific chromosomes with labeled, specific DNA probes (FISH, fluorescent *in situ* hybridization) has allowed translocations to be reliably analyzed.

The analysis of dicentrics and rings in the lymphocytes of exposed humans can be used to assess the

TABLE 4 Human Disorders Affecting DNA Repair[a]

Disorder	Major clinical features	Cancer	Specific cellular hypersensitivity	Proposed DNA repair defect	Number of genes
Ataxia-telangiectasia	Neurological defects, immunodeficiency	Lymphoma	Ionizing radiation, radiomimetic chemicals	Kinase activity	1
Bloom syndrome	Photosensitivity, dwarfism	Various	UVR, some chemicals	DNA helicase	1
Cockayne syndrome	Photosensitivity, dwarfism	No excess	UVR, ionizing radiation?	Preferential repair of transcribed strands	2
Fanconi anaemia	Bone marrow deficiency, skeletal abnormalities	Leukaemia	Bifunctional alkylation agents, ionizing radiation?	Repair of intrastrand cross-links	4
Hereditary nonpolyposis colorectal cancer	Colon and other cancers	Colon and other cancers	None known	Defective DNA mismatch repair	4
Li–Fraumeni syndrome	Cancer excess	Leukemia, sarcoma, breast cancer	Spontaneous genomic instability, ionizing radiation (chromosomal)	Via cell cycle control	>1
Nevoid basal-cell carcinoma syndrome	Skeletal abnormalities, cancer	Basal cell carcinoma	Ultra-violet? ionizing radiation	Defect in repair of potentially lethal ionizing radiation damage?	1
Nijmegen breakage syndrome	Microencephaly, immunodeficiency	Lymphoma	Ionizing radiation, radiomimetic chemicals	?	2
Retinoblastoma	Retinal tumours	Retinoblastoma and others	Ionizing radiation?	Via cell cycle control?	1
Trichothiodystrophy	Photosensitivity, abnormal sulphur-deficient hair	No excess	UVR	Excision repair	2
Werner syndrome	Accelerated ageing	Various	?	DNA helicase	1
Xeroderma pigmentosum	Photosensitivity and cancer of UVR-exposed skin	Squamous-cell carcinoma, basal-cell carcinoma, and melanoma	UVR, some chemicals	Excision repair or daughter strand repair	8

[a]Adapted from R. Cox (personal communication).

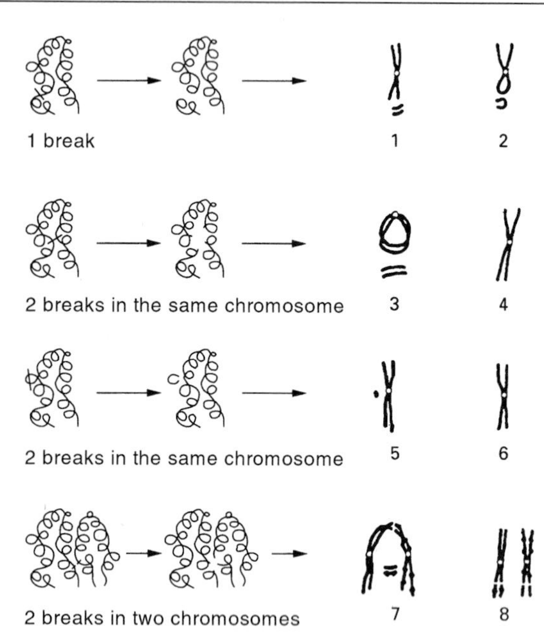

FIGURE 3 Formation of radiation-induced chromsome aberrations. (1) and (2) Chromosome with deletion. (3) Chromosome with a ring and an acentric piece. (5) Two breaks in the same chromosome with a deletion and an acentric. (7) and (8) Translocation of fragments from 2 chromosomes: (7) asymmetric translocation, (8) symmetric translocation. Redrawn after Fritz-Niggli (1959).

received dose (biological dosimetry). Dicentrics, however, disappear gradually with time from peripheral blood as a result of the formation of an anaphase bridge with subsequent cell death or by the loss of the acentric fragment that accompanies a dicentric. In contrast, symmetrical translocations are generally stable at division for a long time and can potentially be used to estimate radiation exposure that occurred years before. Unexposed individuals (controls) have in their blood about 4×10^{-4} dicentrics per cell; after exposure to 1 Gy *in vitro,* this value increases up to 6×10^{-2} dicentrics per cell.

Dicentrics, reciprocal translocations, and rings exhibit a characteristic dose–effect curve. They are produced either by the passage of one track of charged particles going through two chromosomes in close proximity resulting in a linear dose–response curve, or by two chromosomes being damaged by two separate tracks, leading to a quadratic dose–effect curve. Because both one- and two-track processes occur, the overall response is a linear–quadratic function for dicentrics,

$$Y_{\text{dic}} = a\,D + b\,D^2 \qquad (12)$$

where a and b are the one- and two-track coefficients that depend on the types and condition of the irradiation. For example after exposure to densely ionizing radiation with high LET, the linear component a becomes predominant.

Chromosomal aberrations also can be studied by "premature chromosome condensation" (PCC), which allows the analysis of chromosomal structural alterations in interphase shortly after radiation without the need for the chromosomes to proceed to metaphase. Such analyses are important for mechanistic studies. A fast procedure for getting information on the chromosomal structural changes is the analysis of micronuclei, which are fragments of chromosomes liberated from the whole genome. The analysis of micronuclei can be used for biological dosimetry. They do, however, reflect only a fraction of the total induced damage that can be analyzed at metaphase.

Cellular Radiation Biology

Ionizing and nonionizing radiation can, depending upon the dose; produce alterations in a whole range of cellular macromolecules that affect their proper functioning. The relevant parameter for characterizing the biological effects of radiation is radiation-induced cell killing as assessed by the reciprocal effect to cell survival (i.e. the ability of a cell, to form a colony within a certain time; e.g., 14 days in culture).

Survival Curve Parameters

Survival curves are of two basic types when plotted semilogarithmically, exponential or shoulder (Fig. 4). Specific parameters are generally used to describe the type of the survival curve. D_0 is a measure of the slope of the exponential component of the curve and is defined as the dose required to reduce survival from S to $e^{-1}S = 0.37$ S.

The extrapolation number (n) is a measure of the width of the shoulder; the larger the value of n, the broader the shoulder. D_q is a quasithreshold value; it is also the measure of shoulder magnitude and is a rather artificial value. Additional description of survival curves can be found in Hall (1994). A mathematical description of the survival curves is given by

$$S = (1 - (1 - e^{-kD})^n)e^{-\alpha D}, \qquad (13)$$

where α is the initial linear part of the survival rate and k is a general constant. In the upper range of the survival curve, S can also be formulated by

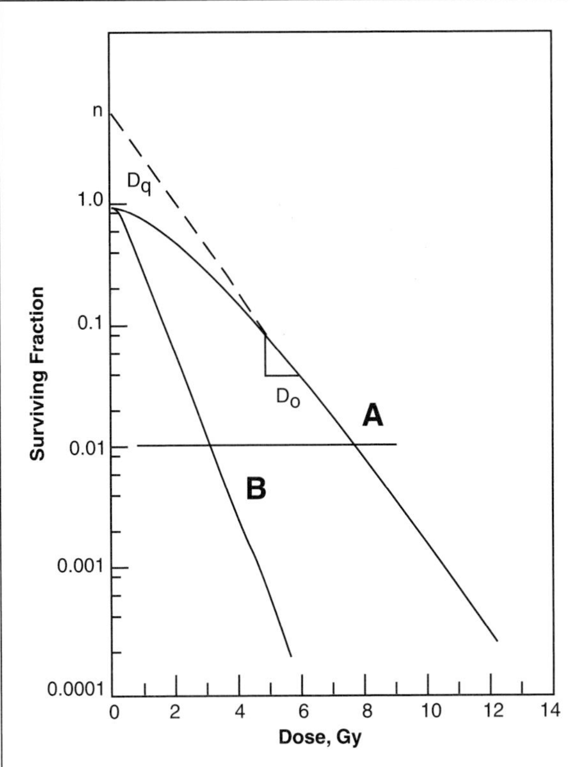

FIGURE 4 Survival curve illustrating descriptive parameters. Single-cell survival curves for low-LET radiation (a) and high-LET radiation (b) plotted on a log-linear format. Relative biological effectiveness (RBE) is the relation of the doses at 1% survival.

$$S = (\exp - (\alpha D + \beta D^2)). \quad (14)$$

Relative Biological Effectiveness (RBE) and Radiation Quality

As previously described, RBE is the ratio of the dose of the radiation of interest compared to the dose of gamma rays that would produce the same level of biological effect. For the purposes of radiation protection the term Q is used instead of RBE to characterize a specified radiation type.

The quality of the radiation can be described by its linear energy transfer (LET), expressed in the amount of energy lost per unit of particle length (e.g., keV/μm). Low LET radiation (X-rays and gamma rays) are considered to be those for which the distance between primary ionizing events is large on the scale of a cell nucleus. In contrast, high LET radiations (alpha particles and neutrons) produce ionizing events that are small in distance, smaller than the cell nucleus.

The RBE depends upon the LET. With low LET radiation, cell-survival curves exhibit an initial shoulder followed by exponential decline (Fig. 4). After exposure to high LET radiation, only an exponential plot is observed. Based on simple target theory, it can be proposed that one track of high LET radiation produces the lethal lesion, whereas in low LET radiation two tracks are frequently involved in the production the lethal lesions (cf. Eq. (14)). With increasing LET values, the RBE will rise as more and more single hits kill the cell until at a certain LET a maximum of the RBE is observed. At further increasing LET, part of the absorbed energy is wasted (more than needed for lethal lesions). The resulting maximum RBE is found at about 100 keV/μm.

Effects of Dose Rate and Dose Fractionation

For low LET radiation, reducing the dose rate, such that the total dose is delivered in hours rather than in minutes, reduces the amount of cell killing and the frequencies of chromosome aberrations and mutations. Similarly, dividing the exposure into two or more fractions, for example, separated by hours, reduces the effect in comparison with a single exposure of the same total dose (Fig. 5). For high LET radiations, in general, lowering the dose rate does not lower the effectiveness of the radiation.

The explanation underlying the dose-rate and dose-fractionation effects involves the mechanism of

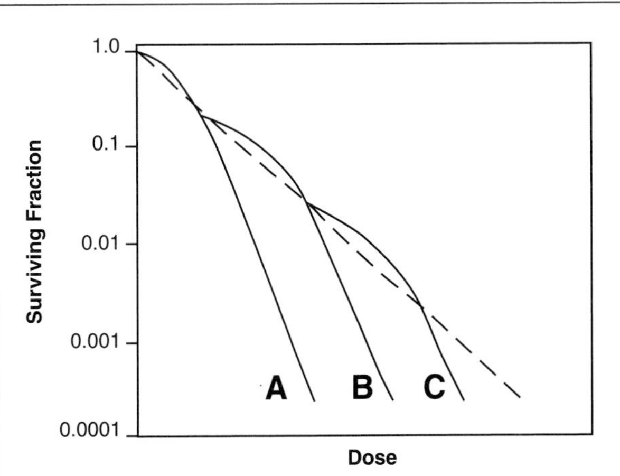

FIGURE 5 Illustrations of survival curves for fractionated exposures. (a) Single acute exposure; (b) exposure to D_f and variable second doses, separated by several hours; (c) exposure to two doses D_f and separated third variable dose. The dotted line is the survival curve for multiple exposures D_f each.

cell killing by chromosome aberrations. As shown above, the majority of chromosome alterations require two lesions (hits) for their formation. The pair of required lesions can be produced by one or two tracks. However, during the extended period for low dose-rate exposure or the period between dose fractions, DNA repair take place such that one lesion is repaired before the second chromosome lesion occurs. Thus, there is a decline of cell killing with increasing protraction or fractionation. For high LET radiation, cell killing and chromosome aberrrations occur mostly by one track; thus no effect of dose protraction or fractionation is observed.

Oxygen Enhancement Ratio (OER)

Generally, low LET radiations are more effective in the presence of oxygen than under anoxic conditions. This relative increase in biological effectiveness is known as the oxygen enhancement ratio (OER), which is defined as the ratio of the hypoxic doses to oxic doses that produce the same level of biological effect. The mechanism of the oxygen effect is based on the higher concentration of radiation-induced peroxy radicals (Eq. (8) in Fig. 1) in the tissue, which cannot be restored as radicals induced in absence of oxygen (cf. Eq. (4)). The OER for X-rays and gamma rays is between 2.5 and 3; for 1 MeV fast neutrons it is about 1.5 and for alpha particles 1.0.

Radiation Pathology and Radiation Syndrome

Acute Radiation Syndrome

The consequences of ionizing radiation on proliferating cells *in vivo* are essentially identical to those shown for cells cultured *in vitro*. Stem cells of renewal tissues, such as bone marrow, skin, and mucous membranes, are inactivated according to the dose relationship that will discussed here. In marked contrast, differentiated cells in tissues that are already postmitotically fixed (e.g., osteocytes, neurocytes, and muscle cells) are affected very little even by relatively large doses. As they are usually able to complete their normal life span; the onset of severe cell depletion and hence of clinical symptoms is related to the tissue turnover time. This divergent responsiveness explains the specific organ and time pattern of acute radiation sequelae as observed after total or partial body irradiation or after local radiotherapy.

The acute radiation syndrome following total body irradiation reflects the failure of several tissues with different radiosensitivities and latent periods. The dominant symptoms therefore depend both on dose and time (Table 5). In bone marrow, several lineages are affected when the dose exceeds 1.5 Gy. Damage to the myeloid line becomes manifest early, due to the short life span of the peripheral granulocyte, and causes increased susceptibility to infection, while thrombopenia occurs later, showing as coagulopathy and petechial bleeding mostly into skin and mucosae. Owing to the long life time of erythrocytes, anemia is usually not observed. In the small intestine, the critical stem cell depletion in the jejunal crypts induced by doses of ≤ 8 Gy translates into villus denudation within a few days; the clinical symptoms correspond to the breakdown of barrier function, such as diarrhea, electrolyte loss, and infection, and are fatal if spontaneous epithelial regeneration is not possible.

The large total doses that are employed in local tumor radiotherapy (equivalent to single doses of 18–20 Gy) induce typical acute damage in a variety of organs. In the skin, the earliest visible changes are erythema (1–2 weeks), epilation, and dry desquamation (3 weeks), usually progressing into exudative desquamation but also followed by rapid reepithelialization. More important is the acute response of oropharyngeal mucosa, a regular side effect of the treatment of head and neck tumors that culminates in

TABLE 5 Acute Radiation Syndrome after Total Body Irradiation

Mean dose	Symptoms
<1 Gy	No specific symptoms
1–2 Gy	Nausea within hours; transient decrease in peripheral white blood cell count to non-critical levels; no specific treatment required
2–4.5 Gy	Vomiting within hours; drop of lymphocyte count to $<1000/\mu l$ within 3 days; critical granulocytopenia in weeks 3–5; with adequate treatment very good prognosis for full recovery
4.5–9 Gy	Severe vomiting within the first hour; drop of lymphocyte count $<500/\mu l$ within 3 days and diarrhea within 2–3 days; septicaemia and diffuse intestinal hemorrhage due to severe granulocytopenia and thrombopenia; epilation within one week; even with adequate treatment prognosis doubtful
9–16 Gy	Severe vomiting, erythema and shock within first hour; life-threatening diarrhea is the major clinical problem; even with intensive care considerable mortality
>16 Gy	Shock, severe diarrhea, circulatory failure, and somnolence; no specific treatment possible

painful patchy or confluent mucositis after 2 to 3 weeks of treatment and may enforce treatment interruption.

Radiation injury to the gonads is inevitable in the irradiation of the pelvic lymph nodes, as routinely given in seminoma patients or patients with disseminated lymphoma (e.g., Hodgkin's disease). Spermatogenesis is highly radiosensitive and (scatter) doses as low as 1 Gy impose temporary aspermia, while doses higher than 3–5 Gy cause permanent sterility (not hormonal castration). Permanent loss of ovary function is induced in about 50% of the patients after doses around 4 Gy, and includes infertility and menopause; the well-documented decrease of ovarian tolerance with age mirrors the spontaneous decline of the oocyte number after birth.

Late Radiation Damage in Normal Tissue

While the pathogenesis of acute radiation sequelae is well explained by proliferative damage and stem cell depletion, chronic side effects are more complex and involve irreversible damage to the vascular-connective tissue as an important component. In contrast to acute effects, they can develop months and years after radiotherapy and progressively lead to a loss of tissue architecture. In the skin, the most frequent chronic damage is fibrotic induration of the dermis and subcutis; also telangiectasia is a characteristic chronic effect, showing progression over more than 5 years. In the gastrointestinal tract, late changes in the bowel wall typically cause loss of motility, ulceration, and stenosis, or even perforation. The lung is a very sensitive organ, in which both radiation pneumonitis (after 2 months) and fibrosis (later) are life-threatening side effects. Other most serious complications concern the kidney (sklerosis and nephrogenic hypertension), the spinal cord (tetraplegia), and the heart. For myocardial damage, the loss of capillaries was shown to be the critical event that leads on to parenchymal degeneration and disseminated fibrosis. A well-known alteration is the opacification of the eye lens, which is distinct from age-related cataract and can be induced by low doses.

Local radiation exposure in children or adolescents often results in compromized organ growth as a late manifestation of stem cell depletion (e.g., the premature closure of the epiphyseal plate after irradiation of growing long bones or vertebrae (scoliosis)). A particularly sensitive organ is the mammary gland, as shown by the failure of breast development in puberty. Growth retardation may result from irradiation of the head, affecting growth hormone production by the pituitary gland.

The dose relationship of both acute and chronic responses is typically "deterministic," with an initial organ-specific threshold followed by a steep sigmoidal curve. The relationship is modified by several factors. Most importantly, tolerance can be increased by splitting the total dose into small dose fractions (Fig. 6). This effect is definitely more pronounced in late-responding tissues where dose fractionation is the most important principle to enhance organ tolerance. High LET radiation, which induces a smaller relative amount of repairable damage, will shift the dose–effect curves to the left. Compared to late responses, acute effects are less dependent on dose fractionation but, in contrast, can be mitigated by dose protraction

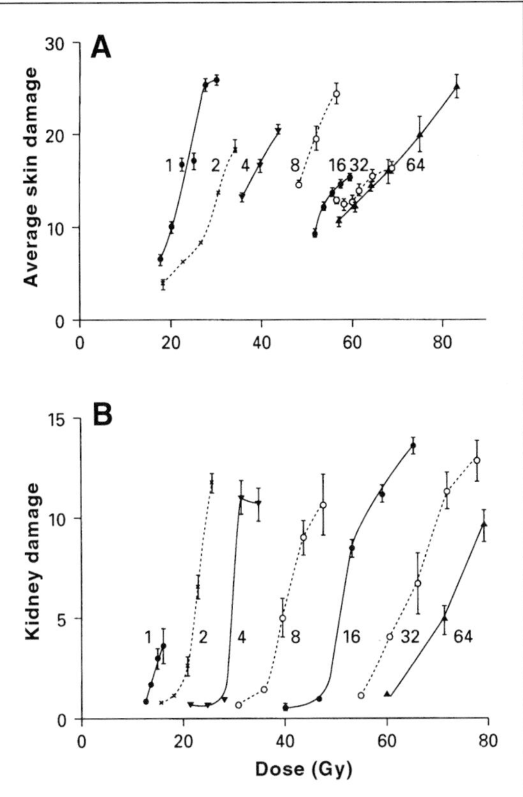

FIGURE 6 Ordinate (i): Average skin score; Ordinate (ii): Kidney damage (% retention of Cr-51-EDTA). Typical deterministic dose–effect curves of normal tissues to single doses or fractionated irradiation, showing a large dose threshold followed by a steep sigmoidal dose–response. (A) Acute skin injury (arbitrary score) demonstrating little additional increase in tolerance when the dose is split into more than 16 fractions. (From Douglas and Fowler, 1976). (B) Functional kidney damage (expressed as the fraction of injected Cr-51-EDTA not excreted) represents a typical late effect with marked tolerance increase up to 64 fractions (Stewart *et al.*, 1984).

because this will give the necessary time for compensatory proliferation.

Radiation Effects on Tumors

The basic mechanism of permanent tumor cure by radiotherapy is the eradication of all clonogenic cells or malignant stem cells; if this is not achieved, the tumor will locally recur after periods ranging from months to years. Stem cells make up only a minor fraction of all tumor cells, but their absolute number in a macroscopic tumor is still high enough (10^5–10^7/g) to necessitate large radiation doses for sterilization. The stringent relationship between stem cell inactivation and local tumor control has convincingly been demostrated in animal experiments with transplantable tumors (Fig. 7).

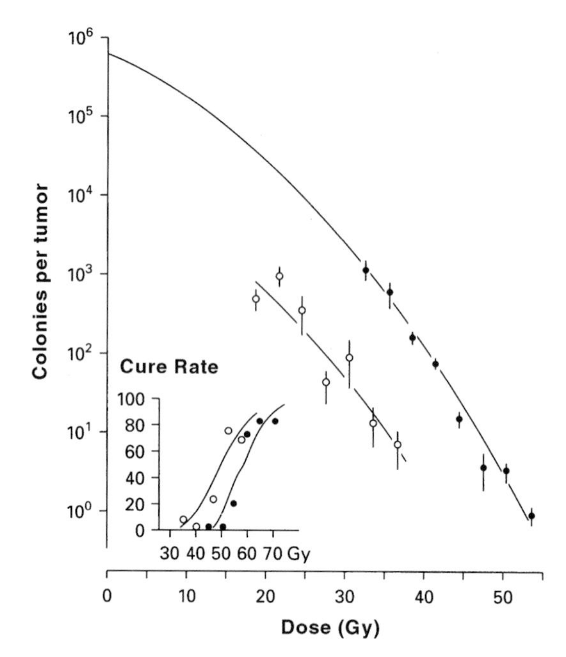

FIGURE 7 Ordinate (i): Clones per 100 mg tumor; Ordinate (ii): percent local tumor control; Abscissa: Radiation dose (Gy). Survival of stem cells in a transplantable mouse mammary carcinoma as a function of single radiation doses given either under normal ambient conditions (o) or during transient tumor anoxia induced by clamping the arterial blood supply (•). Date after ambient irradiation present survival of the spontaneously hypoxic cells approximately 3% of all tumor stem cells). The matching dose–effect curves of permanent tumor control (insert) indicate that a 50% cure probability is achieved when the mean surviving cell number is approximately one. (Data from Kummermehr and Trott, 1997).

It is important to realize that the gradual inactivation of stem cells in the course of fractionated radiotherapy does not correlate with the observed tumor response during treatment. The retarded volume regression is explained by the fact that stem cells constitute only a minority of all cells (typically 0.01–0.1%) and their sterilized descendants can be metabolically active or at least physically present over extended periods before being lysed and phagocytosed. Tumor shrinkage during therapy, hence, has no great prognostic relevance and is not a guide to prescribed dose. The only relevant parameter to describe the clinical radiosensitivity of a tumor is the dose that prevents local recurrence (or achieves local control) in 50% of the cases treated.

Successful clinical radiotherapy is a difficult balance between optimizing the change of tumor eradication and limiting the rate of severe complications in normal tissue. This goal is best achieved by highly fractionated radiotherapy. The standard protocol that has emerged is delivery of 5 × 2 Gy per week over 6 to 8 weeks, up to total doses of 60–70 Gy. Splitting the dose into multiple fractions uses the greater repair capacity of late-responding normal tissue (Fig. 6). In addition, it facilitates reoxygenation and thus the sensitization of the hypoxic cells that exist only in tumors but not in normal tissues. In some tumor entities, it is now clear that their stem cells respond to radiation-induced cell depletion by accelerated proliferation in a way similar to that mentioned for normal renewal tissues, and accelerated treatment is recommended in these cases.

Radiation Exposure by Incorporated Radionuclides

Radiation exposure of humans in our environment is due not only to external radiation but also to incorporated radionuclides. Potassium-40 and the actinides are examples of natural radiation sources. Nuclides from nuclear fission products, formed either by atomic test explosions or in nuclear reactors, also contribute to the internal radiation dose (Table 6).

To evaluate the dose an organism recieves due to incorporated nuclides, the conversion factors from Bequerel (Bq) to the dose in Sv must be known. For example, the potassium-40 activity in adult humans of 4400 Bq leads to an effective dose of only 0.18 mSv/year.

The natural radionuclides in the body are in equilibrium; for the anthropogenic ones the transfer from their source to humans has to be analyzed. Such an evaluation has to consider the metereological conditions during emission and the transfer into air, water, and soil. From these data the activity in plants, animals, and the food chain can be evaluated and finally the radioactive load in humans determined.

The nuclear test explosions in the 1950s and 1960s led to a transport of fission products into the stratosphere and subsequently their descent to Earth, espe-

TABLE 6 Important Radionuclides in the Environment

Compound	Physical half-life	Biological half-life	Deposition
Potassium-40	1.3×10^9 years	Equilibrium	Whole body
Iodine-131	8 days	6–8 days	Thyroid gland
Iodine-129	1.6×10^7 years	50–130 days	Thyroid gland
Caesium-137	33 years	35–100 days	Whole body
Strontium-90	28 years	15 years	Bone
Yttrium-90	64 hours	64 hours	Bone, liver
Plutonium-239	2.41×10^4 years	c. 100 years	Bone, liver
Plutonium-238	88 years	63 years	Lung
Carbon-14	5.7×10^3 years	12 days	Whole body
Tritium	12 years	12 days	Whole body

cially cesium-137 (4 kBq/m^3), strontium-90 (2.5 kBq/m^3), and plutonium-239 (0.1 kBq/m^3). It was estimated that this radioactivity lead to an exposure of 0.4 mSv/person in the Northern Hemiphere in the subsequent years.

In 1986 the ill-fated Unit 4 of the reactor station Chernobyl exploded and 200 tons of burning graphite, together with fission products, were distributed into the air all over Europe. Iodine-131 in the first days, and later cesium-134 and cesium-137 contributed primarily to the radiation exposure in the environment; as to a less extent did strontium-90 and plutonium. In the immediate neighborhood of Chernobyl (the Ukraine and Belarus), the heavy contamination demanded an evacuation of the inhabitants.

Quite another situation is the long-lasting exposure of people to plutonium-239 and strontium-90 in course of plutonium breeding and processing in the southern Urals near Cheljabinsk. Highly radioactive waste was released into the Techa River and evacuation of the villages on the river came too late to prevent individual effective doses above 1 Gy. Due to uncertainties of the dosimetry and the statistical evaluation of health effects, no relevant conclusions can be made about the toxicologic consequences for the population in these areas.

Radon and its decay products contribute to the largest extent to natural radiation exposure, especially to the bronchial epithelium. Radon is emitted from the soil and concentrated in the air of the houses, depending upon the geology of the ground (i.e., primarily rocks or sandy soil). In central Europe, on average, 50 Bq/m^3 radon and 15 Bq/m^3 decay products are measured in the air of living rooms but with great variations. A measurement of 50 Bq/m^3 means that the bronchial epithelium of the lung is exposed with an equivalent dose of 15–20 mSv per year and an effective dose of 1–1.5 mSv. The high radon exposure of miners, combined with inhaled dust and smoking, lead to a high carcinogenic potential for bronchial epithelial carcinomas.

Therapeutic Measures in Radiation Accidents

In the case of life-threatening radiation exposure, a series of measures must be taken to prevent fatal consequences. One is the removal of external or internal radionuclides by decontamination and decorporation. When the absorbed dose makes bone marrow failure a likely event, marrow transplantation may be considered. Yet, while total body irradiation with subsequent bone marrow grafting from a HVA-compatible donor is a well-established curative treatment in leukemia patients, the success rate in radiation victims is poor, as the required clinical work-up and the precise assessment of the (total) conditioning dose are difficult to achieve. Bone marrow transplantation is therefore no longer generally recommended and instead supportive therapy plays the major role, including patient admission to a sterile hospital unit, intensive antibiotic therapy, and the administration of growth factors that stimulate the proliferation of surviving hemopoietic cells. Impending complications from coagulopathy can be treated by platelet infusion. While electrolyte and fluid substitution can counteract some degree of intestinal damage, the extensive depletion of epithelial lining after high abdominal doses is intractable.

A frequent problem is the estimation of the actual dose received, be it for inhomogenous exposure or technical limitations of the common personal dosimeter at high dose levels. The dose-dependent decline of peripheral lymphocyte number, although in itself of no greater clinical bearing, plays an important role as a prognostic indicator and is readily evaluable in the very first days after exposure. Retrospectively, the analysis of chromosomal damage, including micronuclei formation or stable translocations, can be used to reconstruct the individual dose.

If radionuclides are involved, the immediate measures to be taken in order to minimize the dose burden are external decontamination (e.g., showers and hair washes) and internal decorporation (e.g., gastric lavage and laxatives). Radionuclide uptake by gastrointestinal absorption or from wounds may be reduced by administering the appropriate stable nuclides (e.g., iodine for radioiodine, potassium as a "diluent" for cesium), or by applying specific complex-forming agents. This is important with radioisotopes that otherwise are deposited in bone or liver with a very long biological half-life (e.g., Pu-239 or Sr-90). In animal experiments, the oral application of (Zn)-DTPA has been effective if initiated early and extended over-a long period. With humans, there is insufficient experience to assess its effectiveness.

Radiation Risk Assessment

Genetic Effects

The various classes of genetic diseases that contribute to the genetic risk from exposures to ionizing radiations include single-gene disorders, chromosome aberrations, multifactorial and polygenic inheritance, and nontraditional inheritance.

There are two broadly acceptable approaches for deriving estimates of genetic risk to humans following exposures to ionizing radiations. These are the doubling-dose (indirect) method and the direct method. The doubling-dose method is clearly defined in UNSCEAR (1993). When mutations are induced by radiation, they will be additive to the background level and over time a new equilibrium frequency will be reached. The doubling dose used in the calculation is the dose of radiation needed to induce the same frequency of mutations per generation as the background frequency. The data used for calculating a doubling dose are those from mouse studies, particularly involving the mutation assessment for seven specific loci.

The doubling-dose value used for risk-assessment calculations is 1 Gy for low-LET, low-dose-rate irradiation. Using this dose, the risk for different genetic end points can be calculated as

$$\text{Risk per unit dose} = PF_{\text{m}}D_d,$$

where P is the prevalence of a particular disease class, F_{m} the mutational component for that disease and D_d the doubling dose. Table 7 presents the risk estimated for the different genetic-disease classes using the doubling-dose method.

The direct method uses the extent of radiation-induced phenotypic damage in the offspring of exposed persons to estimate the frequency of genetic alterations in a human population. Dominant mutations are presumed to be responsible for all first-generation phenotypic damage. The genetic risk is estimated as

$$\text{Risk per unit dose} = F_dMN.$$

The risk per unit dose is defined as the estimated number of significant, radiation-induced dominant diseases in humans per million live-born in first-generation offspring of irradiated parents. F_d is the frequency of radiation-induced dominant mutations per unit dose obtained from mouse studies; M, the multiplication factor, is the reciprocal of the fraction of total mutations proposed to affect the body system in mice under study (e.g., 10 for skeletal damage and 36.8 for cataracts); N is the number of children born in the population for which risk is being estimated (usually 1 million).

The result is that $15–30 \times 10^{-6}$ radiation-induced mutations occur after exposing males to 0.01 Gy, whereas for exposed females the data are unavailable. In general, the values for dominant mutations obtained by the direct and indirect methods are very similar.

The great majority of data on the assessment of genetic or heritable effects in human populations following exposure to radiation has come from studies of atomic bomb survivors. The following endpoints have been assessed: untoward pregnancy outcomes (major congenital malformation, stillbirth, and neonatal death); sex of child; tumors with onset prior to the age of 20; death of live-born infants through an aver-

TABLE 7 Risk Estimates for Genetic Disease in Humans from 0.01 Gy of Low-LET Radiation Using the Indirect Method[a]

Genetic disease	Incidence (per million live births)	Effect of 0.01 Gy per generation (per million live births)		
		First generation	Second generation	Equilibrium
Autosomal dominant	10,000	15	13	100
Autosomal recessive	2500	0.05	0.05	15
Chromosomal structural anomalies	400	2.4	1	4
Numerical anomalies	3400	Very small	Very small	Very small
Congenital anomalies	60,000		Not estimated	
Multifactorial disease	600,000		Not estimated	

[a]Adapted from UNSCEAR (1993).

age life expectancy of 26.2 years, exclusive of death from malignancy; growth and development of life-born infants; cytogenetic abnormalities; and mutations altering the electrophoretic behavior or function of a selected battery of erythrocyte and blood plasma proteins. There were no significant increases in any of these indicators from a combined parental gonadal equivalent dose of 0.4 to 0.5 Sv.

UNSCEAR (1993) also estimated the acute dose that would, on the average, increase the incidence to twice the background—the doubling dose—as 1.7 to 2.2 Sv. Allowing for chronic exposure, a gonadal dose-reduction factor was applied to give a minimal doubling dose of 4 Sv for genetic effect.

Radiation Carcinogenesis

Mechanisms

Association between Radiation and Cancer Humans have evolved in an environment of radiation. Evolution must have selected for mechanisms that inhibit radiation effects and stimulate repair and recovery of the damage induced. Thus, mechanisms for controlling cell proliferation, programmed cell death, and repair of the damage induced are essential for the development and maintenance of organisms. One of the consequences of misrepair of a variety of genes is that cancer will be induced late in life.

Evidence of an association between radiation in the environment and cancer was recognized in the mines in Saxony in the 16th century. But not until Becquerel's discovery of radioactivity it was possible to associate lung cancer to radon and radon daughters in the mine. The first report of a solid cancer induced by large doses of X-rays was published in 1895. Multiple exposures from a fluoroscope caused radiation burns, radiodermatitis, and skin cancer.

Oncogenes, Tumor Supressors, and Mutator Genes Cancer is characterized by an altered control of cell proliferation in which the replication of cells capable of proliferation is greater than the loss. This is the initial change. Two classes of genes have been identified that roughly meet Boveri's suggestion in the early 1900s that cancer might arise from both positive and negative regulators. Oncogenes, caused by mutations in proto-oncogenes, are recognized as causing "gain-of-function" in the cell carrying the altered gene and to enhance proliferation. The *ras* and *myc* families of genes are examples of this class. Oncogenes are frequently associated with leukemias and lympohomas. Because the products of oncogenes act in a dominant fashion, a single copy may be sufficient to cause neoplastic transformation.

The other class, usually referred to a tumor-suppressor genes, result in loss of function in the gene and a loss of the inhibitory control on cell proliferation when mutated or deleted. Examples of this class are the RB, WTI, APC, p16, and p53 genes. In contrast to oncogenes, tumor-suppressor genes are recessive, so that loss of function involves mutation in both chromosomes. Loss of both suppressor genes can occur also by process known as somatic homozygosity, or one gene could be affected by germ-line mutation and the second gene by a mutation in early life. Retinoblastoma occurs in this way. In tumors, loss of p53 may result in chromosome instability and gene amplification affecting many targets. Most important, overexpression of wild-type p53 induces delayed progression through the cell cycle and/or apoptosis.

The importance of the induction of a mutator gene, especially in cancer induced by single acute exposure to radiation, is clear because the probability of all the genes that appear to be involved in carcinogenesis being hit is extremely low. The discovery of a mutation of hMSH2, the mismatch-repair gene, in cases of hereditary nonpolyposis colorectal cancer (HNPCC) may provide an explation for a cascade of mutations.

Chromosome Aberrations and Cancer Chromosomal translocations are induced by radiation and specific translocations are combined with, in particular, leukemias. The identification of the Philadelphia chromosome was the first association of a consistent chromosome aberration with a malignancy, the chronic myelogenous leukemia. A translocation involving chromosome 9 and 22 is found in pluripotential stem cells that can give rise to both myeloid and lymphoid cells. The abl gene, which is a homolog of a viral oncogene v-abl, is normally located on chromosome 9 but is translocated to chromosome 22 next to the bcr gene, resulting in a product of the fusion of the two genes.

Animal experiments have established that the susceptibility to the induction of tumors by radiation is correlated with the frequency of the specific tumor in control animals. Furthermore, the characteristic chromosome aberration found in radiation-induced myeloid leukemia in mice is the same in the leukemias induced by either gamma rays or neutrons.

The Carcinogenic Process Cancer is not only a disease in which the control of cell proliferation is defective. Tumors do, of course, vary in their growth rate and the size of the growth fraction. For tumors to grow beyond microscopic dimensions, angiogenesis must occcur. This is a complex, sequential process. Fibroblast growth factors are among the most effective stimulators of endothelial proliferation and angiogenesis. There are three oncogenes that encode for proteins with homology with this growth factor. Angiogenesis or neovascularization has not been noted as a direct consequence of radiation; it has to occur for the growth of a cancer and metastasis is the hallmark of lethality. Both loss and activation of gene function are involved in metastasis.

The sequence of events in carcinogenesis suggests four main limiting factors: (1) control of cell proliferation, (2) induction or development of genomic instability, (3) angiogenesis, and (4) development of the capability of invading tissues and vessels. It is probable that single exposures of radiation are more likely to affect the first of these. It is possible that protracted exposures may affect the other limiting factors, but only if the doses are relatively high.

Models of Carcinogenesis The model of carcinogenesis by Armitage and Doll, based on the increase in cancer approximately to the power of one's age, requires six or seven events. Other models are based on stages such as initiation, promotion, and progression and fit the widely held views that cancer is a multistage process. The model for solid cancers in atomic bomb survivors in the light of their two-mutation clonal expansion model consists of initiation, (the first rate-limiting step), malignant conversion (the second), and the clonal expansion of initiatied cells with promotion. The data indicate that it possible that the only effect of acute radiation "is the virtually instantaneous creation of initiated cells."

The question is: How does the induction only of initiation by radiation result in overt cancer? There is experimental evidence that many more cells than cancers are initiated but that only a few neoplastic transformed cells proceed over a considerable period of time to accumulate changes that are expressed as the malignant cell phenotype. Multiple mutations in cancer could arise also from an initial change in a mutator gene that leads to a cascade of mutations in various target genes.

Recently there has been evidence to support the old idea that radiation induces genomic instability, which is a broad term that includes destabilization of chromosomes, gene amplification, and mutation. It seems likely that genomic instability is of importance in tumor progression. Delayed reproductive cell death, cell fusion, altered cell attachment, delayed chromosomal stability, and delayed mutation are some of the findings after irradiation. It is not known what molecular lesion(s) cause genomic instability, but DNA double-strand breaks are a candidate.

Risk Assessment for Tumors

Exposed Populations The assessment of the effects of exposure to ionizing radation and how the data should be applied to radiation protection is a continuing task. The information has come from the study of the populations as follows:

- Workers populations (e.g., nuclear plant workers, miners, radium-dial painters, radiation technologists, and radiologists)
- Medical exposures (e.g., thymic enlargement, benign tumors, tinea capitis, and ankylosing spondylitis)
- Diagnostic examination (e.g., tuberculosis, internal emitters such as iodine-131, and thorotrast)
- Cancer treatment (e.g., cervical cancer, breast cancer, Hodgkin disease, and childhood cancers)
- Atomic bomb survivors (in Hiroshima and Nagasaki, and the Marshall Island)

All of these are cohort studies, which are less prone to bias than other types of epidemiological studies.

The atomic bomb survivors are the main source of data used for the estimated risk on which radiation protection is based. The reasons for the primacy of the data for atomic bomb survivors are the exposures were whole-body, the population size is large, the estimated doses range from 0.0 to greater than 4 Gy, and there has been a meticulous follow-up of the populations exposed in Hiroshima and Nagasaki since 1950 and continuing.

There are 85,500 persons included in the study. Until 1990, the number of estimated excess deaths from solid cancers is 334 and for leukemia about 90, in six dose categories ranging from 0.005–0.1 Sv to greater than 2.0 Sv. About 67% of the excess deaths from solid cancers are in the 0.2–0.5 Sv, 0.5–1.0 Sv and >2.0 Sv groups. There has been a total of 8,040 cancer deaths in the control and exposed groups, of these about 5.2% are associated with radiation exposure.

In addition to the cancer mortality study, the total cancer incidence at seven organ sites have been determined. The excess relative risk per Sv—cancer cases above those expected in the absence of exposure—differs, of course, among sites but on average is 37% higher for cancer incidence (0.63) than for cancer mortality (0.46).

About 50% of the atomic bomb survivors were still living in 1997, including the youngest persons at the time of the bomb. Because this segment of the population is probably the most sensitive to the induction of cancer, much of the data is still to come. Therefore, the life-time risk of cancer must be estimated using a projection model. The model that has been chosen is a constant-excess relative-risk model with a linear nonthreshold dose–response with allowance for gender and for age at exposure. The dependence of the risk on age at exposure and gender is illustrated in Fig. 8.

Epidemiology and Risk Assessment There are a number of uncertainties in the estimates of risk of the atomic bomb survivors: 1) the dosimetry, 2) the shape of the dose–response, and 3) the risk projection model. There are two further uncertainties. The exposure to the atomic bomb radiation was at a very high dose rate, whereas the general and worker populations are exposed at low dose rates. Thus, some dose and dose-rate effectiveness factor (DDREF) must be applied to estimate the risks from the exposures most commonly experienced. A DDREF of two has been selected by the International Commisssion for Radiological Protection. Another uncertainty is the method of transferring the estimates of risk determined for the Japanese population exposed over 50 years ago to other populations.

The estimated excess risk for cancer mortality that is currently used for total body irradiation and for acute high dose-rate exposure to low-LET radiation is 5.00×10^{-2} Sv^{-1}. Different organs contribute, with high (the stomach, colon, and lung; 0.85–1.10), medium (the bone marrow; 0.5), and low (the liver 0.15, thyroid 0.08, and skin 0.2×10^{-2} Sv^{-1}) sensitivity. The corresponding probability coefficient for the worker population is 4.0×10^{-2} Sv^{-1}.

The low excess mortality from thyroid and skin

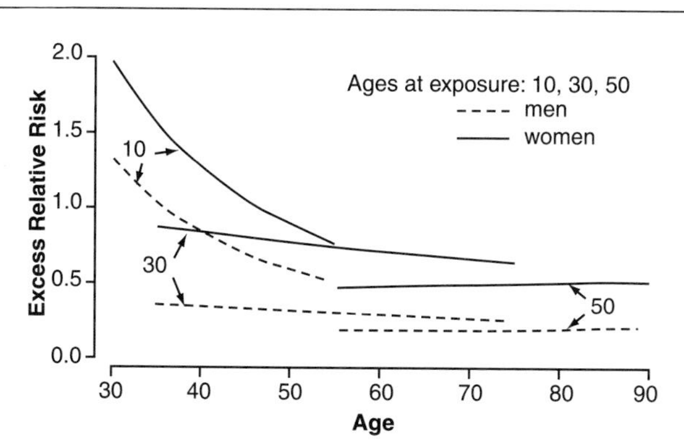

FIGURE 8 Excess relative risk (ERR), solid cancers by age and gender for selected ages at exposure. The figure is based on the ERR modified to allow for decreasing ERR for those under 20 years of age at the time of exposure. The two black dots indicate the constant ERR estimated for 10-year-old children using the cancer model in Pierce *et al.* (1996). (From Preston *et al.*, 1997.)

cancer is related to the fact that these types of cancers have a low mortality. The high risk for cancer in the gastrointestinal tract may be due to its high frequency in the Japanese population in general and is not appropriate for all other populations.

Other studies are also important to determine whether the DDREF of 2 is appropriate for all types of cancer. For example, tuberculosis patients who had frequent fluoroscopic examinations involving multiple small doses of X-rays but relatively high total doses had an excess breast cancer mortality but did not have an excess of lung cancer. The finding indicates that the reduction in the carcinogenic effects of radiation by fractionation differs markedly, a fact long recognized in experimental carcinogenesis.

Recently populations of nuclear workers exposed to radiation in the Unites States, Great Britain, and Canada have been studied to determine the risk from exposures to low doses and low-dose rates. Such risk estimates would obviate the need to extrapolate responses observed at high doses to responses at low doses. Although the numbers of workers in this international combined analysis of radiation workers was large (over 95,000), the average cumulative dose was low (about 0.05 Sv), and only about 5% of the workers had cumulative doses greater than 0.2 Sv. Also, the follow-up period was short and the statistical power low. Nevertheless, the estimates of the excess relative risk Sv^{-1} for the nuclear workers monitored for external radiation are comparable to the data for the atomic bomb survivors (e.g., for leukemia: workers, 2.2, and for the atomic bomb survivors, 3.7 for the linear model and 1.4 for a linear–quadratic model).

In addition to the factors that contribute to the low statistical power of these studies, the uncertainty of the estimates is contributed to by confounding factors. Radiation is not the only agent that may influence of many of the workers, especially in weapons facilities. Chemical agents, especially those known to be leukemogenic, must be considered and, of course, smoking. These agents can confound the studies of the effects of radiation or, more important, can interact with the radiation.

Radon The major current sources of information on the risks from exposure to alpha-particle radiation comes from studies of miners of uranium and other minerals and of radon in the home. About 65,000 miners are included in 11 studies and in this population there were 2,700 cases of lung cancer. Forty percent of these cases were attributed to radiation. For the general population, exposed to radon in their homes, it was estimated that about 8% of all lung cancer should be attributed to radon.

A comparison of the relative risk as a function of radon concentration in the combined miner study and the eight-case control studies of exposure to radon in the home gives the result that the risk of lung cancer from radon in the home is comparable to the linear dose–response obtained from the miner studies. A difficulty in the interpretation of these studies, however, is the fact that smoking is the predominant source of risk for lung cancer and its influence, as well as its interaction with radon, are difficult to take into account with accuracy. There are also conditions in the mines that must be of concern when extrapolating the risk to the environment in the home.

A summary of the various risks estimations for worker and general populations is given in Table 8. It is based on all the epidemiological data, particularly those from the study of the Japanese atomic bomb survivors and taking into account the pertinent radiobiological knowledge.

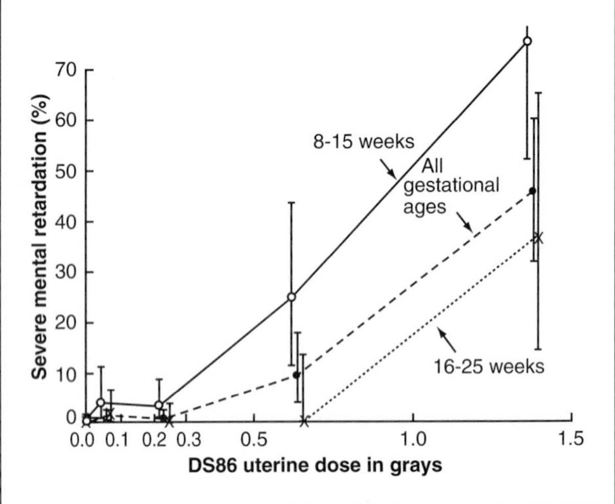

FIGURE 9 Frequency of severe mental retardation and 90% confidence limits by uterine-absorbed dose and post-ovulatory age. (From Otake *et al.*, 1996, with permission.)

Teratogenic Effects due to Prenatal Irradiation

The high radiosensitivity during the development of organisms was established quite early; experimental studies on animals, especially mice, show that the radiation-induced effects depend on the stage of development during the exposure. Irradiation in the preimplantation period leads mostly to cell death. Surviving cells carry, however, chromosome aberrations and micronuclei, which lead to damage of the embryo at later developmental stages.

Irradiation during the stage of organogenesis leads to malformations; this period occurs 8–15 days after conception for mice and 22–70 days for humans. In the studies with mice, the most predominant malformations induced during organogenesis are exencephaly, evisceration, and anencephaly due to a failure of the closure of the ectoderm. Other radiation-induced malformations are found in the skeleton and the eye.

TABLE 8 Nominal Probability Coefficients for Cancer[a]

	Fatal cancer	Nonfatal cancer	Total[b]
Workers	4.0	0.8	4.8
General population	5.0	1.0	6.0

[a]ICRP (1991) and NCRP (1993). Risk coefficients (10^{-2} Sv^{-1}).
[b]When severe genetic effects are included, the total detriment becomes 5.6×10^{-2} Sv^{-1} and 7.3×10^{-2} Sv^{-1} for the worker and general populations, respectively.

Knowledge about the human response to irradiation in the prenatal stage was obtained from the 1566 children exposed *in utero* in Hiroshima and Nagasaki. The principal effects are small head size and severe mental retardation. Other tests, including anthropometric measurements, show a general trend of decline in growth with increasing radiation dose.

The frequency of mental retardation depends strongly on the stage of development, as shown in Fig. 9. The most sensitive stage of human development is the late organogenesis with brain development between 8–15 weeks. Stages before and after this period are less sensitive in this respect. This sensitivity of 50%/Sv is the highest known in radiobiology; for comparison, the risk of carcinogenesis is about 5%/Sv and the genetic risk even smaller.

It is an open question whether there is a threshold dose below which there is no teratogenic effect (i.e., no visible malformations). In animal studies such a threshold can be observed at about 0.25 Sv. Re-analyzing the human data in Fig. 9, a threshold dose of 0.15–0.31 Gy can be assumed.

Of special interest is also the question of whether the radiation exposure *in utero* shows a higher carcinogenic risk than post-natal exposure. There are only a few data available in the cohort of the *in utero* irradiated cases that suggest that the risk for this cohort is in the range of that of the young children cohort (0–5 years age), but there is a need for caution because of the limited data until data from longer observation periods are available.

Radiation Protection Laws

Radiation protection is concerned with a wide range of circumstances, including occupational, medical, and public exposures. The aim is to prevent or limit the deleterious effects without diminishing the benefits of the use of radiation in medicine, scientific research, and industry.

Radiation protection is the prevention of clinically significant deterministic effects, which is possible by limiting exposures to below the relevant thresholds to limit stochastic effects. It is assumed that stochastic effects cannot prevented completely because there is no unequivocal evidence of a threshold. Radiobiological evidence and caution recommend the use of a no-threshold linear dose–response relationship for use in radiation protection. However, the linear response is not a direct interpolation from data obtained at high doses and high-dose rates to effects at the doses of concern in radiation protection.

The International Commission on Radiological Protection (ICRP), founded 1928, has drawn on a wide range of international expertise to consider the effects of ionizing radiation and to make recommendations that can be a consistent basis for national standards. A detailed description of the system of protection can be found in ICRP publication 60 (1991). The most recent recommendation limits the occupational dose to 20 mSv per year, averaged over defined five-year periods. The limit for the public is 1 mSv in a year. It should be pointed out that

1. These limits apply to doses from external exposures and to 50-year committed doses from intakes.
2. The effective dose is the sum of doses, weighted by radiation, in various tissues and organs.
3. Annual exposures that correspond to equivalent doses in the respiratory epithelium in excess of 1 mSv from radon are common in homes. In the U.S., the Environmental Protection Agency (EPA) recommends remedial action at a radon level that corresponds to about 8 mSv annual effective dose to the bronchial epithelium. In Great Britain and Germany the level requiring action is about twice that proposed by the EPA.

In Germany a maximum cumulative life-time equivalent dose of 400 mSv has been recommended and the National Council on Radiation Protection and Measurements in the U.S. (NCRP) has proposed a life-time limit of 10 mSv $\times$ age. To prevent deterministic effects for the lens of the eye and the skin, localized occupational exposures of 150 mSv and 500 mSv should be the limit. The corresponding limits for the public are 15 mSv and 50 mSv.

The principle of restricting exposures to a level "as low as reasonably achievable," referred to as the ALARA principle, has been very successful in reducing exposures, especially in industry.

NONIONIZING RADIATION

Not only do the primary ionization events, as discussed previously, lead to human harm but also radiations that produce biological effects by the absorption of their energy in tissue are harmful. Among these, ultraviolet light is the radiation of most interest.

Ultraviolet Radiation

Biological Effects

In the spectrum of electromagnetic waves, ultraviolet radiation is in the range of 200–400 nm, and is divided in UVC, 200–280nm; UVB, 280–320 nm; UVA, 320–400 nm. UVC from the sun is absorbed by the atmosphere, whereas UVB and UVA are in the sunlight reaching Earth. UVC and UVB can also be produced by artificial sources.

UV light is absorbed by biomolecules, leading to excitation and chemical reactions (photochemistry). Photochemical reactions in the atmosphere occur as the formation of ozone from oxygen and as photolysis of NO_2 (generated from automobiles) with UVA as

$$NO_2 \xrightarrow{h\nu} NO + O\cdot \tag{15}$$

and

$$O\cdot + O_2 \longrightarrow O_3, \tag{16}$$

which oxidizes NO to NO_2. Thus, there is an equilibrium,

$$NO_2 + O_2 \rightleftharpoons NO + O_3. \tag{17}$$

In the stratosphere there is, in contrast, a light-induced degradation of O_3, catalyzed by fluorocarbohydrates. A biologically important photochemical reaction is the formation of vitamin D in the skin.

UV light-induced cell inactivation and mutation are due to the absorption by nucleic acids of energy between 240–280 nm (mostly UVC), but UVB contributes also to the biological effect. Various photoproducts are formed (Fig. 10). Apart from the cyclobutane

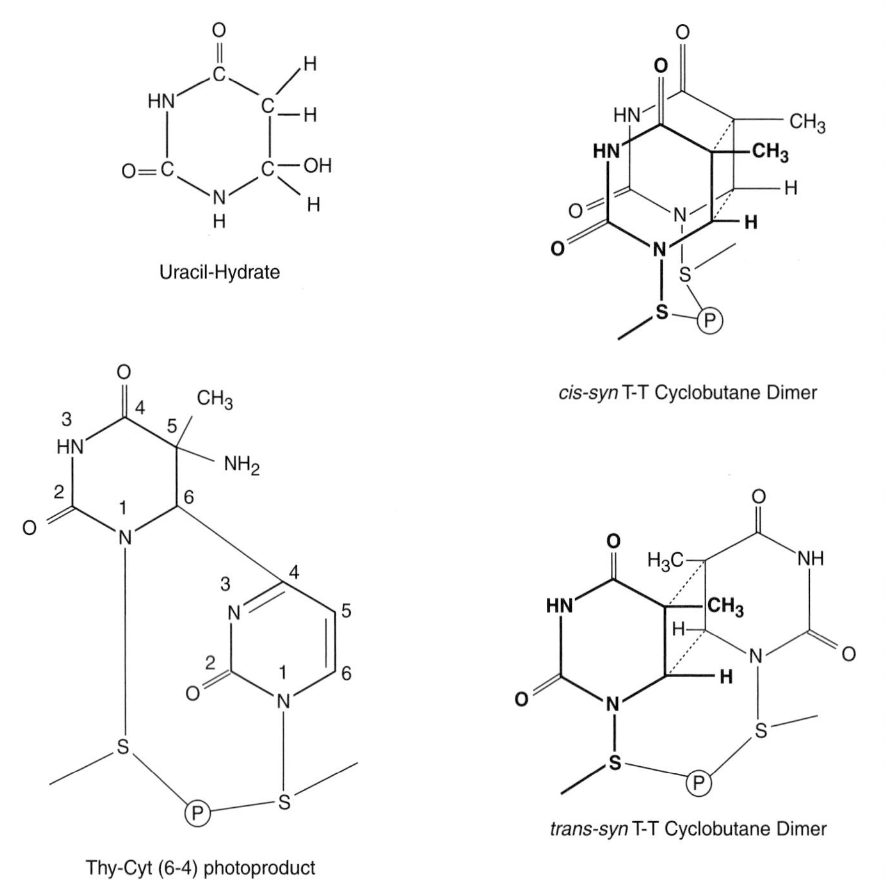

FIGURE 10 Ultraviolet light photoproducts in the DNA.

dimer, the 6-4-pyrimidine-thymine photoproduct is largely responsible for UV-induced mutation. In addition, cross-links between DNA and protein are formed but no DNA strand breaks. UV light-induced DNA damage is repaired in the cell.

The UV light-induced cell inactivation and mutation is most effective in the range of DNA absorption (action spectrum); but there is also a distinct biological effect in the range of >300 nm. In relationship to cell inactivation, the mutagenic potential of UV light is much higher than that of ionizing radiation, possibly due to the fact, that UV light does not produce the DNA strand breaks that contribute to cell killing by ionizing radiation.

Medical Effects and Applications of Ultraviolet Light

Harm from ultraviolet light is observed in the human skin and eye. There are a variety of symptoms of this skin damage, known as sunburn (dermatitis solaris), induced by UVB from 295–315 nm. The symptoms begin 6–12 hours after exposure, with erythema and edematous swelling reaching a maximum at 24 hours. In severe cases, crustaceous and moist stages are observed. The intensity of sunburn depends on the skin type of the individual; persons with fair skin and hair are more sensitive than those with darker skin and hair. In addition, the UVB-induced tanning of the skin (e.g., melanine formation in the basal layer) is greater in persons with dark skin. The UV-induced erythema is used sometimes as a biological dosimeter; a bright sunny day can lead to several erythema units.

A high sensitivity towards UV light is also seen in the eye. Without the protection of sunglasses, a painful keratoconjunctivitis can develop within several hours; exposure from germinating lamps (UVC) are very dangerous in this respect. The treatment of such symptoms is usually successful with glucocorticoids.

Chronic exposure to bright sunlight over many years leads to keratosis and telangiectasia, a basis for precarcinogenesis and malignant tumors. The light-induced superficial melanomas show a high risk for metastases; early diagnostic and medical care are necessary. The lentigo-malignant melanomas are also UV light-induced. There is no exact correlation known between UV dose and the frequency of skin tumors in a population, but it is evident that in countries with high UVB exposure a high incidence of skin tumors is observed, whereas in countries with low UV exposure there is a low incidence. Patients with the genetic disease Xeroderma pigmentosum, show a high sensitivity with cancer proneness discussed previously (see the section on DNA repair).

Light-induced effects from visible light can be induced by the transfer of light-induced exitation from the absorbing molecule to another. Such light-induced dermatosis has to be distinguished from photoallergic reactions. Phototoxic reactions are induced locally by agents such as tar or psoralene or generally by tetracyclines and phenothiacine. The combination of psoralene with low-level UVA radiation is an effective treatment of psoriasis.

Laser Rays

Laser rays (light amplification by stimulated emission of radiation) are strongly monochromatic radiations in the wavelength range of 180–1000 nm. The wavelength depends on the active medium of the laser (solid state, fluid, or gas) producing the amplification of simultaneously oscillating photons. Lasers generate a high intensity of light, which damages tissue by high local temperatures causing local necrosis. This is especially the case for lasers such as the neodymium-ytrium-Al-garnet (ND:YAG) laser (1060 nm) and argon laser (488 and 514 nm), used by surgeons for the coagulation of blood vessels.

The application of laser light, however, is harmful, especially to the eyes, as laser light in the visible range is absorbed in the retina and leads to punctiform necrosis (diameter 10 μm). Limits for the intensity of laser exposure have been evaluated for the protection of the skin and eyes; in any case, safety goggles should be worn during use of laser light. The genotoxic effects of laser light can be excluded by correct person protection procedures.

Radar, Radiowaves, and Microwaves

Radiation at high frequencies is produced by a variety of sources transmitting different energies, ranging from traffic radar (25 mW), radiotelephones (several watts), and microwave ovens (0.3–1.2 kW) up to radiation in megaWs, such as radiotransmitters and military radar installations

The effect of high-frequency radiation on biological objects is mostly due to local heating; the influence on ionic transport across membranes is negligible. The heat effect depends on the energy of the radiation and on the capacity of the organism to dissipate the heat from the exposed tissue via the blood flow. In organs with low blood flow the temperature can increase from 3–5°C. The lens of the eye may be damaged in this case, leading to cataracts.

The increase of temperature in an organ is also the basis for estimating the risk to workers. In the case of a single exposure at 70–280-W high-frequency whole-body irradiation (1–4 W/kg body weight) the exposure should be limited to 1 hour. For exposures of longer duration, a limit of 0.4 W/kg is recommended and for the public 0.1 W/kg. This latter value also applies to microwave ovens, which show only a minimal leaking of radiation intensity of <0.1 W/kg.

Electromagnetic Fields

Electromagnetic fields are formed by the transmission of electric energy and by the use of electrical equipment. Humans or other organisms in such a field change their charge until the surface of the whole organism (body) has reached a stable potential. Thus an electric current will be induced in the body, which may cause biological reactions. For the current density, a "dose" in mA/m^2 is used. Visual and nervous effects are reported in the range of 10–100 mA/m^2. Higher intensities produce dysfunction in excitable tissues, such as the heart with extrasystoles and ventricular fibrillations (electric accidents).

The widespread use of domestic electric power results in an exposure of humans to low-level (50/60 Hz) electric and magnetic fields (EMF). Numerous epidemiological studies have been done on the possible health effects of EMFs on workers (e.g., linemen, electricians, and welders) or people living close to power-transmission lines. There was "some evidence for an association between occupational magnetic field exposure and adult leukemia, but the inconsistencies between and within studies weaken the evidence."

In addition, attempts were made to determine whether an interaction of EMFs with biological material was physically and biological plausible. Studies have shown that the current densities induced at the cellular level by EMFs are more than 1000 times lower than those naturally occurring in cells. In addition, it is nearly impossible to determine reliable values for a "dose" of an exposure to EMFs.

Bibliography

Alapetite, C., Wachter, T., Sage, E., and Moustacchi, E. (1996). Use of the alkaline comet assays to detect DNA repair deficiencies in human fibroblasts exposed to UVC, UVB, UVA and gamma-rays. *Int. J. Radiat. Biol.* **69,** 359–369.

Arlett, C. F. (1992). Human cellular radiosensitivity—the search for the holy grail or a poisoned chalice. *Advan. Radiat. Biol.* **16,** 273–292.

Bauchinger, M., Schmid, E., Zitzelberger, H., and Braselmann H. (1993). Radiation-induced chromosome aberrations analysed by two-color fluorescence *in situ* hybridization with composite whole chromosme-specific DNA probes and a pancentromeric DNA probe. *Int. J. Radiat. Biol.* **64,** 179–184.

Burkart, W. (1996) Radioepidemiology in the aftermath of the nuclear program of the former Soviet Union: Unique lessons to be learnt. *Radiat. Environ. Biophysics* **35,** 565–573.

Cardis, E., Gilbert, E. S., Carpenter, L., Howe, G, Kato, I., Armstrong, V., Beral, V., Cowper, G., Douglas, A., Fix, J., Fry, S. A., Kaldor, J., Lave, C., Salmon, L., Smith, P. G., Voelz, G. L., and Wiggs, L. D. (1995). Effects of low doses and dose rates of external ionizing radiation: Cancer mortality among nuclear industry workers in three countries. *Radiat. Res.* **142,** 117–132.

Delongchamp, R. R., Mabuchi, K., Yoshimoto, Y., and Preston, D. L. (1997). Cancer mortality among atomic bomb survivors exposed in utero or as young children, October 1950–May 1992. *Radiat. Res.* **147,** 385–395.

Douglas, B. G., and Fowler, J. F. (1976). The effect of multiple small doses of X-rays on skin reactions in the mouse and a basic interpretation. *Radiat. Res.* **66,** 401–416.

Feychting, M. (1996) Occupational exposure to electro-magnetic fields and adult leukemia: A review of the epidemiological evidence. *Radiat. Environ. Biophysics* **35,** 237–242.

Fritz-Niggli, H. (1959). "Strahlenbiologie - Grundlagen und Ergebnisse." Georg Thieme Verlag, Stuttgart, Germany.

Hall, E. J. (1994). "Radiobiology for the Radiologist." 4th ed. Lippincott, Philadelphia, PA.

Holley, W. R., and Chatterjee, A. (1996). Clusters of DNA damage induced by ionizing radiation: Formation of short DNA fragments. I. Theoretical modeling. *Radiat. Res.* **145,** 188–199.

International Commission on Radiological Protection (ICRP) (1991). "Recommendations of the ICRP." Publication 60, Annals of the ICRP 21. Pergamon Press, Elmsford, NY.

Kummermehr, J., and Trott, K.-R. (1997). Tumour stem cells. In "Stem Cells" (C. S. Potten, ed.), pp. 363–399. Academic Press, London.

Lubin, J. H., and Boice, J. D., Jr. (1997). Lung cancer risk from residential radon: Meta analysis of eight epidemiological studies. *J. Natl. Cancer Inst.* **89,** 49–57.

Mill, A. J., Wells, J., Hall, S. C., and Butler, A. (1996). Micronucleus iuduction in human lymphocytes: Comparative effects of X-rays, alpha particles, beta particles and neutrons and implications for biological dosimetry. *Radiat. Res.* **145,** 575–585.

Modrich P., and Lahue, R. (1996). Mismatch repair in replication fidelity, genetic recombination, and cancer biology. *Annu. Rev. Biochem.* **65,** 101–133.

Neel, J. V., and Schull, W. J. (eds.) (1991). "The Children of Atomic Bomb Survivors: A Genetic Study." National Academic Press, Washington, D.C.

Otake, M., Schull, W. J., and Lee, S. (1996). Threshold for radiation-related severe mental retardation in prenatal exposed A-bomb survivors: A re-analysis. *Radiat. Res.* **70,** 755–763.

Pierce, D. A., Shimuzu, Y., Preston, D. L., Vaeth, M., and Mabuchi, K. (1996). Studies of the mortality of A-bomb survivors. Report 12. Part I: Cancer: 1950–1990. *Radiat. Res.* **146,** 1–27.

Preston, D. L., Kusumi, S., Tomonaga, M., Izumi, S., Ron, E., Kuramoto, A., Kamada, N., Dohy, H., Matsui, T., Nonaka, H., Thompson, D. E., Soda, M., and Mabuchi, K. (1994). Cancer incidence in atomic bomb surviors. Part III: Leukemia, lymphoma and multiple myeloma 1958–1987. *Radiat. Res.* **137,** S68–S97.

Preston, D. L., Mabuchi, K., Pierce, D. A., and Shimizu, Y. (1997). Mortality among atomic-bomb survivors. In "Implications of New Data on Radiation Cancer Risk." Proceedings No. 18. National Council of Radiation Protection and Measurements. Bethesda, Maryland.

Rydberg, B. (1996). Clusters of DNA damage induced by ionizing radiation: Formation of short DNA fragments. II Experimental detection. *Radiat. Res.* **145,** 200–209.

Salassidis, K., Georgiadou-Schumacher, V., Braselmann, H., Müller, P., Peter, R. U., and Bauchinger, M. (1995). Chromosome painting in highly irradiated Chernobyl victims: A follow-up study to evaluate the stability of symmetrical translocations and the influence of clonal aberrations for retrospective dose estimation. *Int. J. Radiation Biol.* **68,** 257–262.

Sancar, A. (1996). DNA excision repair. *Annu. Rev. Biochem.* **65,** 43–81.

Sankaranarayanan, K. (1993). Ionizing radiation, genetic risk estimation and molecular biology. *Trends Genet.* **9,** 79–84.

Shore, R. E. (1990). Overview of radiation-induced skin cancer in humans. *Int. J. Radiat. Biol.* **57,** 809–827.

Stewart, G. G., Soranson, J. A., Alpen, E. L., Williams, M. V., and Denekamp, J. (1984). Radiation-induced renal damage. The effects of hyperfractionation. *Radiat. Res.* **98,** 407–420.

Thompson, D. E., Mabuchi, K., Ron, E., Soda, M., Tokunaga, M., Ochikubo, S., Sugimoto, S., Ikeda, T., Terasake, M., Izumi, S., and Preston, D. L. (1994). Cancer incidence in atomic bomb survivors. Part II: Solid tumors, 1959–1987. *Radiat. Res.* **137,** 517–567.

United Nations Scientific Commitee on the Effects of Atomic Radiation (1993). "Sources and Effects of Ionizing Radiation: UNSCEAR 1993 Report to the General Assembly." United Nations, New York.

Valberg, P. A., Kavet, R., and Rafferty, C. N. (1997). Review: Can low-level 50/60 Hz electric and magnetic fields cause biological effects? *Radiat. Res.* **148,** 2–21.

Vos, J.-M. H. (ed.) (1995). "DNA Repair Mechanisms: Impact on Human Diseases and Cancer." Springer-Verlag, Heidelberg, Germany.

Wood, R. D. (1996). DNA repair in eukaryotes. *Annu. Rev. Biochem.* **65,** 135–167.

CHAPTER

40

Natural Compounds

J. WESTENDORF
Department of Toxicology, University Medical School, Hamburg, Germany

INTRODUCTION

The use of chemical compounds for defense or attack is common in nature and an important tool of the evolution. Poisons are present in almost all classes of organisms from the most primitive bacteria to the highly developed vertebrates. The variation of natural poisons with respect to their chemical structures and biological action is enormous. The highest concentration of toxic organisms is located at places of maximal population density, such as tropical rain forests and coral reefs. Because a sufficient treatise on the entire field of natural poisons is not possible here, this chapter will only give an overview of the most important principles of action with some selected examples.

The use of plant- and animal-derived toxins by humans has been reported throughout history. Such poisons have been used for hunting purposes (arrow poisons), for occult ceremonies (belladonna, psilocybe, and opium) for executing victims (*Conium maculatum*), as abortives, and especially to treacherously murder people. Although poisons had been used as medicine in antiquity, it was Paracelsus (1493–1451), who recognized the dualistic principle of many poisons of their curative and deadly actions; "dosis sola facit venenum" (only the dose makes the poison). Modern pharmacology is a product of the knowledge of the special biological actions of compounds derived from plants and animals.

ANIMAL VENOMS AND POISONS

Animals use poisons and venoms for defense against potential enemies and to paralyze or kill their prey. In the latter case, the venom is located in special glands and transferred by bite or sting. If the venom or poison is only used for defense, it may be located also in the skin, or inner organs. The toxicity of such animals is often supported by conspicuous colors (e.g., frogs of the Dendrobate family and salamanders) to warn potential enemies "be careful, I am toxic." Some animals contain poisons that are derived from other organisms. This is often the case in aquatic systems, where certain dinoflagellates are the primary source of the toxic compounds, which are transferred to higher organisms by the food chain or via symbiosis.

The chemical composition of animal-derived venoms and toxins is, in most cases, very complex and contains proteins, peptides, glycosides, alkaloids, neurotransmitters, ketones, and even hydrocarbons. The poisons are often highly specialized and target the nervous system very efficiently. The components of complex toxins are often synergistic with respect to their adverse effects. Typical poisons of Hymenoptera, snakes, scorpions, and spiders contain

Amines: histamine, serotonine, acetylcholine, and kinines; these act as inflammatory agents, cause pain, and decrease blood pressure.

Enzymes: hyaluronidase (loosening up connecting tissue); and phospholipases (destroys cell membranes and increases the synthesis of inflammatory compounds, e.g., prostaglandines).

Polypeptides: these act as neurotoxins, myotoxins, and cardiotoxins.

The peptides are often the main toxicants in such complex mixtures and responsible for the death of the victim, whereas the other components act as adjuvans to help the peptides to reach its target (e.g., the nerve system receptors and heart). The protein components may cause allergic reactions after repeated application of the poison, which may also cause lethal anaphylactic-shock reactions.

Aquatic Animals

The aquatic ecosystem is characterized by a great complexity of species, many of which use toxic compounds to survive. The greatest concentration of different and, therefore, toxic species is located at tropical coral reefs. To swim or dive in such regions may be dangerous, especially for inexperienced people. The number of accidents caused by poisonous aquatic animals worldwide is between 40,000 and 50,000. Another 20,000 intoxications are caused by eating poisonous fish or mollusks.

Coelenterata (Coelenterate)

Poisonous representatives can be found among the hydras, jellyfish, sea anemones, and corals, all of which are marine inhabitants of the warm belt between the 30th parallels. In the warm Atlantic Gulf Stream, they can be found up to the 60th parallel. The toxins of these animals are usually polypeptides, which serve to catch prey or to protect against potential voracious enemies.

Upon touching the tentacle of these animals, which are covered with cnidoblasts (nematocysts), a sophisticated apparatus (cnidocile) rushes out. A kind of flagellum with numerous bristles and barbed hooks penetrates the skin, injecting the poison. The most dangerous representatives live in the tropical coral reefs. Among the most dreaded jellyfishes are the Portuguese man-of-war (*Physalia physalis*) and the sea wasp (*Chironex fleckeri*). Contact with these animals is followed by extreme pain caused by histamine, kinines, and prostaglandines, all contents of the poison. The victim may become unconscious because the pain is so violent and drown. Death may also occur by the poison itself. The toxic peptides of these Coelenterates are sodium channel blockers, which cause an extreme prolongation of the action potential of the synapses and neuromuscular endplate, causing very painful muscular contractions, paralysis, shock symptoms, and respiratory arrest. Antidotes do not exist and the treatment is symptomatic. The iv application of calcium, glucocorticoids, and plasma expanders is necessary in cases of shock. Topical application of local anesthetics is helpful because the contact with the poison is very painful. In most cases of accidents with poisonous Coelenterates, no medical care is immediately available. Information about the local situation and avoidance of any contact with such animals is, therefore, most important.

Mollusks (Mollusca)

Among these are the genera for mussels (*Lamellibranchiata*) and snails (*Gastropoda*). Poisoning by these species is, in most cases, caused by ingestion. Dinoflagellates are often the primary source of the toxins. The mollusks concentrate their toxins during their consumption of these organisms. The presentation of these toxins, which occur also in some fish species, is given elsewhere in this book.

Among the active toxic mollusks are Conidae (*Toxoglossa*), inhabiting the tropical marine areas. The animals possess a sophisticated venom apparatus serving as an offensive weapon for the gaining of food. It may also be used to a lesser extent as a defensive weapon. The apparatus consists of a muscular bulb, a venom duct, the radula, and the radular teeth, which are formed like little harpoons from 1 to 10 mm in length. The venom is forced under pressure from the venom duct into the radula and taken up by the radular teeth, which are then transported through the pharynx into the proboscis. The animals use this organ like a gun in shooting toxic arrows into the prey. The different Conidae are specialized to different prey (worms, snails, fish). Only those species preying on vertebrates (fish) are dangerous for humans. The venom contains basic peptides with a chain length of 13 to 29 amino acids. Three main species are distinguishable. α-Conotoxins possess a curare-like action on nicotinergic acetylcholine receptors at the neuromuscular endplate. ω-Conotoxins are calcium channel-blockers in the synapses of the neuromuscular endplate. μ-Conotoxins block sodium channels in muscle cell membranes. The actions of the different peptides are perfectly coordinated in order to block the nerve function with maximum efficiency. Normal prey is paralyzed almost immediately after being attacked by Conidae. This is important because these animals are slowly moving and not able to follow their prey. Some species of Conidae are quite able to kill humans (e.g., *Conus geographus* and *Conus tulipa*).

Conidae live in the shallow regions of tropic marine areas and are often collected as souvenirs because most are very pretty. This should be performed with great care and only dead shells should be picked up. The sting of fish-hunting Conidae results in a local numbness that spreads through the whole body, followed by paralysis of the muscles and finally heart arrest. No specific antidote is available, and the treatment has, therefore, to be symptomatic.

Echinoderms (Echinodermata)

The genus of Echinoderms contains two groups, the *Pelmatozoa* and *Eleutherozoa*. Most of the poisonous species belong to the *Eleutherozoa*. Among these are *Asteroidea* (starfishes), *Ophioidea, Echinoidea* (sea urchins), and *Holothurioidea* (sea cucumbers). Echinoderms are benthic organisms spread all over the oceans. However, most of the toxic species live in tropical areas.

Starfish use their poison most probably for preying on other organisms. For this purpose they produce a toxin located in skin glands, which is released into the water. The toxins are able to paralyze mussels, snails, and shrimps. After one touche a poisonous starfish, the stings may penetrate the skin, causing great pain and local inflammation. The toxins of starfish are steroid glycosides, which act as detergents, similar to the saponines occurring in many plant species. Figure 1 shows the toxic principle of the starfish *Acanthaster planci*. The toxin of this starfish decreases the blood pressure after parenteral application in mammals. This is believed to be mediated by endogenous arachidonic acid metabolites, such as prostacyclin.

Sea urchins cause painful wounds with their pointed stings, which break off after drilling into the skin. The stings of some species contain a venom, that causes great pain and inflammation. Sometimes systemic reactions, such as paresthesia, gastrointestinal symptoms, headache, and allergic reactions occur. Fatal cases are rare. The poisons are not only located in the stings but also in the genital organs. Eating sea urchins is, therefore, not recommended, especially during the spawning period. The chemistry of the sea urchin toxins is unknown. The toxins are most probably high molecular-weight compounds, which decompose during the procedure of isolation.

Among the sea cucumbers there are many poisonous species. Some of their toxins are located in skin glands. More important, however, are special organs, which are called as "Cuvierian tubules." In case of danger these tubules are extruded through the anus, releasing a mixture of toxic compounds that act as repellents for possible predators. The main toxic principles of sea cucumbers are saponins of the lanosterin-type, such as holothurin A (Fig. 1). Skin contact with sea cucumbers may cause painful symptoms, which normally disappear soon. In some Asian countries sea cucumbers are used as food (trepang). This sometimes causes intoxication dominated by gastrointestinal symptoms, such as vomiting and diarrhea. After absorption of considerable amounts of holothurin A, hemolysis and paralysis may occur. Fatal cases have also been reported.

Fishes (Pisces)

Most of the venomous or poisonous fishes live in the area of tropical coral reefs. They are distinguished as active (venomous) and passive (poisonous) species. Some of the poisons are produced by microorganisms living in a symbiosis with the fish.

Venomous fishes have venom glands and stings, which are used for defensive purposes. These fishes are in most cases lazy and stationary. Their toxic nature serves as a substitute for flight from predators. Among the around 200 species living in marine areas are stingrays (Dasyatidae), scorpionfishes (Scorpaenidae), weevers (Trachinidae), catfishes (Siluroideae) and others. The toxins consist of a complex mixture of very unstable proteins. The specific toxicity (LD_{50} in mice) varies between 200 μg/kg (stonefish) and several mg/kg. Stings from these fishes are sometimes extremely painful and cause local inflammation and necrosis with a bad prognosis for healing. The most toxic venomous fish, the stonefish (*Synaceja horrida*) was used by the native Malays on hunting darts.

After systemic application, the toxins exert pronounced myotoxic action. Affected are the heart, the blood circulatory system, and the skeletal muscles. Lethal doses cause a paralysis of the extremities and a circulatory collapse. Most dangerous are the stonefish species *Synaceja horrida* and *Synaceja trachinus*. The animals live in shallow marine areas and spend most of the time buried in the sand waiting for prey. Their color is so perfectly adapted to the neighboring environment that, even if not buried, they are almost invisible. Accidents occur in most cases by stepping on the fish. The dorsal spines penetrate the skin and the venom is injected by the pressure of the victim's weight into the wound. Fatal cases are not rare. Death occurs normally 8–24 hours after the envenomation.

Treatment first consists of removal of the sting fragments and cleaning the wound carefully. The af-

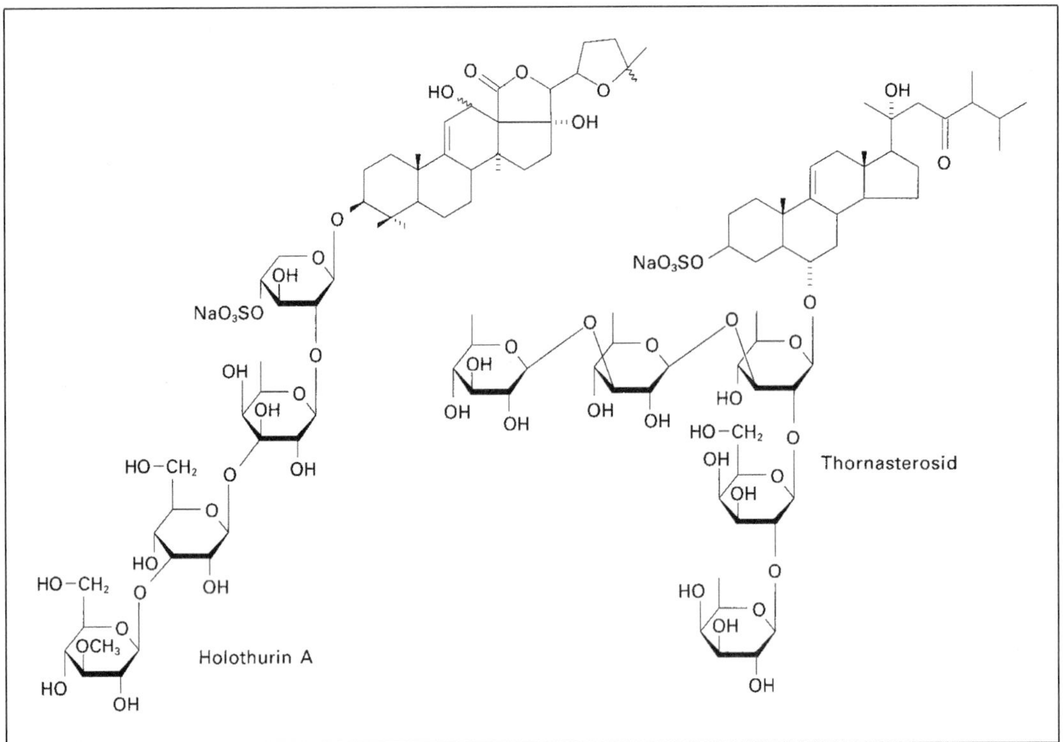

FIGURE 1 Steroidglycosides of Echinodermata. Thornasterosid occurs in *Acanthaster planci,* a starfish living in tropical coral reefs. Holothurin A is a toxin of the cuvierian tubules of sea cucumbers

fected extremity should be treated with hot water (40–50°C) for at least 30 minutes. This results in a decrease in the pain and a partial washout of the venom. In severe cases of intoxication the iv injection of an antivenin is recommended. However, in many cases an antivenin may not be available and the treatment has to be only symptomatic. The best way to prevent complications is to avoid any contact with these fishes. In areas known to be the habitats of stonefishes, the wearing of bathing shoes is recommended.

Other toxic fish species excrete their toxins through the skin. These are called "crinotoxic." An example is the boxfish (*Ostracion lentiginosus*), which excretes a toxin called pahutoxin. It is a choline ester of 3-acetoxyhexadecanoic acid (Fig. 2). Because of its amphophilic character, the compound acts as a detergent. Once released into the water, it has a strong repelling action on fishes, even on sharks, and other aquatic animals. If it is impossible to escape the toxin (e.g., as in an aquarium), the victims develop a decrease in movement, loss of equilibrium and locomotion, and, finally, sporadic convulsions and death. After parenteral application to mammals, the toxin, like other detergents, causes severe hemolysis. The LD_{50} in mice is 200 mg/kg.

Some fish contain toxic gonads, whereas the rest of the body is free from toxins. These fishes are called "ichtyootoxic." Most of these species live in freshwater and only a few live in marine environments. Among these is the Cabezon (*Scorpenichtys marmoratus*), which inhabits the Pacific coastal areas between California and British Columbia. The fish weighs up to 20 pounds and is a valuable food fish. Eating of the roe will cause intoxication with mainly gastrointestinal symptoms. In more severe cases arrhythmia, chest

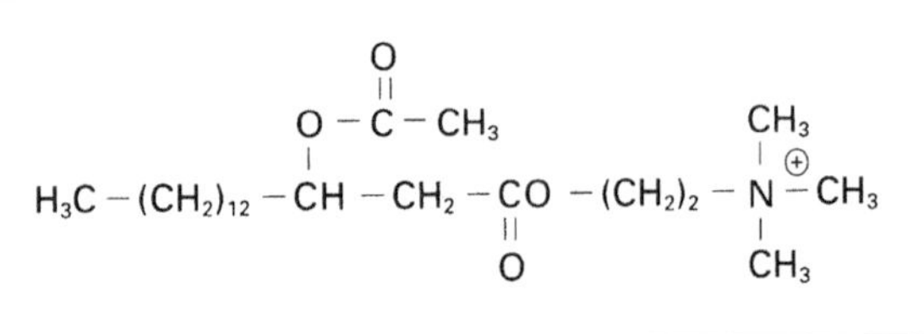

FIGURE 2 Pahutoxin, isolated from the skin of the boxfish (*Ostracion lentiginosus*). The compound is a cholinester of 3-acetoxyhexadecanoic acid.

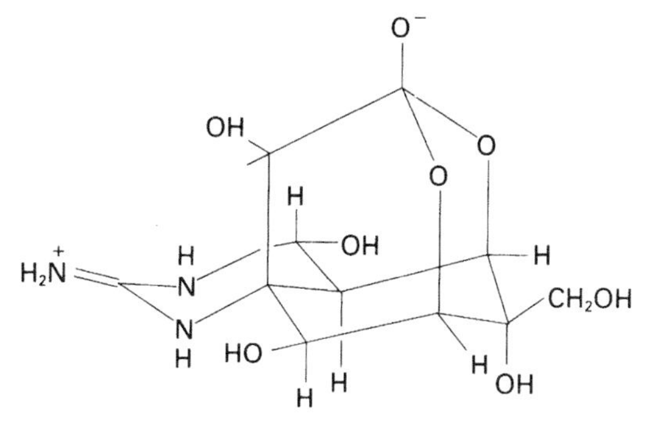

FIGURE 3 Tetrodotoxin.

pain, convulsion, and coma may occur. Lethal events are rare.

Some fishes contain toxins only in their blood and are, therefore, called "ichtyohematoxic." Among these are eels and muraena. Intoxication occurs if greater amounts of blood from these fishes are ingested. Nothing is known about the chemistry of the toxins, except that they are labile upon heating. The eating of cooked fish is, therefore, safe.

Passive toxic fishes contain toxins originally produced by certain microorganisms, such as bacteria, protozoa, or algae. The toxins are sometimes extremely potent and may be present in all tissues or only in certain organs of the fish. The term "ciguatera" characterizes an intoxication caused by eating groupers, barracudas, sharks, and other predatory fishes living in some tropical or subtropical marine areas, mainly near coral reefs. The phenomenon is frequent in certain areas of the Caribbean Sea and the Gulf of Mexico. The term ciguatera is derived from the Spanish word for a snail living on the isle of Cuba, erroneously thought to be responsible for the intoxication. The primary source of the toxin are epiphytic dinoflagellates living on macrophytic algae. The toxin is concentrated in the food chain (dinoflagellate to herbivorous fish to predatory fish). The highest concentrations occur in the gut and liver; however, the concentration of the toxin in muscular tissue is high enough to cause intoxication after eating contaminated fish. It is very hard to predict whether a fish is contaminated with the ciguatera toxin. Certain species of fish should, therefore, not be used for food in areas with a known history of ciguatera intoxication. A more detailed presentation of the symptoms of the ciguatera intoxication follows elsewhere.

A toxin derived from bacteria and concentrated in the gonads and liver of certain pufferfishes is tetrodotoxin (Fig. 3). The pufferfish (*Sphaeroides*), known in Japan as fugu, is very popular because of its delicious meat. The fish is cut into very thin slices and eaten raw. Very strict qualifications are required for cooks preparing the fugu. The problem is to avoid cutting the inner organs, which contain the toxin. Nevertheless about 75 fatal cases of intoxication from fugu are reported every year from Japan alone. Worldwide the number is about 125. Tetrodotoxin occurs not only in pufferfish, but also in other fish species (*Diodontidae, Molidae, Gobius* ssp.) and in other aquatic animals, such as starfish, crab, worms, and blue-ringed octopus, and even in some terrestric animals, such as the amphibians *Taricha torosa* and *Atelopus* ssp.

There is no doubt that tetrodotoxin is synthesized by bacteria, however, the exact species is unknown. An *Alteromonas* species and different marine species of *Pseudomonas* and *Vibrio* have been demonstrated to synthesize tetrodotoxin and the analogs epitetrodotoxin and anhydrotetrodotoxin in culture. It is thought that the bacteria enter the GI tract of the fishes via their food. The toxin is produced by the bacteria in a fish's gut and transported to the liver and the ovary after absorption. The highest concentration of the toxin occurs immediately before spawning. This gives rise to the suggestion that the accumulation process can be controlled by the fish. The toxin is most probably intended to protect the eggs from predators. It was also shown that pufferfish born in aquariums were not toxic. After releasing the fish into the natural environment, they became toxic very soon.

Tetrodotoxin blocks the sodium transport across the axoplasma membrane without influencing the opposite potassium transport. This inhibits the formation of action potentials. The specific side of action at the central nerve conduction is responsible for the extreme potency of the poison. The LD_{50} in mice after ip injection is 10 μg/kg. After oral administration, it is 322 μg/kg, still an extremely low value. If the toxin is taken up by humans via contaminated food, a tingling occurs 5 to 30 minutes later at the lips, tongue, and throat, followed by a paresthesia. The symptoms spread to the extremities. Other symptoms follow; among these are hyperthermia, hypotension, nausea, chest pain, and, for severe intoxication, muscle pain, convulsion, and respiratory arrest, which finally leads to death. Because of the lack of a specific antidote, only symptomatic therapy is possible. Gastric lavage and induction of vomiting is recommended. The oral application of charcoal is intended to bind the toxin still in the lumen and prevent its absorption. Additional treatment consists of oxygen, iv substitution of fluids, and the application of atropine. Some decades ago most of the victims died. Due to the modern intensive care about half of the patients now survive.

Terrestrial Animals

Arthropods

This phylum contains spiders and scorpions (*Arachnoidea*) and insects (*Hexapoda*). The venomous species transfer their venom by sting or bite. Almost all spiders are toxic, but only a few species, most of which are living in tropical areas are dangerous to humans. Most of the scorpions are toxic, too, whereas most insects are not toxic; however, some of the toxic species are responsible for numerous fatal cases, caused by allergic rather than toxic reactions.

Spiders (Araneae)

Around 25,000 species of spiders are known; however, only 1% have fangs (chelizera) long and strong enough to penetrate the skin and are of real danger. Some of the dangerous species live in the Mediterranean area of southern Europe, but most of the fatal cases occur in Central and South America, Africa, and Australia. Among the dangerous genera of spiders are *Atrax* ssp., *Trechona* ssp. (funnel-web spider), *Harpactirella* ssp. (trapdoor spider), *Phoneutria* ssp. (hunting spider), *Loxosceles* ssp. (brown or violin spider), *Lycosa* ssp. (wolf spider), and *Latrodectus* ssp. (widow spiders).

The black widow spider (*Latrodectus mactans*) is the best-known species of its genus and is responsible for most of the spider accidents in the European area. This and other widow spiders are found nearly globally. The name "widow spider" is related to the fact that the females kill and eat their mates after mating. Due to their bigger size (10–18 mm), only the females have fangs (chelizera) large and strong enough to penetrate the human skin when they bite. The venom of the black widow spider contains a variety of peptides, some of which are only toxic to insects. The fraction that is toxic for humans is called α-latrotoxin and consists of a peptide with a molecular weight of 130,000. The animals contain median amounts of 0.22 mg of the toxin. The LD_{50} in mice (iv) is 0.55 mg/kg. The fact that sometimes fatal cases in humans occur (3% of cases) suggests that humans are more sensitive to the toxins than rodents. The symptoms after a bite consists of local inflammation, painful swelling of lymph nodes, spontaneous muscle contractions, hyperthermia, hypertension, headache, and nausea. Fear and hallucinations sometimes occur. At particular risk are patients with diseases of the heart and circulatory system. Death is often caused by a stroke or heart arrest. The best therapy consists of the injection of calcium and *Latrodectus mactans* antivenin. Because the progression of the symptoms is usually slow, there is enough time to start with the antivenin application. One should, however, consider that antivenins sometimes cause anaphylactic reactions. It is, therefore, not recommended that it be used in the less severe cases of intoxication.

The venom of the *Loxosceles* genus causes severe necrotic action. The brown recluse (*Loxosceles reclusa*) contains approximately 70 μg of a toxic protein, composed of different fractions. The LD_{50} for guinea pigs (ip) is 0.43 mg/kg. After bites from Loxosceles ssp., extensive local necroses occur, leaving irreversible tissue damage in most cases. After systemic distribution of greater amounts of the venom, extensive hemolysis occurs resulting in considerable hematuria and, sometimes, kidney failure. After less severe envenomation, the symptoms may be restricted to fever, nausea, vomiting, jaundice, splenic enlargement, and disturbance of coagulation. Similar symptoms are also common after bites of *Lycosa* ssp. Local and systemic application of glucocorticoids are recommended for the treatment of the cytotoxic action of the venom components. Systemic effects have to be treated symptomatically. The use of antivenins is not always successful.

The most toxic spider is the black banana spider (*Phoneutria nigriventer*). Three neurotoxic peptide fractions have been isolated from the raw venom. The LD_{50} for mice is in the range of 50 μg/kg. Severe symptoms of intoxication occur almost immediately. After a bite, mice will be paralyzed almost within seconds. In humans, the first symptoms occur after 10–20 minutes and are dominated by great pain. Central symptoms are fever, heavy sweating, tachycardia, arrhythmia, nausea, vomiting, hypertonia, visual disturbance, heavy convulsions, and, finally, respiratory arrest. Immediate application of an antivenin together with symptomatic treatment is the only sufficient therapy.

Scorpions (Scorpiones)

About 75 of the 800 species of scorpions are dangerous to humans. They live in almost all tropical and subtropical areas. Most of the accidents occur in houses, especially the primitive ones, where it is easy for the scorpion to enter. The animals like to hide themselves in clothing and shoes at the night. In the morning, when people put on this clothing, the scorpions feel attacked and sting. Children are at higher

TABLE 1 Occurrence of Toxic Scorpion Species and Relative Toxicity of Their Venoms

Genus species	Occurrence	LD_{50} of venom (mg/kg mice, sc)
Androctonus spp.	North Africa, Middle East	
A. australis		6.00
A. oeneas oeneas		0.31
A. mauretanicus mauretanicus		0.32
A. crassicauda		0.40
A. amoreuxi		0.75
Buthus spp.	France, Spain, North Africa, Middle East	
B. occitanus tunetanus		0.99
B. occitanus paris		4.15
Buthotus spp.	Africa, Middle East, Central Asia	
B. judaicus		8.00
B. minax		4.25
Centruroides spp.	North America, Central America, South America	
C. limpidus		5.00
Leiurus spp.	North Africa, Middle East	
L. quiquestriatu		0.33
Parabuthus spp.	South Africa	
P. transvaalicus		4.25
Tityus spp.	Central America, South America	
T. serrulatus		1.45
T. bahiensis		9.35
T. trinitatis		2.00

risk than adults because they are less careful and have a lower body weight. Worldwide about 150,000 accidents due to scorpions are registered per year, most occur in Latin America (Mexico) and North Africa. The overall mean mortality is 2%, but among children it is 20%. Some data for medically relevant scorpions are shown in Table 1. The LD_{50} data have been derived from experiments with mice. With respect to the relative toxicity, humans usually are much more sensitive.

The scorpion's venom is composed mainly of neurotoxic peptides with a chain length of 60–70 amino acids. Biogenic amines have been observed in the venom of some species. Stings of scorpions are normally very painful. Numbness may occur after a certain time. The systemic effects consist of convulsions, tachycardia, arrhythmia, nausea, vomiting, visual disturbances, and respiratory distress. Death normally occurs from respiratory arrest. If the victim survives the first 24 hours after the sting, the prognosis is relatively good. The best results are observed after the injection of specific antivenins. It is important that sufficient amounts be given intravenously shortly after the sting (up to 30 ml). Since specific antivenins have become available, the mortality from scorpion stings has decreased dramatically, especially in children.

Insects (Hexapoda)

The insects are the most successful animal class on Earth, contributing to more than 90% of the biomass of terrestrial animals. Many of the numerous species are active or passive toxic. Although the amount of toxin in one individual is not dangerous to humans, many fatal cases occur after insect stings, such as from bees and wasps. In almost all cases, this is due to a systemic allergic reaction, resulting in an anaphylactic-shock reaction. Some species contain a lot of interesting chemically toxins that have structures more common with the plant kingdom rather than with animals. Some myriapods (*millipedes* and *centipedes*) contain repellents consisting of hydrocyanide, nitriles, phenols, quinones, and aromatic nitro compounds. Saturated and unsaturated hydrocarbons, alcohols, esters, and fatty acids were observed in the repellents of bedbugs (*Hemiptera*).

The toxin of the spanish fly (*Lytta vesicatoria*), which is actually a bug, is famous as an aphrodisiac. The active toxin is cantharidin, an inner ether of tetrahydrophtalic acid anhydride (Fig. 4). The compound ex-

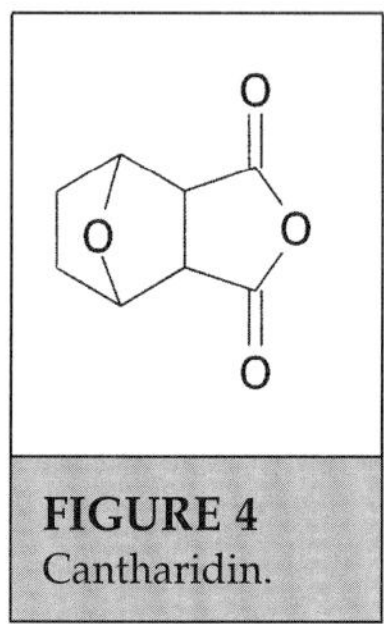

FIGURE 4
Cantharidin.

erts characteristic blisters on the skin and is a strong mucous-membrane irritant. Poisoning in humans are not rare and in most cases is due to an overdose of pulverized bugs. The stimulating action is due to an irritation of the mucous membrane of the urethra, causing spontaneous erections. After oral uptake of toxic amounts of cantharidin, strong irritation occurs in all parts of the intestinal and urogenital tract. The symptoms consist of the formation of blisters on the tongue and throat, accompanied by salivation, nausea, vomiting, and spastic contractions of musculature in the stomach and intestine. The mucous membrane of the urogenital tract gets irritated and hemorrhages. Tachycardia occurs, followed later by bradycardia. Tetanic convulsions, delirium, and coma may also occur. The lesions on the gastric and intestinal epithelium may lead to intraluminal accumulation of fluid followed by a hypovolemic shock. The lethal dose of pulverized spanish flies for an adult is several grams; however, 10 mg of pure cantharidin may be lethal. A case has been reported in which a patient survived 75 mg. In absence of a specific antidote the therapy is symptomatic.

Some insects take up toxic compounds from plants and accumulate it in their bodies. Sometimes the uptake occurs in the larval stage and persists during the metamorphosis. In these cases the adult insects contain the toxins without consuming the toxic plants. This is observed in some species of butterflies, which consume plant leaves in the larval and nectar in the adult stage. Toxic compounds are often found in plant leaves but are rare in plant nectar. The toxins protect the insects against predators. Other insects accumulating toxic plant constituents are bed bugs and some bug species. Their toxic food plants are oleander (cardiac glycosides), *Aristolochia clematitis* (aristolochic acid), and *Senecio* ssp. (unsaturated pyrrolizidine alkaloids).

Hymenoptera

In this genus are ants, bees, wasps, and hornets. The insects have a special venomous apparatus, consisting of a venom gland and an injecting tool, the sting. Stings by bees and wasps can happen to almost everyone once in his or her life. Although the stings are often very painful, they are normally harmless, unless hundreds occur at the same time. Nevertheless, there are no other animals, scorpions and snakes included, that are responsible for so many fatal cases. The reason is that many people develop an allergy to the venom after the first event. The allergic reaction gets worse after every sting and it may result in an anaphylactic-shock reaction. Patients with a known history of an allergy to the stings of bees or wasps should be extremely careful and carry a kit in their pockets containing an antihistamine and epinephrine, in case of a sting from these insects.

The venom of Hymenoptera contains biogenic amines, kinines, peptides, and enzymes, such as phospholipases and hyaluronidase. The amines are responsible for the pain reaction, whereas the enzymes result in a local destruction of tissue connection. Kinines are found only in the venom of wasps and hornets and are responsible for a decrease of the blood pressure.

The venom of bees is well investigated and the structure of the toxic peptides is known. Apamin, making up 2% of the dry weight, consists of 18 amino acids. It acts at the central nervous system (CNS), causing a hypermotility. With 50% of dry weight, mellitin is the main constituent of bee venom. It is a strong basic peptide (pK_a 10) with 26 amino acids. Interestingly the peptide lacks sulfur containing (Cys, Met), aromatic (Phe, Tyr), and heterocyclic (His) amino acids. It acts as a strong detergent and has, therefore, a hemolytic activity. Additionally the toxin damages mast cells and platelets. Mellitin also contracts the smooth muscles. Small doses stimulate the heart, which is inhibited by high doses. The LD_{50} in mice after iv injection is 3.5 mg/kg. The third peptide in bee venom is the mast cell degranulating peptid (MCDR). It contains 22 amino acids and makes up 2% of the bee venom. The LD_{50} (in mice, iv) is 40 mg/kg. This peptid destroys mast cells, which release inflammatory agents, such as histamine, serotonine, and kinines.

Ants (Formicidae)

In this family are biting and stinging representatives. The latter inject their venom, similar to bees and wasps. Ants consist of approximately 6000 species, most of which are harmless to humans. Fire ants (*Solenopsis*), which are endemic in the southern parts of the United States are dangerous. The reaction after a sting may vary from a weak skin rash to a severe dermatitis, accompanied by local inflammation and

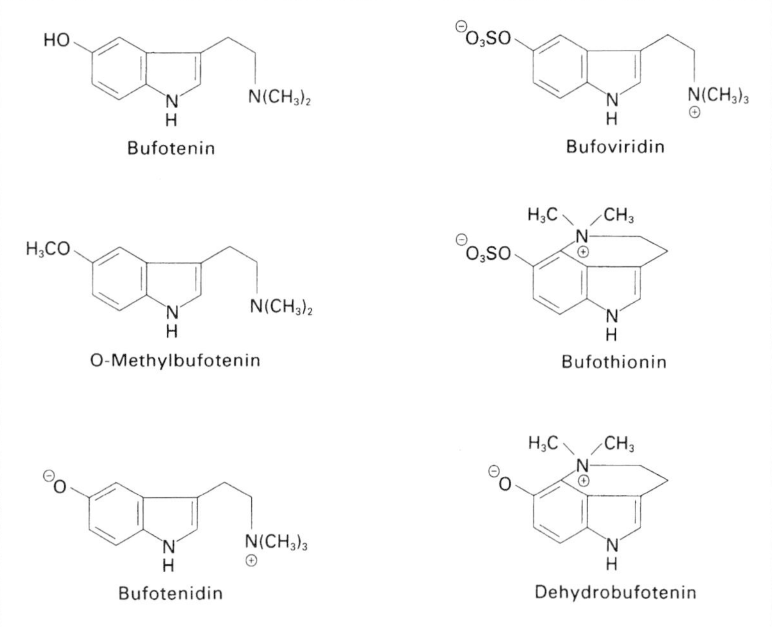

FIGURE 5 Indol derivatives of toads.

necrosis. Anaphylactic reactions may occur after repeated stings. Different toxic piperidine derivatives have been isolated from the venom of fire ants.

Amphibia

Most amphibians are classifiable as toxic. Their toxins are thought to protect their hosts from predators and from skin contamination from microorganisms. The toxins are produced in special skin glands. They are impressive because of their diversity in interesting chemical structures and biological actions. Some amphibians (*Dendrobatidae*) produce the most potent toxins occurring in animals.

Indol derivatives

The skin of some toad species (Bufonidae) contains biogenic amines, related to serotonin. Among these are bufotenin (*N*, *N*-dimethyl serotonin) and its methyl ether. Other compounds are bufotenidine, bufoviridine, and the tricyclic derivatives bufothionine and dehydrobufotenine (Fig. 5).

N-alkylated indol derivatives have a high affinity to serotoninergic (5-HT2-) receptors in the CNS. This is the reason for their psychodelic action. The compounds exert an LSD-like action, with hallucinations and spectral visions. *O*-Methylbufotenin is most active in this regard, with an effective dose of 50 μg/kg. Recently it has been shown that the N-methylation of serotonin takes place in the CNS of mammals under the control of the enzyme indolethylamin-*N*-methyltransferase. It is suggested that the resulting bufotenin plays a role in certain psychotic diseases, such as schizophrenia.

The hallucinogenic action of extracts prepared from toads was known long ago and many witch recipes are based on it. An example is given in the following two text phrases from William Shakespeare's *Macbeth*.

> Third Act:
> . . . Round about the cauldron go; In the poison'd entrails throw. Toad, that under cold stone Days and nights has thirty-one Swelter'd venom sleeping got, Boil thou first i' the charmed pot.
>
> Fifth Act:
> . . . The juice of toad, the oil of adder. Those will make the younker madder.

Obviously it was well known at that time that the slime of toads is rich in compounds acting on the brain.

The toxins of toads are not dangerous to humans under normal circumstances because the penetration through the skin is low after touching the animals. Rodents are less sensitive than humans after systemic application of the toxins. The lethal doses of bufotenin and 5-methylbufotenin in mice (ip) are 290 mg/kg and 115 mg/kg, respectively. Much less sensitive are the amphibians themselves. Frogs tolerate up to 2500 mg/kg without any symptoms, whereas doses of 1 mg/kg are lethal to sheep. Death occurs after a series of tremors and convulsions and, finally, respiratory arrest.

Steroids

The chemical structure of the steroid-like toad toxins is related to cardiac glycosides present in some plant species (e.g., oleander and purple foxglove). The toxins are synthesized in the parotis glands and excreted with the saliva. Representatives of genins (bufotaline) and glycosides (bufotoxin) are shown in Fig. 6. The biological action is mainly targeted on the heart and consists of an inhibition of Na^+K^+-ATPase, resulting in a negatively chronotropic and inotropic action. High doses cause arrest. Beside the action on the heart, the toxins act as local anesthetics. The lethal doses are relatively independent of the species and vary between 200–1000 μg/kg.

An interesting group of steroids with a ring system consisting of seven carbon atoms occurs in some species of salamanders. The benefit for the animals is most likely related to its antibiotic action. A pronounced inhibition of the growth of bacteria and fungi was demonstrated. The compounds are, however, also toxic to higher organisms. The LD_{50} values for most rodents is below several mg/kg. The action is targeted to the CNS. Muscle contractions and arrest of breathing occur after application of the toxins.

Alkaloids

The most toxic amphibians live in the rain forest of Central and South America and belong to the families Dendrobatidae and Phyllobatidae. They are small, very colorful frogs, climbing on branches (Greek *dendros*) or leaves (Greek *phyllos*), where they wait for insects. Because of the pretty colors, which function as a warning signal to their possible predators, they are also called as color frogs; however, they are better known as poison dart frogs, because the Indians of Colombia and Panama use the toxins on hunting darts. The Choco imitate the whistling of the frogs, which attracts the animals. To protect the skin of their palms from the extremely toxic slime, they cover them with leaves before catching the frogs. The animals are then speared on pointed sticks and put near a fire. This extreme stress causes the frogs to excrete lots of their toxin. The toxic slime is spread on the darts by direct contact with the frog's skin. About 50 darts can be toxified by a single frog. The most toxic species (*Phyllobates terribilis*) contains enough poison to kill 20,000 mice or 10 humans.

The toxins belong to the alkaloids and are divided into batrachotoxins (from *Phyllobates aurotaenia*), pumiliotoxins (from *Dendrobates pumilio*), and histrionicotoxins (from *Dendrobates histrionicus*) (Fig. 8). All of these are strong nerve and muscle toxins. Batrachotoxin is among the most potent natural toxins (LD_{50} in mice, sc, 2 μg/kg) known so far. The action is related to an inhibition of the sodium channel of nerve and muscle cells, which is unable to collapse after an action potential occurred. This will result in a permanent depolarization. The action is opposite to that of tetrodotoxin, which inhibits the opening of the sodium channel.

Pumiliotoxin B causes the liberation of Ca^{2+} from intracellular reservoirs of muscle cells and inhibits the reabsorbtion into the endoplasmatic reticulum. This causes long-acting muscular contractions. The spasmogenic action is promoted by an increase of the Ca^{2+} influx into nerve cells, followed by an increase in the liberation of neurotransmitters. Pumiliotoxin C, gephyrotoxin, and the histrionicotoxins inhibit the transmembraneous flux of Na^+ and K^+, initiated by aceteylcholine at the neuromuscular endplate, resulting in a paralysis of the skeletal muscles.

Peptides

The skins of most amphibian species contain a variety of peptides related to biogenic peptides. Among these are physalein, caerulein, and ranatensin. Like other biogenic peptides, present in mammals, such as bradykinin, the compounds contract smooth muscles, decrease the blood pressure, and increase the permeability of capillary walls.

Reptiles

Lizards

Two poisonous species of lizards live in the southern part of the United States and in northern Mexico, *Heloderma suspectum* and *Heloderma horridum*. The animals inject their venom during a bite, which mainly consists of serotonin and a variety of enzymes. Among these are hyaluronidase, phospholipase A, aminooxidase, and proteases. The LD_{50} (in mice, ip) of the raw toxin is 1.4 mg/kg. Fatal cases are very rare. In most cases the victims recover spontaneously a few days to 2 weeks later. If large amounts of venom are injected, the blood pressure and the circulating fluid may decrease, resulting in a responding tachycardia. Death may result from a lack in ventricular contractility. Specific antivenins are not available.

Snakes

Human beings have been fascinated by snakes throughout time, due to the deadly hazard associated

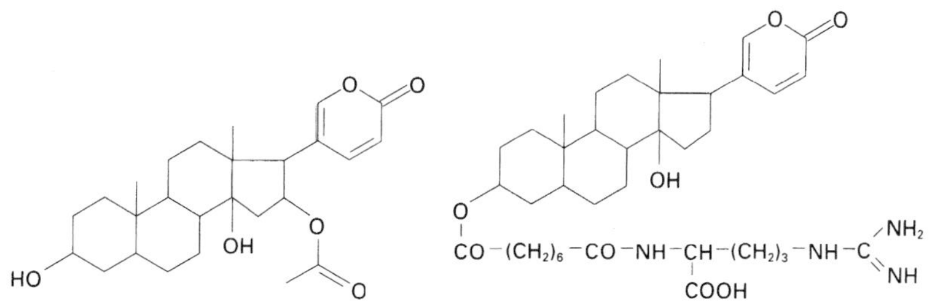

FIGURE 6 Cardiac glycosides from the parotis glands of toads.

with many snake species. Among the 3500 species there are only 375 (i.e., 10%) that are venomous. These snakes are subdivided into four classes.

1. *Elapidae* (e.g., coral snakes, kraits, mambas, and cobras).
2. *Viperidae* (e.g., vipers).
3. *Crotalidae* (e.g., rattlesnakes).
4. *Hydrophiidae* (e.g., seasnakes).

Venomous snakes contain a venom apparatus consisting of venom glands, which are comparable to the parotis glands, and teeth that function like injection needles. Approximately 1.7 million accidents with venomous snakes occur every year worldwide and 40,000 (2.35%) end with the death of the victim. The mortality rate is dependent on the snake species.

European viper (*Vipera berus*)	1%
Indian cobra (*Naja naja*)	32%
Black mamba (*Dendroaspis polylepis*)	≈100%

An overview about the toxicity of snake venoms is given in Table 2. The ratio of the injected amount of venom during one bite and the toxic potential of the venom (the lethality coefficient of a bite) is the same for the Indian cobra and black mamba; however, the lethality observed is different. This is due to the fact that mambas bite preferentially at the head and neck whereas cobras prefer the legs and arms. In the latter case it is possible to prevent the distribution of the venom by tying up the affected extremity. With respect to the lethality coefficient, bites from European adders should not be lethal to humans at all. The few lethal events reported may be due to an unfortunate direct application of venom into a greater blood vessel or an extreme sensitivity of the victim. Repeated bites may also cause in an anaphylactic-shock reaction.

The composition of snake venom is rather complicated. The different components often have a synergistic action. The actually toxic compounds are peptides with a chain length of 60–70 amino acids. The peptides contain numerous disulfide bridges, responsible for the formation of a characteristic three-dimensional structure. Like at all other higher venomous animals, the toxic action of the peptides is directed preferentially against the central and peripheral nerve system. This will result in a fast paralysis of the prey or attacker.

The toxins of *Elapids* and *Hydrophiids* are preferentially directed against acetylcholine receptors at postsynaptic membranes and neuromuscular endplate. β-Bungarotoxin (*Bungarus multicinctus*) acts at the presynaptic membrane, resulting in a gradual depletion

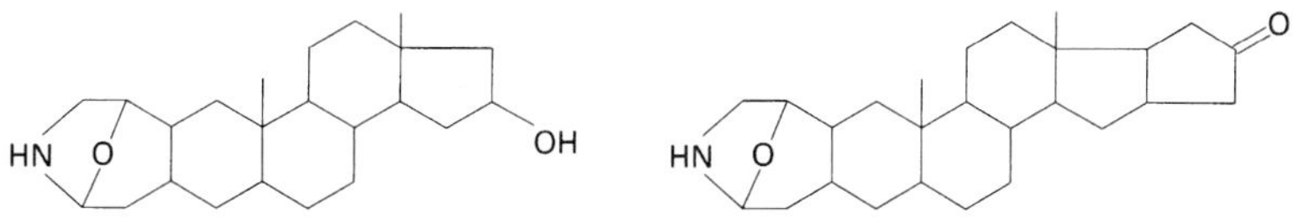

FIGURE 7 Toxins from salamander species (e.g., *Salamandra maculosa*).

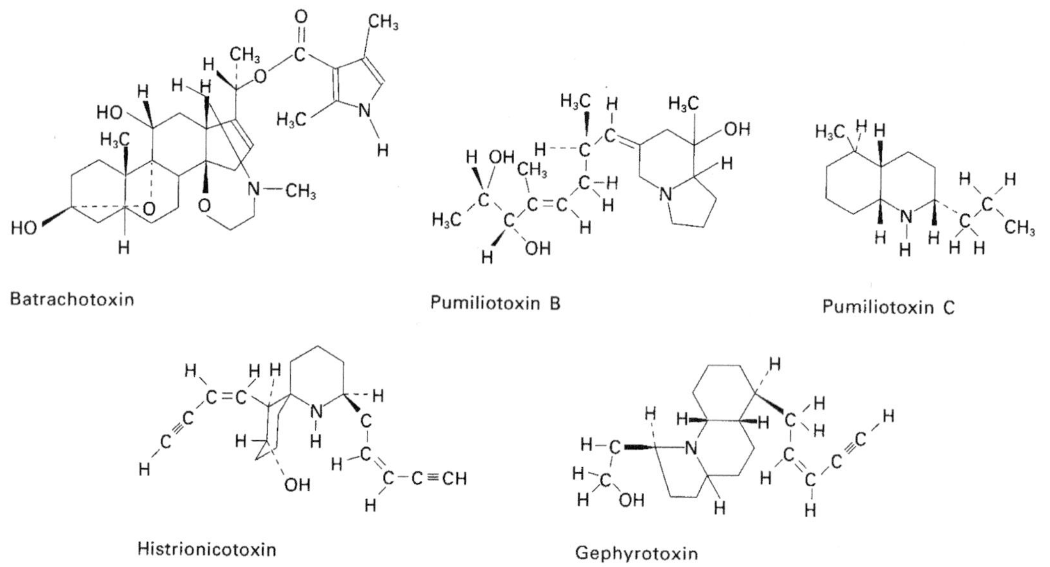

FIGURE 8 Toxins of Dendrobatidae and Phyllobatidae.

of acetylcholine. The toxins of some viper species result in cardiovascular shock. It is suggested that their site of action is located in the medulla oblongata. These toxins are different from the others also in that their chain lengths are shorter (30–40 amino acids). A variety of enzymes occurring in snake venom promote the distribution of the toxic peptides by disintegrating the tissue at the bite side.

About 25 different enzymes have been isolated from snake venom so far. Their catalytic action is categorized into four groups (Table 3).

Proteolytic enzymes catalyze the hydrolysis of proteins. They are mainly distributed in crotalids and responsible for the tissue necrosis reactions often observed after rattlesnake bites. Fewer of these enzymes are present in *Viperides* and the venom of *Elapids* and

TABLE 2 Minimal Lethal Dose of Some Snake Venoms[a]

Species	Ejected amount of venom/bite	Lethal dose for humans
Elapidae		
Naja naja (Indian cobra)	210 mg	15 mg
Naja bungarus (King cobra)	100 mg	12 mg
Bungarus candidus (Malayan krait)	5 mg	1 mg
Bungarus caeruleus (Indian krait)	10 mg	6 mg
Dendroaspis polylepis (Black mamba)	1000 mg	120 mg
Viperidae		
Vipera russeli (Russel's viper)	70 mg	42 mg
Vipera carinatus	12 mg	5 mg
Vipera berus (European viper)	10 mg	75 mg
Crotalidae		
Bothrops neuwiedii (Urutu)	200 mg	200 mg
Trimeresurus gramineus	14 mg	100 mg

[a]According to Habermehl (1994).

TABLE 3 Enzymes Occurring in Snake Venom

Enzyme	Occurrence
Proteolytic enzymes	
Proteinases	*Crotalidae, Viperidae*
Proteases	*Crotalidae, Viperidae*
Peptidases	*Crotalidae, Viperidae*
Endopeptidases	*Crotalidae, Viperidae*
Argininesterhydrolase	*Crotalidae, Viperidae, Hydrophiidae*
Nucleotidases	
Phosphomonoesterase	All venomous snakes (except *Colubrides*)
Phosphodiesterase	All venomous snakes
5′-Nucleotidase	All venomous snakes
NAD-Nucleotidase	All venomous snakes
DNase	All venomous snakes
RNase	Rare (exp. *Naja oxiana*)
Tissue-disintegrating enzymes	
Collagenase	*Crotalidae, Viperadae*
Hyaluronidase	All venomous snakes
Phospholipasen	All venomous snakes
Other enzymes	
Acetylcholinesterase	*Elapidae, Viperidae*
Lactatdehydrogenase	*Elapidae*
L-Aminosäureoxidase	All venomous snakes
Thrombin-like enzymes	*Crotalidae, Viperidae*

Hydrophiids is almost free of it. Especially after bites of seasnakes, no necrotic reactions are observed.

Nucleotide-degrading enzymes are present in almost all snake venoms. They destroy fundamental energy-carrying molecules (ATP), second messengers (cAMP), and redox-coenzymes (NAD, NADH, NADP, NADPH). These enzymes interfere, therefore, with the most fundamental biochemical processes, which makes them strongly cytotoxic. Enzymes, such as acetylcholinesterase, L-aminoacidoxidase, or lactatdehydrogenase, occur in some snake venoms.

Some enzymes act on the connective tissue. Among these are collagenase and hyaluronidase, which cause the tissue next to the bite side to loosen. Phospholipases exert a destructive action on cell membranes. This enables cytotoxic enzymes to enter the cells. The destruction of red blood cells by these enzymes causes a severe hemolysis. The venom of *Viperidae* and *Crotalidae* contains thrombin-like enzymes, causing a clotting of plasma or pure fibrinogen solution *in vitro*.

The clinical course of a snake bite is dependent on a number of variables, such as the age, body weight, and constitution of the victim, as well as the toxicity and size of the snake. The location of the bite is also important. Systemic effects, such as disturbances of the cardiovascular system or CNS, will occur almost immediately if the bite hits a blood vessel. Severe necrosis accompanied by great pain often occurs after bites of *Crotalidae* and *Viperidae*. If a patient has a history of other snake bites, an anaphylactic-shock reaction may occur.

Many patients survive snake bites today because of the availability of specific antivenins. It is, however, most important that not too much time be lost before the beginning of treatment. If the symptoms of the intoxication occur soon, compression of the affected extremity should be initiated if possible. It is important that the compression affects only the veins and lymph drains and not the arteries. The incision of the bite location is not recommended. This will cause lengthy bleeding and promote the invasion of the venom into the bloodstream. The application of a sedative may be useful to decrease the patient's irritation. Peripheral or central analgesics should be given if great pain is present. Because of the possibility of allergic reactions, the infusion of an antivenin should only be performed in serious cases of envenomation (25% of all snake bites). Anaphylactic-shock reactions with fatal outcomes occur in approximately 0.3% of the cases.

The amount of the antivenin is dependent on the amount of the venom injected by the snake and not on the body weight of the patient. It may vary between 10–300 ml. Monovalent as well as polyvalent antivenins are available. If possible, a monovalent antivenin should be used.

TOXINS OF PROTOZOA AND ALGAE

Marine phytoplankton contain numerous species that produce strong toxins. Most belong to the dinoflagellates. Toxins are mainly observed in the genus *Protogonyaulax, Gonyaulax, Pyrodinium, Gambierdiscus, Gymnodinium,* and *Ptychodiscus*. At certain times of the year these algae proliferate enormously ("red tide"). This may result in a considerable loss of the endemic fish fauna. Human poisoning may occur via the food chain from mollusks to shrimps to fish.

Saxitoxin

Dinoflagellates, such as *Gonyaulax tamarensis, Gonyaulax catenella, Gonyaulax excavata, Ptychodiscus (Gymnodinium) breve,* and *Ptychodiscus veneficum*, contain the extraordinarily toxic compound saxitoxin (Fig. 9). This compound is possibly synthesized by bacteria, living in symbiosis with the dinoflagellates. The phy-

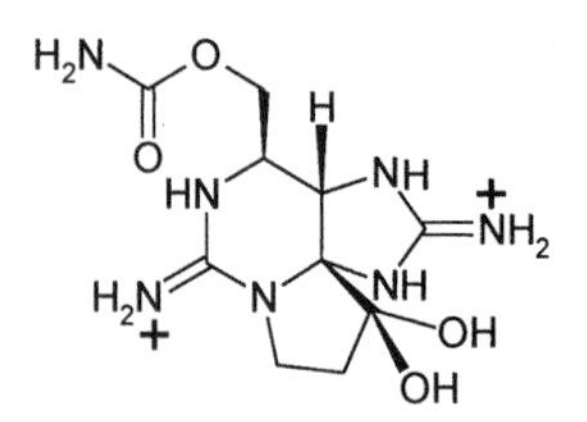

Saxitoxin

FIGURE 9 Saxitoxin is often involved in cases of paralytic shell fish poisoning.

toplankton is then trapped by mussels, which concentrate the toxin. The mussels themselves are not sensitive to the toxic action of the poison. At certain seasons, mainly in the summer, poisoning of humans occurs after they consume the mussels. The disease is known as paralytic shellfish poisoning. The symptoms begin with a prickling of the tongue and lips, followed by a paralysis of the musculature in the mouth. Later the muscle paralysis progresses all over the body. When the paralysis affects the diaphragm, death occurs from suffocation.

The mechanism of the toxicity of saxitoxin is similar to tetrodotoxin. Both compounds are sodium-channel blockers. They inhibit the transmission of excitation signals from pre- to post-synaptic neurons and to muscle cells. The LD_{50} for mice (i.p.) is 10 μg/kg. The lethal dose for humans is approximately 1 mg. This amount may be eventually present in only a few mussels. In the United States and Canada, the limit value is 80 μg/100 g mussel meat. The treatment of saxitonin poisoning consists of gastric lavage and symptomatic treatment, especially artificial respiration.

Brevetoxins

In the Gulf of Mexico a phenomenon occurs at certain times, called "red tide". It is caused by a massive proliferation of the dinoflagellate *Ptychodiscus (Gymnodinium) breve* and accompanied by the death of thousands or millions of fishes. *Ptychodiscus* contains a variety of toxins, which are different from saxitoxin with respect to their chemical structure as well as toxic action. The brevetoxins (Fig. 10) consist of an unusual structure of linearly linked polycyclic ethers. The toxins bind to the lipophilic domain of the sodium channel of the synapses and lead to depolariza-

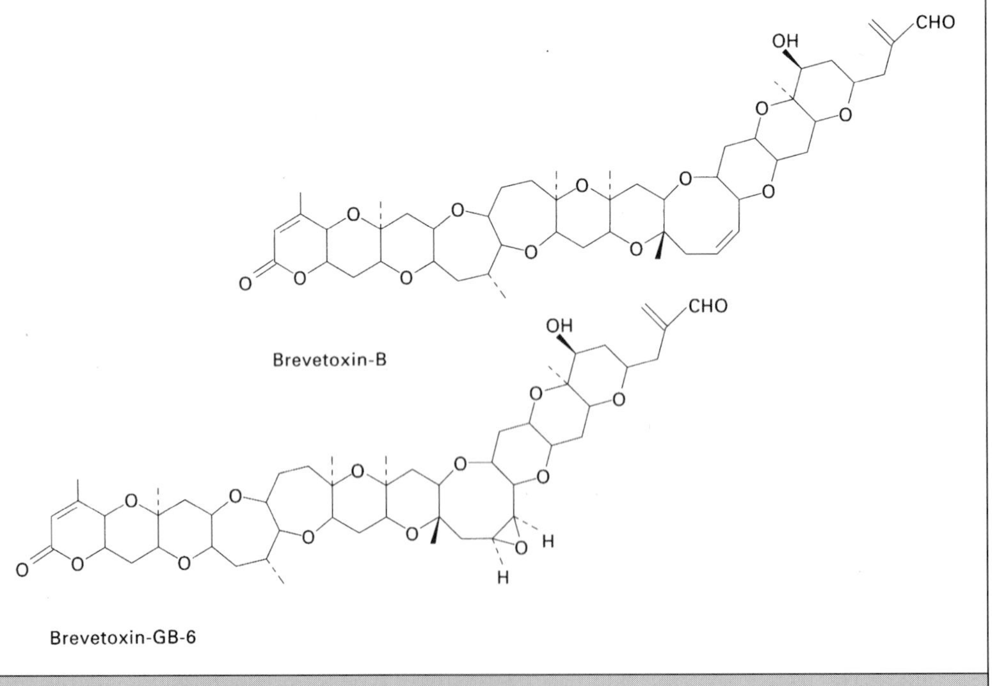

Brevetoxin-B

Brevetoxin-GB-6

FIGURE 10 Brevetoxins consist of a mixture of related compounds. Shown are brevetoxin B and its epoxide (brevetoxin-GB-6).

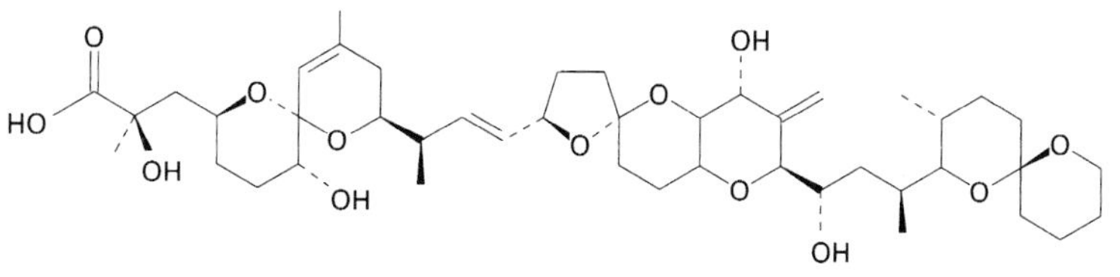

FIGURE 11 Ocadaic acid.

tion. The resulting liberation of acetylcholine at the neuromuscular endplate causes fascicular twitching. If the depolarization persists, the nerves will lose their irritability completely and paralysis occurs. The increased liberation of noradrenalin at the heart causes ventricular arrhythmia and fibrillation. The action of tetrodotoxin and local anesthetics are antagonistic to the depolarizing action of brevetoxin. Related to brevetoxin are the dinophysistoxins and ocadaic acid (Fig. 11), which also occur in dinoflagellates.

Cigateratoxin

Poisonings from edible fishes, such as barracudas, snappers, and sharks, occur in some tropical marine areas. The toxin responsible for these cases is called ciguateratoxin and is found in the dinoflagellate (*Gambierdiscus toxicus*), living epiphytically on macrophytic algae in reef areas. The algae are taken up by herbivorous fishes, which are then consumed by predatory fishes. The poison accumulates via the food chain and is stored in the liver and gonads of these fishes. Considerable amounts of the toxin may, however, also be present in the muscular tissue and cause poisoning after consuming the fishes.

The lethal dose of ciguateratoxin is extremely low (in mice, ip, 45 ng/kg). The structure of the long stretched molecule, which is related to some part to ocadaic acid, is shown in Fig. 12. The action is directed to the sodium channel and consists of an increase of the permeability of Na^+. This will cause excitatory reactions. The action of ciguateratoxin is antagonistic to tetrodotoxin and saxitoxin, both of which inhibit the sodium channel.

The symptoms of ciguatera poisoning begin with irritations of the mucous membranes in the mouth and throat, followed by a generalized weakness, diarrhea, rigor, fever, motion, insomnia, and shortness of breath. If lethal doses are taken up, death occurs by arrest of breathing. After the uptake of sublethal doses, the symptoms may persist for months. In the absence of any causal therapy, the treatment has to be symptomatic. The infusion of mannitol (1g/kg in 45 minutes) may be advantageous. The protective mechanism is possibly due to an inhibition of the formation of edemas in the neuronal tissue.

Another toxin, maitotoxin, often occurs concomitantly with ciguateratoxin. In contrast to ciguateratoxin the action of maitotoxin is directed to the calcium channel. The compound increases the permeability of nerve and muscle cells for Ca^{2+}, resulting in a calcium overload of these cells. This causes the liberation of neurotransmitters in the nerve cells and lead to long-acting muscle contractions and heart arrhythmia.

MYCOTOXINS

The fungi are divided into lower (monocellular) fungi (*Ascomycetae*) and higher (multicellular) fungi (*Basidiomycetae*). About 300,000 species have been characterized so far. Most produce a large spectrum of secondary metabolites. Among these are also many toxic compounds.

Toxins from *Ascomycetae*

Many lower fungi produce toxic metabolites that are distributed in the environment, most probably to inhibit the growth of other microorganisms. Poisoning by mycotoxins is a common phenomenon, because molds of the genus *Aspergillus*, *Penicillium*, and *Fusarium* often contaminate food. In industrial nations, such food will normally go to waste. In many developing countries, however, where food is scarce, people will eat it regardless of mold contamination. The growth of molds is supported in such countries by the often hot and humid climate.

The actions of mycotoxins vary from weak irritation to severe damage. Some of the compounds are even teratogenicic and carcinogenic. A summary of the most important mycotoxins is given in Table 4.

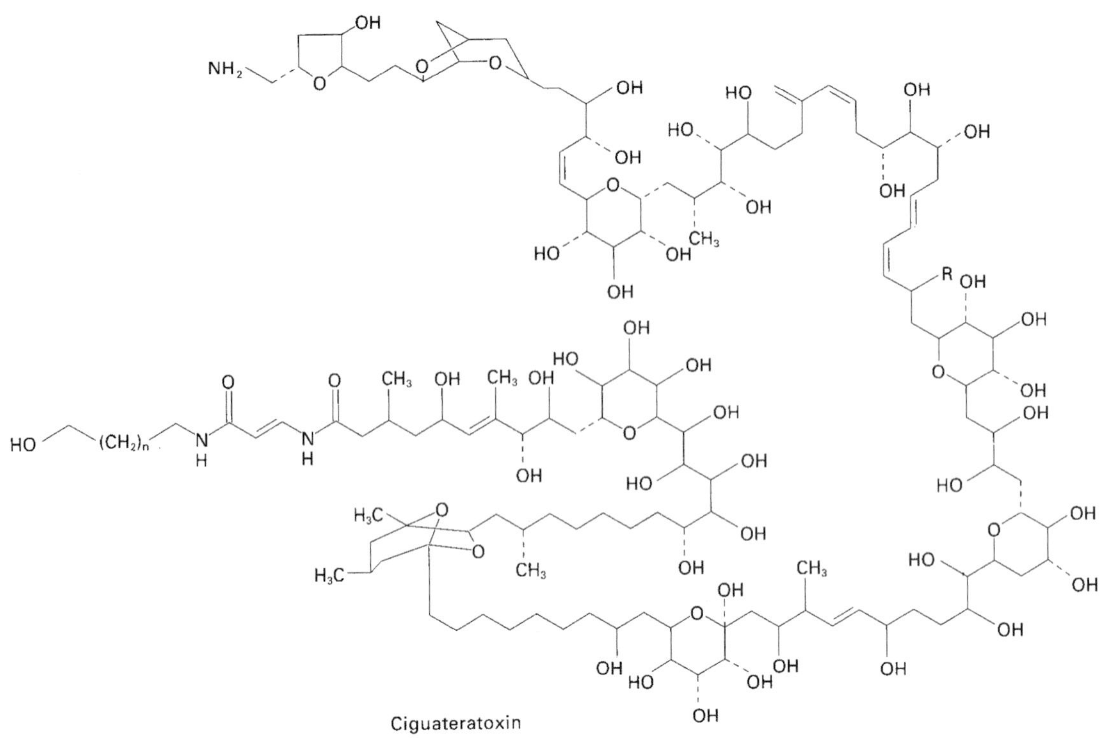

Ciguateratoxin

FIGURE 12 Ciguateratoxin. The toxin is present in marine animals. Among these are also a variety of edible fishes, such as barracudas and groupers.

The presentation of the mycotoxins in the following will be in botanical order, although there are many overlaps in compounds.

Aspergillus Species

Aflatoxins

The fungi *Aspergillus flavus, Aspergillus parasiticus,* and *Aspergillus oryzae* synthesize a variety of related mycotoxins known as aflatoxins (Fig. 13). The fungi often contaminate food, such as peanuts, wheat, rice, corn, and soybeans. The aflatoxins M_1 and M_2 occur also in the milk of cattle and sheep, if the animals' food is contaminated with the fungi. A limit value for the aflatoxin concentration in many countries is 50 ng/liter. Endemic poisoning from aflatoxins occurs in animals as well as in humans. The target organ of most aflatoxins is the liver. The aflatoxins B_1, G_1, and M_1 are converted under the catalytic action of cytochrome P450 to highly reactive epoxides, which then form covalent adducts with nucleophilic molecules of the liver cells. AFB_1 forms C7 adducts with the guanine moieties of DNA and RNA. The saturated aflatoxins G_2 and M_2 are less toxic and not carcinogenic. AFB_2 is, however, partially converted in the liver to the unsaturated and highly toxic AFB_1.

After the uptake of high doses of aflatoxins, liver necrosis occur and the victim may die from liver failure. Damage to the kidney tubules occur sometimes. The lethal dose for humans is approximately 1–10 mg/kg AFB_1. The chronic uptake of smaller doses may cause liver cirrhosis or liver tumors. The daily amount of AFB_1 causing liver cirrhosis in children is 9–18 μg. The sources of the toxin are often contaminated peanuts. Liver damage was also observed in infants whose lactating mothers consumed aflatoxin-contaminated food. AFB_1 is the most potent hepatocarcinogen in rats. Sufficient evidence of the hepatocarcinogenic action in humans was derived from epidemiological studies. A correlation was observed between the excretion of aflatoxins in the urine and the incidence of hepatocarcinomas (HCC) (Fig. 14). Very high incidences of HCC occur in some African countries, such as Mozambique, Swaziland, Kenya, and Uganda, where the aflatoxin contamination of the food is high.

TABLE 4 Mycotoxins

Toxin	Fungi	LD_{50}	Target organ
Aflatoxin B_1	*A. flavus,*	1.7 mg/kg (rat, po)	Hepatotoxic, Nephrotoxic
Aflatoxin B_2	*A. parasiticus,*	84.8 μg/50g (duck, 1 day old, po)	
Aflatoxin G_1	*A. oryzae,*	39.2 μg/50g (duck, 1 day old, po)	Hepatocancerogenic
Aflatoxin G_2	*P. puperulum*	172.5 μg/50g (duck, 1 day old, po)	
Aflatoxin M_1	*A. flavus*	16.6 μg/duck (duck, 1 day old, po)	Hepatotoxic, hepatocancerogenic
Aflatoxin M_2		62 μg/duck (duck, 1 day old, po)	
Aspertoxin	*A. flavus, A. versicolor*	0.7 μg/egg (duck)	Hepatotoxic, hepatocancerogenic
Citreoviridin	*P. citreo-viride*	3.6 mg/kg (rat, sc)	Neurotoxic
Citrinin	*P. citrinum*	67 mg/kg (rat, sc)	Hepatotoxic, nephrotoxic
Cyclochlorotin	*P. islandicum*	470 μg/kg (mice, sc)	Respiration and circulation toxin, hepatotoxic
Cytochalasin A	*Helminthosporium dematioideum*		Damage of cytosceleton, teratogenic
Cytochalasin B			
Cytochalasin C	*Metarrhizium anisopliae*		
Cytochalasin D	*Zygosporium mansonii*	1.9 mg/kg (mice, ip)	
Cytochalasin E	*A. clavatus*	2.6 mg/kg (rat, ip)	
Islanditoxin	*P. islandicum*	338 μg/kg (mice, iv)	Hepatotoxic, hepatocancerogenic
Luteoskyrin		145 mg/kg (mice, ip)	Hepatotoxic, hepatocancerogenic
Maltoryzin	*A. oryzae*	3 mg/kg (mice, ip)	Hepatotoxic, nephrotoxic, neurotoxic
Moniliformin	*Fusarium ssp.*	29 mg/kg (mice, ip)	Local irritatant
Ochratoxin A	*A. ochraceus*	20 mg/kg (rat, po)	Nephrotoxic
Patulin	*Penicillium ssp.*	30 mg/kg (rat, po)	Local irritant
Penicillic acid	*Penicillium ssp.*	100 mg/kg (mice, po)	Hepatotoxic, cytotoxic
Roquefortin	*P. roqueforti*	18 mg/kg (mice, ip)	Neurotoxic
Rubratoxin A	*P. rubrum*	6.6 mg/kg (mice, ip)	Local irritant, mutagenic Teratogenic
Rubratoxin B	*P. rubrum*	3 mg/kg (mice, ip)	Hepatotoxic
Sterigmatocystin	*A. nidulans, A. versicolor*	800 mg/kg (mice, po)	Hepatotoxic, hepatocancerogenic
Trichothecenes	*Fusarium ssp.*		Local irritant, hematotoxic, neurotoxic

Sterigmatocystin

Sterigmatocystin is structurally related to the aflatoxins (Fig. 15), and occurs in *Aspergillus versicolor, Aspergillus nidulans,* and *Aspergillus bipolaris,* which, together with aflatoxin-producing fungi, frequently contaminate food. Although the toxic potency of sterigmatocystin is less than the aflatoxins, the former compound is usually present in much higher concentrations. The mode of action is similar to that of the aflatoxins. The compound damages mainly the liver and, additionally, the kidney and the myocardium. Liver tumors in rats were observed after long-term oral treatment with the compound. The metabolic conversion (hydroxylation) of sterigmatocystin leads to aspertoxin (Fig. 15), which is also toxic.

Patulin

The mold species *Aspergillus clavatus, Aspergillus giganteus, Penicillium patulinum, Penicillium expansum,* and *Penicillium urticae* produce a toxin called patulin (Fig. 16). It was observed in flour, meat, and particularly in apple juice. The toxin has a high affinity to SH groups and damages cell membranes especially. Membrane-bound ATPases are inhibited. Skin contact results in local irritation. Mucous membrane irritation, nausea, vomiting, and diarrhea occur after oral consumption of contaminated food. Edemas and hemorrhages of the lung and brain were observed after oral application of patulin in experimental animals. The amounts usually occuring in human food is not sufficient to cause these symptoms.

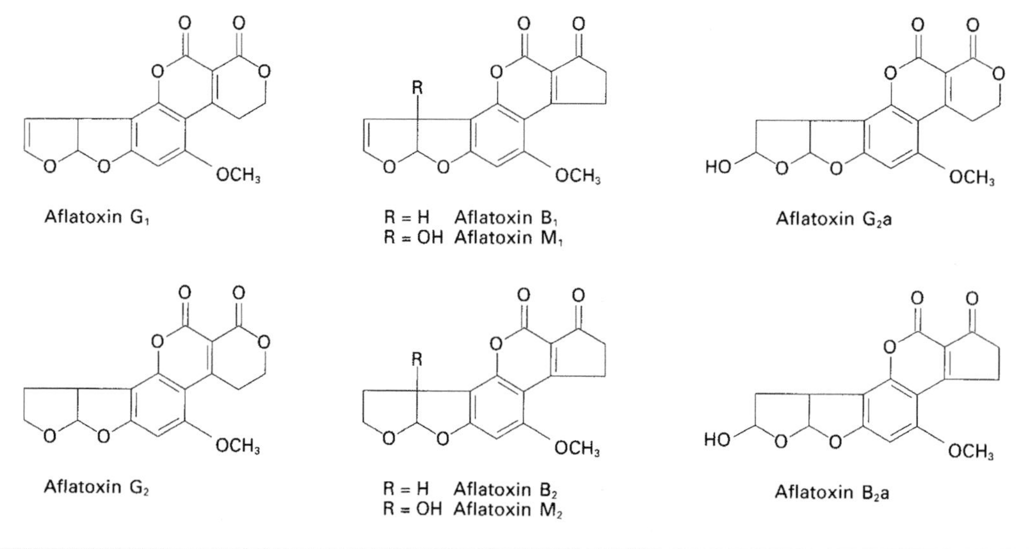

Aflatoxin G_1

R = H Aflatoxin B_1
R = OH Aflatoxin M_1

Aflatoxin G_2a

Aflatoxin G_2

R = H Aflatoxin B_2
R = OH Aflatoxin M_2

Aflatoxin B_2a

FIGURE 13 Structure of aflatoxins. Aflatoxins belong to the most potent carcinogens known. They occur in some *Aspergillus* species, which often contaminate the food of humans and livestock.

A carcinogenic action of patulin could not be demonstrated in laboratory animal after either oral or intraperitoneal application. Sarcomas, observed after s.c. injection of patulin in rats, were more the result of a local irritation rather than a carcinogenic action of the compound. A teratogenic action was observed only in chicken embryos but not in mammals. However, chromosomal aberrations in the bone marrow were observed in Chinese hamsters after treatment with patulin.

Ochratoxin A

Aspergillus ochraceus frequently contaminates cereals, peanuts, and vegetables. The mold synthesizes a variety of structurally related toxins, called ochratoxins. Especially toxic is the chlorine-containing ochratoxin A (Fig. 17). The phenylalanyl moiety of the molecule binds to the enzyme phenylalanyl-*t*-RNA-synthetase, which results in an inhibition of the protein synthesis. This mechanism is most probably responsible for the observed teratogenic action of the compound in mice. Malformations occurred mainly in the CNS. The application of sublethal doses in young chickens leads to damage of the hematopoietic system. Immunosupressive effects were also observed in mice after i.p. application of 10μg/kg ochratoxin A.

The organs especially affected by ochratoxin are the kidneys. Necrosis occurs in the proximal tubules, resulting in severe inhibition of the kidney function, finally leading to anuria. An endemic nephropathia observed in humans and livestock living in some Mediterranian countries (e.g., Bosnia and Croatia) correlated with the ochratoxin A content of the food. Considerable amounts of the toxin were also observed in the meat of pigs.

Ochratoxin A is not genotoxic in *Salmonella* or yeast. However, tumors (adenomas) were observed in the livers and kidneys of mice fed a diet containing 40 ppm of the toxin. In rats only a few kidney but no liver tumors were observed.

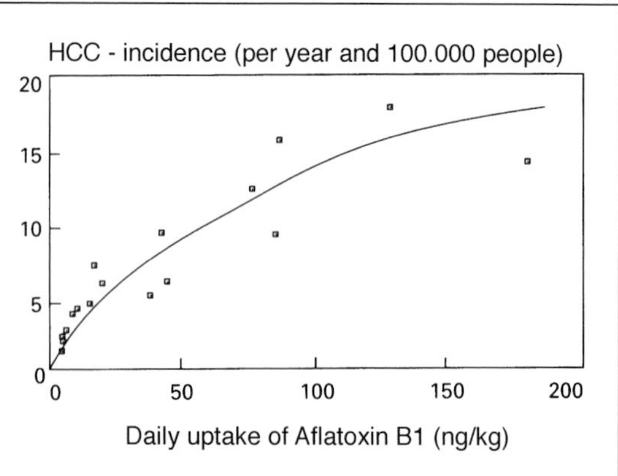

FIGURE 14 Correlation between the incidence of hepatocellular carcinomas and the daily aflatoxin uptake. The analysis of international data shows a dose-dependent increase in the rate of HCC and the aflatoxin concentration in urine. There is a synergistic action of aflatoxins and hepatitis B infections.

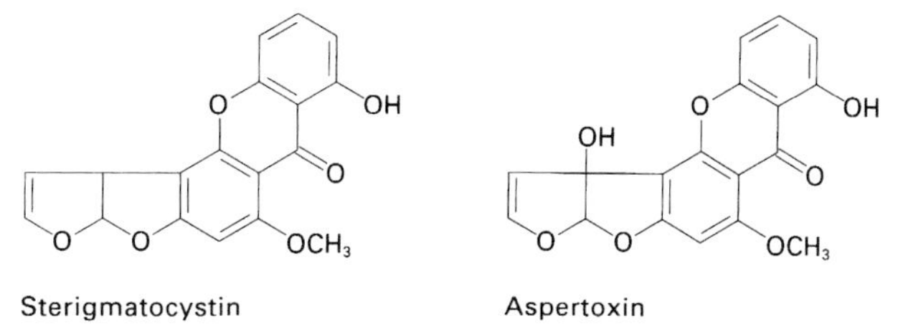

Sterigmatocystin Aspertoxin

FIGURE 15 Structure of sterigmatocystin and aspertoxin.

Maltoryzin and Kojic Acid

The fungus *Aspergillus oryzae* is used in eastern Asia for the fermentation of foods and spices, such as soy sauce, sake, and miso. The fungus synthesizes the mycotoxins maltoryzin and kojic acid (Fig. 18). In the foods the concentration of the mycotoxins remains normally below critical values. Of greater concern is the contamination of food for the livestock. Acute toxic doses result in convulsions and arrest of breathing whereas sublethal doses damage nearly all parenchymatous organs and the CNS. Kojic acid is mutagenic in *Salmonella typhimurium*.

Penicillium Species

Citrinin

Citrinin, an antibiotic active compound (Fig. 19) is synthesized by the fungi *P. citrinum, P. viridicatum, P. expansum, P. notatum, P. citreoviride,* and *P. chrysogenum.* These species prefer moderate temperatures. Therefore, their occurrence is limited to the moderate climate zones. Citrinin is also produced by some *Aspergillus* species (*A. candidus, A. niveus, A. terreus,* and *A. flavipes*). The antibiotic action of the compound is not used therapeutically because of its considerable toxicity. In rats acute toxic doses were demonstrated to cause vasoconstriction, bronchoconstriction, and fascicular twitching. Sublethal doses, especially after chronic administration, lead to damage of the proximal renal tubules, resulting in a progressive renal dysfunction. It is suggested that citrinin is accumulated in the renal tubules by the acid transport carrier. The cytotoxic action is probably based on an inhibition of RNA synthesis.

Damage also occurs after citrinin uptake at other organs, such as liver, spleen, and bone marrow. Teratogenic effects were demonstrated in rats, mice, and chickens. Adenomatous hyperplasias were observed in the liver and kidneys of rats after long-term treatment with citrinin. In tissue culture (V79 cells), the compound produced chromosomal aberrations after the addition of rat liver microsomes (S9).

Penicillic Acid

Penicillic acid is, like patulin, an α,β-unsaturated lactone. The compound (Fig. 19) occurs in numerous *Aspergillus* and *Penicillium* species, which often contaminate human and animal food. The cytotoxic compound has a high affinity for SH groups and depletes glutathion. This is the reason for the hepatotoxic action, observed after higher doses. The administration of glutathion or cystein has, therfore, a protective action against poisoning from penicillic acid. A hepato-

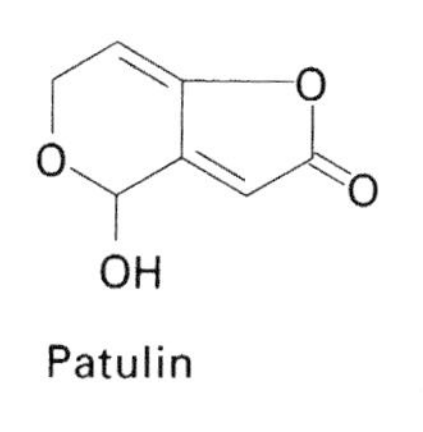

Patulin

FIGURE 16 Chemical structure of patulin.

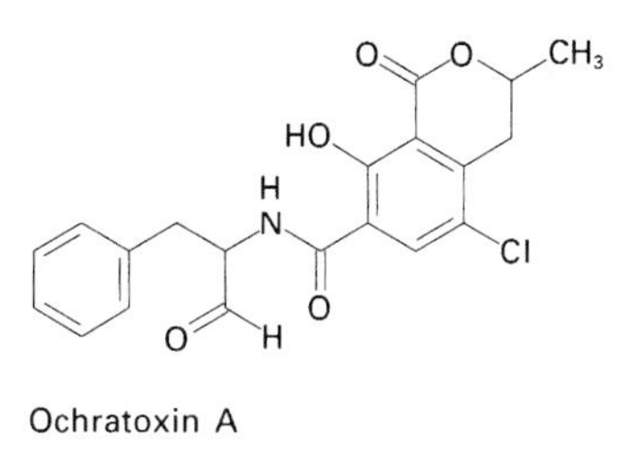

Ochratoxin A

FIGURE 17 Chemical structure of ochratoxin A.

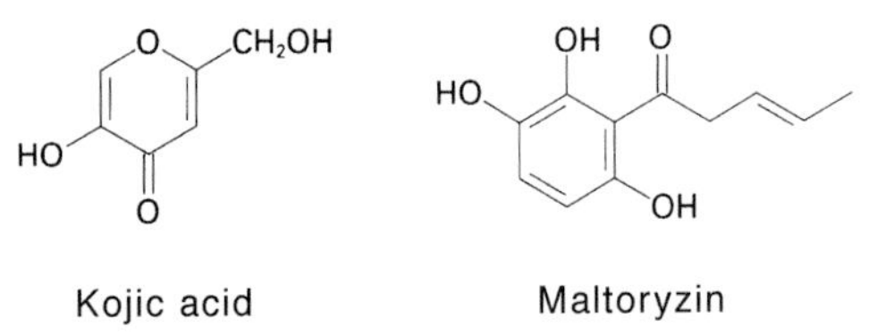

Kojic acid

Maltoryzin

FIGURE 18 Structure of kojic acid and maltoryzin.

carcinogenic action was observed in mice after chronic application of the compound.

Citreoviridin

Rice is often contaminated by the mold *Penicillium citreoviride,* which produces the mycotoxin citreoviridin. The compound (Fig. 19) has a neurotoxic and cardiotoxic potential and is responsible for the endemic occurrence of the heart disease "Cardiac beri beri." Damage of the liver and kidneys have also been correlated with the uptake of citreoviridin. It is suggested that the compound inhibits a mitochondrial ATPase, which is important for the cells, energy support. Especially sensitive are nerve and muscle cells, which have a higher energy requirement to support their electrical potentials.

Luteoskyrin and Rugulosin

Two other molds frequently contaminate rice in Asia, *Penicillium islandicum* and *P. rugulosum.* The color of the rice turns to yellow after being contaminated, which is caused by the mycotoxins luteoskyrin (*P. islandicum*) and rugulosin (*P. rugulosum*). The two bis-anthraquinones (Fig. 20) are hepatotoxic and hepatocarcinogenic in laboratory animals. It is believed that a considerable percentage of liver tumors in Asia is due to food contamination with these compounds. Both compounds have been demonstrated to accumulate to a high degree in the liver. It is believed that luteoskyrin induces liver injuries via the formation of active oxygen species generated in the process of autoxidation of the luteoskyrin semiquinone radical, which is produced in the one-electron redox systems catalyzed by the liver NAD(P)H-dependent cytochrome reductases. Because the mycotoxins are not mutagenic, an epigenetic process via oxidative stress may be responsible for the hepatocarcinogenicity.

Islanditoxin (Cyclochlorotin)

Islanditoxin, a mixture of closely related cyclic peptides (Fig. 20) with a L-dichloroproline moiety, also occurs in *Penicillium islandicum.* The toxin is very potent in mice (LD_{50} of 0.45 mg/kg). The toxicity mainly targets the liver. The mechanism of action is based on a binding of the compound to actin fibers. After contact of the liver cells with islanditoxin, the shape of

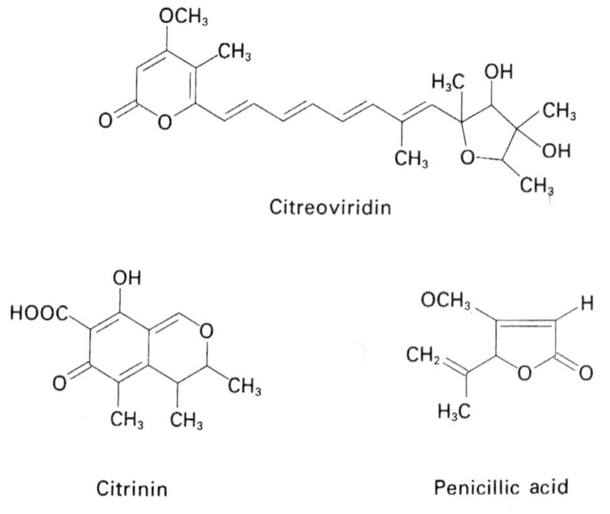

Citreoviridin

Citrinin

Penicillic acid

FIGURE 19 Structures of citreoviridin, citrinin, and penicillic acid.

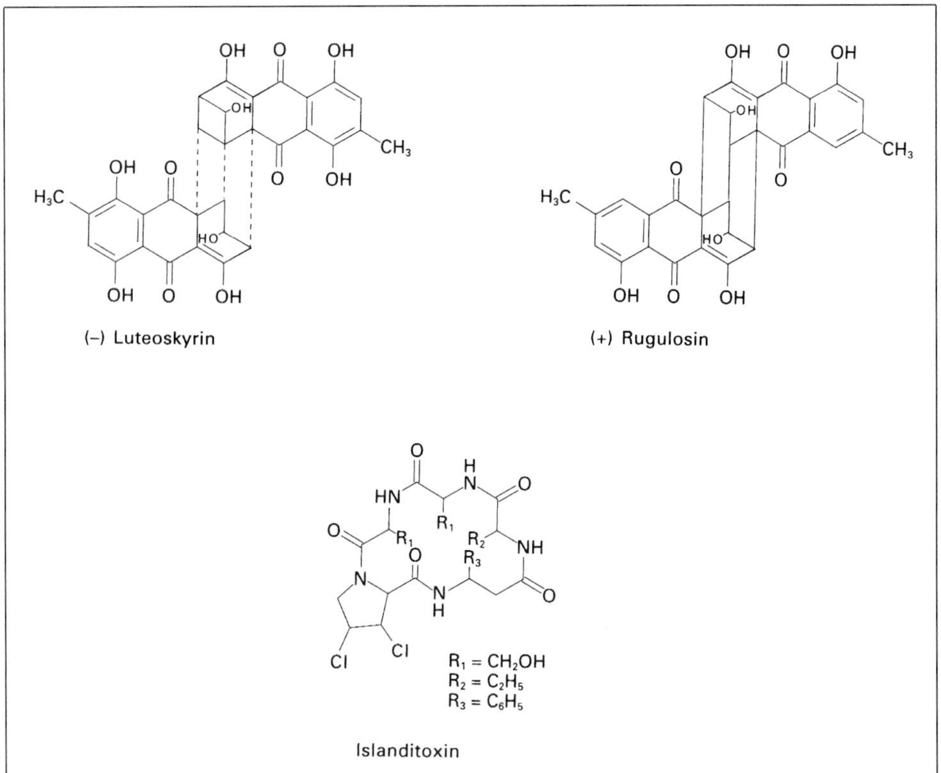

FIGURE 20 Mycotoxines from *Penecillium islandicum.*

the cells changes and numerous blisters occur at the surface of the cell membrane. After rodents are fed 50 μg/kg/day, necroses at periportal liver areas occur, leading to cirrhosis and hepatomas. It has been demonstrated that the presence of chlorine in the molecule is essential for the toxic action.

Cyclopiaconic acid and Penitrem A

The mold *Penicillium cyclobium* frequently contaminates cereal. It produces the neurotoxic compounds cyclopiaconic acid and penitrem A (Fig. 21). The compounds seem to act at presynaptic sites in the CNS and to interfere with the neurotransmitters GABA, glutamic acid, and aspartic acid.

Fusarium Species

Fusarium species are common molds contaminating cereal, hay, and other liverstock food. The fungi produce a variety of extraordinarily toxic compounds,

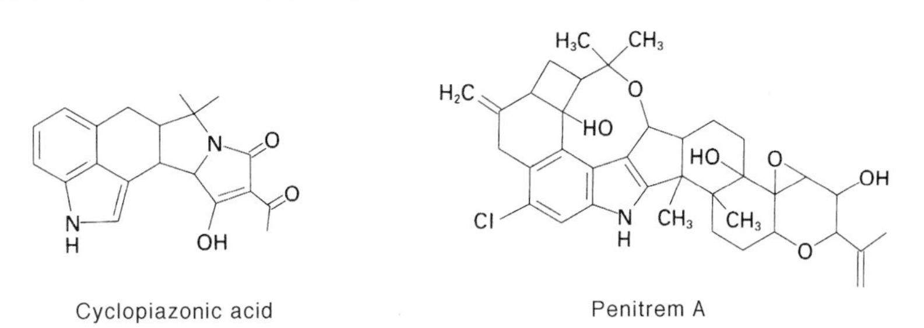

FIGURE 21 Mycotoxins from *Penicillium cyclobium.*

exerting neurotoxic, immunotoxic, and cytotoxic actions.

Trichotecenes

The most important group of fusarian toxins is that of the trichotecenes (Table 5). These compounds form a family with more than 60 structurally related compounds divided into four subclasses. The compounds have in common an epoxy group at C-12, 13 and a double bond between C-8, 9. Some important examples are shown in Fig. 22. The toxic action is related to the nature of the side chain. The fact that the toxicity is almost the same after enteral or parenteral application indicates a good absorption from the GI tract. The toxicity of the derivative diacetoxyscirpenol increases from mice to rats to rabbits to guinea pigs. It is suspected that humans are even more sensitive.

The trichotecenes are cytotoxic compounds that bind to a 60S subunit of eucaryotic ribosomal proteins, resulting in an inhibition of protein synthesis. Procaryotes are much less sensitive. The epoxy group of the toxins is essential for the action. Hydrolysis of this group abolishes the activity. This is an important inactivation pathway, taking place in liver cells. The side chain is important for the affinity of the toxins to the ribosomal-binding proteins. SH groups are involved in the binding process.

The high cytotoxic potential is responsible for the irritation of mucous membranes in the GI tract, causing nausea, vomiting, and severe diarrhea. After absorption, the toxic symptoms are dominated by the cytotoxic action on the bone marrow. The resulting immunosuppression is responsible for many secondary effects observed in humans and livestock after consuming cereal contaminated with *Fusarium* species. Teratogenic actions were observed after the administration of some trichotecenes (T-2 and deoxynivalenol) to laboratory animals. T-2 also induced chromosomal aberrations in the bone marrow of Chinese hamsters. No mutagenic or direct carcinogenic action of trichotecenes could be observed; however, after initiation with DMBA the compounds acted as tumor promotors. Epidemiologic studies in South Africa revealed a correlation between the food content of deoxynivalenol and the incidence of esophagus cancer. The mechanism could be either a tumor-promoting or immunosuppressive action of the trichotecenes. An op-

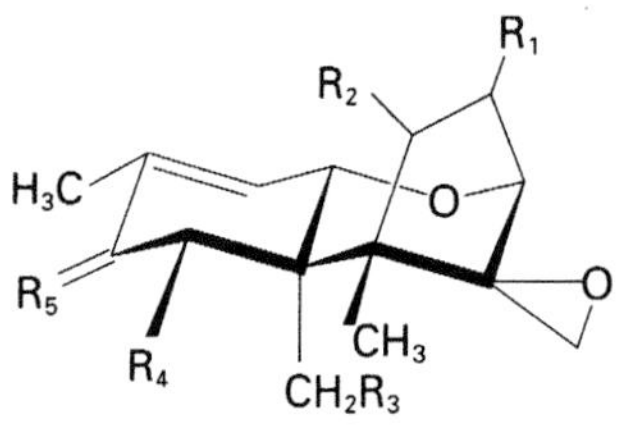

	R$_1$	R$_2$	R$_3$	R$_4$	R$_5$
T2-Toxin	OH	OAc	OAc	H	$(CH_3)_2CHCH_2OCO$
HT2-Toxin	OH	OH	OAc	H	$(CH_3)_2CHCH_2OCO$
Diacetoxyscirpenol	OH	OAc	OAc	H	H
Neosolaniol	OH	OAc	OAc	H	OH
Nivalenol	OH	OH	OH	OH	O
Fusarenon X	OH	OAc	OH	OH	O
Diacetylnivalenol	OH	OAc	OAc	OH	O
Tetraacetylnivalenol	OAc	OAc	OAc	OAc	O
Dehydronivalenol	OH	H	OH	OH	O
Dehydronivalenol	AC	H	OH	OH	O
Trichothecin	H	$CH_3CH{=}CHOCO$	H	H	O
Trichothecolon	H	OH	H	H	O

FIGURE 22 Chemical structure of trichothecenes.

TABLE 5 LD_{50} Values for Some Important Trichothecenes[a]

Group	Trichotecen	Animal	Mode of application	LD_{50} (mg/kg)
A	T-2 toxin	Mouse	ip	5.2
			po	10.5
		Rat	po	5.2
		Guinea pig	iv	1.2
		Chicken	po	4.0
		Trout	po	6.1
	Diacetoxyscirpenol	Mouse	ip	23.0
			po	7.3
		Rabbit	iv	1.0
		Guinea pig	iv	0.37
B	Nivalenol	Mouse	ip	4.1
	Deoxynivalenol	Mouse	po	46.0
		Duck	sc	27.0
	Fusarenon X	Mouse	ip	3.4
			po	4.5
		Rat	po	4.4
		Cat	sc	5.0
C	Crotocin	Mouse	po	1000
			ip	810
D	Roridin A	Mouse	iv	1.0
	Verrucarin A	Mouse	iv	1.5
		Rat	iv	0.87
		Rabbit	iv	0.54
	Verrucarin B	Mouse	iv	7.0
	Verrucarin J	Mouse	ip	0.5

[a]According to Ueno (1985).

erating immune system is important as a natural defense system against cancer.

Moniliformin

Corn is frequently contaminated with *Fusarium moniliforme,* which leads to considerable losses of this cereal. The mold produces several toxins, of which moniliformin is most important. The compound is a cyclobutadiene derivative (Fig. 23) with a high toxic potential. After administration of lethal doses to rats, mice, and chickens, the animals die of arrest of breathing. Sublethal doses lead to myocardial injury. The mechanism of action consists of an irreversible inhibition of the enzyme pyruvat dehydrogenase, resulting in an inhibition of the citric acid cycle and, thus, the energy support of the cells. Muscle, especially cardial, cells have an higher energy requirement than most other cells, which may be the reason for their special sensitivity to these toxins.

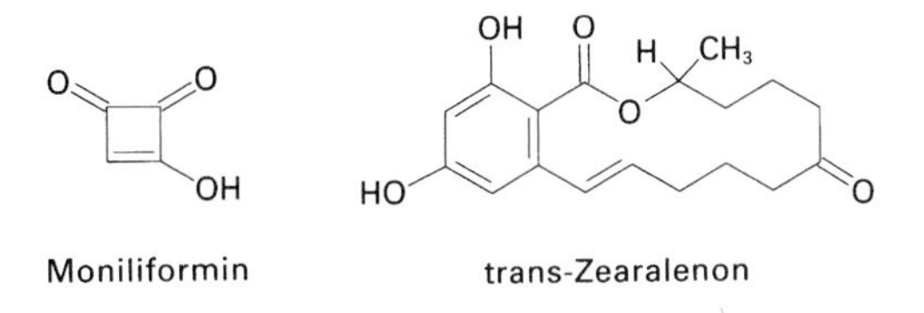

FIGURE 23 Moniliformin and Zearalenon.

Zearalenon

Fusarium gramineum is a mold that not only contaminates corn and hay but also other types of herbal foodstuff. The fungus produces a toxin, zearalenon (Fig. 23), which exerts an estrogenic action. Typical symptoms in female domestic animals consuming contaminated food consist of uterus hyperplasia, vulvovaginitis, and a decrease in fertility (which also effects male animals). The milk of cows consuming contaminated hay may contain considerable amounts of zearalenon. Drinking contaminated milk causes an accelerated maturation of the genital organs in girls, a disturbance of the estrous cycle in adult women, and a decrease of fertility in men.

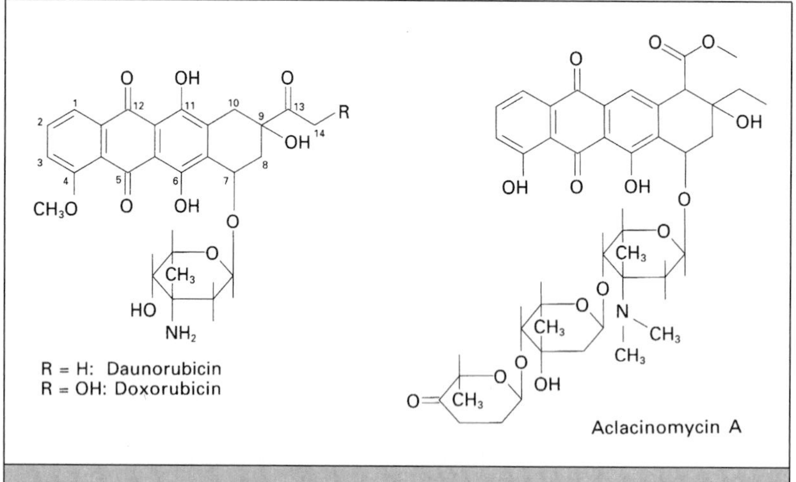

R = H: Daunorubicin
R = OH: Doxorubicin

Aclacinomycin A

FIGURE 24 Structure of anthracycline antitumor antibiotics.

It was shown that zearalenon binds at the intracellular estrogen receptor of the uterus. The compound binds also to estrogen receptors in the hypothalamus and the pituitary gland. This results in a disturbance of the estrogen-feedback mechanism. The use of zearalenon as a substitute for estrogen in post-menopausal women was stopped after the observation of a carcinogenic action in laboratory animals. In the meantime, however, it is well known that estrogen itself promotes the development of breast and uterine tumors. Zearalenon was teratogenic in rats and pigs. The malformations were especially prevalent in the skeleton. With respect to this observation, it should be noted that osteoporosis is a common complication in post-menopausal woman.

Toxins of Other Monocellular Fungi

Cytochalasins

The cytochalsins form a class of structurally related mycotoxins produced by the fungi *Helminthosporium dematioideum* (cytochalasin A and B), *Metarrhizium anisopliae* (cytochalasin C), *Zygosporium mansonii* (cytochalasin D), and *Aspergillus clavatus* (cytochalasin E). Acute toxic doses initiate severe damage of the capillary walls, leading to massive loss of intravasal proteins, systemic edema, and shock. The compounds are useful tools in experimental pharmacology and cell physiology because they bind to and inhibit the function of tubulin and actin.

Antitumor Antibiotics

The red-colored mycotoxins daunorubucin and doxorubicin (Fig. 24) are synthesized by *Streptomyces peucetius* and *S. peucetius var. caesius*, respectively. The compounds belong to the group of anthracyclines and are used therapeutically as antineoplastic agents. Doxorubicin has a broad spectrum of activity and is used for the treatment of leukemia and several solid tumors, whereas daunorubicin is used almost exclusively for the treatment of leukemia. The yellow anthracycline derivative aclacinomycin A (Fig. 24) is produced by *Streptomyces galileus*. This compound is also used for the treatment of leukoblastoses and some solid tumors. Although the biological action of the anthracyclines has been the subject of thousands of papers, the exact mechanism of action is not known. It is most likely the result of a summary of different actions. Among these are the intercalation between the base pairs in the DNA helix the formation of reactive oxygen species, and interactions with the cytoplasmic membrane. Similar to most other antineoplastic agents, the treatment with anthracyclines is accompanied by severe side effects, which are mainly directed against proliferating tissues, such as the epithelium of the GI tract and the bone marrow. Daunorubicin and doxorubicin exert a cardiotoxic action, which is related to radical formation in heart muscle cell mitochondria. The effect is cumulative and limits the total dose used in a treatment schedule. Both anthracyclines are mutagenic in bacterial and mammalian *in vitro* systems and carcinogenic in rodents after a single i.v. injection of a sublethal dose. The primary amino group of the sugar moiety is essential for the genotoxic and carcinogenic action of anthracyclines. Aclacinomycin A, which has a N,N-dimethylated sugar moiety is, therefore, not mutagenic and does not induce tumors in rats.

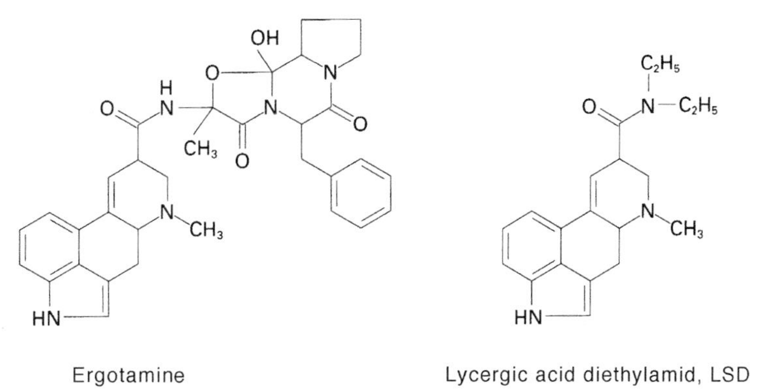

Ergotamine

Lycergic acid diethylamid, LSD

FIGURE 25 Ergot alkaloids and the synthetic hallucinogenic derivative, LSD.

Claviceps Alkaloids

The parasitic fungus *Claviceps purpurea,* also known as *Secale cornutum,* grows parasitically on wheat, rye, and various other grasses. The fungus consists of a long, black, slightly curved body, the sclerotium, which contains a variety of alkaloids, known as "ergot" (Fig. 25). During harvest and threshing, the sclerotia get into the grain. Modern techniques allow the separation of the sclerotia from the grain before it is ground. In recent times, however, endemic poisoning sometimes occurred when a great amount of *Secale* was present in the grain and, thus the flour and bread. Directives of the European Community restrict the ergot content of grain to less than 0.1%.

Two forms of chronical poisoning are known, gangrene ergotism and convulsive ergotism. The latter form causes paresthesias of the extremities and, because of a permanent constriction of the arteries, ischemia and gangrene develop. The affected extremities may become subject to amputation. The convulsive form is characterized by tonoclonic convulsions, which are very painful. Ergot alkaloids act also on the CNS, resulting in psychotic disorders, which may end in dementia. Because of its contractile action on plain muscles, ergot was used in folk medicine as a birth-accelerating drug and an abortive. In modern medicine, the alkaloid ergotamine is used in the therapy of migraine headache.

Lysergic acid is produced after hydrolysis of ergotamine. Its conversion into the *N,N*-diethylamid yields one of the most powerful hallucinogenic drugs, called LSD. The psychogenic action of LSD is accompanied by spectral visions and erotic feelings. The drug, which was first synthesized by the German chemist A. Hofmann at Ciba-Geigy in Basel, Switzerland, was very famous during the "hippie movement," which started in the late 1960s. The effective dose range to cause hallucinations is 0.5–2 μg/kg. Higher doses may lead to a phenomenon known as "horror trip," which is characterized by fear and manic episodes. Sometimes the symptoms last for several weeks. Irreversible parachromatism and schizophrenia have also been observed after the use of high doses of LSD.

Toxins from Mushrooms *(Basidiomycetae)*

Among the higher fungi (mushrooms) are many toxic species, which are responsible for severe, sometimes lethal poisoning in humans. Most of the toxic mushrooms belong to the genus of *Amanita, Inocybe,* and *Cortinarius.* The collection and cooking of toxic instead of edible mushrooms is, in most cases, due to a lack of botanical knowledge. Fortunately, lethal poisonings are rare. However, gastroenteritic discomfort is common after the ingestion of toxic mushrooms. A survey of the most important species of toxic mushrooms follows.

***Amanita* Species (*A. phalloides, A. virosa, A. citrina,* and *A. verna*)**

Up to 90% of the fatalities of mushroom poisoning are caused by *Amanita phalloides* or other *Amanita* species. The toxic principles consist of two groups of cyclic peptides, the amatoxins (Fig. 26) and the phallotoxins (Fig. 27). The amatoxins block the transcription process via an inhibition of the RNA polymerase. This causes an intracellular depletion of mRNA, followed by a gradual depletion of proteins, finally causing cell death. The liver is the main target organ of the toxins, which is due to an intensive first-pass effect. Damage also occurs in the GI tract and the kid-

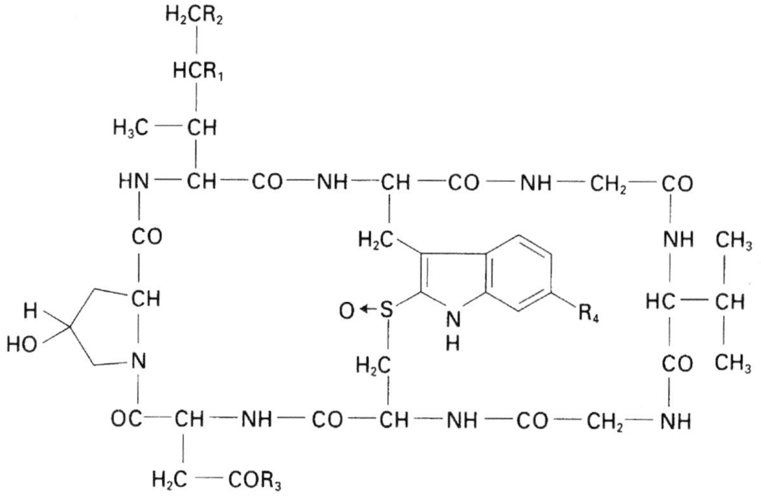

	R_1	R_2	R_3	R_4	LD_{50}(Mice p.o.)
α-Amanitin	OH	OH	NH_2	OH	0.3 mg/kg
β-Amanitin	OH	OH	OH	OH	0.5 mg/kg
γ-Amanitin	OH	H	NH_2	OH	0.2 mg/kg
ε-Amanitin	OH	H	OH	OH	0.3 mg/kg
Amanin	OH	OH	OH	H	0.5 mg/kg
Amanullin	H	H	NH_2	OH	>20 mg/kg

FIGURE 26 Amatoxins.

neys. In most cases of *amanita* poisoning, the hepatotoxic action is first recognized 1–2 days after ingestion. At this time, the degree of liver damage is usually severe and irreversible.

The phallotoxins bind to actin fibers at the cell membrane, resulting in changes of the membrane permeability, which finally leads to cell death. Their action is comparable to that of the cytochalasins. In contrast to the amatoxins, the phallotoxins exert their action a few hours after ingestion. The amatoxins are much more potent than the phallotoxins. If large masses of mushrooms are ingested, the symptoms of intoxication may be dominated by the earlier-acting phallotoxins. The lethal doses for amatoxins and phallotoxins are 0.1 mg and 5–10 mg, respectively. A quantity of 100 g fresh *Amanita phalloides* contains up to 17 mg amatoxins. A single mature mushroom is, therefore, sufficient to kill a whole family.

The symptomatic therapy of amanita poisoning is very complex. Gastric lavage is important to remove undigested material. Ingestion of activated charcoal is helpful to bind toxins that still remain in the GI tract. Infusions of fluid and plasma expanders are essential in cases of shock. Further treatment requires the infusion of high doses of vitamins, fibrinogen, antibiotics, glucocorticoids, and, eventually, cardiac glycosides. Modern intensive care has reduced the lethality rates below 20%. After the severe progression of liver damage, liver transplantation is the last possibility to save the patient's life.

Amanita muscaria and Amanita pantherina

Both of these mushrooms contain the anticholinergic compounds ibotenic acid, also converted into muscimol and the cholinergic compound muscarine (Fig. 28). After the ingestion of the mushrooms, mainly anticholinergic symptoms, such as tachycardia, hyperthermia, and mydriasis, dominate. Parasympathetic symptoms, such as bradycardia, salivation, and miosis, are also sometimes observed. Similar to the anticholinergic compound atropine, ibotenic acid and muscimol enter the CNS and cause reactions, such as dizziness, ataxia, delirium, hallucinations, and erotic feelings. Because of its psychotic actions, the mushrooms have been used historically at cult ceremonies and in the preparation of witch recipes. Lethal intoxication is rare. It sometimes occurs when the toxic

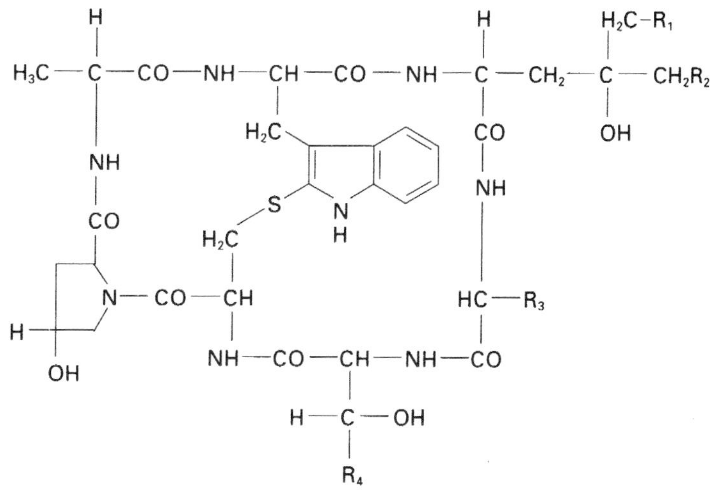

	R_1	R_2	R_3	R_4	LD_{50} (Mice p.o.)
Phalloidin	OH	H	CH_3	CH_3	2.0 mg/kg
Phalloin	H	H	CH_3	CH_3	1.5 mg/kg
Phallisin	OH	OH	CH_3	CH_3	2.5 mg/kg
Phallacidin	OH	H	$CH(CH_3)_2$	COOH	2.5 mg/kg

FIGURE 27 Phallotoxins.

mushroom *Amanita pantherina* (lethal dose, 110 g fresh weight) is mistakenly collected instead of the edible species *Aminita rubescens*. Almost no fatal cases have been reported for *A. muscaria*, which is less toxic than *A. panhterina;* also the intense red color of this mushroom prevents it from being erroneously collected.

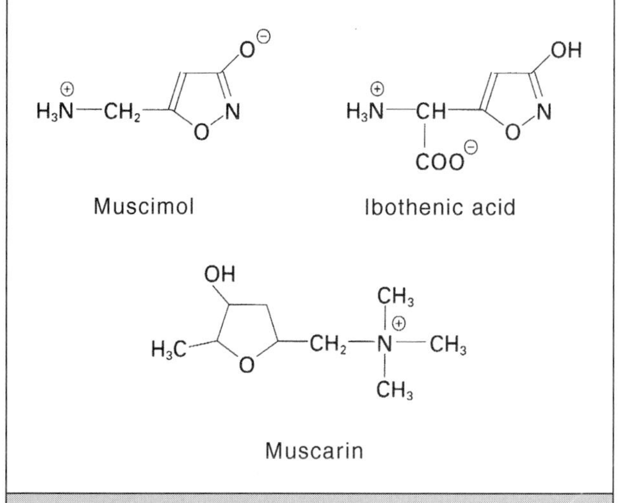

FIGURE 28 Toxins from *Amanita muscaria* and *Inocybe ssp.*

Inocybe Species

Most of the approximately 130 *Inocybe* species are toxic. Some also cause fatal intoxication (e.g., *Inocybe patoulliardi*). The mushrooms contain great amounts of muscarin, which acts on post-synaptic acetylcholinergic (muscarinic) receptors (Fig. 28). The symptoms of intoxication are, therefore, characterized by excessive parasympathetic excitement (salivation, lacrimation, sweating, gastrointestinal spasms, severe diarrhea, bradycardia, and bronchospasm). If medical care is soon available, the prognosis is good, because all the symptoms are reversible after administration of atropine. If no atropine is given, the symptoms progress to coma and respiratory or heart arrest. Further toxic mushrooms are listed in Table 6 (Fig. 29).

PLANT TOXINS

Many plants contain compounds that are toxic to animals and humans. Some of these compounds serve as repellents against herbivorous animals, fungi, or bacteria. Others may be just accidentally, toxic. Toxic plants have been used by humans for different purposes as long as they have existed. Modern methods of chemical analysis made the chemical structures of

TABLE 6 Toxic Mushrooms Responsible for Severe or Fatal Intoxication

Mushroom	Poison	Symptoms
Amanita phalloides	Amatoxins	Hepatotoxic
Amanita verna	Amatoxins	Hepatotoxic
Amanita virosa	Amatoxins	Hepatotoxic
Amanita pantherina	Ibotenic acid	Parasymphatolytic
Amanita muscaria	Ibotenic acid	Parasymphatolytic
Cortinarius ssp.	Orellanines	Nephrotoxic
Galerina ssp.	Amatoxins	Hepatotoxic
Gyromitra esculenta	Gyromitrin	Hepatotoxic
Inocybe ssp.	Muscarin	Parasympathomimetic
Lactarius ssp.	Nectaronon	Gastrointestinal
Omphalotus olearius	Sesquiterpenes	Gastrointestinal
Paxillus involutus	Unknown	Anaphylactic shock

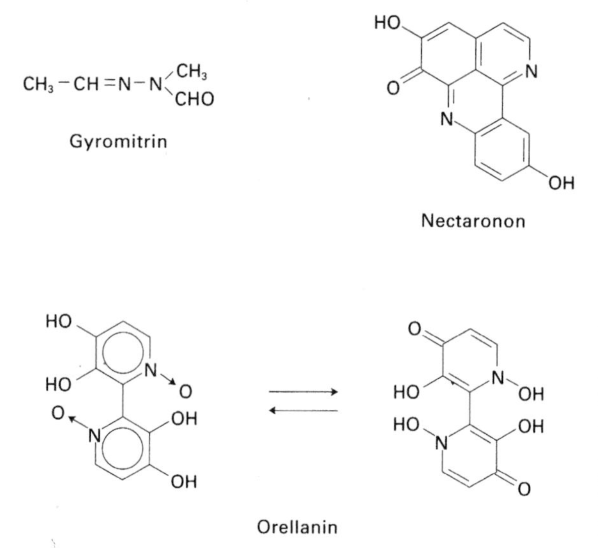

FIGURE 29 Toxins from *Cortinarius ssp.*, *Gyromitra esculenta*, and *Lactarius ssp.*

many toxic plant ingredients available, and their pharmacological and toxicological mechanisms have been investigated.

Poisoning by plants is mainly due to oral ingestion of plants or parts of plants. At special risk are little children, who are more careless than adults and often attracted by the appearance of plants (e.g., the nice color of purple foxglove or the appetizing appeal of the fruits of belladonna). In the case of adults, a lack of botanical knowledge may lead to the mistaken use of toxic plants for food or preparation of phytotherapeutics. Finally, toxic plants are also used as abortives, and in suicides and homicides.

A differentiation of toxic plants by their site of action is difficult, because the toxicity is often the result of a complex mixture of compounds with different modes of action (Table 7). Moreover, individual differences in sensitivity may lead to different symptoms, especially if allergic reactions are involved. Plant toxins are normally less target directed than are animal toxins. Plants also often contain compounds with antagonistic properties, whereas the components of animal toxins act synergistically, in most cases.

Compounds with Action on the Gastrointestinal System

Irritation of the mucous membranes of the GI tract is caused by most plant toxins ingested orally. Some toxins exert their action almost exclusively at this site. Among these are the saponines, a group of glycosidic compounds containing a lipophilic aglycone and a hydrophilic sugar moiety. Their name "saponines" is based on the Latin word for soap (principium saponeum) and characterizes the action of the compounds as detergents. Saponines are widely distributed in the plant kingdom and cause many plants to be inedible. An example for a saponine-containing plant that caused endemic poisoning in past centuries in western Europe is *Argostemma githago* L. The seeds of this plant, which sometimes grows together with cereals, contain the saponine githagin glycoside. The ingestion of bread prepared from flour with *Argostemma*-contamination caused endemic poisoning with many fatal cases. Poisoning was also observed in domestic animals. The toxic dose for humans is approximately 3–5 g of *Argostemma* seeds. Another saponine-containing plant is *Cyclamen purpurescens*, a popular indoor plant. The bulbs contain the triterpenglycoside cyclamin. The purple foxglove (*Digitalis purpurea* L.) contains the saponine digitonin (Fig. 30). A well-known saponine plant is the horse chestnut (*Aesculus hippocastanum* L.). The chestnuts contain a mixture of triterpeneglycosides called aescin. In North America, the American pokeweed (*Phytolacca americana* L.) is used in folk medicine as a remedy against rheumatism. All parts of the plant, especially the roots, contain triterpene glycosides. Poisoning occurred from overdosing from tea preparations made from the roots or leaves of the plant (pokeroot tea). The symptoms are directed mainly to the GI tract. Other saponine-containing plants with rare cases of human poisoning are: *Primula* L. (primrose), *Viola purpurea* L. (violet), *Astragalus glycyphyllos* L. (licorice milkvetch), *Panax ginseng* C. Meyer (ginseng), and *Equisetum arvense* L. (field horsetail).

TABLE 7 Overview of the Most Important Plant Toxins

Compound	Occurrence	Toxicity[a]	Action
Abrin	*Abrus precatorius*	LD_{50} (M ip) 0.02 mg/kg	Cytotoxic, gastroenteritis,
Aconitin	*Aconitum* spp	LD_{50} (M iv) 0.16 mg/kg	Increase nerve excitability, later paralysis
Adonitoxin	*Adonis vernalis*	LD_{50} (M) 191 μg/kg	Heart glycoside
β-Aescin	*Aesculus hipp.*	LD_{50} (M po/iv) 400/2 mg/kg	Oral: gastroenteritis, parenteral: Hämolysis
Aethusin	*Aethusa cynap.*		Spasmogenic
Allylisothiocyanat	*Brassica nigra*	LD_{50} (M po) 108 mg/kg	Mucous membrane irritant
Amygdalin	*Cotoneaster* spp.		Cyanogen, asphyxia
Anabasine	*Nicotiana tabacum*	LD (H) 22 mg	Ganglia blocking
Arecolin	*Areca catechu*	LD_{50} (M sc) 100 mg/kg	Parasympathomimetic
Aristolochic acid	*Aristolochia clematitis*	LD_{50} (M po) 30 mg/kg	Gastroenteritis, carcinogenic
Atropin	*Atropa belladonna*	LD (H) 60–100 mg	Parasympatholytic
Berberin	*Berberis vulgaris*	LD_{50} (M ip) 100 mg/kg	Gastroenteritis, nephritis
Brucin	*Strychnos nux-vomica*	LDlo (H) 30 mg	Spasmogenic
Bulbocapnin	*Corydalis cava*	LD_{50} (M sc) 195 mg/kg	Paralysis, hypnotic
Caffeine	*Coffea arabica*	LD_{50}(R po) 200 mg/kg	Inhibition of phosphodiesterase
Cannabinol	*Cannabis sativa*	LD_{50} (R po) 670 mg/kg	Hallucinogenic
Capsaicin	*Capsicum* ssp.	LDlo (C iv) 1.6 mg/kg	Mucous membrane irritant, hypothermia
Cheirosid A	*Cheiranthus cheiri*		Heart glycoside
Cheirotoxin	*Cheiranthus cheiri*	LDlo (C iv) 0.12 mg/kg	Heart glycoside
Chelidonin	*Chelidonium majus*	LD_{50} (M iv) 35 mg/kg	Mitotic arrest
Chrysarobin	*Andira araroba*	LDlo (M ip) 4 mg/kg	Cytotoxic, tumor promoting
Cicutoxin	*Cicuta virosa*	LDlo (C po) 7 mg/kg	Spasmogenic
Cocaine	*Erythroxylum coca*	LD_{50} (R iv) 17.5 mg/kg	Local anesthetic, exciting
Colchicine	*Colchicum autumnale*	LD (H) 20 mg	Mitotic arrest
Coniine	*Conium maculatum*	LD (H) 500 mg	Paralysis
Convallatoxin	*Convallaria majalis*	LD (F iv) 0.3 mg/kg	Heart glycoside
Cotinine	*Nicotiana tabacum*		Ganglia blocking
Cycasin	*Cycas revoluta*	LD_{50} (R po) 562 mg/kg	Carcinogenic
Cyclamin	*Cyclamen purpurescens*		Gastroenteritis, hemolysis
Cytisin	*Laburnum anagyroides*	LD_{50} (C po) 3 mg/kg	Ganglia blocking
Digitonin	*Digitalis purpurea*		Gastroenteritis, hemolysis
Digitoxin	*Digitalis purpurea*	LD_{50} (C po) 0.18 mg/kg	Heart glycoside
Digoxin	*Digitalis purpurea*	LD_{50} (C po) 0.2 mg/kg	Heart glycoside
Emetin	*Cephaelis ipecacuana*	LD_{50} (R ip) 12 mg/kg	Cytotoxic, gastroenteritis
Ephedrine	*Ephedra vulgaris*	LD (M po) 400 mg/kg	Sympathomimetic
Gitoxigenin	*Digitalis* ssp.	LD_{50} (C iv) 3 mg/kg	Heart glycoside
Hellebrin	*Helleborus* ssp.	LDlo (GP po) 0.6 mg/kg	Gastroenteritis, CNS excitation
L-Hyoscyamine	*Solanaceae*	LD (H) 60–100 mg	Parasympatholytic
Hypericin	*Hypericum* ssp.		Phototoxic, MAO-inhibitor
Khellin	*Ammi visnaga*	LD_{50} (R po) 80 mg/kg	Spasmolytic
Lycorin	*Ammarillaceae*		Gastroenteritis, skin irritating
Mescaline	*Lophophora Williamsii*	LD_{50} (M ip) 212 mg/kg	Hallucinogenic, teratogenic
Morphine	*Papaver somniferum*	LD (H) 300–500 mg	Central analgesic, respiratory depressant
Narcotine	*Papaver somniferum*	LD_{50} (M po) 0.83 mg/kg	Spasmolytic
Nicotine	*Nicotiana tabacum*	LDlo (H) 40 mg	Ganglia blocking
Nornicotine	*Nicotiana tabacum*	LD_{50} (R ip) 23.5 mg/kg	Ganglia blocking
Oenanthotoxin	*Oenanthe crocata*	LD (M ip) 0.83 mg/kg	Spasmogenic
Papaverine	*Papaver somniferum*	LD_{50} (R po) 750 mg/kg	Spasmolytic
Phasin	*Phaseolus vulgaris*		Cytotoxic, hemagglutinine
Phorbolester	*Croton tiglium*		Skin irritant, tumor promoting
Physostigmin	*Physostigma venenosum*	LD_{50} (M po) 3 mg/kg	Inhibition of acetylcholinesterase
Picrotoxin	*Anamirta cocculus*	LD_{50} (M ip) 4 mg/kg	Spasmogenic
Pilocarpin	*Pilocarpus jaborandi*	LD_{50} (R po) 911 mg/kg	Parasympathomimetic
Protoanemonine	*Helleborus* ssp.	LD_{50} (M ip) 190 mg/kg	Gastroenteritis, skin irritant, paralysis
Psilocybin	*Psilocybe* ssp.	LD_{50} (M ip) 275 mg/kg	Hallucinogenic
Psoralen	*Citrus* ssp.		Skin irritant
Quinidine	*Cinchona pubescens*	LD_{50} (C iv) 22 mg/kg	Heart poison
Quinine	*Cinchona pubescens*	LDlo (GP po) 300 mg/kg	Heart poison
Reserpine	*Rauvolfia serpentina*		Antisympathicotonic
Retrorsin	*Senecio* ssp.	LD_{50} (M iv) 59 mg/kg	Hepatotoxic, carcinogenic
Ricin	*Ricinus communis*	LD_{50} (M iv) 12 μg/kg	Cytotoxic, gastroenteritis
Safrol	*Sassafras albidum*	LD_{50} (R po) 1950 mg/kg	Skin irritant, carcinogenic
Scopolamine	*Solanaceae*	LD_{50} (M iv) 163 mg/kgp	Parasympathicolytic
Senecionin	*Senecio* ssp.	LD_{50} (M iv) 64 mg/kg	Hepatotoxic, carcinogenic
Senkirkin	*Tussilago farfara*		Hepatotoxic, carcinogenic
Solanin	*Solanaceae*	LDlo (H) 400 mg	Gastroenteritis, hemolysis, CNS disturbance
Sparteine	*Genista tinctoria*	LDlo (RB iv) 30 mg/kg	Heart arrest
g-Strophantin	*Strophantus* ssp.	LD (C iv) 0.15 mg/kg	Gastroenteritis, heart arrest
Strychnine	*Strychnos nux-vomica*	LDlo (H) 30 mg	Spasmogenic
Tetrahydrocannabiol	*Cannabis sativa*	LD_{50} (R iv) 29 mg/kg	Halluzinogenic
Thujon	*Thuja* ssp.	LD (R ip) 240 mg/kg	Nerve poison
Tubocurarine	*Chondrodendron tomentosum*	LD (H) 50–120 mg	Paralysis of motoric endplate
Urushioles	*Rhus toxicodendron*		Severe skin irritant
Vicin	*Vicia faba*		Hämolytic anemia
Vinblastine	*Catharantus roseus*	LD_{50} (M iv) 17 mg/kg	Mitotic arrest
Vincristine	*Catharantus roseus*	LD_{50} (M iv) 2 mg/kg	Mitotic arrest
Yohimbine	*Pausinystalia yohimba*	LD (H) >1.8 g	Aphrodisiacic, alpha-2-agonistic
		LDlo (M iv) 16 mg/kg	Sympathomimetic

[a] Abbreviations: F = Frog, C = cat, M = mouse, H = human, GP = guinea pig, R = rat, RB = rabbit.

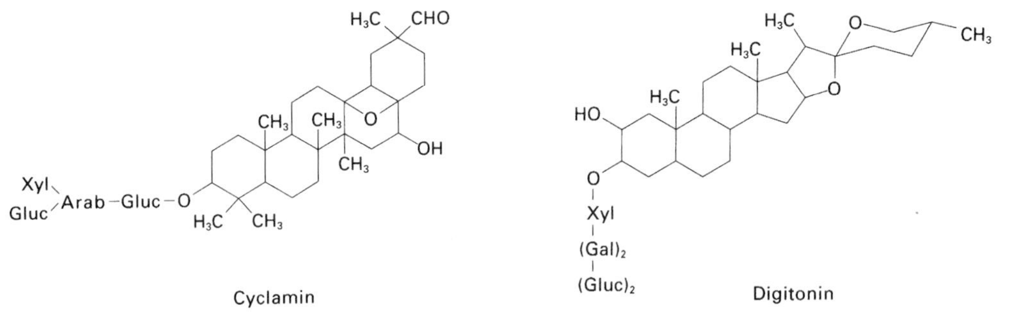

FIGURE 30 Typical representatives of saponines. Cyclamin contains triterpene aglycon, whereas digitonin belongs to the steroids.

Saponines are weakly absorbed by the intestine. Because of their action as a detergent they concentrate in the lipid layer of the cell membranes of the gastric and intestinal epithelium, which is damaged. This causes severe irritation, characterized by burning of mouth and stomach, cough, salivation, and lacrimation; followed by nausea, vomiting, and diarrhea; and sometimes resulting in severe loss of fluids and electrolytes. Reflexes via the autonomic nerve system may cause disturbances to heart function and circulatory system. Death is often the result of shock reaction. Although saponines are normally poorly absorbed, the local irritation of the mucous membranes may enhance the permeability via damage to the intestinal wall. Systemic reactions of saponines after absorption are mainly directed to red blood cells and may consist of severe hemolysis, causing anoxia and kidney failure as secondary reactions.

The therapy for saponine poisoning consists of the oral application of activated charcoal in order to absorb and, thus, inactivate the saponines. Slime preparations of rice and oats or paraffin should be administered as a mucous-membrane protective. The substitution of electrolytes and fluid is essential after extensive episodes of vomiting and diarrhea. If the patient is excited, sedatives should be given and artificial respiration is necessary if arrest of breathing occurs. Due to modern intensive care, fatal poisonings by saponine-containing plants are very rare.

Another group of plant toxins with irritating action on the GI tract are hydroxyanthraquinones (HA). They occur in numerous medicinal plants, most of which are used as laxatives. Anthraquinone-containing drugs are aloe (*Aloe barbadensis* P. Mill. and *A. ferox* Mill.), sennae folium, and sennae fructus (*Cassia angustifolia* Vahl.), rhei radix (*Rheum officinale* Baillon, Chinese rhubarb) and rhamni frangulae cortex (*Rhamnus ssp.*, buckthorn). They contain the anthraquinones rhein, aloe-emodin, chrysophanol, and physcion as free aglycones and as glycosides (Fig. 31). Intestinal bacteria reduce the anthraquinones (glycosides) to very reactive anthrones, which increase the net secretion of fluid into the lumen by irritation of the intestinal wall. This process causes the laxative action. The presence of two hydroxy groups in 1,8-position is essential for the laxative action. Upon chronic use of anthraquinones, its laxative potency decreases, ending up in a vicious circle (Fig. 32).

Some of the anthraquinones (Fig. 31) are genotoxic (e.g., aloe-emodin, and emodin) in a variety of *in vitro* short-term assays. All HA with hydroxygroups in 1,8-position (i.e., laxative active ones) act as tumor promoters in primary liver cell cultures (via induction of mitosis) and in C3H-mouse fibroblasts (via enhancement of malignant transformation after low-dose treatment with an initiating carcinogen). A carcinogenic action in rodents was demonstrated after feeding rats and mice danthron and 1-hydroxyanthraquinone. There is also limited evidence that long-term abuse of anthraquinone laxatives is correlated with colon cancer. The action of the HA is most probably related to oxidative stress.

The toxic proteins ricin, abrin, and phasin occur in the seeds of *Ricinus communis* L (castor bean), *Abrus precatorius* L. (jequirity bean), *Phaseolus vulgaris* L. (kidney bean), and *Phaseolus coccineus* L. (scarlet runner). The compounds, which belong to the lectines, are destroyed upon cooking the plants; however, they are resistant to digestive enzymes. Ricin and abrin are among the most potent plant poisons known. After IV injection into mice the LD_{50} is approximately 0.1 μg/kg. The lethal dose after oral consumption by hu-

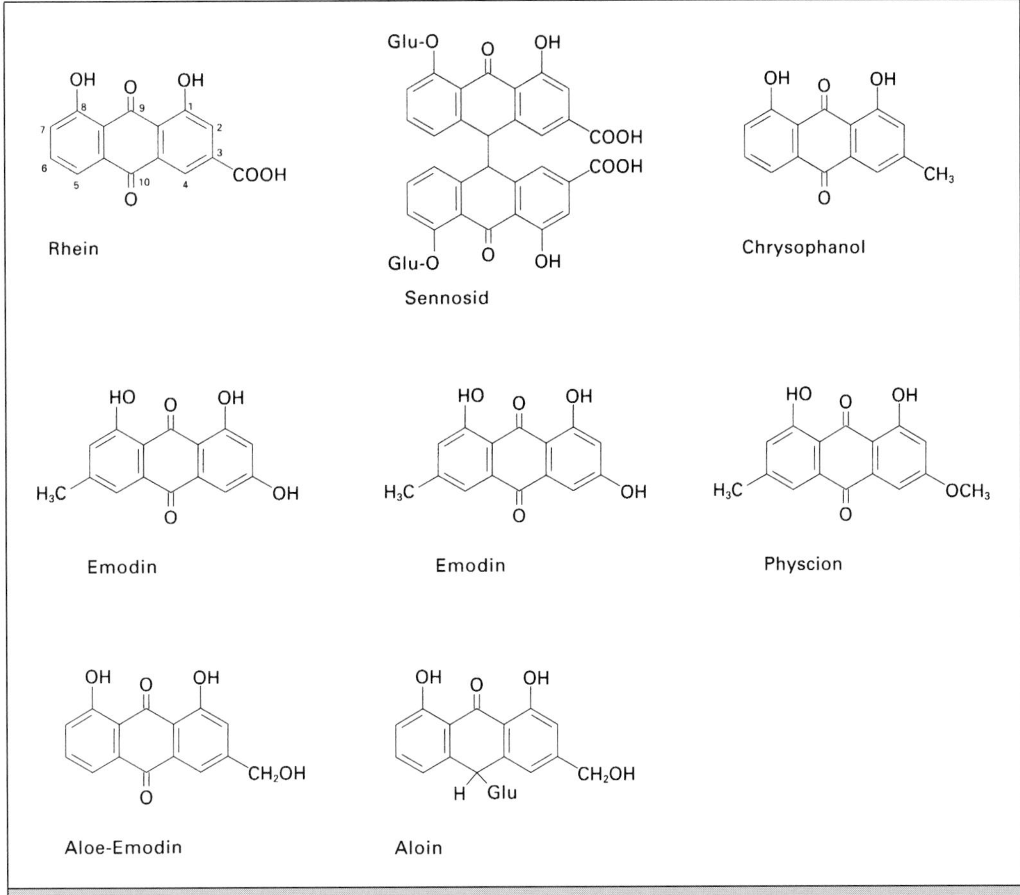

FIGURE 31 Hydroxyanthraquinones and -glycosides occurring in medicinal plants used as laxatives. Two hydroxy groups in 1,8-position are essential for the laxative (and tumor-promoting) action.

mans is approximately 5 $\mu g/kg$. If jequirity beans or castor beans are ingested without chewing, the liberation of the poison is inhibited by the tough skin. After the beans are chewed, however, lethal intoxication may occur. Pulverized jequirity beans were used by jealous Aztec women, who mixed it into the food of their unfaithful husbands. Kidney beans are toxic if ingested raw because of their phasin content. Fatal cases in children occurred after ingestion of 5–6 raw beans.

The toxic lectines consist of two protein chains (A and B), connected by a disulfide bridge. The B-chain binds covalently to the surface of the cell membrane, whereas the A-chain enters the cell and inhibits the ribosomal protein synthesis by splitting off adenine from the rRNA. It is believed that a single molecule of abrin or ricin is sufficient to kill a cell. After oral ingestion of the compounds, the mucosa cells of the GI tract are first damaged. Severe vomiting and diarrhea may lead to death by hypovolemic-shock syndrome. After absorption of the toxic proteins, other organs, especially the liver and kidney, are damaged. The latency period between ingestion of the toxin and death is normally 2–3 days. After parenteral application (caused by contact of the toxin with a predamaged skin) the symptoms soon occur and are not directed to the GI tract.

A local irritation of the GI tract mucosa is also achieved by uptake of capsaicin (Fig. 33), which is in hot spices, such as pepper. The highest amounts (up to 1%) are present in cayenne pepper (*Capsicum frutescens* L.). The burning taste of capsaicin is still detectable after dilution of 1:2,000,000. Mustard and horseradish contain the irritating compound allylisothiocyanate (Fig. 33). After the ingestion of greater amounts of these compounds, severe irritation of the GI tract may cause vomiting and diarrhea. The functions of the heart and kidneys may also be disturbed. A carcinogenic action of the compounds was demonstrated in laboratory animals.

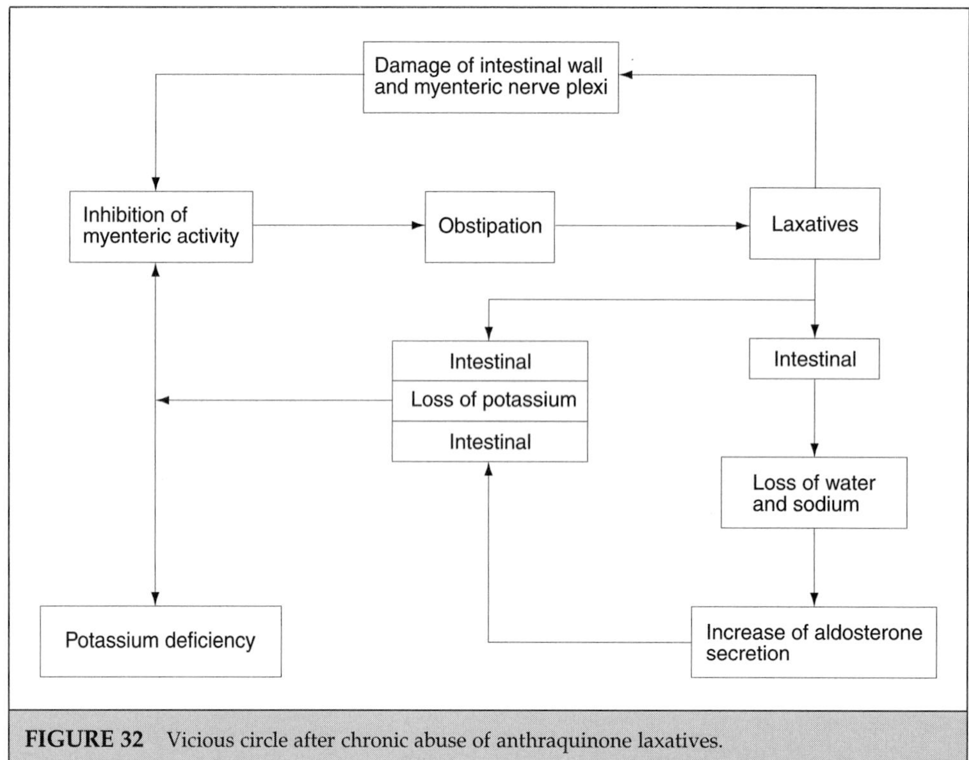

FIGURE 32 Vicious circle after chronic abuse of anthraquinone laxatives.

Compounds with Action on the Heart

Cardiotoxic compounds are glycosides, present in *Digitalis purpurea* L. and *Digitalis lanata* Ehrh. (foxglove species), *Convallaria majalis* L. (European lily of the valley), *Nerium oleander* L. (oleander), *Cheiranthus cheiri* L., *Adonis vernalis* L. (spring pheasant's eye), *Helleborus niger* L. (black hellbore), *Euonymus europaeus* L. (spindle tree), and *Scilla bifolia* L. All cardiac glycosides have similar chemical structures. The main structure consists of a steroid ring system, connected at C17 with a monounsaturated γ-lactone ring (cardenolid group) or a bis-unsaturated δ-lactone ring. Examples for both groups are shown in Fig. 34. Derivatives of the bufadienolid group are also present in the saliva of toads (bufo means toad). The aglycones of the plant-derived cardiac glycosides are linked to sugar moieties, such as D-glucose, D-fructose, D-fucose, L-rhamnose, and some characteristic 2-deoxy- or 3-*O*-methyl sugars.

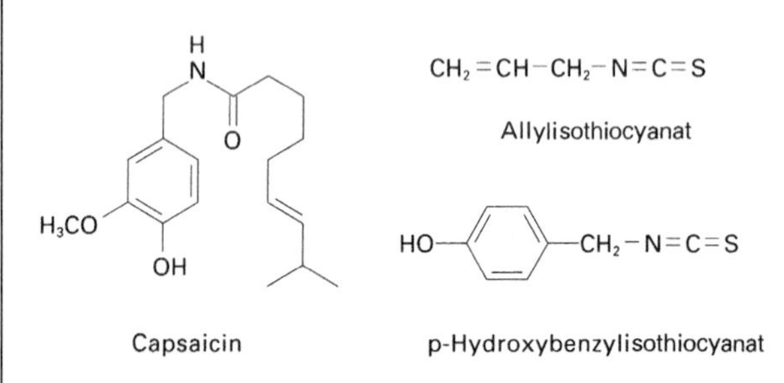

FIGURE 33 Capsaicin is the hot principle of capsicum species. Allylisothiocyanat and *p*-hydroxybenzylisothiocyanat are present in black and white mustard (*Sinapis nigra* L. and *Sinapis alba* L.).

The glycosidic moiety and the lactone rings are not essential for the action of the compounds, although the latter are involved in the potency. The compounds possess a high affinity for the Na^+-K^+-ATPases of the heart muscle cells. Binding results in an inhibition of the active Na^+-K^+ fluxes across the cell membrane and an increase of the intracellular Ca^{2+} concentration. Small doses create a positive inotropic effect, which is therapeutically used in patients with cardiac insufficiency. The therapeutic dose range is narrow. Intoxication may occur at 60% overdose only. Reduction of the blood-potassium level as a result of the use of diuretics, hyperaldosteronism, or diarrhea increases the toxicity of cardiac glycosides.

Intoxication with cardiac glycosides are characterized by a massive intracellular loss of K^+, followed by bradycardia and arrhythmia and, finally, ventricular fibrillation and heart failure. The lethal dose of digi-

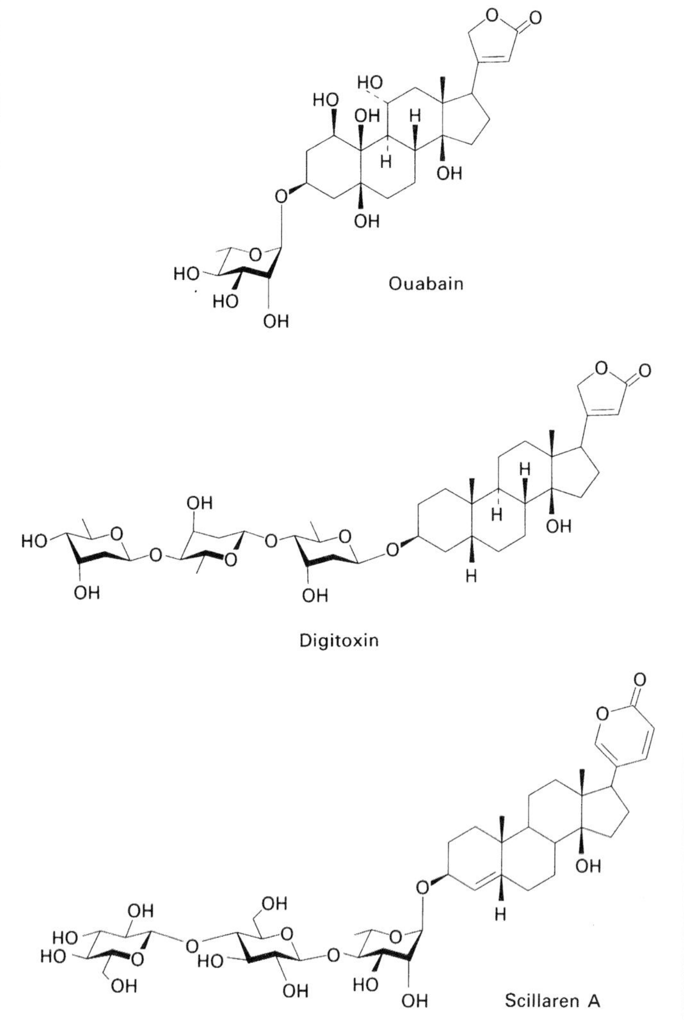

FIGURE 34 Main structures of cardiac glycosides. Cardenolid and bufodienolid structures are represented by digitoxin and scillaren A, respectively.

tonin is approximately 10 mg, occurring in only 2–3 leaves of purple foxglove.

The bark of *Cinchona pubescens* Vahl (quinine) contains the alkaloids quinine and quinidine (Fig. 35). The compounds are used therapeutically for the treatment of malaria and as an antiarrhythmic. Both compounds inhibit the spontaneous contractions of the heart muscles at high doses, finally leading to heart arrest. Similar actions are exerted by the compound spartein, occurring in the genus *Genista* and *Lupinus*.

Taxus baccata L. (yew tree) contains a mixture of related toxic alkaloids, the taxanes (Fig. 36). The poison is present in the needles and the fruit pits of the plant. The fruit pulp is free of poison and edible. Poisoning often occurs in domesticated animals, such as horses, cattle, and pigs. The lethal dose for a horse is approximately 500 g of needles. The toxicity is mainly caused by taxin (Fig. 36), a mixture of two components with strong cardiotoxic activity. After ingestion of toxic amounts of the plant, severe bradycardia occurs leading to diastolic heart arrest. The action is most probably due to an inhibition of the transmembraneous flux of Na^+ and Ca^{2+}.

Compounds with Action on the Liver

The liver is the central detoxification organ. All compounds taken up orally pass through the liver

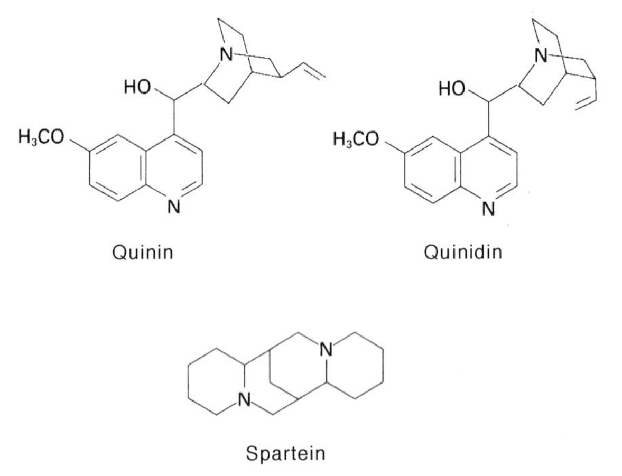

Quinin

Quinidin

Spartein

FIGURE 35 Quinine and quinidine occur in the bark of the quinine tree (*Cinchona pubescens* Vahl). Spartein is a component of plants belonging to the genera *Genista* and *Lupinus*.

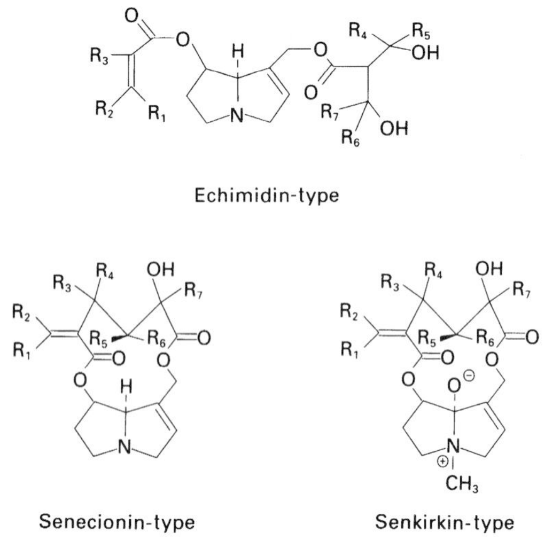

Echimidin-type

Senecionin-type

Senkirkin-type

FIGURE 37 Structures of typical pyrrolizidine alkaloids.

first after absorption from the GI tract. It is, therefore, likely that the liver is also the target for many toxins entering our bodies. However, only a few toxins are liver specific. Among these are secondary toxic compounds, which are activated by the xenobiotic metabolism of the liver cells to highly reactive intermediates that bind almost completely to macromolecules of the liver.

An important group of plant compounds with toxicity to the liver are the pyrrolizidine alkaloids (PA), occurring in about 350 plant species. Among these are numerous medicinal plants, such as *Tussilago farfara* L. (coltsfoot), *Symphytum officinale* L. (comfrey), *Petasites hybridus* (L.) P.G. Gaertn., B. Mey., & Scherb (butterbur, butterfly dock), *Cynoglossum officinale* L. (hound's tongue), and various *Senecio ssp.* (ragwort). The pyrrolizidine alkaloids consist of about 200 derivatives, containing a heterocyclic ring system, the necin base, which is connected with two acid moieties, often part of a macrocyclic two-basic acid. There are two main classes of PAs, a saturated and an unsaturated necin moiety. Only unsaturated PAs are toxic. Fig. 37 shows some typical structures of PA.

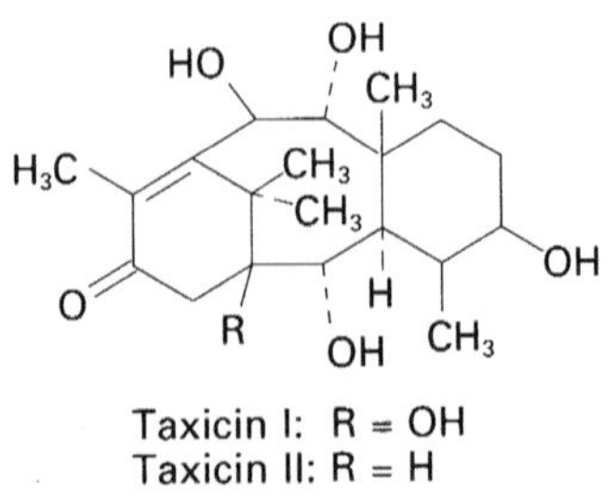

Taxicin I: R = OH
Taxicin II: R = H

FIGURE 36 Toxins of the yew-tree (*Taxus baccata*). The toxic principle taxin is a mixture of two components, taxicin I and taxicin II, differing only with respect to one hydroxy group.

After absorption, the PAs are oxidized by liver mixed functional oxidases to highly reactive pyrrole derivatives, which bind covalently to macromolecules of the liver cells. The ingestion of toxic doses may result in necrotic liver damage, known as veno-occlusive syndrome. In some areas of Central America and the Caribbean islands (e.g., Jamaica), endemic liver cirrhosis was observed in babies and little children treated with "bush teas" made from plants often containing senecio species; these are used as folk medicines against various diseases. Endemic poisoning with PAs was also reported from other parts of the world. Outbreaks of severe liver damage occurred in Afghanistan after the consumption of cereals contaminated with the seeds of *Heliotropium* and *Crotalaria* species. About 100 million sheep in Australia suffer from liver damage caused by ingestion of *Heliotropium* species. The animals normally avoid these plants as long as other (nontoxic) food plants are available, but this is not the case during especially the dry season.

PAs also represent an important class of natural carcinogens. It was demonstrated that PAs, after metabolic activation, bind covalently to liver DNA.

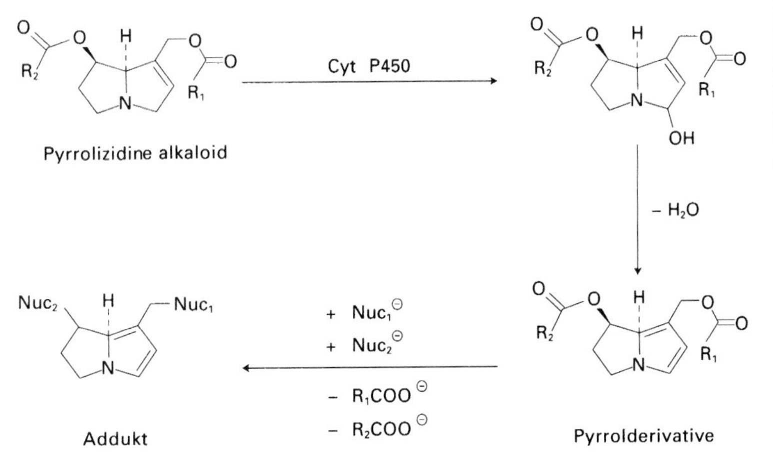

Pyrrolizidine alkaloid → Cyt P450 → (OH derivative) → $-H_2O$ → Pyrrolderivative → $+ Nuc_1^{\ominus}$, $+ Nuc_2^{\ominus}$, $- R_1COO^{\ominus}$, $- R_2COO^{\ominus}$ → Addukt

FIGURE 38 Metabolic activation of pyrrolizidine alkaloids. Proteins, RNA, or DNA may function as nucleophiles undergoing covalent linkages with the electrophilic pyrrole derivatives.

PA diesters are able to cross-link DNA (Fig. 38). The compounds are mutagenic in numerous *in vitro* assays and teratogenic in laboratory animals. Rats developed characteristic tumors of the liver after long-term feeding on PAs or plants containing such compounds.

Compounds with Toxicity on the Kidneys

Many xenobiotic compounds concentrate in the kidneys during the process of excretion. It is, therefore, not surprising that the kidneys are often involved in the toxic action of chemical compounds. Indirect mechanisms may also lead to kidney dysfunction and damage. Severe intravasal hemolysis may cause in a crystallization of heme crystals in the kidney tubules and thus lead to kidney failure. Oligo- and anuria may also be a result of electrolyte-balance disturbances occurring after episodes of severe diarrhea or vomiting, frequent symptoms of poisoning from plants. In this case, kidney failure is the result of an activation of the renin–angiotensin–aldosterone system. Very few plant toxins act specifically at the kidneys.

The seeds of a tree (*Pithecolobium lobatum*) belonging to the plant family of leguminoses contain the sulfur-containing amino acid djencolic acid. The beans of this tree are often eaten on the islands of Java and Sumatra. Djencolic acid is composed of two cysteine moieties bridged by a -S-CH_2-S- chain. The compound is poorly water soluble, leading to crystallization in the kidney tubules during the process of concentration and excretion. The symptoms are related to the amount of the compound ingested and vary from cases of slight oliguria to complete anuria. Similar symptoms are caused by excessive uptake of oxalic acid, which occurs in some vegetable plants, such as rhubarb, spinach, and celery. Damage to the kidney tubules is caused by crystallization of Ca oxalate.

Plants with Hematotoxic Action

Many plants contain saponines that cause hemolysis after absorption. Because of the poor intestinal absorption of saponines, the symptoms of poisoning by such plants are mainly restricted to the GI tract. If considerable amounts are absorbed, severe hemolysis may occur, resulting in cyanosis and kidney failure. The horse chestnut saponin aescin was used clinically for the treatment of or as a prophylactic for post-operative brain edema. Overdosing in children caused some fatal cases in Germany.

Lectines consist of a group of compounds with action on the blood cells. These compounds, which occur in numerous plants, bind to specific sugar moieties of the cell membrane. Ricin, abrin, and phasin have already been discussed. Another lectin is concanavalin A, occurring in the bean *Canavalia ensiformis* (L.) D.C. Lectines cause the agglutination of blood cells. Some derivatives stimulate the mitosis of lymphocytes, acting in a way similar to antigens. The action is, however, not specific. Lectines are also used diagnostically for blood-group determination.

A syndrome called "favism" occurs after the consumption of the edible bean *Vicia faba* L. (horsebean)

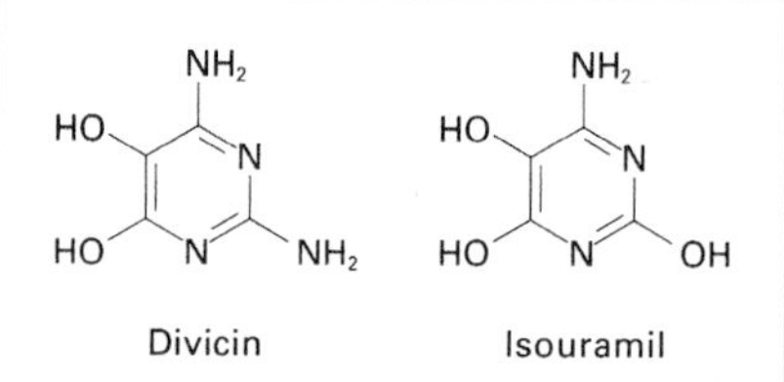

FIGURE 39 Divicin and isouramil occur in the bean *Vicia faba* L. (horsebean). The compounds are responsible for a syndrome known as favism.

by susceptible persons. The patients suffer from massive hemolysis, often with a fatal outcome. The susceptibility is correlated with a recessive X-chromosomal abnormality, leading to a lack of glucose-6-phosphate-dehydrogenase (GPDH) of the erythrocytes. The abnormality is frequent in blacks, Asiatics, and people living in Mediterranean areas. The enzyme is important for the synthesis of NADPH, which regulates the level of reduced glutathione (GSH). A lack of GSH leads to oxidative damage of the erythrocytes followed by hemolysis. Horsebeans contain the compounds divicin and isouramil (Fig. 39), which cause the oxidation of GSH to GSSG. Persons with normal concentrations of GPDH contain enough NADPH to compensate for the oxidative stress due to the toxins. In sensitive persons, however, the GSH concentration of the erythrocytes may be reduced to only 6% of the normal value.

Plant Toxins with Neurotoxic and Myotoxic Action

Numerous plant-derived toxins act on the conduction of the central and autonomic nerve systems and on the skeletal muscles. Most of these compounds belong to the alkaloids, which mimic or inhibit the action of endogenous neurotransmitters. Some compounds act directly on transmembraneous ion fluxes. Such compounds purified from plants, as well as plant extracts or the plants itself, are used for medicinal purposes, such as blood-pressure regulates, spasmolytics, analgesics, analeptics, and psychopharmacons.

Compounds with Action on the Autonomic Nerve System

These compounds are divided into those acting on the sympathetic or parasympathetic nerves and those acting on the autonomic ganglia, influencing the total

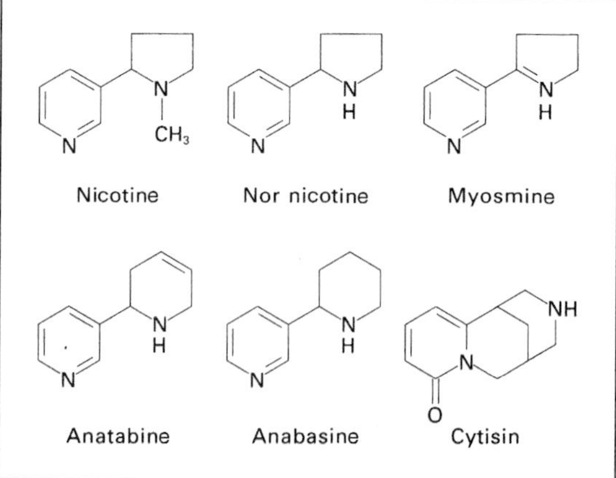

FIGURE 40 Cytisin is the toxic principal of the garden tree *Laburnum anagyroides* Medik. The other alkaloids occur in tobacco (*Nicotiana tabacum* L.).

autonomic nerve system. To the latter ones belong the pyridine alkaloids occurring in tobacco (*Nicotiana tabacum* L.) (Fig. 40). The action is related mainly to nicotine, which leads to a depolarization of all autonomic ganglia. Small doses of nicotine have a stimulating action. The anorectic action is also due to the liberation of epinephrine, which leads to glycogenolysis followed by an increase of the blood-glucose level. Higher doses also cause parasympathetic excitement with symptoms of sweating and intestinal spasms. The lethal dose for adult humans is 40–60 mg nicotine, the content of one-half cigar or two cigarettes. The fact that acute poisoning is normally not observed after smoking is due to the slow uptake of nicotine by the lungs and its rapid metabolic inactivation. Additionally, a nicotine tolerance occurs in heavy smokers. Intoxication is, however, frequently observed after oral ingestion of nicotine, occurring, for example, after the eating of cigarettes by little children. Lethal intoxication may also occur after careless handling or suicidal ingestion of nicotine-based pesticides. Toxic amounts of nicotine may also penetrate the skin after contact with aqueous tobacco extracts. Lethal amounts of nicotine lead to short episodes of convulsions followed by respiratory and cardiac arrest.

Cytisin (Fig. 40), occurring in laburnum species, such as *Laburnum anagyroides* Medik., a popular garden plant, is similar to nicotine with respect to its structure and pharmacological action. The poison is located mainly in the seeds. Ingestion of 15–20 seeds is lethal for an adult, whereas only five seeds may be sufficient to kill a child. Cytisin intoxication was also reported after consuming goat milk. Goats, which are relatively insensitive to the toxic action of cytisin, excrete the compound with their milk after feeding on the plant. The symptoms of a cytisin intoxication are similar to that caused by nicotine; however, the central stimulating effects directed to the medulla oblongata are more pronounced. The symptoms begin with an increase in blood pressure as a result of vasoconstriction and tachycardia, followed by tonoclonic spasms, unconsciousnes, and respiratory arrest. Treatment of the patients is symptomatic after the removal of plant material by gastric lavage.

Pilocarpine (Fig. 41), the active principal of jaborandi leaves (*Pilocarpus jaborandi* Holmes), stimulates the parasympathetic receptor mechanism. The pure compound is used pharmaceutically for the treatment of glaucoma. The symptoms of pilocarpine intoxication consist of an excessive stimulation of the parasympathetic nerve system with symptoms of salivation, sweating, miosis, spasms of the almost all smooth muscles, and bradycardia. Severe intoxication occurs after ingestion of more than 20 mg of pilocarpine. Another compound with action on parasympathetic receptors is muscarine, which occurs in basidiomycte species (see the section on mycotoxins).

Physostigmine, occurring in the African plant *Physostigma venenosum* Balf. (calabar bean) exerts its cholinergic action by a reversible inhibition of the enzyme acetylcholinesterase. This will cause in an excessive accumulation of endogenous acetylcholine. The symptoms consist mainly in parasympathetic reactions. In contrast to the direct-acting compound pilocarpine, physostigmine also causes fascicular twitching of striped muscles. The therapy of intoxication consists of the administration of atropine and diazepam.

Tropa alkaloids act as antagonists on cholinergic receptors. Among such compounds are L-hyoscyamine, its racemate atropine and the atropine epoxide scopolamine (Fig. 42). The compounds occur in different species of the plant family of Solanaceae (nightshade). High concentrations occur in *Atropa belladonna* L. (atropa), *Hyoscyamus niger* L. (black henbane), *Datura stramonium* L. (jimson weed), and *Mandragora officinarum* L. (mandrake). Where the plants grow wild, the black (pseudo-) berries of belladonna and the seeds of datura are often eaten by children. The berries of atropa look appetizing and have an agreeable, slightly sweet taste. Only 2–3 berries may be fatal in children, whereas the lethal dose in adults is about 20 berries. Poisoning with Solanacea plants is also due to overdosing of herbal remedies.

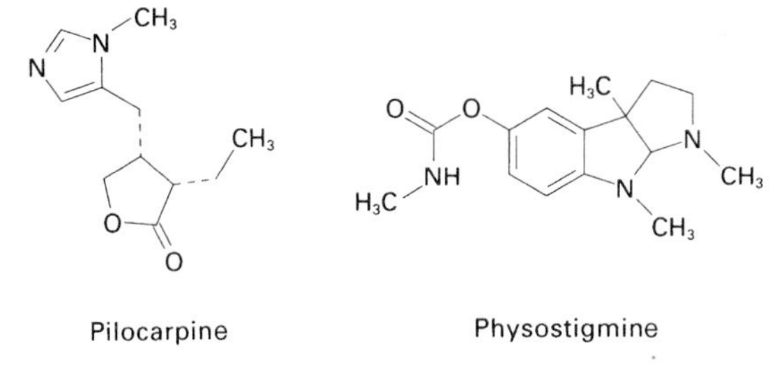

FIGURE 41 Compounds acting directly or indirectly on the parasympathetic nerve system.

After the ingestion of atropa berries (or other sources of atropine), the symptoms of poisoning begin with dryness of the mouth and throat, a scarlet flush of the face, and dialation of the pupils. Symptoms of central excitement occur a little later. The patient is lively, merry, and agitated. Spectral illusions and erotic feeling are often perceived. The condition may then change to an anxious or furious state. The pulse is quick and faint, and the respiration is stertorous. In fatal cases, the symptoms of excitement disappear slowly and deep coma occurs. Death is normally caused by respiratory arrest.

Extracts of Solanacea plants, such as jimson weed, black henbane, and mandrake, were used in Europe in the Middle Ages in the preparation of special ointments by witches. The ointments were applied to the mucous membranes of the genital organs to produce a condition of ecstasy and erotic feeling. Jimson weed was also known to the native people of North and Latin America. The Aztecs worshipped the plant and used it for cult purposes and for punishments. A special application was the insertion of rolled-up leaves into the anus. Beside cult purposes, Solanacea plants have also been extensively used for murdering people.

Plant Toxins with Action on Sympathetic Nerves

The plant *Ephedra distachya* L. (joint fir), which occurs mainly in Mediterranean areas, contains the alkaloid ephedrine (Fig. 43), which acts in a way similar to norepinephrine. The compound is also in the horsetail-like shrub *Catha edulis* (Vahl) Forsskal ex Endl (khat). Because of its stimulating action, chewing of the khat leaves is common in countries of the Middle East and North Africa. The pharmacological action of ephedrine is due to the liberation of norepinephrine in the peripheral nerve endings and of norepinephrine, serotonine, and dopamine in the CNS. This produces an increase in attention and fitness and a decrease in tiredness and hunger. Chronic use of the drug causes addiction and tolerance (tachyphylaxia). Sweating, mydriasis, insomnia, retention of urine, and constipation occur after overdosing on the drug. Toxic

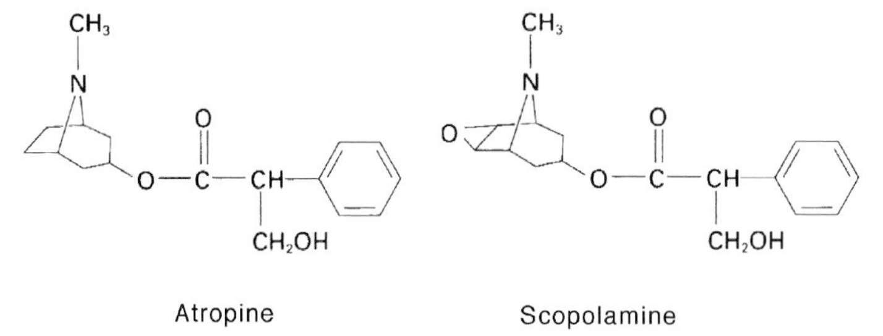

FIGURE 42 Tropa alkaloids.

doses lead to convulsions, shock, and respiratory arrest.

Other plant compounds with action on the sympathetic system are indol alkaloids occurring in *Rauvolfia serpentina* (L.) Benth. ex Kurz (serpentine wood). The most important derivative is reserpine (Fig. 44). The compound acts by an inhibition of the re-uptake of norepinephrine into the vesicles of sympathetic nerve endings, which are gradually depleted. The resulting decrease of sympathetic reactions was used for the treatment of hypertension. Because of the central symptoms, consisting of sedation and depression, the drug was replaced by synthetic compounds with less central side effects. Toxic doses lead to bradycardia, arrhythmia, and finally heart arrest.

Plant-derived compounds with spasmolytic action are papaverine and narcotine, both occurring in *Papaver somniferum* L. (opium poppy) and khellin, a component of *Visnaga daucoides* Gaertn. or *Ammi visnaga* (toothpickweed) (Fig. 45). The compounds, which act as inhibitors of the calcium flux through the membrane of smooth muscle cells, are used pharmaceutically for the treatment of spasms in various smooth-muscle-containing hollow organs. Overdosing causes severe hypotension and heart paralysis.

Plant Toxins with Action on Striped Muscles

These are divided into compounds causing paralysis and those convulsions. Among the paralytic-acting compounds is curare, a mixture of alkaloids occurring in the tropic climber *Chondrodendron tomentosum* Ruiz & Pavon. The active principles (+)- tubocurarin and C-toxiferin I (Fig. 46) act as inhibitors of acetylcholine receptors at the neuromuscular endplate. The Indians in the South American jungles impregnate hunting darts with extracts of the plant. After the toxin has entered the blood stream, the victim is paralyzed almost immediately. Both toxins are very potent. The LD_{50} of tubocurarin in mice after application is 130 μg/kg; it is only 23 μg/kg for C-toxiferin. As quaternary ammonium salts, the compounds are not absorbed after oral ingestion. Animals killed by curare darts are, therefore, edible without danger of being poisonous, as long as the epithelium of the GI tract is

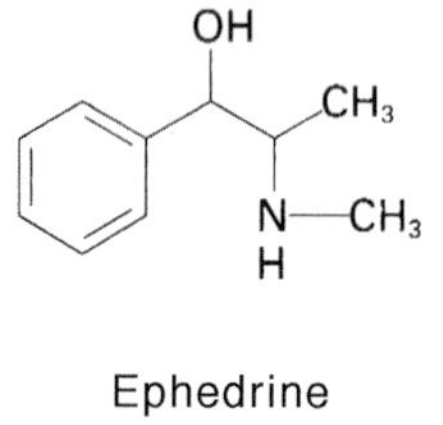

FIGURE 43 Ephedrine, the active principle of *Ephedra distachya* L. (*E. vulgaris*, joint fir).

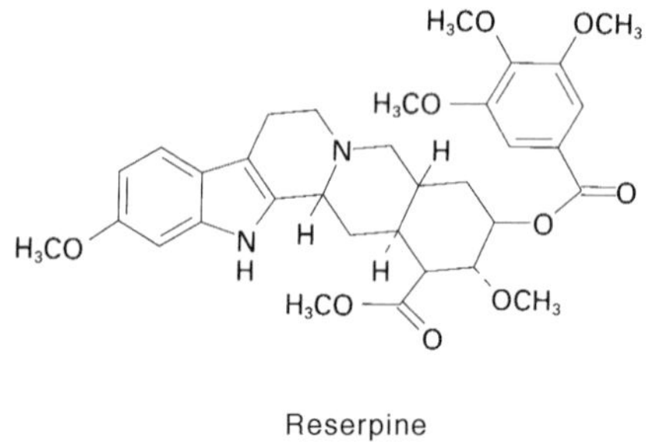

FIGURE 44 Reserpine, the most important indole alkaloid of *Rauvolfia serpentina* (L.) Benth. ex Kurz.

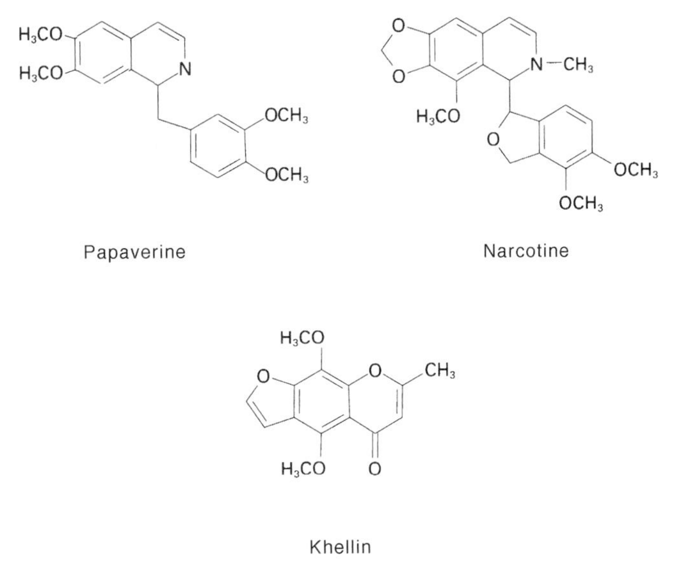

Papaverine

Narcotine

Khellin

FIGURE 45 Compounds with action on the calcium flux of smooth muscle cells.

intact. If sufficient amounts of the toxins enter the circulatory system, a rapid paralysis of all striped muscles occurs. Suffocation occurs as a result of the inability to contract the diaphragm. The use of tubocurarin as a muscle relaxant in surgery was abolished because of the histamine release, leading sporadically to anaphylactic reactions.

Another compound with paralytic action is coniin (Fig. 47), occurring in *Conium maculatum* L. (poison hemlock) and *Aethusa cynapium* L. (fool's parsley). The volatile compound is distributed in all parts of the plants. Concentrations up to 3.5% occur in the seeds of poison hemlock. The bad smell of coniin, which is similar to the urine of mice, prevents the ingestion of the plant by humans in most cases. Intoxication is more common in greasing animals. The ancient Greeks used extracts of the poison hemlock for executions. The most famous case was the execution of Socrates (399 A.D.), precisely reported by his friend Plato. The lethal dose for adult humans is approxi-

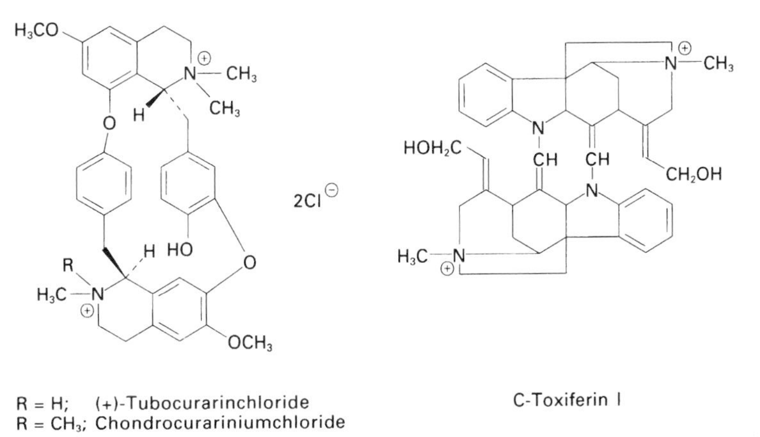

R = H; (+)-Tubocurarinchloride
R = CH_3; Chondrocurariniumchloride

C-Toxiferin I

FIGURE 46 Tubocurarin and c-toxiferin I, the toxic principles of curare.

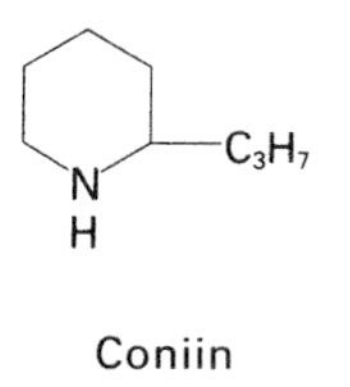

FIGURE 47 Coniin, the toxic principle of *Conium maculatum* L. (poison hemlock) and *Aethusa cynapium* L. (fool's parsley).

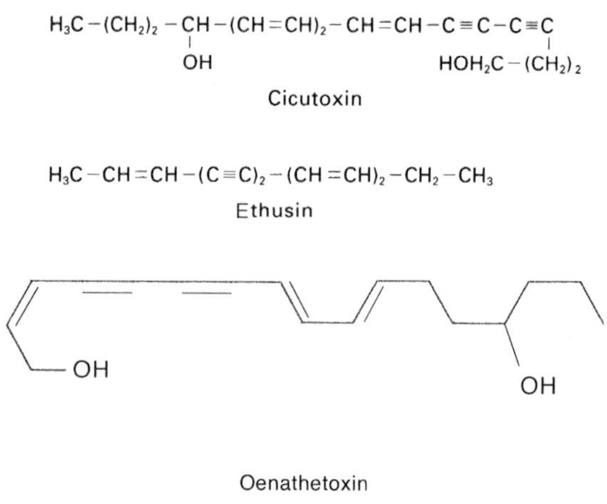

FIGURE 49 Toxic polyinols. Cicutoxin (*Cicuta virosa* L.), Oenanthotoxin (*Oenanthe crocata* L.), Ethusin (*Aethusa cynapium* L.).

mately 500 mg coniin. The compound is easily absorbed by the GI tract and also through the skin. After uptake of toxic doses, the symptoms of intoxication begin with a short period of excitement followed by paralysis, starting at the lower extremities and rising slowly to the head. When the paralysis reaches the diaphragm, death occurs by suffocation. Because consciousness is not affected, the victim experiences all phases of the intoxication until the end. Coniin exerts teratogenic effects in animals.

The convulsive compounds are divided into those acting at the medulla and the spinal cord. Among the central-acting compounds is picrotoxin, occurring in the seeds of the Asiatic climber *Anamirta cocculus* Wight et Arnott (levent berry, cockles). Picrotoxin is a mixture of two components, the toxic compound picrotoxinin and the nontoxic compound picrotin (Fig. 48). Because aquatic animals are extremely sensitive to the toxin, extracts of the plant have been used by native people for catching fish. Picrotoxin is used medicinally as an analeptic. Doses <10 mg stimulate the respiration and the vasomotor center. This effect is

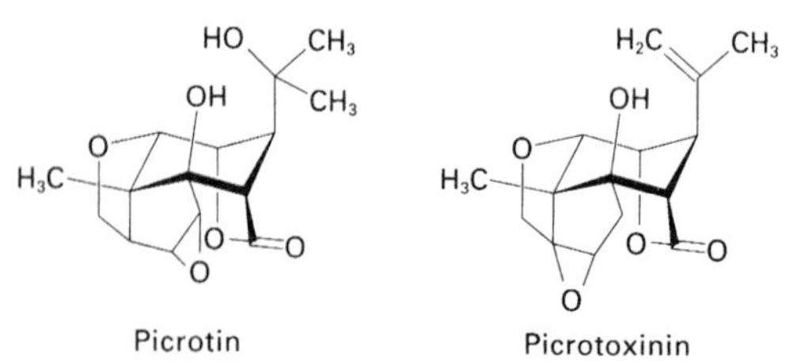

FIGURE 48 Pikrotoxin. The compound is a mixture of two components, picrotin (inactive) and picrotoxinin (toxic).

used for the treatment of beginning respiratory arrest. Toxic doses cause convulsions, similar to epilepsy. The LD_{50} in mice (iv) is 4 mg/kg.

Cicuta virosa L. (Mackenzie's water hemlock) is one of the most toxic plants, growing in swampy areas of the moderate zones. The bulbs, which look similar to celery bulbs, contain a light yellow-orange juice located in caverns. The whole plant, especially the bulb contains the toxic polyinol cicutoxin (Fig. 49). Poisoning occurs mainly by children who mistakenly eat the bulb. The plant was also used for suicide or homicide. Cicutoxin, like picrotoxin, causes excitement of the medulla. A single bite into the bulb of cicuta may be lethal. The symptoms of poisoning are extreme torment. Very painful epileptiform seizures occur every 15–20 minutes and lead to total exhaustion (ATP depletion). Death occurs by heart or respiratory arrest.

The toxic polyinol oenanthotoxin (Fig. 49) is present in *Oenanthe crocata* L. (waterdropwort). The bulbs of this plant have a pleasant pastinak-like taste. The LD_{50} of the toxin for mice (iv) is less than 1 mg/kg. *Aethusa cynapium* L. (fool's parsley) contains an unsaturated aliphatic hydrocarbon, ethusin (Fig. 49), together with the paralyzing toxin coniin. Intoxication sometimes occurs by the erroneous use of the plant instead of parsley (*Petroselinum crispum* L.). The symptoms of intoxication depend on the proportion of the two toxins in the plant and may be either paralysis or convulsion.

Strychnine and brucine (Fig. 50), two related toxins occurring in *Strychnus nux vomica* L. (poison-nut tree) and *Strychnus ignatii* Berg., act at the medulla spinalis.

Like picrototoxin, strychnine is used as an analeptic. Because of the easy access (strychnine was used as a rodenticide) and its toxic potential (the lethal amount is 100 mg for adults and 1–5 mg for children), the toxin was often used in homicide. Strychnine and brucine inhibit post-synaptic inhibitory neurons, thus intensifying central neural impulses. Small doses cause an increase of sensory perceptions, whereas tetanoid convulsions occur after uptake of toxic doses. Episodic convulsions occur either spontaneously or after minimal external stimuli, such as noise, light, or touching. Isolation of the patient in a dark quiet room is, therefore, an essential part of the therapy. Death occurs by central vasomotor or respiratory inhibition.

Compounds with Hypnotic or Psychotropic Action

Hypnotics

The coagulated juice of the incised seed capsules of *Papaver somniferum* L. (opium poppy), known as opium, contains about 20 alkaloids of the phenantrene or isoquinoline type. The spasmolytic-acting isoquinoline derivatives papaverine and narcotine have already been discussed. The phenanthrene derivatives in opium, represented by morphine, codeine, and thebaine (Fig. 51), act as hypnotics, analgesics, and psychotropics. Especially the last property is responsible for the abuse of opium for thousands of years. The use of opium was reported 4000 years ago by the Sumerians and later by the ancient Egyptians, Greeks, and Romans. Paracelsus (1493–1541) named opium "laudanum" and used it for many medicinal purposes. In the 19th century, opium advanced to a fashionable drug, especially among poets. The list of opium users includes Friedrich Schlegel, Novalis, E.T.A. Hoffmann, Edgar Allen Poe, and Charles Baudelair.

Morphine is used in modern medicine as an effective central analgesic, whereas codeine is mainly used as an antitussive agent. Morphine and its derivatives act as agonists of the opioid (endorphine) receptors, which belong to the endogenic analgesic system. Long-time use leads to tolerance and addiction.

Poisoning by opium alkaloids is not rare and mainly due to the widespread abuse of narcotics, especially of the semisynthetic morphine analog heroin (Fig. 51). The diacetylation of the two hydroxygroups in morphine increases the lipophilicity. Heroin, therefore, enters the central nervous system more rapidly than morphine and the psychotropic action is more pronounced. Opium alkaloids easily pass through the placenta, causing tolerance and addiction in the newborn infant. The compounds are also excreted in the milk. It is, however, not clear, whether the doses are high enough to affect the nursling.

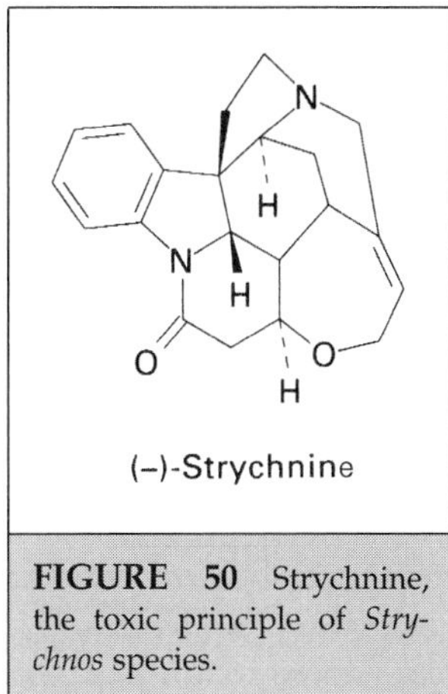

FIGURE 50 Strychnine, the toxic principle of *Strychnos* species.

The symptoms of intoxication occur 30–60 minutes after oral ingestion and almost immediately after the injection of toxic doses of opium alkaloids. They consist of dizziness, drowsiness, general sedation, and increasing depression of respiration. Finally the victim falls into a deep coma. The combination of three symptoms is important for the diagnosis—miosis, respiratory depression, and unconsciousness. The contraction of the pupils is maximal (pin-point pupils) and is released if asphyxia occurs. The sphincters of the intestine and urinary bladder are spastically contracted. Death occurs by central respiratory arrest.

Plant Toxins with Psychotropic Properties

The use of plants with psychotropic properties for ceremonial purposes was common in almost all his-

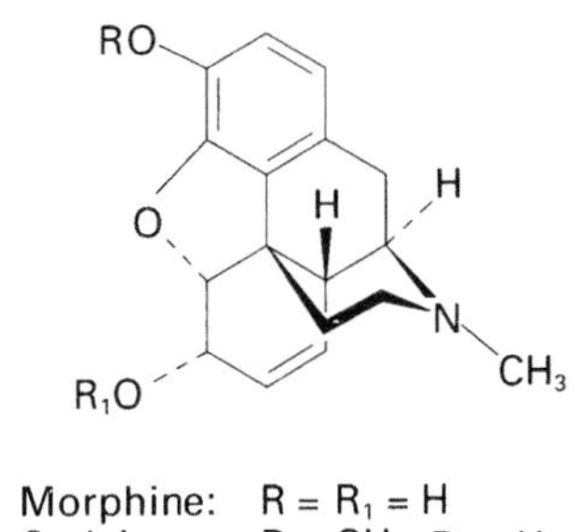

Morphine: $R = R_1 = H$
Codeine: $R = CH_3$; $R_1 = H$
Thebaine: $R = R_1 = CH_3$
Heroin: $R = R_1 = COCH_3$

FIGURE 51 Opium alkaloids, occurring in *Papaver somniferum* L. (opium poppy).

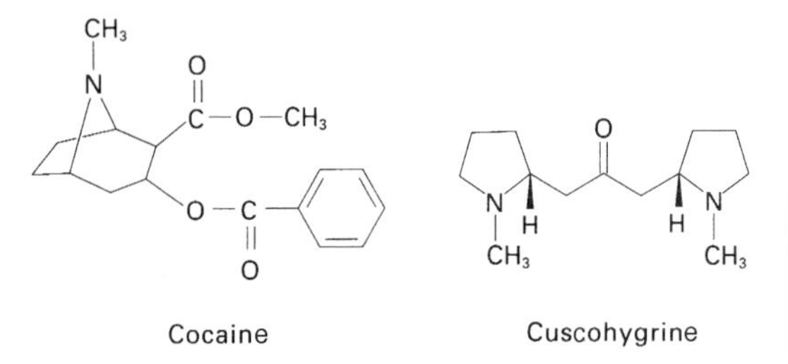

Cocaine Cuscohygrine

FIGURE 52 Coca alkaloids, occurring in *Erythroxylum coca* Lam (coca).

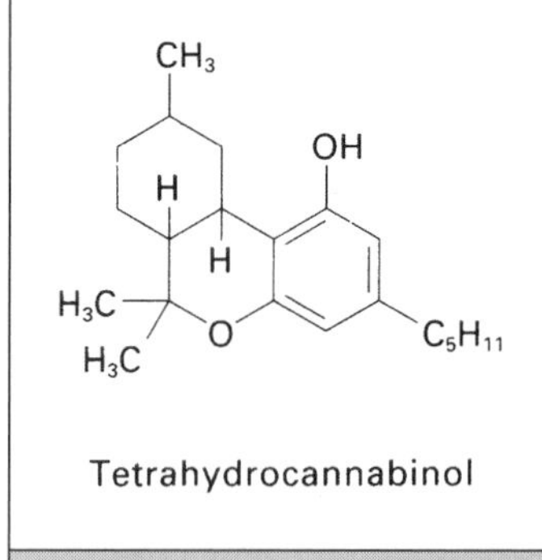

FIGURE 53 Δ-9-10-Tetrahydrocannabinol, occuring in *Cannabis sativa* L. *ssp. indica* (Indian hemp).

torical cultures. The drugs were used help to get into contact with demons and the spirits of deceased relatives. The use of such drugs has never ceased and most modern nations have considerable problems with the abuse of psychotropic drugs. Although the trade in and even the possession of many psychotropic drugs are prohibited, the money earned by illegal trade in such compounds exceeds that of the most legal therapeutics by far.

In the hot and humid highlands of South America and Java grows the shrub *Erytroxylum coca* Lam. (coca). The leaves contain 0.7–2.5% alkaloids, mainly consisting of (-)-cocaine and cuskohygrin (Fig. 52). Although chemically related to atropine, cocaine is devoid of parasympatholytic properties. The compound inhibits the re-uptake of norepinephrine into axonic vesicles and is, therefore, adrenergic. It also inhibits the catecholamine-degrading enzyme monoaminooxidase (MAO). Especially after parenteral application (sniffing), it leads to excitation, euphoria, and hallucinations. The active oral dose is 50 mg, whereas much lower amounts are sufficient if taken by nasal application. The lethal dose is normally 1–2 g; however, fatal cases have been reported after uptake of only 100–200 mg. The LD_{50} (iv) in rats is 17.5 mg/kg. The symptoms of intoxication consist of psychic exitement, convulsions, and, finally, respiratory arrest. On the mucous membranes and after subcutaneous injection, cocaine acts as a local anesthetic. This action is no longer used medicinally, but it is still useful for a simple identification of the drug; cocaine causes a feeling of numbness after contact with the tongue.

Great amounts of cocaine are produced in illegal laboratories. For this purpose, the leaves are used for extraction first with diluted hydrochloric acid. The hydrolyzed ester alkaloids are then isolated, esterified with methanol, and then benzoylated. Great amounts of pure cocaine are produced in Colombia, Bolivia, and Peru, from where it is illegally transported to the black markets of North America and Europe. Cocaine leads to an addiction similar to that of opium alkaloids. Chronic abuse leads to physical and mental destruction. Consuming cocaine during pregnancy increases the incidence of malformations considerably.

The Indians of South America chew coca leaves after mixing them with lime or bone ash. This leads to a hydrolysis of the ester alkaloids. The resulting ecgonin exerts a stimulating effect similar to that of caffeine and decreases the feeling of hunger, which is important for poor people, such as the Indians in South America. In contrast to the parenteral application of cocaine, the chewing of coca does not produce addiction.

Canabis sativa L. ssp, Indica (Indian hemp) is used for the production of the psychedelic drugs marijuana (from the dry tips of the female plant) and hashish (from the brown resin made from the leaves and flowers of the female plant). The main areas of cultivation are the Middle East, India, and Mexico. The psychotropic actions are caused by the compound Δ-9,10-tetrahydrocannabinol (THC) (Fig. 53). The drug is most effectively used as a mixture of marijuana or hashish with tobacco and smoked in cigarettes ("joints") or pipes. A dose of 1 g of marijuana or 0.3 g of hashish, containing 5–20 mg THC, is necessary for one "trip." The drug is also effective after oral ingestion (as a tea); however, greater amounts are necessary because of the less-effective absorption. The action of the drug consists of euphoria and hallucinations. Overdosing may result in long-acting psychiatric disorders and unpredictable reactions ("horror trips"). Whether the drug causes addiction is a matter for discussion; however, marijuana consumers often change to stronger drugs, such as heroine and cocaine.

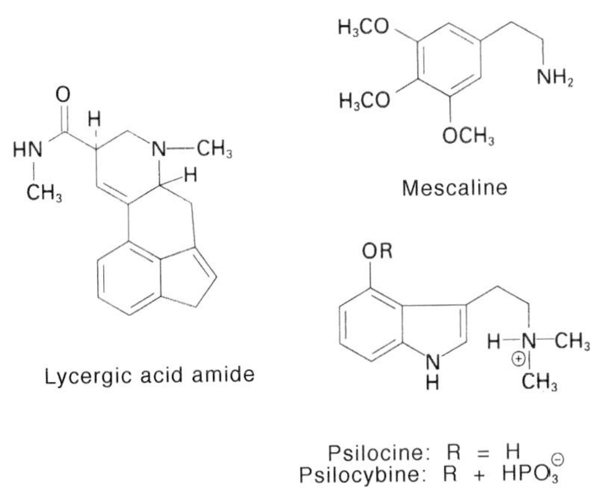

Lycergic acid amide

Mescaline

Psilocine: R = H
Psilocybine: R + $HPO_3^{\ominus}$

FIGURE 54 Psychedelic drugs with tryptaminergic action.

The Indians of North and Central America used a cactus that they called peyotl for cult ceremonies. Its psychotropic action is caused by mescaline (Fig. 54). Because of its relatively simple chemical structure, mescaline was synthesized in great amounts, mainly around 1970 and used instead of the more potent LSD as a psychedelic drug during the "hippie movement" (by the "people of flower power"). The effective dose is 200–500 mg. Today mescaline has been almost completely replaced by much more potent derivatives, such as 4-methyl-2,5,dimethoxy-α-methylphenylethylamine (DOM). The action of mescaline and DOM is comparable to that of LSD and caused by its action on central tryptamine receptors. It consists mainly of spectral and acoustic visions, as well as an increased sense of touch. Mescaline was demonstrated to be teratogenic in animal experiments.

Similar symptoms are produced by psilocybine (Fig. 54), occurring in the mushroom *Psilocybe mexicana* Heims, which grows in Mexico. With an effective dose of 10 mg, psilocybine is much more potent than mescaline. The symptoms after the ingestion of psilocybine are similar to that of mescaline and LSD and are also due to an action on central tryptamine receptors. Like mescaline, psilocybine was shown to be teratogenic in laboratory animals. Other tryptamine derivatives occur in the seeds of a tree growing at the Orinoco river and on the isle of Trinidad. The tree, known by the native people as Yopo (*Piptadenia peregrina* (L.) Benth.), contains the compounds *N,N*-dimethyltryptamin (DMT) *N*-methyltryptamin, 5-methoxy-*N*-methyltryptamin and *N,N*-dimethyl-5-hydroxytryptamin (bufotenin). The Indians pulverize the seeds, mix it with ash, and blow it in breathe through the nose. The seeds of two winding flowers growing in Mexico, *Rivea corymbosa* L. Hall and *Ipomoea tricolor* Car. (morning glory; Nauhaut, coatlxoxouhqui) contain the amide of lysergic acid, which acts similar to, although less potent than, LSD. The effective dose is 2–10 mg. The native people liked to use the plants for cult ceremonies, as well.

Plant Toxins with Cytotoxic Action

Some *plant*-derived compounds with cytotoxic action have already been discussed earlier in this chapter (the lectines ricin, abrin, and phasin). Colchicine (Fig. 55), occurring in *Colchicum autumnale* L. (autumn crocus) acts as an inhibitor of cell mitosis. It is a very potent poison. The lethal dose is 20 mg for adults and 5 mg for children. After ingestion of the plant, the first symptoms of poisoning occur 2–6 hours later and consist of severe gastrointestinal irritation with vomiting and diarrhea. An advancing paralysis occurs af-

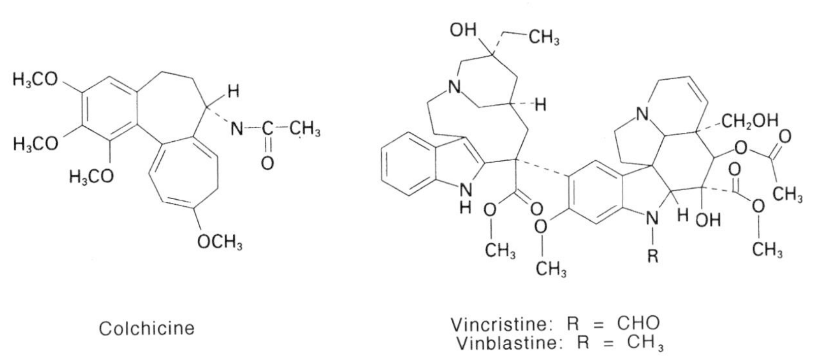

Colchicine

Vincristine: R = CHO
Vinblastine: R = CH_3

FIGURE 55 Plant toxins causing mitotic arrest.

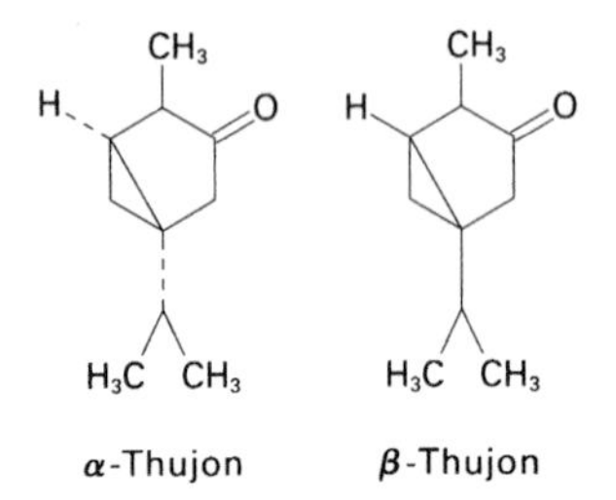

CH3 CH3 H O H O H3C CH3 H3C CH3

α-Thujon β-Thujon

FIGURE 56 Thujon occurring in *Artemisia absinthium* L. (absinthe).

ter the absorption of colchicine. Death occurs after a latent period of 2 days by respiratory arrest. The consciousness is retained until the end. Cochicine reacts with cellular tubulin, causing a depolymerization of the microtubules. The mitosis is inhibited during the anaphase. This property is used in tissue culture for the investigation of chromosomes.

A similar action is caused by the vinca alkaloids (Fig. 55), occurring in the shrub *Catharantus roseus* (L.) G. Don. Vincristine and vinblastine are used as chemotherapeutic agents in the treatment of cancer. Both compounds have severely toxic side effects, consisting mainly in neurotoxic reactions with sometimes irreversible paresthesia. Both compounds cause leukopenia, which is more pronounced after the application of vinblastine and is dose limiting.

Among the monoterpenes there are also compounds with a high cytotoxic potential. Most important is thujon (Fig. 56), present in *Thuja occidentalis* L. (Eastern arborvitae) and *Artemisia absinthium* L. (absinthe) Acute intoxication causes severe irritation of the GI tract, as well as kidney and liver damage. Finally paralysis of the central nervous system occurs. Chronic intoxication was common in the 1800s from the drinking of absinthe, an alcoholic beverage made by the distillation of brandy over vermouth, anise, and fennel. In this case, the symptoms of intoxication consist in the degeneration of the brain, leading to a total mental and physical disintegration. Today the production of and trade in absinthe are prohibited.

Plant Toxins with Skin-Irritating and Allergic Actions

Skin irritation and allergic skin reactions from plants or plant products are common and of growing concern because of the increasing popularity of "natural" cosmetics and skin-care products. Skin-irritating plants cause inflammation reactions without the involvement of immune reactions. These actions are produced, for example, by amines, such as acetylcholine, histamine, or serotonin, occurring in the bristles of *Urtica dioica* L. (stinging nettle). The tips of the silicated bristles break upon contact with the skin and the pointed stalks penetrate the skin. The amines cause erythema and itching. Severe symptoms, even fatal shock reactions, may occur if large areas of the skin are involved.

The milk of several Euphorbiaceae contains compounds that release histamine and other neuroactive amines from endogene reservoirs, such as mast cells. The chemical structures consist mainly in di- and triterpenes. Among these compounds are also the phorbol esters, which are known as potent tumor-promoting agents. Plant-derived enzymes are also able to cause skin irritation. Examples are papain, occurring in the fruit of *Carica papaya* L. (papaya) and bromelin, occuring in *Ananas comosus* L. Merr. (pineapple).

Plants with Allergenic Potential

Contact with such plants causes a sensitizing reaction with participation of T lymphocytes. Lymphokines and cytokines are liberated after repeated contact with plant allergens and are responsible for inflammation reactions and the occurrence of eczema. About 10,000 plant species with an allergenic potential are known so far. Most belong to the family *Asteraceae* (former Compositae). Of special concern are species of the family *Anarcardiaceae.* Some species, such as *Rhus toxicodendron* L. (poison ivy), are among the most potent allergenic plants that exist.

Contact allergies are often caused by garden plants, such as *Primula vulgaris* Huds. (English primrose), *Tulipa sylvestris* L. (tulip), and *Chrysanthemum frutescens* L. (marguerite); food plants, such as *Helianthus annuus* L. (common sunflower), *Humulus lupulus* L. (common hops), and *Cynara scolymus* L. (globe artichoke); and many medicinal plants (see Table 8). The increasing popularity and uncontrolled use of herbal remedies promotes the occurrence of allergies to medicinal plants. An example is *Arnica montana* L. (mountain arnica). Tinctures prepared from the blossoms of the plant are used internally as well as externally for all kinds of injury. The poisonous compounds are sesquiterpene lactones (Fig. 57). Severe skin irritation with bullous blisters may occur after external use of extracts that are too concentrated. Internal overdosing results in irritation of the mucous membranes. After absorption, the sesquiterpene lactones cause headache, and cardiovascular and respiratory disorders.

TABLE 8 Medicinal Plants with Allergenic Potential[a]

Plant	Potency	Frequency of allergy occurrence
Anthemis cotula L. (stinking chamomile)	Strong	Occasional
Arnica montana L. (Mountain arnica)	Strong	Frequent
Cinnamomum zeylanicum (Cinnamon tree)	Moderate	Frequent
Hedera helix L. (English ivy)	Moderate	Occasional
Helianthus annuus L. (sunflower)	Moderate	Occasional
Inula helenium L. (Elecampane inula)	Strong	Occasional
Rhus toxicodendron L. (poison ivy)	Very strong	Rare (in Europe); frequent (in the United States)

[a]According to Hausen (1988).

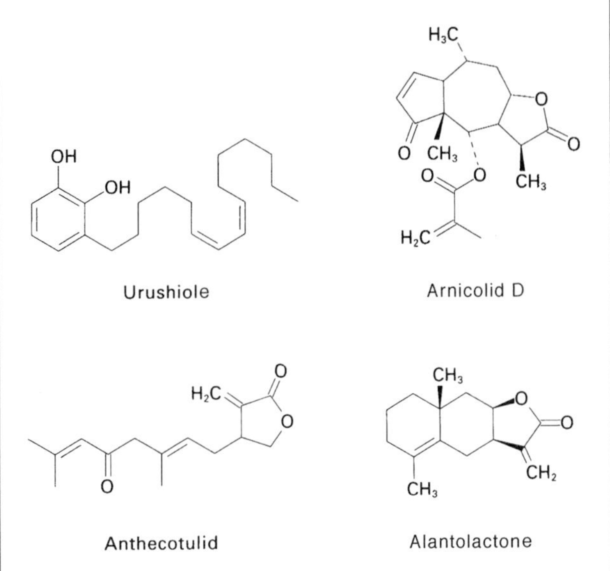

FIGURE 57 Plant-derived compounds that are often subject of contact allergy. Urushioles, a mixture of alkylcatecholes with side chains differing in length and number of double bonds are the toxic principles of *Rhus toxicodendron* L. The example shown is one of the most toxic derivatives. Arnicolid D is the allergenic principle of *Arnica montana* L. Anthecotulid and alantolactone are contents of *Anthemis cotula* L. (*stinking chamomile*) and *Inula helenium* L.

Fatal cases have been reported. Patients who have had allergic reactions to arnica are often allergic to other plants of the Asteraceae family, as well as to sesquiterpen-containing plants, belonging to other families (e.g., *Calophyllum ssp.*, laurel).

The most potent plant allergen is the milky juice of *Rhus toxicodendron* L. (poison ivy). Even contact with the leaves may result in severe eczema. About 60–80% of the North American population is allergic to this plant. After acquiring an allergy, the symptoms may occur even after the use of homeopathic dilution >D6. Urushioles have been recognized as the toxic and allergenic principles. The compounds are catechol derivatives with aliphatic side chains variable in length and double bonds.

Plants Containing Phototoxic Compounds

Some plants contain compounds that cause dermatitis after contact or ingestion. The symptoms occur after exposure to sunlight as a result of the UVA content. Most of the phototoxic compounds belong to the group of furocoumarines (Fig. 58). In Europe, photodermatitis is often produced by *Heracleum mantegazzianum* Somm. et Lev. (giant hogweed) and *Heracleum sphondylium* L. After injury to the plant, a white juice is released that contains a mixture of furocoumarines. The compounds are activated by wavelengths of 310–320 nm and sometimes cause severe itching and bullous dermatitis after contact with the skin. Healing may take several weeks.

Further plants with phototoxic components are *Ruta graveolens* L. (common rue), *Archangelica officinalis* (Moench) Hoffm. or *Angelica archangelica* (Norwegian angelica), *Peucedanum osthruthium* (L.) W. D. J. Koch (masterwort), *Pastinaca sativa* L. (wild parsnip), and *Dictamnus albus* L. (gas plant). Plants containing phototoxic compounds belonging to the group of anthraquinones are *Hypericum perforatum* L. (common St. Johns wort) and *Fagopyrum esculentum* Moench (buckwheat). The former is a popular medicinal plant, used mainly as a mild sedative, whereas the latter is used as a food plant. Photodermatoses occur after the internal use of *Hypericum* extracts and exposure to sunlight. Fatal cases of phototoxicity were also observed in domestic animals (mainly in horses) after ingestion of wild St. Johns wort.

Carcinogenic and Tumor-Promoting Plant Compounds

A considerable percentage of the known carcinogens are of natural origin. Most are produced by fungi, but some are also synthesized by plants. Al-

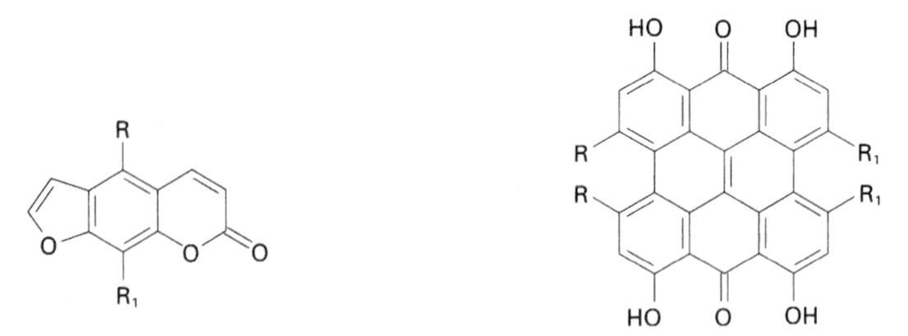

Furocumarine

phototoxic Anthraquinones

Xanthotoxin: R = H, $R_1 = OCH_3$
Bergapten: $R = OCH_3$, $R_1 = H$
Imperatorin: R = H, $R_1 = O{-}CH_2{-}CH{=}C(CH_3)_2$

Fagopyrines: R = OH, $R_1 = CH_2{-}[C_5H_8(CH_3)NO]$
Hypericine: R = OH, $R_1 = CH_3$

FIGURE 58 Plant-derived compounds with phototoxic properties.

most no carcinogens are produced primarily by animals. Natural carcinogens are an important cause of human cancer, possibly exceeding the importance of anthropogenic carcinogens. The occurrence of carcinogenic compounds is not limited to special plant families and extends over the most primitive Pteridophytes (fern) to higher developed Gymnosperms (cycas palms) and the most developed Angiosperms (*Senecio* ssp.). Plant-derived carcinogens also vary greatly with respect to their chemical structures. An overview of the most important compounds is given in Table 9.

Bracken fern (*Pteridium aquilinum* L. Kuhn) is the most important representative of primitive plants with carcinogenic action. The plant is ubiquitous in all temperate and mid-tropic zones of the world and responsible for considerable losses of domestic animals. Many cattle and sheep die after the ingestion of the plant, either from acute poisoning or after the development of esophageal or intestinal tumors. The use of bracken fern as a human food plant was correlated with the incidence of esophageal cancer in Japan. The carcinogenic action is related to aquilide A (Fig. 59). The compound is mutagenic in bacterial systems and carcinogenic in rats.

Cycad plants of the families *Cycas, Zamia, Macrozamia, Bowenia, Enzepaloartos,* and *Stangeria* are endemic in all tropical and subtropical areas of the world. Different parts of the plants are used in the preparation of food and herbal medicine in Africa, Asia, and Central America. The carcinogenic action is related to cycasin (methylazooxymethanol-β-D-gucoside), which occurs especially in some cycas species (*Cycas cirinalis* L. and *Cycas revoluta* Tunb.), used as food plants. Methylazooxymethanol, an ultimate carcinogen, is produced after the cleavage of the glycosidic linkage. The compound, which reacts covalently with DNA, is tumorigenic in laboratory animals after long-term oral treatment. Tumors occur in the liver, kidneys, and intestine.

The chewing of betel quid is popular in Malaya, New Guinea, East Africa, and Madagascar. The total number of betel-chewing people is estimated to about 450 millions. The quid consists of the nuts of the betel palm (*Areca catechu* L.), the green leaves of betel pepper (*Piper betel* L.), and lime ($Ca(OH)_2$). The taste is often refined by the addition of tobacco and spices. Betel-chewing people have an extraordinarily high incidence of esophageal and laryngeal cancer. The action is most probably related to the alkaloid arecoline (Fig. 59), a compound that acts on the parasympathetic nerves. Tannins may also be involved in the carcinogenicity of betel quid.

Alkylbenzene derivatives, such as safrole, isosafrole, estragole, and β-asarone, occur in numerous plants that are used as foods and food additives. Among these are celery, basil, sassafras, anise, carrots, bananas, black pepper, and fermented tobacco. Especially high concentrations of safrole were detected in sassafras oil, produced by steam distillation of the bark and wood of the sassafras tree (*Sassafras albidum* (Nutt) Nees). The addition of safrole or β-asarone to foods or beverages (e.g., root beer and vermouth) is now prohibited. Animal experiments show that the liver is the main target of the carcinogenic action of alkylbenzenes.

Tannin, a mixture of polyphenols, occurs in numerous foods and beverages. High concentrations are usually found in red wine, black tea, and tea prepa-

TABLE 9 Carcinogenic Plant Compounds[a]				
Compound	**Occurrence**	**Species**	**Target organ**	**Source**
Allylisothiocyanat	*Brassica*-ssp.	Mouse	Skin, stomach	Mustard, cabbage, horseradish
Aquilid A	*Pteridium aquilinum*	Rat	Breast, intestine, bladder	Bracken fern
Arecoline	*Areca catechu*	Mouse	Liver, lung, stomach	Betel nuts, drug
Aristolochic acid	*Aristolochia clematitis*	Rat	Stomach, kidney, bladder	Drug
β-Asaron	*Acorus calamus*	Rat	Intestine	Flavoring agent, drug
Asiaticosid	*Centella asiatica*	Mouse	Skin	Externum against wounds
Benzylacetat	*Jasminum* ssp.	Mouse	Forestomach, liver	Perfumes, jasmine tea
Capsaicin	*Capsicum* ssp.	Mouse	Intestine	Chili, red pepper
Crotonoil	*Croton tiglium*	Mouse	Skin	Contact with plant
Coumarin	*Dipteryx odorata, Asperula odorata, Cinammonum cassia Lavendula officinalis*	Rat	Bile duct	Food additive fragrance, drug
Cycasin	*Cycas* ssp., *Zamia* ssp.	Rat	Liver, kidney, intestine, lung, breast, brain, testis	Cycad nuts, starch, drug
		Mouse	Liver, kidney, lung, bone marrow	
		Hamster	Liver, bone marrow	
Estragole	*Artemisia draculuncus Ocimium basilicum, Foeniculum vulgare*	Mouse	Liver	Flavoring agent, fragrance
Gossypol	*Gossypium hirsutum*	Mouse	Skin	Cotton seed oil
Isosafrole	*Cananga odorata*	Rat	Liver, esophagus	Flavoring agent, fragrance
Limonene	*Citrus* ssp.	Mouse	Skin	Citrus oil
Psoralene	*Umbelliferaceae, Rutaceae, Leguminosae, Moraceae, Orchidaceae*	Mouse	Skin	Celery, fig, parsley, drug, cosmetics
(+)Parasorbinic acid	*Sorbus aucuparia*	Rat	Local sarkomas	Jelly
Pyrrolizidinalkaloids				
Clivorine	*Ligularia dentata*	Rat	Liver	
Dehydroheliotridine	*Heliotropium* ssp.	Rat	Multiple organs	Drug
Dehydromonocrotaline	*Crotalaria* ssp.	Mouse	Skin	Drug, food
Dehydroretronecine	*Senecio* ssp.	Rat	Musculature	Drug, food
Heliotrine	*Heliotropium* ssp.	Rat	Pancreas, liver, bladder, testis	Drug
Hydroxysenkirkine	*Tussilago farfara,*	Rat	Brain	Drug, food
Lasiocarpine	*Heliotropium* ssp. *Symphytum* ssp.	Rat	Liver, skin, bone marrow	Drug
Petasitenine	*Petasites japonicus*	Rat	Liver	Drug, food
Isatidine	*Senecio* ssp.	Rat	Liver	Drug, food
Jacobine	*Senecio* ssp.	Chicken	Liver	Drug, food
Lycopsamine	*Amsinckia intermedia*	Rat	Pancreas	Drug, food
Monocrotaline	*Crotalaria* ssp.	Rat	Liver, lung, pancreas	Drug, food
Retronecine	*Senecio* ssp.	Rat	Pituitary, spinal cord	Drug
Retrorsine	*Senecio* ssp.	Rat	Liver, kidney, lung	Drug, food
Riddeline	*Senecio* ssp.	Rat	Liver	Drug, food
Senkirkine	*Tussilago farfara*	Rat	Liver	Drug
Symphytine	*Symphytum officinale*	Rat	Liver, kidney, lung	Drug, food
Reserpine	*Rauvolfia serpentina*	Rat	Liver, adrenal, bone marrow	Drug
Rotenone	*Derris* ssp., *Tephrosia* ssp. *Lonchocarpus* ssp.	Rat	Breast, thyroid gland parathyroid gland	Piscicide, insecticide
Safrole	*Sassafras albidum, Illicium anisatum, Myrisitica fragrans Cinammonum* ssp	Rat	Liver	Root beer
		Mouse	Liver, lung	Sassafras tea, natural drugs, black pepper, nutmeg
Sanguinarine	*Argemone mexicana*	Rat	Bladder	Drug, food oil
Shikimic acid	numerous plants	Mouse	Stomach, bone marrow	Green plants
Sterculic acid	*Sterculia foetida Hibiscus syriacus*	Trout	Liver	Cotton seed oil
Tannines	*Cammellia sinensis, Acacia mollissima, Hammamelis virginiana, Pteridium aquilinum, Areca catechu*	Rat	Liver	Tea, red wine, fruits, vegetables, leather industry
		Mouse	Liver, bladder	
Thiourea	*Laburnum* ssp.	Rat	Liver, thyroid gland	Drug, fungicides
		Mouse	Thyroid gland	Textile-, paper-, photo-industry, cosmetics
		Trout	Liver	

[a] According to Lai und Woo (1987).

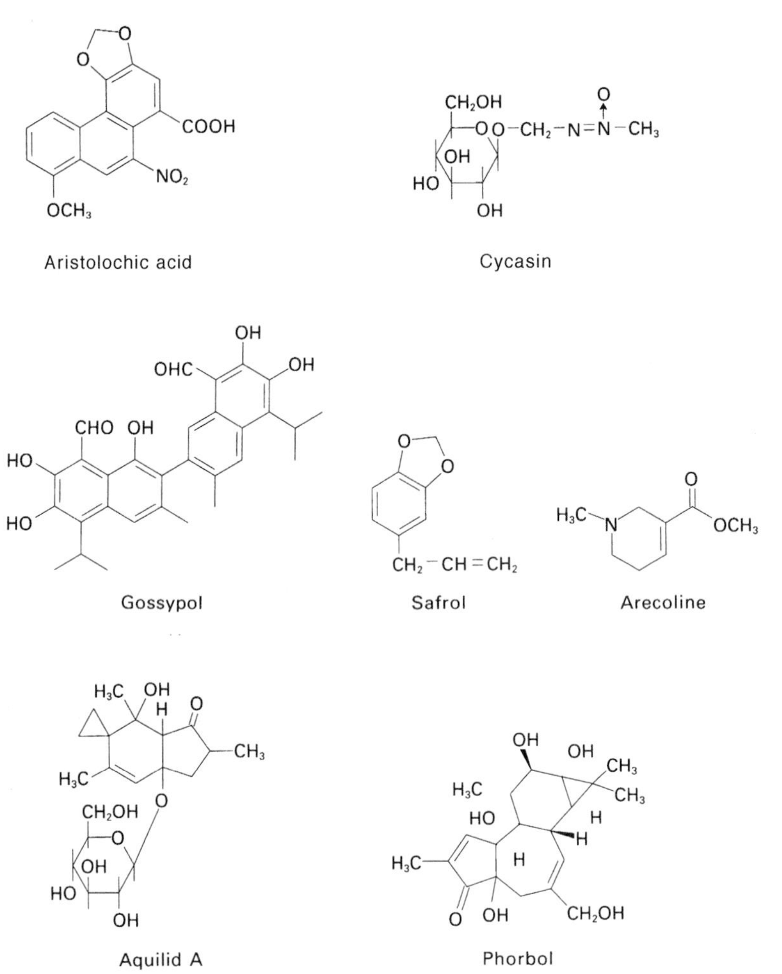

Aristolochic acid

Cycasin

Gossypol

Safrol

Arecoline

Aquilid A

Phorbol

FIGURE 59 Carcinogenic plant compounds. Examples of plant compounds with carcinogenic action in laboratory animals.

rations of mate (*Ilex paraguariensis* A. St. Hil.), cacao (*Theobroma cacao* L.), and khat (*Catha edulis* (Vahl) Forsskal ex Endl.). Numerous epidemiological investigations suggest a correlation between the uptake of tannin and the occurrence of liver and esophageal cancer. The incidence of liver cancer is much higher in countries with a high consumption of red wine (e.g., France, Greece, and Italy), compared with those with a consumption of predominantly white wine (e.g., Germany). The gauchos of Rio Grande do Sul (Brazil) have a high incidence of esophageal cancer. A correlation with the use of mate, a stimulating tea prepared from the leaves of *Ilex paraguariensis* A. St. Hil., rich in tannin, is most probable. A high incidence of esophageal cancer occurs also in people living in East Africa, where the chewing of khat is common. The carcinogenic action of tannin was demonstrated in rats.

Another polyphenol with carcinogenic properties is gossypol (Fig. 59), occurring in cotton seed oil, which is used for cooking in some countries (e.g., Egypt). Gossypol in a dose of 10 mg/day is an effective inhibitor of the spermatogenesis. About 10,000 men in China have been treated experimentally with the compound as a contraceptive. Gossypol was shown to act as a potent tumor promoter in the mouse skin model.

Many medicinal plants contain carcinogenic compounds, for example, pyrrolizidine alkaloid-containing plants, such as *Tussilago farfara* L. (coltsfoot), *Petasites hydridus* L. (pestilence wort), *Symphytum officinale* L. (common comfrey), and many *Senecio* ssp (ragwort). The compounds are metabolized in the liver to toxic pyrrole derivatives, which form covalent adducts with the DNA of liver cells (Fig. 38). The hepatocarcinogenic action of pyrrolizidine alkaloids, such as senkirkine, hydroxysenkirkine, senecionine, lasiocarpine, monocrotaline, dehydromonocrotaline, retrorsine, retronecine, isatidine, riddeline, lycopsamine, intermedine, jacobine, and seneciphylline, was demonstrated in numerous animal studies.

A carcinogenic nitro compound of plant origin is aristolochic acid (Fig. 59), occurring in *Aristolochia clematitis* L. (birthwort), a plant with a long tradition as a herbal medicine. The compound was shown to produce DNA adducts and gastric tumors in rats. The preparation of drugs from birthwort is prohibited in many countries, whereas other medicinal plants with carcinogenic ingredients are still in use. Among these are plants containing pyrrolizidine alkaloids and anthraquinones.

Phorbolesters (Fig. 59) belong to the most powerful tumor-promoting agents known. They occur in plants of the family Euphorbiaceae, especially in the seeds of *Croton tiglium* L. (purging croton). Ingestion of croton oil causes severe irritation of the gastrointestinal mucosa, with vomiting and diarrhea. Irritation also occurs after epidermal contact with croton oil. The ingestion of four seeds of croton may be lethal for humans. The inflammation reactions are mediated by prostaglandins and reactive oxygen species, which are most probably also responsible for the tumor-promoting activity of croton oil.

Bibliography

De Smet P. A. G. M., Keller, K., Hänsel, R., and Chandler, R. F. (eds.) (1993). "Adverse Effects of Herbal Drugs" Vol. I and II. Springer Verlag, Berlin.

Frohne, D. and Pfänder, H. J. (1983). "Giftpflanzen. Ein Handbuch für Apotheker, Artzte, Toxikologen und Biologen," 2nd ed. Wiss. Verlagsgesellschaft, Stuttgart.

Habermehl, G. (1985). "Mitteleuropäische Giftpflanzen und ihre Wirkstoffe." Springer-Verlag, Berlin.

Habermehl, G. (1987). "Gift-Tiere und ihre Waffen" (Toxic Animals and Their Weapons 4th ed. Springer Verlag, Berlin.

Harding, K. A., and Welch, K. R. G. (1980). "Venomous Snakes of the World: A Check List." Pergamon Press, Elmsford, NY.

Hausen, B. (1988). "Allergiepflanzen, Pflanzenallergene. Handbuch und Atlas der allergieinduzierenden Wild- und Kulturpflanzen." Ecomed, Landsberg.

Mebs, D. (1992). "Gifttiere" (*Toxic Animals*). Wissenschaftl Verlagsgesellschaft, Stuttgart.

Lai, D. Y., and Woo Y. (1987). Naturally occurring carcinogens: An overview. *J. Environ. Sci. Ilth.* **C5(2),** 121–173.

Roth, L., Daunderer, M., and Korman, K. (1988). "Giftpflanzen, Pflanzengifte. Vorkommen, Wirkung, Therapie, Allergische und phototoxische Reaktionen," 3rd ed. Ecomed, Landsberg.

Roth, L., Frank, H., and Korman, K. (1990). "Giftpilze-Pilzgifte. Schimmelpilze Mykotoxine. Vorkommen, Inhaltssoffe, Pilzallergien, Nahrungsmittelvergiftungen." Ecomed, Landsberg.

Russel, F. E. (1980). "Snake Venom Poisonining." Lippincott, Philadelphia, PA. (Reprinted Scholium International, Great Neck, NY., 1983).

Ueno, Y. (1985). The toxicology of mycotoxins. *Crit. Rev. Toxicol.* **14,** 99–132.

CHAPTER

41

Bacterial Toxins

HANS BIGALKE, HANS-HERBERT WELLHÖNER

Medical School of Hanover, Department of Pharmacology and Toxicology, Hanover, Germany

INTRODUCTION

Microorganisms produce various kinds of substances not necessary for their own metabolism but which, however, facilitate infiltration into the host and provide advantages over competitors. Not only microorganisms, such as yeast, other fungi, and bacteria, but also the host could be impaired by these products that belong to a wide variety of chemical classes. Many of these compounds have gained entry into the field of practical medicine. Aminoglycosides, for example, inhibit bacterial protein biosynthesis and protect their producers from falling prey to other organisms; they are also valuable antibiotics. Streptokinase, a streptococcal protease, promotes bacterial spread in tissue by cleaving fibrin, which is involved in encapsulating bacterial infiltrations. The capacity for fibrinolysis can also be exploited for therapeutic purposes such as the reopening of clotted blood vessels. Cholera and pertussis toxins from *Vibrio cholera* and *Bordetella pertussis,* respectively, are used in experimental medicine to investigate intracellular signal transfer.

Occasionally, bacteria protect their hosts by preventing them from being consumed by other organisms. They infiltrate the host's tissue with substances that are nontoxic to the host but that may constitute a deadly poison to a careless consumer. In this way, shellfish could be enriched with saxitoxin, which is produced by bacteria living endosymbiotically with the algae upon which shellfish feed. The toxin does not impair the shellfish, but it will endanger the gourmet feasting on them. Similarly, tetrodotoxin, a poison found in the pufferfish, is not produced by the fish itself, but by a species of *Pseudomonas* that infects its skin. Toxic derivatives of this substance are also synthesized by other bacteria, such as *Micrococcus, Alteromonas,* and *Acinetobacter,* living in symbioses with both terrestrial and aquatic animals. The presence of tetrodotoxin in *Atelopus* and *Taricha* protects them from prospective carnivores.

Toxins can also be synthesized by bacterial enzymes in decaying organisms. The most common fish poisoning is due to histamine being formed from histidine by a bacterial decarboxylase released into the fish muscle.

This chapter will deal only with bacterial products that are secreted by the microorganism, are toxic to humans, and have a specific action at the cellular level. Substances of low toxicity, deriving from the extracellular activity of bacterial enzymes, will not be discussed. Toxins produced in animals by endosymbiotic bacteria are described elsewhere.

CLASSIFICATION OF BACTERIAL TOXINS

Bacterial toxins are pathogenic factors. They can be divided into endotoxins and exotoxins.

Endotoxins derive from decaying gram-negative bacteria. They are constituents of the bacterial cell wall and belong to the chemical class of lipopolysaccharides. They provoke nonspecific inflammation by stimulating macrophages to release mediators, such as prostaglandins, thromboxans, free radicals, and interleukins. These mediators cause fever, disseminated intravascular coagulation, and shock. The endotoxins do not directly participate in the toxic reactions, but they induce nonspecific responses of the immune system that are identical for all endotoxins, irrespective of their bacterial origins.

Exotoxins are synthesized and released by some bacterial species. In the majority of cases, these are proteins whose sequences are encoded by a phage or plasmid. The synthesis of the toxins is not essential for the bacteria. Individuals of the same species, which either possess or lack the phage or plasmid, exist side by side, and both are infectious. Various species of bacteria can be transfected with the toxin-encoding phages under laboratory conditions and then become producers of the poison.

Thus, the capability of producing exotoxins can be transferred to other individuals or species, although it is of no vital importance to the organism. In contrast, endotoxins are essential for the integrity of the bacterial cell wall and also responsible for its ability to infect. The classification into endo- and exotoxins is historical and was intended to show the origin of the toxin. Both endo- and exotoxins, however, can be released by perishing bacteria and may induce inflammation and other immune responses.

The exotoxins bind specifically to receptors in the plasma membrane, which, however, are not expressed particularly for these toxins. Rather, they are integral structures of the plasma membrane or receptors for endogeneous substances. In contrast to endotoxins, each exotoxin initiates its own characteristic symptoms, which originate from an alteration of the plasma membrane or interaction with intracellular, mostly regulatory proteins. The clinical symptoms of infectious diseases, irrespective of the causative agent, derive mostly from several pathogenic factors. Nonspecific reactions induced by endotoxins or the bacteria themselves are often superimposed on the specific actions of the exotoxins. In many cases the latter may even be totally concealed. Thus, *Staphylococcus aureus*, through several cell wall antigens and exotoxins, causes a severe necrotizing inflammation. Bacterial dysentery is caused by lipopolysaccharides from the cell wall of *Shigella* as well as by shiga toxins that inhibit protein synthesis.

Both examples demonstrate the necessity of the presence of the pathogenic germ for causing the symptoms. It is the infection that is the centerpiece and not an intoxication with a distinct poison. In cholera, which is also an infectious disease, the severe diarrhea is caused by the cholera toxin. In tetanus, the infection with *Clostridium tetani* is of minor importance; the spasms are evoked by the action of tetanus toxin alone. Botulism is a true intoxication; only the toxin produced and released by the organism, not the organism itself, enters the host's body from the gastrointestinal tract. Similar conditions prevail in the case of food poisoning with staphylococcal toxins. As a rule, however, true intoxications in which a pathogenic organism is not involved occur only under laboratory conditions when purified toxins, such as cholera, diphtheria, or shiga toxins, are administered to experimental animals.

Exotoxins have many characteristics in common. They are peptides or proteins often consisting of several subunits. These subunits serve different functions in pathogenesis. Many toxins have been purified and sequenced. Their mechanisms of action have been elucidated down to the cellular level. In contrast to endotoxins, whose actions are uniform and depend on the reaction of the immune system, each exotoxin has

TABLE 1 Bacterial Protein Toxins

Extracellularly acting toxins
Pore-forming toxins (lysins)
- Alpha-toxin from *Staphylococcus aureus*
- Streptolysin O
- Pneumolysin
- Tetanolysin

Indirectly acting toxins
- Enterotoxins from *Staphylococcus aureus*
- Endotoxins (lipopolysaccharides)

Intracellularly acting toxins
ADP ribosyltransferases
- Diphtheria toxin
- Pertussis toxin
- Cholera toxin
- Botulinum toxin type C_2

Glucosyltransferases
- *Clostridium difficile* toxin
- *Clostridium novyi* alpha-toxin
- *Clostridium sordellii* lethal toxin

Deamidases
- Cytotoxic necrotizing factor from *Escherichia coli*
- Dermonecrotic toxins from *Bordetella* species

Glycosidases
- Shiga toxin
- Shiga-like toxins

Neurotoxic proteases
- Tetanus toxin
- Botulinum toxin types A, B, C_1, D, E, F, G

its own profile of action. They can be divided into several groups (Table 1). In the following, one characteristic representative from each group will be discussed in detail. The clostridial neurotoxins will be more extensively dealt with because they are responsible for typical intoxications. The actions of endotoxins are described in textbooks of immunology.

AGENTS THAT INTERACT WITH THE PLASMA MEMBRANE

This group comprises toxins that exert a cellular action without passing through the plasma membrane. They interact with receptors located in the plasma membrane, causing either active secretion or passive loss of endogenous substances. Endotoxins can be assigned to this group.

Toxins Forming Membrane Pores

Many bacterial toxins have the property of forming pores across the plasma membrane of host cells. Many antibiotics penetrate the cell walls of microorganisms, resulting in their death. In the pathogenesis of infectious diseases, pore-forming toxins play a minor role. However, they are important tools in experimental medicine and research.

Cholesterol-Binding Toxins

A common characteristic of these toxins is their high-affinity binding to cholesterol, whereupon pores are formed whose diameters are in the range of 1–14 nm, depending on the concentration of the toxin (Fig. 1). The toxins in this group are products of *Streptococcus, Clostridium, Listeria,* and many other bacteria and were called "lysins," due to their lytic action. Streptolysin O is the representative most thoroughly investigated.

Streptolysin O is produced and released by *Streptococcus* of type A. A protein of 60 kDa is composed of 538 amino acids. Although human erythrocytes *in vitro* are lysed by 15 molecules of the agent and myocardial cells are also impaired, this toxin participates very little in the pathology of a staphylococcal infec-

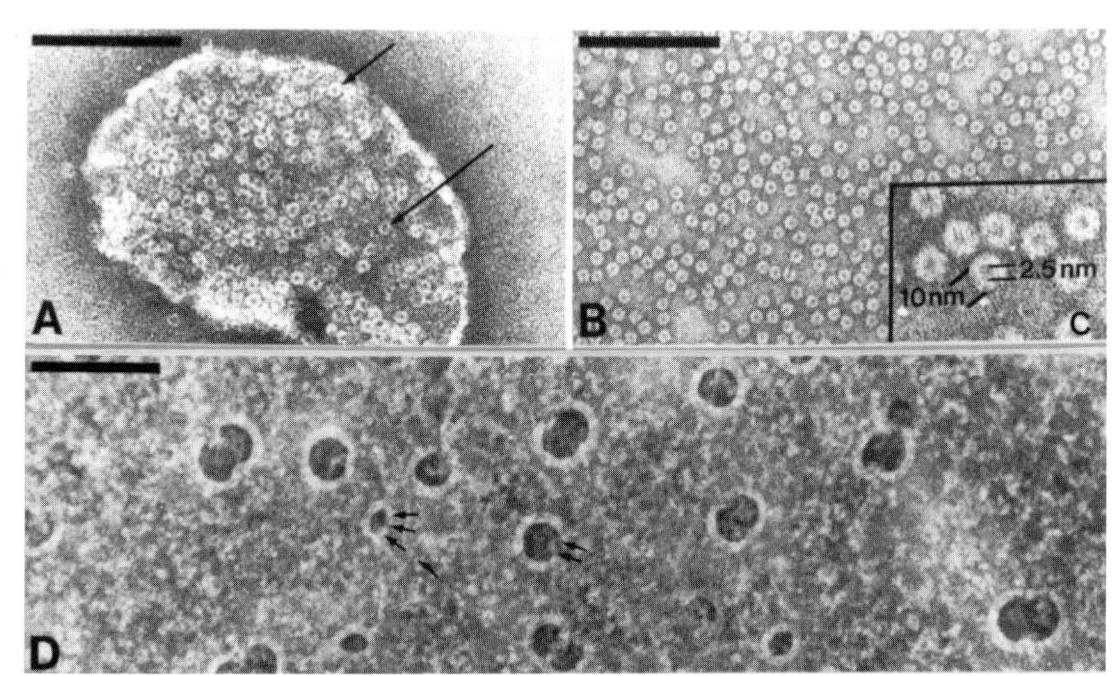

FIGURE 1 Electron micrograph of permeabilized cells. (A) Negative-contrast micrograph of rabbit erythrocytes permeabilized with staphylococcal alpha-toxin. The surface of the cell fragment is covered with circular structures (10 nm in diameter, arrows), enclosing 2.5 nm pores. (B) Toxin hexamers isolated by treatment with a detergent. Inset (C): Part of B at higher magnification. (D) Fragment of an erythrocyte membrane with incorporated oligomers of streptolysine O toxin. Two semicircular oligomers may join to encircle a round pore. (From Bhakdi and Tranum-Jensen, Mechanism of complement cytolysis and the concept of channel-forming proteins. *Philos. Trans. R. Soc. London Ser. B.* **306,** 311–324, © 1984 The Royal Society, with permission.)

tion. The toxin is a strong immunogenic agent. There is always a marked anti-streptolysin O titer following an infection.

The toxin is a tool used in experimental permeabilization of eukaryotic cells. The pores formed allow large molecules to enter the cytosol from the extracellular fluid and enable scientists to change the composition of the cytoplasm. Molecules, such as proteins, can diffuse through those pores, and their intracellular function can be studied.

The pore formation is characterized by a two-step mechanism. Independent of pH and temperature, streptolysion O binds irreversibly to cholesterol. For binding, free disulfide groups are essential. Whether they are involved in an interaction with membrane proteins or whether they are responsible for the steric conformation of the molecule remains to be elucidated.

Pores are formed by oligomers of the toxins (Fig. 1), and they precede lysis. As opposed to binding, pore formation depends on temperature and pH values that must be in the range of 5.5 to 9. How the pores evolve is unclear. The lytic activity is determined by the spectrometric measuring of hemoglobulin release from erythrocytes.

Staphylococcal Alpha-Toxin

This toxin (M_r 30,000) is one of various biologically active proteins produced by *Staphylococcus aureus*. Monomers assemble to form hexamers in the plasma membrane, surrounding a central pore with a diameter of approximately 2.5 nm (Fig. 1). Molecules of less than 3 kD can pass through the pores. The mechanism of lysis is similar to that for streptolysin O. It is unclear which role the toxin plays in necrotizing infections caused by *Staphylococcus*. Probably several pathogenic factors are involved in inducing necrosis. Like streptolysin O, staphylococcal alpha-toxin is also used in research to manipulate the cytosolic composition of eukaryotic cells.

Indirectly Acting Toxins

Staphylococcus aureus produces several enterotoxins which are contained in food contaminated with the organisms. The toxins are devoid of odor and taste and do not change the appearance of comestibles. They are heat-resistant. The organisms grow extremely well in cooked food rich in protein. Their contamination can largely be avoided by cleanliness and strict compliance with the guidelines for hygiene.

Most cases of food poisoning are due to these enterotoxins. After a latent period of approximately 1 to 6 hours, the toxins evoke severe gastroenteritis characterized by vomiting, intestinal spasms, and profuse diarrhea. Recovery is achieved after about 48 hours. A therapy with antibiotics is not effective because this disease is due to an intoxication. Restoring the balance of electrolytes and water is a sufficient therapy in most cases. Enterotoxins are also involved in the pathogenesis of pseudomembraneous enterocolitis, osteomyelitis, septicemia, and inflammation of injured sites.

Seven serotypes of enterotoxins are known. Their molecular mass is in the range of 26 to 28 kDa, and they are made up of 228 to 239 amino acids, A disulfide bridge spans 9 to 19 amino acids near the center of the chain. The sequence is highly homologous.

Enterotoxins of this type are not taken up by cells, they do not form pores, and they are not directly involved in causing the symptoms. Similar to the endotoxins (lipopolysaccharides), they bind to cells of the immune system, especially to macrophages and lymphocytes, and stimulate the release of mediators (e.g., interleukins, leukotrienes, and tumor necrosis factor). These mediators produce a toxic inflammation. In addition, the toxins bind to intestinal receptors that stimulate the emetic center in the medulla oblongata via vagal and sympathetic afferent nerves. The receptors have not yet been identified.

INTRACELLULARLY ACTING TOXINS

All protein toxins that act intracellularly are enzymes. Because under physiological conditions the plasma membrane is an insurmountable barrier to proteins, bacteria have developed sophisticated methods to introduce their toxins into the cytosol. To understand the pathogenesis of diseases caused by bacterial toxins, it is necessary to have a thorough knowledge not only of the toxicodynamics but also of the kinetics of the poisons.

Uptake and Distribution

Almost all toxins acting intracellularly have some structural characteristics in common. They consist of at least two parts; one is the kinetic part, and the other is the dynamic part that is characterized by enzyme activity. Each part by itself, when purified, is nontoxic. Both parts may be connected by covalent bonds or noncovalent forces. The latter is true for anthrax toxin and botulinum toxin type C_2. Usually, the toxins are synthesized as a single-chain protein. Proteases from bacterial or other origins, by limited proteolysis (nicking), sever a distinct, easily accessible location in the chain. In general, nicking enhances toxicity. The kinetic part and the enzyme can still be covalently linked by a disulfide bond between two cysteine residues. This bond will be cleaved by reductases when the toxin is taken up by a cell.

The kinetic part may consist of two functional domains that reside on different parts of the peptide chain. The first domain, always present, binds to the receptor inserted into the plasma membrane, while the second domain, only present sometimes, can become integrated into the membrane if the pH decreases. This takes place in endosomes and may be a prerequisite for the translocation of the toxin into the substrate-containing compartment.

The enzyme is usually highly specific for a single reaction. To activate the enzyme, each covalent bond between the kinetic part and the enzyme has to be split inside the cell. Thus, apart from "nicking," a reduction of the disulfide bonds also has to take place. A portion of the toxin molecules will not be reduced within the cell. They can be released into the extracellular space to be taken up again by neighboring cells. These mechanisms are essential for the pathogenesis of tetanus.

Mode of Action

The symptoms of toxin-induced diseases do not follow solely from the reactions catalyzed by the enzymes (Table 1), but mainly from their high specifity for a single substrate. The enzymatic activities are restricted to only a few reactions. Most toxins transfer ADP-ribose to intracellular protein. This may interrupt intracellular signal transduction, inhibit protein biosynthesis, and destroy the cellular cytoarchitecture (Table 2). Protein biosynthesis can also be inhibited by cleaving ribosomal RNA with glycosidases. In addition to ADP ribosylation, UDP glucosylation and proteolytic cleavage also inactivate proteins. Both toxins from *Clostridium difficile* and products from *Clostridium botulinum* and *Clostridium tetani* interfere with cellular function through these enzymatic pathways. In contrast, proteins may be activated by deamidation, as was shown for Rho proteins that are involved in regulation of the cell cycle.

TABLE 2 ADP Ribosyltransferases

Enzyme	Substrate	Function
Diphtheria toxin	Elongation factor 2	Biosynthesis of proteins
Cholera toxin	G_s	Signal transduction
Pertussis toxin	G_i, G_0, transducin	Signal transduction
Botulinum toxin C_3	Rho proteins	Regulation of various cellular functions
Botulinum toxin C_2	G-actin	Polymerization of actin

ADP-Ribosylating Toxins

These toxins transfer an adenosine diphosphate moiety from nicotinamide adenine dinucleotide to nitrogen in the amino acids arginine, asparagine, cysteine, and diphthamide (Fig. 2), the latter being the product of a posttranslational modification of histidine. Regulatory GTP-binding and cytoskeletal proteins, which are involved in the regulation of cellular pathways and biosynthesis of proteins, are modified by this reaction. ADP ribosylation blocks the function of GTP-binding proteins. Actin, an essential part of the cytoskeleton, conferring shape on the cell, is also involved in the migration of cells and, in addition, enables the intracellular transport of vesicles. Actin filaments are dynamic structures assembling and disassembling continually. ADP ribosylation suppresses the polymerization of actin.

Diphtheria Toxin

Diphtheria toxin is encoded by a corynebacterium phage of type beta$^+$, which infects *Corynebacterium diphtheriae*. The toxin-encoding DNA of the phage is integrated into the bacterial DNA. The bacteria are transmitted among humans through expectorated aerosols and spread over the mucous membranes of the throat. The toxin released produces a severe necrotizing inflammation accompanied by exudation. Cell debris, erythrocytes, and plasma proteins form a characteristic false membrane. Its expansion into the airways impairs respiration. The disease also affects the heart muscle (myocarditis), impulse propagation (arrhythmia), and the nervous system (motor palsy, especially in the pharynx and thorax, affecting swallowing and respiration). Before active immunization was introduced, diphtheria was a fatal disease.

The toxin is produced as a single chain consisting of 535 amino acid residues (M_r 58,342). It is nicked by a serine protease before it enters the cell. The resulting N-terminal (A) and C-terminal (B) fragments are connected by a disulfide bond extending between cysteine^{186} and cysteine^{201}. Fragment B represents the kinetic part with the binding and pore-forming domains. Upon binding to a yet unknown receptor, the toxin is taken up by receptor-mediated endocytosis. The B fragment, aquiring a hydrophobic character at the low endosomal pH, is incorporated into the endosomal membrane while pore formation occurs.

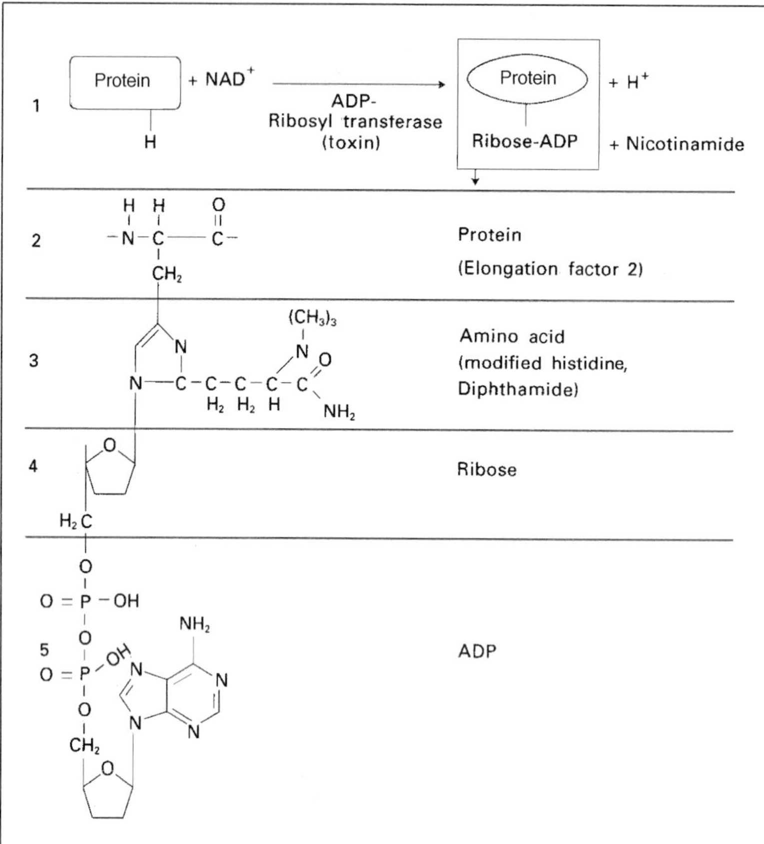

FIGURE 2 ADP-ribosylation of proteins. (1) ADP-ribosyltransferases (toxins) catalyze the translocation of an adenosine diphosphate ribose moiety from nicotinamide adenine dinucleotide to a nitrogen atom in an amino acid of the substrate (protein). The substrate changes its shape and loses its physiological function. (2) The elongation factor 2 is the substrate of diphtheria toxin, which contains (3) diphthamide, an amino acid formed from histidine following translation. The nitrogen atom of the imidazole ring binds ribose (4), which is linked to ADP (5). (Reproduced from Aktories, K., Clostridium botulinum C_2 toxin and C. botulinum C_3 ADP-ribosyl transferase. *In* "Selective Neurotoxicity," (H. Herkin and F. Hucho, eds.), pp. 841–854, © 1992 Springer-Verlag, with permission.)

The disulfide bond is reduced by the intracellular redox systems, which is an essential step to render the enzyme active. The A fragment enters the cytosol where it transfers an ADP-ribose moiety from nicotinamide adenine dinucleotide to a nitrogen atom in the imidazole ring of diphthamide in the elongation factor 2. The ADP-ribosylated GTP-binding protein loses its capability to translocate the ribosome on the mRNA, which results in the discontinuation of protein biosynthesis (Fig. 3). In theory, one molecule of diphtheria toxin should be able to kill a cell. The lethal dose in humans is approximately 100 ng/kg body weight.

Pseudomonas aeroginosa toxin has the same mode of action as diphtheria toxin. Both toxins have highly conserved A fragments, in contrast to their B fragments. The latter are probably responsible for the different diseases caused by these toxins.

Cholera Toxin

Cholera toxin is the prototype of a group of similarly constructed enterotoxins that are produced by various bacteria. The disease erupts epidemically, especially in countries with a low standard of hygiene. The germs are transmitted by contaminated water and food. The disease breaks out suddenly with a severe, watery, and painless diarrhea. The loss of water can amount to as much as 30 liters a day. A successful treatment can usually be achieved with tetracycline antibiotics and the substitution of the lost water

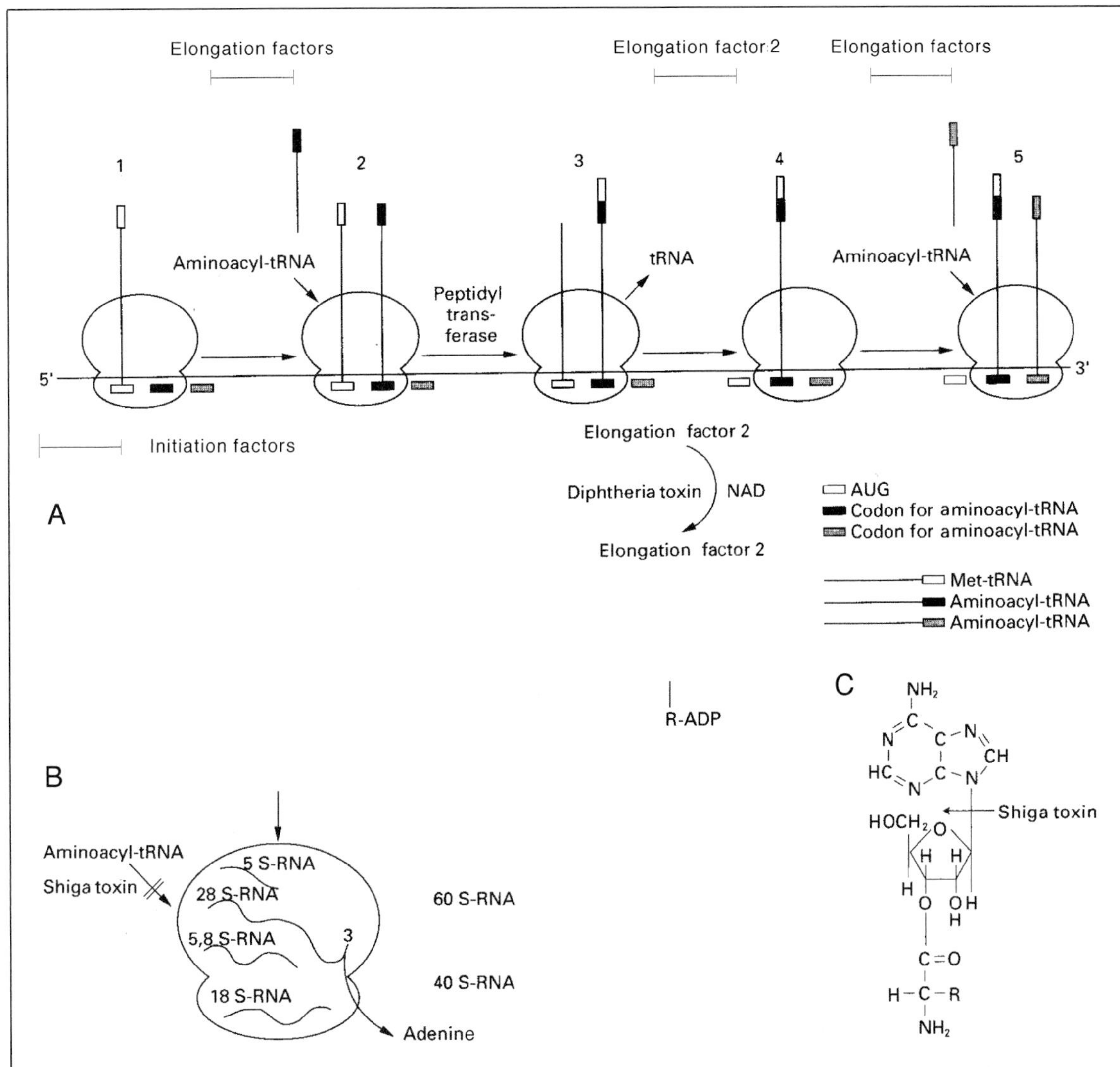

FIGURE 3 Mode of action of diphtheria and Shiga toxins. (A) Methionine-tRNA is docked to the first AUG sequence of the mRNA. Various initiation factors are involved in this reaction (1). Elongation factors transfer aminoacyl-tRNA to the codon of the next amino acid (2). A peptidyl transferase conjugates methionine with the amino acid, and the tRNA is cleaved from its AUG codon (3). Then elongation factor 2 translocates the ribosome to the next base triplet of the mRNA (4). In a next cycle, a further aminoacyl-tRNA will be conjugated with the nascent end of the peptide (5). Elongation factor 2 is the substrate of diphtheria toxin. The ADP-ribosylated form has lost its capability to translocate the ribosome on the mRNA and protein biosynthesis comes to a halt. (B) Shiga toxin cleaves adenine from ribose within the 28-S RNA subunit (C). Aminoacyl-tRNA molecules can bind no longer to this modified ribosome (B), leading to an inhibition of protein biosynthesis.

and electrolytes. Travelers to countries where cholera is endemic should have an active immunization.

Cholera toxin consists of one A subunit that is surrounded by five identical B subunits. They are encoded by two genes, one for each subunit. The genes are located in an operon of the chromosome of *Vibrio cholera*. The B subunits bind to gangliosides of type GM1, while the A subunit is translocated into the cell and cleaved by proteolysis into two fragments, A1 and A2. Their molecular masses are 22 and 5 kDa, respectively. A1 and A2 are linked by a disulfide bond, which has to be cleaved to render fragment A1 active as an ADP ribosyltransferase. It transfers a single ADP-ribose moiety from nicotinamide adenine dinucleotide to an arginine in the α-subunit of the regulatory G protein, G_s, which stimulates adenylate cyclase. Through ribosylation, G_s loses its ability to hydrolyze GTP to GDP, the cyclase thus remaining activated. This leads to an increase in the intracellular content of the second messenger cAMP (Fig. 4). cAMP activates the secretorial transport of ions from the blood into the intestine. Water follows the ions due to the os-

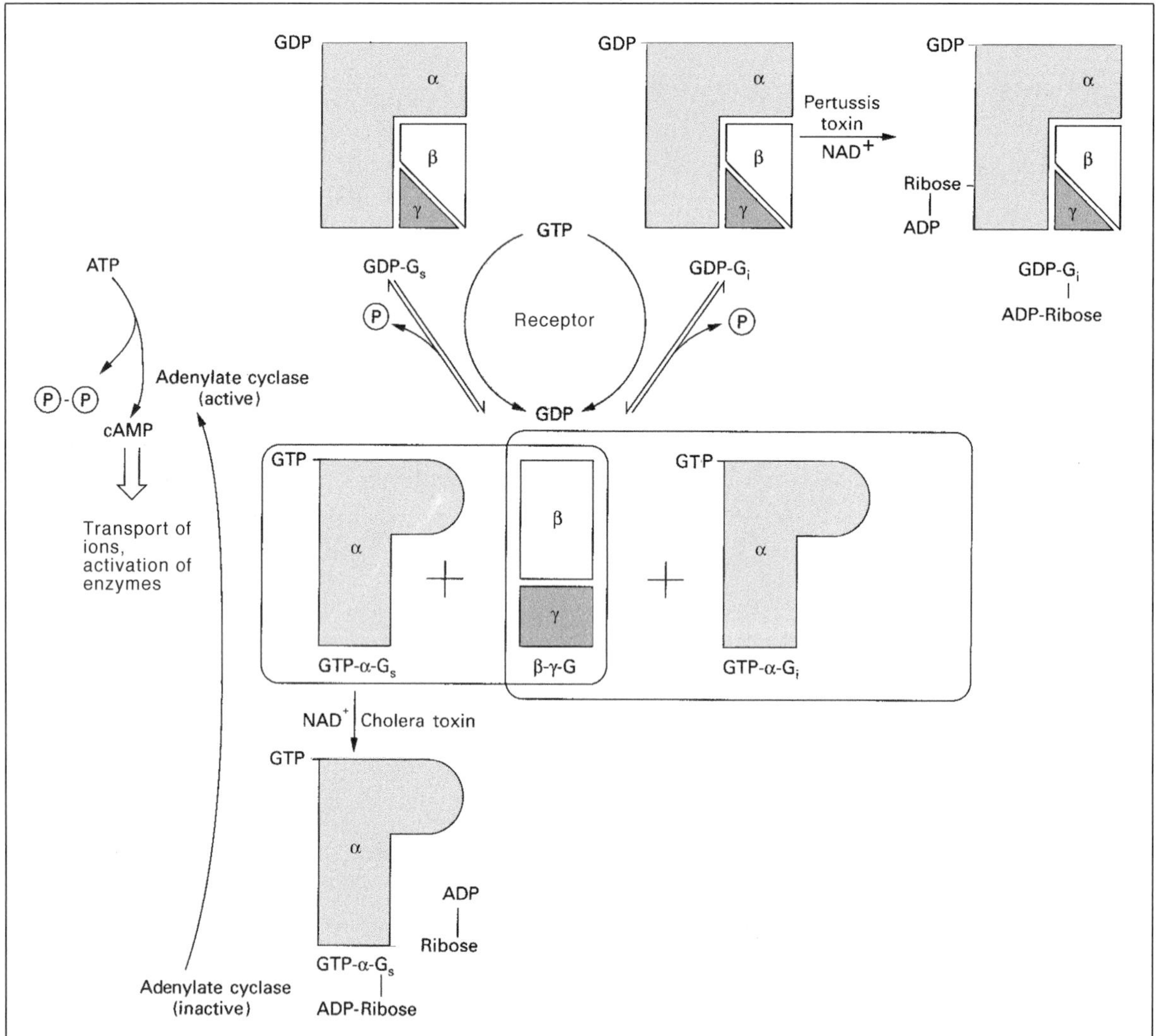

FIGURE 4 Mode of action of cholera and pertussis toxins. G proteins are the substrates of the ADP ribosyltransferases, such as cholera and pertussis toxins. The membrane-anchored, regulatory proteins consist of three subunits, alpha, beta, and gamma. The alpha-subunit binds GDP. Stimulation of a receptor leads to an exchange of GDP for GTP within the alpha-subunit (GTP-alpha-G). GTP-alpha-G_s activates adenylate cyclase which cleaves ATP to cAMP and pyrophosphate. cAMP is a second messenger that regulates many intracellular pathways. Moreover, GTP-alpha-G_s is a GTPase hydrolizing its bond GTP to GDP. Thus the alpha-subunit inactivates itself. Cholera toxin translocates an ADP-ribose unit to GTP-alpha-G_s. GTPase activity decreases completely, while adenylate cyclase remains active, trapped in its activated form. Like the stimulatory G proteins (G_s), inhibitory G proteins (G_i) are composed of three subunits. The beta- and gamma-subunits of the G_s and G_i are identical. The number of G_i molecules is much larger than the number of G_s. If G_i is cleaved into GTP-alpha-G_i and beta-gamma-G, an increasing number of beta-gamma-G molecules will be available for the inactivation of GTP-alpha-G_s. This mechanism of G_s inhibition is blocked by pertussis toxin, which translocates an ADP-ribose moiety to GDP-alpha-G_i. The modified G-protein can bind GTP no longer, leading to a decrease in beta-gamma-G. Although different substrates are involved, both pertussis toxin and cholera toxin up-regulate adenylate cyclase.

motic gradient, and the clinical symptom is a severe diarrhea followed by serious dehydration and electrolyte imbalance.

Pertussis Toxin

Bordetella pertussis causes whooping cough. Pertussis toxin is one of several factors participating in the genesis of the disease; its role, however, has not been clarified. The molecular mass is approximately 105 kDa, and the protein consists of five subunits, S1–S5. S1 is the enzyme that is translocated into the cell by S2–S5. The translocation is initiated by binding to a glycoprotein (M_r 165,000) via a mannose-containing sialic acid. The toxin transfers ADP-ribose to cysteine[352] in the α-subunits of the G proteins, G_o, G_i and transducin, which subsequently become unable to bind GTP and thus remain in their inactive state (Fig. 4).

Pertussis and cholera toxins are potent tools for controlling the activation and inactivation of regulatory G proteins. Both toxins are experimentally used to study signal transduction in eukaryotic cells and to investigate the role of various G proteins in the regulation of cell homeostasis.

Botulinum Toxin Type C_2

When describing the toxicology of botulinum toxins, the most important property of these compounds seems to be their neurotoxicity. Botulinum toxin type C_2, synthesized by *Clostridium botulinum* C, however, is not neurotoxic. It increases vascular permeability, leading to hemorrhage, edema of the lung, and hypotension. Initially, the chromosomally encoded toxin consists of two single proteins. One of these proteins (M_r 74,000) serves as a carrier and binds to an unknown receptor. The other protein, an enzyme (M_r 45,000), recognizes this membrane-bound protein and is taken up by receptor mediated endocytosis (Fig. 5). In the cytosol, it ADP-ribosylates the β- and γ-isoforms of monomeric G-actin in arginine[177]. Physiologically, G-actin cleaves ATP. This ATPase-like activity increases when G-actin is polymerized to F-actin. Ribosylated G-actin, like G-actin, binds to the nascent end of F-actin, thus terminating polymerization. When F-actin depolymerizes to G-actin monomers, the monomers also become ribosylated and lose their ATPase activity. ADP-ribose–G-actin is unable to form polymers (Fig. 5). The cytoarchitecture of the microfilaments is destroyed in cells containig β and γ-actin. Because it differs from β- and γ-actin in its N-terminal region, α-actin is not ribosylated, and, therefore, cannot interact with the toxin. This is the reason why muscle cells, which contain α-actin, are not destroyed by botulinum C_2 toxin.

Clostridium botulinum bacilli of types C and D synthesize not only the neurotoxins and the ADP-ribosylating C_2 toxin but also another ADP ribosyltransferase. This exoenzyme, C_3, is nontoxic because it cannot enter intact cells. Its code resides in the DNA of a phage and has no sequence homologies with the codes of the other clostridial toxins. C_3 is a single-chain enzyme (M_r 26,000) that modifies the small GTP-binding, regulatory Rho proteins (M_r 21,000), Rho A, B, and C, which are involved in the regulation of enzymes and cell cycles, as well as in the control of endocytosis, transcription, apoptosis, and transformation. The Rho proteins, which belong to the superfamily of Ras proteins, act as molecular switches and interfere with various bacterial toxins. They are inactive when bound to GDP. The GTPase cycle of Rho proteins is similar to that of the heterotrimeric G proteins, which also are targets for bacterial toxins (i.e., cholera and pertussis toxins). Transferases acting in a similar manner are produced by *Clostridium limosum, Bacillus cereus,* and *Staphylococcus aureus.* All these enzymes are basic proteins of similar molecular mass and show 30–70% homologies in their amino acid sequences. They modify Rho proteins in asparagin[41] resulting in a blockage of Rho-dependent signal transduction. Although the transferases cannot enter intact cells and their involvement in diseases caused by bacteria is unclear, they serve as useful tools for the investigation of the role of Rho proteins in cell regulation.

UDP-Glucosylating and UDP-Acetylglucosaminylating Toxins

Rho proteins are substrates for the *Clostridium difficile* toxins A and B. Toxin A is responsible for antibiotic-associated diarrhea and colitis, while toxin B shows a much more potent cytotoxicity for eukaryotic cells. The molecular mass of the toxins is approximately 300 kDa. They inactivate the regulatory Rho proteins by translocation of glucose to threonine[37], using uridine diphosphate-glucose (UDP-glucose) as a co-substrate. This leads to an increase in intestinal permeability and a stimulation of chloride secretion. *Clostridium sordellii* lethal and hemorrhagic toxins and *Clostridium novyi* α-toxin affect Rho proteins as well. Both toxins show a different substrate specificity, and the latter toxin translocates *N*-acetylglucosamine (GlcNAc) using UDP-GlcNAc.

Deamidases

Dermonecrotic toxins from *Bordetella* consist of a group of toxins lethal to mice following i.v. application. They also cause atrophic rhinitis in pigs. Their molecular mass, amino acid sequence, and mode of action are similar to those of the cytotoxic necrotizing factors from *Escherichia coli.* The escherichia toxins cause damage to the actin cytoskeleton by increasing the content of F-actin in eukaryotic cells. The substrates of the deamidases are also proteins of the Rho family that are deamidated in glutamine[63]. The modified protein loses its GTPase activity. Thus, in contrast to ADP ribosylation and UDP glucosylation, deamidation of the regulatory proteins turns on the molecular switch that keeps the cell in its activated state. An overview of the toxins acting on Rho proteins is given in Table 3.

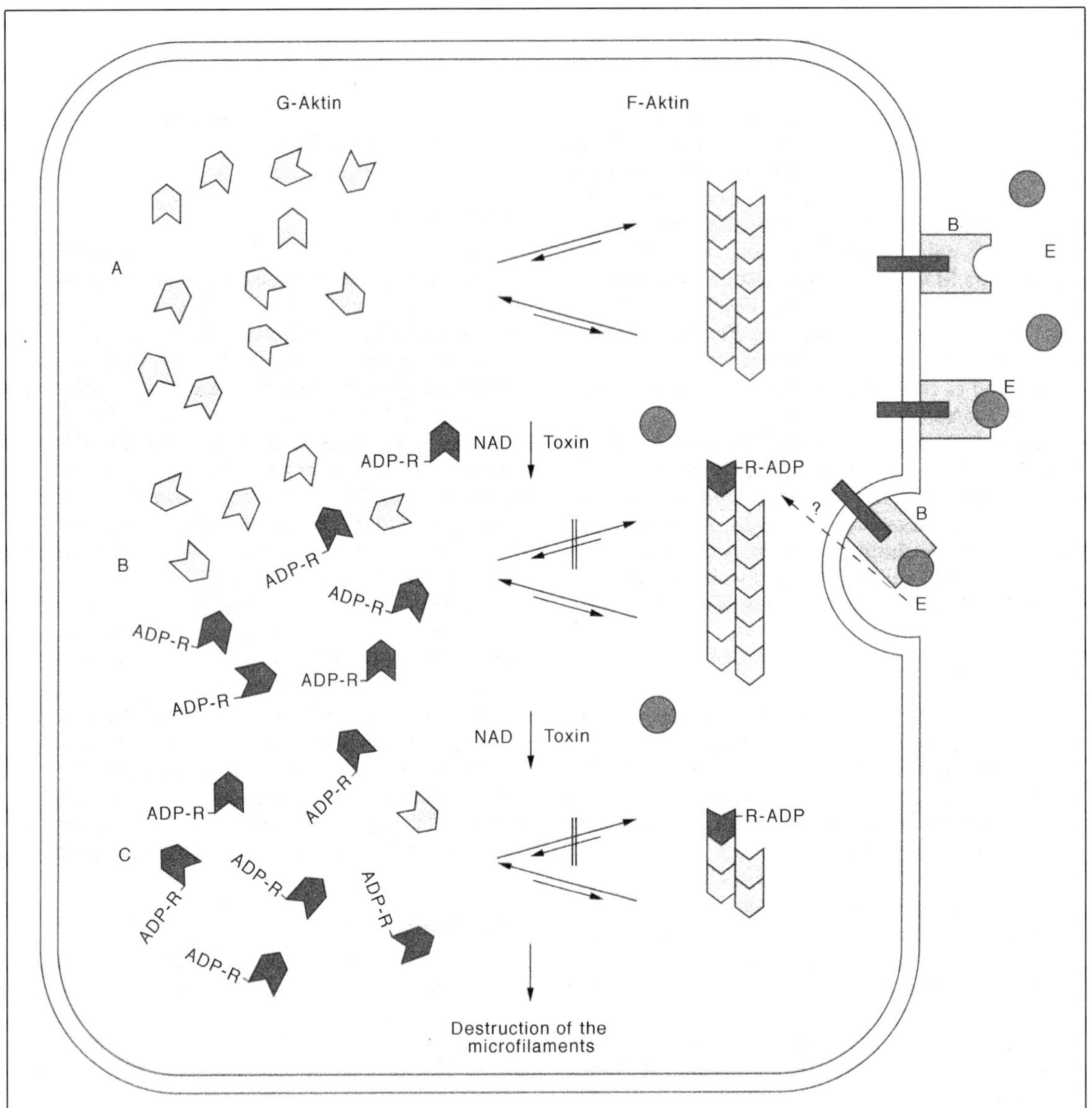

FIGURE 5 Mechanism of the ADP-ribosylation of actin. Botulinum toxin type C_2 consists of a binding (B) and an enzyme (E) unit. E is translocated with the help of B by an unknown route into the cytosol. Here, it ADP-ribosylates G-actin, which physiologically polymerizes to F-actin (A) and depolymerizes to the monomer form again. The ADP-ribosylated G-actin masks the nascent end of F-actin and inhibits polymerization (B). Depolymerizing F-actin continues to release G-actin, which is also ADP-ribosylated and thus inactivated (C). Both events, masking (B) and inactivation (C), are involved in the destruction of the microfilament network by the ADP ribosyltransferase, botulinum toxin type C_2.

Glycosidases

Shiga toxin type 1 is produced by *Shigella dysenteriae.* Being the prototype of a group of similarly acting bacterial toxins synthesized by various strains of *Escherichia coli,* it is a cofactor in the pathogenesis of bacterial dysentery. These shiga-like toxins, as well as the shiga toxin of type 1, consist of a single A fragment (M_r 32,225), which is the biologically active part, and four B fragments (M_r 7691 each), which are the kinetic part. The latter part binds to glycolipids inserted into the plasma membrane. The active part is taken up by adsorptive endocytosis, is cleaved by proteolysis, and is reduced to two subunits, A1 and A2. Subunit A2 is the enzyme. In their amino acid sequence and structure, the toxins show homologies with the plant lectins, abrin and ricin. They cleave a single molecule of adenine from the eukaryotic ribosomal complex, close to the 3′ terminal of the 28-rRNA component. This

TABLE 3 Toxins Modifying Rho Proteins[a]

A	B	C	D
Rho + NAD	ADP ribosyltransferase, type C_3	Rho-ribose-ADP + nicotinamide + H^+	Inactive
Rho + UDP-glucose	Glucosyltransferase, toxins A, B	Rho-glucose + UDP	Inactive
Rho + UDP-GlcNAc	Glucosyltransferase, α-toxin	Rho-GlcNAc + UDP	Inactive
Rho-glutamine + H_2O	Deamidase, bordetella toxins	Rho-glutaminic acid + NH_3	Active

[a]The substrates and co-substrates (A) interact with the respective toxins (B), yielding a modified rho protein (C) that can either be active or inactive (D).

truncated complex can no longer bind aminoacyl-tRNA; the elongation of the peptide is terminated, and protein biosynthesis is inhibited.

Neurotoxic Proteases

Bacteria synthesize various proteases. These specialize in cleaving peptide bonds between particular amino acids, irrespective of the neighboring sequences. Like other bacterial toxins, proteases cannot surmount the barrier of the plasma membrane and do not gain access to the central nervous system. With the help of their kinetic segment, however, the neurotoxic proteases enter nerve cells exclusively and are capable of reaching the spinal cord using neuronal transport systems. Each binds specifically to a particular neuronal protein and cleaves it by limited proteolysis.

Tetanus toxin and the botulinum neurotoxins of types A, B, C_1, D, E, F, and G are neurotoxic proteins. Tetanus toxin is produced by *Clostridium tetani* deep within infected wounds, whence it enters the blood stream by diffusion. Botulinum toxins are synthetized by *Clostridium botulinum* in protein-rich substrates. *Clostridium botulinum*, a gram-(+) bacterium, grows only under anaerobic conditions; for example, insufficiently conserved, sealed food is an excellent substrate. Upon intake in contaminated food, the toxins are absorbed from the intestine. All neurotoxic proteases are susceptible to heat and are inactivated by cooking. Botulinum toxin type A is the most thoroughly investigated botulinum toxin. It consists of hemagglutinins, another nontoxic and nonhemagglutinating protein, and two neurotoxin molecules (M_r 150,000), which together form a complex of approximately 900 kDa. The complex is stable at an acidic pH and protects the neurotoxin from inactivation in the stomach and intestine. All types of botulinum toxins act in a similar manner. Therefore, discussion of these toxins will be restricted to the botulinum A toxin, with the tetanus toxin also mentioned.

Both toxins are taken up by peripheral motor nerve endings. Tetanus toxin reaches the spinal cord by retrograde axonal transport, which is used physiologically to convey metabolites. It leaves the motoneuron, crosses the synaptic cleft, and is endocytosed by the presynaptic nerve endings of inhibitory interneurons. In these neurons it blocks the exocytosis of the inhibitory transmitters, glycine and gamma-amino butyric acid (GABA). Thereupon, the motoneuron lacks inhibitory input, and incoming excitatory signals are transmitted unmodulated to the striated muscles and cause spastic paralysis (Fig. 6). The autonomic nervous system is affected by the same mechanism, resulting in vegetative disturbances. Botulinum toxin, in contrast, remains mostly in peripheral nerve endings, where it inhibits the release of acetylcholine. Therefore, an intoxication with this toxin is characterized by a severe flaccid paralysis accompanied by exhausted vegetative function. The contrasting symptoms of tetanus and botulism result solely from the different toxicokinetic behaviors of the toxins. They can persist for several weeks and may cause death due to a failure of the respiratory muscles.

Despite the difference in toxicokinetics and their differing symptoms, the toxins have some characteristics in common. Their most obvious common feature is the extremely high toxicity, which is about 1 ng/kg body weight. The plasma concentrations in cases of poisoning are so low that they hardly suffice to stimulate the immune system. Therefore, a patient will not acquire immunity should he or she be lucky enough to survive an intoxication.

Furthermore, the toxins have a characteristic structure. Both are synthesized as single-chain proteins of approximately 150 kDa. Tetanus and botulinum G toxins are encoded in plasmids, botulinum C_1 and D toxins in bacteriophages, and botulinum A, B, E, and F toxins in the bacterial chromosome. The single-chain toxins, which are hardly active, are cleaved by bacterial proteases at particular sites (nicking), resulting in the potent double-chain neurotoxins. A disulfide bond

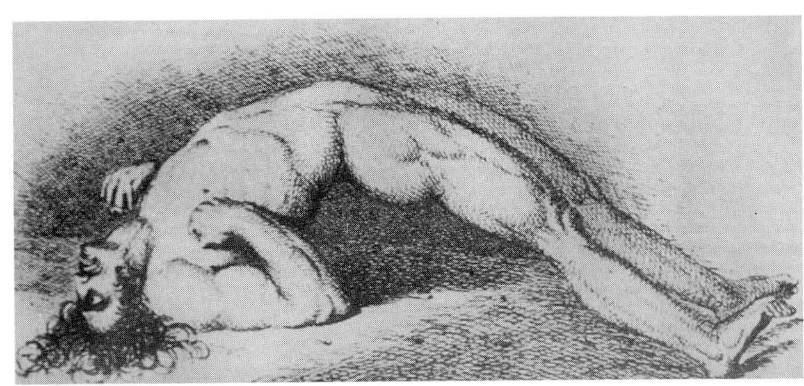

FIGURE 6 Tetanus as viewed by the English physiologist Sir Charles Bell. Sir Charles Bell (1774–1842), the author of "New Idea of Anatomy of the Brain" (known as the "Magna Carta of Neurology"), drew this image of a soldier wounded in the Peninsular War (1808–1814) and suffering from tetanus. Due to his brilliant observation, Bell succeeded in catching the characteristic symptoms of the disease in an artistic manner. All skeletal muscles are in a state of extreme contraction. The contraction of the flexors exceeds that of the extensors. The predominance of the muscles of the neck and back leads to the development of opisthotonus. Trismus and risus sardonicus are evident. These symptoms result from the contraction of the masticatory and facial muscles. Patients afflicted in this manner were destined to die.

and ionic forces tightly link the N-terminal light chain (M_r 50,000) with the C-terminal heavy chain (M_r 100,000). Binding to plasma membrane-located receptors is mediated by the heavy chain. Binding sites for tetanus toxin are gangliosides of types GT1 and GD1b. Botulinum A toxin binds to gangliosides of type GD1a. The occurrence of protein receptors has been proposed and demonstrated for botulinum B toxin, which binds to the vesicular protein, synaptotagmin. This protein protrudes into the synaptic cleft after fusion of the vesicle with the plasma membrane. The occurrence of two different binding sites, a protein and ganglioside, may account for the marked specificity of clostridial toxins for nerve cells. Nonneuronal cells are insensitive because they lack either the specific ganglioside or protein receptors, although they may contain either the substrate itself or a cleavable isoform (e.g., cellubrevin). Cellubrevin is a substrate for the tetanus toxin.

Following binding, the toxin is endocytosed and trapped in endosomes. While tetanus toxin is transported preferentially into the somata of spinal cord motoneurons, botulinum toxin remains mainly in nerve endings. Tetanus toxin leaves the motoneuron by an unknown mechanism and is taken up by interneurons, probably via receptors identical with those in the periphery. Before exocytosis can be blocked, the toxins, in particular their light chains, have to gain access to the cytosol. Their translocation is facilitated by the acidic environment within the endosomes and the pores formed in the endosomal membrane by the N-terminal part of the heavy chains. The interchain disulfide bond of the two chains has to be reduced to render the toxins active, which is done by the cellular thioredoxin system (Fig. 7). Despite these specific sites of actions, tetanus toxin, in addition to its central effect, is able to paralyze striated muscles, whereas BoNT is capable of inhibiting the release of glycine and GABA from interneurons. However, while botulinum toxin at its peripheral site of action is 1000 times more potent than tetanus toxin, the reverse is true with respect to the central effects on interneurons. The inactivation of the toxins, which precedes recovery in patients, is caused by cellular proteases. These enzymes cleave the active proteins into small inactive fragments (Fig. 7). The long duration of the tetanus and botulism diseases probably results from a low activity of cytosolic proteases.

The light chains of all clostridial neurotoxins have highly conserved regions, in particular, a sequence (HELIH) that can be found in many metalloproteases. In cooperation with neighboring amino acids, this motif is capable of binding one molecule of zinc. If chelators compete for zinc, or if the zinc-binding motif

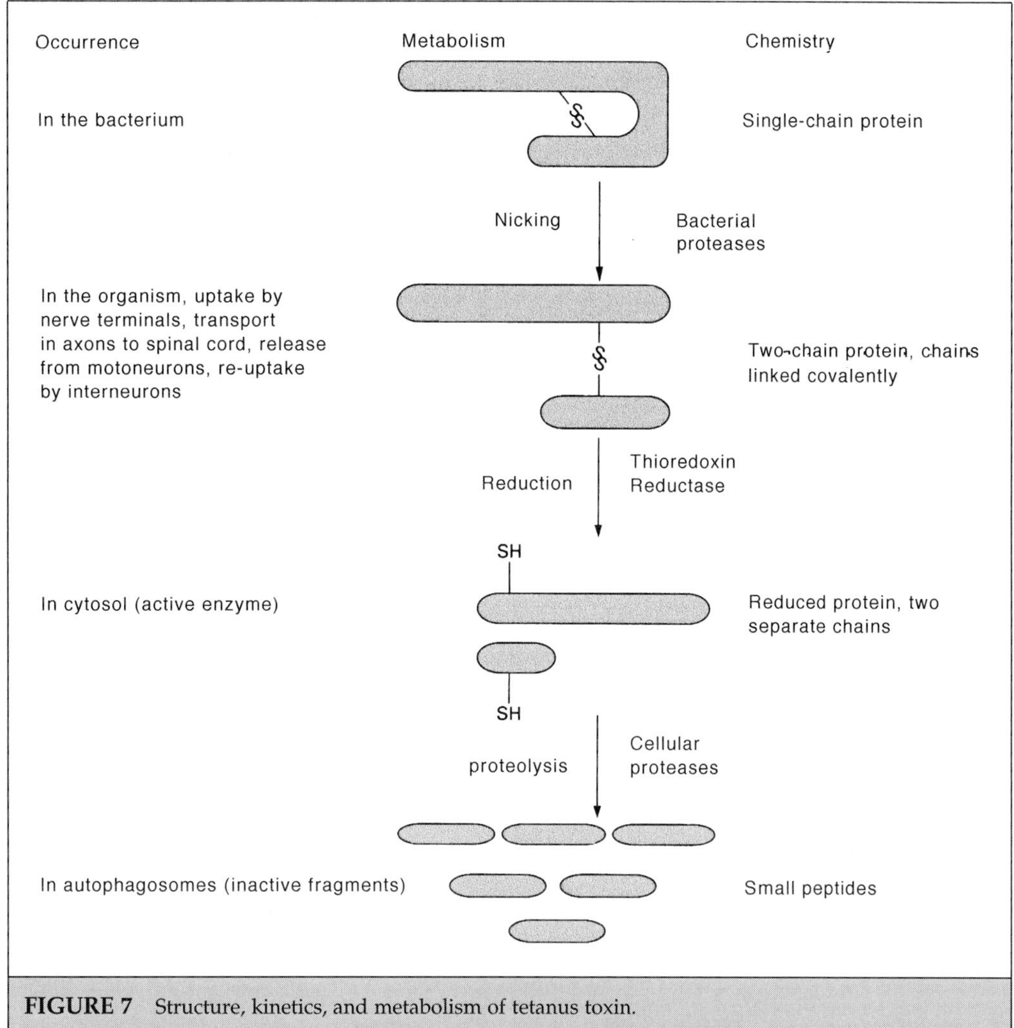

FIGURE 7 Structure, kinetics, and metabolism of tetanus toxin.

has been subject to mutation, the toxins lose their activity. Thus, all clostridial neurotoxins may derive from a single ancestral prototoxin.

The substrates of clostridial neurotoxins have been localized in the membrane of transmitter-containing vesicles, where they form a very stable "fusion complex" consisting of synaptobrevin II, syntaxin, and SNAP 25 (synaptosomal-associated protein of 25 kDa). Synaptobrevin II is cleaved by tetanus toxin and the botulinum toxins of types B, D, F, and G; syntaxin by botulinum C_1 toxin; and SNAP 25 by botulinum A and C_1 toxins (Fig. 8). The formation of the complex is a prerequisite of the calcium-induced fusion of the vesicles with the plasma membrane. If any one of the constituents of the complex is destroyed, fusion with the membrane will be impossible, and transmitter release will cease, even if the concentration of intracellular calcium increases. It is likely that these fusion proteins or their isomers play the same key role not only in neuronal but also in all nonneuronal cells in which exocytotic membrane fusion occurs. Therefore, clostridial neurotoxins may prove to be universal tools for research into the function of fusion proteins and their interaction with each other. They may play a similar role in exploring synaptic transmission as the ADP-ribosylating toxins do in the investigation of intracellular signal transduction.

Clostridial neurotoxins cannot kill single cells. Although exocytosis of neurons is inhibited, the individual nerve cell will finally eliminate the toxin and restore exocytosis if the organism as a whole survives. This lack of cytotoxicity is the prerequisite for the use of botulinum A toxin as a therapeutic agent for the treatment of blepharospasm, torticollis spasmodicus, and spasms of the jaw muscles. Extremely low doses (in the nanogram range) can be injected into the dys-

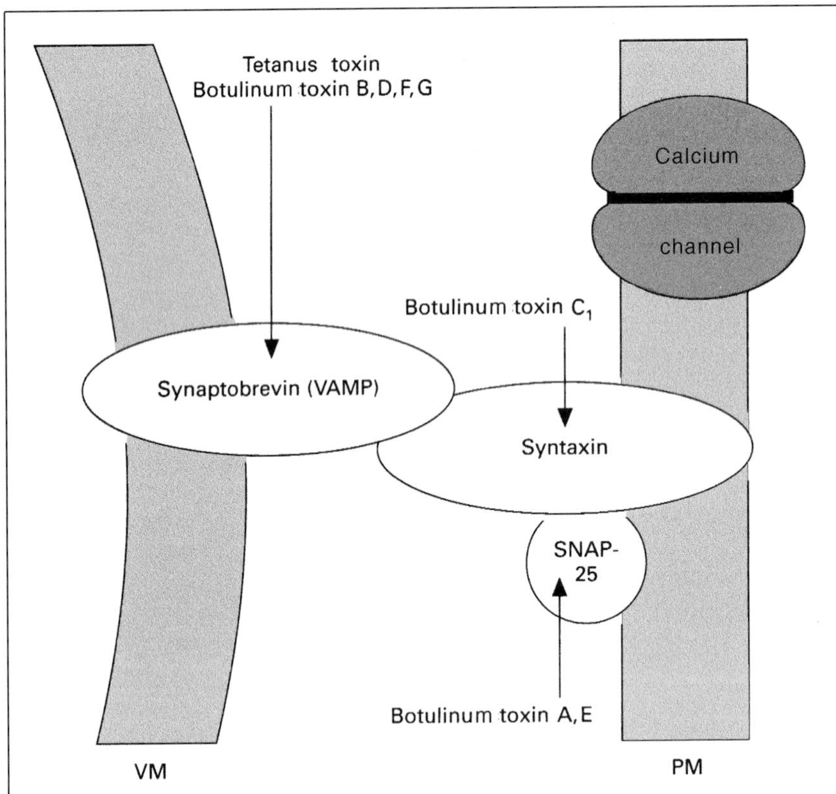

FIGURE 8 The fusion complex is the target of clostridial neurotoxins. The physiological functions of the fusion proteins, synaptobrevin 2, syntaxin, and SNAP 25 (synaptosomal-associated protein of 25 kD a), are not fully understood. They occur in the plasma (PM) and vesicular membranes (VM). In the latter, they form a very stable complex resistent even to SDS. The complex formation precedes the fusion, which is initiated by an influx of calcium ions through the calcium channel. Upon increase of the intracellular calcium concentration, plasma-membrane-docked vesicles fuse with the membrane, releasing their contents into the synaptic cleft. If one of the fusion proteins is destroyed, fusion will not occur and transmitter release will be inhibited. Clostridial neurotoxins proteolyse one distinct substrate each before the formation of the complex occurs. Each toxin cleaves its substrate at a different site, except for tetanus and botulinum B toxins, which cleave synaptobrevin 2 at the same site.

tonic or spastic muscles, which will be paralyzed within 3–5 days, resulting in the disappearance of pain and in an improvement of control of motor function. The protein normally will not stimulate the immune sytem. In rare cases when antibodies are produced and the toxin loses its efficacy, the patients can be treated with one of the other serotypes of botulinum toxin.

Bibliography

Ahnert-Hilger, G., and Bigalke, H. (1995). Molecular aspects of tetanus and botulinum neurotoxin poisoning. *Prog. Neurobiol.* **46,** 83–96.

Aktories, K. (1992). Clostridium botulinum C2 toxin and C. botulinum C3 ADP-ribosyltransferase. *In* "Selective Neurotoxicity" (H. Herken and F. Hucho, eds.), pp. 841–854. Springer Verlag, Berlin-Heidelberg.

Aktories, K. (1997). Rho proteins: Targets for bacterial toxins and regulators of bacterial invasion. *Trends in Microbiology,* (in press).

Bhakdi, S., and Tranum-Jensen, J. (1984). Mechanism of complement cytolysis and the concept of channel-forming proteins. *Philos. Trans. R. Soc. London Ser. B* **306,** 311–324.

Bhakdi, S., and Tranum-Jensen, J. (1988). Damage to cell membranes by pore-forming bacterial cytolysins. *Progress in Allergy* **40,** 1–43.

Bouquet P., and Gill, D. M. (1991). Modulation of cell functions by ADP-ribosylating bacterial toxins. *In* "Sourcebook of Bacterial Protein Toxins" (J. E. Alouf and J. H. Freer, eds.), pp. 23–44. Academic Press, San Diego, CA.

Collier, J. R., and Kaplan, D. A. (1984). Immunotoxins. *Sci. Amer.* **251,** 44–52.

Montecucco, C,. Schiavo, G., Tugnoli, V., de Grandis, D. (1996). Botulinum neurotoxins: Mechanisms of action and therapeutic applications. *Mol. Med.* **46,** 419–424.

Niemann, H. (1991). Molecular biology of clostridial neurotoxins. *In* "Sourcebook of Bacterial Protein Toxins" (J. E. Alouf and J. H. Freer, eds.), pp. 229–344. Academic Press, San Diego, CA.

O'Brien, A. D., Tesh, V. L., Donohue-Rolfe, A., Jackson, M. P., Olsnes, S., Sandvig, K., Lindberg, A. A., and Keusch, G. T. (1992). Shiga toxin: Biochemistry, genetics, mode of action and role in pathogenesis. *Curr. Topics in Microbiol. Immunol.* **180,** 65–116.

Südhof, T. C., and Jahn, R. (1991). Proteins of synaptic vesicles involved in exocytosis and membrane recycling. *Neuron* **6,** 665–677.

Wellhöner, H. H. (1992). Tetanus and botulinum neurotoxins. *In* "Handbook Experimental Pharmacology" (H. Herken and F. Hucho, eds.), pp. 357–417. Springer Verlag, Berlin-Heidelberg.

PART

IV

APPLICATION OF TOXICOLOGY

CHAPTER

42

Biomonitoring in Occupational Medicine

HUGO W. RÜDIGER
Department of Occupational Medicine University of Vienna, Vienna, Austria

INTRODUCTION

Occupational medicine faces some unique conditions, which facilitate the acquisition of scientific information on the health effects of toxic substances and which may be characterized as follows.

- Hazardous substances that may occur in a given working environment are well known.
- There are a few substances, sometimes only a single substance, that are present in large amounts in a work place, in contrast to the situation in the general environment with innumerable substances, each being present in a very small quantity.
- Regulations exist for the health surveillance of exposed workers in most industrial countries. Systematic investigations have been initiated to fulfill these regulatory needs, which have provided a large body of data on the possible health effects, benefits of preventive measures, and conditions of specific individual susceptibilities.
- Occupational diseases have been established, which, by definition, represent health disturbances that are typically related to specific work conditions or particular toxic influences during work. These diseases are the subjects of study of occupational physicians with respect to diagnosis, therapy, rehabilitation, prevention, and expert opinion for compensation.

On the basis of this information it is possible to define threshold values for chemical substances in the work environment "which generally do not have adverse effects on the health of the employee nor cause unreasonable annoyance, even when the person is repeatedly exposed during long periods, given a forty-hour week and an eight-hour working day" (German Commission for the Investigation of Health Hazards of Chemical Compounds at the Workplace, 1997). These threshold limit values have initially been determined for the work place air (MAK values, TLV values); their protective function, however, has limitations (Table 1). To overcome the limitations of air monitoring with respect to an optimal prevention of toxic hazards in the work place, methods have been evaluated to supplement the determination of toxic compounds in the ambient air by analytical procedures in the biologic material. Analyses of the biological material provide information on the various steps inside the exposed individual that bridges the gap between an external exposure to a toxic agent and a possibly resulting occupational or environmental disease (Fig. 1).

According to this concept, biological monitoring encompasses the determination of three general types of markers in the biological material, which in principle have different meanings.

1. Markers of the internal dose with the target dose in critical tissues as an important subfraction.
2. Markers of biologic effects, which in the sequel may cause a disturbed function.
3. Markers of susceptibility, which may play a role in each of the various steps that ultimately may lead to a clinical disease.

SOURCES OF BIOLOGICAL MATERIAL

A variety of sources can be used for biological monitoring in occupational medicine: blood, urine, sa-

TABLE 1 Principal Shortcomings of Ambient Air Monitoring

Uptake depends on the extent of physical work load
Dermal and intestinal uptake is possible and may be independent of the concentration of the substance in the ambient air
Uptake of chemical substance from the ambient air is largely influenced by individual hygiene measures
Individual differences exist in the metabolism of the variant toxic substances
May be a large interindividual variability in the excretion of a genotoxic substance
Substances and metabolites with an uneven compartmental distribution and accumulation in various tissues of the body may lead to toxic internal concentrations even though the concentration in the ambient air is kept within limits; this is noteworthy in particular for metals and for halogenated organic compounds
Chemical substances may interact with one another in the organism and interact with various lifestyle effects in unpredictable ways

liva, epithelial cells, hair, and seminal fluid. Among these, blood and urine are the most predominantly studied materials. Analyzing exhaled air has been proposed for some volatile compounds, such as benzene or ethyl alcohol; standardization, however, is difficult here, and the frequent occurrence of preanalytical errors has prevented its application in a larger scale for routine investigations. Hair, although it can be obtained easily and has been used for metal analysis in environmental studies, especially in children, has not gained a place in occupational toxicology, because the quantitative determinations with this material are very unreliable—washing, dyeing, the location from where it is taken, and even its natural color may affect the test results. Epithelial cells, from mucous membranes in particular, have been used for genotoxic monitoring only. Studies of seminal fluid are confined to reproductive toxicity.

QUALITY ASSURANCE IN THE ANALYTICAL LABORATORY

In contrast to routine assays in clinical chemistry, the analytical parameters in the field of biological monitoring in occupational medicine are used less frequently and the material to be analyzed often must be forwarded to a distant specialized laboratory. This creates a higher risk of preanalytical errors due to contamination. Other sources of preanalytical errors are inappropriate sampling of the material, major delay between the collection and analysis, and inappropriate temperature during the transport (Table 2). Sometimes the disposable plastic tips of semi-automatic pipettes may liberate metal ions that have been used as catalysts during the manufacturing process or as coloring pigments, especially Zn, Fe, Mn, and Cd.

Achieving precision and accuracy in laboratory analyses is a complex task, requiring the identification, estimation, and the elimination of various kinds

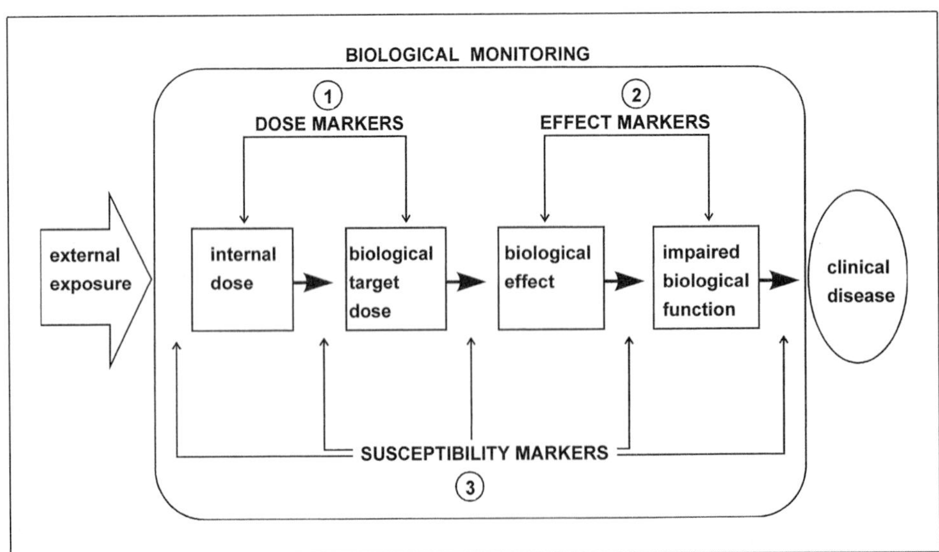

FIGURE 1 Biological monitoring deals with the various steps of the continuum between external exposure and clinical disease. These steps can be grouped as exposure markers, effect markers, and susceptibility markers.

of errors. Within the categories of preanalytical, analytical, and post-analytical errors, three types can be discerned—crude, systematic, and random errors—a clear distinction being difficult in cases where a combination of errors are involved. The main goal of quality control is the elimination of systematic errors that determine the distribution of measurement results from individual laboratories and methods (Table 3).

While the determination of pre- and post-analytical errors may be very difficult, the analytical error, involving the imprecision and inaccuracy of the method, can be monitored with internal control systems and external quality-assessment schemes. To ensure that the required precision is maintained, control samples at different concentration levels should be included at fixed or random positions in each analytical run and the results of measurement must be plotted on control charts. Most quality-control decisions are based on daily observations and each individual laboratory has to define its system for internal quality-control decisions. In any case, the conditions under which a result is obtained must be specified.

The control of accuracy is an important continuing activity in the laboratory's quality-control program in order to assess the adequacy of a measurement method. It is not so much the precision as the trueness of the analyses that needs improvement. It is essential to recognize changes in the calibration curve over a long period of analysis. Reference procedures and reference materials have been widely applied for ensuring correct calibration.

In addition to internal quality control, external proficiency testing is essential for the improvement of the trueness of laboratory methods. It provides an independent validation of internal quality-control systems by an external agency and gives at intervals a comparison of a laboratory's results with those of other laboratories. External quality-control programs include a wide range of analyses and are performed to ensure inter-laboratory comparability and long-term stability of analytical quality.

TABLE 2 Frequent Sources of Pre-analytic Errors
Inappropriate collection of the material
Use of stainless steel needles for the collection of blood may cause contamination from Cr, Co, Ni, and Mn
Residual traces of disinfectants and detergents; presence of softeners liberated from plastic material
Coating of the tubes, anticoagulants, additives, and stoppers may contain large amounts of interfering material in particular metals
Glassware is a major source of metal contamination
Contamination by dust and water (urine collection)
Problems during transport of the samples
Contamination by infectious agents, in particular from buffer substances, such as citrate, phophates, and acetate, which may serve as a fertile soil for bacteria and fungi
Decomposition of labile organic compounds
Evaporation of volatile substances if not collected in gas-tight tubes
Inappropriate temperature during transportation

TABLE 3 Sources of Systematic Errors in the Analytical Laboratory
Inappropriate specification of a chemical.
Inadequate sampling or preparation, e.g., contamination, storage conditions, dilution effects, loss of recovery.
Reagents, e.g., poor quality, wrong storage, inadequate use
Inappropriate reference materials, e.g., differences in sample matrix and reference material, deterioration, background values
Insufficient calibration, e.g., deficient standard solutions, lack of reference materials, measurement error
Method-related error, e.g., low specificity, interferences, measurement beyond the tested range, ignorance of blank values
Insufficient conditions of measurement, e.g., equipment settings, drifting, contamination, deficient maintenance

REFERENCE VALUES IN THE BIOLOGICAL MATERIAL

The systematic evaluation of reference values for occupational toxicants in biological material started in 1971 in Germany. These biological workplace tolerance values (BAT values) of a substance were related to the corresponding maximal tolerance values in the air of the work place (MAK values). BAT values were not intended to control or even correct MAK values but, by definition, represent the ceiling values for the concentration of a substance or of a relevant metabolite for a healthy individual. BAT values are defined for healthy adult persons exposed at work for at most 8 hours a day and 40 hours a week. These values, therefore, must not be used either directly or with a fixed conversation factor to protect other groups or the population in general from adverse health effects caused, for instance, by environmental influences. BAT values do not protect from allergic reactions and may not exclude embryotoxic effects that can occur below the defined threshold level. The German Commission for the Investigation of Health Hazards of Chemical Compounds in the Working Area therefore intends to evaluate the individual substances on the

MAK list in order to determine whether an embryotoxic risk can be excluded by adherence to MAK and BAT values, whether such risk has been reliably proven, and whether it must be assumed as probable according to the existing informations (Deutsche Forschungsgemeinschaft, MAK and BAT values, 1996).

When considering the definition of BAT as an internal ceiling value corresponding to the respective MAK in the working air, it becomes clear that a BAT value does not make sense for substances that are not incorporated at all or that exert their predominant toxic influence by an irritation of the skin, conjunctivae, or mucous membranes. In this case the limit value as defined for the air is sufficient.

In the U.S., reference values for biological monitoring are defined as biological exposure indices (BEI values). The aim of the BEI is similar to that of the BAT values; the definition, however, differs, as BEI do not represent ceiling values but the mean values of a substance, a metabolite, or another relevant indicator found in the biological material at the threshold-limit air value of a substance. Therefore BAT and BEI, although largely in the same range, may differ slightly from one another depending on the different underlying philosophy.

Reference values for the biological material as defined by the German Commission for the Investigation of Health Hazards of Chemical Compounds in the Work Area and by the American Conference of Governmental Industrial Hygienists are listed for comparison in Table 4. No attempt has been made by either commission to distinguish in principle between internal dose markers and biological effect markers.

BIOLOGICAL EFFECT MONITORING

In addition to the determination of an internal dose, it is often desirable to determine whether an incorporated substance has induced a functional impairment or an adverse alteration of the biological structures. This surveillance for biological strain has been called biological effect monitoring, and it is feasible to use it for many toxic compounds in the working environment to supplement the parameters of the internal dose (Table 4). In general, biological monitoring should not be based on a single parameter only and should not rely entirely on internal dose monitoring when biological effect markers are available. The great number of indices that can be monitored in lead-exposed workers provide a good example to illustrate this (Table 5). The following conclusions can be deduced from the data.

- Because lead is accumulated in various tissues, in particular in the bone, a quantitative determination in the bone mirrors the long-term exposure rather than a determination in the blood or urine.
- Various parameters of biological effect monitoring may be considerably altered in lead-exposed workers, even though the lead level in the blood and urine is in the tolerable range. This discrepancy is particularly pronounced with coproporphyrine III (Fig. 2), which in workers chronically exposed to lead may be increased up to four-fold compared to the controls, although the lead level in blood (mean 11.2 vs. 4.5 μg/dl) of these probands was only slightly higher and, on an individual basis, exhibited only a marginal correlation with the coproporphyrine excretion in the urine as determined after HPLC separation.
- Some of the parameters that may indicate biological strain are highly unspecific and may thus be used only in connection with other more specific indices.
- Growing information on the biological effects of an exposure may stimulate the adaptation of the threshold levels of exposure. In particular, the cognitive disturbances that are a consequence of chronic low-level exposure to lead provide a reason to consider a decrease of the maximal allowable concentration in the work place.

Biological Effect Monitoring of Genotoxic Hazards

Biological effect monitoring in exposed workers is performed in particular when safety limits for a substance cannot be defined, as for genotoxic and carcinogenic compounds. The ultimate target of such agents is the genetic substance, DNA. In germ cells, alterations of DNA may lead to germ-line mutations and to genetic diseases in subsequent generations; in somatic cells the relevant endpoint is neoplastic transformation. Indices of a genotoxic effect that have been used in occupational medicine are listed in Table 6.

Most of the indices listed here are very sensitive, but common to all is a very low specificity. This may be considered as an advantage for the purposes of biological monitoring because this low specificity makes it possible to use these tests for the genotoxic surveillance of workers in almost all instances of a supposed genotoxic exposure, even exposures to unidentified agents or complex mixtures. On the other hand, any enhanced values of these unspecific parameters must be interpreted with great caution because they might have been elicited by innumerable influ-

TABLE 4 Threshold Level Values in the Biological Material

Exposure	Measured Parameter	ACGIH[a]			DFG[b]		
		TLV[c]	BEI value[d]	Sampling time	MAK[e]/TRK[f]	BAT[g]/EKA[h] values	Sampling time
Acetone	Acetone (U)	750 ppm	100 mg/liter	b	500 ppm	80 mg/l	b
Acetylcholinesterase inhibitors	Acetylcholinesterase (E)		30% drop	a		30% drop	b, c
Acrylonitrile	Cyanoethylvaline (E)				3 ppm*	420 μg/l*	a
Alkali chromates (VI)	Chromium (E)	0.05 mg/m³ (water-soluble) 0.01 mg/m³ (insoluble)			0.05 mg/m³* CrO_3	17 μg/liter whole blood*	c
	Chromium (U)		30 μ/g creatinine	b		20 μg/liter*	b
	Chromium (U)		10 μg/g creatinine	Increasing g during shift			
Aluminum	Aluminum (U)	10 mg/m³ (Metal dust)	100 μg/l	b	6 mg/m³ (Fine particles)	200 μg/liter	b
Aniline	Free aniline (U)	2 ppm			2 ppm	1 mg/liter	b, c
	Liberated from hemoglobin					100 μg/l	b, c
	Total *p*-aminophenol (U)		50 mg/g	b			
	Methemoglobin (B)		1.5%	b, c			
Arsenic including soluble derivatives	As and As metabolites (U)	0.01 mg/m³; arsine: 0.05 ppm	10 μg/g creatinine	b			
Arsenic trioxide	Arsenic (U) by hydrogenation	0.01 mg/m³	50 μg/g creatinine	b	0.1 mg/m³*	130 μg/liter*	b
Benzene	Benzene (EA) mixed-exhaled	0.3 ppm (intended)	0.08 ppm	d			
	Benzene (EA) end-exhaled		0.12 ppm	d			
	Total phenol (U)		50 mg/g creatinine	b			
	Benzene (B)				1 ppm*	5 μg/liter*	b
	S-Phenyl-mercapturic acid (U)					0.045 mg/g creatinine*	b
	t,t-Muconic acid (U)					2 mg/liter*	b
2-Butoxyethylacetate	Butoxyacetic acid (U)				20 ppm	100 mg/liter	c
2-Butoxyethanol	Butoxyacetic acid (U)				20 ppm	100 mg/liter	c
p-ter-Butylphenol	*p*-ter-Butylphenol (U)				0.08 ppm	2 mg/liter	b
Cadmium and inorganic compounds	Cadmium (B)	0,01 mg/m³ (total dust)	5 μg/liter	a			
	Cadmium (U)		5 μg/g creatinine	a			
Carbon disulfide	4-Thio-4-thiazolidine carboxylic acid (=TTCA) (U)	10 ppm	5 mg/g creatinine	b	10 ppm	8 mg/liter	b
Carbon monoxide	Carboxyhemoglobin (B)	25 ppm	3.5%	b	30 ppm	5%	b
	Carbon monoxide (EA) end-exhaled		20 ppm	b			

continues

		ACGIH[a]			DFG[b]		
Exposure	Measured Parameter	TLV[c]	BEI value[d]	Sampling time	MAK[e]/TRK[f]	BAT[g]/EKA[h] values	Sampling time
Chlorobenzene	Total 4-chlorocatechol (U)	10 ppm	150 mg/g creatinine	b	50 ppm	300 mg/g creatinine	b
	Total 4-chlorocatechol (U)					70 mg/g creatinine	d
	Total *p*-chlorophenol (U)		25 mg/g creatinine	b			
Cobalt	Cobalt (B)	0.02 mg/m^3	1 μg/liter	b	0.1 mg/m^3*	5 μ/liter*	a
	Cobalt (U)		15 μg/1	b		60 μ/liter*	a
Dichloromethane	Dichloromethane (B)	50 ppm			100 ppm	1 mg/liter	b
	Carboxyhemoglobin (B)					5%	b
N,N-Dimethylacetamide	*n*-Methylacetamide (U)	10 ppm	30 mg/g creatinine	b	10 ppm		
Dimethylformamide	*n*-Methylformamide (U)	10 ppm	20 mg/g creatinine	b	10 ppm	15 mg/liter	b
2-Ethyoxyethanol	Ethoxyacetic acid (U)	5 ppm	100 mg/g creatinine	b	5 ppm	50 mg/liter	b, c
2-Ethoxyethyl acetate	Ethoxyacetic acid (U)	5 ppm	100 mg/g creatinine	b	5 ppm	50 mg/liter	b, c
Ethylbenzene	Mandelic acid (U)	100 ppm	1.5 g/g creatinine	b	100 ppm		
Ethylene	Hydroxyethylvaline (E)				50 mg/m^3*	90 μg/liter*	a
Ethylene glycol dinitrate	Ethylene glycol dinitrate (B)				0.05	0.3 μ/liter	b
Ethylene oxide	Ethylene oxide (EA)	1 ppm			1 ppm*	0.24 ppm*	During exposure (> 4 h)
	Hydroxyethylvaline (E)					90 μ/liter*	a
Furfural	Total furoic acid (U)	2 ppm	200 mg/g creatinine	b			
Halothane (2-bromo-2-chloro-1,1,1-trifluoroethane)	Trifluoroacetic acid (B)	50 ppm			5 ppm	2.5 mg/liter	b, c
γ-1,2,4,4,5,6-Hexachlorocyclohexane	γ-1,2,4,4,5,6-Hexachlorocyclohexane (B)	0.5 mg/m^3			0.5 mg/m^3	20 μg/liter	b
	γ-1,2,4,4,5,6-Hexachlorocyclohexane (P/S)					25 μg/liter	b
Hexachlorobenzene	Hexachlorobenzene (P/S)					150 μg/liter	a
n-Hexane	Hexane-2,5-dione and 4,5-Dihydroxy-2-hexanone (U)	50 ppm			50 ppm	5 mg/liter	b
	2,5-Hexanedione (U)		5 mg/g creatinine	b			
Hydrazine	Hydrazine (U)	0.01 ppm			0.1 ppm*	380 μ/g creatinine*	b
	Hydrazine (P)					340 μ/liter*	b
Hydrogen fluoride and inorganic fluorine compounds (fluorides)	Fluoride (U)	2.5 mg/m^3	10 mg/g creatinine	b	3 ppm	7 mg/g creatinine	b
	Fluoride (U)		3 mg/g creatinine	d		4 mg/g creatinine	d

Lead	Lead (B)	0.05 mg/m³	300 μg/liter	a	0.1 mg/m³	700 μg/liter; 300 μg/liter woman <45 year	a
	δ-Aminolevulinic acid (U)					15 mg/liter; 6 mg/liter women <45 y	a
Mercury, metallic and inorganic compounds	Mercury (B)	0.025 mg/m³	15 μg/liter	b	0.08 mg/m³	50 μg/liter	a
	Mercury (U)		35 μg/g creatinine	d		200 μg/liter	a
Mercury, organic compounds	Mercury (B)	0.01 mg/m³ alkylcomp. 0.1 mg/m³ arylcomp.			0.01 mg/m³	100 μg/liter	a
Methyl butyl ketone; 2-hexanone	Hexane-2,5-dione and 4,5-Dihydroxy-2-hexanone (U)	5 ppm			5 ppm	5 mg/liter	b
Methyl ethyl ketone; 2-butanone	2-Butanone (U)	200 ppm	2 mg/liter	b	200 ppm	5 mg/liter	b
Methanol	Methanol (U)	200 ppm	15 mg/liter	b	200 ppm	30 mg/liter	b, c
Methemoglobin inducers	Methemoglobin (B)		1.5%	b, c			
Methyl isobutyl ketone	4-Methyl-2-pentanone (U)	50 ppm	2 mg/liter	b	20 ppm	3.5 mg/liter	b
Nickel	Nickel (U)	0.05 mg/m³			0.5 mg/m³*	45 μg/liter*	c
Nitrobenzene	Aniline (released from hemoglobin-conjugate) (B)	1 ppm			1 ppm	100 mg/liter	c
	Total *p*-nitrophenol (U)		5 mg/g creatinine	b			
	Methemoglobin (B)		1.5%	b			
Nitroglycerin	1, 2-Glycerindinitrate (P/S)				0.05 ppm	0.5 μg/liter	b
	1,3-Glycerindinitrate (P/S)					0.5 μg/liter	b
Parathion	*p*-Nitrophenol (U)	0.1 mg/m³	0.5 mg/g creatinine	b	0.1 mg/m³	500 μg/liter	c
	Cholinesterase (E)		30% drop	a		30% drop	c
Pentachlorophenol	Total PCP (U)	0.5 mg/m³	2 mg/g creatinine	c, d	0.05 mg/m³*	300 μg/liter*	a
	Total-PCP (P/S)					1000 μg/liter*	a
	Free PCP (P)		5 mg/liter	b			
Phenol	Phenol (U)	5 ppm	250 mg/g creatinine	b	5 ppm	300 mg/liter	b
2-Propanol	Acetone (B)				200 ppm	50 mg/liter	b
	Acetone (U)					50 mg/liter	b
Styrene	Mandelic acid (U)	20 ppm	800 mg/g creatinine	b	20 ppm	400 mg/liter	b
			300 mg/g creatinine				
				d			
	Mandelic acid and Phenylglyoxylic acid (U)					500 mg/liter	b
	Phenylglyoxylic acid (U)		240 mg/g creatinine	b			
			100 mg/g creatinine	d			
	Styrene (VB)		0.55 mg/liter	b			

continues

TABLE 4 *(Continued)*

Exposure	Measured parameter	ACGIH[a]			DFG[b]		
		TLV[c]	BEI value[d]	Sampling time	MAK[e]/TRK[f]	BAT[g]/EKA[h] values	Sampling time
Tetramethyl lead, Tetraethyl lead	Diethyllead (U)				0.05 mg/m^3	25 μg/liter (calculated as Pb)	b
	Total lead (U)					50 μg/liter	b
Tetrachloroethylene	Tetrachloroethylene (B)	25 ppm	0.5 mg/liter	c, d	50 ppm	1 mg/liter	d
	Tetrachloroethylene (EA)		5 ppm	c, d		9.5 ml/m^3	d
	Trichloroacetic acid (U)		3.5 mg/liter	b			
Tetrachloromethane	Tetrachloromethane (EA)				10 ppm	1.6 ml/m^3	e: 1 h
	Tetrachloromethane (B)					70 μg/liter	b, c
Tetrahydrofuran	Tetrahydrofuran (U)	200 ppm			50 ppm	8 mg/liter	b
Toluene	Toluene (B)	50 ppm	50 μg/liter (intended)	d	50 ppm	1 mg/liter	b
	o-Cresole (U)					3 mg/liter	b, c
1,1,1-Trichloroethane	1,1,1-Trichloroethane (B)	350 ppm			200 ppm	550 μg/liter	c, d
	1,1,1-Trichloroethane (EA)		40 ppm	c, d		20 ml/m^3	c, d
	Trichloroacetic acid (U)		10 mg/liter	b			
	Total trichloroethanol (U)		30 mg/liter	b			
	Total trichloroethanol (B)		1 mg/liter	b			
Trichloroethylene	Trichloroethanol (U)	50 ppm	4 mg/liter	b		5 mg/liter	b, c
	Trichloroacetic acid (U)		100 mg/g creatinine	b		100 mg/liter	b, c
	Trichloroacetic acid and trichloroethanol (U)		300 mg/g creatinine	b			
Vanadium pentoxide	Vanadium (U)	0.05 mg/m^3	50 μg/g creatinine	b	0.05 mg/m^3 (fine dust)	70 μg/g creatinine	c
Vinyl chloride	Thiodiglycolic acid (U)	5 ppm			2 ppm*	2.4 mg/24 h	c
Xylene (all isomers)	Xylene (B)	100 ppm		b	100 ppm	1.5 mg/liter	b
	Methylhippuric acid (U)		1.5 g/g creatinine	b			b
	Methylhippuric (toluric) acid (U)					2000 mg/liter	b

[a] ACGIH: American Conference of Governmental Industrial Hygienists.
[b] DFG: Commission for the Investigation of Health Hazards of Chemical Compounds in the Work Area (Germany).
[c] TLV: Threshold limit values (U.S.).
[d] BEI: Biological exposure indices (U.S.).
[e] MAK: Maximum concentrations at the workplace (Germany).
[f] TRK: Technical exposure limits (Germany).
[g] BAT: Biological tolerance values (Germany).
[h] EKA: Exposure equivalents for carcinogenic materials (Germany).

TABLE 5 Biological Monitoring of Inorganic Lead Exposure

Parameter/Source	Significance	Specifity
A. Parameters of dose monitoring		
Lead (blood)	most frequently used but questionable correlation with health effects (for instance in central nervous system); is a composite of lead contribution from the environment and from internal stores, primarily bone; cumulative blood lead index provides a good indicator of chronic lead exposure; nonlinear relationship between B-Pb and lead exposure and uptake; nonlinear relationship between different metabolic and toxic effects, such as those on the heme and nucleotide synthesis and B-Pb, therefore not a very good index of either exposure or effects; half life of 30 days	specific
Lead (urine)	similar to blood level determination; dependent on renal function; in low or moderate exposure the lead concentrations are considerably lower in urine than in blood	specific
Lead (bone)	provides a practical technique for lead screening purposes; good indicator of long term lead exposure; helps to assess cumulative lead absorption; correlates well with cumulative blood lead indices and some lead induced CNS-effects; source of internal exposure; has the biggest share of the total body burden; half life of 17 to 25 years	specific
B. Parameters of effect monitoring		specific
1. Synthesis of heme		
δ-aminolevulinic acid	considerable interindividual variation	
δ-aminolevulinic acid dehydratase	begins to decline at very low B-Pb concentrations (10-20μg/dl) and is totally inhibited at moderate levels (70-90μg/dl); inhibition of ALA-dehydratase is the earliest of all known biologic effects of lead; correlates well with B-Pb; sensitive measure for the early determination of increased lead exposure; considerable interindividual variation	specific
Coproporphyrin III	considerable interindividual variation	moderately specific
Erythrocyte protoporphyrin	considerable interindividual variation; close correlations between EP and B-Pb; begins to rise at B-Pb concentrations of 25-30μg/dl; not sufficiently sensitive at lower levels of B-Pb	moderately specific
Hemoglobin	slight drop in the hemoglobin level at B-Pb levels of 50 to 80μg/dl; considerable interindividual variation; at low levels of exposure lead in erythrocytes is associated primarily with hemoglobin	unspecific
Erythrocytes	99% of the lead in blood is associated with erythrocytes; lead shortens the erythrocyte life span; considerable interindividual variation	unspecific
2. Renal function		
β-NAG	impaired tubular function	unspecific
Creatinine clearance	impaired glomerular function	unspecificc
3. Nervous system		
homovanillinic acid (urine)	is a major metabolite of dopamine; is positively correlated with biomarkers of lead exposure (B-Pb, ZPP); is negatively correlated with some neurobehavioral performances	unspecific
a. Peripheral nerves		
Vibration	vibratory thresholds provide a sensitive measure of effects of lead; correlation between current B-Pb and vibratory thresholds	unspecific
Conduction velocity	negative correlation with long-term exposure to lead; slowing motor nerve conduction velocity in workers with blood lead concentrations below 70μg/dl; slowed conduction in the small motor fibers of the ulnar nerve is the most sensitive peripheral index of the neurotoxicity of lead; correlation between B-Pb and sensory and motor conduction velocity of the median nerve	unspecific
Electromyography	fibrillations and diminished numbers of motor units of maximal contraction	unspecific
Tendon reflexes		unspecific
b. Central nervous system	lead induced CNS-effects are age- and dose-dependent; correlation between exposure to lead and diminished neuropsychological performance in asymptomatic workers; subjective symptoms like headache, restlessness, depression or hyperirritability with occur	unspecific

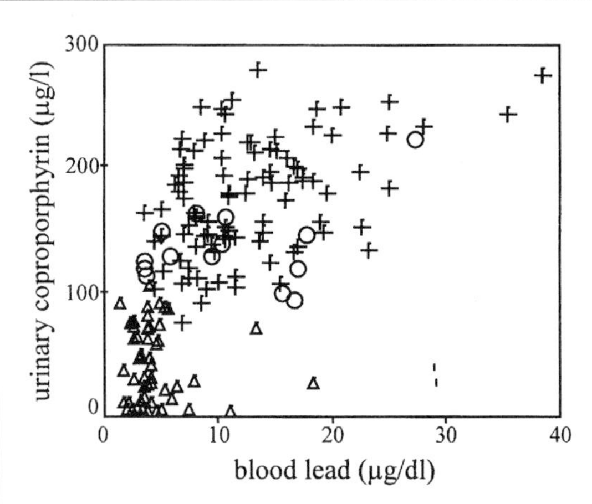

FIGURE 2 Urinary coproporphyrine excretion in workers exposed to lead (+, O) and unexposed control probands (▲) were plotted against the individual blood-lead levels. Although their blood lead was only slightly elevated and below the BAT value of 70 μg/dl, the exposed workers had a markedly enhanced excretion of total coproporphyrine.

ences other than exposure in the work place and may even be increased on the basis of an individual's constitution. The cytogenetic parameters exhibit any especially large interindividual variability that cannot be explained in most cases and that may not be attributed to genotoxic exposure at all. Normal individuals, for instance, may have up to 12 SCE per metaphase and up to 10 micronuclei per 500 double-nucleated cells in PAH-stimulated lymphocytes. In addition, some cytogenetic parameters, in particular, micronuclei, increase with age, and women may have a higher rate than men.

Therefore the following rules should be followed when gentoxic parameters are used for biological monitoring.

1. Each surveillance study with genotoxic markers must include an unexposed control group.
2. All laboratory analyses within the same study preferably should be done by the same investigator and must be blind.
3. Genotoxic markers preferably should be used on a group basis. Determinations in single individuals cannot be interpreted unless actual values are extremely high or pre-exposure values are available for the same individual. In contrast to the use of laboratory parameters elsewhere in medicine, normal values have not been defined here.
4. A detailed history has to be obtained from each proband of a study, which includes lifestyle factors; other genotoxic exposures, such as smoking, medication, alcohol, and exposure to radiation; and intake of possible protective agents, such as vitamins.

DETERMINANTS OF SUSCEPTIBILITY TO TOXIC INFLUENCES

The continuum between exposure and clinical diseases is influenced by susceptibility markers that may specifically be active at each of the various steps that can be determined by biological monitoring. The susceptibility categories listed in Table 7 can be grouped into three classes.

1. Common factors, such as age, gender, and ethnic origin, which are of almost neglectable significance in occupational toxicology. Periods of life such as early childhood or old age are not to be considered in the working environment, and fetotoxic effects are separately evaluated. Reports of an enhanced cancer risk in black coke-oven workers are exposure related and not secondary to ethnic origin because 19% of the black employees, but only 3% of the whites, worked on the top side the coke oven where the exposure to carcinogenic polycyclic aromatic hydrocarbons is highest. Other enhanced rates of susceptibility in ethnic groups can be related to polymorphic alleles, which are known to differ among ethnic groups, such as, for instance, the alcohol dehydrogenase and acetaldehyde dehydrogenase polymorphisms that may cause an alcohol intolerance in individuals of Asian origin. Enhanced lead sensitivity in Caucasians secondary to δ-aminolevoulinic acid dehydratase polymorphism is another example. The increased sensitivity of women to many toxicants can easily be explained by their lower body weight.
2. Susceptibility factors with moderate prevalence, which may have a marked significance. This group consists of the numerous acquired conditions or diseases, chemical environment and lifestyles, genetic polymorphisms, and heterozygous states of some recessive disorders. Most of the recessively inherited diseases are very rare, but according to the Hardy–Weinberg formula of genetic equilibrium in the population, the frequency of heterozygous carriers, even of rare genetic diseases, is surprisingly high. The prevalence of Bloom syndrome, for instance, in the population is $1{:}10^6$, although the frequency of heterozygotes is 1:500.
3. Rare genetic conditions that may strongly increase sensitivity to particular substances in the work place. This category contains a large number of indi-

TABLE 6 Indices Used to Monitor Genotoxic Effects in the Workplace

Method	Advantages, limitations, problems
A. Cytogenetic tests	
1. Chromosome analysis with phytohemagglutinin (PAH) stimulated blood lymphocytes:	
A. Dicentric chromosomes, acentric fragments, ring chromosomes, gaps, breaks by conventional techniques	Rarely applied anymore for a biologic monitoring except dicentrics which are predominantly used to monitor exposure to ionizing radiation. First generation metaphases should be used only.
B. Other structural variations as translocations and inversions by fluorescent *in situ* hybridization (FISH)	May be expensive dependent on the type and the number of the chromosome markers used. Very sensitive. Allows detection of long time cumulative exposure since these cells are not preferentially eliminated in contrast to all other cytogenetic endpoints.
2. Sister chromatid exchange (SCE) with PAH stimulated blood lymphocytes in the presence of 5-bromodeoxyuridine (5-BrUdR)	Less sensitive for clastogenic agents. Smoking may considerably increase SCE and therefore may be an important confounder when this test is used for a biologic monitoring.
3. Micronucleus test (MN) with blood lymphocytes or epithelial cells	Detects clastogenic agents. When PHA stimulated lymphocytes are used, test should be done after the first *in vitro* division. Age dependent; increase of MN must be considered.
B. Induction of DNA strand breaks and crosslinks	DNA crosslinking reduces the extent of DNA breaks which can be detected by the each of the assays listed below
1. Alkaline filter elution with white blood cell DNA	
2. Comet assay, performed with single cells, mostly blood lymphocytes or epithelial cells	
3. Nick translation assay with DNA of blood lymphocytes	
C. Covalent binding of xenobiotics (formation of adducts)	
1. DNA adducts	Several methods have been described with sensitivities being largely different as Gc/MS, immunoassays, fluorescence spectroscopy, or ^{32}P-postlabeling. Detection of 1 adduct in 10^9 base pairs is possible in some cases using ^{32}P-postlabeling.
2. Protein adducts (hemoglobin, albumin)	Principle disadvantage: proteins are not the critical target of genotoxicity. An agent may not reach the nucleus or may be completely removed from DNA by repair.
D. Induction of mutations	
1. In cellular indicator genes mostly of blood cells (HPRT, P_{53}, glycophorin locus)	
2. Induction of revertants in auxotrophic Salmonella strains (Ames test)	Unreliable results because large nutritional influences are possible and because necessary purification procedures may remove critical agents from urine.
E. Induction of DNA repair	Not useful in general when the genotoxic action of an agent is caused at least in part by its interference with DNA repair (for instance arsenic)
1. Unscheduled DNA synthesis in blood lymphocytes (UDS)	
2. SOS chromotest (urine) with genetically engineered microorganisms	

vidual conditions, each of them very rare. This precludes the use of these markers for screening tests in occupational medicine.

The practical value of susceptibility testing has often been questioned. The main reasons for critical reservation are

- The testing can be misused as a general instrument of selection among workers on the basis of particular sensitivities.
- The testing can be misused to discriminate against individuals and groups.
- Application of susceptibility markers may serve as a surrogate for, and therefore delay improvements in, occupational hygiene measures to reduce a toxic exposure.
- Instead of the identification and protection of the individual susceptible worker, attempts should be made to adapt the allowable exposure limits in the work place to the reduced tolerance level of the

TABLE 7 Determinants of Susceptibility to Toxic Influences

Factors	Biologic effect and susceptibility
I. Genetic factors	
Genetic polymorphisms	
Cytochrome P450 gene family in particular CYP1A1, CYP1A2, CYP2D6, CYP2E1, CYP3A4	Increased cancer risk described for extensive metabolizers after exposure to polycyclic aromatic hydrocarbons, heterocyclic amines, aflatoxins, and aromatic amines.
Glutathion-S-transferase gene family GSTa, GSTμ, GST-theta	Decreased detoxification of various epoxides, ethylene oxide, and halogenated aliphatic compounds.
N-acetyltransferase (NAT1, NAT2)	Slow acetylators (ca. 50% Caucasians) are at risk for allylamine-induced cancer of the urinary bladder.
Paraoxonase	Decreased activity possibly associated with enhanced sensitivity to organophosphates and with coronary heart disease.
Aldehyde dehydrogenase gene family Polymorphism of ALDH-1, -2, -5 has been identified	Reduced metabolism of aldehydes generated during the metabolism of various compounds.
Variation of DNA repair	
Heterozygotes BLOOM syndrome	Helicase deficiency. Increased sensitivity to various genotoxic agents.
Xeroderma pigmentosum	Reduced excision repair of thymidine dimers in DNA. Increased sensitivity to ultraviolet radiation.
Ataxia telangiectasia	Impaired DNA repair due to a defective cell cycle checkpoint. Increased sensitivity to ionizing radiation.
O6-alkyl-DNA-alkyltransferase	Decreased activity corresponds with enhanced genotoxic effect of DNA methylating agents.
II. Nongenetic factors	
Acquired conditions or diseases (examples)	
Bone marrow depression	Aplastic anemia by benzene and toluene, chloramphenicol.
Renal tubular dysfunction	Reduced tolerance to lead, cadmium and mercury.
Diseases of the liver	Increased sensitivity to most organic solvents, in particular halogenated organic compounds.
Bronchial hyperresponsiveness	Increased sensitivity to bronchial irritants like NO_x and SO_2.
Chemical environment/lifestyle (examples)	
Smoking	Increased sensitivity to asbestos.
Alcohol	Increased sensitivity to neurotoxic effects of many solvents.

minority, thus eliminating all problems of discrimination and selection.

- The prediction value of a sensitivity marker is dependent on its prevalence in the population. According to Bayes' theorem, it can be calculated that testing for a rare trait of 0.1% prevalence in the population will result in 91% false positives, even under the optimistic assumption that both the sensitivity and the specificity of the test is 99%.

These considerations, although justified in principle, must be weighed against the endeavor of occupational medicine, namely to protect the individual worker and to prevent work-related diseases as effectively as possible. As long as the sensitivity level of the most sensitive worker is not known, nobody will be able to define the level to which current threshold values are to be reduced. Moreover, threshold limit values in the work place in most Western countries are well followed, this means that the average worker should not be endangered at all by an exposure in the work area. This may be not be the case for those who have particular sensitivities for various reasons. Thus the problem of the protection of workers against toxic influences has largely boiled down to the protection of risk groups of minorities with a particular susceptibilities and, therefore, the importance of sensitivity markers is steadily increasing for practical reasons.

In general, biological monitoring in the work place does a lot more than use the worker as a "walking sampling device." Compared to air monitoring of toxic substances, it is much closer to the critical target and, in addition, it may provide a better understanding of the toxic mechanisms of substances and may finally enable us to install the necessary safety measures for individuals.

Bibliography

Badawi, A. F., Stern, S. J., Lang, N. P., and Kadlubar, F. F. (1996). Cytochrome P-450 and acetyltransferase expression as biomarkers of carcinogen n-DNA adduct levels and human cancer susceptibility. *Prog. Clin. Biol. Res.* **395,** 109–140.

Balbus-Kornfeld, J., Stewart, W., Bolla, K., and Schwartz, B. (1995). Cumulative exposure to inorganic lead and neurobehavioral test performance in adults: an epidemiologic review. *Occup. Environ. Med.* **52,** 2–12.

Barton, H. A., Flemming, C. D., and Lipscomb, J. C. (1996). Evaluating human variability in chemical risk assessment: Hazard identification and dose-response assessment for noncancer oral toxicity of trichloroethylene. *Toxicology* **111,** 271–287.

Bartsch, H. (1996). DNA adducts in human carcinogenesis: Etiological relevance and structure-activity relationship. *Muta. Res.* **340,** 67–79.

Bayes, E. T. (1763). An assay toward solving a problem in the doctrine of chance. *Philos. Trans. R. Soc. London (Biol)* **53,** 370–418.

Bielfeld, V., Weichenthal, M., Roser, M., Breitbart, E., Berger, J., Seemanova, E., and Rüdiger, H. W. (1989). Ultraviolet-induced chromosomal instability in cultured fibroblasts of heterozygote carriers for Xeroderma Pigmentosum. *Cancer Genet. Cytogenet.* **43,** 219–226.

Bleecker, M., Lindgren, K., and Ford, P. (1997). Differential contribution of current and cumulative indices of lead dose to neuropsychological performance by age. *Neurology* **48,** 639–645.

Bolt, H. M., and Drexler, H. (1994). Biologische Arbeitsstoff-Toleranzwerte (Biomonitoring), Teil II: Toxikokinetische Grundlagen (Aufnahme, Verteilung, Stoffwechsel, Ausscheidung). *Arbeitsmed, Sozialmed. Umweltmed.* **29,** 206–208.

Bolt, H. M., Riemer, F., and Schaller, K. H. (1994). Biological tolerance values for working materials (biomonitoring), Part IV. *Arbmed. Sozmed. Umwelt.* **65,** 320–323.

Deutsche Forschungsgemeinschaft (1997). *In* "Toxikologisch Arbeitsmedizinische Begründung von BAT-Werten" (H. Greim and G. Lehnert, eds.) VCH Verlagsgesellschaft, Weinheim.

Di-Giorgio, C., De-Meo, M. P., Laget, M., Guiraud, H., Botta, A., and Dumenil, G. (1994). The micronucleus assay in human lymphocytes: Screening for inter-individual variability and application to biomonitoring: *Carcinogenesis* **15,** 313–317.

Farmer, P. B., Sepai, O., Lawrence, R., Autrup, H., Nielsen, P. S., Vestergard, A. B. *et al.* (1996). Biomonitoring human exposure to environmental carcinogenic chemicals. *Mutagenesis* **11,** 363–381.

Gatti, R. A. (1991). Localizing the genes for ataxia-telangiectasia—A human model for inherited cancer susceptibility. *Adv. Cancer Res.* **56,** 77–104.

Greim, H., Csanady, G., Filser, J. G., Kreuzer, P., Schwarz, L., Wolff, T. *et al.* (1995). Biomarkers as tools in human health risk assessment. *Clin. Chem.* **41,** 1804—1808.

Guengerich, F. P., Thier, R., Persmark, M., Taylor, J. B., Pemble, S. E., and Ketterer, B. (1995). Conjugation of carcinogens by theta class glutathione s-transferases: Mechanisms and relevance to variations in human risk. *Pharmacogenetics* **5,** 103–107.

Hanawalt, P. C. (1991). Heterogeneity of DNA repair at the gene level. *Muta. Res.* **247,** 203–211.

Hemminki, K. (1995). DNA adducts in biomonitoring. *J. Occup. Environ. Med.* **37,** 44–49.

Holz, O., Joerres, R., Kaestner, A., Krause, T., and Magnussen, H. (1995). Reproducibility of basal and induced DNA single-strand breaks detected by the single-cell gel elektrophoresis assay in human peripheral mononuclear leukocytes. *Int. Arch. Occup. Environ. Health* **67,** 305–310.

Kadlubar, F. F., and Badawi, A. F. (1995). Genetic susceptibility and carcinogen-DNA adduct formation in human urinary bladder carcinogenesis. *Toxicol. Lett.* **82,** 627–632.

Krause, T., Einhaus, M., Holz, O., Meiáner, R., Baumgartner, E., and Rüdiger, H. W. (1993). A novel technique for the detection of DNA single strand breaks in human white blood cells and its combination with the unscheduled DNA synthesis assay. *Int. Arch. Occup. Environ. Health* **65,** 77–82.

Landrigan, P. (1989). Toxicity of lead at low dose. *Br. J. Indust. Med.* **46,** 593–596.

Lauwerys, R., Bernard, A. M., Roels, H. A., and Buchet, J. P. (1994). Cadmium: Exposure markers as predictors of nephrotoxic effects. *Clin. Chem.* **40,** 1391–1394.

Lewalter, J., and Neumann, H. G. (1996). Biologische Arbeitsstoff-Toleranzwerte (Biomonitoring). *Arbmed. Sozmed. Umwelt.* **31,** 275–280.

Li, W. F., Costa, L. G., and Furlong, C. E. (1993). Serum paraoxonase status: A major factor in determining resistance to organophosphates. *J. Toxicol. Environ. Health* **40,** 337–346.

Nakachi, K., Imai, K., Hayashi, S., and Kawajiri, K. (1993). Polymorphisms of the CYP1A1 and glutathione S-transferase genes associated with susceptibility to lung cancer in relation to cigarette dose in a Japanese population. *Cancer Res.* **53,** 2994–2999.

Natarajan, A. T., Boer, J. J. W. A., Darroudi, F., Van Diemen, P. C. M., Dulout, F., Hande, M. P. *et. al.* (1996). Current cytogenetic methods for detecting exposure and effects of mutagens and carcinogens. *Environ. Health Perspect.* **104,** 445–448.

Neumann, H. G., van Dorp, C., and Zwirner-Baier, I. (1995). The implications for risk assessment of measuring the relative contribution to exposure from occupation, environment and lifestyle: Hemoglobin adducts from amino- and nitro-arenes. *Toxicol. Lett.* **82,** 771–778.

Okkels, H., Sigsgaard, T., Wolf, H., and Autrup, H. (1997). Arylamine N-acetyltransferase 1(NAT1) and 2(NAT2) polymorphisms in susceptibility to bladder cancer: the influence of smoking. *Cancer Epidemiol. Biomarkers Prev.* **6,** 225–231.

Olsen, L. S., Nielsen, L. R., Nexo, B. A., and Wassermann, K. (1996). Somatic mutation detection in human biomonitoring. *Pharmacol. Toxicol.* **78,** 364–373.

Paoletti, P. (1995). Application of biomarkers in population studies for respiratory non-malignant diseases. *Toxicology* **101,** 99–105.

Perera, F. P. (1996). Molecular epidemiology: Insights into cancer susceptibility, risk assessment, and prevention. *JNCI* **88,** 496–509.

Perera, F. P., Tang, D. L., O'Neill, J. P., Bigbee, W. L., Albertini, R. J., Santella, R. *et al.* (1993). HPRT and glycophorin A mutations in foundry workers: Relationship to PAH exposure and to PAH-DNA adducts. *Carcinogenesis* **14,** 969–973.

Rappaport, S. M. (1995). Biological monitoring and standard setting in the USA: A critical appraisal. *Toxicol. Lett.* **77,** 171–182.

Raunio, H., Husgafvel-Pursiainen, K., Anttila, S., Hietanen, E., Hirvonen, A., and Pelkonen, O. (1995). Diagnosis of plymorphisms in carcinogen-activating and inactivating enzymes and cancer susceptibility—a review. *Gene* **159,** 113–121.

Rios, R., Poje, G. V., and Detels, R. (1993). Susceptibility to environmental pollutants among minorities. *Toxicol. Indust. Health* **9,** 797–820.

Risch, A., Wallace, D. M., and Bathers, S. (1995). Slow N-acetylation genotype is a susceptibility factor in occupational and smoking related bladder cancer. *Hum. Mol. Genet.* **4,** 231–236.

Rüdiger, H. W., and Lehnert, G. (1988). Toxikogenetik: Grundlagen, Methoden und Bedeutung für die Arbeitsmedizin. *Arbmed. Sozmed. Pravmed. Sonderheft* 11.

Rüdiger, H. W., Nowak, D., Hartmann, K., and Cerutti, P. (1985). Enhanced formation of Benzo(a)pyrene DNA adducts in monocytes of patients with a presumed genetic risk for lung cancer. *Cancer Res.* **45,** 5890–5894.

Rüdiger, H. W., Schwartz, U., Serrand, E., Stief, M., Krause, T., Nowak, D., Doerjer, G., and Lehnert, G. (1989). Reduced O^6

Methylguanine repair in fibroblast cultures from patients with lung cancer. *Cancer Res.* **49,** 5623–5626.

Schaller, K. H. (1996). Biologische Arbeitsstoff-Toleranzwerte (Biomonitoring). *Arbeitsmed. Sozialmed. Umweltmed.* **31,** 95–106.

Schaller, K. H., and Triebig, G. (1996). Biologische Arbeitstoff-Toleranzwerte (Biomonitoring). *Arbeitsmed. Sozialmed. Umweltmed.* **31,** 504–512.

Skerfving, S., Nilsson, U., Schütz, A., Gerhardsson, I. (1993). Biological monitoring of inorganic lead. *Scand. I. Work Environ. Health* **19,** 59–64.

Smith, C. M., Wang, X., Hu, H., and Kelsey, K. T. (1995). A polymorphism in the d-aminolevulinic acid dehydratase gene may modify the pharmacokinetics and toxicity of lead. *Environ. Health Perspect.* **103,** 248–253.

Tice, R. R., and Strauss, G. H. (1995). The single cell gel electrophoresis/comet assay: A potential tool for detecting radiation-induced DNA damage in humans. *Stem Cells Dayt* **13,** 207–214.

Turk, D., Schonfeld, D., Cullen, M., and Rainey, P. (1992). Sensitivity of erythrocyte protoporphyrin as a screening test for lead poisoning. *N. Engl. J. Med.* **326,** 137–137.

Van Damme, K., Casteleyn, L., Heseltine, E., Huici, A., Sorsa, M., Van Larebeke, N., and Vineis, P. (1995). Individual susceptibility and prevention of occupational diseases: Scientific and ethical issues. *JOEM* **37,** 91–99.

Wetmur, J. G., Kaya, A. H., Plewinska, M., and Desnick, R. J. (1991). Molecular characterization of the human delta-aminolevulinate dehydratase 2 (ALAD2) allele: Implications for molecular screening of individuals for genetic susceptibility to lead poisoning. *Am. J. Hum. Genet.* **49,** 757–763.

CHAPTER

43

Water

RICHARD J. BULL

Pacific Northwest National Laboratory, Richland, Washington 99352

INTRODUCTION

The potential importance of water as a medium of human exposure to toxic chemicals is widely recognized. Public acknowledgement of this perceived hazard has been codified in many statutes and guidelines issued by a large variety of national and international bodies. The complex mixture of natural and human-made chemicals in waters used as sources and the nature of the hazards that do exist are not as widely appreciated.

Contamination of drinking water does not simply involve contamination of water sources. The actual chemical exposures experienced by humans directly consuming the water involves interactions with the physical and chemical processes associated with the treatment and distribution of the water. Therefore, it is dangerous to treat human exposure through drinking water too simplistically.

Following a brief general introduction to problems of water, this chapter will focus on the most important chemicals that are produced and may contaminate drinking water. These chemicals are a problem specific to direct human uses of water. Thus, it provides a concrete example of the complexity of water as a source of human exposure to potentially toxic chemicals.

PATHWAYS OF EXPOSURE INVOLVING WATER

Chemicals in water present complex problems in exposure assessment. The simplest way to conceptualize the problem is in terms of potential point and nonpoint sources that can contribute contaminants to ambient surface waters. These chemicals can be divided into two general categories, those chemicals whose principal pathway to humans is through food chains that are dependent upon a body of water and more direct human uses of water for drinking, food processing, and preparation. Human exposure is indirectly mediated in the former case, but is quite direct in the latter case. The chemicals that impact human health through these two pathways generally have different chemical and physical properties. Some general discussion is provided below to explain these facts. The point at which a chemical is introduced relative to where the water is withdrawn for use, the chemical and physical properties (e.g., pH and hardness) of the water involved, and the matter that may be suspended in the water can easily produce violations of these generalizations.

To reach humans via the aquatic food chain in amounts that present a high potential for inducing harm to health requires that the chemical be bioaccumulated in aquatic organisms to concentrations that are significantly higher than present in the surrounding water. Two types of chemicals have this property, nonpolar organic compounds and certain metals or metalloids. The extent to which an organic chemical bioaccumulates is primarily a function of their oil–water partition coefficient. Compounds with high oil–water partition coefficients accumulate in the fatty portions of the organism to high concentrations. Once deposited there, they back-diffuse very slowly and as a result accumulate in the body. Bioaccumulation of nonpolar organic chemicals is therefore largely a passive process. It is important to note that an ability to bioaccumulate does not, in itself, imply that a chemical is extremely toxic. However, some chemicals that bioaccumulate are extremely toxic (e.g., 2,3,7,8-tetrachlorodibenzodioxin, TCDD), while others have much lower intrinsic toxicity despite their being efficiently bioaccumulated.

The bioaccumulation of some metals can also be related to oil water partition coefficients (e.g., methyl mercury) or other specific physical and chemical properties (e.g., thallium, cadmium, and lead). More generally, the accumulation of metals involves specialized transporter systems that have developed to facilitate the absorption and distribution of essential trace metals and/or binding proteins that sequester metals in forms that will prevent their participation in free radical chemistry that could be destructive to cells.

The nonpolar compounds described and to a large extent toxic heavy metals tend to not stay in the water column but become associated with bottom sediments. It is there that they are first taken up by benthic organisms and begin the process of bioaccumulation in the food chain. It is this property that also makes them infrequent problems in drinking water. Their adsorption to suspended solids and the desire on the part of most water utilities to produce aesthetically pleasing water virtually guarantees that sediments will be removed before the water is distributed in a public water supply.

Chemicals can also contaminate groundwater. The properties of chemicals that do so are generally quite different from those that are associated with surface waters. In general, ground water contaminants are very mobile in soils, meaning that they are generally of low molecular weight, less nonpolar, or even very polar. Ordinarily, chemicals that are very nonpolar are not mobile and tend to stick to soil components. Solvents are perhaps the most representative of chemicals that are mobile in soils. They range from polar to fairly nonpolar in character, but have less complex structures and are generally smaller than very nonpolar chemicals such as dioxins, polychlorinated biphenyls, and organochlorine pesticides. Other pesticides are much more mobile in soils and are of more concern (e.g., atrazine and aldicarb). The contamination of groundwater by metals and metalloids very much depends on the properties of the individual metal. Certain soil types have a tremendous absorptive capacity for nonpolar compounds and many metals.

Chemicals that occur in drinking water arise from many different sources. To this point only the source of the water used for producing drinking water has been considered. However, many of the chemicals most frequently found in drinking water are introduced during its treatment and distribution. Considerable recent attention has focused on the by-products of the disinfection of drinking water. It is important to recognize that chemicals are also used in water treatment for the purposes of aiding filtration, reducing color, and preventing corrosion in the distribution system, as well as for disinfection (discussed more fully later). Adhesives and sealants are often components of the equipment used in the treatment of water; these may be found in drinking water. Water necessarily contacts a lot of surfaces in the course of its distribution and treatment. These surfaces may contribute metals, particulates, or organic compounds to the drinking water. For example, lead in drinking water almost exclusively comes from lead pipes or lead-containing solder that was used in the installation of copper pipe. For these reasons, lead solder has been banned in the United States and most European countries. However, minor fittings and faucets frequently have lead components that can result in reasonably high concentrations of lead in the water that is first withdrawn in the morning after sitting in the household plumbing overnight. Various plastic pipes can contribute monomers, stabilizers, or solvents to water, particularly when first installed. In most countries, there is no direct legislative authority to require the approval of the products used in treatment or that contact water during its distribution. As a consequence, sets of industry standards have been developed for certifying direct and indirect (unintentional) additives to drinking water (ANSI/NSF, 1996) that are similar in concept to existing product registration laws administered by agencies such as the U.S. Food and Drug Administration or Environmental Protection Agency.

BY-PRODUCTS ASSOCIATED WITH THE DISINFECTION OF WATER

Chlorine has been employed in the disinfection of drinking water since 1902, when it was introduced in Middelkerke, Belgium. The effectiveness of this treatment (especially when combined with filtration) gradually became apparent through associated decreases in the incidence of waterborne infectious disease. For example, in the United States the typhoid death rate decreased from 36 per 100,000 population per year in 1900 to 20/100,000 in 1910 and 3/100,000 in 1935, largely reflecting improvements in drinking water treatment.

In 1974 two groups independently reported that trihalomethanes were produced as a result of the reaction of chlorine with organic material that occurs in natural waters. Advances in analytical chemistry suddenly opened up the question of whether one of the most effective public health measures of all time was safe or not. These initial observations have lead to the identification of a very wide range of chemicals that are formed following chlorination and this knowledge is rapidly expanding to the more difficult task of identifying the by-products of disinfectants that do not add a telltale chlorine to an organic matrix. Now the question is beginning to focus more clearly on whether the trace amounts of these chemicals really represent a health hazard of sufficient proportion to warrant the replacement of disinfection by other methods of water treatment. This is not a trivial question because one of the advantages of chemical disinfection is that it is easily applied in small systems as well as large systems. It can also be employed in remote areas where the economic base does not support the development of sophisticated water treatment facilities. Thus, a combination of the factors of effectiveness, uncomplicated use and low cost make chlorine difficult to discard in favor of alternative treatments without a clear case being made that the risk is unacceptable. However, this should not be construed to mean that there are not good alternative approaches to dealing with waterborne infectious disease if an unacceptable risk were to be clearly demonstrated.

The original concern with chlorination by-products arose from the concurrent finding by the National Cancer Institute that chloroform treatment produced an increased incidence of liver cancer in B6C3F1 mice and kidney tumors in male Osborne–Mendel rats. This result stimulated a series of epidemiological studies and further testing of other disinfectant by-products in experimental animals.

Epidemiological Associations between Chlorination of Drinking Water and Cancer

Epidemiological investigations have associated several target organs for cancer with chlorinated drinking water in humans, with most work focusing on the urinary bladder and the colon and rectum. Associations with bladder cancer have been most consistently observed. In general, these studies have found small increases in the odds ratio (OR $\cong$ 1.4–2.5) in populations that consume chlorinated water. Increased risks appear to be confined to populations that have consumed such water in excess of 30 years. The risks of colorectal cancer have been reported to be of a similar magnitude. Again these risks appeared to be elevated only in cases where exposure was quite protracted. While these studies have been more or less consistent in their findings, there are weaknesses in the designs that prevent broad acceptance of these small odds ratios as indicative of there being a causal relationship between chlorinated water and increased risk of cancer. The most important reservations relate to the accuracy of exposure assessments, inconsistent interactions with cigarette smoking between studies, and apparent protective effects of exposures of less than 30 years.

Research since the 1970s has continued to identify additional by-products of chlorination and other forms of disinfection (Table 1). While most by-products appear to be associated with chlorination, this is in part due to the relative ease of identifying chemicals that have chlorine added to them. A large number of chemicals are relatively straightforward oxidation

TABLE 1 Classes of Disinfectant By-products Found in Municipal Drinking Water

Disinfectant	Inorganic	Organic
Chlorine gas		Trihalomethanes Haloacetates
Hypochlorite	Chlorate	Other haloacids
Chloramine		Haloacetonitriles Haloaldehydes Haloketones Halohydroxyfuranones Cyanogen chloride Aldehydes Ketones Carboxylic acids
Chlorine dioxide	Chlorite Chlorate	Poorly characterized Aldehydes
Ozone	Bromate	Bromoform Bromoacetates Bromoaldehydes Bromoketones Bromohydrins Aldehydes Ketones Carboxylic acids Epoxides

products, and many of these chemicals are seen with all forms of chemical disinfection. These include aldehydes, ketones, and organic acids. Moreover, halogenated compounds are not unique to chlorination, but are formed with nonhalogenated disinfectants such as ozone under the right circumstances.

The types of by-product that are formed with disinfection are not simply dependent upon the disinfectant that is used. The amount of organic carbon that is in the water is a major determinant of the amount of the organic by-product that is formed. However, the type of by-product formed also depends upon the bromide concentration and pH of the treated water. Ammonia suppresses the formation of halogenated by-products by serving as a substrate for the formation of chloramines and other haloamines. Then there

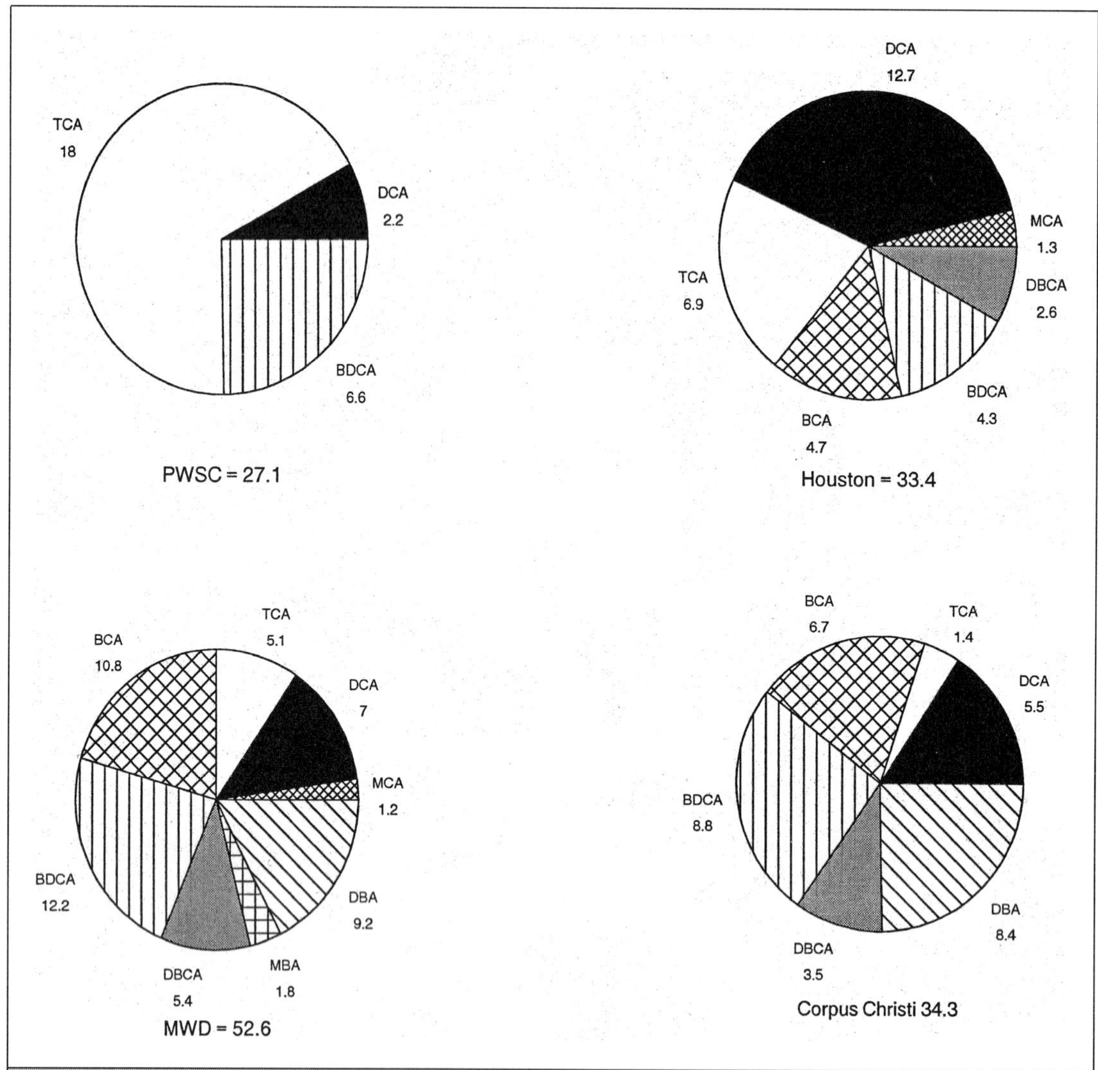

FIGURE 1 Distribution of brominated and chlorinated haloacetates in different water systems in the United States. DCA = dichloroacetate, BCA = bromochloroacetate, DBA = dibromoacetate, TCA = trichloroacetate, BDCA = bromodichloroacetate, DBCA = dibromochloroacetate. The total organic carbon (TOC), Br^- and total haloacetate concentrations, respectively, were as follows: PWSC = 2.6 mg/liter, 51 μg/liter, 27.1 μg/liter; Houston = (4.8 & 8.8 mg/liter), (72 & 134 μg/liter), 33.4 μg/liter; MWD = 3.3 mg/liter, 220 μg/liter, 52.6 μg/liter; Corpus Christi = 4.7 mg/liter, 412 μg/liter, 34.3 μg/liter. Data adapted with permission from Cowman and Singer (1996).

is the special chemistry of certain disinfectants that appear to lead to unique by-products, such as chlorite with chlorine dioxide and bromate with ozone. More recently, chlorate has been a by-product that has been specifically associated with the use of hypochlorite solutions rather than chlorine gas for disinfection; previously, chlorate had been thought only to be associated with the use of chlorine dioxide as a disinfectant. In the end, the amounts and types of by-products observed in the water consumed by humans is a complex interaction of the type of disinfectant used and the chemical characteristics of the water that is being treated. As discussed later, these factors can result in the formation of different by-products in different locations, even when the same disinfectant is employed. Different by-products are likely to exhibit differing toxicological properties. This could serve to dilute the associations between disinfectant by-products and particular adverse effects, thus more precise information about exposure must be obtained to make sense of the epidemiological data. It also makes apparent that the solution of this complex problem cannot be obtained from epidemiological studies alone.

Toxicological Evidence

Research has also resulted in an expanded list of the number of by-products of disinfectants that have been shown to be carcinogenic in experimental animals.

Factors that Influence the Nature of By-Products That Are Formed with Disinfectants

The amount of organic by-product produced is dependent upon the organic carbon concentration in the treated water. Humic and fulvic acids (humic substances, collectively) are of natural origin and make up a large share of the organic substrate with which disinfectants react to form by-products. There is some variation in the amount of by-product depending upon chemical character of humic substances. However, the nature of the by-products and their relative yields per unit concentration of humic substances does not vary significantly.

Other variables in the source water are more influential on the chemical nature of the by-products that are formed. The reactions of strong oxidants in water result in the conversion of bromide and iodine into a form capable of adding bromine or iodine to particular carbons in organic compounds. Bromide and to a lesser extent iodine in sources used for drinking water treatment are most often present in direct proportion to the salinity of the water. In coastal areas, this problem usually originates from the intrusion of seawater into the groundwater. However, even in the heartland of North America, there are traces of underground remnants of seas that can contribute bromide. Almost all waters contain some bromide; for example, bromodichloromethane is found in almost all waters surveyed. As the bromide concentration in the treated water increases relative to the organic carbon present, the proportion of halogenated by-products that the water contains will increase in bromine content. The fraction of the haloacetates that are brominated varied from as little as 25% in Philadelphia Suburban Water Co. (PSWC) to about 80% in Corpus Christi, and the relative levels of the total trihaloacetates (trichloroacetate, TCA; bromodichloroacetate, BDCA; dibromochloroacetate, DBCA; and tribomoacetate, CTBA also vary significantly between sites, making up from about 90% of the total haloacetic acid concentrations to as little as 30% (Fig. 1). Notice that this occurs without there being significant differences in the total haloacetate concentrations between these cities. This change in the haloacetic acids will be paralleled in all classes of halogenated organic by-products in particular drinking waters.

The other major variable that affects the type of by-product that will be formed is the pH of the water that is being treated. The final concentration of trichloroacetate formed in a solution of fulvic acids is greatly decreased as pH decreases (Fig. 2). This decrease in trichloroacetate is in large part balanced by the enhanced formation of chloroform. In contrast to trichloroacetate, dichloroacetate concentrations do not vary with pH. Chloral hydrate, however, parallels the behavior of trichloroacetate. Mutagenic activity produced from chlorination reactions also tends to decrease as the pH of the treated water increases, although some forms of mutagenic by-products seem to be stabilized at alkaline pH. Finally, alkaline pH appears to be necessary to convert hypobromous acid formed with ozone to be further oxidized to bromate. This appears to be related to the higher concentrations of hydroxyl radicals that are generated by ozone at alkaline pH.

Basically, these variables indicate that chlorination of drinking water does not produce a consistent set of by-products. Some variability has been demonstrated for other disinfectants, but the issue has not been as well documented.

Summary of Toxicological Data

A large number of disinfectant by-products have been identified. The data available are too sparse to

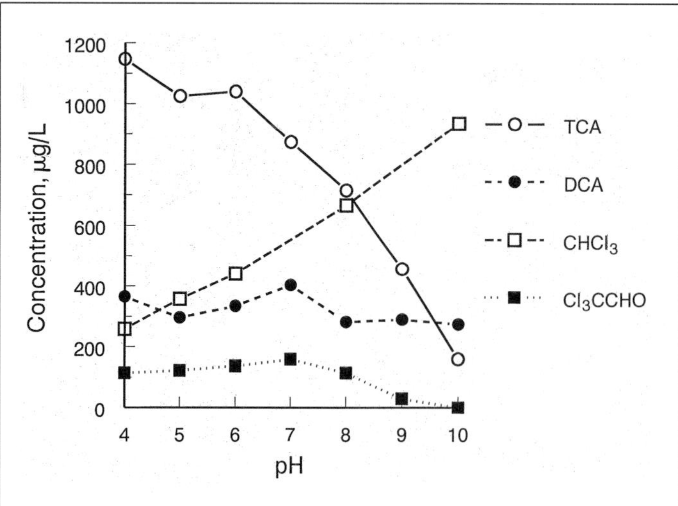

FIGURE 2 The effect of pH on the concentrations of different by-products of chlorination. Reactions were carried out in an artificial system containing elevated concentrations of fulvic acid. TCA = trichloroacetate; DCA = dichloroacetate; $CHCl_3$ = chloroform; and Cl_3CHO = chloral hydrate. Reprinted from *Journal AWWA 85(1)* (January 1993), by permission. Copyright © 1993, American Water Works Association.

project the distribution of the concentrations of most by-products. The most extensively studied are compounds in the trihalomethane, haloacetic acid, and haloacetonitrile classes of organic by-products. Concerns about inorganic by-products focus primarily on bromate, chlorite, and chlorate; these compounds can be produced at significant concentrations when ozone, chlorine dioxide, or chlorine are used as disinfectants, respectively. The key question is not simply whether these chemicals are toxic but whether they are present in drinking water in concentrations sufficient to produce adverse health effects in humans. Four of the five trihalomethanes that have been studied appear to be carcinogenic in at least one organ system of at least one rodent species. These included chloroform, bromodichloromethane, dibromochloromethane, and bromoform. Iodoform (triiodomethane) is the only member of the class tested in both rats and mice that was apparently not carcinogenic. Although the trihalomethanes are generally regulated as total trihalomethanes, they differ significantly in their carcinogenicity potency. Experimental data are now convincing that the carcinogenic responses to chloroform in the mouse liver and rat kidney are largely, if not entirely, dependent on its ability to induce cytotoxic responses followed by reparative hyperplasia. Because chloroform has been largely negative in both *in vitro* and *in vivo* tests for mutagenic effects, it would appear that it would present little carcinogenic hazard at the low concentrations found in drinking water. Its other toxic effects, including liver and kidney toxicity, require doses in excess of 10 mg/kg to produce. This would be equivalent to an adult human consuming 700,000 µg/per day, whereas intakes of more than 100 µg/day would be very unusual in individuals drinking chlorinated drinking water. In contrast to chloroform, brominated trihalomethanes appear to be mutagenic in various test systems. Mutagenic activity carries implications for low-dose effects not inherent in compounds that act strictly by cytotoxicity and reparative hyperplasia. In addition, two of the trihalomethanes, bromodichloromethane and bromoform, target the colon of the rat. There is little suggestion that the target organs of chloroform are associated with the consumption of chlorinated drinking water by humans. In contrast, as indicated above, colon cancer is one of the tumor sites most frequently associated with chlorinated drinking water. While this association may be suggestive, it falls far short of constituting proof that these compounds account for the association that has been observed epidemiologically. On average, the bromodichloromethane and bromoform are present in drinking water at lower concentrations than chloroform in chlorinated drinking water. The combination of likely doses and the potency of these by-products suggest that it is unlikely that these compounds could account for the association by themselves.

While the trihalomethanes have other toxicological properties, none would seem to be any more important than carcinogenicity at the doses that could be reasonably be derived from chlorinated drinking water.

Trichloroacetate and dichloroacetate have been the members of the haloacetic acid class that have received the most attention experimentally. Their toxicological effects are more diverse than the trihalomethanes, but carcinogenic responses have received the most study. Both compounds induce liver tumors in mice, but only dichloroacetic acid has been shown to also induce liver tumors in rats. Despite the fact that these compounds are closely related chemically, they appear to produce liver cancer by somewhat different mechanisms. Dichloroacetate has been suggested to be weakly mutagenic. However, the acidification of media was not controlled in these studies. Subsequent studies suggest neither compound is mutagenic. Moreover, there is strong evidence that both compounds have promoting activities that are probably more important than any small mutagenic effects that might be present.

Both dichloroacetate and trichloroacetate have been demonstrated to promote liver tumors initiated by*N*-methyl-*N*-nitrosourea. The dose–response relationships for these responses are very similar to that produced when the compounds are administered alone. These responses match very closely with the compounds effects on cell replication rates within normal liver and preneoplastic lesions. Both trichloroacetate and dichloroacetate appear to increase the replication rates of normal hepatocytes for brief periods, but this appears to be inhibited with continued treatment. Trichloroacetate does appear to act primarily as a peroxisome proliferator, a response that appears to occur only in rats and mice. Dichloroacetate has this same property, but the induction of liver tumors occurs at doses lower than those inducing peroxisome proliferation. The difference between the compounds is that trichloroacetate does not affect the replication rates in tumor cells, simply providing a negative selection environment for initiated cells. Dichloroacetate at high doses approximately doubles the rate of replication in cells of hyperplastic nodules that express high levels of protein that are immunoreactive to antibodies to c-Jun and c-Fos proteins. This stimulation of replication of a particular phenotype appears to be responsible for the much more rapid induction of liver tumors by dichloroacetic acid when administered at high doses. In the case of both dichloroacetate and trichloroacetate, however, the differential effects on cell replication rates of normal and initiated cells is very closely associated with their tumorigenic activity. In contrast, there is no evidence that genotoxic effects of either compound play a role in tumorigenesis.

Brominated haloacetates share many of the properties of dichloroacetate and trichloroacetate. Like the brominated trihalomethanes, the brominated haloacetates have additional toxicological properties that may be of concern at low doses. Those brominated haloacetates that have been tested (bromochloroacetate, dibromoacetate acid, and bromodichloroacetate) all produce liver tumors in B6C3F1 mice. However, they also appear to affect other target organs. Specifically, bromodichloroacetate appears to increase the incidence of lung tumors and lymphoma in mice. Preliminary data has shown that dibromoacetate induces an increased frequency of aberrant crypt foci in the colon of rats with as little as 8 weeks of treatment. These lesions are thought to be precursors of colon cancer. In addition to having a more diverse set of target organs, the brominated haloacetic acids are also more likely to damage DNA. It was demonstrated recently that the formation of 8-hydroxy-2-deoxyguanosine results in nuclear DNA of liver following the administration of brominated haloacetonitriles. While dichloroacetate produced a similar but smaller response to a large acute dose, it did not sustain an increased steady-state level of the adduct with drinking water treatments, as was demonstrated with the brominated analogs. In addition, the varying phenotypes of the liver tumors induced by brominated and chlorinated haloacetates suggests that there is more than one mechanism responsible for inducing tumors. It is not clear that these different mechanisms are capable of inducing carcinogenic responses at the very much smaller amounts of haloacetates consumed by humans in drinking water.

While this review has focused on the carcinogenic effects of haloacetates and haloacetonitriles, these compounds also have reproductive and developmental effects. In particular, the haloacetates and haloacetonitriles have been shown to induce developmental defects in the heart. Dibromoacetate also interferes with spermatogenesis. These effects appear to be less important for the development of drinking water standards because the assumptions used in the extrapolation of carcinogenic effects to low doses are much more conservative than for other types of toxic responses. However, there are reasons to be concerned, based on the potential interactions in the metabolism of disinfectant by-products that are discussed later.

The production of mutagenic compounds by water disinfection has been an intense area of research since the early 1980s. Members of the haloacetonitrile, halogenated aldehyde, halogenated ketone, and simple aldehyde classes have been identified as mutagenic. By far the most potent mutagenic compounds identified has been 3-chloro-4-(dichloromethyl)-5-hydroxy-2(5*H*)-furanone, commonly referred to as MX. While preliminary data suggest that several of these other compounds could also be carcinogenic, only MX has been sufficiently well studied to establish its ability to act independently as a carcinogen. A chronic study has shown it is capable of inducing thyroid tumors and cholangiomas in both male and female rats and mammary tumors in female rats. Doses in the 0.4 to 6.6 mg/kg per day range were sufficient to induce these cancers.

MX is found in drinking water at concentrations approximately 20 ng/liter. If it is assumed that the average adult human consumes approximately 2 liters of water per day, 40–50 ng per day is the expected exposure level. Thus, the average dose would be something less than 1 ng/kg per day. Carcinogenic doses in rats are approximately 1 million times higher than this intake. As a comparison, the concentrations of bromodichloromethane are less than 10 μg/liter, giving rise to an average dose to humans of about 0.3 μg/kg per day and doses of about 50 mg/kg per day to induce tumors. Thus, this compound is present at about 1/200,000 the dose required to produce tumors. Although MX may be the most potent carcinogen identified among disinfectant by-products, these rough calculations suggest that it is no more likely to account for human cancer than other disinfectant by-products.

A comparison of the potency of bromate as a carcinogen to its concentrations in drinking water suggests that it is present at the highest effective concentrations of all disinfectant by-products. Bromate induces renal tumors in rats. It also induces mesothelioma in hamsters. To date, it appears that ozone is the only disinfectant that causes bromate to be formed. Until better data with which to estimate cancer risk are available, this finding may limit the use of ozone in bromide-containing water.

Mixtures of Disinfectant By-Products

The number of carcinogenic by-products identified with the chlorination of drinking water continues to grow. Individually, the combination of concentrations and potency of the chemicals identified are not sufficiently great to account for the levels of risk that seem to be suggested by epidemiological studies. This brings up the inevitable question of whether synergisms between the by-products could be responsible for the cancer risk. There are clearly a variety of mechanisms of action represented by the different by-products. Diverse mechanisms can result in synergistic effects.

Research has raised the possibility that some disinfectant by-products can have very large effects on their own metabolism and that of other disinfectant by-products. Dichloroacetate administered to rats at concentrations of $\geq$20 mg/liter inhibits its own metabolism and that of other disinfectant by-products. A similar inhibition has been observed in human subjects who were administered doses of dichloroacetate therapeutically. The nature of enzymatic activity has yet to be established, but it is glutathione-dependent and can have dramatic effects on the disposition of other disinfectant by-products, such as bromodichloroacetate. Depending upon the specific identity of the enzyme, it is possible that dichloroacetate could interfere with the metabolism of trihalomethanes, MX, and haloacetonitriles. All of these compounds are metabolized, at least in part, by glutathione-dependent processes. Such interactions can affect the disposition of the active forms of disinfectant by-products within the body. In particular, low levels of the dihaloacetic acids are metabolized almost completely before they reach the systemic circulation in animals not previously exposed to dichloroacetate. Loss of this enzyme activity dramatically increases the amount of dihaloacetates that are delivered by the blood to other organs. Such interactions could change the target organs normally found when animals are treated with a single compound. In turn, this could account for the differing target organs identified in studies of individual by-products in experimental animals and those identified in the epidemiological studies.

Whether a particular mixture of disinfectant by-products is responsible for the epidemiological associations of chlorination with carcinogenic effects is an important research question. However, the nebulous concern over such possibilities cannot be allowed to drive policy judgments in the near term. Hasty policy decisions could be dangerous because one potential outcome could be a more serious increase in the risk from waterborne infectious disease. It needs to be recognized that there are lower limits to the doses at which interactions can occur between chemicals. Extending synergisms that are observed at high doses to the very low doses that humans encounter in drinking water is premature.

Two related issues also have to be recognized.

1. Humans could simply be more sensitive than experimental animals to the carcinogenic effects of a particular by-product.
2. There could be a very potent, as yet unindentified carcinogen present in chlorinated drinking water.

The first possibility can only be dealt with by establishing this point experimentally, probably by employing human cells in culture and comparing their sensitivity to rodents in cells derived from the appropriate target organs (e.g., bladder epithelium or cells derived from the colon). The latter possibility simply means that less well characterized disinfectant by-products need to be studied for carcinogenic activity.

SUMMARY

This discussion provides some indication of the complex basis of human exposure to chemicals in drinking water. Although covered in a cursory fashion, the issues surrounding disinfectant by-products illustrate that many of the problems involved in the provision of safe drinking water to both large and small populations can be complex. With respect to the disinfectant by-products, the following conclusions can be drawn.

1. The risk of cancer and other risks from disinfected drinking water remain to be clearly established.
2. The benefits of chemical disinfection are sufficiently large to make it irrational to discard the practice casually.
3. If there is a risk for cancer from consuming chlorinated water, it cannot be derived from the toxicological potency of the chlorinated by-products that have been identified and studied.
4. The contributions of less well studied and/or mutagenic by-products need to be explored with respect to the cancer sites suggested by epidemiological studies.
5. It is important to focus research on whether chemically disinfected water produces significant health hazards to the consuming public. While it is essential to understand the toxicological properties of individual by-products before one can understand the mixture, even research work on individual by-products needs to explicitly recognize this larger question.
6. Sufficient information has been developed on individual by-products to pursue the question of whether epidemiological results can be duplicated by examining specific mixtures of disinfectant by-products that can be reasonably postulated to be synergistic.
7. An alternate hypothesis to 6 is that humans are uniquely sensitive to one or more disinfectant by-products. These questions can be addressed by the careful comparison of the response of primary cells from target organs of human donors to disinfectant by-products with those of test species, *in vitro*.

Toxicology can contribute knowledge that is essential for making decisions about the safety of chemicals or chemical processes. The critical judgment is recognizing at what point *sufficient* information is available to make an informed decision. If a critical process such as disinfection is to be judged on safety, it is more important to be accurate in the assessment of human risk than to introduce a new chemical product that simply replaces other safe alternatives. The clear benefits that accrue from the chemical disinfection of drinking water at low cost and the very large number of people who are directly exposed demand more of toxicology than simple routine tests. This problem requires hypothesis-driven research directed at resolving the differences between animal and human results. These hypotheses need to be based on the available information on the mechanisms that these chemicals use to induce cancer. Such research can be very expensive, if it is not properly directed.

Bibliography

Akin, E. W., Hoff, J. C. and Lippy, E. C. (1981). Waterborne outbreak control: Which disinfectant? *Environ. Health Perspect.* **46,** 7–12.

ANSI/NSF (1996). "Standard 60 Drinking Water Treatment Chemicals—Health Effects." NSF International, Ann Arbor, MI.

ANSI/NSF (1996). "Standard 61 Drinking Water System Components–Health Effects." NSF International, Ann Arbor, MI.

Austin, E. W. and Bull, R. J. (1997). The effect of pretreatment with dichloroacetate and trichloroacetate on the metabolism of bromodichloroacetate. *J. Toxicol. Environ. Health* **52,** 367–383.

Bellar, T. A., Lichtenberg, J. J., and Kroner, R. C. (1974). The occurrence of organohalides in chlorinated drinking waters. *J. AWWA* **66,** 703–706.

Bolyard, M., Fair, P. S., and Hautman, D. P. (1993). Sources of chlorate ion in US drinking water. *J. AWWA* **85,** 81–88.

Bull, R. J., Meier, J. R., Robinson, M., Ringhand, H. P., Laurie, R. P., and Stober, J. A. (1985). Evaluation of the mutagenic and carcinogenic properties of brominated and chlorinated acetonitriles By products of chlorination. *Fundam. Appl. Toxicol.* **5,** 1065–1075.

Bull, R. J., Sanchez, I. M., Nelson, M. A., Larson, J. L., and Lansing, A. L. (1990). Liver tumor induction in B6C3F1 mice by dichloroacetate and trichloroacetate. *Toxicology* **63,** 341–359.

Bull, R. J., Birnbaum, L. S., Cantor, K. P., Rose, J. B., Butterworth, B., E., Pegram, R., and Tuomisto, J. (1995). Symposium overview: Water chlorination: Essential process or cancer hazard. *Fundam. Appl. Toxicol.* **28,** 155–166.

Cantor, K. P., Hoover, R., Hartge, P. *et al.* (1987). Bladder cancer, drinking water source, and tap water consumption: A case-control study. *J. Nat. Cancer Inst.* **79,** 1269–1279.

Cowman, G. A., and Singer, P. C. (1996). Effect of bromide ion on haloacetic acid speciation resulting from chlorination and chloramination of aquatic humic substances. *Environ. Sci. Tech.* **30,** 16–24.

DeAngelo, A. B., Daniel, F. B., McMillan, L., Wernsing, P., and Savage, R. E., Jr. (1989). Species and strain sensitivity to the induction of peroxisome proliferation by chloroacetic acids. *Toxicol. Appl. Pharmacol.* **101,** 285–298.

Epstein, D. L., Nolen, G. A., Randall, J. L., Christ, S. A., Read, E. J., Stober, J. A., and Smith, M. K. (1992). Cardiopathic effects of dichloroacetate in the fetal Long-Evans rat. *Teratology* **46,** 225–235.

Fox, A. W., Yang, X., Murli, H., Lawlor, T. E., Cifone, M. A., and Reno, F. E. (1996). Absence of mutagenic effects of sodium dichloroacetate. *Fundam. Appl. Toxicol.* **32,** 87–95.

Gonzalez-Leon, A., Schultz, I. R., and Bull, R. J. (1997). Pharmacokinetics and metabolism of dichloroacetate in the F344 rat after prolonged administration in drinking water. *Toxicol. Appl. Toxicol.* **146,** 189–195.

IARC (1991). Chlorinated drinking water; chlorination by-products. *In* "IARC Monographs on the Evaluation of Carcinogenic Risks To Humans, Vol. 52, Chlorinated Drinking Water; Chlorination By-Products; Some other Halogenated Compounds; Cobalt and Cobalt Compounds," pp. 45–298 Lyon: International Agency for Research on Cancer.

Komulainen, H., Kosma, V.-M., Vaittinen, S.-L., Vartiainen, T., Kaliste-Korhonen, E., Lotjoinen, S., Tuominen, R. K. and Tuomisto, J. (1997). Carcinogenicity of the drinking water mutagen 3-chloro-4-(dichloromethyl)-5-hydroxy-2(5*H*)-furanone. *J. Natl. Cancer Inst.* **89,** 848–856.

Kurokawa, Y., Maekawa, A., Takahashi, M., and Hayashi, Y. (1990). Toxicity and carcinogenicity of potassium bromate—A new renal carcinogen. *Environ. Health Perspect.* **87,** 309–335.

Larson, J. L., Templin, M. V., Wolf, D. C., Jamison, K. C., Leininger, J. R., Mery, S., Morgan, K. T., Wong, B. A., Conolly, R. B., and Butterworth, B. E. (1996). A 90-day chloroform inhalation study in female and male B6C3F1 mice: Implications for cancer risk assessment. *Fundam. Appl. Toxicol.* **30,** 118–137.

Linder, R. E., Klinefelter, G. R., Strader, L. F., Narotosky, M. G., Suarez, J. D., Roberts, N. L., and Perreault, S. D. (1995). Dibromoacetic acid affects reproductive competence and sperm quality in the male rat. *Fundam. Appl. Toxicol.* **28,** 9–17.

McCauley, P. T., Robinson, M., Daniel, F. B. and Olson, G. R. (1995). The effects of subchronic chlorate exposure in Sprague-Dawley rats. *Drug Chem. Toxicol.* **18,** 185–199.

Meier, J. R. (1988). Genotoxic activity of organic chemicals in drinking water. *Mutat. Res.* **196,** 211–245.

Miller, J. W., and Uden, P. C. (1983). Characterization of non-volatile aqueous chlorination products of humic substances. *Environ. Sci. Technol.* **17,** 150–157.

NCI (1976). "Report on the Carcinogenesis Bioassay of Chloroform." NTIS PB-264-018, National Cancer Institute, Bethesda, MD.

NCI (1978). "Bioassay of Iodoform for Possible Carcinogenicity." NCI-CG-TR- 110, DHEW Publication No. (NIH) 78-1365. National Cancer Institute, Bethesda, MD.

NTP (1985). "Toxicology and Carcinogenesis Studies of Chlorodibromomethane in F344/N Rats and B6C3F1 Mice (Gavage Studies)." NTP Technical Report Series No. 282. U.S. Dept. Of Health and Human Services, National Toxicology Program, National Institutes of Health, Research Triangle Park, NC.

NTP (1987). "Toxicology and Carcinogenesis Studies of Bromodichloromethane in F344/N Rats and B6C3F1 Mice." NIH Publication 88-2537, NTP TR 321. U.S. Dept. Of Health and Human Services, National Institutes of Health, National Toxicology Program, Research Triangle Park, NC.

NTP (1989). "Toxicology and Carcinogenesis Studies of Tribromomethane (Bromoform) in F344/N Rats and B6C3 F1 Mice (Gavage Studies)." NTP Technical Report Series No. 350. U.S. Dept. Of Health and Human Services, National Toxicology Program, National Institutes of Health, Research Triangle Park, NC.

NTP (1990). "Draft Technical Report on the Toxicology and Carcinogenesis Studies of Chlorinated and Chloraminated Water in F344/N Rats and B6C3F1 Mice." Technical Report Series No. 392, NIH Publication No. 91-2847. Research Triangle Park, NC: National Toxicology Program.

Parrish, J. M., Austin, E. W., Stevens, D. K., Kinder, D. H., and Bull, R. J. (1996). Haloacetate-induced oxidative damage to DNA in the liver of male B6C3F1 mice. *Toxicology* **110,** 103–111.

Pegram, R. A., Andersen, M. E., Warren, S. H., Ross, T. M., and Claxton, L. D. (1997). Glutathione S-transferase-mediated mutagenicity of trihalomethanes in Salmonella typhimurium: Contrasting results with bromodichloromethane and chloroform. *Toxicol. Appl. Pharmacol.* **144,** 183–188.

Pourmoghaddas, H., Stevens, A. A., Kinman, R. N., Dressman, R. C., Moore, L. A., and Ireland, J. C. (1993). Effect of bromide ion on formation of HAAs during chlorination. *J. AWWA* **85,** 82–87

Robinson, M., Bull, R. J., Olson, G. R. and Stober, J. (1989). Carcinogenic activity associated with halogenated acetones and acroleins in the mouse skin assay. *Cancer Lett.* **48,** 197–203.

Siddiqui, MS, Amy, GL, and Rice, RG. (1995). Bromate ion formation: A critical review. *J. AWWA* **87,** 58–70.

Smith, M. K., Randall, J. L., Tocco, D. R., York, R. G., Stober, J. A., and Read, E. J. (1988). Teratogenic effects of trichloroacetonitrile in the Long-Evans rat. *Teratology* **38,** 113–120.

Smith, M. K., Randall, J. L., Stober, J. A., and Read, E. J. (1989). Developmental toxicity of dichloroacetonitrile: A by-product of drinking water disinfection. *Fundam. Appl. Toxicol.* **12,** 765–772.

Smith, M. K., Randall, J. L., Read, E. J., and Stober, J. A. (1992). Developmental toxicity of dichloroacetate in the rat. *Teratology* **46,** 217–223.

So, B-J, and Bull, RJ (1995). Dibromoacetate (DBA) acts as a promoter of abnormal crypt foci in the colon of F344 rats. *Toxicologist* **15,** 1242.

Stauber, A. J., and Bull, R. J. (1997). Differences in phenotype and cell replicative behavior of hepatic tumors inducted by dichloroacetate (DCA) and trichloroacetate (TCA). *Toxicol. Appl. Pharmacol.* **144,** 235–246.

Toth, G. P., Kelty, K. C., George, E. L., Read, E. J., and Smith, M. K. (1992). Adverse male reproductive effects following subchronic exposure of rats to sodium dichloroacetate. *Fundam. Appl. Toxicol.* **19,** 57–63.

Young, T. B., Wolf, D. A., and Kanarek, M. S. (1987). Case-control study of colon cancer and drinking water trihalomethanes in Wisconsin. *Int. J. Epidemiol.* **16,** 190–197.

CHAPTER

44

Risk Assessment in Environmental Remediation

THOMAS E. RODRIGUEZ,* DENNIS J. PAUSTENBACH†

*McLaren/Hart, Inc. Lester, Pennsylvania

†Exponent, Menlo Park, California

INTRODUCTION

The role that toxicology and risk assessment have played in environmental remediation has evolved considerably since the 1970s. In the United States, the early days of the "environmental movement" were strongly influenced by the response to the incident at Love Canal and a decade of pondering the significance of *Silent Spring*. The result was the development of a national priority to clean up industrial waste, and to control (or ban) the production and/or release of industrial chemicals into the environment.

As early as the mid 1970s, efforts to understand and control industrial chemicals relied upon three skill sets or professions. Toxicologists identified the hazardous properties that chemicals possessed, risk assessors quantified the exposures to these chemicals and calculated appropriate cleanup levels, and engineers developed the appropriate, hopefully cost-effective solutions. Although all three professions were needed and played important roles in dealing with the problems generated during the post-war era, in general, the degree of interaction among these parties was minimal or nonexistent, even in the 1980s.

Fortunately, since about 1992, significant advances have been made in the quality and quantity of dialog among toxicologists, risk assessors, and environmental engineers. The benefits of these communications have been improved sampling plans, which now focus on the chemicals that pose the greatest hazard; more accurate exposure assessments; and better fate and transport models developed by engineers. The product of these efforts is evidenced by the emergence of the term "risk-based approach" within environmental remediation. That is, the sampling methods, number of samples, media to be sampled, and chemicals to be studied are a function of the human or environmental toxicity of the chemical rather than some arbitrary standard or guideline. This approach is finally enjoying support among regulatory agencies and within the regulated community.

This chapter examines the roles of toxicology and risk assessment in environmental science and engineering as applied to environmental remediation. It describes how toxicological data and risk assessment concepts can be applied at various stages of the assessment and remediation process, from the initial site characterization, through establishing cleanup goals, selecting remedies, and confirming that cleanup has been effective.

HISTORY OF ENVIRONMENTAL REMEDIATION

Environmental remediation can be described as the process of identifying, characterizing, and abating anthropogenic effects on otherwise "natural" environmental systems to achieve societal objectives. Humans are not the first or only species to profoundly impact our surrounding environment to the detriment of other species and ourselves. Humans, however, have the unique ability to comprehend the adverse impacts on the environment and devise remedies that correct both the damages and the behaviors that cause them.

The fundamental objectives of environmental intervention (e.g., remediation) have been understood and used throughout most of human history. Ancient farming cultures understood the importance of crop rotation to allow overworked land a chance to reestablish its viability. Similarly, it has long been understood that sanitary management of human waste is fundamental to preventing epidemics such as cholera. It was not until the mid-1970s, however, that a specialty section of environmental engineering began to evolve whose purpose was to address the problems that had been caused by the improper disposal of chemical wastes. Fortunately, society is now coming to view environmental issues as something requiring a long-term strategy. As a result, there has been increased focus during the 1990s on issues such as recycling, waste minimization, and manufacturing process design. At the same time, there has been an increase in the use of risk assessment methods to prioritize the problems.

Most environmental regulations at the federal and state levels make it clear that the goals of environmental remediation are to protect human health and the environment. The National Oil and Hazardous Substance Pollution Contingency Plan (NCP), for example, states that "The NCP applies to and is in effect for . . . releases into the environment of hazardous substances, and pollutants or contaminants which may present an imminent and substantial danger to public health or welfare." In most instances, it was the intent of these regulations to achieve these goals by using sound scientific methodologies to evaluate the risks to humans and ecological systems posed by chemicals present in different environmental media (e.g., soil, groundwater, surface water, sediments, and air), and to mitigate excess risks to socially acceptable levels by reducing the concentrations and/or exposure to humans or wildlife. This intent to use sound and current science is consistent with U.S. EPA's commitment to ensure that "national efforts to reduce environmental risks are based on the best available scientific information communicated clearly to the public."

In general, social and regulatory priorities for mitigating *perceived* risks have for the past 25 years exceeded the capacity of science to accurately characterize the *actual* risks posed by low concentration contamination. Further, in an attempt to ensure that the responsible parties fulfilled their obligations to restore sites to an acceptably clean condition, authorities have enforced environmental laws on a site-by-site basis. This has resulted in significantly diverging approaches to remediation, as well as different degrees of cleanup. The use of risk assessment methods should help make risk management decisions more balanced.

RISK-BASED REMEDIAL INVESTIGATIONS

A remedial investigation is generally described as a mechanism for collecting data to characterize site conditions, determine the nature of the chemicals in environmental media, assess the risk to human health and the environment, and evaluate and select alternative remedial actions. A risk-based remedial investigation (RBRI) focuses this process on collecting primarily those data that allow a complete understanding of the risks rather than simply characterizing the magnitude and extent of contamination. The difference between this approach and the standard one is that most sampling is focused on those media to which persons or wildlife may be exposed, and on those chemicals that pose the greatest threat to health or the environment.

Perhaps the earliest and best-documented applications of a risk-based site investigation involved a site in Illinois. Residents were allegedly exposed to high concentrations of pesticides due to suspected aerial deposition from a cyclodiene bagging and distribution facility. At a fraction of the cost of a full-scale remedial investigation, a limited yet statistically representative number of samples were collected from surface soils, home-grown vegetables, airborne particles, and groundwater in the residential areas adjacent to the facility as well as outside the town (background conditions). Using the resulting data set, a risk assessment showed that the risks to humans in the area due to aerial deposition from the facility were insignificant relative to background quantities of cyclodienes, which were present due to historical agricultural and residential applications. The community and the governing regulatory agency agreed with these conclusions, and a decision of no action was reached.

Using a similar approach, it was shown that concentrations of volatile organic compounds in groundwater beneath a former hazardous waste-treatment facility presented no incremental risk to human health when measured at the up-gradient and down-gradient property boundaries. Using a risk-based approach, the site investigation was designed to focus initially on determining if the cumulative impact to groundwater from all potential releases at the site produced an unacceptable increase in risk relative to background. The intent was to then focus the investigation on characterizing individual potential releases within the site if the incremental risks due to all potential releases combined were found to be unacceptable. The risk assessment found no incremental risk due to releases of volatile organic compounds to groundwater from the site, when compared to background, and no further action was required.

In Europe, the risk-based approach to site investigation and site remediation has also become common. For example, the government of Jena decided in 1994 that an abandoned coal gasification facility needed to be remediated. Unlike many prior efforts in Germany, where cleanup to background concentrations was the goal, the objective at this site was to identify the most cost-effective approach to reduce the human and ecological hazards to insignificant levels. Because literally hundreds of different chemicals were present in the soil, especially the polycyclic aromatic hydrocarbons (PAHs), a risk assessment approach was used to select the number and location of soil and groundwater samples.

The originally proposed approach suggested that grid sampling of the soils be conducted and that follow-up sampling then be used to better understand the most highly contaminated areas. This approach was estimated to be costly and to require 3–4 years of effort. A risk-based approach that relied upon stratified random sampling was eventually adopted and the estimated cost was expected to be about 50% of the original approach. The primary difference between the two programs was that the risk-based approach recognized that the PAHs would be the chemicals that would dictate the degree of clean-up and that only about 4% of the site was likely to be contaminated with this chemical; therefore, the bulk of the samples were collected in the areas likely to be contaminated with PAHs. Likewise, although many different chemicals were in the groundwater, it was clear that the benzene from a lagoon would dictate the severity of the water hazard; therefore, the delineation of this plume was the focus of that effort. Ultimately, by remediating the chemicals of the most toxicological importance, rather than attempting to reduce the concentration of most or all chemicals to background, the site will be made acceptable for nearly any use at a fraction of the original cost estimates.

The following section describes the components of an RBRI. The formulation of data quality objectives, development of a site conceptual model, identification of chemical fate and transport mechanisms, and assorted sampling strategies for obtaining representative data sets are discussed. Phased sampling and data evaluation, which are integral components of the risk-based remedial investigation process, are also presented.

Establishing Data Quality Objectives

Data Quality Objectives (DQOs) are intended to eliminate unnecessary, duplicative, or overly precise data, while at the same time ensuring that the data are of a sufficient quality and quantity to support defensible decision making. The DQO process is a strategic planning approach that should be used to formulate data collection activities by clarifying study objectives, defining appropriate types of data and sampling conditions, and specifying tolerable limits on decision. The process involves the following seven iterative steps.

Step 1. State the problem. Review prior studies and existing information to gain a sufficient understanding of the site so the problem can be concisely described.
Step 2. Identify the decision. Identify the questions the study will attempt to resolve, and what actions may result based on various outcomes (Fig. 1).
Step 3. Identify the inputs to the decision. Identify the information that must be obtained and the measurements that must be collected to answer the questions.
Step 4. Define the study boundaries. Specify the time periods and spatial area to which decisions will apply. Determine when and where data should be collected.
Step 5. Develop a decision rule. Define the statistical parameter of interest, specify the action level (i.e., the numeric value of the selected parameter that will trigger the decision to pursue a specific action), and integrate the previous DQO outputs into a single statement that describes the logical basis for choosing among alternative actions.
Step 6. Specify tolerable limits on decision factors.
Step 7. Optimize the data-collection design. Evaluate information from the previous steps and generate alternative data-collection designs.

Steps 1 through 6 result in the development of specific DQOs, while step 7 develops a resource-efficient data collection program.

The Site Conceptual Model

The first step in the DQO process involves the development of a problem statement that forms the basis of the remedial investigation. An important aspect of this step is the evaluation of existing information

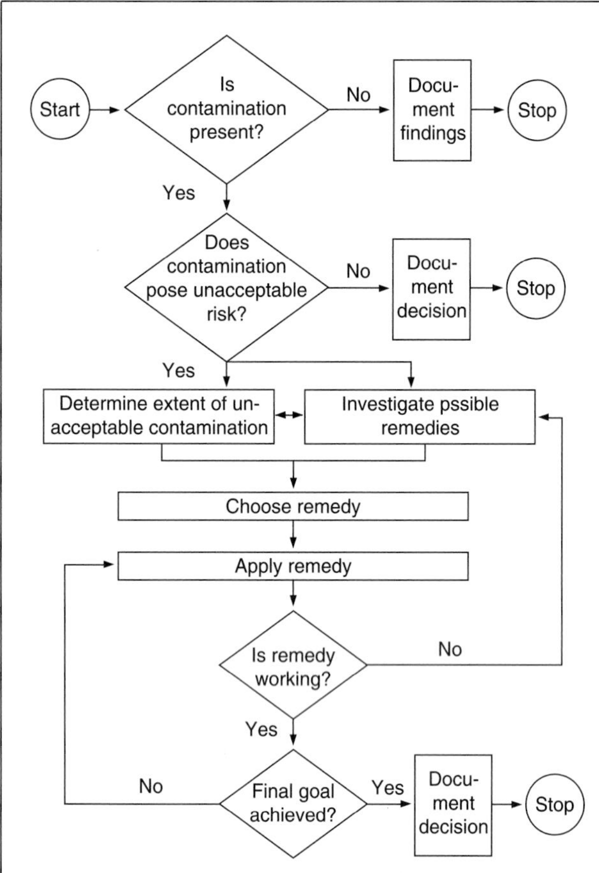

FIGURE 1 A multiple decision flow chart applicable to the risk-based remediation process. As depicted here, risk-based decision making is based on the risks presented by contaminants in the environment, not solely on the existence of contamination. Note that the determination of unacceptable risk should be made prior to the decision to delineate the extent of the contamination. (From: USEPA, 1994.)

about the site. For example, it would be logical to conduct soil sampling using a grid that is based on the results of a model that shows where the deposition of airborne toxics likely occurred. It would also be appropriate to use existing monitoring wells and review existing data regarding background concentrations before embarking on a comprehensive sampling program.

In simplest terms, a site conceptual model (Fig. 2) is a compilation of all the available information regarding the sources, pathways, and potentially exposed humans and wildlife at a site that is required to evaluate the potential incremental risks to human health and the environment. The site conceptual model should include known or suspected sources of chemicals, types of chemicals and their physical properties, affected media, geology and hydrogeology data, known and potential migration routes, fate and transport mechanisms, and known or potentially affected human populations and environmental systems. The model should be prepared as the first stage in the remedial investigation process and be continually revised as additional information becomes available. If, for example, it is found that a new and relatively toxic chemical is being detected in some media, then the model should be revised and the sampling plan adjusted accordingly.

Representative Sampling Strategies

In the remedial investigation process, samples of environmental media are generally collected for one or more reasons, including the determination of natural physical and chemical characteristics of the environmental media, definition of source areas, delineation of the extent of chemicals in affected media, determination of fate and transport characteristics that control how the chemicals move, and determination of the rate of formation of degradation products, if any.

One of the most frequently debated issues in risk-based remedial investigations is how much delineation is needed regarding chemicals in various media to which persons or wildlife are unlikely to be exposed. U.S. EPA's guidance for conducting remedial investigations and feasibility studies under the Comprehensive Environmental Response, Compensation, and Liability Act (CERCLA) states that a field investigation should characterize the nature and extent of contamination so that informed decisions can be made as to the level of risk presented by the site and the appropriate types of remedial response. Some regulatory jurisdictions require the delineation of all chemicals in all media to nondetectable concentrations in all directions (horizontally and vertically) or until background concentrations are observed, regardless of exposure potential. Other agencies in the United States accept delineation via extrapolation of directional concentration trends defined by two or more samples along a vector.

Regardless of the media being sampled or the type of data that is being collected, sampling designs for data acquisition fall into a number of general categories, including simple random sampling, stratified random sampling, simple systematic sampling, and sequential random sampling. The type of sampling program selected for a given site will depend upon the data quality objectives and the type of statistics that will be used to evaluate the data.

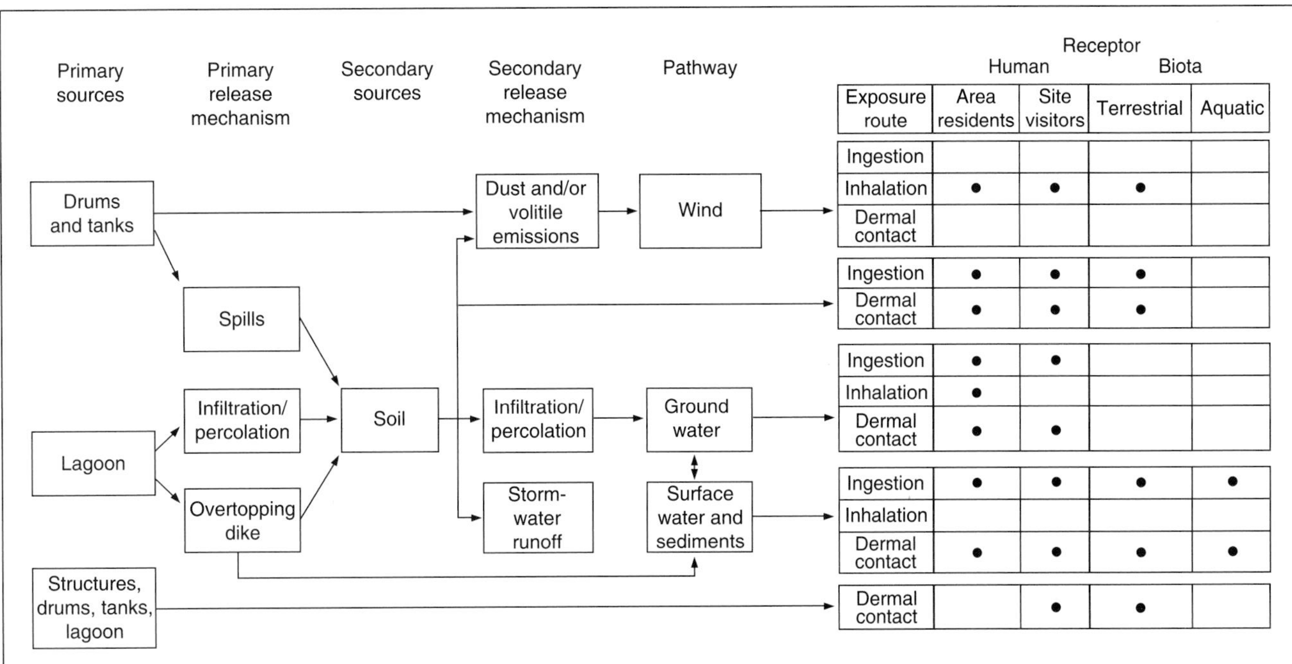

FIGURE 2 Site conceptual model. This example of a site conceptual model shows the gamut of potential sources, release mechanisms, migration pathways, and potentially exposed human and biologic populations. (From USEPA, 1988a.)

Random, systematic, and stratified sample arrays are illustrated (Fig. 3). In general, a randomized sampling plan is necessary to allow for probability or confidence statements about the results of the sampling. In contrast, sample selection using the judgement of the sampler has no randomization. Judgment sampling may be justified during the preliminary assessment and site investigation stages if the sampler has substantial knowledge of the sources and history of contamination. However, judgement samples should not be used to determine compliance with media cleanup criteria when assessing the need for or effectiveness of remediation.

A random sampling plan requires that each sample be selected independent of the location of all other samples, and no pattern is expected in the distribution of sample points. A pure random sampling presents the possibility that many samples could be clustered in one or two quadrants of the site, although this is less probable in larger sample arrays. For this reason, purely random sampling is rarely conducted. Systematic sampling, on the other hand, will usually distribute the sample locations relatively uniformly across the site, but may provide less than adequate data in key areas of the site.

The most popular approach that avoids the possible problem of clustering in random sample arrays is a stratified random sampling plan. In this approach, the sampling locations are still chosen at random, but a minimum number of samples in each quadrant are collected. This sampling methodology usually improves the precision of statistical estimates by controlling the variability due to soil type, location, characteristics of the terrain, and so on. This approach will normally work well at those sites that have only a few sources of contamination. Factors that can be used to divide strata include sample depth, chemical concentration levels (if known in advance), physiography and topography, previous cleanup attempts, and source area history. As a rule, the strata must not overlap and the sum of the sizes of the strata must account for the entire area being sampled.

Finally, sequential sampling is a process whereby statistical analysis is performed on the data set over and over as each new sample is obtained. The need to collect additional samples is reevaluated after each round of sampling. The objective of sequential sampling is that sampling in less-contaminated areas can be completed early in the process as the statistical criteria are met, while the more contaminated or hazardous areas may require a greater number of samples to achieve the required statistical criteria. One benefit of sequential sampling is that it minimizes the potential for oversampling when attempting to con-

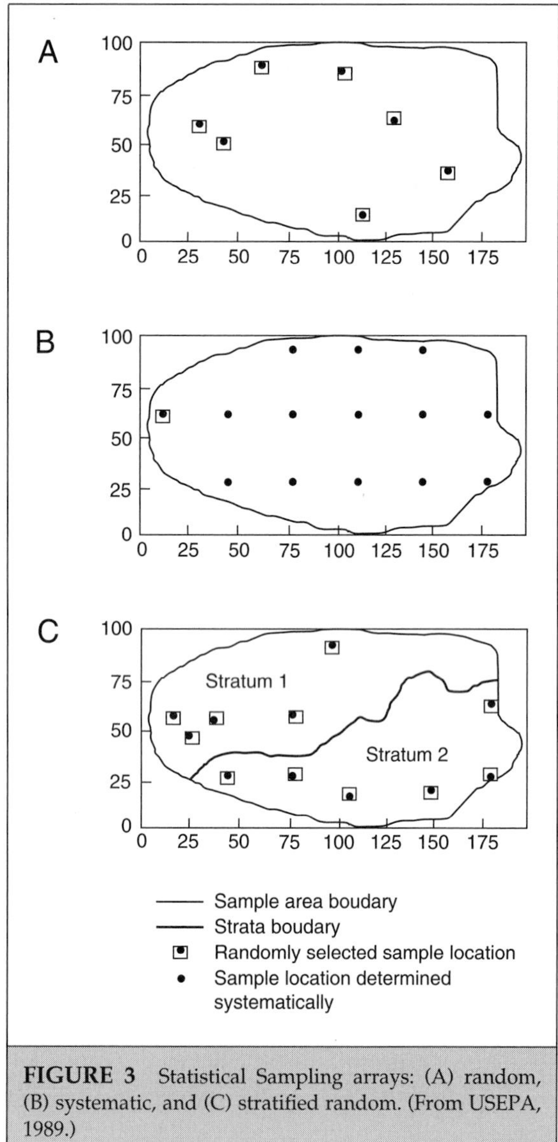

FIGURE 3 Statistical Sampling arrays: (A) random, (B) systematic, and (C) stratified random. (From USEPA, 1989.)

firm that the attainment of cleanup standards has been achieved, or that the area is generally consistent with background concentrations.

Evaluating Chemical Fate and Transport Mechanisms

Understanding how chemicals move and change (i.e., degrade or metabolize) in the environment is a fundamental objective of a remedial investigation. Without this understanding, it is impossible to assess or predict the magnitude of the risks of a chemical at a given location. Factors that affect the fate and transport of chemicals in the environment include the characteristics of the chemicals and the characteristics of the environmental media.

Some examples of chemical-specific characteristics that affect fate and transport in the environment include boiling point, melting point, molecular weight, specific gravity, acid dissociation constant, octanol/water partition coefficient, organic carbon partitioning coefficient, water solubility, vapor pressure, Henry's law constant, and ultraviolet spectrum. Some examples of environmental factors include naturally occurring sources and/or concentrations of the chemical in question, release mechanisms from anthropogenic sources, and characteristics of environmental media, such as geology and hydrogeology, surface water flow and suspended sediment load, soil vegetative cover, wind speed and direction, pH, oxygen, presence of electron acceptors, concentration of free radicals, organic carbon content, particle size, clay mineral composition, and cation-exchange capacity.

An understanding of these chemical-specific and environmental factors will enable the evaluation of various dispersive and degradative processes, such as advective transport, biodegradation, abiotic degradation (photolysis, oxidation, reduction, and hydrolosis), bioaccumulation, soil adsorption, volatilization, diffusion, and dispersion. The results of such evaluations can then be used to model or predict chemical concentrations at the location of exposure.

The Phased Approach to Site Characterization and Remediation

Most regulations and guidance documents suggest that the remedial investigation process should be performed in an interactive and iterative fashion with the risk assessment and feasibility study. For example, the RI/FS model for Superfund (Fig. 4) establishes a framework for the evaluation of risk and alternative risk-reduction measures concurrently with the remedial investigation, with the scope and need for complete site characterization and/or remediation being contingent upon the results of the risk assessment. In the United States and Canada, this process is generally referred to as risk-based corrective action (RBCA).

The American Society of Testing and Materials (ASTM) in 1995 standardized the RBCA process because the risk-based intent of environmental regulations was generally thought to have been lost or significantly hampered by the regulatory enforcement process. Due to the clear benefits of this approach and the clarity of the guidance, the RBCA process has since been adopted, mimicked, or cited by most regulatory agencies as a fundamental approach to environ-

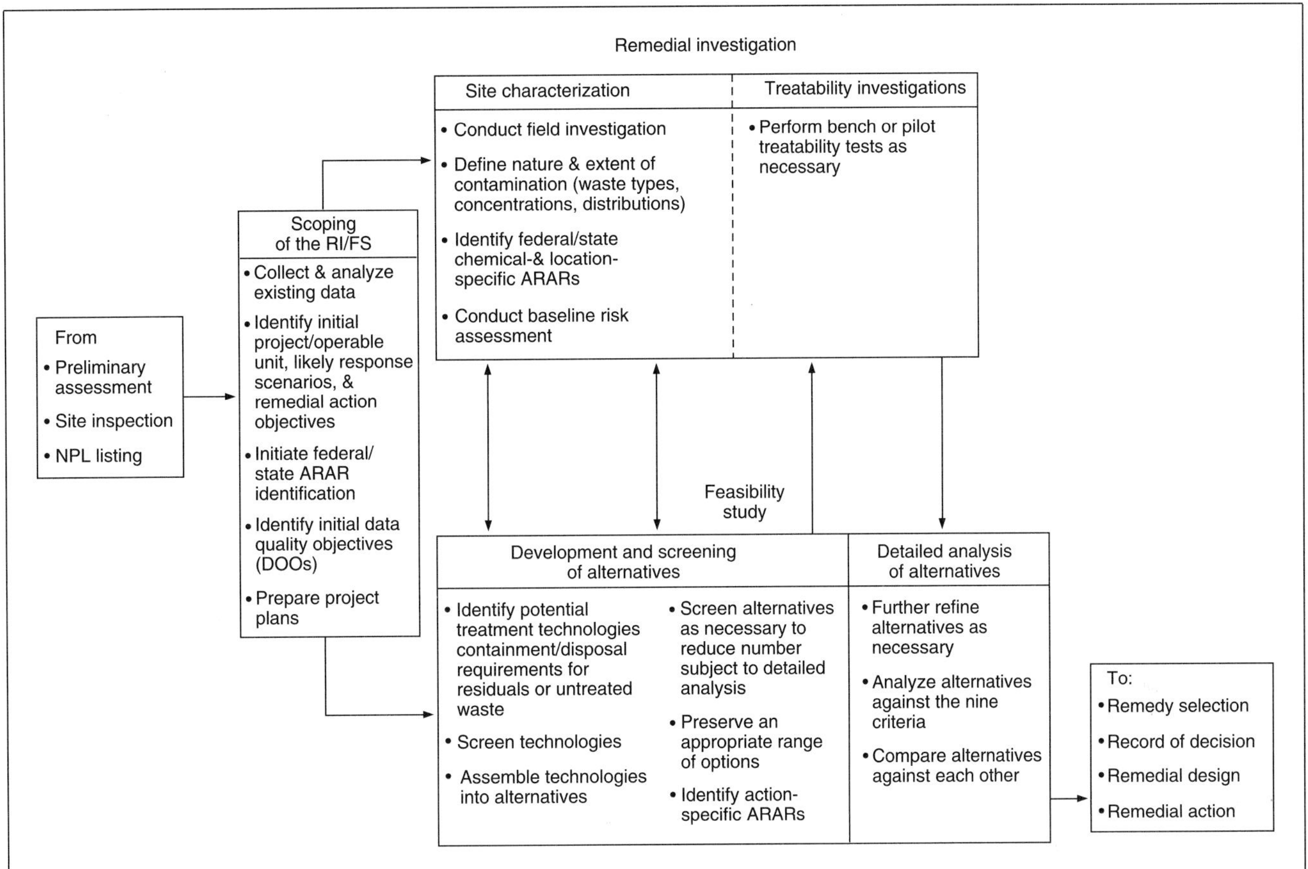

FIGURE 4 The remedial investigation and feasibility study (RI/FS) process. The RI/FS process under the U.S. Superfund program is intended to be an interactive and iterative process wherein site characterization and risk assessment are performed interactively with the evaluation of appropriate remedial alternatives. (From USEPA, 1988a.)

mental remediation for petroleum and other chemicals.

The RBCA process comprises up to 10 stages, beginning with an initial site assessment that is followed by a site classification and the implementation of appropriate initial response actions. Initial response actions vary in magnitude depending on the severity of the risks identified and may range from the evacuation of people to the monitoring of the natural attenuation of the identified contaminants. Consistent with the Data Quality Objectives process described previously (Fig. 1), these two preliminary stages may then be followed by up to three "tiers," involving progressively more detailed acquisition and evaluation of site-specific data. The final two stages of the RBCA process are the final remedial action and the confirmation of effective remediation. This iterative process of collecting progressively more detailed site-specific information, and evaluating the likely human health or ecological risks and prospective remedial actions, ensures that the data collected will be only that which is necessary to identify and mitigate risks. The RBCA process also provides for the development of risk-based screening levels and target cleanup levels that can be refined as more site-specific exposure information becomes available during successive tiers of the investigation.

RISK-BASED CLEANUP CRITERIA

Many regulatory agencies in the United States and Europe have developed numerical criteria that define for regulatory purposes the acceptable concentrations of various chemicals in various environmental media. Remedial action is typically not required at sites where the mean or 95% upper confidence limit on the mean concentration of the toxicant falls below these criteria, and a certain "peak" concentration is not exceeded.

Historically there has been a wide disparity in the methods that were followed to generate these criteria. In the 1970s and 1980s, many agencies in the United States and in Europe adopted a quest for "pristine" or "pre-industrial" conditions—a goal that proved problematic, especially in areas with a century or more of industrialization. For example, the average lead concentration in soil in and around Baltimore or Philadelphia, and in some parts of London, exceeds the national background concentration by up to 100-fold. In an effort to impart some guidance in the 1970s, some agencies adopted the same criteria for soil and groundwater quality that had been established for food and tap water, while others based their cleanup criteria on technical considerations via the results achievable through "best available technology" (BAT). In short, most cleanup criteria lacked a good scientific basis until the early 1990s.

Serious efforts to develop well-founded guidance for developing risk-based cleanup goals began in the mid-1980s, nearly a decade after the passage of the Resource Conservation and Recovery Act (RCRA) in 1977. At that time, EPA completed one of the first meaningful attempts to provide guidance for the development of alternate concentration levels (ACLs) for groundwater ("alternate" in the context of the default tap-water quality criteria that otherwise apply) using a legitimately risk-based approach. In its more recent *Soil Screening Guidance* released in 1996, EPA also proposed specific soil cleanup guidelines for many chemicals, and set forth a method of calculating cleanup criteria for those chemicals not listed. In many cases, EPA's approach was a result of the successful approaches used by the Dutch, who began issuing soil quality criteria more that 15 years ago. Elsewhere, the process for setting cleanup levels continues to evolve, but most methods for setting cleanup goals derived from Dutch, U.S., or German guidelines.

Background Cleanup Criteria

The concept of "cleaning up to background" essentially means reducing the concentrations of chemicals in the affected media to the concentrations that most likely existed prior to their release into the environment. Requirements to achieve "background" levels are usually applied to naturally occurring inorganic constituents, such as lead, mercury, and zinc. However, using background as a cleanup standard has, at times, been suggested for some synthetic organic chemicals in industrialized areas. Background concentrations of various metals in soil at particular sites can often be obtained from published sources, or they can be determined through site-specific sampling to determine the concentrations outside the affected area. In recent years, few agencies have decided that cleaning sites to background concentrations could be economically justified.

Generic Health-Based Cleanup Criteria

A generic health-based cleanup criterion for a particular chemical, in contrast with a site-specific cleanup criterion, is defined as the maximum concentration at which that chemical can exist in a given environmental medium without posing unacceptable risks to exposed humans or wildlife. The bases for criteria form the definition of "acceptable risk," and they vary among different countries and within the various agencies and regions of these countries.

In the United States, generic health-based cleanup criteria for suspected human carcinogens are generally established so that exposure to humans will not pose a theoretical increased life-time cancer risk greater than one in one million ($1 \times 10^{-}$) to one in ten thousand (1×10^{-4}). For systemic toxicants (the noncarcinogens), health-based criteria are concentrations that should not produce adverse effects within exposed populations, including sensitive subgroups, following either acute or chronic exposure. Usually, safe or acceptable concentrations are defined as those that will not produce an absorbed dose greater than the EPA reference dose (RfD) or, in some regulatory jurisdictions, one-tenth that value.

Generic health-based criteria are generally developed using the methodologies described in the U.S. EPA's 1991 *Risk Assessment Guidance for Superfund (RAGS), Human Health Evaluation Manual Part B,* in which the equations for calculating carcinogenic and noncarcinogenic risks at a given chemical concentrations are rearranged to calculate permissible chemical concentrations based on target risk levels and/or hazard indexes. The equations contained in RAGS Part B for the inhalation of volatiles and fugitive dust have recently been revised and these can be found in EPA's 1994 *Final Soil Screening Guidance* document.

In Europe, the approach to setting soil cleanup guidelines has varied with each country and it has changed over time since the 1980s. For example, in the mid-1980s, it was not uncommon for a number of European nations, as well as Australia and New Zealand, to adopt the Dutch soil guidelines because they had been established upon reasonable principles. Beginning in about 1995, various countries accelerated their efforts to formalize their own approaches to setting both soil and drinking water standards.

In Europe and in most other industrialized areas of the world, the cleanup criteria for the noncarcinogens have since the 1960s been established using the standard toxicological approach; that is, the no observed effect level (NOEL) in chronic animals studies was divided by a factor of about 100 in order to identify a likely "safe dose" in humans (the safety factor approach). However, unlike in the United States, where mathematical models were used to identify safe levels of exposure to carcinogens beginning in 1976, the European countries and others have continued to divide the NOEL from life-time rodent bioassays by a factor of 100–200 to identify a safe level of exposure for humans. Interestingly, after having used low-dose models since the 1970s, in 1996 the U.S. EPA suggested in its new policy for chemical carcinogens that for the nongenotoxic carcinogens, and perhaps others, it was no longer necessary to rely exclusively on the models and that the safety factor approach was likely to be considered acceptable.

Soil Cleanup Criteria for Protection of Groundwater

Since the 1970s, soil cleanup criteria have been generally intended to protect humans who might be in contact with the soil via inhalation, ingestion, or dermal contact. Since the early 1990s, however, a priority has also been placed on cleaning soils to protect the quality of underlying groundwater and nearby surface water. The migration of chemicals from the soil to groundwater can be envisioned as a two-stage process. Chemicals in soil are first released into a soil leachate, and then the leachate is transported through the underlying soil, into the underlying aquifer, and eventually to humans and/or wildlife.

Soil cleanup criteria for groundwater protection are usually developed by back-calculating from acceptable groundwater concentrations. First, an acceptable target groundwater concentration for a given chemical is identified at a point of compliance (e.g., the site boundary) or point of exposure (e.g., a wetland or a household tap) as appropriate. This target groundwater concentration is then multiplied by a dilution fact or to obtain an acceptable leachate concentration within the soil source area. For example, if through groundwater modeling the dilution factor is determined to be 10, and the acceptable groundwater concentration is 0.05 mg/liter at the point of compliance, the target leachate concentration would be 0.5 mg/liter. Soil-to-water partitioning equations are then used to calculate the soil concentration that corresponds to the target leachate concentration. Because the conditions that affect intermedia partitioning differ from site to site, generic soil quality criteria for the protection of groundwater are generally developed using the following assumptions.

1. Infinite source duration (i.e., source is not diminished via leaching).
2. Uniform chemical distribution within the source area.
3. Soil source is in contact with the water table (i.e., no clean zone beneath source).
4. No attenuation due to chemical, biological, or physical factors in source area.
5. Soil/water partitioning is instantaneous and linear throughout soil zone.
6. Groundwater point of compliance is at the edge of the soil source area.
7. Groundwater exists in an unconfined and unconsolidated aquifer.
8. The aquifer is homogenous and isotropic.
9. No attenuation due to chemical, biological, or physical factors in groundwater.
10. No nonaqueous phase liquids (NAPL) present at the site.

The soil cleanup levels developed for any specific site using this generic method are expected to be reevaluated as additional information becomes available during the remedial investigation and is in lieu of the default assumptions.

Site-Specific Risk-Based Cleanup Criteria

Site-specific risk-based cleanup criteria are generally computed in the same fashion as generic cleanup criteria and soil-to-groundwater criteria. The major difference is that site-specific information, fate, and transport factors, as well as exposure data, are used in lieu of the default assumptions and generic exposure criteria to calculate cleanup levels. Because generic and default assumptions are designed to be very conservative, site-specific risk-based cleanup criteria are generally less stringent than generic health-based cleanup criteria.

In many instances, site-specific exposure conditions reflect various land-use patterns, and these conditions may change if the use of the affected site changes (e.g., if a manufacturing plant were some day decommissioned and used as the site of an elementary school and playground). For this reason, it has been proposed that as many as seven soil cleanup standards should be developed for each major chemical contaminant in soil; one for each of seven kinds of site use or exposure scenario (agricultural, residential, industrial, recreational, groundwater protection, wildlife protection, and runoff and erosion of particles to waterways).

Improving Site-Specific Risk-Based Cleanup Criteria

The risk-based approach to conducting remedial investigations and developing site-specific cleanup criteria is receiving a high level of acceptance in the regulatory and regulated communities. However, the methods for establishing site-specific risk-based criteria for any contaminated medium can fall short of supporting true risk-based remediation decisions due to their failure to account for five important factors:

1. The appropriateness or validity of the one-in-one-million cancer risk criterion.
2. Inadequacies in the toxicity data.
3. Scientific uncertainties in the techniques for extrapolation from laboratory rodents to humans.
4. Several layers of conservative exposure assumptions, which result in the overestimation of risk, and the expression of these risk estimates as single-point estimates.
5. Failure to communicate the risk characterization in a transparent manner to the public.

To overcome these possible deficiencies, the following additional suggestions should be considered when developing site-specific risk-based cleanup goals.

1. Carefully evaluate the appropriateness of the one in one million benchmark for acceptable excess cancer risk in humans. This risk criterion (10^{-6}) does not imply that science has the ability to accurately predict if one person in a population of one million people may develop cancer sometime during his or her life time due to exposure to a particular substance or assemblage of substances. Indeed, when considered against the background life time cancer risk of one in four, estimated by the American Cancer Society, an incremental increase in cancer occurrence of one in one million cannot be detected using epidemiological methods for human populations exposed to any single contaminated site.

2. For each chemical of interest at a given site, evaluate the adequacy of the toxicity data used in the hazard identification and dose–response assessments. If necessary, supplement this data set with more recent or complete data and reevaluate the appropriateness of the cancer slope factors and noncancer reference doses.

3. For each chemical of interest, evaluate the adequacy of the methods used to extrapolate from observed dose–response relationships in laboratory rodents to humans. If necessary, recalculate the predicted human dose–response relationship using the most recent developments in physiologically based pharmacokinetic (PB-PK) modeling.

4. Use probabilistic or Monte Carlo techniques when analyzing complex exposure scenarios. Present the risk estimates associated with the resultant cleanup goals using a probability distribution rather than a point estimate. Avoid using multiple conservative exposure assumptions in setting cleanup goals.

5. Communicate the ranges and probabilities of the potential risk associated with targeted cleanup goals in terms that can be readily understood.

Demonstrating Attainment of Cleanup Standards

Once established, risk-based cleanup standards define the objectives of site remediation in numerical terms. Before a site can be termed "closed" or "remediated," it is necessary to demonstrate that these objectives have been met. For this reason, soil cleanup criteria can be viewed as having three components:

1. Numerical component. The soil cleanup level should be protective of human health and the environment.
2. Attainment sampling. The types, numbers, and locations of the post-remediation samples needed for proof of compliance must be described.
3. Demonstrate attainment. The statistical method that will be used to compare the attainment sampling data to the numerical cleanup criteria needs to be described.

A risk-based cleanup standard that is developed only as a numerical component, such as 25 milligrams of trichloroethylene (TCE) per kilogram of soil, without a description of attainment sampling and demonstration criteria, has little practical utility.

Perhaps the most critical factor in evaluating attainment involves the selection of the appropriate statistical parameter from the post-remedial data set for comparison to the cleanup standard. Comparisons typically use the mean, median, or upper proportion or percentile of the comparison data set. Some guidance specifies limits on the proportion of sample results that can exceed the cleanup standard, and the maximum permissible exceedances, expressed as a multiple of the cleanup standard. For example, the 70/10 rule used by the state of Pennsylvania states that 70% of the sample results must fall below the standard, and that no single result may exceed the standard by a factor of 10, regardless of whether the mean, median, or upper proportion or percentile will be used for comparison. It should be noted that numerous different attainment criteria have been used since the 1970s and, regrettably, there is no "best approach."

Factors affecting the selection of the appropriate statistical criteria for proving that the site has been cleaned include the criteria used to develop the risk-based standard, whether the effects of the chemical being measured are acute or chronic, the relative sample sizes required, the likelihood of detecting concentrations below the cleanup standard, and the range of the confirmation data. For example, if the cleanup criterion is a risk-based standard based on toxicity studies that relied on the mean concentration, it is to be compared to the mean of the confirmation data. However, if the cleanup standard is developed for extreme concentrations that should rarely be exceeded, it may be more appropriate to establish criteria that focus on the upper percentile of the distribution of the compliance data set.

USING RISK ASSESSMENT TO OPTIMIZE REMEDY EVALUATION AND SELECTION

The purpose of the remedy selection process is to identify the measures that will eliminate, reduce and/or control risks to human health and the environment that are due to the presence of contaminants in certain environmental media. For the most part, the target risk-reduction criteria have been no adverse effects to human populations, including sensitive subgroups, due to life-time exposure to systemic toxicants; and the theoretical life-time incremental cancer risk should be between 10^{-4} and 10^{-6}.

Overview of the Feasibility Study Process

Most regulatory authorities require that prospective remedies first be identified through an initial screening process that evaluates effectiveness, implementability, and cost. Viable remedial options identified are then subjected to a more detailed analysis, which is based on meeting the following criteria.

1. Overall protection of human health and the environment. The remedy needs to adequately protect human health and the environment over both the short term and long term by eliminating or reducing contaminants, or by controlling exposures to contaminants.
2. Compliance with applicable or relevant and appropriate requirements. The remedy needs to meet most applicable or relevant and appropriate requirements (ARARs) under the given legislative situation.
3. Long-term effectiveness and permanence. The remedy needs to prove successful over the long term, including the consideration of the magnitude of residual risk remaining from untreated wastes or waste residuals, and the adequacy and reliability of long-term engineering and institutional controls such as caps, slurry walls, and land-use restrictions.
4. Reduction of toxicity, mobility, or volume through treatment. The remedy should quantitatively characterize the specific treatment processes and materials limitations; that is, the amount of material to be treated; degree of reduction of volume, toxicity, and/or mobility; irreversibility; characteristics of residuals; and ability to reduce the inherent hazards of the site.
5. Short-term effectiveness. An evaluation of the time required to achieve targeted risk reduction levels must be performed, and the short-term risks that may be posed to the community and/or the environment during or as a result of remedy implementation.
6. Implementability. The implementability the remedy with respect to technical feasibility, administrative feasibility, and availability of services and materials should evaluated.
7. Cost. A complete description of all costs, including net present value of capital costs and annual operations and maintenance costs, should be developed.
8. Jurisdictional acceptance. The remedy must be acceptable not only to the regulatory agency overseeing the cleanup, but to all regulatory agencies having jurisdiction over the site.
9. Community acceptance. An evaluation of the components of each alternative remedy that is being considered should be shared with the community or community members.

It is clear from this basic decision framework that risk assessment plays a major role in the remedy selection process in terms of the overall risk associated with the conduct of the remediation, as well as the reduction of human and environmental risks following remediation. In addition, the long-term effectiveness and permanence of risk reduction, the specific risk-reduction mechanisms (i.e., toxicity, volume, and mobility of contaminants), and risks that may be created during remedy implementation should be described and shared with the public.

Technologies Based on Volume Reduction

Achieving risk reduction through the reduction of the volume of contamination in environmental media depends upon the ability to physically remove the contaminants from the affected medium, thereby reducing or eliminating residual concentrations and the possible exposure of humans and wildlife. All technologies that can produce a reduction of the in-place volume of contamination get high marks in the area of overall risk reduction. Generally, the long-term effectiveness and permanence of risk reduction at these sites is also achieved following remediation. However, there can be important short-term risk factors due to temporary increases in contaminant mobility and/or toxicity during and following remediation.

Most contaminant removal techniques rely on temporarily *increasing* the mobility of the contaminants to facilitate their extraction from the affected medium. For example, soil flushing with surfactants desorbs contaminants from soils, and other techniques often promote the release of contaminants into an airstream for subsequent collection (e.g., thermal desorption, vapor extraction, air stripping, and air sparging). Thus, inadequate collection and handling methods can result in the spread of contaminants into surrounding media or previously unaffected areas, and the increased exposure of workers. Further, the process of contaminant removal typically results in a waste product that requires subsequent treatment, storage, and/or disposal.

Technologies Based on Toxicity Reduction

Achieving risk reduction through the reduction of the toxicity of contaminants in environmental media depends upon the ability to chemically or biologically alter or destroy the contaminants within the affected medium. In recent years, toxicity reduction techniques are those most favored by regulatory agencies and society at large (with the exception of incineration) because they represent ultimate destruction and therefore complete elimination of risk, as opposed to a transfer of risk to another location (some volume-reduction techniques) or time (some techniques that reduce mobility or exposure). Although incineration offers many advantages over other techniques, the concerns about the toxicity of the airborne emissions and the ash has halted most new construction except in Japan.

The short-term effectiveness associated with toxicity reduction techniques are varied. Incineration, for example, could be highly effective as a risk-reduction process, but it requires extensive air-emissions controls. In general, the historical environmental or safety problems associated with incineration have been resolved in modern facilities. However, this technology is not being promoted.

Low-temperature processes of oxidation and reduction and biodegradation usually involve mobilizing contaminants in soils prior to, or concurrently with, degradation. Depending on the physical characteristics of the media being treated, it is not unusual for this increase in mobility to exceed the capacity for degradation and produce a short-term increase in intermedia contaminant migration and/or migration of the contaminants beyond the area being targeted for remediation. This should be anticipated and closely monitored, particularly in saturated soils where the increased contaminant mobility could cause increases in the concentrations of contaminants in groundwater.

By far, the most popular and socially acceptable process of reducing contaminant toxicity is bioremediation. Bioremediation has gained attention and acceptance in the mid 1990s as research, development, and application continue to reveal a much broader realm of effectiveness. For example, bioremediation methods are now accepted in nearly every case involving remediation of petroleum hydrocarbons. Emerging research continues to expand the envelop of recalcitrant and persistent organic compounds that are treatable via microbial metabolic processes, and metals that can be taken up and metabolized by plants in a process termed "phytoremediation."

Technologies Based on Mobility Reduction

Achieving risk reduction through the reduction of the mobility of contaminants in environmental media depends upon the ability to physically prevent the contaminants from moving out of the affected medium. These processes fall into the categories of stabilization and fixation. Stabilization is the process of preventing contaminants from dissolving or otherwise migrating into surrounding media by bonding them in place through the addition of a binding agent, such as Portland cement. Vitrification (melting the soil matrix to bind or encapsulate the contaminants in a glass-like matrix) is another type of stabilization that has proven difficult and expensive to implement and thus has largely fallen out of favor. Recently, melting soils at extremely high temperatures in vats, the "molten metals" technology, is well accepted with radioactive wastes, but this is the most expensive technology.

Fixation is the process of chemically altering contaminants to render them immobile, insoluble, or otherwise reduce their movement into the environment. Examples of fixation include the adsorption of heavy metals onto fly ash and the conversion of soluble metal salts into insoluble elemental forms. Some fixation techniques also have the benefit of reducing the toxicity of contaminants.

Processes that reduce contaminant mobility generally achieve favorable results for overall risk reduction, although their long-term effectiveness and permanence continues to be debated. Despite positive laboratory and field testing results, stabilization and fixation techniques that do not also chemically alter the contaminants and reduce their toxicity are less favored by regulators and society at large than those techniques that involve destruction. The concern is that toxic chemicals that are "bound up" could one day be released. Nonetheless, from a toxicological standpoint, the rate at which stabilized or fixed chemicals would be released under most plausible circumstances will generally be so low that the resultant risks will usually be negligible.

Mobility-reduction processes often have short-term effectiveness questions that stem from the possible risks associated with worker exposure during remedy implementation in *ex situ* applications. Because stabilization and fixation alter the physical state and/or chemistry of the media in which the contaminants are contained, *in situ* applications may have negative impacts on ecological systems. For example, the resulting change in the physical nature of the soils may alter groundwater flow patterns and/or prevent rooting and plant growth within the stabilized area.

Technologies Based on Exposure Reduction

The fourth approach to risk reduction is the elimination or reduction of exposure to the contaminants by humans and wildlife via the use of engineering and/or institutional controls. Engineering controls physically restrain contaminants and prevent them from moving into or through the environment, but without altering their form or state, or changing their inherent mobility or solubility (e.g., slurry walls, sheet piling, liner systems, caps, leachate collection systems, and groundwater recovery trenches and wells for plume containment). Institutional controls are measures that limit or prohibit certain activities that may result in exposure to contaminants (e.g., fences, signs, and land-use restrictions).

When applied as a sole remedy, exposure control measures are considered by many regulators and environmentalists as being little more than deferments of environmental problems to be solved by future generations. This is not an unfair assessment, although the concept of effectively managing our historical and future contamination problems through these measures is growing in social acceptance. Regrettably, many exposure control measures have been known to fail due to flaws in design or craftsmanship.

The short-term effectiveness of exposure control measures are varied. Institutional controls are virtually instantaneous in their ability to achieve targeted risk-reduction levels, and it is rare that adverse risks are created as a result of their implementation. Engineering controls require a longer time period for implementation. Engineering controls often have significant worker exposure considerations that need to be addressed in remedial action health and safety plans. Many engineering controls cause significant impacts to surrounding ecosystems that often out-weigh any perceived benefits of the remediation in terms of overall risk reduction. For example, soil capping programs designed to prevent human exposure that also destroy established ecological habitats, or groundwater extraction systems designed to prevent plume migration that also result in the de-watering of adjacent wetlands areas.

Natural Attenuation

Many of the remedial technologies discussed that serve to reduce contaminant volume, toxicity, and/or mobility are enhancements of physical, chemical, and biological processes that occur to some degree in nature, while others (e.g., surfactant flushing and electro-osmosis) do not typically occur naturally. The concept of using naturally occurring degradative processes, with little to no enhancement, in an attempt to reduce the volume, toxicity, and/or mobility of contaminants in environmental media is termed "natural attenuation," and it has received significant acceptance by the scientific and regulatory communities.

Naturally occurring processes include nondestructive processes, such as sorption (reduction of mobility), dispersion, dilution, and volatilization (reduction of the volume of contaminant per unit volume of the affected medium). Natural attenuation also involves destructive processes, such as biodegradation (aerobic and anaerobic) and abiotic oxidation/reduction reactions, which serve to reduce contaminant toxicity through chemical or biochemical alteration.

It is apparent that natural attenuation is not a remedial approach, but rather a category of processes that occur in nature and, given time, may attain risk reduction goals without substantive enhancement. The single largest obstacle to embracing natural attenuation as a viable remedial concept by the regulatory community and society at large has been the misconception that "natural attenuation" is synonymous with the "no action" or "do nothing" alternative. This is certainly not the case, and this misconception has been largely dissipated since 1995 as a result of social pressures on regulators to limit the spending of large sums of money on ineffective remedies that, over time, would not need to be implemented.

Because natural attenuation is a category of the degradative processes and not a process in itself, it is not possible to apply the same evaluation of the risk factors involved in remedy selection, as for the other processes. Rather, a natural attenuation remedy must specify in the same level of detail and rigor each of the nine remedy evaluation criteria discussed earlier.

RISK-BASED REMEDIATION IN BROWNFIELDS REDEVELOPMENT

As society moves into the 21st century, the environmental movement is reacquainting itself with the fundamental concepts of risk assessment, risk reduction, and risk management upon which it was formed in the 1970s. Experience has revealed some of the financial and societal costs of overly aggressive implementation of environmental policies. The problems associated with "moving too quickly" have forced a reevaluation of long-term priorities and social objectives in most developed countries, including Great Britain, Japan, Germany, France, Canada, the United States, Sweden, and Australia.

Perhaps the single most significant unintended problem of the environmental movement in the United States has been the introduction of the legal postulate that the owner of a property should and can be held liable for contamination that occurred on the property prior to his or her ownership. As a result of this, most prospective landowners and developers have avoided purchasing properties that have had historical industrial activity, due primarily to the potential cost of environmental remediation. Thus, hundreds of thousands of acres of farmland and open spaces have been developed for industrial purposes while former industrial properties remain vacant.

These abandoned properties are collectively referred to as "brownfields" (as opposed to pristine rural land commonly referred to as "greenfields"). In the past 3 or 4 years, many regulatory agencies in the United States and Germany have passed legislation geared toward facilitating the reuse of brownfields properties by limiting the liability assumed by purchasers and financial lending institutions, and establishing funding sources to help pay for remediation. These "brownfields redevelopment" programs use a risk-based decision-making process that tailors the cleanup objectives for a given property to the intended end use of the property. The future for this approach looks quite attractive.

COMPARING THE UNITED STATES APPROACHES TO THOSE USED IN OTHER COUNTRIES

Since the 1960s, the United States almost certainly had the most aggressive program for regulating the production, release, and disposal of industrial chemicals of the industrialized countries. Since about 1994, the United States spent about $165 billion annually on environmental issues. During this same period, virtually every other country was also initiating and implementing fairly thorough regulatory programs; however, they were different in that they were less prescriptive. That is, the various emitters of chemicals were given a goal, but they were not told how to achieve it and the timeline for achievement was less rigid than is usually called for in the United States.

As discussed previously, the specific goal established by the various countries varied considerably. For example, in Germany and Switzerland, it was not unusual for the firm responsible for the pollution to be required to remediate the lands to pre-industrial conditions (e.g., to nearly background concentrations). In the Netherlands, this approach was considered too onerous, so risk-based approaches were adopted. The methods for identifying acceptable soil or water concentrations were the same for carcinogens and noncarcinogens; that is, the no observed effect level (NOEL) from a long-term animal study was divided by a factor of 100–500 and then risk assessment calculations were used to identify safe concentrations for humans. In Japan, depending on the situation, either Dutch or U.S. cleanup values were often adopted. In Australia and New Zealand, committees were formed to evaluate all of the various values promulgated by the various countries and to identify some "reasonable" concentration after weighing the work of the other nations.

CONCLUSIONS

Although at the beginning of the environmental movement it was attractive to adopt national goals that required returning contaminated properties to nearly pristine conditions, this objective soon proved to be too costly for most nations to initiate. Over the years, toxicology or risk-based approaches have generally been brought into the regulatory arena because they tend to identify concentrations that, although not "as low as background concentrations" or not necessarily "as low as technologically feasible," achieve the goal of protecting humans and the ecology, and tend to be much less expensive.

It is quite likely that the social pressures to continually improve the environment will exist in virtually every developed or developing country in the world for the foreseeable future. At the same time, there will be increasing pressures to find the optimal point in the cost–benefit relationship, so that "safe conditions" will occur as a result of cleanup efforts while spending the least amount of money to achieve this goal. Thus far, most scientists and regulators seem to believe that risk-based approaches to studying contaminated sites and remediating them offers the most promise for accomplishing these goals. Although this chapter serves only as an introduction to the topic, it can be a springboard to developing new and better ways of improving future cleanup activities.

Bibliography

Ames, B. N., and Gold, L. S. (1995). The causes and prevention of cancer. *In* "The True State of the Planet" (R. Bailey ed.), pp. 142–175. Free Press, New York.

ASTM. (1995a). "Guide for Developing Conceptual Site Models for Contaminated Sites." E1689-95. American Society of Testing and Materials, Philadelphia, PA.

ASTM. (1995b). "Standard Guide for Risk-Based Corrective Action Applied at Petroleum Release Sites." E 1739-95. American Society of Testing and Materials, Philadelphia, PA.

ASTM. (1996). "New Standard Guide for Remediation by Natural Attenuation at Petroleum Release Sites." E50.01 (96-01). American Society of Testing and Materials, Philadelphia, PA.

ATSDR (1992). Public Health Assessment Guidance Manual. Lewis Publishers. Ann Arbor, Michigan.

Burmaster, D. E., and Harris, R. N. (1993). The magnitude of compounding conservatism in superfund risk assessments (essay). *Risk Anal.* **13(2),** 131–134.

Carson, R. (1962). "Silent Spring." Houghton Mifflin, New York.

Chiras, D. D. (1992). An inquiry into the root causes of the environmental crisis. *Environ. Carcino. Ecotox. Rev.* **C10(1),** 73–119.

Colten, C. E., and Skinner, P. N. (1996). "The Road to Love Canal: Managing Industrial Waste before EPA." University of Texas Press, Austin.

Conway, R. A. (1984). "Environmental Risk Analyses for Chemicals." Van Nostrand, New York.

El Saadi, O., and Langley, A. (1991). The Health Risk Assessment and Management of Contaminated Sites. South Australian Health Commission. Adelaide, Australia.

Errampalli, D., Trevors, J. T., Lee, H., Leung, K., Cassidy, M., Knoke, K., Marwood, Shaw, K., Blears, M., and Chung, E. (1997). Bioremediation: A perspective. *J. Soil Contamination.* **6(3),** 207–218.

Finley, B. L., and Paustenbach, D. J. (1990). Using risk assessment to design cost-effective remedial investigation: A case study. *Econ.* **5(1),** 57–59.

Finley, B. L., and Paustenbach, D. J. (1994). The benefits of probabilistic exposure assessment: Three case studies involving contaminated air, water, and soil. *Risk Analysis* **14(1),** 53–73.

Finley, B. L., Scott, P., and Paustenbach, D. J. (1993). Using an Uncertainty Analysis of Exposure to Contaminated Tapwater to Evaluate Health-Protective Cleanup Goals. *Regul. Toxicol. Pharmacol.* **18,** 438–455.

Fox, R. D. (1996). Physical/Chemical Treatment of Organically Contaminated Soils and Sediments. *J. Air & Waste Management Assoc.* **46,** 391–413.

Gilbert, R. O. (1987). "Statistical Methods for Environmental Pollution Monitoring." Van Nostrand Reinhold, New York.

Graham, J. D., and Weiner, J. B. (1995). Risk vs Risk Tradeoffs in Protecting Health and the Environment. Harvard University Press, Cambridge, Massachusetts.

Graham, J. D. (1993). The legacy of one in a million. *Risk in Perspective* **1(1),** 1–6.

Hawkins, N. C. (1991). Conservatism in maximally exposed individual predictive exposure assessments: A first-cut, analysis. *Regul. Toxicol. Pharmacol.* **14,** 107–117.

Judge, C., Kostecki, P., and Calabrese, E. (1997). State summaries of soil and groundwater cleanup standards. *Soil & Groundwater Cleanup* **Nov.,** 10–34.

Lawrence Livermore National Laboratory (1995). "Recommendations to Improve the Cleanup Process for California's Leaking Underground Fuel Tanks." University of California, Livermore.

Lloyd, K. J., Thompson, K. M., and Burmaster D. E. (1992). Probabilistic techniques for back-calculating soil cleanup targets. *In* "Superfund Risk Assessment in Soil Contamination Studies" (K. B. Hoddinott and G. D. Knowles, eds.). ASTM STP 1158. American Society for Testing and Materials, Philadelphia, PA.

McCord, C. P. (1931). "Industrial Hygiene for Engineers and Managers." Harper and Brothers, New York.

McKone, T. E. (1991). Human exposure to chemicals from multiple media and through multiple pathways: Research overview and comments. *Risk Anal.* **11,** 5–10.

National Research Council (1996a). "Commission of Risk Assessment and Risk Management (CRAM) Risk Assessment and Risk Management in Regulatory Decision-Making." National Academy Press, Washington, D. C.

National Research Council (1996b). "Understanding Risk: Informing Decisions in a Democratic Society." National Academy Press, Washington, D.C.

Page, N. P., Singh, D. V., Farland, W., Goodman, J. I., Conolly, R. B., Andersen, M. E., Clewell, H. J., Frederick, C. B., Yamasaki, H., and Lucier, G. (1997). Implementation of EPA revised cancer assessment guidelines: Incorporation of mechanistic and pharmacokinetic data. *Fundam. Appl Toxicol* **37(1),** 16–36.

Paustenbach, D. J. (1984). Risk assessment . . . and engineering in the 80s. *Mech. Eng.* **106,** 54–59.

Paustenbach, D. J. (1995). The practice of health risk assessment in The United States (1975–1995): How the U.S. and other countries can benefit from that experience. *Human and Ecological Risk Assessment* **1(1),** 29–79.

Paustenbach, D. J., and DuFour, J. T. (1984). The engineer's role in protecting human health: Legal aspects. *Mech. Eng.* **106,** 62–69.

Paustenbach, D. J., Finley, B. L., and Long, T. F. (1997). The critical role of house dust in understanding the hazards posed by contaminated soils. *Int. J. Tox.* **16,** 339–362.

Paustenbach, D. J., Jernigan, J. D., Bass, R. Kalmes, R., and Scott, P. (1992). A proposed approach to regulating contaminated soil: Identify safe concentrations for seven of the most frequently encountered exposure scenarios. *Reg. Toxicol. Pharmacol.* **16,** 21–56.

Rodriguez, T. E., Russell, K. E., Walker, L. B., and D'Alleinne, C. P. (1994). Assessing real human health risks in the RCRA corrective action program by overcoming common pitfalls in the exposure assessment process. *In* "Proceedings of the Air & Waste Management Association Conference." Cincinnati, Ohio. 94-WP75B.03, pp. 374–384.

Ruckelshaus, W. D. (1984). Science, risk, and public policy. *Science* **221,** 1026–1031.

Sanders, P. F. (1995). Calculation of soil cleanup criteria for volatile organic compounds as controlled by the soil-to-groundwater pathway: Comparison of four unsaturated soil zone leaching models. *J. Soil Contamination* **4(1),** 1–24.

Smith, E. (1848/1949). The contribution of engineering to industrial hygiene. An address at the closing session of the Congress. *In* "The Proceedings of the Ninth International Congress on Industrial Medicine." John Wright and Sons, Ltd, Bristol, England.

Smith, R. L. (1996). Development of risk-based concentrations. "EPA Region III Risk-Based Concentration Table." EPA Region III, Philadelphia, Pennsylvania, pp. 1–148.

Thibodeaux, L. J. (1979). "Chemodynamics. Environmental Movement of Chemicals in Air, Water, and Soil." John Wiley and Sons, New York.

Travis, C. C., Richter, S. A., Crouch, E. A., Wilson, R., and Wilson, E. (1987). Cancer risk management. A review of 132 federal regulatory decisions. *Environ. Sci. Technol.* **21(5),** 415–420.

USEPA (1987). "Alternate Concentration Limit Guidance; Part I." EPA/530-SW-87-017. Washington, DC.

USEPA (1988a). "Guidance for Conducting Remedial Investigations and Feasibility Studies under CERCLA." Interim Final OWSER Directive 9355.3-01. Office of Emergency and Remedial Response, Washington, D.C.

USEPA (1988b). "Alternate Concentration Limit Guidance; Part II". EPA/530-SW-87-031. Washington, DC.

USEPA. (1989). "Methods for Evaluating the Attainment of Cleanup Standards, Vol. 1, Soil." EPA 230/02-89-042. Washington, D.C.

USEPA (1991a). "National Oil and Hazardous Substance Pollution Contingency Plan." 40 CFR 300. Washington, DC.

USEPA (1991b). "Risk Assessment Guidance for Superfund: Volume 1. Human Health Evaluation Manual (Part B; Development of Risk-Based Preliminary Remediation Goals)." Interim Publ. 9285.7-01B. Office of Emergency and Remedial Response, Washington, DC.

USEPA (1994). "Final Guidance for the Data Quality Objectives Process." EPA QA/G-4. Washington, DC.

USEPA (1995a). "The Brownfields Economic Redevelopment Initiative." EPA/540/R-94/068. Washington, D.C.

USEPA (1995b). "Draft Proposed Guidelines for Ecological Risk Assessment." EPA/630/R-95/002. Washington, DC.

USEPA (1996). "Soil Screening Guidance: Technical Background Document." EPA/540/R-95/128. U.S. Environmental Protection Agency, Office of Solid Waste and Emergency Response, Washington, DC.

USEPA (1997). "Policy for Use of Probabilistic Analysis in Risk Assessment. Technical Guidance Manual Risk Assessment." Guiding Principles for Monte Carlo Analysis EPA/630/R/-97/001. Washington, D.C.

Williams, C. A., James, R. C., and Freeman, R. W. (1995). Using the EPC approach to develop health-based soil and water screening concentrations for environmental chemicals. *Reg. Toxicol. Pharmacol.* **22,** 64–75.

CHAPTER

45

Ecotoxicology

HEIDI FOTH

Institute of Environmental Toxicology, Martin Luther University of Halle/Wittenberg, Halle, Germany

INTRODUCTION

The pollution of water, soil, and air with chemicals increased dramatically when industrial and economic development started. Because of technical demands, many naturally occurring compounds such as metals, coal, oil, sulfur, and phosphorus are taken from their fossil storage sites and new anthropogenic chemicals are released into the environment. In agriculture, synthetic biocides are distributed over the soil in large quantities to promote the growth of useful plants, suppress wild plants, and control pests. Chemicals are released unintentionally into the environment from permeable deposits at landfill sites and by the combustion of fuel and burning or heating during industrial production. As a consequence of our industrial and technical standard, the cycling of nutrients and of natural chemicals is enhanced and new material is brought into the system. In part, natural life cycles are interrupted, for example, by the eutrophication of small inland lakes. In other cases new processes that are started deplete resources that cannot be renewed within a reasonable time, such as the production of energy using fossil resources. The question is thus raised whether the degree of pollution of our environment with natural and anthropogenic chemicals might extinguish our co-inhabitants and whether industrial evolution and our need for new industrial space will push out wildlife. A debate has started about whether it is possible to cover the economic demands for health and social welfare of today's humans and also maintain the sustainability of development and availability of nonrenewable resources for future generations.

Ecotoxicology is concerned with the harmful effects of chemicals upon ecosystems, that is, the chronic effects of anthropogenic chemicals, chemical mixtures, and natural substrates on organisms, structures within ecosystems, diversity of organisms, populations, and communities. Ecotoxicology thus combines knowledge from many disciplines, such as toxicology, biology, chemistry, and geology. The aim is to understand the regulation of ecosystems in detail and to recognize anthropogenic influences on this process within this wide field. Environmental devastation caused by human activity is to be blocked, harmful events should be predicted correctly, and concepts are to be developed that will maintain the organisms of ecosystems within their ranges of tolerance.

SPECIFIC ASPECTS OF ENVIRONMENTAL TOXICITY

The basic toxicological concepts of how chemicals act on the physiological functions of cells, organs, and individuals, acutely or chronically exposed, can also be applied to the understanding of the harmful effects of chemicals on ecosystems. Important determinants for the outcome are therefore the amount of release (total input), the mechanism of action (toxicodynamics), and the fate of the foreign compounds in the entire ecosystem, which takes into account distribution, retention, and decomposition (toxicokinetics). However, some events are specific to ecosystems and cannot be recognized using classic methods to test chemicals for toxicity.

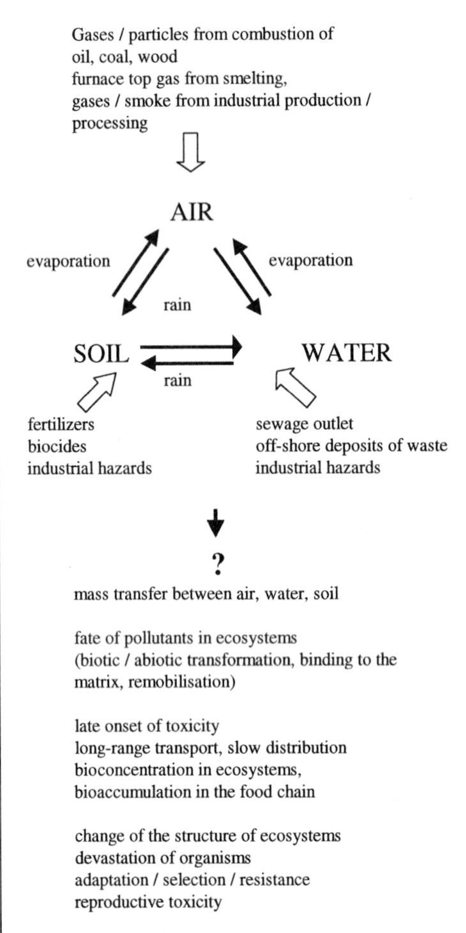

FIGURE 1 Aspects of ecotoxicity by pollutants. Compounds are released directly into air or water or onto soil. In most cases, the pollutants vanish from the place of entry by dilution and by transport into other spaces. Ecotoxicity may occur at large distances from the points of release, may mainly affect organisms at higher trophic levels, and may change the topography of communities and populations in ecosystems. In particular, the risk assessment of ecotoxicity requires information on the effect of pollutants on the structure of ecosystems, the fate of pollutants within ecosystems, and long-term effects of compounds and complex mixtures on organisms from different trophic levels.

All ecosystems together form the biosphere and all persistent chemicals that are brought into the biosphere by human activity will remain there. The ice of the polar regions is relatively highly contaminated with environmental compounds that are deposited in this area by condensation from the air. This environment is an important archive and reflects how environmental contamination by geochemical and human activity has developed. Apart from this long-range movement of chemicals into regions far away from industrial settings, another important point is that the harmful effects on the environment cannot be simply stopped when the causative agents are recognized. Remediation of enviromental pollution is a complex problem (Fig. 1). Furthermore, the contamination of ecosystems often involves many unnatural compounds and detection of the most important contaminant within the complex mixture constitutes a problem. However, strategies for remediation aim at detecting the leading compound with respect to the activity and the area that is most contaminated before efforts that may be limited in time and cost can be investigated.

The risk for environmental toxicity is particularly high for compounds that have high biological activity, are persistent in ecosystems, and can be bioconcentrated because of their lipophilicity and stability against metabolic inactivation. These compounds are accumulated in the fat and lipid-rich tissue of consumers and may be bioconcentrated along the food chain. The ecotoxicological importance, for example, of tetrachlorodibenzo-p-dioxin (TCDD) and polycyclic aromatic hydrocarbons (PAHs) is caused by their ability to induce gene expression and to initiate events leading to tumors. Certain pesticides remain persistent in the soil and undergo long-range movement, together with the transport of other substrates in the ecosystems. Lipophilic persistent compounds remain in the aquatic and terrestrial food chains and finally accumulate substantially, especially in organisms at high trophic levels. As a consequence, high concentrations of these pollutants are present in the tissue and milk of predators that are at the top of the food chain pyramid. This bioconcentration factor is very high for some pollutants (e.g., 10^5 for DDT).

In conclusion, a specific feature of persistant pollutants is that they are distributed over almost the entire biosphere, but they are not uniformly concentrated or diluted. Due to interactions between biotic and abiotic components, some pollutants are trapped within sediments, bioconcentrated within tissues, and concentrated at particular places. Although many compounds are spread within ecosystems, some of them have specific biological activities and can be considered to be leading compounds of ecotoxicological importance. Assessment of the risk for environmental toxicity demands that information on many different levels of the ecosystem be provided.

Pollution of Ecosystems

A characteristic of pollutants is their mobility, which results from the intense mass transport between the aquatic and terrestrial systems and the air. Gaseous pollutants, such as CO_2, SO_2, NO_x, methane; volatile compounds or compounds absorbed to particles, such as VOCs (volatile organic compounds); pesticides; PCBs (polychlorinated biphenyls); and PAHs, are transferred by circulation in the atmosphere. In the troposphere (the lower part of the atmosphere, up to 10–11 km), the main circulation in air is predominantly a horizontal stream, and the vertical transfer of air mass between the troposphere and stratosphere is low. As a consequence, pollutants in air undergo relatively fast long-range movements, whereas the vertical diffusion of volatile compounds is very slow. This is a main reason for the destroying effect of flourohydrocarbons on the ozone layer in the stratosphere having become visible only years after the release of these reactive pollutants. Despite the fact that the use of fluorohydrocarbons has been banned or at least restricted, these ecotoxic effects still persists because these compounds have already been released into the lower layer of the atmosphere and will now continue to diffuse vertically. It is unknown what effects might be caused by modern space technology through which hydrazine, hydrazine products, and metals, mostly aluminum, are released, especially into the upper layer of the atmosphere.

Chemicals in the air are washed out by rain or are deposited with particles and reach surface water or the soil. Many persistent water-soluble compounds are washed from the land and reach the aquatic system. The aquatic systems are contaminated also by deposition from the air but the burden comes from direct input from the offshore deposition of chemicals and from the outfall of sewage. The main precautionary measure to reduce environmental toxicity by dumping of waste into the sea is dilution which is still commonly applied to acids, bases, highly toxic chemicals sealed into containers, and sealed radioactive waste. In case the waste is released, the huge mass of seawater is thought to prevent the compounds from exerting (human) toxicity.

Soils are polluted mainly by the direct application of herbicides, insecticides, and fertilizers and their contaminants during modern agriculture. In regions where the mining and smelting of metal ores are common, landfill sites are used to deposit the overburden, smelting slag, and remnants of poor ore. Another source of contamination of soils is particles and dust from chimneys and washout from deposits of industrial and municipal waste. Water-soluble compounds, metal (oxides), mineral salts, and remnants from the chemical industry are brought into the upper layer of soils. This burden of contaminants is often retained there by complexation with mostly inorganic components or by absorption to the organic matter of soils. These stores can be remobilized when the local conditions are changed (e.g., by acidification, change in the water content, access to oxygen, or shift in the structure of microorganisms). Afterward, this fraction can be taken up by the roots and enter the biosphere through the terrestrial food chain via plants.

Fate of Pollutants in Ecosystems

Local concentrations of pollutants in soil or water are strongly dependent on many parameters: the type of release (e.g., gaseous compounds from chimneys, leakage from waste deposits, and washout from agricultural land), the amounts that have been released, the frequency (permanently, periodically, or by acute incidents), and the physicochemical features (e.g., volatility, affinity for being adsorbed onto a surface, and partition coefficient between phases). Important factors from the ecosystem are the temperature, pH, reduction–oxidation conditions, density of particles, sedimentation, and type of normal nutrient cycling.

The tendency of molecules to escape from a particular phase or compartment (fugacity) leads finally to a widespread, sometimes even global, distribution of persistent pollutants within the ecosystems. Fugacity models describe the distribution of environmental chemicals. Equilibrium is reached when the chemical has the same fugacity in all phases. However, in fact, pollutants are not uniformly distributed between and within soil, water, and air because formation of insoluble complexes, incorporation into organisms, deposition into sediments, or transfer along the food chain may lead to only temporary retention of compounds, which may be remobilized when the local conditions have changed accordingly. The availability of chemicals in ecosystems is terminated by abiotic and biotic transformation or almost permanent complexation with ligands. Altogether, the real exposure may be highly variable, which is an important point when the monitoring of pollution is designed.

Molecular modifications of environmental pollutants occur in ecosystems by abiotic transformations due to photolysis, hydrolysis, and redox reactions or by biotic transformations. Abiotic photolysis is initiated in the atmosphere either by direct absorption of light or by reaction with photooxidants, such as hydroxyl radicals, peroxy radicals, singlet oxygen, or radicals originating from chemicals in the air or water. Hydrolytic decomposition occurs particularly in water systems and depends strongly on temperature and in some cases also on pH. Redox reactions are mediated biotically as well as abiotically and lead to molecular transformation, mainly by oxidation of the pollutant. Reduction occurs mainly in anaerobic sediments and soils and leads, for instance, to the dechlorination of chemicals.

In most cases pollutants are deactivated by molecular transformation. Many examples demonstrate that there are important exceptions where the transformation reactions in the environment produce species that are more active. The biotic methylation of metals raises the toxic activity for mercury, lead, and tin. Dechlorination of DDT to DDE produces a metabolite that is still active and persists even longer in the ecosystem than the mother substrate. Oxidation in phase I metabolisms leads to the production of reactive metabolites, for instance, in the case of organophosphorous insecticides, such as dimethoate, diazinon, malathion, disulfoton, chlorpyriphos, or to the production of carcinogens, as in the cases of benzo(*a*)pyrene, aflatoxin, and vinyl chloride. Alkylphenolpolyethoxylates, formerly used in washing powders, are transformed to nonylphenol and octylphenol, which are compounds suspected of participating in estrogenic effects observed in fish in moving surface waters where the outlet of sewage is released.

The example of ozone demonstrates that ecotoxicologic effects are often relatively complex. Many years after their release into the atmosphere, fluorochlorohydrocarbons diffuse from the troposphere into the stratosphere where a complex chemical reaction is initiated by dechlorination, which results in the scavenging of ozone molecules by reactive species. The rate of ozone production by natural chemical and physical reactions in the atmosphere cannot renew the ozone layer. The "ozone holes" show a periodicity in dimension and are located mainly at the polar region of the southern hemisphere. The consequences of this effect for ecosystems are genotoxic and mutagenic effects in animals and plants that result from the increase in UV radiation, which is now much less filtered. The main effect in humans is expected to be an increased incidence in malignant melanoma of the skin. On the other hand, close to the surface ozone is a gaseous oxidant pollutant of substantial environmental significance. Ozone is generated in the air by sunlight radiation and a high concentration of nitrogen oxides released from the combustion of fuel. The local concentrations of ozone show a typical periodicity during days and between months. The highest values are observed at noon or early afternoon on hot summer days. The levels decrease on weekends when the traffic is less. The regional distribution between urban and rural regions is a paradox; the ozone concentrations are lower in cities, where ozone is generated, compared to regions of low traffic. The explanation for this effect is that a certain fraction of ozone is scavenged by particles and pollutants in cities. However, the microclimate, which is determined by the intensity of solar radiation, the density of traffic, and the circulation of air, determines that the actual concentration of ozone differs substantially even within cities. Polluted places have relatively high ozone concentrations, at least temporarily reaching levels that are relevant to human toxicity.

Changes in Populations and Communities

A well-documented example concerning the color of the peppered moth (*Biston petularia*) clearly indicates that environmental changes caused by pollution initiate selective pressure on a population, which leads to adaptation. The pollution of the air with fine particulate carbon coated almost all surfaces with a black layer. The peppered moth is normally adapted to the background of its preferred habitat, the bark of birch trees, by mottled white, silver, and grey pigmentation, which provides perfect camouflage. Once the background was changed by pollution, the wild-type moth was captured by predators and the population changed toward the rare dark phenotype, which was now at an advantage (industrial melanism). Later, when the pollution ceased, this adaptation reversed and the normal structure within the population appeared, again driven by the advantage of not being captured for the best-adapted phenotype. Populations and communities are able to adapt to pollution within certain limits, as long as there is enough genetic diversity and population size.

An acute incident leading to the severe contamination of a region may destroy all life in this habitat or even in the ecosystem. An example of this event is contamination with crude oil in shipwrecks. Another case happened in the Rhine River when pesticides were drained off in large amounts after a fire in a large storehouse for chemicals was extinguished. This wave of pesticides caused acute fish toxicity downstream from the point of release. As the water flow diluted the pollutant, this effect happened only within certain distances. In most cases of sudden destruction of the population, the ecosystems regenerate, mostly by immigration from the proximity. It is essential of course that the population size of the species be large enough.

When the biological effect of pollutants involves the induction of reproductive toxicity, the consequences for ecosystems are severe. Early life stages of fish are highly sensitive to the acidification of water. In small lakes with weak buffering capacities, acid rain induced a pH shift toward the acidic range, which as a consequence induced a change in the structure of the fish population toward adults. Finally these lakes became fishless, a process that could have been interrupted. These effects are documented from epidemiological studies, as well as from progressive experimental acidification of a small lake. Many lakes in Scandinavia, Canada, and the northeastern United States have already faced this problem. Organotin compounds from antifouling paints of boats are responsible for the imposex phenomenon observed in dog whelk in many harbors used for recreational boating. In this case, the female individual undergoes virilization and, as a consequence, the population becomes infertile. A dramatic decrease in the population size has been observed for fish otter and beluga whale (white whale), which is considered to be due mostly to reproductive toxicity because the populations do not recover despite strict protection.

Almost all levels of organisms within ecosystems are able to adapt to environmental conditions within certain limits of stress response. The development of resistance is mainly caused by avoidance, a decreased rate of absorption, increased elimination, and an increase in binding to intracellular ligands. On the cellular level, the adaptation is due to the induced expression of high-affinity metal-binding proteins, induction in transporter activity (mdr transporter), or induction of phase I and phase II enzymes. Resistant species of organisms may be used as biomarkers in order to recognize the response of organisms to contamination in the environment and to relate the response to the degree of pollution. The phenomenon of resistance to toxic chemicals will more or less selectively lead to the loss of the nonresistant species and this will decrease the diversity between species and within the gene pool. However, knowledge of the mechanism of resistance may offer new methods for the remediation of polluted areas or new techniques for sewage treatment, which might be advantageous compared to conventional methods with respect to the energy supply, the production of toxic waste, or the need for material.

ECOSYSTEMS

Basics of Ecology

Ecology deals with all questions concerned with the interrelationships between organisms and their environments and therefore also deals with problems regarding substrate and energy supply. The biosphere is identical to the space where all microorganisms, plants, animals, and humans live. It includes the air close to the ground, the soil where the roots of plants are present, caves, and all surface-water systems, including the depths of the ocean. Ecosystems are part of the biosphere and are connected to each other by immense transfers of mass and substrates. The biosphere is divided into aquatic systems (hydrobiosphere) and terrestrial systems (geobiosphere). The lower part of the atmosphere, in which flying animals are prevalent and where substrates are transferred by the wind, is also part of the biosphere in a wider sense.

The organisms living in the biosphere are classified according to their endogenous metabolism and energy transfer. Phototrophic organisms use light as a source of energy needed in endogenous metabolism. Chemotrophic organisms use reduction–oxidation reactions from their nutrient substrates to supply energy. Lithotrophic organisms use inorganic compounds (H_2O, H_2S, Fe^{2+}, NH_4^+) as H donors. Organotrophic organisms are dependent on organic compounds as H donors. Autotrophic organisms gain carbon for the synthesis of organic compounds from carbon dioxide. Heterotrophic organisms are dependent on the supply of organic compounds from nutrient substrates. Green plants, algae, and blue-green algae are photoautotrophic organisms, which need H donors, gain oxygen by photosynthesis, and release oxygen into the atmosphere. Some sulfur bacteria use hydrogen sulfide as an H donor and their photosynthesis yields sulfur. Chemoautotrophic bacteria oxidize NH_4^+, Fe^{2+}, H_2, and H_2S, and carbon dioxide is incorporated into organic compounds by oxidation–reduction reactions. Heterotrophic organisms are chemotrophic and need organic compounds for their energy supply. Some chlorophyl-less plants and most bacteria, fungi, and animals belong to this group (Fig. 2). Autotrophic organisms are able to produce organic material from inorganic precursors using external energy sources (e.g., sunlight). These organisms are termed primary producers and the organic material that they produce can be used as an energy supply and is the basis of existence for the organisms of all other levels.

Cycling of Compounds

When the form of energy turnover is considered, ecosystems represent open systems that use external light and thermal energy. The required dynamic stability of ecosystems and the close connection between ecosystems and the biosphere are guaranteed by typical substrate flow and material flow. Rain and the evaporation of water, as well as water uptake and excretion by individual organisms, maintain permanent water transport within a global water cycle. Oxy-

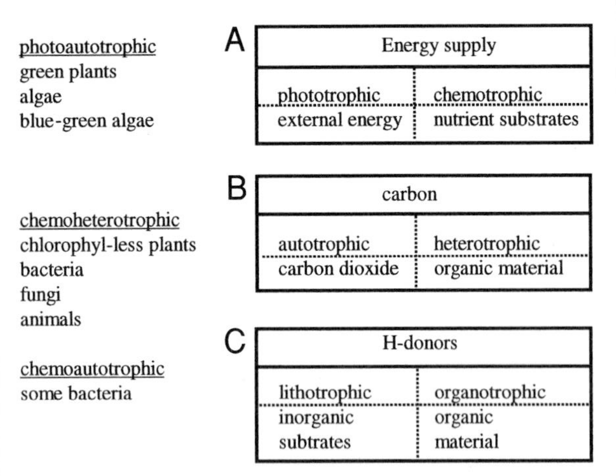

FIGURE 2 Classification of organisms in the biosphere. The main criteria for the classification of organisms within the biosphere are (A) the source of energy (light or thermal energy versus nutrient substrates), (B) the main source of carbon for the synthesis of organic material (carbon dioxide versus organic material) and (C) the type of substrates used as H donors (inorganic compounds such as Fe^+, NH_4^+, H_2S, and H_2O versus organic compounds).

gen is consumed by the vast majority of organisms in order to gain energy via the oxidation of nutrient substrates. The end products are carbon dioxide and water. Green plants and blue-green algae produce oxygen in the course of photosynthesis. The rate of production is higher than the demand, and therefore oxygen is released to the pool in the atmosphere.

In typical substrate cycles, elements such as carbon, nitrogen, phosphorus, sulfur, and calcium are used by primary producers and are introduced into organic substrates, which are used in the food chain. During this process, the compounds are transformed step by step into inorganic forms by mineralization. Ecosystems release substrates into the biosphere and atmosphere and, on the other hand, receive substrates from the biosphere. Therefore ecosystems are stabilized systems open to external influence and are connected to a global circulation of material. These global cycles of nutrient substrates are accelerated (carbon cycle), overloaded (phosphorous and nitrogen), or more or less initiated (metal) under anthropogenic influence.

Carbon is taken up by autotrophic primary producers as carbon dioxide and used for the synthesis of organic compounds. Via the food chain, the fraction fixed in organic form reaches all other organisms and is released as carbon dioxide. In most cases, a more or less significant fraction is retained in long-living organisms or in waste products that can be degraded only slowly. This fraction is, in fact, taken from the carbon cycle. Fossil stores of coal and oil are currently being used for the production of energy, which is needed in large quantities. The final product of burning or combustion is carbon dioxide, which leads to an unnatural input of CO_2 into the atmosphere. In principle, it must be predicted that an increase of CO_2 concentration will raise the activity of photosynthesis, but this increase in global CO_2 has been related, together with other compounds such as methane, to the global warming effect. Biogeochemical effects due to the increase in CO_2 are the acidification of rain, fog, water, and soil. However, other products of burning and combustion, such as SO_2 and NO_x, are much more active in this respect.

The phosphate cycle in the biosphere is determined mostly by dissolution in water systems or adsorption onto particles (Fig. 3). Phosphates are transported to the sea and are finally sedimented in immense phosphate deposits. Back-cycling to terrestrial ecosystems occurs via the feces of fish-eating birds. Another important input comes from the weathering of rocks; most important in this respect are apatite-containing materials. Phosphates are taken up by the roots of plants and introduced into the phytophage food chain. The residues from dead material are decomposed by autolysis and the phosphate content can be reused from this pool. In surface-water systems, phosphate is the key factor in the growth rate of algae. An overload of the phosphate cycle occurs from fertilizers drained from the land or, formerly, by supplements in washing powders that led to blooms of algae in many lakes, even those of large size. The algae and the bacteria dealing with the decay consumed vast amounts of oxygen, resulting in the destruction of the living bases for other organisms, and finally the aquatic systems shifted to anaerobic or low-oxygen conditions without normal aquatic life.

Nitrogen is cycled by processes that are much more complicated than those concerning carbon or phosphorus. Briefly described, nitrate (NO_3) and ammonium compounds (NH_4^+) are used by primary producers for the synthesis of organic compounds (e.g., amino acids) and are introduced into the food chain. Via the destructor–saprophage chain, many organic nitrogen compounds are transferred into ammonium in the dead material. The details of the nitrogen cycles in aquatic systems are much more complex, but nitrate and ammonium compounds are key factors in the trophic state of lakes (oligotrophic, mesotrophic, or eutrophic). In general, freshwater lakes naturally

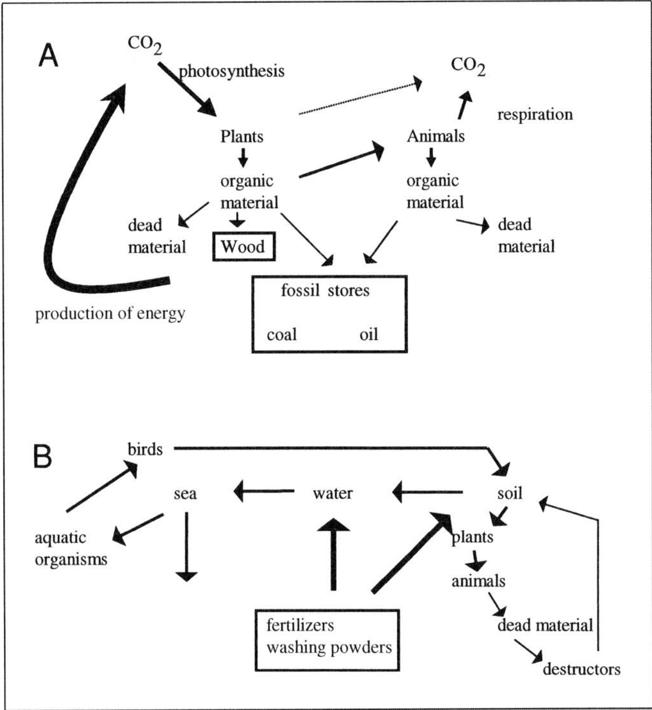

FIGURE 3 Anthropogenic influence on the (A) carbon and (B) phosphate cycles. Simplified scheme of the main human influence on important substrate cycles because of the need for the production of energy by the combustion of fuel and because of the use of phosphates as fertilizers for agriculture.

change from the oligotophic to the eutrophic state and finally to anaerobic forms, such as bogs.

Structure of Ecosystems

Primary producers synthesize organic material from inorganic compounds and need external light or thermal energy. Chemoautotrophic forms are much more important by far than photoautotrophic organisms from a quantitative point of view. Heterotrophic organisms consume organic material in order to supply for energy and synthesize new organic material for their own growth. Some aquatic organisms, such as protozoa and parasites, take up dissolved substrates from water. Most animals consume particles in order to supply essential requirements.

Consumers are classified according to their habit of food intake into predator–prey relationships, plant-eating animals, and parasites. Consumers of the first level eat material from plants (phytophage consumers). Consumers of the second level feed on living and just-dead material from animals (zoophage consumers, such as raptors). Consumers of level three and four present the next steps of the food pyramid. Pantophage animals feed on material from plants and animals and from time to time on dead material (Fig. 4).

Contrary to the habits of consumers of living material, the users of dead material feed on dead organic compounds and with this step finally close the substrate cycles in the biosphere. The users of dead material in the groups fungi and bacteria are termed saprophytes. These particular forms of heterotrophic organisms are also classified as destructions. They are important, in particular, for the recycling of organic compounds, providing the basis for the almost total availability of energy stemming from photosynthesis by producers.

Some physical–chemical parameters are key factors in the sustainability and stability of ecosystems. These are the oxygen content of aquatic systems and soils, the phosphate content and nitrate concentration of surface water, and the pH of soil and water. Any change in these factors as a result of human activity may have dramatic consequences for the natural dynamics that determine the structure of ecosystems. This is not identical to a toxic event. The living conditions for some organisms, such as steady-state con-

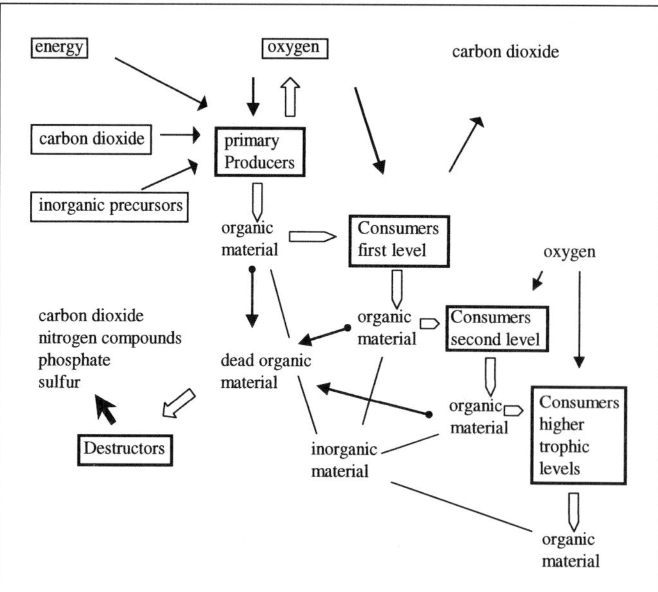

FIGURE 4 Substrate cycles by producer–consumer–destructor relationships. Ecosystems are linked together within the biosphere by complex cycles of inorganic substrates and the intense use of organic material as an energy supply. Primary producers (plants) use external energy, carbon dioxide, and inorganic substrates in photosynthesis for energy and the synthesis of organic matter. Consumers are dependent on oxygen and nutrient substrates for energy and for the synthesis of organic material. In the destructor–saprophage chain, the organic material is finally degraded to inorganic substrates, which are available for the next cycle.

ditions between predators and prey or the availability of preferred types of food in plant-eating animals, may substantially affect ecosystems. Many examples demonstrate that interference with the living basis (e.g., reproductive toxicity in fish, birds, and marine mammals) and devastation of the habitats of specialized organisms (e.g., large mammal predators of terrestrial systems) may lead step by step to a dramatic shift in the structure and internal stability of ecosystems. Ecosystems change permanently by natural processes and, therefore, it is the task of ecotoxicology to recognize which processes are substantially influenced by human activity and to detect the causative agents within the complex mixtures of foreign compounds in ecosystems.

POLLUTION OF ECOSYSTEM AND FATE OF POLLUTANTS

Air

Pollutants are discharged into the atmosphere in the gaseous state from the combustion of fuel, open fires, industrial processing of metals, gasoline, synthetic chemicals, and the domestic energy supply, as droplets and particles or adsorbed to particles. Important components of atmospheric pollution are carbon dioxide (CO_2), sulfur dioxide (SO_2), oxides of nitrogen (NO_x), volatile organic compounds such as benzene and toluene, polycyclic aromatic hydrocarbons such as benzo(*a*)pyrene, hydrogen fluoride, and chlorofluorocarbons. Many organic compounds are released from chimneys as smoke particles. Despite the fact that the majority of particles are filtered out, a substantial proportion still enter the atmosphere and carry many toxic compounds in association. The small components of less than 10-μm particle size (PM 10 fraction) are retained by the mammalian lung and thus may enter the body. Natural compounds, such as carbon dioxide and methane, are also released from anthropogenic sources and the question is to what extent these additional amounts will influence the global climate.

Serious pollution of the lower atmosphere with SO_2 resulted from the burning of sulfur-rich coal and oil. The smoke from chimneys of industrial and domestic premises is distributed over a long range, depending on the atmospheric conditions and the height and the form of the chimneys. SO_2 has high solubility in water and is therefore dissolved in rain. Together with nitrogen oxides, it is the main component of acid rain and is one of the causative agents of forest die-back and acidification of freshwater lakes. The control of emissions by the substitution of sulfur-rich coal and oil and by use of filter devices in industrial chimneys was effective with respect to the concentration of sulfur dioxide in air. A main source of nitrogen oxides in the atmosphere is internal-combustion engines in land vehicles, airplanes, and ships. The primary product of combustion is NO, which is oxidized in the atmosphere to NO_2. The mixture of both is termed the NO_x fraction. Nitrogen oxides are oxidant gases that easily dissolve into water and the water surfaces of epithelia. The inhalation of nitrogen oxides is therefore dangerous with respect to respiratory toxicity. The concentration of these pollutants in the urban air often surmounts the threshold limits for chronic toxicity in animal studies at certain places, at least for a short time.

The combustion of fuel in engines also produces carbon monoxide; inorganic lead compounds; organic molecules such as polycyclic aromatic hydrocarbons, aldehydes, ketones; and organolead compounds that arise from tetraethyl lead, formerly used as an antiknock agent. Many of these toxic compounds are not originally present in the fuel, but are generated during the operation of engines. The control of emissions from traffic vehicles by the introduction of catalytic converters and filters and the improvement in design of modern engines and the optimization of engine performance have considerably decreased the pollution of the air. However, a significant loss of hydrocarbons and of volatile tetraethyl lead occurs by evaporation from the fuel tank, around the pistons, and from the engines (mostly the crankcase).

Gaseous pollutants can be transported over considerable distances by air movement, which on the global scale is very complex. The layer of air close to the surface undergoes particular turbulence and localized air flow. Smoke from large open fires demonstrates very clearly that pollutants released within the lower layer are likely to return to the ground quickly. Particulate matter is transported only over a short distance. The gaseous and volatile components of the smoke are distributed over a larger area and can be smelled from larger distances. Pollutants that reach greater heights may be transported over considerable distances, depending on the main stream of circulation in air. SO_2 pollution in Sweden originates mostly from SO_2 release in England. Traces of persistant pollutants have been detected in the ice of polar regions and in the food and tissues of animals living there, although these regions are far away from the places where these compounds are released. Radioactive contamination by Chernobyl fallout outside the area of release has been most persistent in Scandinavia and northwestern Europe. Cesium contamination of the soil and plants of these nutrient-poor regions leads to significant levels of cesium in the tissue and milk of sheep and reindeer. The latter are adapted to consume lichens during the vegetation-poor wintertime and these are still highly contaminated with radiocesium due to retention by complexation. However, the Chernobyl fallout in 1986 could be monitored by radioactive contamination almost everywhere in the northern hemisphere. This clearly demonstrates that one problem of air pollution is long-range movement of compounds leading to almost global distribution. On the other hand, another problem is that toxic compounds are heterogenously deposited, resulting in substantial pollution of certain areas. Locally, a pollutant will be diluted quickly by the mixing of air under warm and clear conditions. The current of warm air, the stream of cold air that replaces it, and side winds produce convection currents and carry pollutants from chimneys away from the initial point of release. When the air cools in the evening, a layer of mist or fog may form and trap the layer of cold air beneath it, unless there is sufficient air flow. Under certain conditions the sun will not warm the air the following morning, thus preventing the dispersal of pollution from chimneys and traffic.

About 99% of the total air mass is distributed in the lower atmosphere (extending about 35 km above the surface), which is divided into the troposphere (extending to 10–11 km) and the stratosphere. The circulating air mass in the troposphere follows strong vertical mixing and horizontal surface winds. The main surface winds are termed the northeast and southeast trade winds. Another important direction of wind flow is determined by hot air rising and cooling in the upper part of the troposphere. The air flow then subsides and begins to flow towards the surface, thus completing the cycle. The air mass is readily mixed in a vertical direction in this layer of the atmosphere, while in the stratosphere above it little vertical mixing occurs. The boundary between these layers is termed the tropopause. As a consequence, the vertical movement for small, stable, and volatile molecules from the troposphere to the stratosphere is slow. The stratosphere contains a layer of high ozone concentration that absorbs ultraviolet light. Chlorofluorocarbons and fluorocarbons are suspected of reducing this ozone layer after their photochemical activation in the stratosphere to hydrocarbon radicals that react with ozone molecules and scavenge them. Chlorofluorocarbons are released from aerosol containers, coolants in refrigerators, and foam packaging. Because of the slow distribution of the causative agents into the strato-

TABLE 1 Ecotoxicity by Pollution of Air, Water, and Soil

Event of release	Compounds	Ecotoxic effect of pollution
	Pollution of air	
Combustion of fuel	SO_2, CO_2, NO_x	Acid rain
Open fire	Benzene, toluene	Acidification of soil, small inland lakes
Processing of petrol	Polycyclic aromatic hydrocarbons	Damaged ozone layer
Processing of metals	Hydrogen fluoride, chlorofluorocarbons	Increase in UV radiation
Chemical industry	Aldehydes, ketones	
Fallout of nuclear power stations	Radionuclides	
	Organolead compounds	
	Metals	
	Pollution of soil	
Leachates from industrial and municipal waste	Nitrates, phosphates	Remobilization of metals
Use of biocides, fertilizers	Biocides	Devastation of soil organisms
Deposits from rain and smoke	Metals (lead, copper, zinc, cadmium)	Loss of essential elements to lower soil layers
Industrial hazards	Detergents	Induced growth rates of plants and leaves
Sewage disposal	Synthetic chemicals	Adaptation of (destructor) microorganisms
Offshore dumping	Heavy metals, detergents	Acute fish toxicity
Release from shipwrecks	Inorganic, organic chemicals	Acute lethal effects on aquatic organisms
Run-off from agricultural and industrial land	Oil	Delayed lethal effects via food chain
Industrial hazards	Fungicides, pesticides, chlorophenols	Bloom of algae
	Synthetic organic compounds	Eutrophication of small inland lakes
	Organochlorine compounds	Fishless lakes (after acidification)
	Radionuclides	Topographic changes in zooplankton and phytoplankton
	Pollution of water	
Sewage disposal	Heavy metals, detergents	Acute fish toxicity
Offshore dumping	Inorganic, organic chemicals	Acute lethal effects on aquatic organisms
Release from shipwrecks	Oil	Delayed lethal effects via food chain
Run-off from agricultural and industrial land	Fungicides, pesticides, chlorophenols	Bloom of algae
Industrial hazards	Synthetic organic compounds	Eutrophication of small inland lakes
	Organochlorine compounds	Fishless lakes (after acidification)
	Radionuclides	Topographic changes in zooplankton and phytoplankton

sphere, the damaging of the ozone layer continues, although the use of these compounds has been restricted.

Volatile molecules move through the air by diffusion and mass transport. Diffusion may be driven by concentration differences and by thermal processes. A large fraction of pollutants in the air will be deposited into the marine and freshwater systems and will also be transferred from the water into the air by evaporation due to thermal diffusion. Pollutants exist also as droplets or particles or are incorporated into and adsorbed onto particles. Particles and droplets normally move only over short distances before they are deposited onto the ground. Soluble gases, such as SO_2 and NO_x, or other pollutants may be incorporated into rain droplets either during the formation of clouds or during the course of precipitation.

The transport of pollutants by air is an important type of transfer between terrestrial and aquatic ecosystems. Some events initiated by pollution specifically target the atmosphere. One example that has already been mentioned is the reduction of the ozone layer, which increases exposure to ultraviolet radiation. The level of CO_2 in the atmosphere has increased over the past decades due to massive burning of coal and oil. Despite the fact that CO_2 is absolutely necessary for photosynthesis by plants and is thus a requisite for the first step in the production of organic material, this anthropogenic influence on the composition of the atmosphere is expected to lead to a global change in the climate. Apart from the increased rate of production, the level of carbon dioxide is also influenced by the decreased rate of consumption due to a substantial reduction in the area of forest land. Other compounds, such as methane, which is released as a waste product from metabolism, for instance, by cattle and rice plants, are also suspected of contributing to a warming of the atmosphere. Pollutants that affect plants and slow down the use of CO_2 for photosynthesis are examples of indirect action on atmospheric CO_2 (Table 1).

Terrestrial Ecosystems

The contamination of land may be deliberate due to the disposal of wastes at landfill sites or due to the control of pests or vectors during farming. The dumping of wastes occurs on domestic and general industrial premises. Toxic waste from other sources requires other forms of safe storage, but often any form of landfill site is debated. The use of sewage sludge as a fertilizer on agricultural land brings nitrates, phosphates, detergents, and heavy metals into the soil. Accidental contamination of land results from the dry deposition of particles from the air or from rain and humidity, flooding of surface water, or collision of vehicles carrying toxic chemicals. Another important source is metalloferous deposits of metals from mining activity, which in some areas have accumulated over centuries, and leachates of into which water are an ecotoxicological problem. Substantial influence results from synthetic organic chemicals that are persistent or from biocides that contain metals. Furnace gas from smelting works is an important source of contamination of the surrounding region with lead, copper, zinc, and cadmium. Inorganic materials such as arsenite, which forms stable complexes within copper or silver containing clays, are often also contaminants in areas of copper mining and smelting works. An important source of lead contamination is the combustion of lead-containing fuel. The extensive use of leaded gasoline has led to widespread contamination of urban soils. Long-range movements of the metal have occurred by transportation in air and elevated levels can be detected in regions far from industrial areas.

The main effect of heavy aerial deposition of cadmium is a reduction in the decomposition rate of dead vegetation. Organisms such as earthworms, woodlice, and millipedes are absent in cadmium-contaminated soils. The initial fragmentation of leaf litter cannot take place and the dead organic material accumulates on the surface as a thick layer. Metal contamination of soils has a long residence time because metals cannot be biodegraded and the soil will retain substantial amounts because of a large binding capacity. Metal–ligand complexes are sensitive to changes in pH and, therefore, metals, especially aluminum, can be remobilized into the soil after acidification. Generally, the acidification of soil also decreases the binding of essential elements, which are leached to lower soil layers. Thus, uptake of essential elements (e.g., magnesium) by the roots of trees may be impeded. Due to the high input of nitrogen compounds, the growth rate of leaves is induced. Altogether, the trees are seriously stressed (lending to forest die-back in Germany and Scandinavia).

Soils are complex associations among living organisms, mineral particles, and organic matter. The clay fraction of minerals and the humus present a large surface area. When organic compounds are spread onto the soil, they become distributed between soil water, soil air, and the available surfaces of minerals and organic matter. Pesticides are applied as formulations dissolved in water, emulsified concentrates, or wettable powder. The distribution of organic compounds in soil is dependent upon their solubility, vapor pressure, and chemical stability. Organic compounds are degraded by hydrolysis, oxidation, isomerization, and photolysis. Polar compounds tend to be soluble in water and are absorbed into the soil only to a limited degree. The herbicide paraquat binds strongly to the negatively charged sites of mineral clays. Compounds of high vapor pressure tend to be distributed between the soil, air, and atmosphere. Chemically stable lipophilic compounds have long half-lives in the soil and are metabolized very slowly. Hydrophilic compounds are readily available to soil organisms and are often very rapidly metabolized by these organisms. Some hydrophilic compounds (carbofuran) induce the development of adapted strains of microorganisms that can then metabolize these compounds. As a consequence, the kinetics in soil become faster after a period of time. In most cases, the decay of biocides in soil increases with temperature and humidity.

Some soil organisms, such as earthworms, may acquire pollutants from ambient water. The major route for terrestrial vertebrates is uptake of contaminants from ingested food and water. The passage of organic pollutants and their stable biotransformation products, as well as of lipophilic metal compounds, along the food chain is important for the toxicity of anthropogenic compounds in terrestrial ecosystems. The highest concentrations are found in organisms at the highest trophic level in the food pyramid. Although relatively high levels of persistent organochlorine compounds and methyl mercury are reported for terrestrial predators, this does not necessarily lead to substantial bioaccumulation even for highly persistent compounds. A well-known example is that of grain-eating birds acquiring lethal doses of dieldrin when they fed on dressed grain. The exposure of animals of the same species in areas where dieldrin was not used was almost zero. These compounds were not transferred along the food chain because the concentration in the first step was already high and the first consumer had fed on selectively contaminated grain (Table 1).

Aquatic Ecosystems

Aquatic systems represent by far the largest part of the environment, covering most of the surface of the planet and about 70% of all organisms live within these systems. Generally, the aquatic ecosystem consists of the freshwater (surface-water) systems of small lakes and rivers, and the marine systems of the large oceans. All parts are closely connected with one another by water flow and water circulation via rain and humidity. Chemicals are discharged into the water systems by sewage disposal, outfalls from commercial premises, run-off from land, deposition from air, offshore dumping at sea, and release from oil rigs and shipwrecks. The pollution of marine systems is terminated in most cases by dilution and this concept is used for the disposal of highly toxic liquids and compounds sealed in containers. However, experience has shown that the organisms living in oceans, especially, can substantially bioconcentrate many pollutants in the aquatic food chain.

The major source of pollution of surface water is the discharge of sewage from domestic and industrial waste. The type of pollution in domestic waste is soap, detergents, and chelating agents—some of the last (ethylenediamine tetraacetic acid) are chemically stable and cannot effectively be cleaned during sewage treatment. Detergents that are extensively used in industrial as well as domestic premises have given rise to serious pollution problems. The components of industrial effluents are heavy metals from mining and smelting works, chlorophenols, fungicides with pump mills, insecticides, a variety of organic chemicals, and radionuclides in case of outfalls from nuclear power stations. The offshore extraction of oil and manganese nodules has led to the direct release into the sea.

Pollutants present in the air, such as insecticides, organochlorine compounds, and hydrocarbons, are precipitated, together with dust or rain and snow, or enter surface-water systems by partition from the air. Generally, this is an important source of pollution because of the immense dimension of the surface. Sludge from sewage, acids, sealed radioactive waste, and highly toxic chemicals sealed in containers are damped offshore into the marine system. Sometimes a substantial fraction of pesticides intended for the use on soil are accidentally sprayed onto surface water or are trapped in water droplets in humid air. These compounds are often highly toxic to aquatic organisms. Biocides have also been used directly in surface waters in order to control invertebrates, plants, aquatic weeds, fish parasites, or pests in watercress beds. Tributyl tin fungicides have been used in antifouling paints on boats and leaked into the water of harbors in freshwater systems and the sea. A further problem is the input of gasoline hydrocarbons into the marine system by marine tanker operations, discharges from industrial and municipal wastes, shipwrecks, and incidents such as their release during the Gulf War.

Metals or pesticides are washed from the land surface by heavy rainfall and enter the water systems of rivers, lakes, streams, and oceans. The concentration of pollutants released into moving surface water is diluted and, therefore, biological effects are most likely to occur at or near the point of release. After a fire incident in a chemical store at Schweizerhalle, the Rhine River was highly polluted with pesticides, which were drained with the water used for extinguishing the fire. Acute lethal effects were observed in fish in that part of the river. Ducks were poisoned some months later via their food. This ecosystem regenerated within a relatively short time. In fast-flowing rivers, the dilution effect is marked and pollutants are unlikely to reach high concentrations a certain distance below the outfall. However, persistent pollutants, such as heavy metals, are moved over a long range and precipitate downstream into the sediment of the rivers. The sludge from this part of a river is heavily contaminated with metals and insoluble complexes of chemicals with inorganic and organic material in the sediment. Oceans can effectively dilute pollutants that are spilled into surface waters. Of greater concern in this respect are lakes and small inland seas because they have no effective outlet. Pollution tends to build up in these systems, depending on the rate of input of polluted water, the water evaporation, and the degradation or precipitation of pollutants. The fate of organic compounds entering aquatic ecosystems depends on their lipophilicity, vapor pressure, and stability. Pollutants that are hydrolyzed seldom present problems unless their transformation products are toxic. Volatile compounds tend not to persist in water, and lipophilic compounds, on the other hand, tend to become associated with the particulate matter of sediments. The availability of metals in the sediment is strongly dependent on the pH. When the pH is decreased by acidification, the speciation of heavy metals changes towards water-soluble ionized forms and the metals are remobilized from the sediment. A decrease in pH also affects the toxicity of inorganic pollutants, such as cyanides, metal cyanides, and H_2S. The fraction of the undissociated forms that have a bioavailability higher than that of the dissociated forms increases. The toxicity of the nitrogen compounds ammonia (NH_3) and ammonium ion (NH_4^+), which are important components of the natural nitrogen cycle, is also dependent on the pH of water. In this case, the toxic species is the ammonium ion, which has a pK_a of 9.6. Therefore, the fraction of the toxic compound rises with high levels of pH. About 10% of the total content of nitrogen fixed in the ammonium system is NH_4^+ at a temperature of 20°C and a pH of 8.5. The main sources of ammonium nitrogen in surface water are rain that has drained from areas with intensive cattle farming and effluent of sewage works from domestic and agricultural waste.

The acidification itself is an important factor for aquatic communities in the surface water. Acidification comes from rain in which the pH is decreased to values of 3–4, due mainly to the solution of SO_2 and NO_x. As a consequence, the pH in weakly buffered lakes tends towards levels below 6, which may have a dramatic effect on the fish population. Juveniles are generally more sensitive than adults, and there is a difference in the sensitivity among species. Fishless lakes have been observed, for instance, in Scandinavia, Canada, and the northeastern United States. Field experiments with the progressive acidification of an oligotrophic lake provided data that phytoplankton communities and zooplankton communities are changed predominantly with respect to topographic parameters, mainly by the disappearance of acid-sensitive organisms. The littoral zones were altered in that green algae became the dominant species and that biochemically the nitrogen cycle was disrupted. The most prominent effect was the diappearance of almost all juvenile forms of fish. Secondary problems may be caused by the sunlight that reaches deeper areas of the water and thus increases UV radiation.

Inland lakes undergo a normal shift from the oligotrophic state to the mesotrophic to the eutrophic state and will finally change to the final anaerobic level, the bog. Each state has its own structure in community and ecosystem and in the dynamics of nutrient supply. Nitrate fertilizers, which are extensively used in agriculture, are released into the adjacent watercourse by being drained with rain and by the decomposition of dead plant material. Freshwater systems are enriched with available nitrogen, which causes a bloom in algae populations. The natural process of eutrophication is dramatically increased and the oxygen content declines. Oxygen-dependent benthal microorganisms disappear and the oxygen content in the sediment is finally changed toward anaerobic conditions. Similar problems of eutrophication can also arise from phosphates used as fertilizers and, formerly, also as components in washing powders. The main pollution of surface waters comes from rain drained from agricultural land and from outfalls from sewage works. The availability of phosphate is a key factor for the development of algae populations. Consequently, a bloom of algae also may occur after pollution with phosphates when the oxygen content in the water systems falls below critical levels.

The water systems of the oceans are considered the ultimate sink that dilutes almost any pollutant to concentrations that cannot cause toxic effects. However, organic pollutants may be adsorbed onto particles of sediments and living organisms and enter the aquatic food chain. Residue levels of persistent organochlorine compounds have been observed in organisms of almost all trophic levels and in almost all places. There is a strong relationship between the [log] concentrations of the residues and the trophic level of the organisms. The lowest levels are in plants (brown algae) and the highest are in predators of trophic levels 4 and 5. Bioaccumulation and biomagnification occur at every stage of the food chain, assuming that most of the pollutant burden comes from food. Fish-eating birds bioaccumulate substantial levels of persistent organochlorine compounds because they have low activities of the monooxygenase system, which is mainly responsible for the detoxication. A deficiency in the detoxication system and the high contamination of prey favors bioaccumulation. Apart from the organochlorine insecticides, persistent polychlorinated biphenyls (PCBs), polychlorinated dibenzodioxines (PCDDs), and polychlorinated dibenzofuranes (PCDFs) have been shown to bioaccumulate substantially, especially in the aquatic food chain. Lipophilic compounds, which are extensively metabolized and have relatively short half-lives, do not pass along the food chain. Some invertebrates of the lower trophic level bioconcentrate them because the rate of degradation by metabolism is low. On the other hand, individuals of the next trophic level, such as fish, birds, and mammals, metabolize them rapidly via the mono-oxygenase system. A consequence of this may be metabolic activation toward genotoxic and cancerogenic intermediates (Table 1).

EFFECTS OF POLLUTANTS—SELECTED EXAMPLES

Almost all ecosystems are contaminated by a more or less complex mixture of chemicals from anthropogenic source; many of these are synthetic chemicals. This does not necessarily mean that all of them will trigger a biological response or possibly harmful effects. The risk of ecotoxicity increases for compounds used in large amounts that are persistent, concentrate in the abiotic and biotic matter of ecosystems, are lipophilic, and are highly active. The following examples briefly describe the fate and effect of a few pollutants from natural sources (metals and oil), biocides (atrazine and DDT), and organochlorine compounds (PCBs, PCDDs, and PCDFs) intended only for technical use.

Metals

Cadmium, mercury, lead, copper, tin, and aluminum are pollutants in the environment because the global cycles of metals are increased through human activity, mainly mining and smelting. Metals are geochemically bound in ore in complexes with other inorganic material and metals that are also deposited in landfill sites. Metals are nondegradable and remain in the biosphere unless they are again complexed. Although some of them are essential elements that are needed as an integral part of nutrient substrate in animals, plants, and microorganisms, it is well known that metals exert ecotoxicity.

Apart from toxicity from metals at workplaces, metals are incorporated into plants and enter the aquatic and terrestrial food chains. Cadmium contamination of rice fields has caused serious intoxications (e.g., itai itai disease and osteoporosis in post-menopausal women). The release of inorganic mercury into the sea led to serious toxicity in human and animals from methyl mercury via fish. Metals appear in ecosystems in different chemical state (speciation). They may be dissolved in water as free aqueous ions, bound to inorganic or organic ligands forming soluble complexes, or adsorbed onto suspended particles, or may form insoluble complexes with ligands in the sediment.

The toxic effects in ecosystems are determined by the concentration of free metals in surface water or in the water phase in soils. The solubility is strongly dependent on the pH, the salinity of water, and the concentration of ligand. Synthetic ligands, such as EDTA, have the main influence and are released by municipal and industrial waste. At low pH, metals are more soluble in water and their toxicity for aquatic organisms increases. In mining areas, the water flow is often acidic and, as a consequence, the surface water contains high concentrations of dissolved metals. As the streams become diluted with uncontaminated water further downstream, the pH rises and metals are precipitated onto the sediment. Acid deposition in downstream areas is a problem for the Rhine River, which contains a potent cocktail of metals and organic chemicals in the sludge in its bed close to the North Sea. Acid deposition also occurs with snow and this leads to a sudden short increase of acidity in moving water during the spring thaw.

An important problem in metal toxicity by acidification of water or soils is aluminum, which is mobilized from terrestrial stores, especially in regions of weak buffering capacity and low carbohydrate content. Aluminum forms complexes with fluoride, silicate, and sulfate and is tightly bound at neutral pH. Aquatic life (e.g., fish, due to the precipitation of aluminum on the gills) is sensitive to Al^{3+}-induced toxicity. Other factors in water, such as the content of carbohydrates, organic ligands, ligands containing chlorine and sulfuric residues, and dissolved organic compounds such as humic acid, are critical with respect to the water solubility of metal. Mercury, cadmium, zinc, and lead form stable complexes in water and, therefore, the toxicity of cadmium is decreased by a rise in pH and the high content of chloride in saltwater. The amount of dissolved lead in drinking water decreases with a high content of hydrogen carbonate.

Metals are nondegradable and are eliminated only by precipitation, incorporation into organisms, and metabolic transformation, for example, by oxidation or methylation. In aquatic systems, metals are adsorbed onto particles and are eliminated by deposition in sediment or incorporation into algae or zooplankton. This metal store in the sediment of rivers and the sea may be remobilized a long time later. Microorganisms in the sediment perform oxidation, depending on local factors, which in some cases can increase the availability of metals in pores of the sediment. The biotic transformation of metals by alkylation or incorporation into organic complexes often promotes the transfer of metals into the biosphere by evaporation or an increase in bioavailability. A well-documented example is methyl mercury intoxication as a result of consuming fish from Minimata Bay, Japan.

Organotin compounds are released into ecosystems due to their use as components in antifouling paints on boats (mostly tributyl tin compounds), as fungicides in agriculture (triphenyl tin compounds), or as stabilizers or catalysts for chemical industry (in the production of PVC and polyurethanes). The main burden of organotin compounds reaches aquatic systems by sewage outlets, leakage from paints, or drainage from agricultural land. Aquatic toxicity became evident in oyster farms, dog whelk populations, and other aquatic organisms (e.g., shell species and tadpoles) in many harbors for recreational boating in freshwater systems or on the seacoast of England toward the canal. Many marine species, such as algae, zooplankton, or oysters, underwent increased mortality and other species, e.g., the dog whelk population, also suffered from severe reproductive toxicity due to the imposex phenomenon—the virilization of female dog whelk. The bioaccumulation factor for organotin compounds is dependent on the pH of the water. The pK_a of tributyl tin, for example, is 6.2–6.5 and, therefore, the fraction of tributyl tin hydrochloride increases under slightly alkaline conditions. Thus, tributyl tin is much better absorbed at a pH of 8 than under slightly acidic conditions.

Some ecosystems show adaptation when exposed to sublethal concentrations of metals. Metal-resistant phenotypes and ecotypes are selected in communities of plants and lichen. The mechanism of gaining resistance is mostly intracellular complexation to metal-binding proteins and peptides, for instance, by the increased expression of metallothionein or the enhanced synthesis of phytochelatines in plants and fungi. Also, some fish species (estuarian fish) develop adaptations or limited tolerance to mercury when exposed to mercury during their early life stages. However, the normal growth rate of the exposed fish is decreased. This effect can also be explained by an induction of metallothionein expression shown in the livers and kidneys of exposed individuals. Copper(2+), zinc(2+), cadmium(2+), and mercury(2+) are also external factors that upregulate metallothionein expression in several experimental systems and, therefore, the phenomenon of tolerance to metals may occur also under other circumstances.

Oil

Oil is released into the marine water system by the normal operations of tankers, oil rigs and filling stations and also from shipwrecks and larger incidents. Oil is a natural product with a complex mixture of aliphatic and aromatic hydrocarbons with a very broad range of volatility. In cases of release into water, oil spreads as a layer on the water surface, depending on the local conditions of air circulation and water movement. About 25% of the oil evaporates into the air; this fraction increases under hot air and when the fraction of volatile hydrocarbons in the crude oil is high. A fraction of about 10% is dissolved in the water or is degraded by photolyses. About 30% of the oil contamination undergoes biotic transformation by microorganisms. In some incidents, enhancement of this process by adding fertilizers to the water was attempted. A fraction of about 15% is deposited into the sediment of the sea and about 20% is moved to the land. After oil contamination, almost all aquatic life of the benthal and littoral zones is devasted. Birds lose thermoregulation and are orally intoxicated during their efforts to clean their plumage. Almost all spawn of fish are destroyed and the catch quota of the contaminated region is dramatically decreased. Fish that are chronically exposed to hydrocarbon in their habitats have induced levels of cytochrome P-450 (CYP) in the liver, which is used as a biomarker for the contamination of their ecosystem.

Polycyclic Aromatic Hydrocarbons (PAHs)

PAHs reach the biosphere through contamination by oil, combustion of fuel in engines, and burning of coal, oil, and wood. PAHs are moved over long ranges and almost globally contaminate the air, water, and soil of ecosystems. These compounds are ecotoxicologically important mostly due to their high bioavailability and their high biological activity, in inducing enzymes and initiating genotoxic and cancerogenic events. PAHs are highly lipophilic and are trapped on particles in air or organic particles in water and deposited onto the surfaces of plants and soil. PAHs can be taken up from the soil by the roots of plants and incorporated. A substantial contamination of nutrient plants occurs at PAH concentrations in the soil of about 1 mg/kg. PAHs are relatively persistent in soil but are effectively metabolized by many organisms at higher trophic levels. Therefore, PAHs are not bioaccumulated via the food chain. The ecotoxicological risk results from their being bioactivated by CYP, which occurs in almost all physiologically highly developed organisms. The induction of CYP1A, the formation of adducts with DNA, and the rate of tumors within the liver of different species, including fish and birds, are used as biomarkers for contamination with PAHs and PCBs in the organisms of an ecosystem. In particular, fish in close contact with the sediment in their habitat develop liver tumors with a relatively high incidence when the sediment is polluted with PAHs and PCBs.

Biocides

Atrazine

Atrazine is a herbicide with a relatively low vapor pressure under normal conditions and a small Henry's law constant, which leads to a broad distribution when the compound is used. Atrazine is relatively persistent because its rate of abiotic transformation and its affinity for binding to the soil and to particles, which would increase its contact with microorganisms are low. A substantial fraction of atrazine is drained off with the rain because the compound is easily soluble in water. Especially in agricultural areas in which mostly corn is grown, relatively high atrazine concentrations are present in the surface water of small rivers and lakes. In aquatic systems, particularly the communities of phytoplankton up to higher green plants are affected by atrazine toxicity. The other organisms of the ecosystems, such as zooplankton, benthal organisms, and fish, are secondarily targeted by a lack of nutrients. The NOEC (no observed effect concentration) for atrazine in test systems using model ecosystems is about 20 $\mu g/ml$. At about five-fold higher levels, the structure of the species and communities of aquatic ecosystems is shifted, which also affects the availability of food for organisms of higher trophic levels. Test systems for chronic toxicity have shown that effects are induced in fish at concentrations below the NOEC in model ecosystems.

Dichlorodiphenyltrichloroethane (DDT)

Organochlorine pesticides are the best examples of substances with a high risk of inducing environmental toxicity that is not recognized in toxicity testing over short periods of time. The insecticidal activity is high and the toxicity for most vertebrates is low. Furthermore, chemical synthesis is not expensive and, therefore, DDT was distributed in large amounts to control plant pests and vectors for tropical diseases. The high potency of DDT in initiating environmental toxicity is caused by the long persistence of DDT and its metabolite DDE in soil and water, its large bioaccumulation factor, and its biologically high activity in certain species, especially in fish-eating birds and predatory birds of high trophic level. The bioconcentration factor of DDT in the aquatic and terrestrial food chains amounts to 10^5 from water to consumers of levels 4 and 5.

The first evidence of DDT toxicity was obtained several years after the intense use of DDT as an insecticide when a dramatic decrease in the population of peregrine falcons and of other raptors, as well as of fish-eating birds, was recognized. Extensive epidemiological studies demontrated that this decline in number was caused by low success of the birds in raising their broods, which was associated with eggshell thinning. This phenomenon was observed in many predator and prey bird species, such as falcons, peregrines, brown pelicans, double-crested cormorants, eagles and sparrowhawks, but it was most devastating for these species when there were also alterations in their preferred environment. Raptors that were at the top of the food chain accumulated a large body burden of these insecticides and their persistent metabolites and thus the association of eggshell thinning and ingestion of DDT appeared likely. DDT was banned for use in many countries and the populations of most bird species recovered.

Experimental injection of DDT into the eggs of quail also produced reproductive toxicity. DDT and DDE induce eggshell thinning, increased mortality of embryos, neurotoxicity, behavorial changes during breeding of the offspring, and estrogenic effects in adults. Estrogenic activity has been shown for several pesticides, including those of different chemical structures. Laboratory bird species most commonly used for *in vivo* toxicity tests (e.g., quail, pheasant, and chicken) are much less sensitive or almost completely insensitive to the uptake of DDT-contaminated food. Therefore it is questionable whether this feature of DDT might have been recognized by testing. However, the potential for bioaccumulation and biomagnification in the food chain would have been identified.

Organochlorine Compounds

Polychlorinated Biphenyls (PCBs)

Synthetic organochlorine chemicals, such as PCB, and polybromated biphenyls (PBBs) demonstrate high thermal and chemical stability and can be mixed with, for example, technical liquids and oils. PCBs were widely used as components in hydraulic liquids; as coolant-insulation fluids; as plasticizers in paints, resins, and plastics; and in fire extinguishers (PBBs). A substantial amount of PCBs, about 30% of the total production, was unintentionally released into the environment, although these compounds were intended only for technical use. Despite the fact that PCBs are widely banned for use, they still escape technical systems and contaminate the environment. PCBs are slowly disintegrated by photolysis or biotic dechlorination. Their main chemical characteristic is their high persistance in the environment. Commercial PCBs are a mixture of many congeners that differ with respect to their toxicological activity. Their fate in ecosystems is determined by the activity of microorganisms that perform biotic transformation, which depends upon the stereochemical structure of the congeners. Therefore, the pattern of congeners varies between different samples of soil, water, or organism, which must be kept in mind when the toxic risk in the environment is to be assessed. Apart from this factor, the biological activity of the mixture also is based on polychlorinated dibenzodioxines (PCDDs) and polychlorinated dibenzofuranes (PCDFs), which are by far the most potent inducers of CYP. PCDDs and PCDFs are generated together with PCBs during chemical synthesis and are present in PCB mixtures in trace amounts.

Several incidents with PCB-contaminated food have occurred, which demonstrates that these chemicals have relevant human toxicity by oral ingestion. Rice oil was contaminated with PCBs during production and was ingested by humans in the case of the Yusho intoxication (in 1968 in Japan) and the Yu-Cheng intoxication (in 1979 in Taiwan). The symptoms were variable, including loss of weight, skin disease (chloracne), loss of hair, increased rate of infection, increased liver size, and increased activity of liver enzymes in serum. Generally the acute toxicity of PCBs in mammals is low, but chronic toxicity is relevant and is associated with the persistance of these compounds in the ecosystems and their bioconcentration along the food chain. The highest burden is found in lipid-enriched tissues or in species with a naturally high content of lipids in the tissue (e.g. the eel). Predators at the top of the food chain are the most severely exposed and undergo chronic toxic effects. One species that is at risk of being extirpated is the fish otter, which almost exclusively consumes fish. In some large habitats, these animals are already extinct and this is explained mostly by reproductive toxicity due to bioaccumulation of organochlorine chemicals and only to a lesser extent to alterations in preferred environment.

Polychlorinated Dibenzodioxines (PCDDs) and Polychlorinated Dibenzofuranes (PCDFs)

PCDDs and PCDFs are generated unintentionally during the chemical synthesis of PCBs and are formed during burning or heating of almost any kind of material in the presence of chlorine. PCDDs and PCDFs are released from chimneys into the air, followed by long-range movement. The main source for terrestrial and aquatic systems is dry and wet deposition onto soils and water surfaces. These compounds are ecotoxicologically important because of their high biological activity, long persistence in the environment, and bioconcentration along the food chain. Highly chlorinated congeners that have a low rate of evaporation are predominantly deposited into the sediment, whereas volatile tetra- and hexachlorinated congeners are distributed over a larger area. The bioavailability of congeners deposited in sediment is relatively low due to their tight binding to particles. About 25–30% of the tetra- and hexachlorinated congeners are remobilized from the sediment. In polar regions, the dust and humidity of the air are condensed and therefore the ice and snow are also contaminated with PCDDs and PCDFs. Relatively high concentrations are therefore present in the tissue and milk of predators of the highest trophic level.

The acute toxicity of PCDDs and PCDFs in mammals has been documented from incident cases where large amounts of TCDD were released. These cases have shown that the most important feature of TCDD is its activity to induce CYP by the Ah receptor mechanism. The biological activity and metabolism of TCDD differ substantially between species. The elimination half-lives range from several days and months (in many mammals) to several years (in adult humans). Considering that exposure to TCDD always involves many biologically active congeners, it is not possible to extrapolate clearly the risk of TCDD for environmental toxicity. One approach is to use the concept of dioxin equivalents in order to express and compare the effect of complex mixtures. The activity of the most powerful compound, 2,3,7,8-TCDD, is set at one and the potencies of the other compounds are calculated for their ability to induce CYP. Next, the composition of PCDDs and PCDFs in the mixture must be considered. This concept is based on the assumption that all compounds exert additive effects, have almost the same mechanism of action, and have the same dose–response curve, only shifted in parallel. Therefore, this method can only be used to approximate the real situation, although the problem of complex mixtures is considered.

METHODS OF RECOGNIZING ECOTOXICITY BY POLLUTANTS

Ecotoxicology is concerned with potential hazards and risks associated with the exposure of individual organisms, populations, communities, and structures within ecosystems to environmental chemicals. The basic concepts of toxicity elicited by chemicals demand that data be provided on the quantity of the chemical to which an organism is exposed, on the dose–response relationship, on the nature of the toxic effects, and on the individual sensitivity of the organisms within ecosystems. Many hazards associated with environmental chemicals have clearly shown that an important aim of ecotoxicology must be to recognize risks and potential hazards in an early stage. A further problem is to discriminate correctly between anthropogenic influences and natural changes within the biosphere. Finally, due to limited work forces, time, and finances, it is mandatory to recognize priorities and to concentrate on causative agents and processes that destabilize most.

The strategies for recognizing environmental risks involve screening tests for the fate and action of chemicals, on-line monitoring of the concentrations of a certain battery of pollutants, identifying biomarkers for pollution in ecosystems, *in situ* biological monitoring, and modeling of data from population studies. Each level has its special advantages and limitations and, therefore, different methods must be taken into account. Most approaches, to environmental risk assessment rely on testing the target trophic level instead of the target species. An important point is that the test must be standardized and must be sensitive. On-line montoring of pollution in moving surface waters and air is an important method of recognizing hazards early and offers insight into the extent of pollution for a limited number of compounds at the place from which the sample was taken. It provides data on the distribution of pollution within that particular environment. Screening methods in aquatic toxicity testing or in systems with terrestrial organisms measure more or less crude endpoints (e.g., fraction of survivors and rate of development) and are standardized within specific limits. Common methods for aquatic toxicity are acute testing in algae (growth rate and photosynthesis), in bacteria (luciferase reaction and respiration), in zooplankton, such as daphnia, (survivors), and in fish. The last are restricted to those species that can be maintained and cultivated in laboratories, that is, mostly species adapted to warm water. Subacute toxicity tests have also been established for aquatic organisms (daphnia and fish) in which the rate of reproduction and development of juvenile forms are measured. Early lifestage tests follow growth rate, mortality, and malformation of juvenile fish because experience has shown that many fish species are sensitive to chemicals and environmental factors, especially in early stages of their lives. The disadvantage of these tests is that only the limited number of species for which enough data are available for standardization can be used. The lifecycle test covers the development of the exposed species for several generations and provides information on the chronic toxicity of the test compounds. A general question is how the test compounds should be applied in order to gain information useful for the assessment of environmental risk.

Toxicity testing is much less prevalent for terrestrial organisms than for aquatic systems. The test battery includes tests with invertebrates, plants, and birds in order to cover different trophic levels. Exposure is performed via the gut but also via the external medium. The measure for acute toxicity testing is, again, the fraction of survivors or the growth rate or the rate of photosynthesis. Functional measures in samples from soil are the rate of CO_2 production, nitrification, or enzymic conversion of model compounds by the microorganisms in the soil. It is almost impossible to standardize this type of test because the normal distribution of microorganisms is highly variable between soils.

The biomarker approach aims to measure a biological response to a chemical as a parameter that provides information on exposure and on adverse effects that sometimes happen. Biomarkers are initiated in organisms at various organizational levels and cover events due to exposure via the environment and not in the laboratory. Examples of different levels of biomarkers are TCDD binding to Ah receptor, induction of mono-oxygenases, formation of vitellogenin, eggshell thinning, feminization of embryos, and behavorial changes (e.g., food searching activity and breeding offspring). Biomarkers are of value in hazard assessment, although they range from highly specific to highly nonspecific responses. Although the term "response" is not identical to "adverse effect," it is clearly useful to be able to relate biomarkers to the decision about remediation of contaminations.

In situ biological monitoring attempts to analyze various parameters of natural populations that reflect the situation in the field. The approaches involve the description of the community (e.g., number and species composition), the concentrations of pollutants in indicator organisms, the assessment of the effects on a concentration–effect basis, and the detection of genetically different strains in which resistance has evolved. The latter effect is of specific interest for actual concepts on remediation using plants (phytoremediation) or microorganisms. Finally, in population dynamics, an effort is made to interpret data on the number and development of populations with respect to cause and effect. This demands complex modeling of the data using parameters and information that are generated more or less specifically from the other levels of toxicity testing, field observations, and natural development of populations in the biosphere.

Bibliography

Ahman, B., and Ahman, G. (1994). Radiocaesium in swedish reindeer after the Chernobyl fallout: Seasonal variations and long-term decline. *Health Physics* **66,** 503–512.

Babich, H., and Borenfreund E. (1991). Cytotoxicity and genotoxicity assays with cultured fish cells: A review. *Toxicol. In Vitro* **5,** 91–100.

Bester, K., Hühnerfuss, H., Brockman, U., and Rick, H. J. (1995). Biological effects of triazine herbicide contamination on marine phytoplankton. *Arch. Environm. Contam. Toxicol.* **29,** 277–283.

Bick, H. (1998). "Grundzüge der Ökologie, 3." Auflage Fischer, Stuttgart, Germany.

Bucheli, T.D., and Fent, K. (1995). Induction of cytochrome P-450 as a biomarker for environmental contamination in aquatic ecosystems. *Crit. Rev. Environ. Science Technol.* **25,** 201–268.

Edwards, C.A. (1994). Chernobyl [*sic*]. *National Geographic* **186,** 100–115.

Erickson, R.J., Benott, D.A., Mattson, V.R., Nelson, H.P., and Leonard, E.N. (1996). The effects of water chemistry on the toxicity of copper to fathead minnows. *Environ. Toxicol. Chem.* **15,** 181–193.

Ernst, W.H.O., Verkleij, J.A.C., and Schat, H. (1992). Metal tolerance in plants. *Acta Botanica Neerlandica* **41,** 229–248.

Fangmeier, A., Hadwiger-Fangmeier, A., Van der Erden, L., and Jaeger, H.J. (1994). Effects of atmospheric ammonia on vegetation—A review. *Environ. Pollution* **86,** 43–82.

Fent, K. (1996). Ecotoxicology of organotin compounds. *Crit. Rev. Toxicol.* **26,** 1–117.

Fent, K. (1998). "Ökotoxikologie. Umweltchemie, Toxikologie, Ökologie." Thieme-Verlag, Heidelberg, Germany.

Freedman, B. (1995). "Environmental Ecology: The Environmental Effects of Pollution, Disturbance and Other Stresses," 2nd ed. Academic Press, San Diego, CA.

Manahan, E.E. (1994). "Environmental Chemistry," 6th ed. Lewis, Boca Raton, FL.

Nimrod, A.C., and Benson, W.H. (1996). Environmental estrogenic effects of alkylphenol ethoxylates. *Crit. Rev. Toxicol.* **26,** 335–364.

Parlar, H., and Angerhoefer, D. (1995). "Chemische Ökotoxikologie." Springer-Verlag, Berlin.

Peakall, D.B., and Bart, J.R. (1983). Impacts of aerial application of insecticides on forest birds. *Crit. Rev. Environ. Control* **13,** 117–165.

Peakall, D.B., and Shugart, L.R. (1993). "Biomarkers. Research and Application in the Assessment of Environmental Health." Springer-Verlag, Berlin.

Posthuma, L., and Van Straalen, N.M. (1993). Heavy metal adaptation in terrestrial invertebrates: A review of occurrence, genetics, physiology and ecological consequences. *Comp. Biochem. Physiol.* **106C,** 11–38.

Safe, S. (1990). Polychlorinated biphenyls (PCBs), dibenzo-*p*-dioxins (PCDDs), dibenzofurans (PCDFs), and related compounds: Environmental and mechanistic considerations which support the development of toxic equivalency factors (TEFs). *Crit. Rev. Toxicol.* **21,** 51–88.

Salt, D.E., Smith, R.D., and Raskin, I. (1998). Phytoremediation. *Annu. Rev. Plant Physiol. Plant Mol. Biol.* **49,** 643–668.

Sanders, B.M. (1993). Stress proteins in aquatic organisms: An environmental perspective. *Crit. Rev. Toxicol.* **23,** 49–75.

Schindler, D. W., Curtis, P. J., Parker, B. R., and Stainton, M. P. (1996). Consequences of climate warming and lake acidification for UV-B penetration in North American boreal lakes. *Nature* **379,** 705–708.

Shaw, I.C., and Chadwick J. (1998). "Principles of Environmental Toxicology." Taylor & Francis, London.

Solomon, K.R., Baker, D.B., Richards, P., Dixon, K.R., Klaine, S.J., La Point, T.W., Kendall, R.J., Weiskopf, C.P., Giddings, J.M., Giesy, J.P., Hall, L.W., and Williams, W.M. (1996). Ecological risk assessment of atrazine in North American surface waters. *Environ. Toxicol. Chem.* **15,** 31–76.

Walker, C.H., Hopkin, S.P., Sibly, R.M., and Peakall, D.B. (1996). "Principles of Ecotoxicology." Taylor & Francis, London.

Wolfe, D.A., Hameedi, M.J., Galt, J.A., Watabayashi, G., Short, J., O'Claire, C., Rice, S., Michel, J., Payne, J.R., Braddock, J., Hanna, S., and Sale, D. (1994). The fate of the oil spilled from the Exxon Valdez. *Environ. Sci. Technol.* **28,** 561A–568A.

CHAPTER

46

Food Toxicology: Legal Aspects

DAVID G. HATTAN,* ALAN M. RULIS†

*Division of Health Effects Evaluation and †Office of Premarket Approval, US FDA Center for Food Safety and Applied Nutrition, Washington, DC

HISTORICAL PERSPECTIVE

The unique subdiscipline of food toxicology exists at the nexus of chemistry, toxicology, nutrition, law, and regulation. To better understand this subject area, it is helpful to briefly review the history of food safety regulation in the United States. That history begins in the last decades of the 19th century. In 1883, Dr. Harvey Washington Wiley of Purdue University was named Chief Chemist of the U.S. Department of Agriculture (USDA). That era saw the beginning of numerous debates about the use of chemical preservatives, such as benzoates and salicylates; flour-bleaching agents, such as nitrites and nitrogen peroxide; artificial sweeteners, such as saccharin; and synthetic coal-tar dyes used for coloring foods. The issues raised in those debates formed the basis for the development of food toxicology during the 20th century.

Under Dr. Wiley's leadership, the U.S. government addressed the safety of a range of substances in food and helped to develop approaches to the issues of food adulteration in general. One of the era's unique institutions was the "poison squad." This group of a dozen or so healthy men was recruited by Dr. Wiley to ingest various foods containing additives and chemical preservatives under controlled conditions to test their purported effects on the health of the volunteers. Wiley's efforts against the use of inappropriate food chemicals soon culminated in the passage by the U.S. Congress of the Food and Drugs Act of 1906. That law declared a food to be adulterated if it contained "any added poisonous or other added deleterious ingredient which may render such article injurious to health." At that time, however, there was no clear concept of how to establish "safe" levels of intakes of defined chemical substances added to any food. The concept of "safe per se" was assumed, and the aphorism of Paracelsus that the "dose makes the poison" seems not yet to have been rediscovered.

Throughout the following decades of the 20th century, the science of toxicology as applied to food developed further. The USDA Bureau of Chemistry eventually evolved into the Food and Drug Administration (FDA) during the 1920s. During the 1930s toxicologists relied mainly on acute studies in animals (to quantify the lethal dose in one-half the animals or LD_{50}) with little, if any, reliance on longer term and chronic studies designed to examine the subtler effects of chemicals in the diet over the life time of the animal species tested.

The 1940s and the period just after the Second World War saw the burgeoning simultaneously of the food industry and the chemical industry. The U.S. population grew and was concomitantly becoming more urbanized. There was a need for the use of more pesticides on agricultural crops, and the need for more shelf-stable processed foods for people living in larger cities. Consumers demanded a wider range of prepared foods. During this era when chemical pesticides were being developed, the science of toxicological testing was invoked to ascertain the safety of these agents. The newly amended Food, Drug, and Cosmetic Act of 1938 clarified the regulation of poisonous and deleterious substances in foods. Foods under this statute are considered adulterated if they contain added poisonous or deleterious substances that "may render the food injurious to health." In case a substance is not added but is naturally present, the food would be adulterated only if the substance present "ordinarily renders" the food injurious.

During the post-World War II period, the discipline of food toxicology in the FDA advanced within the Division of Pharmacology under the leadership of Dr. O. Garth Fitzhugh. The field made use of the results of acute toxicological tests to determine the LD_{50} and longer term subacute studies conducted at somewhat lower doses, and also chronic (i.e., life-time studies) in animals. During the 1950s, Dr. Arnold J. Lehman, the new director of the Division of Pharmacology published experimental programs and guidelines for appraising the safety of chemical components of foods, drugs, and cosmetics. In that program, the FDA established an organized approach to reaching safety decisions on food ingredient substances. Subsequently, in 1959, the FDA published the document *Appraisal of the Safety of Chemicals in Foods, Drugs and Cosmetics.*

Also during the 1950s the Joint FAO/WHO Expert Committee on Food Additives (JECFA), under the guidance of Professor Rene Truhaut, began developing the concept of "acceptable daily intake."

In 1982, the FDA Center for Food Safety and Applied Nutrition (CFSAN) (then known as the Bureau of Foods) published a document titled *Toxicological Principles for the Safety Assessment of Food Additives and Color Additives Used in Food,* sometimes referred to as the FDA "Redbook." This document provides a scheme for determining the minimum configuration of toxicological studies likely to be needed for establishing the safety of a food additive, depending on the chemical structure of the additive and on the likely exposure levels to consumers of foods containing the additive. The document provides general guidance on protocols for toxicological studies deemed appropriate for the safety assessment of food additives. The specific toxicological guidelines presented in this document will be outlined more fully below.

On the international level, in 1987 the World Health Organization with cooperation from the International Programme for Chemical Safety and the JECFA, published the document Environmental Health Criteria 70, *Principles for the Safety Assessment of Food Additives and Contaminants in Food.* This document represents the most up-to-date consensus of a number of international experts in food-ingredient safety evaluation, brought together under the auspices of the WHO and under the IPCS to give guidance on safety-testing criteria for food ingredients.

CURRENT U.S. FOOD LAW

The regulatory tools used by the U.S. FDA Center for Food Safety and Applied Nutrition (CFSAN) to evaluate the safety of food and of food additives derive primarily from the Food, Drug and Cosmetic Act (the Act) and its various amendments, most recently the Food Additives Amendment of 1958. (Parallel statutory provisions applying to food colors are found in the Color Additive Amendments of 1960.)

Food Additives

Section 201(s) of the 1958 Food Additives Amendment defines the term "food additive" very broadly. The term "food additive" means

> . . . any substance the intended use of which results or may reasonably be expected to result, directly or indirectly, in its becoming a component or otherwise affecting the characteristics of any food (including any substance intended for use in producing, manufacturing, packing, processing, preparing, treating, packaging, transporting, or holding food; and including any source of radiation intended for any such use), if such substance is not generally recognized, among experts qualified by scientific training and experience to evaluate its safety, as having been adequately shown through scientific procedures (or, in the case of a substance used in food prior to January 1, 1958, through either scientific procedures or experience based on common use in food) to be safe under the conditions of its intended use . . .

The Food Additives Amendment covers both substances added directly to food intentionally to exert a technical effect in the food itself, the "direct" food additives, and substances whose intentional use brings them into contact with food (via use in fabricating food containers or in food processing), but which become components of food only unintentionally, the "indirect" food additives.

Title 21 of the Code of Federal Regulations (21 CFR) Part 172 refers to direct additives added deliberately to food for a specific technical purpose; such substances usually remain in food as consumed (Food and Drug Administration, 1997a). 21 CFR Part 173 describes secondary direct additives added to food or food components during the manufacture or processing, but which are usually removed from the food before the product is consumed. Small amounts of these processing aids may remain in the final food. 21 CFR Part 174 governs indirect additives, which are substances that may become components of food, such as materials that may migrate from food contact surfaces during production, manufacturing, packing, processing, preparing, treating, packaging, transporting, or holding food. To be approved, a food additive must be demonstrated to be safe at levels of requested use (Act, Section 409(c)(3)(A)). In addition, the actual addition of a substance to food should be at levels no higher than necessary to fulfill the desired technical effect, even if the safety data support a higher level of exposure (21 CFR 171.1(c)(C)).

In creating the broad definition for food additives, Congress realized that many common food ingredients, such as butter, eggs, salt, milk, vinegar, and sugars, had a long history of safe use in food; they were *g*enerally *r*ecognized *a*s *s*afe (GRAS), and if considered food additives they would have had to undergo rigorous premarket safety review. Because of this, the definition of "food additive" above excludes GRAS substances, exempting them from the usual food additive premarket approval process. Current FDA regulations (21 Part 170.30) state that general recognition of safe for food ingredients can be supported by the views of experts qualified by "scientific training and experience." GRAS status may be based on either a safe history of "common use in food prior to 1958" or the satisfaction of "scientific procedures" that demonstrate safety.

Through regulation, the FDA has provided the sponsor of a food ingredient the option of obtaining affirmation by the FDA of the general recognition of safety of the use of a substance. To obtain FDA affirmation of the GRAS status of the use of a food ingredient, the sponsor may voluntarily petition the agency to review and confirm that the available data establish that, under the proposed conditions of use, the material is safe and that safety is generally recognized by qualified experts. The determination of GRAS status based on scientific procedures requires the same quality and quantity of data as that required for a food additive. In order to satisfy the requirement that the data supporting safety be widely available, it is usually required that such data be from published studies, although the results from unpublished studies and other information can be used to corroborate the published findings.

The Code of Federal Regulations (CFR) in section 21 CFR 182.1 (a) explains certain aspects of the listing of GRAS substances. It points out that it is impractical to list all of the substances that are either components of food or added to food that are GRAS for example, materials such as salt, pepper, sugar, vinegar, baking powder, and monosodium glutamate are safe for their intended use. In this section are included substances for certain purposes that the U.S. FDA commissioner considers GRAS when these materials are used according to good manufacturing practices. Other parts of 21 CFR that are relevant to this discussion are Section 184, for food components that are considered GRAS from their long history of use in food, and Section 186.1, listing those substances affirmed to be GRAS by specific consideration by the U.S. FDA.

New Proposals for Determining the GRAS Status of Food Ingredients

On April 17, 1997, the FDA proposed sweeping changes in the manner in which sponsors of food ingredients can assert the GRAS status of their ingredients. In the proposal, the FDA stated that it intended to do away with the process for submitting and reviewing GRAS affirmation petitions and move to a notification system in which a sponsor would provide to the FDA in writing its determination that a given use of a food ingredient is GRAS. The FDA would evaluate the basis for the determination and then respond as appropriate without reviewing the sponsor's data in depth. The thrust of the new proposal is to more clearly define the scientific and toxicological basis for the GRAS status of common food ingredients and to make it possible for sponsors to go to the market more quickly with safe products, while at the same time notifying the FDA of their intentions. The FDA can call into question any uses of new food ingredients marketed in this way, but will be in a better position to allocate its limited resources to only those that it determines are worthy of its focused attention. Rapid risk assessments of generic categories of food ingredients will be necessary to implement this new process, and FDA is currently defining the necessary regulatory tools and procedures to implement this new approach (Food and Drug Administration, 1997c).

Color Additives

In a manner analogous to the food additives amendment, Congress in 1960 passed the Color Additive Amendments. This part of the statute requires color additives that are added to food, drugs or cosmetics be demonstrated to be safe prior to marketing. While color additives are added to food much like food additives, they are defined separately in Section 201(t) of the Act. Title 21 of the CFR, Section 70.3(f) further defines color additives as follows.

> A "color additive" is any material, not exempted under section 201(t) of the Act, that is a dye, pigment, or extracted, isolated, or otherwise derived with or without intermediate or final change of identity, from vegetable, animal, mineral, or other source and that, when added or applied to a food,

> drug, or cosmetic or to the human body or any part thereof, is capable (alone or through reaction with another substance) of imparting a color thereto. Substances capable of imparting a color to a contaimer for foods, drugs, or cosmetics are not "color additives" unless the customary or reasonably foreseeable handling or use of the container may reasonably be expected to result in the transmittal of the color to the contents of the package or any part thereof. Food ingredients such as cherries, green or red peppers, chocolate, and orange juice which contribute their own natural color when mixed with other foods are not regarded as color additives; but where a food substance such as beet juice is deliberately used as a color, as in pink lemonade, it is a color additive.

For certain color additives, namely those that are of synthetic chemical origin and which may contain harmful impurities that can be detected in the color itself, but not easily when added to food, Section 706 of the Act require "batch certification." FDA chemists analyze the color material batch-by-batch to certify that no more than tolerable amounts of the impurities are present. Once a batch has been chemically analyzed and certified, the color is then labeled as a Food, Drug, and Cosmetic (FD and C) color or Drug and Cosmetic (D and C) color. For example, tartrazine that has undergone batch U.S. FDA certification is labeled "FD and C Yellow No. 5." Uncertified tartrazine is not allowed for addition to foods, drugs, and cosmetics that are to be sold in the United States.

Recall that before the passage of the 1958 Act, the safety of food was based on the concept that food and food additives should be "harmless per se". The idea that a food additive had to be harmless at any level of exposure was, and is, of course, impractical and impossible. Virtually any material administered in sufficiently high doses will elicit some toxicity. In spite of the general scientific agreement concerning this latter observation, there was no consideration of thresholds of toxicity at that time.

Safety Standards

The current safety standard for food and color additives in the United States is "reasonable certainty of no harm." The "harmless per se" concept suggested that if a material were added to the food supply, and it was poisonous and deleterious, then the food was determined to be "adulterated" and should not be consumed. The FDA had the burden of proving the poisonous nature of the material. Before the 1958 Food Additives Amendment, food processors could add substances to the food supply without prior safety review and approval by the FDA. The responsibility for marketing safe food was entirely on industry's shoulders; the FDA had the burden to prove whether a certain food additive was poisonous or deleterious.

Even before 1958, however, firms sought the FDA's concurrence on the acceptability of adding new substances to the food supply. FDA scientists evaluated the scientific data supplied by the manufacturers and issued advisory opinions on the safety of the newly added substances. If the FDA agreed that a substance was safe, it issued an advisory opinion to that effect. Today these written opinions are called "prior sanctions," and provide a legal basis for marketing uses of substances without the requirement of a premarket safety review.

Section 409 of the 1958 Food Additives Amendment states that before a food additive can be added to food, it must be demonstrated to be safe under its intended conditions of use. This statute is the foundation of the premarket approval of food additives. Under this statute, for a new food additive to be legally added to foods, it must first be precleared. This process of premarket approval requires the submission of a petition to the U.S. FDA, as outlined in the provisions of 21 CFR 171.1. FDA scientists review the data and information in the petition in support of the safe use of the new additive and, objectively and independently of the petitioner, determine whether the intended use of the new additive is consistent with the safety standard of reasonable certainty of no harm. Once the FDA determines that the intended use of the food additive is safe, it issues a regulation permitting the addition of the new food additive to food.

Congress did, however, realize that it is impossible to assure the absolute safety of food additives under all circumstances, no matter how extreme. Thus, Section 409 states that:

> Safety requires proof of *a reasonable certainty* that *no harm* will result from the intended use of an additive. It does not—and cannot—require proof beyond any possible doubt that no harm will result under any conceivable circumstance. The safety of the use of a given additive involves the informed judgment based on educated estimates by scientists of the anticipated level of ingestion of an additive by man or animals under likely patterns of use (U.S. Senate, 1958).

Toxicological Testing Recommendations for Food Additives

The discipline of food toxicology is concerned with the safety of both the food itself and the chemicals that are purposefully or inadvertently added to food for various technical effects. Because of the very large number of components that make up food, the structural diversity of those food components, and the chemicals added to food as GRAS ingredients, food additives, and color additives, this discipline is unique and complex compared to the study of the potential toxicity of a single substance, as in the study of drugs.

The scientific data and other information submitted in food additive petitions should contain "full reports of investigations made with respect to the safety of the Food Additive." These submissions should be complete reports of the detailed data from studies that clearly and completely describe the methods used and the results obtained. Any results from scientific investigations must be included unless the petitioner adequately explains and justifies why the lack of these results will not bias the safety assessment of the food additive under consideration. These submissions of scientific data and other information should be the result of the conduct of adequate toxicological tests as discussed in the following.

As noted previously, in 1982 the FDA first published its toxicological testing recommendations for food additives in *Toxicological Principles for the Safety Assessment of Direct Food Additives and Color Additives Used in Food,* the Redbook. This document lays out the basic array of minimum toxicological data normally needed for evaluating the safety of the use of direct food additives.

The Redbook defines the needed toxicological testing for food ingredients based on the chemical structure of the material being tested and its projected level of human exposure. This consideration of both structure and exposure determines the minimal toxicological testing for any given food additive. The two factors, structure and exposure, are used in an algorithm that defines a concern level to which the substance is assigned.

Structure–activity relationships assign the additive to one of three structure categories. Food additives that appear to have a low toxicological potential are assigned to Category A; those with intermediate or unknown toxicological potential are assigned to category B; and those with structural elements that imply a high degree of toxicological concern are placed in Category C. For example, a substance that is observed to be a common component of food or that is generated by endogenous metabolism, such as fatty acids, would be placed in Category A; a substance that is structurally similar to a known carcinogen (such as ethylenethiourea) would be classified in Category C; and a substance with structural components of unknown toxicological significance would be entered into Category B. An example of this last category might be a food additive with a novel molecular structure that does not possess structurally alerting elements for carcinogenicity.

TABLE 1 Category Assignments to Determine Toxicologic Testing

Structure Category A	Structure Category B	Structure Category C	Concern level
<0.05 ppm	<0.025 ppm	<0.0125 ppm	I
0.05 ppm	0.025 ppm	0.0125 ppm	II
1.0 ppm	0.5 ppm	0.25 ppm	III

The estimated human dietary exposure to a food additive is the major factor in the assessment of the degree of initial toxicological testing recommended. Each one of the three chemical structural categories, when combined with estimates of the probable human exposure to the additive, results in the assignment of an additive into one of three concern levels I, II, or III. Table 1 summarizes how structure categories and estimated dietary exposure to the additive combine to determine the initial minimum toxicological testing. From Table 1 we see that if the exposure to a food additive of structure Category C is projected to be greater than 0.25 parts per million (ppm) in the diet, then that compound falls into Concern Level III and should be subjected to the minimum set of toxicological testing appropriate for that Concern Level. If, on the other hand, the exposure is estimated to be less than 0.0125 ppm, the same compound would be assigned to toxicological Concern Level I.

It can be seen from the table that much more emphasis is placed on the probable exposure to the additive than on the structure category assessment in determining the amount of toxicological testing that is recommended. This is an acknowledgment that the state of the art in the assessment of presumptive toxicological activity based on structure is still an imprecise one.

Each concern level is associated with a different level of initial toxicological testing. Listed in the Table 2 are the recommended initial testing batteries for substances assigned to Concern levels I, II, and III, as presented in the FDA Redbook. For concern level I compounds, the concept is to assure that the substance is not acutely toxic at low levels of dietary exposure and to allow some idea of which organ system(s) might be affected by the compound. In addition, Level I tests provide information on the range of

TABLE 2 Recommended Initial Testing Based on Concern Level Assignment

Type of study	Concern level I	II	III
Short-term feeding study (usually of 28-day duration)	X	X	X
Battery of short-term test for carcinogenic potential	X	X	X
90-day feeding study in a rodent		X	X
90-day feeding study in a nonrodent		X	X
Multigeneration reproduction study (two generations) with teratology phase		X	X
Carcinogenicity study in two rodent species			X
Chronic feeding study of 1 year in rodent (usually combined with the carcinogenicity study)			X

doses to be used for longer duration tests of those substances with higher dietary exposures.

The battery of short-term tests for concern level II compounds is designed to assess whether longer tests (e.g., carcinogenicity bioassays) may be necessary. The data obtained from reproduction studies are meant to assist in determining the need for additional reproduction and teratology testing or to suggest whether an *in utero* phase needs to be added to the feeding studies being performed. Additives that fall into concern level III ought to be subjected to the most extensive set of toxicological testing, as outlined in Table 2. Table 2 shows that for food additives that have widespread exposure in the food supply and entail significant and/or frequent dietary use, long-term or lifetime studies in rodents are recommended. It should be emphasized that the testing regimens in Table 2 are the *minimum* testing recommendations; more extensive testing may be needed with certain substances to resolve scientific questions that may arise during research and development.

While testing in human subjects may not be required for the safety assessment of many food additives, there are certain circumstances or scientific issues that arise that may profit from this type of testing. In these situations, the FDA encourages this kind of study when it is appropriate and ethically supported. As discussed above in the section dealing with GRAS substances, the presence of data documenting common use in food can reduce the amount of safety testing needed or may affect the size of the safety factor used to make the safety decision. Metabolism and pharmacokinetic studies may usefully guide the selection of the species used to most reliably assess the safety of a food additive. In addition, the species that metabolizes a food additive in the manner most like humans can provide the most accurate reflection of toxicological effect in human subjects.

The FDA expects that any toxicological testing that is conducted to provide data to support the safety of food additives will comply with its regulations entitled *Good Laboratory Practice for Nonclinical Laboratory Studies* that are found in 21 CFR 21.58. A "nonclinical laboratory study" is an *in vivo* or *in vitro* experiment in which the food additive is given prospectively to test systems under controlled laboratory conditions. The term does not apply to human testing or to studies performed to characterize the physical or chemical properties of the food additive. As a part of the system of assuring the integrity and orderliness of data collection, specially trained and authorized FDA employees conduct periodic inspections of facilities specializing in the conduct of toxicological studies. These inspections verify that the reports provided describing the conduct of the studies accurately reflect how these studies were conducted.

NOAELs, Safety Factors, and ADIs

The outcome of the toxicological testing of a food additive is focused on determining the acceptable daily intake (ADI) of the additive. This quantity, when compared to the estimated daily intake (EDI) of the additive, then determines whether the proposed use of the additive falls within the bounds of "reasonable certainty of no harm."

The ADI is but a single numerical estimate, but it is the result of a complex process of evaluation of *all* the appropriate data collected on a specific food additive. Commonly the FDA uses the longest duration study in the most appropriate animal species to establish a no observed adverse effect level (NOAEL) for the substance. The NOAEL is the highest dose that causes no observed adverse effects in the animal species under the toxicological test. To this NOAEL, a safety factor is applied and the ADI is calculated us-

$$\text{ADI} = \frac{\text{NOAEL}}{100}$$

FIGURE 1. Calculation of the ADI for food additives.

ing the equation in Fig. 1. The particular safety factor chosen for a specific ADI calculation will vary with the nature of the food additive, the intensity of toxicological testing, the quality of data submitted to support the safety of the compound, and the nature of the toxicological effect found. In many instances, however, a safety factor of 100 is used.

This application of safety factors to the NOAEL provides a satisfactory margin of safety to human consumers. It has traditionally been applied to account for an estimated 10-fold variation in the sensitivity of different species to the test agent and the manifestation of toxic effects (humans are assumed to be more sensitive than the animal model), and another 10-fold variation to account for varying sensitivities to toxic effects from the compound due to subpopulation characteristics, for example, differences in the rates of metabolism based on the age and state of maturity of the human subject or differences in the state of health of individuals.

The 100-fold safety factor has proven to be especially useful for many of the traditionally regulated food additives substances for which only a very small amount of the substance is required to fulfill the technical effect. In other instances, for example, micronutrient materials, vitamins, and minerals, it is not possible to apply a 100-fold safety factor to a NOAEL and have an adequate dietary intake to allow them to fulfill their physiological roles. In the other extreme, there are newly developed and proposed substances, called "macroingredients," that are ingested as appreciable percentages of the diet and thus do not permit the use of 100-fold safety factors. In both of these instances, 10-fold or lower safety factors are not uncommon. The safety assessment of macroingredients is discussed later.

For materials that fall in concern level II, where the longest-duration studies typically provided are subchronic studies (this is often the case for indirect food additives), the FDA may apply a 1000-fold safety factor to the NOAEL. The additional 10-fold factor is applied because these shorter-duration studies ordinarily possess a lower degree of toxicological sensitivity than chronic studies.

The FDA does not apply traditional safety factors to substances that have been demonstrated to be carcinogenic in humans or animals. The Delaney Clause prohibits the addition of carcinogenic food additives to the food supply. One limited exception to this prohibition involves the carcinogenic impurities of noncarcinogenic additives. This will be discussed in the section "Quantitative Low-Dose Extrapolation for Carcinogen Risk Assessment" later. Recently an article presented a compendium of NOAELs for over 600 chemical substances and related their NOEL ranges to chemical structure classes.

Dietary Exposure Assessment for Food Additives

In the process of deciding the concern level for a food additive as described above, the FDA must determine an estimate of the level of dietary exposure. This determination is referred to as the estimated daily intake or EDI for the additive. Three factors combine to provide an estimate of additive intake—the concentration of the additive in food; the amount of the food containing the additive that is eaten during an eating occasion (the portion size); and the frequency with which the food containing the additive is eaten over a defined time period. Usually the EDI is based on the amount of food ingested daily, but a good estimate of chronic intake of an additive requires that the data be based on time periods that are multiples of one day. In actual practice, this determination is difficult to make because the food additive may be added to a number of foods. This means that one must measure or estimate the frequency of ingestion and portion size of a given food in a given time period and multiply that value times the concentration in that food. The estimation of the total exposure to a food additive can thus be complicated if it is added to a number of different types of food products.

Practically speaking how does one measure how much is added to each of the food categories, and what are the food categories and how are they defined? The amount of food additive necessary to perform its intended technical function is known from research performed by the food additive manufacturer. All the uses of the additives must be consistent with good manufacturing practice, as defined in FDA regulations (21 CFR 110). According to this regulation, a manufacturer should use the miminum amount of an additive necessary to achieve the intended technical effect, for example, only the amount of antioxidant required to protect the specific food product from oxidative deterioration. Food manufacturers are inter-

TABLE 3 Typical Surveys Used in Estimating Food Intakes

Databases	Organization
The Nationwide Food Consumption Survey	USDA[a]
Continuing Survey of Food Intakes by Individuals	USDA
Estimates of Daily Intake from Food Industry Surveys	NAS/NRC[b]
The FDA Total Diet Study	FDA[c]

[a]United States Department of Agriculture.
[b]National Academy of Sciences/National Research Council (Abrams, 1992).
[c]Food and Drug Administration (Pennington and Gunderson, 1987).

ested in knowing this quantity because it limits the cost of production of the food to which the substance is added.

Estimates of the amounts of food from the various food categories eaten by U.S. consumers are provided by the federal government and various private bodies. The databases most often used by FDA in determining food intakes are listed in Table 3. These databases provide various estimates of food intakes; some for a short, 3-day period, and some for a more prolonged, 14-day period; and some provide a detailed profile of intakes based on various subpopulation characteristics, for example, in children or the elderly, or by ethnic group. The actual database used in the estimation of intakes depends on the needs of the intake estimator. In many cases, the FDA will desire both general population estimates of intakes and breakdowns along various age categories, 2–5 years or greater than 5 years.

Safety Assessment: Comparison of ADI to EDI

Traditionally, the safety decision for a food additive is based on a comparison of the ADI to the EDI for the proposed use. Typically, if the EDI in mg/kg body weight/day is less that the acceptable daily intake (ADI) in the same units, the use of the additive is considered to lie within the bounds of "reasonable certainty of no harm," and the food additive may be approved for its proposed use in food.

Indirect Food Additives

As noted previously, some materials are legally food additives because they may become components of food inadvertently, when their intentional use in food-contact situations results in their migration to the food itself. These materials are often referred to as indirect food additives. They migrate from the surfaces of food-contact materials used to hold, package, and transport food while in the distribution chain or from food-processing equipment. Because they are considered food additives, the FDA requires petitions for their use. These petitions are evaluated in much the same way as for direct food ingredients; an ADI is necessary from appropriate toxicological studies and this needs to be compared to an EDI. Because the presence of the additive in food is a result of inadvertent migration, the FDA requires data to allow it to estimate the amount of migration likely to take place. The FDA recommends the use of specialized techniques, often including measurements of the levels of extraction of the additive into food-simulating solvents. The food simulants used in cases where an additive may contact fatty foods characterize the degree of lipophilicity of food—8% ethanol, 50% ethanol, and corn oil. The conditions used to measure migration depend on the intended uses of the packaging materials. For example, if a packaging material is to be subjected to retorting, extractions would need to be performed for 2 hours at 275°F (135°C).

The extraction data are used to estimate the human exposure to migrants from the packaging materials. In performing this calculation, the FDA uses estimates of the fraction of the U.S. diet that comes into contact with different types of food-contact surfaces—glass; metal; coated and uncoated; paper, coated and uncoated; and polymers. Each one of these classes has an assigned "consumption factor," that is, the fraction of the total diet that comes into contact with these types of materials. The EDI for an indirect additive is calculated by multiplying the consumption factor times the proportion of food types (e.g., aqueous, alcoholic, or fatty) times an appropriate value for the total daily food consumption, usually 3 kg/day to account for the consumption of fluid beverages.

For additives with extremely small levels of migration (less than 50 ppb) or exposure, only acute toxicity data are recommended. The acute toxicity data are meant to preclude only the possibility of a very toxic substance entering the food. If the migration studies show that greater than 50 ppb, but less than 1 ppm, enter the food, then the U.S. FDA recommends subchronic feeding studies in a rodent and nonrodent species and, with demonstrated need, that reproduction studies in rodents be conducted to assure the safety of these materials. If significant migration (i.e., greater than 1 ppm exposure) is demonstrated, then long-term toxicological data from studies of carcinogenicity and chronic toxicity of at least 1-year duration in rodents and two-generation reproduction studies with a teratology phase in rodents are recommended by the U.S. FDA. As with direct additives, additional studies may be indicated if unresolved toxicity issues remain following the recommended set of initial tests.

Threshold of Regulation

On July 17, 1995, the FDA published a final rule putting in place a new policy and procedures for exempting indirect food additive situations from full-blown premarket evaluation and petition review in cases where the likely dietary exposure to humans from the migrating substances is below 0.5 parts per billion. This Threshold of Regulation policy is based upon the notion that below certain dietary exposure levels, additives migrating into food will present only negligible risk. The policy is intended only for substances not known to be carcinogenic, but is based upon the presumption that even if a migrating substance were inadvertently a carcinogen, the upper-bound risk of cancer from exposure to the substance at the low levels permitted would be negligible. The policy is based upon a systematic analysis of the potencies of numerous carcinogens and noncarcinogens, and today provides a basis for exempting approximately 40 food indirect additive petitions per year from the rigors of full-blown petition review.

Carcinogenicity Testing and Assessment

According to the Delaney Clause of the Act (Sections 409(c)(3)(A) and 706(b)(5)(B)), no food or color additive may be intentionally added to food that has been "found to induce cancer when ingested by man or animals." The most widely accepted method for determining the carcinogenic potential of a chemical substance is the rodent-based carcinogenicity bioassay. Following the exposure of the test animals to the test material by an appropriate route of exposure for an appreciable portion of the test animal's life span, either an increase in the incidence of neoplasms or a decrease in the latency period for the induction of neoplasms is considered predictive of carcinogenesis in humans. The following is a brief discussion of some of the important design considerations for carcinogenicity testing.

Test Material

Prior to the initiation of the carcinogenicity bioassay, certain critical data should be obtained for the material to be tested—for example, the chemical structure and purity, method of analysis, possible contaminants or impurities, sources of supply, stability on storage, water/octanol coefficient, and a projection of the daily human exposure. The availability of adequate amounts of the test material to conduct the entire study precludes the need of repeatedly reestablishing the substance's chemical characteristics.

Route of Administration

While there are several routes of administration used in chronic bioassays (the oral, dermal, and inhalation routes are most often used), the route considered most appropriate for the evaluation of food additives is the oral route. There are variations on the oral route—for example, gavage dosing for volatile or distasteful substances, and solution in the drinking water if the material is sufficiently stable. The simplest and most frequently used route is admixture in the dietary ration.

Dose Selection

In the process of selecting doses to be used in the chronic bioassay, data from the subchronic toxicity study, as well as pharmacokinetic and metabolism results from specialized studies, are the best means to determine the doses to be used in the chronic bioassay. The collection of an adequate base of information early in the process can help alleviate concerns about choosing a range of test doses that are either too high or too low to achieve regulatory objectives.

The usual procedure is to exaggerate the dose, especially the high dose, in hopes of increasing the sensitivity of carcinogenicity detection and to avoid a false negative result. One must remain aware of the need, however, to not produce excess toxicity in the animals in the study and thereby inadvertently induce toxicity that would substantially impair the life span of the animals from effects other than tumors. The lowest dose administered should not interfere with normal growth and development; ideally it should not cause any non-tumor-related toxicity. The intermediate dose should be approximately midway between the high and low doses, depending, of course, on the results of absorption, distribution, metabolism, and elimination (ADME) characteristics of the test compound. Multiple dose levels are very important in providing dose–response information that can be used to rationally interpret the results of the study. A recent review of the difficulties of dose selection and recommendations for addressing them is available (Foran, 1997).

Study Duration

Tumor expression is a toxicity manifesting a late onset. For this reason, the study design should provide for early post-natal initiation of the study (6–8 weeks) and be carried out until the rodents have been tested for 24–30 months (for rats) and 18–24 months (for mice). If the food additive is to be used widely in the food supply with significant dosage, the FDA recommends an *in utero* testing phase. In this instance, the dam is exposed before and during mating and during gestation and lactation, with the pups' exposure continued throughout their normal life span. The rationale for this procedure is to allow longer overall exposure to the test material and to determine whether any of the perinatal organ systems are more susceptible to carcinogenicity than those of the adult animal. While this phase of testing is controversial, there are examples of food additives (e.g., saccharin) that have expressed tumors with perinatal exposure and not expressed tumors with adult-only exposure. It is noted that food additives are ingested by virtually every age, physical condition (e.g., during pregnancy and infancy), and pathophysiologic state (e.g., diabetes, heart disease, and irritable bowel syndrome) that occur in humans.

Size of Treatment Groups

Due to the high cost of life-time maintenance of animals and of histopathology procedures, it is not possible to enter extremely large numbers of animals (e.g., hundreds per treatment group) in the test. The generally accepted number for studies is currently 50 males and 50 females per treatment group (Food and Drug Administration, 1982). A control group should be included with every study and all test subjects should be cared for and treated in the same manner, except that the controls do not receive the test substance.

Test Observations

The following outcomes and characteristics are routinely observed or measured during the chronic bioassay: body weight, organ weights, food consumption, behavior, and gross and microscopic pathology. It is very important that animals be necropsied as soon as possible and that moribund animals be sacrificed and subjected to a timely postmortem examination. The microscopic examination is the linchpin of the carcinogenicity bioassay. Thus, it is important for the technicians performing the sample collection to be very well trained and adequately supervised by a qualified pathologist who is familiar with the species being examined. The FDA Redbook recommends the following for a minimum microscopic examination:

1. All grossly visible tumors or lesions should be examined in all groups.
2. All preserved organs and tissues of all animals that die or are killed during the study and animals of the highest-dose group and control group should be examined.
3. If a significant difference is observed between the highest dose and control groups in the incidence of hyperplastic, preneoplastic, or neoplastic lesions at a particular site, the organs or tissues at that site should be examined for all animals in the study.
4. If the results indicate a substantial reduction in the animals' normal life span or the expression of results that might affect the neoplastic response, the next lower dose also should be examined.

Analysis of Statistics

The advice of a statistician should be sought when designing the chronic bioassay. The statistician will provide tools to adequately randomize the assignment of animals to treatments and assist the investigator in determining the appropriate number of test animals for the study. In addition, the statistician can provide an appropriate statistical analysis of the test results, for example, the appropriate size of the p value in the determination of statistical significance for pairwise comparisons and for trend analysis.

Analysis of Carcinogenicity Bioassay Data

In the process of analyzing the data derived from carcinogenicity bioassays, the expertise of a number of disciplines is necessary. The pathologist examines the slides and provides a diagnosis of the lesions to determine the number and type of tumors from the study. The statistician conducts analyses to determine the statistical significance of the comparative incidences of tumors between the substance-treated and control groups. The chemist provides valuable insight into the chemical characteristics of the substance. The toxicologist assesses whether the tumor is related to treatment by analyzing all the pertinent data on other target organ toxicity, such as the occurrence of preneoplastic lesions.

Some of the factors that are important in determining whether tumor incidences are biologically as well as statistically significant are:

1. The historical rate of tumor development in this species and strain in this particular laboratory.
2. The comparative survival of the treated and control groups.
3. The patterns of tumor incidence. (Was there a dose–response relationship?)
4. The biological interpretation of the results. (Was there consistency across studies? Was there occurrence in the target tissue?)
5. The reproducibility of the effect across species, strains, and genders.
6. Evidence of hyperplasia, metaplasia, or other signs of an ongoing carcinogenic process.
7. Evidence of increase in the types of tumors or progression of severity.
8. Strength of the evidence for increased tumor incidence. (What is the size of the p value for pairwise comparisons and for trend?)
9. Results of short-term tests for carcinogenic potential.
10. Evidence for a structure–activity relationship with other substances of similar structure.

Quantitative Low-Dose Extrapolation for Carcinogen Risk Assessment

As noted above, the Delaney Clause of the Act prohibits the FDA from approving any food additive shown to induce cancer in humans or animals. This prohibition does not apply, however, if the food additive in question is not a carcinogen but rather contains only a carcinogenic contaminant or impurity. Since April 2, 1982, the FDA has implemented a policy, the carcinogenic "constituents" or carcinogenic "impurities" policy, to evaluate the safety of additives that may contain carcinogenic impurities. Carcinogenic impurities may be permitted to be present in noncarcinogenic additives so long as the overall risk assessment of the use of the additive along with its carcinogenic impurities is consistent with reasonable certainty of no harm. This can happen if a carcinogenic impurity is present at a low-enough level in the additive or its potency is low enough to support the conclusion that it is safe in spite of the potential carcinogenic effect. The determination of a safe level of a carcinogenic constituent relies on the quantitative extrapolation of carcinogenic risk at low doses.

The quantitative risk-assessment process involving low-dose extrapolation of risk for carcinogens has been useful in implementing the constituents (impurities) policy. The FDA uses quantitative risk-assessment procedures, where appropriate, to determine the upper bound limit of life-time risk to the consumer from the presence of the carcinogenic contaminant or constituent chemical. In 1984, the U.S. sixth Circuit Court of Appeals unanimously agreed with this interpretation by the FDA.

The quantitative risk assessment (QRA) process for establishing upper-bound risk estimates for carcinogenic risk is a relatively new technique developed since the 1970s. One of the most frequently quoted descriptions of the overall process that serves as the basis for QRA has been presented by the National Research Council's report entitled *Risk Assessment in the Federal Government: Managing the Process*. In this report, the NRC states that the ideal risk-assessment process contains all or part of the following four steps.

1. Hazard identification. The determination of whether a particular chemical is or is not causally linked to particular health effects.
2. Dose–response assessment. The determination of the relationship between the magnitude of exposure and the probability of occurrence of the health effects in question.
3. Exposure assessment. The determination of the extent of human exposure before or after application of regulatory controls.
4. Risk characterization. The description of the nature, and often the magnitude, of human risk, including the attendant uncertainty.

A further delineation of principles underlying risk assessment for carcinogens was published by the Office of Science and Technology Policy (OSTP) and entitled *Chemical Carcinogens; A Review of the Science and Its Associated Principles*. Part I of this document describes 31 principles that are relevant to the evaluation of the role of chemicals in carcinogenesis. Part II provides a discussion of current information in different areas of science useful to the process of risk assessment. One of the topics discussed by the OSTP document is that of QRA. Among the principles that support QRA are that there are threshold levels for the toxicity of chemicals, that carcinogenicity is dose-dependent, and that the exposures to carcinogens are additive.

Safety Assessment of Macroingredient Food Additives

In recent years, food manufacturers have begun to introduce certain food additives into the food supply that are somewhat different than the more traditionally incorporated potent substances. These new additives are intended to replace macronutrients, such as fats, in the diet. They are added to food in appreciable quantities in order to effect their technological purpose, which, in some cases, is to replace traditional sources of nutrients. Here a number of factors are discussed that should be considered in designing the research and development program for macroingredients.

One example of this type of food additive is olestra, a fat-replacement substance in which the sucrose molecule is esterified with 6–8 fatty acids (thus, the chemical name of sucrose polyester). This chemical modification results in a substance that is very lipid-like in appearance and mouth feel, but which cannot be digested by the lipases in the gastrointestinal tract. The overall result is that foods containing olestra retain the desirable taste and texture characteristics of lipids in food, but without adding calories or fat to the diet.

In the toxicological testing of traditional food additives or microingredients in feeding studies, one can expect to observe 100-fold or greater dose margins between the ADI and the EDI for a food additive. This magnitude of dose margin is, in many cases, not possible with macroingredients and it is possible to see less than 10-fold margins between the doses that are fed to animals and the expected levels of consumption with a macroingredient. In the case of olestra, animals were fed up to approximately 6 g/kg body weight/day and the human 90th percentile intake of olestra for just one food category, snack foods, is 0.33 g/kg body weight/day. In the clinical-testing phase of olestra, doses as high as 32 g/person/day or approximately 0.5 g/kg body weight/day were used.

Various authors have proposed toxicological testing methods for macroingredients. Most of these testing plans involve a step-wise progression of toxicity testing. First, the physical–chemical characteristics of the substance must be carefully ascertained. This includes information on lipid versus water solubility, melting point, molecular structure and size, composition and purity, source or the synthetic process used in production, manufacturing specifications, and stability during production, storage, and use. The quantities of use are sizeable enough to require a consideration of the nature and amounts of the impurities and they may have to be tested separately if they are present in sufficient quantities and are inadequately characterized.

At the next stage of testing, it is important to determine the absorption, distribution, metabolism, and excretion characteristics of the new substance. If, after using a radiolabeled substance of sufficient purity and specific activity, there is compelling evidence that the material is essentially not absorbed, then the demands of the ADME profile assessment are substantially lessened. Factors then to be investigated are the potential adverse effects of unabsorbed materials on the gastrointestinal epithelium, the lymphatics, microbial populations, and metabolism and pharmacokinetics of the bile acids. In addition, it is necessary to consider and assess the influence of the macroingredient on the absorption of fat-soluble vitamins, the digestion and utilization of macronutrients (e.g. carbohydrates, fats, and proteins), and the bioavailability of lipid-soluble drugs, especially those used in very low doses and/or to treat serious diseases and disorders.

It should be noted that the overall safety assessment of macroingredients involves two distinctly different kinds of testing. First, the material must be fed to a suitable animal model to evaluate the potential for direct or cellular toxicity. The duration of testing and animal model to be used in the traditional feeding study must consider the results of the ADME and physicochemical testing. Second, the material must be fed to animals and to human subjects to screen for indirect toxicity (e.g., possible antinutrient activity). In the case of olestra, its ingestion was shown to interfere with the absorption of fat-soluble vitamins and an extensive series of both animal and human studies were required to measure the absorption impairment and then to determine how much of the fat-soluble vitamins was needed to be added to the olestra containing foods in order to compensate for this adverse effect.

The results of testing olestra also point out the importance of using different types of diets to feed animals and different levels of micronutrients administered with those diets. Thus, in studies designed to detect direct toxicity, an excess of micronutrients is acceptable, even desirable, to assure that any effects observed are due to the toxicity of the compound and not secondary to inadequate nutrition. On the other hand, in those studies designed to assess the potential influence of the macroingredient on nutrition, it is important to provide only the minimum daily intakes of micronutrients recommended by authoritative bodies (e.g., the American Institute of Nutrition) to maintain normal growth and development.

This design element is incorporated into the nutrition studies to model those human subjects who may eat less-nutritious diets and in anticipation of detecting any capacity of the macroingredient to interfere with the absorption or utilization of micronutrients. Finally, while it is acceptable to feed the subjects in a traditional toxicity study chow diets, it is not recommended for the nutrition studies. It is standard practice for the nutritionist to specify a chemically defined diet in which a carefully measured quantity of vitamin and mineral mix has been added and then confirmed by direct measurement. In this manner, it is possible to know which nutrients and amounts have been ingested by the experimental subjects. It became clear in studies conducted on mice that olestra was impairing either absorption or utilization of vitamin K in the test animals when, a few weeks into a feeding study, several of the mice died of hemorrhagic events with no other signs of toxicity. This problem disappeared when supplemental vitamin K was added to the diets of the mice. To alleviate concern about this phenomenon, the FDA required that olestra contain compensatory levels of vitamin K. Olestra exerted similar effects on the other fat-soluble vitamins, A, E, and D. Compensatory levels were determined for each of these other fat-soluble vitamins when used in foods and these compensatory levels must also be added to olestra.

International Developments

With the creation of the World Trade Organization (as a result of the Uruguay Round of negotiations under the General Agreement on Tariffs and Trade, GATT, and the signing of that treaty by many nations, including the United States in January 1995), the safety evaluation and regulation of food additives has taken on an international dimension. A central purpose of the WTO is to enable and enhance trade between participating member states. One important aspect of this is to remove technical trade barriers and create a consensus on safety standards for the international exchange of goods. The WTO agreements on Technical Barriers to Trade (the TBT agreement) and the Sanitary and Phytosanitary (SPS) agreement provide a basis for progress in this area. In the area of food, including processed foods containing chemical additives, the SPS agreement under the WTO refers to the Codex Alimentarius Commission of the United Nations as the reference body for determining safety standards for international trade.

One particular Codex Committee, the Codex Committee on Food Additives and Contaminants, is currently creating general standards for both food additives and contaminants in foods. The general standard for food additives (GSFA) currently contains 170 additives that may be added to food under only the restriction of "good manufacturing practice." In time, the GSFA will grow to contain hundreds of food additives, with appropriate maximum levels of use in specifically defined food categories. No additive may be listed on the GSFA unless it has been reviewed and has received an appropriate sanction (usually an ADI) from the Joint FAO/WHO Expert Committee on Food Additives. Thus, the field of food toxicology has progressively become one of international dimensions, where the determinations of safety performed in one country increasingly need to be seen in the context of similar determinations made in all other countries within their individual systems for safety evaluation.

Similar changes are occurring for determining the acceptable levels of many of the ubiquitous contaminants in food, such as heavy metals and mycotoxins, as the same Codex Committee develops the General Standard for Contaminants.

Recent U.S. Legislative Changes

The Food and Drug Administration Modernization Act of 1997 was signed into law on November 21, 1997. Under that statute, a process was created that permits food-contact substances (indirect food additives) to be marketed 120 days after proper notification of the FDA, unless the FDA objects. This significantly streamlined process for permitting new indirect food additives places the burden of objecting on the FDA and requires a much more rapid appraisal of the toxic potential of such substances than before. Under these circumstances FDA must review the data it receives and come to conclusions about the safety of proposed uses very rapidly, in comparison to the previous situation. To do this the agency must design effective means of referring to past decisions and accessing the existing toxicological information to determine whether the situation currently before it presents a potential risk to which it must object. The agency developed procedures for handling premarket notifications for food contact substances during a period of 18 months following the signing of the legislation into law.

CONCLUSION

The field of food toxicology is firmly rooted in a long tradition. The safety assessment of food and food components using the science of toxicology undergirds food-safety policy and regulation throughout the 1900s. Nevertheless, the field has seen many changes and developments in the last half of the

1900s. With the advent of the chronic bioassay, animal testing has risen to new levels of detail and complexity, allowing regulatory authorities to focus on ever more subtle toxic endpoints. However, the tried and true methodology of applying safety factors to no effect levels and comparing ADIs and EDIs has still proven essential for decision making. Making use of quantitative risk extrapolation, regulatory authorities have found ways to set priorities and make decisions about the safety of carcinogens in the food supply. The challenge of developing rational international standards has begun. The expectations for more rapid and consistent regulatory decision making are high, even in the face of these growing complexities. In light of the changes imposed by scientific developments, modifications to legislative mandates for regulatory agencies and other authoritative bodies, and the changes in the nature of food additive materials themselves, food toxicology has been presented with an unprecedented opportunity for redefining and redesigning itself to meet these important and sometimes conflicting demands.

Bibliography

Abrams, I. J. (1992). Using the menu census survey to estimate dietary intake-Postmarket surveillance of aspartame. *In* "Food Safety Assessment" (J. W. Finley *et al.*, eds.), pp. 201–213. American Chemical Society, Washington, DC.

Borzelleca, J. F. (1992). Macronutrient substitutes: Safety evaluation. *Reg. Toxicol. Pharmacol.* **16,** 253–264.

Codex Alimentarius Commission (1997a). "Report of the Twenty-Ninth Session of the Codex Committee on Food Additives and Contaminants." Joint FAO/WHO Food Standards Programme, Rome.

Codex Alimentarius Commission (1997b). "Twenty-Second Session of Codex Alimentarius Commission." Joint FAO/WHO Food Standards Programme, Rome.

Flamm W. G., Kotsonis, F. N., and Hjelle, J. J. (1994). Threshold of regulation: A unifying concept in food safety assessment. *In* "Nutritional Toxicology" (F. N. Kotsonis *et al.*, eds.), pp. 223–233. Raven Press, New York.

Food and Drug Administration (1975). "Appraisal of the Safety of Chemicals in Foods." Drugs and Cosmetics, Editorial Committee of the U. S. EDA, Washington, D.C.

Food and Drug Administration (1982a). "Toxicological Principles for the Safety Assessment of Direct Food Additives and Color Additives Used in Food (the Redbook)." U.S. EDA, Washington, DC.

Food and Drug Administration. (1982b). Policy for Regulating Carcinogenic Chemicals in Food and Color Additives; Advance Notice of Proposed Rulemaking. *Federal Register,* Vol. 47, April 2, U.S. Government Printing Office, Washington, DC.

Food and Drug Administration. (1988). Recommendations for chemistry data indirect food additive petitions. Chemistry Review Branch. Washington, DC.

Food and Drug Administration (1993). "Principles for the Safety Assessment of Direct Food Additives and Color Additives Used in Food (the Redbook), Draft Revision." U.S. FDA, Washington, DC.

Food and Drug Administration (1995). Food additives: Threshold of regulation for substances used in food-contact articles. *Federal Register,* **60,** 36582–36596.

Food and Drug Administration (1996). Food additives permitted for direct addition to food for human consumption: Olestra; final rule. *Federal Register* **61,** 3118–3173.

Food and Drug Administration (1997a). Food additives. "Code of Federal Regulations, Title 21, Food and Drugs," Parts 170–199. U.S. Government Printing Office, Washington, DC.

Food and Drug Administration (1997b). "Food and Drug Administration Modernization Act of 1997" Public law 105–115. Superintendent of Documents, U.S. Government Printing Office, Washington, DC.

Food and Drug Administration. (1997c). Substances generally recognized as safe; proposed rule. *Federal Register* **62,** 18938–18964.

Foran, J. A. (ed.) (1997). "Principles for the Selection of Doses in Chronic Rodent Bioassays." International Life Sciences Institute, Washington, DC.

Junod, S. W. (1994). "Chemistry and Controversy: Regulating the Use of Chemicals in Foods, 1883–1959." Ph.D. thesis, Emory University, Atlanta, GA.

Kokoski, C. J., and Flamm, W. G. (1984). Establishment of acceptable limits of intake. *In* "Proceedings of the Second National Conference for Food Protection," pp. 61–72. DHHS, Washington, DC.

Kokoski, C. J., Henry, S. H., Lin, C. S., and Ekelman, K. B. (1989). Methods used in safety evaluation. *In* "Food Additives" (A. L. Branen *et al.*, eds.), pp. 579–616. Dekker, New York.

Kotsonis, F. N., Burdock, G. A., and Flamm, W. G. (1996). Food toxicology. *In* "Toxicology: The Basic Science of Poisons" (L. J. Cassaret and J. Doull, eds.), pp. 909–949. MacMillan, New York.

Lawrence, C. E., and Paulson, A. S. (1981). Cigarette smoke: Cancer risk at low dose. *In* "The Analysis of Actual Versus Perceived Risks" (V. Covello *et al.*, eds.), p. 169. Plenum, New York.

Lehman, A. J., and Fitzhugh, O. G. (1954). 100-Fold margin of safety. *Q. Bull. Assoc. Food Drug Office U.S.* **18,** 33–35.

Lehman, A. J., Laug, E. P., Woodward, G., Draize, J. H., Fitzhugh, O., Garth, G., and Nelson, A. A. (1995). Procedures for the appraisal of the toxicity of chemicals in foods. *Food Drug and Cosmetic Law J.* **10,** 679.

Munro, I. C. (1990). Issues to be considered in the safety evaluation of fat substitutes. *Food Chem. Toxicol.* **28,** 751–753.

Munro, I. C., Ford, R. A., Kennepohl, E., and Sprenger, J. G. (1996). Correlation of structural class with no-observed-effect levels: A proposal for establishing a threshold of concern. *Food Chem. Toxicol.* **34,** 829–867.

National Research Council. (1983). "Risk Assessment in the Federal Government: Managing the Process." National Academy of Sciences Press, Washington, DC.

Paracelsus (1564). "Carinthian Trilogy; The Third Defense." A. Byrckmann, Cologne.

Pennington, J. A. P., and Gunderson, E. L. (1987). History of the Food and Drug Administration total diet study—1961–1987. *J. Assoc. Off. Anal. Chem.* **70,** 772.

Poulsen, E. (1995). Rene Truhaut and the acceptable daily intake: A personal note. *Terat. Carcin. and Mutat.* **15,** 273–275.

Rulis, A. M. (1989). Establishing a threshold of regulation. *In* "Risk Assessment in Setting National Priorities" (J. J. Bonin, and D. E. Stevenson, eds.), pp. 271–278. Plenum, New York.

Rulis, A. M. (1992). Threshold of regulation; Options for handling minimal risk situations. *In* "Food Safety Assessment" (J. W. Finley *et al.*, eds.), American Chemical Society Symposium Series 484. ACS, Washington, DC.

U.S. Court of Appeals (1984). Court of Appeals 6th Circuit Constituent Policy, Scott vs. FDA, 728 F. 2d. 322.

U.S. Office of Science and Technology Policy (1985). "Chemical Carcinogens; A Review of the Science and Its Associated Principles."

U.S. Senate (1958). Senate Report No. 2422, August 16. p.6. Superintendent of Documents, U.S. Government Printing Office, Washington, DC.

Vanderveen, J. E., and Glinsmann, W. H. (1992). Fat substitutes: A regulatory perspective. *Annu. Rev. Nutr.* **12**, 473–87.

World Health Organization (1987). "Principles for the Safety Assessment of Food Additives and Contaminants in Food." Environmental Health Criteria, No. 70. World Health Organization, Geneva, Switzerland.

CHAPTER

47

Food

Compound-Related Aspects

WERNER GRUNOW
Federal Institute for Health Protection of Consumers and Veterinary Medicine, Germany

INTRODUCTION

At first glance, the expression "food toxicology" seems to be a contradiction in terms. Food is meant for nutrition and should not be toxic under any circumstances. It is a fact, however, that in some cases the consumption of food can indeed lead to intoxication and disease. Such food-attributed intoxications are caused mainly by microbial toxins but can also be a result of toxic substances occurring naturally in some food.

Another important field of food toxicology is the toxicological assessment of food additives and constituents, and also of contaminants and residues of various kinds. The assessment is based on the results of toxicological studies on the substances concerned; it includes the identification of hazards and the characterization of potential risks of these substances when taken in with food. If feasible, the assessment will establish tolerable levels of intake.

TOXINS FORMED BY MICROBES

The main reasons for microbial food poisoning are toxins formed by bacteria. Most frequently involved are the enterotoxins derived from staphylococci (*Staphylococcus aureus*), which may contaminate food during preparation. These toxins are proteins that are not inactivated by heat. They induce food poisoning characterized by vomiting and diarrhea. Similar cases of poisoning are caused by toxins derived from *Clostridium perfringens* and *Bacillus cereus.*

The most dangerous cases of poisoning are those caused by toxins derived from *Clostridium botulinum* (botulism). These cases are rare, but sometimes take a deadly course. The characteristic symptoms are visual disturbances and neuroparalysis. They are predominantly caused by consumption of home-made canned food that has turned bad, but also by consumption of insufficiently cured or smoked meat. Botulinus toxins are a group of neurotoxic proteins that resemble tetanus toxin. Their extremely high toxicity is remarkable. In humans, even 10 μg of orally taken botulinus toxin A can be deadly.

Poisoning with bacterial toxins, however, should not be confused with food infections, such as salmonellosis, which also have their origin in bacteria and lead to a feverish inflammation of the bowel.

Scombroid poisoning is of microbial origin, too. It is associated with headache, nausea, redness of the face, and urticaria, and occurs occasionally after the consumption of mackerel fish (*Scombridae*) and sardines. This can be attributed to histamine and other biogenic amines (e.g., tyramine, phenylethylamine, cadaverine, and putrescine) formed from amino acids by microbial decarboxylation when fish and fish products turn bad.

Biogenic amines are also formed in fermented food, such as cheese, wine, and sauerkraut. Hard cheese especially may contain high levels of histamine and tyramine. With the exception of patients taking monoamine oxidase inhibitors, however, incompatibilities with cheese due to the content of biogenic amines have rarely been reported. Obviously, the threshold dose for incompatibility reactions is higher in this case than with intake from other foods. This might be ex-

TABLE 1 Mycotoxins in Food

Mycotoxin	Source
Aflatoxins	Nuts, peanuts, corn, soybeans
Ochratoxin A	Cereals, coffee beans
Citrinin	Cereals
Sterigmatocystine	Cereals
Patulin	Apple juice
Zearalenone	Corn
Trichothecenes	Cereals
Fumonisines	Corn
Ergot alkaloids	Rye

plained by slower release of amines from cheese in the gastrointestinal tract.

Molds, too, can form dangerous toxins in food and thus lead to poisoning (mycotoxicosis). A classic example is the infestation of rye with *Claviceps purpurea,* which leads to the formation of ergot alkaloids. In earlier centuries, mass poisonings (ergotism) occurred frequently; in present days, ergot poisoning no longer plays a role.

Other mycotoxins associated with certain diseases are formed in food by strains of *Aspergillus* and *Penicillium.* For instance, in some tropical countries of Africa, as well as in regions of Thailand and China, where food is frequently infested with molds, the intake of aflatoxin B_1 is significantly correlated with the incidence of liver cancer, which is much more frequent in these regions than in Europe. Balkan nephropathy, which occurs endemically in certain regions in Yugoslavia, Bulgaria, and Romania, seems to be caused by the contamination of cereals with ochratoxin A.

Many other food-contaminating mycotoxins (Table 1) have considerable toxic potential. In humans, however, diseases have so far been observed only in exceptional cases, for example, with the consumption of cereals heavily infested with strains of *Fusarium* and *Cladosporium* in East Siberia (Kashin–Beck disease and toxic aleukia).

Toxins formed by algae (phycotoxins) can also lead to severe cases of food poisoning. These occur relatively often after the consumption of mussels and oysters, which filter and accumulate toxic algae, mainly dinoflagellates, from the water. The toxins that are distinguished are PSP (paralytic shellfish poisoning), DSP (diarrhetic shellfish poisoning), ASP (amnesic shellfish poisoning), and NSP (neurotoxic shellfish poisoning) toxins; these cause paralysis, diarrhea, impaired memory, and neurotoxic symptoms, respectively. The group of water-soluble PSP toxins consists of more than 10 structurally similar tetrahydropurine derivatives, of which saxitoxin is known best. The fat-soluble DSP toxins are derivatives of ocadaic acid. Domoic acid, a toxic amino acid, was identified as a toxin of the ASP group. In several countries, tolerance limits were established at 80 μg PSP toxin/100 g mussel meat, and DSP toxins must not be detectable by certain methods. Ciguatera fish poisoning is also caused by toxins derived from dinoflagellates. The ciguatera toxins (ciguatoxin and maitotoxin) accumulating in tropical fish species do not play a role in Europe; in the Caribbean and in the Oceania–Pacific region (coral-reef areas), however, they cause more than 50,000 cases of poisoning with gastrointestinal and neurotoxic symptoms every year. Characteristic signs are muscular weakness, tingling and burning sensations in hands and oral mucosa, and an altered perception of temperature.

TOXIC FOOD CONSTITUENTS

Apart from toxins formed by microorganisms, normal food constituents can also be toxic (Table 2) and may possibly cause poisoning or incompatibilities.

Many plants contain cyanogenic glycosides. These are hydrolyzed by glycosidases, enzymes that also

TABLE 2 Toxic Constituents of Food Plants

Constituents	Source
Cyanogenic glycosides	
Amygdalin	Bitter almonds, fruit stones and kernels
Dhurrin	Sorghum
Linamarin	Linseed, cassava (manioc), lima beans
Erucic acid	Rapeseed
Glycyrrhizic acid	Licorice root
Gossypol	Cottonseed
Hemagglutinines	Beans
Isoflavone glucosides (genistin, daidzin)	Soybeans
Myristicin	Nutmeg
Neurotoxic amino acids	Seeds of *Lathyrus* species ("lathyrism")
Psoralens	Celery, pastinak, parsley root
Solanine	Potatoes
Thioglucosides (e.g., sinigrin)	Cabbage, mustard, horseradish
Vicine, convicine	Fava beans (*Vicia faba*) ("favism")

occur in the plants or are present in the intestinal tract and that release hydrocyanic acid. Vegetable foods containing such glycosides include bitter almonds and other fruit stones and kernels (amygdalin), linseed, cassava or manioc, and lima beans (linamarin), sorghum (dhurrin), and bamboo sprouts. Eating 60 bitter almonds is said to cause deadly poisoning in adults, and eating just 5–10 bitter almonds will do the same in small children. But the involuntary uptake of such amounts is prevented by the bitter taste. In the other cases, the traditional methods of food preparation ensure the extensive elimination of hydrocyanic acid and destruction of the glycosidase. Manioc roots, for example, are peeled, washed for extended periods of time, and then cooked. Lima beans and sorghum are crushed, soaked, and cooked in an open container in water that is then discarded. Nevertheless, poisonings from cassava, sorghum, and lima beans in tropical countries have been reported frequently. Poisoning with bamboo sprouts also occurs, and the import of lima beans (*Phaseolus lunatus*) to Europe led to many deaths during World War I.

However, the statement found in earlier literature that linseed meal may lead to deadly poisoning is incorrect. The enzyme linase found together with linamarin in linseed is obviously inactivated under the physiological conditions in the stomach. Even in the absence of stomach acid, the slow release of hydrocyanic acid from linamarin is compensated for by the fast-acting detoxification processes.

The consumption of fava beans (*Vicia faba*) may lead to hemolytic anemia (favism). This disease is causally connected with the β-glucosides, vicine and convicine, from which—in the beans themselves or in the digestive tract—the pyrimidines, divicine and isouramil, are released as aglycones. They are able to oxidize glutathione, thereby inducing hemolytic anemia. In more severe cases, the symptoms of the disease are fever, hemoglobinemia, jaundice, and hepatosplenomegaly. The clinical picture is observed particularly in Mediterranean countries and occurs after the consumption of fresh or, less frequently, cooked beans. It can even be induced by pollen. An important factor in the occurrence of favism is glucose-6-phosphate dehydrogenase deficiency, which is widespread in the population of the Mediterranean area. In favism, this enzyme is reduced in the erythrocytes to 6% or less, leading to a decreased level of reduced glutathione. If the remaining glutathione is then oxidized by pyrimidines from fava beans, the normal cell metabolism of the erythrocytes is disturbed and hemolysis occurs.

Lathyrism is a food-induced disease that occurs in response to the regular consumption of food in which at least one-third consists of chickpeas (*Lathyrus sativus*). It no longer plays a role in Europe, but in 1958, about 25,000 cases were observed in a region in India. Two forms are distinguished, osteolathyrism, which is observed only in animals, and neurolathyrism. In the latter, the neurological disturbances in humans include spastic paralysis of the lower extremities, paralysis of the bladder and intestine, and cerebral damage. These neurotoxic effects are due to a number of toxic amino acids occurring in chickpeas and other *Lathyrus* species, for example β-cyanalanine. In contrast, β-aminopropionitrile and β, β'-iminodipropionitrile are responsible for osteolathyrism.

Toxic constituents, however, do not only occur in more or less exotic foods or in foods that are only consumed regionally or occasionally; they are present even in a widely used staple food, the potato. As do other members of the nightshade family, particularly immature or green and sprouting potatoes contain solanine, a mixture of the two glycoalkaloids α-chaconine and α-solanine. Because the peels and sprouts are removed from the potato tubers and the cooking water is discarded, poisoning is rare and runs a relatively mild course; it is associated with burning or tickling sensations in the throat, headache, vomiting, and diarrhea. When left unpeeled, most of the potato varieties contain 2 to 10 mg of solanine per 100 g. If the content rises to 40 mg/100 g, poisoning may occur. In humans, the toxic dose of solanine is said to be 25 mg and the lethal dose 400 mg.

FOOD ADDITIVES

An important field of food toxicology is the testing and safety evaluation of food additives. Food additives are defined as substances added to food for technological reasons during production, processing, preparation, treatment, packaging, transport, and storage. The purpose of their use is to avoid the induction of microbial, chemical, or physical changes in food or to improve appearance, consistency, and taste (Table 3). In some countries, the definition of additives varies, so that certain nutrients and flavors are either excluded from or included in this definition.

In principle, food additives are only allowed if their use is considered safe. To ensure this, additives have to be approved, and proof of their safety must be provided by appropriate studies.

The type and extent of toxicological studies required for proof of safety and the principles of safety evaluation have been described in detail by the Joint FAO/WHO Expert Committee on Food Additives (JECFA) and by the Scientific Committee on Food

TABLE 3 Purposes for Food Additives

Purpose of treatment	Food additive
Protection against changes caused by microbes	Preservatives
Protection against chemical changes	Antioxidants, acids, and acidity regulators
Protection against physical changes	Humectants, antifoaming agents, anticaking agents
Improvement of appearance	Colors, color stabilizers, glazing agents (including lubricants)
Improvement of consistency	Emulsifiers, gelling agents, firming agents, anticaking agents, thickeners, stabilizers
Improvement of taste	Sweeteners, flavors, flavor enhancers

(SCF) of the European Union. Food additives must be tested in two animal species for acute, subchronic, and chronic toxicity. In addition, studies have to be performed in at least two generations of laboratory animals to test whether there are any effects on reproduction and offspring and whether a teratogenic potential exists. Furthermore, whether the substances in question have genotoxic and/or carcinogenic properties must be investigated. Included in the test program are also studies on the absorption, distribution, metabolism, and excretion (ADME) and possible tissue deposition (toxicokinetics). Of particular importance is the inclusion of observations in humans following occupational exposure, from epidemiological findings, from reports of poisonings, and from self-experiments or clinically monitored studies in volunteers.

The purpose of the studies to be carried out is to toxicologically characterize the substances tested, to identify toxic and unwanted effects and their dosage relationships, and to establish the highest dose that does not cause a detectable effect (no observed effect level, NOEL).

The Food and Drug Administration (FDA) in the United States divides additives into three groups (concern levels I–III), based on the anticipated exposure and the potential toxicity estimated from chemical structure. The test requirements are reduced in the least-suspect structure category at exposure levels below 50 μg/kg body weight and, even further, below 2.5 μg/kg body weight. In the most suspect structure category, the extent of toxicity testing is only reduced when the exposure is below 12.5 or more extensively below 0.62 μg/kg body weight.

The safety evaluation of food additives is done according to the principle of acceptable daily intake (ADI) developed by the JECFA for food additives and pesticide residues. The NOEL is determined in chronic feeding experiments by taking into consideration as many parameters of observation as possible and by testing substances in the most sensitive or most suitable animal species. The ADI is then derived from the NOEL by including a safety factor. Hence, the ADI is lower by the safety factor than the NOEL determined in animal experiments. It is defined as the amount of a food additive, expressed in mg/kg body weight, that can be ingested daily over a life time without appreciable health risk.

Usually, a value of 100 is chosen as safety factor. This is supposed to cover by a factor of 10 the possible differences in sensitivity between laboratory animals and humans, and by another factor of 10 the variability in sensitivity within the heterogenous human population (due to genotype, sex, age, state of nutrition, and health).

A numerical ADI value is not always allocated; the term "ADI not specified" is used instead. However, this happens only when the additive is of such minor toxicity that the possible total intake with food does not represent a health risk. Such an additive must be used according to good manufacturing practice; that is, "it should be used at the lowest level necessary to achieve the technological effect, it should not conceal inferior food quality or adulteration, and it should not create a nutritional imbalance" (WHO, 1987).

The ADI values can guarantee safety only according to the current state of knowledge and testing procedures. For this reason, ADI values are frequently altered due to new findings; in some cases, they have been even dramatically reduced. Furthermore, it has to be noted that the values set by different committees are not always identical.

"Generally recognized as safe" (GRAS) is another term characterizing the safety of substances added to food. This term is used in the United States for substances and groups of substances (e.g., many salts, spices, flavors, vegetable gums, and baking powder) that are excluded from the approval process and, hence, from the associated formal requirements for food additives. The condition is that a consensus has been formed among qualified experts about the safety of the substance for its intended use.

In the past, research has shown in a number of cases that food additives carried potential hazards that need to be taken seriously. Examples are the dye butter yellow and the sweetener dulcin, both of which showed carcinogenic effects in animal experiments. These substances have been excluded from use in food. The use of other additives, such as boric acid, erythrosine, and canthaxanthin, has been restricted due to their toxic properties.

For other food additives, the effects observed in animal experiments have been recognized to be irrelevant to their safety. That is the case with adrenal and renal hyperplasia and accompanying nephrocalcinosis associated with higher doses of polyols (such as isomaltol, lactitol, maltitol, mannitol, sorbitol, and xylitol). The bladder tumors observed in male rats after the chronic administration of higher doses of saccharin are also considered irrelevant to the use of this sweetener.

FOOD CONTAMINANTS

Another subject of food toxicology is the evaluation of substances that get into food as contaminants. According to the definition of the Codex Alimentarius of the Joint FAO/WHO Food Standard Programme, food contaminants include "any substance not intentionally added to food, which is present in such food as a result of the production (including operations carried out in crop husbandry, animal husbandry and veterinary medicine), manufacture, processing, preparation, treatment, packing, packaging, transport or holding of such food, or as a result of environmental contamination." This definition includes not only totally unintentional contaminants but also residues from the deliberate use of pesticides, veterinary drugs, feed additives, and substances migrating from "food contact material."

The most important food contaminants are environmental chemicals that originate from industrial and other human activities and get into food via soil, water, air, and the food chain. Among other substances, the environmental contaminants include heavy metals, such as lead, cadmium, and mercury; polycyclic aromatic hydrocarbons and halogenated organic compounds, such as polychlorinated biphenyls; and the group of polychlorinated dibenzo-*p*-dioxins and dibenzofurans.

Many of these environmental contaminants are very toxic and have carcinogenic potential. In addition, some of them tend to bioaccumulate, leading to their accumulation in the food chain. They represent a potential risk to human health when taken in quantities exceeding the tolerable limits.

In a number of cases, the contamination of food with these substances has led to large-scale poisoning. In Japan, for example, the consumption of rice with an increased cadmium content was responsible for the appearance of the "itai-itai" disease. For years, the pit water from a lead–zinc–cadmium mine had been directed into a river used for irrigating rice fields. Two hundred people fell ill and suffered from severe pain in their bones and joints and from extreme osteomalacia, which often had a fatal outcome. Also in Japan, more than one hundred fishermen and their families who lived in the Minamata Bay contracted a nervous disorder that clearly could be traced back to the consumption of fish and shellfish containing high concentrations of methyl mercury. The cause of the mercury contamination was a chemical plant using mercury oxide as a catalyst in the production of acetaldehyde from acetylene and directing the effluent into the bay, so that marine animals caught in the area had a mercury content of up to 100 mg/kg.

Such extremely high contaminations, however, occur only rarely. Normally, the contamination of food by environmental chemicals is relatively low. For instance, the average intake of lead from food in most estimates is far below 300 μg/day. If there is no appreciable supply from other sources, the critical blood level of about 30 μg/dl in adults is not reached. Children, however, are more at risk than adults. They have a higher absorption rate and are more sensitive to lead with regard to the effects on the central and peripheral nervous systems. In fetuses and small children, a blood level of only 10 μg/dl has to be considered as the lowest observed adverse effect level (LOAEL). In children of up to 6 years of age, such a blood level corresponds to an intake with food of only 60 μg/day.

The average intake of cadmium with food is estimated to be approximately 10 to 50 μg/day. Cadmium is characterized by an extremely long half-life period and accumulates especially in the kidneys, where it induces renal dysfunction and cellular damage. The critical concentration in the renal cortex is estimated to be 200 mg Cd/kg and is reached with an intake of approximately 200 μg Cd/day over 45 yrs. The average intake with food is clearly lower. However, there is wide variation in both the cadmium content of food and, depending on consumption habits, the actual intake. Therefore, recommendations have been made to restrict the consumption of food with relatively high levels of cadmium, such as the livers and kidneys from old slaughtered animals, as well as certain mushrooms.

The main source of mercury intake in the form of methyl mercury is fish and fish products. The average daily intake has been estimated to be 2.4 μg methyl mercury and does not represent a risk. Blood levels of 200 μg/liter and hair contents of 50 μg/g, which are associated in adults with the risk of early neurological effects, can only occur when large amounts of heavily contaminated fish are consumed.

Like the heavy metals, the polychlorinated biphenyls (PCB), polychlorinated dibenzo-*p*-dioxins, and dibenzofurans (PCDD/PCDF), including the particularly toxic 2,3,7,8-tetrachlorodibenzo-*p*-dioxin (TCDD), are widely distributed throughout the environment and accumulate in the food chain. They occur especially in fish, meat, and milk. In adults, the average daily intake with food is estimated to be 0.005–0.2 μg PCB/kg body weight and 1–2 pg TCDD equivalents/kg body weight. Due to their accumulation in body fat, this leads to a relatively high content in human milk. For infants in the breastfeeding period, an average daily intake of 2–12 μg PCB/kg body weight and 150 pg TCDD equivalents/kg body weight has been reported. In animal experiments, very low doses of these substances have been shown to affect reproduction and to be carcinogenic. However, the induction of tumors is attributed to the tumor-promoting activity of these substances and the sensitivity of humans seems to be lower than that of the experimental animals used. Nevertheless, the introduction of these substances into the environment and, hence, their presence in food should be avoided as much as possible.

The establishment of tolerable levels of intake for environmental contaminants, if feasible at all, is based not only on toxicological studies in laboratory animals but also preferably, on epidemiological findings and known cases of poisoning. The natural occurrence of many contaminants and the possible total intake of the substances from all conceivable sources must be taken into account. The evaluation is made difficult when accumulation in the organism has to be expected and the difference between the toxic dose and unavoidable intake is relatively small.

Instead of the acceptable daily intake (ADI) used for additives, a provisional tolerable weekly intake (PTWI) is established for contaminants accumulating in the body. It is deliberately called "provisional" because of the uncertainties in deriving tolerable exposure levels. For contaminants that do not accumulate in the body, the provisional maximum tolerable daily intake (PMTDI) is used.

The residues of pesticides are another type of food contaminants with a considerable risk potential. Therefore, pesticides are subject to approval and maximum residue limits are established. As with additives, the toxicologically acceptable levels of pesticide intake are derived primarily from animal experiments and include safety factors. Because of the higher toxic potential of these substances, the resulting ADI values are much lower than in the case of additives. The average intake of pesticide residues, however, is generally much lower still, and no risk must be expected as long as the residues do not exceed the maximum limits.

Among pesticides, the group of persistent organochlorine compounds, such as aldrin, dieldrin, chlordane, DDT, heptachlor, hexachlorobenzene, and hexachlorocyclohexane (HCH), poses a particular toxicological problem. These compounds are minimally biodegradable, remain in the soil, and accumulate in the food chain. They are deposited in human fat tissue and, therefore, are found in human milk. Apart from γ-HCH (lindane), the use of these substances has been prohibited in many countries.

Finally, veterinary drugs and feed additives must be mentioned as contaminants occurring in meat, milk, and eggs. Like pesticides, they are only approved if the expected residue intake with food is shown not to exceed the ADI.

In the case of these contaminants, the waiting periods that have to follow the last administration play an important role in making sure that critical residues are no longer present at the time of slaughter or when milk and eggs are collected.

FOOD-CONTACT MATERIALS

Food contaminants also include substances that pass into food from containers, packaging material, kitchen utensils, and dishes. In the past, containers made of metal and ceramics caused food poisoning from time to time because of the release of metal ions. However, containers and packaging made of plastics can also release components into food, such as the residues of nonpolymerized starting materials (monomers), auxiliary agents for the polymerization process (cross-linking agents and catalysts), and additives for influencing the properties of the plastics (stabilizers, plasticizers, lubricants, flame retardants, fillers, dyes, and propellants). The high-molecular material in plastics cannot pass into food because it is insoluble and, therefore, does not represent a toxicological problem. However, the low-molecular starting materials, adjuvants, and additives do represent a potential hazard and, therefore, require toxicological testing and evaluation.

The toxicological evaluation of plastic components is based on migration, that is, on the analytical measurement of their transfer into food or food simulants (such as deionized water, 3% acetic acid, 15% ethanol, and olive oil). From the migration values, which are material-dependent parameters, the exposure is estimated and compared to the toxicological properties of these substances. As these are often unknown, toxicological studies are required depending on the level of exposure. Their results must demonstrate the safety of these substances when they are used in plastics.

In the European Union, food-contact plastic materials are regulated on the community level, and the toxicological evaluation of plastic components is done by the Scientific Committee on Food (SCF). In this committee's approach, the extent of toxicological studies with plastic components depends on the degree of exposure; the exposure level is derived from the surface-based migration, assuming that 1 kg food is in contact with 600 cm^2 (83 in^2) of plastic surface and that an adult of 60 kg body weight consumes 1 kg of such food daily.

For substances migrating in amounts of more than 5 mg/kg food, the required tests are one 90-day feeding study, three *in vitro* mutagenicity tests (gene mutations in bacteria, chromosomal aberrations in mammalian cells, and gene mutations in mammalian cells), studies on toxicokinetics, reproduction toxicity, and teratogenicity, and one long-term toxicity and carcinogenicity study. In certain circumstances, studies in one animal species may be considered sufficient. Within the migration range of 0.05–5 mg/kg food, which is equivalent to a maximum intake of 0.1 mg/kg body weight/day, the test requirements are lower. In general, they are limited to one 90-day-feeding study, three mutagenicity tests, and data on the potential for bioaccumulation (octanol–water distribution coefficient). In the case of migration in amounts below 0.05 mg/kg food, the maximum possible intake is only about 1 μg/kg body weight/day. Therefore only three mutagenicity tests are required.

Based on the knowledge obtained in toxicological studies, the Scientific Committee on Food has grouped the components of plastics coming into contact with food into categories. Once sufficient information is available, safe levels of intake can be quantified. In analogy with the ADI values for direct food additives, these are called TDI values (tolerable daily intake). Under the assumption discussed, these are transformed into migration limits called SML values (specific migration limit) (Table 4). For certain substances, additional restrictions in food or maximum permitted quantities in the material (QM) have been established. Approximately 1200 monomers and 1000 additives had been classified according to this system by 1991.

In the United States, certain substances used in food-contact materials have been excluded from regulation by the FDA (threshold of regulation). This means that there will be no requirement for testing them at all, if, among other things, these substances are not carcinogenic or the chemical structure does not give reason to suspect carcinogenic effects. Above all, their content in food should not exceed 0.5 ppb; under the assumptions usually applied in the United States, this corresponds to a maximum intake of 1.5 μg/day.

The risk evaluation of unsaturated monomers with carcinogenic potential and genotoxic activity is a special problem. Examples of such monomers are acrylamide, acrylonitrile, 1,3-butadiene, vinyl chloride, and vinylidene chloride. Because of the irreversible and cumulative effect of minute doses, no threshold can be established for such substances. As a general principle, therefore, the minimization rule applies, according to which exposure should be completely avoided or, if this is not feasible, restricted as far as possible. This means that the residues of such monomers in plastics should be minimized so that, with accepted sensitive methods, no transfer can be demonstrated in food coming into contact with such plastics.

TREATMENT AND PREPARATION OF FOOD

In the widest sense, food contaminants also include substances present in food as a result of treatment and preparation. These contaminants pose a number of toxicological problems as well.

One example for the formation of toxic reaction products in food is the treatment of wheat flour with nitrogen trichloride (agene process), which was customary in the past. This treatment gave rise to methionine sulfoximine, which was responsible for epileptic seizures occurring in dogs fed with such flour. Another example affecting feed is the formation of *S*-(1,2-dichlorovinyl)-L-cysteine during the extraction of soybean flour with trichloroethylene, which caused hemorrhagic disorders in cattle and aplastic anemia in horses and sheep.

Reaction products formed by a treatment process were also considered to be responsible when, in 1960, erythema occurred in the Netherlands in more than 100,000 individuals. The disorder was attributed to the consumption of a new variety of margarine (Planta margarine) and was described as margarine disease; however, its cause could not be clarified unambiguously.

The formation of hydroperoxides and epoxides of unsaturated fatty acids during the heating of fats is problematic as well. Together with other substances formed in overheated fats, these oxidation products are the cause of toxic effects observed in laboratory animals fed with large quantities of overheated fats. However, the risks to humans are thought to be negligible because food prepared in overheated fats is rarely consumed. Except in extreme circumstances,

TABLE 4 Tolerable Daily Intake (TDI) and Specific Migration Limits (SML) of Monomers and Additives of Plastics for Food Contact[a]

Compound	TDI (mg/kg body weight)	SML (mg/kg of food or food simulants)
Acrylonitrile	—	Not detectable (detection limit: 0.02)
Bis(2-ethylhexyl) phthalate (DEHP)	0.05	3
Bisphenol A	0.05	3
1,3-Butadiene	—	Not detectable (detection limit: 0.02)
Caprolactam	0.25	15
Di-*n*-octyltin compounds	0.0003 (as tin)	0.018 (as tin)
Terephthalic acid	0.125	7.5
Tetrahydrofuran	0.01	0.6
Vinyl chloride	—	Not detectable (detection limit: 0.01)

[a]As established by SCF.

only small amounts of oxidation products are formed and many of them are destroyed in the intestinal tract rather than being absorbed.

Another conversion of fat occurs when vegetable proteins that still contain some fat from the raw material are hydrolyzed with hydrochloric acid. Part of the glycerol contained in the fat reacts by forming chloropropanols, which have mutagenic and carcinogenic properties.

When sugars are heated at high temperature, they caramelize. In the presence of amino acids or amines, the carbonyl groups of the sugars react with the amino groups by forming various compounds, which causes the browning of food (Maillard reaction). Furthermore, the complex reaction can lead to amino acid imbalances and a decrease in the quality of protein, as certain amino acids—such as the essential amino acid, lysine—are no longer fully available. However, the occurrence of Maillard products in the human diet does not seem to be toxicologically relevant.

During the heating of meat, heterocyclic amines are formed from amino acids. These include pyrolytic products that have the structure of aminopyridoindoles and -imidazoles (e.g., Trp-P-1, Trp-P-2, Glu-P-1, Glu-P-2) and, under milder conditions and participation of creatine present in the meat, aminoimidazoquinolines (IQ, MeIQ), -quinoxalines (MeIQ$_x$), and -pyridines (PhIP). These compounds have an extremely high mutagenic potential, and feeding experiments in mice and rats have shown that they are carcinogenic. Special target organs are the liver and the forestomach.

Furthermore, polycyclic aromatic hydrocarbons (PAHs), such as benzo(*a*)pyrene, are formed when meat is fried and especially when it is barbecued, in the latter case mainly by fat dripping into the fire; toxicologically, they have to be taken into account mainly because of their carcinogenicity. PAHs are generally formed during incomplete combustion and pyrolysis of organic material; they also contaminate food through their ubiquity and during drying (direct heating) and preparation of smoked food.

Important contaminants in food are also the *N*-nitroso compounds formed in cured meat products—particularly during the heating of breakfast bacon—from nitrite pickle and amines or amides present in food. The most frequently demonstrated have been *N*-nitrosodimethylamine (NDMA), *N*-nitrosopyrrolidine, and *N*-nitrosopiperidine, which are particularly noteworthy for their carcinogenic effects. In the past, an important source of NDMA was the contact of nitrogen oxides with barley malt during kiln drying. Since then, the resulting contamination of beer with an average of 2–3 μg NDMA/liter and an extreme value of 68 μg NDMA/liter has been significantly reduced through technological measures (indirect heating).

Furthermore, the process of food irradiation has raised toxicological questions. Based on the findings of irradiation chemistry and numerous feeding experiments involving irradiated food, it is assumed today that food components are not significantly altered under the usual conditions of irradiation. However, as with other procedures, such as heating, the conversion products formed in small amounts are only partially known.

CONFUSION OF FOOD WITH TOXIC PRODUCTS AND ADULTERATIONS

The confusion of food with products not intended as food can cause severe poisoning. This includes not only the consumption of poisonous mushrooms and plants by mistake, but also, for example, the consumption of seed dressed with fungicides, which has happened occasionally in the past.

The literature reports over 10 episodes of poisoning in which seeds treated with mercury compounds, hexachlorobenzene, or thallium sulfate were consumed. In some cases, this affected several thousand people. A tragic mass epidemic occurred in Iraq in the winter of 1971–1972 when bread was baked from seeds dressed with fungicides containing methyl mercury. Over 6500 were taken to the hospital and 459 died. A mass poisoning of similar magnitude occurred in Turkey in the years 1955–1959. In this case, cereals had been dressed with hexachlorobenzene used as a fungicide. A characteristic symptom was cutaneous porphyria.

In canteens and restaurants, there have been repeated confusions of powder-like food (such as milk powder or sodium chloride) with pesticides of similar appearance, especially with sodium fluoride-containing rodenticides. The worst case of poisoning of this kind happened in 1942 in a hospital in Oregon when sodium fluoride was mistaken for milk powder during the preparation of scrambled eggs; 263 people were affected and 47 died.

In 1984, in Michigan, there was an incident of considerable magnitude when magnesium oxide, which was supposed to be added to animal feed, was confused with the fire retardant polybromobiphenyl (PBB). The confusion attracted attention only when cows began producing less milk and many animals died. The contaminated milk had been consumed for a long period. Many farmers who were directly affected showed the apparent signs of poisoning, such as memory loss, muscle weakness, headaches, and stomach complaints.

The catastrophic mass poisoning that occurred in Spain in the spring of 1981, and which has been described as toxic oil syndrome, must be attributed to the adulteration of food. The first symptoms of the disorder were atypical pneumonia with fever, exanthema, and distinct eosinophilia; it often changed later into a chronic phase with severe neuromyopathy, vasculitis, and diverse skin manifestations. It affected approximately 20,000 people, 11,000 of whom were taken to hospitals and over 500 died. Epidemiologically, a close connection was found between the appearance of this disorder and the consumption of adulterated cooking oil, which was derived from rapeseed oil that had been denatured with aniline for industrial purposes and was then sold by street vendors.

The confusion of ethyl alcohol (ethanol) with methyl alcohol (methanol) and the deliberate adulteration of alcoholic beverages with methanol have claimed many victims. The lethal dose of pure methanol has been reported to be in the range of 30 to 100 ml. But the toxic effects, particularly visual disturbances including loss of vision, can be observed after the intake of only a few milliliters. As the simultaneous intake of ethanol is counteractive, it is difficult to establish which concentration of methanol—also occurring naturally in alcoholic beverages—must be regarded as detrimental to health. Contents up to 150 mg/liter white wine and 300 mg/liter red wine, the limits recommended by the International Wine Office, and 13.5 g/liter pure alcohol in fruit brandies, the maximum level tolerated at present in the European Union, are considered to be harmless.

Another adulteration is the addition of diethylene glycol to wine, which happened recently in Austria. Although contents up to 48 g/liter have been found and the lowest dose for toxic effects of diethyleneglycol was estimated to be 3–6 g in adults, no cases of demonstrated poisoning following the consumption of the adulterated wine have become known.

CARCINOGENIC SUBSTANCES IN FOOD

A central problem in food toxicology is the assessment of risks derived from carcinogenic substances in foods. It is unanimously assumed that the risk of cancer is considerably influenced by nutrition. According to Doll and Peto (1981), 35% of all cancer deaths in the United States have nutritional causes. Although the most important risk factors are seen to be overnutrition, high fat consumption, and other dietary patterns, the question is whether carcinogenic substances taken in with food also contribute to the development of cancer.

Substances that are carcinogenic in animal experiments occur in food as natural constituents, contaminants, or residues and, in certain cases, are even added to food. The relevance for health of their intake with food varies widely from substance to substance, depending on the mechanism of action and the carcinogenic potential of the substances in question, and also on the level of intake.

It is now undisputed that alcoholic beverages have carcinogenic potential. Epidemiological evidence is growing that not only the pronounced abuse of alcohol can lead to cancer, but even a relatively moderate consumption of alcohol poses a risk as well. However, the carcinogenicity of ethyl alcohol has not yet been experimentally demonstrated.

Beyond that, a connection between the presence of carcinogenic substances in food and an increase in cancer incidence in humans has been demonstrated or made plausible only in exceptional circumstances.

TABLE 5 Intake of Genotoxic Carcinogens from Food

Substance	Daily intake (DI) (μg/kg body weight/day)	LOEL (μg/kg body weight/day)	LOEL/DI
Heterocyclic aromatic amines	1.5	8000 (mean TD_{50} in mice)	5000 (TD_{50}/DI)
Ethylcarbamate	0.02 0.2[a]	100	5000 500[a]
Nitrosodimethylamine	0.008	8	1000
Benzo(*a*)pyrene	0.004	150	37,000
Ochratoxin A	0.0009	70	80,000
Aflatoxin B_1	0.00025	0.05	200

[a]Including a weekly consumption of 50 ml brandy from stone fruits.

This is the case with aflatoxin B_1, which correlates with the incidence of primary liver cancer in some tropical countries, where food is often infested with molds and heavily contaminated with aflatoxins. Similarly, the high intake of ochratoxin A in some Balkan countries seems to be responsible for endemic nephropathy and the kidney tumors associated with it. Higher concentrations of *N*-nitroso compounds in food in some Asian countries have also been connected with an increased incidence of tumors (esophagus and stomach cancer). However, a causal relationship between these substances and the development of cancer has not been demonstrated for the much lower levels of intake outside the heavily contaminated areas.

For toxicological risk assessment, one must distinguish, in principle, between genotoxic and nongenotoxic carcinogens. No threshold doses can be established for genotoxic carcinogens, which either per se or following metabolic activation react with the genetic material of the cell and thereby may initiate tumor formation. However, as with other substances, their effect is dose-dependent. The magnitude of their potential risk can be demonstrated by comparing the daily intake with the TD_{50} values (the daily doses leading to 50% tumor incidence) determined in animal experiments, or—as another measure for the carcinogenic potential—with the lowest doses for which a carcinogenic effect has been demonstrated (lowest observed effect level, LOEL).

Such comparisons (Table 5) show that the daily levels of intake are considerably below the effective doses observed in animal experiments. For example, the total intake of heterocyclic aromatic amines from heated protein-rich food is estimated to be 1.5 μg/kg body weight/day. Although this intake is relatively large compared to other genotoxic carcinogens, it is lower by a factor of 5000 than the mean TD_{50} of this group of substances, namely 8000 μg/kg body weight/day in mice. When compared to the lowest effective doses, the differences are, of course, smaller. For example, in the United States, the average exposure to aflatoxin B_1 from peanuts is 0.25 ng/kg body weight/day and, therefore, only lower by a factor of 200 than the dose of 50 ng/kg body weight/day, which was apparently carcinogenic in rats. Far greater, however, is the factor between the lowest dose still apparently carcinogenic and the average intake with food for ochratoxin A (80,000) and for benzo(*a*)pyrene (37,000). Benzo(*a*)pyrene, however, always occurs together with other polycyclic aromatic hydrocarbons and therefore the total intake of this group of substances is significantly higher.

Apart from genotoxic carcinogens, some foods contain carcinogenic substances that are not genotoxic or have only secondary genotoxic effects (Table 6). These compounds do not react with the cell's genetic material nor are they converted to genotoxic metabolites. Their action is based on other mechanisms, such as acceleration of normal cell proliferation, cytotoxicity, or induction of oxygen radicals. Once threshold doses have been determined for these primary effects, NOELs for secondary tumor formation can be derived. Some primary effects worth mentioning are the formation of bladder stones after chronic administration of xylitol or terephthalic acid, accumulation of α-2μ-globulin in the renal tubules of male rats (hyalin droplet nephropathy) induced by *d*-limonene, and peroxisome proliferation with increased oxygen radical formation due to the plasticizer di(2-ethylhexyl) phthalate (DEHP) and di(2-ethylhexyl) adipate (DEHA).

TABLE 6 Intake of Nongenotoxic Carcinogens from Food

Substance	Daily intake (DI) (μg/kg body weight/day)	NOEL (μg/kg body weight/day)	NOEL/DI
Caffeic acid	$\sim 10^3$	10^6 (LOEL)	1,000 (LOEL/DI)
d-Limonene	$\sim 10^3$	7.5×10^4 (LOEL)	75 (LOEL/DI)
Saccharin	3×10^3	5×10^5	167
DEHP	3×10^{-1}	5×10^3	16,700
TCDD	1.3×10^{-6} (TCDD equivalent)	10^{-3}	800

Once the NOELs of these substances are known, or when the corresponding mechanism of action is obviously not relevant to humans, tolerable levels of intake can be established by including suitable safety factors. Thus ADI values for *d*-limonene (ADI not specified) and saccharin (0–5 mg/kg body weight/day) have been established by the Joint FAO/WHO Expert Committee on Food Additives. For DEHP, a TDI value of 0.05 mg/kg body weight/day has been established by the Scientific Committee on Food of the EU.

Polychlorinated dibenzo-*p*-dioxins and dibenzofurans also belong to those substances that do not have genotoxic properties. Based on what is known about the Ah receptor-mediated mechanism of their action, they seem to be tumor promoters for which threshold values should exist. Because of their extraordinarily high carcinogenic potential, however, their NOELs are extremely low, for example, 0.001 μg/kg body weight/day in the case of TCDD. Based on this NOEL and depending on the safety factor used, tolerable levels for the intake of TCDD equivalents in the range of 1–10 pg/kg body weight/day have been established.

Bibliography

Ames, B. N., Magaw, R., and Gold, L. S. (1987). Ranking possible carcinogenic hazards. *Science* **236,** 271–280.

Branen, A. L., Davidson, P. M., and Salminen, S. (eds.) (1990). "Food Additives." Dekker, New York.

Classen, H. G., Elias, P. S., and Hammes, W. P. (1987). "Toxikologisch-hygienische Beurteilung von Lebensmittelinhalts- und -zusatzstoffen sowie bedenklicher Verunreinigungen." P. Parey, Berlin.

Concon, J. M. (1988). "Food Toxicology." Dekker, New York.

Doll, R., and Peto, R. (1981). The causes of cancer: Quantitative estimates of avoidable risks of cancer in the United States today. *J. Natl. Cancer Inst.* **66,** 1191–1309.

FAO/WHO (1994). "Summary of Evaluations Performed by the Joint FAO/WHO Expert Committee on Food Additives (JECFA)." FAO/WHO, Geneva.

Ferrer, A., and Cabral, R. (1991). Toxic epidemics caused by alimentary exposure to pesticides: A review. *Food Additives and Contaminants* **8,** 755–776.

Fülgraff, G. (1989). "Lebensmittel-Toxikologie." E. Ulmer, Stuttgart.

Gibson, G. G., and Walker, R. (eds.) (1985). "Food Toxicology—Real or Imaginary Problems?" Taylor and Francis, London.

Knudsen, I. (ed.) (1986). "Genetic Toxicology of the Diet." A. R. Liss, New York.

Lindner, E. (1990). "Toxikologie der Nahrungsmittel," 4th ed. Thieme, Stuttgart.

Lutz, W. K, and Schlatter, J. (1992). Chemical carcinogens and overnutrition in diet-related cancer. *Carcinogenesis* **13,** 2211–2216.

Macholz, R., and Leverenz, H. J. (eds.) (1989). "Lebensmitteltoxikologie." Springer, Berlin.

Miller, S. A. (1991). Food additives and contaminants. *In* "Casarett and Doull's Toxicology" (M. O. Amdur *et al.,* eds.), 4th ed., Pergamon Press, New York, pp. 819–863.

National Research Council, Committee on Food Protection (1973). "Toxicants Occurring Naturally in Foods," 2nd ed. National Academy of Sciences, Washington, DC.

Rechcigl, M., Jr. (1983). "CRC Handbook of Naturally Occurring Food Toxicants." CRC Press, Boca Raton, FL.

Schauder, P. (Ed.) (1991). "Ernährung und Tumorerkrankung." Karger, Basel.

Teuscher, E., and Lindequist, U. (1994). "Biogene Gifte," 2nd ed. Fischer, Stuttgart.

Watson, D. H. (ed.) (1987). "Natural Toxicants in Food. Progress and Prospects." VHC Verlagsgesellschaft, Weinheim; Ellis Horwood, Chichester.

WHO (1987). "Principles for the Safety Assessment of Food Additives and Contaminants in Food." Environmental Health Criteria 70. World Health Organization, Geneva.

CHAPTER

48

Evaluation of Methods for the Registration of Chemicals

HEINZ-PETER GELBKE*, BERNARD HILDEBRAND*, EDWARD J. KERFOOT†

*Department of Toxicology, BASF Aktiengesellschaft, Ludwigshafen, Germany
†Product Regulations and Toxicology, BASF Corporation, Southgate, Michigan

For many years, toxicological studies have been required by regulatory authorities for the registration of pharmaceuticals, crop protection products, and the notification of intent to manufacture new chemical substances. Detailed protocol compilations regarding the scope and conduct of toxicological studies of pharmaceuticals are described by authors such as Hess (1991). Testing requirements for chemicals in general, and specifically for the registration of crop protection products, food additives, and cosmetics, will be described in this chapter.

Originally, there were considerable differences in the toxicological testing requirements among different national regulatory agencies. Therefore, the OECD (Organization for Economic Cooperation and Development) started negotiations to harmonize toxicological test methods at the end of the 1970s. Thus, uniform international guidelines were gradually developed to incorporate state-of-the-art test methods to fulfill the regulatory requirements. These international guidelines had to be adopted as practical methods that could be applied to reflect the broad interests of preventive health protection.

In 1981, this initiative resulted in a description of test methods for the whole range of studies from acute toxicity to carcinogenicity. According to an "OECD decision" (Annex to OECD Guidelines for Testing of Chemicals), the OECD member states agreed to mutually recognize toxicological studies if they had been carried out in accordance with the OECD principles and Good Laboratory Practices (GLPs).

The regulation of test guidelines has advantages and disadvantages. A positive aspect is the legal status that is given by the statutory registration and notification processes. It also ensures that different products are comparably evaluated in different countries or at different times. However, there is a danger that such regulations are not flexible enough to allow the incorporation of new methodology into these international guidelines and other regulations in a timely manner. Because these international test guidelines have gained great importance, they will serve as the basis of the following descriptions of the various toxicological test methods.

The regulatory requirements for the registration of new chemicals in the United States are primarily affected by federal legislation that is administrated by the U.S. EPA. This federal legislation includes the Toxic Substances Control Act (TSCA) and the Federal Insecticide, Fungicide, and Rodenticide Act (FIFRA). Other federal agencies play supporting roles in the approval process of chemicals, depending on the nature of the chemical and its intended use. These agencies/organizations include the Food and Drug Administration (FDA), Occupational Safety and Health Administration (OSHA), and National Institute of Occupational Safety and Health (NIOSH), which operate under separate legislation. This chapter provides a general background on the TSCA, FIFRA, and the Federal Food, Drug, and Cosmetic Act (FDCA) toxicological testing methods required for the registration of chemicals.

GENERAL CONSIDERATIONS

Good Laboratory Practice (GLP)

Today, all toxicological studies for the registration of chemical substances (including pharmaceuticals and crop protection products) must be carried out in compliance with GLP regulations. These regulations evolved in the 1970s under the FDA due to some serious irregularities in safety evaluations that resulted in a need for stricter adherence to appropriate laboratory animal practices and record-keeping. The circumstances at some contract toxicology testing laboratories were highly irregular, casting doubt on the validity of study results on substances that were being submitted for registration. Many of these studies were later audited and some had to be repeated.

Therefore, among the objectives of the GLP regulations are the elimination of disruptive factors in the conduct of the studies, transparency of the studies, integrity of the data, verification of the results, and official control of the testing facility. Regulations were issued for a satisfactory study design, the use of qualified personnel, appropriate instruments and laboratory rooms, complete documentation of all findings, a highly structured study report, and the safe storage of all associated documents. Thus, the GLP guidelines provide general quality assurance requirements, but they do not directly affect the scientific or methodical basis of a study. Some examples provided here will clarify the purpose of the GLP requirements. The reliable record keeping of all data is of central importance. It must be quite clear who obtained the data and at what time. The findings must be recorded in permanent documents; records in pencil are expressly forbidden because they could be altered at a later date. If corrections are necessary, there are detailed instructions as follows:

1. The original entry must still be recognizable after the correction.
2. The reason for each correction must be given in writing.
3. The correction must be dated.
4. The person making the correction has to sign it.

The GLP regulatory value depends on the control measures implemented. Thus, a quality assurance unit has to be established for toxicology laboratories, and this unit should report solely to the head of the institute, independently of the study director. This internal enforcement unit has to systematically monitor the GLP regulations. Furthermore, toxicological testing facilities now have to regularly comply with official controls. The introduction of GLPs involved a considerable increase in the costs of toxicological studies. Operating procedures were formalized; monitoring mechanisms, including the quality assurance unit, had to be established, and extensive written documentation led to an increase in controls and other administrative activities. Today, however, GLP is a trust-building bridge between regulatory agencies and industry. Thus, the authorities know that industry must ensure that the results of its studies are verifiable, and industry must be prepared for governmental inspections at any time. GLP has also led to a considerable improvement in the quality of the reports of toxicological studies because it assures a safeguard against the loss, falsification, or erroneous transmission of data, which is of particular importance in modern toxicity studies that frequently contain several hundred thousand separate pieces of data.

Concomitant Chemical Analysis

The GLP principles of the OECD and of various authorities worldwide require extensive analytical investigations before and during ongoing toxicological studies. In addition to the characterization of the identity, stability, and homogeneity of the test and reference substances, investigations must be carried out to determine the correctness, stability, and homogeneity of the substance itself, as well as the substance in mixtures in the carriers, such as feed, drinking water, or other solvents and suspension agents. In long-term feeding or drinking water studies, concentration control analyses are spot-checked at prolonged intervals. In contrast, in inhalation studies, the substance–air mixtures that are generated have to be monitored regularly (i.e., several times a day or continuously during exposures). The conduct of these analytical investigations is to some extent also subject to the GLP regulations. If the analytical investigations reveal a substantial deviation ($\geq 10\%$) from the nominal doses or concentrations used in a study, it must be taken into consideration when evaluating the toxicological results.

Alternatives to Animal Testing

For some time, there has been a strong movement to reduce the number of animals being used for testing. Many animal rights organizations have demonstrated that some of the animal testing conducted today is no longer needed. This concern is justified in part because occasionally the acute toxic effects of a test chemical can be accurately predicted without animal data. Toxicologists have recognized this fact and alternatives to animal testing are under development or already implemented. On the one hand, the use of *in vitro* test systems, such as cellular and tissue preparations, is constantly being explored to replace some of the screening methods requiring the use of live animals. On the other hand, the use of animal studies is in some cases, such as pregnancy, the only means of obtaining accurate and specific data for a substance with regard to its hazardous potential in humans. Therefore, there is a need to qualify the available test methodologies.

Maintenance of Test Animals

The maintenance of animal facilities must comply with all regulations of the various animal protection acts. A distinction is made between "open" and "closed" maintenance systems, depending on the hygiene status. In recent years, maintenance facilities under suitable "optimal hygienic conditions" (ohc) provided assurance that certain technical factors and conditions of personnel hygiene are observed. In closed or barrier systems, the animals are strictly isolated from the environment. Entry to or exit from the system is only possible via personnel airlocks with obligatory showering and/or change of clothes. Material is introduced via autoclaves or immersion tanks. Particular attention must be paid to the air conditioning and the processing of materials used in the construction of the building. However, this maintenance system is currently used mainly for toxicological studies in SPF (Specific Pathogen Free) animals and in breeding laboratories.

Air-conditioned animal facilities must guarantee an air exchange of at least 10 to 15 air changes per hour, depending on the number of animals in the room. The air pressure in the animal rooms must be higher than outside in order to avoid contamination by microorganisms (about 50 Pa = 5 mm water column). The air flow rate between the racks of animal cages in the rooms should not be more than 0.3 m/s in order to prevent the animals from being exposed to drafts. The air entering and leaving the rooms must also be filtered. Up to three-stage suitable filtration equipment, consisting of prefilters, fine filters, absolute filters or suspended matter filters, is required. A dust filter before the exhaust air ducts is also recommended in the animal rooms in order to prevent the contamination of the duct system.

Adult animals (rats, mice, and hamsters) should be kept at a room temperature of 22 ± 3°C with a relative humidity of 30–70%. Daylight is undesirable in the animal rooms because uncontrollable fluctuations in the intensity and duration of illumination may affect the study results. The rooms must be equipped with natural daylight, or with artifical warm-tone fluorescent lights, which at the same time must ensure that the rooms are illuminated uniformly. As a rule, the dark–light cycle is 12 h, but may be regulated depending on the objective of the study. A light intensity of 300–450 lux, measured about 1 m above the floor, has proved to be sufficient for work place and animal room illumination. The level of noise from equipment should not exceed 50 dB(A) in empty animal rooms. In the event that some of the supply facilities should fail, the technical equipment of the building must guarantee a minimum safety level of 50% operation in order to be able to maintain an emergency service. Today, an automatic data acquisition system with appropriate alarm systems is generally used for monitoring such facilities.

Selection of Test Animals

Depending on the study objective, it must be decided whether inbred or outbred animals are used. With inbred test animals, a homozygotic genotype is reached after about 20 generations of systematic mating between siblings. This means that a substantial degree of homozygosis is achieved and the animals may be expected to react more uniformly in the studies.

In the case of outbred animals, where relatives are prevented from mating with one another, heterozygosis must be retained. The reaction of these test animals in a toxicity study is determined by various genetic parameters and is thus more diverse. Inbred animals are frequently very prone to external influences (stress and infection), whereas outbred animals are more hearty. In some cases, the advantages of inbreeding (uniformity of the reaction) and outbreeding (robustness) may be combined by hybridizing two inbred strains. During randomization of the study groups, attempts should be made to establish biological variability among the dose groups. All pheno- and genotypical features should, if possible, be represented in each of the test groups.

Today, SPF animals are used for toxicological studies wherever possible. In other words, animals are examined regularly and found to be free from specified pathogens. The investigators decide what specific requirements regarding the hygiene status are necesary for the animals when defining objectives and maintenance conditions. It may be necessary, especially in long-term studies, to examine the animals at regular intervals for virus-neutralizing antibodies, not only to check the health of the animals in an ongoing study, but also to yield valuable diagnostic information for the interpretation of potential organ changes. Such investigations may also be carried out for spontaneous bacterial infections or parasitic invasions.

Identification

Test animals must be specifically identified in accordance with GLP guidelines. Even when animals are singly housed, the identification of the cage only is not sufficient. Albino animals can be uniquely identified by ear tattoo (e.g., consecutive numbering system on ear tags) and pigmented animals may be identified by metal or plastic ear tags (with care taken due to the danger of injury). From an animal protection perspective, ears should only be notched or punched in exceptional cases. For some years now, an electronic identification system with implantable transponders has been successfully used. The transponder is injected under the skin and is activated eletromagnetically by means of a reading device and the coding is made visible on the readout. This method is fairly expensive, but has already proved to be valuable in practice.

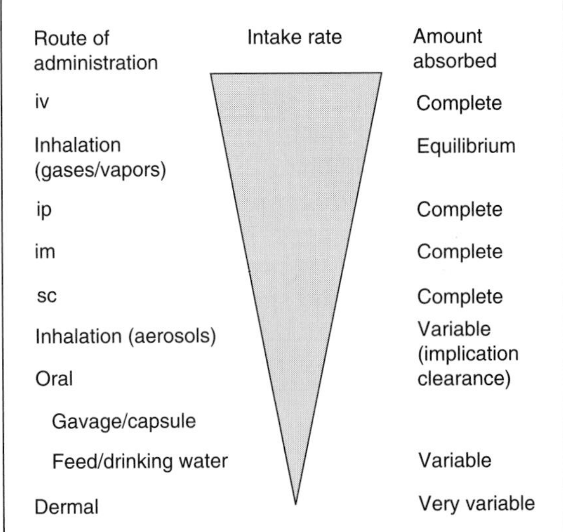

FIGURE 1 The rate of bioavailability frequently drops in the order intravenous > intraperitoneal > intramuscular > subcutaneous > oral > dermal. In the case of the inhalation of gases and vapors, there is in most cases a rapid passage into the total organism; in the case of the inhalation of aerosols, the bioavailability is determined by the solubility of the test substance and by the localization of the precipitate in the respiratory tract (impaction) and may be very low.

Feeding and Watering

Depending on the study objective, feeding is generally ad libitum; a formulated feed is offered as pellets or meal. The latter is particularly suitable in mice and rat studies for administering test substances that are mixed with the feed. Animal drinking water provided by the public water supply system must satisfy the criteria of the drinking water regulations. Apart from watering ad libitum (rodents and dogs) via automatic systems, rodents in particular can be provided with drinking water bottles in order to monitor the daily water consumption. Under GLPs, feed and drinking water are subject to strict quality criteria and checks that are carried out regularly to ensure that these criteria are being met.

Routes of Administration

As a rule, the administration of the test substance in animal studies should correspond to the route of human exposure because the result of the study will significantly depend on the route of administration. Depending on the type of administration, there may be considerable differences in the amount and rate of test substance that is absorbed by the organism (Fig. 1).

In the case of parenteral routes of administration (intravenous, intraperitoneal, intramuscular, and subcutaneous), the dose administered is, of course, directly available in the organism. Depending on the solubility of the material, considerable delays may occur after intramuscular and subcutaneous administration, due to a depot effect. A large proportion of the administered chemical is also taken up by the whole organism upon inhalation of gases and vapors in accordance with the phase equilibrium. Poorly soluble aerosols, however, are taken up from the alveoli into the blood only in small amounts, whereas the residual amounts may be removed from the lungs by mucociliary clearance. In the case of oral and dermal administration, the bioavailability of chemicals may differ considerably depending on their physicochemical properties.

Due to the importance of the oral intake of chemicals, the major variants (diet, drinking water, by gavage or in capsules) will be dealt with in more detail. Administration via the feed or drinking water is preferred, especially in long-term studies because less work is involved. However, these vehicles cannot be used if the test substance is unstable in the carrier, due either to chemical instability or to a reaction with components in the feed or with water. If the test material has an unpleasant taste, the animals may consume less feed or drinking water due to unpalatability. In such cases, daily gavage or administration by capsules is necessary in spite of the additional work involved. Small rodents cannot vomit and this is a particular advantage to dosing. When substances are administered by gavage that are lipophilic or susceptible to hydrolysis, preparations in edible oil are frequently used, although this may lead to a caloric imbalance. When the test substance is administered via feed or drinking water, the uptake of the test substance increases with feed uptake during the night, the active metabolic phase of the animals. The administration of the test substance by gavage or in capsules, however, can put an abrupt strain on the organism. Therefore, depending on the route of administration, considerable differences in pharmacotoxicokinetics may be observed. In the case of dietary administration, a "slow release"-like plasma concentration is measured, whereas after administration by gavage or capsule, a typical peak concentration is observed. These mode of entry differences can have profound effects on the outcome of toxicity studies.

GROUPS OF TOXICOLOGICAL STUDIES

The main purpose of studies for registration or marketing approval of chemicals, crop protection agents, or pharmaceuticals by governmental regulatory authorities is to assess the hazard potential and risk to humans. Safety evaluation studies can be roughly classified with regard to the duration of exposure of the animals (Fig. 2).

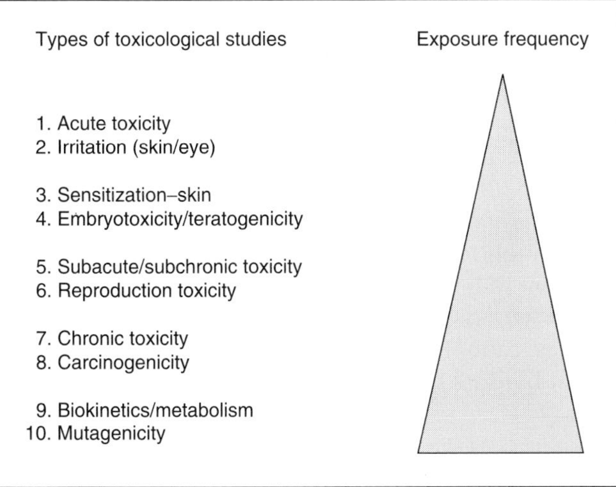

FIGURE 2 In the study types listed, the exposure frequency and duration increases in an inverse sequence from acute toxicity to carcinogenicity. Studies in types 9 and 10 are designed to mainly clarify mechanistic questions.

One type of study is a single administration, such as the testing of acute toxicity or of irritation to the skin and eye. The purpose is to reveal information about the toxic effects after a single high-dose exposure. This type of testing simulates possible risks that may occur in the work place if there are unwanted releases from production units, leaks, spills or cleaning operations, transport accidents, or an intoxication by suicidal intent. At the other end of the scale, there are studies involving the major portion of the animals' life span, such as chronic toxicity and carcinogenicity studies. Here, the potential risk of long-term intake is investigated because no single dose on its own would elicit any detectable effect. The studies for subacute and subchronic toxicity and for reproduction toxicity elicit the toxic risk between these two endpoints.

Some objectives, such as skin sensitization, embryotoxicity, and teratogenicity, cannot be clearly assigned to this dosing scheme. In some cases, single exposures may elicit damage. However, in the case of skin sensitization, at least one additional exposure challenge is necessary to provoke clinical signs. In most instances, definite findings are obtained after repeated exposures. Finally, studies on mutagenicity, pharmacotoxicokinetics and metabolism are required. These studies are primarily designed to clarify mechanistic questions.

TEST METHODS

Acute Toxicity

Acute toxicity means the single administration of a substance to the test animals, usually rodents. The route of administration of a test substance should correspond to the expected route of human exposure. In practice, however, oral administration is the most common method. In the industrial handling of compounds, inhalation and dermal contamination must also be taken into consideration. In the case of pharmaceuticals, parenteral administration routes (intravenous or intramuscular) are commonly used.

In oral-dosing studies, the test substance is most commonly administered by gavage. In dermal studies, the chemical is applied to the skin under occlusive conditions for 24 h. Inhalation studies usually involve a single 4-h exposure at defined concentrations in "nose-only" facilities. Depending on the regulatory requirements, the selected doses may lead to definite toxic lesions, but are not lethal. A lethal dose-50 (LD_{50}) determination is frequently required to classify chemicals and crop protection agents. Therefore, doses in the lethal range have to be administered. The admin-

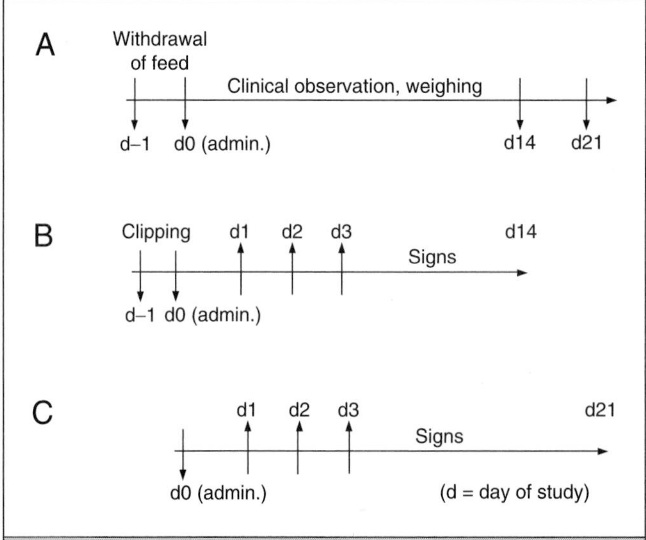

FIGURE 3 OECD methods. Diagrammatic time schedule of studies with a single administration. (A) Acute toxicity studies with different routes of administration and the schedules of studies on (B) skin and (c) eye irritation.

istration of the test substance is followed by an observation period of at least 14 days, which may be extended if the signs of toxicity continue. During this period, the toxic signs and the body weight must be checked regularly. At the end of the study, the animals undergo necropsy and the organs are examined for any gross lesions (Fig. 3). In case of specific objectives, histopathological examinations may also be required.

Skin Irritation

Skin-irritation studies are usually carried out on albino rabbits or guinea pigs. The fur is first clipped, and 24 h later the test substance is applied to the skin for 4 hours, generally under semi-occlusive conditions. The skin is evaluated for manifestations of irreversible tissue damage, such as erythema, edema, or necroses at 1, 2, and 3 days following application. If the reversibility of the effects cannot be estimated adequately, the observation period must be extended; as a rule, 14 days are sufficient (Fig. 3).

Eye Irritation

Albino rabbits are also generally used for eye-irritation studies. Approximately 100 μl of the test chemical (as a liquid or bulk volume of solids) is applied to the lower conjunctival sac of the eye. Observations are recorded after 1, 2, and 3 days of, for example, the effects on the conjunctivae (redness or edema), on the cornea (opacity to corrosion), and on the iris (inflammation caused by chemicals). An extension of the observation period may be necessary. As a rule, 21 days are sufficient in order to clarify the reversibility of more serious findings (Fig. 3).

It should be emphasized that the studies on skin and eye irritation are particularly sensitive. For example, it has been shown that the skin of albino rabbits has a particularly high sensitivity in comparison to that of primates and humans. The exposure procedures are much more stringent than the conditions under which human exposure would occur. For example, animal testing involves semi-occlusive and long-term (4-hour) contact of the test substance with the skin. In the case of the ocular-sensitivity evaluation, the large amount of test substance (100 μl) and the close contact with the cornea and conjunctivae via application to the conjunctival sac provide conditions unlikely to be encountered by humans. These studies reflect worst-case scenarios and the results of these studies cannot be extrapolated without considering the individual situation of humans carefully.

Skin Sensitization

Skin-sensitization studies, which are generally carried out on guinea pigs, simulate the course of an immunological reaction in its three phases.

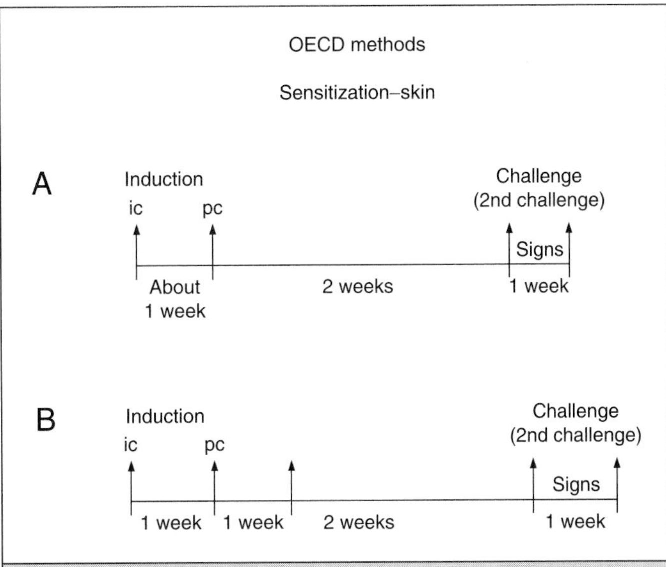

FIGURE 4 OECD methods, skin sensitization. In (A) the maximization test, the skin barrier is penetrated by intracutaneous (ic) injection. Induction in (B) the Buehler test is carried out by repeated percutaneous (pc) induction (wk. = week).

1. Induction of immunologically competent cells.
2. Rest phase for the proliferation of the immunologically competent cells.
3. Challenge to unmask any change in the immune response.

The conditions during the induction phase are of particular importance. During its course, the sensitivity of the animal model may be increased, for example, by the occlusive percutaneous contact of the test substance, multiple exposures, long-term skin contact, or penetration of the skin barrier by intracutaneous injection of Freund's adjuvant to stimulate the immune system. The various combinations of these marginal conditions led to the development of numerous test models. The Buehler test and the maximization test, in particular, have become internationally established (Fig. 4). The maximization test was designed for the highest possible sensitivity in order to enable it to detect weaker and moderately potent sensitizers. With adequate sensitivity, the Buehler test is based on the possibility of exposures in the real world and is particularly suitable for testing mixtures and formulations.

In the maximization test, the test substance is injected intracutaneously together with Freund's adjuvant for optimal induction and administered again 1 week later percutaneously (48 hours occlusively). As far as possible, a minimal- to definite-irritant dose concentration of the test chemical is chosen. In the Buehler test, induction is carried out by administering irritant concentrations of the test chemical percutaneously (6 hours under occlusive conditions) three times at weekly intervals. A 2-week rest period follows in both methods. The challenge is then carried out with the highest nonirritant concentration of the test chemical. Should skin changes (e.g., erythema and edema) occur under these conditions, the outcome is interpreted as evidence of an earlier sensitization. If the results are inconclusive, the reaction may be checked 1 week later with a second challenge.

Toxicity after Repeated Administration

Animal studies with repeated administrations are useful in answering a series of questions. Initial range-finding studies to clarify the toxicity profile of substances that have not yet been investigated are generally carried out following oral administration to rats for 28 consecutive days. This type of evaluation is part of the base set in the EU guidelines for new chemicals. Subacute studies involving an administration period of 14–28 days are also usually conducted to define a suitable dose range for further investigations. Although subacute evaluations are not routinely required, they are necessary to clarify the route of administration and the dose range for long-term studies. A dose of 1000 mg/kg body weight has commonly become established as the upper limit for all types of studies with repeated oral administration (OECD limit tests). In the case of food additives, a 5% concentration in the feed is an accepted upper limit (e.g., the FDA's "Redbook"). If preliminary observations reveal that not enough test substance will be taken up, these upper limits or definite signs of toxicity are not going to be achieved. In this case, if the administration via the feed or drinking water is interrupted due to a taste aversion (limited palatibility), different routes of administration must be chosen, such as daily gavage or inhalation, if there is specific human exposure by that route. Rarely is dermal exposure selected for determining the toxic profile.

In inhalation exposure to dusts, lung clearance may be explored in preliminary studies in which the animals are exposed for 14 or 28 days and are then observed for various periods up to 12 months without any further treatment. The retention time of the substance in the lungs can then be evaluated. Knowledge of the threshold concentration at which the physiological clearance of inhaled particles is impaired is of particular importance for long-term inhalation studies in order to avoid overload phenomena, which may occur at concentrations with no practical exposure situation relevance.

The determination of the irritation threshold after repeated dermal applications is the primary objective of preliminary studies over a period of 5 to 30 days (in exceptional cases even up to 90 days), depending on the purpose of the subsequent studies. Systemic toxicity after dermal application is generally determined based on 21-day studies in rats or rabbits. The information is used for risk assessment of occupational dermal exposure (e.g., in crop protection production). Extended preliminary evaluations are recommended before the main skin painting is carried out, to determine the carcinogenic potential. These studies may be conducted over the life span of various mouse strains.

The typical 90-day studies have proved suitable for assessing the risk of numerous different exposure scenarios and are firmly established in regulatory requirements. In addition to obtaining a reliable toxicity profile from such broadly based studies, which should cover all organ systems and body functions, the determination of a no observed adverse effect level (NOAEL) is among the objectives of this study. The results of 90-day studies are also used to determine the highest dose for subsequent long-term studies on carcinogenicity that adopt the concept of the "maximum tolerable dose" (MTD).

Risk assessment from chronic toxicity studies are particularly suitable for compounds intended for chronic treatment (drugs) or when a potential long-term exposure of the general public is possible. The latter include food additives, residues of crop protection products, and solvents widely used in consumer products. The duration of treatment specific in the different testing guidelines varies between 12 and 24 months for rodents (generally rats) and for nonrodents (commonly dogs).

The carcinogenic potential of substances is investigated in life-time studies in rats or mice. Depending on the objective, several nontoxic doses of the test substance may be administered by gavage, via the feed or drinking water, by inhalation (6 to 24 h, 5 to 7 days per week) and by skin painting or dripping (2 to 5 times per week). The route of administration should reflect the expected human exposure route to facilitate use of the data for a reasonable risk assessment.

During these studies with repeated administration, the body weight gain or loss of the test animals must be monitored regularly. The exposure to the test substance must be determined by measuring the feed and drinking water consumption, as well as the test article concentration in the case of oral administration and by monitoring the air concentrations in the chamber as frequently as possible or continuously. In inhalation studies, the exposure data are usually given in mg/m^3 or ppm, or in ml/m^3 for vapors and gases. In oral studies, doses are given in mg/kg body weight. In skin painting studies, the concentration of the test substance in the solvent and the absolute amount applied per animal is decisive. Studies using other routes of administration, such as intraperitoneal injection, intratracheal instillation, and subcutaneous or intramuscular injection or implantation, may be used as screening studies or for answering specific questions, for example, about mechanisions of toxicity. However, there is usually insufficient data for determining risk assessments in humans. Further parameters are evaluated during physical examinations, clinical chemistry tests, hematology, and other investigations.

Where clinical findings are obtained at least once a week by examining the animals thoroughly, other parameters in studies of up to 90 days are determined by blood sampling or urine collection at least once per study and in long-term studies, as a rule, at half-year intervals. The choice of parameters for such examinations will be adapted to the known or assumed profile of the test substance. However, most parameters have now become more routinely established for these examinations, due to the increasing availability of automation in clinical chemistry and hematology (Table 1).

All studies with repeated administration provide results for a thorough gross pathological examination during necropsy. The scope of other examinations,

TABLE 1 Minimum Scope of Parameters to be Examined in Hematological and Clinicochemical Investigations

	Blood examinations	
Hematology and differential blood count	Hemoglobin Hematocrit Mean corpuscular volume Mean corpuscular hemoglobin concentration Reticulocytes	Erythrocytes Mean corpuscular hemoglobin Platelets Leukocytes Differential blood count
Clotting analysis	Hepato Quick's test	
Blood chemistry	Total bilirubin Urea Potassium Albumin Inorganic phosphate Chloride Cholesterol	Creatinine Sodium Total protein Glucose Calcium Triglycerides
Enzymes	Alanine aminotransferase Alkaline phosphatase	Aspartate aminotransferase
	Urinalysis	
pH	Protein	Glucose
Ketones	Bilirubin	Blood
Nitrite	Urobilinogen	Sediment microscopy

such as the determination of organ weights or the histopathological evaluation of various organs, may vary substantially depending on the duration of the study. The histopathological examination of macroscopically visible changes and of known or assumed target organs is always required. The examinations in the range-finding studies for determining the toxic profile are restricted to the large parenchymatous organs and selected organs of reproduction and of the nervous and immune systems. The whole spectrum of the different tissues should be examined in the subsequent studies (>90 days) (Table 2).

The overall goal of the assessment of the data from all toxicity studies is to describe the toxic profile, determine a NOAEL, and finally, identify potential carcinogenic effects. In long-term studies, a large number of animals, at least 50 animals per group and sex, are used, although the first signs of a possible carcinogenic effect may have already been obtained in shorter studies. Particularly, nongenotoxic substances showing special morphological and biochemical features may also be manifested in subacute and subchronic studies. These data should be regarded as the indicators of potential cell proliferation of target tissues.

Of particular importance in animal studies with repeated administration are the appropriate hygienic and logistic conditions, including a detailed study de-

TABLE 2 Minimum Scope of the Organs and Tissues to Be Examined Histopathologically in Toxicological Studies for 90 Days and Longer

Brain, duodenum	Adrenals	Pancreas
Pituitary	Esophagus	Testes and ovaries
Thyroids (with cecum parathyroids)	Stomach	Accessory
Thymus	Skeletal muscle	Female mammary gland
Lungs, uterus	Jejunum	Skin
Trachea	Ileum	Peripheral nerve
Heart, lymph nodes	Colon	Spinal cord (cervical, thoracic and lumber cords)
Salivary glands	Rectum	Sternum with marrow
Liver (with gall bladder)	Femur with joint	Eyes
Spleen, genital organs	Urinary bladder all gross lesions	Target organs
Kidneys		

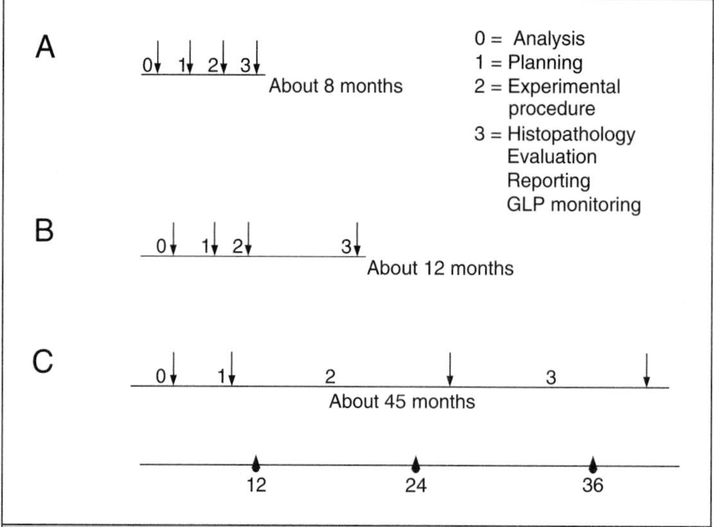

FIGURE 5 Time schedule, toxicity after repeated administration (A) subacute, (B) subchronic, and (C) chronic or carcinogenic. The duration of phase 3 within the toxicological studies, which determines the time in addition to the actual experimental procedure, is especially dependent on the number of animals per study and the number of tissues to be examined histopathologically.

sign (protocol), organized cooperation between various disciplines in toxicology (chemistry, animal maintenance, clinical chemistry, hematology, pathology, histology, and biostatistics), and a realistic time schedule (Fig. 5). As shown in the time schedules of the various studies, the evaluation of the data, and especially the histotechnical processing and histopathological assessment of the organs, may take several months, depending on the number of animals in the study. The evaluation of carcinogenicity studies with 400 to 600 rodents is particularly lengthy and expensive. The evaluation of chronic studies with dogs is less intensive because the minimum number of animals required in most testing guidelines is only four dogs per dose and sex. In subacute rodent studies, there are at least five animals per dose and sex, and in subchronic studies there are usually 10 animals per dose and sex. Here the evaluation times are correspondingly shorter. It should be taken into consideration that the shorter studies must be completely evaluated before the subsequent long-term studies with the same test substance can be started. This is necessary for not only planning the lowest dose in the chronic toxicity study for obtaining a NOAEL, but also for finding the highest dose for carcinogenicity studies, defined as MTD. This means that for an entire toxicological program with a consistent schedule, a total time period of about 60 months is necessary. Because carcinogenicity studies are always required for the registration of crop protection products, this study determines the start of the preparation of the toxicological registration dossier.

Reproduction Toxicity

The purpose of reproduction toxicity studies is to determine the potential adverse effects of chemicals in the male and female reproduction systems. Generation studies are designed to determine adverse effects by the test substance on the gonadal function, estrous cycle, mating behavior, fertilization, fertility, course of pregnancy, parturition, and postnatal development of the offspring. However, possible teratogenic effects of a substance (i.e., gross structural changes), in particular, can only be revealed to a limited extent in generation studies. Therefore, embryotoxicity studies are suitable, in which the test substance is administered to the dam during organogenesis, the most sensitive phase of embryonic development.

Multigeneration Studies

Multigeneration studies are carried out to assess the risks, especially of food additives and pesticides, to which humans may be exposed for prolonged periods. The design of such studies may vary depending on the requirements of the registration authority. Today, two-generation studies are carried out according to the guidelines of the OECD, EPA/FIFRA, EPA/TSCA, and JAPAN/MAFF. However, depending on specific requirements, the test substance may be administered over only one, two, or more than two parent generations. In the following, the design and course of a typical two-generation study in rats will be given.

Most official guidelines recommend the use of rats, and rarely mice, in two-generation studies. However, other mammalian species may also be employed if the fertility rate is adequate. Rats and mice are particularly suitable for such studies due to their high fertility, relatively shorter gestation periods, and simple maintenance and handling. Furthermore, the reproduction physiology of the two species is well-known and the reproduction parameters exhibit more or less constant values in the rat strains used.

All statutory guidelines require at least three dose groups and one control group for two-generation studies. A test group should consist of at least 20 pregnant females and a corresponding number of males. The highest dose should be toxic for the treated animals, but not cause mortalities, if possible. The lowest dose should not elicit any toxic effects in the test animals. As a rule, the relationship between the doses should be a geometrical series. The intermediate dose, on the one hand, may elicit marginal effects in the parents and/or pups, or, on the other hand, this dose may even prove to be the no effect dose. The correct selection of doses is a decisive factor in planning such a study. The results from preliminary studies, specific range-finding, or reliable data from other toxicological studies are absolutely necessary. For practical reasons, the test substance is administered most frequently via the feed or drinking water. In a two-generation study, F_1 pups are obtained by mating the first parents (F_0). Selected F_1 pups are reared as the second parent (F_1) generation, and then, are mated with each other to produce F_2 pups (Fig. 6).

The administration of the test substance to the animals of the first parent (F_0) generation begins at an age of 5–9 weeks. There is a constant exposure for all following generations that descend from the F_0 generation or from the subsequent generation.

Before mating, the F_0 parent animals are generally exposed for 8–10 weeks and the F_1 parent animals for about 14 weeks. An exception to this procedure are the OECD guidelines, which recommend that the female F_0 parent animals should be pretreated merely for a period of at least two estrous cycles (i.e., 8–10 days). Here the males and females are mated with each other in a ratio of 1:1 or 1:2 until mating has taken place or 3 weeks have elapsed. Successful mating may be determined by the presence of a copulation plug in the female or by a vaginal smear. If further litters are needed from the same parent generation (e.g., in order to check whether the effects observed in the first litter are caused by the test sub-

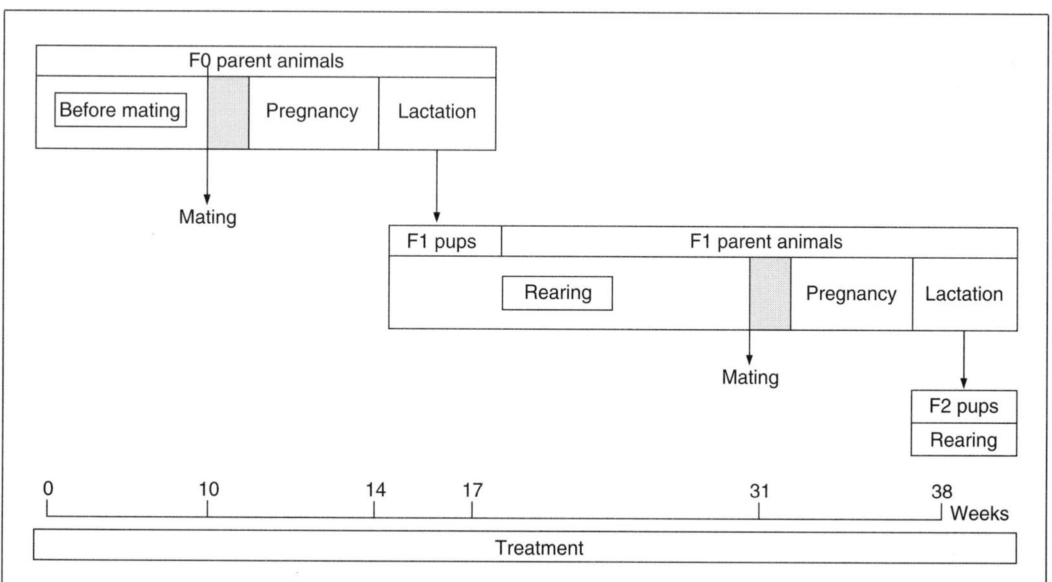

FIGURE 6 In the two-generation study in rats, the parents and the offspring are exposed for two generations in the same way to concentrations of the test substance constantly maintained during all phases of reproduction.

stance or are of spontaneous genesis), mating takes place again about 10–15 days after the pups have been separated from the dam. Mating between siblings must definitely be avoided.

The pregnant female F_0 and F_1 parent animals deliver the pups spontaneously and rear them for 3 weeks. Then the pups are removed from the dam (weaning of the pups) and are either sacrificed or used for further breeding. In order to reduce the impact of litter size on the development of the pups, some guidelines recommend a reduction of the litter size on the 4th day after delivery to four male and four female pups.

Immediately after parturition and during the lactation period, the live, dead, and malformed pups are recorded. The body weight of the live pups is periodically determined and recorded, along with their behavior, physical development, and clinical appearance. Dead pups are macroscopically examined, as are those sacrificed on the 4th day after birth to standardize the size of the litters and those sacrificed after weaning on the 21st day.

During the study, not only are the usual toxicological parameters (e.g., feed consumption, body weight gain, clinical findings, and mortality) assessed in the parent animals, but also the mating-specific behavior, fertility, and the behavior of dams during pregnancy, parturition, and lactation. After their pups have been reared, the F_0 and F_1 parent animals are sacrificed and necropsied. Primarily, the reproductive organs and the accessory gonads are subjected to a thorough gross pathological examination. Tissue from these organs and other target organs with macroscopically visible pathological changes are then processed and examined histopathologically, always in the control and highest dose groups. In the other groups, histopathology is performed if there are substance-induced lesions. Furthermore, all parent animals that died during the study must be subjected to gross pathological and complete histopathological examinations. Blood sampling for specific hematological and/or clinical chemistry may be carried out on the weaned pups or their parents.

Embryotoxicity Studies

The development of the embryo is the most sensitive stage of the whole reproduction cycle. The effect of exogenous factors, such as chemicals, during this period may lead to fetal death, malformations, and growth retardation, as well as to postnatal damage to the offspring. In teratogenic studies, the compound is administered during the sensitive organogenesis phase of the embryo. The fetuses are removed from the uterus shortly before parturition and examined. Two species, a rodent (rats or mice) and a nonrodent (rabbits), are normally used in order to obtain reliable information on the prenatal toxicity of a substance.

In general, these studies are performed using at least three dose groups and a control group, each with at least 20 pregnant female rats or mice and 12 pregnant rabbits. If the compound is known to be less toxic, a limit test may be carried out with only one dose of ≥1000 mg/kg body weight/day and one control group. Preliminary studies are critical for a reliable selection of the doses because a massive impairment of the dams' health, even without any specific effect of the test substance, may cause the death of the fetuses or induce malformations. In an embryotoxicity study conducted under the test guidelines, the highest dose should only elicit a slight toxic effect (e.g., slight loss of weight) in the dams. The lowest dose should not elicit any substance-induced effects, whereas the intermediate dose should be the geometrical mean.

The test substance is administered daily from days 6 to 18 of gestation, generally by gavage, to pregnant female rats and mice at about the time of implementation up to the end of the embryonic phase (Fig. 7). The repeated administration of the compound is necessary because the specific developmental stage of the embryo during which it is maximally affected by the test substance is not known. The embryotoxicity of a compound is of particular relevance when observed at doses that are not maternally toxic. The body weight and feed consumption (sometimes the drinking water consumption as well) of the dams are determined for the whole duration of the study. The general status of the animals is observed daily with special attention given to any indications of intrauterine fetal death (vaginal hemorrhages and abortions).

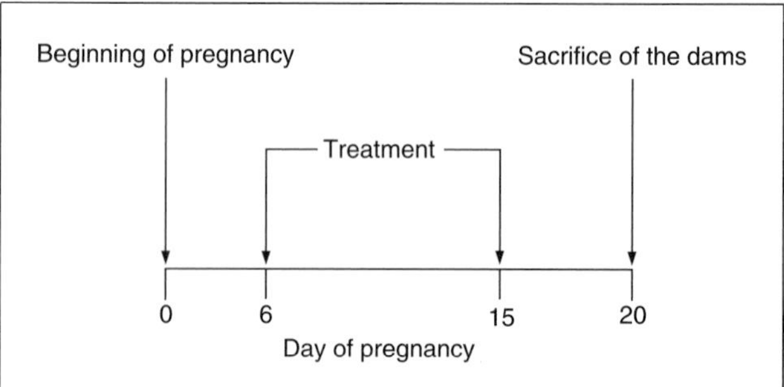

FIGURE 7 In an embryotoxicity study in rats, the dams are treated during the organogenesis of the embryos. The important examinations are carried out in the fetuses, which are removed from the uterus of the sacrificed dams shortly before parturition (day 20).

Clinical chemistry, hematological examinations, and organ-weight determinations are not usually carried out here because it is often done in the preliminary studies.

Approximately 1 day before the expected date of parturition (in rats approximately on day 20; in rabbits approximately on day 30 after fertilization), the dams are sacrificed and their uteri are removed with the ovaries. This procedure prevents the dams from cannibalizing their malformed or stillborn offspring. Furthermore, the developmental defects attributed to the test substance and an abnormal gestation period cannot be compensated for by a prolonged gestation period and thus remain undiscovered. When the uterus has been removed from the abdominal cavity, the dams are subjected to a gross pathological examination to determine any compound-related effects.

The uterus is then opened and the live and dead fetuses are counted, weighed, and the determination of their sex and the date of death of the fetuses that have already been resorbed during gestation is estimated based on their development (early or late resorptions). The corpora lutea on the ovaries are also counted. After the examination of all fetuses for any visible changes, the fetuses are also examined for malformations of the skeleton and/or soft tissues. In rabbits, all fetuses are evaluated for skeletal and organ changes, while only about half of rat or mouse fetuses are used for skeletal examinations and the other half for soft tissue examinations. In order to assess the skeletons of the fetuses, they are generally stained with Alizarin Red after all soft tissues have been macerated in caustic soda or potash solution and assessed microscopically using Dawson's method (1926). The organs of the rabbit fetuses are generally examined in a nonfixed state immediately after being removed from the uterus, while the soft tissues of the rat and mouse fetuses are usually assessed after being fixed in Bouin's solution.

Various methods may be used to examine rat, mouse, and rabbit fetuses according to Wilson's method (1985). Cross sections of the fixed fetuses about 1 mm thick are prepared and assessed or according to Barrow and Taylor (1969). The thoracic and abdominal cavities of the fetuses are opened to study the natural position of the organs in question before further examinations are conducted. The gross structural, visible skeletal, and organ effects observed are frequently divided into malformations (i.e., rare findings and/or findings inconsistent with life), such as cleft palate and hydrocephalus; variations (minor deviations from normal that are consistent with life and may also occur in controls), such as the primordium of an additional rib; and retardations (retardations in the development), such as the retarded ossification of bone elements. Because such findings may also occur spontaneously, it is essential for a final evaluation that the historical control data collected from earlier studies also be used in the assessment. This characteristic data for the animal species and strain provides information about the appearance and frequency of occurrence of spontaneous changes. By comparing the historical and actual control data with the findings in the treatment groups, it is possible to estimate the teratogenic properties of a compound more reliably.

Genotoxicity

There are over 100 test methods available for testing genotoxic effects *in vitro* (in bacteria, yeasts, fungi, and mammalian cells) and *in vivo* on somatic and germ cells (*Drosophila,* mouse, hamster, and rat). These test systems may be used for detecting the various genetic endpoints of point mutations, chromosome aberrations, genome mutations, and DNA damage and repair. Although many of these test methods are continuously being modified, the majority of them are not sufficiently standardized or validated to be required by the agencies.

Uniform testing guidelines establishing minimal criteria were prepared for the most common test methods through the international harmonization of the OECD at the end of the 1970s. These methods, valid in principle for all substances to be investigated, were generally adopted by the EU and are being continuously modified to adapt them to the current state-of-the-art methodology. Testing guidelines were also issued in the United States by the EPA and in Japan by various authorities. However, these guidelines are only collections of methods and do not contain a recommendation for a suitable choice and interpretations of the results.

In the meantime, genotoxicity studies have become a strict regulatory requirement in many countries for authorizing the marketing of chemicals, pharmaceuticals, and crop protection agents. The objective of such investigations is not merely limited to detecting a genotoxic effect, but they may also be used to screen for a possible carcinogenic potential. Two tests are required as a minimum by most authorities; one test has to be carried out for the detection of point mutations and another one for the determination of chromosome changes.

The most common methods are:

1. Point mutations. Point mutation test in *Salmonella typhimurium* and/or *Escherichia coli;* point mutation test in mammalian cells *in vitro.*

2. Chromosome aberrations. Chromosome aberration test in mammalian cells *in vitro; in vivo* studies in the bone marrow of mammals; micronucleus test; and chromosome analysis.

Further batteries of tests may be required, depending on the results of the preliminary mutagenicity studies, on the production volume, and on the intended application of a substance and the possible exposures. Test methods to detect an *in vivo* point mutation and DNA damage and repair have only played a minor role in requirements of the agencies. Similarly, investigations for "genome mutations" are not usually required because sufficient validated test methods are not available. Indications of genome mutations (aneuploidies and polyploidies) must, therefore, be cytogenetic studies (e.g., chromosome analysis and micronucleus test).

EXTRAPOLATION AND CORRELATION OF ANIMAL DATA

From the various toxicological investigations, the toxicologist must extrapolate and correlate the data for assessing the risk of human exposures; the results from animal studies are extrapolated to predict a response in humans. Sometimes, it is difficult to elicit the same response in humans because of ethical reasons or because the selected animal species is not a suitable model. The target tissue dose is not always directly related to the dose administered because of different absorption, distribution, metabolism, and elimination processes. Conventional pharmacokinetic models have been of great use in examining the consequences of nonlinear processes on tissue dosimetry, but have been of less value in extrapolating the effects after dosages some orders of magnitude lower than in animal experiments. In physiologically based pharmacokinetic models, compartments are related to specific organs or tissue groups and attempt to describe a simulation of the physiological characteristics and pathways for compound metabolism and disposition. These models are readily amenable to high-dose to low-dose, dose-route, interspecies, and exposure scenario extrapolations of tissue dosimetry, but have to be used with experience and the necessary precautions.

RISK ASSESSMENT AND RISK MANAGEMENT

Risk assessment and risk management are the processes used to evaluate and control risks associated with exposure to toxic substances. Risk assessment information from existing toxicology, epidemiology, environmental fate, and potential exposures are used to describe the likely health hazards to humans or the environment. The guidelines established by the EPA uses a three-step process for regulatory decisions and action—research, risk assessment, and risk management.

The research element of the process uses laboratory and field observations, toxicological studies, and field measurements. It begins with laboratory and field observations of adverse health effects and exposures to particular agents. This information is used later as a basis for making a hazard identification. From animal toxicological studies, information is extrapolated from high- to low-dose studies and from animals to humans. Field measurements to estimate and characterize the population exposures are the last step in the research process.

Following the research phases, the procedures of hazard identification, dose–response assessments, and exposure assessments are used to characterize the risk. Hazard identification attempts to determine whether the agent causes an adverse effect using laboratory and field observations. From the hazard identification, a dose–response assessment is made from the toxicological investigations. Extrapolations and correlations are then made from the various tests for potential human consequences. Exposure assessments under different conditions are very critical in determining the total risk. The toxicity and potential exposures are then evaluated to characterize the risk.

From an industrial perspective, once a risk is properly assessed and characterized, it can be managed. The management of the risk may involve the elimination of the risk in some cases or, more commonly, reducing the risk by various control measures. Risk management, from a regulatory perspective, involves the development of regulatory options incorporating the public health, economic, social, and political consequences of these regulatory alternatives. From these options and evaluations of the risk characterization, a regulatory agency should be able to make accurate and reasonable regulatory decisions on managing the risk. These actions should result in realistic scientific regulations with which the regulated community can comply and that the agency can reasonably enforce.

Decisions regulating the use, manufacture, and disposal of a chemical can have far-reaching effects economically and socially. These regulatory decisions are often based on a risk characterization that uses health-based risk estimates. There is considerable interest in understanding the dynamics of risk assessment and risk management as practiced by the agencies, along with a concomitant concern for improving the process. Through effective risk assessment and risk characterization to reduce the uncertainty factors, there is a definite need to identify the research needs. This feedback allows for a better understanding of the mechanistic linkages between toxicity, exposure, and response. To develop pertinent mechanistic information, for example, a four-pronged multidisciplinary research approach is used, involving *in vitro* studies with cells and tissues from both laboratory animals and humans, *in vivo* studies using laboratory animals, the use of whatever data are available from clinical investigations and epidemiological studies of human populations, and the use of information on the physical and chemical properties of chemicals. Biomathematical and computer models are frequently used to integrate data from the four types of studies, especially to facilitate assessments of human risk.

PRODUCT SAFETY AND PRODUCT STEWARDSHIP

The chemical industry is concerned with the safety of the thousands of chemical substances in commerce today and their potential effects on its employees, its customers, and the environment. Product safety has been a major concern and effort for the chemical industry over the years, and there is also much more emphasis directed toward this area on an international basis.

Laboratory testing to learn more about toxicity and potential exposures has greatly expanded. Many highly sophisticated methods to test for a variety of possible health effects caused by exposure to chemicals are more readily available. This testing is done by companies in their own laboratories, contract facilities, universities, or private institutes. The studies are sponsored by individual companies or are jointly sponsored by groups of companies.

This research-testing effort will help the industry reevaluate the safety of many long-accepted chemical compounds. Regulations, such as those under the Toxic Substances Control Act (TSCA), are designed to ensure that new and existing chemicals do not constitute an unreasonable risk. Together, this product safety effort is focusing on developing toxicological information for safe handling of chemicals that is useful by all people involved with the product's life cycle, from research, manufacturing, and transportation to end-use and disposal. This philosophy is the basis for product stewardship.

Product stewardship, however, goes beyond regulation. Responsible chemical companies today conduct testing not only to comply with regulations, but to adequately charcterize these substances for the product's life cycle. Research efforts are currently underway to provide mechanistic information for linking sources of chemicals to human exposure, the dose delivered to critical biological targets, and the potential health responses that may be produced.

Bibliography

Ames, B., McCann, J., and Yamasaki, E. (1975). Methods for detecting carginogens and mutagens with the salmonella/mammalian microsome mutagenicity test. *Mutat Res.* **31,** 347–364.

Barrow, M. V., and Taylor, W. J. (1969). A rapid method for detecting malformations in rat fetuses. *J. Morphol.* **127,** 291–306.

Buehler, E. V. (1965). Delayed contact hypersensitivity in the guinea pig. *Arch. Dermatol.* **91,** 171–177.

Calabrese, E. J. (1983). "Principles of Animal Extrapolation." Wiley, New York.

Dawson, A. B. (1926). A note on the staining of the skeleton of cleared specimens with Alizarin Red S. *Stain Technol.* **1,** 123–124.

Dearfield, K. L., Auletta, A. E., Cimino, M. C., and Moore, M. M. (1991). Considerations in the U.S. Environmental Protection Agency's testing approach for mutagenicity. *Mutat. Res.* **258,** 259–283.

Draize, J. H., Woodard, G., and Calvery, H. O. (1944). Methods for the study of irritation and toxicity of substances applied typically to the skin and mucous membranes. *J. Pharmacol. Exp. Ther.* **82,** 377–390.

Hess, R. (ed.) (1991). "Arzneimitteltoxikologie: Anforderungen, Verfahren, Bedeutung." Georg Thieme Verlag, Stuttgart.

Hildebrand, B., Ashby, J., Grasso, P., Sharrat, M., Bontinck, W. J., and Smith, E. (eds.) (1991). Early indicators of non-genotoxic carcinogenesis. *Mutat. Res.* **248,** 211–374.

Kästner, W. (1977). Zur Speziesabhängigkeit der Hautverträglichkeit von Kosmetik-Grundstoffen. *J. Soc. Cosmet. Chem.* **28,** 741–754.

Kerfoot, E. J. (1995). Industrial toxicology. *In* "Handbook of Highly Toxic Materials Handling and Management" (S. S. Grossel and D. A. Crowl, eds.), pp. 21–59. Dekker, New York.

Kerfoot, E. J., Klosowski, M., Steinmetz, D., and Kovalic, J. (1990–1991). A chemical company's compliance experience and outlook with the Toxic Substances Control Act. *Environ. Carcinog. Rev. J. Environ. Sci. Health* **C8,** 379–390.

Magnusson, B., and Kligman, A. M. (1969). The identification of contact allergens by animal assay. The guinea pig maximisation test. *J. Invest. Dermatol.* **52,** 268–272.

McKenna, W., and Cuneo, G. (1997). "TSCA Handbook," 3rd ed. Government Institute, Rockville, MD.

Wilson, J. G. (1985). Methods for administering agents and detecting malformations. *In* "Teratology, Principles and Techniques" (J. G. Wilson and J. Warkany, eds.), pp. 251–277. University of Chicago Press, Chicago.

CHAPTER

49

In Vitro Methods

HORST SPIELMANN*, ALAN M. GOLDBERG†

*National Center for Documentation and Evaluation of Alternatives to Animal Experiments, BgVV, Berlin, Germany 12277

†Center for Alternatives to Animal Testing, Johns Hopkins University Baltimore, Maryland 21202

INTRODUCTION

During the 20th century, the field of toxicology has evolved from describing the consequences of exposure to chemicals, to studying xenobiotics in animals, to mechanistically based studies of both animals and cell or tissue cultures. During the 1990s, *in vitro* studies of cell and tissue cultures, such as the Ames mutagenicity assay, have become important approaches used to understand the consequences of exposure and to assign risk.

In both U.S. and European laboratories, scientists have vigorously pursued the development of *in vitro* methods to advance their science. Since the 1970s, the considerable and significant advances in tissue culture methodology, the use of chemically defined cell and tissue culture media, and the availability of human cells have transformed *in vitro* methods from a new technology to a valuable research tool.

In product development, drug discovery, and safety evaluation, the use of *in vitro* tests has become commonplace, resulting almost exclusively from the evolution of science rather than any fundamental change in philosophy. Yet all *in vitro* methods are alternatives to animal testing.

THE THREE Rs CONCEPT OF RUSSELL AND BURCH

The term "alternative" emerged following the publication of a now-classic book by William Russell and Rex Burch, *The Principles of Humane Experimental Technique*. The authors suggested that proper experimental design should consider methods that *refined* current techniques to lessen pain or distress, *reduced* the number of animals necessary for a particular test, or *replaced* animals with non-whole-animal models, such as *in vitro* cell cultures. The concept of refinement, reduction, and replacement became known as the "Three Rs," and methods that incorporated one or more of the Three Rs were considered "alternative" methods.

Refinement alternatives are methods that either eliminate or minimize pain and distress to the animal or enhance the animal's well-being. The assessment of pain in animals is difficult, but generally one can recognize that an animal is in pain or predict that if a procedure would be painful to humans it would be painful to animals. Just recognizing this can change experimental design. Animal well-being can be enhanced by using appropriate handling techniques and cage sizes, as well as by environmental enrichment techniques well known to the psychological field.

Reduction alternatives are those methods that provide the correct number of data for an experimental design. It is important to recognize that statistical input must be provided at the earliest stages of experimental design and not only after the data have been collected. This not only will provide better science, but also will result in using the correct number of animals—generally, fewer than when guessing what the correct number should be.

Replacement alternatives are methods that do not use whole live animals, or that replace an animal

TABLE 1 ***In Vitro* Tests Replacing Testing in Animals in the Quality Control of Biological Drugs and in Toxicology**

In vitro method	Animal test	Degree of replacement	Regulatory authorities acceptance
	Quality control—biological drugs		
Pregnancy test; immune assay	Frog test	Complete replacement	Worldwide
Pyrogenicity test; limulus-(LAL)-test	Rabbit test	Replacement for protein-free solutions	U.S.-, EU- and Japan-Pharmacopoe
Vitamins and hormones (oxytocin, sexual hormones); HPLC, immune assays	Bioassay in chicken, rats & mice	Complete replacement	EU-Pharmacopoe
Insulin determination; HPLC	Convulsion test mouse	Complete replacement	U.S.- and EU-Pharmacopoe
Insulin determination; HPLC	Blood glucose determination mouse and rabbit	Complete replacement	U.S.- and EU-Pharmacopoe
	Toxicity testing		
Eye irritation; HET-CAM test, BCOP test, isolated chicken eye, isolated rabbit eye	Draize test in rabbit's eye	Replacement for severely irritating materials	EU, according to OECD Guideline 405 Germany Belgium Netherlands U.K.
Skin corrosion; "artificial" human skin cultures	Corrosivity testing on rabbit skin	Complete replacement for corrosive materials	U.S. Department of Transportation, Transport Canada
Delayed neurotoxicity of organophosphates; NTE-esterase determination in neuroblastoma cells	OECD neurotoxicity test of organophosphates in chicken	Partial replacement for esterase inhibitors	Worldwide, according to OECD Guidelines 418 and 419

method with physical or chemical models and/or human studies, when ethically appropriate. These include the use of *in vitro* methods (Table 1).

According to Russell and Burch (1959), the incorporation of the Three Rs into experimental design has led not only to more humane research, but also to better science. *The Principles of Humane Experimental Technique* became the foundation of all animal welfare legislation in both the United States and Europe. In 1995 the Three Rs concept was reviewed and its importance and usefulness was confirmed.

There are centers throughout the world that focus on the development, validation, and use of alternatives in the biomedical sciences including toxicology. As the science behind *in vitro* technology advances, and as results from new methods are shown to be both transferable and reproducible, these alternatives continue to gain acceptance. In addition, the scientific community has responded to the substantial public outcry for a decrease in animal use by considering the advantages and limitations of alternatives.

Information about alternatives is widely available through journals, databases, and sites on the World Wide Web devoted to the Three Rs. However, the word "alternative" has become politicized, and for many in the scientific or animal activist community, it conjures up an image very different from the thoughtful, human experimental science proposed by Russell and Burch. As a result, at the 1995 meeting on the Three Rs, it was decided that the word "alternative" would, when appropriate, have one of the Three Rs in front of it (i.e., replacement alternative, refinement alternative, or reduction alternative), or be used as the phrase "the Three Rs of alternatives."

Methods for increasing the awareness and use of alternatives in the United States and Europe complement each other and, at the same time, demonstrate differences in the political and scientific approaches to effecting change on each side of the Atlantic.

In Europe, since 1990, EU Directive 86/609/EEC on the use of laboratory animals has required the replacement of testing on animals with nonanimal procedures. This directive has resulted in the establishment of ECVAM (European Center for the Validation of Alternative Methods) at the EU Joint Research Centre (JRC) in Ispra (Italy), which is coordinating the validation of *in vitro* methods in toxicology for regulatory purposes. The current focus is on the application of *in vitro* alternatives for safety testing of cosmetics.

In the United States, animal welfare laws have forced institutions to establish ethical review committees and have encouraged the development of refinement procedures through these ethical committees. However, U.S. regulatory agencies, such as the Food and Drug Administration (FDA) and the Environmental Protection Agency, have only very recently—and on an almost entirely voluntary basis—begun to learn about the need to evaluate programs with regard to their use of alternatives. The FDA has taken the most active role and encouraged the development and use of alternatives. In 1993, the U.S. Congress passed the NIH Revitalization Act, which resulted in the formation of the Interagency Coordinating Committee for the Validation of Alternative Methods (ICCVAM). The U.S. government has provided almost no funding for this process, and most of the real advances in validation in the United States occur through the private sector. In contrast, both the private sector and European governments have provided substantial financial support to the development of alternatives in Europe.

VALIDATION AND VALID METHODS

Political pressure to decrease animal testing has created a rush in recent years to get *in vitro* methods into the regulatory acceptance process. At the same time, the potential for many *in vitro* methods to be commercially profitable has resulted in a push to bring inadequately developed methods to the commercial market. As a result, validation has suffered from something of a "cart before the horse" phenomenon. Only recently has it been universally recognized that there is a need for a terminology of validation and a coordinated set of approaches.

The scientific community always has required that new methods be proven to be reproducible, published in peer-reviewed journals, and subjected to additional independent studies before becoming accepted for wide use, or as valid method. There are, of course, different experimental approaches to proving that an *in vitro* method provides the same information as an established animal test. To reach international consensus in both the scientific and regulatory communities, an agreement was reached on the validation process for toxicity test procedures. Studies that were conducted according to these recommendations, predominantly in Europe, have produced significant and useful information, but have failed to provide validated methods that are accepted by the regulatory community. However, the effort provided ECVAM with valuable practical experience in creating a validation process.

The OECD (1996), ECVAM (1995), and ICCVAM (1997) have developed sets of criteria that describe the set of information needed before regulatory acceptance can be considered and also have provided criteria for the regulatory acceptance of methodology. Once these criteria gain international acceptance within the scientific community, it is anticipated that regulatory acceptance will occur. The next stage of development is to identify the minimum set of criteria that have to be met to gain regulatory acceptance.

CURRENT USE OF *IN VITRO* METHODS IN TOXICOLOGY TESTING

In vitro methods are routinely used by all industries and regulatory bodies in toxicity testing, safety assessment, and risk evaluation, and they offer unique advantages (Table 2). The greatest use of *in vitro* methods, however, is for elucidating mechanisms of toxicity and/or demonstrating the biological processes involved in toxic responses to xenobiotics, including drugs. With the development and widespread use of the Ames mutagenic assay, nonanimal testing became routine in both industry and regulatory laboratories.

Within the cosmetics industry, the 1990s have seen a remarkable change in the approach to safety evaluation. Although the ingredients of finished cosmetic products have been tested in animals, most of the finished products now on the market have generally been tested in *in vitro* toxicity tests, which are sufficient for safety evaluations.

TABLE 2 Advantages and Limitations of *In Vitro* Toxicity Testing

Advantages
Controlled testing conditions
Reduction of systemic effects
Reduction of variability between experiments
Same dose range can be tested in a variety of test systems (cells and tissues)
Time-dependent studies can be performed and samples taken
Testing is fast and cheap
Very small amount of test material is required
Limited amount of toxic waste is produced
Human cells and tissues can be used
Transgenic cells carrying human genes can be used
Reduction of testing in animals
Limitations
General side effects cannot be assessed (e.g. weight reduction)
Systemic effects cannot be evaluated
Interactions between tissues and organs cannot be tested
Pharmacokinetic effects cannot be evaluated
Specific organ sensitivity cannot be assessed
Chronic effects cannot be tested

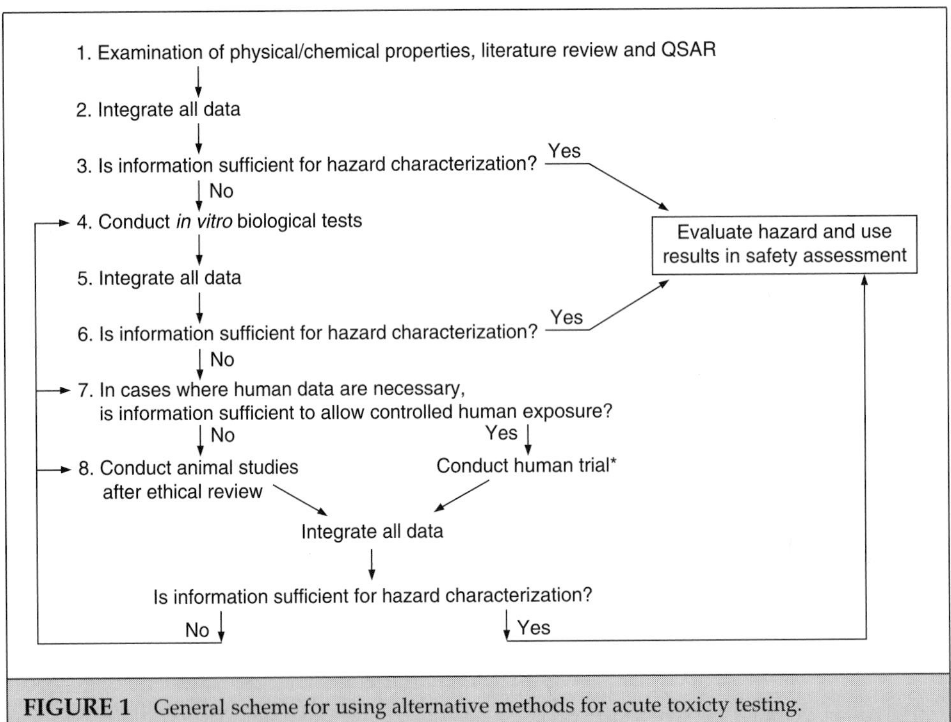

FIGURE 1 General scheme for using alternative methods for acute toxicty testing.

Within the chemical and pharmaceutical industries, *in vitro* methods are used in a very different context. *In vitro* methods are used to screen compounds for their biological effects and to understand why a specific *in vivo* response has been obtained in one species and may not be seen in another. Additionally, screens are used to determine the presence or absence of a specific biological effect within a chemical class and to identify the mechanism of action of a chemical or group of chemicals. It is being recognized that with advances and changes in chemical synthesis (e.g., combinatorial chemistry), more sophisticated and predictive *in vitro* tests will be required.

With advances in genetics and genetic screening approaches, future development for these industries clearly will include the use of either genetically altered cells or integrated biological and silicon-chip systems and other complex and sophisticated systems yet to be envisioned.

WHERE DO *IN VITRO* METHODS FIT?

In the past, *in vitro* methodology has been used as the last approach in product development in order to identify the underlying biology of undesired effects and, in some limited cases (e.g., receptor binding), to assist in product development. In the United States, the Toxic Substances Control Act (TOSCA) incorporated *in vitro* methods into the last stages of compound characterization. Only in the late 1990s has this approach been questioned so that, *in vitro* methods are used at earlier stages of chemical evaluations.

The Scientific Group on Methodologies for the Safety Evaluation of Chemicals (SGOMSEC) has recognized that, at least in acute toxicity testing, *in vitro* methods could play a much more important role in the risk assessment process (Fig. 1).

Acute Oral Toxicity (LD_{50})

The late Gerhard Zbinden, in his numerous important contributions to *in vitro* alternatives, suggested that one did not have to find an alternative to the LD_{50}, one just had to stop using it. In actual fact, the classical LD_{50} that required 60+ animals has essentially become extinct. It remains necessary, however, to determine acute oral toxicity for a series of related but independent reasons. At present, the OECD has accepted two approaches to determining acute oral toxicity, a fixed-dose procedure (FDP) and the acute toxic class method (ATC) procedure.

The fixed-dose procedure, developed in Great Britain by the British Toxicological Society, has several features that demonstrate its applicability and dependence upon the Three Rs concept of alternatives. First, animals are killed as soon as the first toxic signs are observed. In addition, the experimental design reduces the number of animals considerably. The worldwide validation study of the FDP was accepted by the OECD in 1992.

The ATC method has been developed and validated in Germany since 1988. It is based on a sequential dosing scheme in which one dose group is used at a time. Depending on the outcome of testing, in the next step the dose is either decreased or increased. A worldwide validation trial confirmed the biostatistical prediction that the number of animals per test chemical can be reduced to an average of seven in the ATC method without losing the accuracy of the LD_{50} test. In 1996, the ATC method was accepted by the OECD after it had been shown that it can be used for all types of classification schemes currently established in OECD member countries.

Structure–Activity Relationships

As was pointed out earlier, acute toxicity testing as envisioned in the SGOMSEC Workshop requires that a series of physicochemical approaches, databases, and structure–activity relationships be evaluated prior to any biological testing. During the 1990s, there have been remarkable and rapid changes in structure–activity relationship studies.

In the case of therapeutics, rational drug design is clearly a major approach. In the area of toxicology, both commercial and noncommercial databases have been developed to explore structure–activity relationships. Derek and TOPKAT are two systems based on quantitative structure–activity relationships (QSARs) uses and limitations of which have been documented extensively.

Skin Sensitization

In the area of skin sensitization, incredible progress has been made by using quantitative structure–activity relationships for corrosivity and skin-sensitization testing. Although these methods are not 100% predictive, in the area of corrosivity and skin-sensitization studies the success rates are quite remarkable. Coupled with other physicochemical methodologies and with *in vitro* studies, these QSARs may eliminate the need for animal testing in the future.

Photoirritation and Photosensitization

Photosensitization is used to describe the reaction of the skin to an exogenous chemical and UV or visible radiation. The term includes both phototoxic and photoallergic reactions. Phototoxicity is an acute reaction that can be induced by a single treatment with a chemical and UV or visible radiation. In contrast, the term photoirritation is used to describe phototoxic reactions in skin produced with topically applied substances combined with exposure to light. To date, no standard guidelines for the testing of photoirritation potential either *in vivo* or *in vitro* have been accepted for regulatory purposes at the international level by the OECD.

In 1991, the European Commission (EC) and COLIPA (the European Cosmetics, Toiletry and Perfumery Association) established a joint program on developing and validating *in vitro* photoirritation tests. The first phase was designed as a prevalidation study to identify *in vitro* test procedures for a formal validation trial under blind conditions (Table 3). In the second phase, the most promising *in vitro* photoirritation tests were validated with 30 carefully selected chemicals in 11 laboratories in a blind trial. In the 3T3 NRU PT test, mouse fibroblasts, cell line 3T3, are exposed to chemicals in the absence and presence of UVA. An increase in cytotoxicity (Neutral Red Uptake test, NRU) was used to assess the photoirritation potential of chemicals.

The results obtained in this *in vitro* test under blind conditions were reproducible, and the correlation be-

TABLE 3 Methods for *In Vitro* Photoirritation Testing[a]

Screening tests for photoirritation
Bacteria, algae, yeast
Primary cell cultures: human keratinocytes, lymphocytes, and mast cells
Permanent cell lines: mouse fibroblasts (e.g., BALB/c 3T3 fibroblasts)[b]
Skin organ culture models: artificial human epidermis and skin models
Identification of specific mechanisms of photoirritation
Effects on the nucleus: yeast
Effects on the cell membrane: erythrocyte photohemolysis test
Energy transfer to biologically active molecules: hemoglobin oxidation
Formation of reactive molecules in lipids, proteins, and DNA: histamine release from mast cells, induction of DNA strand breaks and of DNA synthesis and degradation; histidin binding

[a]Exposure to UVA.

[b]The 3T3 Neutral Red Uptake Photoirritation (3T3 NRU PI) test has successfully undergone a formal validation in an EU/COLIPA validation study from 1992–1997 (Spielmann *et al.*, 1997).

TABLE 4 ***In Vitro* Alternatives to the Draize Eye Test**[a]

Name of test	Material tested	Duration of testing
Cell culture methods		
Cytotoxicity test	BALB/c 3T3 mouse fibroblasts	Exposure for 24 h
Fluorescein leakage	Epithelial cells (e.g., MDK cells)	Exposure for 30 min
Microphysiometer	pH determination in single epithelial cells	Continuous monitoring
Organ culture techniques		
Rabbit eye, isolated	From sacrificed rabbits	Exposure for 1–4 h
Chicken eye, isolated	From the abattoir	Exposure for 1–4 h
Bovine cornea[b] (BCOP test)	From the abbattoir	Exposure for 1–4 h
HET-CAM-test[c]	Embryonated chicken egg	Exposure for 5 min
Artificial human skin and epidermis	High-quality commercial products	Exposure for 5–20 min

[a]These *in vitro* tests have been evaluated and validated in the EU Home Office validation trial of *in vitro* alternatives to the Draize eye test. None of the *in vitro* tests is able to replace the Draize eye test for all aspects of eye irritation and all types of chemicals. The conclusions of this study were that no test is better than any other test and that no test was validated (Balls *et al.*, 1995).

[b]Accepted by some European governments for classifying severely irritating materials.

[c]Accepted by the French and German government for testing of finished cosmetic products.

tween *in vitro* and *in vivo* data was almost perfect. In an additional blind trial of UV filter chemicals, the phototoxic potential of all of the 20 test chemicals was predicted correctly. The Commission of the EUs, therefore, in 1998 accepted the 3T3 NRU PT test as the first experimentally validated *in vitro* toxicity test for regulatory purposes and, in addition, officially applied to the OECD for worldwide acceptance of this *in vitro* toxicity test.

Eye Irritation

The general public has protested the Draize eye test more than any other procedure used on animals, so,

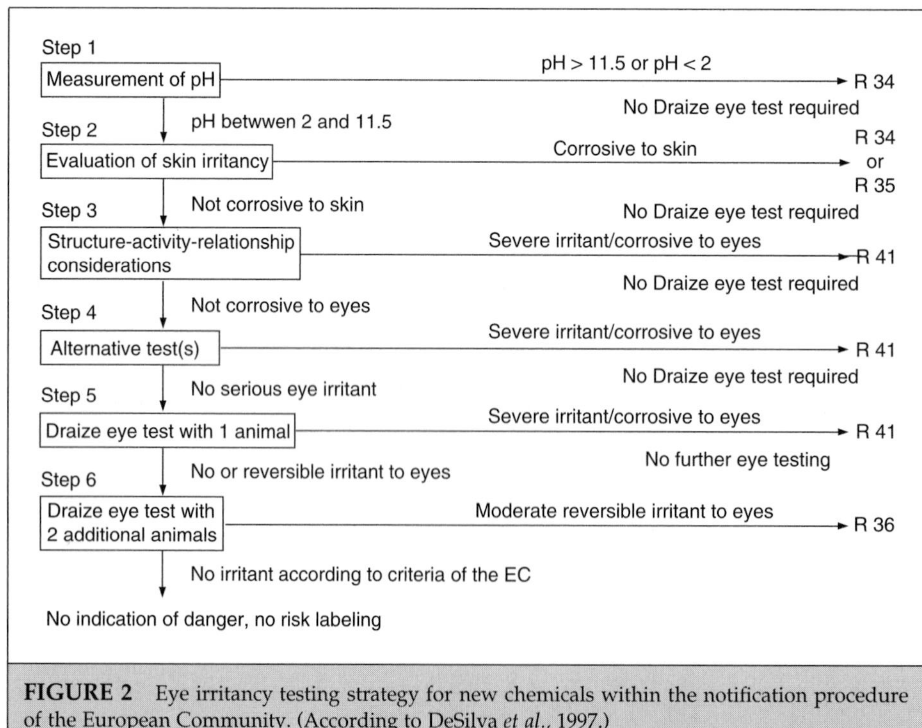

FIGURE 2 Eye irritancy testing strategy for new chemicals within the notification procedure of the European Community. (According to DeSilva *et al.*, 1997.)

not surprisingly, scientists in the alternatives field have devoted more time and attention to finding an alternative to this test than to any other. The Draize eye test is easy for the public to understand and difficult for scientists to justify if strong irritants and corrosives are not eliminated from the testing protocol. Unfortunately, replacing the Draize test has proven to be more difficult than anticipated. This is due to the lack of knowledge about the biology of eye irritation, the lack of standardized and adequate human data, and the lack of *in vitro* models to evaluate appropriate tests. A series of alternatives to the Draize eye test have been evaluated in Europe (Table 4). None is able to replace the Draize eye test for all aspects of eye irritation and all types of chemicals.

AN INTEGRATED *IN VITRO* AND *IN VIVO* TESTING STRATEGY

Today, several organizations are attempting an integrated strategy. The approach (Fig. 2) eliminates animal testing for eye irritancy if certain structure–activity or other nonanimal tests indicate the compound would be a severe irritant or corrosive. The only time that animals are to be used is when there is the expectation that the compound is not corrosive or a severe irritant.

German regulatory authorities and the U.S. EPA developed a stepwise strategy for eye-irritation testing that takes into account the escape clause of the OECD guideline for eye-irritation testing. In this procedure the data from a sequence of physicochemical data and the results obtained in toxicity testing *in vivo* and *in vitro* are taken into consideration in evaluating eye irritation potential of new chemicals (Fig. 2). In this procedure, only chemicals that are positive may be classified and labeled "risk of severe damage to eyes." All chemicals that are found negative have to undergo *in vivo* testing in the Draize eye test in rabbits. This approach is used in several EU member states according to experience gained in validation trials at the national level, but it is not used in the United States and other OECD member countries.

Bibliography

Atterwil, C. K., and Steele, C. E. (eds.) (1987). "*In Vitro* Methods in Toxicology." Cambridge University Press, Cambridge.

Balls, M., Blaauboer, B. J., Brusik, D., Frazier, J., Lamb, D., Pemberton, M., Reinhardt, C., Roberfroid, M., Rosenkranz, H., Schmid, B., Spielmann, H., Stammati, A.L., and Walum, E. (1990). Report and recommendations of the CAAT/ERGATT workshop on the validation of toxicity test procedures. *ATLA* **18,** 313–337.

Balls, M., Blaauboer, B. J., Fentem, J., Bruner, L., Combes, R. D., Ekwal, B., Fielder, R. J., Guillouzo, A., Lewis, R. W., Lovell, D. P., Reinhardt, C. A., Repetto, G., Sladowski, D. Spielmann, H., and Zucco, F. (1995). Practical aspects of the validation of toxicity test procedures. The report and recommendations of ECVAM Workshop 5. *ATLA* **23,** 129–147.

Balls, M., Bridges, J., and Southee, J. (eds.) (1991) "Animals and Alternatives in Toxicology: Present Status and Future Prospects." Macmillan Academic and Professional Ltd., London.

Barratt, M. D. (1996a). Quantitative structure–activity relationships (QSARs) for skin corrosivity of organic acids, bases and phenols: Principal components and neural network analysis of extended datasets. *Toxicology In Vitro* **10,** 85–94.

Barratt, M. D. (1996b). Quantitative structure–activity relationships for skin irritation and corrosivity of neutral and electophilic organic chemicals. *Toxicology In Vitro* **10,** 247–256.

Basketter, D.A., Scholes, E.W., Chamberlain, M., and Barratt, M.D. (1995). An alternative strategy to use guinea pigs for the identification of skin sensitization hazard. *Food Chem. Toxicol.* **33,** 1051–1056.

Castell, J. V., and Gomez-Lechon, M. J. (1997). "*In Vitro* Methods in Pharmaceutical Research." Academic Press, San Diego, CA.

De Silva, O., Cottin, M., Dami, N., Roguet, R., Catroux, P., Toufic, A., Sicard, C., Dossou, K. G., Gerner, I., Schlede, E., Spielmann, H., Gupta, K. C. and Hill, R. N. (1997). Evaluation of eye irritation potential: Statistical analysis and tier testing strategies. *Food Chem. Tox.* **35,** 159–164.

Frazier, J. M. (ed.) (1992). "*In Vitro* Toxicity Testing: Applications to Safety Evaluation." Dekker, New York.

Gad, S. C. (ed.) (1994). "*In Vitro* Toxicology." Raven Press, New York.

Goldberg, A. M. (ed.) (1983–1995). "Alternative Methods in Toxicology," Vol. 1–11. The Johns Hopkins Center for Alternatives to Animal Testing. Mary Ann Liebert, New York.

Goldberg, A. M. and Libowitz, L. A. Altweb—The Alternatives to Animals Testing Web Site of the Johns Hopkins Center for Alternatives to Animal Testing (http://altweb.jhsph.edu).

Goldberg, A. M., and Van Zutphen, L. F. M. (1995). "Alternative Methods in Toxicology, Vol. 11, World Congress Proceedings." Mary Ann Liebert, New York.

NIEHS (1997). "NIEHS Validation and Regulatory Acceptance of Toxicological Test Methods: A Report of the Ad Hoc Interagency Coordinating Committee on the Validation of Alternative Methods." NIH Publication No. 97-3981. NIEHS, Research Triangle Park, NC.

OECD (Organisation for Economic Cooperation and Development) (1996). "Final Report of the OECD Workshop on Harmonisation of Validation and Acceptance Criteria for Alternative Toxicological Test Methods." ENV/MC/CHEM/TG(96)9. OECD Publications Office, Paris.

O'Hare, S., and Atterwil, C. K. (eds.) (1995). "*In Vitro* Toxicity Testing Protocols." Humana Press, Totowa, NJ.

Rougier, A., Goldberg, A. M., and Maibach, H. (eds.) (1994). "Alternative Methods in Toxicology, Vol. 10, *In Vitro* Skin Toxicology." Mary Ann Liebert, New York.

Russell, W. M. S., and Burch, R. L. (1959). "The Principles of Humane Experimental Technique." Methuen & Co. Ltd., London.

SGOMSEC (Scientific Group on Methodologies for the Safety Evaluation of Chemicals (1998). Alternative testing methodologies. *Environ. Health Perspect.* **106** (Suppl. 2), 403–620.

Spielmann, H., Balls, M., Dupuis, J., Pape, W. J. W., de Silva, O., Holzhütter, H. G., Gerberick, F., Liebsch, M., Lovell, W. W., and Pfannenbecker, U. (1998). A study on UV filter chemicals from Annex VII of Euroepan Union Directive 76/768/EEC, in the *in vitro* 3T3 NRU phototoxicity test. *ATLA* **26,** 679–708.

Spielmann, H., Balls, M., Dupuis, J., Pape, W. J. W., Pechovitch, G., de Silva, O., Holzhuetter, H. G., Clothier, R., Desolle, P., Gerberick, F., Liebsch, M., Lovell, W. W., Maurer, T., Pfannenbecker, U., Potthast, J. M., Sladowski, D., Steiling, W., and Brantom, P. (1998). The international EU/COLIPA *in vitro* phototoxicity validation study: Results of phase II (blind trial): The 3T3 NRU phototoxicity test. *Toxicology in Vitro* **12,** 305–327.

Van Zutphen, L. F. M., and Balls, M. (1997). "Proceedings of the Second World Congress on Alternatives: Animal Alternatives, Welfare and Ethics." Elsevier, Amsterdam.

CHAPTER

50

Regulatory Toxicology

ARPAD SOMOGYI,* GIO B. GORI,† KLAUS E. APPEL*

*Federal Institute for Health Protection of Consumers and Veterinary Medicine, Berlin, Germany

†The Health Policy Center, Bethesda, Maryland

INTRODUCTION

Toxicology—the science of poisons—meets real life when asked to help regulate and restrict the attending risks in a social context through appropriate norms. The framework of regulatory toxicology will depend as much on the philosophical premises and the cultural and ethical values of the society it is to serve as on the scientific objectivity and experimental verifications that define poison hazards. It follows that regulatory toxicology is interpreted differently in different countries, even when they profess to share the common social model of a liberal democracy. The differences account for often subtle nuances in what is considered the permissible reach of government's paternalism and on historically diverse levels of autonomy that public officials are granted in different societies. In seeking some common ground, we shall here assume a somewhat ideal social model generally protective of the rights to self-determination of citizens, who in turn accept mutual limitations on their liberties as social norms. What could be the philosophical and ethical underpinnings for regulatory toxicology in this model?

The model's philosophy is fundamentally libertarian, although it allows a limited authority of regulatory intervention to the state. In practice, the bounds of these limitations are not fixed by general consensus but are modulated by continuing arguments pitting statist and libertarian views around such pristine questions as what could justify a coercive government interest in fostering longevity per se, in restricting voluntary risk taking, and in preventing risks whose existence often appear to be merely hypothetical. Corollary arguments have raised additional questions about the potential conflicts of interest in the delegation of regulatory autonomy to unelected officials who—ostensibly free of most checks and balances—are expected at once to define hazards and risks, to produce the related normative writ, and to enforce the same with power of police, imposing fines, and even detention.

At the same time, it is undisputable that the essence of government is regulation and that elected legislators generally lack technical expertise and cannot be expected to shoulder the volume and detail of work required to fulfill the regulatory needs and expectations of complex societies. These requirements have been universally construed to justify regulatory administrations with the authority to formulate and execute policies, usually restrained by the continuing oversight of elected representatives and the allowance of legal actions by citizens and organizations for or against specific regulation.

Necessary as it is, the legitimacy and the bounds of the regulatory apparatus continue to raise philosophical questions and debate in modern societies. A detailed survey of such questions is beyond the scope of the present analysis, which will focus rather on the technical issues of regulation, although selected aspects of these questions will surface from time to time in the following pages.

Getting closer to more practical aspects of regulation, our ideal social model would recognize that risks posed by hazards are inevitable attributes of living, that the attainment of a risk-free society is Utopian and could not be the goal of regulation, and that risk taking usually has a utilitarian counterpart. At the same time, a distinction is drawn between risks and costs that are voluntarily accepted and risks or costs that are suffered involuntarily, the latter being either naturally occurring or caused by the hazardous activities of other members of society. Because of utilitarian implications, the model recognizes the implicit value—however idiosyncratic—of voluntary risk taking to individuals (e.g., rock climbing), as well as the value to individuals and to society of certain hazardous activities that may subject members of society to involuntary risks or costs (e.g., pesticide uses).

The understanding of regulatory toxicology would be incomplete without a clear vision of the different interests of toxicology as a science and of regulatory agencies as political constructs. While toxicologists should be interested in the experiment-driven truth-seeking of science, regulators are under pressure to accommodate a variety of demands and expectations, which include the often idealistic intransigence of statutes under which they operate, their own institutional interests, the insistence of assorted advocates, the reactions of the regulated, and the inadequacy of toxicology and epidemiology in providing reliably objective input. In this regard, uncertainties frequently give regulators no alternative but to extend the meaning of tentative toxicological evaluations in order to justify the often exacting demands of legislation and the pressures of public anxieties.

All things considered, it should not be surprising that attempts to accommodate various tensions have resulted in a regulatory practice based on contrasting and even contradictory principles and guidelines, the upshot of which has deeply affected toxicology. Regulatory agencies have developed their own toxicological laboratories and are a major source of funding for academic toxicology, a situation that has put increasing pressures on the profession to comply with the requirements of the agencies. The same agencies have provided guidelines for toxicological research to suit their needs and prescribe how toxicological investigations should be conducted, while the research supported by the agencies focuses on the solutions to problems and directions that the agencies perceive as useful to their goals and needs.

The regulated industries develop toxicology usually in compliance with regulatory guidelines but also with confrontational aims, in a manner that also exerts a profound influence on research methods and priorities. Thus, in the end, it is inevitable that the administrative imposition of technical and scientific standards in the service of regulation eventually should affect the professional and intellectual Weltanschauung of toxicologists, many of whom are actually employed by regulatory agencies and the regulated industries. This becomes especially evident when considering that regulators must act in a real time framework and cannot postpone until some distant research might (perhaps) provide better answers. They have to make decisions "here and now" on the basis of actually available knowledge. In principle and by necessity, regulators focus on moving targets and remain flexible and open to emerging new evidence, but at any given time they must seek definite and even particular answers, even though the scientific reality may permit only a range of more or less plausible conjectures.

THE SCOPE OF REGULATORY TOXICOLOGY

Over the years, the scope of regulation and toxicology has expanded parallel to the development of global industries, which has multiplied the potential hazards to the environment, to health, and safety. In the United States, the European Union, and most other developed areas, regulatory toxicology covers most aspects of manufacturing, trade, and the environment. The following are some of the main areas of interest.

Foods

The model for most food regulation in the world has been the 1906 Food and Drug Act of the United States, the basic language of which is unchanged today; it bars the marketing of food that contains added substances that may render it injurious to health, or that contains natural agricultural commodities that may be ordinarily injurious to health (FDCA, 1938). Regulations are usually applied to functional additives (e.g., colorants, sweeteners, tenderizers, emulsifiers, and bulking agents), and nonfunctional or indirect additives (e.g., residues of drugs used in animals, pesticide residues, and contaminants) that migrate to foods from contact with manufacturing tools and packaging.

Medicinal Substances

Medicines for human use are the most stringently regulated substances in most countries. Unlike other substances, medicines are generally required to pass safety and efficacy tests in human clinical trials, usually after extensive preclinical experimentation in animals. For most medicines, approval depends on how favorable the ratio is between therapeutic efficacy and undesirable side effects, and their dispensation and use are regulated under strict medical supervision. Equally stringent requirements are applied to medical devices and veterinary medicines, particularly when the latter result in residues in foods for human consumption.

Toxic Substances

Many countries regulate the production, storage, packaging, distribution, disposal, and use of substances that could pose hazards to health and safety. Agricultural and environmental pesticides are a special class of toxic substances that are usually more stringently regulated because they end up in the food and drinking water supplies. Here, too, economic considerations generally require risk–benefit considerations to enter in all regulatory decisions that may limit exposures.

Work Place Safety

Permissible exposures of workers to toxic substances are regulated in many countries with widely different criteria and safety standards, and usually with decisive reliance on risk–benefit considerations.

Air and Water Pollutants

Legislation in various countries has been directed at reducing toxic emissions from stationary sources (e.g., manufacturing plants, mines, agricultural activities and runoffs, aquifers, and potable waters) as well as from mobile sources, such as cars and other transport. Given that the sources of pollution derive from activities of significant economic value, most regulations in this area rely on and are profoundly affected by risk–benefit considerations. Regulations may impose limits of emission for stationary sources and motor vehicles; quality standards for urban air, drinking water, rivers, and lakes; and controls for contamination levels in hazardous waste sites.

Substances of Abuse

Psychotoxic, addictive, and other substances that can be abused are usually prohibited, although many are permitted under strict regulation when they may have significant therapeutic efficacy.

Cosmetics

In the past, the regulation of cosmetics has followed a more relaxed interpretation of the general guidelines of food and medicines regulation. More recently in most countries, notably the United States, cosmetic colorants are handled under the strict guidelines that regulate potential carcinogenic substances. In the European Union, the Directive on cosmetic products includes a list of substances whose use is prohibited as cosmetic ingredients. In addition, it lists the substances that are allowed to be used only in certain areas of application or up to a specified maximum quantity. Three annexes list preservatives, UV filters, and coloring agents that have obtained final or limited authorization and specify the area of application, as well as maximum concentrations.

Consumer Products

Consumer products, from toys to automobiles, are regulated in certain countries by agencies that evaluate their ultimate safety at point of use. In addition to sources of mechanical injury, these agencies focus on potential toxic, radioactive, corrosive, explosive, and flammable hazards, often joining forces with agencies that regulate other substances under different statutes. Here too, regulations are heavily influenced by risk–benefit considerations.

PROCEDURAL FRAMEWORKS OF REGULATION

Different statutes create different regulatory philosophies in different agencies. Fundamental differences can arise in regard to "burden of proof" issues, that is, whether the statute requires the regulating agency or the regulated parties to provide proof of the safety of a product or procedure. In the United States, for instance, the Food and Drug Administration (U.S. FDA) regulates under the former requirement, but the Occupational Safety and Health Administration (U.S. OSHA) observes the latter approach. Similar situations prevail in other countries.

Mandates for No-Risk Tolerance

Often, governing statutes mandate a strict no-risk approach to regulation. The notorious precedent for this approach is the Delaney clause, introduced in the United States into the Food, Drug, and Cosmetic Act (FDCA) in 1958; this clause has influenced similar concepts in other countries. The clause is found in sections 409 and 412 of the FDCA and reads in part "that no additive shall be deemed to be safe if it is found to induce cancer when ingested by man or animal, or if it is found after tests which are appropriate for evaluation of safety of food additives to induce cancer in man or animal" (FDCA, 1958). Such a no-risk approach has been directed specifically at potentially carcinogenic substances, based on the overpowering public emotions on the subject of cancer and the resulting urge of legislators and regulators to adopt default assumptions that negate—at least in principle and theory—the possibility of safe levels for carcinogens. Because the Delaney clause would be triggered merely by carcinogenic results in animal tests, it has the potential of forbidding many of the significant products of science and technology. This is because animal tests for carcinogenicity have been designed to maximize positive outcomes and usually succeed in doing so in more than half the tests. In fact, positive carcinogenic responses in animals can be elicited by most common foods under favorable if extreme experimental conditions. In the United States, all sorts of compromises and legal and administrative stratagems have been devised, largely on the basis of explicit or implicit risk–benefit considerations, to permit the use of countless substances, from foods to medicines to pesticides, food additives, industrial chemicals, and their consumer derivatives.

In the United States again, the clause has been partially neutralized by the existence of other "flow-through" provisions of the FDCA. Section 402, for instance, provides for the regulation of pesticides in raw agricultural commodities at tolerances specified in section 408, but also permits pesticides in processed foods if the levels do not exceed those set out in section 408 for raw commodities. This statutory equivocation has been the source of some confusion, but at the same time it has been of much practical use as a counter to an absolute no-risk Delaney clause with the potential of causing impossible hardship to the overall food supply.

Substances in Traditional Use

Regulation in the United States and other countries recognizes the implicit safety of substances that have been in traditional human use for long time, especially foods and common dietary components. In the United States, these are listed in the class of substances generally recognized as safe (GRAS). The regulatory recognition and approval of safety is specific for traditional uses but not for uncommon ones, so that a GRAS substance could be used freely in foods but not for medicinal or other uses (U.S. FDA, 1997).

Approved Tolerances

In theory, approved tolerances are issued for hazards that are not carcinogenic, although—as discussed—carcinogens too could be approved within certain limits of use. For noncarcinogens, approved tolerances are defined by first determining a no observable adverse effect level (NOAEL), initially measured by animal tests and then transformed into human equivalents by suitable formulas. A further reduction of NOAEL values is obtained by the application of safety factors that cover a discretionary range from 10 to 10,000, depending on the uncertainties, cost benefit considerations, and the judgment of regulators. For instance, safety factors may be higher in the case of items for child use, or lower for occupational situations. Approved tolerances have different denominations in different regulatory settings. For foods, they are usually expressed as "acceptable daily intake" (ADI) levels; for occupational situations they could be "threshold limit values" (TLV) and "permissible exposure limits" (PEL) for peak exposures, or "short-term exposure limit" (STEL) and "time-weighted averages" (TWA) for prolonged exposures. Also used in occupational settings are acute warning levels, such as the IDLH, "immediately dangerous to life or health."

Threshold or *De Minimis* Regulation

The concept that regulation should focus only on significant hazards has been around for a long time under the legal maxim that *de minimis non curat lex*. It has often surfaced in various regulatory settings as the concept of tolerable risk, variously defined as a 10^{-6} risk or similar definition. Although discussed and proposed for decades the concept has been adopted only in 1995 by the U.S. FDA with the promulgation of threshold of regulation guidelines (U.S. FDA, 1995a). The guidelines exempt from regulation certain indirect contact food additives that could migrate from packaging or processing equipment, if their concentration does not exceed 0.5 ppb in the total daily diet. The effectiveness of this procedure continues to be tested, but it holds a promise of relieving much of the delay in regulatory decisions due to the administrative gridlock that trivial issues are known to cause.

Risk–Benefit Considerations

In considering approval, regulators are usually required by law or compelled by circumstances to relax or restrict evaluation criteria based on cost–benefit tradeoffs. In the United States, for instance, the U.S. OSHA may only consider a standard that "most adequately assures, to the extent feasible . . . that no employee will suffer material impairment . . . (U.S. OSHA, 1970). U.S. OSHA's test of feasibility depends on whether risk-reducing technology may be available, and whether it can be economically provided. The U.S. Environmental Protection Agency (U.S. EPA) is required to conduct extensive risk and benefit balances before acting under the U.S. Toxic Substances Control Act (TSCA, 1976). Similarly the control of pesticides by the U.S. EPA under the U.S. Federal Insecticide, Fungicide, and Rodenticide Act (FIFRA, 1972) is limited by the obvious advantages of their use in producing adequate food supplies, so that restrictions are applied only if the pesticide use may cause "unreasonable adverse effects on health or the environment."

Risk–benefit considerations usually command the last word in actual regulation and could prevail over any other concern. A clear example is that of drinking water, where chlorine has been used to control bacterial contamination. The practice results in vanishing but measurable traces of chloroform, which is carcinogenic in animals under certain conditions and could trigger a strict regulatory ban under Delaney criteria. The benefits of an otherwise safe drinking water override this last injunction in favor of a threshold approach. In the United States, for instance, the U.S. EPA issues a "maximum contaminant level goal" (MCLG) for potable water as a nonenforceable ideal objective, coupled with an enforceable "maximum contamination level" (MCL) that is higher than the goal and is periodically revised to reflect what is technologically attainable.

REGULATORY INFLUENCES IN TOXICOLOGY

Because of their legal authority, regulatory agencies have exerted a profound influence on the practice of toxicology, both with the imposition of testing protocols, and with the design and funding of research to discover novel toxicological hazards and the methods for their detection and evaluation. In general, agencies that require approval before a substance is produced and marketed (premarketing approval) have had the most profound influence and in many countries this has resulted in the promulgation of standard test guidelines. Because of different statutory objectives and language, different regulatory agencies may produce somewhat conflicting guidelines, even within the same country. National coordination committees have been instituted in many countries to mitigate the problem, usually with modest success. At the international level, various attempts at harmonization have been in place for many years through such organizations as the OECD, FAO, and others.

Although the globalization of trade continues to be a force for international harmonization of regulatory policy, a strong reason behind the reluctance of major players to adopt uniformity is that differing regulatory prerogatives and incentives have been traditionally used to secure advantages in trade. For the moment, the only widely shared protocols are those of good laboratory practices (GLP), which refer to generic standards of experimentation, i.e., cleanliness, environmental variables, and animal care and handling (GLP, 1989). A major contribution of GLP standards is the requirement of impeccable record-keeping to safeguard technical integrity and to prevent misconduct and abuses. Still, toxicologists in different countries may use similar GLP standards, but will design and evaluate experiments by often quite different methods and purposes, usually as prescribed by their own regulatory laws, policies, and agencies.

In certain countries much of toxicology research in and out of academia is funded directly by regulatory agencies, or by the regulated industries that anticipate or respond to regulatory requirements. As a consequence, toxicology research is constrained by practical necessities more often than not. In general, such pressures emphasize the development of testing methods over the study of more fundamental mechanistic processes of toxicity, and the search for novel hazards that may expand the reach of regulatory agencies.

It should be emphasized that health and safety regulations are influenced equally by animal tests and by clinical and epidemiological studies in humans. For ethical reasons, studies in humans cannot be proactive but seek answers about potential hazards that are already in use, except for clinical trials of new medicines. Strict guidelines have been accepted and practiced only for clinical trials, whereas the rest of epidemiology operates generally without standards of conduct and practice for study design, conduct, and interpretation. Such laxity and other incurable uncertainties have not prevented epidemiology from having a strong regulatory influence, a situation that could considerably improve if guidelines of good epidemiologic practice were to be issued and enforced. It would be most desirable that efforts in this direction—pioneered by the Association of French Speaking Epidemiologists—should be rapidly considered and adopted worldwide (ADELF, 1997).

Guidelines for animal tests as surrogates of human risk detection have been issued by many countries and international agencies, and all share common features. The most stringent and controversial guidelines are those for the testing of potential carcinogenic agents, which theoretically aim at maximizing the chance of obtaining positive results. With this in mind, those tests require maximum tolerated doses, ostensibly to make up for the statistical disparity between a few hundred test animals and the much larger human populations they are supposed to represent. Still, high doses have no rational justification as surrogates of statistical power, while the toxicity they inevitably produce is known to induce secondary effects that can induce cancer responses not specifically linked to the agent tested.

It is known that susceptibility varies from species to species. Hence results can be further skewed by requirements that the most susceptible animals be used. For instance, there is a wide disparity of response from rats to mice, the latter being especially prone to develop hepatomas, and especially under marginal liver toxicity.

Further complications arise when guidelines give priority to positive reports or require the pooling of benign and malignant lesions: problematic issues in view of the often contrasting judgments of different pathologists. Other dilemmas arise when agents appear to protect animals against certain tumors while enhancing others. Overall, the conclusion seems inescapable that guidelines result in tests that are unreliable predictors of cancer risks in humans and perhaps in animals. Nevertheless, lacking better means, animal tests are universally required under the standard default assumptions of conservative prudence.

RISK ASSESSMENT, CHARACTERIZATION, AND MANAGEMENT

The inputs of both toxicology and epidemiology are the initial considerations of the regulatory process, which then proceeds with the evaluation of potential risks, and finally with the regulations that are intended to manage those risks. Although data might be fairly well documented and reliable for most toxicological endpoints, they become much less so in the case of carcinogens, a situation that results in the most contentious policies and regulatory outcomes. Here, inescapable difficulties are encountered at the initial stages because direct human toxicological data are seldom available and because epidemiologic studies are seldom verified according to the standard scientific criteria of verification—namely through experiments that account for biases and confounders, that compare groups that are the same except for the variable being measured, and that are repeated and repeatable under controlled conditions to yield the same or equivalent results.

In epidemiology, for instance, most studies of diseases of multifactorial origins (such as cancer, cardiovascular, and other chronic diseases) compare nonrandomized groups that differ in many more than the variables being studied, which generally excludes the possibility of an adequate control for confounding variables. As a norm, such studies are observational surveys which are not replicable under controlled conditions and which often yield contrasting outcomes. Sir Richard Doll, a prominent epidemiologist, noted that "epidemiological observations . . . have serious disadvantages . . . . They can seldom be made according to the strict requirements of experimental science and therefore may be open to a variety of interpretations . . . . These disadvantages limit the value of observations in humans . . . ."

Randomization of the epidemiologic studies might improve the situation, but prospective experimental studies of cancer causation in human subjects are clearly unethical, which leaves animal experiments as the only surrogates for the testing of potential carcinogens. Unfortunately, reliably objective ways of translating carcinogen bioassay results in terms of human risk are not available, and regulators have had no other option but to adopt certain assumptions (default assumptions) even though they may be conjectural or may conflict with the available evidence. The main assumptions are that humans are as susceptible or more susceptible than the test animals to the agents tested; that physiological, immunological, repair, metabolic, and clearance patterns are similar in test animals and humans; that kinetics of response are independent of dose and follow identical (linear) kinetics in test animals and humans; that human routes of exposure can be reproduced in test animals; and that maximum tolerated doses are necessary to evaluate the carcinogenic risks of chemicals, although they do not reflect the potential exposures in humans.

As a consequence, carcinogenicity bioassays and their interpretation may use sophisticated protocols and technologies, but in the end their interpretations inevitably reflect value judgments. Just as with epidemiology, this unhappy situation has led to the admission that ". . . a correlation between carcinogenicity in animals and possible human risk cannot be made on a scientific basis."

The absence of objective evidence is not unique to carcinogens but extends to a variety of pathologic and hazard endpoints that do not depend on single causes—as in the case of infectious diseases—but on complex multifactorial mechanisms that prevent pinpointing the individual responsibility of associated risk factors. Some of these endpoints include teratogenicity, reproductive toxicity, genotoxicity, immunotoxicity, neurotoxicity, and other complex outcomes that may target specific tissues, organs, and systems. The specific case of carcinogens is simply the most discussed, probably on account of the visceral fears that cancer evokes in public perceptions and, by reflection, in legislative concerns and regulatory statutes around the world.

Uncertainties notwithstanding, it is an axiom of health and safety regulation that the worst is to be assumed unless demonstrated otherwise. In this context, the lack of reliable toxicological and epidemiological evidence has had the effect of imposing judgmental approaches to regulation, which in time have given rise to ever more complex methodologies, with the intent of compensating for the absence of objective data and the straightforward regulatory decisions they would enable. Despite their apparent complexity and numerical sophistication, there is wide recognition among experts—but not necessarily in the public opinion—that current approaches to the regulation of most agents remain judgmental.

Indeed, the regulatory process can be relatively straightforward when risks can be identified with a degree of certainty that compels all parties—the regulated, advocacy groups, and the law—to face reality and to accept suitable regulatory standards. Yet, in the case of potential carcinogens and other hazards that are not objectively definable, regulators are facing potential risks that might or might not exist. Here, the regulatory intent can only be prudential, and addresses not realities but "what if" questions. The inevitable arbitrary nature of such decisions has been uncomfortable, and has persuaded different regulators to adopt different regulatory approaches, here summarized as two extremes.

Some countries have adopted closed and strictly administrative regulatory procedures that at most admit the confidential participation of outside experts, as was the case in Europe at one time, and which still is the case in Japan, Canada, and other countries. Elsewhere, and notably in the United States, the potential for controversial decisions has persuaded regulators to adopt the open process of a political dialog with the participation of experts and other interested parties—a move intent on easing the responsibilities of regulators and securing public acceptance, but often ending up in heightened tensions. This approach usually culminates in a public hearing, known in the United States as a "rule-making" hearing. In any event, both the closed and open regulatory models advance through the progressive phases of hazard identification, usually by animal bioassay and dose–response and exposure assessment; characterization of population risk; risk–benefit considerations; and finally risk management leading to regulatory standards.

Hazard Identification

The first step is to define the toxic mode(s) of a particular agent, generally by experimentation that may supply information on cytotoxicity, mutagenicity, developmental toxicity, neurotoxicity, other specific organ and biochemical effects, carcinogenicity, and mortality. The data usually derive from exploratory animal experimentation, at times motivated by clinical or epidemiological observations. Participants in this phase are technical experts alone.

Dose–Response Assessment

Information about the intensity of an effect in relation to dose and duration of exposure is seldom obtained by direct human observations in clinical or epidemiological settings. This information is usually extrapolated from animal experiments, which require maximum tolerated doses in the contentious case of carcinogens. Even in animals, response effects at low exposures cannot be experimentally detected and are unknown, which has prompted regulators to use a variety of mathematical models to extrapolate from a few high-dose observations to unobservable low-dose projections.

Regulation usually admits threshold models and extrapolations when thresholds are observed, but in the case of carcinogens the prevailing official policies usually disregard thresholds, even if experimentally observed, and require nonthreshold extrapolation models. For carcinogens, various mechanistic assumptions have been used, The single hit (one mutation = one cancer cell) and multi-hit (multiple mutations = one cancer cell) assumptions result in nonthreshold Poisson distribution models that in time have been superseded by linearized multistage (LMS) models, which assume multiple hits and transformation stages before a cell becomes cancerous. Although LMS models are the most commonly used, other models that are still employed are the Probit and Logit distributions, and the time-to-tumor variants of the Weibull and Cox models. Both cancer and noncancer models extrapolate to presumed low-dose effects, and require a further step for scaling from animals to humans, most often using empirical formulas, such as

$$\frac{KW^{2/3}}{100S},$$

where K is a constant peculiar to the animal

species, W is the weight in kg, and S is the body surface in m^2. Another widely used scaling formula is simply $W^{3/4}$ (U.S. EPA, 1992).

In estimating potential cancer risks to humans from animal data, additional uncertainties often occur when a compound may be carcinogenic in one species but not in another, or when the tumors observed may be peculiar to the animals in the test, as is often the case for hepatomas in mice. Much has been made of the possible use of mechanistic data, but until reliable knowledge about cancer causation and development is available, such an approach remains largely speculative. More often, the mechanistic approach is limited to physiologically based pharmacokinetic considerations (PBPK) regarding the absorption, distribution, metabolism, and excretion (ADME) of a substance, but those considerations also may have unknown relevance to the final objective of human risk determinations. Conversely, some use of certain physiological and pathological peculiarities have been used to disregard the regulatory significance of certain animal effects, as in the cases of *d*-limonene and isophorone and kidney tumors mediated by $\alpha_{2\mu}$-globulin in male rats; red No.3, ethylenethiourea, sulfametazine and rat thyroid tumors induced by imbalances in thyroid hormones; glass beads, melanine, or oxalate crystals and bladder tumors in rodents, possibly induced by mechanical injury; and butylhydroxytoluene and propionic acid and forestomach tumors in rodents mediated by epithelial irritation.

In the end, and despite the vast amount of mathematical expertise and ingenuity that these models have inspired, it is widely understood and conceded that such exercises cannot claim the verifiable superiority of one over the others, all being structured around conjectural assumptions with no verifiable links to actual human conditions.

Risk Characterization

Technical experts have exclusive competence in the preceding phases of risk assessment and, despite scientific and rational injunctions against human risk inferences from most animal data, they provide such inferences routinely on the basis of policies and procedures that have the effective weight of law. Reflecting fundamental uncertainties, in general such procedures lack well-defined rules and rely heavily on judgmental criteria, such as the strength and specificity of endpoint measures, consistency among different animal tests, and biological plausibility in humans.

When the available information is epidemiological, equivocal, and short of exposure–responses data, often other considerations have resulted in the much-used weight-of-evidence approach, theoretically aimed at consolidating in a final judgment all available evidence. Here, too, the potential for elastic and selective interpretations of available reports has prompted the exploration of analytical methodologies, the most notable of which is the statistical procedure of meta-analysis. This method combines endpoints from different studies into single estimates, usually by combining the mean of relative risks or odds ratios of different studies, each weighted by the inverse of their variance. The procedure has been especially popular and useful in summarizing the results from randomized clinical trials, but it has been extended in epidemiology to the synthesis of results from disparate observational studies, with less than satisfactory outcomes.

The obstacle is that the combined studies must be homogeneous—usually a salient feature of clinical trials that share common protocols—whereas observational studies in epidemiology are inevitably heterogeneous because of the lack of randomization and differences in biases and confounders in the study design and protocols and in the ways data are collected. Further difficulties can be introduced by a bias favoring the publication of data that sustain popular hypotheses, or by the intentional selection or exclusion of available reports in ways that could be dangerously close to scientific fraud.

Risk determinations resulting from animal or epidemiological sources are often introduced uncritically in the risk characterization phase, where an additional initial step is also left to the sole competence of technical experts. This step involves estimating what fractions of a population might be exposed to a hazard, at what concentrations, and for how long. The procedure is inherently problematic because it lacks empirical inputs, given that it usually deals with exposures that are new or whose distributions are poorly understood. Various approaches to these estimates have been proposed, the most recent one by the U.S. EPA, which favors a Monte Carlo probabilistic elaboration of demographic assumptions and market and distribution inferences. Regardless of their numerical sophistication, these methodologies are open to criticism, as they are likely to compound the uncertainties derived from dose–response inferences.

Risk–Benefit Considerations

Procedures for risk–benefit analysis have been widely discussed as providing useful generic guidance, but they generally recommend approaches that are tailor-made to the specific issues at hand. Regulators or specialized advisors execute the necessary analyses at least in a preliminary mode, to be further refined and stabilized in policy hearings and debates.

Rule-Making Hearings

Especially in the United States, regulators have felt the necessity to open up the rule-making process and to share responsibilities through a formal open hearing that invites public dialog. Usually, this phase extends the evaluation of a problem under "what if" assumptions, introducing a crossover of ethical and risk–benefit considerations to decide what level of protection the regulation should target. The tolerance of a one in one million adverse event has often been mentioned as a standard objective, but considerable departures have applied if the target population are children, or workers, or expectant mothers, or the elderly, and so on. Thus, risk characterization in open hearings ends up being a deliberative and often confrontational process.

Risk Management

Risk management is the last phase of regulation and entails the promulgation of regulations that reflect risk characterization decisions and, subsequently, their policing and enforcement.

Regulation and the Courts

Often regulators are challenged by court actions that either demand specific regulatory attentions or that challenge regulatory outcomes. Seldom have regulators been forced to initiate regulatory proceedings as a result of court injunctions, but it has not been unusual for the courts to deny, reverse, or to require modification of issued regulations, especially in the United States.

Postregulatory Surveillance

Many regulations are the product of over-conservative assumptions and defaults that tend—at least in principle—to ensure the virtual absence of risks. Still, when cost–benefit considerations or other reasons of need have been the major determinants of regulations that cannot cancel residual risks, the necessity of monitoring the effectiveness of those regulations becomes obvious. Programs to assess post-regulatory effectiveness are routinely established, especially in occupational situations, for approved medicines and food additives, and for certain environmental norms likely to affect large fractions of a population, such as drinking water, air quality, and vehicle safety.

CONCLUSION

When toxicology or epidemiology objectively identifies strong hazards, their input is unquestionably normative and directly results in regulation. However, it is apparent that hazard signals that are weak or not scientifically verifiable are handled differently. In the political context of regulation, they simply raise warning signals of different strengths, which are then considered in a "what if" context of prudence. In that context, the original toxicological or epidemiological reports that raised the warning signal are overcome by a value-laden political dialog that considers how much costly societal "prudence" could be applied.

Toxicological or epidemiological inputs to the process acquire a symbolic truth in the political debate of the risk characterization process, even though they may have been obtained on the basis of assumptions and extrapolations from animal data that are not objectively interpretable in equivalent human terms, or from highly uncertain epidemiological reports. Toxicologists and epidemiologists dealing with regulatory issues need to be alert to the fact that their reports are usually taken at face value by nonscientists, so that the results of a political dialog of risk characterization often are made to appear more solid than they actually are and could result in debatable regulation. Even in countries where the regulatory procedure is strictly administrative and without public participation, the regulatory outcomes may not be better, although in such situations regulators have the discretion of discarding *ex officio* weak toxicological signals that are not worthy of consideration before they can arouse unjustified public anxieties. Yet, such discretionary power carries potential risks too, as the evolving BSE (bovine spongiform encephalopathy) saga has shown.

It is clear that the combined pressures of scientific progress, of uncertainty, and of the political dialog will continue to make sure that health and safety regulation will not be a static paradigm of fixed rules and policies. It should also be apparent that toxicology and epidemiology have most likely already discovered the major health and safety risks that can be incontrovertibly verified on objective scientific grounds. What will continue to interest regulation are the potential risks that might derive from novel uses of human-made or naturally occurring agents whose chronic effects cannot be tested ethically in humans, leaving the usually vague epidemiological observations and animal tests as possible detectors. Advancing research in molecular biology and genetics carries the promise of mechanistic understandings of direct relevance to human risk assessment, although their practical availability is not in sight.

Epidemiology will continue to be a source of equivocal frustrations, given that nonexperimental observational studies can be expected to continue providing hints of increasingly smaller potential risks, whose interpretation will be made extremely problematic by complex tangles of multifactorial associations that are virtually impossible to sort out. Although the potential risks flagged by animal tests and epidemiological reports will likely get smaller and more uncertain, they still will not be ignored in open societies that by design and inclination rely on the adversarial confrontation of different interests.

In all probability, such realities will make life progressively harder on regulators, who already find themselves a natural target of fire from all directions and who will encounter mounting difficulties in reaching consensual solutions under the added prospect of increasing legal challenges.

What are the promising directions that regulators might take to ease these pressures? Seeking consensus, regulators might seek to adopt the open U.S. model of public hearings and participation in the rulemaking process, but such a move would raise new reservations because the introduction of more dialectic and emotional issues could further distance the regulatory process from objective scientific benchmarks and could result in increased tensions rather than consensus.

In a more promising direction, regulators may be compelled to face a wider problem also looming on the horizon, namely how to set regulatory priorities in a context of limited resources. Until now, and notwithstanding the requirements for risk–benefit considerations, a philosophy of safety at all costs has been the implicit regulatory ideal in affluent developed societies driven by the allied interests of advocacy groups, media, public opinion, and legislators. Soon, however, this philosophy may no longer be sustainable, as advocacy and popular exigencies are likely to press for the regulation of increasingly smaller and more uncertain risks, whose hypothetical prevention would carry costlier and costlier price tags. Hence the need for priorities.

Both at the national and global levels, the evidence will mount that an efficient use of scarce resources calls for setting defensible priorities among the many warning signals and the public anxieties that animal tests and epidemiological reports will continue to foster. Regulators will be increasingly challenged with the responsibility of grading potential "what if" hazards and of proposing which ones may deserve regulatory priority and the expenditures of costly measures of prudence. Credible procedures for ranking the uncertainty of risks are not available and need to be formalized: an effort also likely to demand the attention of regulators, who while relentlessly pursuing their inalienable mission of protecting the public from harm emanating from toxic chemicals, must increase their level of alertness to the consequences of their actions on overall economic and cultural values.

This would be a new, unfamiliar, and as yet untested role for toxicologists and epidemiologists who may participate in setting regulatory priorities. Both professions could gain much from a chance to represent themselves forthrightly as the purveyors not of absolute evidence but of credible prudent choices about possible risks. The affirmation of Paracelsus that the dose makes the poison is still fundamental, and it matches the common observation that life endures against all but the most extraordinary odds. Thus, in time, toxicologists, epidemiologists, and regulators might come to find it desirable to adopt changed attitudes and a new role in public education—that of persuading a well-informed public to demand regulatory policies that are always solidly based on the best available science and grounded in realities, and to resist both economically motivated pressure and conjectural anxieties leading to unwarranted excesses of hypothetical prudence.

Bibliography

ADELF (Association des Épidemiologistes de Langue Française) (1997). "Deontologie and bonnes pratiques en epidemiologie. Recommandations de l'Association des Épidemiologistes de Langue Française." ADELF, Paris.

AFL-CIO v. American Petroleum Institute, 448 US 607, 1980.

Bensel, R. F. (1990). "Yankee Leviathan: The Origins of Central State Authority in America, 1859–1877." Cambridge University Press, New York.

Blair, A., Burg, J., Foran, J. *et al.* (1995). Guidelines for application of meta-analysis to environmental epidemiology. *Regul. Toxicol. Pharmacol.* **22,** 189–197.

Doll, R., and Peto, R. (1981). The causes of cancer. *J. Natl. Cancer Instit.* **66,** 1192–1312.

FAO (1995). "Procedural manual. Codex Alimentarius Commission." 9th ed. Food and Agriculture Organization, United Nations, Rome.

FDCA (1938). "US Federal Food, Drug, and Cosmetic Act 21," USC, § 402(a).

FDCA (1958). "US Federal Food, Drug, and Cosmetic Act. Food additive amendments to the Federal Food, Drug & Cosmetic Act 21," USC § 348 et seq.

FIFRA (US Federal Insecticide, Fungicide and Rodenticide Act 7) (1972). USC.

Gaylor, D. W., Axelrad, J. A., Brown, R. P., Cavagnaro, J. A., Cyr, W. H., Huleback, K. L., Lorentzen, R. J., Miller, M. A., Mulligan, L. T., and Schwetz, BA. (1997). Health risk assessment practices in the U.S. Food and Drug Administration. *Regul. Toxicol. Pharmacol.* **26,** 307–321.

Girardeau, J. L. (1995). "The Federal Theology: Its Import and Its Regulative Influence." A Press, Greenville, SC.

GLP (1989). "US Good Laboratory Practice Standards 21," CFR, Part 58.

Gulf South Insulation v. CPSC, 701 F.2d 1137, 5th Cir., 1983.

IARC (International Agency for Research on Cancer Working Group) (1980). An evaluation of chemicals and industrial processes associated with cancer in humans based on human and animal data. *Cancer Res.* **43,** 1–52.

ILO (1990). "Safety in the Use of Chemicals at Work." Convention No. 170. International Labor Organization, Geneva.

Krimsky, S., and Golding, D. (eds.) (1992). "Social Theories of Risk." Praeger, New York.

Lu, F. (1988). Acceptable daily intake: Inception, evolution and application. *Regul. Toxicol. Pharmacol.* **8,** 45–60.

NRC (National Research Council) (1983). "Risk Assessment in the Federal Government: Managing the Process." National Academy Press, Washington, DC.

NRC (National Research Council) (1996). "Understanding Risk: Informing Decisions in a Democratic Society." National Academy Press, Washington, DC.

OECD (Organization for Economic Cooperation and Development) (1987). "Guidelines for testing chemicals." Paris.

Russell, R., Schmalensee, V., Smith, K., and Stavins, R. N. (1996). "Benefit-Cost Analysis in Environmental, Health, and Safety Regulation: A Statement of Principles." American Enterprise Institute, The Annapolis Center, Resources for the Future, Washington, DC.

Shapiro, S. (1998). Is meta-analysis a valid approach to the evaluation of small effects? *In* "Epidemiological Practices in Research on Small Effects (H. Hoffmann *et al.,* eds.). Springer Verlag, Berlin.

Shrader-Frechette, K. S. (1985). "Science, Policy, Ethics, and Economic Methodology." Reidel Publishing, Boston, MA.

Slovic, P. (1993). Perceived risk, trust, and democracy. *Risk Analysis* **13,** 675–681.

Teich, A. H., and Frankel, M. S. (1992). "Good Science and Responsible Scientists: Meeting the Challenge of Fraud and Misconduct in Science." AAAS publication 92-13S. American Association for the Advancement of Science, Washington, D.C.

TSCA (Toxic Substances Control Act 15) USC, 1976.

U.S. CPSC (U.S. Consumer Products Safety Commission) "Summary of Guidelines for determining chronic toxicity." Code of Federal Regulations 16 CFR 1500.135.

U.S. EPA "Health Effects Testing Guidelines. Subchronic Exposure." Code of Federal Regulations 40 CFR 798.

U.S. EPA "Health Effects Testing Guidelines. Chronic Exposure" Code of Federal Regulations 40 CFR 798.

U.S. EPA "Health Effects Testing Guidelines. Genetic Toxicity." Code of Federal Regulations 40 CFR 798.

U.S. EPA (1992). A cross-species scaling factor for carcinogen risk assessment based on equivalence of $mg/kg^{3/4}/day$. *Federal Register* **57,** 24152–24173.

U.S. EPA (1996). US Environmental Protection Agency. Proposed guidelines for carcinogen risk assessment. *Federal Register* **61,** 17960.

U.S. EPA (1997). Guidelines for reproductive toxicity risk assessment. *Federal Register* **61,** 56273.

U.S. EPA (1998a). Guidelines for ecological risk assessment. *Federal Register* **63,** 26845.

U.S. EPA (1998b). Guidelines for neurotoxicity risk assessment. *Federal Register* **63,** 26925.

U.S. FDA (1982). "Toxicological principles for the safety assessment of direct food additives and color additives used in food." U.S. Food and Drug Administration, Washington DC.

U.S. FDA (1995a). Threshold of regulation for substances used in food contact articles. *Federal Register* **60,** 36582. (Also 21 CFR 170.39.)

U.S. FDA (1995b). Guidelines for the assessment of systemic exposure in toxicity studies. *Federal Register* **95,** 11263.

U.S. FDA (1996). International conference on harmonization. Guidelines on testing for carcinogenicity of pharmaceuticals. *Federal Register* **61,** 43298–3300.

U.S. FDA (1997). Substances generally recognized as safe. *Federal Register* **62,** 18937.

U.S. OSHA, "Occupational Safety and Health Standards." Code of Federal Regulations, 29 CFR 1910.

U.S. OSHA (Occupational Safety and Health Act. 29) USC, 1970.

Van DeVeer, D. (1986). "Paternalistic Intervention: the Moral Bounds of Benevolence." Princeton University Press, Princeton.

WHO (1987). "IPCS Environmental Health Criteria 70. Principles for the Safety Assessment of Food Additives and Contaminants in Food." Geneva, World Health Organization.

WHO (1990). "IPCS Environmental Health Criteria 104. Principles for the Toxicological Assessment of Pesticide Residues in Food." Geneva, World Health Organization.

WHO (1994). "IPCS Environmental Health Criteria 170. Assessing Human Health Risks of Chemicals: Derivation of Guidance Values for Health-based Exposure Limits." Geneva, World Health Organization.

Wilson, B. S. (1987). Legislative history of the Pesticide Residues Amendment of 1954 and the Delaney Clause of the Food Additives Amendment of 1958. *In* "Regulating Pesticides in Foods. The Delaney Paradox," pp. 161–173. National Research Council, National Academy Press, Washington, DC.

PART V

RISK ASSESSMENT

CHAPTER

51

Risk Assessment and Preventive Hazard Minimization

DIETHER NEUBERT

Institute of Clinical Pharmacology and Toxicology, Benjamin Franklin Medical Center, Free University Berlin, Berlin, Germany

INTRODUCTION

The assessment of toxicological risk is a difficult process. Evaluation of the necessary clinical and experimental data requires a high degree of toxicological and medical expertise, including a solid medical education and toxicological experience acquired over many years.

The assessment of the probability of adverse effects of an agent on the mammalian organism, and especially on humans, is performed in a sequence of steps, and a number of prerequisites must be fulfilled for meaningful conclusions. The initial extent of complete uncertainty gradually decreases with a growing relevant database (Fig. 1), and, ideally, data both from observations in humans and from experimental animal studies should be available. Data from human trials or appropriate epidemiological studies carry the highest weight.

For many agents the database available has been far from satisfactory. In such cases, statements on possible toxic effects to be expected in humans are not substantiated and must remain largely speculative. Therefore, it would be fair to state the degree of uncertainty associated with a toxicological statement. However, this is rarely done. This leads to considerable confusion for the general public because well-founded conclusions, on one hand, and mere speculations, on the other hand, cannot be distinguished.

This chapter will focus on medical toxicology, and predominantly substance-induced effects will be discussed. However, the general principles of toxicology are also valid in the field of veterinary medicine, and they also apply to physical agents, such as ionizing radiation. Risk assessments for certain ecosystems will only be discussed with respect to human exposure because otherwise this field requires special expertise and different priorities must be considered.

Up to 1993 about 12 million chemicals were known and described in the literature. It is fair to state that there is either no or only an insufficient database for the vast majority of these substances. To change this situation would necessitate more, and not less, animal experimentation or a drastic reduction of the number of substances we are exposed to (thus eliminating the need for toxicological testing). However, citing the number of known chemicals is misleading from a toxicological point of view for several reasons:

- Humans are not exposed to many of the known substances because many have never left the laboratory or are not present in the environment.
- Human exposure to the majority of substances is not at a toxic dose level. This holds especially true for the thousands of natural nutritional substances. In addition, there is certainly a vast number of substances not clearly recognized in our food.

Most adverse health reactions in Europe or North America are caused by overdoses or unfavorable combinations of medicinal drugs. Therefore, a solid knowledge of pharmacology forms the basis for un-

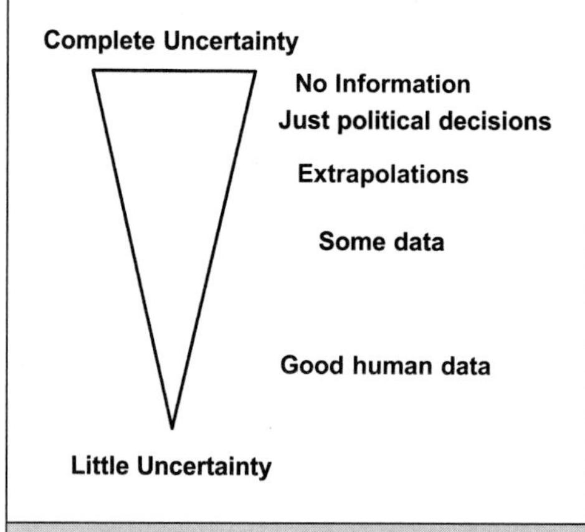

FIGURE 1 Degree of uncertainty with respect to toxic effects in humans, depending on the database. With increasing information, "complete uncertainty" is shifted to "little uncertainty."

derstanding of many toxic effects, and many misinterpretations occurred because of ignorance in this field.

In most industrialized countries, toxic reactions in humans are rarely caused by environmental chemical or physical agents, such as exposure to anthropogenic pesticides, organic solvents, or heavy metals, despite the fact that some political parties, self-elected "environmental" groups and a few regulatory agencies exaggerate this problem. Accidental events associated with very high exposures to chemical or physical agents may create problems, and in former times occupational exposures at various insufficiently protected work places frequently caused chronic and acute intoxications. However, the frequency of such poisonings has considerably decreased with the progress made in preventive health protection.

Most adverse health effects caused by natural or human-made environmental agents are allergic reactions, which should be clearly distinguished from toxic effects. Clear-cut diseases for which environmental agents are jointly responsible often have a multifactorial cause (including genetic factors), for example, as in carcinogenesis co-triggered by environmental factors such as smoking.

Toxicological problems are, as are those of medicine in general, quite different in various regions of the world. Furthermore, the priorities of toxicology change with time. Yesterday's problems may be irrelevant today. This is largely due to preventive measures taken once a problem has been recognized. In some countries, the excessive use of pesticides by unskilled persons still creates problems that have not existed in industrialized countries for decades. In some countries, suicidal poisonings, (e.g. by organophosphates) which are largely unknown in other countries are frequently seen. The rich industrialized countries have the responsibility of performing risk assessments that also have relevance for the residents of the developing countries with continuing excessive chemical exposure and considerable problems in medical toxicology.

Toxicological science attempts to provide the basis for keeping the risk reasonably small, that is, tolerable or acceptable. "Acceptable" is not a scientific but a pragmatic or political term. We must always take certain risks in life, and this will not change in the future. Because absolute safety is impossible to achieve in all aspects of life, this pretension can not be fulfilled in toxicology either. Zero risk cannot be associated with exposure to any agent because it is impossible to prove a "negative."

Toxicological investigations can only attempt to reduce the degree of uncertainty as much as possible. For any attempt in this direction, the quality and size of the database are critical. Uncertainty is maximal when toxicological data are lacking. This is still the case for a multitude of chemicals, and this will continue for decades to come. The chance of a meaningful toxicological evaluation increases when the database grows larger, with respect to both experimental and clinical information. The uncertainty in risk assessment becomes minimal when extensive data from observations in humans are available (Fig. 1).

It makes little sense to evaluate possible toxic effects without considering other factors simultaneously acting on the organism. Organ functions fluctuate permanently, adapting to many exogenous and endogenous variables, such as nutrition, respiration, other exposures, and psychological effects. The organism is not at all static, but is a very dynamic system undergoing numerous adaptative changes. Additional toxic effects will be greatly modified by the usual environmental factors, and the resulting alterations must be clearly outside the physiological fluctuations, with respect to extent and length of time, to be medically significant.

What Is a Poison?

The terms "toxic" and "poisonous" are synonymous. From a medical and a scientific point of view there are no "poisons." Every agent may be harmful if acting on an organism at a high enough dose. The statement made by Paracelsus in 1538 in his "Dritte Defension" is still valid after more than 450 years. Out of all the mystics of that time and in his own publications, the fundamental and quite "modern" sentences stand out and may be translated as: . . . All things are poison, and nothing is without poison. Solely the dose makes that a thing is no poison. . . . This indicates that all things could be toxic, if a high enough dose is applied.

It is now well established that the statement that all agents may be toxic at appropriate dose levels may be reversed. A low enough dose of any agent will cause no or negligible toxicity. This includes carcinogenicity, and it is the basis for all attempts to reduce the possible toxic influences from the environment. Interestingly, Paracelsus not only rejected the term "poison" as a label for an agent, but also predicted for the first time the existence of "no effect ranges."

Nevertheless, in daily life sometimes the term "poison" is used in association with a substance. We use terms such as snake poison, bee poison, poisonous mushroom, and poisonous plants or berries. What is meant by such a designation is that adverse health effects may occur from such agents at exposure levels achievable in daily life. However, with all such agents it is again the dose that is essential. There are always dose ranges at which no adverse health effects occur. This can be illustrated with a few examples. Several berries of deadly nightshade (*Atropa belladonna,* a "poisonous" plant) ingested by children may induce toxic symptoms, and even death when the number of berries is high enough. However, the use of appropriately low doses of atropine is quite safe in medicine, and a single dose (e.g., 1 μg atropine/kg body weight or less) will certainly not induce any adverse effects in adult persons. Another example is a possible poisoning with overdoses of *Digitalis* leaves, but the ingredients with the toxic potential may be safely used in medicine. Here again, even chronic doses of 0.1 μg digoxin/kg body weight or less will not induce any toxic symptoms in adults. The agent with one of the highest toxic potencies known, botulinus toxin from *Clostridium botulinum,* has been used to treat spasmodic torticollis and strabismus. Thus, toxicity is relative and not absolute.

TOXICOLOGICAL RISK BY HUMAN-MADE VERSUS NATURAL CHEMICALS

Interestingly and without any justification, there is the general belief among a considerable part of the population that human-made chemicals are *a priori* loaded with adverse health risks while all naturally occurring chemicals are "good and healthy." As a consequence of this, many believe in "health food," instead of preferring a balanced diet, and presume that a product with the prefix "bio" added to its name automatically becomes "atoxic," as exploited by many manufacturers.

A similar situation exists in therapeutical medicine. All "biological" and most often poorly defined preparations are *a priori* considered safe, and only newly developed and extensively (in preclinical and in clinical trials) tested chemicals developed by the pharmaceutical industry are suspected of being loaded with undesired "side effects." It must be taken into account that many groups of modern medicinal drugs are highly effective, and it should be agreed that highly active substances at appropriate dose levels also have the capability of inducing additional and thereby undesirable health effects. When reading the extensive lists of possible untoward effects attached to a medicinal drug, the consumer can quite understandably become confused, especially because the frequencies of such adverse effects are rarely indicated. As a consequence, especially in Europe, patients are less willing to accept therapeutic risks much smaller than those they take all the time during everyday life. The stage has been reached where the informational value of such instructions for the consumer may be seriously questioned, and the statements are predominantly aimed at protecting the producer from liability for possible damages.

On the other hand, the undesired effects of undefined "biological" mixtures are rarely elaborated on—mostly they have not even been elucidated—and highly questionable claims of therapeutical effectiveness are given special emphasis. If the therapeutic value is doubtful, as with most of such preparations, even small health risks are not acceptable. This holds especially true when allergic reactions are also taken into account.

Favoring undefined "biological" extracts and mixtures, often containing considerable amounts of alcohol, must be considered a step backward. One of the great achievements of modern pharmacology and the pharmaceutical industry is the isolation of active principles out of an undefined and highly variable mixture of hundreds of components, and the possibility of exactly defining the dose of the active ingredients. If old folk medicine presents us with beneficial components, and it often does, these constituents should be isolated and clinically tested according to today's well-established standards.

The rather naive assumption that all natural components are per se harmless is plainly wrong, and it is contrary to the opinion of experts in the field of toxicology. In fact, the substances with the highest toxic potential are invented by nature, and it is a basic principle of biology to take advantage of many organisms' capability to produce substances with a toxic potential aimed at other species. This principle has culminated in the production of antibiotics produced by defined microorganism (e.g., fungi), to achieve growth and living advantages over other organisms (e.g., bacteria). While humans have used substances formed according to this principle in a few cases to develop remedies against infectious diseases (e.g., penicillin), the vast majority of the hundreds of thousands of such antibiotics occurring in nature have a far too toxic potency for mammals to be used in medicine. Over the centuries, humans have experienced the beneficial effects of natural ingredients, such as food or remedies. Even more of the toxic actions of many components in our natural environment produced by plants, animals, and microorganisms, have been found by trial and error.

Compared with the possible harm from defined human-made or natural substances, it is quite likely that in the long run more individuals in our industrialized countries will become sick or die because of an unhealthy life style—eating too much and improper food (e.g., consuming too much undesirable animal fat in their diet), and doing too little exercise. Subsequently, often the attempt is made to compensate for the resulting unfavorable situations by using a multitude of medicinal drugs. Toxicity is relative, and an excess of the relatively "atoxic" glucose may easily kill a diabetic person. However, in their general linguistic uses, animal fat or glucose are not designated as "toxic."

DEFINITION OF TOXICITY, HAZARD, AND RISK

Even scientists trained in fields not far from toxicology often use nomenclature that is quite unacceptable to experts. Unfortunately, vague nomenclature often triggers blurred thinking. This starts with the simple terms "toxic" and "poison", as well as "risk" and "hazard."

Definition of "Toxicity"

As mentioned before, toxicity per se is not a property of a substance but of the dose. There are no toxic substances but only toxic doses of a given substance. Although simple, this is the main secret of toxicology. The absolute toxic dose for different substances will vary over many orders of magnitude. For some substances many grams are required to produce toxic effects, for others nanogram quantities are sufficient.

There are two variables governing the toxicological potency of a given substance.

- The toxic potential of the substance.
- The dose (or exposure level).

This can be illustrated by an example. If botulinus toxin, the substance with the highest toxic potency known, is kept in a sealed ampoule on a table, the resulting toxicity is zero because the exposure is zero. If the ampoule is dropped and shatters, a potentially dangerous situation arises. If it only spills on the shoes and these are burned, no toxicity will arise. If some of the substance is ingested, the resulting effect will depend on the amount taken up, ranging from no effect to serious poisoning or death.

The potential to induce death is also not a property of a given substance, but again a function of the dose. There are no "deadly poisons," and a lethal effect may be induced by any agent, if it is possible to administer a high enough dose.

Most agents induce a certain pattern of toxicity. This means that not all agents are capable of inducing all possible types of adverse effects. This special susceptibility of certain organ systems to a defined chemical is designated "organotropy." It is the aim of animal experiments in toxicology to reveal such a pattern of adverse effects for the substance under investigation. This is one justification for applying overdoses that have little or no relevance to the situation in humans. It is hoped that the specific toxicity profile of the special substance can be recognized by such an approach. Recognition of the pattern of the toxic potential per se will not allow any kind of quantitative risk assessment for humans.

Definition of "Hazard" and "Risk"

Unfortunately, the terms "hazard" and "risk" are not used uniformly by different agencies and scientists in various countries. This has led to considerable confusion. Within the frame of this book we shall use a definition agreed upon by most experts as being most appropriate.

Hazard indicates the potential (i.e., the possibility) of inducing adverse health effects under appropriate conditions. It is a qualitative expression. Appropriate conditions could occur during everyday life with one substance, or may be reached only at extreme exposure scenarios with another agent. Hazard gives information neither on the probability of the induction of an effect under defined conditions of exposure nor on the likelihood that it occurs at all in humans.

Risk, in general, is a quantitative expression. It characterizes the incidence of a defined adverse effect at given exposure levels (doses). Risk is identical with the dose–response relationship, sometimes confined to a single dose. Because from a medical point of view we are only interested in humans, the term only or preferentially refers to a risk for humans. This definition *a priori* excludes extrapolations from animal studies.

To provide an example, a certain agent may exhibit a mutagenic hazard. The risk for the human germ line is not defined by this statement, and it will be extremely small, if it is present at all. Still, we might not like to have an agent with such a potential around in our environment, if this can be avoided. This would be a political not a medical decision. However, substances with a mutagenic potential might be associated with the induction of certain human cancers. In this respect, mutagenicity may provide a hint to a possible carcinogenic potential. The hazard expressed does not give any information on whether increased cancer rates might occur in humans at relevant exposures, and what the incidence might be. This means that no risk for humans can be assessed. This is only possible by conducting epidemiological studies on exposed humans. Such studies are difficult because there are many confounding factors. There is rarely a unifunctional cause, and humans must have been exposed previously. When a risk assessment for humans is demanded, no primary prevention is possible. These two strategies contradict each other. If, in the course of preventive hazard minimization, exposure of humans is avoided, we will never know whether there really has been a risk or not.

The above-mentioned nomenclature for hazard and risk will be used in this chapter, and considerable confusion could be avoided if clear definitions were used throughout the entire toxicological literature, resulting in by far fewer misinterpretations by the general public.

TOXICOLOGICAL RISK ASSESSMENT VERSUS PREVENTIVE HAZARD MINIMIZATION

The greatest confusion in toxicology for the general public as well as for many persons working actively in this field comes from the term "risk." This expression is frequently used for two quite different strategies, which differ from each other like day and night. The intentions of these two strategies are quite different, and the only common aspect is that both attempt to recognize and reduce adverse health effects in humans. To distinguish the two strategies from each other, we designate them here as (Fig. 2):

- Human risk assessment.
- (Administrative) preventive hazard minimization.

The first strategy relies entirely on observations in humans; the second is highly restricted to extrapolations from animal data. While the first approach endeavors to quantitatively characterize adverse health effects from human data, the second one seeks to define acceptable or tolerable exposure levels by extrapolations from animal studies. We have to recall that extrapolations are *per definitionem* "speculations" the correctness of which cannot be recognized. If the true incidence could be assessed, no extrapolations would be necessary.

Toxicological risk assessment itself is not an area of scientific research but an activity pursued by experts evaluating the available scientific data with respect to quality and predictive value in order to draw conclusions about human health risks after chemical or physical exposure. It must be distinguished from risk management, which may or may not take scientific data into account in order to reach political decisions for protecting the health of the public.

Stepwise Approach to Risk Assessment or Hazard Minimization

It has been proposed that risk assessment be divided into a number of steps, such as:

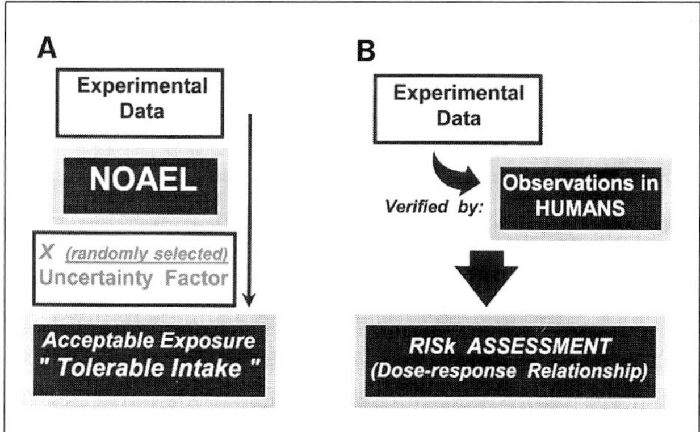

FIGURE 2 Two strategies for revealing and preventing adverse health effects in humans, (A) preventive hazard minimization versus (B) clinical risk assessment. The concepts have little in common except that both are aimed at recognizing and preventing (primary and secondary prevention) adverse health effects.

1. Hazard identification. Determination of whether an adverse effect can be caused by the agent of interest.
2. Dose–response evaluation. Determination of the relationship between dose and the incidence and severity of resulting adverse effects.
3. Human exposure evaluation. Determination of the size and the duration of the dose received by the population.
4. Risk characterization. Integration of the information from the first three steps to provide an estimate of the magnitude of the risk incurred by the population.

From a pragmatic point of view, such a strategy is quite unrealistic and barely in accordance with the general situation in toxicology. The following sequence is more representative of the everyday situation in the assessment of toxicity:

1. Selection of a substance and of the endpoints to be tested.
2. Deciding whether human studies on toxicological endpoints are feasible or not. Quantification of human exposure and establishment of data on kinetics and metabolism in experimental animals and in humans.
3. Selection of appropriate methods and conducting the studies (experimental experiments and human trials).
4. Interpretation and quantification of the data obtained and decision whether further studies are needed.
5. Summarizing all data available and attempting toxicological risk assessment or toxicological preventive hazard minimization.

The sequential procedure outlined has the advantage that it is similar whether studies in humans or experimental animal are to be performed.

Considerations at the first level are important, because it is feasible neither to study all the substances in our environment, nor to use all the toxicological test systems available. Therefore, the selection of the substances to be studied and the endpoints to be evaluated are largely pragmatic. Hazard recognition is not possible as a first step in the sequence because the toxicological profile is often (e.g., at the early stages of developing a new substance) completely unknown. The first step may be designated "problem recognition" because the decision must be made whether a risk assessment or hazard minimization will be attempted at all for the given chemical. This decision is easy in the case of potential medicinal substances and pesticides because a toxicological evaluation is always required by law, but the selection of the endpoints to be evaluated out of a large repertoire very much depends on the type of substance. New medicinal drugs are toxicologically investigated rather extensively. On the other hand, toxicological testing for other environmental chemicals is generally done on an extremely low level with quite limited toxicological test systems. The amount of the chemical released into the environment or first hints of possible adverse effects may govern the decision to do testing or not. The majority of substances in our environment (e.g., food ingredients) are not toxicologically studied at all. This does not imply at all that they are safe for human health at overdoses.

The most important point during a toxicological evaluation is at the second level, the recognition of whether observations in humans are possible and essential or cannot be performed. Here the distinction is made whether a clinical risk assessment with relevance for humans can be attempted or the toxicological evaluation must remain at the much lower and actually unsatisfactory level of a preventive hazard minimization (i.e., limited to extrapolations from animal data).

Kinetic data are compiled at the third level of the evaluation. It is advisable to generate such kinetic data as soon as possible during studies on pharmacology and toxicology. The design of many of the experimental studies greatly profits from the availability of data on kinetics and metabolism, from both experimental animals and humans.

The forth level is not solely to establish dose–response data, because quantitative data may not be required for all endpoints; if for example, mutagenicity is revealed in several systems, it may be decided at this level to stop further development of the chemical. At this level the aim is to compile whatever information is available and to decide which types of further studies should be initiated. A data pool sufficiently large to allow a decision on various types of toxicity must be established. Depending on the class of substance, a limited number of experimental studies are selected out of the great variety of possible test systems. At this level interpretation and quantification of the experimental and, if possible, clinical data are also attempted. The aim is to derive the no observed adverse effect levels (NOAEL) for the various toxicological endpoints in experimental studies, or at incidences of adverse health effects in clinical trials.

At the fifth and final level, an overall interpretation of the results is attempted. An evaluation is meaningful only if it takes all the information available into account. However, often the decisions are no longer scientifically based, but may be largely political or pragmatic. They may be the result of a risk–benefit evaluation. While often based on an extensive database, such decisions need not necessarily be at the end of laborious scientific investigations, but a negative decision may be reached at any step in the strategy described, possibly even at step 1 of the toxicological evaluation (then based entirely on political arguments). The management of risk assessment or hazard minimization is not the result of one-time brain storming, but of decisions that must continuously be adapted to the current level of knowledge. For medicinal drugs, such a stage may only be reached after decades of use and the exposure of hundreds of thousands of persons.

Toxicological Risk Assessment with Relevance for Humans

As pointed out before, toxicological risk for humans can only be assessed from observations in humans. This has been established during the extensive use of medicinal drugs. Substances used for therapy are the domain of human toxicological risk assessment, and this is the most important area of such investigations. Admittedly, clinical data sufficient for a human risk assessment are not available for the majority of chemicals outside the area of therapeutics. Therefore, no risk assessment is possible for most of the environmental substances, and we have to be content with a preventive hazard minimization.

Preventive Hazard Minimization

Protection of humans from agents outside the medical use is also required. Because of the lack of human data, only the second of the mentioned strategies can be pursued. Whenever possible, the extrapolations must be supplemented with observations in humans. Most often this is only possible following massive exposures (occupationally or after accidents) resulting in the occurrence of pronounced adverse health effects. In the past such adverse effects have been observed with many chemicals. Older clinical observations often form the basis of human risk assessment for such agents.

It must be stressed that preventive hazard minimization based on animal data has nothing to do with clinical human risk assessment. If a quantitative risk evaluation were the intention, animal experimentation should be abandoned at once because we know very well that this goal cannot be approached in this way. Preventive hazard minimization serves a quite different purpose, which is to recognize and subsequently prevent presumed toxicological hazards for humans as much as possible. The severe limitations of such an approach are obvious.

Scientific Conclusions versus Political Decisions

Toxicological preventive hazard minimization is ultimately a mixture of scientific evaluations and political–administrative decisions. It is often impossible to recognize where the former ends and the latter starts. For this reason, it would be appropriate to clearly indicate which statements are mostly political or administrative, with little or even no acceptable scientific background. Unfortunately, this is not the case, unavoidably confusing the public and also many "experts." It has become habit to base political decisions on pseudoscientific arguments. Although scientists must recognize their political responsibility, science should not be prostituted for purely political reasons.

Political or administrative influences always begin when scientific data are manipulated. For this reason, the use of "safety factors" or of mathematical models for extrapolating results to lower exposure levels than the ones used in the experiments is always nonscientific. This does not mean that the conclusions based on such assumptions and that administrative extrapolation procedures cannot be helpful or even reasonable and essential. Most often they are quite pragmatic and logically justified. However, they are not backed up by sufficient scientific evidence or measurable data in the species of concern, humans. If such data were available, no extrapolations would be necessary.

The importance of distinguishing between conclusions based on scientific data and those based predominantly or entirely on political decisions is twofold:

- The predictive value for humans is fundamentally different. It is extremely poor in the case of entirely political decisions, and may be very high when sufficient observations in humans are available.
- As a consequence, exposure levels somewhat higher than those limited by political decisions or by preventive hazard minimizations are likely to be without much harm, but the results of risk assessments must be taken much more seriously because they often refer to true incidences.

Placebo Effects and Toxicophobia

Many physiological and pathological situations in human life are altered by psychological influences.

These important factors should not be ignored. Various psychological effects could be both beneficial and adverse to human health. Foreign influences and autosuggestion are the predominant modifying factors. Confidence, faith, belief, and also fear are important and powerful modulators in this respect.

Significance of Placebo and Nocebo Effects

Placebo effects play an important role in therapy, both within the frame of established medicine and in "alternative" medicine. It must be stressed that the extent of placebo effects depends very much on the types of therapeutic intervention, although the boundaries are not strict. Sedative, hypnotic, analgesic or antiemetic effects are strongly modulated by various placebo attempts, which may be associated either with the application of remedies (devoid of true pharmacological actions) or by other means. In some trials, response rates of up to 50% have been reported, for example, with headache or other pains as an endpoint. Responses mediated by the vegetative nervous system seem to respond especially easily to placebo. Some other organ systems and body functions are apparently much less susceptible to unspecific influence (e.g., cardiac insufficiency, failure of renal function, or effects of antibiotics). With increasing scientific knowledge, some placebo effects may now be better understood; for example, links between the CNS and the immune system are becoming evident, and the release of opioid-type cytokines has been reported after acupuncture.

Placebo effects are true effects. The resulting alterations of body functions may be impressive. In contrast to clear-cut specific effects causally linked to defined chemical or physical means, placebo remedies act unspecifically, and the resulting effect is not specifically linked to an active ingredient. Many established drug-induced therapeutic results are composed of a mixture of both clearly pharmacological actions and placebo actions.

Placebo effects are not clearly definable and reproducible actions, but are highly variable with respect to extent, duration, and response in different persons. Even the same individual may react to a placebo differently at various times and occasions. We must remember that pain perception is a complex cerebral phenomenon and not simply a neurological event. Reports of soldiers severely wounded but feeling no pain for hours in a war-time stress situation are well documented. One might argue that endogenous opioid-type cytokines are liberated during such a psychological situation.

The belief of the efficacy of an effect or skepticism toward it are essential confounding factors. It will make a great difference whether one tells a patient suffering from a headache that he or she is receiving a new and powerful drug (which is not true!), or communicates that no effect is to be expected because the preparation is ineffective anyhow. Therefore, the doctor will always be the most efficient placebo. This is common knowledge in medicine. For this reason, reports on placebo effects vary over a wide range with respect to the incidence within a study group.

There is no doubt that unspecific effects may also affect human health adversely. The term "nocebo" (Latin "I want to harm") has been suggested for this type of action. Although mostly of a mild type, such unwanted effects may occasionally be drastic, even fatal. In hundreds of clinical trials this approach has routinely been used to reveal adverse effects clearly attributable to the drug treatment in question (Table 1). Only adverse effects clearly above the placebo rate are considered as drug-induced.

For the reasons mentioned, the true pharmacological and toxic effects of new medicinal drugs are evaluated in double-blind placebo-controlled trials. If the use of a placebo group is not possible for ethical reasons, an established drug therapy is used as a reference group in such clinical trials.

It is self-explanatory that such an evaluation, differentiating between true effects and secondary psychological alterations, cannot be achieved in the case of environmental agents. Strong psychological superposition must be expected in individuals who know they have been highly exposed to an environmental agent, whether toxic effects are expected or not.

Significance of Toxicophobia

Due to massive campaigns by the media and certain political parties in many industrialized countries, many people have been convinced that they live in a heavily polluted world with considerable impact on their health. This has created a massive toxicophobia, and it may be asked whether more damage is done by this mass hysteria, often induced by deliberate misinformation, than by the corresponding agents and industries themselves. Dioxins, passive smoking, wood preservatives, waste incinerators, and nuclear power plants are a few examples. This has distracted attention away from the real problems, and it has prevented a balanced and realistic discussion of public health and the possible dangers of environmental agents. It may be safely stated that "environmental medicine" plays a minor role in all industrialized countries, especially when the general population is concerned. Most problems are politically induced, and medical pseudo-arguments are used as an excuse.

TABLE 1 Examples of the Frequency of Desired or Undesired Placebo Effects as Revealed in Clinical Trials[a]

Symptom or disease	Percentage of "beneficial" placebo effects			Percentage of adverse placebo (nocebo) effects[b]
	N	Mean	Range	
Headache	4588	62%	46–95%	30%
Migraine	4908	32%	20–58%	
Anxiety, neuroses	135	34%	0–61%	25%
Dysmenorrhea	88	24%	11–60%	24%
Dizziness				24%
Fatigue				30%
Nausea				20%
Diarrhea				19%
Impaired vision				18%
Skin rash				4%
Angina pectoris	346	18%	0–57%	
Gastrointestinal symptoms	284	38%	21–56%	
Rheumatic diseases	358	49%	14–84%	
Arterial hypertension	240	17%	0–60%	

[a]Beneficial and adverse effects were not evaluated in the same trials. Exemplified values for favorable effects were from three to ten studies, examples for adverse effects from one study. Because percentages will be extremely variable, depending on the circumstances, they should not be taken at its face value.

[b]From Schindel (1967).

PHARMACOLOGICAL AND TOXICOLOGICAL PRINCIPLES RELEVANT TO RISK ASSESSMENT

Both toxic (i.e., undesired) and pharmacological (i.e., therapeutically beneficial) effects are governed by the same general principles. There is a difference in that some toxic manifestations are more or less irreversible, while pharmacological effects generally only persist during the period of treatment. From a scientific point of view, chemically induced biological effects are neutral, and their classification according to benefits for humans under certain conditions is artificial. Because many exaggerated pharmacological effects may be considered toxic, the distinction between "good" and "bad" is entirely anthropocentric, as is medicine by and large.

The Three Dogmata of Pharmacology and Toxicology

Pharmacology and toxicology are governed by three fundamental principles. These principles hold true independent of the chemical in question.

- All pharmacological or toxic effects occur dose-dependently.
- When the dose is increased, more effects are observable.
- Only pronounced effects can be verified in humans or animal tests.

Although so extremely simple, it seems to be very difficult for most laymen and also for a number of "experts" to bear these principles in mind and to consider them. It is the essence of these dogmata that a desired specific pharmacological effect can only be obtained during a certain dose interval. Below this dose level, no effect can be expected. The same holds true for most toxic manifestations.

Dose-Dependency of Toxic Effects

All toxic effects occur dose-dependently, but the shape and slope of the dose–response curves may be different for various agents and endpoints. Modifying factors include:

- Species differences. Susceptibility, kinetics, slope and shape of the dose response will be expected to differ in various species.
- Pharmacogenetics. Inter- and intraspecies genetic differences will modify the dose response.
- Endpoints. Dose–response curves will be different for various toxic manifestations.

- Complexity of effects. Agents may exhibit more than one effect, and complex situations may result (e.g., induction of their own metabolism), especially when acute and chronic exposures are compared.
- Interferences by mixtures. Components present in mixtures may influence one another's effects (additive, overadditive, or antagonistic).

More Toxic Manifestations at Higher Doses

According to the second dogma, adverse health effects are bound to occur when the dose required for a beneficial therapeutic effect is drastically increased. Additional effects will manifest themselves, and it is very unlikely that those will be beneficial with respect to a medicinal substance highly selected for a defined therapeutic purpose. Some of the effects occurring at overdoses will be incompatible with life. This is why there is a lethal dose for almost any chemical or physical agent.

Impossibility of Detecting Borderline Effects

In the entire field of medicine it is impossible to verify or clearly define "borderline effects." Toxicology is no exception. There are a number of reasons that this is true:

- "Normality" in almost all instances is not a constant but a fluctuating range, and "abnormality" continuously confluxes into the normal range.
- Small deviations from the normal range can usually not be considered as clearly pathological, in the sense of "disease."
- Very small deviations from a reference range can often not be confirmed in subsequent studies. Typically, out of several trials, some turn out to be positive and some negative. Therefore, data from single studies are quite unreliable, unless very pronounced effects are documented.
- "Statistical significance" and "medical significance" are not synonymous. Many minor statistical differences are biologically and medically meaningless.

Although very small deviations from a reference range, as revealed in studies in humans or animals, cannot be interpreted or even verified and are, in general, without medical significance, they often trigger the most vivid discussions. It is typical of such effects that contradictory results are reported in several publications on the same topic. Much of the interest in such postulated effects is not understandable from a scientific or medical point of view, but such a matter provides an excellent platform for often fruitless political discussions and ideological persuasions.

Exposure, Intake, and Uptake into the Organism

A prerequisite for a biological action is that the agent reaches the target inside the organism. For this purpose, a sufficient dose must be offered to the organism (exposure), and the agent must penetrate the organism (Fig. 3). With respect to chemical substances, this is designated "absorption." "Exposure" is defined as concentration at the borders of the organism. This includes the skin, gut, and lungs. If an oral

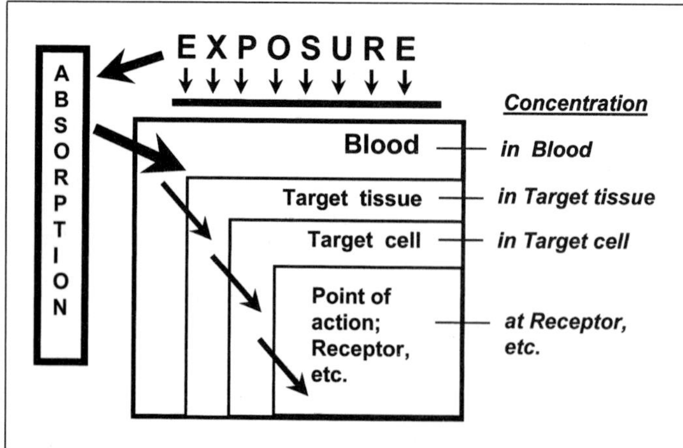

FIGURE 3 Difference between exposure and body burden. Exposure is defined as dose (concentration) at the outer body surface (including uptake). Body burdens are a function of the degree of absorption (intake) and the speed of elimination (e.g., elimination half-life). The concentration at the point of action cannot be assessed, and plasma concentrations are often taken as a surrogate marker.

exposure to a substance is not associated with an absorption from the intestinal tract, no systemic effect will result. Similarly, if an inhaled substance or particle is not absorbed from the lung, it cannot induce a systemic effect, although local irritations may result.

The effective dose is sometimes designated the "internal dose," or, better, the "body burden." It is best defined as the concentration within a given tissue. Because this evaluation can often not be achieved in humans, concentrations in blood plasma are accepted as a surrogate. It is assumed, often rightly, that an equilibrium exists between the blood and resulting tissue concentrations. This does not mean identical concentrations in the blood and various tissues. An extreme situation exists when a substance is bound to a defined tissue component (e.g., bone trabecula), resulting in a considerable discrepancy between the concentrations in the blood and the storing tissue. Bone and liver cancers and leukemia induced by certain radioactive substances (e.g., thorium or plutonium) are good examples.

Although a certain concentration in the target tissue is the prerequisite for biological effects, the predominant manifestations need not necessarily occur in the tissues with the highest concentration of the xenobiotic. The affinity for a special target (e.g., a receptor) is the crucial factor, and numerous unspecific bindings are common events. Highly lipophilic substances are predominantly stored within the adipose tissue. This is generally not the target tissue. Extensive storage within the body fat may even effectively decrease target tissue concentrations. Thus, adverse health effects may be greatly diminished. There is evidence that this behavior may be responsible for the relatively small toxic effects induced by tetrachlorodibenzo-*p*-dioxin (TCDD) in humans.

A special situation exists with respect to the possible effects on the conceptus. The rate of transfer to the embryo or fetus may vary considerably during gestation, and the membranes do certainly not constitute a strict obstacle for certain agents. Larger molecules (e.g., IgG) or polar substances may reach the conceptus, quite in contrast to functions of the blood–brain or the blood–testes barrier.

Dose–Response Relationships of a Defined Toxic Action

As described, all toxic and pharmacological actions occur dose-dependently. However, such a dose response does not continue indefinitely. A maximum of a defined effect is always reached, unless limited by other overriding manifestations, such as death. This means that the dose–response curve levels off at a certain maximal dose range. With respect to different toxicological endpoints, the slope of the dose–response curves for various organ manifestations cannot be expected to be identical (Fig. 4).

The phenomenon of approaching a maximal effect can be explained in the case of a pharmacological effect in terms of receptor saturation or maximal

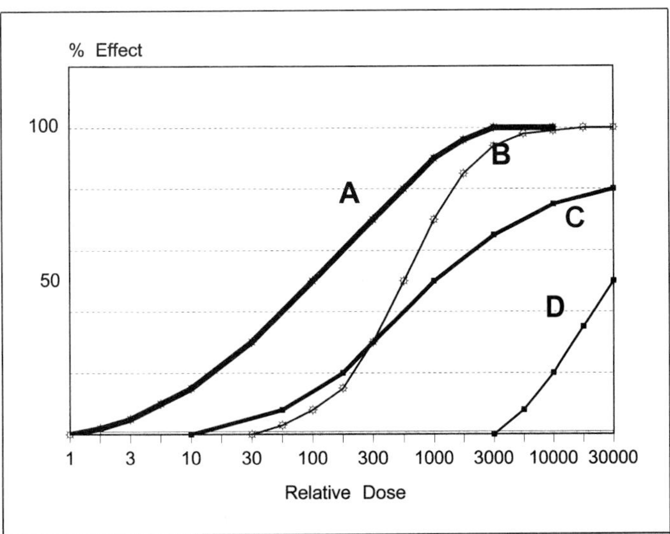

FIGURE 4 Examples of dose–response curves. (A) shows the effect to be considered. When increasing the dose, more effects will occur, with different slopes of the corresponding dose–response curves. At one of the doses the effects will no longer be compatible with life.

inhibition of an enzyme, or the maximal contraction or relaxation of a muscle.

With respect to toxic or pharmacological effects two types of manifestations may be distinguished.

- Variable magnitude of an effect on an individual or on a defined organ endpoint.
- Effects on an increasing number of individuals within a given population.

The outcome of the first case is a graded response. In the second case, a certain incidence of an effect will result. It is important to remember that dose–response relationships hold true for both of these manifestations.

There is no strict rule with respect to the shape of the dose–response curve. The steepness may also vary considerably for different effects and in various species. A dose of zero is always correlated with no effect. A no effect level will often be reached at clearly measurable doses. A dose response is best defined as the 50% effective dose (ED_{50} or LD_{50}). At this response rate of the S-shaped curve, the confidence interval is especially narrow.

Lowest Observed Effect Level and No Observed Effect Level

For most toxicological or pharmacological evaluations, the ED_{50} is not the most convenient estimate. In pharmacological evaluations, the dose inducing the highest beneficial response with little or no adverse health effects is desired. In toxicological evaluations, the lowest dose inducing an undesired effect (lowest observed adverse effect level, LOAEL) or, even better, inducing no detectable effect (no observed adverse effect level, NOAEL) has the greatest significance.

It should be remembered that LOAEL and NOAEL refer to a defined experiment. Repeating the study is not likely to provide the same number. Furthermore, the reliability of a LOAEL and NOAEL critically depends on a number of aspects.

- Spacing of the doses in the study. Smaller differences between the doses give a greater confidence.
- Steepness of the dose–response curve.
- Number of individuals used per dose group. Larger numbers give a greater confidence.

Although otherwise pragmatically used, LOAEL and NOAEL are not well-defined numbers. They exhibit a confidence interval, depending on the factors mentioned.

Opposite Effects at Low Exposure Levels

The dose dependency of exogenously induced effects has been verified in thousands of studies, in experimental animals as well as in humans. It represents the basis for any attempt at environmental protection and at an effective medical drug treatment.

There has been a claim that effects opposite of those observed at high doses are regularly induced at lower dose levels. Such "homeopathic" effects have been speculated to occur within a dose range of many orders of magnitude, up to dilutions in which no molecule of the substance is left. Of course, this dogmatic belief has not been proven over a period of more than 100 years. Surprisingly, an increasing number of individuals in many countries confess to this belief. It must be stressed that accepting the principles of toxicology is incompatible with believing in homeopathy!

There is some evidence that opposite responses are possible within certain areas of a dose–response curve. Such U-shaped areas of a dose–response curve only occur over a narrow range (Fig. 5). With a further lowering of the dose they rapidly convert into no effect. The reversal of the induction of precarcinogenic hepatic lesions by TCDD or similar effects of the same substance on defined immunological components are good examples.

Opposite effects may also be observed with substances exhibiting dual functions. This could occur by simultaneously acting on more than one receptor. Epinephrine acting on adrenergic α- and β-receptors may serve as an example. The simultaneous applica-

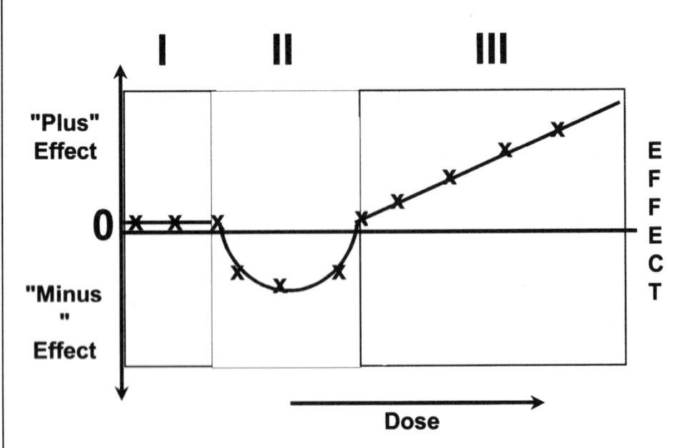

FIGURE 5 Biphasic (U-shaped) dose–response curve. A similar shape was reported for the tumor-promoting property of TCDD, and for effects induced by this substance on immunological components. This has a profound influence on attempts to extrapolate to lower dose levels. Closer analysis may reveal similar curves for other agents.

tion of an α-adrenergic blocking agent will induce the well-known "epinephrine reversal" on blood pressure.

Opposite effects of a special type are also well known when an excess of a vital substance is applied. While vitamin A is essential for normal pregnancy, an excess of this substance will induce malformations. In this case a lack of this vitamin will also induce abnormal development.

The phenomena described are special situations. They are not related in any way to the general principle of homeopathy but rather contradict it.

TOXICOLOGICAL RISK ASSESSMENT FROM HUMAN DATA

Adequate human data carry the highest weight with respect to toxicological evaluations. They are the only data usable for a proper human risk assessment. Conclusions on causal relationships are only possible when clear-cut and pronounced effects are evaluated.

For an appropriate risk assessment, the database should be as large as possible. Data on the chemical reactivity are required as well as data from preclinical studies (Table 2).

TABLE 2 Database for the Medical–Toxicological Evaluation of a Substance

Data on the chemistry of the substance (e.g., functional groups, possibly parallels to already known substances, chemical reactivity)
Toxicological data from animal experiments (e.g., results of studies on acute and chronic toxicity, symptoms of intoxication, data on organ toxicity, reproductive toxicity, mutagenicity, carcinogenicity, local tolerance, effects on the immune system including sensitization)
Data on *in vitro* studies (e.g., on mutagenicity, additional studies on abnormal prenatal development, studies on sensitization)
Data on pharmacokinetics and the metabolism of the laboratory animal species used (absorption, tissue distribution, elimination, active and inactive metabolites after single and multiple application, question of cumulation, enzyme induction, interactions)
Data on pharmacokinetics in humans
Data on biological and toxic effects in humans (e.g., acute exposure, long-term exposure, medical studies, small to extremely large groups of exposed persons
Data on kinetics of the *in vitro* studies (e.g., concentration of the free substance in the medium, concentration in the explant, formation of reactive metabolites)
Data of model studies (e.g., biologically based pharmacokinetic models)

Types of Information in Humans

There are several types of observations for detecting toxicological effects. Such an observation may be made either by chance or during systematic trials or evaluations. Three types of observations in humans may be distinguished:

1. Case reports. Defined symptoms are observed and associated with a chemical exposure. Often several exposures occur simultaneously and many other factors may modify a response. Cause-and-effect relationships can rarely be proven. A better causal relationship may be established with multiple case reports in which pronounced effects were observed. The teratogenicity of thalidomide was revealed in this way. Deliberate reexposure may be another possible way to strengthen the correlation. This is often used in revealing the cause of allergic reactions.

2. (Placebo-) controlled double-blind clinical trials. These use defined exposures to single agents and evaluate one or a few clearly defined endpoints. This is the highest level of human evaluation, used extensively for medicinal drugs.

3. Epidemiological studies. These are evaluations of greatly differing quality on human data. It is one principle of epidemiology that such single studies do not allow us to prove a causal relationship. From the results of a single epidemiological investigation, a hypothesis may be advanced. The validity of such a hypothesis must be assessed in further independent studies. Thus, all types of epidemiological studies are, with regard to design and predictive power, much inferior to well-performed clinical trials. Three types of epidemiological studies may be distinguished.

(a) Prospective studies, or cohort studies. From all types of epidemiological evaluations these are the ones with the highest predictive power. It is possible to recognize incidences of abnormal outcome in the exposed group compared with an appropriate reference group (relative risks).

(b) Retrospective studies, or case-control studies. Although some information may be obtained with such a study design, this type of exploration is loaded with compromises. It is impossible to recognize incidences. Unless a very pronounced effect is observed, the study design gives no unequivocal results. No risks are detectable, but odds ratios assessed among the groups. Often the number of exposed persons per group is assessed with respect to a special endpoint rather than the frequency of effects within a well-defined exposed group.

(c) Intervention studies. Sometimes it is possible to reveal a deficiency as possible cause of a pathological situation. In another situation, a defined antagonistic action is feasible. By supplementation or antagonistic measures, one may succeed in counteracting the deleterious situation and thereby the pathological outcome. This type of study will predominantly be a prospective design. The prevention of neural tube defects by maternal folate supplementation during pregnancy and counteracting the induction of gastric cancer by vitamin supplementation (with the aim of preventing nitrosamine formation) are examples of such approaches.

Predictive Power of Different Types of Studies

The descriptions of the study designs indicate that the predictive power with respect to revealing cause-and-effect relationships must be very different for the various types of observations in humans. The sensitivity and specificity of the test are critical. Because the spontaneous rate will vary considerably under different conditions (Table 3), the prevalence of an outcome also is of considerable importance (Table 4). There are also examples of a yearly fluctuation of the spontaneous malformation rate, depending on the number of evaluated mother–child pairs (Table 5).

For a satisfactory conclusion, a number of criteria must be met. If several of these criteria are not fulfilled, the predictive value of a toxicological evaluation will be doubtful.

1. Exposure or, better, the body burdens of the exposed individuals must be proven to be unambiguously increased (Fig. 6). Living in a contaminated area or being at a contaminated work place is often an insufficient criterion. The quantification of the resulting individual body burden (e.g., from a certain work place) is optimal. Calculations of exposure scenarios are generally unsatisfactory. In retrospective studies, it is often impossible to satisfy this demand.
2. Exposure should be to a single well-defined agent. Multiexposure only allows conclusions with respect to the exposure situation (e.g., a certain work place or smoking) but not to a single agent. Not satisfying this criterion is a drawback of many studies.
3. The study design should allow us to distinguish between acute and chronic manifestations.
4. A well-defined single endpoint (or a few endpoints) should be evaluated. A clear hypothesis should be formulated before the study is initiated. Assessing a multiplicity of endpoints only allows us to generate possible hypotheses for further studies. It is not capable of recognizing cause-and-effect relationships.
5. The reference group should be well defined and representative of a comparison with the exposed group. Inevitable variations within reference groups should be taken into account. Statistically significant differences may critically depend on

TABLE 3 Example of Difficulties in the Interpretation of Data from a Large Experimental Series on Embryotoxicity Testing in Mice[a]

Group	Viable fetuses/litters	Resorptions (%)/ implantation sites	Cleft palates/fetuses	Cleft palates/litters
Experimental series to be evaluated				
Experimental (1)	350/28 = 12.5	35/385 = (9.1%)	6/350 = 1.71%	6/28 = 21.4%
Concurrent controls (2)	686/58 = 11.8	40/726 = (5.5%)	3/686 = 0.44%	3/58 = 5.2%
Statistical test: (1) → (2)	Cleft palates per fetuses	$\chi^2 = 4.39$ significant difference		
Statistical test: (1) → (2)	Cleft palates per litter	$\chi^2 = 5.33$ significant difference		
Statistical test: (1) → (2)	Resorptions	$\chi^2 = 5.13$ significant difference		
Historical reference data				
(3)	441/37 = 11.9	37/478 = (7.7)	3/441 = 0.68%	3/37 = 8.1%
(4)	297/24 = 12.4	22/319 = (6.9)	5/297 = 1.68%	5/24 = 20.8%
(5)	294/24 = 12.3	23/317 = (7.3)	3/294 = 1.02%	3/24 = 12.5%
Sum 2–5 (6)	1718/143 = 12.0	122/1840 = (6.6)	14/1725 = 0.82%	14/141 = 9.9%
Sum 3–5 (7)	1032/85 = 12.1	85/1114 = (7.6)	11/1032 = 1.07%	11/85 = 12.9%
χ^2 test: (2) → (4) Cleft palates per fetus	$p = 4.00$	significant difference		
χ^2 test: (2) → (4) Cleft palates per litters	$p = 4.73$	significant difference		
All other tests:		no significant difference		

[a]Does the dose of the substance (1) increase the incidence of embryofetomortality or of malformations (cleft palates) as compared to controls (2–5)?

TABLE 4 Two Examples of the Influence of the Prevalence on the Predictive Value of a Test[a]

	Number of cases in which the effect is								
	Present			Absent					
		I	II		I	II	Sum	
Prevalence		5%	(28%)		5%	(28%)		
Number of *positive* test cases	(*a*)	50	(49)	(*b*)	28	(4)	78	(53)
Number of *negative* test cases	(*c*)	5	(5)	(*d*)	917	(117)	922	(122)
Sum		55	(54)		945	(121)	1000	(175)

	I	II
n =	1000	(175)
Prevalence[b] =	5%	(28%)
Sensitivity[b]	91%	(91%)
Specificity[b]	97%	(97%)
Correct prediction of the effect[c]	64%	(93%)
Correct prediction of a missing effect[c]	99%	(96%)

[a]Two examples are given (second example in parenthesis). According to Sackett *et al.* (1991).
[b]Prevalence = $a + c/a + b + c + d$. Sensitivity = $a/a + c$. Specificity = $d/b + d$.
[c]Predictive value of a positive test result = $a/a + b$. Predictive value of a negative test result = $d/c + d$.

TABLE 5 Fluctuation of the Yearly Incidence of Anencephaly in Humans, Depending on Size of the Study Group[a]

Year of observation	Absolute number of cases[b]	Incidence per 10,000 births: Sweden	Incidence per 10,000 births: United States
1974	42/111,000	3.8	4.4
1975	29/104,000	2.8	4.3
1976	38/99,000	3.8	4.2
1977	37/97,000	3.8	3.7
1978	18/94,000	1.9	3.7
1979	23/97,000	2.4	3.6
1980	17/98,000	1.7	3.3
1981	11/95,000	1.2	3.5
1982	14/93,000	1.5	3.3
1983	17/92,000	1.8	3.0
1984	10/94,000	1.1	2.6
1985	7/99,000	0.7	2.7
1986	13/102,000	1.3	2.6
1987	20/105,000	1.9	2.0
1988	8/113,000	0.7	2.1

[a]Evaluation of 0.5–1.2 million births/year from the USA (1974–1988), but only about 0.1 million births/year from Sweden. Data from International Clearinghouse (1991).
[b]Malformations/total births.

the references chosen, especially when the effect is not very pronounced. It is poor strategy to use several reference groups in order to find one providing statistical significance.

6. The results obtained should be plausible with respect to outcome and known mechanisms of action (e.g., with data from animal studies and kinetic data).
7. The effect observed should be pronounced. It is impossible to assess borderline effects. Generally, odds ratios in epidemiological studies of <2 are difficult to interpret and prone to misinterpretations. Case-and-effect relationships are not convincing. Confounding factors cannot be controlled and will often not even be recognized. This limitation in the interpretation of the results also holds true when the difference was shown to be "statistically significant."

It is obvious that these criteria may be fulfilled in controlled clinical trials. Most often corresponding experimental conditions cannot be chosen in epidemiological studies, especially in retrospective ones. This *a priori* limits the predictive power of such studies.

Surrogate Markers versus Endpoints of Real Medical Interest

Especially in clinical trials, the endpoints evaluated are often surrogate markers. When assessing the pos-

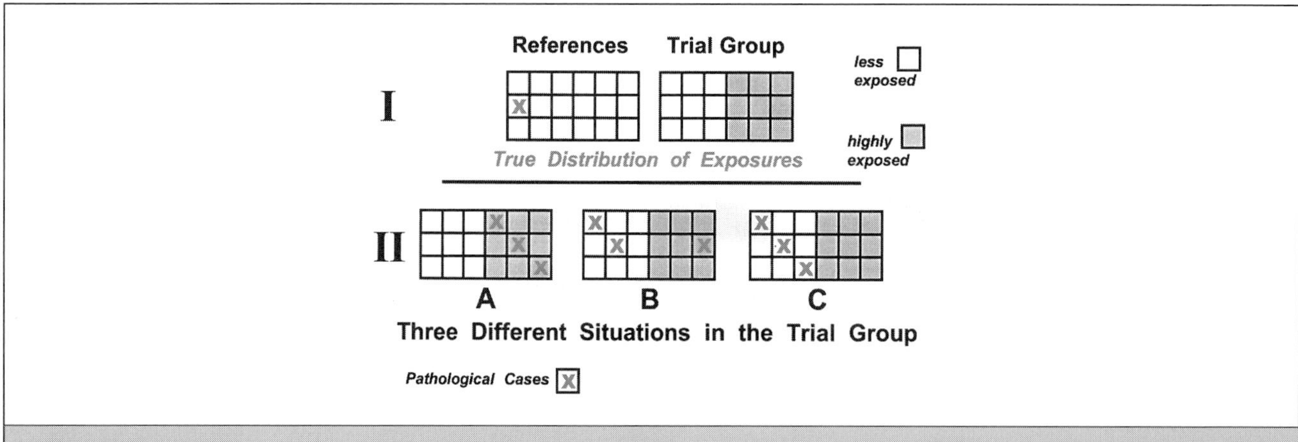

FIGURE 6 Uncertainty in epidemiological studies (especially case-control studies) when the individual body burden (i.e., the true distribution of exposures within a group) is unknown, as is usually the case. In the example illustrated each box represents 10 volunteers (sum: 180 exposed, and 180 reference persons). The spontaneous incidence in the reference group is 10/180 = 6%. In the exposed group it is 30/180 = 17% (χ^2, $p < 0.05$). Within the trial group, the exposure of 50% of the volunteers was heavy, that of the rest negligible. The distribution of volunteers among these exposure subgroups must remain unknown to the investigator, and it cannot be distinguished among the following three hypothetical situations.

	Incidence of pathological cases among highly exposed persons	Real situation with respect to exposure	Incidence measured in the study
Situation A	30/90	Excellent correlation; good dose–response; true risk will even be underestimated in the study!	30/180
Situation B	10/90	Poor correlation; no dose–response; true risk will be overestimated in the study!	30/180
Situation C	0/90	Pseudo-correlation; reversed dose–response; pathological cases probably due to confounding factors	30/180

sible benefits of blockers of cholesterol biosynthesis, cholesterol levels in the blood are monitored. However, we are not interested in high or low cholesterol levels, unless these are correlated with a reduction of cardiovascular diseases. Thus, the surrogate marker may or may not be correlated with the incidence of the ultimate disease in question. In the long run, the effectiveness of the agent in reducing the incidence of the disease is the relevant aspect, and not the "cosmetics" of laboratory values. Therefore, trials are essential to verify the effectiveness with respect to the most relevant medical endpoint.

There are numerous examples of assessments in which only a surrogate marker was evaluated, and data on the effect of real interest are lacking. Because any effective therapy is associated with some risk of adverse effects, the proof of effectiveness against the disease in question is crucial for any attempt at a risk–benefit evaluation. The much easier use of surrogate markers can only be a first step toward such a goal, especially when no convincing effect on this marker is obtained.

The percentage of persons who benefit from a given treatment is essential. If few persons benefit and the treatment involves a nonnegligible toxic risk, the overall evaluation of such a procedure may not be favorable. With the limited resources available, cost–benefit may also play a role.

Associations by Chance and Nonsense Correlations

Because it is impossible to control all possible confounding factors in an experiment or clinical trial, associations by chance must occur. Such associations may well be statistically significant. This indicates that a blind belief in statistics will be dangerous in medicine, and especially in a toxicological evaluation. Evaluating medical significance, not assessing statistical significance, is the final goal.

Associations by chance are bound to occur. Uncertainties caused by multiexposure have been mentioned. When a multiplicity of endpoints are evaluated without stating a clear-cut hypothesis before initiating the study, the impossibility of a toxicological interpretation is preprogrammed. This type of "all-around epidemiology" is largely worthless from a toxicological point of view. Only hypotheses may be generated. Generally, the crucial follow-up studies are not performed, and there is no intention of performing them. The benefit may only be the overall medical examination of a certain subpopulation.

Even in well-designed large multicenter studies nonsense associations will be found when multiple endpoints, such as laboratory data, various cancers, and malformations, are evaluated simultaneously, preferentially when different confounding conditions are present. In contrast to other associations occurring by chance, nonsense correlations are easily recognized as such. Some examples of such obviously false associations are found in the excellent "Boston Study" on 56,000 mother–child pairs (Table 6). The chance of stumbling over a false association is especially pronounced when small relative risks or odds ratios are found. Reason always demands that we be cautious of conclusions when such ratios are ≤2.

Risk for Individuals or for a Population

We may distinguish between a toxicological risk for an individual and a risk within an exposed group of a population. The result of these two types of evaluation may be quite different. Although there could be a small risk for an individual, the number of severe pathological cases within the population may be considered unacceptable. For example, if an agent caused a 1:100 incidence of having a child with pronounced mental retardation, this would be a small individual risk. If 5000 pregnant women were exposed, this risk of 50 handicapped children may constitute a considerable burden to society. (A possible spontaneous rate is ignored in this example.)

The probability of a risk for an individual, depending on the calculated relative risk, is shown in Table 7. Even with a relative risk of 2.0, there is, per definitionem, only a 50% chance that the outcome was caused by the exogenous factor in question. For all relative risks <2.0, the outcome will not be caused by the agent in the majority of the cases. Therefore, relative risks of <2.0 are considered by many investigators as highly unreliable in epidemiological studies, considering the many confounding factors.

The absolute number of adverse health effects induced by an agent in a population depends on the toxic potential of the agent and the number of exposed persons (Table 8). When an incidence of 1:1000 is induced by an agent and 50 persons are exposed, it is very unlikely that a single adverse health effect will be observed within this subgroup. Furthermore, the percentage increase will be high when a rare specific endpoint is affected (exposed 3:100 versus 1:100 of references). A pronounced effect may be hidden when an overall incidence (e.g., the overall malformation or

TABLE 6 Examples of Probable Correlations by Chance, or Nonsense Correlations[a]

Substance class or factor	Defect evaluated	Incidence: Observed/ expected	SRR[b]	95% CI
Local antimicrobial substances	Musculoskeletal	30/20.4	1.5	(1.10–1.96)
Local antimicrobial substances	CNS	7/14.8	0.5	(0.19–0.98)
	Clubfoot	19/11.2	1.7	(1.03–2.65)
Cetalconium	Clubfoot	9/3.1	2.9	(1.33–5.47)
Meclicine	Eye or ear	7/2.5	2.8	(1.23–5.73)
Antidepressants	Funnel chest	5/12.5	0.4	(0.13–0.95)
Nitrofurazone	Gross malformations	1/6.7	0.2	(0.00–0.82)
Phenazopyridine	Gross malformations	1/6.2	0.2	(0.00–0.89)
Progesterone	Malformations	7/14.6	0.5	(0.19–0.98)
Never smoked	Down syndrome	31	1.6	
Weight of placenta unknown	Down syndrome	10	2.1	
Weight gain unknown	Down syndrome	5	2.5	
Other than Protestant religion	Down syndrome		1.7	
Catholic	Malformations		1.4	

[a]Studies of drug-induced effects during pregnancy. Data modified from Heinonen *et al.* (1977).
[b]SRR, standardized relative risk. CI, confidence interval.

TABLE 7 Probability of a Substance-Related Risk for an Individual Based on the Outcome of Well-Conducted Human Studies[a]

Relative risk found	Pathological cases found[b]	Assumed 95% CI[c]	Probability: Induced by the substance	Probability: Induced spontaneously	Substance-induced risk
1.2	12/10	0.7–2.5[d]	(17%)	(83%)	Cannot be verified as "effect"
1.5	15/10	0.9–2.5[d]	(33%)	(67%)	Cannot be verified as "effect"
4.0	40/10	0.9–6.5[d]	(75%)	(25%)	Cannot be verified as "effect"
1.2	12/10	2.1–2.5	17%	83%	Might be increased
1.5	15/10	1.1–2.5	33%	67%	May be increased
2.0	20/10	1.6–4.5	50%	50%	Equal to spontaneous risk
4.0	40/10	2.1–6.5	75%	25%	Clearly increased
10.0	100/10	3.1–25	90%	10%	Convincingly increased

[a]In the case of a "positive" manifestation in an individual (e.g., cancer or malformations) the probability of the outcome being caused by the agent or may have occurred spontaneously is indicated.
[b]Exposed/references, if exposed and reference groups are of equal size.
[c]CI: confidence interval.
[d]If the first value is <1.0, the claimed apparent increase is likely to have occurred by chance.
[e]Purely hypothetical values, because an "effect" cannot be verified, are in parentheses.

cancer rate), including many possible adverse effects, is used as a criterion (Table 9).

New Lifestyle Drugs and Health Risks

A new dimension of possible health risks will be initiated by the mass consumption of newly developed lifestyle drugs, which have recently been marketed with the tremendous help of the mass media and accepted by regulatory agencies in most industrialized countries. These drugs have not been designed to treat clear-cut diseases but are aimed at improving certain body functions, such as sexual potency, or at improving the results of the excesses of a modern lifestyle, such as being overweight from overfeeding, or minor disabilities, such as being bald.

Even though such drugs may exhibit few undesirable toxic effects, they will, on the one hand, lead to hitherto unknown levels of health risks and, on the other hand, may even reduce the well-known risks of undesired symptoms and side effects of the associated medical treatments. The mass consumption of such substances by individuals considered as largely healthy from a medical point of view is rather new. Being bald may be a social problem, but it is certainly not a medical one.

The definition of a "lifestyle drug" remains difficult because the borders between this type of substance and medicinal drugs proper are anything but clearly defined. The mass use of hormones by women all over the globe to prevent pregnancy can certainly not

TABLE 8 Absolute Number of Adverse Effects in a Population Depending on the Toxic Potential of the Substance and the Number Exposed

Size of exposed population	Incidence of adverse effects	Number of persons affected
80,000,000	1:100,000	800
800,000	1:1000	800
80,000	1:100	800
8,000	1:10	800

TABLE 9 Overall Consequence of the Thalidomide Disaster (1961) on the Total Malformation Rate in the Federal Republic of Germany

	Rough estimates
Birth rate per year at that time in the Federal Republic of Germany	≈1,000,000
Number of total severe malformations per year (rate: 3% of live births)	≈30,000
Number of severe limb reduction defects per year (rate: 0.01% of live births)	≈100
Number of additional limb reduction defects due to thalidomide per year	≈2,000
Increase of limb reduction defects due to thalidomide per year	0.01 to 0.2%
Increase of total severe malformations due to thalidomide per year	from 3 to 3.2%

be designated as a typical medical treatment because pregnancy is not a disease. It may rather be looked on as part of a social revolution and perhaps also the desire to reduce the overpopulation of this planet. However, there are well-known health risks associated with undesired pregnancies, and thus some medical aspect cannot be denied. It is more difficult to separate lifestyle drugs from the many chemicals or biological "medical" preparations, long overwhelmingly advertised and excessively consumed in the past (mostly with the false promises of prolonging the life span), but of doubtful effectiveness and benefit. Garlic, ginseng, melissa spirit, and hundreds of other preparations belong into this group.

Among the lifestlye drugs on the market are compounds capable of facilitating male sexual intercourse. This may be of some therapeutic value in selected patients. However, this indication was probably not the main intention of the manufacturer. The mass use of such a highly effective chemical by older men in whom special risk problems are bound to arise may be expected to increase the incidence of cardiovascular diseases and of deaths due to additional and unusual stress situations. There are numerous problems associated with this new type of risk caused by this category of substance:

- The normal prevalence of serious diseases or deaths in this group of senior persons due to excessive sexual activity is largely unknown, but it does not appear to be negligible. It will, at present, be difficult to reveal an additional incidence caused by the use of a lifestyle drug and to clearly establish a cause–effect relationship.
- This type of substance will be freely available ("restricted" by prescription laws or not). It will be almost impossible to relate heart attacks or deaths to the use of such drugs because their use will often not be disclosed.
- Without medical supervision the drug may be taken by patients with diseases contraindicating its use.
- Although the producer may issue warnings because of possible adverse health effects due to interactions with other medications (e.g., with nitro preparations), it is typical that many users will not read and obey these warnings.

Despite these objections, the use and misuse of such drugs will continue. It is doubtful whether possible regulatory measures will be effective in the case of these types of substances. It may be expected that in the near future many similar lifestyle drugs will be developed and used for mass experiments in humans. The danger is that many of such drugs will be highly effective. This could create a hitherto unknown dimension of medicinal risks and public health problems, with little experience to deal with them.

It is impossible to predict a low incidence of severe adverse health effects of an agent from the relatively few, mostly healthy, persons exposed at the beginning of the marketing of a new substance. When the exposure of a large proportion of a population is intended, a "human mass experiment" is necessary for a reliable toxicological risk assessment. The outcome of such an experiment in humans cannot be predicted. The first example of this type of exposure was the use of hormonal anticonceptive drugs in millions of women when virtually nothing was known about the possible health risks with respect to cardiovascular diseases or cancer incidence associated with such a long-term exposure. We were lucky that the outcome of this "experiment" with female sex hormones was comparatively favorable. One should not count on such luck in all cases, and unpleasant surprises are bound to occur in such a game of Russian roulette.

However, it would be a one-sided story to only concentrate on the possible adverse health effects. The opposite is also feasible. If a lifestyle drug designed to help to reduce body weight with little adverse effects of its own is effective, complications like diabetes type II or cardiovascular diseases may be prevented. Furthermore, if the specific drug treatment for such resulting secondary diseases is no longer required, the adverse effects associated with such therapeutic attempts will also be reduced.

These examples illustrate the impact a large-scale use of lifestyle drugs will have on toxicological problems. Many of these problems are not anticipated when the use of such drugs is initiated.

PREVENTIVE HAZARD MINIMIZATION FROM ANIMAL DATA

For several reasons it is impossible to quantitatively predict the occurrence of all possible toxic effects in humans exclusively from animal data. Therefore, preventive hazard minimization always remains a compromise because a toxicological risk assessment proper (i.e., an evaluation on the basis of information from humans), cannot be achieved.

Preventive hazard minimization is aimed at recognizing, from a series of animal studies, a typical pattern of toxic effects characteristic of a given agent. It is presumed that this toxic potential is relevant to the situation in humans, and by appropriate administrative measures the chance of such an adverse health effect in humans is minimized. Administrative actions

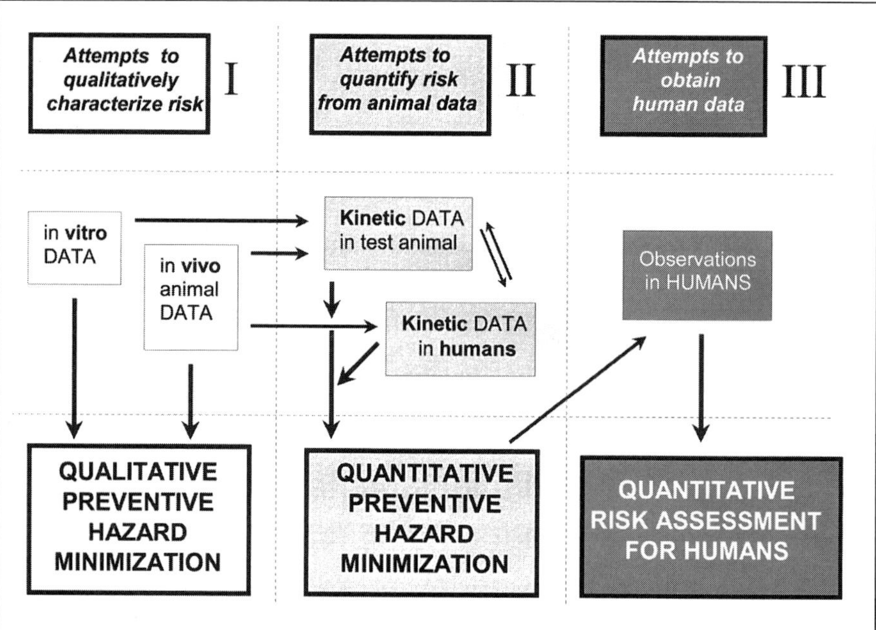

FIGURE 7 Scheme for attempting a preventive hazard minimization or a clinical risk assessment with relevance to humans. Attempts at hazard minimization (I and II of the scheme), and medical a risk assessment for humans (III of the scheme) must be clearly distinguished because they have little in common. The first (primary or secondary hazard minimization) relies on *extrapolations* based on animal data, the second is the real description of medical risk for humans on the basis of *observations* or *measurements* in humans. Evaluations of environmental substances are most often limited to extrapolations. Quantitative preventive hazard minimization is impossible without kinetic data.

range from the restriction of human exposure up to the complete banning the use of the substance.

The idea of a hazard minimization on the basis of animal data is primary prevention. It attempts to preclude the occurrence of human adverse health effects by avoiding or minimizing human exposure to this agent. The decision is most often made on the grounds of a single type of toxic effect, and it is of little interest whether the agent may exhibit other types of toxic manifestations at higher doses.

The goal of animal tests in toxicology is not to predict qualitatively or quantitatively effects that occur with high probability in humans. The results of animal studies extrapolated to the situation in humans are always restricted to suspicions, the validity of which cannot be verified. Thus, these studies are not aimed at a (always quantitative) risk assessment for humans (Fig. 7). On the other hand, primary prevention is not possible on the basis of toxicological information in humans because an exposure of humans must have taken place for obtaining such data. Thus, both strategies have their place in the course of a toxicological evaluation.

There are two situations in which preventive hazard minimization must be performed because risk assessment based on human data is not feasible:

1. Evaluation of chemicals for which the availability of human data is unlikely, but for which prevention of the relevant presumed hazards is desirable and primary prevention advisable.
2. Additional evaluations for special endpoints in the case of substances (e.g., medicinal drugs) for which risk assessment with respect to other endpoints is quite possible. Such additional endpoints may be carcinogenicity or developmental toxicity, for which human data will not become available for several years or decades.

General Testing Strategy

A number of prerequisites should be fulfilled to allow meaningful extrapolations from one species, in this case the experimental animal, to another, in this case the human. It is well established by an extensive body of information that these demands can only be fulfilled to a very limited extent.

The prerequisites essential for a meaningful extrapolation between species include:

- High sensitivity of the test. A specific toxic effect likely to occur at a relevant exposure of humans should be recognizable in the animal tests.
- High specificity of the test. A specific toxic manifestation irrelevant to humans should not be signaled by the animal test.
- Same toxicodynamic behavior in both species. The experimental animal chosen should respond to the chemical in the same or nearly the same way, qualitatively and quantitatively, as humans. For example, it should show the same receptor affinity and the importance of the impaired reaction for overall health should be comparable.
- No substantial differences in the kinetics of the substance (e.g., tissue distribution and elimination half-life). The kinetics should be similar in the animal tests and in humans. Doses used in the animal tests should give rise to similar concentrations of the chemical in the target tissue (or at least in the blood). Tissue distribution should be similar. Alternatively, species differences in kinetics have been recognized and are taken into account during comparative evaluation.
- No relevant differences in the metabolism of the substance, including kinetics of the relevant metabolites. Bioconversion and the metabolic profile of the chemical should be similar in the test animal and in humans. Alternatively, appropriate additional tests must be performed to consider the possible toxicological profile of the relevant metabolites.
- Rare types of adverse effects in humans should be revealed in animal studies. All relevant adverse health effects of the substance should be revealed by the animal tests applied, and no important manifestation should be missed.
- Unimportant endpoints should not be signaled. The animal tests should not indicate effects that are irrelevant to humans or for which the significance cannot be interpreted.

None of these seven prerequisites is absolutely fulfilled when performing animal tests and extrapolating the results to situations presumed to exist in humans. Although humans belong to the animal kingdom, animals are not humans. This touches on the significance of animal studies in general. Numerous animal experiments have revealed identical, or at least very similar, responses in physiology, biochemistry, and pathology between mammalian experimental animals and humans. However, it is equally well established that in toxicology species differences are the major problem.

One can attempt to address the problem of species differences in toxicology by using more than one experimental animal species as a model for conclusions with respect to humans. If experimental animals did indeed respond like humans, this would be a completely unnecessary approach, opposing all attempts at animal protection.

Although somewhat oversimplified, it may be stated that the sensitivity of animal tests, as they are applied today, is high, possibly too high. The specificity is certainly quite deficient and completely inadequate for a toxicological risk assessment relevant to humans, especially with respect to low dose levels.

What is the justification for animal tests, and what is their usefulness? From a huge data base, mostly coming from medicinal drugs, it can be concluded that many types of typical toxic manifestations of a given substance may be qualitatively recognized in animal studies. Although many of such manifestations will not be relevant to humans at the usual exposure levels, it will be advisable, according to the strategy of primary prevention, to further minimize the dose levels to which humans are exposed. The value of such a preventive measure will never be revealed, unless the chemical is much more toxic in humans than in the test animals. Without any doubt, the preventive measures will often be unnecessary or the acceptable intake for humans set much too low, but we would rather be on the safe site. There is no "too low" from a toxicological point of view when "no effect" in humans is the goal with respect to avoidable environmental chemicals. This does not mean that an extremely low acceptable exposure level is always required.

Strategy of Using Several Animal Species

The fact that in many toxicological studies the effects in more than one animal species are evaluated clearly indicates that the prediction of the real situation in humans is not the goal (human risk assessment) but rather the strategy is a "worst case" recognition.

By using several animal species, the attempt is to reveal a profile of toxic potentials characteristic of the specific chemical. Typically, one of two responses will result.

- An undesired effect is observed in several of the animal species used.
- An undesired effect is observed in one species only (but not in others).

If a toxic effect is reconfirmed in several mammalian species (preferentially also in nonhuman primates), there is a good chance that it may be inducible in most of them, including humans. In such a case, there is a good argument, although by no means any proof, that humans may be endangered if they are exposed to a high enough dose. For many reasons, toxicodynamic as well as kinetic ones, animal studies alone will not provide any clue to the critical dose level in humans. Therefore, it is prudent to use a suitable "uncertainty factor" for attempts at an extrapolation.

If a toxic effect is confined to one mammalian species and not reproducible in other animals, the situation is muddled. In drawing conclusions from the most susceptible species used, it is understood that a defined adverse effect might also have some relevance to humans. This is a characteristic worst-case assumption—without knowing better one is inclined to assume the worst and to react accordingly. There is no proof whatsoever that this type of toxic effect will ever occur in humans at any reasonable exposure condition, and probably we shall never acquire any knowledge on this matter.

What Are the Criteria for Selecting Experimental Species?

The best criterion for selecting a test animal would be that the response of the animal species selected is identical, or at least very similar, to that of humans. This ideal situation is rarely achieved because it would imply the knowledge of the human response to the agent in question. There is no doubt that such a similarity revealed for one agent will not hold true for all the other different chemicals. If this level of similarity were known in a special case, no animal data would be required.

The selection of the animal species for routine studies in toxicology is highly pragmatic and by no means governed by scientific considerations. Even if whale or elephant were ideal species, they would not be preferred for this purpose, for reasons easy to understand.

The rat has a number of advantages for toxicological testing, but most humans would disprove of being considered a large rat. This already illustrates the problem involved in comparing human beings with rats. As an advantage, the usual laboratory rodents (rats and mice) are small, easy to breed and handle, and can be standardized to some extent with regard to strain and health status (e.g., spf status), and a multiplicity of data on physiology, biochemistry, toxicology, and pathology have been accumulated. Thus, it is mostly convenience and experience that rule the selection. Certainly the reason is not because rats are especially similar to humans.

In tests for general toxicity, especially for long-term organ toxicity, most regulatory agencies require the use of one rodent (mostly the rat) and one nonrodent animal species (mostly the dog). Again there is little scientific rationale for this selection, not for using two species (why not three or four?) nor for selecting rats and dogs. There are certain animal species for which the most experience has been accumulated in toxicological research (Table 10), and it would not be wise for an investigator to choose some other odd species for this type of testing, although it is not forbidden by most guidelines.

The concept of using a rodent and a nonrodent species is consequently not pursued in other areas of toxicology, and testing for a carcinogenic potential is most often performed in rats and mice, two rodent species.

In tests of developmental and reproductive toxicity, usually the rat and rabbit are selected as experimental species. Again the rabbit, not selected for other toxicological studies, is not used because of its special suitability for this purpose, but for historical reasons. Some strains had shown a certain susceptibility to thalidomide.

Mice have been used in the majority of immunological studies. When, in the future, immunotoxicological

TABLE 10 Common Selection of Species for the Evaluation of Different Toxicological Endpoints

Toxic effect	First species	Second species	Third species
Acute toxicity	Rat	Other species	
Long-term (organ) toxicity	Rat	Dog	Primates
Reproductive toxicity	Rat	Rabbit (mouse)	Primates
Carcinogenicity	Rat	Mouse	Hamster
Mutagenicity (*in vivo*)	Hamster	Mouse	Rat
Immunotoxicity	Rat, mouse	Guinea pig	Primates

studies are included more extensively in toxicological evaluations, this might be the preferred species. In this respect, rats have been found to be less sensitive to a number of substances. However, because mice are not the favorite species for tests on general toxicity, it is difficult to incorporate such evaluations of immunological variables within the existing tests for subchronic toxicity.

Summarizing, some species seem to be more suitable as experimental animals for defined purposes in toxicological research than others. However, to use a variety of species for special areas in toxicology creates the disadvantage that a comparison of various endpoints is made difficult and manifold accompanying kinetic studies are required. Using only one species to reveal the possible effects on the divergent toxicological endpoints increases the comparability of the numerous data, but increases the chance for missing special adverse effects. No way out of this discrepancy has been found so far.

Emotional Aspects in Selecting Experimental Species

Because many persons are emotionally attached to dogs and cats as pets, the use of these species in toxicological research has been criticized more than the use of employing rats for the same purpose. There has been considerable discussion on whether the second species, the dog, is really needed in long-term studies to reveal organ toxicity. It has been argued that there are only a few instances in which additional severe and crucial adverse health effects were revealed in dog when compared to those observed in long-term rat studies. Altogether, this problem has not been solved.

"Goodness" of Data and Documentation

There are two aspects governing the "goodness" of data from experimental animal studies and their documentation:

1. Shortcomings, or even mistakes, in performing the studies in different research laboratories.
2. Limitations intrinsic to the strategy of testing used.

To minimize the first aspect, various guidelines have been published. Besides good laboratory practice (GLP), the study design has been standardized for many types of toxicological experiments. Investigators are not compelled to exactly follow these rules. However, it may be somewhat foolish to completely ignore the suggestions.

There is a considerable problem with the second aspect. None of the procedures routinely used in toxicological testing are ideal. The scientific soundness of many procedures may be questioned; an example is the long-term testing for revealing a carcinogenic potential. However, no better strategies are available or generally accepted.

Problem of Overdoses and Small Number of Individuals

In many toxicological investigations overdoses that are irrelevant to the situation in humans are used. The rationale for this is the attempt to recognize a pattern of toxic manifestations. In evaluating the results of such studies, it is often ignored that many of the effects observed may not be relevant to the situation in humans. It is stated that a substance is "nephrotoxic" or "teratogenic," although such an effect may never occur with human exposure.

Another problem is the use of a limited number of individuals in animal studies. The number per dose group is usually 10–20 (or even lower with dogs or primates), and almost never exceeds 50 per gender. This strategy only allows the recognition of rather frequent events. Overdosing is used to compensate for this limitation.

Problems with Concurrent and Historical Controls

The greatest problem in toxicologic experimental research, very similar to the problem in epidemiology, is the selection of an appropriate control group. Persons with little experience in experimental research are inclined to assume that controls are something constant. This is certainly not the case. Depending on the number of individuals involved, control values fluctuate within certain, more or less pronounced, limits. It is unlikely that in different studies the control values will be identical. If one performs an experimental study with 10 simultaneous control groups (with 15 individuals per group), differences between the groups are likely to occur. Such differences may well be statistically significant. The variability of controls will be due to many reasons.

The fluctuation of control values is obvious when historical controls are evaluated. The interpretation of a toxicological study must be affected by this variability of controls, especially when the deviation in the treated group is not too pronounced. This phenomenon is especially pronounced when certain deviations occur spontaneously within the controls. Tumor formation, teratogenicity, and other embryotoxic effects are good examples. The evaluation of the relevance of

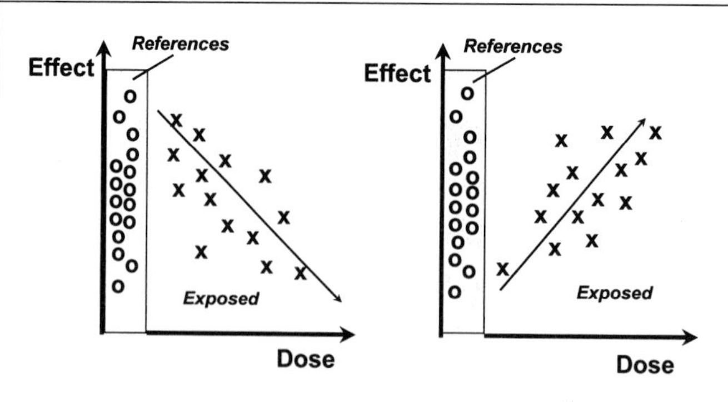

FIGURE 8 Apparent dose-dependency of experimental or clinical data located within a defined reference range. There is a statistically significant positive or negative regression if the reference data are not included in the calculation.

the data of such studies may not be possible without taking historical controls into account.

Substance-Induced Effects within the Reference Range

There are ample examples in the literature of studies in which a dose-dependent effect was claimed to occur, but in which all values stayed within the reference range (Fig. 8). In several of such evaluations, the statistically significant "effect" occurred because the control values were not included in the regression analysis. In such cases the claims of a chemically induced effect are not justified. The data were improperly evaluated. However, it may be possible that the values of exposed individuals are in the lower limits of the reference range. A certain dose dependency may result. The interpretation of such data is difficult. When all values of the exposed individuals stay within the reference range, no substance-induced effect has occurred. It cannot be excluded that at even higher doses the values of the exposed group may be outside the references. However, this cannot be proven from the data. Further studies with higher doses are required to answer the question.

Is It Sufficient to Provide M ± SE Values?

It has become fashionable to provide only mean values and errors of the mean of data in publications on toxicology. This is quite unsatisfactory when small deviations from the reference range are reported. For very clear-cut effects, statistical calculations are unnecessary anyhow. Documentation of M ± SE values is insufficient for several reasons. Biological data are seldom randomly distributed. The mean values, range (minimal and maximal values), and possibly some percentiles (e.g., Q_1 and Q_3) are more informative. Additionally, one would like to evaluate how many data stay within the reference range and how many deviate from it. This is best shown in a box-plot or a dot-plot providing all the experimental data. Then, what is specific about the individuals showing deviating values from the references should be analyzed. Because reference values are often defined as 5 to 95% percentiles, some outliers from this range are bound to occur. These are not necessarily pathological data.

Reliability of Experimental Data and Their Documentation

At present there is a tremendous difference between the quality of the performance of routine studies and of the documentation of data in industrial or contract laboratories, on the one hand, and information published by many investigators from university institutes and some government institutions all over the world, on the other. While industrial or contract laboratories are forced to perform experiments according to the strict rules of good laboratory practice (GLP) and to follow the recommendations of several guidelines, information published by other laboratories is often of quite limited quality with respect to the number of animals used, quality of housing and maintenance, and the quality of the investigations performed. Furthermore, the documentation of the experimental conditions is often poor and the reporting of the results limited to mean values and standard deviations. Because of these shortcomings in quality, it is often difficult or impossible to evaluate the significance of some of the published data. On the other hand, the details of the results obtained in industrial or contract laboratories are normally not accessible outside regulatory agencies, and available information is filtered through the perspective of such agencies or through short information leaflets from industry. Because an expert opinion can most often only be obtained from reviewing the raw data, independent judgment of the validity of the data and of the conclusions drawn is generally impossible.

TYPES OF EXTRAPOLATION

When one intends to extrapolate toxicological information from animal studies to the situation possibly relevant to human exposure, three types of extrapolation are attempted:

- Extrapolation from high to low doses in the same species.
- Extrapolation from one species (experimental animal) to another (humans).
- Taking intraspecies variability into account.

There may be some rationale for the first type of extrapolation when the attempts are confined to doses close to the lowest experimental values and a sufficient number of data points are available. There is virtually no scientific basis for the second and third type of extrapolation, especially when a quantitative assessment is the goal. For this reason, a considerable extent of uncertainty must remain, especially with respect to the last two types of extrapolation. This limitation is often hidden when only the final results of an extrapolation are presented.

Extrapolations to Lower Doses in the Same Species

In many toxicological studies rather high doses are used. The evaluation of a possible hazard at relevant, and mostly much lower, human exposures must include an extrapolation to the lower dose levels. Generally, no effects can be measured under these conditions in the animal studies. Thus no verification of this extrapolation enterprise is possible.

A quantitative extrapolation may be expected to provide reasonably reliable results when two prerequisites are fulfilled (Fig. 9):

- Information on dose–response relationships is available.
- The extrapolation is restricted to a dose range rather close to the experimental data.

Not fulfilling these criteria will render the extrapolation largely speculation. The shape and slope of the

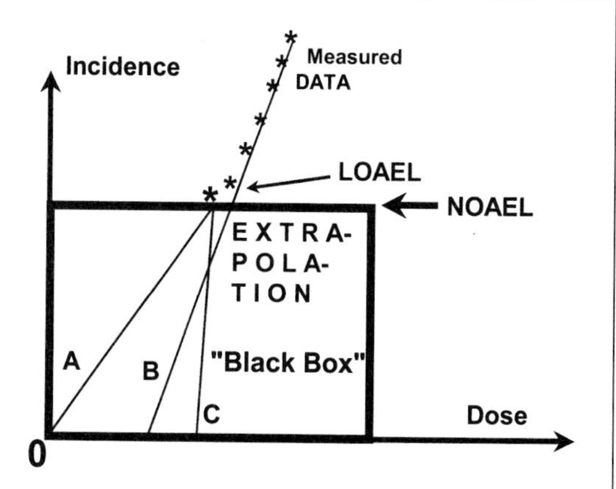

FIGURE 9 Extrapolation into a "black box" when attempting to draw conclusions from much lower doses than those used in the experimental study. The shape of the dose–response curve must remain completely unknown. Extrapolated values greatly depend on the mathematical model used.

dose–response curve in areas without experimental data are completely unknown.

Many mathematical procedures have been presented and extensively used for this type of extrapolation. Most of these are worst-case assumptions, the validity of which cannot be assessed. It should be stressed that lack of data and ignorance of dose–response relationships cannot be compensated for by any kind of mathematics.

There is one principle that alone governs toxicological hazard minimization, and this is the dogma of dose relationship. The key issue is the faith in the rule that the probability of an adverse effect will be reduced with declining doses, and the hazard will finally become insignificant. Any method of hazard minimization, whether relying on a mathematical transformation of the data or using safety factors, is based on this principle. When the margin between experimental data (e.g., LOAEL or NOAEL) and human exposure becomes large enough, the incidence of possible adverse health effects becomes negligible. The hazard is considered to be "tolerable" or "acceptable." However, the risk proper cannot be assessed with confidence.

Extrapolations from One Species to Another

It must be remembered that overall there is no reliable scientific basis for this second type of extrapolation. Numerous examples of pronounced species differences are documented in the toxicological literature. It is well established that these differences can rest in one of the following:

- Toxicokinetics and metabolism.
- Toxicodynamics.

An interspecies comparison of chemically induced toxic effects is facilitated when the doses are based on kilograms of body weight. An even better comparison seems to be possible when the species differences in surface area are taken into account. Some orientating comparative calculations were performed with cytostatic agents. These data might suggest that the error in recognizing known adverse effects in humans through animal experiments does not exceed one order of magnitude (Table 11). This would support a safety factor of about 10 for this type of extrapolation. However, these data are highly selected and generalizations on the basis of so few data would be daring. Differences in drug-metabolizing capacity are known to even occur among primates (Table 12), thus illustrating the difficulties.

The reliability of an extrapolation between species is strengthened when special experimental conditions are achieved:

- A defined effect has been found to be inducible in several experimental species at similar dose levels.
- Comparative kinetic data (from the experimental animal species and humans) are available.
- Information on the mechanism of the toxicity has been obtained. Comparative data on the susceptibility of the target tissue in different species (experimental animals and humans) can be obtained.

If an effect can be demonstrated in several experimental species and in both sexes at a similar dose level, the chance that it may be relevant to the situation in humans is increased. An even better criterion is the inducibility of an adverse reaction at comparable serum levels in several species.

Extrapolation on the basis of doses is known to be a poor strategy. Such extrapolations have been performed for several decades, for examples, for establishing ADI (acceptable daily intake) or similar values. The results of such calculations were quite unreliable. Considerable species differences with respect to kinetics are well known to be the rule rather than the exception. For this reason, extrapolations on the basis of comparative kinetic data (from experimental animals and humans) must be preferred. They constitute the present scientific standard.

The most important aim of animal studies is to recognize a possible mechanism of a toxic action. Such information may suggest that a corresponding mechanism may also be relevant for humans at appropriate dose levels.

TABLE 12 Constitutive Expression of Hepatic Cytochrome P450 Isozymes in Various Species and Enhanced Expression after Enzyme Induction[a]

	CYPIA1[b]	CYPIA2[c]
Constitutive expression		
Rat	Ø	+
Cynomolgus monkey	Ø	Ø
Marmoset monkey	Ø	+
Humans	Ø	+
After pretreatment with TCDD		
Rat	↑↑	↑↑
Cynomolgus monkey	↑↑	(↑)
Marmoset monkey	(↑)	↑↑

[a]Symbols: Ø, activity not present; +, activity present; ↑, increased enzyme activity.
[b]This CYP is also expressed in extra-hepatic tissue (e.g., lung, intestine, and placenta).
[c]Expression of this CYP is confined to liver.

TABLE 11 Comparative Data on General Toxicity of Some Cytostatic Agents in Humans[a] and in Experimental Animals (LD_{10}), Based on Body Surface[b]

	General toxicity compared to humans[c]			
Substance	Rat	Rhesus	Dog	Human
Methotrexate	0.2	2.3	0.1	1.0
6-Mercaptopurine	0.3	0.6	0.4	1.0
5-Fluorouracil	0.2	0.4	0.3	1.0
5-Fluorodeoxyuridine	0.4	0.6	0.7	1.0
Nitrogen mustard	0.3	0.3	1.2	1.0
Cyclophosphamide	0.2	1.7	0.6	1.0
Thiotepa	1.9	1.6	2.8	1.0
Busulfan	0.8	2.8	4.6	1.0
Carmustine[d]	0.4	0.7	0.5	1.0
Dactinomycin	0.8		1.0	1.0

[a]Maximally tolerated dose.
[b]Dose in mg/m^3 body surface. Calculations from Freireich *et al.* (1966).
[c]Ratio of corresponding doses of animal/human. Values <1.0 indicate that the animal species is more sensitive. Values >1.0 indicate that humans are more sensitive.
[d]1,3-Bis(2-chloroethyl)-1-nitrosourea.

Susceptibility of Different Human Populations

In contrast to experimental animal strains, which are purposely rather uniform, humans are genetically heterogeneous. Furthermore, there may be certain subgroups more susceptible than others or than the general population. This may refer to children, elderly persons (Table 13), different genders, and persons with special diseases. When attempting to extrapolate from experimental animals to humans, these deviations from the "norm" can seldom be taken into account. There is no proper way of considering such possible differences because they are not obligatory and uniform, and they may not be of significance for all the agents.

There is no way to cope with this problem with respect to a selected agent and the sole availability of animal data. Again, only applying an additional uncertainty factor may be a pragmatic solution in the attempt at extrapolation that considers such proposed differences in susceptibility. However, such an additional preventive measure will direct a hazard minimization attempt further away from a risk assessment proper.

Metabolic and Kinetic Differences in Humans (Polymorphisms)

Intraspecies differences with respect to kinetics and xenobiotics metabolism have two consequences.

- The area under a plasma concentration curve (AUC) is not identical in different individuals because, for example, elimination half-lives are not constant. A remarkable variability exists within a population.
- The rate of metabolic conversion of a given xenobiotic and the resulting metabolic pattern are not constants either, and different metabolic pathways may be used by individuals.

Many of these differences in kinetics and metabolism are genetically determined. Individuals deviating from the "norm" may be rather frequent within a population, or the special behavior may occur at a very low prevalence, often with considerable ethnic differences. While fast and slow acetylators (polymorphism of acetyltransferase type 2) are about equally frequent within the Caucasian race, only 10% or fewer persons of Asian descent are slow acetylators. With respect to the best-investigated debrisoquine polymorphism, responsible for numerous oxidative drug-metabolizing reactions and linked to CYP2D6, slowly metabolizing persons constitute 1–10% of various ethnic populations.

It is obvious that the risk of undesired reactions in such groups with polymorphisms may deviate considerably from that of the average population. Many such polymorphisms are known, and many more, especially very rare ones, are suspected to exist but have not sufficiently been investigated. Therefore, it cannot be assumed that human risk assessment can be pinned down to a single dose level. While being satisfactory for the majority of persons, there will always be a smaller or even larger special group with a higher susceptibility, due to genetic peculiarities. From this point of view, rare adverse health effects due to defined exogenous agents will never be completely avoidable, unless exposure is excluded.

TABLE 13 Physiological Age-Dependent Changes of Creatinine Clearance[a]

Age (years)	Weight (kg)	Assumed serum creatinine (mg/dl)	Calculated renal clearance (ml/min)
20	70	1.0	117
20	70	1.5	78
80	70	1.0	58
80	70	1.5	39

[a]Calculated using the equation:

$$Cl_{creat.} = \frac{(140 - \text{age}) \times \text{weight}}{72 \times \text{serum creatinine}}$$

Male persons.

Extrapolations from *In Vitro* Data

Interspecies extrapolations are already loaded with difficulties. It is obvious that the number of these uncertainties is further increased when attempting to extrapolate results from *in vitro* data to the situation in humans.

If one is satisfied with qualitative extrapolations, some conclusions with respect to risk minimization may be possible. Positive results in *in vitro* mutagenicity tests may signal a high chemical reactivity of the agent. It could be concluded that the substance is undesirable for the purpose intended (e.g., as a headache remedy). Quantitative extrapolations are impossible when no kinetic data are available. Such an assessment may be attempted with limited validity when kinetic data from humans have been obtained. Additionally, it is necessary to establish kinetic data for the *in vitro* studies. Most often, no linear kinetic is obtained *in vitro* when data are based on the dissolved substance, especially when protein binding is involved. In such a situation bovine serum may behave differently compared with human plasma proteins.

SPECIAL PROBLEMS IN CERTAIN FIELDS OF TOXICOLOGY

The general principles of risk assessment and preventive hazard minimization are independent of the type of agent. However, there are specific problems connected with some areas of toxicology.

Special Situation of Revealing Acute Toxicity

Although it is one of the most extensively used routine procedures in toxicological studies, it is not easy to define the role of testing for acute toxicity within the frame of a risk assessment with relevance to humans. No single test may provide sufficient information for risk assessment. Multiple information from a variety of observations is always essential to complete the puzzle of the possible toxic potential or potency of an agent.

The significance of testing for acute toxicity is limited if it is not combined with pharmacokinetic studies. Nevertheless, the following reasons may be imagined to form a basis for testing for acute toxicity.

- To obtain some information of the dose required to induce general adverse health effects in the animal.
- To serve as a basis for further experimental studies on toxicity (e.g., multiple-dosing studies and tests on teratogenicity or carcinogenicity).
- To obtain qualitative information on symptoms to be expected following massive exposures of humans (e.g., during accidents).
- To serve as a basis for the classification of agents with respect to their toxic potency (with relevance to humans).

Few of these arguments are really convincing.

Obtaining some information on the dose required to induce adverse health effects may be considered by many to be the main reason for performing such tests. It is assumed that the dose found in animal studies may be similar to that required in humans (on the basis of kilograms of body weight or square meter of surface area) for inducing toxic effects. Because there are many species differences, this is a daring assumption.

Results obtained in studies on acute toxicity might serve as a basis for further studies on toxicity (e.g., multiple dosing, teratogenicity, carcinogenicity). However, longer-term dose-finding studies are much more appropriate for this purpose.

Some information on toxic symptoms is obtained from such studies. Again, information on organ toxicity is much better revealed by longer-term studies with multiple exposures. If it is hoped that solid information on the symptoms to be expected following massive exposures of humans (e.g., during accidents) is deducible from such studies, the results will be disappointing. If this were really the main reason for acute toxicity testing, the procedures used in many laboratories are largely unsuited to serve the purpose. The endpoints routinely evaluated, and often observed by a technician, are too crude to give the required information. All the relevant recent publications on this subject demand that a close observation of the symptoms and the revealing of more subtle variables should be the goal of acute toxicity testing. No clear-cut suggestions have been made on this matter and there is no agreed upon procedure on how to obtain this additional information. The reproducibility of recognizing toxic effects in various laboratories is far from being optimal. Furthermore, while it holds true that in numerous cases it has been shown that symptoms seen in humans after massive exposure and poisoning are very similar to those observed after acute exposure in laboratory animals, poisoning of humans (e.g., either as suicide or at a working place) is rare and in general not the predominant toxicological problem. It is questionable whether this reason would justify the sacrifice of an enormous number of experimental animals.

Animal data on acute toxicity, and especially LD_{50} values, are used for the classification and labeling of agents with respect to their toxic potency, with relevance to humans. Again, this assumption has turned out to be too optimistic for most of the substances. Assessments have always been attempted on the basis of dose. The correlation between doses toxic in experimental animals and those toxic in humans has been found to be, in general, rather poor. One reason is that kinetics and metabolism in the experimental species and humans are seldom identical.

Problems with LD_{50} Estimates

When mortality is evaluated in an animal experiment, LD_{50} values provide the greatest confidence of all points of a dose–response curve. For this reason, LD_{50} values have long been used for characterizing the overall toxicity of an agent. In most cases, data from rat studies were used.

There are three aspects that greatly limit the applicability of such data:

- LD_{50} values do not provide any information on the slope of the dose–response curve.
- In order to clearly characterize the LD_{50} values a considerable number of animals must suffer and die.
- LD_{50} values as calculated from rat data have a very limited value for assessing the toxicity in humans.

The course of a dose–response curve is much better characterized by providing LD_{05} and LD_{95} values than LD_{50} values. However, values close to zero or to 100% of the S-shaped curve are difficult to measure, and the variability is considerable.

Considerable efforts were made to reduce the number of animals needed for estimating LD_{50}. It was demonstrated that an "approximate LD_{50}" is sufficient for all purposes. Such an approximate value may be calculated from data using very few animals. This is the best example showing that a reduction of the number of experimental animals can effectively be achieved by a collaboration of scientists from universities, industry laboratories, and regulatory agencies.

LD_{50} values, almost exclusively from rat studies, are also increasingly used for labeling of substances as "very toxic", "toxic", and so on. Because such rat data have relatively little relevance to the situation in humans, this is a political exercise of rather questionable value.

Special Situation of Revealing Organ Toxicity

Assessing a possible organotropic action of an agent is an important issue in preclinical animal testing. With respect to medicinal substances, results from such studies provide valuable clues for suspicions to be considered in the subsequent clinical trials in humans. These human studies provide information on whether the suspicion raised from preclinical studies is relevant to humans. If under the human-exposure conditions, that is, at risk assessment proper, the corresponding adverse effects are not confirmed, the preclinical information is obsolete.

The situation is different when the subsequent evaluation in humans is not possible. Then these data will be used in the course of a preventive hazard minimization, that is, an extrapolation to a situation postulated to exist in humans.

Special Situation of Revealing Mutagenicity

Although some types of mutagenicity tests can be performed with human tissue (e.g., lymphocytes), an evaluation of mutagenic actions in humans is the exception. Studies of chromosomal aberrations in lymphocytes have been performed in patients treated with cytostatic agents, and in a few instances after occupational exposure.

Hereditary mutagenic effects have so far not been found in humans after exposure to mutagenic agents, including ionizing radiation. The reason is that the expected incidence with respect to malformations or inborn errors of metabolism would be so small that very large numbers of volunteers would have to be examined. Such large subpopulations are rarely exposed to the adequate agents. Furthermore, additional effects would have to be evaluated against a background of spontaneous effects of the same kind, which can only be approximately assessed and is complicated by considerable fluctuations.

The direct value of mutagenicity tests is, rather, to provide some clue to the possible carcinogenic potential of the agent. For certain groups of substances, this clue may be sufficient to abandon the use of such an agent.

Special Situation of Revealing Carcinogenicity

This is a most difficult area of research because there is much concern about the potential of chemical carcinogenicity as a possible cause of human cancers, although evidence is accumulating that human cancer diseases are not predominantly caused by exogenous mutagenic substances. Routine experimental animal testing is still largely confined to effects caused by initiating agents, and they are not especially designed to reveal tumor promoters.

Epidemiological studies with respect to carcinogenic risk assessment in humans are difficult to perform, time-consuming, and expensive. Furthermore, almost all studies in this area are retrospective (case-control studies), with ample possibilities for criticism. There is no doubt that only pronounced effects can be revealed with reasonable certainty. For these reasons, the number of well-established human carcinogens is still very small, despite considerable efforts.

TABLE 14 Qualitative Evaluation Categories of the International Agency for Research on Cancer[a]

Category	Carcinogenicity to humans	Information of carcinogenicity of agent: In humans	In animals
1	Existing	Sufficient	Sufficient
2A	Probable	Limited	Sufficient
2B	Possible	Limited	Insufficient
3	Not classifiable	Inadequate	Inadequate
4	Probably not	No effect	No effect

[a]From: IARC Monograph, Supplement 7, 1987.

Consequently, information on possible carcinogenic effects will largely rely on data from animal studies, with all the intrinsic limitations and difficulties of interpretation of the results. A risk assessment proper is not possible for almost all agents, and attempts at preventive hazard minimization must rely on extrapolations. The assessment is largely of a qualitative nature (Table 14), such as the categories used by the International Agency for Research on Cancer (IARC of WHO).

In many instances, the performance of long-term animal studies of carcinogenic potentials and the interpretation of the resulting data are loaded with difficulties. This starts with the selection of the test animals. In contrast to the strategy of species selection in long-term toxicity studies (one rodent species and one nonrodent species), two rodent species (rats and mice or hamsters) are generally used in carcinogenicity tests. Furthermore, the strains selected of these species will have a considerable impact on the outcome of the studies. In addition, there is a trend to use animals especially susceptible to the action of carcinogens. The relevance of the outcome of such studies is doubtful, especially when any kind of quantitative evaluation is attempted.

Often, different results are obtained when varied species are used for such long-term studies (Table 15). This may even be the case when different animal strains are used (Table 16). Usually, the unfavorable results obtained in the most susceptible species are used for hazard minimization. Of course, it is completely unknown whether humans respond similarly to the susceptible or the not susceptible test species. Furthermore, often differences in the carcinogenic response of the genders are observed, and again the more susceptible gender is used for hazard minimization attempts. Most often it cannot be assumed that the gender differences observed in animal studies will also hold true for humans.

Revealing mechanistic information on a carcinogenic action is helpful for attempts at hazard minimization. In a number of cases it has been possible to

TABLE 15 Examples of Controversial Results of Carcinogenicity Studies

Substance	Rat: Male	Rat: Female	Mouse: Male	Mouse: Female
Chlordan	Negative	Negative	Positive	Positive
4-Chlor-*o*-toluidin	Negative	Negative	Positive	Positive
p,p′-DDE	Negative	Negative	Positive	Positive
Nitrofen	Negative	Negative	Positive	Positive
N,N′-Diethylthiourea	Positive	Positive	Negative	Negative
Azobenzene	Positive	Positive	Negative	Negative
N-Nitrosodiphenylamine	Positive	Positive	Negative	Negative
2,4-Dinitrotoluol	Positive	Positive	Negative	Negative
p-Nitrosodiphenylamine	Positive	Negative	Positive	Negative
Isophosphamide	Negative	Positive	Negative	Positive
Trimethylphosphate	Positive	Negative	Negative	Positive
Tretachlorvinvos	Negative	Positive	Positive	Positive
2,4,6-Trichlorophenol	Positive	Negative	Positive	Positive
2,4-Diaminotoluol	Positive	Positive	Negative	Positive
Dicofol	Negative	Negative	Positive	Negative
2-Nitro-*p*-phenylendiamine	Negative	Negative	Negative	Positive

[a]Positive indicates tumor incidence increased in the study; negative indicates tumor incidence not increased. Data from Envir. Health Perspect. 101, Suppl. 1 (1993).

TABLE 16 Difference in Carcinogenic Effect[a] of Diethylnitrosamine (DEN)[b] plus Phenobarbital (PB) in Mouse Strains[c]

Study group		Mouse strain CH3	DBA	C57Bl
Vehicle	36–52 weeks	0/10	0/10	0/10
PB	after 36 weeks	0/10	0/10	0/10
PB	after 36 weeks	2/10	0/10	0/10
PB	36–52 weeks	4/10	0/10	0/10
DEN	after 24 weeks	2/10	0/10	0/10
DEN	after 36 weeks	5/10	1/10	1/10
DEN	36–52 weeks	9/10	4/10	2/10
DEN + PB	after 24 weeks	7/10	9/10	1/10
DEN + PB	after 36 weeks	10/10	9/10	0/10
DEN + PB	36–52 weeks	10/10	10/10	3/10

[a]Liver tumors.
[b]Dose: 90 mg DEN/kg body wt ip; 2 weeks after initiation, 0.05% PB in the drinking water.
[c]Data from Diwan *et al.* (1986).

provide evidence that an effect observed in experimental animals has little or no relevance for the situation in humans. The rat, for example, is very susceptible to the induction of thyroid tumors by substances enhancing thyreotropic hormone (TSH) formation (Fig. 10). Such a mechanism of tumor induction apparently is of little significance for the situation in humans.

The present strategy used for revealing a carcinogenic potential of an agent is acceptable as a qualitative preventive means of protecting humans. If the goal is to minimize the exposure to agents with postulated carcinogenic properties, this strategy is expensive but acceptable from a pragmatic point of view. It has been stressed that many of these rodent carcinogens will not be relevant as human carcinogens. Thus, the sensitivity of the test is high; the specificity is probably very low.

Can One Molecule Cause Cancer?

A stochastic event is one governed by chance. In this case, the probability of an effect decreases, dose-dependently, when the dose is reduced. Assume you are shooting at a target disk with a shotgun. At a given distance, a defined number of the bullets will, in a random fashion, reach the target. Increasing the distance means that fewer balls will hit the target. At a certain greater distance the number of hits will be zero.

The assumption that mutagenic chemical or physical carcinogenesis (initiation) is caused by a stochastic process has caused considerable confusion, especially among lay persons. It was concluded that with decreasing doses the incidence would decrease more or less linearly, and that one or a few molecules could

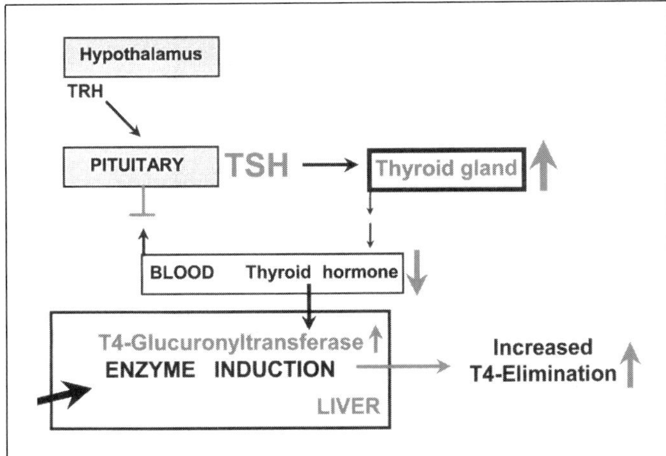

FIGURE 10 Proposed mechanism of inducing neoplastic lesions in rats by chronic stimulation of the thyroid gland via the TSH/T_4 regulatory circle. Enzyme induction of hepatic glucuronyl transferase (T_4-UDGP) facilitates T_4 elimination and results in a compensatory TSH formation and chronic stimulation of the thyroid gland. Hypothyroidism is not a risk factor for the induction of thyroid tumors in humans.

induce biological effects and thereby cancer. Although this is obviously nonsense, this false argument is so deeply rooted that it is hard to eliminate.

It is a fact that chemical or physical carcinogenesis caused by initiating and by promoting agents is strictly dose-dependent. This implies that when the exposure is reduced, the incidence will decrease, until at extremely low exposures the incidence becomes negligible.

The absurdity of the statement that one molecule is able to induce cancer can be demonstrated by an extremely conservative intellectual experiment, containing many worst-case assumptions:

- *Assume* there is a chemical (molecular mass of 300 Da) inducing, at a single dose of 300 pg (10^{12} moles), tumors in all exposed humans (such a substance is, of course, not known and very unlikely to exist). This dose would correspond to 6×10^{11} molecules.
- *Assume* there is a linear dose–response relationship down to zero without any threshold (again an extremely unlikely assumption). Then the probability of the occurrence of cancer at a dose of 1 molecule would be 1:6×10^{11} persons.
- *Assume* Earth's population is 6×10^9 persons. The probability of inducing cancer would be 1:100 Earth-populations.
- *Assume* the exposure is to even 1000 molecules. The probability would still be virtually nil (10 in Earth's population) under these extremely unlikely assumptions.

The following have not been considered:

1. There is only a very small chance that the one molecule will reach a DNA molecule because it is much more likely to react before unspecifically or with protein, which is known to exhibit a much higher adduct rate.
2. It is assumed that no repair takes place, but repair is known to revert most preneoplastic lesions.
3. Even if a single mutation occurred, this might not lead to cancer because only a small percentage of mutations can be associated with malignant transformation.
4. Most carcinogens must be metabolically activated, and it is unlikely that this just happens to this single molecule.
5. Cancer cannot be induced by any agent in all possible organs, and it must be assumed that the organotropy is just right, and the molecule reaches the right and susceptible tissue.

These considerations illustrate the absurdity of the one-molecule assumption. A statement such as "Cancer may also be induced by the smallest dose of an agent," always needs the continuation "but at an extremely low, practically negligible, probability." It should be remembered that additional cancer incidences induced by a defined chemical would have to be judged against the background of rather variable spontaneous rates. No specific effect and causal relation with a special exposure can be postulated when the incidence is within the fluctuation of this spontaneous prevalence.

Rodent but Not Human Carcinogens and Teratogens

There are few examples of clear-cut toxic effects observed in humans that have not been revealed in animal studies (Table 17). Thus, the sensitivity of the test systems appears to be rather high. However, the most important question is: What is the significance of "rodent" carcinogens or teratogens for humans? Is the specificity of our test systems so low that many agents are labeled "carcinogens" or "teratogens" that do not exhibit such capabilities in humans at relevant exposures?

We must recall that it is not the aim of animal tests to reveal human carcinogens. All tests performed to reveal such a capability in animals will only detect the corresponding potential of the test substance. At that stage there is no evidence that this capability is relevant to humans at reasonable exposures. It is a political and not a scientific decision whether substances with such a potential should be banned or drastically restricted in its use. Because most scientists have refused to define "safe" doses of carcinogens, it appears a justified political strategy to label such substances and avoid human contact as much as possible.

From a scientific point of view, it is almost impossible to define the term "carcinogen." An agent may be capable of increasing the incidence of tumors above that of a reference group in a certain species under defined experimental conditions. These conditions include the constant daily dose, the defined treatment period, the chosen animal strain, and defined maintenance conditions. No increased tumor frequency may occur under different experimental conditions. Specifying the conditions under which an agent increases the spontaneous frequency of tumors provides a scientifically correct statement, without rubber-stamping. It will be recognized that the selected experimental conditions will often differ drastically from the relevant exposure conditions of humans.

Carcinogens and Anticarcinogens

A good example of a chemical inducing *in vivo* carcinogenic and anticarcinogenic effects at different locations, simultaneously at the same dose group of

TABLE 17 Predictive Value of Animal Studies for Recognizing Established Carcinogenic and Teratogenic Effects in Humans[a]

Substance	Effect in humans	Qualitatively detectable in animal studies?	
		Yes/no	Species
Aflatoxin	Carcinogenic	Yes	Multiple species
Arsenic	Carcinogenic	Difficult	Usual rodent species
Asbestos	Carcinogenic	Yes[b]	Usual rodent species
Benzidine	Carcinogenic	Yes	Usual rodent species
Chromium (6-valent)	Carcinogenic	Yes[b]	Usual rodent species
Cyclophosphamide	Carcinogenic Teratogenic	Yes Yes	Usual rodent species Usual laboratory species
DES	Carcinogenic	Difficult[b]	Usual rodent species
Folic acid antagonists	Teratogenic	Difficult	Usual laboratory species
2-Naphthylamine	Carcinogenic	Yes	Usual rodent species
Nickel	Carcinogenic	Yes[b]	Usual rodent species
Retinoids	Teratogenic	Yes	Multiple species
Thalidomide	Teratogenic Teratogenic	No Yes[b]	Usual rodent species All primate species
Vinyl chloride	Carcinogenic	Yes	Usual rodent species
Warfarin	Teratogenic	Difficult	Usual laboratory species

[a]Usual rodent species for carcinogenicity testing are rats and mice. Usual laboratory species for testing on developmental toxicity are rats and rabbits. Information from IARC Monograph, Supplement 7 (1987).

[b]Comparatively easy when attempting to verify after the effect was observed in humans.

animals, is TCDD (Table 18). The opposite effects of increasing the frequency of precancerous changes (liver foci) at high doses and reducing the frequency at low dose levels were also observed with this chemical in further studies. Thus, an agent may increase the tumor incidence at high doses and reduce it at lower exposure levels. Or it may increase the frequency of one type of tumor and decrease the prevalence of tumors at other locations. Should it be labeled as a "carcinogen" or as an "anticarcinogen?"

A similarly difficult situation exists with respect to some tumor promoters. They may exaggerate the tumor formation induced by certain agents at defined locations. However, they may reduce the effectiveness of other tumor initiators, if they induce xenobiotic metabolizing reactions. Again, this has been demonstrated in the case of TCDD.

With respect to polychlorinated dibenzo-*p*-dioxins and dibenzofurans, another situation exists that is typical for several environmental chemicals. These agents exist as mixtures of congeners with apparently very similar properties, but greatly varying potencies. For these substances the concept of toxic equivalency factors (I-TE factors) has been proposed and extensively used by regulatory agencies. The potency of the different congeners is expressed relative to the most active member of this family (Table 19). Although pragmatic, this strategy has been criticized from a scientific point of view. The procedure becomes highly problematic when some of the congeners exhibit more than one action or they induce different effects, as is the case for polychlorinated biphenyls (PCBs). Furthermore, such TE factors are chosen almost because of convenience when the results from various test systems indicate quite different potencies (Tables 20–21).

At our present stage of knowledge, or ignorance, it would be daring to predict the carcinogenic potency of PCDD–PCDF congeners with the help of TE factors. This holds especially true when such attempts are made for dioxin-like PCB (non-*ortho*-PCB or mono-*ortho*-PCB). Agonistic and antagonistic effects have been observed in combinations of different PCBs, and of PCB and dioxins.

TCDD also is a good example of the pronounced species differences with respect to kinetics (Fig. 11).

TABLE 18 Examples of Increases and Decreases in Tumor Incidence in Male and Female Sprague–Dawley Rats after a 2-Year Application Period of TCDD in Their Feed[a]

Tumor type	Organ	Male	Female
Adenoma	Liver	=(↓)	↑↑
Carcinoma	Liver	=(↓)	↑
Carcinoma	Palate, nose, tongue	↑	↑
Carcinoma	Lung	=	↑
Adenoma	Adrenal cortex	↑	=(↑)
Phaeochromocytoma	Adrenal gland	↓↓	=(↓)
Adenoma	Pancreas	↓↓	=
Benign tumors	Uterus		↓↓
Benign tumors	Mammary gland	=	↓↓
Carcinoma	Mammary gland	=(↓)	↓↓
Adenoma	Pituitary gland	=(↓)	↓↓

[a]Only selected data are presented. Symbols for tumor incidence: ↑, increased; ↓, decreased; =(↓), certain tendency towards decrease; =, no statistically significant change as compared with controls. Data from Kociba *et al.* (1978).

These differences of several orders of magnitude must be taken into account in preventive hazard minimization. However, within the past decade sufficient human data have accumulated to attempt a risk assessment proper for some of the relevant endpoints.

Special Situation of Revealing Prenatal Toxicity

Revealing the teratogenic potential of an agent is of interest because the experience with thalidomide has shown that a relatively short exposure to therapeutic doses may induce severe malformations. This is quite in contrast to the conditions leading to carcinogenesis. However, thalidomide-type teratogenicity has turned out to be the exception rather than the rule. Only a few additional types of substances have been found to react in a similar fashion, that is, inducing malformations at short-term exposure with therapeutic doses. Some therapeutically used retinoids are an example.

Similar to the situation with respect to carcinogenicity, teratogenic effects must be judged against a background of spontaneous occurrences. Furthermore, single and defined malformations are rare events, necessitating the evaluation of a great number of mother–child pairs. Given a certain size of a study, the statistical power of detecting a significant increase in the incidence over background may only be sufficient with respect to the sum of all severe malformations, but not for single types of abnormalities (Table 22). In addition, many confounders and problems with recall bias complicate the situation.

With regard to hazard minimization, which endpoint of embryotoxicity is chosen will make a differ-

TABLE 19 Example of a calculation of the International TCDD Toxicity Equivalencies of a mixture of PCDD and PCDF

Congener	Measured amount (ppt)	I-TE factor	I-TEq (ppt)
2,3,7,8-TCDD	3.0	1.0	3.0
1,2,3,7,8-P5CDD	9.6	0.5	4.8
1,2,3,4,7,8-H6CDD	7.8	0.1	0.8
1,2,3,6,7,8-H6CDD	36	0.1	3.6
1,2,3,4,6,7,8-H6CDD	6.3	0.1	0.6
1,2,3,7,8,9-H7CDD	42	0.01	0.4
1,2,3,4,6,7,8,9-OCDD	192	0.001	0.2
2,3,7,8-TCDF	1.6	0.1	0.2
1,2,3,7,8-P5CDF	0.5	0.05	0.03
2,3,4,7,8-P5CDF	26	0.5	13
1,2,3,4,7,8-H6CDF	7.2	0.1	0.7
1,2,3,6,7,8-H6CDF	6.8	0.1	0.7
2,3,4,6,7,8-H6CDF	3.2	0.1	0.3
1,2,3,4,6,7,8-H7CDF	5.9	0.01	0.06
1,2,3,4,6,7,8,9-OCDF	1.5	0.001	0.002
Sum			28.4 ppt I-TEq

[a]Abbreviations: I-TEq, International TCDD Equivalencies (NATO/CCMS, 1988); ppt, ng/kg. Example of a breast milk sample. Data from Beck *et al.* (1996).

TABLE 20 Variability of TE Factors for Coplanar and Mono-*ortho* (Coplanar)-PCB with Agonistic Activity at the *Ah*-Receptor[a]

IUPAC #	PCB congener	Range of relative potency in various systems[b]	Difference	Suggested TE factor
77	3,3′,4,4′-Tetra-CB[c]	0.000007–0.1	19,000 ×	0.0005
126	3,3′,4,4′,5-Penta-CB[c]	0.008 –0.8	260 ×	0.1
105	2,3,3′,4,4′-Penta-CB	0.00003 –0.001	35 ×	0.01
118	2,3′,4,4′,5-Penta-CB	0.000009–0.0003	30 ×	0.0001
123	2′,3,4,4′,5-Penta-CB	0.00001 –0.0001	10 ×	0.0001
114	2,3,4,4′,5-Penta-CB	0.00005 –0.0004	10 ×	0.0005
169	3,3′,4,4′,5,5′-Hexa-CB[c]	0.0006 –1.1	1,900 ×	0.01
156	2,3,3′,4,4′,5-Hexa-CB	0.00001 –0.001	85 ×	0.0005
157	2,3,3′,4,4′,5′-Hexa-CB	0.00006 –0.0006	10 ×	0.0005

[a]According to a survey from Ahlborg *et al.* (1994).
[b]Compared with TCDD.
[c]Coplanar (non*ortho*) PCB.

ence for quantitative extrapolation. The steepness of the various dose–response curves certainly is not identical (Table 23). An advantage is that the dose–response curves for teratogenic effects generally are rather steep. Thus, a comparatively small safety factor (e.g., of 10) should provide a considerable degree of safety.

Special Situation of Revealing Immunotoxicity

Basic research on immunology has been performed predominantly with mice. In routine studies on general toxicity, rats have been the preferred species. There is evidence that the immune system of rats is less susceptible to toxic response than that of mice.

Until now, no universally agreed upon routine strategy for immunotoxicity testing has been accepted. There have been suggestions that tests on immunotoxicity be integrated within the usual longer-term toxicity studies in rats. However, the validity of such an approach is doubtful. The question of whether studies with nonhuman primates are essen-

TABLE 21 Some Prerequisites for the Scientific Acceptance of Toxicity Equivalence Factors[a]

All congeners should exhibit the same toxicologic pattern
The effects of the congeners should be strictly additive
There should be only one receptor or limiting reaction in different organs and species
Dose–response curves for different endpoints should run parallel
Dose–response curves for one endpoint in different species should run parallel
Pharmacokinetics in different species should be identical or comparable.
The pattern of effects should be identical at a high- and a low-dose range
Effects observed in experimental animals must be relevant for humans

[a]According to Neubert *et al.* (1992).

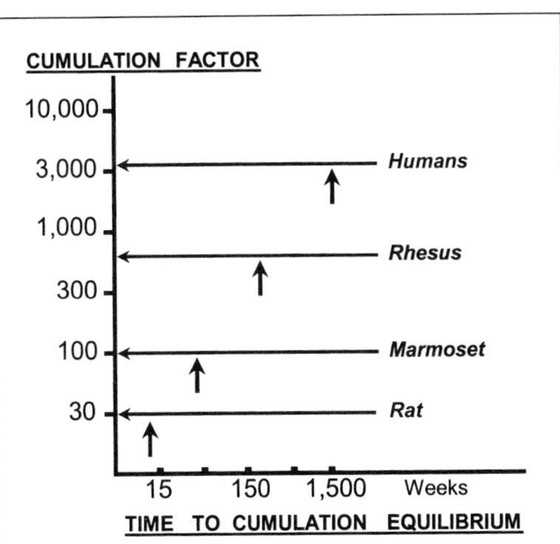

FIGURE 11 Influence of kinetic variables on risk assessment. Due to extreme differences in the elimination half-life, the same daily doses will accumulate about 30-fold in rats (elimination half-life ≈ 3 weeks) and about 3000-fold in humans (elimination half-life ≈ 7 years), up to the equilibrium. Similarly, the equilibrium in the body burden is reached much faster in rats than in humans.

TABLE 22 Predictive Power of Data on Frequency of Malformations in the Contaminated Seveso Area and Minimal Recognizable Odds Ratios Deduced[a]

Abnormalities	Spontaneous risk for nonexposed	Recognizable relative risk		
		Zone A	Zone AB	Zones ABR
All defects	4%	4.5[b]	1.7	1.3
Hemangioma	1.4%	8.0	2.2	1.5
Cardiac defects	0.4%	20.0	3.5	2.1
Diaphragmatic hernia	0.03%	140	14.0	5.8
Esophageal atresia	0.03%	140	4.0	5.8

[a]It must be stressed that the corresponding defects were not observed. Data from Mastroiacovo *et al.* (1988).

[b]Due to the small number of births from exposed women, only a four- to fivefold increase in the total malformation rate would have been recognizable in highly exposed residents of zone A.

tial for revealing immunotoxic effects has not yet been answered. There is evidence that the response of the human immune system to several chemicals is more similar to that of nonhuman primates than to that of rodents. Because many facets of the immune system have been well studied in nonhuman primates, the use of such species for toxicological tests is quite feasible.

As is true for all types of toxicity, humans are also the best test species for revealing immunotoxicity. Many immunological components and functions can be studied with modern technology in humans. So far, insufficient advantage has been taken of this possibility.

TABLE 23 Steepness of Dose–Response Curves for Different Abnormalities in the Same Experiment

Affected organ	Type of defect	Steepness of the dose–response curve (tangent α)
Tail	Lacking	16
Anterior limbs	All defects	15
	No fingers	11
Palate	Cleft	10
Skull	All defects	9
Sternum	All defects	8
Vertebrae	Drumstick-like	5

[a]Application of hydroxyurea in rat, day 11 of pregnancy. According to Neubert *et al.* (1987).

VERIFICATION OF PRECLINICAL DATA IN HUMANS

It is the purpose of preclinical data to provide information on the toxicological pattern of a given substance based on animal tests. From these data, suspicions are raised as to the potential adverse effects that the agent may also induce in humans. When exposure of humans is intended (e.g., in the case of medicinal drugs), this information must be used to specifically monitor the possibility of the occurrence of such effects in humans. This is the clinical risk assessment. In well-planned clinical trials, such suspicions must be verified or excluded for the human species. When evaluating the significance of such a suspicion, three questions must be answered in order to attempt a risk assessment:

- Can this endpoint be studied in humans?
- Is the adverse effect likely to occur at the exposure level of humans?
- What is the incidence of the effect as it occurs under realistic conditions in humans?

Not all endpoints can be studied easily in clinical trials or short-term observations in humans (Table 24). For several toxicological effects, long-term exposure of a sufficient number of individuals is necessary, and epidemiological studies, with all their *a priori* limitations, must be performed.

Because any risk assessment rests on a quantitative evaluation, the second question is the crucial one. Even if the adverse effect seen in animal studies may occur in humans, its relevance at a defined exposure level must be assessed. The toxicological outcome

TABLE 24 Verification of Preclinical Data in Humans

Type of animal study	Result confirmed in humans
Acute toxicity	Not relevant[a]
Organ toxicity	Yes
Immunotoxicity	Yes
Mutagenicity	No
Carcinogenicity	No[b]
Teratogenicity	No[b]

[a]Qualitative and quantitative acute toxicity in animals has little relevance to human acute toxicity.
[b]In special cases only, and after many years of use.

may be irrelevant at the intended exposure. If it occurs at the defined dose level, the incidence of its induction should be assessed. When the use of the given agent is continued, final information on all its adverse effects may not be revealed until after many years of application, and only after many individuals have been exposed.

Again, the success of the attempted risk assessment greatly depends on the type of substance. There is a good chance that many, certainly not all, adverse effects will be revealed after a reasonable period of time in the case of medicinal drugs. In contrast, even after many years of application, a risk assessment is not possible for a variety of environmental agents. We shall be content with the much lower level of a preventive hazard minimization, based entirely on animal data and extrapolations.

Bibliography

Ahlborg, U. G., Becking, G. C., Birnbaun, I. S., Brouwer, A. Derks, H. J. G. M., Freeley, M., Golor, G., Hanberg, A., Larsen, J. C., Liem, A. K. D., Safe, S. H., Schlatter, C., Wærn, F., Younes, M., and Yrjänheikki, E. (1994). Toxic equivalency factors for dioxin-like PCBs. *Chemosphere* **28,** 1049–1067.

Albert, R. E. (1994). Carcinogen risk assessment in the U.S. environmental agency. *Crit. Rev. Toxicol.* **24,** 75–85.

Ames, B. N., and Gold, L. S. (1990). Too many rodent carcinogens: Mitogenesis increases mutagenesis. *Science* **249,** 970–971.

Ashby, J., and Elliott, B. M. (1997). Reproducibility of endocrine disruption data. *Reg. Toxicol. Pharmacol.* **26,** 94–95.

Bailar, J. C., Needleman, J., Berney, B. L., and McGinnis, J. M. (1993). "Assessing Risk to Health." Auburn House, London.

Bass, R., Henschler, D., König, J., Lorke, D., Neubert, D., Schütz, E., Schuppan, D., and Zbinden, G. (1982). LD_{50} versus acute toxicity. Critical assessment of the methodology currently in use. *Arch. Toxicol.* **51,** 183–186.

Bass, R., Neubert, D., Stötzer, H., and Bochert, G. (1985). Quantitative dose–response models in prenatal toxicology. *In* "Methods for Estimating Risk of Chemical Injury: Human and Non-human Biota and Ecosystems" (V. B. Vouk *et al.*, eds.), pp. 437–453. SCOPE, 26, John Wiley and Sons, Ltd, Sussex, England.

Beck, H., Heinrich-Hirsch, B., Koss, G., Neubert, D., Roβkamp, E., Schrenk, D., Schuster, J., Wölfle, D., and Wuthe, J. (1996). Anwendbarkeit von 2,3,7,8-TCDD-TEF für PCB für Risikobewertungen. *Bundesgesundheitsblatt* **39,** 141–147.

Blackwell, B., Bloomfield, S. S., and Buncher, C. R. (1972). Demonstration to medical students of placebo responses and non-drug factors. *Lancet* **II,** 1279–1282.

Bradford, Hill A. (1965). The environment and disease: Association or causation? *Proc. Royal Soc. Med.* **58,** 295–300.

Brown, N.A., and Fabro, S. (1983). The value of animal teratogenicity testing for predicting human risk. *Clin. Obstetr. Gyn.* **26,** 467–477.

Cohrssen, J. J., and Covello, V. T. (1989). "Risk Analysis: A Guide to Principles and Methods for Analyzing Health and Environmental Risks." National Technology Information Service, U.S. Department of Commerce, Washington D.C.

Concato, J., Feinstein, A. R., and Holford, T. R. (1993). The risk of determining risk with multivariable models. *Ann. Inter. Med.* **118,** 201–210.

Crouch, E., and Wilson, R. (1979). Interspecies comparison of carcinogenic potency. *J. Toxicol. Environ. Health* **5,** 1095–1118.

Daston, G. P., Rogers, J. M., Versteeg, D. J., Sabourin, T. D., Baines, D., and Marsh, S. S. (1991). Interspecies comparison of A/D ratios: A/D ratios are not constant across species. *Fundam. Appl. Toxicol.* **17,** 696–722.

Diwan, B. A., Rice, J. M., Ohshima, M., and Ward, J. M. (1986). Interstrain differences in susceptibility to liver carcinogenesis initiated by N-nitrosodiethylamine and its promotion by phenobarbital in C57BL/6NCr, C3H/HeNCr^{MTVV-} and DBA/2NCr mice. *Carcinogenesis* **7,** 215–220.

Dourson, M. L., Teuschler, L. K., Durkin, P. R., and Stiteler, W. M. (1997). Categorical regression of toxicity data: A case study using aldicarb. *Reg. Toxicol. Pharmacol.* **25,** 121–129.

ECOTOC (1992). "Toxic to Reproduction" Guidance on Classification," (EC 7th amendment). ECOTOC Technical Report #47 (ISSN-0773-8072-47), Brussels.

Editorial (1996). Social position and health. *Ann. Epidemiol.* **6,** 21–23.

Environm. Health Perspect. (1993). **101,** suppl. 1.

Frankos, V. H. (1985). FDA perspectives on the use of teratology data for human risk assessment. *Fundam. Appl. Toxicol.* **5,** 615–625.

Freireich, E. J., Gehan, E. A., Rall, D. P., Schmidt, L. H., and Skipper, H. E. (1966). Quantitative comparison of toxicity of anticancer agents in mouse, rat, hamster, dog, monkey, and man. *Cancer Chemother. Rep.* **50,** 219–244.

Greenland, S. (1994). A critical look at some popular meta-analytic methods. *Am. J. Epidemiol.* **140,** 290–296.

Habermann, E. (1995). Vergiftet ohne Gift. *Skeptiker* **8,** 92–100.

Haseman, J. (1985). Issues in carcinogenicity testing: Dose selection. *Fundam. Appl. Toxicol.* **5,** 66–78.

Heinonen, O. P., Slone, D., and Shapiro, S. (1977). "Birth Defects and Drugs in Pregnancy." Science Group Inc, Littleton, MA.

IARC Monograph (1987). Supplement 7, International Agency for Research on Cancer, WHO, Lyon.

International Clearinghouse (1991). "Congenital Malformations Worldwide. A Report from the International Clearinghouse for Birth Defects Monitoring Systems." Elsevier, Amsterdam.

IPCS/OECD (1996). "IPCS/OECD Joint Project on the Harmonization of Chemical Hazard/Risk Assessment Terminology." IPCS, Geneva.

Kayajanian, G. (1997). Dioxin is a promotor blocker, a promotor, and a net anticarcinogen. *Reg. Toxicol. Pharmacol.* **26,** 134–137.

Kociba, R. J., Keyes, D. G., Beyer, J. E., Carreon, R. M., Wade, C. E.,

Dittenber, D. A., Kaknins, R. P., Frauson, L. E., Park, C. N., Barnard, S. D., Hummelk, R. A., and Humiston, C. G. (1978). Results of a two-year chronic toxicity and oncogenicity study of 2,3,7,8-tetrachlorodibenzo-*p*-dioxin in rats. *Toxicol. Appl. Pharmocol.* **46,** 279–303.

Lasagna, L., Mosteller, F., von Felsinger, J. M., and Beecher, H. K. (1954). A study of the placebo response. *Am. J. Med.* **16,** 770–779.

Lima, B. R., Pai, S., Toledo, V., Caris, L., Haro, J. M., Lozano, J., and Santacruz, H. (1993). Emotional distress in disaster victims, a follow-up study. *J. Nervous. Mental. Dis.* **181,** 388–393.

Lorke, D. (1983). A new approach to practical acute toxicity testing. *Arch. Toxicol.* **54,** 275–287.

Löscher, W., and Marquardt, H. (1993). Sind Ergebnisse aus Tierversuchen auf den Menschen übertragbar? *Dtsch. Med. Wschr.* **118,** 1254–1263.

Lynch, J. W., Kaplan, G. A., Cohen, R. D., Tuomilehto, J., and Salonen, J. T. (1996). Do cardiovascular risk factors explain the relation between socioeconomic status, risk of all-cause mortality, cardiovascular mortality, and acute myocardial infarction? *Am. J. Epidemiol.* **144,** 934–942.

Mastroiacovo, P., Spagnolo, A., Marni, E., Meazza, L., Bertoleini, R., and Segni, G. (1988). Birth defects in the Seveso area after TCDD contamination. *JAMA* **259,** 1668–1672.

Mordenti, J. (1985). Pharmacokinetic scale-up: Accurate prediction of human pharmacokinetic profiles from animal data. *J. Pharmaceut. Sci.* **74,** 1097–1099.

Nakachi, K., Imai, K., Hayashi, S., and Kawajiri, K. (1993). Polymorphism of the *CYP1A1* and glutathione S-transferase genes associated with susceptibility to lung cancer in relation to cigarette dose in a Japanese population. *Cancer Res.* **53,** 2994–2999.

NATO/CCMS (1988). Pilot study on international information exchange on dioxins and related compounds. International toxicity equivalency factors (I-TEF). Method of risk assessment for complex mixtures of dioxins and related compounds. *NATO/CCMS Report* **176,** 1–26.

Nellis, R. (1997). Human liver cell studies can predict the metabolism of toxic chemicals in people. *CIIT Impact* August, Research Triangle Park.

Neubert, D. (1992). TCDD toxicity-equivalencies for PCDD/PCDF congeners: Prerequisites and limitations. *Chemosphere* **25,** 65–70.

Neubert, D. (1998). Reflections on the assessment of the toxicity of "dioxins" for humans, using data from experimental and epidemiological studies. *Teratog. Carcinog. Mutagen* **17,** 157–215.

Neubert, D., Bochert, G., Platzek, T., Chahoud, I., Fischer, B., and Meister, R. (1987). Dose-response relationships in prenatal toxicology. *Cong. Anom.* **27,** 275–302.

Neubert, D., Kavlock, R. J., Merker, H.-J., Klein, J. (eds.) (1992). "Risk Assessment of Prenatally-Induced Adverse Health Effects." Springer-Verlag, Berlin.

OECD (1995). "Report of the Workshop on Environmental Hazard/Risk Assessment." OECD Environmental Monograph # 105, Paris.

Phillips, D. H., Hewer, A., Martin, C. N., Garner, R. C., and King, M. M. (1988). Correlation of DNA adduct level in human lung with cigarette smoking. *Nature* **336,** 790–792.

Pitot, H. C., Goldsworth, T. L., Moran, S., Kennan, W., Glauert, H. P., Maronpot, R. R., and Campbell, H. A. (1987). A method to quantitate the relative initiating and promoting potencies of hepatocarcinogenic agents in their dose-response relationships to altered hepatic foci. *Carcinogenesis* **8,** 1491–1499.

Platzek, T., Bochert, G., Meister, R., and Neubert, D. (1993). Embryotoxicity induced by alkylating agents: 7. Low dose prenataltoxic risk estimation based on NOAEL risk factor approach, dose–response relationships, and DNA adducts using methylnitrosourea as a model compound. *Teratogenesis Carcinogen. Mutagen.* **13,** 101–125.

Potter, J. D. (1997). Hazards and benefits of alcohol. *N. Engl. J. Med.* **337,** 1763–1764.

Reynolds, P., and Kaplan, G. A. (1990). Social connections and risk for cancer: prospective evidence from the Alameda County Study. *Behavioral Med.* **16,** 101–110.

Roth, W. T., Clarc, D. B., Sheikh, J., Agras, S., and Taylor, C. B. (1991). How "blind" are double-blind studies? *J. Consult. Clin. Psychol.* **59,** 184–187.

Sackett, D. L., Haynes, R. B., Guyatt, G. H., and Tugwell, P. (1991). "Clinical Epidemiology, A Basic Science for Clinical Medicine," 2nd ed. Little, Brown, Boston.

Salsburg, D. (1989). Does everything cause cancer; an alternative interpretation of the "carcinogenesis" bioassay. *Fundam, Appl. Toxicol.* **13,** 351–358.

Schindel, L. (1967). Placebo and placebo-effects in the clinic and research [in German]. *Arzneimittelforsch.* **17,** 892–917.

Schütz, E., and Fuchs, H. (1982). A new approach to minimizing the number of animals used in acute toxicity testing and optimizing the information of test results. *Arch. Toxicol.* **51,** 197–220.

Skrabanek, P., and McCormick, J. (1993). "Torheiten und Trugschlüsse in der Medizin", 3rd ed. Verlag Kirchheim, Mainz.

Smialowicz, R. J., Riddle, M. M., Williams, W. C., Copeland, C. B., Luebke, R. W., and Andrews, D. L. (1992). Differences between rats and mice in the immunosuppressive activity of 2-methoxyethanol and 2-methoxyacetic acid. *Toxicology* **74,** 57–67.

Smith, G. D., Neaton, J. D., Wentworth, D., Stamler, R., and Stamler, J. (1996). Socioeconomic differentials in mortality risk among men screened for the multiple risk factor intervention trial: I white men. *Am. J. Public Health* **86,** 486–496.

Stavric, B., and Gilbert, S. G. (1990). Caffeine metabolism: A problem in extrapolating results from animal studies to humans. *Acta Pharm. Jugosl.* **40,** 475–489.

Somogyi, A., Appel, K. G., and Katenkamp, A. (eds.) (1992). "Chemical Carcinogenesis. The Relevance of Mechanistic Understanding in Toxicological Evaluation." BGA Schriften 3, MMV Medizin Verlag, Munich.

Storey, A., Thomas, M., Kalita, A., Harwood, C., Gardiol, D., Mantovani, F., Breuer, J., Leigh, I. M., Matlashewski, G., and Banks, L. (1998). Role of p53 polymorphism in the development of human papilloma-virus-associated cancer. *Nature* **393,** 229–234.

Taubes, G. (1995). Epidemiology faces its limits. *Science* **269,** 164–169.

Thun, M. J., Peto, R., Lopez, A. D., Monaco, J. H., Henley, S. J., Heath, C. W., and Doll, R. (1997). Alcohol consumption and mortality among middle-aged and elderly U.S. adults. *N. Engl. J. Med.* **337,** 1705–1714.

Williamson, D. F., Parker, R. A., and Kendrick, J. S. (1989). The box plot: A simple visual method to interpret data. *Ann. Intern. Med.* **110,** 916–921.

Wogan, G. N. (1992). Aflatoxins as risk factors for hepatocellular carcinoma in humans. *Cancer Res.* **52,** 2114–2118.

C H A P T E R

52

Toxicity Equivalents and Their Use in Hazard and Risk Assessment

STEPHEN SAFE

Department of Veterinary Physiology and Pharmacology, Texas A&M University, College Station, Texas

INTRODUCTION

Halogenated aromatic hydrocarbons are industrial compounds or by-products formed during the combustion of organic material containing a source of chlorine. Some of these chemicals include polychlorinated dibenzo-*p*-dioxins (PCDDs), dibenzofurans (PCDFs), biphenyls (PCBs), naphthalenes (PCNs), and terphenyls (PCTs). Halogenated aromatic hydrocarbons vary with respect to their degree of chlorination and chlorine substitution pattern, and there are 75, 135, and 209 possible PCDD, PCDF, and PCB congeners, respectively. They are stable lipophilic compounds that have been detected throughout the environment, including air, water, fish, wildlife, food, and human adipose tissue, serum, and milk. Hazard and risk assessment of halogenated aromatic hydrocarbons initially focused on emissions and exposure to the most toxic member of this class of chemicals, namely 2,3,7,8-tetrachlorodibenzo-*p*-dioxin (TCDD); however, this compound is often a minor component of many environmentally relevant halogenated aromatic hydrocarbon mixtures.

TOXICOLOGY AND MECHANISM OF ACTION

TCDD and related compounds induce a number of common toxic and biochemical responses, including a wasting syndrome; reproductive and developmental toxicity; neurotoxicity; hepatotoxic effects, including porphyria; immune suppression; modulation of endocrine responses; chloracne; induction of drug-metabolizing enzymes; and both induction and suppression of diverse genes and/or their related activities. The aryl hydrocarbon (Ah) receptor was identified as the initial intracellular target for halogenated aromatic hydrocarbons and many other classes of anthropogenic and natural compounds. The Ah receptor is a ligand-induced transcription factor that initially binds ligand and forms a nuclear heterodimeric transcription factor with the Ah receptor nuclear translocator (Arnt) protein. Subsequent interaction of the nuclear Ah receptor complex with dioxin or xenobiotic responsive elements (DREs and XREs) located in the 5′-promoter region of target genes results in the transactivation of this gene. Interaction of the nuclear Ah receptor complex with DREs, which contain only the GCGTG core binding sequence (inhibitory DREs), also can lead to the inhibition of target gene expression.

STRUCTURE–ACTIVITY RELATIONSHIPS AND DEVELOPMENT OF TOXIC EQUIVALENCY FACTORS (TEFs)

Structure–activity relationships for halogenated aromatics showed that the most toxic PCDDs and PCDFs were substituted in all four lateral 2, 3, 7, and 8 positions (Fig. 1). The removal of a lateral Cl group or the introduction of an additional nonlateral (1, 4, 6, or 9) Cl substituent into a 2,3,7,8-substituted congener resulted in both decreased activity and binding affinity for the Ah receptor. Similar structure–activity relationships were also derived for the PCBs. The most active coplanar congeners, 3,4,4′,5-tetraCB, 3,3′,4,4′-

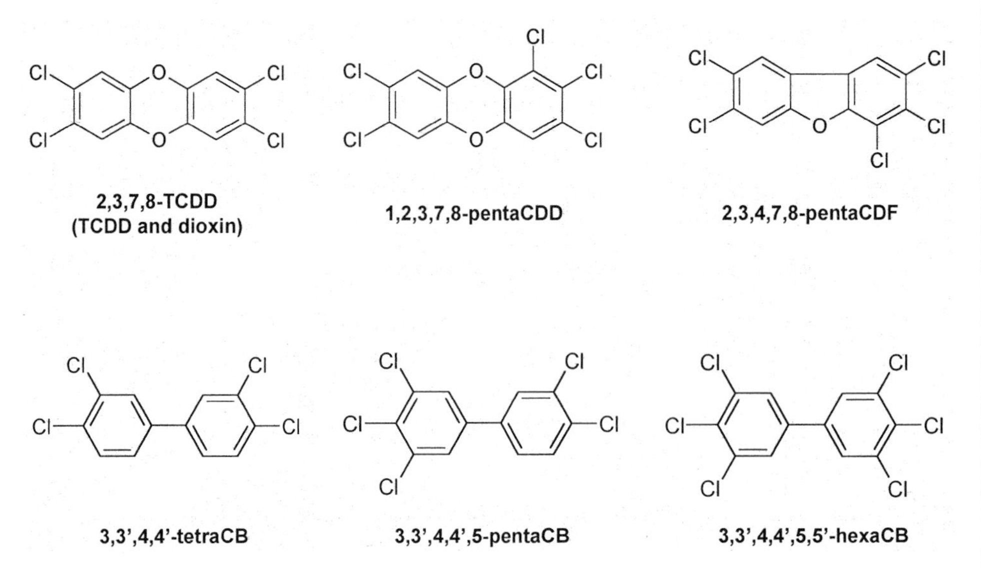

2,3,7,8-TCDD (TCDD and dioxin)

1,2,3,7,8-pentaCDD

2,3,4,7,8-pentaCDF

3,3',4,4'-tetraCB

3,3',4,4',5-pentaCB

3,3',4,4',5,5'-hexaCB

FIGURE 1 Structures of toxic halogenated aromatic compounds.

tetraCB, 3,3′,4,4′,5-pentaCB, and 3,3′,4,4′,5,5′-hexaCB, were substituted in both the para and 2 or more meta positions (Fig. 1). In addition, the monoortho derivatives of coplanar PCBs were also Ah receptor agonists with lower activities than the nonortho-substituted analogs. Initial studies indicated that the effects of submaximal doses or concentrations of some halogenated aromatic hydrocarbon mixtures were related to the potency and concentrations of the individual congeners. Toxic equivalency factors for PCDD and PCDF congeners were derived by comparing their potencies relative to TCDD (TEF = 1.0) and values were assigned only for the 2,3,7,8-substituted compounds which are known to persist in environmental samples (Table 1). Individual toxic equivalency factors were selected from a range for each compound; selection was based on "scientific judgment," which gave more credence to data obtained from longer term feeding experiments or studies with endpoints such as cancer, developmental toxicity, and reproductive toxicity.

Initially, bioassay-derived toxic equivalency factors were used for the coplanar and monoortho coplanar PCB congeners and showed that for fish, wildlife, and human samples the coplanar and monoortho-substituted PCBs were major contributors to the TCDD-like toxicity of halogenated aromatic hydrocarbons in environmental samples. Initially, toxic equivalency factors for PCBs were proposed and then a World Health Organization working group recommended toxic equivalency values for the more important toxic and environmentally relevant PCB congeners (Table 1). These values have not been adopted officially by regulatory agencies; however, they are routinely used to estimate the toxicity or TCDD equivalents in various environmental extracts.

USE OF TOXIC EQUIVALENCY FACTORS

The major application of toxic equivalency factors is to estimate toxic equivalents for any mixture where

$$\mathrm{TEQ} = \Sigma[\mathrm{PCDD}_i] \cdot \mathrm{TEF}_i + \Sigma[\mathrm{PCDF}_i] \cdot \mathrm{TEF}_i + \Sigma[\mathrm{PCB}_i] \cdot \mathrm{TEF}_i + \cdots \quad (1)$$

and the i value denotes the concentration and TEF for an individual congener in a mixture. This approach assumes that at submaximal doses of an halogenated aromatic hydrocarbon mixture, the contribution of individual components are essentially additive.

The validation of the toxic equivalency approach for the hazard assessment of halogenated aromatic mixtures has also been reported for some *in vitro* and *in vivo* responses in which the calculated toxicity of a mixture (Eq. 1) is compared to the experimentally derived toxic potency of a mixture (e.g., the EC_{50} value) relative to that of TCDD for the same response (and response intensity). The comparative acute toxicity of four PCDD congeners was determined (TCDD, 1,2,3,7,8-pentaCDD, 1,2,3,4,7,8-hexaCDD, and 1,2,3,4,6,7,8-heptaCDD) and a mixture of these com-

TABLE 1 Proposed Toxic Equivalency Factors for the 2,3,7,8-Substituted PCDDs and PCDFs and the Monoortho and Coplanar PCBs

Congener	TEF
PCDDs	
2,3,7,8-TCDD	1.0
1,2,3,7,8-PentaCDD	0.5
1,2,3,4,7,8-HexaCDD	0.1
1,2,3,6,7,8-HexaCDD	0.1
1,2,3,7,8,9-HexaCDD	0.1
1,2,3,4,6,7,8-HeptaCDD	0.01
OCDD	0.001
PCDFs	
2,3,7,8-TCDF	0.1
2,3,4,7,8-PentaCDF	0.5
1,2,3,7,8-PentaCDF	0.1/0.05
1,2,3,4,7,8-HexaCDF	0.1
2,3,4,6,7,8-HexaCDF	0.1
1,2,3,6,7,8-HexaCDF	0.1
1,2,3,7,8,9-HexaCDF	0.1
1,2,3,4,6,7,8-HeptaCDF	0.01
1,2,3,4,7,8,9-HeptaCDF	0.01
OCDF	0.001
PCBs	
3,3′,4,4′,5-PentaCB	0.1
3,3′,4,4′,5,5′-HexaCB	0.01
3,3′,4,4′-TetraCB	0.0005
2,3,3′,4,4′-PentaCB	0.0001
2,3,3′,4,4′,5-HexaCB	0.0005
2,3′,4,4′,5-PentaCB	0.0001
2,3,3′,4,4′,5′-HexaCB	0.0005
2′,3,4,4′,5-PentaCB	0.0001
2,3,4,4,5-PentaCB	0.0005

pounds in the Sprague–Dawley rat, and the results indicated that the toxicity of the mixture was due to additive contributions of individual congeners. Additive interactions for complex halogenated aromatic mixtures have also been observed using various induction (CYP1A1-dependent) skin cell keratinization, receptor binding, and *in vivo* bioassays.

The utility of this approach for PCB mixtures has been validated in both *in vivo* and *in vitro* studies. Based on induction-derived toxic equivalency factors obtained for coplanar and monoortho-substituted PCB congeners and their concentrations in Aroclor 1242, 1254, and 1260, the toxic equivalency values could be calculated for these mixtures. Because the ED_{50} values for the induction of hepatic CYP1A1-dependent aryl hydrocarbon hydroxylase (AHH) and ethoxyresorufin *O*-deethylase (EROD) activities by TCDD was known (1.29 and 0.97 μg/kg, respectively), the ED_{50} values for the PCB mixtures can be calculated. A comparison of the ED_{50} (observed)/ED_{50} (calculated) indicates that with one exception the ratios varied from 0.80 to 1.76, indicating a good correspondence between the experimentally derived and calculated ED_{50} values. Similar results were also observed for Aroclor mixtures in rat hepatoma H4IIE cells. Induction toxic equivalents have also been correlated with adverse effects in wildlife exposed to halogenated aromatic hydrocarbon mixtures.

LIMITATIONS OF THE TOXIC EQUIVALENCY FACTOR APPROACH FOR RISK ASSESSMENT

Range of Values

The number of response-specific toxic equivalency factors for 2,3,7,8-substituted PCDDs and PCDFs, and nonortho- and monoortho-substituted PCBs is continually expanding. Values for compounds such as 3,3′,4,4′-tetraCB, which are readily metabolized, range from 0.000007 to 0.13. The mean value for 19 responses was 0.017 ± 0.030, and the toxic equivalency factor assigned by the WHO working group was 0.0005. It was recently reported that in the resistant male and female Hann–Wistar rat strain, the order of toxic potency was 1,2,3,4,7,8-hexaCDD > 1,2,3,4,6,7,8-heptaCDD > 1,2,3,7,8-pentaCDD > TCDD. 1,2,3,4,6,-7,8-HeptaCDD was more acutely toxic than TCDD in Hann–Wistar rats, whereas in other rat strains and the guinea pig, TCDD is at least 100 times more toxic than 1,2,3,4,6,7,8-heptaCDD. These results indicate the experimentally derived toxic equivalency factors did not correlate with assigned values (Table 1).

Nonadditive Interactions Associated with PCBs

In most environmental matrices, levels of non- and monoortho coplanar congeners and the more toxic lower chlorinated (tetra-hexachloro) PCDDs and PCDFs are relatively low compared to other PCBs such as 2,2′,4,4′,5,5′-hexaCB, which exhibit minimal to nondetectable aryl hydrocarbon receptor agonist activity. Several groups have investigated the nonadditive interactions of PCB mixtures and congeners with TCDD and other aryl hydrocarbon receptor agonists and have shown that PCBs and some PCDFs antagonize several aryl hydrocarbon receptor-mediated responses including fetal cleft palate, hydronephrosis, and immunotoxicity in mice; embryotoxicity in chick embryos; and induction of CYP1A1-dependent activities in several *in vivo* and *in vitro* systems.

TABLE 2 Examples of Antagonistic Interactions of Halogenated Aromatics: Inhibition of TCDD or 3,3′,4,4′,5-PentaCB-Induced Responses

Antagonists	Response (animal cell)	Source
1,3,6,8-TetraCDF,2,4,6,8-tetraCDF, Aroclor 1254	AHH/EROD activities (H4IIE cells)	(Keys *et al.* (1986); Bannister *et al.* (1987); Tysklind *et al.* (1995)
2,2,4,4′,5′,6-HexaCB	EROD activity (chick embryo hepatocytes)	Bosveld *et al.* (1995)
2,2′,5,5′-TetraCB	Luciferase activity (mouse and rat cell lines)	Aarts *et al.* (1995)
Aroclors 1232, 1242, 1248, 1254 and 1260; reconstituted PCB mixtures; 1,3,6,8-tetraCDF, 2,3,3′,4,4′,5-hexaCB; 2,3,3′,4,5,5′-hexaCB; 2,3,3′,4,5′-pentaCB, 2,3,4,4′,5,6-hexaCB; 2,2′,4,4′,5,6′-hexaCB; 2,2′,4,4′,6,6′-hexaCB; 2,2′,4,4′,5,5′-hexaCB	Splenic plaque-forming cell response to sheep red blood cells or trinitrophenyl-lipopolysaccharide (mouse strains)	Bannister *et al.* (1987); Davis and Safe (1988, 1989, 1990); Harper *et al.* (1995)
2,2′,4,4′,5,5′-HexaCB	Serum IgM units (mice)	Harper *et al.* (1994)
Aroclor 1254; 2,2′,4,4′,5,5′-hexaCB; 2,2′,5,5′-tetraCB	Fetal cleft palate and hydronephrosis (mice)	Haake *et al.* (1987); Biegel *et al.* (1989); Morrissey *et al.* (1992); Zhao *et al.* (1997a)
2,2′,4,4′,5,5′-HexaCB	Chick embryotoxicity (malformations, edema, liver lesions)	Zhao *et al.* (1997b)

Table 2 summarizes the antagonistic interactions of various aryl hydrocarbon receptor agonists, including TCDD, 2,3,4,7,8-pentaCDF, 3,3′,4,4′,5-pentaCB, and 3,3′,4,4′-tetraCB, with diverse antagonists or inhibitors.

The dose-dependent immunotoxicity of Aroclors 1260, 1254, 1248, and 1242 and the major nonortho- and monoortho-substituted PCBs were investigated in B6C3F1 mice immunized with trinitrophenyl-lipopolysaccharide (TNP-LPS). Toxic equivalency factors were derived for the nonortho- and monoortho-PCB congeners; toxic equivalents were calculated using immunotoxicity-derived toxic equivalency values; and ED_{50} values could be readily calculated for the commercial PCB mixtures. A comparison of the calculated versus observed ED_{50} values and their ratios indicated that for Aroclors 1254, 1248, and 1242, the observed ED_{50} values were significantly higher than expected (5.9- to 22-fold; i.e., lower potency) indicating that the toxic equivalency approach would significantly overestimate the immunotoxicity of these PCB mixtures. The failure to observe nonadditive interactions with Aroclor 1260 may be due to the relatively low levels of the potent nonortho-substituted coplanar PCBs in this mixture compared to Aroclors 1242, 1248, and 1254. Most environmental mixtures contain 2,3,7,8-substituted PCDDs and PCDFs and coplanar PCBs, and it is likely that their interactions in the immunotoxicity assay would be similar to those observed for the lower chlorinated Aroclors. It was reported that 2,2′,4,4′,5,5′-hexaCB markedly enhanced TCDD-induced hepatic porphyrin levels in rats. Porphyria is an aryl hydrocarbon receptor-mediated response; however, this effect is also induced by other compounds through aryl hydrocarbon receptor-independent pathways, and it is likely that the synergistic interaction between TCDD and 2,2′,4,4′,5,5′-hexaCB may involve more than one pathway.

Nonadditive antagonist interactions between halogenated aromatic hydrocarbons (Table 2) represent important limitations of the toxic equivalency approach for the risk assessment of these compounds, and the ratio of antagonist/agonist required for inhibitory responses (usually $>1000/1$) are observed in many environmental mixtures. The antagonistic interactions have all been observed at relatively high doses or concentrations of both agonist and antagonist, and the importance of these interactions at lower environmental exposure levels is unknown.

Dioxins versus Natural Ah Receptor Agonists

The average dietary toxic equivalents intake from PCDDs and PCDFs is approximately 79 to 188 pg/day for Germany, North America, and The Netherlands, and if PCBs are included, the overall values may be approximately 300 pg/day. Tolerable daily intakes (ADIs and TDIs) for most countries, derived from a safety factor approach, range from 1 to 10 pg/

TABLE 3 Dietary Intakes and Toxic Equivalents Values for PCDDs and PCDFs and Some Natural Ah Receptor Agonists[a]

Compounds	Dietary intake (pg/day)	Toxic equivalency factor (relative potency)	Toxic equivalents (pg/day)
Antiestrogenicity			
PCDDs and PCDFs	1000–2000	—	120
Indole-3-carbinol	735,000,000	0.0001	73,500
Polynuclear aromatic hydrocarbons	1.2–5 × 10^6	0.001	1200–5000
Immunotoxicity			
PCDDs and PCDFs	1000–2000	—	120
Indole-3-carbinol	735,000,000	0.0001	73,500
Polynuclear aromatic hydrocarbons	1.2–5.0 × 10^6	0.0001	120–500

[a]Safe (1995b).

kg. In contrast, the U.S. Environmental Protection Agency has treated TCDD and related compounds as complete carcinogens (no threshold) and has recommended a virtually safe dose of 0.01 pg/kg toxic equivalents. Moreover, in its recent document, which reassessed the hazards and risks associated with PCDDs/PCDFs, it stated that, "Based on all of the data reviewed in this reassessment and scientific inference, a picture emerges of TCDD and related compounds as potent toxicants in animals with the *potential* to produce a spectrum of effects. Some of these effects may be occurring in humans at very low levels and some may be resulting in adverse impacts on human health."

Hazard and risk assessment of any class of toxicants should also consider the contributions of naturally occurring chemicals in foods, which elicit the same class-specific toxic responses. This type of approach has been used for carcinogens, estrogens, and Ah receptor agonists (natural versus xenodioxins). For example, the relative carcinogenic potencies of industrially derived compounds were calculated (including halogenated aromatic hydrocarbons) and natural food-derived carcinogens in the diet using a human exposure/rat potency (HERP) dose index. This ratio has been used to rank possible carcinogenic hazards in the diet. For example, the HERP (%) value for beer (12 oz) based on its alcohol content was 2.8, whereas the value for PCBs (0.2 μg/day) was 0.0002. Similar results were obtained using TCDD, suggesting that the carcinogenic contributions of dietary halogenated aromatics were minimal compared to natural carcinogens in the diet. Using a toxic equivalency factor approach, a similar argument has also been made for xenoestrogens versus "natural estrogens" in the diet, such as lignans, fungal estrogens, flavonoids, and related compounds.

The human diet also contains Ah receptor agonists, and these compounds include indole-3-carbinol and related compounds in vegetables, polynuclear aromatic hydrocarbons, and aromatic amines that are formed during cooking. Table 3 compares estimated dietary intake of both dioxins and natural Ah receptor agonists, and it is apparent that mass intake of natural Ah receptor agonists ≫PCDDs and PCDFs. Moreover, several studies indicate that natural Ah receptor agonists elicit responses in humans.

1. Consumption of pan-fried hamburger cooked at >250°C induced CYP1A2-dependent caffeine metabolism in humans, and this response is associated with cooking-derived polynuclear aromatic hydrocarbons, aromatic amines, and related compounds.
2. Humans consuming indole-3-carbinol exhibit higher excretion rates of catechol estrogen (CYP1A2-dependent 2-hydroxylation).
3. Caffeine metabolism was not induced in workers occupationally exposed to phenoxy herbicides compared to a control group; in contrast, analysis of TCDD-exposed and control groups as smokers or nonsmokers showed that there was a significant increase in caffeine metabolism only in the former group.
4. Polynuclear aromatic hydrocarbons, which act through the Ah receptor, exhibit anti-estrogenic activity in both rodent and cell-culture models, and this correlates with the lower incidence of en-

dometrial cancer in smokers and the potential *in vivo* anti-estrogenic effects of polynuclear aromatic hydrocarbons in humans. These data complement studies on women in Seveso accidentally exposed to TCDD who have a decreased incidence of both breast and endometrial cancer.

These data demonstrate that natural Ah receptor agonists can induce Ah receptor-mediated responses in humans and, at least in the liver, the induction of CYP1A2 by polynuclear aromatic hydrocarbons can be observed at levels that are in the range of dietary exposures for some groups (e.g., high meat eaters and smokers). In contrast, no significant induction was observed in workers with high serum levels of TCDD.

In utero exposure of pregnant rats on gestation day 15 to low doses of TCDD (<1 μg/kg) resulted in several adverse effects in male offspring, including decreased anogenital distance, delayed testicular descent, decreased testicular parenchymal weight, reduced spermatogenesis and epididymal sperm reserves, and decreased accessory gland weights. Recent studies compared the effects of prenatal treatment of female Sprague–Dawley rats on gestation day 15 with a single oral dose of TCDD (1.0 μg/kg) or indole-3-carbinol (1 mg/kg). Both compounds altered anogenital distance, anogenital distance/body weight ratio, crown-to-rump length, and crown-to-rump length/body weight ratio at days 1 or 5. In 62-day-old offspring, seminal vesicle weight, prostate weight, daily sperm production/g testicular parenchyma, and daily sperm production/testis were also decreased by both compounds. TCDD also significantly decreased total number of sperm in the epididymis, and this was primarily due to decreased sperm in the tail of the epididymis. In contrast, prenatal exposure to indole-3-carbinol did not affect any of these parameters. TCDD also decreased epididymal transit time of the sperm through the tail of the epididymis, whereas indole-3-carbinol significantly increased the total epididymal transit time. These studies showed that prenatal exposure of pregnant rats to indole-3-carbinol, a "natural" Ah receptor agonist, caused some reproductive abnormalities in male rat offspring, which resembled those observed for TCDD and other adverse effects that were Ah receptor-independent. Based on dietary exposures (Table 3), the results suggested that indole-3-carbinol, a natural component in cruciferous vegetables, would constitute the major risk for *in utero* exposure to Ah receptor agonists in rats.

In summary, humans are exposed to both natural Ah receptor agonists and antagonists and to PCDDs and PCDFs with significantly higher intake of the former group of compounds (Table 3). The use of toxic equivalency factors for risk assessment of a specific class of chemicals that act through a common pathway (e.g., Ah receptor) must consider contributions from both xeno and natural analogs and their possible interactions. This type of approach suggests that at least for some responses, the effects of dioxins may be significantly lower than for natural Ah receptor agonists. While it is clear that toxic equivalents for halogenated aromatics are useful for predicting some adverse effects in wildlife populations, the specific responses in humans, who are preferentially impacted by PCDDs and PCDFs, should be further investigated.

Bibliography

Aarts, J. M. M. J. G., Denison, M. S., Cox, M. A., Schalk, M. A. C., Garrison, P. M., Tullis, K., De Haan, L. H. J., and Brouwer, A. (1995). Species-specific antagonism of Ah receptor action by 2,2′,5,5′-tetrachloro- and 2,2′,3,3′,4,4′-hexachlorobiphenyl. *Eur. J. Pharmacol.* **293,** 463–474.

Ahlborg, U. G., Brouwer, A., Fingerhut, M. A., Jacobson, J. L., Jacobson, S. W., Kennedy, S. W., Kettrup, A. A. F., Koeman, J. H., Poiger, H., Rappe, C., Safe, S. H., Seegal, R. F., Tuomisto, J., and Van den Berg, M. (1992). Impact of polychlorinated dibenzo-*p*-dioxins, dibenzofurans, and biphenyls on human and environmental health with special emphasis on application of the toxic equivalence factor concept. *Eur. J. Pharmacol.* **228,** 179–199.

Bannister, R., Davis, D., Zacharewski, T., Tizard, I., and Safe, S. (1987). Aroclor 1254 as a 2,3,7,8-tetrachlorodibenzo-*p*-dioxin antagonist: effects on enzyme activity and immunotoxicity. *Toxicology* **46,** 29–42.

Biegel, L., Harris, M., Davis, D., Rosengren, R., Safe, L., and Safe, S. (1989). 2,2′,4,4′,5,5′-Hexachlorobiphenyl as a 2,3,7,8-tetrachlorodibenzo-*p*-dioxin antagonist in C57BL/6J mice. *Toxicol. Appl. Pharmacol.* **97,** 561–571.

Bosveld, A. T. C., Verhallen, E., Seinen, W., and Van den Berg, M. (1995). Mixture interactions in the *in vitro* CYP1A1 induction bioassay using chicken embryo heptocytes. *Organohalogen Compounds* **25,** 309–312.

Davis, D., and Safe, S. (1988). Immunosuppressive activities of polychlorinated dibenzofuran congeners: quantitative structure-activity relationships and interactive effects. *Toxicol. Appl. Pharmacol.* **94,** 141–149.

Davis, D., and Safe, S. (1989). Dose-response immunotoxicities of commercial polychlorinated biphenyls (PCBs) and their interaction with 2,3,7,8-tetrachlorodibenzo-*p*-dioxin. *Toxicol. Lett.* **48,** 35–43.

Davis, D., and Safe, S. (1990). Immunosuppressive activities of polychlorinated biphenyls in C57BL/6 mice: Structure-activity relationships as Ah receptor agonists and partial antagonists. *Toxicology* **63,** 97–111.

Gold, L. S., Slone, T. H., Stern, B. R., Manley, N. B., and Ames, B. N. (1992). Rodent carcinogens: setting priorities. *Science* **258,** 261–265.

Haake, J. M., Safe, S., Mayura, K., and Phillips, T. D. (1987). Aroclor 1254 as an antagonist of the teratogenicity of 2,3,7,8-tetrachlorodibenzo-*p*-dioxin. *Toxicol. Lett.* **38,** 299–306.

Halperin, W. E., Kalow, W., Sweeney, M. H., Tang, B. K., Fingerhut, M., Timpkins, B., and Wille, K. (1995). Induction of P-450 in workers exposed to dioxin. *Occup. Environ. Med.* **52,** 86–91.

Harper, N., Connor, K., Steinberg, M., and Safe, S. (1994). An ELISA specific for antibodies to TNP-LPS detects alterations in serum immunoglobulins and isotype switching in C57BL/6 and DBA/2 mice exposed to 2,3,7,8-tetrachlorodibenzo-*p*-dioxin and related compounds. *Toxicology* **92,** 155–167.

Harper, N., Connor, K., Steinberg, M., and Safe, S. (1995). Immunosuppressive activity of polychlorinated biphenyl mixtures and congeners: Non-additive (antagonistic) interactions. *Fundam. Appl. Toxicol.* **27,** 131–139.

Harris, M., Zacharewski, T., and Safe, S. (1993). Comparative potencies of Aroclors 1232, 1242, 1248, 1254 and 1260 in male Wistar rats—Assessment of toxic equivalency factor (TEF) approach for polychlorinated biphenyls (PCBs). *Fundam. Appl. Toxicol.* **20,** 456–463.

Kannan, N., Tanabe, S., Wakimoto, T., and Tatsukawa, R. (1987). Coplanar polychlorinated biphenyls in Aroclor and Kanechlor mixtures. *J. Assoc. Offic. Anal. Chem.* **70,** 451.

Kannan, N., Tanabe, S., and Tatsukawa, R. (1988a). Toxic potential of non-*ortho* and mono-*ortho* coplanar PCBs in commercial PCB preparations: 2,3,7,8-T_4CDD toxicity equivalence factors approach. *Bull. Environ. Contam. Toxicol.* **41,** 267–276.

Kannan, N., Tanabe, S., and Tatsukawa, R. (1988b). Potentially hazardous residues of non-*ortho* chlorine substituted coplanar PCBs in human adipose tissue. *Arch. Environ. Health* **43,** 11–14.

Keys, B., Piskorska-Pliszczynska, J., and Safe, S. (1986). Polychlorinated dibenzofurans as 2,3,7,8-TCDD antagonists: In vitro inhibition of monooxygenase enzyme induction. *Toxicol. Lett.* **31,** 151–158.

Krishnan, V., Porter, W., Santostefano, M., Wang, X., and Safe, S. (1995). Molecular mechanism of inhibition of estrogen-induced cathepsin D gene expression by 2,3,7,8-tetrachlorodibenzo-*p*-dioxin (TCDD) in MCF-7 cells. *Mol. Cell. Biol.* **15,** 6710–6719.

Morrissey, R. E., Harris, M. W., Diliberto, J. J., and Birnbaum, L. S. (1992). Limited PCB antagonism of TCDD-induced malformations in mice. *Toxicol. Lett.* **60,** 19–25.

Pohjanvirta, R., Unkila, M., Lindén, J., Tuomisto, J. T., and Tuomisto, J. (1995). Toxic equivalency factors do not predict the acute toxicities of dioxins in rats. *Eur. J. Pharmacol.* **293,** 341–353.

Poland, A., Glover, E., and Kende, A. S. (1976). Stereospecific, high affinity binding of 2,3,7,8-tetrachlorodibenzo-*p*-dioxin by hepatic cytosol: Evidence that the binding species is receptor for induction of aryl hydrocarbon hydroxylase. *J. Biol. Chem.* **251,** 4936–4946.

Safe, S. (1984). Polychlorinated biphenyls (PCBs) and polybrominated biphenyls (PBBs): Biochemistry, toxicology and mechanism of action. *C.R.C. Crit. Rev. Toxicol.* **12,** 319–395.

Safe, S. (1986). Comparative toxicology and mechanism of action of polychlorinated dibenzo-*p*-dioxins and dibenzofurans. *Annu. Rev. Pharmacol. Toxicol.* **26,** 371–399.

Safe, S. (1990). Polychlorinated biphenyls (PCBs), dibenzo-*p*-dioxins (PCDDs), dibenzofurans (PCDFs) and related compounds: Environmental and mechanistic considerations which support the development of toxic equivalency factors (TEFs). *C.R.C. Crit. Rev. Toxicol.* **21,** 51–88.

Safe, S. (1994). Polychlorinated biphenyls (PCBs): Environmental impact, biochemical and toxic responses, and implications for risk assessment. *C.R.C. Crit. Rev. Toxicol.* **24,** 87–149.

Safe, S. (1995a). Modulation of gene expression and endocrine response pathways by 2,3,7,8-tetrachlorodibenzo-*p*-dioxin and related compounds. *Pharmacol. Therap.* **67,** 247–281.

Safe, S. (1995b). Environmental and dietary estrogens and human health—Is there a problem? *Environ. Health Perspect.* **103,** 346–351.

Sawyer, T., and Safe, S. (1982). PCB isomers and congeners: induction of aryl hydrocarbon hydroxylase and ethoxyresorufin *O*-deethylase enzyme activities in rat hepatoma cells. *Toxicol. Lett.* **13,** 87–94.

Stahl, B. U., Kettrup, A., and Rozman, K. (1992). Comparative toxicity of four chlorinated dibenzo-*p*-dioxins (CDDs) and their mixture. Part I: Acute toxicity and toxic equivalency factors (TEFs). *Arch. Toxicol.* **66,** 471–477.

Tysklind, M., Bosveld, A. T. C., Andersson, P., Verhallen, E., Sinnige, T., Seinen, W., Rappe, C., and Van den Berg, M. (1995). Inhibition of ethoxyresorufin-*O*-deethylase (EROD) activity in mixtures of 2,3,7,8-tetrachlorodibenzo-*p*-dioxin and polychlorinated biphenyls. *Environ. Sci. Pollut. Res.* **4,** 211–216.

U.S. EPA. (1994). "Health Assessment for 2,3,7,8-TCDD and Related Compounds." External Review Draft. EPA/600/BP-92/001a-c. Washington, DC.

Van Birgelen, A. P. J. M., Fase, K. M., Van der Kolk, J., Poiger, H., Brouwer, A., Seinen, W., and Van den Berg, M. (1996). Synergistic effect of 2,2′,4,4′,5,5′-hexachlorobiphenyl and 2,3,7,8-tetrachlorodibenzo-*p*-dioxin on hepatic porphyrin levels in the rat. *Environ. Health Perspect.* **104,** 550–557.

Zhao, F., Mayura, K., Harper, N., Safe, S. H., and Phillips, T. D. (1997a). Inhibition of 3,3′,4,4′,5-pentachlorobiphenyl-induced fetal cleft palate and immunotoxicity in C57BL/6 mice by 2,2′,4,4′,5,5′-hexachlorobiphenyl. *Chemosphere* **34,** 1605–1613.

Zhao, F., Mayura, K., Kocurek, N., Edwards, J. F., Kubena, L. F., Safe, S. H., and Phillips, T. D. (1997b). Inhibition of 3,3′,4,4′,5-pentachlorobiphenyl-induced chicken embryotoxicity by 2,2′,4,4′,5,5′-hexachlorobiphenyl. *Fundam. Appl. Toxicol.* **35,** 1–8.

PART

VI

APPENDIX

Threshold Values and Recommendations

INGA OLLROGE
Department of Labor, Health, and Social Welfare, Division of Health and Environment, Hamburg, Germany

GENERAL REMARKS

The substances mentioned in this book can be present in the work place, or as residues or contaminants in environmental media (e.g., air, water, and food) and in cosmetics. Threshold values and recommendations have been set to protect humans, as well as flora and fauna and the biosphere. In this appendix, only values concerning the protection of humans are listed, using standards of general importance developed by the World Health Organization (WHO), several institutions of the United States, and by the European Union (EU). As the different organizations or institutions sometimes use different chemical names for the same substance, the tables contain the chemical name mentioned in the corresponding list. These lists cannot be expected to be complete; predominantly, the values refer to substances mentioned in this book. The tables contain the available values as of March–October 1997 and parts of fall 1998.

REFERENCE DOSES

Acceptable Daily Intakes (ADI) and Provisional Tolerable Weekly Intakes (PTWI) from the World Health Organization (WHO)

Various programs of WHO have evaluated the ADIs for pesticides, food additives, and veterinary drugs. The ADI is defined as "the daily dosage of a chemical which, during an entire lifetime, appears to be without appreciable risk . . . ." The toxicological assessments for pesticides were carried out by the Joint FAO (Food and Agricultural Organization)/WHO Meeting on Pesticide Residues (JMPR) and the ADIs are listed in Table 1. For those pesticides that appear as contaminants (not residues) in food because their agricultural use is restricted, the ADI is converted to provisional tolerable daily intake (PTDI). In addition to the ADIs evaluated by JMPR, the tolerable daily intakes (TDI) estimated by a WHO ad hoc group for the development of guideline values for drinking water are cited in Table 1.

For environmental contaminants other than pesticides and some relevant mycotoxins, the Joint FAO/WHO Expert Committee on Food Additives (JECFA) has established PTWIs (Table 2). At the beginning of 1972, PTWIs were derived for metals that accumulate in the human body as a consequence of their ubiquitous distribution. As dietary habits may lead to enhanced daily intake of no importance, the tolerable intake is expressed in a weekly dose. The term "provisional" indicates that a reevaluation should take place if new data are available. Later the concept was also used for substances that do not accumulate and get into food by migration from food-contact material. For substances that are essential for humans but for which the margin between the dietary requirement and toxic dose is very narrow, PTDIs were developed.

Reference Doses for Oral (RfD) and Inhalative (RfC) Intake from the U.S. Environmental Protection Agency (U.S. EPA)

Reference doses were derived for nongenotoxic substances and are defined as an estimate (with uncertainty spanning perhaps one order of magnitude)

TABLE 1 Recommendations of ADIs (WHO) and RfDs/RfCs (U.S. EPA)[a]

Substance	ADI[b] (mg/kg/day)	RfD (mg/kg/day)	RfC (mg/m³)
Abamectin (Avermectin B1)	0.001 (1995)	0.0004 (1989)	
Acenaphthene		0.06 (1994)	
Acetaldehyde			0.009 (1991)
Acetone		0.1 (1993)	
Acetonitrile		0.006 (1996)	
Acetophenone		0.1 (1989)	
Acrolein			0.00002 (1993)
Acrylamide		0.0002 (1991)	
Alachlor		0.01 (1993)	
Aldicarb	0.003 (1992)	0.001 (1993)	
Aldicarb-sulfone		0.001 (1993)	
Aldrin	0.0001 PTDI[c] Aldrin + Dieldrin (1994)	0.00003 (1988)	
Amitrole	0.0005 T[d] (1993)		
Ammonia			0.1 (1991)
Aniline			0.001 (1993)
Anthracene		0.3 (1993)	
Antimony	0.00086 TDI	0.0004 (1991)	
Antimony trioxide			0.0002 (1995)
Arsenic	See Table 2	0.0003 (1993)	
Arsine			0.00005 (1994)
Atrazine	0.0005 TDI	0.035 (1993)	
Azinphos-methyl	0.005 (1991)		
Barium	0.051 TDI	0.07 (1990)	
Benomyl	0.1 (1995)	0.05 (1989)	
Benzaldehyde		0.1 (1988)	
Benzidine		0.003 (1995)	
Benzoic acid		4 (1993)	
Beryllium		0.002 (1998)	
1,1-Biphenyl	0.125 (1967)	0.05 (1989)	
Bisphenol A		0.05 (1993)	
Boron	0.088 TDI	0.09 (1995)	
Bromide ion	1.0 (1988)		
Bromodichloromethane		0.02 (1991)	
Bromoform	0.0179 TDI	0.02 (1991)	
Bromomethane	1.0, as bromide ion (1966)	0.0014 (1991)	0.005 (1992)
n-Butanol		0.1 (1990)	
Cadmium	See Table 2	0.0005 (1994)	
Camphechlor (toxaphene)	No ADI (1973)		
Carbaryl	0.003 (1996)	0.1 (1988)	
Carbofuran	0.002 (1996)	0.005 (1987)	
Carbon disulfide	No ADI (1965)	0.1 (1990)	0.7 (1995)
Carbon tetrachloride	0.000714 TDI	0.0007 (1991)	
Chloral hydrate	0.0016 TDI		
p-Chloraniline		0.004 (1995)	
Chlordane	0.0005 PTDI (1994)	0.0005 (1998)	0.0007 (1998)
Chlorine	0.150 TDI	0.1 (1994)	
Chlorine dioxide		0.0002 (1990)	
Chloroacetophenone			0.00003 (1991)
Chlorobenzene	0.0867 TDI	0.02(1993)	
1-Chloro-1,1-difluoroethane			50 (1995)
Chlorodifluoromethane			50 (1993)
Chloroform		0.01 (1992)	
2-Chlorophenol		0.005 (1993)	
o-Chlorotoluene		0.02 (1990)	
Chloral		0.002 (1996)	
Chlorpyrifos	0.01 (1982)	0.003 (1988)	

(*continues*)

TABLE 1 *(Continued)*

Substance	ADI[b] (mg/kg/day)	RfD (mg/kg/day)	RfC (mg/m^3)
Chlorpyrifos-methyl	0.01 (1982)		
Chromium III, insoluble salts		1 (1988)	
Chromium VI		0.005 (1996)	
Cresol, *o*-, *m*-		0.05 (1990)	
Cumene		0.01 (1997)	0.4 (1997)
Cyanide, free	0.012 TDI	0.02 (1993)	
Cyanogen bromide		0.09 (1988)	
Cyclohexylamine		0.2 (1988)	
Cyfluthrin	0.02 (1987)	0.025 (1988)	
Cyhexatin	0.007 (1994)		
Cypermethrin	0.05 (1981)	0.01 (1990)	
2,4-D	0.01 (1996)	0.01 (1988)	
2,4-DB	0.03 TDI	0.008 (1992)	
DBCP			0.0002 (1991)
DDT	0.02 PTDI (1994)	0.0005 (1996)	
Deltamethrin	0.01 (1982)		
Demeton	No ADI (1984)	0.00004 (1988)	
Demeton-*S*-methyl	0.0003 (1989)	0.00004 (1986)	
1,2-Dibromoethane	No ADI (1994)		
Dibutyl phthalate		0.1 (1990)	
o-Dichlorobenzene	0.429 TDI	0.09 (1991)	
p-Dichlorobenzene	0.107 TDI		0.8 (1996)
Dichlorodifluoromethane		0.2 (1995)	
1,2-Dichloroethane	No ADI (1994)		
1,1-Dichloroethylene	0.009 TDI	0.009 (1989)	
trans-1,2-Dichloroethylene	0.017 TDI	0.02 (1989)	
Dichloromethane	0.006 TDI	0.06 (1988)	
2,4-Dichlorophenol		0.003 (1988)	
1,2-Dichloropropane	0.00714 TDI		0.004 (1991)
1,3-Dichloropropene		0.0003 (1990)	0.02 (1991)
Dichlorprop	0.0364 TDI		
Dichlorvos	0.004 (1993)	0.0005 (1993)	0.0005 (1994)
Dicofol	0.002 (1992)		
Dieldrin	0.0001 PTDI (1994)	0.00005 (1990)	
Diesel engine emissions			0.005 (1993)
Diethyl phthalate		0.8 (1993)	
Di(2-ethylhexyl)adipate	0.280 TDI	0.6 (1992)	
Di(2-ethylhexyl)phthalate	0.025 TDI See also Table 2	0.02 (1991)	
1,1-Difluoroethane			40 (1994)
Dimethoate	0.002 (1996)	0.0002 (1990)	
N,N-Dimethylaniline		0.002 (1988)	
N,N-Dimethylformamide			0.03 (1990)
Dimethyl terephthalate		0.1 (1995)	
m-Dinitrobenzene		0.0001 (1988)	
2,4-Dinitrophenol		0.002 (1991)	
2,4-Dinitrotoluene		0.002 (1993)	
Diphenylamine	0.02 (1984)	0.025 (1990)	
Diquat	0.002 (1993)	0.0022 (1995)	
Dithiocarb		0.03 (1988)	
Diuron		0.002 (1988)	
Endosulfan	0.006 (1989)	0.006 (1994)	
Endrin	0.0002 PTDI (1994)	0.0003 (1991)	
Epichlorohydrin	0.000143 TDI	0.001 (1992)	
2-Ethoxyethanol			0.2 (1991)
Ethyl acetate		0.9 (1988)	
Ethylbenzene	0.0971 TDI	0.1 (1991)	1 (1991)
Ethylene glycol		2 (1989)	

(continues)

TABLE 1 (*Continued*)

Substance	ADI[b] (mg/kg/day)	RfD (mg/kg/day)	RfC (mg/m³)
Ethylenethiourea (ETU)	0.004 (1993)	0.00008 (1996)	
Fenamiphos	0.0005 (1987)	0.00025 (1990)	
Fentin compounds	0.0005 (1991)		
Fenvalerat (Pydrin)	0.02 (1986)	0.025 (1992)	
Ferbam	0.003 (1996)		
Fluoranthene		0.04 (1993)	
Fluorene		0.04 (1990)	
Fluorine		0.06 (1989)	
Formaldehyde	0.15 TDI	0.2 (1990)	
Heptachlor	0.0001 PTDI (1994)	0.0005 (1991)	
Heptachlor epoxide	0.0001 PTDI (1994)	0.000013 (1991)	
Hexachlorobenzene	Conditional ADI, withdrawn (1978)	0.0008 (1991)	
Hexachlorobutadiene	0.0002 TDI		
Hexachlorocyclopentadiene		0.007 (1990)	
Hexachloroethane		0.001 (1991)	
Hexachlorophene		0.0003 (1991)	
1,6-Hexamethylene diisocyanate			0.00001 (1994)
n-Hexane			0.2 (1993)
Hydrogen chloride			0.02 (1995)
Hydrogen cyanide	0.05 (1965)	0.02 (1993)	0.003 (1994)
Hydrogen phosphide (phosphine)	ADI not necessary (no residue in food) (1966)	0.0003 (1993)	0.0003 (1995)
Hydrogen sulfide		0.003 (1988)	0.001 (1995)
Isobutyl alcohol		0.3 (1991)	
Lindane (γ-Hexachlorocyclohexane)	0.008 (1989)	0.0003 (1988)	
Linuron		0.002 (1990)	
Malathion	0.02 (1966)	0.02 (1992)	
Mancozeb	0.03 (1993)		
Maneb	0.03 (1993)	0.005 (1992)	
Manganese		0.14 (1996)	0.00005 (1993)
MCPA (2-Methyl-4-chloro-phenoxyacetic acid)	0.0005 TDI	0.0005 (1991)	
MCPP (α-2-Methyl-4-chlorophenoxy) propionic acid)		0.001 (1990)	
Mercuric chloride	See Table 2	0.0003 (1995)	
Mercury, elemental			0.0003 (1995)
Metiram	0.03 (1993)		
Methamidophos	0.004 (1990)	0.00005 (1991)	
Methanol		0.5 (1993)	
Methomyl	0.03 (1994)	0.025 (1991)	
Methoxychlor	0.1 (1977)	0.005 (1991)	
2-Methoxyethanol			0.02 (1991)
Methylmercury	See Table 2	0.0001 (1995)	
Mirex		0.0002 (1992)	
Molybdenum		0.005 (1993)	
N,N-Dimethylaniline		0.002 (1988)	
Nickel, soluble salts		0.02 (1996)	
Nitrate		1.6 (1991)	
Nitrilotriacetic acid	0.01 TDI		
Nitrite		0.1 (1992)	
Nitrobenzene		0.0005 (1991)	
2-Nitropropane			0.02 (1991)
Omethoate	ADI withdrawn (1996)		
Paraquat	0.004 (1986)	0.0045 (1991)	
Parathion	0.004 (1995)		
Parathion-methyl	0.003 (1995)	0.00025 (1991)	
PCB			
Aroclor 1254		0.00002 (1996)	
Aroclor 1016		0.00007 (1996)	
Pentachlorobenzene		0.0008 (1988)	

(*continues*)

TABLE 1 (*Continued*)			
Substance	**ADI[b] (mg/kg/day)**	**RfD (mg/kg/day)**	**RfC (mg/m^3)**
Pentachlorophenol	0.003 TDI	0.03 (1993)	
Permethrin	0.05 (1987)	0.05 (1986)	
Phenol		0.6 (1992)	
m-Phenylenediamine		0.006 (1991)	
Phenylmercuric acetate	ADI withdrawn (1967)	0.00008 (1996)	
Phosphoric acid			0.01 (1995)
Phosphorus, white		0.00002 (1993)	
Potassium cyanide		0.05 (1996)	
Propham	No ADI (1992)	0.02 (1987)	
Propineb	0.007 (1993)		
Propoxur (Baygon)	0.02 (1989)	0.004 (1992)	
Pyrene		0.03 (1993)	
Pyrethrins	0.04 (1972)		
Resmethrin	0.03, bioresmethrin (1991)	0.03 (1988)	
Selenium		0.005 (1991)	
Silver		0.005 (1996)	
Strontium		0.6 (1996)	
Strychnine		0.0003 (1988)	
Styrene	0.0077 TDI	0.2 (1990)	1 (1993)
2,4,5-T (2,4,5-Trichlorophenoxyacetic acid)	0.03 (1981) 0.003 TDI	0.01 (1989)	
1,2,4,5-Tetrachlorobenzene		0.0003 (1991)	
1,1,1,2-Tetrachloroethane		0.03 (1996)	
Tetrachloroethylene	0.014 TDI	0.01 (1988)	
2,3,4,6-Tetrachlorophenol		0.03 (1992)	
Tetraethyl-lead	See Table 2	0.0000001 (1988)	
1,1,1,2-Tetrafluoroethane			80 (1995)
Thallium acetate		0.00009 (1990)	
Thallium chloride		0.00008 (1990)	
Thiabendazole	0.1 (1992)		
Thiophanate-methyl	0.02 (1995)	0.08 (1992)	
Thiram	0.01 (1992)	0.005 (1992)	
Toluene	0.223 TDI	0.2 (1992)	0.4 (1991)
2,4,5-TP (Fenoprop)	0.003 TDI	0.008 (1988)	
Tributyltin oxide	0.00025 TDI	0.00003 (1993)	
Trichloroacetic acid	0.0178 TDI		
1,2,4-Trichlorobenzene	0.0077 TDI, all isomers	0.01 (1996)	
1,1,1-Trichloroethane	0.580 TDI		
1,1,2-Trichloroethane		0.004 (1995)	
Trichloroethylene	0.0238 TDI		
2,4,5-Trichlorophenol		0.1 (1988)	
1,1,2-Trichloropropane		0.005 (1988)	
1,2,3-Trichloropropane		0.006 (1990)	
1,1,2-Trichloro-1,2,2-trifluoroethane		30 (1996)	
Trifluralin	0.0075 TDI	0.0075 (1989)	
1,3,5-Trinitrobenzene		0.03 (1997)	
2,4,6-Trinitrotoluene		0.0005 (1995)	
Uranium, soluble salts		0.003 (1989)	
Warfarin		0.0003 (1988)	
Vinyl bromide			0.003 (1994)
Xylenes	0.179 TDI	20 (1987)	
Zinc and compounds		0.3 (1992)	
Zineb	0.03 (1993)	0.05 (1988)	
Ziram	0.003 (1996)		

[a]For ADI values, the year of evaluation is given in parentheses. For RfD and RfC values, the year of last revision is given in parentheses.

[b]For some substances, for which no ADI has been developed by JMPR, the tolerable daily intake (TDI) is noted. These TDIs were calculated as the basis for the guideline values for drinking water (WHO, 1993).

[c]PTDI, provisional tolerable daily intake.

[d]T, temporary ADI.

TABLE 2 Provisional Tolerable Weekly Intake (PTWI) and Other Endpoints[a]

Substance	PTWI
Acrylonitrile	Provisional acceptance[b]
Aflatoxins	Lowest practicable level[c]
Aluminium	7
Arsenic	0.015
Cadmium	0.007
Copper	[0.05–0.5][d]
Di(2-ethylhexyl)phthalate	Provisional acceptance[b]
Iodine	[0.017]
Iron	[0.8]
Lead	0.025
Mercury, total	0.005
Methyl mercury	0.0033
Ochratoxin A	0.0001
Patulin	[0.0004]
Styrene	[0.04]
Tin	14
Zinc	[0.3–1][d]

[a]Values are in mg/kg/week. Bracketed values are provisional maximum tolerable daily intake (PMTDI) in mg/kg/day.

[b]The use of food-contact materials from which the substance may migrate is provisionally accepted, on the condition that the amount of the substance migrating into the food is reduced to the lowest level technologically attainable.

[c]Presence in food should be reduced to irreducible level.

[d]The first number is the daily dietary requirement; the second number is the maximum tolerable daily intake (MTDI).

of the daily exposure to the human population (including sensitive subgroups) that is likely to be without an appreciable risk of deleterious effects during a lifetime. The concept has been published by Barnes and Dourson in 1988 and is part of the U.S. EPA's risk assessment guidelines. The term "reference dose" should avoid the conclusion that an intake exceeding this level might be unacceptable, which is implied by the term "ADI." RfDs and RfCs form the basis for developing regulating doses (e.g., in connection with the Clean Air Act, the Clean Water Act, the Safe Drinking Water Act, and the Federal Insecticide, Fungicide, and Rodenticide Act).

Minimal Risk Levels (MRL)

The U.S. Agency for Toxic Substances and Disease Registry (ATSDR) developed MRLs for hazardous substances that are listed on the CERCLA (Comprehensive Environmental Response, Compensation, and Liability Act) National Priority List (NLP). They should be used as screening levels to identify potential health risks at hazardous waste sites. The MRLs are listed separately in Table 3 because, in contrast to the RfDs/RfCs, they are derived for acute, subacute, and chronic intake (oral and inhalative).

WORKPLACE

Permissible Exposure Limits (PEL) of the U.S. Occupational Safety and Health Administration (OSHA); Threshold Limit Values (TLV) from the American Conference of Governmental Industrial Hygienists (ACGIH); Recommended Exposure Limits (REL) from the U.S. National Institute for Occupational Safety and Health (NIOSH)

The PELs listed in Table 4 are the legal standards in the United States for occupational exposure in general industry. The task of NIOSH is to evaluate the scientific information about a substance. The derived RELs are transmitted to OSHA, which decides whether to promulgate them as legal standards. As not all recommendations are adopted by OSHA, some states of the United States use the more protective values as recommended by NIOSH or ACGIH (Table 4). Table 4 contains only values for a selection of substances taken from the Registry of Toxic Effects of Chemical Substances (RTECS, 3198); further information should be taken from the original documents.

Indicative Limit Values (91/322EEC; 96/94/EC) of the European Union

Indicative limit values (Table 5) must be applied by the EU member states if they adopt provisions for the protection of workers.

Biological Exposure Limits (BEI) from ACGIH

BEI can be found in Chapter 42 (Biomonitoring in Occupational Medicine).

DRINKING WATER

Guidelines for Drinking Water Quality from the World Health Organization (WHO)

The guidelines were published in 1993 and can be used as basis for developing national standards. The guideline values (Table 6) were derived from tolerable

TABLE 3 Minimal Risk Levels (MRL) for Selected Substances

Substance[a]	Duration[b]	Oral MRL (mg/kg/day)	Inhalative MRL (ppm)
Acenaphthene (1995)	int.	0.6	
Acetone (1994)	acute		26
	int.	2	13
	chronic		13
Acrolein (1991)	acute		0.00005
	int.		0.000009
	chronic	0.005	
Acrylonitrile (1991)	acute	0.1	0.1
	int.	0.01	
	chronic	0.04	
Aldrin (1993)	acute	0.002	
	chronic	0.00003	
Ammonia (1991)	acute		0.5
	int.	0.3	
	chronic		0.3
Anthracene (1995)	int.	10	
Arsenic (1993)	chronic	0.0003	
Benzene (1995, draft)	acute		0.05
Boron (1993)	int.	0.01	
Bromomethane (1993)	acute		0.05
	int.	0.003	0.05
	chronic		0.005
Cadmium (1993)	chronic	0.0007	0.0002 mg/m^3
Carbon disulfide (1996)	acute	0.01	
	chronic		0.3
Carbon tetrachloride (1994)	acute	0.02	0.2
	int.	0.007	0.05
Chlordane (1994)	acute	0.001	
	int.	0.0006	0.0002 mg/m^3
	chronic	0.0006	0.00002 mg/m^3
Chlorobenzene (1991)	int.	0.4	
Chloroform (1995, draft)	acute	0.3	1
	int.	0.1	0.05
	chronic	0.01	0.02
Chloromethane (1991)	acute		0.5
	int.		0.4
	chronic		0.4
Chlorpyrifos (1995, draft)	acute	0.003	
	int.	0.003	
Chromium, hexavalent (1993)	int.		0.00002 mg/m^3
	chronic		0.00002 mg/m^3
Cobalt (1993)	int.		0.00003 mg/m^3
Cresol, *m*-, *o*-, *p*- (1993)	acute	0.05	
Cyanide (1995, draft)	int.	0.05	
DDT, *p,p'*- (1994)	acute	0.0005	
	int.	0.0005	
Diazinon (1996)	int.	0.0002	0.009 mg/m^3
Di-*n*-butyl phthalate (1991)	int.	0.6	
1,4-Dichlorobenzene (1993)	int.	0.1	0.2
1,1-Dichloroethane (1994)	int.		0.02
	chronic	0.009	
1,2-Dichloroethane (1994)	acute		0.2
	int.	0.2	
	chronic		0.2
1,2-Dichloroethene, *cis*- (1996)	acute	1	
	int.	0.3	
1,2-Dichloroethene, *trans*- (1996)	acute		0.2
	int.	0.2	0.2

(continues)

TABLE 3 (*Continued*)

Substance[a]	Duration[b]	Oral MRL (mg/kg/day)	Inhalative MRL (ppm)
Dichlorvos (1995, draft)	acute	0.004	0.002
	int.	0.003	0.0003
	chronic		0.00006
Dieldrin (1993)	acute	0.00007	
	chronic	0.00005	
Di (2-ethylhexyl) phthalate (1993)	acute	1	
	int.	0.4	
Diethyl phthalate (1995)	acute	7	
	int.	6	
1,1-Dimethylhydrazine (1994, draft)	int.		0.000009
	chronic		0.000009
1,2-Dimethylhydrazine (1994, draft)	int.	0.0008	
1,3-Dinitrobenzene (1995)	acute	0.008	
	int.	0.0005	
4,6-Dinitro-*o*-cresol (1995)	acute	0.004	
	int.	0.004	
2,4-Dinitrophenol (1995)	acute	0.01	
2,4-Dinitrotoluene (1990)	acute	0.06	
	int.	0.05	
	chronic	0.002	
2,6-Dinitrotoluene (1990)	int.	0.04	
Di-*n*-octyl phthalate (1994, draft)	acute	2	
Endosulfan (1993)	int.	0.002	
	chronic	0.002	
Endrin (1996)	int.	0.002	
	chronic	0.0003	
Ethyl benzene (1991)	int.		0.3
Ethylene glycol (1993, draft)	chronic	2	
Ethylene oxide (1991)	int.		0.09
Fluoranthene (1995)	int.	0.4	
Fluorene (1995)	int.	0.4	
Fuel oil no. 2 (1995)	acute		0.02 mg/m^3
Hexachlorobenzene (1996)	acute	0.008	
	int.	0.0003	
	chronic	0.00002	
Hexachlorobutadiene (1994)	int.	0.0002	
Hexachlorocyclohexane, β- (1994)	int.	0.0003	
Hexachlorocyclohexane, γ- (1994)	acute	0.01	
	int.	0.00004	
Hexamethylene diisocyanate (1996, draft)	int.		0.00003
	chronic		0.00001
Hydrazine (1994, draft)	int.		0.0002
Kepone (1995)	acute	0.01	
	int.	0.0005	
	chronic	0.0005	
Kerosene (1995)	int.		0.01 mg/m^3
Manganese (1993)	chronic		0.0003 mg/m^3
Mercury (1994)	acute		0.00002 mg/m^3
	chronic		0.000014 mg/m^3
Mercury, inorganic (1994)	acute	0.007	
	int.	0.002	
Methoxychlor (1994)	acute	0.02	
	int.	0.02	
Methyl parathion (1993)	chronic	0.0003	
Methylene chloride (1993)	acute		0.4
	int.		0.03
	chronic	0.06	

(*continues*)

TABLE 3 (*Continued*)

Substance[a]	Duration[b]	Oral MRL (mg/kg/day)	Inhalative MRL (ppm)
Methylmercuric chloride (1994)	acute	0.00012	
	int.	0.00012	
1-Methylnaphthalene (1995)	chronic	0.07	
Mirex (1995)	chronic	0.0008	
Naphthalene (1995)	acute	0.05	
	int.	0.02	
	chronic		0.002
Nickel (1995, draft)	int.		0.0001 mg/m^3
n-Nitroso-di-*n*-propylamine (1990)	acute	0.095	
2,3,4,7,8-Pentachlorodibenzofuran (1994)	acute	0.000001	
	int.	0.00000003	
Pentachlorophenol (1994)	acute	0.005	
	int.	0.001	
Phenol (1990)	acute	0.6	
Polybrominated biphenyls (1995)	acute	0.01	
Polychlorinated biphenyls (1995, draft)	chronic	0.00002	
Propylene glycol dinitrate (1995)	acute		0.003
	int.		0.00004
	chronic		0.00004
Selenium (1996)	chronic	0.005	
Styrene (1993)	int.	0.2	
	chronic		0.06
2,3,7,8-Tetrachlorodibenzo-*p*-dioxin (1989)	acute	0.0000001	
	int.	0.000000001	
	chronic	0.000000001	
1,1,2,2-Tetrachloroethane (1996)	int.	0.6	0.4
	chronic	0.04	
Tetrachloroethylene (1995, draft)	acute	0.05	0.2
	chronic		0.04
Titanium tetrachloride (1994, draft)	chronic		0.001 mg/m^3
Toluene (1994)	acute	0.8	3
	int.	0.02	
	chronic		1
Toxaphene (1996)	acute	0.005	
	int.	0.001	
1,1,1-Trichloroethane (1995)	acute		2
	int.		0.7
1,1,2-Trichloroethane (1990)	acute	0.3	
	int.	0.04	
Trichloroethylene (1995, draft)	acute	0.5	2
	int.	0.002	0.1
2,4,6-Trichlorophenol (1991)	int.	0.04	
2,4,6-Trichlorotoluene (1995)	int.	0.0005	
Vanadium (1993)	acute		0.0002 mg/m^3
	int.	0.003	
Vinyl acetate (1993)	int.		0.01
Vinyl chloride (1995, draft)	acute		0.5
	int.		0.03
	chronic	0.00002	
m-Xylene (1995)	int.	0.6	
p-Xylene (1995)	acute	1	
Xylenes, total (1995)	acute		1
	int.	0.2	0.7
	chronic		0.1
Zinc (1994)	int.	0.3	
	chronic	0.3	

[a]The year the value was set is given in parentheses.
[b]Acute (1–14 days); intermediate (15–364 days); chronic (>364 days).

TABLE 4 Legal Standards and Recommendations for Workplace Exposure[a]

<table>
<tr><th></th><th colspan="2">PEL (OSHA)</th><th></th><th colspan="2">TLV (ACGIH) [REL (NIOSH)]</th></tr>
<tr><th>Substance</th><th>TWA (ppm | mg/m^3)</th><th>STEL (ppm | mg/m^3)</th><th>CC</th><th>TWA (ppm | mg/m^3)</th><th>STEL (ppm | mg/m^3)</th></tr>
<tr><td>Acetaldehyde</td><td>200 | 360</td><td></td><td>A3</td><td></td><td>C25 | C45</td></tr>
<tr><td>Acetic acid</td><td>10 | 25</td><td></td><td></td><td>10 | 25
[10 | 25]</td><td>15 | 37
[15 | 37]</td></tr>
<tr><td>Acetone</td><td>1000 | 2400</td><td></td><td>A4</td><td>500 | 1188
[250 | 590]</td><td>750 | 1782</td></tr>
<tr><td>Acetonitrile</td><td>40 | 70</td><td></td><td>A4</td><td>40 | 67
[20 | 34]</td><td>60 | 101</td></tr>
<tr><td>Acetophenone</td><td></td><td></td><td></td><td>10 | 49</td><td></td></tr>
<tr><td>Acrolein</td><td>0.1 | 0.25</td><td></td><td></td><td>0.1 | 0.23
[0.1 | 0.25]</td><td>0.3 | 0.69
[0.3 | 0.8]</td></tr>
<tr><td>Acrylamide (skin)</td><td>— | 0.3</td><td></td><td>A3</td><td>— | 0.03
[— | 0.03]</td><td></td></tr>
<tr><td>Acrylonitrile (skin)</td><td>20 | 45</td><td></td><td>A2</td><td>2 | 4.3
[1 | —]</td><td>[10 | —]</td></tr>
<tr><td>Adipic acid</td><td></td><td></td><td></td><td>— | 5</td><td></td></tr>
<tr><td>Aldrin (skin)</td><td></td><td></td><td>A3</td><td>— | 0.25
[— | 0.25]</td><td></td></tr>
<tr><td>Aluminium</td><td></td><td></td><td></td><td></td><td></td></tr>
<tr><td>metal dust</td><td>— | 15</td><td></td><td></td><td>— | 10
[— | 10]</td><td></td></tr>
<tr><td>Pyro powders, welding fumes, as A1</td><td>— | 5</td><td></td><td></td><td>— | 5
[— | 5]</td><td></td></tr>
<tr><td>soluble salts, as A1</td><td></td><td></td><td></td><td>— | 2
[— | 2]</td><td></td></tr>
<tr><td>Aluminium oxide, total dust</td><td>— | 15</td><td></td><td>A4</td><td>— | 10</td><td></td></tr>
<tr><td>Amitrole</td><td></td><td></td><td>A3</td><td>— | 0.2
[— | 0.2]</td><td></td></tr>
<tr><td>Ammonia</td><td>50 | 35</td><td></td><td></td><td>25 | 17
[25 | 18]</td><td>35 | 24
[35 | 27]</td></tr>
<tr><td>Aniline and homologus (skin)</td><td>5 | 19</td><td></td><td>A3</td><td>2 | 7.6
[lowest feasible concentration]</td><td></td></tr>
<tr><td>Antimony and compounds, as Sb</td><td>— | 0.5</td><td></td><td></td><td>— | 0.5
[— | 0.5]</td><td></td></tr>
<tr><td>Arsenic, elemental and inorganic compounds (except arsine), as As</td><td>— | 0.5</td><td></td><td>A1</td><td>— | 0.01</td><td>[— | C0.002]</td></tr>
<tr><td>Arsine</td><td>0.05 | 0.2</td><td></td><td></td><td>0.05 | 0.16</td><td>[— | C0.002]</td></tr>
<tr><td>Asbestos, all forms</td><td></td><td></td><td>A1</td><td>2 fibers (>5 μm) | cc
[0.1 fiber | cc, 100 min TWA]</td><td></td></tr>
<tr><td>Atrazine</td><td></td><td></td><td>A4</td><td>— | 5
[— | 5]</td><td></td></tr>
<tr><td>Azinphos-methyl (skin)</td><td>— | 0.2</td><td></td><td>A4</td><td>— | 0.2
[— | 0.2]</td><td></td></tr>
<tr><td>Barium and soluble compounds, as Ba</td><td>— | 0.5</td><td></td><td>A4</td><td>— | 0.5
[— | 0.5]</td><td></td></tr>
<tr><td>Barium sulfate</td><td></td><td></td><td></td><td></td><td></td></tr>
<tr><td>total dust</td><td>— | 15</td><td></td><td></td><td>— | 10
[— | 10]</td><td></td></tr>
<tr><td>respirable fraction</td><td>— | 5</td><td></td><td></td><td>[— | 5]</td><td></td></tr>
<tr><td>Benomyl</td><td></td><td></td><td>A4</td><td>0.84 | 10</td><td></td></tr>
<tr><td>total dust</td><td>— | 15</td><td></td><td></td><td></td><td></td></tr>
<tr><td>respirable fraction</td><td>— | 5</td><td></td><td></td><td></td><td></td></tr>
<tr><td>Benzene (skin)</td><td></td><td></td><td>A1</td><td>— | 1.6
[0.1 | 0.32]</td><td>— | C8
[C1 | C3.2]</td></tr>
<tr><td>Benzoyl peroxide</td><td>— | 5</td><td></td><td>A4</td><td>— | 5
[— | 5]</td><td></td></tr>
<tr><td>Benzo[a]pyrene</td><td>— | 0.2</td><td></td><td>A2</td><td></td><td></td></tr>
</table>

(continues)

<table>
<tr><th colspan="6">TABLE 4 (Continued)</th></tr>
<tr><th></th><th colspan="2">PEL (OSHA)</th><th></th><th colspan="2">TLV (ACGIH) [REL (NIOSH)]</th></tr>
<tr><th>Substance</th><th>TWA (ppm | mg/m³)</th><th>STEL (ppm | mg/m³)</th><th>CC</th><th>TWA (ppm | mg/m³)</th><th>STEL (ppm | mg/m³)</th></tr>
<tr><td>Benzyl acetate</td><td></td><td></td><td>A4</td><td>10 | 61</td><td></td></tr>
<tr><td>Beryllium and compounds, as Be</td><td>— | 0.002</td><td>— | C0.005</td><td>A2</td><td>— | 0.002
[— | 0.0005]</td><td></td></tr>
<tr><td>Bismuth telluride, as Bi_2Te_3</td><td>— | 15</td><td></td><td>A4</td><td></td><td></td></tr>
<tr><td>undoped</td><td></td><td></td><td></td><td>— | 10
[— | 10]
— | 5</td><td></td></tr>
<tr><td>Se-doped</td><td></td><td></td><td></td><td>— | 5</td><td></td></tr>
<tr><td>Borates, tetra, sodium salts</td><td></td><td></td><td></td><td></td><td></td></tr>
<tr><td>anhydrous</td><td></td><td></td><td></td><td>— | 1
[— | 1]</td><td></td></tr>
<tr><td>decahydrate</td><td></td><td></td><td></td><td>— | 5
[— | 5]</td><td></td></tr>
<tr><td>pentahydrate</td><td></td><td></td><td></td><td>— | 1
[— | 1]</td><td></td></tr>
<tr><td>Bromine</td><td>0.1 | 0.7</td><td></td><td></td><td>0.1 | 0.66
[0.1 | 0.7]</td><td>0.2 | 1.3
[0.3 | 2]</td></tr>
<tr><td>1,3-Butadiene</td><td>1000 | 2200</td><td></td><td>A2</td><td>2 | 4.4
[lowest feasible concentration]</td><td></td></tr>
<tr><td>Butane</td><td></td><td></td><td></td><td>800 | 1900
[800 | 1900]</td><td></td></tr>
<tr><td>n-Butanol (skin)</td><td>100 | 300</td><td></td><td></td><td></td><td>C25 | C76[b]
[C50 | C150]</td></tr>
<tr><td>sec-Butanol</td><td>150 | 450</td><td></td><td></td><td>100 | 303
[100 | 305]</td><td>[150 | 455]</td></tr>
<tr><td>tert-Butanol</td><td>100 | 300</td><td></td><td>A4</td><td>100 | 303
[100 | 300]</td><td>[150 | 450]</td></tr>
<tr><td>n-Butyl acrylate</td><td></td><td></td><td>A4</td><td>10 | 52</td><td></td></tr>
<tr><td>Cadmium and compounds, as Cd</td><td></td><td></td><td>A2</td><td>— | 0.01
[lowest feasible concentration]</td><td></td></tr>
<tr><td>Calcium carbonate</td><td></td><td></td><td></td><td></td><td></td></tr>
<tr><td>total dust</td><td>— | 15</td><td></td><td></td><td>— | 10
[— | 10]</td><td></td></tr>
<tr><td>respirable fraction</td><td>— | 5</td><td></td><td></td><td>[— | 5]</td><td></td></tr>
<tr><td>Calcium cyanamide</td><td></td><td></td><td>A4</td><td>— | 0.5
[— | 0.5]</td><td></td></tr>
<tr><td>Calcium silicate (synthetic)</td><td></td><td></td><td></td><td></td><td></td></tr>
<tr><td>total dust</td><td>— | 15</td><td></td><td>A4</td><td>— | 10
[— | 10]</td><td></td></tr>
<tr><td>respirable fraction</td><td>— | 5</td><td></td><td></td><td>[— | 5]</td><td></td></tr>
<tr><td>Camphor, synthetic</td><td>— | 2</td><td></td><td>A4</td><td>2 | 12
[— | 2]</td><td>3 | 19</td></tr>
<tr><td>Caprolactam</td><td></td><td></td><td>A4</td><td></td><td></td></tr>
<tr><td>dust</td><td></td><td></td><td></td><td>— | 1
[— | 1]</td><td>— | 10
[— | 3]</td></tr>
<tr><td>vapor</td><td></td><td></td><td></td><td>5 | 23
[0.22 | 1]</td><td>3 | 46
[0.66 | 3]</td></tr>
<tr><td>Carbaryl</td><td>— | 5</td><td></td><td>A4</td><td>— | 5
[— | 5]</td><td></td></tr>
<tr><td>Carbofuran</td><td></td><td></td><td>A4</td><td>— | 0.1
[— | 0.1]</td><td></td></tr>
<tr><td>Carbon black</td><td>— | 3.5</td><td></td><td>A4</td><td>— | 3.5
[— | 3.5]</td><td></td></tr>
<tr><td>Carbon dioxide</td><td>5000 | 9000</td><td></td><td></td><td>5000 | 9000
[5000 | 9000]</td><td>30000 | 54000
[30000 | 54000]</td></tr>
<tr><td>Carbon disulfide (skin)</td><td>20 | —</td><td>C30 | —</td><td></td><td>10 | 31
[1 | 3]</td><td>[10 | 30]</td></tr>
</table>

(*continues*)

TABLE 4 (*Continued*)

Substance	PEL (OSHA) TWA (ppm ∣ mg/m³)	PEL (OSHA) STEL (ppm ∣ mg/m³)	CC	TLV (ACGIH) [REL (NIOSH)† TWA (ppm ∣ mg/m³)	TLV (ACGIH) [REL (NIOSH)† STEL (ppm ∣ mg/m³)
Carbon monoxide	50 ∣ 55			25 ∣ 29	
				[35 ∣ 40]	[C200 ∣ C229]
Carbon tetrabromide				0.1 ∣ 1.4	0.3 ∣ 4.1
				[0.1 ∣ 1.4]	[0.3 ∣ 4]
Carbonyl fluoride				2 ∣ 5.4	5 ∣ 13
				[2 ∣ 5]	[5 ∣ 15]
Catechol (skin)			A3	5 ∣ 23	
				[5 ∣ 20]	
Cellulose					
total dust	— ∣ 15			[— ∣ 10]	
respirable fraction	— ∣ 15			[— ∣ 5]	
Chlordan (skin)	— ∣ 0.5		A3	— ∣ 0.5	
				[— ∣ 0.5]	
Chlorine		C1 ∣ C3	A4	0.5 ∣ 1.5	1 ∣ 2.9
				[0.5 ∣ 1.45]	[1 ∣ 3]
Chlorine dioxide	0.1 ∣ 0.3			0.1 ∣ 0.28	0.3 ∣ 0.83
				[0.1 ∣ 0.3]	[0.3 ∣ 0.9]
α-Chloroacetophenone	0.05 ∣ 0.3		A4	0.05 ∣ 0.32	
				[0.05 ∣ 0.3]	
Chloroacetyl chloride (skin)				0.05 ∣ 0.23	0.15 ∣ 0.69
				[0.05 ∣ 0.2]	
Chlorobenzene	75 ∣ 350		A3	10 ∣ 46	
o-Chlorobenzylidene malononitrile (skin)	0.05 ∣ 0.4		A4		C0.05 ∣ C0.39
					[C0.05 ∣ C0.4]
Chlorobromomethane	200 ∣ 1050			200 ∣ 1060	
				[200 ∣ 1050]	
Chlorodifluoromethane			A4	1000 ∣ 3540	
				[1000 ∣ 3500]	[1250 ∣ 4375]
Chloroform		C50 ∣ C240	A3	10 ∣ 49	[2 ∣ 9.78, 60 min]
β-Chloroprene (skin)	25 ∣ 90			10 ∣ 36	[C1 ∣ C3.6]
o-Chlorotoluene				50 ∣ 259	
				[50 ∣ 250]	[75 ∣ 375]
Chlorpyrifos (skin)			A4	— ∣ 0.2	
				[— ∣ 0.2]	[— ∣ 0.6]
Chromium, metal, and inorganic compounds, as Cr					
metal and Cr III compounds	— ∣ 1		A4	— ∣ 0.5	
				[— ∣ 0.5]	
water-soluble Cr VI compounds (NOC)		— ∣ C0.1	A1	— ∣ 0.05	
insoluble Cr VI compounds (NOC)			A1	— ∣ 0.01	
carcinogenic Chromium (VI)				[— ∣ 0.001, 10-hr]	
Coal dust					
respirable dust				— ∣ 2	
<5% SiO_2	— ∣ 2.4				
>5% SiO_2	— ∣ 10				
Coal tar pitch volatiles, as benzene solubles	— ∣ 0.2		A1	— ∣ 0.2	
				[— ∣ 0.1]	
Cobalt, elemental, and inorganic compounds, as Co	— ∣ 0.1		A3	— ∣ 0.02	

(*continues*)

TABLE 4 *(Continued)*

Substance	PEL (OSHA) TWA (ppm ǀ mg/m³)	PEL (OSHA) STEL (ppm ǀ mg/m³)	CC	TLV (ACGIH) [REL (NIOSH)] TWA (ppm ǀ mg/m³)	TLV (ACGIH) [REL (NIOSH)] STEL (ppm ǀ mg/m³)
Cobalt metal, dust, and fume				[— ǀ 0.05]	
Copper					
fume	— ǀ 0.1			— ǀ 0.2 [— ǀ 0.1]	
dusts and mists, as Cu	— ǀ 1			— ǀ 12 [— ǀ 1]	
Cresol, all isomers (skin)	5 ǀ 22			5 ǀ 22 [2.3 ǀ 10]	
Crotonaldehyde	2 ǀ 6		A3	2 ǀ 5.7 [2 ǀ 6]	
Cumene (skin)	50 ǀ 245			50 ǀ 246 [50 ǀ 245]	
Cyanamide				— ǀ 2 [— ǀ 2]	
Cyclohexane	300 ǀ 1050			300 ǀ 1030 [300 ǀ 1050]	
Cyclohexylamine			A4	10 ǀ 41 [10 ǀ 40]	
2,4-D	— ǀ 10		A4	— ǀ 10 [— ǀ 10]	
DDT	— ǀ 1		A3	— ǀ 1 [— ǀ 0.5]	
Demeton (skin)	— ǀ 0.1			0.01 ǀ 0.11 [— ǀ 0.1]	
Diazinon (skin)			A4	— ǀ 0.1 [— ǀ 0.1]	
Diazomethane	0.2 ǀ 0.4		A2	0.2 ǀ 0.34 [0.2 ǀ 0.4]	
1,2-Dibromoethane (ethylene dibromide) (skin)	20 ǀ —	C30 ǀ —	A3	[0.045 ǀ —]	[C0.13 ǀ —]
Dibutyl phthalate	— ǀ 5			— ǀ 5 [1 ǀ 5]	
Dichloroacetylene			A3	— ǀ —	C0.1 ǀ C0.39 [C0.1 ǀ C0.4]
1,2-Dichlorobenzene (skin)		50 ǀ 300	A4	25 ǀ 150	50 ǀ 301 [C50 ǀ C300]
1,4-Dichlorobenzene	75 ǀ 450		A4	10 ǀ 60	
Dichlorodifluoromethane	1000 ǀ 4950		A4	1000 ǀ 4950 [1000 ǀ 4950]	
1,1-Dichloroethane	100 ǀ 400		A4	100 ǀ 405 [100 ǀ 400]	
1,2-Dichloroethane (ethylene dichloride)	50 ǀ —	C100 ǀ —	A4	10 ǀ 40 [1 ǀ —]	[2 ǀ —]
1,2-Dichloroethylene (acetylene dichloride)	200 ǀ 790			200 ǀ 793 [200 ǀ 790]	
1,1-Dichloroethylene (vinylidene chloride)			A3	5 ǀ 20 [lowest feasible concentration]	20 ǀ 79
Dichlorofluoromethane	1000 ǀ 4200			10 ǀ 42	
Dichloromethane (methylene chloride)	500 ǀ —	C1000 ǀ —	A3	50 ǀ 174 [lowest feasible concentration]	
1,2-Dichloropropane	75 ǀ 350		A4	75 ǀ 347 [lowest feasible concentration]	110 ǀ 508
1,2-Dichloro-1,1,2,2-tetra-fluoroethane	1000 ǀ 7000		A4	1000 ǀ 6990 [1000 ǀ 7000]	
Dichlorvos (skin)	— ǀ 1		A4	0.1 ǀ 0.90 [— ǀ 1]	

(*continues*)

TABLE 4 *(Continued)*

Substance	PEL (OSHA) TWA (ppm ǀ mg/m³)	PEL (OSHA) STEL (ppm ǀ mg/m³)	CC	TLV (ACGIH) [REL (NIOSH)] TWA (ppm ǀ mg/m³)	TLV (ACGIH) [REL (NIOSH)] STEL (ppm ǀ mg/m³)
Dieldrin (skin)	— ǀ 0.25		A4	— ǀ 0.25 [— ǀ 0.25]	
Diesel exhaust particles				[lowest feasible concentration]	
Diethylene triamine (skin)				1 ǀ 4.2 [1 ǀ 4]	
Di(2-ethylhexyl)phthalate (DEHP)	— ǀ 5		A3	— ǀ 5 [— ǀ 5]	— ǀ 10 [— ǀ 10]
Diisopropylamine (skin)	5 ǀ 20			5 ǀ 21 [5 ǀ 20]	
Dimethylaniline (skin)	5 ǀ 25		A4	5 ǀ 25 [5 ǀ 25]	10 ǀ 50 [10 ǀ 50]
Dimethylformamide (skin)	10 ǀ 30		A4	10 ǀ 30 [10 ǀ 30]	
1,1-Dimethylhydrazine (skin)	0.5 ǀ 1		A3	0.01 ǀ 0.025	[C0.06 ǀ C0.15, 120 min]
Dimethyl sulfate (skin)	1 ǀ 5		A3	0.1 ǀ 0.52 [0.1 ǀ 0.5]	
1,2-Dinitrobenzene (skin)	— ǀ 1			0.15 ǀ 1.0 [— ǀ 1]	
Dinitrotoluene (skin)	— ǀ 1.5		A3	— ǀ 0.2 [— ǀ 1.5]	
1,4-Dioxane (skin)	100 ǀ 360		A3	25 ǀ 90	[C1 ǀ C3.6]
Diphenyl	0.2 ǀ 1			0.2 ǀ 1.3 [0.2 ǀ 1]	
Diphenylamine	— ǀ 10		A4	— ǀ 10 [— ǀ 10]	
Diphenylmethane-4,4′-diisocyanate (MDI)	0.02 ǀ 0.2			0.005 ǀ 0.051 [0.005 ǀ 0.050]	[C0.020 ǀ C0.200, 10 min]
Diquat (skin)			A4	— ǀ 0.5 [— ǀ 0.5]	
Disulfiram			A4	— ǀ 2 [— ǀ 2]	
Endosulfan (skin)	— ǀ 0.1		A4	— ǀ 0.1 [— ǀ 0.1]	
Endrin (skin)	— ǀ 0.1		A4	— ǀ 0.1 [— ǀ 0.1]	
Epichlorohydrin (1-chloro-2,3-epoxypropane) (skin)	5 ǀ 19		A3	0.5 ǀ 1.9 [lowest feasible concentration]	
2,3-Epoxy-1-propanol	50 ǀ 150		A3	2 ǀ 6.1 [25 ǀ 75]	
Ethanol	1000 ǀ 1900		A4	1000 ǀ 1880 [1000 ǀ 1900]	
2-Ethoxyethanol (EGEE) (skin)	200 ǀ 740			5 ǀ 18 [0.5 ǀ 1.8]	
2-Ethoxyethyl acetate (EGEEA) (skin)	100 ǀ 540			5 ǀ 27 [0.5 ǀ 2.7]	
Ethyl acetate	400 ǀ 1400		A4	400 ǀ 1440 [400 ǀ 1440]	
Ethyl acrylate	25 ǀ 100		A2	5 ǀ 20	15 ǀ 61
Ethyl benzene	100 ǀ 435			100 ǀ 434 [100 ǀ 435]	125 ǀ 543 [125 ǀ 545]
Ethyl bromide (skin)	200 ǀ 890		A3	5 ǀ 22	

(continues)

TABLE 4 *(Continued)*

<table>
<tr><th rowspan="2">Substance</th><th colspan="2">PEL (OSHA)</th><th rowspan="2">CC</th><th colspan="2">TLV (ACGIH) [REL (NIOSH)]</th></tr>
<tr><th>TWA (ppm | mg/m³)</th><th>STEL (ppm | mg/m³)</th><th>TWA (ppm | mg/m³)</th><th>STEL (ppm | mg/m³)</th></tr>
<tr><td>Ethylene chlorohydrin (skin)</td><td>5 | 16</td><td></td><td>A4</td><td></td><td>C1 | C3.3
[C1 | C3]</td></tr>
<tr><td>Ethylene oxide</td><td></td><td></td><td>A2</td><td>1 | 1.8
[0.1 | 0.18]</td><td>[C5 | C9]</td></tr>
<tr><td>Ethyleneimine (skin)</td><td></td><td></td><td>A3</td><td>0.5 | 0.88</td><td></td></tr>
<tr><td>Ethyl ether</td><td>400 | 1200</td><td></td><td></td><td>400 | 1210</td><td>500 | 1520</td></tr>
<tr><td>Ferbam</td><td>— | 15</td><td></td><td>A4</td><td>— | 10
[— | 10]</td><td></td></tr>
<tr><td>Fluorides, as F</td><td>— | 2.5</td><td></td><td>A4</td><td>— | 2.5
[— | 2.5]</td><td></td></tr>
<tr><td>Fluorine</td><td>0.1 | 0.2</td><td></td><td></td><td>1 | 1.6
[0.1 | 0.2]</td><td>2 | 3.1</td></tr>
<tr><td>Formaldehyde</td><td></td><td></td><td>A2</td><td>
[0.016 | —]</td><td>C0.3 | C0.37
[C0.1 | —]</td></tr>
<tr><td>Formic acid</td><td>5 | 9</td><td></td><td></td><td>5 | 9.4
[5 | 9]</td><td>10 | 19</td></tr>
<tr><td>Gasoline</td><td></td><td></td><td>A3</td><td>300 | 890</td><td>500 | 1480</td></tr>
<tr><td>Glutaraldehyde</td><td></td><td></td><td></td><td></td><td>C0.05 | C0.2
[C0.2 | C0.8]</td></tr>
<tr><td>Glycerin mist</td><td>— | 15</td><td></td><td></td><td>— | 10</td><td></td></tr>
<tr><td>Halothane</td><td></td><td></td><td>A4</td><td>50 | 404</td><td>[C2 | C16.2, 60 min]</td></tr>
<tr><td>Heptachlor and heptachlor epoxide (skin)</td><td></td><td></td><td>A3</td><td>— | 0.05</td><td></td></tr>
<tr><td>Heptachlor</td><td>— | 0.5</td><td></td><td></td><td>[— | 0.5]</td><td></td></tr>
<tr><td>Heptane (n-heptane)</td><td>500 | 2000</td><td></td><td></td><td>400 | 1640
[85 | 350]</td><td>500 | 2050
[C440 | C1800]</td></tr>
<tr><td>Hexachlorobenzene (skin)</td><td></td><td></td><td>A3</td><td>— | 0.02</td><td></td></tr>
<tr><td>Hexachlorobutadiene (skin)</td><td></td><td></td><td>A3</td><td>0.02 | 0.2
[0.02 | 0.24]</td><td></td></tr>
<tr><td>Hexamethylene diisocyanate</td><td></td><td></td><td></td><td>0.005 | 0.034
[— | 0.035]</td><td>
[— | C0.14, 10 min]</td></tr>
<tr><td>Hexane (n-hexane)</td><td>500 | 1800</td><td></td><td></td><td>50 | 176
[50 | 180]</td><td></td></tr>
<tr><td>other isomers</td><td></td><td></td><td></td><td>500 | 1760
[100 | 350]</td><td>1000 | 3500
[C510 | C1800]</td></tr>
<tr><td>2-Hexanone (skin)</td><td>100 | 410</td><td></td><td></td><td>5 | 20
[1 | 4]</td><td></td></tr>
<tr><td>Hydrazine (skin)</td><td>1 | 1.3</td><td></td><td>A3</td><td>0.01 | 0.013</td><td>[C0.03 | C0.04, 120 min]</td></tr>
<tr><td>Hydrogen chloride</td><td></td><td>C5 | C7</td><td></td><td></td><td>C5 | C7.5
[C5 | C7]</td></tr>
<tr><td>Hydrogen cyanide (skin)</td><td>10 | 11</td><td></td><td></td><td></td><td>C4.7 | C5
[4.7 | 5]</td></tr>
<tr><td>Hydrogen fluoride, as F</td><td>3 | —</td><td></td><td></td><td>
[3 | 2.5]</td><td>C3 | C2.3
[6 | 5.0]</td></tr>
<tr><td>Hydrogen peroxide</td><td>1 | 1.4</td><td></td><td>A3</td><td>1 | 1.4</td><td></td></tr>
<tr><td>Hydrogen sulfide</td><td></td><td>C20 | —</td><td></td><td>10 | 14</td><td>15 | 21
[C10 | C15, 10 min]</td></tr>
<tr><td>Hydroquinone</td><td>— | 2</td><td></td><td>A3</td><td>— | 2</td><td>[— | C2, 15 min]</td></tr>
<tr><td>Iodine</td><td></td><td>C0.1 | C1</td><td></td><td></td><td>C0.1 | C1.0
[C0.1 | C1.0]</td></tr>
<tr><td>Iodoform</td><td></td><td></td><td></td><td>0.6 | 10
[0.6 | 10]</td><td></td></tr>
<tr><td>Iron oxide, dust and fume</td><td>— | 15</td><td></td><td>A4</td><td>— | 10
[— | 5]</td><td></td></tr>
<tr><td>Isopropyl alcohol</td><td>400 | 900</td><td></td><td></td><td>400 | 983
[400 | 980]</td><td>500 | 1230
[500 | 1225]</td></tr>
</table>

(continues)

<table>
<tr><th colspan="6">TABLE 4 (Continued)</th></tr>
<tr><th></th><th colspan="2">PEL (OSHA)</th><th></th><th colspan="2">TLV (ACGIH) [REL (NIOSH)]</th></tr>
<tr><th>Substance</th><th>TWA (ppm | mg/m^3)</th><th>STEL (ppm | mg/m^3)</th><th>CC</th><th>TWA (ppm | mg/m^3)</th><th>STEL (ppm | mg/m^3)</th></tr>
<tr><td>Lead elemental, and inorganic compounds, as Pb</td><td></td><td></td><td>A3</td><td>— | 0.05
[— | <0.1]</td><td></td></tr>
<tr><td>Lindane (skin)</td><td>— | 0.5</td><td></td><td>A3</td><td>— | 0.5
[— | 0.5]</td><td></td></tr>
<tr><td>Lithium hydride</td><td>— | 0.025</td><td></td><td></td><td>— | 0.025
[— | 0.025]</td><td></td></tr>
<tr><td>Magnesium oxide fume</td><td>— | 15</td><td></td><td></td><td>— | 10</td><td></td></tr>
<tr><td>Malathion (skin)</td><td>— | 15</td><td></td><td>A4</td><td>— | 10
[— | 10]</td><td></td></tr>
<tr><td>Manganese, elemental, and inorganic compounds, as Mn</td><td></td><td>— | C5</td><td></td><td>— | 0.2
[— | 1]</td><td>[— | 3]</td></tr>
<tr><td>Mercury, as Hg (skin)</td><td></td><td></td><td></td><td></td><td></td></tr>
<tr><td>alkyl compounds</td><td>— | 0.01</td><td></td><td></td><td>— | 0.01
[— | 0.01]</td><td>— | 0.03
[— | 0.03]</td></tr>
<tr><td>aryl compounds</td><td>— | 0.01</td><td></td><td></td><td>— | 0.1</td><td>[— | C0.1]</td></tr>
<tr><td>inorganic forms including metallic mercury vapor</td><td></td><td>— | C0.1</td><td>A4</td><td>— | 0.025
[— | 0.05]</td><td>[— | C0.1]</td></tr>
<tr><td>Methanol (skin)</td><td>200 | 260</td><td></td><td></td><td>200 | 262
[200 | 260]</td><td>250 | 328
[250 | 325]</td></tr>
<tr><td>Methomyl</td><td></td><td></td><td>A4</td><td>— | 2.5
[— | 2.5]</td><td></td></tr>
<tr><td>2-Methoxyethanol (skin)</td><td>25 | 80</td><td></td><td></td><td>5 | 16
[0.1 | 0.3]</td><td></td></tr>
<tr><td>2-Methoxyethyl acetate (skin)</td><td>25 | 120</td><td></td><td></td><td>5 | 24
[0.1 | 0.5]</td><td></td></tr>
<tr><td>Methyl acetate</td><td>200 | 610</td><td></td><td></td><td>200 | 606
[200 | 610]</td><td>250 | 757
[250 | 760]</td></tr>
<tr><td>Methyl acrylate (skin)</td><td>10 | 35</td><td></td><td>A4</td><td>2 | 7
[10 | 35]</td><td></td></tr>
<tr><td>Methylamine</td><td>10 | 12</td><td></td><td></td><td>5 | 6.4
[10 | 12]</td><td>15 | 19</td></tr>
<tr><td>Methyl bromide (skin)</td><td></td><td>C20 | —</td><td>A4</td><td>1 | 3.9
[lowest feasible concentration]</td><td></td></tr>
<tr><td>Methyl chloride (skin)</td><td>100 | —</td><td>C200 | —</td><td>A4</td><td>50 | 103
[lowest feasible concentration]</td><td>100 | 207</td></tr>
<tr><td>2-Methylcyclopentadienyl manganese tricarbonyl, as Mn (skin)</td><td></td><td></td><td></td><td>— | 0.2
[— | 0.1]</td><td></td></tr>
<tr><td>Methyl demeton (skin)</td><td></td><td></td><td></td><td>— | 0.5
[— | 0.5]</td><td></td></tr>
<tr><td>4,4′-Methylene bis (2-chloro-aniline) (MBOCA) (skin)</td><td></td><td></td><td>A2</td><td>0.01 | 0.11
[— | 0.003]</td><td></td></tr>
<tr><td>4,4′-Methylene dianiline (skin)</td><td></td><td></td><td>A3</td><td>0.1 | 0.81
[lowest feasible concentration]</td><td></td></tr>
<tr><td>Methylisocyanate (skin)</td><td>0.02 | 0.05</td><td></td><td></td><td>0.02 | 0.047
[0.02 | 0.05]</td><td></td></tr>
<tr><td>Methylmethacrylate</td><td>100 | 410</td><td></td><td>A4</td><td>100 | 410
[100 | 410]</td><td></td></tr>
<tr><td>Methylparathion (skin)</td><td></td><td></td><td>A4</td><td>— | 0.2
[— | 0.2]
[0.01 | 0.092]</td><td>[0.03 | 0.27]</td></tr>
<tr><td>Mevinphos (skin)</td><td>— | 0.1</td><td></td><td></td><td>0.01 | 0.092</td><td>0.03 | 0.27</td></tr>
<tr><td>Mineral wool fiber</td><td></td><td></td><td></td><td>— | 10
[3 million fibers/m^3]</td><td></td></tr>
</table>

(*continues*)

TABLE 4 (Continued)					
	PEL (OSHA)			TLV (ACGIH) [REL (NIOSH)]	
Substance	TWA (ppm ǀ mg/m³)	STEL (ppm ǀ mg/m³)	CC	TWA (ppm ǀ mg/m³)	STEL (ppm ǀ mg/m³)
Molybdenum, as Mo					
soluble compounds	— ǀ 5			— ǀ 5	
insoluble compounds	— ǀ 15			— ǀ 10	
Monochlorobenzene	75 ǀ 350		A3	10 ǀ 46	
Morpholine (skin)	20 ǀ 70		A4	20 ǀ 71 [20 ǀ 70]	 [30 ǀ 105]
Naphthalene	10 ǀ 50		A4	10 ǀ 52 [10 ǀ 50]	15 ǀ 79 [15 ǀ 75]
Nickel					
metal	— ǀ 1			— ǀ 1 [— ǀ 0.015]	
insoluble compounds, as Ni	— ǀ 1			— ǀ 0.1 [— ǀ 0.015]	
soluble compounds, as Ni	— ǀ 1		A4	— ǀ 0.05 [— ǀ 0.015]	
Nickel carbonyl, as Ni	0.001 ǀ 0.007			0.05 ǀ 0.12 [0.001 ǀ 0.007]	
Nicotine (skin)	— ǀ 0.5			— ǀ 0.5 [— ǀ 0.5]	
Nitric acid	2 ǀ 5			2 ǀ 5.2 [2 ǀ 5]	4 ǀ 10 [4 ǀ 10]
Nitric oxide	25 ǀ 30			25 ǀ 31 [25 ǀ 30]	
p-Nitroaniline	1 ǀ 6		A4	— ǀ 3 [— ǀ 3]	
Nitrobenzene (skin)	1 ǀ 5		A3	1 ǀ 5 [1 ǀ 5]	
p-Nitrochlorobenzene (skin)	— ǀ 1		A3	0.1 ǀ 0.64 [lowest feasible concentration]	
Nitrogen dioxide		C5 ǀ C9	A4	3 ǀ 5.6	5 ǀ 9.4 [1 ǀ 1.8]
Nitrogen trifluoride	10 ǀ 29			10 ǀ 29 [10 ǀ 29]	
Nitromethane	100 ǀ 250			20 ǀ 50	
1-Nitropropane	25 ǀ 90		A4	25 ǀ 91 [25 ǀ 90]	
2-Nitropropane	25 ǀ 90		A3	10 ǀ 36 [lowest feasible concentration]	
Nitrotoluene, (*o*-, *m*-, *p*-) (skin)	5 ǀ 30			2 ǀ 11 [2 ǀ 11]	
Nitrotrichloromethane	0.1 ǀ 0.7		A4	0.1 ǀ 0.67 [0.1 ǀ 0.7]	
Nitrous oxide			A4	50 ǀ 90 [25 ǀ 30]	
Oil mist, mineral	— ǀ 5			— ǀ 5 [— ǀ 5]	— ǀ 10 [— ǀ 10]
Osmium tetroxide, as Os	— ǀ 0.002			0.0002 ǀ 0.0016 [0.0002 ǀ 0.002]	0.0006 ǀ 0.0047 [0.0006 ǀ 0.006]
Oxalic acid	— ǀ 1			— ǀ 1 [— ǀ 1]	— ǀ 2 [— ǀ 2]
Ozone	0.1 ǀ 0.2				[C0.1 ǀ C0.2]
heavy work				0.05 ǀ 0.1	
moderate work				0.08 ǀ 0.16	
light work				0.10 ǀ 0.2	
Paraquat					
total dust				0.5 ǀ —	
respirable fraction	— ǀ 0.5 (skin)			0.1 ǀ — [— ǀ 0.1]	0.1 ǀ —

(*continues*)

<table>
<tr><th colspan="6">TABLE 4 (Continued)</th></tr>
<tr><th></th><th colspan="2">PEL (OSHA)</th><th></th><th colspan="2">TLV (ACGIH) [REL (NIOSH)]</th></tr>
<tr><th>Substance</th><th>TWA (ppm | mg/m³)</th><th>STEL (ppm | mg/m³)</th><th>CC</th><th>TWA (ppm | mg/m³)</th><th>STEL (ppm | mg/m³)</th></tr>
<tr><td>Parathion (skin)</td><td>— | 0.1</td><td></td><td>A4</td><td>— | 0.1
[— | 0.05]</td><td></td></tr>
<tr><td>Particulates not otherwise classified (PNOC)</td><td></td><td></td><td></td><td></td><td></td></tr>
<tr><td>inhalable particulate</td><td></td><td></td><td></td><td>— | 10</td><td></td></tr>
<tr><td>respirable particulate</td><td></td><td></td><td></td><td>— | 3</td><td></td></tr>
<tr><td>PCB Arochlor 1242 (skin)</td><td>— | 1</td><td></td><td></td><td>— | 1
[— | 0.001]</td><td></td></tr>
<tr><td>Pentachlorophenol (skin)</td><td>— | 0.5</td><td></td><td>A3</td><td>— | 0.5
[— | 0.5]</td><td></td></tr>
<tr><td>Pentane (all isomers)</td><td>1000 | 2950</td><td></td><td></td><td>600 | 1770
[120 | 350]</td><td>750 | 2210
[C610 | C 1800]</td></tr>
<tr><td>Phenol (skin)</td><td>5 | 19</td><td></td><td>A4</td><td>5 | 19
[5 | 19]</td><td>
[C15.6 | C 60]</td></tr>
<tr><td>Phenothiazine (skin)</td><td></td><td></td><td></td><td>— | 5
[— | 5]</td><td></td></tr>
<tr><td>o-Phenylenediamine</td><td></td><td></td><td>A3</td><td>— | 0.1</td><td></td></tr>
<tr><td>m-Phenylenediamine</td><td></td><td></td><td>A4</td><td>— | 0.1</td><td></td></tr>
<tr><td>p-Phenylenediamine (skin)</td><td>— | 0.1</td><td></td><td>A4</td><td>— | 0.1
[— | 0.1]</td><td></td></tr>
<tr><td>Phenylhydrazine (skin)</td><td>5 | 22</td><td></td><td>A3</td><td>0.1 | 0.44</td><td>[C0.14 | C0.6, 120 min]</td></tr>
<tr><td>Phosgene (carbonyl chloride)</td><td>0.1 | 0.4</td><td></td><td></td><td>0.1 | 0.40
[0.1 | 0.4]</td><td>
[C0.2 | C0.8]</td></tr>
<tr><td>Phosphine</td><td>0.3 | 0.4</td><td></td><td></td><td>0.3 | 0.42
[0.3 | 0.4]</td><td>1 | 1.4
[1.0 | 1.0]</td></tr>
<tr><td>Phosphoric acid</td><td>— | 1</td><td></td><td></td><td>— | 1
[— | 1]</td><td>— | 3
[— | 3]</td></tr>
<tr><td>Phosphorus (yellow)</td><td>— | 0.1</td><td></td><td></td><td>0.02 | 0.1
[— | 0.1]</td><td></td></tr>
<tr><td>Phosphorus oxychloride</td><td></td><td></td><td></td><td>0.1 | 0.63
[0.1 | 0.6]</td><td>
[0.5 | 3.0]</td></tr>
<tr><td>Phosphorus pentachloride</td><td>— | 1</td><td></td><td></td><td>0.1 | 0.85
[— | 1]</td><td></td></tr>
<tr><td>Phosphorus pentasulfide</td><td>— | 1</td><td></td><td></td><td>— | 1
[— |1]</td><td>— | 3
[— | 3]</td></tr>
<tr><td>Phosphorus trichloride</td><td>0.5 | 3</td><td></td><td></td><td>0.2 | 1.1
[0.2 | 1.5]</td><td>0.5 | 2.8
[0.5 | 3.0]</td></tr>
<tr><td>Phthalic anhydride</td><td>2 | 12</td><td></td><td>A4</td><td>1 | 6.1
[1 | 6]</td><td></td></tr>
<tr><td>Platinum</td><td></td><td></td><td></td><td></td><td></td></tr>
<tr><td>metal</td><td></td><td></td><td></td><td>— | 1
[— | 1]</td><td></td></tr>
<tr><td>soluble salts, as Pt</td><td></td><td></td><td></td><td>— | 0.002
[— | 0.002]</td><td></td></tr>
<tr><td>Potassium cyanide (skin)</td><td>— | 0.02</td><td></td><td></td><td></td><td>— | C5</td></tr>
<tr><td>Potassium hydroxide</td><td></td><td></td><td></td><td></td><td>— | C2
[— | C2]</td></tr>
<tr><td>Propane</td><td>1000 | 1800</td><td></td><td></td><td>[1000 | 1800]</td><td></td></tr>
<tr><td>β-Propiolactone</td><td></td><td></td><td>A3</td><td>0.5 | 1.5</td><td></td></tr>
<tr><td>Propionic acid</td><td></td><td></td><td></td><td>10 | 30
[10 | 30]</td><td>
[15 | 45]</td></tr>
<tr><td>Propoxur</td><td></td><td></td><td>A3</td><td>— | 0.5
[— | 0.5]</td><td></td></tr>
<tr><td>n-Propyl alcohol (skin)</td><td>200 | 500</td><td></td><td></td><td>200 | 492
[200 | 500]</td><td>250 | 614
[250 | 625]</td></tr>
<tr><td>Propylene glycol monomethyl ether</td><td></td><td></td><td></td><td>100 | 369
[100 | 360]</td><td>150 | 553
[150 | 540]</td></tr>
</table>

(*continues*)

TABLE 4 (*Continued*)					
	PEL (OSHA)			TLV (ACGIH) [REL (NIOSH)]	
Substance	**TWA (ppm I mg/m³)**	**STEL (ppm I mg/m³)**	**CC**	**TWA (ppm I mg/m³)**	**STEL (ppm I mg/m³)**
Propylene oxide	100 I 240		A3	20 I 48 [lowest feasible concentration]	
Pyrethrum	— I 5		A4	— I 5 [— I 5]	
Pyridine	5 I 15			5 I 16 [5 I 15]	
Quinone	0.1 I 0.4			0.1 I 0.44 [0.1 I 0.4]	
Resorcinol			A4	10 I 45 [10 I 45]	20 I 90 [20 I 90]
Rhodium			A4		
metal	— I 0.1			— I 1 [— I 0.1]	
insoluble compounds, as Rh	— I 0.1			— I 1 [— I 0.1]	
soluble compounds, as Rh	— I 0.001			— I 0.01 [— I 0.001]	
Rotenone (commercial)	— I 5		A4	— I 5 [— I 5]	
Rubber solvent (Naphtha)	100 I 400			400 I 1590 [100 I 400]	
Selenium and compounds, as Se	— I 0.2			— I 0.2 [— I 0.2]	
Silica, amorphous					
diatomaceous earth (uncalcined)	— I 80			— I 10 — I 6	
precipitated silica and gel	— I 80			— I 10 [— I 6]	
fume				— I 2	
Silica, crystalline					
cristobalite	— I 5			— I 0.05 [— I 0.05]	
fused	— I 10			— I 0.1 [— I 0.05]	
quartz	— I 10			— I 0.1 [— I 0.05]	
tridymite	— I 5			— I 0.05 [— I 0.05]	
tripoli	— I 10			— I 0.1 [— I 0.05]	
Silicon					
total dust	— I 15			— I 10 [— I 10]	
respirable fraction				[— I 5]	
Silicon tetrahydride				5 I 6.6 [5 I 7]	
Silver					
metal	— I 0.01			— I 0.1 [— I 0.01]	
soluble compounds, as Ag				— I 0.01 [— I 0.01]	
Sodium azide					
as sodium azide			A4		— I C0.29 [— I C0.3]
as hydrazoic acid vapor			A4		C0.11 I — [C0.1 I —]

(*continues*)

TABLE 4 *(Continued)*

Substance	PEL (OSHA) TWA (ppm | mg/m³)	PEL (OSHA) STEL (ppm | mg/m³)	CC	TLV (ACGIH) [REL (NIOSH)] TWA (ppm | mg/m³)	TLV (ACGIH) [REL (NIOSH)] STEL (ppm | mg/m³)
Starch					
total dust	—	15		A4	—	10 [—	10]	
respirable fraction	—	5			[—	5]	
Strontium chromate, as Cr		—	C0.1	A2	—	0.0005	
Strychnine	—	0.15			—	0.15 [—	0.15]	
Styrene, monomer (skin)	100	—	C200	—	A4	20	85 [50	215]	40	170[b] [100	425]
Sucrose					
total dust	—	15		A4	—	10 [—	10]	
respirable fraction	—	5			[—	5]	
Sulfur dioxide	5	13		A4	2	5.2 [2	5]	5	13 [5	10]
Sulfuric acid	—	1		A2	—	1 [—	1]	—	3
Talc (containing no asbestos fibers)	—	20 mppcf		A4	—	2 [—	2	
Tellurium and compounds, as Te	—	0.1			—	0.1 [—	0.1]	
Terephthalic acid				—	10	[C05	C5]
Terphenyls		C1	C9			C0.53	C5
1,1,1,2-Tetrachloro-2,2-difluoroethane	500	4170			500	4170 [500	4170]	
1,1,2,2-Tetrachloro-1,2-difluoroethane	500	4170			500	4170 [500	4170]	
1,1,2,2-Tetrachloroethane (skin)	5	35		A4	1	6.9 [1	7]	
Tetrachloroethylene	100	—	C200	—	A3	25	170 [lowest feasible concentration]	100	685
Tetrachloromethane (skin)	10	—	C25	—	A2	5	31	10	63 [2	12.6, 60 min]
Tetraethyl lead, as Pb (skin)	—	0.075		A4	—	0.1 [—	0.075]	
Tetramethyl lead, as Pb (skin)	—	0.075			—	0.15 [—	0.075]	
Tetranitromethane	1	8		A3	0.005	0.04 [1	8]	
Thallium, soluble compounds, as Tl (skin)	—	0.1			—	0.1 [—	0.1]	
Thioglycolic acid (skin)				1	3.8 [1	4]	
Thiram	—	5		A4	—	1 [—	5]	
Tin					
metal	—	2			—	2	
oxide and inorganic compounds, except SnH_4, as Sn	—	2			—	2 [—	2]	
organic compounds, as Sn (skin)	—	0.1		A4	—	0.1 [—	0.1]	
Titanium dioxide	—	15		A4	—	10 [lowest feasible concentration]	
Toluene (skin)	200	—	C300	—	A4	50	188 [100	375]	[150	560]

(continues)

TABLE 4 (*Continued*)

Substance	PEL (OSHA)		CC	TLV (ACGIH) [REL (NIOSH)]	
	TWA (ppm ∣ mg/m³)	STEL (ppm ∣ mg/m³)		TWA (ppm ∣ mg/m³)	STEL (ppm ∣ mg/m³)
Toluidine (*o*-, *p*-) (skin)	5 ∣ 22		A3	2 ∣ 8.8 [lowest feasible concentration]	
m-Toluidine (skin)	5 ∣ 22		A4	2 ∣ 8.8	
Toxaphene (skin)	— ∣ 0.5		A3	— ∣ 0.5 [lowest feasible concentration]	— ∣ 1
Tributyl phosphate	— ∣ 5			0.2∣ 2.2 [0.2 ∣ 2.5]	
Trichloroacetic acid			A4	1 ∣ 6.7 [1 ∣ 7]	
1,2,4-Trichlorobenzene					C5 ∣ C37 [C5 ∣ C40]
1,1,1-Trichloroethane	350 ∣ 1900		A4	350 ∣ 1910	450 ∣ 2460 [C350 ∣ C1910]
1,1,2-Trichloroethane (skin)	10 ∣ 45		A4	10 ∣ 55 [10 ∣ 45]	
Trichloroethylene	100 ∣ —	C200 ∣ —	A2	50 ∣ 269 [25 ∣ —]	100 ∣ 537 [C2 ∣ —, 1 hr] [C1000 ∣ C5620]
Trichlorofluoromethane	1000 ∣ 5600		A4		C1000 ∣ C5620
Trichloromethane		C50 ∣ C240	A3	10 ∣ 49	[2 ∣ 9.78, 60 min]
Trichloronitromethane	0.1 ∣ 0.7		A4	0.1 ∣ 0.67	
2,4,5-Trichlorophenoxyacetic acid (2,4,5-T)	— ∣ 10		A4	— ∣ 10	
1,1,2-Trichloro-1,2,2-trifluoro-ethane	1000 ∣ 7600		A4	1000 ∣ 7670 [1000 ∣ 7600]	1250 ∣ 9590 [1250 ∣ 9500]
Triethanolamine	25 ∣ 100			— ∣ 5	
Trimethylamine (skin)			A4	5 ∣ 12 [10 ∣ 24]	15 ∣ 36 [15 ∣ 36]
Trimethyl phosphite				2 ∣ 10 [2 ∣ 10]	
2,4,6-Trinitrophenol (skin)	— ∣ 0.1			— ∣ 0.1 [— ∣ 0.1]	[— ∣ 0.3]
2,4,6-Trinitrotoluene (skin)	— ∣ 1.5			— ∣ 0.1 [— ∣ 0.5]	
Triorthocresyl phosphate (skin)	— ∣ 0.1		A4	— ∣ 0.1 [— ∣ 0.1]	
Triphenyl phosphate	— ∣ 3		A4	— ∣ 3 [— ∣ 3]	
Uranium (natural)	— ∣ 0.05		A1		
soluble compounds				— ∣ 0.2 [— ∣ 0.05]	— ∣ 0.6
insoluble compounds				— ∣ 0.2 [— ∣ 0.2]	— ∣ 0.6 [— ∣ 0.6]
Vanadium pentoxide, as V_2O_5, respirable dust or fume		— ∣ C0.5	A4	— ∣ 0.05	[— ∣ C0.05]
Vinyl bromide			A2	5 ∣ 22 [lowest feasible concentration]	
Vinyl chloride			A1	5 ∣ 13 [lowest feasible concentration]	
4-Vinylcyclohexene (skin)			A3	0.1 ∣ 0.44	
Warfarin	— ∣ 0.1			— ∣ 0.1 [— ∣ 0.1]	

(*continues*)

TABLE 4 (*Continued*)

Substance	PEL (OSHA) TWA (ppm ∣ mg/m³)	PEL (OSHA) STEL (ppm ∣ mg/m³)	CC	TLV (ACGIH) [REL (NIOSH)] TWA (ppm ∣ mg/m³)	TLV (ACGIH) [REL (NIOSH)] STEL (ppm ∣ mg/m³)
Wood dust (certain hardwoods, such as beech and oak)			A1	— ∣ 1 [— ∣ 1]	
Wood dust, softwoods				— ∣ 5 [— ∣ 1]	— ∣ 10
Xylene (*o*-, *m*-, *p*-isomers	100 ∣ 435		A4	100 ∣ 434 [100 ∣ 435]	150 ∣ 651 [150 ∣ 655]
Xylidine (mixed isomers) (skin)	5 ∣ 25		A3	0.5 ∣ 2.5 [2 ∣ 10]	
Yttrium metal and compounds, as Y	— ∣ 1			— ∣ 1 [— ∣ 1]	
Zinc oxide					
fume	— ∣ 15			[— ∣ 5] — ∣ 5	[— ∣ 10] — ∣ 10
dust	— ∣ 15			— ∣ 10 [— ∣ 5]	[— ∣ C15]

[a]Abbreviations: PEL, permissible exposure limits; TLV, threshold limit value; REL, recommended exposure limit; CC, categories for carcinogenicity (ACGIH)—A1, confirmed human carcinogen; A2, suspected human carcinogen; A3, animal carcinogen; A4, not classifiable as a human carcinogen; TWA, time-weighted average (concentration for a conventional 8-hour (REL: 10-hour) workday and a 40-hour work week); STEL, short-term exposure limit (15 minute TWA exposure, which should not be exceeded during a workday even if the 8-hour TWA is within the TLV–TWA); C, ceiling (concentration that should not be exceeded during any part of the working exposure); NOC, not otherwise classified.

daily intakes (TDI, see Table 1) for nongenotoxic substances by accounting for 10% (with some exceptions) of the TDI for the daily intake of drinking water (2 liters) by an adult (60 kg body weight). In some cases the guideline values are based on the consumption of 1 liter (or 0.75 liter by a 10-kg) child (or 5-kg infant). For genotoxic substances, the concentration in drinking water is associated with an estimated excess lifetime cancer risk of 10^{-5}.

National Primary Drinking Water Standards from the U.S. Environmental Protection Agency (U.S. EPA)

U.S. EPA drinking water standards are health-related values with legal character in the United States (Table 6).

Council Directive on Water Quality (EU)

The new Council Directive 98/83/EC (Table 6) of the EU concerning the quality of water intended for human consumption must be adopted by the national legislatures of the member states within a fixed period of time.

AIR

Emergency Response Planning Guidelines (ERPG) from the American Industrial Hygiene Association (AIHA, 1996)

The ERPGs are recommendations that have been developed for short-time exposures of not more than 1 hour, as may occur in emergency situations.

Air Quality Guidelines for Europe (WHO)

Air quality guidelines developed by the World Health Organization (WHO), revised in 1996 are values for short-term, long-term, and lifetime exposures. They are recommendations that can be used by national and international authorities as background information and for setting standards. They are intended to protect human health and do not differentiate between indoor and outdoor air (Table 7).

National Ambient Air Quality Standards (NAAQS) (U.S. EPA)

The "Primary Standards" of the National Ambient Air Quality Standards (NAAQS) are health-related

TABLE 5 Indicative Limit Values of the European Union[a]

Substance	TWA (pp ǀ mg/m³)	STEL (ppm ǀ mg/m³)
Acetic acid	10 ǀ 25	
Acetonitrile	40 ǀ 70	
Allyl alcohol (skin)	2 ǀ 4.8	5 ǀ 12.1
Amylacetate, *tert*-	50 ǀ 270	100 ǀ 540
Barium (soluble compounds as Ba)	— ǀ 0.5	
Bromine	0.1 ǀ 0.7	
Calcium dihydroxide	— ǀ 5	
Carbon dioxide	5000 ǀ 9000	
Chlorodifluoromethane	1000 ǀ 3600	
Cresols (all isomers)	5 ǀ 22	
Cumene (skin)	20 ǀ 100	50 ǀ 250
Cyanamide	— ǀ 2	
Diethylamine	10 ǀ 30	
N,N-Dimethylacetamide (skin)	10 ǀ 36	20 ǀ 72
Dimethylamine	2 ǀ 3.8	5 ǀ 9.4
Diphosphorus pentaoxide	— ǀ 1	
Diphosphorus pentasulfide	— ǀ 1	
Ethylamine	5 ǀ 9.4	
Formic acid	5 ǀ 9	
Heptan-2-one (skin)	50 ǀ 238	100 ǀ 475
Hydrogen bromide	— ǀ —	2 ǀ 6.7
Hydrogen chloride	5 ǀ 8	10 ǀ 15
Hydrogen selenide	0.02 ǀ 0.07	0.05 ǀ 0.17
Isopentylacetate	50 ǀ 270	100 ǀ 540
Lithium hydride	— ǀ 0.025	
Mesitylene	20 ǀ 100	
Methanol	200 ǀ 260	
2-Methoxy-1-methylethylacetate (skin)	50 ǀ 275	100 ǀ 550
1-Methylbutylacetate	50 ǀ 270	100 ǀ 540
(2-Methoxymethylethoxy)propanol (skin)	50 ǀ 308	
Naphthalene	10 ǀ 50	
Nicotine	— ǀ 0.5	
Nitrobenzene	1 ǀ 5	
Nitrogen monoxide	25 ǀ 30	
Oxalic acid	— ǀ 1	
3-Pentylacetate	50 ǀ 270	100 ǀ 540
Pentylacetate	50 ǀ 270	100 ǀ 540
Phosphoric acid	— ǀ 1	— ǀ 2
Phosphorus pentachloride	— ǀ 1	
Picric acid	— ǀ 0.1	
Platinum (metallic)	— ǀ 1	
Propionic acid	10 ǀ 31	20 ǀ 62
Pyrethrum	— ǀ 5	
Pyridine	5 ǀ 15	
Resorcinol	10 ǀ 45	
Silver (soluble compounds as Ag)	— ǀ 0.01	
Tin (inorganic compounds as Sn)	— ǀ 2	
1,2,4-Trichlorobenzene (skin)	2 ǀ 15.1	5 ǀ 37.8
1,2,3-Trimethylbenzene	20 ǀ 100	
1,2,4-Trimethylbenzene	20 ǀ 100	

[a]See Table 4.

TABLE 6 Guidelines for Drinking Water Quality (WHO), National Primary Drinking Water Standards (U.S. EPA), and Proposed Directive Concerning the Quality of Water Intended for Human Consumption (EU)[a]

Parameter	WHO	U.S. EPA MCL	U.S. EPA MCLG	EU
Inorganic constituents (mg/liter)				
Antimony	0.005 (P)	0.006	0.006	0.005
Arsenic	0.01[b]	0.05 (I)	0.05 (I)	0.01
Asbestos	U	7 MFL	7 MFL	—
Barium	0.7	2	2	—
Beryllium	NAD	0.004	0.004	—
Cadmium	0.003	0.005	0.005	0.005
Chromium	0.05 (P)	0.1	0.1	0.05
Copper	2 (P)	TT[c]	1.3	2
Cyanide	0.07	0.2	0.2	0.05
Fluoride	1.5	4.0	4.0	1.5
Lead	0.01	TT[d]	Zero	0.01
Manganese	0.5 (P)	—	—	—
Mercury (total)	0.001	0.002 (inorganic)	0.002 (inorganic)	0.001
Nickel	0.02	0.1	0.1	0.02
Nitrate (as NO_3^-)	50	10	10	50
Nitrite (as NO_2^-)	3 (P)	1	1	0.5
Selenium	0.01	0.05	0.05	0.01
Thallium	—	0.002	0.0005	—
Organic constituents (μg/liter)				
Acrylamide	0.5[e]	TT	Zero	0.1
Benzene	10[e]	5	Zero	1
Carbon tetrachloride	2	5	Zero	—
1,2-Dichlorobenzene	1000	600	600	—
1,4-Dichlorobenzene	300	75	75	—
1,2-Dichloroethane	30[e]	5	Zero	3
1,1-Dichloroethene	30	7	7	—
1,2-Dichloroethene	50	70 100	*cis*: 70 *trans*: 100	—
Di(2-ethylhexyl)adipate	80	400	400	—
Di(2-ethylhexyl)phthalate	8	6	Zero	—
Dichloromethane	20	5	Zero	—
Dioxin	—	0.00003	Zero	—
Edetic acid (EDTA)	200 (P)	—	—	—
Epichlorohydrin	0.4 (P)	TT	Zero	0.1
Ethylbenzene	300	700	700	—
Hexachlorobutadiene	0.6	—	1	—
Monochlorobenzene	300	100	100	—
Nitrilotriacetic acid	200	—	—	—
Polyaromatic Hydrocarbons (PAH)				0.1[f]
Benzo[*a*]pyrene	0.7[e]	0.2	Zero	0.01
PCBs	—	0.5	Zero	—
Styrene	20	100	100	—
Tetrachloroethene	40	5	Zero	—
and trichloroethene	—	—	—	10
Toluene	700	1000	1000	—
Tributyltin oxide	2	—	—	—
Trichlorobenzenes (total)	20	—	—	—
1,2,4-Trichlorobenzene		70	70	
1,1,1-Trichloroethane	2000 (P)	200	200	—
1,1,2-Trichloroethane	—	5	3	—
Trichloroethene	70 (P)	5	Zero	—
and Tetrachloroethene	—	—	—	10
Vinyl chloride	5[e]	2	Zero	0.5
Xylenes	500	10,000	10,000	—

(*continues*)

TABLE 6 *(Continued)*

Parameter	WHO	U.S. EPA MCL	U.S. EPA MCLG	EU
Pesticides (μg/liter)				0.1[g] (Σ0.5[h])
Alachlor	20[e]	2	Zero	
Aldicarb	10	3	1	
Aldicarb sulfone	—	2	1	
Aldicarb sulfoxide	—	4	1	
Aldrin/Dieldrin	0.03	—	—	0.3
Atrazine	2	3	3	
Carbofuran	5	40	40	
Chlordane	0.2	2	Zero	
Chlorotoluron	30	—	—	
2,4-D	30	70	70	
2,4-DB	90	—	—	
DDT	2	—	—	
1,2-Dibromo-3-chloropropane (DBCP)	1[e]	0.2	Zero	
Dichlorprop	100	—	—	
Diquat	—	20	20	
Endrin	—	2	2	
Fenoprop	9	—	—	
Glyphosate	—	700	700	
Heptachlor	0.03	0.4	Zero	0.3
Heptachlor epoxide	0.03	0.2	Zero	0.3
Hexachlorobenzene	1[e]	1	Zero	
Lindane	2	0.2	0.2	
MCPA	2	—	—	
Mecoprop	10	—	—	
Methoxychlor	20	40	40	
Pentachlorophenol	9 (P)	1	Zero	
Permethrin	20	—	—	
Propanil	20	—	—	
2,4,5-T	9	—	—	
Toxaphene	—	3	Zero	
Trifluralin	20	—	—	
Disinfectants (mg/liters)				
Chlorine	5	—	—	—
Disinfectant by-products (μg/liter)				
2,4,6-Trichlorophenol	200[e]	—	—	—
Bromate	25[e] (P)	—	—	10
Chloral hydrate	10 (P)	—	—	—
Chlorite	200 (P)	—	—	—
Dibromoacetonitrile	100 (P)	—	—	—
Dichloroacetic acid	50 (P)	—	—	—
Dichloroacetonitrile	90 (P)	—	—	—
Formaldehyde	900	—	—	—
Trihalomethanes (THM)[i]		100 (I, sum)	Zero	100 (sum)
Chloroform	200[e]			
Bromoform	100			
Bromodichloromethane	60[e]			
Dibromochloromethane	100			
Trichloroacetic acid	100 (P)	—	—	—
Trichloroacetonitrile	1 (P)	—	—	—

[a] Abbreviations: MCLG, maximum contaminant level goal; MCL, maximum contaminant level; P, provisional guideline value; NAD, no adequate data to permit recommendation of a health-based guideline value; U, unnecessary to recommend a guideline value; I, interim standard; TT, treatment technique requirement; MFL, million fibers per liter (>10 μm).

[b] For excess skin cancer risk of 6×10^{-4}.

[c] Action level 1.3 mg/liter.

[d] Action level 0.015 mg/liter.

[e] For excess cancer risk of 10^{-5}.

[f] Sum of benzo[*a*]pyrene, fluoranthene, benzo[*b*]fluoranthene, benzo[*k*]fluoranthene, benzo[*ghi*]perylene, and indeno[1,2,3-*cd*]pyrene.

[g] The parametric value applies to each individual pesticide except aldrin, dieldrin, heptachlor, and heptachlor epoxide.

[h] "Pesticides" means organic insecticides, herbicides, fungicides, nematocides, acaricides, algicides, and related products (growth regulators).

[i] For WHO, the sum of the ratio of the concentration of each to its respective guideline value should not exceed 1.

TABLE 7 Air Quality Guidelines for Europe (WHO), National Ambient Air Quality Standards (U.S. EPA), and Air Quality Limit Values (EU)[a]

	WHO (Europe)	U.S. EPA	EU
Classic air pollutants			
Carbon monoxide	100 mg/m^3 (15 min)		
	60 mg/m^3 (30 min)		
	30 mg/m^3 (1 hour)	40 mg/m^3 (1 hour)	
	10 mg/m^3 (8 hour)	10 mg/m^3 (8 hour)	
Ozone	120 $\mu g/m^3$ (8 hour)	235 $\mu g/m^3$ (1 hour)	
health protection threshold			110 $\mu g/m^3$ (8 hour)
information threshold			180 $\mu g/m^3$ (1 hour)
warning threshold			360 $\mu g/m^3$ (1 hour)
Nitrogen dioxide	200 $\mu g/m^3$ (1 hour)		200 $\mu g/m^3$ (1 hour)[b]
	40 $\mu g/m^3$ (annual)	100 $\mu g/m^3$ (annual)	
Sulfur dioxide	500 $\mu g/m^3$ (10 min)		
	125 $\mu g/m^3$ (24 hour)	365 $\mu g/m^3$ (24 hour)	
	50 $\mu g/m^3$ (annual)	80 $\mu g/m^3$ (annual)	80 $\mu g/m^3$ if TSP >150 $\mu g/m^3$ (annual)[c]
			120 $\mu g/m^3$ if TSP ≤150 $\mu g/m^3$ (annual)[c]
			130 $\mu g/m^3$ if TSP >200 $\mu g/m^3$ (winter)[c]
			180 $\mu g/m^3$ if TSP ≤200 $\mu g/m^3$ (winter)[c]
			250 $\mu g/m^3$ if TSP >350 $\mu g/m^3$[d]
			350 $\mu g/m^3$ if TSP ≤350 $\mu g/m^3$[d]
Particulate matter (PM_{10})	Effect–response[e]	150 $\mu g/m^3$ (24 hour)	
		50 $\mu g/m^3$ (annual)	
Organic pollutants			
Benzene	6×10^{-6} $(\mu g/m^3)^{-1}$ (UR/lifetime)		
1,3-Butadiene	No guideline		
Dichloromethane	3 mg/m^3 (24 hour)		
Formaldehyde	0.1 mg/m^3 (30 min)		
PAH (BaP)	8.7×10^{-5} $(ng/m^3)^{-1}$ (UR/lifetime)		
Styrene	0.26 mg/m^3 (1 week)		
Tetrachloroethylene	0.25 mg/m^3 (24 hour)		
Toluene	0.26 mg/m^3 (1 week)		
Trichloroethylene	4.3×10^{-7} $(\mu g/m^3)^{-1}$ (UR/lifetime)		
Inorganic pollutants			
Arsenic	1.5×10^{-3} $(\mu g/m^3)^{-1}$ (UR/lifetime)		
Cadmium	5 ng/m^3 (annual)		
Chromium (VI)	4×10^{-2} $(\mu g/m^3)^{-1}$ (UR/lifetime)		
Fluoride	No guideline		
Lead	0.5 $\mu g/m^3$ (annual)	1.5 $\mu g/m^3$ (quarterly)	2 $\mu g/m^3$ (annual)
Manganese	0.15 $\mu g/m^3$ (annual)		
Mercury	1.0 $\mu g/m^3$ (annual)		
Nickel	3.8×10^{-4} $(\mu g/m^3)^{-1}$ (UR/lifetime)		

[a] Type of average given in parentheses. Abbreviations: TSP, total suspended particles; UR, unit risk.
[b] 98th percentile of mean values per hour throughout the year.
[c] Median of daily mean values.
[d] 98th percentile of all daily mean values throughout the year.
[e] A level below which no effect would be expected could not be established.

TABLE 8 Selected Substances That Cosmetic Products Must Not Contain, Except Subject to Restrictions (EU)

Substance	Restrictions: Field of application	Restrictions: Maximum authorized concentration in finished cosmetic product
Ammonia		6% as NH_3
Chlorates of alkali metals	Toothpaste	5%
	Other uses	3%
Diaminophenols	Oxidizing coloring agents for hair dyeing	10% calculated as free base
Dichloromethane		35% (when mixed with 1,1,1-trichloroethane, total concentration must not exceed 35%)
Fluoride (aluminium-, ammonium-, calcium-, potassium-, sodium-, stannous-)	Oral hygiene products	0.15%, as F
Formaldehyde	Nail hardener	5%
Hydrogen peroxide, and other compounds or mixtures that release hydrogen peroxide, including carbamide peroxide and zinc peroxide	Hair-care preparations	12% H_2O_2
	Skin-care preparations	4% H_2O_2
	Nail-hardening preparations	2% H_2O_2
	Oral hygiene products	0.1% H_2O_2
Hydroquinone	Oxidizing coloring agent for hair dyeing	2%
	Agents for localized skin lightener	2%
Methanol	Denaturant for ethanol and isopropyl alcohol	5% calculated as percent of ethanol and isopropyl alcohol
6-Methylcoumarin	Oral hygiene products	0.003%
Methylphenylenediamines, their *N*-substituted derivatives, and their salts, except 4-Methyl-*m*-phenylenediamine and its salts	Oxidizing coloring agents for hair dyeing	10% calculated as free base
Monofluorophosphate (ammonium-, calcium-, potassium-, sodium-)	Oral hygiene products	0.15%, as F
α-Naphthol	Coloring agent for hair dyeing	0.5%
Nitromethane	Rust inhibitor	0.2%
Oxalic acid, its esters, and alkaline salts	Hair-care products	5%
Phenol and its alkali salts	Soaps and shampoos	1%, as phenol
m- and *p*-Phenylenediamines, their *N*-substituted derivatives, and their salts; *N*-substituted derivatives of *o*-phenylenediamines	Oxidizing coloring agents for hair dyeing	6% calculated as free base
Resorcinol	Oxidizing coloring agent for hair dyeing	5%
	Hair lotions and shampoos	0.5%
Selenium disulfide	Anti-dandruff shampoos	1%
Silver nitrate	Solely for products intended for coloring eyelashes and eyebrows	4%
Strontium hydroxide	pH regulator in depilatory products	3.5%, as strontium
Thioglycollic acid and its salts (as thioglycollic acid)	Depilatories	5%
	Other hair-care products that are removed after application	2%
Thioglycollic acid, its salts, and esters (as thioglycollic acid)	Hair-waving or -straightening products	
	general use	8%
	professional use	11%
Zinc 4-hydroxybenzene sulfonate	Deodorants, antiperspirants and astringent lotions	6%, as anhydrous substance

TABLE 9 Selected Preservatives Allowed (EU)

Substance	Maximum authorized concentration
Benzoic acid, its salts, and esters	0.5% (acid)
Formaldehyde and paraformaldehyde	0.2% (except for products for oral hygiene) 0.1% (products for oral hygiene)
Formic acid and its sodium salt	0.5% (acid)
Glutaraldehyde	0.1%
4-Hydroybenzoic acid, its salts, and esters	0.4% (acid) for 1 ester 0.8% (acid) for mixtures of esters
Phenylmercuric salts (including borates)	0.007% (as Hg)
Propionic acid and its salts	2% (acid)
Salicylic acid and its salts	0.5% (acid)
Sorbic acid and its salts	0.6% (acid)

standards (Table 7) in contrast to the "Secondary Standards," which are welfare related and not listed here. They have been developed by the U.S. Environmental Protection Agency (U.S. EPA) and have the character of threshold values in the United States.

Council Directives on Air Quality (EU)

In the European Union, limit values for air pollutants are regulated in various council directives that must be adopted by the member states (Table 7).

FOOD

There are extensive regulations for pesticide residues in food. As the threshold values differ depending on the individual food items, it would go beyond the scope of this appendix to list all these values. Interested readers are referred to the source documents mentioned here.

United States

Action Levels for Poisonous or Deleterious Substances in Human Food and Animal Feed have been established by the Food and Drug Administration (FDA) in 1992. These action levels, as well as tolerances, represent legal standards and concern the following substances: aflatoxin, aldrin and dieldrin, benzene hexachloride (hexachlorocyclohexene), cadmium, chlordane, chlordecone (kepone), crotalaria seeds, dicofol, DDT, DDE, TDE, dimethylnitrosamine and other *N*-nitrosamines, endrin, ethylene dibromide

TABLE 10 Limit Values for Heavy-Metal Concentrations in Soil and in Sludge for Use in Agriculture (EU)

Substance	Limit values in soil (mg/kg dry matter, soil pH 6 to 7)[a]	Limit values in sludge (mg/kg dry matter)[a]	Limit values for amounts added to agricultural land[b] (mg/ha/year)
Cadmium	1–3	20–40	0.15
Copper[c]	50–140	1000–1750	12
Lead	50–300	750–1200	15
Mercury	1–1.5	16–25	0.1
Nickel[c]	30–75	300–400	3
Zinc[c]	150–300	2500–4000	30

[a]The use of sludge is prohibited if the concentrations are exceeded.
[b]Added annually, based on a 10-year average.
[c]Member states may permit the limit values they fix to be exceeded with respect to these parameters in soil with a pH consistently higher than 7. The maximum authorized concentrations of these heavy metals must in no case exceed those values by more than 50%. Member states must also seek to ensure that there is no resulting hazard to human health or to the environment, particularly to groundwater.

(EDB), heptachlor and heptachlor epoxide, lead, lindane, mercury, methyl alcohol, mirex, paralytic shellfish toxin, polychlorinated biphenyls (PCBs), and toxaphene.

European Union

Maximum levels for pesticide residues in and on cereals and foodstuffs of animal origin, respectively (Council Directives 86/362/EEC, 86/363/EEC, 93/57/EEC, 94/29/EC, 96/33/EC).

Maximum levels for pesticide residues in and on fruit and vegetables (Council Directive 76/895/EEC).

Maximum levels for pesticide residues in and on certain products of plant origin, including fruit and vegetables (90/642/EEC, 93/58/EEC, 94/30/EC).

COSMETICS

United States

In the United States, cosmetic products are regulated by the Food and Drug Administration (FDA). But there are no threshold limits or guideline values for cosmetic ingredients. Except for color additives and those ingredients that are prohibited or restricted by regulation from use in cosmetics, a manufacturer may essentially use any ingredient in the formulation of a cosmetic provided that the ingredient and the finished cosmetic are safe, the product is properly labeled, and the use of a specific substance does not otherwise cause the cosmetic to be adulterated or misbranded. Colorants used in cosmetics are specifically allowed by color additive regulations (Title 21, Code of Federal Regulations, Part 1-99).

European Union

The European Union has regulated that substances may not form part of a cosmetic product (Annex II), as well as the maximum concentrations of cosmetic ingredients and preservatives (Annex III and VI) by the Cosmetic Directive 76/768/EEC. Table 8 contains a choice of substances and the corresponding restrictions, including all the amendments to the directive published to August 30, 1996. Table 9 contains regulations for preservatives.

SOIL

European Union

The Council Directive 86/278/EEC of the European Union "on the protection of the environment, and in particular of the soil, when sewage sludge is used in agriculture" contains limit values for heavy-metal concentrations in soil and sludge (Table 10).

Index

C

D

F

G

H

J

K

M

P

Q

S

T

U

V

W

X

Y

Z